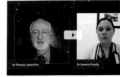

McMaster Internal Medicine

Euthyroid women, TPO antibodies, a... thyroid supplementation

Roman Jaeschke, Serena Gundy

References

Roman Jaeschke, MD: Good morning, welcome to another edition of McMaster... Today I would like to introduce to you Doctor Serena Gundy, who is our expert... conditions and diseases surrounding pregnancy. Serena, there is something... thyroid status in pregnancy. Could you expand? The field is yours.

Serena Gundy, MD: Thank you very much. Some new evidence has come o... of women with recurrent miscarriages and infertility, particularly looking at th... thyroid peroxidase (TPO) antibody positivity. Miscarriage is obviously a very c... complication for women who conceive, occurring in almost 1 out of 5 pregnan... very devastating for both women and their partners, particularly when it is re...

The data has been mixed in the last years, looking at the association of these... infertile women or women who have adverse reproductive outcomes, but their... association with these consequences in women with TPO antibody positivity e... absence of thyroid dysfunction.

This has led a lot of fertility specialists and endocrinologists to consider testing... for TPO antibody positivity and even if they are euthyroid to consider the addi... levothyroxine supplementation in those with a history of recurrent pregnancy... a sentiment that is reflected even in the most recent American Thyroid Associa... thyroid guidelines from 2017.

This study in particular set out to look at this question in further detail. It was... published in the New England Journal of Medicine. It was a multicenter, doubl... placebo-controlled trial. The authors screened about 19,000 women with a hi... miscarriage or infertility and then tested them for their TPO status and those...

McMaster Internal Medicine

New leadless devices enable ventricular stimulation and are useful to avoid lead-related problems.

Late **complications** of pacemaker implantation include lead dislodgement or damage affecting pacing or sensing/detection, pacemaker damage, pacemaker-induced tachycardia, increased pacing threshold, pacemaker syndrome (AV dissociation in patients with VVI pacemakers, which leads to reduced cardiac output and atrial contractions while AV valves are closed, consequently resulting in syncope, dizziness, fatigue, and neck... infection, infective endocarditis related to a foreign body (cardiac device-re... endocarditis), and very rarely sepsis.

▶ FIGURES

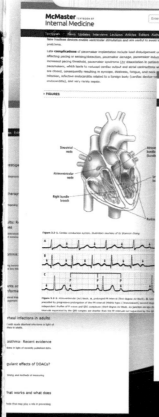

Sinoatrial node

Atrioventricular node

Right bundle branch

Atrial bundle (Bundle...

Le...

Purkin...

Figure 3.3-1. Cardiac conduction system. Illustration courtesy of Dr Shannon Zhang.

Figure 3.3-2. Atrioventricular (AV) block. **A**, prolonged PR interval (first-degree AV block). **B**, inter... preceded by progressive prolongation of the PR interval (Mobitz type I [Wenckebach]) second-degr... independent (buffer of P waves and QRS complexes [third-degree AV block, AV junction escape rhy... intervals separated by the QRS complex are shorter than the PP interval not subtended by the QR...

rheal infections in adults
...t with acute diarrheal infections in light of
...has in adults.

asthma: Recent evidence
...dates in light of recently published data.

gulant effects of DOACs?
...iming and methods of measuring

...hat works and what does
...eds that may play a role in preventing

McMaster Internal Medicine

▌Diagnostic Criteria

1. **Primary hypothyroidism:**
   1) **Overt:** Low serum FT_4 and elevated se...
   2) **Subclinical:** Normal serum FT_4 (often serum FT_4 and mildly elevated serum...
2. **Secondary and tertiary hypothyroid...** levels.
3. **Myxedema coma:** Low serum FT_4 and v... diagnosis depends primarily on clinical m... coma.

▌Differential Diagnosis

Differential diagnostic algorithm for hypoth... differential diagnose of primary hypothyroid... exposure to iodine or i... previous thyroid surge... several years earlier).... other underdose glands... insufficiency before init... cavities, hypercholest... pernicious anemia, an...

In patients hospitalize... not related to the thyro... remain <20 mU/L. Ca... dobutamine, glucocorti... impaired synthesis, th... illness, which leads to... low, although method... levels increase; the ris... nonthyroidal illness as... but is not commonly u... laboratory abnormaliti... thyroid hormone leve... the pituitary-thyroid in... function tests should b... thyroid dysfunction.

Patient on thyroid hor...

Serum TSH and FT_4

Hold treatment for 3-6 weeks[a]

– TSH normal – FT_4 normal	– TSH slightly elevated – FT_4 normal	– TSH high – FT_4 low	– TSH normal or low – FT_4 low
Normal thyroid function	**Subclinical hypothyroidism**	**Primary hypothyroidism**	**Secondary or tertiary hypothyroidism[b]**

[a] If the diagnosis of hypothyroidism is questionable.
[b] A thyrotropin-releasing hormone test is sometimes useful in differentiating these conditions from primary hypothyroidism.

FT_4, free thyroxine; TSH, thyroid-stimulating hormone.

Figure 6.6-1. Diagnostic algorithm of hypothyroidism based on TSH and FT_4 levels.

▶ TREATMENT

Overt hypothyroidism i... lifelong.

▌Long-Term Hormone Replacement Therapy

Monotherapy with **levothyroxine ($L-T_4$)** is the treatment of choice. Fixed combinations of $L-T_4$ and liothyronine ($L-T_3$) are not recommended, as T_4 is converted to T_3. Dosage: once daily, 30 to 60 minutes before the first meal or at bedtime 4 hours after the last meal. The daily dose is estimated on an individual basis: in adults usually ~1.7 microg/kg/d; in the elderly use lower doses, even as low as 1 microg/kg/d. In the majority of patients the dose range is 100 to 150 microg/d (TSH levels should be within the reference range, optimally 1-3 mIU/L). In young healthy adults initiating treatment with full replacement doses is suggested.... For patients >50 to 60 years without evidence of coronary heart disease, you...

McMaster TEXTBOOK OF
Internal Medicine

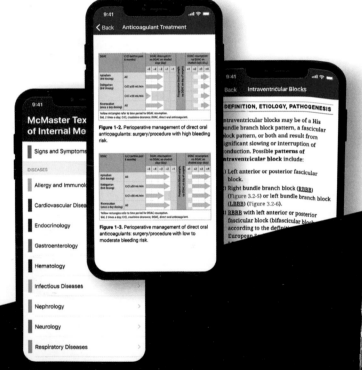

GET IT ON
Google play

DOWNLOAD ON THE
App Store

mcmastertextbook.com/**app**

collagenous colitis, functioning endocrine tumors (carcinoid, VIPoma, gastrinoma, villous adenoma of the colon, medullary thyroid carcinoma, mastocytosis). **Drugs**: The most frequent causes are contact laxatives (bisacodyl, anthranoids, aloe vera) and other laxatives (as in acute diarrhea), antiarrhythmics (quinidine, digoxin), auranofin, caffeine, calcitonin, carbamazepine, and chemotherapeutic agents. Other potential causes include cimetidine, misoprostol, metformin, NSAIDs, simvastatin, theophylline, levodopa/benserazide, and cholinesterase inhibitors.

b) **Osmotic diarrhea**: Certain food and confectionery products that contain fructose, sorbitol, mannitol, or xylitol; lactase deficiency (lactose intolerance) and other types of disaccharidase deficiency (primary [congenital; eg, adult-type hypolactasia] or secondary [eg, to intestinal infection or inflammation]); short bowel syndrome; intestinal fistula and enteral feed. **Drugs**: Osmotic laxatives (magnesium sulfate, polyethylene glycol, lactulose); antacids (magnesium hydroxide); orlistat, acarbose, cholestyramine, ampicillin, clindamycin, neomycin, phosphates, prebiotics, quinidine, propranolol, hydralazine, ACEIs, procainamide, biguanides, methyldopa.

c) **Steatorrhea**: Maldigestion (exocrine pancreatic insufficiency [chronic pancreatitis, pancreatic cancer, cystic fibrosis], bacterial overgrowth syndrome, cholestatic liver disease), malabsorption (celiac disease, giardiasis, Whipple disease, bowel ischemia, abetalipoproteinemia, intestinal lymphangiectasia, and other causes of protein-losing enteropathy).

d) **Inflammatory diarrhea**: IBD (Crohn disease, ulcerative colitis); microscopic, ischemic, or radiation-induced colitis (eg, after radiotherapy to the abdominal region); food hypersensitivity; primary and secondary immunodeficiency; intestinal tumors (eg, colon cancer); intestinal protozoal infections (*Giardia intestinalis, Entamoeba histolytica, Cryptosporidium parvum, Isospora* spp, *Cyclospora* spp) and helminthic infestation.

e) **Drugs**: Antibiotics (clindamycin, ampicillin, amoxicillin, cephalosporins), auranofin, carbamazepine, etanercept, flutamide, cytotoxic agents, cyclosporine (INN ciclosporin), NSAIDs, statins, mercaptopurine, mycophenolate mofetil, olmesartan, oral contraceptives, penicillamine, rituximab, selective serotonin reuptake inhibitors (SSRIs), sodium phosphate, ticlopidine, tyrosine kinase inhibitors, H_2 blockers, ticlopidine, proton pump inhibitors (PPIs), gold salts, and laxatives.

f) **Accelerated GI transit** (ie, increased motility): IBS, thyrotoxicosis, carcinoid, and diabetes mellitus. **Drugs**: Prokinetic agents (metoclopramide, cisapride), acetylcholinesterase inhibitors (tacrine), cholinergic agents (bethanechol), irinotecan, macrolides (erythromycin), ticlopidine, thyroid hormones, colchicine.

Selected aspects of diarrhea in patients with cancer: In patients receiving palliative care, diarrhea is most frequently due to:

1) Overtreatment with laxatives (often in patients with inadequately treated constipation).

2) GI infections.

3) Cytotoxic agents (most frequently fluorouracil, irinotecan, mitomycin) and radiotherapy to the abdomen or pelvis.

4) Enteral nutrition.

5) Insufficient pancreatic exocrine secretion (steatorrhea) in patients with pancreatic head tumors.

6) Bile acid and carbohydrate malabsorption (disaccharidase deficiency) a ileal resection. In such patients diarrhea is caused by excessive infl water and electrolytes into the colonic lumen.

7) Insufficient water absorption in the small intestine following total resection of the large intestine (ileostomy).

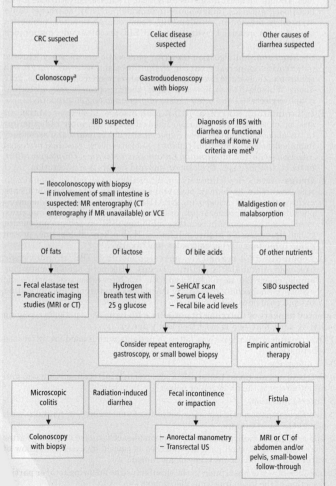

Clinical assessment
- History: Duration of diarrhea, stool frequency and appearance, alarming symptoms, and risk factors suggestive of organic disease (blood in stool, nocturnal diarrhea, involuntary weight loss)
- Physical examination (including rectal)

Initial tests:
- Blood tests: CRP, CBC (including ferritin in case of anemia), thyroid function, and serologic tests specific for celiac disease
- Stool tests: Parasitology, *C difficile*, fecal calprotectin, FIT

As necessary:
- Serum B_{12}, folate, calcium, and albumin
- Immunodeficiency testing: Immunoglobulins, HIV testing

CRC suspected	Celiac disease suspected	Other causes of diarrhea suspected
Colonoscopy[a]	Gastroduodenoscopy with biopsy	

IBD suspected	Diagnosis of IBS with diarrhea or functional diarrhea if Rome IV criteria are met[b]

- Ileocolonoscopy with biopsy
- If involvement of small intestine is suspected: MR enterography (CT enterography if MR unavailable) or VCE

Maldigestion or malabsorption

Of fats	Of lactose	Of bile acids	Of other nutrients
- Fecal elastase test - Pancreatic imaging studies (MRI or CT)	Hydrogen breath test with 25 g glucose	- SeHCAT scan - Serum C4 levels - Fecal bile acid levels	SIBO suspected

Consider repeat enterography, gastroscopy, or small bowel biopsy	Empiric antimicrobial therapy

Microscopic colitis	Radiation-induced diarrhea	Fecal incontinence or impaction	Fistula
Colonoscopy with biopsy		- Anorectal manometry - Transrectal US	MRI or CT of abdomen and/or pelvis, small-bowel follow-through

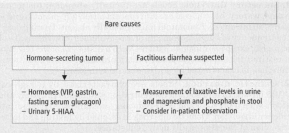

a If no organic changes in the large intestine are found, include assessment of the distal small intestine with collection of biopsy specimens of unchanged colon mucosa to evaluate for microscopic colitis.
b Consider bile acid malabsorption if clinically suspected.

5-HIAA, 5-hydroxyindoleacetic acid; C4, 7α-hydroxy-4-cholesten-3-one (bile acid precursor); CBC, complete blood count; CRC, colorectal cancer; CRP, C-reactive protein; CT, computed tomography; FIT, fecal immunochemical test; HIV, human immunodeficiency virus; IBD, inflammatory bowel disease; IBS, irritable bowel syndrome; MR, magnetic resonance; MRI, magnetic resonance imaging; SeHCAT, 75selenium homotaurocholic acid testing; SIBO, small intestinal bacterial overgrowth; US, ultrasonography; VCE, video capsule endoscopy; VIP, vasoactive intestinal peptide.

Figure 5-2. Algorithm for the diagnosis of chronic diarrhea. *Adapted from Gut. 2018;67(8):1380-1399.*

→ DIAGNOSIS

Assess the severity of dehydration in every patient.

If no characteristic manifestations are seen and the patient's history does not suggest a noninfectious cause (eg, drugs), assume that **acute diarrhea** is caused by a GI infection or food poisoning. If symptoms persist or worsen despite appropriate treatment and diarrhea persists for >10 days or diarrheal episodes recur frequently, consider causes of chronic diarrhea and perform appropriate workup (→Figure 5-2). Also →Chapter 6.1.3.5.2. In the case of **chronic diarrhea**, evaluate the appearance of stools and determine the type of diarrhea, which will be helpful in narrowing down the list of possible causes. The patient should remain fasting to determine the type of diarrhea.

For every patient with **chronic diarrhea**, consider testing stools for ova and parasites, fecal leukocytes, or fecal lactoferrin/calprotectin (testing for inflammation in IBD); *Clostridium difficile* toxin assay; and stool pH. Stool may be examined for fat (qualitative or quantitative 3-day fecal fat; if steatorrhea is considered, 3-day fecal fat collection is usually performed). Consider investigations for lactase deficiency (hydrogen breath tests or impact of a lactose-free diet if lactase deficiency is a possibility). Certain tests (eg, complete blood count, thyroid function tests) may be of value in diagnosis while other (eg, electrolytes, renal function) should be done as required to assess the consequences of diarrhea. Further testing depends on the suspected etiology and clinical course and may include investigations towards, for example, pancreatic insufficiency, bacterial overgrowth, or laxative abuse. Colonoscopy with or without biopsy may be valuable in certain situations (→Figure 5-2).

Exclude **spurious diarrhea**, which is frequent passage of small amounts of liquid brown stool, typically accompanied by fecal incontinence. It is related to overfilling and distention of the colon caused by fecal impaction in the rectum in patients with severe constipation or by narrowing of the sigmoid colon (less frequently of the rectum) due to organic causes, including tumors.

Fecal osmotic gap is expressed in mOsm/L and may be either measured (s osmolality $- 2 \times [\mathrm{Na_{stool}} + \mathrm{K_{stool}}]$) or estimated ($290 - 2 \times [\mathrm{Na_{stool}} + \mathrm{K_{stool}}]$) rarely used in clinical practice.

1. Secretory diarrhea: Stools are typically abundant (up to several liters a day), watery, have a fecal sodium concentration >70 mmol/L and low osmotic gap (<50 mOsm/L). Abdominal pain is usually absent. Fasting does not reduce the frequency of bowel movements or stool volumes (diarrhea wakes the patient at night); exceptions include patients with a history of bowel resection and with intestinal fistulas (anatomic or functional short bowel syndrome) in whom diarrhea is exacerbated by oral or enteral nutrition.

2. Osmotic diarrhea: Stools are characterized by a high osmotic gap (>125 mOsm/L) and sodium concentration <70 mmol/L. Foamy and explosive stools with a pH <5.5 and fecal reducing substances >0.5% indicate disaccharide maldigestion. Osmotic diarrhea is stopped by fasting and by withholding ingestion of the osmotically active substance.

3. Steatorrhea: Stools are fatty, shiny, sticky, difficult to flush, and foul smelling. If steatorrhea is confirmed, further investigations towards pancreatic insufficiency may be needed.

4. Inflammatory diarrhea: This may be manifested by the presence of blood in stool, high fecal white blood cell count, or positive fecal lactoferrin test. It may be accompanied by systemic manifestations of inflammation (fever, elevated acute-phase protein [eg, C-reactive protein] levels, elevated erythrocyte sedimentation rate) or peripheral eosinophilia (eg, in allergic diarrhea) and hypoalbuminemia.

5. Dehydration is the key complication of acute and chronic diarrhea. The severity of dehydration determines the techniques and intensity of rehydration therapy (oral or IV, outpatient or inpatient, volume of administered fluids). The most accurate assessment of the severity of dehydration is based on comparing the patient's current body weight with the most recent weight before the onset of diarrhea. The severity of dehydration is expressed as a percentage of body weight loss, which determines the volume of fluid that needs to be administered during the rehydration phase. Dehydration can also be estimated on the basis of clinical manifestations and is classified approximately as:

1) **No clinical manifestations of dehydration** (loss of <3% of body weight): No signs or symptoms of dehydration.

2) **Mild dehydration** (loss of 3%-5% of body weight): Increased thirst (absent in elderly patients with impaired sensation of thirst) and dry oral mucosa.

3) **Moderate dehydration** (loss of >5%-9% of body weight): Markedly increased thirst, dry oral mucosa, sunken eyes, oliguria, postural hypotension, prolonged capillary refill time (for >2 seconds apply pressure to a nail bed until it blanches, then release; the pink color normally reappears within <1.5 seconds of releasing pressure), delayed skin fold recoil (assessed on the abdomen) and dry skin (dry axilla increases the odds of moderate dehydration ~3-fold).

4) **Severe dehydration** (loss of ≥9% of body weight): Manifestations of moderate dehydration accompanied by features of hypovolemic shock.

→ **TREATMENT**

Symptomatic Treatment

1. Indications for hospitalization (IV rehydration necessary): Severe dehydration, manifestations of dehydration in an elderly patient (these patients often have no sensation of thirst and drink insufficient amounts of fluids), conditions precluding oral rehydration (persistent vomiting or adynamic ileus), and failure of oral rehydration (signs and symptoms of dehydration worsening despite receiving seemingly appropriate amounts of oral rehydration solutions [ORSs] or difficulty drinking the required amounts of liquids).

2. Rehydration therapy is the mainstay of symptomatic treatment of diarrhea. Most patients with mild to moderate dehydration (loss of ≤9% of body weight) may be managed using an outpatient or home oral rehydration therapy. It is usually sufficient to take regular fluids (water, juices, isotonic drinks, soups) and table salt (eg, salt crackers). For hydration in children and the elderly with severe diarrhea, commercial glucose-electrolyte ORSs are available. Frequent administration of small portions of cold (refrigerated) ORS improves the patient's tolerance. Fluid therapy consists of 2 phases:

Replacement of deficits (rehydration): For the first 3 to 4 hours, administer ORS only. The volume of ORS should be equal to the estimated weight loss (the patient should drink freely to quench thirst):

1) No signs of dehydration: Up to ~20 mL/kg.

2) Mild dehydration: ~40 mL/kg.

3) Moderate dehydration: ~70 mL/kg.

4) Compensate for ongoing fluid loss by adding 5 mL/kg to the calculated volume after each diarrheal stool or episode of vomiting.

Patients with severe dehydration, signs of shock, or evidence of bowel obstruction require immediate hospitalization and IV administration of crystalloids. After the patient's condition has stabilized (normalization of vital signs, improved level of consciousness, resolution of signs of intestinal obstruction), replace the estimated fluid deficit. Depending on the degree of improvement, continue IV rehydration or switch to oral rehydration using ORS (→above). Frequent reassessment is crucial.

Maintenance therapy: Continue ORS to replace the water and electrolytes lost with stool and emesis (→above) and start oral nutrition (realimentation). In addition, the patient should drink ORS or neutral fluids (in unlimited amounts until thirst is quenched) in the amount equal to the basic daily fluid requirement (after subtracting the volume of ingested foods). ORS should be administered until the resolution of diarrhea.

3. Management of other abnormalities: If necessary (usually in patients with severe dehydration), treat metabolic acidosis, hypernatremia, hyponatremia, hypokalemia, hypocalcemia, and hypomagnesemia (→Chapter 4). Isotonic dehydration is most frequently seen in patients with diarrhea. In patients with chronic diarrhea, also treat malnutrition, vitamin deficiencies, and trace element deficiencies.

4. Antidiarrheal agents:

1) Oral **loperamide** is an opioid derivative that decreases bowel peristalsis, increases water absorption, and decreases the number of bowel movements. It should be considered as supportive treatment in patients with watery diarrhea without fever or with mild fever. Loperamide is well tolerated in adolescents and adults and is associated with low risk of adverse reactions. Start from 4 mg followed by 2 mg after each diarrheal stool (up to 16 mg/d). Loperamide is contraindicated in patients with bloody diarrhea and in those with high fever.

2) **Diosmectite** is an intestinal content absorbent. The usual dose is 3 g orally bid to tid.

3) **Octreotide** is used for symptomatic treatment of diarrhea associated with chemotherapy, Zollinger-Ellison syndrome, carcinoid tumor, ileostomy, fistula, bowel obstruction, and for symptomatic treatment of chronic diarrhea in patients with AIDS. Octreotide reduces visceral blood flow, inhibits intestinal secretion, and normalizes intestinal peristalsis. It is administered as subcutaneous or intermittent injections, usually at a dose of 300 to 600 µg/d.

4) **Diphenoxylate/atropine** (trade name Lomotil; activator of opioid receptors): 5 mg qid until control achieved (maximum dose of diphenoxylate, 20 mg/d) then reduce the dose as needed. Maintenance doses may be as low as 25% of the initial daily dose required for achieving control.

5) Oral **bismuth**: ~524 mg every 30 to 60 minutes or 1050 mg every 60 min as needed for up to 2 days (maximum, ~4200 mg [8 doses of regular str or 4 doses of maximum strength] per 24 hours).

6. Dyspepsia

→ **DEFINITION**

Dyspepsia is a complex of symptoms that includes epigastric pain or burning, abdominal fullness after meals (an unpleasant sensation of food retention in the stomach), and early satiety (feeling full that is disproportionate to the amount of consumed food and prevents the patient from finishing the meal). Dyspepsia **does not include heartburn** (a retrosternal burning sensation); although heartburn is often present in addition to dyspeptic symptoms, it cannot be the dominant problem.

→ **CAUSES AND PATHOGENESIS**

1. Undiagnosed dyspepsia: Patients presenting with dyspepsia symptoms that have not had investigations to determine whether the cause is organic or functional.

2. Organic dyspepsia: Gastroesophageal reflux disease (GERD); drug-induced gastric, duodenal, or esophageal mucosal injury (acetylsalicylic acid and other nonsteroidal anti-inflammatory drugs [NSAIDs], certain oral antibiotics [mainly doxycycline, erythromycin, ampicillin], digitalis, theophylline, iron or potassium salts, calcium channel blockers, nitrates, glucocorticoids, bisphosphonates); peptic ulcer disease; diseases of the biliary system; hepatitis; pancreatitis; pancreatic pseudocysts; malignancy (gastric, pancreatic, colorectal); intestinal ischemia; and abdominal aortic aneurysm.

3. Functional dyspepsia: Dyspepsia lasting ≥3 months (with onset of symptoms ≥6 months prior to diagnosis) with no organic cause identified on upper gastrointestinal endoscopy. Symptoms do not resolve on bowel movement and are not associated with changes in the frequency of bowel movements or the appearance of stool (features of irritable bowel syndrome).

→ **DIAGNOSTIC WORKUP**

1. History and physical examination: Determine:
1) How long the symptoms have been present.
2) Whether they are accompanied by bloating (this may suggest irritable bowel syndrome) or heartburn and regurgitation of acid (suggestive of GERD).
3) Whether the frequency of bowel movements and stool consistency are normal (any abnormalities and resolution of pain after bowel movements are suggestive of irritable bowel syndrome).
4) What medications the patient is taking (identify drugs that cause dyspepsia, particularly NSAIDs).
5) Whether there are any **alarming symptoms**, or **red flags** (unintended weight loss, abdominal pain waking the patient, jaundice, gastrointestinal bleeding, dysphagia, recurrent vomiting, epigastric mass).

2. Diagnostic studies: Perform the following to confirm or exclude an organic cause:
1) Complete blood count (CBC) (iron deficiency anemia is a red flag suggestive of an organic cause).
2) Abdominal ultrasonography (to be performed in patients with red flags).
3) Upper gastrointestinal endoscopy (not always necessary but usually warranted in patients aged ≥60 years in areas of low risk of gastric cancer and younger ages in countries where gastric cancer is more common. Red flags may prompt endoscopy in younger age groups but this depends on the

concern regarding cancer. For example, a 5-kg weight loss may not be of a major concern in a 20-year-old patient with dyspepsia but it may prompt endoscopy in a 55-year-old person.

→ MANAGEMENT

1. Undiagnosed dyspepsia: A noninvasive test for *Helicobacter pylori* followed by treatment if infected (→Chapter 6.1.2.4) is the recommended approach for young patients with dyspepsia. If the patient is *H pylori*–negative or does not respond to successful eradication therapy, then empiric proton pump inhibitor (PPI) therapy should be offered. Endoscopy should not be done routinely in young patients with dyspepsia. The definition of "young" will vary by country according to gastric cancer risk. In low-risk countries endoscopy is not necessary in those <60 years of age.

2. Organic dyspepsia: Treat the underlying condition and, if possible, discontinue the drugs that cause dyspepsia. In patients with coexisting heartburn and dyspepsia, the preliminary diagnosis is GERD, and empiric treatment with PPIs is started (agents and dosage: →Chapter 6.1.2.4). If dyspepsia persists despite appropriate treatment, GERD is an unlikely diagnosis. Of note, some European experts include a positive *H pylori* status among causes of organic dyspepsia.

3. Functional dyspepsia: By definition, if the patient has had an endoscopy and histology, they should have *H pylori* testing. If the test result is positive, start eradication therapy (→Chapter 6.1.2.4). If the test is negative or eradication therapy fails, treat the patient with a PPI. You may try amitriptyline 10 to 25 mg taken at bedtime for 8 to 12 weeks (if effective, continue for ~6 months). Instruct the patient to stop smoking, avoid foods and drinks that cause or worsen the symptoms, and eat frequent small meals. Prokinetic therapy, such as domperidone, may be tried if available in the country of practice. Psychotherapy may also be useful.

7. Dysphagia

→ DEFINITION AND ETIOLOGY

Dysphagia is a symptom of progressive or intermittent swallowing difficulty in the passage of solids and liquids from the oral cavity to the stomach due to a structural abnormality or esophageal motility disorder. Dysphagia may present as difficulty with swallowing, drinking, chewing, eating, sucking, controlling saliva, taking medication, or protecting the airway. It is usually related to underlying medical or physical conditions but occasionally may have a psychological component.

Oropharyngeal dysphagia refers to difficulty in the formation of a food bolus, propulsion of the bolus towards the pharynx, and initiation of swallowing movements. **Esophageal dysphagia** refers to difficulty in transition of the food bolus through the esophagus to the stomach. **Globus sensation** is a functional disorder manifested by a sensation of a lump, tightness, or retained food bolus in the pharyngeal or cervical area in the absence of major organic causes (esophageal dysmotility and association with gastroesophageal reflux disease [GERD]). **Functional dysphagia** is a sense of solid and/or liquid food lodging, sticking, or passing abnormally through the esophagus without evidence of objective abnormalities. **Odynophagia** refers to pain with swallow

Dysphagia-associated symptoms may include heartburn, regurgitation, food or fluid retention in the oral cavity, sensation of food "sticking", coughing during or right after eating or drinking, weight loss, chest di or pain, hematemesis, anemia, and respiratory symptoms. Food impaction is the most common cause for acute onset of dysphagia in adults. Aging-related mild esophageal dysmotility is rarely symptomatic.

1. Causes of oropharyngeal dysphagia:

1) Structural: Inflammation (stomatitis, pharyngitis, tonsillitis, abscess, syphilis), tumors (of the pharynx, tongue, floor of the mouth), compression by the surrounding structures (goiter, lymphadenopathy), severe degenerative lesions of the spine, or foreign bodies.

2) Neuromuscular disorders: Most frequently cerebrovascular disorders (ischemic stroke, thrombosis, intracranial bleeding), bulbar and pseudobulbar palsy, brain tumors, head trauma, sedating medications. Less frequently tabes dorsalis, neurodegenerative diseases, extrapyramidal syndromes (Parkinson disease, Huntington disease, tardive dyskinesia), peripheral neuropathy (diabetes mellitus, sarcoidosis, Sjögren syndrome, amyloidosis), connective tissue disease (systemic sclerosis, systemic lupus erythematosus, dermatomyositis), Guillain-Barré syndrome, diphtheria, botulism, radiation, poliomyelitis, myasthenia and myasthenic syndromes, or myopathy (oculopharyngeal muscular dystrophy, facioscapulohumeral muscular dystrophy, mitochondrial myopathy, myotonic dystrophy).

2. Causes of esophageal dysphagia:

1) Esophageal stricture: Erosive esophagitis (GERD, Zollinger-Ellison syndrome), eosinophilic esophagitis, carcinoma of the esophagus or cardia; esophageal diverticula (eg, Zenker diverticulum), caustic ingestions, postsurgical resection for esophageal or laryngeal cancer, drugs (eg, KCl, salicylates), radiation therapy for tumors located in the proximity of the esophagus, esophageal ring (Schatzki ring) or web, foreign bodies, lymphocytic esophagitis, or healing of pressure ulcers caused by a long-term indwelling nasogastric tube.

2) Esophageal motility disorders: Achalasia (type I, II, and III), esophagogastric junction outflow obstruction, distal esophageal spasm, hypercontractile esophagus (Jackhammer esophagus), ineffective esophageal motility, absent contractility due to systemic sclerosis or Sjögren syndrome, esophageal dysmotility due to diabetes mellitus, Chagas disease, or drugs (nitrates, calcium channel blockers, estrogens, methylxanthines).

3) Compression of the esophagus by the surrounding structures: Mitral valve disease, retrosternal goiter, mediastinal or bronchial tumor, paraesophageal hiatal hernia, or history of cardiac or thoracic surgery.

→ **DIAGNOSIS**

Dysphagia is an alarming symptom, especially if it has recently developed in an elderly patient and is rapidly worsening; in such cases promptly exclude cancer of the esophagus or cardia.

1. History and physical examination: Determine the type of dysphagia:

1) Oropharyngeal dysphagia is characterized by difficulty in the formation of a food bolus, its passage towards the pharynx, initiation of swallowing of liquids and solids, and sensation of residual food remaining in the pharynx or cervical region. Associated symptoms include dry cough, choking, throat discomfort, nasopharyngeal regurgitation, and aspiration. Pharyngeal dysfunction–induced dysphagia may be accompanied by dysphonia, sneezing, and lacrimation. Oral dysfunction–induced dysphagia may be associated with pain during swallowing, drooling, food spillage, sialorrhea, piecemeal swallows, and dysarthria.

2) Esophageal dysphagia is manifested by a sensation that food (initially solid food) is being obstructed at the suprasternal notch or retrosternal level for several seconds after initiating a swallow, distension or pressure in the

chest, vomiting, cough and expectoration of saliva, and in some cases also by pain on swallowing.

2. Diagnostic procedures:

1) Upper gastrointestinal endoscopy is essential to confirm or exclude structural changes of the esophagus, esophagogastric junction, and stomach with histologic examination.

2) Barium radiography is performed to identify the cause of oropharyngeal dysphagia (fluoroscopic examination of the process of swallowing) and esophageal motility disorders, such as Zenker diverticulum, achalasia, Jackhammer esophagus, hiatal hernia, and GERD.

3) Esophageal high-resolution manometry with or without impedance study can confirm the diagnosis of esophageal motility disorders, such as different types of achalasia and Jackhammer esophagus.

4) Ambulatory esophageal pH monitoring with or without impedance study is used to exclude GERD. It also provides information on whether dysphagia is associated with acid exposure of the esophagus.

→ COMPLICATIONS AND CONSEQUENCES

Malnutrition and dehydration, aspiration pneumonia, compromised general health, chronic lung disease, choking, and even death may be a consequence of dysphagia. Morbidity related to dysphagia is a major concern. Adults with dysphagia may also experience lack of interest in or less enjoyment of eating or drinking and embarrassment or isolation in social situations involving eating. Dysphagia may increase burden to caregivers and require significant lifestyle alterations for the patient and the patient's family.

→ TREATMENT AND PROGNOSIS

The treatment and prognosis of dysphagia depend on the nature of underlying condition.

8. Dyspnea: General Considerations

→ DEFINITION

Dyspnea is a subjective sensation of breathlessness or difficulty breathing. Dyspnea can be characterized by its acuity and association with exertion and positioning as:

1) Acute, intermittent or paroxysmal, and chronic dyspnea.

2) Dyspnea at rest and exertional dyspnea.

Dyspnea severity scales help quantify breathlessness or disability associated with breathlessness. Examples:

1) Modified Medical Research Council (mMRC) dyspnea scale (available at mdcalc.com): A 4-point scale for evaluating activities that generate dyspnea as ranging from strenuous exercise (0 points) through walking up a slight hill (1 point), walking slower than peers (2 points), running out of breath after a few minutes' walk on level ground (3 points), to getting dyspneic when dressing (4 points).

2) Borg scale (0, no dyspnea; 5, severe dyspnea; 10, maximal dyspnea).

3) Disease-specific scales: The New York Heart Association (NYHA) scale to evaluate dyspnea in heart failure (→Chapter 3.8, Table 8-3), rangin

dyspnea with strenuous exertion (stage 1) through dyspnea with ordinary physical activity (stage 2) to dyspnea with less than ordinary activity (stage 3) and dyspnea at rest (stage 4).

Orthopnea refers to dyspnea occurring in the recumbent position and improving when sitting or standing. Platypnea refers to dyspnea increasing in the sitting or standing position.

→ CAUSES AND PATHOGENESIS

1. Causes of dyspnea according to the underlying pathophysiology: The pathophysiology of dyspnea is complex and often involves interaction between pulmonary and extrapulmonary (cardiovascular, neuromuscular, and oxygen delivery) systems. Underlying mechanisms can be broadly categorized as impaired gas exchange (both at the level of the lungs and tissue) or impaired ventilatory drive, in either case leading to perception of breathlessness.

1) **Pulmonary**: Abnormal gas exchange may arise from dysfunction at the level of the alveoli, bronchi, lung parenchyma, pleura, or pulmonary vasculature. Alveolar disease processes may include infection, inflammation, and alveolar fluid (eg, in congestive heart failure). Bronchial disease processes include inflammatory conditions such as chronic obstructive pulmonary disease (COPD) and asthma. Examples of parenchymal disease include infection, inflammatory or collagen vascular diseases, malignancy, and interstitial lung disease. Pleural disease includes pleural effusions and malignancy, while pulmonary arterial diseases include pulmonary hypertension and pulmonary embolism.

2) **Extrapulmonary**:

   a) **Cardiovascular**: Dyspnea in cardiovascular disease is often driven by decreased cardiac output (shock or heart failure). Further categorization of specific causes includes cardiac ischemia, cardiac arrhythmia, valvular disease, and myopericardial disease.

   b) **Neuromuscular**: This predominantly affects ventilatory drive and effort in the absence of gas exchange abnormalities. Neuromuscular causes of hypoventilation can arise at the level of the muscle (myopathy or respiratory muscle/diaphragmatic weakness), neuromuscular junction (neuromuscular conduction abnormalities such as myasthenic crisis) or nerve conduction abnormalities (Guillain-Barré syndrome). Other etiologies of hypoventilation and hypercapnia include mechanical causes such as chest wall deformities, obesity hypoventilation syndrome (OHS), and metabolic causes outlined below.

   c) **Metabolic**: This includes sensation of breathlessness caused by nonrespiratory acidosis (eg, lactic acidosis, diabetic ketoacidosis, renal tubular acidosis), thyrotoxicosis, stimulation of the respiratory center by endogenous toxins (toxins originating in the liver, uremic toxins) and exogenous toxins (salicylates).

   d) **Other**: Abnormal tissue gas exchange can result from impaired oxygen binding by hemoglobin (eg, carbon monoxide poisoning and methemoglobinemia) or decreased cellular oxygen utilization (eg, with cyanide poisoning). Anxiety and strenuous exercise in healthy individuals are more benign considerations.

2. Causes of specific presentations of dyspnea:

1) **Acute dyspnea** (and differential diagnosis): →Table 8-1.

2) **Chronic dyspnea** (initially exertional, subsequently also at rest): COPD, bronchiectasis, chronic heart failure, interstitial lung disease, posttuberculous lesions in the lungs, primary and secondary lung tumors, anemia, neuromuscular disorders.

3) **Paroxysmal nocturnal dyspnea and orthopnea**: Left ventricular failure; chronic pulmonary diseases causing impaired sputum evacuation during sleep (COPD, bronchiectasis), ventilation abnormalities increasing in the recumbent

Table 8-1. Differentiation of causes of dyspnea based on its onset and accompanying symptoms

Onset	
Sudden onset of dyspnea, often with severe chest pain	Pneumothorax, pulmonary edema; foreign body aspiration; MI; pulmonary embolus
Dyspnea progressing over minutes to hours, often with wheezing	Asthma (history of asthma attacks); exacerbation of COPD, acute left ventricular failure (eg, in acute MI)
Dyspnea progressing over hours to days, often with fever and expectoration	Pneumonia; acute bronchitis
Accompanying symptoms	
Stridor	Tumor in trachea; foreign body aspiration, anaphylaxis
Chest pain	Angina pectoris or MI, pulmonary embolism; aortic dissection; cardiac tamponade
Pleural pain	Pneumonia or pleurisy; early phase of pleural effusion accumulation; pulmonary embolism, pneumothorax
Sputum expectoration	Bronchiectasis; chronic bronchitis; left ventricular failure; pneumonia, pulmonary abscess
Hemoptysis	Lung tumor; pulmonary embolism; chronic bronchitis; systemic vasculitis, tuberculosis, bronchiectasis, pulmonary abscess
Muscle weakness, neurologic symptoms	Myasthenia gravis (myasthenic crisis); amyotrophic lateral sclerosis; Guillain-Barré syndrome, diaphragmatic weakness (phrenic nerve injury)
Expiratory wheeze	Asthma; COPD (acute exacerbation); bronchiectasis; left ventricular failure

COPD, chronic obstructive pulmonary disease; MI, myocardial infarction.

position (interstitial lung disease) or increase in airway resistance during sleep (obstructive sleep apnea, in some cases asthma or COPD).

4) **Platypnea**: Dyspnea in the upright position that is relieved in the recumbent position. This is usually related to intracardiac or intrapulmonary (eg, hepatopulmonary syndrome) shunting (→Chapter 6.2.2.5.).

Also →Chapter 11.1.

DIAGNOSIS

Assess the vital signs (temperature, respiratory rate, oxygen saturation, heart rate, blood pressure) and take a history. Perform physical examination (differential diagnosis based on the time of onset of dyspnea and accompanying symptoms: →Table 8-1), blood gas analysis, complete blood count, and chest radiography. Depending on the suspected cause, perform further cardiovascular (electrocardiography [ECG], echocardiography, venous ultrasonography, chest computed tomography [CT] angiography) or respiratory (pulmonary function tests, chest CT) investigations. Additionally, measure serum levels of electrolytes, glucose, ketones, and lactate, and perform renal function tests (especially in patients with acidosis), liver function tests, tests for hemoglobinopathy, neurologic examination when appropriate.

→ TREATMENT

Treatment of dyspnea depends on the underlying etiology. For most causes, there are disease-specific treatments that are discussed in relevant chapters.

In patients with acute hypoxemia, starting oxygen therapy is warranted, even before establishing the cause. If patients are not hypoxic there may be no role for supplemental oxygenation. We recommend avoiding oxygen supplementation achieving saturation >94% to 96%.🗹🗙 Caution is warranted when administering oxygen to patients with chronic carbon dioxide retention; in such situations the goal of supplemental oxygen should be to achieve an oxygen saturation level between 88% and 92%. Patients with hypoxia, hypoventilation, or hypercarbia may require noninvasive positive-pressure ventilation (high-flow nasal oxygen, continuous positive airway pressure [CPAP], or bilevel positive airway pressure [BiPAP]). In patients in whom noninvasive ventilation has failed or those who are unable to maintain their airway, endotracheal intubation and mechanical ventilation may be warranted.

9. Edema

→ DEFINITION AND PATHOGENESIS

Edema (swelling) is the accumulation of fluid in the tissue interstitium.

1. Mechanism: There are 4 major mechanisms that fundamentally lead to edema. Frequently ≥1 mechanism is present.

1) Increased hydrostatic pressure at the venous end of the capillary bed (eg, in patients with congestive heart failure or venous valve incompetence).

2) Decreased plasma oncotic pressure (due to hypoalbuminemia).

3) Increased capillary wall permeability (most frequently due to inflammation).

4) Impaired lymphatic drainage (eg, in patients with severe lymphadenopathy, with a recent history of lymphadenectomy or radiotherapy, or with filariasis).

2. Location and distribution:

1) **Local edema**: Inflammation, allergy (eg, Quincke edema), impaired venous drainage (eg, deep vein thrombosis [DVT]), impaired lymphatic drainage (eg, malignancy-related lymphadenopathy, erysipelas, filariasis).

2) **Generalized edema**: Due to cardiac causes (eg, heart failure), hepatic causes (eg, cirrhosis), renal causes (eg, nephrotic syndrome), endocrine causes (eg, hypothyroidism), malnutrition (eg, protein deficiency, vitamin B_1 deficiency), pregnancy; drug-induced (eg, glucocorticoid treatment); idiopathic.

→ DIAGNOSIS

Assess the extent and location of edema (local or generalized).

1. Localized edema: Local inflammatory edema is characterized by pain, warming, and erythema. Edema due to impaired venous drainage is usually asymmetric (except for superior vena cava syndrome) and painless. Clinical examination may reveal features of DVT. Prolonged venous edema leads to trophic changes in the skin. Allergic edema develops rapidly, is pale and painless, and resolves quickly. If venous obstruction is a possibility (based on the patient's history and physical examination), compression ultrasonography (CUS) may be used for initial evaluation. If there is a suggestion of obstruction within the pelvis, computed tomography (CT) may be of use.

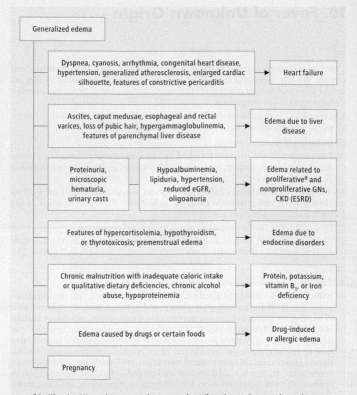

Generalized edema

Dyspnea, cyanosis, arrhythmia, congenital heart disease, hypertension, generalized atherosclerosis, enlarged cardiac silhouette, features of constrictive pericarditis → Heart failure

Ascites, caput medusae, esophageal and rectal varices, loss of pubic hair, hypergammaglobulinemia, features of parenchymal liver disease → Edema due to liver disease

Proteinuria, microscopic hematuria, urinary casts | Hypoalbuminemia, lipiduria, hypertension, reduced eGFR, oligoanuria → Edema related to proliferative[a] and nonproliferative GNs, CKD (ESRD)

Features of hypercortisolemia, hypothyroidism, or thyrotoxicosis; premenstrual edema → Edema due to endocrine disorders

Chronic malnutrition with inadequate caloric intake or qualitative dietary deficiencies, chronic alcohol abuse, hypoproteinemia → Protein, potassium, vitamin B₁, or iron deficiency

Edema caused by drugs or certain foods → Drug-induced or allergic edema

Pregnancy

[a] Proliferative GNs can have many other nonrenal manifestations and may not have edema.

CKD, chronic kidney disease; eGFR, estimated glomerular filtration rate; ESRD, end-stage renal disease; GN, glomerulonephritis.

Figure 9-1. Differential diagnosis of generalized edema.

2. Generalized edema: Significant generalized edema occurs in patients with advanced heart failure, nephrotic syndrome, or acute or chronic liver disease. These conditions cause major fluid retention and significant weight gain, which may be accompanied by pleural effusion or ascites. In patients who are able to walk, edema usually starts in the lower limbs, while in bedridden patients it affects the sacral area. The edema is usually pitting (applying pressure with a finger produces a pit that disappears slowly). Diagnostic workup depends on the clinical situation.

Generally, the history and physical examination are very helpful in differentiating various organ diseases that manifest with generalized edema. Initial laboratory and imaging findings include (if available) attaining a urine dipstick to evaluate for proteinuria, serum albumin level, thyrod-stimulating hormone (TSH) level, and measures of renal and liver function. Chest radiography, ultrasonography, and echocardiography can also be of use.

Differential diagnosis of generalized edema: →Figure 9-1.

10. Fever of Unknown Origin

→ DEFINITION AND ETIOLOGY

Fever of unknown origin (FUO) is a clinical entity that may have various causes. Its key feature is fever that does not resolve spontaneously, persists longer than an average infectious disease, and whose cause remains unknown despite routine investigations.

Classic FUO is diagnosed if all of the 3 following criteria are met:

1) Fever >38.3°C that persists or recurs on several occasions.

2) Duration of fever >3 weeks.

3) The cause has not been established or remains uncertain despite routine diagnostic investigations continued for ~1 week (≥3 days in the hospital or ≥3 outpatient visits).

In hospitalized patients (after ≥2 days of hospitalization) as well as patients with neutropenia or HIV infection, FUO is diagnosed if the following criteria are met:

1) Fever >38.3°C that persists or recurs on several occasions.

2) The cause has not been established or diagnosis remains uncertain despite routine inpatient diagnostic investigations continued for 3 to 5 days.

Causes

1. The most important causes of classic FUO:

1) **Infection** (the longer the duration of FUO, the more unlikely the infectious etiology): Most frequently pulmonary and extrapulmonary tuberculosis (TB), abscess (intraabdominal, subphrenic, perinephric, pelvic), infectious endocarditis, cytomegalovirus (CMV) infection, toxoplasmosis, typhoid fever, paratyphoid fever, chronic prostatitis; less frequently systemic fungal infection or zoonotic diseases (mostly travel-associated infections, particularly those linked to travelling to tropical countries), such as malaria, leptospirosis, brucellosis, tularemia, psittacosis, rickettsial infections (spotted fevers, typhus), Q fever, anaplasmosis, ehrlichiosis, bartonellosis, and cat-scratch disease.

2) **Inflammatory diseases**: Systemic connective tissue diseases (most frequently adult-onset Still disease, polyarteritis nodosa, systemic lupus erythematosus) and inflammatory bowel disease (particularly Crohn disease). In elderly patients more frequent causes are temporal arteritis, polymyalgia rheumatica, and rheumatoid arthritis.

3) **Cancer**: Most frequently hematologic and lymphatic malignancies (Hodgkin lymphoma, non-Hodgkin lymphoma, leukemia, myelodysplastic syndrome), clear cell renal cell carcinoma, hepatic adenoma, liver cancer, pancreatic cancer, colorectal cancer, primary central nervous system (CNS) malignancies.

4) **Drugs (usually polytherapy)**: Most frequently penicillins, sulfonamides, vancomycin, amphotericin B, salicylates, bleomycin, interferons, quinidine derivatives, phenothiazine derivatives (promethazine, thiethylperazine), barbiturates, phenytoin, methyldopa, haloperidol (malignant neuroleptic syndrome), tricyclic antidepressants, and lithium. Drug-induced fever is more frequent in the elderly. It usually develops within 1 to 2 weeks of starting treatment (although it may occur at any point of treatment) and resolves spontaneously within 48 to 72 hours (later in patients with liver disease or renal failure). Fever may be accompanied by erythematous, macular, or maculopapular rash and increased eosinophil counts. The pattern of fever is not significant. Relative bradycardia is often present.

5) **Other**: Alcoholic hepatitis, thyroiditis, pulmonary embolism (generally recurrent and undetected, without severe clinical symptoms), and hematomas.

2. Causes of FUO based on the risk group:

1) **FUO in a hospitalized patient**: Most frequently caused by abscess (intra-abdominal or pelvic), sinusitis (due to prolonged presence of a nasotracheal tube), catheter-associated bloodstream infection (long-term indwelling catheter in a large vessel), infective endocarditis (associated with invasive diagnostic procedures, catheterization of large vessels, or surgery), pseudomembranous colitis (*Clostridium difficile*), drugs, septic thrombophlebitis, pulmonary embolism, pancreatitis, retroperitoneal hematoma.

2) **FUO in a patient with neutropenia**: Primary bacteremia, catheter-associated bloodstream infections (long-term indwelling catheter in a large vessel), fungemia (eg, *Candida* spp), hepatosplenic candidiasis, invasive fungal infection (eg, *Aspergillus* spp), pelvic abscess (perirectal or located between the rectum and sacral bone), drugs, metastases to the CNS or liver.

3) **FUO in a patient with HIV infection**: TB and non-TB mycobacterial infection are the most common causes. Less frequent are pneumocystosis, CMV infection, herpes simplex virus (HSV) infection, toxoplasmosis, salmonellosis, fungal infection, lymphoma, Kaposi sarcoma, and drugs (eg, sulfamethoxazole/trimethoprim). HIV alone is rarely responsible for FUO.

4) **FUO in a patient returning from tropical regions**: Malaria (incubation period up to 6 weeks, although in cases of *Plasmodium vivax* and *Plasmodium ovale* it may be up to several months or years); other tropical parasitic infestations (amebiasis, leishmaniasis, trypanosomiasis, cryptosporidiosis, filariasis, tropical pulmonary eosinophilia, schistosomiasis, paragonimiasis); typhoid fever (incubation period up to 6 weeks); viral hemorrhagic fevers, most frequently dengue fever (incubation period 3-8 days).

→ DIAGNOSIS

Basic diagnostic studies used in the evaluation of FUO:

1) **Laboratory tests**: Complete blood count (CBC) with differential count; erythrocyte sedimentation rate (ESR); serum levels of electrolytes, bilirubin, liver enzymes, urea/blood urea nitrogen (BUN), creatinine, and uric acid; urinalysis; rheumatoid factor; antinuclear antibodies; microbiologic studies: blood cultures (2-3 cultures in a patient not treated with antibiotics), urine cultures, tuberculin skin test, serologic studies (HIV, CMV, Epstein-Barr virus [EBV]). Some clinicians use procalcitonin as an aid in differentiation between bacterial infections and other causes of fever, but the clinical utility of the test in this setting is unclear.

2) **Imaging studies**: Abdominal ultrasonography, chest radiography, abdominal and pelvic computed tomography (CT) or magnetic resonance imaging (MRI); if necessary (symptoms or signs of CNS involvement), also CT or MRI of the head.

Take a detailed history and repeatedly perform thorough physical examinations. Make sure that body temperature is measured and interpreted correctly (→below). The combination of localizing signs and symptoms accompanying FUO (potential diagnostic clues) together with the results of key diagnostic studies provide the basis for preliminary diagnosis and guide further investigations. If the patient's condition is stable, the preliminary diagnostic workup may be performed in an outpatient setting.

If the condition is not life-threatening and the patient is hospitalized, you m consider watchful waiting and use targeted diagnostic studies to confirr exclude the most probable causes in a given risk group (eg, patients retur from a tropical country; hospitalized patients; patients with neutro patients with HIV infection; patients aged >50 years). Start with noninvasive studies and add invasive studies when necessary. If the patient is severely ill, simultaneously exclude probable causes. In febrile patients with a recent history of travel to areas endemic for malaria, promptly exclude malaria (prophylactic treatment with antimalarial agents during travel does not exclude the possibility of infection).

If drug-induced fever is suspected, start by discontinuing all drugs used by the patient (including over-the-counter agents) or reduce their number to the necessary minimum. Check if the patient has used drugs of abuse (including designer drugs) or unapproved weight-loss products. Drug-induced fever usually resolves within 48 to 72 hours following discontinuation of the offending agent.

In justified cases some experts suggest empiric treatment if specific but unconfirmed diseases are suspected; most frequently, this involves TB (if clinically suspected, start TB treatment after obtaining specimens for culture), infective endocarditis (if suspected based on the Duke criteria [→Chapter 3.10, Table 10-1], start antimicrobial therapy after obtaining appropriate blood cultures), temporal arteritis, or other systemic connective tissue diseases (exclude infection, then consider glucocorticoids and nonsteroidal anti-inflammatory drugs [NSAIDs]). Resolution of fever and other symptoms in response to therapy confirms the preliminary diagnosis. In the case of transient improvement, consider investigation for malignancy, particularly if low-grade or high-grade fever is accompanied by systemic manifestations or lymphadenopathy.

Differential Diagnosis

1. Incorrect measurement of body temperature: To meet the criterion of a body temperature elevation >38.3°C, it is necessary to establish how the measurement was made, including the type of thermometer (mercury, electronic, LCD, infrared), site of measurement (mouth, forehead, axilla, ear, rectum), time of day, frequency of measurements, and conditions and technique of measurement. You may ask patients to demonstrate how they measure their temperature and handle the thermometer. The least accurate measurements are made in the axilla (results are ~0.8°C lower than the core body temperature) and ear (results are highly variable, depending on the presence of cerumen and other factors). Oral temperature is ~0.5°C lower and rectal temperature is ~0.5°C higher than the core temperature. Chewing gum immediately before the measurement increases temperatures measured in the mouth or ear, while smoking has a similar effect on the temperature measured in the mouth. Measure body temperature preferably several times a day over a few days of diagnostic hospitalization with monitoring of pulse rate, which eliminates measurement errors and may be used to assess the patterns of fever and pulse. Note that the reference ranges for body temperatures are variable and change depending on the time of day, season, phase of the menstrual cycle, and nutrition status.

2. Factitious fever: It is generally chronic and accompanied by varied changing symptoms. The course is inconsistent. The patient's history reveals numerous hospitalizations. A chronic fever of this type is generally not accompanied by weight loss and patients are in good general condition. Antipyretic drugs are usually ineffective. Most patients have psychiatric or personality disorders; somatic disorders are often seen. Hospitalized patients generally refuse their consent for supervised body temperature measurements and certain diagnostic tests. If body temperature is taken using a mercury thermometer, the recorded values are usually very high and show no diurnal variation. The skin is cold. Relative bradycardia is present. You may ask the patient to provide a urine sample after body temperature measurement and immediately measure the sample's temperature (it is always slightly higher than the oral or axillary temperature).

→ TREATMENT

Symptomatic Treatment

1. Antipyretic agents:

1) First-line agents: Oral or rectal **acetaminophen** (INN paracetamol) 500 to 1000 mg, repeated if necessary every 6 hours (up to 4 g/d). If oral or rectal administration is not possible, 500 to 1000 mg may be administered IV every 6 hours (maximum, 4 g/d). In patients with severe renal failure (creatinine clearance <10 mL/min), increase the dosing interval to every 8 hours. In patients with cirrhosis, limit acetaminophen to a maximum dose of 2 g/d. Acetaminophen overdose leads to acute liver failure (this may occur even with 8 g/d; the risk is highest in patients who are fasting or abuse alcohol). Management of acetaminophen overdose: →Chapter 15.1.

2) Alternative antipyretics: **NSAIDs:**

   a) Oral **ibuprofen** 200 to 400 mg, repeated if necessary every 5 to 6 hours (maximum, 2 g/d).

   b) Oral **acetylsalicylic acid** 500 mg, repeated if necessary every 5 to 6 hours (maximum, 2.5 g/d). Contraindicated in patients with peptic ulcer disease, bleeding disorder, or aspirin-induced asthma.

2. Techniques of physical cooling: These are used in patients with a very high fever (>40°C) not responding to antipyretic agents.

11. Fingers, Deformed

11.1. Clubbing

→ ETIOLOGY AND PATHOGENESIS

Clubbing of the fingers (with their shape resembling drumsticks) develops due to the proliferation of the connective tissue of the dorsal aspect of distal phalanges of the fingers or less frequently of the toes, which leads to elevation of the nail (→Figure 11-6). Periungual erythema is commonly present. The angle between the nail bed and the nail fold is ≥180° (a normal angle is ~160°). The underlying mechanism of clubbing is unknown.

Causes:

1) Pulmonary: Pulmonary neoplasms (non–small cell lung cancer, mesothelioma, adenocarcinoma), pulmonary fibrosis, subacute or chronic inflammatory or infectious conditions (eg, empyema, lung abscesses, bronchiectasis, tuberculosis), cystic fibrosis, sarcoidosis.

2) Cardiac: Congenital cyanotic heart disease, infective endocarditis, left atrial myxoma.

3) Gastrointestinal: Crohn disease, ulcerative colitis, cirrhosis (biliary and portal).

4) Endocrine: Graves disease, thyrotoxicosis.

5) Idiopathic clubbing.

Bilateral clubbing is characteristic for central cyanosis. Clubbing limited to one limb is a result of impaired arterial perfusion in the affected limb due to patent ductus arteriosus, aneurysm (eg, of the aorta or subclavian artery) arteriovenous fistula (in patients treated with hemodialysis), or arteritis. may also occur in the course of **hypertrophic osteodystrophy** (pai subperiosteal formation of new bone), which is additionally character by periosteal thickening palpable over surfaces of the bones not cove muscles (around the ankles and wrists) and tenderness in these locations, as well as edema, joint pain, and features of joint effusion (most frequently affecting the knees, ankles, and elbows). In primary hypertrophic osteodystrophy generalized cutaneous thickening may occur, with the skin becoming folded. The most frequent (>90%) cause of secondary hypertrophic osteodystrophy is paraneoplastic, occurring in lung cancer, commonly known as hypertrophic pulmonary osteoarthropathy (HPOA). However, other pulmonary infections, cystic fibrosis, right to left cardiac shunting, and lymphomas have also been associated with HPOA.

→ DIAGNOSIS

A detailed history and physical examination are required to identify the underlying etiology. Further diagnostic workup should be performed depending on the suspected organ system involved.

If HPOA is suspected, radiographs of the epiphysis of long bones (revealing periosteal thickening) can be obtained. Bone scintigraphy can be helpful in excluding skeletal involvement. Because of the association of this disorder with pulmonary malignancies, chest radiographs and computed tomography (CT) may be necessary.

11.2. Fingers in Rheumatic Diseases

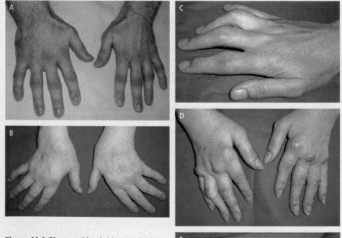

Figure 11-1. Rheumatoid arthritis. **A**, early changes: symmetric swelling of the metacarpophalangeal and proximal interphalangeal joints. **B**, ulnar deviation of the fingers and subluxation of the metacarpophalangeal joints. **C**, boutonnière deformity (fingers III and IV). **D**, swelling of the metacarpophalangeal and proximal interphalangeal joints, subluxation of the metacarpophalangeal joints, numerous rheumatoid nodules around the joints. **E**, swan-neck deformity of the little finger.

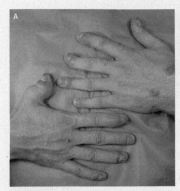

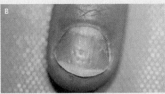

Figure 11-2. Psoriatic arthritis. A, psoriatic lesions on the skin of the outer aspect of both hands, telescopic finger I of the right hand, characteristic involvement of the distal interphalangeal joints, subluxation of the distal phalanx of finger III of the left hand, sausage-shaped finger II of the right hand. B, nail pitting.

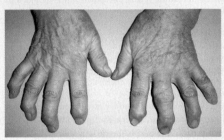

Figure 11-3. Osteoarthritis of the hand: Heberden nodes (over the distal interphalangeal joints) involving most fingers of both hands, a Bouchard node (over the proximal interphalangeal joint) on finger III of the left hand.

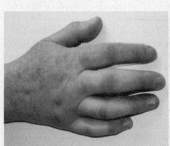

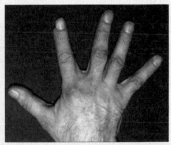

Figure 11-4. Systemic sclerosis. The skin on the digits is shiny, hardened, and limits full extension and full flexion of the fingers.

Figure 11-5. Polymyositis and dermatomyositis. Bluish papules over the interphalangeal and metacarpophalangeal joints (Gottron papules).

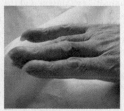

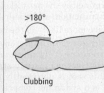

Figure 11-6. Clubbing.

12. Hematuria

→ DEFINITION

Hematuria is defined as an increased number of red blood cells (RBCs) in urine, namely, >3 RBCs per high-power field (HPF) in a centrifuged urine sample. In **microscopic hematuria** the color of urine is unchanged. In **gross hematuria** the color of urine suggests the presence of blood.

→ CAUSES AND PATHOGENESIS

Causes of hematuria: The following classification is based on the origin of RBCs in the urinary tract:

1) **Glomerular hematuria** (caused by glomerular disease): All types of acute or chronic glomerulonephritis, including IgA nephropathy, anti–glomerular basement membrane disease, and immune complex glomerulonephritis; hereditary causes, such as Alport syndrome; and benign causes, such as thin basement membrane disease.

2) **Nonglomerular hematuria**:

   a) Upper urinary tract: Nephrolithiasis, renal cysts, cancer (renal parenchyma, renal pelvis, renal calyces, ureter), hypercalciuria, hyperuricosuria, pyelonephritis, renal trauma, renal papillary necrosis, renal infarct, renal vein thrombosis, renal tuberculosis.

   b) Bladder: Cystitis, cancer, polyp, trauma, bladder stones, endometriosis.

   c) Urethra: Urethritis, trauma, stricture, cancer, foreign body.

   d) Prostate: Cancer, benign prostatic hyperplasia, prostatitis.

3) **Other**: Strenuous exercise, fever, sexual intercourse, bleeding disorder, admixture of menstrual blood, unknown cause.

Nonglomerular hematuria accounts for ~90% of all cases of hematuria.

The color of urine suggestive of hematuria may be due to the presence of pigments contained in foods (beetroot, rhubarb, certain mushrooms (*Lactarius deliciosus* or "saffron milk cap"), synthetic food dyes, or medications (senna, rifampin [INN rifampicin], phenolphthalein).

→ DIAGNOSTIC WORKUP

A positive urine dipstick result for the presence of blood should always be confirmed by microscopic examination (positive result may be due to the presence of hemoglobin or myoglobin). Take a medical history and perform a physical examination with initial diagnostic studies (urinalysis including microscopic examination of the urine sediment; complete blood count; serum levels of creatinine, sodium, potassium, and calcium; coagulation parameters if bleeding disorder is suspected). The scope of diagnostic evaluation and the sequence of tests are determined by the most likely causes of hematuria based on the patient's history, examination, and results of diagnostic studies above:

1) Nonglomerular causes are more likely in the case of gross hematuria.

2) Glomerular causes are suggested by the presence of proteinuria (>0.5 g/24 h) and RBC casts. The presence of dysmorphic RBCs in urine sediment detected using phase-contrast microscopy strongly suggests glomerular hematuria (although this test is not readily available in many centers). **Nephritic syndrome** is a syndrome comprising signs of nephritis or inflammation within the glomeruli. Glomerular hematuria (or active urine sediment), proteinuria, elevated creatinine, and hypertension may be

present. The diagnostic workup for nephritic syndrome would entail sending bloodwork for complements, antinuclear antibodies, extractable nuclear antigens, rheumatoid factor, cytoplasmic antineutrophil cytoplasmic antibodies, perinuclear antineutrophil cytoplasmic antibodies, anti–glomerular basement membrane antibodies, quantitative immunoglobulins, antistreptolysin O titers, hepatitis B and C serology, cryoglobulins, and HIV in at-risk individuals. Renal biopsy may be considered if clinically indicated after consultation with a nephrologist. In patients with microscopic or gross hematuria without other features strongly suggestive of glomerular etiology, a complete diagnostic workup should be performed, including imaging studies of the kidneys (ultrasonography or high-resolution computed tomography [HRCT]), upper urinary tract (intravenous urography or HRCT urography), cystoscopy, and cytologic examination of urine. In women gynecologic examination should be also considered. In patients receiving anticoagulation treatment, persistent hematuria requires a diagnostic evaluation.

No further evaluation is usually necessary if hematuria has occurred:

1) In a young woman with typical clinical features of cystitis, confirmed urinary tract infection (significant bacteriuria), and hematuria resolving after antibiotic treatment.

2) In the case of strenuous exercise, fever, menstruation, or potential urinary tract injury (eg, sexual intercourse) if follow-up urinalysis obtained >48 hours after resolution of the potential precipitant reveals no hematuria.

13. Hemoptysis

→ DEFINITION AND ETIOLOGY

Hemoptysis refers to expectoration of frank blood or blood-tinged sputum.

Massive hemoptysis refers to bleeding from the respiratory tract, usually >200 mL over 24 hours, which may be life-threatening and lead to respiratory failure.

Bleeding can originate from two sources: bronchial arteries or the pulmonary vasculature. Nearly the entire cardiac output traverses through the low-pressure pulmonary arteries, while the bronchial arteries are under much higher pressure but carry only a small fraction of the total cardiac output. Bleeding from high-pressure bronchial vessels is the cause, particularly in the setting of massive hemoptysis, as the bronchial arteries are the vascular supply of the large airways. Mechanisms of bleeding include:

1) Inflammation and proliferation of vessels prone to bleeding (bronchiectasis, tuberculosis).

2) Infiltration and angiogenesis in pulmonary malignancies.

3) Pulmonary vascular disorders: Increased left atrial pressure (mitral stenosis, left ventricular failure), pulmonary hypertension, pulmonary embolism.

4) Bleeding diathesis that is either congenital, acquired, or iatrogenic.

5) Parenchymal disorders including infection and inflammatory conditions including capillaritis (→Chapter 14.23).

6) Neoplasm with direct invasion into bronchial arteries or pulmonary arteries

Causes of hemoptysis:

1) Frequent causes: Bronchitis, bronchiectasis, lung cancer, bacterial pneumonia, tuberculosis (in some geographic locations).

2) Moderately frequent causes: Pulmonary embolism (thrombotic, less commonly septic and fat), left ventricular failure, aspergillosis, vasculitis including granulomatosis with polyangiitis [formerly Wegener granulomatosis], connective tissue disease (anti–glomerular basement membrane disease [formerly Goodpasture syndrome], systemic lupus erythematosus), lung trauma (including iatrogenic trauma caused by bronchoscopy, lung biopsy, chest tubes or central line insertions, and thoracotomy).

3) Rare causes: Bleeding disorder, mitral stenosis, parasitic infestations, pulmonary artery pseudoaneurysm (Rasmussen aneurysm), drugs (anticoagulant agents, fibrinolytic agents, acetylsalicylic acid, cocaine), foreign body aspiration, hemosiderosis, amyloidosis, trauma related to performing right heart catheterization.

The most frequent causes of massive hemoptysis: Malignancy, bronchiectasis, tuberculosis, trauma, bleeding disorder.

→ **DIAGNOSIS**

1. History and physical examination: Establish the cause on the basis of:
1) **Characteristics of hemoptysis and accompanying signs and symptoms**:
   a) Massive expectoration of blood-stained sputum is suggestive of bronchiectasis.
   b) Purulent and bloody sputum: Bronchitis, bronchiectasis; if accompanied by fever, pneumonia or pulmonary abscess.
   c) Pink frothy sputum: Left ventricular failure, mitral stenosis.
   d) Expectoration of pure blood: Lung cancer, tuberculosis, arteriovenous malformations, pulmonary embolism.
2) **History**:
   a) Smoking, recurrent hemoptysis: Suggestive of lung cancer.
   b) Sudden-onset hemoptysis with severe chest pain and dyspnea: Pulmonary embolism.
   c) Chest trauma, invasive diagnostic procedures: Trauma-induced hemoptysis.
   d) Vasculitis or connective tissue disease: Hemoptysis and manifestations of the underlying systemic condition.
   e) Considerable weight loss: Lung cancer, tuberculosis, systemic inflammatory condition.
   f) Paroxysmal nocturnal dyspnea or exertional dyspnea: Left ventricular failure, mitral stenosis.

2. Diagnostic studies:
1) Chest radiography or computed tomography (CT) depending on the suspected cause (CT angiography if pulmonary embolism is suspected).
2) Complete blood count (CBC) and blood coagulation tests (international normalized ratio [INR], activated partial thromboplastin time [aPTT], and other).
3) Bronchoscopy for diagnostic purposes, particularly if lung cancer, diffuse alveolar hemorrhage, or infection is suspected; therapeutic bronchoscopy (→Treatment, below).
4) Ear, nose, and throat (ENT) examination if upper respiratory tract bleeding is suspected.
5) Other tests depending on the clinical suspicion (eg, testing for tuberculosis, antinuclear antibody, extractable nuclear antigen, antineutrophil cytoplasmic antibody, glomerular basement membrane antibody, urinalysis).

→ TREATMENT

Management of Massive Hemoptysis

1. Maintain the airway and secure IV access. Transfer the patient to a monitored unit with frequent vital signs assessment. In patients with severe shortness of breath, poor gas exchange, hemodynamic instability, or rapid ongoing bleeding, resuscitation procedures should be initiated and the patient should be intubated with a large-bore endotracheal tube. Consider placing the tube in the main bronchus of the opposite lung, allowing separate ventilation and isolation of the affected lung. Placement of a double-lumen tube is an alternative solution.

2. Start oxygen therapy. Maintain oxygen saturation (SaO_2) >90%.

3. Identify which side is bleeding. If the bleeding site has been identified, place the patient in a recumbent position on the side of the affected lung.

4. Collect blood samples for blood type, cross-matching, complete blood count (CBC), and blood coagulation parameters. Perform portable chest radiography.

5. Correct any coagulation abnormalities, anemia, and hypovolemia.

6. Exclude bleeding from the upper respiratory and gastrointestinal tracts.

7. Bronchoscopy can serve both diagnostic and therapeutic purposes in the management of massive hemoptysis. First, it can identify the source of bleeding. Second, bronchoscopy techniques may assist in controlling pulmonary hemorrhage through balloon tamponade, iced saline lavage, application of topical vasoconstrictive agents, cryotherapy, and guiding double-lumen endotracheal tube positioning.

8. If bleeding persists, arteriography may be performed, which allows for diagnosis and therapeutic embolization. High-resolution CT of the chest with contrast can be performed if bronchoscopy is nondiagnostic and arteriography is not indicated (ie, bleeding has stopped).

9. Unilateral uncontrollable bleeding should warrant thoracic surgery consultation for consideration of resection of the affected lobe of the lung if the conventional measures outlined above are not successful.

14. Hiccups (Singultus)

→ DEFINITION AND PATHOGENESIS

Hiccups (singultus) are involuntary synchronous contractions of the intercostal muscles and the diaphragm that cause sudden inspiration. This leads to closure of the glottis and is accompanied by a characteristic sound.

Hiccups are triggered by stimulation of the vagus nerve, phrenic nerve, and sympathetic nerves innervating the chest, abdomen, ear, nose, and pharynx, or by stimulation of the hiccup center in the central nervous system (CNS). The hiccup rate may be from 2 to 60 per minute. Episodes of hiccups are usually brief (lasting several minutes) and are most frequently associated with rapid or excessive gastric distension. **The vast majority of episodes of hiccups are short, self-terminating, and inconsequential, requiring no investigation.**

Persistent hiccups (>48 hours) may result in exhaustion, discomfort, weight loss (due to interference with food intake), insomnia, and depression.

Causes of persistent hiccups:
1) CNS disorders: Vascular, inflammatory, neoplastic, multiple sclero drocephalus.

2) Metabolic disorders: Diabetes mellitus, uremia, hyponatremia, hypocalcemia, hypocapnia.

3) Toxins and drugs: Alcohol, nicotine, barbiturates, benzodiazepines, etoposide, dexamethasone.

4) Neck and chest disorders: Tumor, lymphadenopathy, lung cancer, pneumonia with pleural inflammation, myocardial infarction, esophageal cancer, mediastinal tumors, diaphragmatic hernia, gastroesophageal reflux disease (GERD).

5) Abdominal disorders: Gastric cancer, peptic ulcer disease, gastric distension (a very common cause), gastrointestinal (GI) bleeding, pancreatic cancer, pancreatitis, hepatomegaly, splenomegaly, ascites, cholelithiasis, intestinal obstruction, peritonitis.

6) Psychogenic causes.

→ D I A G N O S I S

Diagnostic Workup of Persistent Hiccups

A thorough history and physical examination often elucidate the etiology of persistent hiccups. Routine supplemental investigations may include laboratory investigations (eg, complete blood count [CBC] and levels of creatinine and electrolytes including calcium), electrocardiography (ECG), and chest radiography.

Depending on clinical presentation, additional tests may be performed: Abnormal chest radiographs should be followed by computed tomography (CT) of the chest. Neurologic findings on physical examination or in history may warrant CT or magnetic resonance imaging (MRI) of the head, and possibly lumbar puncture or electroencephalography. Referral to an ear, nose, and throat (ENT) specialist should be considered to evaluate identified abnormalities of the head and neck. GI findings may be further investigated with liver function tests, endoscopy, or abdominal ultrasonography and CT. For patients with respiratory abnormalities, spirometry and bronchoscopy may be appropriate.

→ T R E A T M E N T

The initial approach to management should aim to treat the underlying condition. Pharmacologic therapy can be used for symptomatic treatment; however, no high-quality evidence exists to guide this therapy. Antipsychotic agents are considered first-line treatment. **Chlorpromazine** is the only US Food and Drug Administration (FDA)-approved therapy for hiccups. The initial oral dose is 25 mg tid for up to 7 days titrated up to 50 mg qid as needed. Slow IV administration of the same dose is appropriate for more severe cases. Other options include **metoclopramide** 5 to 10 mg IV or 10 mg orally every 6 hours for up to 5 days. **Baclofen**, a skeletal muscle relaxant, may be used as a second-line agent, 5 to 10 mg tid orally (up to 40 mg/d). IV infusion of **midazolam** may be effective in controlling refractory hiccups; however, some data suggest benzodiazepines may precipitate or worsen hiccups.

Numerous other agents have been reported in small case reports or case series to be effective treatments for intractable hiccups, sometimes in the palliative setting. These include anticonvulsant agents (eg, **gabapentin** up to 300-900 mg/d, **pregabalin** 100-300 mg/d, **valproic acid**, **carbamazepine**), neuroleptic agents (eg, **haloperidol** IM or orally, **olanzapine**), stimulants (eg, **methylphenidate**), and other miscellaneous drugs including **nifedipine**, **quinidine**, **lidocaine** (as IV infusion [2 mg/min, up to 1.5 mg/kg], subcutaneous infusion [up to 480 mg per day] or oral viscous solution), and **nefopam**.

Surgical treatments have been described in extreme cases of intractable hiccups. These include implantation of a diaphragmatic pacemaker and phrenic nerve ablation.

15. Hirsutism

→ DEFINITION AND ETIOLOGY

Hirsutism refers to excessive male-pattern hair growth in androgen-dependent areas, such as the upper lip, chest, abdomen, back, buttock, and inner thighs, where women typically have little to no hair. It may be idiopathic, caused by androgen excess, or drug induced.

Virilization occurs with severe androgen excess and includes hirsutism, male-pattern hair loss (starting above the temple and visible also around the top of the head), acne, deepening of the voice, increased muscle mass, reduced breasts and uterus size, and clitoromegaly.

Hypertrichosis refers to generalized excessive hair growth not limited to locations sensitive to androgens and not caused by hyperandrogenemia. It may be hereditary, idiopathic, or drug induced (phenytoin, penicillamine, diazoxide, minoxidil, cyclosporine [INN ciclosporin]). It also occurs in women with hypothyroidism, anorexia nervosa, porphyria, or dermatomyositis.

Causes of androgen excess in women:

1) **Ovarian dysfunction**: Polycystic ovary syndrome (PCOS) (most common), androgen-secreting ovarian tumor, hyperthecosis (hyperplasia of the theca interna of the ovary leading to increased production of androgens).

2) **Adrenal gland dysfunction**: Androgen-secreting adrenal tumor, Cushing syndrome, congenital adrenal hyperplasia caused by 21-hydroxylase or 11β-hydroxylase deficiency.

3) **Other endocrinopathies**: Hyperprolactinemia, acromegaly, insulin resistance.

4) **Drugs**: Androgens, anabolic steroids, danazol, oral contraceptives containing androgenic progestogens, valproic acid.

5) **Idiopathic hirsutism**.

→ DIAGNOSIS

Take a medication history as well as history of dysmenorrhea and galactorrhea. Establish the time of onset and rate of progression of hirsutism (sudden-onset, rapidly developing hirsutism not coinciding with puberty and virilization may suggest an ovarian or adrenal tumor, which may be malignant). Assess the type and distribution of hair in all androgen-sensitive locations; look for the features of Cushing syndrome). In patients with PCOS hirsutism may be associated with menstrual irregularities and obesity with insulin resistance.

Hair distribution and type are indicators of the degree of androgen excess. Hirsutism may be assessed with the Ferriman-Gallwey score (→Figure 15-1). This score considers 9 androgen-sensitive areas. The criteria for identifying hirsutism are arbitrary and vary among different ethnic groups, from 2 in Asian through 9 in white to 10 in the Mediterranean populations, although scores much lower than 9 may be associated with androgen excess.

Diagnostic algorithm for hirsutism: →Figure 15-2.

→ MANAGEMENT

Address the underlying cause. Discontinue any potentially responsible medications if possible.

Assess the impact of hirsutism on the patient and whether treatment is desire

If the patient has PCOS, assess for associated conditions, such as metab
risk factors (obesity, insulin resistance, impaired glucose tolerance [

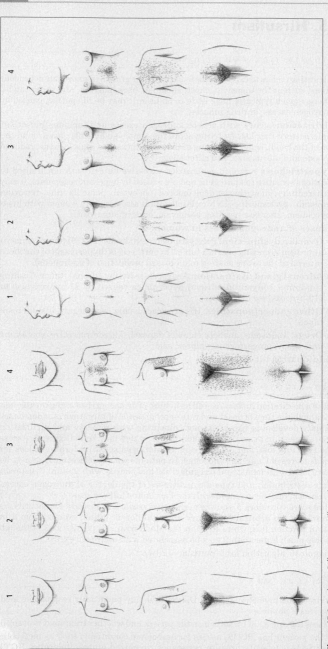

Figure 15-1. Ferriman-Gallwey score. Illustration courtesy of Dr Shannon Zhang.

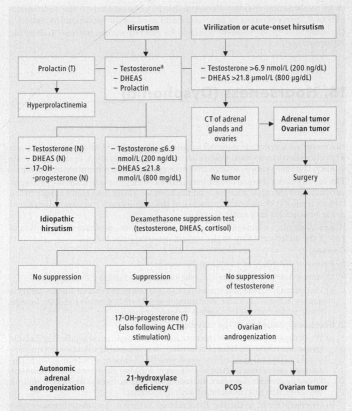

Figure 15-2. Diagnostic algorithm for hirsutism and virilization.

dyslipidemia) and anovulatory infertility. Counsel on lifestyle changes including diet and weight loss, as this may decrease insulin resistance, lower serum androgen levels, and improve fertility. Consider metformin in patients with obesity, insulin resistance, and IGT or impaired fasting glucose (IFG). Referral to specialists who regularly deal with these conditions (eg, endocrinologists, gynecologists, infertility specialists) may be needed.

First-line pharmacologic therapy for hirsutism is an oral estrogen-progestin contraceptive if the risk for venous thromboembolism is considered acceptable. If oral contraceptives are contraindicated or response to this therapy is adequate after 6 months, spironolactone may be considered as monothe or in combination therapy. Patients should be counseled on the teratogenic effects of spironolactone in pregnancy and need for adequate contraception.

Consider direct hair removal methods for mild hirsutism with no underlying endocrinopathies.

16. Hoarseness (Dysphonia)

→ **DEFINITION, ETIOLOGY, PATHOGENESIS**

Hoarseness is a symptom reported by patients that refers to alteration in the voice. This alteration can be vocal weakness, tremor, pitch alteration, or change in voice quality. Dysphonia refers to impaired voice generation as recognized by clinicians.

The larynx is made up of several structures, which include a set of cartilages, extrinsic and intrinsic muscles, and the mucosal lining. The nerve supply to the larynx is mostly done by the branches of the vagus nerve (recurrent laryngeal nerve or superior laryngeal nerve).

Hoarseness can be caused by damage, inflammation, or abnormal function of any of the structures that make up and innervate the larynx.

Causes:

1) Primary disorders of the larynx:
   a) Acute: Laryngopharyngitis, epiglottitis, laryngotracheitis, croup.
   b) Chronic: Occupational voice overuse, exposure to tobacco smoke, pharyngeal or laryngeal cancer, gastroesophageal reflux disease (GERD), foreign body, endotracheal intubation–related trauma.

2) Secondary disorders of the larynx:
   a) Weakness or paralysis of the extrinsic or intrinsic muscles: Bulbar palsies (polio, amyotrophic lateral sclerosis), demyelinating diseases, brainstem strokes (lateral medullary syndrome/Wallenberg syndrome), hypothyroidism, myasthenia gravis, long-term inhaled glucocorticoid treatment. Other neurologic disorders, including Parkinson disease and motor neuron diseases, are also associated with dysphonia.
   b) Cricoarytenoid arthritis: Rheumatoid arthritis, systemic lupus erythematosus, gout.
   c) Recurrent laryngeal nerve damage: Iatrogenic (most commonly following thyroid surgery), cancer (esophageal cancer, lung cancer, mediastinal tumors, metastatic spread to the mediastinal lymph nodes), neuropathy (diabetic neuropathy), marked enlargement of the left atrium, or dilation of the main pulmonary artery (Ortner syndrome).
   d) Other: Laryngeal amyloidosis, which may be isolated or associated with systemic amyloidosis.

3) Functional disorders: No organic cause.

→ **DIAGNOSIS**

The most important tests for detection of the underlying etiology are laryngeal evaluation with laryngoscopy or videostroboscopy (a special form of laryngoscopy that uses strobe lights, which allows for assessment of laryngeal vibration). There is role for laboratory evaluation if a specific etiology is expected on the basis of history and physical examination (eg, metastatic malignancy, amyloidosis, thyroid diseases, diabetes).

An ear, nose, and throat (ENT) assessment is necessary if hoarseness is not related to the common cold or influenza, has been present for >2 weeks, or is accompanied by other alarming symptoms, such as dyspnea, hemoptysis, pain on speaking, dysphagia or odynophagia, neck masses, or serious problems with articulation persisting for more than several days.

17. Jaundice

→ DEFINITION, ETIOLOGY, PATHOGENESIS

Jaundice (icterus) is yellow or yellowish coloration of the sclera, mucous membranes, and skin caused by the accumulation of bilirubin in tissues.

Jaundice becomes visible at bilirubin levels >43 μmol/L (~2.5 mg/dL), first in the sclera, then on the skin. It resolves in the reverse order. Bilirubin, an end product of heme metabolism, is conjugated in the liver, excreted in the biliary tree, and stored in the gallbladder. Excess heme degradation, disruption to bile flow, or disruption of any step in the bile metabolism may result in hyperbilirubinemia (predominantly unconjugated or conjugated hyperbilirubinemia, depending on etiology) and clinically manifest as jaundice.

Classification based on etiology:

1) **Predominately unconjugated (indirect) hyperbilirubinemia** is usually due to excess hemoglobin destruction or its compromised stability and survival. Specific causes:

   a) Extravascular or intravascular hemolysis: Congenital hemolytic anemia, immune hemolytic anemia, erythrocyte damage (artificial heart valves, march hemoglobinuria, thrombotic thrombocytopenic purpura, hemolytic uremic syndrome, disseminated intravascular coagulation, sickle cell anemia), infection (sepsis, malaria, toxoplasmosis), severe burns, hypersplenism, and paroxysmal nocturnal hemoglobinuria.

   b) Impaired conjugation of bilirubin with glucuronic acid: Gilbert syndrome or Crigler-Najjar syndrome.

2) **Predominately conjugated (direct) hyperbilirubinemia or mixed hyperbilirubinemia** is usually due to cholestasis (obstructive jaundice):

   a) Intrahepatic cholestasis: Primary biliary cholangitis, hepatotoxicity (acute alcoholic hepatitis, biologic toxins [fungi, plant alkaloids] or inorganic toxins [carbon tetrachloride, alcohol]), malignancy (lymphoma, liver tumors), sepsis, viral infection without inflammation and with extensive necrosis of hepatocytes (yellow fever and other hemorrhagic fevers), bacterial infections (leptospirosis, secondary and congenital syphilis), infiltrative diseases (sarcoidosis and amyloidosis), inherited disorders (Dubin-Johnson syndrome, Rotor syndrome), chronic liver disease of any etiology, and pregnancy.

   b) Extrahepatic cholestasis: Choledocholithiasis, malignancy (pancreatic cancer, lymphoma, cholangiocarcinoma, extrinsic compression from other malignancies), sclerosing cholangitis, HIV cholangiopathy, infection (parasitic).

→ DIAGNOSIS

Take a history and perform physical examination. Jaundice is often associated with pruritis, dark urine, and pale stool, all of which are nonspecific. Clinicians should seek information regarding liver toxicity or injury secondary to prescribed medications and over-the-counter (herbal) supplements. It also important to assess for viral hepatitis risk factors (IV drug use, h' -risk sexual activity, HIV status), occupation, travel history, family histo

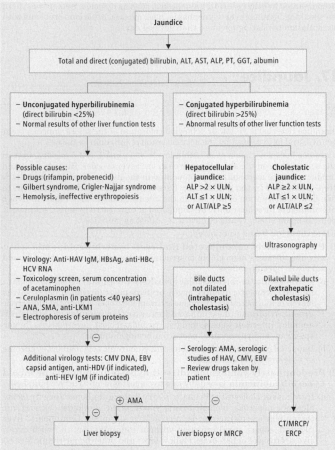

ALP, alkaline phosphatase; ALT, alanine aminotransferase; AST, aspartate aminotransferase; ALT/ALP (de Ritis ratio), ratio of ALT to ALP, expressed as a multiple of the upper limit of normal; AMA, antimitochondrial antibodies; ANA, antinuclear antibodies; anti-LKM1, antibodies to liver-kidney microsomal type 1 antibodies; CMV, cytomegalovirus; CT, computed tomography; EBV, Epstein-Barr virus; ERCP, endoscopic retrograde cholangiopancreatography; GGT, γ-glutamyl transferase; HAV, hepatitis A virus; HBc, hepatitis B core; HBcAg, hepatitis B core antigen; HBsAg, hepatitis B surface antigen; HCV, hepatitis C virus; HDV, hepatitis D virus; HEV, hepatitis E virus; MRCP, magnetic resonance cholangiopancreatography; PT, prothrombin time; SMA, anti–smooth muscle antibodies; ULN, upper limit of normal.

⊕ Positive result. ⊖ Negative result.

Figure 17-1. Diagnostic algorithm of jaundice.

liver disease or hemoglobinopathies, previous intraabdominal surgeries, and history of chronic liver disease. In addition, jaundice should be evaluated in the context of other presenting clinical signs and symptoms including sepsis and malignancy (eg, weight loss, night sweats).

The Courvoisier sign (a palpable nontender gallbladder in patients presenting with jaundice) may be a sign of underlying malignancy. Jaundice in the context of end-stage liver disease/cirrhosis (eg, ascites, splenomegaly, spider angiomas, nail clubbing) may be suggestive of acute-on-chronic decompensation of liver disease. Infection should be strongly considered in patients who present with signs of sepsis (possibly with right upper quadrant abdominal pain).

Differential diagnosis of jaundice: →Figure 17-1. In the differential diagnosis of yellowish coloration of the skin, consider excess β-carotene in the skin (carotenemia) associated with excessive intake of preparations containing carotene or drinking large amounts of carrot juice.

18. Lymphadenopathy

→ DEFINITION AND ETIOLOGY

Depending on the cause, lymphadenopathy (enlarged lymph nodes) is a result of an increased number of normal or neoplastic lymphocytes, inflammatory cells, or both. In adults lymph nodes ≥1 cm in diameter are considered significantly enlarged.

Etiology:

1) Infections: Bacterial (tuberculosis, syphilis, staphylococcal infection, streptococcal infection, brucellosis, tularemia, diphtheria, leprosy, cat-scratch disease), viral (cytomegaly, infectious mononucleosis, HIV, herpes simplex virus, varicella-zoster virus, herpes zoster virus, rubella, measles, viral hepatitis), protozoal (toxoplasmosis), fungal (histoplasmosis, coccidiomycosis, blastomycosis, sporotrichosis, torulosis), rickettsiosis.

2) Immunologic diseases: Systemic lupus erythematosus, rheumatoid arthritis, mixed connective tissue disease, dermatomyositis, Sjögren syndrome, serum sickness, drug hypersensitivity reactions (phenytoin, hydralazine, primidone, gold salts, carbamazepine), primary biliary cholangitis, graft-versus-host disease.

3) Tumors: Primary tumors of the lymphopoietic system (Hodgkin lymphoma, non-Hodgkin lymphoma, chronic lymphocytic leukemia, acute lymphoblastic leukemia), metastasis of solid tumors.

4) Storage diseases: Gaucher disease, Niemann-Pick disease, Fabry disease.

5) Other: Thyrotoxicosis, sarcoidosis, Castleman disease, Kawasaki disease, Langerhans cell histiocytosis.

→ DIAGNOSIS

After confirming lymphadenopathy in a certain area, examine all the lymph nodes accessible for palpation. Assess the lymph nodes for:

1) **Location**: Localized lymphadenopathy (limited to one group of lymph nodes) suggests a local cause (exceptions are the following systemic disorders: tularemia, yersiniosis, non-Hodgkin lymphoma), while generalized lymphadenopathy suggests systemic disease, including malignancy of the lymphatic system.

2) **Texture**: Firm lymph nodes suggest metastases, lymphoma, or chronic lymphocytic leukemia. Relatively soft lymph nodes are found in acute leukemia. Soft lymph nodes, sometimes fluctuant, are found in tuberculos acute lymphadenitis, and diphtheria (fistulas communicating with the s may be present).

3) **Tenderness**: Pain on palpation suggests rapidly progressive enlargement, typical of inflammation; less frequently, it may be associated with bleeding to the lymph node, immune reaction, or malignancy.

4) **Mobility of the lymph node relative to the skin and surrounding tissues**: Fixed lymph nodes and conglomerates of lymph nodes are found in patients with chronic inflammation or with malignancy.

Lymph nodes that are inaccessible to physical examination (mediastinal and retroperitoneal) can be assessed using imaging studies (radiography, ultrasonography, computed tomography [CT], magnetic resonance imaging [MRI], scintigraphy). In equivocal cases histologic examination of the lymph node is necessary and achieved through biopsy or excisional removal.

19. Meningeal Irritation Signs

→ **DEFINITION AND ETIOLOGY**

Signs of meningeal irritation are nonspecific reactions that may occur in a patient with meningeal irritation.

Meningism is defined as signs of meningeal irritation occurring without other features of meningitis or noninflammatory meningeal involvement (eg, in a patient with high-grade fever unrelated to a central nervous system [CNS] disorder).

Causes: Infectious meningitis (bacterial or viral), subarachnoid hemorrhage, neoplasms of the brain and meninges, extensive stroke affecting an area adjacent to the spaces with cerebrospinal fluid.

→ **DIAGNOSIS**

1. Physical examination:

1) **Neck stiffness**: Make sure the patient does not have cervical spine instability (eg, due to trauma or rheumatoid arthritis) and is not at risk of cerebral herniation. Place the patient in the supine position. Support the patient's chest with one hand, slide your other hand under the patient's occiput, and try to move their chin towards the sternum. In patients with neck stiffness, the reflex contraction of the muscles of the neck prevents the patient's chin from touching their chest, causing resistance and pain. The distance between the chin and the sternum is a measure of the severity of neck stiffness. In extreme cases, tension of the long paraspinal muscles is high enough to cause spontaneous posterior flexion of the neck and anterior arching of the trunk (opisthotonus). Neck stiffness needs to be differentiated from other causes of limited neck flexion (cervical spine degeneration, parkinsonism, cervical lymphangitis, severe throat infection). Neck stiffness has a sensitivity of ~70% for meningitis, although this is based on low-certainty evidence.

2) **Brudzinski sign**:
   a) Upper: Movement of the chin towards the chest while assessing for neck stiffness causes reflex flexion of the lower limbs at hips and knee joints.
   b) Lower: The same lower limb flexion is produced upon exerting pressure on the pubic symphysis.

3) **Kernig sign**: Place the patient in the supine position. Flex the patient's hip to 90°, then attempt to extend a knee. In patients with a positive Kernig sign, reflex muscle contraction prevents extension of the knee, which manifests as resistance and pain. Kernig sign is bilateral (as opposed to Lasègue sign in sciatica).

The sensitivity of signs of meningeal irritation in diagnosing meningitis is moderate, although lower in infants and elderly patients. Brudzinski sign has good sensitivity but poor specificity while Kernig sign has good specificity and poor sensitivity. Because of the implications of misdiagnosis and the ability to perform lumbar puncture to definitively confirm or exclude meningitis in those with moderate to high likelihood of this disease, the degree to which the presence or absence of those signs dictates further management is limited. For those with low pretest probability, the absence of these signs may provide a degree of reassurance, whereas their presence should dictate further investigations.

Other manifestations of meningitis: →Chapter 8.5.3.

2. Other diagnostic tests: Lumbar puncture (measurement of the opening pressure; cytologic, biochemical, and microbiologic examination of cerebrospinal fluid [direct microscopy, cultures, polymerase chain reaction]); neuroimaging (computed tomography [CT], magnetic resonance imaging [MRI]).

20. Pain Management: Basic Principles

DEFINITIONS

Pain is an unpleasant sensory and emotional experience that results from actual (eg, trauma) or potential tissue damage (eg, tissue ischemia). Pain can be purely nociceptive, purely neuropathic, or mixed.

Nociceptive pain is caused by active tissue damage. It can be visceral (cardiac ischemia, renal colic) or somatic (skin laceration, fractured bone).

Neuropathic pain is associated with nervous system disease (diabetic neuropathy) or damage (severed nerves after surgery, compression by tumor).

Myofascial pain is either localized in or referred to a muscle. Myofascial pain is characterized by the presence of trigger points (an area of the muscle that fails to relax, forming a hard spindle-shaped nodule or band that is tender on palpation). Myofascial pain is both nociceptive and neuropathic in nature.

Breakthrough pain (incident pain) refers to a sudden and transient exacerbation of pain that occurs in spite of adequate management of background pain. Breakthrough pain can be nociceptive or neuropathic in origin.

CAUSES

In **patients with cancer** causes of pain include:
1) Infiltration or compression of various tissues or organs by tumor.
2) Complications of cancer (eg, pathologic vertebral fractures due to skeletal metastases).
3) Cancer treatment (eg, radiation-induced plexopathy, postmastectomy pain syndrome, chemotherapy-induced neuropathy).
4) Non–cancer-related pain (eg, primary headache, angina).

Noncancer pain is caused by injury or compression of various tissues or organs. Mechanisms of this include external trauma, ischemia, or toxins (both external, such as chemical burns, and internal, such as neuropathy caused by uremia).

TREATMENT

Principles of Pharmacotherapy

1. Use oral analgesics whenever possible, as this route of administration the least invasive. If oral treatment is not possible (due to nausea, vomit dysphagia), subcutaneous or transdermal administration should be

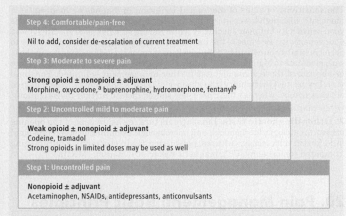

[a] Oxycodone is considered a weak opioid when used in combination with another dose-limiting drug.
[b] Transdermal fentanyl should not be initiated in opioid-naive individuals.

NSAID, nonsteroidal anti-inflammatory drug.

Figure 20-1. The World Health Organization analgesic ladder.

Transdermal absorption can be unpredictable in patients with edema or reduced peripheral blood flow (including those actively dying). Initiation of transdermal medications should be avoided in such situations. However, if patients are already receiving these medications at the end of life and find them effective, there is no need to stop this therapy. Subcutaneous injections, when appropriate for selected medication, are preferred over IV injections for patients at home and for those using long-term parenteral analgesics. Repeated IM injections are painful and offer no benefits over the subcutaneous or IV route.

2. Use analgesics in accordance with the World Health Organization (WHO) analgesic ladder (→Figure 20-1). In patients with mild pain, start treatment with acetaminophen (INN paracetamol), nonsteroidal anti-inflammatory drugs (NSAIDs), and other nonopioid medications, unless contraindicated. If results are unsatisfactory, move up to the next step of the analgesic ladder. Patients with severe pain generally need an opioid regardless of the underlying mechanism of pain; there is no reason to start at the bottom step if pain is severe. On each step of the analgesic ladder coanalgesics and nonopioid medications improve analgesia, reduce opioid requirements, and inhibit the development of opioid tolerance.

3. In patients with ongoing pain analgesics should be administered on a regular basis (around the clock) at intervals adjusted to the pharmacokinetics of a specific agent. Regular dosing provides more consistent pain control than intermittent (as-needed) dosing.

4. Patients with ongoing pain should receive immediate-release breakthrough analgesics for incident pain. Incident or breakthrough pain is pain that occurs despite the regular administration of analgesics. Patients receiving analgesics on the around-the-clock basis should receive immediate-release doses of analgesics to relieve this pain. Patients with only incident pain may achieve good pain control with a breakthrough analgesic alone.

5. Controlled-release (long-acting) opioid formulations should be used only after stable dosing is achieved with immediate-release formulations. Controlled-release opioids provide analgesia with longer intervals between doses, allowing for patient convenience. They have a slower onset of action and cannot be titrated as fast as immediate-release formulations. Pain control may be poor for the first several hours or days of use of a long-acting opioid and the patient will require an immediate-release breakthrough medication. The full effect of a controlled-release medication can take several hours or days to be reached and toxicity can develop if the agent is titrated quickly. Controlled-release formulations should not be used in opioid-naive patients.

6. Always use lower starting doses in the elderly and those with renal or hepatic impairment. Opioid metabolism is slower in the elderly, increasing the risk of adverse events and toxicity. Most opioids and their metabolites are excreted by the kidneys (hydromorphone and fentanyl are notable exceptions), requiring lower doses in patients with renal failure. Patients with significant hepatic impairment are particularly sensitive to neurologic adverse effects of opioids.

Nonopioid Analgesics

1. Acetaminophen has a rapid onset (15-30 minutes) and short duration of action (up to 4-6 hours). The maximum daily dose in adults (>12 years) who are not at increased risk of hepatotoxicity is 3 to 4 g/24 h. Doses ≤2.6 g/d are recommended in the elderly and even lower doses are recommended in those with liver disease or alcohol abuse.

2. NSAIDs, with analgesic and anti-inflammatory properties, have the most potent analgesic effect in bone pain, myofascial pain, and pain caused by inflammation. The onset and duration of action varies by formulation and includes ibuprofen with a rapid onset (15-30 minutes) and short duration (4-6 hours) and celecoxib with a slower onset (3 hours) and long duration (14 hours). Before using NSAIDs, the risk of cardiovascular, gastrointestinal, and renal adverse effects must be evaluated. Use of selective cyclooxygenase-2 (COX-2) inhibitors, proton pump inhibitors (PPIs), or both will reduce (but not eliminate) the risks of gastrointestinal bleeding. There is no evidence that COX-2 inhibitors have a reduced renal or cardiac risk compared with nonselective COX inhibitors.

Weak Opioid Analgesics

The provided trade (brand) names are valid for Canada.

Weak opioids are so named not because they are inherently less effective than other opioids. At equianalgesic doses, they are just as effective as stronger opioids, such as fentanyl or morphine. Rather, they are called weak opioids because they are commonly combined with other medications that limit the maximum daily dose. When used alone (without the dose-limiting presence of another drug), weak opioids could be considered strong opioids. The distinction between weak and strong opioids is thus, to a certain degree, arbitrary.

1. Codeine: Start immediate-release oral codeine 15 mg to 30 mg every 4 to 6 hours. If necessary, titrate the dose up to a maximum of 240 mg/d. Immediate-release and controlled-release formulations are available. Immediate-release formulations contain codeine alone or combined with acetaminophen (marketed as Tylenol with codeine) or acetylsalicylic acid (previously available as 222's), limiting the maximum daily dose. Oral formulations are the only formulations available in Canada. Codeine should not be used in moderate or severe renal failure, as metabolites accumulate, causing sedation and altered level of consciousness.

2. Dihydrocodeine (not available in Canada): Start from 60 mg orally every 12 hours. If necessary, titrate the dose up to 120 mg every 12 hours. Dihydrocodeine is a synthetic opioid. Immediate-release formulations are available as dihydrocodeine alone or combined with acetaminophen, aspirin, ibuprofen, antihistamines, or decongestants, limiting the maximum daily dose.

3. Oxycodone: Start from 5 mg every 4 hours. Titrate the dose to achieve an adequate analgesic effect. Immediate-release and controlled-release formulations are available. Immediate-release formulations contain oxycodone

Table 20-1. Analgesic equivalencies

Drug	PO dose	To convert to PO morphine equivalent multiply by:	To convert from PO morphine equivalent multiply by:	To convert PO to SC or IV[a] (same drug) multiply by:
Codeine	100 mg	0.1	10	0.5 (SC only; IV not available in Canada)
Morphine	10 mg	–	–	0.5
Oxycodone	7.5 mg	1.5	0.75	Not available in Canada
Hydromorphone	2 mg	5	0.2	0.5
Methadone and tramadol	Morphine dose equivalence not reliably established			
Buprenorphine	5 µg/h patch = 30 mg morphine PO (daily dose) 10 µg/h patch = 30-80 mg morphine PO (daily dose) Higher doses (35, 52.5, 70 µg/h) available is some countries			
Fentanyl	Should be reserved for monitored settings (IV formulations) and opioid-experienced patients (PO, buccal, transdermal formulations)			

[a] SC dosing limited to 2 mL per injection site. If concentration of the drug does not allow for this, >1 injection site or conversion to IV dose is required.

Adapted from Canadian Guideline for Safe and Effective Use of Opioids for Chronic Non-Cancer Pain. Canada: National Opioid Use Guideline Group (NOUGG); 2010. Available from: http://nationalpaincentre.mcmaster.ca/opioid/ and Health Canada. Important Changes to the Dose Conversion Guidelines for Fentanyl Transdermal Systems – For Health Professionals. http://healthycanadians.gc.ca/recall-alert-rappel-avis/hc-sc/2009/14548a-eng.php. Published January 7, 2009.

IV, intravenous; PO, oral; SC, subcutaneous.

alone (in which case it should be considered a strong opioid) or combined with acetaminophen (marketed as Percocet), limiting the maximum daily dose. Oral formulations only in Canada. Oxycodone is available in combination with naloxone (in Canada marketed as Targin), which helps to minimize the adverse effect of constipation.

4. Tramadol: The usual starting dose is 25 to 50 mg every 4 hours in an immediate-release oral formulation. Titrate the dose as needed at a rate no faster than 25 mg every 3 days up to a maximum of 400 mg/d. Tramadol works through opioid receptors and serotonin receptors. Nausea and vomiting are common at the beginning of treatment. Immediate-release and controlled-release formulations are available. Immediate-release formulations contain tramadol alone or combined with acetaminophen (marketed as Tramacet), limiting the maximum daily dose. Oral formulations are the only formulations available in Canada. Caution and lower initial doses are needed in the elderly and in those with renal or hepatic failure. Do not use in patients with poorly controlled seizure disorders. Tramadol is associated with serotonin syndrome.

Strong Opioid Analgesics

At equianalgesic doses, weak and strong opioids have the same level of effect. Some weak opioids are actually more potent than certain strong opioids. Examples of drug conversions: →Table 20-1, →Table 20-2.

Table 20-2. Dosage conversion guidelines for transdermal fentanyl[a] by Health Canada

Current analgesic	Daily dose (mg/d)						
Morphine PO	60-134	135-179	180-224	225-269	270-314	315-359	360-404
Morphine IM/IV[b]	30-66	67-90	91-111	112-134	135-157	158-179	180-202
Oxycodone PO	30-66	67-90	91-112	113-134	135-157	158-179	180-202
Codeine PO	150-447	448-597	598-747	748-897	898-1047	1048-1197	1198-1347
Hydromorphone PO	8-16	17-22	23-28	29-33	34-39	40-45	46-51
Hydromorphone IV	4-8.4	8.5-11.4	11.5-14.4	14.5-16.5	16.6-19.5	19.6-22.5	22.6-25.5
Recommended FTS dose	25 µg/h	37 µg/h	50 µg/h	62 µg/h	75 µg/h	87 µg/h	100 µg/h

Conversion method for adult patients taking opioids or doses not listed here: →Table 20-1.

This table **should not be used for conversion in the other direction (from FTS to other opioids)**, because this conversion to FTS is conservative. Its use for conversion to other analgesics can overestimate the dose of the new agent and result in overdosage.

[a] The usual starting dose is 25 µg/h. Lower doses could be occasionally used if considered required. FTS at any dose is contraindicated in opioid-naive patients.

[b] Calculation in this table is based on a 1:2 ratio of parenteral to PO morphine doses. For some patients, a 1:3 parenteral to PO dose ratio may be more appropriate (10 mg parenteral morphine = 30 mg PO morphine).

FTS, fentanyl transdermal system; IM, intramuscular; IV, intravenous; PO, oral.

Source: Health Canada. Important Changes to the Dose Conversion Guidelines for Fentanyl Transdermal Systems – For Health Professionals. http://healthycanadians.gc.ca/recall-alert-rappel-avis/hc-sc/2009/14548a-eng.php. Published January 7, 2009.

1. Morphine: Start from 5 to 10 mg orally every 4 hours. Titrate the dose to achieve adequate analgesia or based on adverse effects. Immediate-release and controlled-release formulations are available. Oral, rectal, subcutaneous, and IV formulations in Canada (conversion between routes of administration: →Table 20-1, →Table 20-2). Morphine and its active metabolites are excreted by the kidneys. Not advised in patients with renal failure.

2. Hydromorphone: Start from 0.5 mg to 1 mg orally every 4 hours. Titrate the dose to achieve adequate analgesia or based on adverse effects. Immediate-release and controlled-release formulations are available. Oral, subcutaneous, and IV formulations in Canada (conversion between routes of administration: →Table 20-1, →Table 20-2). Hydromorphone is a semisynthetic (morphine-based) opioid. Patients with a true allergy to morphine should try a different fully synthetic opiate where there is no known cross-reactivity. Hydromorphone has relatively inert metabolites that are excreted by the kidneys. It can be safely used in patients with renal failure.

3. Buprenorphine: An intermediate-acting opioid available in Canada in transdermal form only. Buccal and sublingual formulations are available outside of Canada. Dosing is based on prior exposure to opioids. Buprenorphine can be used in opioid-naive patients at low doses with caution. Conversion from other opioids: →Table 20-1. All routine dosing of alternative opioids should be stopped when buprenorphine is started. Intermittent breakthrough opioids can be used to prevent increases in pain or symptoms of withdrawal. Buprenorphine is safe for use in patients with renal failure.

1) Transdermal patches (up to 20 µg/h) are changed every 7 days. Dose adjustments should occur only after 3 to 7 days. Higher-dose preparations of transdermal patches (from 35 µg/h) changed every 3 to 4 days are used in some European countries.

2) Buccal film and sublingual tablets are taken every 12 hours. Dose adjustments should occur no quicker than every 4 days. Lower doses and slower titration are advised in patients with oral lesions.

3) Sublingual tablets that contain both buprenorphine and naloxone are available in 2 dosage forms but currently in Canada these are approved only for use in opioid addiction.

4. Fentanyl: A strong opioid reserved for opioid-tolerant patients. Immediate-release (buccal and IV) and controlled-release formulations (transdermal patches) are available. Starting doses depend on prior opioid use. Not recommended for patients using <45 mg to 60 mg of morphine (or equivalent) per day. IV dosing should be reserved for monitored settings, such as operating rooms and intensive care units. Patients using controlled-release formulations will need breakthrough analgesics for incident pain. Controlled-release formulations should be titrated no quicker than once a week because of their long half-life. When a patch is removed, drug levels may be found in blood for up to 1 day. Conversion from alternative opioids to fentanyl is not as exact as in other opioid conversions. Deaths have occurred in Canada when opioid-naive patients started using fentanyl patches, even the smallest doses possible. Prescription of fentanyl patches should be reserved for practitioners experienced in opiate dosing. It is suggested that for critically ill patients, transdermal fentanyl dosing can be converted directly to IV (and back again when the patient's condition improves and they are able to take oral formulations) at a 1:1 ratio.☉○ This should be done in a monitored setting. Fentanyl is safe for use in patients with renal failure.

5. Methadone: An intermediate-acting opioid used in opioid-tolerant patients. Only oral formulation is available. Dosing is based on use of other opioids and goals of therapy (pain management or addiction therapy). Methadone may be used in patients with end-stage renal disease. It is safe for use in patients with renal disease. Methadone prolongs the cardiac QT interval. It must be used with caution in patients taking other medications.

6. Oxycodone: Described in the weak opioids section (→above), it can be considered a strong opioid when administered without dose-limiting medications. The starting doses and rate of titration are the same with and without additional medications.

Management of Adverse Effects of Opioids

1. Sedation (manifesting as daytime somnolence) usually occurs at the beginning of opioid treatment or after a considerable dose increase and resolves within several days. If somnolence persists or worsens, the dose of opioid can be decreased to the lowest dose that ensures pain control. Other causes of sedation (eg, other medications, dehydration, renal failure, disease progression, hypercalcemia) should be excluded and treated where possible. Persistent somnolence may be an indication for switching to another opioid. Patients should be advised not to drive or operate heavy equipment until they are aware how their opioids will affect them (in some countries driving when using opioids is not allowed).

2. Nausea and vomiting may develop in the first days of starting an opioid or following a dose increase and usually resolve spontaneously. Opioids can elicit nausea and vomiting through direct effects on the vomiting center in the brain or by way of reduced gut motility (with or without constipation). Always inform the patient about the risk of nausea or vomiting (or both) and explain these are likely to be transient (to prevent patients from discontinuing the drug on their own). Consider providing the patient with an antiemetic agent to be used at home in case of nausea or vomiting associated with opioid treatment. Other causes of nausea and vomiting (eg, other medications, renal failure, disease progression, constipation) should be excluded and treated where possible. Opioid-induced nausea and vomiting respond best to prokinetic antiemetics (metoclopramide) or dopamine antagonists (haloperidol). If nausea and vomiting cannot be managed medically, consider rotation to a different opioid or to another form of the medication (eg, long-acting, transdermal).

3. Constipation is the most frequent adverse effect of opioids. Patients using opioids on a regular basis should be provided with prophylactic laxative therapy. Opioid-induced constipation often requires a combination of medications. Stimulant (senna) and osmotic (lactulose) laxatives are most effective.

4. Delirium may occur with initiation of opioids, dose changes, or accumulation of metabolites (ie, acute renal failure). Subtle cognitive changes may occur in the absence of clinically evident delirium. Cognitive changes are often caused by opioid metabolites rather than the given opioid itself. Cognitive changes can be reduced by decreasing opioid dose to the lowest dose that provides adequate pain control. Opioid rotation, particularly to one with minimally active metabolites (hydromorphone, fentanyl), may reduce cognitive effects. Delirium that does not resolve or is distressing can be treated with low doses of a dopamine antagonist (haloperidol 0.125 to 1 mg orally or subcutaneously). Other causes of cognitive impairment (eg, other medications, renal failure, disease progression, or hypercalcemia) should be excluded and treated where possible.

5. Hyperalgesia: Opioid-induced hyperalgesia is a poorly understood phenomenon where use of opioids leads to overstimulation of nociceptors and sensation of pain. Typically hyperalgesia develops simultaneously with neurotoxicity. Patients with hyperalgesia experience no pain relief with increasing opioid doses. Opioid-induced hyperalgesia is a diagnosis of exclusion, and alternative causes of pain such as disease progression must be ruled out. Hyperalgesia should be managed urgently by decreasing opioid dose (typically by a third or half) to reduce stimulation of the opioid receptor. Opioid rotation (including a dose decrease) and careful use of opioid-sparing analgesics can be helpful as well.

6. Neurotoxicity: Opioid-induced neurotoxicity is a clinical syndrome in which the given opioid or its metabolites cause neurologic adverse effects. Symptoms can include hallucinations, delirium, somnolence, myoclonus, dysesthesia, and hyperalgesia. Opioid neurotoxicity does not appear to be mediated through opioid receptors and thus does not respond to opioid antagonists such as naloxone. Management of opioid-induced neurotoxicity requires reduction of opioid dosing and hydration to assist in the clearance of metabolites. Severe cases may require switching to an alternative opioid. Specific symptoms can be managed with directed therapies, such as benzodiazepines (myoclonus); these therapies must be used with care as they will contribute to the altered cognitive status of the patient.

7. Overdose: Features of opioid overdose include depressed respiratory rate, depressed mental status, decreased bowel sounds, and constricted pupils. Overdose can occur with one large dose or as metabolites accumulate in patients with dehydration or renal failure. Management of a mild overdose includes reduction of opioid dosing and IV fluids to assist in the clearance of metabolites. Low doses of naloxone (0.05-0.1 mg IV, intranasally, or subcutaneously) can be used if necessary but often this is not needed.

Management of a severe opioid overdose (respiratory depression, airway compromise, unresponsiveness) requires reduction of opioid dosing, IV fluids, and an opioid antagonist (naloxone). Initial doses of 0.4 to 1 mg of naloxone IV, intranasally, or subcutaneously are advised. As the half-life of naloxone is shorter than that of therapeutic opioids, many patients require a continuous infusion of naloxone to provide support until clearance of all metabolites is achieved.

Of note, patients at the end of life have symptoms similar to those of opioid toxicity (→Chapter 11.2). As long as death is not related to opioid toxicity, it is important not to give naloxone to actively dying patients, as this will caus' pain and distress and not reverse the symptoms.

8. Other adverse effects: Dry mouth, pruritus, urinary retention, and sweating commonly occur and can be treated symptomatically. With long-term use, suppression of luteinizing hormone, follicle-stimulating hormone, adrenocorticotropic hormone, and growth hormone secretion can occur and can be associated with osteoporosis.

Opioid Rotation

Opioid rotation (switching from one opioid to another) is used in patients who develop unacceptable refractory adverse effects to or tolerance of a certain opioid. Opioid rotation is also used when patients are no longer able to swallow opioids that come only in oral formulations. The method of rotation needs to account for the type of opioid the patient is taking (controlled-release or immediate-release formulation) and the dose of the opioid. Opioid receptors have incomplete cross-tolerance for opioids and tend to take up a novel opioid with greater affinity than the one the patient has been using for some time. As a result, guidelines suggest calculating equianalgesic doses of the new medication and then decreasing this dose by as much as a third to a half. A breakthrough immediate-release opioid can be used to improve analgesia during the transition period. Consultation with a palliative care or pain medicine specialist is recommended for opioid rotation.

Coanalgesics

Coanalgesics are agents that are not classified as analgesics but in certain types of pain have inherent analgesic effects or enhance the effects of analgesics. When appropriate, coanalgesics should be used at all steps of the WHO analgesic ladder.

1. Antiepileptic drugs:

1) **Gabapentin**: Originally designed as an anticonvulsant, gabapentin is now approved in Canada for treatment of neuropathic pain. The usual starting dose is 200 to 300 mg (100 mg in elderly patients and those with renal impairment) in the evening, with the dose titrated up every 2 to 3 days by 200 to 300 mg/d (100 mg/d in the elderly) until an adequate analgesic effect is achieved or adverse effects develop. Similarly to opioids, there is no maximum dose, although benefits from increases beyond 1200 mg tid are minimal. The goal should be the lowest dose (in a bid or tid dosing) that achieves pain control and minimizes adverse effects. Somnolence is the most common adverse effect that limits the rate at which the dose may be increased. Unsteady gait and falls are common.

2) **Pregabalin**: Pregabalin is an analgesic designed to mimic the neuropathic analgesic properties of gabapentin. Start from 75 mg bid (25 mg bid in the elderly and those with renal impairment). If necessary, titrate the dose up by 25 to 50 mg every 3 to 7 days. The maximum recommended effective dose is 300 mg bid (total daily doses of 50 mg may be effective in patients with renal impairment and in the elderly). Common adverse effects include confusion and volume overload (from sodium and water retention). These effects can be severe and require discontinuation of the medication. The mechanism of action mimics that of gabapentin, thus there is no reason to use these two medications at the same time.

3) **Carbamazepine**: An anticonvulsant with analgesic effects as a neuropathic agent. Start from 50 to 100 mg bid. The dose can be titrated up to a maximum of 800 to 1200 mg/d. Lower doses are needed in those with renal impairment and in the elderly. The main adverse effect is sedation, which can be managed with dose reduction. Carbamazepine is the first-line therapy recommended for trigeminal neuralgia. The effectiveness of analgesia is not related to drug levels, unlike when it is used as an anticonvulsant. There is no need to regularly measure drug levels unless toxicity is suspected (based on the clinical situation or high drug doses).

2. Tricyclic antidepressants (TCAs): This class of medications has been shown to be effective in the management of migraine, arthritis, chronic low back pain, postherpetic neuralgia, fibromyalgia, and diabetic neuropathy. The adverse effect profile of TCAs is that of anticholinergic medications (eg, sedation, dry mouth, constipation, urinary retention, or confusion) and will often limit dosing.

1) **Amitriptyline**: Starting dose 10 mg at bedtime, increased to 25 mg after 3 to 7 days, and then increased by 25 mg/d every 1 to 2 weeks. Effective analgesia (or adverse effects) can often develop with doses <50 mg/d.

2) **Nortriptyline**: Starting dose 10 mg at bedtime, increased to 25 mg after 3 to 7 days, and then increased by 25 mg/d every 1 to 2 weeks. Effective analgesia (or adverse effects) can often develop with doses <75 mg/d.

3. Other antidepressants: Other antidepressants have been shown to have coanalgesic effects. They modulate this effect through management of comorbid mood disorders as well as through mechanisms not yet understood. Evidence suggests that selective serotonin reuptake inhibitors (SSRIs) and serotonin norepinephrine reuptake inhibitors (SNRIs) have inferior efficacy in neuropathic pain management when compared with TCAs. However, the adverse effect profile of SSRIs and SNRIs is better tolerated by most patients, making these agents a suitable option to consider for the management of neuropathic pain.

Duloxetine: The only SNRI officially approved in Canada for management of diabetic neuropathy, fibromyalgia, and chronic musculoskeletal pain. The starting dose of 30 mg is effective in some patients. Others need to have their dose increased to a maximum of 60 mg daily after 1 week of treatment with the starting dose. Duloxetine should not be used in patients with end-stage renal disease or cirrhosis.

4. Other coanalgesics: There are many other agents used as coanalgesics in specific situations.

1) **Glucocorticoids** (dexamethasone) provide pain relief in the setting of inflammatory conditions and when pain is caused by compression, stretch, or infiltration by tumor. They are useful for pain management in patients with rheumatologic disease, solid tumor, or lymphoma.

2) **Bisphosphonates** help to reduce bone pain associated with malignant infiltration through inhibition of osteoclast activity. Not sufficient as a single analgesic agent.

3) **Topical lidocaine** and **capsaicin** are effective in treating localized pain due to neuropathy, vasculitis, or trauma.

Nonpharmacologic Management

An in-depth analysis of nonpharmacologic interventions of pain management is beyond the scope of this chapter. However, in many situations they can be an adjuvant to pharmacologic therapy.

1. Nerve blocks and neurodestructive procedures: Use anesthetic agents to temporarily anesthetize or alcohol to permanently destroy the nerve plexus at the source of pain. Performing such procedures with imaging guidance improves success rates. The availability of interventional procedures is site--dependent and not all clinics and hospitals are able to provide such services.

1) Celiac plexus neurolysis may be used in the treatment of pain caused by pancreatic, gastric, liver, gallbladder, intestinal, or renal cancers; retroperitoneal metastases; or splenomegaly.

2) Hypogastric plexus neurolysis or blocks may be used in patients with pelvic pain secondary to malignant and nonmalignant causes, tenesmus secondary to radiation therapy to the rectum, or malignancy-related rectal pain.

3) Blocks of the stellate ganglion, lumbar sympathetic trunk, and ganglion impar (ganglion of Walther) can be used to ease pain in the limbs, face, and pelvic region.

4) Continuous central neuraxial blocks (subarachnoid and epidural) are most commonly performed when systemic administration of opioids is ineffective or results in unacceptable adverse effects. These blocks can be used to tre

1

intractable neuropathic and nociceptive pain. The most significant benefit of continuous spinal opioid delivery is typically in the reduction of adverse effects rather than in improved pain control.

5) Peripheral nerve blocks are often used for procedures and interventions. A long-term anesthetic effect could be achieved through alcohol lysis of the same nerves.

6) Trigger point injections are injections of an anesthetic agent with or without glucocorticoid into a muscle knot (trigger point). The exact mechanism of pain control is not clear but improvement in local pain has been shown in patients with myofascial pain and fibromyalgia.

2. Radiotherapy is first-line treatment for localized pain associated with metastatic bone disease and direct nerve injury from solid tumor growth. The number of treatments and total size of radiation dose varies based on the nature of pain and the type of cancer.

3. Surgery can be a useful method of pain relief. Prophylactic and postfracture bone fixation provides rapid and profound pain control. Spinal decompression, vertebroplasty, and kyphoplasty have shown mixed results in the management of pain from degenerative disc disease and vertebral compression fractures.

4. Transcutaneous electrical nerve stimulation (TENS) uses electrical stimulation applied to the skin to stimulate nerve endings, in this way altering or eradicating pain. This form of analgesia is easily performed in the outpatient setting. Results are most beneficial when TENS is used for acute and subacute pain from injury or surgery.

5. Physiotherapy, including massage, and exercise are most effective in the management of bone, soft tissue, and neuropathic pain. Physiotherapy is important in maintaining mobility despite ongoing pain and disease.

6. Occupational therapy does not directly provide analgesia. Thanks to modifications in behavior, gait aids, and tools, occupational therapy can indirectly reduce pain through altered body mechanics and minimization of ongoing injury.

7. Cognitive behavioral therapy and behavior therapy have been shown to have very small benefits in overcoming disability, managing mood, and reducing catastrophic thinking associated with chronic pain. It is not clear at this time how long the therapy should be continued or which patients benefit most from such interventions.

21. Respirations

→ DEFINITION AND ETIOLOGY

1. Respiratory cycle:

1) **Respiratory rate** (in adults normal respiratory rates at rest range from 12-20 breaths/min):

   a) **Tachypnea** (increased respiratory rate): Caused by anxiety or panic disorder, pain, exertion, elevated body temperature, sepsis, pregnancy, acidosis, anemia, endocrine disease (hyperthyroidism, pheochromocytoma, hypocalcemia), pulmonary disease, cardiovascular disease, primary myopathy or neuromuscular disorders, and deconditioning (rates >30 breaths/min are often associated with the onset of respiratory failure in patients with pulmonary or cardiovascular disorders).

   b) **Bradypnea** (decreased respiratory rate): Caused by central nervous system (CNS) disorders (eg, elevated intracranial pressure, disorders of the brain stem), opioid or benzodiazepine overdose, hypothyroidism, metabolic alkalosis.

2) **Depth of breathing** (depth of inspiration):

a) **Hyperpnea** (increased volume with or without an increased respiratory rate) may develop in patients with metabolic acidosis. **Kussmaul breathing** involves a deep, gasping, and labored respiratory pattern (increased frequency and tidal volume) that is often seen in severe metabolic acidosis (often associated with diabetic ketoacidosis but can also occur in toxic alcohol ingestion, lactic acidosis, renal failure, or salicylate toxicity).

b) **Hypopnea** (shallow breathing) may develop in patients with respiratory failure, particularly in the case of exhaustion of the respiratory muscles (this is followed by gasping and apnea). Chest wall disorders and neuromuscular weakness can also result in a shallow breathing pattern. **Agonal breathing** is slow and very shallow breathing that may develop in patients with anoxic brain injury of any cause and may lead to apneas.

c) **Hyperventilation** is overventilation (increase in the rate or tidal volume) that is necessary for elimination of carbon dioxide. It leads to hypocapnia. Causes: acidosis, stress, anxiety or panic disorder, high altitude, brain injury, stroke, anemia, pulmonary or cardiovascular disorders as described above.

d) **Hypoventilation** is underventilation that is required for adequate gas exchange. It leads to hypercapnia. Causes: obesity, stroke involving brainstem, medication overdose (benzodiazepines and narcotics), alkalosis.

3) **Inspiration-to-expiration ratio**: Under normal conditions expiration is slightly longer than inspiration. **Prolonged expiration** occurs in patients with exacerbation of obstructive lung diseases (asthma, chronic obstructive pulmonary disease [COPD]).

4) **Other abnormalities**:

a) **Cheyne-Stokes respiration**: An irregular breathing pattern described as a cyclical crescendo-decrescendo pattern with periods of central apnea. Respirations gradually increase in depth and rate and then become less frequent and shallow with periods of apnea. Causes: heart failure, stroke, metabolic or drug-induced encephalopathy, traumatic brain injury, brain tumor, carbon monoxide poisoning, altitude sickness, and sometimes at the end of life.

b) **Biot respirations**: A rapid, shallow, irregular breathing pattern with increasing episodes of apnea (10-30 seconds). Causes: elevated intracranial pressure, CNS lesion at the level of the medulla oblongata, drug-induced coma (opioids). This breathing pattern is sometimes lumped with ataxic breathing, which refers to irregular frequency and tidal volumes intermixed with unpredictable episodes of apneas.

c) **Breathing interrupted by deep inspirations** (sighing respirations): Isolated deep inspirations and expirations occurring between normal breathing cycles, often with audible sighing. Causes: anxiety and psycho--organic disorders.

d) **Apnea and shallow breathing during sleep** (→Chapter 13.11).

2. Mechanism of breathing: The mechanism of breathing is complex and regulated by 2 anatomically distinct but functionally integrated elements involving central (brainstem, metabolic) and voluntary respiratory control centers. Rhythmic control is regulated by central and peripheral chemoreceptors sensing carbon dioxide, pH, and oxygen, as well as lung mechanoreceptors (eg, pulmonary stretch receptors). In the medulla, the dorsal respiratory group is responsible for generating inspiratory impulses while the ventral respiratory group triggers expiration. The pons contains 2 additional respiratory areas: the pneumotaxic center has an inhibitory effect on inspiration while the apneustic center has an excitatory function. Breathing effectors include diaphragm, intercostal muscles, and abdominal and accessory muscles. The diaphragm is the principle muscle of respiration.

1) **Thoracic breathing** uses external intercostal muscles and is more fre quent in women. In patients with severe ascites, large abdominal tum

and diaphragm paralysis, as well as in advanced pregnancy, it is the only breathing mechanism.

2) **Abdominal (diaphragmatic) breathing** uses the diaphragm and is more common in men than in women. It is most frequently seen in patients with ankylosing spondylitis, paralysis of the intercostal muscles, and severe pleural pain.

3. Mobility of the chest:

1) **Unilateral impairment of chest mobility** (with normal mobility on the contralateral side): Caused by unilateral disease process including airway obstruction, pulmonary edema or fibrosis, pleural disease (significant effusion or fibrosis [fibrothorax]), structural immobility or defect (thoracoplasty or rib fracture), and diaphragmatic paralysis.

2) **Paradoxical chest movement**: Recession of the thoracic wall on inspiration. Causes: trauma leading to fracture of >3 ribs in >2 places (so-called flail chest) or fracture of the sternum causing paradoxical mobility of a part of the thoracic wall. Flail chest associated with respiratory failure is the only indication for consideration of rib fracture fixation. Paradoxical chest movement may occasionally occur in patients with respiratory failure due to other causes.

3) **Paradoxical diaphragmatic movement** (diaphragmatic paradox or paradoxical breathing) occurs during respiration when the abdominal and chest wall move in opposite directions. Normally during inspiration the chest wall expands and the diaphragm moves downwards, causing outward expansion of the abdominal wall. Diaphragmatic weakness (paresis or exhaustion) results in its passive upward movement into the chest, especially in the setting of high negative intrathoracic pressure (respiratory effort), and consequently abnormal inward movement of the abdominal wall on inspiration.

4) **Increased work of accessory muscles of respiration** (sternocleido-mastoid, trapezius, scalene muscles): This is found in patients in whom the external intercostal muscles and diaphragm are not sufficient to maintain normal gas exchange (causes as in dyspnea). On physical examination intercostal retractions are visible and the patient may assume a tripod position, which involves stabilizing the shoulder girdle by resting the upper limbs against a hard surface (eg, edge of the bed). In patients with chronic respiratory failure, hypertrophy of the accessory muscles of respiration may occur, as can be seen in patients with COPD and neuromuscular weakness.

22. Respiratory Sounds

→ DEFINITION AND PATHOGENESIS

1. Normal respiratory sounds:

1) **Normal lung or "vesicular" sounds** are soft, nonmusical, and audible over almost entire peripheral lung zones during inspiration and early expiration. They are produced by turbulent air flow through lobar and segmental bronchi. In disease states, there may be diminished intensity due to decreased generation of sound energy, impaired sound transmission, or both. Decrease in sound generation may be due to impaired respiratory drive or impaired flow of air to the peripheral airways (foreign body or obstructive airway diseases). Impaired transmission of sounds may be due to the presence of fluid or air in the pleural space, consolidated lung, large bullae in patients with emphysema, or by chest wall deformities.

2) **Normal tracheal sounds** are hollow nonmusical sounds with a wide spectrum of frequencies that are clearly heard at the suprasternal notch or the lateral neck in both respiratory cycles. **Pathologic tracheal or "bronchial" sounds** are audible over peripheral lung areas and may suggest lung consolidation (due to inflammation, infection, hemorrhage, protein, or malignancy). In patients with upper airway obstruction, tracheal sounds may become musical and can present as either stridor or localized wheeze.

2. Abnormal respiratory sounds:

1) **Crackles** are nonmusical, short (<0.25 seconds), explosive respiratory sounds heard mostly during inspiration, caused by the sudden equalization of gas pressures between two areas of the lung. They occur during the opening of previously closed small airways. Crackles may be transiently apparent in healthy people but disappear after a few deep inspirations.

   a) **Fine crackles,** formerly termed crepitations or "velcro rales," are heard mid-to-late inspiration mostly in dependent lung regions, uninfluenced by cough or body position, and not transmitted to the mouth. These high-pitched sounds may be due to pulmonary fibrosis, congestive heart failure, or pneumonia. Of note, fine crackles are minimal or absent in sarcoidosis, as the disease affects mostly central lung zones.

   b) **Coarse crackles** are heard early in inspiration and throughout expiration, can be transmitted to the mouth, and can change with cough, but they are not influenced by changes in body position. These low-pitched sounds are commonly observed in the setting of bronchiectasis and other conditions characterized by secretions in the airways.

2) **Wheezes** and **rhonchi** are musical continuous breath sounds (>0.25 seconds), which may be high-pitched (wheezes) or low-pitched (rhonchi) and are generally audible during expiration. Wheezes (hissing, whistling sounds) are produced by the turbulent flow of air through narrowed airways, while rhonchi are mainly caused by secretions present in the airways. **Expiratory wheeze** is mostly caused by narrowing of the airways within the chest, which can occur in the setting of asthma, chronic obstructive pulmonary disease, aspiration of gastric contents, or heart failure. Of note, localized wheeze may be due to a focal process, including a tumor, foreign body, or mucous plug.

3) **Stridor** is a particularly loud, high-pitched, continuous sound, more clearly heard on inspiration over the upper airways or sometimes even without a stethoscope. This sound is caused by large airway narrowing and may indicate obstruction of the larynx or trachea. Stridor may be heard in patients with vocal cord dysfunction, epiglottitis, airway edema, anaphylaxis, laryngotracheitis, extrinsic compression of the trachea, or a foreign body.

4) **Squawk, also known as "squeak,"** is a mixed sound consisting of short wheezes accompanied by crackles that are heard in the middle to the end of inspiration. Squawks are most frequently present in patients with hypersensitivity pneumonitis and less often in patients with other interstitial lung diseases, bronchiectasis, or pneumonia.

5) **Pleural friction rub** is caused by the rubbing of the parietal and visceral layers of the pleura due to the deposition of fibrin in the course of an inflammatory or neoplastic process. This is generally biphasic in nature and heard best in basal and axillary regions.

→ DIAGNOSIS

History and physical examination (differential diagnosis of respiratory diseases: →Table 22-1). Diagnostic studies include mainly chest radiography, which may be supplemented with computed tomography (CT) of the thorax and pulmonary function tests (spirometry and others). In patients with dyspnea it is useful perform pulse oximetry and, if abnormal, arterial blood gas measuremen

Table 22-1. Differential diagnosis of respiratory diseases based on physical findings

Lesion	Chest movements	Percussion	Vocal fremitus[a]	Breath sounds	Displacement of the mediastinum[b]
Infiltrate	Asymmetric, motion impaired on the side of infiltrate	Dull	Increased	Bronchial breathing, crackles	No
Atelectasis	Asymmetric, motion markedly impaired on the side of atelectasis (if large)	Dull	– Reduced (atelectasis caused by airway obstruction) – Increased (atelectasis caused by airway compression)	– Reduced lung sounds – Occasional crackles – Bronchial breathing may be audible	Towards the side of atelectasis in setting of lobar collapse
Fibrosis (bilateral)	Slightly impaired symmetrically	Slightly dull	Slightly reduced	– Reduced lung sounds – Crackles	No
Pleural effusion	Asymmetric, motion impaired on the side of effusion	Dull	Reduced	Absent breath sounds; in the setting of small pleural effusions pleural friction may be audible	Away from the side of effusion (if large)
Pneumothorax	Asymmetric, motion impaired on the side of pneumothorax	Hyperresonant	Absent	Absent breath sounds	Away from the side of lesion (especially if tension pneumothorax)
Airway obstruction	– Symmetrically increased – Work of accessory respiratory muscles usually seen	Usually normal	Unchanged or reduced	– Wheezes and rhonchi – Prolonged expiratory phase – Normal lung sounds, may be reduced with occasional crackles	No

[a] Transmission of spoken words while listening with a stethoscope (eg. "blue balloons," "toy boat").

[b] Displacement of the trachea may sometimes be observed on physical examination of the neck.

23. Thirst

> DEFINITION AND ETIOLOGY

1. The sensation of thirst and the role of serum osmolality: The human body needs to maintain a serum osmolality between 280 and 295 mOsm/kg. This physiologic necessity is achieved by a combination of the sensation of thirst, secretion of antidiuretic hormone (ADH) (also referred to as arginine vasopressin [AVP]), and renal response to AVP. Thirst and AVP release are controlled by the central nervous system (CNS). The involved areas of the CNS lack the blood-brain barrier, which allows for direct sensing of the osmolality of circulating blood, so that large fluctuations can be detected and avoided or corrected if they occur.

If serum osmolality rises to ~285 mOsm/kg, below which AVP is essentially undetectable, AVP is released by neurons in the hippocampus. The exact serum osmolality that triggers thirst is debated but is thought to share the same threshold as AVP. Thirst leads to increased consumption of free water and AVP release leads to increased uptake of free water from the kidneys, both eventually resulting in lowering of serum osmolality to the narrowly controlled range. Abnormalities involving any of these steps (thirst, AVP release, or resistance to AVP at the kidney level) can lead to serious derangements in serum sodium levels and osmolality. It is difficult to establish volumes of fluid intake and output that would be considered abnormal, as this may depend on the personal and environmental factors (imagine a long-distance runner in a warm climate).

2. Etiology: Most frequently increased thirst is due to loss of water. Less often it results from a primary disturbance of water intake or reabsorption at the level of the kidneys. Excessive water loss may lead to hypertonic dehydration or less frequently to isotonic or hypotonic dehydration (→Chapter 4.3.1).

1) Water loss through the skin, gastrointestinal (GI) tract, or respiratory tract: Vomiting, diarrhea, fistulas (various enteric and pancreatic fistulas; surgical and nonsurgical), excessive sweating, fever.

2) Water loss through the kidneys due to osmotic (solute) diuresis: Diabetes mellitus and new sodium-glucose cotransporter 2 (SGLT-2) inhibitors, urea diuresis (a mechanism partially responsible for increased water loss in recovering acute tubular necrosis in addition to tubular dysfunction in this condition), increased tissue catabolism, high-protein diet or feeds, administration of urea as treatment of syndrome of inappropriate antidiuretic hormone secretion (SIADH), sodium diuresis (administration of IV fluids and postobstructive diuresis), or mannitol.

3) Primary disturbance of water intake: Psychogenic polydipsia, drug-induced xerostomia (mirtazapine, thioridazine, chlorpromazine, anticholinergic agents).

4) Water loss through the kidneys caused by arginine vasopressin deficiency or resistance: Neurogenic diabetes insipidus, nephrogenic diabetes insipidus.

> DIAGNOSIS

Any diagnostic workup should start with a detailed history and physical examination. If an obvious cause is found, treating the underlying etiology or modification of pharmacotherapy can be considered. Additional studies: plasma and urine osmolality; urinalysis; plasma levels of creatinine, urea, glucose, sodium, potassium, total protein and calcium; urinary levels of sodium; complete blood count (CBC).

A detailed history, physical examination, and results of diagnostic studies are usually sufficient to diagnose polydipsia caused by water loss through the GI tract, skin, or lungs, or through the kidneys due to osmotic diuresis. Once these causes have been excluded, nephrogenic or neurogenic diabetes insipidus or psychogenic polydipsia should be suspected and further testing performed (water deprivation test, vasopressin stimulation test [→Chapter 5.3.1]).

1. Allergic Rhinitis

→ **DEFINITION, ETIOLOGY, PATHOGENESIS**

Allergic rhinitis (AR) is an inflammation of the nasal mucosa related to an allergy, most frequently IgE-dependent.

1. **Classification**:

1) **Based on the duration of signs and symptoms**:
   a) **Intermittent AR**, lasting <4 days a week or <4 weeks.
   b) **Persistent AR**, lasting >4 days a week and >4 weeks.

2) **Based on the severity of signs and symptoms**:
   a) **Mild AR**, in which none of the following criteria are met.
   b) **Moderate or severe AR**, in which ≥1 of the following criteria are met: sleep disturbance; impairment of daily activities, leisure, and sport; impairment of school or work; troublesome symptoms.

3) **Based on causative allergens**:
   a) **Seasonal AR**, caused by seasonal allergens.
   b) **Perennial AR**, caused by allergens present in the environment throughout the year.

2. **Etiologic factors**:

1) **Inhaled allergens**:
   a) Pollens (particularly of anemophilous plants): Most frequently pollens from trees such as birch or *Ficus benjamina* (the weeping fig), grasses and weeds such as ragweed, and other plants such as mugwort.
   b) House dust mites, cockroaches.
   c) Dander, epidermis, and secretions (saliva, urine) of cats, dogs, rodents (eg, rabbits, guinea pigs, hamsters, rats, mice), horses, and cattle.
   d) Molds (eg, *Alternaria* spp, *Cladosporium* spp) and yeasts (eg, *Candida albicans*, *Saccharomyces cerevisiae*, *Saccharomyces minor*, *Pityrosporum* spp).

2) **Food allergens**: Nasal symptoms may accompany anaphylaxis caused by food allergens; cross-reactivity may occur between foods and inhaled allergens (oral allergy syndrome; →Chapter 2.4). In addition, if foods are crushed or boiled and then aerosolized, they may cause respiratory symptoms if the patient is allergic to the food (eg, when shrimp is boiled, it may cause respiratory symptoms in individuals allergic to shrimp; when large loads of soybeans are dumped off a ship in a harbor, the resulting aerosolized soybean powder may cause respiratory symptoms).

3) **Occupational allergens**: Latex (most frequently from latex gloves); high--molecular-weight substances, including plant and animal proteins (eg, allergens of laboratory and farm animals, grain dust, tobacco, red pepper, tea, coffee, cocoa, dried fruit, enzymes present in cleaning products or used in pharmaceutical manufacturing, fish, shellfish); low-molecular-weight substances (eg, nickel and platinum salts, dyes, acid anhydrides); bacterial enzymes used industrially for manufacturing soaps and detergents.

→ **CLINICAL FEATURES AND NATURAL HISTORY**

Typical manifestations: Watery nasal discharge (rhinorrhea); sneezing, frequently paroxysmal; nasal congestion and thick mucous discharge; nasal itching, frequently also conjunctival itching (and injection), itching of the ears, palate, or throat; partial loss of smell (hyposmia); dry oral mucosa; some-times systemic signs and symptoms, including sleep disturbance, impaired concentration and learning abilities, low-grade fever, headache, and depressed mood. Rhinorrhea and sneezing as dominant symptoms suggest seasonal AR, while nasal congestion is usually a dominant feature of perennial AR. In 70% of patients symptoms worsen at night and in the early hours of the morning.

Symptoms are present during exposure to a particular allergen and may be seasonal (eg, during a pollination season in patients with pollen allergy) or perennial (eg, in patients with house dust mite allergy). In both situations symptoms may be persistent or intermittent.

In some patients with AR signs and symptoms improve or resolve spontaneously after several years.

AR, particularly when chronic, may block sinus ostia, result in inflammation in the sinus, or both; the inflammation increases the risk of bacterial sinusitis. AR is also associated with a 3- to 8-fold increase in the risk of asthma development and with worsening of preexisting asthma control.

The following signs and symptoms are usually associated with a condition other than AR (seek an alternative diagnosis): unilateral symptoms, nasal congestion without other accompanying symptoms, mucopurulent nasal discharge, postnasal drip (with thick mucus, without rhinorrhea, or both), facial pain, recurrent epistaxis, and complete loss of smell (anosmia).

→ DIAGNOSIS

Diagnostic Tests

1. Studies confirming the diagnosis of allergy: Positive skin prick tests with inhaled allergens (the most sensitive, quickest, and cheapest diagnostic tests in AR), increased serum levels of specific IgE levels (not recommended as screening, as it is more expensive and less sensitive). In exceptional cases of conflicting results and unclear diagnosis, nasal challenge may be performed.

2. Anterior rhinoscopy and nasal endoscopy reveal bilateral (although not always symmetric) mucosal edema with watery discharge covering the mucosa (in patients with chronic AR the discharge is thick). The mucosa is pale or bluish but may also be hyperemic. Sometimes polyps are present.

3. Cytology of nasal smear reveals an increased percentage of eosinophils (≥2%, usually during exacerbations), mast cells or basophils, and goblet cells (>50%). However, these results are not specific for AR and are similar in patients with nonallergic rhinitis.

4. Computed tomography (CT) of the nose and sinuses is indicated in selected cases where surgery is being considered. It allows for reliable assessment of sinusitis that may coexist with AR.

Diagnostic Criteria

In most cases the diagnosis of AR can be established on the basis of typical symptoms and signs from the patient's history and physical examination, which may be aided as needed by skin prick tests and specific IgE measurements.

Differential Diagnosis

1. Other types of rhinitis:

1) Infectious rhinitis: Caused by viruses (differential diagnosis with common cold: →Table 1-1), bacteria, or fungi.

2) Drug-induced rhinitis: Edema of the nasal mucosa, most frequently caused by the overuse of topical sympathomimetics, or less frequently by acetylsalicylic acid, other nonsteroidal anti-inflammatory drugs (NSAIDs), pyrazolones, angiotensin-converting enzyme inhibitors, antidepressants, reserpine, methyldopa, α-adrenergic antagonists, drugs used in erectile dysfunction, and chlorpromazine.

Table 1-1. Differential features of common cold and allergic rhinitis

Manifestation	Common cold	Allergic rhinitis
Watery nasal discharge	Frequent	Frequent
Nasal congestion	Frequent, usually severe	Frequent, variable
Sneezing	Usual	Frequent
Nasal itching	Never	Usual
Nasal pain	Usual	Never
Ocular itching	Rare	Frequent
Cough	Frequent	Quite frequent
Fever	Rare	Never
Generalized pain	Minor	Never
Fatigue, weakness	Minor	Occasional, minor
Sore throat	Frequent	Never
Palatal and pharyngeal itching	Never	Sometimes
Duration	3-14 days	Weeks or months

Adapted from: National Institute of Allergy and Infectious Diseases. Is It a Cold or an Allergy? https://nccih.nih.gov/health/allergies. Accessed September 9, 2019.

3) Hormonal rhinitis: This may occur during the menstrual cycle, puberty, pregnancy, in women using oral contraceptives or hormone replacement therapy, and in patients with hypothyroidism.

4) Atrophic rhinitis: Progressive atrophy of the nasal mucosa and underlying bone with widening of nasal cavities that are filled with crusts. The disease leads to nasal obstruction, hyposmia, and a constant sensation of bad taste in the mouth. It usually occurs in elderly patients.

5) Idiopathic rhinitis (formerly known as vasomotor rhinitis): Caused by an exaggerated response to chemical and physical factors (eg, dry and cold air or concentrated chemicals). Hot spicy foods may cause rhinorrhea (gustatory rhinitis), probably because of stimulation of sensory nerves and vagal nerve reflex, whereas foods, dyes, and preservatives may cause rhinitis mediated by unknown nonallergic mechanisms. Alcohol may cause nasal congestion by directly degranulating mast cells.

6) Eosinophilic rhinitis with or without NSAID hypersensitivity (nonallergic rhinitis with eosinophilia syndrome [NARES]): Characterized by the presence of eosinophils in the nasal mucosa, perennial symptoms, and absence of features of atopy (although atopy may also be present).

7) Rhinitis caused by intranasal cocaine use: This may cause rhinorrhea, hyposmia, and perforation of the nasal septum.

2. Other conditions: Nasal polyps; polyps of the sinuses; sinusitis; nasal septal deviation; turbinate, tonsillar, or (usually) adenoid hypertrophy; nasal foreign body; nasal neoplasms; abnormalities of the ciliary structure or function; cerebrospinal fluid leakage; granulomatosis with polyangiitis (Wegener granulomatosis) and eosinophilic granulomatosis with polyangiitis (formerly Churg-Strauss syndrome).

→ TREATMENT

General Measures

1. Avoiding allergens: This may involve, for instance, limiting open air exercise during pollen seasons of suspected plants, keeping windows closed or using window filters, and removing pets from home. Combining these with techniques of house dust mite control may be beneficial. Consider using websites or mobile apps providing pollen calendars.

2. Clearing the nose with isotonic or hypertonic saline or with sea water.

3. Indications for referral to an ear, nose, and throat (ENT) specialist: Suspected complications or chronic sinusitis not responding to empiric treatment, recurrent otitis media, unilateral or treatment-resistant symptoms, recurrent epistaxis, nasal septal deviation and other anatomical abnormalities, nasal polyps.

4. Indications for considering surgical treatment: Lower turbinate hypertrophy resistant to pharmacologic treatment, nasal septal deviation affecting nasal function, complications of AR.

Pharmacologic Treatment

According to the 2016 Allergic Rhinitis and its Impact on Asthma (ARIA) guidelines, intranasal glucocorticoids may be used to treat seasonal AR, either alone or in combination with an oral or nasal antihistamine. In perennial AR, treatment with an intranasal glucocorticoid alone is suggested, without the addition of an antihistamine (oral or nasal).

1. Glucocorticoids:

1) **Intranasal glucocorticoids: Beclomethasone, budesonide, ciclesonide, fluticasone furoate, mometasone furoate, fluticasone propionate**: One to 2 doses are administered to each nostril once daily or bid. These are the most effective agents in AR that improve all signs and symptoms (including ocular manifestations). The onset of action is 7 to 12 hours after administration, and the maximum effect is observed after 2 weeks of treatment. Long-term treatment with intranasal glucocorticoids appears to be safe. The main adverse effects are mucosal dryness and minor bleeding from the nasal mucosa.

2) **Oral glucocorticoids**: For instance, **prednisone** 0.5 mg/kg once daily in the morning may be used for a few days in severe AR when treatment with intranasal glucocorticoids and antihistamine drugs has been ineffective.

2. Antihistamines (H_1 antagonists):

1) **Oral antihistamines** (agents and dosage: →Table 1-2): Particularly beneficial in patients with conjunctivitis. The preferred antihistamines are agents that cause less sedation and concentration impairment, are not cardiotoxic, and cause fewer interactions with other drugs or with foods.

2) **Intranasal antihistamines**: Azelastine, levocabastine. These have only topical effects on the nose and are indicated in mild AR. One to 2 doses are administered to each nostril bid. The onset of action is 15 to 20 minutes after administration.

3) **Intraocular antihistamines**: Azelastine, emedastine, epinastine, ketotifen, olopatadine.

4) **Combination intranasal glucocorticoids and intranasal antihistamines** are also available. Fluticasone propionate and azelastine have been combined in one nasal spray to be given bid.

3. Antileukotrienes: Oral montelukast (10 mg once daily), pranlukast, or zafirlukast may be used in patients with seasonal AR, but intranasal glucocorticoids and antihistamines are more effective.

4. Cromones: Intranasal **cromolyn** (INN cromoglicic acid) qid, and 1 to 2 drops intraocularly 4 to 6 times a day in case of ophthalmic symptoms. It is less effective than intranasal glucocorticoids and antihistamines but safe.

Table 1-2. Newer-generation oral antihistamines (H$_1$ antagonists) used in allergic rhinitis

Agents	Usual dosage
Cetirizine	10 mg once daily
Desloratadine	5 mg once daily
Fexofenadine[a]	120 mg once daily
Levocetirizine	5 mg once daily
Loratadine	10 mg once daily
Rupatadine	10 mg once daily
Bilastine	20 mg once daily

[a] In patients with chronic idiopathic urticaria use 180 mg once daily.

5. Decongestants may be used for quick relief of nasal congestion. They are administered intranasally (ephedrine, phenylephrine, naphazoline, xylometazoline, oxymetazoline, tetrahydrozoline [INN tetryzoline], tymazoline; use no longer than for 5 days because of the risk of drug-induced rhinitis) or orally (ephedrine, phenylephrine, pseudoephedrine; do not use in pregnancy, in patients with hypertension, cardiovascular disease, thyrotoxicosis, prostatic hypertrophy, glaucoma, psychiatric disorders, and in patients treated with β-blockers or monoamine oxidase inhibitor inhibitors; in many patients these agents cause insomnia).

6. Anticholinergic agents administered intranasally reduce nasal secretions. They are beneficial in idiopathic rhinitis.

7. Specific allergen immunotherapy is the most effective treatment of AR caused by inhaled allergens. It reduces or eliminates signs and symptoms of the disease, reduces medication use, prevents sensitization to other allergens, and reduces the risk of asthma by two-thirds. It is available for subcutaneous injection or as sublingual tablets. The beneficial effects of therapy may persist for some time after its completion.○

2. Anaphylaxis and Anaphylactic Shock

→ DEFINITION, ETIOLOGY, PATHOGENESIS

Anaphylaxis is a severe, life-threatening, generalized or systemic rapid-onset hypersensitivity reaction (allergic or nonallergic).

Anaphylactic shock is a severe rapidly progressing anaphylactic reaction (anaphylaxis) resulting in a life-threatening drop in blood pressure.

The most frequent causes of anaphylaxis:

1) **Allergic:**

   a) Drugs: Most commonly β-lactam antibiotics, cytotoxic agents.

   b) Hymenoptera venoms.

   c) Proteins administered via parenteral routes, including blood and its products, enzymes (eg, streptokinase), sera (eg, tetanus immunoglobulin), allergens used for in vivo diagnosis and immunotherapy.

d) Foods: In adults most commonly fish, seafood, peanuts.

e) Inhaled allergens, for instance, animal dander.

f) Latex.

g) Dialysis membranes sterilized with ethylene oxide.

h) Vaccines grown on chick embryo culture, which may contain egg protein.

2) **Nonallergic:**

a) Direct release of mediators from mast cells: Opioids, muscle relaxants, colloids (eg, dextran, hydroxyethyl starch, human albumin), hypertonic solutions (eg, mannitol), physical exercise.

b) Immunologic complexes: Blood and its products, immunoglobulins, animal sera, vaccines, dialysis membranes.

c) Alterations of arachidonic acid metabolism: Hypersensitivity to acetyl-salicylic acid (ASA) and other nonsteroidal anti-inflammatory drugs (NSAIDs).

d) Histamine and tyramine present in foods (this makes an anaphylactic reaction more severe).

e) Other mechanisms: Radiologic contrast media, food contaminants and preservatives, or unknown causes.

Nonallergic reactions are not mediated by immunologic mechanisms, and therefore shock may occur even at the first exposure to a certain factor. In ~30% of cases the causative factor remains unknown despite a thorough diagnostic workup (idiopathic anaphylaxis). However, the most frequent mechanism of anaphylaxis is an IgE-related reaction, while nonimmune reactions are less prevalent. Their common feature is degranulation of mast cells and baso-phils. The released mediators, such as histamine, tryptase, arachidonic acid metabolites, platelet activating factor, or nitric oxide, cause bronchial and gastrointestinal (GI) smooth muscle contraction and vasodilation, increased vascular permeability, stimulation of sensory nerve endings, recruitment of inflammatory cells, and activation of the complement, coagulation, and fibri-nolysis cascades. Increased vascular permeability and rapid fluid transfer to extravascular compartment may lead to the loss of as much as 35% of effective circulating blood volume within ~10 minutes.

→ CLINICAL FEATURES AND NATURAL HISTORY

Signs and symptoms of anaphylaxis most often occur within seconds or minutes of exposure to a trigger (although in some cases they may develop later, even after several hours):

1) **Skin and subcutaneous tissue**: Urticaria/angioedema and erythema occur in up to 90% of patients.

2) **Respiratory system**: Upper airway edema, hoarseness, stridor, cough, wheezing, respiratory compromise, rhinitis.

3) **GI system**: Nausea, vomiting, abdominal pain, diarrhea.

4) **Systemic reactions**: Hypotension and other symptoms of shock occur in 30% of patients; they may occur simultaneously with other signs and symptoms of anaphylaxis or (usually) develop shortly after their onset.

5) Less frequent: Dizziness or headache, uterine cramps, anxiety, feeling of impending doom.

The more rapidly the symptoms develop, the higher the risk of severe and life-threatening anaphylaxis; however, it should be noted that symptoms that are initially mild (eg, limited to the skin and subcutaneous tissue) may also rapidly become life-threatening if adequate treatment is not started promptly. Delayed or biphasic reactions may occur, with symptoms developing or relapsing over 3 to 8 hours. Symptoms of anaphylaxis may last for hours or even days despite adequate treatment.

Signs and symptoms of anaphylactic shock (regardless of the trigger) include cold and pale skin, sweating, collapsed subcutaneous veins, hypotension, oliguria or anuria, loss of bowel control, and loss of consciousness. Circulatory arrest may occur.

→ DIAGNOSIS

According to the 2011 World Allergy Organization guidelines, anaphylaxis is highly likely when any of the following criteria is fulfilled:

1) **Acute onset of an illness** (minutes to several hours) with involvement of the skin, mucosal tissue, or both (eg, urticaria, itching, lips-tongue-uvula edema), which is accompanied by either (or both):

   a) Respiratory compromise (eg, dyspnea, stridor, wheeze-bronchospasm, hypoxemia).

   b) Reduced blood pressure or associated symptoms of end-organ dysfunction (eg, hypotonia, syncope, incontinence).

2) **Exposure to a likely allergen for a patient is rapidly followed by ≥2 of the following** (within minutes to several hours):

   a) Involvement of the skin-mucosal tissue (eg, urticaria, itching, lips-tongue--uvula edema).

   b) Respiratory compromise (eg, dyspnea, stridor, wheeze-bronchospasm, hypoxemia).

   c) Reduced blood pressure or associated symptoms (eg, hypotonia, syncope, incontinence).

   d) Persistent GI symptoms (crampy abdominal pain, vomiting).

3) **Decreased blood pressure following exposure to a "known allergen"** (within minutes to several hours):

   a) Infants and children: Low systolic pressure (age-related) or a decrease >30% in systolic blood pressure. (In children low systolic blood pressure is defined as <70 mm Hg from 1 month to 1 year; <[70 mm Hg + 2 × age] from 1-10 years; and <90 mm Hg from 11-17 years.)

   b) Adults: A systolic blood pressure <90 mm Hg or decline by >30% compared with baseline.

Infants are more likely to have respiratory compromise than hypotension or shock, and in this age group, shock is more likely to be manifested initially by tachycardia than by hypotension.

Diagnostic Tests

1. Assays measuring levels of histamine or methylhistamine are not widely available, not specific for anaphylaxis, and not routinely used.

2. Assaying **total tryptase levels** has become more common. Tryptase should be measured within 2 hours of the onset of symptoms and then repeated 24 hours after the symptoms have resolved to get a basal level. The minimal elevation in the acute total tryptase level that is considered to be clinically significant has been suggested as ≥2 + 1.2 × baseline tryptase levels. However, tryptase may not be elevated in a third of patients and its usefulness in excluding diagnosis is thus limited, if any.◗

3. Where there is a clear causative agent, it is best to simply avoid exposure rather than confirm the cause by performing a challenge test. Often sensitivity may be lost over time, and where alternative agents cannot be used, cautious challenge under close observation and after a full discussion with the patient could be considered. Such an attempt to establish the allergic cause of anaphylaxis with skin tests should be made, if considered essential, no earlier than 3 to 4 weeks after the episode. Generally, challenge tests are not recommended after anaphylactic shock. Assessing the levels of IgE specific to suspected allergens may be helpful.

→ TREATMENT

Immediate Treatment

1. Assess airway, breathing, circulation (ABC), and level of conscious-ness. Establish and maintain the airway if necessary. In case of respiratory or cardiac arrest, start cardiopulmonary resuscitation (→Chapter 3.3). In patients with stridor or significant edema of the face and upper airways (tongue, oral and throat mucosa, hoarseness), consider immediate endotracheal intubation. If delayed, it may be progressively more difficult, and unsuccessful intubation attempts may further aggravate the edema. If the edema causes life-threatening airway obstruction and attempts of endotracheal intubation have been unsuc-cessful, perform cricothyroidotomy.

2. Stop exposure to the suspected antigen (eg, stop infusion of a drug or blood transfusion).

3. Administer epinephrine as soon as possible once anaphylaxis is recognized:

1) In patients with a history of anaphylaxis who carry an epinephrine autoin-jector, immediately administer 1 dose of IM epinephrine in the lateral thigh in case of even minor symptoms suggestive of anaphylaxis.

2) In patients without cardiac arrest, **administer IM epinephrine in the lateral thigh in a dose of 0.01 mg/kg of a 1:1000 (1 mg/mL) solution to a maximum of 0.5 mg in adults (0.3 mg in children).**

Record the time of injection and repeat in 5 to 15 minutes as necessary. Most patients respond to 1 to 2 doses. Patients who do not respond to an IM injec-tion of epinephrine and fluid resuscitation (shock is imminent or has already developed) should receive epinephrine in a slow IV infusion; the dose should be titrated on the basis of the effect of treatment on blood pressure assessed using continuous noninvasive monitoring. In adults the starting dose is 2 to 10 µg/min in an IV infusion (0.1 mg/mL; 1:10,000 solution contains 100 µg/mL or 1000 µg in a 10 mL syringe).

4. Place the patient on the back, or in a different position of comfort and safety if there is respiratory distress or vomiting, and elevate the lower extrem-ities, as this may be helpful in the management of hypotension. Do not let the patient sit or stand up suddenly or be placed in an upright position.

5. Administer oxygen 6 to 8 L/min via a face mask. This is indicated in patients in whom it was necessary to administer several doses of epinephrine, patients with respiratory distress, signs and symptoms of myocardial ischemia, or chronic diseases of the respiratory system.

6. Establish peripheral IV access with 2 large-bore needles (optimally ≥1.6-1.8 mm [14-16 gauge]) and use infusion kits allowing for rapid fluid administration.

7. Administer IV fluids: In patients with a substantial decrease in blood pressure who do not respond to IM epinephrine, administer a rapid IV infusion of 1 to 2 L of isotonic crystalloid (eg, in adults 5-10 mL/kg of 0.9% saline over the first 5 to 10 minutes [10 mL/kg in children]).

8. Monitor blood pressure and, depending on the clinical situation, also electrocardiography (ECG), oxygen saturation (SpO_2), or arterial blood gases.

Adjunctive Treatment

1. In patients receiving β-blockers who do not respond to epinephrine, consider administration of IV **glucagon** 1 to 5 mg in a slow infusion over ~5 minutes and then in a continuous IV infusion 5 to 15 µg/min, depending on the clinical response. Nausea, vomiting, and hyperglycemia are frequent adverse effects.

2. IV H_1 **antihistamines** are recommended in case of itching, urticaria, angioedema, and nasal and ocular symptoms (diphenhydramine 25-50 mg [1 mg/kg; maximum, 50 mg in children]). H_1-receptor blockers do not prevent or relieve upper airway obstruction, hypotension, or shock, and they should never be substituted for epinephrine.⊘○

3. Consider an IV **H$_2$ antagonist** in case of hypotension: ranitidine 50 mg every 8 to 12 hours or 150 mg orally bid.⊘○

4. Give an IV **glucocorticoid**,⊘⊖ eg, methylprednisolone 1 to 2 mg/kg, then 1 mg/kg/d, or hydrocortisone 200 to 400 mg, then 100 mg every 6 hours, for a maximum of 3 days; although this is not effective in treatment of the acute phase of anaphylactic shock, it may prevent the late phase of anaphylaxis. As in asthma, if there is wheezing, glucocorticoids may potentiate the β-agonist receptors. In the case of anaphylaxis without signs and symptoms of shock, airway edema, or respiratory compromise, an oral glucocorticoid, eg, prednisone 0.5 mg/kg/d, may be used.

5. Inhaled bronchodilators should be used if wheezing, coughing, and shortness of breath are not relieved by epinephrine; preferably use nebulized albuterol (INN salbutamol) 2.5 or 5 mg in 3 mL 0.9% saline or 2 to 4 puffs with an Aerochamber if the patient is able to follow instructions. Inhalation may be repeated when necessary. Bronchodilators reduce airway obstruction but do not prevent or relieve laryngeal symptoms, hypotension, or shock and should never be used instead of epinephrine.

6. Admit the patient to an intensive care unit without delay if anaphylaxis is refractory to treatment.

→ FOLLOW-UP

Follow-up after the resolution of signs and symptoms of anaphylaxis:

1) Monitor the patients for 8 to 24 hours for a possible late-phase reaction or protracted anaphylaxis. Extend the monitoring to 24 hours in patients with severe anaphylaxis of unknown etiology, slow onset of symptoms, severe asthma, or severe bronchospasm, or if continued exposure to the triggering allergen is probable, as well as in patients with a history of biphasic anaphylactic reactions.

2) Patients in whom the symptoms of anaphylaxis do not recur within 8 hours of completed treatment may be discharged. They should be advised of the possibility of recurrent symptoms and instructed how to act in such situations. Patients should receive a prescription for an epinephrine autoinjector, written anaphylaxis emergency action plan, and medical identification (bracelet, necklace) indicating that they have a history of anaphylaxis and specifying the responsible agent (if known). Educate the patient and family or caregivers on the usage of epinephrine autoinjector and emergency action plan.

3) Refer the patient to an allergy specialist to confirm the diagnosis and suspected triggers and to plan prevention strategies and further management (→below).

→ PREVENTION

In patients with a history of suspected anaphylaxis or an episode diagnosed as anaphylaxis, establish whether it was actually anaphylaxis and whether the suspected trigger was a true trigger of the reaction. Investigations of the putative trigger should be performed not earlier than 3 to 4 weeks after the episode. Initial evaluation and management in patients with a history of suspected anaphylaxis: →Figure 2-1.

Primary Prevention

1. Measures used to reduce the risk of anaphylactic shock:

1) **Administration of drugs**: If possible, administer drugs orally rather than parenterally. Always ask about allergies when taking history, particularly

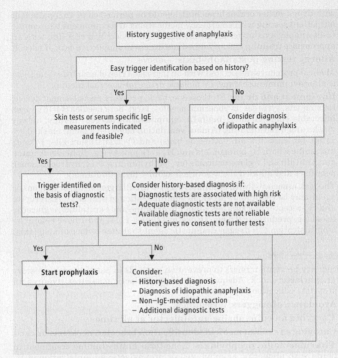

Figure 2-1. Algorithm of initial evaluation and management in patients with suspected anaphylaxis. *Adapted from Ann Allergy Asthma Immunol. 2015;115(5):341-84*

prior to IV drug administration. Never ignore notes added by other physicians or the patients' opinion on drug hypersensitivity. Follow the recommended testing for hypersensitivity and administration of the drug that may trigger anaphylaxis. If the drug is administered IM or subcutaneously, make sure that the needle has not been introduced into a blood vessel. Monitor the patient for 30 to 60 minutes after the administration of a drug that may potentially induce anaphylaxis.

2) **Administration of vaccines or sera**:

   a) Antiviral vaccines: Take a history on hypersensitivity to egg proteins.

   b) Antitoxins (eg, tetanus, diphtheria, or botulinum toxoids, or snake venom serum): Administer human serum. If human serum is not available and allergy to animal serum is suspected, administer both H_1-receptor and H_2-receptor blockers and an oral or IV glucocorticoid prior to the administration of the serum.

3) **Allergy diagnostic testing**: Whenever possible, skin prick tests should be performed before proceeding to intradermal tests. Since intradermal tests are about 1000 times as potent as skin prick tests, if the skin prick test is negative, use a 1:100 dilution of the reagent used for skin prick testing to perform an intradermal test that is then 10 times as potent as the skin prick test. Intradermal tests are used for diagnosis of anaphylaxis to venoms and drugs such as penicillin. For pollen-allergic patients, skin prick tests are usually sensitive enough and can be performed at any time. Challenge tests

with drugs, either oral or bronchial, should be performed in an inpatient or outpatient setting with emergency medications and equipment to promptly treat anaphylaxis under direct medical supervision by a clinician with an appropriate training and an immediate access to supportive care, if needed.

4) **Allergy testing postanaphylaxis**: →above.

2. Medical procedures associated with an increased risk of anaphylaxis (eg, specific allergen immunotherapy, IV biologic drugs, or contrast media):

1) **Equipment and drugs**: Stethoscope, blood pressure measurement device; tourniquets, syringes, hypodermic needles, large-bore needles (14-16 gauge); injectable epinephrine (1 mg/mL); equipment for oxygen therapy; airway masks and a self-inflating (Ambu) ventilation bag with a facial mask; 0.9% saline (at least 500 mL bottles or bags) and IV transfusion kits; IV antihistamines: both H_1 antagonists and H_2 antagonists (eg, diphenhydramine and ranitidine); IV glucocorticoids (eg, methylprednisolone, hydrocortisone); nebulizer and inhaled short-acting β-agonist (eg, salbutamol);

2) The risk associated with administration of an allergen, drug, or diagnostic agent may be reduced by previous administration of oral or IV H_1-receptor and H_2-receptor blockers (eg, diphenhydramine and ranitidine), a glucocorticoid (eg, prednisone 0.5 mg/kg orally 3 times: 12, 7, and 1 hour before the administration of a drug or diagnostic agent that may induce anaphylaxis), or both.

Secondary Prevention

Secondary prevention refers to prevention methods in patients with a history of anaphylactic shock. Adequate use of prophylactic measures requires an appropriate education of patients.

1. Avoidance of triggers, if identified.

2. Carrying an epinephrine autoinjector at all times.

3. Carrying a relevant medical identification bracelet, necklace, or card.

4. Pharmacologic prophylaxis: Long-term antihistamine treatment in patients with idiopathic anaphylaxis, or prophylactic administration of H_1 and H_2 antihistamines, a glucocorticoid, or both prior to expected exposure to a trigger (eg, before contrast-enhanced imaging [→above]). This is not effective in exercise-induced anaphylaxis.

5. Specific allergen immunotherapy, if possible (eg, specific immunotherapy in patients with an allergy to hymenoptera venom or specific immunotherapy for a drug allergy), or immune tolerance induction (in patients with hypersensitivity to drugs, eg, chemotherapeutic agents, monoclonal antibodies, antibiotics, ASA).

1) Oral desensitization to a specific food, such as milk, eggs, or peanuts, can be achieved in carefully selected patients monitored by physicians.⊘● Adverse effects, sometimes requiring the administration of epinephrine, occur during oral desensitization, especially during the initial dose escalation.

2) An anti-IgE antibody given subcutaneously can increase the margin of protection against inadvertently ingested foods (and other allergens) for patients at risk of anaphylaxis.⊘⊖ This is still an experimental strategy.

3) For anaphylaxis triggered by a medication, if it is not possible to substitute an alternative drug, physician-supervised desensitization strategies with the offending agent are effective and safe, particularly for β-lactam or other antibiotics, aspirin, other NSAIDs, and chemotherapy agents.⊘⊖ Desensitization lasts as long as the medication is regularly administered; however, immunologic tolerance does not occur, and if the medication is discontinued for a time, symptoms recur when it is restarted.

4) Stinging insect venom anaphylaxis can be prevented by desensitization in most patients who receive a 3- to 5-year course of subcutaneous immunotherapy to the relevant venoms.⊘●

3. Angioedema

Angioedema is edema of the subcutaneous or submucosal tissue resulting from vasodilation and increased vascular permeability. Most frequently it develops over several minutes to hours and is well demarcated and asymmetric. Angioedema is typically located on the eyelids, lips (→Figure 3-1), genital area, distal limbs, and in the mucosa of the upper respiratory and gastrointestinal (GI) tracts.

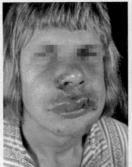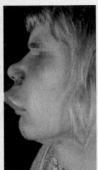

Figure 3-1. Angioedema.

1. Angioedema associated with urticaria:

1) **Allergic**: Drugs (penicillin, sulfonamides), foods (particularly peanuts, walnuts, seafood, milk, eggs, products containing allergens cross-reacting with latex [kiwi, bananas, avocado, chestnuts]), latex, insect venoms.

2) **Nonallergic**: Nonsteroidal anti-inflammatory drugs (NSAIDs), radiologic contrast media, idiopathic eosinophilia/hypereosinophilic syndrome, physical factors (associated with vibratory urticaria, cold urticaria, cholinergic urticaria, or solar urticaria), idiopathic angioedema.

2. Angioedema without urticaria:

1) **Acquired angioedema (AAE)**.

   a) Of unknown etiology: Responding to antihistamine treatment—histaminergic angioedema (idiopathic histaminergic acquired angioedema [IH-AAE]); or not responding to antihistamine treatment—nonhistaminergic angioedema (idiopathic nonhistaminergic acquired angioedema [InH-AAE]).

   b) Associated with angiotensin-converting enzyme inhibitors (ACEI-AAE): Due to inhibition of bradykinin degradation.

   c) Acquired C1 inhibitor deficiency (C1-INH-AAE): Decreased C1-INH levels due to systemic diseases, lymphoproliferative disorders, or antibodies against C1-INH.

2) **Hereditary angioedema (HAE)**:

   a) Associated with C1-INH deficiency (C1-INH-HAE): Type I has low levels of C1-INH due to an autosomal dominant or a new mutation. Type II has low activity and normal levels of C1-INH.

   b) Associated with mutations of factor XII (FXII-HAE) (autosomal dominant).

   c) Of unknown origin (U-HAE) (unknown familial mutation).

1. Angioedema associated with urticaria may appear in any location, although it most frequently affects the face, extremities, and genital areas. In severe cases edema of the tongue, pharynx, or larynx may lead to life-threatening acute respiratory insufficiency. Symptoms of nonallergic angioedema (eg, induced by NSAIDs) are the same as in allergic angioedema.

2. C1-INH-HAE or C1-INH-AAE: C1-INH-HAE type I or type II usually presents in the first or second decade of life and is recurrent. Signs and symptoms may appear spontaneously, but in ~50% of patients they are triggered by an inducing factor: stress, minor trauma (eg, dental procedure), menstruation, pregnancy, use of certain drugs (eg, oral contraceptives, ACEIs), or infection. The majority of patients have prodromal symptoms (mood changes, anxiety, fatigue).

Usually a solitary, well-demarcated, focal edema is present, but less frequently there may be a few small lesions. About half of the patients develop a red rash that may be confused with erythema marginatum. The skin in the edematous area is usually pale. Edema extends slowly over 12 to 24 hours and resolves spontaneously within 8 to 72 hours. Pruritus is absent.

Even the first episode of submucosal edema of the tongue, pharynx, or larynx (presenting as sensation of a lump in the throat, hoarseness, dysphagia, and dyspnea) may cause acute respiratory insufficiency and be life-threatening. Acute edema of the intestinal wall may cause abdominal pain, nausea, vomiting, and subsequent diarrhea. A sudden pain attack may resemble acute abdomen (improvement with administration of C1-INH concentrate allows one to differentiate acute abdomen from angioedema).

Symptoms of C1-INH-AAE are the same as in C1-INH-HAE, but there is no history of familial occurrence and symptoms of angioedema may precede other features of systemic disease for several months.

3. FXII-HAE affects mainly women. Symptoms develop in puberty, after starting hormonal contraceptives or hormone replacement therapy, or in pregnancy. With age, symptoms become less frequent and less severe and may resolve completely at the age of 70 to 80 years.

4. ACEI-AAE develops in 0.3% of patients receiving ACEIs and in 0.13% of patients receiving angiotensin receptor blockers (ARBs). It more often affects women and persons aged >65 years and is 3 to 4 times more frequent in black patients compared with white patients. In ~50% of individuals ACEI-AAE occurs during the first week of treatment and is not related to the type or dose of the ACEI/ARB. It can occur even after a year of being on therapy. Edema usually involves the entire face, mouth, tongue, and respiratory tract; it may also affect the GI mucosa. For patients who develop angioedema when taking an ACEI, the risk of development of any subsequent angioedema when taking an ARB is between 2% and 17%; for confirmed angioedema, the risk is from 0% to 9.2%.◐

→ DIAGNOSIS

Diagnostic workup in angioedema associated with urticaria (urticaria excludes the diagnosis of C1-INH-HAE and C1-INH-AAE, although it is possible to have both conditions): →Chapter 2.7. In patients without concomitant urticaria, it is necessary to establish whether any ACEIs, ARBs, or NSAIDs are currently used. Take a careful history, including familial occurrence of angioedema. Diagnostic workup in suspected C1-INH deficiency: →Figure 3-2.

In patients aged >30 years consider malignancy (the most common types for given age and sex) and systemic connective tissue disease.

Diagnostic Tests

In patients with suspected C1-INH-HAE or C1-INH-AAE, measure C4 concentration (normal values exclude C1-INH-HAE types I and II as well as C1-INH--AAE, although it can rarely be normal between attacks). In patients with C4 <0.1 g/L, measure the concentration and activity of C1-INH.

Differential Diagnosis

It is crucial to exclude acute anaphylaxis and laryngeal edema.

Other conditions that could be considered include hormonal disturbances in women (symmetric edema of the face and hands), heart failure (pitting edema of limbs), superior vena cava syndrome (chronic facial edema), acute allergic contact dermatitis, erysipelas or facial cellulitis, lymphedema, herpes zoster, Crohn disease of the oral cavity and lips, and systemic connective tissue diseases (eg, dermatomyositis).

→ **TREATMENT**

Acute Treatment

Treatment of an angioedema attack depends on the location of edema. Edema situated peripherally (hands, feet, genital area) may not require urgent treatment.

1. In case of risk of acute respiratory insufficiency: In patients with stridor or significant edema of the face and upper airways (edema of the tongue, oral mucosa, and throat mucosa; hoarseness), consider urgent endotracheal intubation. In angioedema associated with urticaria, management is the same as in anaphylaxis unless the patient also has HAE (→below). Patients with acute edema of the pharynx and upper airways should be monitored for ≥24 hours.

2. Angioedema associated with urticaria (eg, after the administration of NSAIDs): →Chapter 2.7.

3. IH-AAE: Administer IV or oral glucocorticoids and IM epinephrine. Use antihistamines as prophylaxis.

4. InH-AAE: Antihistamines, glucocorticoids, and epinephrine are ineffective (but should be used if the type of angioedema is unknown). As prophylaxis, consider administering oral tranexamic acid up to 3 g/d. There are case reports of plasma-derived C1-INH (pdC1-INH) and icatibant being effective and these could be tried if angioedema is life threatening (→below).

5. C1-INH-HAE type I and type II, C1-INH-AAE: Epinephrine, antihistamines, and glucocorticoids are not effective unless the patient also has atopy and the event was triggered by an allergic reaction (however, they should be used if the type of angioedema is unknown). Treatment depends on the severity of angioedema:

1) **pdC1-INH** (brand names: Berinert, Cinryze) is the treatment of choice in life-threatening angioedema (mainly in laryngeal angioedema). It may be also considered in patients with severe intestinal wall edema. One unit of pdC1-INH is an equivalent of the amount of C1-INH in 1 mL of human plasma. Dosage: Berinert 20 U/kg in a rapid IV infusion is used in the treatment of HAE types I and II in adults, children, and infants; Cinryze 1000 U in a rapid IV infusion is approved for use prophylactically in HAE types I and II in patients aged >12 years.

   In patients >12 years you may also use conestat alfa, a recombinant human C1-INH analogue. Dosage: In individuals <84 kg, use 50 U/kg IV; in individuals ≥84 kg, administer 4200 U as a single IV injection.

2) **Kinin pathway modulators**:

   a) Ecallantide is a recombinant, selective, highly potent plasma kallikrein inhibitor, not approved in the European Union. The onset of action is 30 minutes to 4 hours after administration.

   b) Icatibant is a selective bradykinin B_2 receptor antagonist. A dose of 30 mg subcutaneously is approved for HAE types I and II in patients >18 years old. The median time to 50% symptom reduction for icatibant is 2 to 2.3 hours. There are case reports showing it is helpful for other forms of angioedema and a study showing benefit for ACEI-associated angioedema.

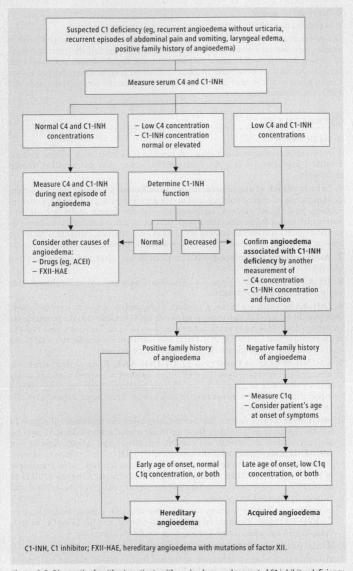

C1-INH, C1 inhibitor; FXII-HAE, hereditary angioedema with mutations of factor XII.

Figure 3-2. Diagnostic algorithm in patients with angioedema and suspected C1 inhibitor deficiency.

3) **Attenuated androgens**: **Stanozolol** up to 16 mg/d, oral **danazol** up to 600 mg/d. These agents may be used preventatively. There are no studies in which they were used acutely to treat attacks. In the majority of patients symptoms may be controlled with danazol 50 to 200 mg administered

daily or every 2 days. Attenuated androgens may be used in patients with peripheral edema or intestinal wall edema to accelerate the regression of symptoms. Do not use them in the first and second trimesters of pregnancy or in children.

4) **Fresh frozen plasma (FFP)** 400 mL may be used only in exceptional cases when C1-INH concentrate is not available. Paradoxically, it may aggravate the symptoms of angioedema by providing more substrate.

6. FXII-HAE: Resolution of angioedema within 1 to 2 hours of the administration of icatibant has been reported. Data on the efficacy of danazol are contradictory.

7. ACEI-AAE: Discontinue the ACEI and consider using an ARB, especially in case of cough.◕ If angioedema occurs in a patient receiving an ARB, discontinue the agent. There is inconsistent experimental evidence that icatibant may result in decreasing time to resolution of symptoms◔ and case reports suggesting pdC1-INH may be helpful.

Long-Term Treatment

1. Angioedema associated with urticaria: →Chapter 2.7.

2. C1-INH-HAE type I and type II:

1) **Avoidance of inducing factors**.

2) **Short-term prophylaxis in patients undergoing minor surgical or dental procedures**:

   a) Prophylaxis is not necessary if C1-INH concentrate is directly available for acute use, but it could be administered.

   b) In other cases use danazol 2.5 to 10 mg/kg/d (maximum, 600 mg/d) starting 5 days before the procedure and continuing until 2 days after the procedure.

3) **Short-term prophylaxis in patients undergoing major surgical procedures**:

   a) C1-INH concentrate IV 1 hour before the procedure (dosage the same as in acute treatment of HAE [→above]). The next dose may be administered during surgery, if necessary. Injections may be repeated once daily until the risk of edema is reduced.

   b) If C1-INH concentrate is not available, use danazol (dosage: →above); if this is also not available, administer FFP (10 mL/kg, 2 U of 400 mL in an adult) ≥1 hour before surgery.

4) **Long-term prophylaxis**: Use androgens (eg, danazol) or tranexamic acid (less effective than androgens). If these drugs are not available but C1-INH can be obtained, the patient may self-administer C1-INH concentrate in case of prodromal symptoms or regularly twice weekly to prevent attacks. A recent study showed pdC1-INH given subcutaneously in doses of 40 U/kg and 60 U/kg significantly reduced attacks.

   Note: Long-term use of androgens may lead to increased body weight, disturbances of the menstrual cycle and masculinization in women, decreased libido, acne, fatigue, headache, hypertension, cholestasis, and liver dysfunction. Monitor liver function and plasma lipid levels regularly. Do not use androgens during pregnancy, lactation, in patients with prostate cancer, or in children who have not reached Tanner stage 3.

3. FXII-HAE: Women cannot use estrogens (contraceptives, hormone replacement therapy).

4. C1-INH-AAE: Treatment is the same as in C1-INH-HAE types I and II (→above). Treatment of the underlying disease is necessary. In some patients plasmapheresis and administration of cytotoxic drugs, androgens, and tranexamic acid may be required.

4. Food Hypersensitivity

Food adverse reactions are recurrent signs or symptoms that are caused by ingestion of particular foods or food components in amounts tolerated by healthy individuals.

Classification of food adverse reactions:

1) **Immune-mediated reactions (hypersensitivity, also referred to as allergy)**:

   a) IgE-mediated reactions (eg, acute urticaria, oral allergy syndrome, anaphylaxis): Incidence is highest in infancy but adult-onset disease is common. Designation of priority food allergens differs by country.

   b) Non–IgE-mediated reactions (eg, celiac disease, food protein–induced enterocolitis, food protein–induced allergic proctocolitis).

   c) Mixed reactions (IgE-mediated and non–IgE-mediated, eg, eosinophilic gastroenteritis and eosinophilic esophagitis, atopic dermatitis).

   d) Cell-mediated reactions (eg, allergic contact dermatitis).

2) **Non–immune-mediated reactions (primary intolerances)**:

   a) Metabolic reactions (eg, lactose or fructose intolerance).

   b) Pharmacologic reactions (eg, to tyramine [cheese, pickled herring], caffeine, theobromine [chocolate, tea, cola]), histamine [fish, sauerkraut], tryptamine [tomato, plum]).

   c) Toxic reactions (eg, to toxins produced by the *Scombridae* fish).

   d) Other, idiopathic, or unclassified (eg, to sulfites).

In Canada, in infants and children the foods that most commonly cause hypersensitivity reactions are cow's milk, hen's egg, peanut, and tree nuts. About 70% to 80% of patients lose their allergies to milk, soy, or egg by the age of 10 years. In adults the most frequent causes of food hypersensitivity are fish, shellfish, milk, peanut, and tree nuts.

Highly cross-reactive tree nuts are cashew with pistachio (~2 out of 3 of cashew allergic reactions are to pistachio), walnut with pecan (~2 out of 3 walnut allergic reactions are to pecan), and possibly almond with hazelnut, although almond allergy is less common than previously thought. As further discussed below, there are sparse data on the cross-reactivity between almond and hazelnut because almost all individuals sensitized to either almond (~98%) or hazelnut (~77%) tolerate the food despite having positive IgE. Common cross-reactivities: →Table 4-1.

In **oral allergy syndrome** symptoms most commonly occur following ingestion of raw fruits or vegetables and are caused by cross-reactivity with pollens in pollen-allergic patients (most frequently birch, grass, ragweed, or mugwort pollen). The responsible allergens are degraded during extensive heating or processing, thereby leading most patients with oral allergy syndrome to be able to tolerate cooked forms of these fresh fruits or vegetables. However, systemic reactions due to cross-reactivity can occur and are thought to be due to heat-stable fruit or vegetable allergens of the lipid transfer protein family. These reactions are referred to as **systemic pollen-food syndrome**.

The clinical features depend on whether the allergy is immediate or delayed (→Table 4-2).

1. In **immediate hypersensitivity (IgE-mediated)** the reaction typically develops within 30 to 60 minutes after ingestion:

1) Mucocutaneous: Urticaria, angioedema.

2) Respiratory: Upper (rhinitis) or lower (wheeze, bronchoconstriction).

Table 4-1. Common cross-reactivities between various allergens

Food	Cross-reaction	Percentage of reactions
Animal-source foods		
Chicken/hen's egg	Poultry	<5%
Cow's milk	Veal/beef	~10%
Cow's milk	Goat's milk	~90%
Fish	Other fish	~50%
Plant-source foods		
Peanuts	Legumes	<10%
Soy	Legumes	<5%
Wheat	Other cereals	~25%

Table 4-2. Manifestations of food allergies[a]

Reaction	Clinical manifestations	Diagnostic tests
IgE-dependent		
Anaphylactic reaction (IgE-dependent)	Onset (typically in 30 min) of urticaria, angioedema, abdominal pain, nausea, vomiting, diarrhea, rhinitis, wheeze, syncope, hypotension	– SPT and/or sIgE – ± Oral challenge
Oral allergy syndrome (IgE-dependent)	Minutes after exposure of oral mucosa: pruritus; tingling; erythema and/or mild edema of lips, tongue, oral mucosa, and pharyngeal mucosa	– SPT with fresh fruits/vegetables (prick-prick test) and/or sIgE – ± Oral challenge (positive with fresh and negative with cooked fruits/vegetables)
IgE-dependent and non–IgE-dependent		
Eosinophilic esophagitis	Chronic or intermittent reflux, vomiting, dysphagia	Endoscopy (rings, furrows, edema, microabscesses, strictures, crepe paper appearance) and biopsy (>15 eosinophils/HPF)
Eosinophilic gastroenteritis	Chronic or intermittent abdominal pain, vomiting, irritability, anorexia, malnutrition, weight loss, anemia, protein-losing enteropathy	– CBC (elevated eosinophils in 80%) – CT – Endoscopy with biopsy showing increased eosinophilic infiltration

[a] Celiac disease and less common conditions are not included.

CBC, complete blood count; CT, computed tomography; HPF, high power field; sIgE, serum-specific IgE; SPT, skin prick test.

3) Gastrointestinal (GI): Oral or pharyngeal pruritus (or both), abdominal pain.
4) Cardiovascular: Presyncope or syncope, hypotension, shock (anaphylactic).
Anaphylaxis is recognized in the case of (1) involvement of ≥2 organ systems after a likely allergen exposure or isolated hypotension after a known allergen

exposure, or (2) a sudden onset of mucocutaneous and either respiratory or cardiovascular involvement.

2. In **delayed hypersensitivity (typically non–IgE-mediated)** the reaction occurs hours to days after exposure:

1) Food protein–induced enterocolitis syndrome (FPIES): Profuse repetitive vomiting 2 to 6 hours after ingestion, most commonly due to cow's milk, soy, or grains.

2) Food protein–induced enteropathy (FPE): Chronic nonbloody diarrhea in the first year of life due to small bowel injury and malabsorption with possible failure to thrive. Implicated foods include cow's milk, soy, wheat, and egg.

3) Allergic proctocolitis: Blood or mucus in stool (or both) in otherwise healthy newborns and infants.

4) Heiner syndrome (pulmonary hemosiderosis): A rare manifestation of allergy to cow's milk leading to cough, rhinitis, recurrent fever, wheeze, hemoptysis, hematochezia, or failure to thrive, almost always with pulmonary infiltrates due to hemosiderosis.

5) Celiac disease and dermatitis herpetiformis (DH): A gluten-sensitive enteropathy leading to small intestinal inflammation, villous atrophy, and malabsorption with symptoms of abdominal pain, bloating, diarrhea, and possible weight loss. DH typically causes clustered pruritic papulovesicular eruptions over extensor surfaces, such as the elbows or lower back.

6) Eosinophilic esophagitis: Dysphagia to solid foods, liquids, or both associated with comorbid aeroallergen sensitization. The most common allergens are cow's milk, soy, wheat, and egg.

→ DIAGNOSIS

Establishing diagnosis can be difficult. The diagnosis of food hypersensitivity can be suspected on the basis of history (including a history of atopy in close relatives or causal relationship between a particular food and symptoms developing consistently after its repeated ingestion), results of skin tests, in vitro immunologic tests, as well as elimination diets and challenge tests.

Diagnostic Tests

1. Immediate hypersensitivity reactions:

1) **Skin prick test**: A mean wheal diameter ≥3 mm than the diameter of the saline control is positive. However, testing does not yield strictly binary results. The size of the skin test correlates with the probability of allergy and not with its severity, and the false-positive rate is high. For this reason, this test alone is not diagnostic and should not be used as a screening tool in the absence of a history of allergic reaction after food ingestion.

2) **Serum-specific IgE (sIgE)**: This can help identify foods that provoke an IgE-mediated reaction, particularly those due to interfering medications (eg, ongoing antihistamine use) or in patients who cannot undergo skin testing for some reason (eg, no immediate access to an allergist; nonallergic skin disease prevents skin testing). Similarly to the skin prick test, this test identifies sensitization, that is, the presence of a specific IgE antibody whose level indicates the probability of a true underlying allergic disease. Asymptomatic sensitization is common. Diagnostic thresholds for both skin testing and sIgE vary by population studied, age, and food allergen. Among both symptomatic and asymptomatic patients with GI or food allergic concerns, there is no diagnostic value of serum-specific IgG testing to foods, which is frequently marketed directly to public without health-care provider counselling or request. Professional medical societies around the world have made statements denouncing such testing; in fact, these tests often cause unnecessary and potentially harmful food elimination.

2. Delayed hypersensitivity reactions:

1) **Histologic examination of GI mucosal biopsy specimens**: The presence of >15 eosinophils per high power field (HPF) on esophageal biopsies is consistent with eosinophilic esophagitis.

2) **Elimination diet**: If symptoms resolve after potentially harmful foods have been eliminated from the patient's diet, it may be assumed that there is a causal relationship between the foods and the symptoms (a 6-week elimination period is required for non–IgE-mediated reactions; however, these findings have to be confirmed by a challenge test. Skin tests typically used for evaluation of IgE-mediated allergies, blood IgE testing, and patch tests are not reliable for guiding elimination diets in eosinophilic esophagitis.

3. Challenge tests for immediate and delayed hypersensitivity reactions: Graded allergen ingestion in a controlled (supervised) setting can be done, as it is the reference standard for diagnosis of immediate-type food allergy. However, as of now no universally accepted protocols exist and there is a risk eliciting severe life-threatening reactions (deaths have been reported). Hence, extensive training and emergency preparedness is required, along with informed consent to perform the challenge. Oral food challenge tests are often done for indeterminate or discordant results of skin or blood allergy testing or to differentiate asymptomatic sensitization from food allergy.

➡ MANAGEMENT

1. Elimination diets (avoiding foods causing hypersensitivity reactions) are the primary way to prevent recurrent food allergic reactions. Care must be taken to avoid nutritional compromise. The treatment approach varies depending on the specific food the patient is allergic to and the type of food allergy. Tolerance to allergens may occur over time. Monitoring of symptoms and laboratory values may assist in identifying when to safely reintroduce certain foods. For some delayed hypersensitivity reactions, such as eosinophilic esophagitis, it may be necessary to use an elemental diet if empiric elimination of the most common allergens is not effective.

2. Anaphylaxis preparedness: Inform patients with allergic hypersensitivity reactions about early recognition of allergic symptoms and management in case of an anaphylactic reaction. Precisely who should or should not carry an epinephrine autoinjector is not standardized globally. In North America most patients with food allergy are given an epinephrine autoinjector, whereas in the United Kingdom and Australia prescription may be determined by the severity of previous allergic reactions or whether the patient has comorbid asthma. However, it should be kept in mind that the severity of previous reactions does not reliably predict the severity of future reactions and previously mild reactions can be subsequently fatal. Many professional societies advocate for health-care providers to develop a written anaphylaxis action plan in case of accidental consumption of a harmful allergen. Also →Chapter 2.2.

3. Symptomatic treatment:

1) Management of anaphylaxis: →Chapter 2.2.

2) Antihistamines (→Chapter 2.2) may result in partial improvement in patients with oral allergy syndrome and IgE-mediated reactions but do not inhibit systemic reactions. They are only adjuncts, not first-line therapy, for anaphylaxis.

3) In patients with eosinophilic esophagitis:

   a) Proton pump inhibitors (PPIs) improve symptoms and eosinophilia. Given the safety profile and benefits, a trial of PPIs is recommended for inducing and maintaining remission.

   b) Topical glucocorticoids are administered orally and swallowed by the patient (budesonide nebulization suspension 2 mg/d mixed with sucralose 5 mg, or fluticasone via a metered-dose inhaler 440-880 µg bid). This treatment is routinely continued for 8 weeks, and in patients with no response it may be repeated at the same or higher doses.

c) Elimination diets: An elemental diet with total elimination of all food allergens or 4-food or 6-food elimination diet (removing soy, egg, milk, wheat, possibly peanut or tree nuts, and all seafood).

d) Esophageal dilation may be necessary for symptoms of dysphagia in patients who develop strictures.

e) Prevention.

4) Oral or parenteral **glucocorticoids** should be limited in their use to treat delayed hypersensitivity reactions as they have transient beneficial effects and significant adverse effects.

→ PREVENTION

Primary prevention of food allergy may be considered in infancy. It is critical to separate interventions during infancy to prevent food allergies from those associated with other benefits (eg, nutrition, maternal-infant bonding, brain development).

1. There are no specific diets or supplements for mothers that have been shown to influence the development of food allergy in their offspring.

2. Appropriate infant nutrition:

1) Currently available evidence, which is generally low quality, shows no association between breastfeeding and prevention of food allergies. The World Health Organization (WHO) guidelines recommend exclusive breastfeeding for all infants up to 6 months of life for its nutritional and other benefits, including the uncertain possibility of reduced incidence of infant wheeze, atopic dermatitis, and asthma.

2) If breastfeeding is not possible, consider formulas. Note that hydrolyzed formulas do not protect against cow's milk allergy.

3) Elimination diets in breastfeeding mothers are not recommended.

Introduction of foods other than breast milk within 4 to 6 months of life while still breastfeeding is not associated with food allergies⊖ and may reduce the incidence of IgE-mediated allergy to certain foods such as milk, egg, or peanut.

5. Immunodeficiency Disorders

→ DEFINITION, ETIOLOGY, PATHOGENESIS

Immunodeficiency disorders are associated with dysfunctions of the immune system. They are classified as:

1) **Primary (hereditary) immunodeficiencies (PIDs)**: Rare conditions caused mostly by genetic defects of the immune system that can lead to an abnormal production of antibodies (most frequently common variable immunodeficiency), abnormal cellular response, abnormal phagocytosis, deficiencies in the complement system, or immune dysregulation. The overall prevalence of PID is estimated at ~1 in 2000. Over 300 distinct disorders have been identified.

2) **Secondary immunodeficiencies caused by external factors or diseases**: These are usually mixed (including an impaired specific immune response [humoral and cellular] and impaired nonspecific immune response [eg, abnormalities of the complement system]). Key etiologic factors include

medications (anticonvulsants, nonsteroidal anti-inflammatory drugs, immunosuppressive treatment, and chemotherapy), infections (HIV, measles, herpes simplex virus, bacterial infections [including mycobacteria], parasitic infections [malaria]), malignancy (chronic lymphocytic leukemia, Hodgkin lymphoma, monoclonal gammopathies, solid tumors), metabolic disturbances (diabetes mellitus, renal failure, liver failure, malnutrition), autoimmune diseases (systemic lupus erythematosus, rheumatoid arthritis, Felty syndrome), burns, environmental exposure (ionizing radiation, chemicals), pregnancy, stress, asplenia, splenic dysfunction, cirrhosis, and aging.

→ CLINICAL FEATURES

Immunodeficiency disorders manifest as **frequent chronic and recurrent infections**. The infections are severe, frequently atypical and prolonged, and sometimes resistant to antimicrobial treatment. They may be due to pathogens that rarely cause serious infections in immunocompetent persons, such as *Mycobacterium avium*, *Cryptosporidium parvum*, cytomegalovirus, or *Candida albicans*. For humoral immunodeficiencies, recurrent respiratory tract and paranasal sinus infections caused by encapsulated bacteria (eg, *Haemophilus influenzae*, *Streptococcus pneumoniae*) are characteristic. The diagnosis is frequently obscured by false-negative results of serologic studies.

Another important presentation is **systemic autoimmunity**. This can manifest as autoimmune cytopenias, vasculitis, gut disease, or cutaneous involvement. Allergic reactions to antimicrobial agents and food allergens are frequently observed.

Clinical symptoms and signs of PIDs usually appear in childhood, but it is not uncommon for the diagnosis to be made in adulthood.

→ DIAGNOSIS

Immunodeficiency should be suspected in every person with recurrent or severe viral or bacterial infections, or with opportunistic infections. Unexplained evidence of autoimmunity can act as an additional clue. In such patients perform the studies reviewed below to assess the specific aspects of immune response, beginning with screening tests and proceeding towards more specialized studies. Once suspected, the diagnosis and management of immunodeficiency frequently requires the guidance and expertise of specialized centers.

Warning signs of PID for adults:

1) Six signs by the European Society for Immunodeficiencies (2008):
   a) At least 4 infections requiring antibiotics within a year (otitis, bronchitis, sinusitis, pneumonia).
   b) Recurring infections or an infection requiring prolonged antibiotic therapy.
   c) At least 2 severe bacterial infections (osteomyelitis, meningitis, septicemia, cellulitis).
   d) At least 2 radiologically proven episodes of pneumonia within 3 years.
   e) Infection with an unusual localization or unusual pathogen.
   f) PID in the family.
2) Ten signs by the Jeffrey Modell Foundation endorsed by Immunodeficiency Canada:
   a) At least 2 new ear infections within a year.
   b) At least 2 new sinus infections within a year in the absence of allergy.
   c) One pneumonia episode per year for >1 year.
   d) Chronic diarrhea with weight loss.
   e) Recurrent viral infections (colds, herpes, warts, condylomata).

f) Recurrent need for intravenous antibiotics to clear infections.

g) Recurrent deep abscesses of the skin or internal organs.

h) Persistent thrush or fungal infection on skin or elsewhere.

i) Infection with normally harmless tuberculosis-like bacteria.

j) A family history of PID.

Diagnostic Tests

1. Assessment of humoral immune response:

1) **Screening tests**: Complete blood count (CBC) with differential cell count; basic liver and kidney function tests; serum protein electrophoresis (to exclude monoclonal gammopathies); serum immunoglobulin (IgG, IgM, IgA) levels; titers of specific antibodies (against antigens of vaccines administered in childhood); HIV testing.

2) **Specialized studies**: Measurement of titers of specific antibodies before and after vaccinations (including assessment of the response to polysaccharide and protein vaccines); IgG subclass measurement; assessment of B-cell counts (subpopulations) using flow cytometry; assessment of in vitro immunoglobulin synthesis in response to mitogens.

2. Assessment of cellular immune response:

1) **Screening tests**: CBC with differential cell count; assessment of T-cell, B-cell, and NK-cell counts (subpopulations) using flow cytometry; skin tests to assess delayed cutaneous hypersensitivity (response to intradermal administration of antigens, eg, BCG, purified protein derivative); radiologic studies of the thymus; HIV testing.

2) **Specialized studies**: Determination of the type of T-cell or NK-cell dysfunction (or both; levels of adenosine deaminase and purine nucleoside phosphorylase); assessment of NK-cell cytotoxic activity; in vitro proliferation in response to mitogen or antigen stimulation; cytokine synthesis and secretion in response to mitogen or antigen stimulation; expression of surface markers after mitogen stimulation; assessment of 22q11 and 10p11 deletions using a fluorescence in situ hybridization assay; genetic analysis (including whole genome sequencing in selected cases).

3. Assessment of phagocyte function:

1) **Screening tests**: CBC with differential cell count; microscopic assessment of neutrophils using standard staining.

2) **Specialized studies**: Dihydrorhodamine reduction assay or nitroblue tetrazolium reduction assay (to assess oxidative processes in phagocytes); assessment of adhesive molecules using flow cytometry; chemotaxis studies; phagocytosis studies using flow cytometry; cytochemical studies performed to assess activity of granulocyte peroxidase and glucose-6-phosphate dehydrogenase; bone marrow aspiration with a quantitative and morphological assessment of the myeloid lineage.

4. Assessment of the complement system:

1) **Screening tests**: Total hemolytic complement activity (CH50); activity of the complement alternative pathway (AH50).

2) **Specialized studies**: Concentrations or activities of respective complement components (serum C1-C9 levels, C1 esterase inhibitor).

➡ **TREATMENT**

General recommendations: →Table 5-1.

1. Avoid situations associated with a high risk of infection.

2. Treat the underlying condition in patients with secondary immunodeficiency.

3. **Administer intravenous immunoglobulins (IVIGs)** in patients with immunodeficiency associated with hypogammaglobulinemia or agammaglobulinemia. The half-life of IgG is ~21 days, so it is recommended to administer IVIG every 21 to 28 days to maintain protective IgG levels ($\geq$500 mg/dL). In patients with agammaglobulinemia or severe IgG deficiency (<200 mg/dL), consider administering a loading dose of 1 g/kg. Protective IgG levels are achieved in the majority of patients who receive IVIG 300 to 600 mg/kg every 3 weeks or 400 to 800 mg/kg every 4 weeks. However, the doses of IVIG necessary to maintain protective IgG levels and to achieve clinical improvement vary greatly among patients. **Subcutaneous immunoglobulins (SCIGs)** may also be used, usually once a week, until the protective IgG levels are achieved and subsequently at lower maintenance doses.

Common adverse effects that can be anticipated with parenteral immunoglobulins include local injection site reactions, systemic allergic reactions, and headache (including aseptic meningitis). Premedication with intravenous fluids, acetaminophen (INN paracetamol), and antihistamines may be helpful in preventing these reactions.

4. **Prophylactic antimicrobial therapy**: Amoxicillin (500 mg/d or 250--500 mg bid), sulfamethoxazole/trimethoprim (160 mg of trimethoprim once daily or 80-160 mg bid), or azithromycin 500 mg once weekly. If these agents are ineffective, use clarithromycin 500 mg/d or amoxicillin + clavulanic acid 875 mg or 1000 mg once daily. Prophylactic antimicrobial therapy is indicated in patients with severe or moderate hypogammaglobulinemia in whom administration of IgG does not prevent frequent infections and in patients with severe deficiency of IgA or subclasses of IgG causing frequent infections. Prophylaxis of *Pneumocystis jiroveci* infections is recommended in patients with combined immunodeficiency displaying significantly defective leukocyte function and in patients undergoing intensive immunosuppressive treatment.

5. **Hematopoietic growth factors** (granulocyte colony-stimulating factor [G-CSF] and granulocyte and macrophage colony-stimulating factor [GM-CSF]) are used in patients with severe neutropenia (absolute neutrophil count <0.5×10^9/L). These agents may reduce the duration of neutropenia of various etiologies (including severe congenital neutropenia, cyclic neutropenia, and AIDS) and reduce the severity and duration of infections. They should be considered in patients with neutropenia and poor performance status who are at high risk of infectious complications, particularly if they have previously undergone anticancer treatment and developed complications in the form of infection or febrile neutropenia. Dosage of hematopoietic growth factors for G-CSF: filgrastim 3.45 to 11.5 µg/kg/d subcutaneously, lenograstim 150 µg/m^2; for GM-CSF, use 250 µg/m^2/d IV or subcutaneously.

6. **Interferon α and interferon γ** are used in patients with congenital defects of humoral response, cell-mediated immune response (abnormalities of the interleukin-12/interferon-γ axis), or phagocytosis.

7. **Allogeneic hematopoietic stem cell transplantation** is used in selected patients with severe (and usually combined) PID.

8. **Vaccinations in patients with immunodeficiency**: Vaccination with attenuated viruses (such as measles, mumps, and rubella) should be avoided in patients with defective cellular immunity. Every patient with asplenia or hyposplenism should receive vaccines against encapsulated bacteria (*S pneumonia*, *Neisseria meningitidis*, *H influenzae* type b) and yearly vaccination against influenza. Recommend vaccination of close contacts of an immunodeficient patient against most common infectious diseases (in particular against influenza).

9. **Transfusions of blood cell concentrates**: In patients with defects of cell-mediated immune response, transfuse only irradiated packed red blood cells or platelet concentrates from cytomegalovirus-negative donors (irradiation is used to reduce lymphocyte counts in the concentrate).

10. **Treatment of febrile neutropenia.**

Table 5-1. General recommendations on treatment of primary immunodeficiency disorders

Type of immunodeficiency	IVIG/SCIG	Allogeneic HSCT	Other treatments	Approximate prevalence (selected examples)
Immunodeficiency affecting predominantly antibodies	+	– (+ for selected cases of CVID)	– Avoidance of live vaccines (except SIGAD, IGGSD, THI) – Antibiotic prophylaxis: All immunodeficiencies of this type if infections continue despite IVIG – Immunomodulators: CVID – Pneumococcal vaccination: SIGAD, IGGSD, SAD	SIGAD, 1:200 CVID, 1:20,000 XLA, 1:200,000
Combined immunodeficiency (including well-defined immunodeficiency syndromes)	+	+	– Avoidance of live vaccines: All immunodeficiencies of this type – Avoidance of nonirradiated blood or products: All immunodeficiencies of this type – Avoidance of CMV-positive blood or cells: All immunodeficiencies of this type – Antibiotic prophylaxis: All immunodeficiencies of this type – Antifungal prophylaxis: SCID, HIGM, HIES, ICD4L – Splenectomy: WAS – Glucocorticoids: WAS – Thymus transplantation: DGS – G-CSF, GM-CSF: ICD4L, HIGM – Gene therapy for IL2RG, ADA deficiency, WAS	SCID, 1:50,000 WAS, 1:100,000 DGS, 1:5000 HIES, 1:100,000 HIGM, 1:500,000 ICD4L, very rare
Immunodysregulation disorders	+	+	– Avoidance of live vaccines: All immunodeficiencies of this type – Antibiotic prophylaxis: All immunodeficiencies of this type – Chemotherapy (as in lymphoproliferative neoplasms): XLP, GS – Chemotherapy (associated with allogeneic HSCT): CHS	XLP, 1:1,000,000

Phagocyte defects	−	+	– Avoidance of live vaccines: All immunodeficiencies of this type – Antibiotic prophylaxis: All immunodeficiencies of this type – IFN-γ: CGD, disorders of IL-12/IFN-γ axis – Surgical or dental debridement: CGD, LAD – Antifungal prophylaxis: CGD, LAD – G-CSF: Neutropenia – Antituberculous agents: Disorders of IL-12/IFN-γ axis	CGD, 1:200,000 LAD, very rare
Primary immunodeficiencies of the innate immune system	− (+ for WHIM)	+	– Avoidance of live vaccines: All immunodeficiencies of this type – Antibiotic prophylaxis: All immunodeficiencies of this type – G-CSF and GM-CSF: WHIM – Antifungal agents: CMCC – Antiviral agents: NK-cell deficiency	CMCC (diverse group of diseases), up to 1:10,000 WHIM, very rare
Complement deficiencies	−	−	– Antibiotic prophylaxis: All complement deficiencies – Pneumococcal vaccine: Deficiency of C1a, C1r, C2, C3, C4 – Meningococcal vaccine: Deficiency of C5, C6, C7, C8, C9 – Immunomodulators (IFN-γ): Deficiency of C1a, C2, C4, factors H and I	C2 deficiency, 1:20,00 C4 deficiency, very rare C5–C9 deficiency, variable, up to 1:2000

Adapted from J Allergy Clin Immunol. 2015;136(5);1186-205.

ADA, adenine deaminase; CGD, chronic granulomatous disease; CHS, Chédiak-Higashi syndrome; CMCC, chronic mucocutaneous candidiasis; CMV, cytomegalovirus; CVID, common variable immunodeficiency; DGS, DiGeorge syndrome; G-CSF, granulocyte-colony stimulating factor; GM-CSF, granulocyte-macrophage colony stimulating factor; GS, Griscelli syndrome; HIES, hyper-IgE syndrome; HIGM, hyper-IgM syndrome; HSCT, hematopoietic stem cell transplantation; ICD4L, idiopathic CD4 lymphocytopenia; IFN-γ, interferon γ; IGGSD, IgG subclass deficiency; IL, interleukin; IL2RG, IL2 receptor γ; IVIG, intravenous immunoglobulin; LAD, leukocyte adhesion deficiency; SAD, specific antibody deficiency; SCID, severe combined immunodeficiency; SCIG, subcutaneous immunoglobulin; SIGAD, selective IgA deficiency; THI, transient hypogammaglobulinemia of infancy; WAS, Wiskott-Aldrich syndrome; WHIM, warts, hypogammaglobulinemia, immunodeficiency, and myelokathexis; XLA, X-linked agammaglobulinemia; XLP, X-linked lymphoproliferative syndrome.

6. Serum Sickness

Serum sickness is a reversible systemic reaction due to the formation of immune complexes with a foreign antigen present in circulation.

"Classic" serum sickness results from the formation of immune complexes due to immunization of a human host with a foreign protein. **Serum sickness–like reactions** refer to a constellation of symptoms clinically resembling classic serum sickness but typically caused by drugs, and less frequently by infection. The pathogenesis of these reactions is not understood.

Causes:

1) Serum sickness:

   a) Foreign proteins: Equine diphtheria antitoxin, botulinum antitoxin, rabies antitoxin, snake antivenom, antithymocyte immunoglobulin (rabbit), chimeric monoclonal antibodies (eg, rituximab, infliximab), streptokinase.

   b) Case reports have implicated humanized monoclonal antibodies, allogenic human plasma, insect stings, mosquito salivary protein, vaccinations, and allergen immunotherapy extracts.

2) Serum sickness–like reactions:

   a) Drugs: Most commonly antibiotics—specifically penicillin, amoxicillin, cefaclor, and sulfamethoxazole/trimethoprim—although a wide range of medications have been implicated.

   b) Viral infections, for example, acute hepatitis B.

Signs and symptoms typically start 7 to 14 days after exposure to the causative agent, though they can occur earlier on subsequent exposures. They last between 1 and 2 weeks and resolve spontaneously, provided the offending exposure has been removed. Typical symptoms include:

1) **Fever**: Fever occurs in virtually all patients and is typically >38.5°C. In serum sickness–like reactions, it tends to be present but less severe.

2) **Dermatologic findings**: Approximately 95% of patients have a pruritic rash, which is most commonly urticarial but can be macular erythematous, papular, or morbilliform. The rash is typically symmetric and does not involve the mucous membranes. Initially, the rash is present on the hands, feet, and trunk (→Figure 6-1) but later may spread to the whole body. If the antigen was

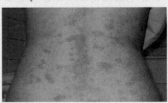

Figure 6-1. Skin lesions in serum sickness.

injected subcutaneously or intramuscularly, the first signs may appear at the injection site. When urticarial lesions appear, they may be atypical in that they last longer than 24 hours. Other possible dermatologic findings include small-vessel vasculitis involving the skin, lesions suggestive of erythema multiforme (sparing the mucous membranes), palmar erythema, and atypical maculopapular lesions located on lateral surfaces of fingers and toes or following a ribbon-like pattern along the external surfaces of the soles.

3) **Other symptoms**: Joint pain and tenderness, edema and erythema of the periarticular area (rare), muscle pain, lymphadenopathy and splenomegaly (in 10%-20% of patients; rare in serum sickness–like reactions), edema of

the lips and eyelids, nausea, vomiting, abdominal cramps, diarrhea, headache and visual disturbances, peripheral neuropathy, neuritis, meningitis and encephalitis, Guillain-Barré syndrome, myocarditis and pericarditis, dyspnea.

→ DIAGNOSIS

Diagnostic Criteria

Diagnosis is based on a characteristic pattern of signs and symptoms associated with exposure to a probable causative agent.

Diagnostic Tests

1. Blood tests: No abnormalities are specific to serum sickness. Frequent findings include elevated erythrocyte sedimentation rate and C-reactive protein levels, lymphocytosis, eosinophilia, transient elevation of alanine aminotransferase and aspartate aminotransferase levels, low levels of C3 and C4 complement components, low levels of total hemolytic complement activity (CH50), and elevated levels of circulating immune complexes (elevated levels of immune complexes and low levels of C3 or C4 are rarely observed in serum sickness–like reactions).

2. Urinalysis: Proteinuria, hyaline casts, and erythrocytes in the sediment.

3. Histologic examination of skin biopsy material (performed only in case of diagnostic difficulties): Leukocytoclastic angiitis, deposits of immunoglobulins and C3 in the vessel walls.

Differential Diagnosis

Rash associated with viral infections, arthritis (including rheumatic fever), polymyositis or dermatomyositis, erythema multiforme, angioedema, urticarial vasculitis, systemic vasculitis, drug reactions with eosinophilia and systemic symptoms.

→ TREATMENT

There are no evidence-based guidelines or high-quality controlled trials on which to base therapy. The general approach is as follows:

1) **Discontinue the drug causing the reaction**.
2) Symptomatic management:
   a) Use **antihistamines** for relief of pruritus.
   b) Use **nonsteroidal anti-inflammatory drugs** for relief of joint symptoms.

   In patients with severe arthritis, high fever, or severe generalized rash, short courses of **systemic glucocorticoids** may be used. A typical approach would be oral prednisone 0.5 to 1 mg/kg once daily, with dose tapering to discontinuation over 1 to 2 weeks.

Symptoms typically resolve in 1 to 2 weeks once the offending trigger has been removed but can persist for months in a minority of cases. Long-term sequelae are uncommon.

→ PREVENTION

The suspected trigger should be avoided. If the use of the drug suspected of causing serum sickness is indispensable, antihistamines and systemic glucocorticoids can be coadministered.

7. Urticaria

→ **DEFINITION, ETIOLOGY, PATHOGENESIS**

Urticaria is a condition characterized by transient wheals (hives), angioedema, or both. Various triggers can lead to the final common pathway of skin mast cell activation. When this occurs, histamine and other mediators are released, leading to local cell recruitment (eg, lymphocytes), vasodilation, increased vascular permeability, and sensory nerve activation. Wheals result from edema of the upper and mid dermis, and angioedema involves a similar change in the lower dermis and subcutis.

Based on the duration of symptoms, urticaria may be classified as **acute urticaria** (≤6 weeks; two-thirds of cases) or **chronic urticaria** (>6 weeks).

Acute urticaria must be differentiated from anaphylaxis. If wheals or angioedema occur with changes in other organs besides the skin, such as the cardiovascular system (hypotension), nervous system (presyncope or syncope), respiratory distress, or gastrointestinal upset (emesis/diarrhea), then anaphylaxis should be suspected.

Acute urticaria may be categorized based on etiology:

1) IgE-mediated allergy, such as allergy to a food (common allergenic foods are tree nuts, peanuts, fish, shellfish, wheat, eggs, dairy, soy, or sesame), medication, or Hymenoptera sting.

2) Non–IgE-mediated reaction:

   a) Foods, for example, those containing proteases, or fish of the Scombridae family (tuna, mackerel) containing histamine-producing bacteria.

   b) Medications, particularly acetylsalicylic acid (ASA) and other nonsteroidal anti-inflammatory drugs (NSAIDs), and direct mast cell activators such as opioids, skeletal muscle relaxants, and radiocontrast dye.

   c) Infection: Commonly viral illnesses.

3) Idiopathic.

4) Early presentation of chronic urticaria (causes: →below).

Chronic urticaria may be further classified as:

1) Chronic spontaneous urticaria (CSU), which involves a spontaneous appearance of wheals, angioedema, or both lasting >6 weeks because of an unknown or known cause, such as:

   a) Autoimmunity mediated by autoantibodies against the high-affinity IgE receptor or directly against IgE.

   b) Bacterial, viral, parasitic, and fungal infections.

   c) Serum sickness.

   d) Autoimmune disease (eg, Hashimoto thyroiditis, systemic lupus erythematosus, or mixed connective tissue disease).

   e) Malignancy (eg, lymphoproliferative disorders; →Differential Diagnosis, below).

   f) Causes of acute urticaria (→above).

   g) Idiopathic (most common).

2) Inducible (or physical) urticaria:

   a) **Dermatographism**, caused by pressure applied to the skin. Wheals appear 1 to 5 minutes after the stimulus (occurs in ~5% of the general population).

   b) **Cold urticaria**, caused by cold air, water, wind. Cold urticaria can be associated with anaphylaxis if there is systemic cold exposure (eg, aquatic activities).

c) **Delayed pressure urticaria**, caused by pressure on the skin. Wheals and edema of deeper skin layers usually appear after 4 to 6 hours (but up to 12-24 hours) and may be painful.

d) **Vibratory angioedema (vibratory urticaria)**, caused by, for instance, vibrations of a lawnmower or pneumatic hammer.

e) **Heat urticaria**, caused by a local source of heat.

f) **Solar urticaria**, caused by ultraviolet or visible light.

g) **Exercise-induced anaphylaxis (EIA) and urticaria**, provoked by exercise and occurring as a manifestation of anaphylaxis. It develops within minutes of starting exercise. The patient can experience any symptoms of anaphylaxis (cutaneous, gastrointestinal, respiratory, cardiovascular).

h) **Cholinergic urticaria**, associated with elevated core body temperature, for instance, after exercise or heating the body. It manifests as "pinpoint" hives from 1 to 3 mm in diameter that appear after 2 to 20 minutes of exposure. The condition is not related to anaphylaxis and occurs in ~11% of the general population.

i) **Aquagenic urticaria**, caused by contact with water, independent of temperature.

j) **Contact urticaria**, following exposure to, for instance, latex, foods (tree nuts, fish, shellfish), chemical agents (formaldehyde present in clothes, resins, animal saliva, ammonium persulfate in cosmetics and foods).

Currently **urticarial vasculitis** is not classified as urticaria.

→ CLINICAL FEATURES AND NATURAL HISTORY

Wheals are usually itchy (sometimes causing pain or a burning sensation), porcelain-white or pink, almost always surrounded by erythema, and elevated over the surrounding skin. They develop and usually also resolve rapidly (<24 hours). Wheals may become confluent, forming different shapes, and may cover extensive areas of the skin. Angioedema is nonpitting, nondependent, erythematous or skin-colored swelling of the lower dermis and subcutis or mucous membranes that is present in 40% of patients with chronic urticaria; 10% have angioedema alone.

Some **characteristic features of the wheals** may suggest the etiology of urticaria:

1) **Appearance** (size, shape): For instance, wheals that are initially small (1-3 mm) and have a wide red halo suggest cholinergic urticaria, whereas very large wheals may indicate exercise-induced or contact urticaria.

2) **Location**: Wheals developing at the site of contact with an allergen suggest contact urticaria. Wheals on uncovered skin areas exposed to cold or sunlight indicate cold or solar urticaria. Wheals at the site of compression are associated with delayed pressure urticaria.

3) **Time from contact with the causative factor to the onset of urticaria**: Lesions developing after several minutes to several hours are suggestive of allergic or physical urticaria. Lesions developing after 3 to 12 hours suggest pressure urticaria. Lesions appearing after several days may indicate urticaria in the course of serum sickness.

4) **Duration of lesions**: Lesions lasting from 1 to 4 hours are associated with allergic urticaria; 30 minutes to 2 hours, with most of physical urticarias; from 6 to 12 hours, with pressure urticaria.

Acute urticaria may appear suddenly, within a few minutes or hours. Typically lesions resolve rapidly. In chronic urticaria lesions may develop daily or periodically (eg, once a week or month); spontaneous remissions frequently occur within a year, but urticaria may also be periodic and last several years.

→ DIAGNOSIS

Diagnostic Criteria

The diagnosis of urticaria is based on typical cutaneous features (→Clinical Features and Natural History, above), identifying triggers of exacerbation or underlying causes, and exclusion of differential diagnoses. The cause of chronic urticaria can be established only in ~20% of patients.

As acute urticaria is usually self-limiting, it usually does not require a diagnostic workup. However, if there is suspicion for an IgE-mediated food allergy or existence of eliciting factors (eg, NSAIDs), allergy testing and patient education on avoidance measures may be undertaken.

History plays a crucial role in establishing the cause of chronic urticaria. Key questions include:

1) Timing (onset, duration, frequency): Typical individual lesions do not last more than 24 to 48 hours.
2) Lesion characteristics (distribution, shape, size, pruritic or painful, residual pigmentation): Typical lesions are pruritic and do not leave pigmentation after resolution of the initial lesions (except from excoriation).
3) Associated angioedema: Typical urticaria can occur with or without angioedema.
4) Other associated features that may suggest atypical causes (eg, arthralgias or arthritis, fever, abdominal cramps, family history).
5) Triggers:
   a) Allergic, for instance, medications, foods, insect bites or stings.
   b) Physical stimuli, for instance, scratching, cold, heat, sweating.
   c) Cofactors, for instance, infection.
6) Response to therapy: Typical lesions should respond to antihistamines.

Physical examination is the next step in diagnosis.

Diagnostic Tests

Diagnostic testing should be guided by the patient's history. In acute urticaria routine testing is not recommended. Testing would be appropriate to establish a cause suggested by history (eg, skin testing or specific IgE testing for a suspected allergen).

For CSU, the recommended routine diagnostic tests are a complete blood count with differential count as well as erythrocyte sedimentation rate (ESR) or C-reactive protein (CRP) levels (or both).

Extensive general screening is not advised in typical cases of CSU. If the etiology is important and in doubt or the history suggests atypical features, referral to a specialist in allergology, clinical immunology, or dermatology is advised. One important consideration is **lesional biopsy**, especially in suspected urticarial vasculitis (dark-red or violet wheals lasting >24 hours, frequently painful).

In cases of suspected inducible (physical) urticaria, the history is key. Provocation testing may also be considered. For example, **dermatographism** may be elicited by stroking the skin with moderate pressure using a smooth item (eg, a wooden spatula) and **cold urticaria** may be elicited by placement of an ice cube in a thin plastic bag on the skin for 5 minutes.

Differential Diagnosis

Start from excluding serious diseases that may present with urticaria (→Definitions, Etiology, Pathogenesis, above). Other conditions that should be part of differential diagnosis:

1) Maculopapular cutaneous mastocytosis (also known as urticaria pigmentosa): Rubbing the red-brown papules can produce bead-like wheals (Darier sign).
2) Urticarial vasculitis.

3) Bradykinin-mediated angioedema.

4) Anaphylaxis.

5) Cryopyrin-associated periodic syndromes, which can present with urticarial rash, recurrent fever attacks, arthralgia or arthritis, ocular inflammation, fatigue, and headaches. Examples include familial cold autoinflammatory syndrome and Muckle-Wells syndrome.

6) Schnitzler syndrome, which can present with recurrent urticarial rash, monoclonal gammopathy, recurrent fever, bone or muscle pain, arthralgia or arthritis, and lymphadenopathy.

7) Gleich syndrome, which features episodic angioedema with eosinophilia.

8) Wells syndrome, which features granulomatous dermatitis with eosinophilia (eosinophilic cellulitis).

9) Bullous pemphigoid.

10) Mild erythema multiforme: Patients often have prodromal symptoms (weakness, fever, sore throat, myalgia, arthralgia) followed by annular lesions on the hands, feet, outer surfaces of extremities, and oral mucosa.

→TREATMENT

General Measures

1. Avoidance of causative factors (allergens, physical factors), if identified.

1) In case of food-induced urticaria, an elimination diet should be used.

2) Patients with cold urticaria are at increased risk of anaphylaxis and should be advised to exercise caution with aquatic activities (and completely avoid cold bodies of water), avoid cold foods and beverages, and their IV fluids should be prewarmed. If they are undergoing surgery, the surgical team should be made aware of their condition and they must be kept warm throughout the procedure.

2. Avoidance of nonspecific factors inducing or worsening urticaria: Drugs (ASA, NSAIDs, opioids), alcohol, stress.

3. Treatment of the underlying condition in secondary urticaria.

Pharmacotherapy

1. Antihistamines are the mainstay of symptomatic treatment in the majority of patients. Administer modern second-generation H_1 **antihistamines** (dosage: →Table 1-2); if this is not effective, higher doses of second-generation antihistamines can be used (up to quadruple of the standard dose).◐◯ In chronic urticaria continuous treatment with H_1 antihistamines is strongly recommended (rather than intermittent use). The only exception is some forms of inducible (physical) urticaria, where on-demand treatment may be more useful, such as 2 hours prior to cold exposure in patients with cold urticaria.

Antihistamines with documented efficacy in treatment of urticaria are bilastine, cetirizine, desloratadine, fexofenadine, levocetirizine, loratadine, and rupatadine. Do not use multiple antihistamines in combination.

Standard treatment with one antihistamine agent is effective in <50% patients with CSU; in one-fourth to one-third of such patients, the urticarial lesions relapse despite treatment with high doses of antihistamines.

2. Other drugs listed below should be considered in patients with urticaria resistant to treatment with high-dose modern second-generation H_1 antihistamines:

1) Omalizumab, a monoclonal antibody against IgE. A dose of 150 to 300 mg/mo is effective—regardless of baseline serum IgE levels—in treatment of CSU, pressure urticaria, heat urticaria, solar urticaria, and cold urticaria. It is generally well tolerated. The strongest evidence of efficacy is present for CSU.◐●

2) If the above treatments are ineffective, then cyclosporine (INN ciclosporin) should be considered as the next step in treatment. Although often effective, it is reserved for more resistant urticaria because of its adverse effects.

3. The following drugs may also be considered in treatment of urticaria:

1) Glucocorticoids may be considered for acute urticaria and acute exacerbations of CSU. A short course of prednisone at 20 to 50 mg/d (continued, eg, up to 10 days) can often be quite effective. Due to significant adverse effects, frequent use should be avoided and long-term use is not recommended outside of specialty clinics.

2) Montelukast 10 mg in the evening may be effective in treatment of CSU (efficacy data are equivocal).

3) Dapsone has been removed from recent urticaria guidelines but may be considered in addition to H_1 antihistamines (efficacy data are equivocal)

4) H_2 antihistamines have been removed from recent urticaria guidelines but may be considered in addition to H_1 antihistamines (efficacy data are equivocal)

→ **SPECIAL CONSIDERATIONS**

Cold-Induced Urticaria

An epinephrine auto-injector and anaphylaxis action plan should be considered in these patients given their risk of anaphylaxis.

1. Anticoagulant Treatment

1.1. Anticoagulant Agents

1.1.1. Direct Thrombin Inhibitors

1. Mechanism of action: Thrombin inhibitors block the catalytic site or the substrate recognition site in the thrombin molecule. Oral **dabigatran** is used for prevention of venous thromboembolism. Agents used for other indications include recombinant hirudin (lepirudin, IV desirudin) and synthetic analogues of hirudin (**bivalirudin**, IV argatroban).

2. Monitoring of the anticoagulant effect is not necessary in patients treated with dabigatran. Within 1 to 3 hours of the administration of dabigatran, corresponding to the peak anticoagulant effect, a slightly prolonged prothrombin time and a prolonged activated partial thromboplastin time (aPTT) (up to 50-65 seconds) can be seen in the majority of patients; the thrombin time is markedly prolonged, frequently beyond the limit of quantification. In patients planned for urgent invasive procedures, determine the aPTT; values >40 seconds suggest a sustained anticoagulant effect. More reliable and precise methods of measuring the anticoagulant effect of dabigatran include the dilute thrombin time (using the Hemoclot assay that is approved for use in the European Union) and ecarin clotting time. The anticoagulant effects of bivalirudin can be monitored using the activated clotting time (this is used in patients with an acute coronary syndrome) or aPTT.

3. Contraindications are the same as in the case of heparins (except for heparin-induced thrombocytopenia) and additionally include pregnancy and breastfeeding. Dabigatran is contraindicated in patients with a glomerular filtration rate (GFR) <30 mL/min, patients with severe liver failure, as well as in patients treated with dronedarone, azole antifungal agents (ketoconazole, itraconazole, voriconazole, posaconazole), rifampin (INN rifampicin), phenobarbital, carbamazepine, phenytoin, and hypericum (St John's wort). The dose of dabigatran should be reduced in patients >80 years, patients with renal failure and a GFR 30 to 50 mL/min, and in patients treated with amiodarone or verapamil. The concomitant use of dabigatran and other anticoagulants (except for unfractionated heparin at doses used to maintain the patency of a central venous or arterial catheter), antiplatelet agents, thrombolytic agents, or dextran may be associated with an increased risk of bleeding.

4. Discontinuation of treatment before surgical procedures: →Chapter 3.1.3.

5. Complications: Mainly bleeding, dyspepsia (in the case of dabigatran). Idarucizumab is an antidote that neutralizes the anticoagulant effect of dabigatran; it should be considered in selected patients who have serious or life--threatening bleeding or who require an emergency (ie, within 6 hours) surgery or procedure. Administer 5 g IV in two 2.5 g doses over 15 minutes. The anticoagulant effect of dabigatran may be neutralized by a prothrombin complex concentrate (PCC) 25 IU/kg (the dose may be repeated twice) or activated PCC 50 IU/kg (maximum, 200 IU/kg/d). Bivalirudin, argatroban, and dabigatran can be eliminated from blood by hemodialysis (without an anticoagulant) or hemoperfusion.

1.1.2. Factor Xa Inhibitors

1. Mechanism of action: Fondaparinux (subcutaneous or IV) is a synthetic pentasaccharide that binds only to antithrombin; **rivaroxaban** (oral), **apixaban** (oral), **edoxaban** (oral), and **betrixaban** (oral) cause factor Xa inhibition that is not mediated by antithrombin.

2. Monitoring of the anticoagulant effect is not necessary. However, within 2 to 4 hours of the administration of rivaroxaban, a prolonged prothrombin time (international normalized ratio [INR]) typically occurs (the effect is less pronounced after the administration of apixaban). Rivaroxaban, apixaban, and edoxaban have little or no effect on the activated partial thromboplastin time and thrombin time. In patients planned for urgent invasive procedures associated with a high risk of bleeding, the prothrombin time may be used to provide a crude estimate of the anticoagulant effect of rivaroxaban, edoxaban, and, to a lesser extent, apixaban. More reliable measures of the anticoagulant effects of rivaroxaban, apixaban, and edoxaban require the use of anti–factor Xa assays specific to these agents.

3. Contraindications are the same as with heparins and additionally include pregnancy and breastfeeding; do not use these agents in patients with creatinine clearance <15 mL/min, patients with severe liver failure, or in combination with other anticoagulants, dual antiplatelet therapy, thrombolytic agents, and drugs that can potentiate or impede the anticoagulant effect (eg, azole antifungal agents, and HIV protease inhibitors). Blood levels of rivaroxaban increase in patients receiving concomitant clarithromycin, erythromycin, cyclosporine (INN ciclosporin), tacrolimus, or fluconazole. Rifampin (INN rifampicin), phenobarbital, carbamazepine, phenytoin, and hypericum (St John's wort) reduce the efficacy of rivaroxaban and apixaban.

4. Discontinuation of treatment before surgical procedures: →Chapter 3.1.3.

5. Complications: Mainly bleeding (in contrast to heparins, factor Xa inhibitors are not known to cause heparin-induced thrombocytopenia), allergic reactions. Andexanet-α is available is some jurisdictions to neutralize the anticoagulant effect but is expensive and not widely available. The anticoagulant effect of oral factor Xa inhibitors may be neutralized by a 4-factor prothrombin complex concentrate (PCC) 25 IU/kg (the dose may be repeated twice). The role of other prohemostatic agents, which include tranexamic acid, cryoprecipitate, and recombinant factor VII, in bleeding management is uncertain but can be considered in cases of bleeding that is refractory to administration of reversal agents. In addition, there is uncertainty about the potential prothrombotic effects of all prohemostatic agents in this clinical setting.

1.1.3. Heparins

Both intravenous and subcutaneous **unfractionated heparin (UFH)** as well as subcutaneous **low-molecular-weight heparins (LMWHs)** are used.

➡ **C O N T R A I N D I C A T I O N S**

1. Absolute contraindications:
1) Active clinically significant bleeding (in exceptional cases heparin may be considered in treatment of some forms of disseminated intravascular coagulation [DIC]).
2) Acute intracranial bleeding, spontaneous or posttraumatic subarachnoid hemorrhage (usually an anticoagulant may be started at prophylactic doses after 5-10 days, and at therapeutic doses after ≥2 weeks).
3) Uncontrolled congenital or acquired bleeding disorder.
4) Hypersensitivity to the drug.
5) A positive history of heparin-induced immune thrombocytopenia (HIT). In selected circumstances (eg, need for cardiac surgery), patients with prior HIT may be re-exposed to heparin if repeat HIT antibody testing is negative. Consultation with a hematologist is recommended.

2. Other clinical conditions associated with an increased risk of bleeding (relative contraindications): In these circumstances, the decision to use or not use anticoagulant therapy is based on an assessment of the risks versus the benefits of anticoagulation in individual patients.

1) Recent gastrointestinal (GI) bleeding or a GI condition associated with a high risk of bleeding.

2) Symptomatic portal hypertension.

3) Kidney failure: Creatinine clearance <30 mL/min (this applies to LMWHs and direct oral anticoagulants both direct thrombin and direct factor Xa inhibitors).

4) Severe liver failure.

5) Acute postinfarction pericarditis.

6) Uncontrolled hypertension: Systolic pressure >180 mm Hg or diastolic pressure >110 mm Hg.

7) Recent brain, spinal cord, or eye surgery (brain or spinal surgery, particularly in patients with additional risk factors for venous thromboembolism, is an indication for prophylaxis, often started as early as on the first day after surgery).

8) Brain tumor.

9) Diagnostic or therapeutic lumbar puncture.

10) ≤24 hours after surgery, organ biopsy, or artery puncture (up to 4 days in patients with abnormal hemostasis during surgery).

11) Aortic dissection.

12) Diabetic retinopathy.

The risk of bleeding is increased in patients simultaneously treated with antiplatelet and anticoagulant agents; however, such combination therapy may be indicated (eg, in acute coronary syndromes).

→ FOLLOW-UP

1. UFH: Measure the **activated partial thromboplastin time (aPTT)**. In patients in whom the target aPTT cannot be achieved despite the use of high--dose UFH, measure anti-Xa activity and adjust the dose of UFH or switch from UFH to LMWH based on the results.

2. LMWH: It is not necessary to monitor the anticoagulant effect by measuring **anti-Xa activity** except for pregnant patients receiving therapeutic doses of LMWHs, patients with severe obesity (eg, >150 kg), and patients with creatinine clearance <30 mL/min; it may be considered in individuals with a history of a thromboembolic event or major bleeding in the course of LMWH treatment, particularly in the elderly. The anticoagulant effect (measured 4 hours after the administration of the drug) is considered satisfactory if anti-Xa levels are 0.6 to 1 IU/mL in a patient receiving LMWH every 12 hours or 1 to 1.3 IU/mL in a patient receiving LMWH every 24 hours.

→ COMPLICATIONS

Bleeding

Subcutaneous injections very frequently cause ecchymosis at the site of injection. Cases of life-threatening or health-threatening bleeding (most frequently GI, intracranial, or retroperitoneal) are rare; they require treatment to neutralize the anticoagulant effect of heparin.

1. Neutralization of the effects of UFH:

1) **For every 100 IU of UFH, administer 1 mg IV protamine** (eg, for 5000 IU of UFH, administer 50 mg of protamine). The injection should be slow (over 1-3 minutes) to avoid hypotension and bradycardia,

2) Due to the short half-life of UFH (60-90 minutes) when calculating the dose of protamine in patients receiving UFH by IV infusion take into account only the amount of UFH administered in the last 3 hours (eg, in a patient receiving an infusion of 1250 IU/h, administer 40 mg of protamine).

3) Monitor the effects of treatment by measuring aPTT (it should become shorter in the course of the treatment).

2. Neutralization of the effects of LMWHs: No established method exists. If the patient has received LMWH within the prior 8 hours, administer 1 mg of IV **protamine** for every 100 IU of anti-Xa (eg, 1 mg of enoxaparin or 150 IU of anti-Xa nadroparin); in patients who received LMWH >8 hours before, use a lower dose (eg, 0.5 mg of protamine). If bleeding persists, you may administer an additional 0.5 mg of IV protamine for every 100 IU of anti-Xa.

Heparin-Induced Thrombocytopenia

1. Types of HIT:

1) **Non–immune-mediated (type I) HIT** is usually associated with a mild reduction in the platelet counts (generally not falling $<100 \times 10^9$/L) observed in 10% to 20% of patients during the first 2 to 4 days of UFH treatment. This causes no clinical manifestations and the platelet count returns to normal despite continued treatment with heparin.

2) **Immune-mediated (type II) HIT**, usually referred to simply as HIT, involves a reduction in platelet counts by >50% (usually to 30×10^9/L to 50×10^9/L, although in 10% of patients platelet counts are $>150 \times 10^9$/L, and in 5% of patients [most often with DIC], $<20 \times 10^9$/L). It usually occurs after 4 to 10 days of UFH/LMWH treatment in 0.1% to 3% of patients receiving UFH (in <0.1% of those treated with LMWHs) and is associated with a 20-fold to 40-fold increase in the risk of venous or arterial thrombosis (not bleeding!), which develops in 30% to 75% of patients with HIT.

2. Risk of HIT and the need for monitoring platelet counts:

1) **High risk (>1%)**: Patients after surgery receiving UFH at prophylactic or therapeutic doses for >4 days (particularly after cardiac, vascular, or orthopedic surgery) and patients with cancer. In these patients, monitor platelet counts at least **every 2 to 3 days** for the first 14 days of heparin treatment or until its discontinuation if the treatment lasts <14 days.

2) **Moderate risk (0.1%-1%)**: Medical patients and pregnant women receiving UFH for >4 days; patients after surgery receiving LMWH for >4 days; patients after surgery or patients requiring intensive care in whom UFH is used to flush a central venous catheter; medical patients and pregnant women receiving LMWHs who have previously received at least one dose of UFH. In these groups monitor platelet counts at least **every 2 to 3 days**, from day 4 until day 14 of treatment, or until its discontinuation if lasting <14 days.

3) **Low risk (<0.1%)**: All patients receiving UFH for <4 days; medical patients and pregnant women receiving LMWH regardless of the time since the start of the treatment, and medical patients in whom UFH is used to flush a central venous catheter. In these groups **it is not necessary to monitor platelet counts**.

When starting treatment with UFH/LMWH in patients who have received UFH in the prior 100 days or in whom such information cannot be obtained, assess the platelet count before starting UFH/LMWH and 24 hours afterwards. Assess the platelet count and compare it with previous results in every patient who develops fever, respiratory failure, heart failure, neurologic symptoms, or any other unexplained clinical symptoms within 30 minutes of an IV injection of UFH.

3. The course of HIT: After the discontinuation of heparin, the platelet count usually increases within a few days; serum antibodies against heparin-PF4 complexes remain elevated for several weeks or months. The most frequent cause of death in patients with HIT is pulmonary embolism, less commonly myocardial infarction or stroke.

4. Diagnosis: You may use the 4T's pretest probability score (→Table 1-1) to predict HIT. It should be suspected in patients after cardiac surgery and in those who have been treated with heparin (usually for ≥5 days) or have recently received heparin if the decrease in the platelet count is due to an unexplained cause. Another clinical sign that is associated with HIT is skin necrosis at the heparin injection sites. Do not delay appropriate treatment until the diagnosis is confirmed by laboratory test results (antiheparin antibodies). A useful indicator for the diagnosis is a characteristic increase in the platelet count observed after the discontinuation of heparin.

5. Treatment:

1) In the case of a strong suspicion of HIT based on clinical symptoms, **immediately discontinue heparin** (including flushing of intravenous catheters).

2) Continue anticoagulant treatment with one of the following drugs: bivalirudin, lepirudin, argatroban (administered IV), fondaparinux (usually 7.5 mg subcutaneously once daily), or a DOAC (preferably rivaroxaban 15 mg orally bid for 21 days followed by 20 mg once daily thereafter).

3) If the patient is receiving a vitamin K antagonist (VKA) at the time of diagnosis of HIT, discontinue the VKA (use of VKAs in the early phases of treatment of HIT complicated by deep vein thrombosis increases the risk of limb necrosis). Do not resume VKAs until the platelet count increases to >150 × 10^9/L; start with a low dose (2-4 mg of acenocoumarol, 3-5 mg of warfarin) in combination with a nonheparin parenteral anticoagulant (preferably fondaparinux), which may be discontinued after 5 days if the platelet counts stabilize and the international normalized ratio (INR) has been maintained within the therapeutic range for 2 consecutive days. Alternatively, a DOAC (preferably rivaroxaban) can be administered alone.

4) In patients with no active bleeding, transfusion of platelet concentrates is not recommended.

6. Management of patients requiring cardiovascular surgery, cardiac catheterization or percutaneous coronary intervention: In individuals with acute HIT or with a history of HIT (with no antibodies), replace heparin with one of the following anticoagulants: bivalirudin, argatroban, or lepirudin.

Other Complications

1. Osteopenia and osteoporosis: In patients treated for >3 months with UFH or (less commonly) LMWH, bone mineral density (BMD) usually decreases by a few percent (in rare cases a greater decrease is observed in patients treated with UFH). BMD usually returns to baseline values within a few months after the discontinuation of heparin. The risk increases with longer heparin administration (particularly >6 months) and with age.

2. Skin necrosis: This occurs rarely, usually after deep subcutaneous injections, typically in the abdominal wall.

3. Other: Allergic reactions (usually urticaria), hyperkalemia (inhibition of the aldosterone effect by UFH), headache, increase in serum aminotransferase levels, alopecia.

1.1.4. Vitamin K Antagonists

1. Mechanism of action of vitamin K antagonists (VKAs): Acenocoumarol and **warfarin** inhibit the posttranslational modification of coagulation factors II, VII, IX, and X, as well as protein C and protein S, which are necessary for the normal activity of the factors. The anticoagulant effect develops after 3 to 5 days; it depends on the dose as well as on the genetic factors, diet, concomitant drugs (→Table 1-2), and comorbidities (due to the reduction of the endogenous sources of vitamin K, a more potent anticoagulant effect is achieved in the course of long-term antibiotic therapy, in patients with diarrhea, and in patients treated with liquid paraffin).

2. Differences between acenocoumarol and warfarin: The most important differences include the time necessary to achieve maximum blood levels (2-3 hours and 1.5 hours, respectively) and half-life (8-10 hours and 36-42 hours). In patients with intolerance of acenocoumarol (eg, due to an allergic reaction)

Table 1-1. Modified 4T's pretest HIT probability score

Only one option in each category may be selected	2 points	1 point	0 points
Thrombocytopenia: Compare the highest and the lowest platelet counts to calculate the% fall of platelet counts	– >50% fall in platelet counts and nadir $\geq 20 \times 10^9$/L in a patient who has not undergone surgery within prior 3 days	– >50% fall in platelet counts and surgery within prior 3 days, or – Any other combination of platelet count fall and nadir not fulfilling the other criteria	– <30% fall in platelet counts, or – Any fall in platelet counts with a nadir <10 × 10^9/L
Timing of the platelet count fall or thrombosis	– Onset within 5-10 days of starting heparin, or – Onset within 1 day of starting heparin if heparin exposure within past 5-30 days	– Unconfirmed onset within 5-10 days of starting heparin (eg, some platelet count results are lacking) – Onset within 1 day of starting heparin if heparin exposure within past 31-100 days – Onset after day 10	Onset of thrombocytopenia within ≤4 days with no heparin exposure (day 0 is the first day of most recent exposure to heparin) within past 100 days
Thrombosis or other clinical sequelae	– Documented new thrombosis (arterial or venous) – Skin necrosis at site of injection – Anaphylactic reaction after IV heparin administration – Adrenal hemorrhage	– Recurrent VTE in a patient treated with anticoagulants at therapeutic doses – Documented thrombosis (still to be confirmed by imaging studies) – Erythematous skin lesions at heparin injection sites	Suspected thrombosis
Other causes of thrombocytopenia not evident	No other evident causes for platelet count fall	Possible other causes are evident: – Sepsis with no microbiologically confirmed etiologic factor – Onset of thrombocytopenia associated with start of mechanical ventilation	Possible other causes: – Within 72 h of a surgical procedure – Documented bacteremia/fungemia – Chemotherapy or radiotherapy within prior 20 days – DIC caused by conditions other than HIT – Posttransfusion thrombocytopenia – Platelet count <20 × 10^9/L in a patient who has received a drug known to cause immune thrombocytopenia[a] – Nonnecrotic skin lesions at LMWH injection sites (delayed hypersensitivity)

Pretest probability of HIT:
   Score 6-8: High probability
   Score 4-5: Intermediate probability
   Score 0-3: Low probability

[a] Selected agents that may cause immune thrombocytopenia:
 – Relatively frequently: GP IIb/IIIa antagonists (abciximab, eptifibatide, tirofiban), quinine, quinidine, sulfonamides, carbamazepine, vancomycin.
 – Relatively infrequently: Actinomycin, amitriptyline, piperacillin, nafcillin, cephalosporins (cefazolin, ceftazidime, ceftriaxone), celecoxib, ciprofloxacin, esomeprazole, fexofenadine, fentanyl, fusidic acid, furosemide, gold salts, levofloxacin, metronidazole, naproxen, oxaliplatin, phenytoin, propranolol, propoxyphene, ranitidine, rifampin (INN rifampicin), suramin, trimethoprim.

Adapted from J Thromb Haemost. 2010 Jul;8(7):1483-5.

DIC, disseminated intravascular coagulation; HIT, heparin-induced thrombocytopenia; INN, international nonproprietary name; IV, intravenous; LMWH, low-molecular-weight heparin; VTE, venous thromboembolism.

or difficulties in maintaining stable international normalized ratio (INR) values, you may consider replacing it with warfarin (the daily dose of warfarin is usually 1.5-2 times higher than that of acenocoumarol).

→ CONTRAINDICATIONS

Contraindications are the same as in the case of heparins (except for heparin--induced thrombocytopenia) and additionally include pregnancy. Breastfeeding is allowed during treatment with VKAs. Pregnant patients with implanted mechanical heart valves should be referred to a specialist center.

→ FOLLOW-UP

Determine the **prothrombin time (PT)**, which is expressed as **INR**.

→ GENERAL PRINCIPLES OF TREATMENT

Starting Treatment
1. If achieving a rapid anticoagulant effect is necessary (eg, in patients with acute deep vein thrombosis/pulmonary embolism), start with a VKA in combination with heparin or fondaparinux. Otherwise, start treatment with a VKA alone (eg, in patients with uncomplicated atrial fibrillation).

2. Start treatment with the administration of acenocoumarol 6 mg on day 1 and 4 mg on day 2, or warfarin 10 mg on day 1 and 5 mg on day 2 (do not use "loading doses," ie, >6 mg of acenocoumarol and >10 mg of warfarin). On day 3, determine the INR and adjust the dose. In patients who are elderly, malnourished, have severe comorbidities (eg, heart failure), or receive multiple drugs (thus being at risk of drug interaction), start with acenocoumarol 4 mg or warfarin 5 mg. If the VKA was started simultaneously with heparin/fondaparinux, the latter agents may be discontinued once the INR has been maintained in the therapeutic range for 2 consecutive days.

Management of Patients Receiving Long-Term VKA
1. Patient education (→Table 1-3), regular INR determination and follow-up visits, providing the patients with appropriate information on the INR values and the resulting VKA dose adjustments.

Table 1-2. Clinically significant interactions with VKAs (acenocoumarol, warfarin)

Drug/sub-stance class	Effects on VKA anticoagulant activity	
	Potentiation	**Inhibition**
Antimicrobials	A: Ciprofloxacin, erythromycin, fluconazole, isoni-azid (600 mg/d), sulfamethoxazole/trimethoprim, metronidazole, miconazole,[a] voriconazole B: Amoxicillin + clavulanic acid, azithromycin, itraconazole, ketoconazole, clarithromycin, levoflox-acin, ritonavir, tetracycline	A: Griseofulvin, nafcillin, ribavirin, rifampicin B: Dicloxacillin, ritonavir
Cardiovascular drugs	A: Amiodarone, diltiazem, fenofibrate, clofibrate, propafenone, propranolol, sulfinpyrazone[b] B: Quinidine, fluvastatin, acetylsalicylic acid, ropin-irole, simvastatin	A: Cholestyramine B: Bosentan, spirono-lactone
Analge-sics, anti--inflammatory and immuno-modulatory drugs	A: Phenylbutazone B: Interferon, acetylsalicylic acid, acetaminophen (INN paracetamol), tramadol	A: Mesalamine B: Azathioprine
Central nervous system drugs	A: Alcohol (in patients with coexisting liver disease), citalopram, entacapone, sertraline B: Disulfiram, chloral hydrate, fluvoxamine, phenyt-oin,[c] tricyclic antidepressants (amitriptyline, clomip-ramine), benzodiazepines	A: Barbiturates, carba-mazepine B: Chlordiazepoxide
Gastrointesti-nal drugs and foods	A: Cimetidine,[c] mango, fish oil, omeprazole B: Grapefruit juice, prokinetic agents (particularly cisapride)	A: Avocado (in large quantities), foods rich in vitamin K_1,[d] enteral nutrition B: Soy milk, sucralfate
Other drugs	A: Anabolic steroids, zileuton, zafirlukast B: Fluorouracil, gemcitabine, levamisole with fluo-rouracil, paclitaxel, tamoxifen, tolterodine, thiama-zole, L-thyroxine	A: Mercaptopurine B: Raloxifene, multi-vitamin supplements, influenza vaccines, chelating agents

A, causation is highly probable. **B**, causation is probable.

[a] Oral topical gel and vaginal suppositories.

[b] Initial potentiation followed by inhibition.

[c] Applies to warfarin.

[d] For instance, kale, spinach, different varieties of cabbage (Chinese, mustard greens, sauer-kraut), beet leaves, Brussels sprouts, broccoli, dandelion (leaves), various types of lettuce, green parsley, asparagus, onions (spring onions and shallots), chicory. Frozen foods are usually richer in vitamin K than fresh foods. One cup (~250 mL) of the foods listed in the table contains ≥80 µg of vitamin K_1 (daily requirement, 80-120 µg).

Adapted from Arch Intern Med. 2005;165(10):1095-106.

INN, international nonproprietary name; VKA, vitamin K antagonist.

2. In adequately educated patients, INR self-determination using a **portable coagulometer** (eg, CoaguChek, INRatio2) and adjustment of the VKA dose by the patient may be allowed. The use of the devices should be considered

---

Table 1-3. Education of patients treated with VKAs (or their caregivers)

– Explain reasons for using the anticoagulant treatment

– List all generic and trade names of the used anticoagulant(s) and discuss how they reduce the risk of thrombosis and its complications

– Explain the expected duration of treatment

– Explain why it is necessary to determine the INR

– Explain the target INR values recommended for the patient and the narrow therapeutic range

– Emphasize the need for frequent and regular INR determinations in order to reduce the risk of bleeding or thrombosis. Inform the patient about the possibility of self-monitoring of the INR in capillary blood using a portable coagulometer (eg, CoaguCheck)

– Describe the most common symptoms of bleeding and the appropriate management

– Describe how to avoid injuries and bleeding

– Describe the most common symptoms and management in case of deep vein thrombosis or pulmonary embolism

– Discuss the effect of foods containing vitamin K_1 on the anticoagulant effect of VKAs (→Table 1-2)

– Discuss the effects of taking certain drugs (both prescription and over-the-counter) on the anticoagulant effect of VKAs (→Table 1-2) and the management when switching drugs

– Discuss the increased risk of bleeding associated with concomitant treatment with antiplatelet drugs

– Discuss the need for limiting or refraining from alcohol consumption

– In female patients likely to become pregnant, discuss the risks associated with using VKAs

– Explain the reason and emphasize the need to inform doctors, dentists, and other medical professionals about the use of VKAs

– Explain at what time of day a VKA should be taken and discuss what to do in case of missing a dose

– Suggest that the patient carries relevant information concerning the use of VKAs (eg, medical information cards together with an ID, a bracelet)

– Document discussing these topics with the patient and/or his/her caregiver in the medical records

Adapted from Ann Pharmacother. 2008;42(7):979-88.

INR, international normalized ratio; VKA, vitamin K antagonist.

---

particularly in patients at high risk of thromboembolism, patients who probably would discontinue the VKA because of disability, living far from the clinic, or due to other factors (eg, type of occupation), as well as in patients in whom lifelong anticoagulant treatment is indicated.

3. In patients receiving long-term VKA treatment, the **intake of foods rich in vitamin K_1** (→Table 1-2) should remain at a relatively constant level.

4. Determine the INR at least once every 4 weeks in patients receiving a constant VKA dose (8 weeks is acceptable in selected patients who have shown consistently therapeutic INR values), and more frequently (every 1-2 weeks) if the INR values fluctuate and fall outside the therapeutic range, or in patients concomitantly treated with antiplatelet drugs and patients with heart failure (New York Heart Association class II-III). Determine the INR in the case of concomitant use of drugs that may interact with VKAs (particularly antibiotics and anticonvulsants) for more than 5 to 7 days.

5. If any INR result in a patient with previously stable INR values is ≤0.5 below or above the therapeutic range, continue using the VKA at the current dose and determine the INR within 1 to 2 weeks.

Table 1-4. Management of patients with INR values above the therapeutic range

Clinical situation	Management
4.5 <INR <6.0 without bleeding	1) Discontinue VKA until the INR is 2.0-3.0[a] 2) Do not administer vitamin K_1 routinely
INR 6.0-10.0 without bleeding	1) Discontinue VKA until the INR is 2.0-3.0 2) You may administer 2.5-5 mg of PO[b] vitamin K_1[c]
INR >10.0 without bleeding	1) Discontinue VKA 2) Administer 2.5-5 mg of PO[b] vitamin K_1
Severe bleeding associated with VKA	1) Discontinue VKA 2) Immediately neutralize the anticoagulant effect by administering a 4-factor prothrombin complex concentrate[d] rather than fresh-frozen plasma[e] 3) In the case of refractory life-threatening bleeding, consider a recombinant factor VIIa concentrate 4) Additionally administer 2.5-5 mg of vitamin K_1 in a slow IV infusion

[a] Discontinuation of the treatment for 1-2 days is usually sufficient.

[b] Use of high doses of vitamin K_1 may cause resistance to VKAs lasting ~7 days.

[c] Some experts (including the American College of Chest Physicians) do not recommend the routine administration of vitamin K_1.

[d] In patients with an INR >6.0, administration of a prothrombin complex concentrate in a dose 50 U/kg usually results in INR normalization within 10-15 minutes; such treatment is necessary particularly in patients with intracranial or other life-threatening bleeding.

[e] The optimum dose of fresh frozen plasma has not been established; the usual dose is 10-15 mL/kg (1 U corresponds to ~200 mL). Time to INR normalization is much longer than in the case of a prothrombin complex concentrate.

Based on Chest. 2012; 141 (2 Suppl): e1S–e801S.

INR, international normalized ratio; VKA, vitamin K antagonist (acenocoumarol, warfarin); PO, oral.

Management of Patients With INR Below Therapeutic Range

1. You can increase the dose by 5% to 20%, using the total weekly dose as the basis.

2. Alternatively, you can determine the INR more frequently and wait for the values to return to the therapeutic range without adjusting the dose of the drug.

3. Make sure that the patient is compliant with the dietary recommendations. A reduction in the intake of green vegetables with a high vitamin K content is usually associated with an increase in the INR by an average of 0.5. In practice, a significant reduction in the INR may be caused by carbamazepine; other drugs rarely cause a significant reduction in the anticoagulant effect.

4. Do not use routine add-on heparin treatment in patients with previously stable INR values in whom this parameter was found to be below the therapeutic range on one occasion; in such cases, repeat INR determination after 7 days.

Management of Patients With INR Above Therapeutic Range
→Table 1-4.

Patients Treated with VKAs and Antiplatelet Agents

1. Duration of antiplatelet therapy after stenting in patients with atrial fibrillation treated with VKAs: Treatment should be tailored to perceived risk of thrombotic versus bleeding events. Recent data indicate that it is safe to use a combination of a VKA and clopidogrel instead of triple antithrombotic therapy (VKA, acetylsalicylic acid [ASA], and clopidogrel).

An increasingly used option is the combination of a direct oral anticoagulant (DOAC) with antiplatelet therapy, usually up to 1 year. Possibilities include low-dose rivaroxaban, 10 to 15 mg daily, combined with clopidogrel or apixaban, 5 mg bid, combined with clopidogrel. ⊘ ●

2. Factors that increase the risk of bleeding in patients treated with VKAs in combination with antiplatelet agents:

1) Age >75 years.

2) Female sex.

3) Chronic kidney disease (creatinine clearance <30 mL/min).

4) History of severe bleeding.

5) INR above the therapeutic range.

3. Radial artery access is recommended during coronary angiography, particularly in patients at high risk of bleeding (eg, with a history of severe bleeding).

Switching to Another Oral Anticoagulant

1. Patients treated with VKAs may be **switched to an oral factor Xa inhibitor** if the INR value is ≤2.0. This may be attained by stopping the VKA and waiting 2 to 3 days to start the oral factor Xa inhibitor.

2. Switching **from an oral factor Xa inhibitor or thrombin inhibitor** to a VKA requires the initial concomitant administration of the VKA and the new anticoagulant until an INR value of ≥2.0 is reached.

Discontinuation of VKAs Before Invasive Procedures

Also →Chapter 3.1.3.

1. The decision to discontinue a VKA before the procedure is made jointly by physicians (usually a surgeon and an anesthesiologist) and the patient after having considered the following:

1) The decision to use a bridging heparin treatment depends on the **risk of thromboembolic complications associated with the discontinuation of VKA** (→Table 1-5).

   a) **Low risk**: Bridging anticoagulation is usually not required.

   b) **Moderate risk**: Bridging anticoagulation is usually not required; alternatively consider prophylactic doses of subcutaneous UFH or LMWH.

   c) **High risk**: Consider a therapeutic dose of subcutaneous LMWH (the preferred option); alternatively IV UFH may be used.

2) **Risk of bleeding associated with the procedure**:

   a) **High risk**: Major vascular surgery, major orthopedic surgery, abdominal or thoracic surgery (including cardiac surgery), neurosurgery, prostatectomy, bladder surgery, polypectomy, implantation of a cardiac pacemaker or implantable cardioverter-defibrillator, biopsy of an organ/tissue than cannot be compressed (eg, liver, prostate, bronchus, bone marrow), and puncture of an artery that cannot be effectively compressed. In these cases it is usually necessary to discontinue the anticoagulant treatment.

   b) **Low risk**: Dental procedures (eg, extraction of 1-2 teeth), arthrocentesis, minor skin surgery (eg, excision of a mole), coronary angiography, selected diagnostic endoscopy (eg, without multiple biopsies, polypectomy), and cataract surgery. In these situations it is usually not necessary to discontinue the anticoagulant treatment. After tooth extraction you may recommend rinsing the mouth with tranexamic acid and applying an ice pack to the cheek for 30 minutes after the surgery. Stitching after tooth extraction does not reduce the risk of bleeding.

2. Temporary discontinuation of VKA:

1) Discontinue acenocoumarol for 2 to 3 days and warfarin for 5 days before the procedure to allow for the normalization of INR values.

2) If despite the discontinuation of the VKA the INR is ≥1.5, you may administer 1 to 2 mg of oral vitamin K_1 1 to 2 days before the procedure.

Table 1-5. Risk stratification of venous or arterial thromboembolism in patients receiving long-term VKA treatment

Indications for VKA treatment	Estimated risk of thromboembolism		
	Low	Moderate	High
Mechanical heart valve	Mechanical bileaflet aortic valve with no additional stroke risk factors	Mechanical bileaflet aortic valve and one of the following risk factors: atrial fibrillation, history of stroke/TIA, hypertension, diabetes mellitus, congestive heart failure, age >75 years	– Mechanical mitral valve; old-type mechanical aortic valve (caged-ball, tilting-disc) – History of stroke or TIA in prior 6 months
Atrial fibrillation	CHADS$_2$ score 0-2 and no history of stroke or TIA	CHADS$_2$ score 3-4	– CHADS$_2$ score 5-6 – History of stroke or TIA in prior 3 months – Rheumatic heart disease
VTE	History of one VTE event >12 months ago, currently no other risk factors for VTE	– History of VTE in the prior 3-12 months or recurrent VTE – Milder forms of thrombophilia (eg, heterozygotes for prothrombin G20210A gene or factor V Leiden) – Cancer (treatment in prior 6 months or palliative therapy)	– History of VTE in prior 3 months – Severe thrombophilia (eg, antithrombin, protein C or protein S deficiency, APS, several coexisting conditions)

CHADS$_2$ score: →Table 4-3.

APS, antiphospholipid syndrome; TIA, transient ischemic attack; VKA, vitamin K antagonist; VTE, venous thromboembolism.

3) When a rapid neutralization of the anticoagulant effect of the VKA becomes necessary before an emergency invasive procedure, use 2.5 to 5 mg of vitamin K$_1$ orally or IV. If the anticoagulant effect must be neutralized immediately, you may additionally administer fresh-frozen plasma, prothrombin complex concentrate, or recombinant factor VIIa concentrate.

3. The use of bridging heparin therapy during the period of discontinuation of VKA:

1) In patients receiving subcutaneous LMWHs at therapeutic doses, administer the last LMWH injection 24 hours before the invasive procedure at a dose amounting to approximately half the daily dose of LMWH.

2) In patients receiving IV UFH, stop the infusion ~4 hours before the procedure.

4. Resuming the anticoagulant treatment after the procedure:

1) In patients undergoing minor invasive procedures who have been receiving subcutaneous LMWHs at therapeutic doses during the period of discontinuation of the VKA, you may resume the administration of the LMWH ~24 hours after the surgery as long as adequate hemostasis is ensured.

2) In patients undergoing major invasive procedures or procedures associated with a high risk of postsurgical bleeding who have been receiving subcutaneous LMWHs or IV UFH at therapeutic doses during the period of discontinuation of the VKA, administer subcutaneous LMWH or IV UFH at therapeutic doses 48 to 72 hours after the surgery as long as adequate hemostasis is ensured. Alternatively, you may use subcutaneous LMWH or UFH at prophylactic doses. It is acceptable not to use heparin immediately after the procedure.

3) VKA treatment may be resumed 12 to 24 hours after the surgery (eg, on the evening of the same day or the next morning) as long as adequate hemostasis is ensured. However, it may be resumed later if necessary because of the patient's clinical condition.

Pregnancy in Women Receiving Long-Term Anticoagulants

1. In women receiving long-term VKA treatment who plan to become pregnant, a recommended safe and convenient management regime is frequent pregnancy testing based on the assumption that VKAs can safely be used during the first 4 to 6 weeks of pregnancy. Once the patient becomes pregnant, she should be switched from VKA to LMWH or UFH.

2. An alternative approach is to switch from VKA to LMWH before attempting to become pregnant.

3. According to the American College of Chest Physicians guidelines, in women receiving long-term VKA treatment because of an implanted mechanical heart valve it is recommended either to switch from VKA to LMWH (while monitoring anti-Xa activity) or to UFH at therapeutic doses for the entire pregnancy, or to use LMWH or UFH for the first 13 weeks of pregnancy and then switch to VKA, which should be used until approximately week 36 of an uncomplicated pregnancy. However, according to the European Society of Cardiology guidelines, it is preferable to continue the use of VKAs throughout the pregnancy due to their superior efficacy compared with LMWHs in the prevention of prosthetic valve thrombosis.

→ COMPLICATIONS

1. Bleeding: Management: →Table 1-4.

2. Teratogenic effects: Acenocoumarol and warfarin cross the placenta and impair γ-carboxylation of proteins in the bones, thus posing a risk of chondrodysplasia punctata and nasal hypoplasia in children whose mothers have received VKAs between weeks 6 and 12 of pregnancy. Nervous system defects have also been reported in children whose mothers used VKAs in the first (after 6 weeks) and second trimesters of pregnancy.

3. Skin necrosis: Rare (more common in individuals with protein C or protein S deficiency), usually develops on the trunk in female patients between days 3 and 8 of VKA treatment. Skin necrosis is caused by thrombosis in the capillaries and small veins of the subcutaneous adipose tissue. If it develops, replace VKA with heparin for a few days or weeks (depending on the severity of the necrosis). If the patient requires long-term anticoagulant treatment, resume VKA starting with a low dose and gradually titrating it up. In severe cases of patients with protein C deficiency, administer protein C concentrate. Reports have been published on the safe use of dabigatran in the case of skin necrosis in patients with protein C deficiency.

4. Allergic reactions: Most often urticaria.

5. Liver damage: This occurs in ~1% of cases, mostly in patients with latent liver disease, such as chronic viral hepatitis. An increase in plasma aminotransferase levels is transient and normalizes within 2 weeks of the discontinuation of VKAs.

6. Warfarin nephropathy (→Chapter 9.1).

7. Alopecia.

1.2. Anticoagulant Treatment and Regional Anesthesia

1. Perispinal hematoma (hematoma of the spinal canal) after a central blockade (ie, epidural or spinal anesthesia) is a rare but serious complication of anticoagulant treatment and antithrombotic prophylaxis.

Table 1-6. Timing of procedures in patients treated with antithrombotic drugs[a]

Agent	Lumbar puncture (with or without introduction of catheter)	Removal of epidural or spinal catheter in patients treated with anticoagulants[b]	Starting antithrombotic prophylaxis after spinal or epidural anesthesia
Acetylsalicylic acid	No restrictions	No restrictions	No restrictions
Clopidogrel	≥7 days from discontinuation of the drug	–	After catheter removal
Ticlopidine	≥14 days from discontinuation of the drug	–	After catheter removal
Vitamin K antagonist[c]	4 days from the discontinuation of the drug + normal INR	When INR <1.5	After catheter removal
Unfractionated IV heparin	4 h after discontinuation of IV infusion and normalization of aPTT	4 h after discontinuation of infusion and normalization of aPTT	– >2 h after removal of catheter – Defer by 12 h in case of bloody puncture (applies to intraoperative use of IV UFH)
SC UFH	4 h after SC injection of prophylactic dose	4 h after SC injection of prophylactic dose	1 h after removal of catheter
SC LMWH	– 10-12 h after standard prophylactic dose – 24 h after last therapeutic dose and after normalization of anti-Xa activity	– 10-12 h after last dose and 4 h before next dose – 24 h after last dose (with doses administered every 24 h)	– 2-4 h after removal of catheter – Defer by 24 h in case of bloody puncture (applies to therapeutic dose)
Fondaparinux	– 24-36 h after standard prophylactic dose (2.5 mg SC every 24 h) – 48-72 h after standard therapeutic dose (7.5 mg SC every 24 h)	36-42 h after last dose (no data available on safety of fondaparinux in patients with indwelling spinal or epidural catheters; other anticoagulants should be used)	– 6-12 h after removal of catheter in patients receiving prophylactic doses (2.5 mg SC every 24 h) – 12-24 h after removal of catheter in patients receiving therapeutic doses (7.5 mg SC every 24 h) or in patients at high bleeding risk
Oral factor Xa inhibitor[d]	Hold day of procedure and 2 days prior (>48 h after last dose)	Hold day of procedure and 2 days prior (>48 h after last dose)	6-12 h after removal of catheter in patients starting prophylactic doses[f] ≥24 h after removal of catheter in patients resuming therapeutic doses[g]
Oral direct thrombin inhibitor[e]	Hold day of procedure and 2 days prior (>48 h after last dose) (hold 4 days if CrCl <50 mL/min)	Hold day of procedure and 2 days prior (>48 h after last dose) (hold 4 days if CrCl <50 mL/min)	6-12 h after removal of catheter in patients starting prophylactic doses[h] ≥24 h after removal of catheter in patients resuming therapeutic doses[i]

[a] No high-quality data is available for oral direct factor Xa inhibitors or thrombin inhibitors.
[b] Applies to patients with normal renal function.
[c] Acenocoumarol and warfarin.
[d] Apixaban, edoxaban, and rivaroxaban.
[e] Dabigatran.
[f] Apixaban 2.5 mg bid, edoxaban 30 mg once daily, or rivaroxaban 10 mg once daily.
[g] Apixaban 5 mg bid, edoxaban 60 mg once daily, or rivaroxaban 20 mg once daily.
[h] Dabigatran 150-220 mg once daily.
[i] Dabigatran 110-150 mg twice daily.

aPTT, activated partial thromboplastin time; bid, 2 times a day; CrCl, creatinine clearance; INR, international normalized ratio; LMWH, low-molecular-weight heparin; SC, subcutaneous; UFH, unfractionated heparin.

Risk factors: Impaired hemostasis (including procedures performed at the time of full anticoagulant activity), anatomic abnormalities of the spine, catheter use, traumatic or repeated attempts to introduce a needle or catheter into the spinal canal, and catheter removal at the time of anticoagulant activity.

2. Timing of lumbar puncture, removal of an epidural or spinal catheter, and start of anticoagulant prophylaxis after an epidural or spinal anesthesia in patients treated with anticoagulants: →Table 1-6. Also →Chapter 3.1.3.

1.3. Perioperative Direct Oral Anticoagulant (DOAC) Management

The perioperative management of patients who are receiving a direct oral anticoagulant (DOAC) and require an elective surgery or invasive procedure is a common clinical problem. In assessing these patients, the task of the clinician is (1) to determine if DOAC interruption is needed, and (2) to provide advice on how to interrupt and resume DOACs perioperatively.

→ INDICATIONS

There are several minor procedures, classified as being **minimal bleeding risk**, where DOACs can be continued without complete interruption (→Figure 1-1). These procedures consist of dental extractions, endodontic (root canal) procedures, skin biopsies, phacoemulsification (cataract) surgery, and selected colonoscopies. Implantation of a cardiac pacemaker or internal defibrillator (ICD) as well as cardiac catheterization can be done without stopping DOACs (→Table 1-7). However, there are several points to note in the management of such patients:

1) Any of these procedures could be considered as having a higher bleeding risk, warranting full anticoagulant interruption. For example, a tooth extraction in a patient with poor dental or gingival hygiene or cataract surgery with retrobulbar instead of topical anesthesia may not be considered minimal bleeding risk.

2) It is suggested to skip the morning DOAC dose just before the procedure, because if a DOAC is taken on the day of the procedure the peak anticoagulant effect—occurring 1 to 3 hours after intake—may coincide with the timing of the procedure and may increase the risk for bleeding.

3) In patients having coronary angiography using a femoral approach, continuing DOACs may not be advisable as such patients are at increased risk for developing an inguinal hematoma or false aneurysm.

4) In patients having a colonoscopy, DOACs can be continued in situations where the need for polypectomy is unlikely, whereas interruption would be

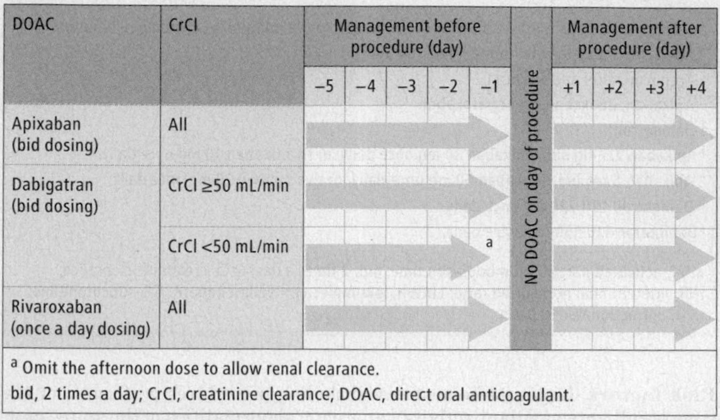

DOAC	CrCl	Management before procedure (day)					No DOAC on day of procedure	Management after procedure (day)			
		−5	−4	−3	−2	−1		+1	+2	+3	+4
Apixaban (bid dosing)	All										
Dabigatran (bid dosing)	CrCl ≥50 mL/min										
	CrCl <50 mL/min					a					
Rivaroxaban (once a day dosing)	All										

a Omit the afternoon dose to allow renal clearance.
bid, 2 times a day; CrCl, creatinine clearance; DOAC, direct oral anticoagulant.

Figure 1-1. Perioperative management of direct oral anticoagulants: surgery/procedure with minimal bleeding risk. See text for exceptions.

required if the likelihood of polypectomy is higher. A discussion with the clinician performing the colonoscopy can ensure optimal anticoagulant management.

5) In dental procedures oral tranexamic acid mouthwash can be used just before and 2 to 3 times daily for 1 to 2 days after the procedure to reduce bleeding, since such bleeding may not be clinically important but may cause distress to patients.

➡ MANAGEMENT

In patients who are receiving a DOAC and require treatment interruption for an elective surgery or invasive procedure, patient management depends on the bleeding risk associated with the surgery or procedure. The thromboembolic risk is less important because DOACs have a rapid offset and onset of action (cessation and resumption of the therapeutic effect), and a short (2-4 days) interruption interval perioperatively is unlikely to substantially increase the risk for thromboembolism.

A **high-bleeding-risk surgery or procedure** comprises major abdominal surgery (eg, cancer resection); major thoracic surgery; major orthopedic surgery; and any cardiac, spinal, or intracranial surgery. Any patient having **neuraxial anesthesia is classified as high bleeding risk** because of the small but important risk for epidural hematomas, which can cause lower limb paralysis. A **low- to moderate-bleeding-risk surgery or procedure** includes most surgeries that typically are <1 hour in duration and do not involve neuraxial anesthesia.

1. Preoperative management:

1) Patients having a **high-bleeding-risk surgery or procedure** should discontinue DOACs for 2 full days (ie, ≥48 hours) before the procedure, which in most cases corresponds to a 60- to 68-hour interval between the last DOAC dose and the time of surgery (→Figure 1-2). For example, if a patient is having a high-bleeding-risk surgery or procedure on a Monday at 8:00 and takes their last DOAC dose at 18:00 on the preceding Friday, this represents a 62-hour interval between the last dose and the surgery. With this interruption interval, there would be minimal or no residual anticoagulant effects at the time of the surgery, given the 12- to 15-hour half-life of DOACs.

Table 1-7. Perioperative bleeding risk categories[a]

Surgery/procedure	Minimal bleeding risk	High bleeding risk
Gastrointestinal and genitourinary procedures	– Colonoscopy[b] – Gastroscopy[b] – Sigmoidoscopy[b] – Capsule endoscopy[c] – Push enteroscopy – Barrett esophagus ablation	Major abdominopelvic surgery: hepatobiliary cancer resection, pancreatic cancer or pseudocyst resection, colorectal and gastric cancer resection, diverticular disease resection, inflammatory bowel disease resection, renal cancer resection, bladder cancer resection, endometrial cancer resection, ovarian cancer resection, radical prostatectomy
Cardiac procedures	– Permanent pacemaker implantation or battery change – Internal cardiac defibrillator implantation or battery change – Atrioventricular node ablation – Coronary artery angiography (radial approach)	Major cardiac surgery (coronary artery bypass, valve replacement or repair)
Major thoracic surgery		– Lobectomy, pneumonectomy – Esophagectomy
Major vascular surgery		– Aortic aneurysm repair – Aortobifemoral bypass, popliteal bypass – Carotid endarterectomy
Major orthopedic surgery		– Hip arthroplasty or hip fracture repair – Knee arthroplasty or tibial osteotomy – Shoulder arthroplasty – Metatarsal osteotomy
Other major cancer or reconstructive surgery		– Head and neck cancer surgery – Reconstructive facial, abdominal, or limb surgery
Dental procedures	– Tooth extraction (≤2 extractions) – Endodontic (root canal) procedure	
Skin procedures	Skin biopsy	
Eye procedures	Phacoemulsification (cataract)	
Neuraxial anesthesia		Any surgery requiring neuraxial anesthesia or injection (including epidural)
Intracranial or neuraxial surgery		– Brain cancer resection – Laminectomy or neuraxial tumor resection – Intracranial (subdural, epidural) bleeding evacuation

[a] Examples of surgeries with minimal and high risk of bleeding. A **low- to moderate-bleeding-risk surgery or procedure** includes most surgeries that typically are <1 hour in duration and do not involve neuraxial anesthesia.

[b] Assuming no polypectomy is expected.

[c] Assuming no sphincterotomy is expected.

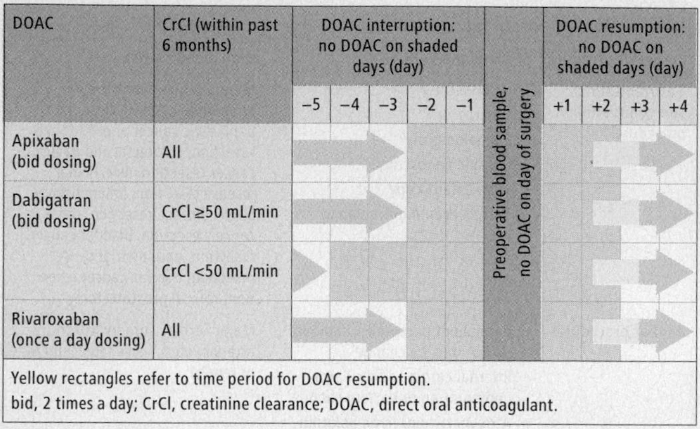

DOAC	CrCl (within past 6 months)	DOAC interruption: no DOAC on shaded days (day)					Preoperative blood sample, no DOAC on day of surgery	DOAC resumption: no DOAC on shaded days (day)			
		−5	−4	−3	−2	−1		+1	+2	+3	+4
Apixaban (bid dosing)	All										
Dabigatran (bid dosing)	CrCl ≥50 mL/min										
	CrCl <50 mL/min										
Rivaroxaban (once a day dosing)	All										

Yellow rectangles refer to time period for DOAC resumption.
bid, 2 times a day; CrCl, creatinine clearance; DOAC, direct oral anticoagulant.

Figure 1-2. Perioperative management of direct oral anticoagulants: surgery/procedure with high bleeding risk.

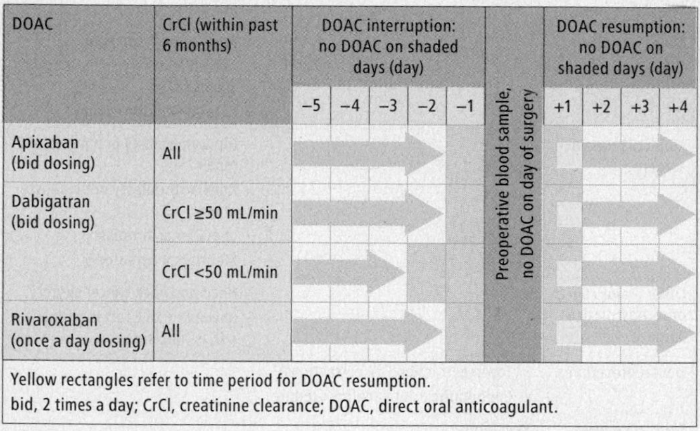

DOAC	CrCl (within past 6 months)	DOAC interruption: no DOAC on shaded days (day)					Preoperative blood sample, no DOAC on day of surgery	DOAC resumption: no DOAC on shaded days (day)			
		−5	−4	−3	−2	−1		+1	+2	+3	+4
Apixaban (bid dosing)	All										
Dabigatran (bid dosing)	CrCl ≥50 mL/min										
	CrCl <50 mL/min										
Rivaroxaban (once a day dosing)	All										

Yellow rectangles refer to time period for DOAC resumption.
bid, 2 times a day; CrCl, creatinine clearance; DOAC, direct oral anticoagulant.

Figure 1-3. Perioperative management of direct oral anticoagulants: surgery/procedure with low to moderate bleeding risk.

2) Patients having a **low- to moderate-bleeding-risk surgery or procedure** should discontinue DOACs for 1 full day before the procedure, which would correspond to a 36- to 42-hour interval between the last DOAC dose and the surgery (→Figure 1-3).

3) Patients having a **minimal-bleeding-risk surgery or procedure** in most situations should not take DOACs on the day of the procedure. Alternatively, one can defer that day's dose until the evening (in the case of a once-daily regimen) or just skip the morning dose and resume the evening dose (in the case of a twice-daily regimen).

In all patients no DOAC is taken on the day of the surgery or procedure. The exception to this approach is patients who are receiving dabigatran and have moderately to severely impaired renal function (creatinine clearance

<50 mL/min): Because dabigatran is excreted mainly by the kidney (80%), a longer interruption interval of 4 days is needed before a high-bleeding-risk surgery or procedure and 2 days before a low- to moderate-bleeding-risk surgery/procedure.

2. Postoperative management: After the surgery or procedure, the resumption of DOACs should, in effect, mirror the preoperative interruption. After a low- to moderate-bleeding-risk surgery or procedure, ≥24 hours should elapse before resuming DOACs (ie, resume the day after the surgery/procedure) and 48 to 72 hours should elapse before resuming DOACs after a high-bleeding-risk surgery/procedure.

The overall management approach can be summarized as: "1 day off before and after a low- to moderate-bleeding-risk surgery/procedure and 2 days off before and after a high-bleeding-risk surgery/procedure." The exception to this approach is patients who are receiving dabigatran with a creatinine clearance <50 mL/min, as they require an additional 1 to 2 days of interruption before a surgery or procedure to allow adequate time for drug clearance.

There are some points to note about postoperative DOAC management:

1) The 48- to 72-hour resumption interval can be extended if the postoperative bleeding is more than expected, which is important because the full anticoagulant effect of DOACs is almost immediate after oral intake.

2) In patients who are unable to take medications by mouth and who are at high risk for venous thromboembolism, low-dose subcutaneous low-molecular-weight heparin (LMWH) can be given for the first 1 to 3 postoperative days.

2. Automaticity and Conduction Disorders

→ DEFINITION

Cardiac conduction system: →Figure 2-1.

Disorders of automaticity and conduction include **sinus node dysfunction**, **atrioventricular (AV) block**, and **intraventricular block**. Disturbances may occur at one or more levels, may be acute or chronic, and may be sustained or recurrent. Bradycardia is classified according to the European Society of Cardiology guidelines as persistent or intermittent (either documented by electrocardiography [ECG] or suspected [undocumented by ECG]).

→ CLINICAL FEATURES

Clinical manifestations depend mainly on the type and severity of bradycardia, age, presence of structural heart disease, and physical activity. Symptoms may range from reduced exercise tolerance or presyncope to syncope and sudden cardiac death. **Symptoms of persistent bradycardia** include easy fatigability, fatigue, irritability, concentration impairment, apathy, cognitive impairment, memory impairment, vertigo or dizziness, dyspnea, symptoms of heart failure, and reduced exercise tolerance (chronotropic incompetence). **Symptoms of intermittent bradycardia** include presyncope, syncope (Adams-Stokes attack), vertigo or dizziness, blurred vision, sudden dyspnea and chest pain unrelated to exercise, and palpitations. Symptoms occurring during an Adams-Stokes attack are suggestive of asystole duration: Visual disturbances and dizziness occur after 3 to 5 seconds, loss of consciousness follows after 10 to 15 seconds, and seizures develop after 20 to 30 seconds. More severe symptoms are usually associated with advanced second-degree or third-degree AV block, particularly occurring in the distal conduction system.

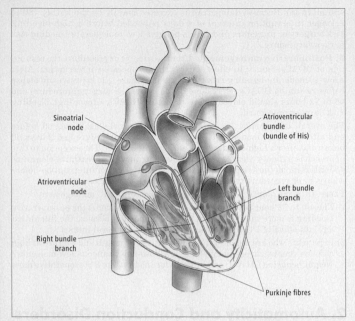

Figure 2-1. Cardiac conduction system. *Illustration courtesy of Dr Shannon Zhang.*

→ DIAGNOSIS

1. ECG, Holter monitoring or ECG recorders, and implantable recorders are used in patients with infrequent but severe symptoms. Patterns of abnormalities:

1) AV block: →Figure 2-2.
2) Right bundle branch block and left bundle branch block: →Figure 2-3.

2. Electrophysiologic study (EPS) is used in case of diagnostic uncertainties.

→ TREATMENT

1. Management of symptomatic bradycardia: →Figure 2-4.

2. Long-term management: Cardiac pacing is electrical cardiac stimulation. A pacemaker consists of a pulse generator and one or many leads. Pacing may be intermittent or continuous. Pacemakers have several programmable parameters (such as heart rate, shock voltage and duration, and thresholds for pacing).

Pacemakers are marked with an **international letter-coding system**. Consecutive letters in the code denominate:

1) Chambers paced (A, atrium; V, ventricle; D, dual).
2) Chambers sensed (A, V, D, as above; O, absence of sensing).
3) Response to sensing (I, inhibited; T, triggered; D, dual; O, no response).
4) Rate modulation, for instance, to exercise (O, none; R, rate modulation).
5) Multisite pacing (A, atrium; V, ventricle; D, dual; O, no multisite pacing).

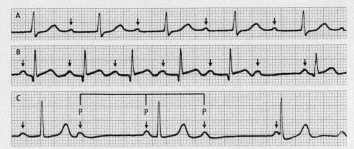

Figure 2-2. Atrioventricular (AV) block. **A**, prolonged PR interval (first-degree AV block). **B**, loss of the QRS complex preceded by progressive prolongation of the PR interval (Mobitz type I [Wenckebach] second-degree AV block). **C**, independent rhythm of P waves and QRS complexes (third-degree AV block, AV junction escape rhythm). The PP intervals separated by the QRS complex are shorter than the PP intervals not separated by the QRS complex (arrows indicate P waves).

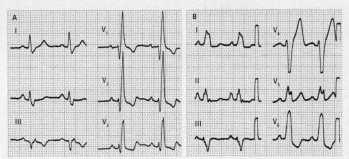

Figure 2-3. A, right bundle branch block. **B**, left bundle branch block.

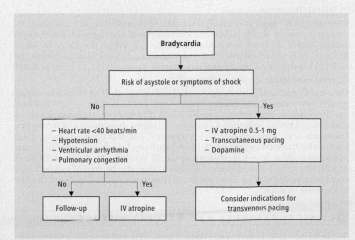

Figure 2-4. Management of bradycardia

The most frequently used pacing modes:

1) **VVI**: Ventricular inhibited pacing (pacing inhibited by a sensed ventricular event).

2) **AAI**: Atrial inhibited pacing (pacing inhibited by a sensed atrial event).

3) **VDD**: Ventricular pacing synchronized with atrial rhythm and inhibited by ventricular rhythm.

4) **DDD**: Dual-chamber pacing and sensing with inhibition and tracking.

New leadless devices enable ventricular stimulation and are useful to avoid lead-related problems.

Late **complications** of pacemaker implantation include lead dislodgement or damage affecting pacing or sensing/detection, pacemaker damage, pacemaker--induced tachycardia, increased pacing threshold, pacemaker syndrome (AV dissociation in patients with VVI pacemakers, which leads to reduced cardiac output and atrial contractions while AV valves are closed, consequently resulting in syncope, dizziness, fatigue, and neck pulsation), local infection, infective endocarditis related to a foreign body (cardiac device–related infective endocarditis), and very rarely sepsis.

2.1. Atrioventricular Blocks

→ DEFINITION, ETIOLOGY, PATHOGENESIS

Atrioventricular (AV) block is an impairment or a blockade of conduction from the atria to the ventricles.

Types of AV block:

1) **First-degree AV block**: Every atrial impulse is conducted to the ventricles but the conduction time is prolonged >200 milliseconds.

2) **Second-degree AV block**: Some impulses are not conducted to the ventricles.

3) **Third-degree (complete) AV block**: No atrial impulses are conducted to the ventricles. The atria and ventricles are controlled by independent pacemakers with a ventricular escape rhythm that is slower than atrial rhythm.

Classification of AV blocks on the basis of location:

1) **Proximal**: At the level of the AV node.

2) **Distal**: Below the AV node.

First-degree AV block may result from abnormal conduction in the atrium, AV node, or (rarely) in the His bundle and Purkinje fibers. Mobitz type I (Wenckebach) second-degree AV block is almost always located within the AV node, while Mobitz type II second-degree block or advanced heart block is located below the node. Third-degree AV blocks may be proximal (located in the AV node) or distal.

Cardiac conduction system: →Figure 2-1.

Causes: Congenital blocks, myocardial infarction (MI) or ischemia, degenerative processes of the conduction system (Lenègre disease, Lev disease), cardiomyopathy, myocarditis, complications of surgery or intravascular procedures, heart tumor, systemic disease (particularly sarcoidosis and connective tissue disease), drugs (β-blockers, verapamil and diltiazem, digitalis, class I antiarrhythmic drugs [→Table 4-1], amiodarone), hypothyroidism, autonomic dysfunction, hyperkalemia, ablation of the AV junction. First-degree AV block and Mobitz type I second-degree AV block may also be caused by increased vagal tone, which is often observed in athletes and occasionally also in healthy individuals at night.

→ CLINICAL FEATURES AND NATURAL HISTORY

AV blocks may be transient (eg, following acute MI), paroxysmal, or permanent.
Signs and symptoms: →Chapter 3.2. In third-degree AV block physical

examination may reveal variable intensity of the first heart sound. In proximal third-degree AV block heart rates are 40 to 60 beats/min and increase during exercise; in distal third-degree AV blocks heart rates are usually lower (typically 20-40 beats/min).

→ DIAGNOSIS

Diagnostic Criteria

Electrocardiography (ECG):

1) In patients with **first-degree AV block**, the PR interval is >200 milliseconds (→Figure 2-2).

2) In patients with **Mobitz type I (Wenckebach) second-degree AV block**, there is progressive PR interval prolongation for several beats preceding the nonconducted P wave. In the following P-QRS complex the PR interval is shorter (normal or near-normal) than the PR interval before the block. This occurs periodically, creating the appearance of "grouped beating" (→Figure 2-2). In patients with **Mobitz type II second-degree AV block**, the block occurs without the prior progressive PR interval increase and the following PR interval remains unchanged. In patients with **advanced second-degree AV block**, the block is sustained for ≥2 cycles (ie, 2 consecutive P waves with no QRS). A special form of second-degree AV block is the **2:1 block**, which may be Mobitz type I or type II block; if the PR interval of the conducted P wave is prolonged and the QRS complex is narrow and has normal morphology, Mobitz type I second-degree AV block is more likely. In 70% of cases second-degree AV block with a narrow QRS complex is proximal in the conducting system, while 80% of cases of second-degree AV block with a wide QRS complex are distal and associated with a high risk of progression to third-degree AV block.

3) In patients with **third-degree AV block**, P waves and QRS complexes are independent and ventricular rate is slower than atrial rate. In proximal block the origin of escape rhythm is located above the His bundle bifurcation, QRS complexes are narrow, and their rate is 40 to 60/min (→Figure 2-2). In a distal block QRS complexes are wide, may be polymorphic, and their rate is 20-40/min; rhythm is less stable and episodes of torsades de pointes may occur.

→ TREATMENT

1. Management of symptomatic bradycardia: →Figure 2-4.

2. Chronic first-degree AV block and Mobitz type I second-degree AV block usually require no treatment. Attempt to discontinue drugs that increase the AV conduction time, particularly in patients with a PR interval >240 to 260 milliseconds. Repeated follow-up is recommended.

3. Indications for pacemaker implantation:

1) Persistent bradycardia: Third-degree AV block or Mobitz type II second--degree AV block, regardless of symptoms.

2) Periodic or paroxysmal third-degree or second-degree AV block (including AF with slow or regular conduction to ventricles).

3) The recommendation is weaker in Mobitz type I second-degree AV block that is symptomatic or has been located below the His bundle using electrophysiologic study. The recommended first-choice pacing mode is DDD, or VVI in patients with AF. Before making the decision to implant a pacemaker, make sure that the AV block is not caused by a transient or reversible cause, such as myocardial infarction, electrolyte disturbances, drugs, perioperative hypothermia, or myocarditis.

2.2. Intraventricular Blocks

→ DEFINITION, ETIOLOGY, PATHOGENESIS

Intraventricular blocks may be of a His bundle branch block pattern, a fascicular block pattern, or both and result from significant slowing or interruption of conduction. Possible **patterns of intraventricular block** include:

1) Left anterior or posterior fascicular block.

2) Right bundle branch block (RBBB) (→Figure 2-5) or left bundle branch block (LBBB) (→Figure 2-6).

3) RBBB with left anterior or posterior fascicular block (**bifascicular block**; according to the definition by the European Society of Cardiology, isolated LBBB is also a bifascicular block).

Trifascicular block refers to simultaneous or alternate conduction impairment in all fascicles. This term is also sometimes used in the case of bifascicular block with first-degree atrioventricular (AV) block, but the definition is not accurate, as PR prolongation in such patients could be related to the AV node and not to a block in the remaining fascicle. Simultaneous impairment in all 3 fascicles presents as complete heart block.

Causes of RBBB: Congenital heart disease (most commonly atrial septal defect), ischemic heart disease (IHD), or idiopathic fibrosis. This is frequently an isolated pathology. Features of a pseudo-RBBB with ST-segment elevation are observed in Brugada syndrome.

Causes of LBBB: Structural heart disease: IHD, cardiomyopathy (particularly dilated cardiomyopathy), myocarditis, congenital or acquired heart disease, connective tissue disease, myocardial infiltrates in the course of various conditions, idiopathic fibrosis, or calcifications.

Intraventricular blocks may be caused by antiarrhythmic drugs, particularly class I drugs (→Table 4-1) and amiodarone. Bundle branch blocks are more frequent in patients with tachycardia and less common in patients with bradycardia.

→ CLINICAL FEATURES AND NATURAL HISTORY

Intraventricular blocks without advanced AV block are usually asymptomatic. In patients with LV dysfunction and heart failure, LBBB worsens the LV dysfunction and mitral regurgitation, and thus also heart failure.

Patients with bifascicular and trifascicular blocks are at risk of slow progression to advanced or complete AV block (this should be suspected in patients with new-onset syncope). Note the risk of ventricular tachycardia.

→ DIAGNOSIS

Diagnosis is based on electrocardiographic (ECG) criteria.

1. Left fascicular block:

1) Left axis deviation $>-30°$ (anterior fascicular block) or right axis deviation $>+90°$ (posterior fascicular block).

2) QRS complex <0.12 seconds.

3) Waves:

   a) A dominant S wave in leads II, III, and aVF, a small Q wave and a dominant R wave in leads I and aVL: Anterior fascicular block.

   b) A dominant S wave in leads I and aVL, a dominant R wave in leads II, III, and AVF: Posterior fascicular block.

2. Bundle branch block:

1) QRS complex ≥0.12 seconds.

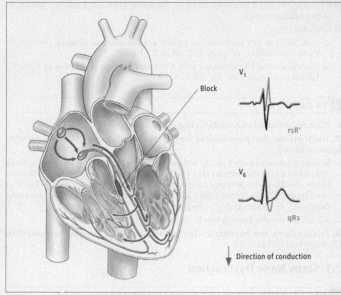

Figure 2-5. Right bundle branch block. *Illustration courtesy of Dr Shannon Zhang.*

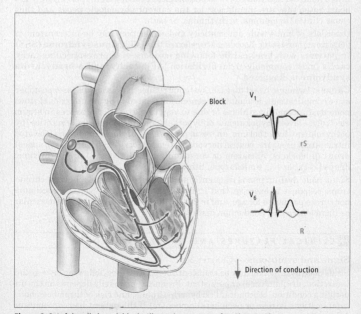

Figure 2-6. Left bundle branch block. *Illustration courtesy of Dr Shannon Zhang.*

2) ST segments and T waves are usually discordant from the dominant deflection of the QRS complex.

3) QRS pattern:

   a) rsR, rSR, or rsr patterns, or rarely a wide-notched R-wave pattern in V_1 to V_2: RBBB (→Figure 2-3). rS in V_1: LBBB.

   b) Monophasic QRS complexes with a notched or biphasic R wave in V_5 to V_6: LBBB (→Figure 2-3). Rs, RS in V_6: RBBB.

→ TREATMENT

1. Management of the underlying condition.

2. Indications for pacemaker implantation in patients with bundle branch block:

1) Syncope, bundle branch block, and positive electrophysiologic study findings defined as a His-ventricular (HV) interval ≥70 milliseconds (conduction time below the AV node) or triggering second-degree or third-degree AV block in the His bundle/Purkinje fibers during atrial stimulation with increasing frequency or pharmacologic challenge.

2) Alternate bundle branch block, regardless of symptoms.

3. Indications for biventricular pacing (cardiac resynchronization therapy): →Chapter 3.8.2.

2.3. Sinus Node Dysfunction

→ DEFINITION, ETIOLOGY, PATHOGENESIS

Sinus node dysfunction refers to pathologies resulting in inappropriately low heart rates that are insufficient for the current physiologic needs and thus cause clinical symptoms, arrhythmias, or both.

Disorders of sinus node automaticity and conduction may be intermittent or persistent; persistent disorders are referred to as **sick sinus syndrome (SSS)**. In patients with bradycardia following episodes of supraventricular tachycardia (most commonly atrial fibrillation [AF]), **tachycardia-bradycardia syndrome** is diagnosed.

Causes: Ischemic heart disease, systemic connective tissue disease, postoperative complications, idiopathic degeneration related to aging, functional sinus node dysfunction (in athletes or due to vagal reflexes, disturbances in serum electrolyte levels [hypokalemia or hyperkalemia], metabolic abnormalities [hypothyroidism, hypothermia, anorexia nervosa], neurologic conditions [elevated intracranial pressure, central nervous system tumors], obstructive sleep apnea), drugs (β-blockers, diltiazem or verapamil, digitalis, class I antiarrhythmic drugs [→Table 4-1], amiodarone, lithium).

Sinus node dysfunction is frequently accompanied by loss of a normal chronotropic response to exercise, that is, inability to achieve 85% of the maximum heart rate predicted for age, and in 20% to 30% of patients, by atrioventricular or intraventricular conduction disturbances.

→ CLINICAL FEATURES AND NATURAL HISTORY

Signs and symptoms: →Chapter 3.2.

Sinus node dysfunction may be transient/intermittent (eg, following myocardial infarction, drug induced) or persistent. Prognosis primarily depends on the underlying condition, concomitant tachyarrhythmias, and risk of thromboembolic complications (stroke or peripheral embolism) if the patient has concomitant AF (→Chapter 3.4.2.2.1).

→ DIAGNOSIS

Diagnostic Criteria

Electrocardiography (ECG):

1) **Sinus bradycardia**: Sinus rhythm with heart rates <50 beats/min when awake.

2) **Sinus pause**: No sinus P wave in a period longer than 2 PP intervals of baseline rhythm. The pause is not a multiplication of the normal PP intervals.

3) **Sinoatrial (SA) block**:

   a) **Mobitz type I (Wenckebach)**: A progressive increase in the SA conduction time until one beat is blocked, which is reflected in a progressive reduction of PP intervals (and prolongation of PR intervals) with a P wave eventually nonconducting to the ventricle.

   b) **Mobitz type II**: Periodic loss of AV conduction at a 2:1 or 3:1 ratio. The resulting pause is a multiplication of baseline sinus rhythm and may result in an escape atrial, nodal, or (less commonly) ventricular contraction.

4) **Tachycardia-bradycardia syndrome**: Commonly seen as a prolonged postconversion pause after an episode of AF transitioning to sinus rhythm.

The diagnosis of SSS requires documented symptoms during an episode of bradycardia <40 beats/min or pauses >3 seconds; however, documentation is often difficult. Prolonged Holter monitoring is the best diagnostic tool. Atrial flutter and AF may mask sinus node dysfunction, which is revealed only after cardioversion.

Differential Diagnosis

Other causes of syncope (→Chapter 10.4.2).

→ TREATMENT

1. Management of symptomatic bradycardia: →Figure 2-4.

2. Long-term management:

1) In the case of patients involved in sports, **stop training**, perform a follow up assessment, and decide about the possible continuation of training based on the results.

2) **Optimize treatment of the underlying condition and discontinue drugs causing bradycardia.**

3) **Theophylline** may be useful in some patients but it is rarely suitable for long-term therapy and not used in Canada.

4) **Implantation of a cardiac pacemaker** (→Chapter 3.2) in patients with persistent bradycardia causing unequivocally documented symptoms or with intermittent bradycardia caused by sinus pauses or SA block. The recommended first-line mode of stimulation is DDDR (or DDD in patients with persistent bradycardia and no chronotropic incompetence) with delayed ventricular stimulation.

3. Cardiac Arrest

→ DEFINITION, ETIOLOGY, PATHOGENESIS

Cardiac arrest refers to cessation of cardiac mechanical function characterized by the absence of palpable pulse, lack of the patient's response to stimulation, and apnea or agonal respirations. If not rapidly reversed by cardiopulmonary

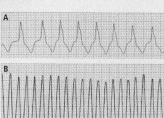
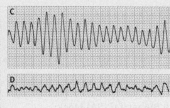

Figure 3-1. Ventricular arrhythmia. **A**, monomorphic ventricular tachycardia. **B**, ventricular flutter. **C**, polymorphic ventricular tachycardia. **D**, ventricular fibrillation.

resuscitation (CPR), defibrillation, cardioversion, or pacing, sudden cardiac arrest progresses to cardiac death.

Primary cardiac arrest is caused by or associated with a principal cardiac condition, such as:

1) **Coronary artery disease** (eg, acute coronary syndrome [ACS]/ischemic heart disease, coronary vasospasm, spontaneous coronary artery dissection).

2) **Cardiomyopathies** (eg, ischemic cardiomyopathy, nonischemic dilated cardiomyopathy, hypertrophic cardiomyopathy, infiltrative disorders such as amyloidosis or sarcoidosis, arrhythmogenic right ventricular cardiomyopathy, ventricular noncompaction, myocarditis).

3) **Congenital arrhythmogenic heart diseases** (eg, long QT syndrome, short QT syndrome, Brugada syndrome, catecholaminergic polymorphic ventricular tachycardia, idiopathic ventricular fibrillation).

4) **Structural heart disease** (eg, severe aortic stenosis, mitral valve prolapse, anomalous coronary artery circulation, Wolff-Parkinson-White syndrome, sinus node disturbances, atrioventricular conduction disturbances).

5) **Other** (eg, cardiac tamponade, commotio cordis, aortic dissection).

Secondary cardiac arrest occurs due to noncardiac causes, such as pulmonary embolism, respiratory arrest, multisystem trauma, hemorrhage, acute intracerebral hemorrhage, intoxication, seizures, or near-drowning.

Rhythms in cardiac arrest:

1) Ventricular fibrillation (VF) or flutter (→Figure 3-1).

2) Pulseless ventricular tachycardia (VT).

3) Asystole: Lack of electrical and mechanical activity of the heart (also diagnosed at a heart rate <10 beats/min).

4) Pulseless electrical activity (PEA): Lack of a hemodynamically effective mechanical contraction of the heart despite preserved organized electrical activity.

Asystole and PEA commonly result from secondary cardiac arrest or more prolonged primary cardiac arrest (degenerated from VF or pulseless VT) and therefore always require a search for reversible causes.

→ MANAGEMENT

Basic Life Support

Basic life support (BLS): →Figure 3-2.

CPR refers to interventions (chest compressions and ventilation) aimed at maintaining circulation and oxygenation of blood in an individual with cardiac arrest. High-quality CPR is essential to improving survival rates. The steps described below are followed in the course of BLS.

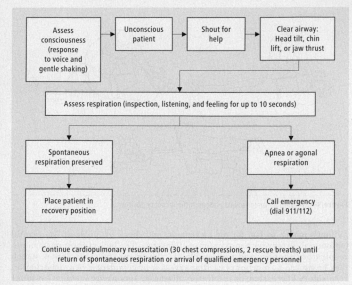

Figure 3-2. Basic life support algorithm. *Adapted from Resuscitation. 2010;81(10):1219-76.*

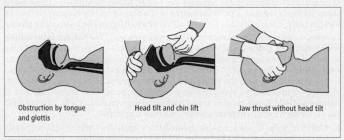

Obstruction by tongue and glottis

Head tilt and chin lift

Jaw thrust without head tilt

Figure 3-3. Clearing the airway.

1. Make sure the patient and you (as well as other rescuers) are safe. Control possible hazards (as necessary, call the police, fire department, or other emergency agency for additional assistance).

2. Assess the patient's consciousness. If the patient does not respond to voice and gentle shaking, assume that they are unconscious.

3. Shout or phone for help.

4. Clear the airway (→Figure 3-3). Place the unconscious patient on their back. Then tilt the head backwards (this maneuver is contraindicated in individuals with suspected cervical spine injury) and examine the mouth, removing any visible foreign bodies. Proceed to chin lift or jaw thrust; these two maneuvers may be performed in patients with suspected cervical spine injury, provided that the head is stabilized in a neutral position without tilting.

5. Assess respirations. Look for chest movements, listen at the patient's mouth for the sounds of inspiration and expiration, place your cheek near the

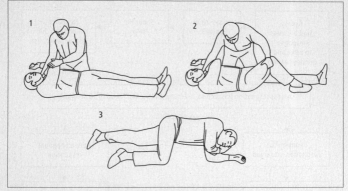

Figure 3-4. Placing an unconscious patient in the recovery position.

patient's mouth to feel for air movement, and check for pulse at the carotid (or femoral) artery for a maximum of 10 seconds. The lack of chest movements, respiratory sounds, and perceptible air movement indicates apnea, which may be caused by a primary cardiac arrest or by complete airway obstruction, respiratory depression, or respiratory diseases. Agonal respirations (residual, single sighs) are treated as apnea. Other sounds accompanying respiration may indicate partial obstruction of the respiratory tract: (1) gurgling due to liquid or semiliquid content in the airways (ie, vomit, blood, respiratory tract secretions); (2) snoring due a partial closure of the throat by the tongue, palate, or foreign body; (3) stridor due to obstruction or swelling at the level of the glottis.

In some cases it may be necessary to clear the airway. If the patient is breathing spontaneously, place them in the recovery position (→Figure 3-4). If a pulse is definitely present in a patient who is not breathing spontaneously, deliver ventilations at the rate of 10 breaths/min without chest compressions (→below). Every 2 minutes check the pulse and look for signs of circulation. Absence of signs of circulation (ie, spontaneous movements, coughing, breathing) and of carotid pulse indicate cardiac arrest and require immediate CPR. During CPR check for signs of circulation and pulse every 2 minutes.

6. Call for help. If you are alone, immediately upon discovering apnea, grossly abnormal breathing, or lack of pulse call for expert assistance if at all practical, even if you have to briefly leave the patient for this purpose. When away from the hospital, call local emergency services. Hospitals should have an emergency extension or phone number known to and available for all employees. Exception: In the case of children and infants, before calling for help proceed with CPR for ~1 minute (perform 5 rescue breaths, then 15 sternal compressions, then another 2 breaths and 15 compressions).

7. Start chest compressions. Place the patient in the supine position on a hard surface and compress the center of the sternum. In adults compress from 5 to 6 cm deep at a rate of 100 to 120 compressions/min (~2 compressions/s), in children compress the sternum with one hand, and in infants compress with 2 fingers to one-third the depth of the sagittal dimension of the chest (or 4 cm deep for infants and 5 cm deep for children). To perform compressions in adults, place the heel of one hand in the center of the patient's chest and the heel of your other hand on the top of the first hand, interlock the fingers of your hands, and keep your arms straight and your shoulders directly over the patient's chest, all without leaning on the patient's ribs. Completely release the pressure without taking your hands off the chest; the duration of a compression

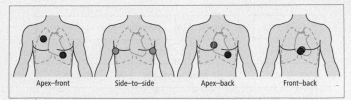

Figure 3-5. Recommended placement of electrodes for defibrillation. Location on the front (red), side (green), and back (blue) of the chest.

and a release should be identical. In adults start with 30 chest compressions followed by 2 rescue breaths, then continue with chest compressions and rescue breaths, maintaining a ratio of 30:2 in nonintubated adult patients or 15:2 in pediatric patients.

8. Continue ventilation, giving mouth-to-mouth rescue breaths while pinching the patient's nose if more than one responder is available. In infants perform mouth-to-mouth-and-nose rescue breaths. A lone rescuer should focus on compressions and should not interrupt compressions to provide rescue breaths. One breath should last ~1 second (2 rescue breaths [inspiration plus expiration] should last <5 seconds). Make sure the chest rises during inspiration and allow for its complete fall during exhalation. Chest compressions should not be interrupted for >10 seconds while rescue breaths are being delivered. If the rescue breaths are ineffective (ie, the chest does not rise), change the position of the head and jaw and repeat a maximum of 2 ventilation attempts. In children start CPR from 5 rescue breaths; maintain a 15:2 ratio of chest compressions to rescue breaths (with a lone rescuer, a 30:2 ratio is acceptable).

9. Defibrillate using an automated external defibrillator (AED). Use an AED immediately when available. Defibrillation of a shockable rhythm within 3 to 5 minutes of a cardiac arrest can increase survival rates by up to 50% to 70%. For each minute that defibrillation is delayed, the likelihood of survival to hospital discharge is reduced by 10% to 12%. Switch on the AED and attach the pads to the chest (one below the right clavicle along the sternum and the other below and to the left of the left nipple in the midaxillary line: →Figure 3-5). Keep away from the patient for the time the AED is assessing the rhythm and when the shock is being delivered. Charge the AED and trigger the shock whenever indicated by the AED. After 1 defibrillation immediately start CPR and continue for 2 minutes before the AED reevaluates the heart rhythm.

Advanced Life Support or Advanced Cardiovascular Life Support

Advanced life support (ALS) or advanced cardiovascular life support (ACLS): →Figure 3-6.

ALS or ACLS refers to procedures performed by a team of appropriately equipped professional rescuers that are aimed at restoring spontaneous circulation using CPR, advanced airway management (eg, endotracheal intubation, laryngeal mask), defibrillation/cardioversion, and administration of medications.

1. Safety assessment (removal of threats) and diagnosis of cardiac arrest: →Basic Life Support, above.

2. Perform CPR: →Figure 3-2. Minimize the time necessary for other activities (intubation performed as quickly as possible, preferably <10 seconds; defibrillation <5 seconds; continue CPR while charging the defibrillator [→below]). If possible, the rescuers performing chest compressions should change every 2 minutes.

3. Assess the mechanism of cardiac arrest and defibrillate when indicated. If a defibrillator is immediately available and ready for discharge and cardiac arrest occurred in the presence of rescuers or in the hospital,

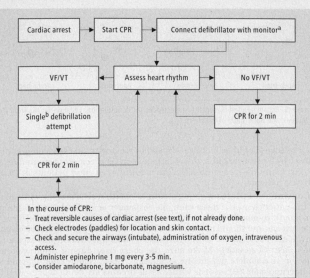

Figure 3-6. Advanced life support algorithm. *Adapted from Resuscitation. 2010;81(10):1219-76.*

defibrillation may be attempted before starting CPR. Connect a manual defibrillator and monitor the patient for arrhythmia eligible for defibrillation (VF or pulseless VT). After turning on the defibrillator, make sure that the lead selector is appropriately set to either paddles or standard electrodes (leads I, II, III). Then attach the 3 electrodes to the chest and connect them to the defibrillator (North American electrode placement: white on the right, red on the left lower chest, and black on the left upper chest; European electrode placement: red on the right shoulder, yellow on the left shoulder, green on the left midaxillary line at the costal margin). In the event of asystole on the monitor, check the connections of the defibrillator (monitor), settings of the signal amplification (gain), and readings from another lead. If in doubt whether the patient is in asystole or low-voltage VF, do not defibrillate and continue CPR. During CPR reassess the heart rhythm every 2 minutes.

Defibrillation using a manual defibrillator:

1) **Apply gel** (or, more often, defibrillation pads) on the skin of the chest where the paddles are to be placed or on the paddles themselves (self-adhesive defibrillation pads require no gel). Self-adhesive defibrillation pads have several advantages over manual paddles and should be used preferentially when available.

2) Most commonly adhesive pads are placed in the **sternal-apical position**, as in manual paddles. Depending on the patient's anatomy and other cardiac arrest features, other acceptable pad positions include (1) bilateral lateral chest walls (biaxillary); 2) one pad at the standard apical position and the other on the right upper back; 3) one pad anteriorly over the left precordium

and the other posteriorly just inferior to the left scapula. If adhesive pads are not available and paddles are used, apply the paddles with a force of ~10 kg or attach defibrillation pads to the chest (one below the right clavicle along the sternum and the other below and to the left of the left nipple: →Figure 3-5).

3) **Assess the rhythm** on the defibrillator monitor (after applying the paddles or electrodes temporarily stop CPR). The indication for delivering a shock is VF or pulseless VT. Resume CPR while the defibrillator charges (remove the paddles from the chest for that time).

4) **Set the shock energy**:

   a) **Adults:** When using **biphasic defibrillators**, providers should use the manufacturer's recommended energy dose (ie, initial energy of 120-200 J). If the dose range is unknown, the provider may use a maximal dose of 200 J. The first shock is usually **150 J**. The energy of subsequent shocks may be increased to **a maximum of 200 J**. In **monophasic defibrillators** the first and subsequent shocks are **360 J**.

   b) **Children:** 4 J/kg (first and subsequent shocks).

5) **Charge** the defibrillator (press "charge").

6) Order all rescuers to **move away and stay clear** of the patient. Make sure no one is touching either the patient or any objects that are in contact with the patient. At this point stop CPR; if using paddles, place them back in the areas of the chest previously covered with gel.

7) **Deliver the shock** (press and hold the "discharge" or "shock" button).

After delivering the shock, **immediately restart CPR** for 2 minutes; stop if signs of circulation appear (coughing, breathing, movements). Then **reassess the rhythm** and if the first shock has not been effective, deliver subsequent shocks every 2 minutes for shockable rhythms. Continue CPR between shocks. Next, establish vascular access (intravenous or intraosseous), intubate the patient when possible (if not done already), and administer medications (→Figure 3-6). Tracheal intubation should not delay defibrillation attempts and may be deferred until return of spontaneous circulation is achieved. A series of 3 shocks at intervals <2 minutes may be used in the case of a cardiac arrest occurring during cardiac catheterization or shortly after a surgical cardiac procedure, or in the case of a witnessed cardiac arrest in a patient already connected to a manual defibrillator. Following the first 2 (American Heart Association [AHA] guidelines) or 3 (European Resuscitation Council [ERC] guidelines) ineffective shocks, administer IV epinephrine 1 mg. After 3 ineffective shocks, administer IV amiodarone 300 mg (→below) before delivering the fourth shock. Do not stop CPR for the time the drugs are being administered. If the fourth shock is also ineffective, deliver subsequent shocks every 2 minutes and administer epinephrine 1 mg every 3 to 5 minutes. Consider administration of another 150 mg of amiodarone and look for reversible causes of cardiac arrest (→below). Consider changing position of the defibrillator paddles to a front-to-back position (→Figure 3-5) or to the opposite middle axillary lines.

In the case of a witnessed cardiac arrest—in particular during electrocardiography (ECG) monitoring that shows VF or pulseless VT—if a defibrillator ready to trigger off a discharge is not immediately available, you may hit the precordial area (sternum) with a clenched fist, delivering a precordial blow or "thump." This is an attempt to defibrillate with low energy, which is sometimes effective within 30 seconds of the onset of VF or pulseless VT. However, the precordial thump should not delay CPR and defibrillation.

Other Interventions and Tasks

1. Clear the airway. Perform **endotracheal intubation** if the provider is sufficiently skilled in this procedure (this should be completed within 10 seconds). Note: **CPR and prompt defibrillation have priority over intubation.** If endotracheal intubation is unsuccessful, you may try an esophageal-tracheal tube (Combitube), laryngeal mask, or laryngeal tube. Alternatively, insert an oropharyngeal or nasopharyngeal airway.

2. Ventilate the patient using a self-inflating bag (with a valve) that is connected to a reservoir bag and high-flow oxygen (>10-15 L/min) to achieve the highest possible levels of oxygen in the inhaled air (close to 100%). Before intubation (and also when an oropharyngeal or nasopharyngeal airway is used) ventilate the patient using a face mask, delivering 30 chest compressions followed by 2 rescue breaths. After successful intubation ventilate the patient via the endotracheal tube at a rate of approximately 8 to 10 breaths/min; synchronization with chest compressions is not necessary. Asynchronous CPR may be also attempted once the airway has been secured using supraglottic airway devices. The ventilation volumes are 6 to 7 mL/kg (500-600 mL) over 1 second. If capnography (measurement of the end-expiratory CO_2 levels) is available, it can be used to additionally confirm endotracheal intubation, effectiveness of ventilation, and return of spontaneous circulation, and to assess the quality of chest compressions.

3. Look for and treat reversible causes of cardiac arrest, particularly in the event of asystole or PEA but also in the case of VF or pulseless VT not responding to defibrillation. Take a history from witnesses and perform a quick targeted physical examination and diagnostic tests during CPR. Reversible causes can be remembered by **H's and T's**; if suspected or confirmed, they should be corrected immediately:

1) **H**ypoxia.
2) **H**ypovolemia (eg, hemorrhage, diarrhea).
3) **H**ydrogen ion or acidosis.
4) **H**ypothermia.
5) **H**yperkalemia, **h**ypokalemia, or other severe electrolyte disturbances (→Chapter 4.2).
6) **T**amponade (cardiac; →Chapter 16.7).
7) **T**ension pneumothorax.
8) **T**hrombosis (→Chapter 3.19.3).
9) **T**hrombosis (myocardial infarction).
10) **T**oxins (eg, drug overdose, poisoning).
11) **T**rauma.

4. Administer medications: After every IV drug administration during CPR, use an additional 20 mL of 0.9% NaCl to flush the IV catheter. In patients without venous access, medications may be delivered via the intraosseous route.

1) **Epinephrine**. Indications: Asystole, PEA, VF, or pulseless VT not responding to the first 2 (AHA) or 3 (ERC) shocks. Dosage: 1 mg IV in 10 mL 0.9% NaCl (or nondiluted) every 3 to 5 minutes (in children 10 µg/kg).

2) **Amiodarone**. Indications: VF or VT not responding to the first 3 shocks. Dosage: 300 mg in 20 mL of 5% glucose (dextrose) as an IV bolus (5 mg/kg in children). In case of persistent VF or VT, an additional 150 mg may be administered; then consider 900 mg/d in a continuous IV infusion.

3) **Sodium bicarbonate**. Indications: Hyperkalemia and tricyclic antidepressant overdose. Outside of these indications, routine use of sodium bicarbonate is not recommended. Dosage: 50 mmol (50 mL of 8.4% solution) IV; repeat as considered necessary according to the clinical condition and serial blood gas measurements.

4) **Magnesium sulfate**. Indications: Torsades de pointes (polymorphic VT with prolonged QT; →Figure 3-1). Magnesium is not likely to be effective in terminating polymorphic VT with a normal QT interval. Dosage: 1 to 2 g diluted in 10 mL of 5% glucose IV over 1 to 2 minutes; repeat after 10 to 15 minutes if necessary.

5) **Calcium chloride**. Indications: Hyperkalemia, hypocalcemia, and overdose of calcium channel blockers. There are no data supporting beneficial effects of the use of calcium chloride in other causes of cardiac arrest; in some cases it may be harmful. Avoid calcium chloride in patients with suspected digoxin toxicity and severe hyperphosphatemia. Dosage: 10 mL of a 10% $CaCl_2$ solution as an IV bolus; repeat as necessary.

6) **Fibrinolysis** should not be used routinely in cardiac arrest. You may consider fibrinolytic therapy when the arrest was caused by proven or suspected pulmonary embolism in the absence of absolute contraindications (→Chapter 3.19.3). Consider continuation of CPR for 60 to 90 minutes following the administration of a fibrinolytic agent.

7) **Other drugs**:

   a) IV glucose. Indications: Hypoglycemia.

   b) IV glucagon. Indications: Hypoglycemia (1 mg) and overdose of β-blockers or calcium channel blockers (5-10 mg).

   c) Antihistamines (H_1 and H_2 antagonists) and IV glucocorticoids. Indications: Anaphylaxis (→Chapter 2.2).

   d) IV fluids. Indications: Hypovolemia, anaphylaxis, or undifferentiated shock (→Chapter 3.16).

   e) Blood products (eg, red blood cells, frozen plasma, platelet concentrates). Indications: Hemorrhage (at the same time make attempts to stop the hemorrhage as soon as possible), coagulopathy.

   f) Naloxone. Indications: Opioid poisoning or overdose.

   g) Lipid emulsion therapy. Indications: Poisonings involving certain lipophilic medications (overdoses of calcium channel blockers, β-blockers, some tricyclic antidepressants, local anesthetics, and chlorpromazine). Before using lipid emulsion therapy, it is recommended to consult a poison control center or toxicologist. Dosage: 20% lipid emulsion (1-1.5 mL/kg bolus followed by a continuous IV infusion at a rate of 0.25-0.5 mL/kg/min). If cardiovascular stability has not been restored after 5 minutes, the 1.5 mL/kg bolus may be repeated a maximum of 2 times.

5. Cardiac pacing. Electrical pacing during cardiac arrest is generally considered ineffective and therefore is not recommended for routine use. Pacing may be considered for recurrent polymorphic VT when precipitated by bradycardia or pauses or early after cardiac surgery in patients with asystole. Pacing can be done via transcutaneous pads or a temporary transvenous wire.

Management After Restoring Spontaneous Circulation

1. Placement of the unconscious patient with preserved spontaneous breathing in the recovery position (this does not apply to intubated patients; →Figure 3-4) unless there is an immediate history of suspected trauma, particularly spine injury.

2. Prompt transfer to an intensive care unit (ICU) or high acuity bed. The patient should be transported to the hospital by an ambulance with the appropriate CPR equipment and CPR-competent personnel and moved around the hospital when attended by a hospital resuscitation team, ideally with a connected defibrillator, continuous oxygen therapy with a saturation target ≥92%, secured airway (in unconscious patients), and continued ventilation.

3. Hospitalization in the ICU or an equivalent unit for a period of time deemed necessary, usually ≥24 hours.

1) **Continuous monitoring** of ECG, pulse oximetry, blood pressure, and urine output, when deemed necessary supplemented by the use of the central line as well as hemodynamic monitoring with an intra-arterial line.

2) **Treatment** of arrhythmias (eg, ventricular and supraventricular tachycardias, bradycardia), shock, heart failure, ACS, respiratory failure.

3) **Determination of the cause** of cardiac arrest and further diagnostic workup and treatment:

a) A repeated broader **history and physical examination** (if the patient cannot provide information on their own, ask the rescuers, witnesses of the cardiac arrest, family, and other persons living with or close to the patient, and use the available medical records).

b) **12-lead ECG**, other diagnostic tests of ACS (cardiac troponin and echocardiography, when necessary), and appropriate treatment if the diagnosis of ACS is established (including revascularization and medical therapies).

c) **Chest radiographs** looking for evidence of various conditions as dictated by clinical situation, for example, pneumothorax, pneumonia, atelectases, pericardial or pleural effusion, or venous congestion. Verify the positioning of the endotracheal tube, gastric tube, and intravenous catheters.

d) **Arterial blood gas measurements** and treatment of acid-base disturbances and respiratory insufficiency (administer oxygen when necessary to maintain an arterial hemoglobin oxygen saturation of 92%-96%). Hyperoxia (saturation >96%) may be harmful.⊘⊖

e) **Measurements of serum electrolyte levels** and treatment of electrolyte disturbances. Measurements of **blood glucose levels** (if >10 mmol/L [180 mg/dL], administer continuous IV insulin).

f) Looking for signs of **active bleeding** (particularly gastrointestinal bleeding; start appropriate prophylaxis), complete blood count (CBC) measurements (look for anemia and transfuse packed red blood cells when necessary).

g) **Kidney and liver function tests**.

h) Basic **coagulation tests**.

i) **Toxicology tests** in the case of suspected poisoning with appropriate treatment when indicated.

j) **Other investigations** to assess for the cause of the arrest as dictated by the clinical situation (eg, chest computed tomography [CT] for suspected pulmonary embolism, echocardiography for suspected ACS or pericardial effusion).

4) **Consider bronchoscopy** to clear the airway in patients with suspected or documented aspiration.

5) **Consider imaging studies of the head** in unconscious patients or those with neurologic symptoms to assess for intracranial hemorrhage, ischemic stroke, cerebral edema, or other significant intracranial pathology.

6) In patients who remain comatose (Glasgow Coma Scale <8 [→Chapter 10.3, Table 3-2] or inability to respond to verbal commands) following the return of spontaneous circulation after a VF or pulseless VT arrest, it is recommended to initiate **targeted temperature management (TTM)** to help improve neurologic prognosis, including improved survival with a good neurologic outcome.⊘⊖ Lower-level evidence exists for the use of TTM in cardiac arrest survivors of nonshockable rhythms.◯. European and American guidelines recommend cooling to 32°C to 36°C for ≥24 hours. Canadian guidelines recommend 33°C to 36°C. TTM is usually accomplished using ice packs or specialized equipment (eg, cooling blankets, cooling suits, or intravascular cooling devices). As an adjunct, an infusion of up to 30 mL/kg of cold (4°C) 0.9% NaCl or Ringer lactate may be considered to lower body temperature, initially by up to 1.5°C. After the cooling period, increase body temperature slowly (0.25°C-0.5°C/h). There is a strong suggestion of similar effects of cooling to 33°C and 36°C⊖ and no benefits of cooling with a cold saline infusion before arrival at the hospital.

4. Cardiac Arrhythmias

→DEFINITION

1. Supraventricular arrhythmias:

1) **Supraventricular premature beats (SPBs)** originate outside the sinus node. They are either premature or escape beats and may be single or multiple. They may occur randomly or in an organized pattern after every normal sinus beat (**bigeminy**) or after every 2 normal sinus beats (**trigeminy**).

2) **Supraventricular tachycardia (SVT)** is any tachycardia >100 beats/min that originates above the bundle of His, including:

   a) **Atrioventricular nodal reentrant tachycardia (AVNRT).**

   b) **Atrioventricular reentrant tachycardia (AVRT).**

   c) **Atrial tachycardia (AT).**

3) **Atrial flutter (AFL).**

4) **Atrial fibrillation (AF).**

2. Ventricular arrhythmias originate from the ventricles:

1) **Ventricular premature beats (VPBs)** may be premature or escape beats. They may also be monomorphic or polymorphic and single or complex. They may occur after every normal sinus beat (**bigeminy**) or after every 2 normal sinus beats (**trigeminy**).

2) **Ventricular tachycardia (VT)** is caused by >3 consecutive VPBs. **Nonsustained VT** will last <30 seconds. **Sustained VT** is defined as lasting >30 seconds or shorter if it causes hemodynamic compromise.

3) **Ventricular fibrillation (VF).**

→CLINICAL FEATURES AND NATURAL HISTORY

1. Supraventricular arrhythmias: Signs and symptoms depend on the ventricular rate, underlying heart disease, arrhythmia duration, and patient's individual sensitivity to arrhythmia. While SVT is more commonly seen in normal hearts and younger patients, AF and AFL usually occur in hypertensive or structural heart disease and in older individuals. Symptoms include palpitations, dizziness, chest discomfort, dyspnea, and near-fainting or syncope. SVT is usually paroxysmal (characterized by a sudden onset and resolution) and can recur with varying frequency. AFL and AF can progress from the paroxysmal form into a more persistent and permanent form (the patient is mainly in AF instead of sinus rhythm). AF and AFL also carry a risk of embolic stroke. Rarely, persistent supraventricular arrhythmia with rapid ventricular rates may cause tachycardia-induced cardiomyopathy and heart failure symptoms.

2. Ventricular arrhythmias: Ventricular arrhythmias in the form of VPBs or nonsustained VT can be asymptomatic. However, patients may have symptoms like palpitations, dizziness, chest discomfort, dyspnea, and near-fainting or syncope. There is an inconsistent correlation between the amount of ectopic beats (percentage of VPBs or nonsustained VT of all beats) and symptoms. In structurally normal hearts even a sustained episode of VT can cause no symptoms; however, the majority of sustained VT episodes are symptomatic and can cause syncope or cardiac arrest. VF is a terminal arrhythmia unless the patient is resuscitated.

→DIAGNOSIS

The key for the diagnosis of an arrhythmia is its electrocardiographic (ECG) appearance. Nevertheless, a proper physical examination can be essential for diagnosis when assessing for pulse rate, rhythm, and signs of structural heart disease (eg, valvular disease, heart failure). At times, a few other diagnostic tests can be useful.

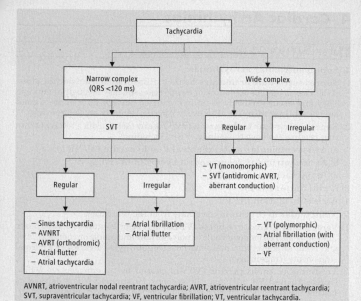

AVNRT, atrioventricular nodal reentrant tachycardia; AVRT, atrioventricular reentrant tachycardia; SVT, supraventricular tachycardia; VF, ventricular fibrillation; VT, ventricular tachycardia.

Figure 4-1. Simplified categorization of arrhythmias.

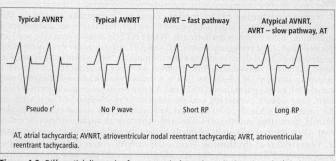

AT, atrial tachycardia; AVNRT, atrioventricular nodal reentrant tachycardia; AVRT, atrioventricular reentrant tachycardia.

Figure 4-2. Differential diagnosis of supraventricular tachycardia based on the relationship of P waves and QRS complexes.

The ECG appearance of arrhythmia can lead to a correct diagnosis (→Figure 4-1). When analyzing the ECG, the following should be taken into consideration:
1) Assess the rate (tachycardia vs bradycardia).
2) Assess the QRS-complex width (wide vs narrow).
3) Assess regularity. If the rhythm is irregular, is there a pattern?
4) Look for P waves:
   a) Assess the relation of P waves to QRS complexes.
   b) If the relation is 1:1, assess the timing of P waves in relation to the previous QRS complex (short RP versus long RP; →Figure 4-2).

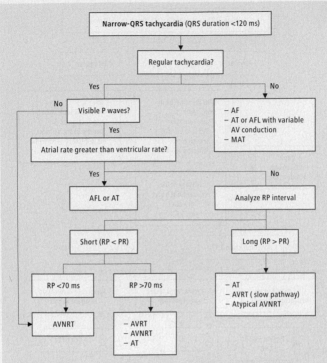

Note: Tests that may be helpful in differential diagnosis of narrow-QRS tachycardia include **response to adenosine** (rapid IV injection of adenosine 6 mg reduces sinus rhythm and AV node conduction) and **carotid sinus massage**; sudden termination of tachycardia suggests possible AVNRT, AVRT, reentrant sinus node tachycardia, or (less frequently) AT. Persistent atrial tachycardia with transient AV block suggests AFL or AF.

AF, atrial fibrillation; AFL, atrial flutter; AV, atrioventricular; AVNRT, reentrant AV node tachycardia; AVRT, reentrant AV tachycardia; MAT, multifocal atrial tachycardia.

Figure 4-3. Differential diagnosis of narrow-QRS tachycardia. *Adapted from guidelines by the American College of Cardiology, American Heart Association, and European Society of Cardiology.*

Diagnostic Tests

1. ECG:

1) **12-lead resting ECG.**

2) **Continuous ECG monitoring** is useful in patients with frequent episodes of arrhythmia. For outpatients, Holter monitors can accumulate continuous ECG information from 24 hours and up to a week. The data are then downloaded and arrhythmias are identified offline. This can also aid in assessing the amount of ectopic beats (SPBs or VPBs in 24 hours), their type (single or complex, nonsustained or sustained VT), and the circadian pattern, and is useful in assessing for slow heart rates (bradycardia) and pauses. Holter monitors are also helpful in the evaluation of QT-segment prolongation, Brugada syndrome ECG patterns, and numerous investigational prognostic markers in structural heart disease (eg, heart rate variability). Inpatients can be monitored by

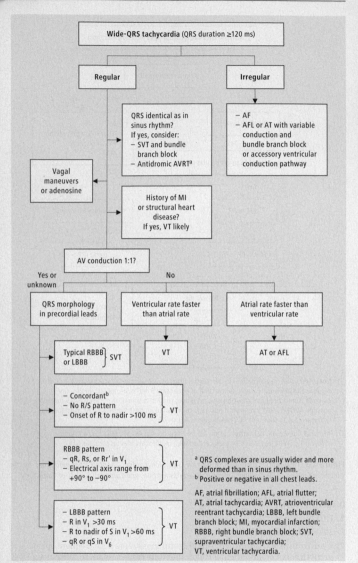

Figure 4-4. Differential diagnosis of wide-QRS tachycardia. *Adapted from guidelines by the American College of Cardiology, American Heart Association, and European Society of Cardiology.*

continuous telemetry ECG monitoring; some of these systems offer storing and processing of data on top of real-time alerting for arrhythmias.

3) **Long-term ECG recorders** come in the form of loop or event recorders. These devices will keep on recording and deleting a few minutes of ECG

Table 4-1. Vaughan Williams classification of antiarrhythmic drugs

Class	Action	Drugs
I	Sodium channel blockade	
Ia	Moderate phase 0 depression, prolonging of action potential	Quinidine, procainamide, disopyramide
Ib	Minimal effect on phase 0, no change in duration of action potential	Lidocaine, mexiletine
Ic	Marked phase 0 depression, conduction slowing, little effect on repolarization	Flecainide, propafenone
II	β-Adrenergic blockade	Propranolol, metoprolol, atenolol, esmolol, bisoprolol
III	Potassium channel blockade	Amiodarone, sotalol, bretylium, ibutilide
IV	Calcium channel blockade	Verapamil, diltiazem

unless an arrhythmia is detected. Usually when using a remote device, the patient can also instruct it to store an episode of ECG when symptomatic, even after regaining consciousness from a fainting spell. The last few minutes of the ECG are thus stored and can also be transmitted over the phone. These devices can be external (using ECG electrodes on the chest skin similar to a Holter device) or internal (implantable loop recorder [ILR]) and are used for detecting arrhythmias in patients with infrequent symptoms. Implantable recorders can last for a few years.

4) **ECG stress testing** is used in the diagnosis of arrhythmias in patients with symptoms that are either related to or exacerbated on exertion.

2. Electrophysiologic study (EPS) is an invasive study, usually combined with a therapeutic intervention, used for making a detailed diagnosis of arrhythmia. Electrodes (catheters) are introduced into the heart via the venous (usually) or arterial approach.

3. Echocardiography is often used to assess for structural heart disease (eg, cardiac function, hypertrophy, valvular disease), which can help in the identification of causes or complications of an arrhythmia (eg, tachycardia-induced cardiomyopathy).

Differential Diagnosis

SVT: →Figure 4-2. Narrow-QRS tachycardia: →Figure 4-3. Wide-QRS tachycardia: →Figure 4-4.

→TREATMENT

It is imperative to make the right diagnosis and to treat an identifiable cause or underlying condition. Treatment of specific arrhythmias may include the following:

1) **Interventions aimed at increasing vagal tone** (eg, carotid sinus massage, Valsalva maneuver). This at times can also aid in diagnosis.
2) **Antiarrhythmic drugs**: Different antiarrhythmic drugs can be used for different indications (→Table 4-1, →Table 4-2).
3) **Electrical cardioversion** and **electrical defibrillation**.
4) Insertion of an **implantable cardioverter-defibrillator (ICD)**, a device that can detect tachyarrhythmia and terminate it in order to prevent sudden cardiac death (→Chapter 3.4.3.6).

Table 4-2. Antiarrhythmic agents

Agent	Dosage		Contraindications
	Acute[a]	Long term	
Adenosine (IV)	6 mg in rapid IV injection followed by 12 or 18 mg after 1-2 min when necessary	–	Sinus node dysfunction, second-degree or third-degree AV block,[b] VT, asthma. Use with caution in AF or AFL with suspected accessory pathway, prolonged QT, severe HF, or hypotension
Amiodarone (IV, PO)	5 mg/kg (most often 300 mg) IV over 15-30 min (infusions over 60-120 min are safer) followed by 360 mg (1 mg/min) over 6 h and then by 540 mg (0.5 mg/min) over 18 h; max, 1200 mg/d (sometimes up to 2000 mg/d)	Loading dose: 200 mg (in selected cases 400 mg) tid for 7-14 days followed by 200 mg bid for 7-14 days Maintenance dose: usually 200 mg/d, in selected cases 100 or 300-400 mg/d	Sinus node dysfunction, second-degree or third-degree AV block,[b] prolonged QT, drug hypersensitivity, thyrotoxicosis, liver disease, pregnancy, breastfeeding
Digoxin (IV, PO)	0.25 mg IV every 2 h; max total dose, 1.5 mg	0.125-0.375 mg/d	Bradycardia,[b] second-degree or third-degree AV block,[b] sick sinus syndrome,[b] carotid sinus syndrome, hypertrophic cardiomyopathy with outflow tract obstruction, preexcitation syndromes, hypokalemia, hypercalcemia, planned electrical cardioversion
Diltiazem (PO)	–	90-240 mg/d	HF, second-degree or third-degree AV block[b]
Dronedarone (PO)	–	400 mg bid	Second-degree or third-degree AV block,[b] sick sinus syndrome,[b] HF or asymptomatic LV dysfunction, permanent AF
Flecainide (IV, PO)	2 mg/kg IV bolus (max, 150 mg)	50-150 mg PO bid	Structural heart disease (in particular heart failure), CAD, sinus node dysfunction, second-degree or third-degree AV block[b]
Lidocaine (IV)	50 mg IV over 2 min; can be repeated every 5 min up to total of 200 mg followed by infusion of 1-4 mg/min; dose should be tapered off	–	Hypersensitivity to local anesthetic drugs

Metoprolol (IV, PO)	5 mg IV every 5-10 min up to total of 15 mg	50-200 mg/d	Second-degree or third-degree AV block,[b] symptomatic bradycardia, symptomatic hypotension, sick sinus syndrome, decompensated HF, asthma
Procainamide (IV)	Loading dose: 100-200 mg/dose or 15-18 mg/kg; do not exceed 50 mg/min; can be repeated every 5 min if required; do not exceed 1 g Maintenance dose: 1-4 mg/min IV infusion	–	Sinus node dysfunction, second-degree or third-degree AV block,[b] prolonged QT, drug hypersensitivity
Propranolol (IV, PO)	1-5 mg IV (in selected cases 10 mg); administer 1 mg over 1 min	20-40 mg every 8 h	Second-degree or third-degree AV block,[b] symptomatic bradycardia, symptomatic hypotension, sick sinus syndrome, decompensated HF, asthma
Propafenone (IV, PO)	1-2 mg/kg IV over 5 min	150-300 mg every 8-12 h	Structural heart disease (in particular HF), CAD, sinus node dysfunction, second-degree or third-degree AV block[b]
Sotalol (PO)	80-160 mg every 12 h	80-160 mg every 12 h	Sinus node dysfunction, second-degree or third-degree AV block,[b] prolonged QT, asthma, renal failure (creatinine clearance <40 mL/min)
Verapamil (IV, PO)	5-10 mg IV over 1-2 min	120-360 mg/d	HF, second-degree or third-degree AV block[b]

[a] Monitor electrocardiography and blood pressure.
[b] In patients without an implanted pacemaker.

AF, atrial fibrillation; AFL, atrial flutter; AV, atrioventricular; bid, 2 times a day; CAD, coronary artery disease; HF, heart failure; IV, intravenous; LV, left ventricle; PO, oral; tid, 3 times a day; VT, ventricular tachycardia.

5) **Catheter or surgical ablation**: Catheter ablation involves destruction of the critical anatomical region of the cardiac tissue that is responsible for the generation or propagation of an arrhythmia. The procedure is performed percutaneously by introducing catheters into the heart via veins or arteries. Surgical ablation is done using thoracic surgery. Ablation can be applied for the treatment of AF, AFL, SVT, and VT.

4.1. Sudden Cardiac Death

➡ **DEFINITION, ETIOLOGY**

Sudden cardiac death (SCD) is defined as death due to cardiac causes preceded by a sudden loss of consciousness in a patient in whom a change in clinical status heralding cardiac arrest was observed ≤1 hour prior to SCD.

Causes: SCD is usually triggered by malignant ventricular arrhythmias that may be caused by ischemic heart disease (IHD), any type of cardiomyopathy, congenital heart disease, or genetic channelopathy. IHD is the most common cause (in 80% of patients). Severe left ventricular dysfunction significantly increases the risk of SCD.

➡ **PREVENTION**

1. Prevention of ischemia in IHD patients.

2. Prevention of specific triggers according to the disorders listed above (eg, QT--prolonging drugs in patients with long QT syndrome).

3. Placement of an **implantable cardioverter-defibrillator (ICD)** for prevention of SCD is recommended in high-risk patients with life expectancy >1 year and good functional status, in jurisdictions where the device is available. High-risk patients include:

1) Patients ≥40 days after myocardial infarction (MI) with a left ventricular ejection fraction (LVEF) ≤35%.
2) Patients with dilated nonischemic cardiomyopathy with an LVEF ≤35% and New York Heart Association (NYHA) class II or III heart failure (→Table 8-3).

➡ **TREATMENT**

ICD implantation in survivors of SCD unless a reversible cause (eg, acute phase of MI, drug-related QT prolongation, bradycardia-induced polymorphic ventricular tachycardia) or noncardiac cause is documented.

4.2. Supraventricular Arrhythmias

4.2.1. Supraventricular Premature Beats

➡ **DEFINITION, ETIOLOGY, PATHOGENESIS**

Supraventricular premature beats (SPBs) originate outside the sinus node, in the atrium and in the veins draining to the atria. They are classified as premature or escape beats. SPBs are most frequently single but may be also multiple and have the form of nonsustained supraventricular tachycardia (usually atrial tachycardia). They are common in healthy individuals.

SPBs are frequently transitory and associated with a transient triggering factor, such as emotions, stimulants (alcohol, caffeine, drugs of abuse), electrolyte disturbances, infection, or thyrotoxicosis.

➔ CLINICAL FEATURES AND NATURAL HISTORY

SPBs are usually asymptomatic, although sometimes patients may experience irregular heartbeats or pauses. Nonconducted SPBs can lead to effective bradycardia, as some do not produce an effective stroke volume. Multiple SPBs may affect the quality of life and increase the risk of atrial fibrillation.

➔ TREATMENT

1. Treatment is rarely necessary. However, the triggering factors should be eliminated.

2. In patients with severe symptoms, multiple SPBs, or short episodes of atrial fibrillation, consider a β-blocker or calcium channel blocker (verapamil or diltiazem), or rarely a class I antiarrhythmic agent (→Table 4-1).

4.2.2. Supraventricular Tachycardias

➔ DIAGNOSIS

Key points for electrocardiographic (ECG) identification of supraventricular tachycardias (SVTs):

1) The ventricular rate should be classified as regular or irregular. An irregular ventricular rate suggests atrial fibrillation, multifocal atrial tachycardia, or atrial flutter with variable conduction.

2) If the atrial rate exceeds the ventricular rate, then atrial flutter or atrial tachycardia are usually present.

3) If the SVT is regular, this may represent atrial tachycardia with 1:1 conduction or an SVT that involves the atrioventricular node (atrioventricular nodal reentrant tachycardia [AVNRT], atrioventricular reentrant tachycardia [AVRT]).

4) In atrial tachycardia ECG will typically show a P wave with a morphology that differs from a sinus morphology.

5) In a typical AVNRT the retrograde atrial activation is nearly simultaneous with the QRS complex (P wave will be invisible or will deform the last portion of QRS). In orthodromic AVRT a retrograde P wave (coming from the ventricle to the atrium through the accessory pathway) is usually seen in the early part of the ST segment (→Chapter 3.4.2.2.5). Both AVNRT and orthodromic AVRT are forms of short-RP tachycardias. A long-RP tachycardia is usually an atrial tachycardia or rarely an uncommon form of AVRT or atypical AVNRT.

➔ TREATMENT

Classification of antiarrhythmic drugs: →Table 4-1.

Antiarrhythmic agents: →Table 4-2.

Acute Management of SVT of Unknown Origin

1. Irregular SVT: Manage as atrial fibrillation.

2. Regular SVT:

1) Vagal maneuvers, adenosine, or both.

2) If these are ineffective or not feasible, proceed according to the patient's hemodynamic situation:

  a) Stable: IV β-blockers; IV diltiazem or IV verapamil. We suggest not to mix IV β-blockers with IV calcium antagonists, especially if cardiac function is unknown.

  b) Unstable: Synchronized cardioversion.

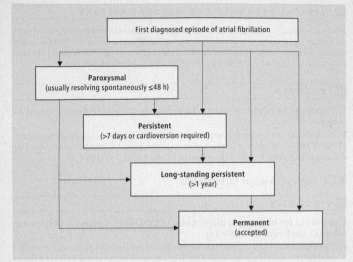

Figure 4-5. Classification of atrial fibrillation. *Based on the 2010 European Society of Cardiology guidelines.*

Ongoing Management of SVT of Unknown Origin

1. Preexcitation present in sinus rhythm:

1) Consider electrophysiologic study (EPS) and ablation.

2) If ablation is unavailable or refused by the patient, consider:

   a) Flecainide or propafenone in the absence of structural heart disease.

   b) Amiodarone or sotalol in patients with structural heart disease.

2. Without preexcitation in sinus rhythm:

1) Consider EPS and ablation.

2) If ablation is unavailable or refused by the patient, consider β-blockers, diltiazem, or verapamil.

4.2.2.1. Atrial Fibrillation

→DEFINITION, ETIOLOGY, PATHOGENESIS

Atrial fibrillation (AF) is the most common supraventricular tachyarrhythmia (prevalence in adults, 1%-2%). It is characterized by fast (350-700 beats/min) and irregular atrial activation, which results in the loss of hemodynamic effectiveness of atrial contractions and a concomitant irregular ventricular rhythm. Ventricular rate depends on the electrophysiologic features of the atrioventricular (AV) node, autonomic function, and effects of drugs; it may be normal (resting heart rates, 70-90 beats/min), fast (tachyarrhythmia), or slow (bradyarrhythmia).

AF classification: →Figure 4-5. In patients with episodes of AF that may be classified as different categories, consider the predominant type of AF.

Risk factors: A variety of cardiac and extracardiac conditions increase the risk of developing AF, including valvular heart disease (primarily mitral valve disease), heart failure irrespective of its cause, cardiomyopathies, hypertension

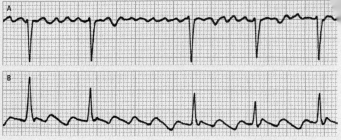

Figure 4-6. Atrial fibrillation and atrial flutter. A, polymorphic F waves replacing P waves during atrial fibrillation. B, monomorphic biphasic F waves replacing P waves during atrial flutter.

(and other cardiac risk factors), thyrotoxicosis, pulmonary diseases, chronic kidney disease, and obstructive sleep apnea. However, AF can also be observed in individuals without structural heart disease.

→ CLINICAL FEATURES AND NATURAL HISTORY

Symptoms may include palpitations, weakness, poor exercise tolerance, syncope, or dizziness. Patients may also be asymptomatic.

The European Heart Rhythm Association (EHRA) score used for the classification of AF-related symptoms:

1) EHRA class I: Asymptomatic.
2) EHRA class II: Mild symptoms not affecting normal daily activity.
3) EHRA class III: Severe symptoms affecting daily activity.
4) EHRA class IV: Disabling symptoms.

Signs include grossly irregular heart rate, irregular pulse, and pulse deficit (not every ventricular contraction, especially if occurring shortly after the previous one, may be sufficiently strong to transmit an arterial pulse wave through the peripheral artery).

A detailed history and analysis of the available medical records are important. **Paroxysmal AF** is self-limiting and resolves within 7 days. **Persistent AF** does not resolve spontaneously, lasts >7 days, or both. **Long-standing persistent AF** refers to uninterrupted AF lasting >1 year. **Permanent AF** refers to situations where efforts to restore sinus rhythm have either failed or been forgone. These categories are not mutually exclusive and it is common for patients with one type of AF to exhibit overlapping features of another type.

→ DIAGNOSIS

Diagnostic Tests

1. Electrocardiography (ECG): A grossly irregular rhythm, P waves absent or not clearly identifiable (→Figure 4-6).

2. Holter ECG monitoring: Long-term monitoring (24 hours to 14 days) may be useful in the identification of episodes of paroxysmal AF.

3. Echocardiography: This is useful in the identification of structural heart disease and assessing left ventricular function and left atrium size. The larger the left atrium, the less likely it is to achieve a stable sinus rhythm.

Differential Diagnosis

Supraventricular tachycardia: →Figure 4-2.

❚TREATMENT

Classification of antiarrhythmic drugs: →Table 4-1.
Antiarrhythmic agents: →Table 4-2.

Acute Management

The management of paroxysmal AF depends on episode duration, symptoms, and hemodynamic status:

1) **AF <48 hours**:
   a) In patients with symptomatic AF lasting <48 hours, an acute rhythm control strategy should be favored in order to avoid left atrial remodeling due to persistent AF.
   b) If a rhythm control strategy is chosen, cardioversion may be achieved either **pharmacologically** or **electrically**. In patients with no structural heart disease and no contraindications, consider oral flecainide 300 mg plus an oral dose of an AV nodal blocker, like a β-blocker, diltiazem, or verapamil; or propafenone 600 mg as a single dose (no need to add an AV nodal blocker). In all other cases consider IV amiodarone but remember that conversion to sinus rhythm usually takes longer (8-12 hours).⊙⊖ In **patients with significant hemodynamic disturbances or severe chest pain caused by rapid AF**, perform urgent electrical cardioversion.
   c) Elderly patients with comorbidities and mild symptoms may benefit from a rate control strategy. For rate control, consider β-blockers, diltiazem, or verapamil. Digoxin is usually not considered in monotherapy but combined with any of the other medications.

2) **AF >48 hours**:
   a) When considering either electrical or pharmacologic cardioversion of AF, patients should receive adequate anticoagulation treatment to prevent thromboembolic complications. The risk of thromboembolism is the same whether conversion is achieved electrically or pharmacologically (→Complications, below).
   b) In case of an AF episode lasting >48 hours, as an alternative to adequate anticoagulation (duration ≥3 weeks), transesophageal echocardiography may be performed to exclude a left atrial appendage thrombus, which would be a contraindication to cardioversion.

Long-Term Management

General Considerations

1. Paroxysmal AF:

1) Eliminate risk factors that may have triggered the arrhythmia, such as alcohol, sleep apnea, or uncontrolled hypertension.
2) If episodes are infrequent and short-lasting, follow up with no antiarrhythmics or consider rate-control medications. If episodes are more frequent but still <1 episode per week, patients with no structural heart disease may be treated with the "pill-in-the-pocket" approach: a single dose of propafenone 600 mg (450 mg in patients <70 kg) or flecainide 300 mg plus an AV nodal blocker (eg, metoprolol, bisoprolol, diltiazem, or verapamil),⊙⊖ provided the efficacy and safety of the drug have been previously confirmed in a hospital setting. There is no need to add a nodal blocker on top of propafenone.
3) Patients with frequent episodes should receive daily medications according to their profile. In young patients with no heart disease, flecainide or propafenone is preferred for a rhythm control strategy. In patients with coronary artery disease, sotalol or dronedarone could be an option. In patients with left ventricular dysfunction or contraindications for other antiarrhythmics, amiodarone should be considered.

2. In patients with **persistent AF**, choose a management strategy:

1) **Rhythm-control strategy**: Restore sinus rhythm either electrically or pharmacologically and attempt to maintain sinus rhythm with antiarrhythmic agents, ablation, or both.

2) **Rate-control strategy**: Do not attempt to restore sinus rhythm but ensure **optimal control of the ventricular rate during AF** using an exercise test or Holter monitor to maintain an average 24-hour heart rate of <110 beats/min and no symptoms. Rate control can be achieved with one or more of β-blockers, diltiazem, verapamil, and digoxin, or with ablation of the AV node (and pacemaker implantation).

3) **Asymptomatic patients with persistent AF** can be managed effectively with a rate control strategy, as studies show there may be no benefit to a rhythm control approach in terms of mortality, morbidity, or quality of life. In young patients with no structural heart disease, usually rhythm control is preferred, while in elderly patients with dilated left atriums, structural heart disease, or both, a rate control approach is preferred.

3. Permanent AF: The goal of treatment is ventricular rate control. The target is to maintain a heart rate <110 beats/min. If left ventricular dysfunction is present, the target for rate control should be more stringent.

Pharmacotherapy

Algorithm for drug selection: →Figure 4-7.

Invasive Treatment

1. Catheter ablation: The key method is isolation of the pulmonary veins using radiofrequency or cryoablation. It is recommended in patients with symptomatic paroxysmal AF in whom treatment with ≥1 class I or class III antiarrhythmic agents has been unsuccessful and in patients who prefer to avoid medication. Catheter ablation has shown superior efficacy in maintaining sinus rhythm when compared with antiarrhythmic drugs.⊘⊖

2. Surgical ablation: An option in patients undergoing cardiac surgery, commonly with mitral valve disease, who have persistent AF.

3. Catheter ablation of the AV junction with pacemaker implantation: This may be considered as a last resource in patients with paroxysmal or permanent AF who remain symptomatic despite other treatment strategies. This is a final rate-control strategy.

→ COMPLICATIONS

The most significant complications of AF include **thromboembolic events**, mainly ischemic stroke. They are associated with the formation of a thrombus in the left atrium (most commonly in the left atrial appendage).

1. Long-term prevention of thromboembolism: In every patient with AF assess the risk of thromboembolic complications using the CHA_2DS_2-VASc score (congestive heart failure, hypertension, age ≥75 years [doubled], diabetes, stroke/transient ischemic attack/thromboembolism [doubled], vascular disease [prior myocardial infarction, peripheral artery disease, aortic plaque], age 65-74 years, sex category [female]). Long-term anticoagulation is recommended in patients with a CHA_2DS_2-VASc score ≥1 except if the single risk factor is female sex (→Table 4-3) or if there is a high risk of intracranial bleeding (→Table 4-4). Recommended prophylaxis: →Figure 4-8.

2. Prophylactic antithrombotic treatment in patients treated with cardioversion:

1) **Patients with AF lasting ≥48 hours or of unknown duration**: Before attempting to restore sinus rhythm (electrical or pharmacologic cardioversion), use a vitamin K antagonist (VKA) for ≥3 weeks before cardioversion and 4 weeks after the procedure (maintain an international normalized

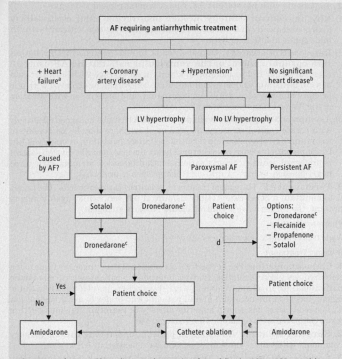

Figure 4-7. Selection of long-term antiarrhythmic treatment in patients with atrial fibrillation. *Adapted from the 2012 European Society of Cardiology guidelines.*

ratio [INR] of 2.0 to 3.0; note that in some patients longer anticoagulation may be indicated; consider risk factors for thromboembolic complications). Dabigatran, rivaroxaban, or apixaban may be used instead of VKAs. If a left atrial appendage thrombus has been excluded with transesophageal echocardiography, it would be safe to proceed with cardioversion before completing 3 weeks of anticoagulation. In any case, 4 weeks of anticoagulation are needed after cardioversion.

If **urgent cardioversion is required** in patients with AF lasting ≥48 hours or of unknown duration, exclude the presence of a thrombus using transesophageal echocardiography, if available. Before cardioversion administer IV unfractionated heparin (or subcutaneous low-molecular-weight heparin). After cardioversion use an oral anticoagulant for ≥4 weeks, depending on the risk factors for thromboembolism (CHA$_2$DS$_2$-VASc score; →above).

Table 4-3. Assessment of the risk of stroke in patients with atrial fibrillation not associated with valvular heart disease

Risk factor	Score	
	CHADS$_2$	CHA$_2$DS$_2$-VASc
Congestive heart failure or left ventricular dysfunction[a]	1	1
Hypertension	1	1
Age ≥75 years	1	2
Diabetes mellitus	1	1
History of stroke, transient ischemic attack, or thromboembolism[a]	2	2
Vascular disease[b]	–	1
Age 65-74 years	–	1
Female sex	–	1

[a] Left ventricular dysfunction and other thromboembolic event are included only in the CHA$_2$DS$_2$-VASc score.
[b] History of myocardial infarction, peripheral artery disease, or atherosclerotic plaque in aorta.

Table 4-4. HAS-BLED bleeding[a] risk score in patients with atrial fibrillation

Clinical characteristic	Points
Hypertension[b]	1
Abnormal renal[c] and liver function[d]	1 or 2
Stroke	1
Bleeding[e]	1
Labile INRs[f]	1
Elderly (age >65 years)	1
Drugs[g] or alcohol	1 or 2

Interpretation:
  Score ≥3 points: High risk

[a] Severe bleeding, that is, intracranial, requiring hospitalization, associated with >20 g/L decrease in hemoglobin levels, or requiring transfusion.
[b] Systolic blood pressure >160 mm Hg.
[c] Chronic dialysis or renal transplantation or serum creatinine >200 μmol/L.
[d] Chronic liver disease (eg, cirrhosis) or biochemical evidence of significant liver derangement (eg, bilirubin >2 × ULN + ALT/AST/alkaline phosphatase >3 × ULN).
[e] History of bleeding, predisposition to bleeding, or both (eg, bleeding diathesis, anemia).
[f] Unstable/high INR or INR frequently (eg, >40% of test results) outside the therapeutic range.
[g] Concomitant treatment with antiplatelet agents or NSAIDs.

ALT, alanine aminotransferase; AST, aspartate aminotransferase; INR, international normalized ratio; NSAID, nonsteroidal anti-inflammatory drug; ULN, upper limit of normal

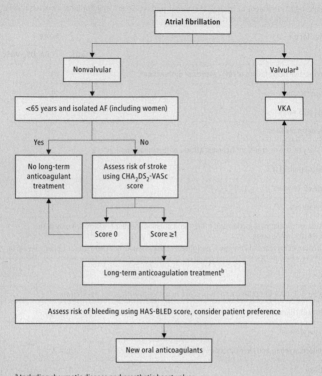

Figure 4-8. Algorithm for prevention of thromboembolism in patients with atrial fibrillation. *Adapted from the 2012 European Society of Cardiology guidelines.*

2) **In patients with AF of documented duration <48 hours,** pharmacologic or electrical cardioversion may be performed immediately after the administration of heparin. Oral anticoagulation should be started immediately for ≥4 weeks, depending on the risk factors for thromboembolism (CHA_2DS_2-VASc score; →above).

3. Prevention of thromboembolism in patients with AF after percutaneous coronary intervention (PCI): This field is rapidly changing and no uniform strong recommendations are relevant in all patients. More recently, dual therapy with modified direct oral anticoagulant (DOAC) doses (in the range of 25%-75% of the full anticoagulation dose) plus clopidogrel have been reported to be noninferior to triple therapy with a VKA with respect to the risk of thromboembolic events, with fewer bleeding events than in the case of triple therapy. Selection of dual therapy (a DOAC or warfarin plus clopidogrel) or triple therapy is based on the presence of clinical and angiographic high-risk features. Prasugrel and ticagrelor should be avoided in conjunction with DOACs.

4.2.2.2. Atrial Flutter

→ DEFINITION, ETIOLOGY, PATHOGENESIS

Atrial flutter (AFL) is a macroreentrant arrhythmia (spinning around a large circuit in the atrium) characterized by a regular atrial rate (usually 250-300 beats/min) and a constant P wave morphology. Paroxysmal AFL can occur in patients with no apparent structural heart disease, whereas chronic AFL is usually associated with preexisting conditions, such as valvular or ischemic heart disease or cardiomyopathy. Those at the highest risk of developing AFL are men, older adults, and individuals with preexisting heart failure or chronic obstructive pulmonary disease. In ~60% of cases AFL occurs as part of an acute disease process.

In >90% of patients with AFL, the AFL circuit involves the cavotricuspid isthmus (CTI), which is the critical area for sustaining the flutter and where efforts to ablate may be directed. AFL can occur in clinical settings similar to those associated with atrial fibrillation (AF) and may be triggered by atrial tachycardia (AT) or AF. Non–CTI-dependent flutter is called **atypical** and is commonly seen in patients with previous AF ablation, severe left atrial disease, or previous atrial surgery.

→ CLINICAL FEATURES AND NATURAL HISTORY

AFL is frequently recurrent and attacks are usually accompanied by tachyarrhythmia. Some patients may be asymptomatic in chronic AFL. Antiarrhythmic drugs and heart rate medications are less effective in AFL than in other types of supraventricular arrhythmias and thus a general recommendation is to either combine atrioventricular (AV) nodal blockers if rate control is intended or consider electrical cardioversion.

In individuals with AF treated with class Ic drugs (→Table 4-1), there is a small risk of AF organizing into AFL, and this is the reason why flecainide should always be associated with an AV nodal blocker. This is not the case for propafenone.

Clinical signs and symptoms largely depend on the type and severity of the underlying condition and include palpitations (most commonly), dyspnea, weakness, or chest pain. Some patients may be asymptomatic. Heart rates are fast (~150 beats/min) and regular.

→ DIAGNOSIS

Diagnostic Tests

Electrocardiography (ECG): Typical AFL (CTI-dependent, counterclockwise rotation around the tricuspid valve) is characterized by dominant negative flutter waves in the inferior leads and a positive P wave in lead V_1. Reverse typical AFL (CTI-dependent, counterclockwise rotation around the valve) shows the opposite pattern, with a positive flutter wave in the inferior leads and a negative P wave in lead V_1. Carotid sinus massage or adenosine can be useful to transiently increase the degree of the AV block and facilitate diagnosis.

Differential Diagnosis

Supraventricular tachycardia: →Figure 4-2. Narrow-QRS tachycardia: →Figure 4-3. Wide-QRS tachycardia: →Figure 4-4.

→ TREATMENT

Classification of antiarrhythmic drugs: →Table 4-1.

Antiarrhythmic agents: →Table 4-2.

AFL treatment algorithm: →Figure 4-9.

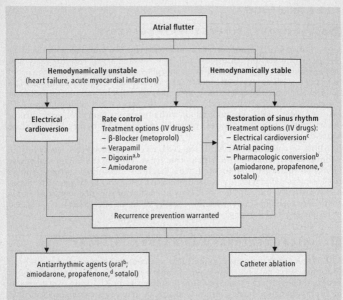

Figure 4-9. Treatment of atrial flutter. *Adapted from guidelines by the American College of Cardiology, American Heart Association, and European Society of Cardiology.*

Acute Management

1. Electrical cardioversion: AFL does not respond well to drugs in general. Electrical cardioversion should be considered early in the management of patents with AFL. Usually a low-energy (50-100 J) shock is used. Prevention of thromboembolism is used as in AF (→Chapter 3.4.2.2.1).

2. Pharmacologic treatment: →Figure 4-9.

Long-Term Management

Guidelines for drug selection (→Figure 4-9) are similar to those used in AF, but the effectiveness of antiarrhythmic drugs is significantly inferior to ablation and lower than when used for AF. Rate control may also be difficult to achieve in AFL. In CTI-dependent AFL, **catheter ablation** has a high success rate with a very low complication rate and may be offered even to patients after a first well-tolerated AFL attack. In atypical AFL, ablation is a more complex procedure with higher recurrence rates and should be considered depending on the patient's profile.

➡ COMPLICATIONS

AFL increases the risk of thromboembolic complications, including ischemic stroke. Therefore, thromboembolism prevention is required, as in patients with AF (→Chapter 3.4.2.2.1).

4.2.2.3. Atrial Tachycardia

→ **DEFINITION, ETIOLOGY, PATHOGENESIS**

Atrial tachycardia (AT) is a paroxysmal or sustained tachycardia originating in the atrium outside the sinus node. **AT may be divided into 2 types:**

1) **Focal AT**: An accelerated (100-250 beats/min) regular rhythm originating in the atrium with a stable P wave morphology. It can occur in patients with or without heart disease.

2) **Multifocal AT**: An irregular rhythm with varying morphology of the P waves. It is commonly seen in patients with cardiac or lung disease and metabolic or electrolytic disturbances.

→ **CLINICAL FEATURES AND NATURAL HISTORY**

Symptoms range from mild or nonexistent to severe, depending on the heart rate during tachycardia and presence of an underlying condition. AT sustained over a long period may lead to tachycardia-induced cardiomyopathy. AT does not cause thromboembolic complications but it may trigger atrial fibrillation (AF).

→ **DIAGNOSIS**

Diagnostic Tests

1. Electrocardiography (ECG): In patients with focal AT, P waves are identical and their shape depends on the location of the anatomical focus (they can also resemble sinus rhythm if coming from a close-by location). In multifocal AT the rhythm is grossly irregular and several morphologies of P waves are seen.

2. Electrophysiologic study (EPS): This is used to establish the exact location of the AT focus and to perform ablation.

Differential Diagnosis

Supraventricular tachycardia: →Figure 4-2. Narrow-QRS tachycardia: →Figure 4-3. Wide-QRS tachycardia: →Figure 4-4.

→ **TREATMENT**

Treatment is more difficult than in the case of atrioventricular nodal reentrant tachycardia and atrioventricular reentrant tachycardia. Effective management of underlying conditions is important.

Acute Management

1. IV β-blockers, diltiazem, or verapamil are useful in hemodynamically stable patients.

2. Synchronized cardioversion is recommended for acute treatment in hemodynamically unstable patients.

3. Adenosine can be useful in the acute setting to either restore sinus rhythm (some atrial arrhythmias respond to adenosine) or diagnose the tachycardia mechanism. In the case of AT, atrial arrhythmia may continue during the atrioventricular block induced by adenosine, making the P waves clearly visible. It is important to record an ECG strip during adenosine administration.

Long-Term Management

1. In patients with **symptomatic focal AT**, catheter ablation is recommended as an alternative to pharmacologic treatment.

2. In patients with **focal AT**, oral β-blockers, diltiazem, or verapamil are recommended for ongoing management.

3. Flecainide or propafenone can be effective in patients with no structural heart disease.

4. In **multifocal AT** catheter ablation is less effective. Oral verapamil or diltiazem are recommended in this case.

4.2.2.4. Atrioventricular Nodal Reentrant Tachycardia

➡ DEFINITION, ETIOLOGY, PATHOGENESIS

Atrioventricular nodal reentrant tachycardia (AVNRT) is a paroxysmal tachycardia that occurs in patients with dual atrioventricular (AV) node physiology, as they have both a fast nodal pathway with a longer refractory period and a slow nodal pathway with a shorter refractory period. It is most commonly observed in individuals with no underlying structural heart disease.

Types of AVNRT:

1) Typical and most common type of AVNRT: Anterograde conduction (from the atrium to the ventricle) proceeds over the slow pathway and retrograde conduction (from the ventricle to the atrium) proceeds over the fast pathway (**slow-fast AVNRT**).

2) Atypical AVNRT: Anterograde conduction proceeds over the fast pathway and retrograde conduction proceeds over the slow pathway (**fast-slow AVNRT**).

➡ CLINICAL FEATURES AND NATURAL HISTORY

AVNRT usually occurs in young patients, causing paroxysmal palpitations that abruptly start and stop. The palpitations are usually relatively well tolerated, as no concomitant structural heart disease is found and the heart rates are usually ≤170 to 180 beats/min. Patients may describe a sensation of rapid regular pounding in the neck during tachycardia. The attacks may be frequent (up to several a day) and may require emergency care.

➡ DIAGNOSIS

Electrocardiography (ECG): Typical AVNRT is characterized by the absence of evident P waves, which are hidden in or present immediately after the QRS complex (short RP interval) but may distort the terminal portion of the QRS by mimicking an S wave in the inferior leads or an r wave in lead V_1. In atypical AVNRT the RP interval is long (RP interval > PR interval). In both typical and atypical AVNRTs the P waves are negative in the inferior leads.

➡ TREATMENT

Classification of antiarrhythmic drugs: →Table 4-1.

Antiarrhythmic agents: →Table 4-2.

Acute Management

1. Termination of an AVNRT attack:

1) Vagal maneuvers (eg, Valsalva,⊘◯ carotid massage, and facial immersion in cold water) should be initiated to terminate the arrhythmia or to modify AV conduction.

2) IV adenosine as a bolus of 6 mg. If not effective, 12 or 18 mg can be given after 1 to 2 minutes.

3) IV β-blockers, diltiazem, or verapamil are a reasonable option in stable patients.

4) Direct current cardioversion should be performed for acute treatment in hemodynamically unstable patients.

2. Recurrence prevention:

1) In patients with **frequently recurring AVNRT attacks who prefer long--term oral treatment to ablation**, use diltiazem, verapamil, or a β-blocker.

2) In patients with **no structural heart disease who do not respond to drugs that inhibit AV node conduction** (→above), use flecainide or propafenone.

3) In **minimally symptomatic patients with AVNRT**, clinical follow-up without pharmacologic therapy or ablation is reasonable.

4) In patients with **poorly tolerated AVNRT, recurrent attacks, and significant symptoms, as well as in those with mild and well-tolerated symptoms who wish to achieve a complete cure of AVNRT**, catheter ablation of the slow pathway is indicated. This is the most successful treatment method, although associated with a low risk (0.5%-1%) of AV block requiring pacemaker implantation.

4.2.2.5. Manifest and Concealed Accessory Pathways

→ DEFINITION, ETIOLOGY, PATHOGENESIS

Preexcitation syndromes refer to a form of congenital arrhythmias resulting from the presence of accessory pathways, that is, muscle fibers bypassing the physiologic conduction system and causing an early activation of a part of the ventricle. The most common type is **Wolff-Parkinson-White (WPW) syndrome**, which refers to the presence of an accessory pathway in association with supraventricular tachycardia (SVT).

Tachyarrhythmias observed in patients with WPW syndrome:

1) **Orthodromic atrioventricular reentrant tachycardia (AVRT)** (>85% of patients): A narrow-QRS tachycardia with anterograde conduction (from the atrium to the ventricle) over the atrioventricular (AV) node and retrograde conduction (from the ventricle to the atrium) over the accessory pathway.

2) **Antidromic AV tachycardia**: A wide-QRS tachycardia with anterograde conduction over the accessory pathway and retrograde conduction over the AV node or another accessory pathway.

3) **Preexcited atrial fibrillation (AF)**: AF with rapid ventricular response, usually with varying degrees of preexcitation (different QRS widths). This may develop in patients with an accessory pathway capable of fast conduction.

→ CLINICAL FEATURES AND NATURAL HISTORY

Symptoms (mainly palpitations) are seen in ~50% of patients with electrocardiographic (ECG) features of preexcitation and usually start during childhood; a new diagnosis of preexcitation in older individuals is rare. The presenting event may be ventricular fibrillation or sometimes syncope requiring hospital admission. Compared with healthy population, the risk of sudden cardiac death is increased particularly in symptomatic patients.

→ DIAGNOSIS

Diagnostic Tests

1. ECG:

1) **Features of ventricular preexcitation during sinus rhythm**: A shortened PR interval (<0.12 seconds) and a wide QRS with a delta wave in the first portion of the QRS. If preexcitation is not clear, one option is to repeat

the ECG during IV administration of adenosine to block the AV node and reveal the accessory pathway (→Figure 4-10).

2) **ECG recorded during SVT:**

a) **Orthodromic AVRT**: A regular narrow QRS, a retrograde P wave usually visible in the first portion of the ST segment (short-RP tachycardia).

b) **Antidromic AVRT**: A regular wide QRS of a fully preexcited morphology (morphology resembles preexcitation during sinus rhythm but QRS is wider).

c) **Preexcited AF**: An irregularly irregular rhythm with varying widths of QRS depending on the degree of preexcitation. At times there is a very rapid ventricular response.

2. Electrophysiologic study (EPS) is used to confirm the presence of an accessory pathway, establish the number and location of the pathways, assess their refractory periods, and to induce tachyarrhythmia to confirm the diagnosis.

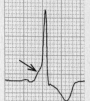

Figure 4-10. Preexcitation syndrome: short PR interval, delta wave on the ascending arm of the R wave (arrow), ST segment and T wave discordant with the QRS complex.

Differential Diagnosis

SVT: →Figure 4-2. Narrow-QRS tachycardia: →Figure 4-3. Wide-QRS tachycardia: →Figure 4-4.

An abnormal QRS shape resulting from preexcitation may mimic myocardial infarction (MI), bundle branch blocks, or ventricular hypertrophy.

→ TREATMENT

Acute Management

Termination of SVT:

1) **Orthodromic (narrow-QRS) AVRT:**

a) Same as for AVNRT (→Chapter 3.4.2.2.4).

b) Vagal maneuvers.

c) IV adenosine, diltiazem, verapamil, or β-blockers can be used.

d) Synchronized cardioversion should be considered in hemodynamically unstable patients and in stable patients when pharmacologic therapy is ineffective or contraindicated.

e) IV ibutilide or IV procainamide is beneficial for acute treatment in patients with preexcited AF. If not available, IV amiodarone could be considered.

2) **Antidromic (wide-QRS) AVRT**: Administer antiarrhythmic drugs that act on the accessory pathway (eg, procainamide, amiodarone, flecainide, propafenone) or perform cardioversion. If preexcited AF has been excluded, a trial of adenosine or nodal blockers is an acceptable choice.

3) **Preexcited AF**: Adenosine and nodal blockers (calcium antagonists, β-blockers) should not be used, as they may predispose to rapid ventricular rates and trigger ventricular fibrillation.

Long-Term Management

1. Patients with **asymptomatic preexcitation**:

1) EPS is reasonable to evaluate the risk for arrhythmic events. If the EPS identifies a high risk for arrhythmic events, catheter ablation is recommended.

2) The finding of abrupt loss of conduction over a manifest pathway during an exercise test or ambulatory monitoring is useful to identify patients at low risk of preexcited AF (the pathway would not be able to conduct at a very high heart rate during AF).

2. In patients with **WPW syndrome causing symptomatic but well-tolerated arrhythmia**, catheter ablation is considered first-line therapy, as it is highly effective and carries a low risk of complications. Medications are generally stopped after a successful procedure.

3. In patients with **AVRT but without preexcitation on their resting ECG**, oral β-blockers, diltiazem, or verapamil are indicated for ongoing management. The confirmation of AVRT if preexcitation is not present on ECG during sinus rhythm can only be made with an EPS.

4. In patients with **preexcitation and SVT who are not candidates for ablation**, treat with flecainide or propafenone to block conduction through the accessory pathway. If not available or contraindicated, amiodarone or sotalol may also be considered.

5. In patients with **WPW syndrome causing AF with fast conduction or poorly tolerated AVRT**, catheter ablation is highly recommended.

4.2.2.6. Sinus Tachyarrhythmias

→ DEFINITION, ETIOLOGY, PATHOGENESIS

Sinus tachyarrhythmias comprise various arrhythmias associated with different mechanisms, natural history, and prognosis.

1. Physiologic sinus tachycardia: A fast sinus rhythm (>100 beats/min) in response to a physiologic stimulus (exercise, stress) or pathologic condition (fever, hypovolemia, anemia, heart failure, thyrotoxicosis, pheochromocytoma, drugs).

2. Inappropriate sinus tachycardia: A sustained fast sinus rhythm (>100 beats/min) unrelated or disproportionate to the stimulus. It results from increased automaticity of the sinus node and its abnormal autonomic regulation. Most commonly observed in young women.

→ CLINICAL FEATURES

Inappropriate sinus tachycardia has variable clinical features and may range from being entirely asymptomatic to completely disabling. The most common symptoms include palpitations, chest pain, dyspnea, dizziness, and presyncope.

→ DIAGNOSIS

Inappropriate Sinus Tachycardia

1. Exclude underlying systemic conditions. Electrocardiography (ECG) reveals persistent daytime sinus tachycardia (>100 beats/min) and P waves of the same morphology as in sinus rhythm. Response to daily activities is exaggerated and heart rate normalizes at night.

2. Tilt table testing can help to identify inappropriate sinus tachycardia that can lead to fainting, also known as postural tachycardia syndrome (POTS).

→ TREATMENT

1. Classification of antiarrhythmic drugs: →Table 4-1.

2. Antiarrhythmic agents: →Table 4-2.

3. β-Blockers are the first-line drugs in inappropriate sinus tachycardia. In patients not responding to this treatment, consider ivabradine. Catheter ablation to modify the sinus node is rarely required.

4.3. Ventricular Arrhythmias

➡ **DEFINITION, ETIOLOGY**

Ventricular tachycardias (VTs) are wide-QRS rhythms (QRS complex >120 milliseconds) that originate in the ventricle. Depending on the presence and type of structural heart disease, they are classified into 3 main types:

1) Idiopathic VT.
2) VT following myocardial infarction.
3) VT in nonischemic cardiomyopathy.

4.3.1. Brugada Syndrome

➡ **DEFINITION, ETIOLOGY**

Brugada syndrome (BrS) is a rare autosomal dominant disease that is 8 times more prevalent in men than in women; it is also more frequent in eastern Asia, where it affects 0.05% to 0.1% of the general population. Disease onset is usually between the age of 20 and 40 years but sometimes may occur earlier, particularly in patients with malignant arrhythmias.

➡ **CLINICAL FEATURES**

Key clinical features include syncope caused by fast polymorphic ventricular tachycardia (VT), cardiac arrest, or sudden cardiac death (SCD). SCD typically occurs at night. Syncope may be a preliminary symptom.

➡ **DIAGNOSIS**

Electrocardiography (ECG) during sinus rhythm has a distinctive pattern and is characterized by an ST-segment elevation of $\geq$2 mm with a negative T wave in $\geq$1 right precordial leads (V_1-V_3) positioned in the fourth, third, or second intercostal space. This Brugada ECG pattern can be transient and is typically apparent in patients with high fever. Sodium channel blocker antiarrhythmic drugs (flecainide, procainamide, ajmaline) can unmask the pattern.

There are 3 described ECG patterns but only the type 1 morphology is diagnostic of BrS. In case of clinical suspicion of BrS in the absence of a spontaneous type 1 ST-segment elevation, a pharmacologic challenge using a sodium channel blocker is recommended. When a type 1 ST-segment elevation is unmasked using a sodium channel blocker, the diagnosis of BrS should require that the patient also present with 1 of the following: documented ventricular fibrillation (VF) or polymorphic VT, syncope of a probable arrhythmic cause, family history of SCD at <45 years with negative autopsy, coved-type ECG in family members, or nocturnal gasping. The diagnosis of BrS can be challenging.

Differential Diagnosis

Differential diagnosis of right precordial ST-segment elevation includes atypical right bundle branch block, early repolarization, acute myocardial ischemia, arrhythmogenic right ventricular cardiomyopathy, and pectus excavatum.

➡ **TREATMENT**

Classification of antiarrhythmic drugs: →Table 4-1.

Antiarrhythmic agents: →Table 4-2.

1. Implantable cardioverter-defibrillator (ICD) is the first-line therapy for patients with BrS presenting with aborted SCD or documented VT or VF. ICDs can be used prophylactically in BrS patients with a spontaneous manifest ECG pattern (type 1) and unexplained syncope.

2. Asymptomatic patients with a Brugada ECG pattern (type 1), either sponta-neous or induced by sodium channel blockers, can be closely followed without an ICD after seeking expert advice.

3. Quinidine may be considered, if available, in BrS patients presenting with electrical storm or frequent ICD shocks. It may also be useful in patients who qualify for an ICD but the device is unavailable, refused, or contraindicated.

4.3.2. Catecholaminergic Polymorphic Ventricular Tachycardia

→ DEFINITION, ETIOLOGY

Catecholaminergic polymorphic ventricular tachycardia (CPVT) is a rare genetic disorder characterized by symptomatic ventricular tachycardia (VT) associated with adrenergic activation in patients with no structural heart disease.

→ CLINICAL FEATURES

More than 60% of patients have an episode of syncope or cardiac arrest before the age of 20 years. Life-threatening arrhythmias are recurrent. In addition to malig-nant VT, patients may have other types of arrhythmia, such as atrial fibrillation.

The key symptoms include syncope caused by fast polymorphic VT, cardiac ar-rest, or sudden cardiac death, most commonly triggered by exercise or emotions.

→ DIAGNOSIS

Diagnosis is based on identifying the arrhythmia typical for CPVT: a fast, polymorphic, frequently bidirectional VT (beat-to-beat changes in the QRS polarity from negative to positive or vice versa), which is most easily triggered by an exercise test.

→ TREATMENT

Classification of antiarrhythmic drugs: →Table 4-1.

Antiarrhythmic agents: →Table 4-2.

Avoidance of exercise, treatment with β-blockers. Placement of an implantable cardioverter-defibrillator (ICD) is indicated in patients with a history of car-diac arrest as well as in those with syncope or VT despite β-blocker treatment.

4.3.3. Congenital Long-QT Syndrome

→ DEFINITION, ETIOLOGY, PATHOGENESIS

Congenital long-QT syndrome (LQTS) refers to genetic abnormalities of ion channels (channelopathies) characterized by a long QT interval with an in-creased risk of polymorphic ventricular tachycardia (VT) (torsades de pointes) and sudden cardiac death (SCD). Overall, 13 types of LQTS caused by >500 mu-tations have been identified. The most common clinical types are types 1, 2, and 3 (LQT1, LQT2, LQT3).

→ CLINICAL FEATURES AND NATURAL HISTORY

Most patients are asymptomatic. Syncope can occur, commonly caused by ventricular tachyarrhythmia or ventricular fibrillation (VF). Episodes may be triggered by emotions, exercise, or noise. Family history includes syncope or SCD, particularly at a young age. The condition is associated with an elevated risk of SCD, especially in patients with a history of syncope, QTc >500 milliseconds, documented polymorphic VT, prior cardiac arrest, and when combined with syndactyly or deafness syndromes.

→ DIAGNOSIS

Diagnostic Criteria

Diagnosis is based on clinical symptoms, history, genetic studies, and electro-cardiography (ECG) results: The normal upper limit for QTc is 470 milliseconds in adult men and 480 milliseconds in adult women, with a significant overlap between the normal spectrum and genetically affected individuals with no or only mild QT prolongation. Concealed long QT may be unmasked by either an exercise test or epinephrine challenge. The occurrence of torsades de pointes depends on the degree of QT prolongation and most of the times is triggered by a short—long—short sequence (ventricular premature beat [VPB]—pause after the VPB—another VPB and tachycardia).

Genetic studies play an important role in the diagnosis of LQTS as well as in prognosis assessment and therapeutic decision-making.

Differential Diagnosis

Acquired LQTS may present with syncope, SCD, or polymorphic VT (torsades de pointes). Causes include electrolyte disturbances (hypokalemia, hypomagnesemia, hypocalcemia) or drugs such as antiarrhythmic agents (amiodarone, sotalol), antihistamines (hydroxyzine, loratadine, terfenadine), antimicrobial agents (erythromycin, clarithromycin, moxifloxacin, trimethoprim), antimalarial drugs (chloroquine), or psychiatric drugs; a complete list of agents can be found at crediblemeds.org. Symptoms of acquired LQTS are very similar to those of congenital LQTS, with ECG also showing prolonged QT intervals. A thorough history including all drugs taken by the patient and measurements of serum potassium, magnesium, and calcium are crucial for diagnosis.

→ TREATMENT

Classification of antiarrhythmic drugs: →Table 4-1.

Antiarrhythmic agents: →Table 4-2.

1. Avoid drugs causing QT prolongation.

2. Correct electrolyte disturbances.

3. Eliminate triggers (strenuous activity in patients with LQT1).

4. β-Blocker treatment at the maximum tolerated doses is indicated, particularly in patients with LQT1 and LQT2. The preferred agents are nadolol and propranolol. In patients with LQT3, flecainide may be effective.

5. Placement of an **implantable cardioverter-defibrillator (ICD)** is indicated after seeking expert advice for secondary prevention of SCD in patients with a history of cardiac arrest as well as malignant syncope, VT, or both despite β-blocker therapy. Prophylactic implantation of an ICD may be advisable in patients at high risk of SCD, (eg, with extremely long QT, congenital deafness, double mutations, or mutations associated with a particularly high risk of SCD). In patients in whom β-blockers are contraindicated, poorly tolerated, or ineffective, surgical removal of the left stellate (sympathetic) ganglion is an option.

6. Pacemaker implantation may be useful in patients with congenital or acquired LQTS where ventricular arrhythmias are related to pauses or bradyarrhythmia.

4.3.4. Idiopathic Ventricular Fibrillation

→ DEFINITION, ETIOLOGY

Idiopathic ventricular fibrillation (IVF) is a spontaneous ventricular fibrillation in individuals without an identified structural heart disease, genetic arrhythmic disorder, or other obvious cause (eg, drug overdose). IVF is responsible for ~5% of cases of cardiac arrest.

→ DIAGNOSIS

Exclude structural heart disease on the basis of history (including family history), physical examination, laboratory studies, electrocardiography, and echocardiography. Cardiac magnetic resonance imaging may be a useful tool to rule out subtle structural disease. Ischemic cardiomyopathy should be excluded taking into consideration the clinical presentation and risk factors (consider exercise testing, coronary computed tomography scan, and cardiac catheterization with coronary angiography). Exclude the administration of drugs causing long-QT syndrome, electrolyte disturbances, alcohol, and drugs of abuse. Electrophysiologic study is of no prognostic value and is not routinely recommended.

→ TREATMENT

Placement of an implantable cardioverter-defibrillator (ICD) is recommended in all survivors.

4.3.5. Idiopathic Ventricular Tachycardia

→ DEFINITION, ETIOLOGY, PATHOGENESIS

Idiopathic ventricular tachycardias (VTs) include 2 types of focal arrhythmias: outflow tract VT and fascicular VT (left septal VT) in patients without structural heart disease. These arrhythmias are idiopathic and generally associated with a good prognosis. They may present as frequent premature ventricular contractions (PVCs) or episodes of sustained VT.

→ CLINICAL FEATURES AND NATURAL HISTORY

Symptoms range from none (asymptomatic) to paroxysmal palpitations. Symptom severity depends on the hemodynamic significance of the arrhythmia. Patients with very frequent PVCs (>30% of total beats in 24 hours) may develop cardiomyopathy. Symptoms are frequently exacerbated by stress or exercise.

→ DIAGNOSIS

Electrocardiography (ECG):
1) **Outflow tract VT**: The most common type, either in the form of monomorphic PVCs or monomorphic VT. The hallmark is an inferior axis on ECG (positive QRS in the inferior leads; →Figure 4-11).
2) **Fascicular VT**: The most common origin is the left posterior fascicle of the left bundle branch. ECG during tachycardia reveals a slightly widened QRS (usually <140 milliseconds, not as wide as in other VTs) with right bundle branch block (RBBB) and a left axis deviation (negative QRS in the inferior leads).

Differential Diagnosis

Differential diagnosis should include other types of VT or supraventricular tachycardia with aberrancy. It is important to exclude structural heart disease and to analyze QRS morphology during the arrhythmia. VT in arrhythmogenic right ventricular cardiomyopathy can resemble benign right outflow tachycardia; determination of the nature of ventricular arrhythmia in this case is an evolving field requiring expert input.

→ TREATMENT

Classification of antiarrhythmic drugs: →Table 4-1.
Antiarrhythmic agents: →Table 4-2.

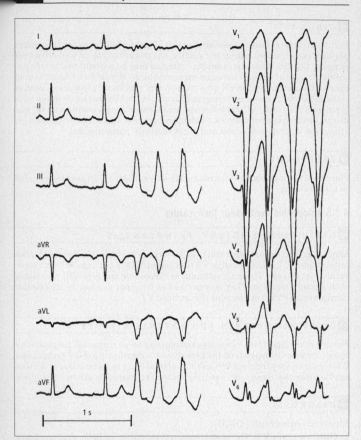

Figure 4-11. Episode of monomorphic right ventricular outflow tract tachycardia.

1. Fascicular VT commonly responds to verapamil (IV or oral).

2. When outflow tract VT/PVCs are suspected, β-blockers, diltiazem, or verapamil should be considered. This type of VT may also respond to class Ic antiarrhythmics.

3. Catheter ablation is indicated in patients with symptomatic right ventricular outflow tract VT or fascicular VT who do not respond to antiarrhythmic drugs, are not willing to take medications on a long-term basis, or cannot tolerate the drugs.

4.3.6. Ventricular Arrhythmia Following Myocardial Infarction

→ DEFINITION, ETIOLOGY, PATHOGENESIS

Patients after myocardial infarction (MI) can develop a myriad of ventricular arrhythmias. **Polymorphic ventricular tachycardia (VT) or ventricular fibrillation (VF)** can develop in the acute phase of MI or during periods of acute ischemia at a later stage. Scar-related arrhythmia (chronic phase of ischemic cardiomyopathy) is usually manifested as **monomorphic VT**, either nonsustained (NSVT) or sustained. Sustained monomorphic VT usually develops in patients with more extensive necrosis and depressed left ventricular (LV) function; this type of VT is related to a reentrant circuit within the myocardial scar.

➔ CLINICAL FEATURES AND NATURAL HISTORY

NSVT may be asymptomatic. However, sustained VT occurring in this group of patients, particularly during faster rhythms (>150-170 beats/min), may cause significant hemodynamic abnormalities leading to hypotension, chest pain, heart failure, syncope, or cardiac arrest (VT can transform into VF).

➔ DIAGNOSIS

Electrocardiography (ECG): →Figure 3-1. Polymorphic VT or VF is manifested as a chaotic ventricular rhythm. Sustained monomorphic VT presents as a wide-complex tachycardia and needs to be differentiated from supraventricular tachycardia with aberrancy and from antidromic atrioventricular reentrant tachycardia. The morphology of the VT can help define the origin (myocardial earliest activation point). For example, in a patient with a previous apical MI (the left anterior descending artery [LAD] territory), a monomorphic VT would have predominantly negative QRS in the precordial leads.

➔ TREATMENT

Classification of antiarrhythmic drugs: →Table 4-1.
Antiarrhythmic agents: →Table 4-2.

Acute Management
→Chapter 3.11.1.2 and →Figure 4-12.

Long-Term Management

1. Optimize ischemic heart disease treatment, including revascularization and treatment of LV dysfunction or heart failure. All patients should receive a β-blocker unless contraindicated.

2. Antiarrhythmic medications: Patients who had VT or VF while on β-blocker therapy may be considered for a trial of amiodarone to prevent arrhythmia recurrence. Although sotalol is less effective, it is still an option for patients who cannot use amiodarone.

3. Catheter ablation of VT was shown to reduce recurrent episodes of VT, particularly in patients already receiving amiodarone.

4. Implantable cardioverter-defibrillator (ICD): This is indicated for secondary prevention of sudden cardiac death (SCD) in patients who have survived VF or VT causing hemodynamic instability unless the episode occurred in the setting of acute ischemia with a treatable cause. The primary indication (individuals at risk for SCD who have not had an episode yet) includes patients >40 days after MI with an LV ejection fraction ≤30 to 35%. If ICD implantation is not possible despite indications (lack of patient consent, contraindications, lack of resources), administer amiodarone or sotalol.

4.3.7. Ventricular Tachycardia in Patients With Nonischemic Cardiomyopathy

➔ DEFINITION, ETIOLOGY, PATHOGENESIS

Cardiomyopathies with or without depressed left ventricular (LV) function may be associated with ventricular arrhythmias, most commonly paroxysmal monomorphic ventricular tachycardia (VT).

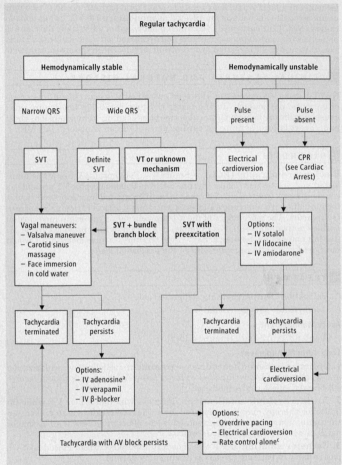

Figure 4-12. Acute management of patients with regular tachycardia. *Adapted from guidelines by the American College of Cardiology, American Heart Association, and European Society of Cardiology.*

Patients with dilated or hypertrophic cardiomyopathy can present with monomorphic VT or with ventricular fibrillation (VF) usually coming from the LV. In arrhythmogenic right ventricular cardiomyopathy, monomorphic VT is most frequently originating in the right ventricle, thus having a left bundle branch block (LBBB) appearance.

➡ CLINICAL FEATURES AND NATURAL HISTORY

Clinical features depend on the VT rate and severity of cardiomyopathy. VT episodes may be recurrent and increase the risk of sudden cardiac death (SCD).

➡ DIAGNOSIS

Like in patients after myocardial infarction (MI), the myocardial origin of the monomorphic VT can be generally assessed by the electrocardiographic (ECG) appearance (right bundle branch block [RBBB]-like vs LBBB-like when coming from the left or right ventricle, respectively) and the axis (superior or inferior).

Bundle branch reentrant VT is a rare type of VT that can occur in patients with cardiomyopathy and abnormal His-Purkinje conduction (wide baseline QRS). It is a circuit that uses both bundle branches. Usually the myocardium is activated by the right bundle, which is why the VT has an LBBB appearance.

➡ TREATMENT

Classification of antiarrhythmic drugs: →Table 4-1.

Antiarrhythmic agents: →Table 4-2.

1. Treatment includes β-blockers and antiarrhythmics. Ablation may reduce the burden of VT, although results are not as good as in ischemic VT ablation. An implantable cardioverter-defibrillator (ICD) is almost always indicated in patients who have had VT or VF episodes and in specific populations as a prophylactic indication (based on LV ejection fraction). Indications for prophylactic ICD implantation in patients with cardiomyopathy to prevent SCD: →Chapter 3.4.1.

2. In patients with **bundle branch reentrant VT**, the recommended treatment is catheter ablation. Patients may require pacemaker insertion after the procedure. Antiarrhythmic therapy is usually ineffective.

5. Cardiac Tamponade

➡ DEFINITION, ETIOLOGY, PATHOGENESIS

Cardiac tamponade represents the most severe and urgent clinical presentation of pericardial effusion. It occurs when pericardial fluid accumulation exceeds the elastic limit of the pericardium, resulting in significantly elevated intrapericardial pressures. Cardiac tamponade is a life-threatening condition resulting from a slow or more rapid compression of cardiac chambers due to the accumulation of pericardial inflammatory/malignant exudates, pus, blood, clots, or gas.

Causes:

1) Pericarditis (eg, idiopathic; viral; other infectious, including tuberculous pericarditis in developing countries where tuberculosis is endemic).

2) Iatrogenic (eg, invasive procedure–related, as in the case of complications related to percutaneous coronary intervention, atrial fibrillation ablation, pacemaker lead insertion; postpericardiotomy syndrome after cardiac surgery).

3) Neoplasm/malignancy (eg, metastatic breast or lung cancer, lymphoma, melanoma).

4) Trauma.

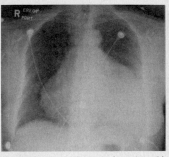

Figure 5-1. Chest radiograph of a patient with cardiac tamponade before pericardiocentesis.

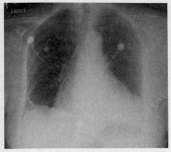

Figure 5-2. Chest radiograph of a patient with cardiac tamponade after pericardiocentesis.

5) Systemic autoimmune disease (eg, systemic lupus erythematosus, rheumatoid arthritis, scleroderma).

6) Post–myocardial infarction.

7) Radiation-induced.

8) Uremia.

9) Myxedema/hypothyroidism.

10) Aortic dissection.

→ CLINICAL FEATURES AND NATURAL HISTORY

1. Symptoms: Dyspnea; reduced exercise tolerance; sometimes cough, dysphagia, syncope or presyncope.

2. Signs: Most common signs include tachycardia (in patients with hypothyroidism or uremia it may be absent), pulsus paradoxus with a systolic arterial pressure drop >10 mm Hg with inspiration, an enlarged cardiac silhouette on chest radiography (before pericardiocentesis: →Figure 5-1; after pericardiocentesis: →Figure 5-2), and jugular venous distention. Other signs include diminished or muffled heart sounds, hypotension, and tachypnea.

3. Natural history: Slowly accumulating effusions cause gradual distension of the pericardium, which allows the accumulation of large pericardial effusions (often ≥1 L). In the case of rapidly accumulating effusions or reduced pericardial elasticity, the intrapericardial pressures increase promptly and lead to cardiac tamponade with as little as a few hundred mL of fluid. Cardiac tamponade can lead to obstructive shock and cardiac arrest.

→ DIAGNOSIS

Diagnostic Tests

1. Electrocardiography (ECG) may occasionally be normal but usually reveals sinus tachycardia. Other potential findings include low QRS voltage (<5 mm in limb leads and <10 mm in precordial leads) and/or electrical alternans of the QRS complex. The end-stages of tamponade are associated with bradycardia, and death is due to pulseless electrical activity (PEA).

2. Chest radiography: Enlargement of the cardiac silhouette without features of pulmonary congestion. In patients with acute cardiac tamponade, the cardiac silhouette may be normal.

3. Echocardiography is the key diagnostic study for evaluating cardiac tamponade, as recognizing tamponade ultimately remains a clinical diagnosis.

In those suspect of having pericardial tamponade, an echocardiogram should be performed without delay. Transthoracic echocardiography can evaluate for the presence of pericardial fluid, and if present, evaluate the size (>20 mm is considered large [→Figure 5-3]) and hemodynamic consequences. Echocardiographic signs of tamponade physiology include:

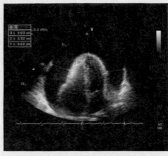

1) Late diastolic and early systolic right atrial collapse.

2) Early diastolic right ventricular free wall collapse (this may be absent in patients with a marked right ventricular hypertrophy or elevated right ventricular diastolic pressures).

Figure 5-3. Transthoracic echocardiogram showing the apical 4-chamber view and a large pericardial effusion.

3) A "swinging heart" within pericardial fluid.

4) Dilation of the inferior vena cava (with loss of the inspiratory collapse).

5) Doppler echocardiography shows exaggerated respiratory variability in mitral and tricuspid inflow velocity.

4. Computed tomography (CT) reveals pericardial effusion. In patients with chylopericardium it may help to locate a connection between the thoracic duct and the pericardium (especially when combined with lymphography).

5. Analysis of the pericardial fluid is used in case of equivocal etiology.

Diagnostic Criteria

Cardiac tamponade is diagnosed on the basis of clinical features and imaging studies, mainly echocardiography.

Differential Diagnosis

Clinical signs of cardiac tamponade should be differentiated from acute right ventricular myocardial infarction and other causes of right ventricular dysfunction.

→ TREATMENT

1. IV fluid bolus may be attempted to temporize (this is not a substitute for definitive treatment); however, only ~50% of patients will have a favorable stroke volume/hemodynamic response to fluid loading.

2. Pericardiocentesis is a life-saving procedure in those with clinical/echocardiographic pericardial tamponade (note that large pericardial effusions do not always cause tamponade, and therefore a clinical and hemodynamic assessment is required). Needle pericardiocentesis with or without pericardial tube insertion using echocardiographic guidance is the preferred method of pericardial fluid drainage if technically feasible.

3. Surgical approaches can be considered if effusion is not amenable to percutaneous needle drainage as well as in case of purulent effusions, recurrent effusions from malignancy requiring pericardial window creation, or hemopericardium with clotted blood.

4. Treatment of chylopericardium depends on the etiology and volume of the lymph in the pericardium. In patients in whom chylopericardium is a postoperative complication, use pericardiocentesis and a diet containing medium-chain triglycerides. If the lymph continues to accumulate, use surgical treatment.

6. Cardiomyopathy

→DEFINITION AND CLASSIFICATION

Cardiomyopathies are myocardial disorders in which the myocardium is structurally and functionally abnormal in the absence of significant coronary artery disease, hypertension, valvular heart disease, or congenital heart disease. These 4 conditions can cause left ventricular dysfunction from volume or pressure overload and are excluded from the classification scheme of cardiomyopathies by the European Society of Cardiology and the American Heart Association.

While classification schemes vary, cardiomyopathies are typically classified according to morphologic phenotypes, which can be further divided into familial or nonfamilial forms.

Classification:

1) **Dilated** cardiomyopathy.
2) **Hypertrophic** cardiomyopathy.
3) **Restrictive** cardiomyopathy.
4) **Arrhythmogenic right ventricular** cardiomyopathy.
5) **Unclassified** cardiomyopathy.

Each of the above 5 types of cardiomyopathy can be further classified as:

1) **Familial** (genetic) cardiomyopathy: Occurrence in more than one family member of a phenotype caused by the same genetic mutation or a de novo mutation in an index patient that can be transmitted to offspring.
2) **Nonfamilial** (nongenetic) cardiomyopathy: Either idiopathic (of an unknown cause) or acquired (associated with toxins, infections, other diseases).

6.1. Arrhythmogenic Right Ventricular Cardiomyopathy

→DEFINITION, ETIOLOGY, PATHOGENESIS

Arrhythmogenic right ventricular cardiomyopathy (ARVC) is a genetic disease involving mainly the right ventricle. It is caused by the gradual replacement of myocardial fibers by fatty and fibrous tissue, particularly in the right ventricular inflow, outflow, and apex, which leads to a propensity to ventricular arrhythmias and sudden cardiac death. Morphologic and functional changes can also occur in the left ventricle (LV), producing a phenotype similar to dilated cardiomyopathy.

Causes: Gene mutations, which are usually autosomal dominant.

→CLINICAL FEATURES AND NATURAL HISTORY

1. History: ARVC usually presents in young adult men. The first symptom is a brief loss of consciousness caused by ventricular arrhythmia. Sudden cardiac death may occur.

2. Risk factors of sudden cardiac death include a young age, history of syncope, cardiac arrest or hemodynamically significant ventricular tachycardia, LV involvement, significant right ventricular damage, sudden cardiac death in a relative aged <35 years, and an epsilon wave on electrocardiography (ECG).

3. Symptoms include palpitations, dizziness, and presyncope or syncope. In more advanced disease, features of right ventricular heart failure develop.

→DIAGNOSIS

Diagnostic Tests

1. ECG: Findings may be transient or invoked upon stress. They may reveal right bundle branch block (RBBB), inverted T waves in right precordial leads,

QRS widening >110 milliseconds in leads V_1 to V_3 and III, S-wave widening >50 milliseconds in leads V_1 to V_3, and an epsilon wave on the descending arm of the QRS complex (this feature is found only in a quarter of patients and is almost pathognomonic for ARVC). Ventricular arrhythmia with LBBB morphology of the QRS complex is frequently seen.

2. Echocardiography reveals impaired right ventricular wall motion and enlargement of the right ventricle.

3. Magnetic resonance imaging (MRI) reveals fatty infiltrates and focal fibrosis in the right ventricular wall. This study is of limited value in the diagnosis of ARVC because of high rates of false-positive results.

Diagnostic Criteria

ARVC is diagnosed on the basis of imaging studies and the presence of severe ventricular arrhythmia. Endomyocardial biopsy is rarely performed because of its low sensitivity.

Differential Diagnosis

ARVC should be differentiated from idiopathic left ventricular outflow tract ventricular tachycardia, Brugada syndrome, Uhl anomaly, right ventricular myocardial infarction, and dilated cardiomyopathy.

→ T R E A T M E N T

1. Symptomatic treatment targets arrhythmia and includes mainly **sotalol**, β-blockers, or **amiodarone**. Agents and dosage: →Table 4-2.

2. Radiofrequency ablation is used in case of intolerance or ineffectiveness of antiarrhythmic agents in patients with life-threatening arrhythmia.

3. Implantable cardioverter-defibrillators (ICDs) are used to prevent sudden cardiac death in patients with severe ventricular arrhythmia and syncope and in patients with a family history of sudden cardiac death.◐○

6.2. Dilated Cardiomyopathy

→ D E F I N I T I O N , E T I O L O G Y , P A T H O G E N E S I S

Dilated cardiomyopathy (DCM) is a disease of the myocardium characterized by dilatation of the left ventricle (LV) and typically global LV systolic dysfunction. In some cases right ventricular dilatation and dysfunction may also be present.

DCM can be familial (eg, muscular dystrophies, mitochondrial cytopathies, inherited metabolic diseases) or acquired from infection (eg, viral myocarditis, Chagas disease), inflammatory causes (eg, systemic lupus erythematosus), toxins (eg, alcohol, cocaine, chemotherapy drugs such as doxorubicin and trastuzumab), nutritional deficiencies (eg, thiamine or carnitine deficiency), endocrinopathies (eg, thyroid disease, acromegaly), tachycardia-induced cardiomyopathy, or peripartum cardiomyopathy. However, in many patients DCM is idiopathic.

→ C L I N I C A L F E A T U R E S A N D N A T U R A L H I S T O R Y

DCM most frequently causes symptoms of heart failure of varying severity (→Chapter 3.8.2). The dynamics of the disease may vary from prolonged asymptomatic periods to rapidly progressive heart failure.

→ D I A G N O S I S

Diagnostic Tests

1. Chest radiographs reveal an enlarged cardiac silhouette and features of pulmonary congestion.

2. Echocardiography usually reveals LV dilatation, eccentric hypertrophy, and systolic dysfunction. Other echocardiographic findings may include functional mitral regurgitation, abnormal LV diastolic function, left atrial dilatation, pulmonary hypertension, and right ventricular dysfunction.

3. Cardiac catheterization is not necessary to make the diagnosis of DCM. However, coronary angiography may be performed to exclude ischemic heart disease as an etiology.

4. Endomyocardial biopsy is rarely indicated and mainly used to exclude active myocarditis in patients with rapidly progressive heart failure.

5. Cardiac magnetic resonance imaging (MRI) may be useful to quantify biventricular function and establish the etiology of the cardiomyopathy.

Diagnostic Criteria

DCM is diagnosed on the basis of history, physical examination, and echocardiography after other causes of LV dilatation have been excluded.

Differential Diagnosis

DCM should be differentiated from cardiomyopathy secondary to ischemia, valvular disease, or prolonged hypertension.

→ TREATMENT

Treatment is the same as in chronic heart failure.

→ SPECIAL CONSIDERATIONS

1. Cardiomyopathy associated with neuromuscular disorders occurs particularly in patients with muscular dystrophy (eg, Duchenne dystrophy, Becker dystrophy, limb-girdle muscular dystrophy, myotonic dystrophy) and Friedreich ataxia. Cardiac complications can include conduction abnormalities, arrhythmias, and sudden cardiac death.

2. Metabolic cardiomyopathy develops in the course of certain endocrine diseases (thyrotoxicosis, hypothyroidism, diabetes mellitus, acromegaly, pheochromocytoma, adrenal insufficiency, severe obesity) or vitamin deficiency (eg, B_1 deficiency causing beriberi). Treatment of the underlying condition may reverse the cardiomyopathy.

3. Peripartum cardiomyopathy (PPCM): The diagnosis is made when LV systolic dysfunction (LV ejection fraction [LVEF] <45%) develops at the end of pregnancy, usually in the third trimester, or within 5 months of delivery in a patient with no prior heart disease and in whom other causes of DCM have been excluded. Risk factors include mothers of a very young age or >30 years, family history of PPCM, multiple births, multiple pregnancy, history of eclampsia or preeclampsia, tobacco smoking, diabetes mellitus, hypertension, poor nutrition, and long-term β-blocker treatment. PPCM resolves spontaneously in ~50% of patients but it may progress to DCM.

Women with peripartum cardiomyopathy have generally been excluded from clinical trials and evidence for treatment is generalized mainly from trials recruiting older patients with mixed cardiomyopathies and heart failure with reduced ejection fraction. Pregnant patients with heart failure should receive the same evidence-informed therapies as those with other causes bearing in mind the medications that are contraindicated during pregnancy and breastfeeding. During pregnancy angiotensin-converting enzyme inhibitors (ACEIs), angiotensin receptor blockers (ARBs), and angiotensin receptor neprilysin inhibitors (ARNIs) are contraindicated and may be substituted with hydralazine and nitrates for afterload reduction. β-Blockers, preferably $β_1$-selective, can be used if tolerated (avoid atenolol). Mineralocorticoid-receptor antagonists are contraindicated during pregnancy. Diuretics should be used only in case of pulmonary edema or congestion.

After delivery, initiation and up-titration of standard heart failure medications are recommended until LVEF normalizes. In breastfeeding patients, the preferred ACEIs are captopril, enalapril, and benazepril. Patients should be cautioned about future pregnancies if the LVEF has not recovered.

4. Alcoholic cardiomyopathy can occur as a result of direct cardiotoxic effects of alcohol. It may have an insidious course with atrial fibrillation often being the presenting feature, but other types of arrhythmia may also be seen. Abstinence from alcohol is recommended in alcoholic cardiomyopathy, as this may lead to a resolution of early cardiomyopathy, while continued alcohol consumption worsens the prognosis.

5. Cardiomyopathy associated with stimulant use: Cocaine, methamphetamine, ecstasy, and bath salts containing cathinone can have significant cardiotoxic effects on the heart. Acute use of cocaine in particular may cause a coronary artery spasm and acute ischemia in addition to direct myocardial damage from the long-term use. Abstinence is certainly recommended. Cardioselective β-blockers are to be avoided for treating cocaine-induced cardiomyopathy and noncardioselective β-blockers are preferred.

6. Tachycardia-induced cardiomyopathy is found in <1% of patients with chronic supraventricular tachycardia (eg, atrial fibrillation or atrial flutter with a rapid ventricular rhythm of 130-200 beats/min) or ventricular tachycardia, mainly sustained. Achieving control of arrhythmia usually leads to the resolution of myocardial dysfunction within ≤3 months.

7. Chemotherapy-induced cardiomyopathy is caused by the toxic effect of drugs on the myocardium. The most commonly involved drugs are chemotherapeutic agents, such as anthracyclines and antibodies to the human epidermal growth factor receptor 2 (HER2). Baseline and serial monitoring of LVEF with echocardiography is recommended during administration of cardiotoxic chemotherapy; discontinuation of the cardiotoxic chemotherapeutic agent may be considered if there is a drop in LVEF >5% or to <55% with concomitant heart failure, or if there is an asymptomatic drop in ejection fraction >10% or to <50%. Anthracyclines may have cardiotoxic effects months or years after administration.

8. Cardiomyopathy associated with sarcoidosis of the heart: Sarcoidosis is a noncaseating granulomatous systemic disease. Cardiac sarcoidosis may precede, occur concurrently with, or follow other organ involvement. Manifestations include ventricular arrhythmias, conduction abnormalities, valve disease, cardiomyopathy, and cor pulmonale. On imaging, sarcoid cardiomyopathy may mimic the appearance of myocardial infarction due to the presence of regional wall motion abnormalities and scar tissue. If diagnosed, glucocorticoid therapy is usually used.

9. Cardiomyopathy associated with HIV: Myocardial changes in HIV are caused by various factors, including HIV viremia, myocarditis, cardiac autoimmunity, and drug toxicity. Treatment is directed at suppressing HIV viremia.

6.3. Hypertrophic Cardiomyopathy

▶ DEFINITION, ETIOLOGY, PATHOGENESIS

Hypertrophic cardiomyopathy (HCM) is a disease of the myocardium that is characterized by an increased left ventricular (LV) wall thickness (>15 mm in any myocardial segment) not explained by conditions that augment LV afterload. HCM is an autosomal dominant disease typically due to genetic mutation or mutations of the sarcomeric proteins causing myocardial disarray.

Patterns of hypertrophy seen in HCM include:

1) **Asymmetric hypertrophy of the interventricular septum**, defined as a septal to posterior wall thickness ratio >1.3 in normotensive individuals or

>1.5 in hypertensive individuals. This may result in systolic anterior motion (SAM) of the mitral valve and dynamic obstruction of the left ventricular outflow tract (LVOT).

2) **Concentric (symmetric) hypertrophy**, defined as an increase in LV wall thickness of all walls not explained by LV loading conditions or infiltrative disease.

3) **Midventricular hypertrophy**, which can give a "dumbbell" appearance to the LV and cause midcavitary obstruction, sometimes resulting in LV apical dilatation and aneurysm.

4) **Apical hypertrophy**, defined as apical wall thickness >15 mm or an apical to basal wall thickness ratio >1.3, can give a "spade" appearance to the LV.

➡ CLINICAL FEATURES AND NATURAL HISTORY

1. Symptoms: Exertional dyspnea, angina, palpitations, dizziness, syncope or presyncope (particularly in patients with LVOT obstruction).

2. Signs: In hypertrophic obstructive cardiomyopathy (HOCM) a systolic murmur may be heard over the left sternal border with radiation towards the right upper sternal border and the apex. The murmur can intensify with a decrease in preload (eg, during the Valsalva maneuver; after standing from a sitting, lying, or squatting position; or following the administration of nitroglycerin/amyl nitrite) and soften with an increase in afterload (passive elevation of a lower extremity, sitting, squatting, or clenching both fists).

3. Natural history depends on the type and severity of myocardial hypertrophy, LVOT gradient, and propensity for ventricular arrhythmia. Most patients have a good prognosis and do not experience complications. Those who do develop complications generally fall into one of 3 pathways: sudden cardiac death/ventricular arrhythmias, heart failure, or paroxysmal/chronic atrial fibrillation.

4. Risk factors for sudden cardiac death: Younger age at diagnosis, non-sustained ventricular tachycardia, LV myocardial thickness ≥30 mm, a family history of sudden cardiac death at a young age (<40 years), unexplained syncope, enlarged left atrial diameter, LVOT gradient >50 mm Hg, abnormal blood pressure response (drop) to exercise (in individuals aged ≤40 years). A calculator for the assessment of the risk of sudden cardiac death in the next 5 years, HCM Risk-SCD Calculator, can be found at www.doc2do.com/hcm/webHCM.html.

➡ DIAGNOSIS

Diagnostic Criteria

HCM is diagnosed morphologically on the basis of results of echocardiography or magnetic resonance imaging (MRI) showing features of myocardial hypertrophy ≥15 mm in a segment of a nondilated LV that cannot be explained only by an increased cardiac load. Genetic testing can be used to confirm the diagnosis and to assess for the presence of HCM in family members.

Diagnostic Tests

1. Electrocardiography (ECG): Nonspecific changes; pathologic Q waves, especially in inferior and lateral leads; left axis deviation; abnormal P waves (indicative of enlargement of the left atrium or both atria); in some patients, deep T-wave inversions in V_2 to V_4; features of LV hypertrophy; ventricular and supraventricular arrhythmias.

2. Holter ECG monitoring is performed to detect ventricular tachycardia, supraventricular tachycardia, and atrial fibrillation (particularly in patients with enlargement of the left atrium). It is also used to establish the need for an implantable cardioverter-defibrillator (ICD) in patients with symptoms of palpitations, dizziness, or unexplained syncope.

3. Echocardiography reveals myocardial hypertrophy, which may either be asymmetric involving the septum, concentric, midventricular, or apical. It should be noted that genotype-positive individuals, including those experiencing sudden cardiac death, may not have significant hypertrophy on imaging. In patients with asymmetric septal hypertrophy (ASH), there may be elongation of the mitral leaflets, SAM of the mitral apparatus, and LVOT gradient. HCM is considered obstructive when the peak gradient across the LVOT at rest or with provocation (eg, Valsalva maneuver, amyl nitrite) is >30 mm Hg. While there is typically impairment in systolic longitudinal function (detected using Doppler imaging or strain), the overall LV ejection fraction (LVEF) may be preserved. LV diastolic function is typically abnormal.

Echocardiography is recommended not only for an initial assessment of every patient suspected of having HCM but also—with ECG—as a screening study in relatives of patients with HCM. A stress echocardiogram may be undertaken to assess LVOT gradients in patients who do not have significant obstruction at rest and after the Valsalva maneuver or administration of amyl nitrite.

4. ECG stress testing can be performed in patients with unexplained syncope or with symptoms of heart failure particularly to assess for systolic blood pressure decrease during exercise.

5. MRI is recommended when echocardiography results are equivocal. MRI can evaluate the morphology of the LV, LV size, diastolic impairment, and degree of myocardial fibrosis.

6. Computed tomography (CT) is recommended when echocardiography results are equivocal in patients with contraindications to MRI.

7. Coronary angiography is recommended in patients with a history of cardiac arrest, with sustained ventricular tachycardia, and in all patients ≥40 years of age in whom invasive treatment of hypertrophy of the interventricular septum is planned.

8. Genetic testing is recommended in all patients with HCM as well as in first-degree relatives of patients with HCM.

Differential Diagnosis

HCM should be differentiated from hypertensive heart disease and athletic heart. Differential diagnosis includes also infiltrative cardiomyopathies (eg, amyloidosis), iron overload, metabolic disorders (eg, Fabry disease, mitochondrial cytopathies, glycogen or lysosomal storage diseases), neuromuscular disease (eg, Friedreich ataxia), or syndromic disorders (eg, Noonan syndrome, LEOPARD syndrome).

→ TREATMENT

Pharmacotherapy

1. Asymptomatic patients: Follow-up.

2. Symptomatic patients: Cardioselective β-blockers in maximum tolerated doses, especially in patients with a postexercise LVOT gradient. The doses should be titrated on the basis of the observed efficacy and treatment tolerance. If β-blockers are not tolerated or contraindicated, use verapamil in a dose gradually titrated up to a maximum tolerated dose. If symptoms persist with target-dose β-blockers or verapamil, consider adding disopyramide at the maximum tolerated dose (while monitoring the QTc interval).⊘◯ Do not use vasodilators (including nitrates and phosphodiesterase inhibitors) and digitalis in patients with LVOT obstruction.

3. Patients with heart failure and LVEF >50% without LVOT obstruction: Consider a β-blocker, verapamil, or diltiazem.

4. Patients with heart failure and LVEF <50%: Consider an angiotensin--converting enzyme inhibitor in combination with a β-blocker. If symptoms and LVEF <50% persist, consider adding a mineralocorticoid-receptor antagonist.

5. Patients with concomitant atrial fibrillation: This may be poorly tolerated hemodynamically and restoration and maintenance of normal sinus rhythm using **electrical or chemical cardioversion** may be necessary. For chemical cardioversion, amiodarone is the treatment of choice. Management of anticoagulation in those patients follows the usual principles, although newer agents have not been studied in this specific population.

Invasive Treatment

1. Septal myectomy: This is performed to relieve LVOT outflow obstruction. Indications include patients with severe symptoms who have a resting or postexercise peak LVOT gradient ≥50 mm Hg despite receiving maximal tolerated medical therapy. In patients with indications for a simultaneous valve repair (eg, mitral valve repair), septal myectomy is preferred.

2. Percutaneous alcohol septal ablation: This is performed by injecting absolute alcohol into a septal perforating arterial branch to induce infarction in a portion of the interventricular septum. Indications are the same as in septal myectomy, and clinical efficacy is similar.

3. Dual-chamber pacing (to facilitate cardiac synchrony) may be considered in patients who have refractory symptoms despite maximal medical therapy and in whom myectomy or alcohol septal ablation cannot be performed.⊘○

4. ICD implantation is recommended in patients at high risk of sudden cardiac death (→Clinical Features and Natural History, above) and in patients who have survived cardiac arrest or have recurrent sustained ventricular tachycardia.⊘○

5. Heart transplantation is indicated in patients with end-stage heart failure or ventricular arrhythmia that does not respond to treatment.

→FOLLOW-UP

1. In stable patients perform ECG, echocardiography, and 48-hour Holter monitoring every 12 to 24 months.

2. In patients with sinus rhythm with left atrial dimension ≥45 mm or new palpitations, perform 48-hour Holter monitoring every 6 to 12 months.

3. In patients with progressive symptoms, consider a symptom-limited ECG stress test yearly or every 2 to 3 years in those who are stable.

4. In asymptomatic patients with a gene mutation, perform evaluation (including ECG and transthoracic echocardiography) every 2 to 5 years in adults and every 1 to 2 years in children.

6.4. Restrictive Cardiomyopathy

→DEFINITION, ETIOLOGY, PATHOGENESIS

Restrictive cardiomyopathy (RCM) is a disease of the myocardium characterized mainly by left ventricular (LV) diastolic dysfunction. RCM may be familial (eg, inherited defects in desmin or troponin I) or caused by systemic disorders (eg, amyloidosis, sarcoidosis, scleroderma, carcinoid disease, radiation, and endomyocardial fibrosis caused by hypereosinophilic syndrome or drugs such as serotonin or ergotamine).

→CLINICAL FEATURES AND NATURAL HISTORY

Manifestations of RCM include dyspnea, fatigue, and in more advanced disease also features of right ventricular dysfunction. The natural history of RCM largely depends on its etiology and severity of myocardial changes.

→ DIAGNOSIS

Diagnostic Tests

1. Electrocardiography (ECG) may reveal abnormal P waves, a low R-wave amplitude, flat T waves, and supraventricular arrhythmias, especially atrial fibrillation. In amyloid cardiomyopathy, ECG typically has low voltages due to infiltration of amyloid.

2. Echocardiography may reveal normal or increased LV wall thickness, enlargement of both atria with relatively small ventricles, normal or slightly impaired systolic function of the ventricles, and diastolic LV dysfunction. Tissue Doppler echocardiography can be useful to differentiate between RCM and constrictive pericarditis.

3. Heart catheterization is performed in case of difficulties in differentiating between RCM and constrictive pericarditis.

4. Endomyocardial biopsy is performed in the case of suspected myocardial infiltrates caused by amyloidosis, sarcoidosis, idiopathic eosinophilia, or hemochromatosis.

5. Cardiac magnetic resonance imaging (MRI) may be useful in differentiating underlying etiologies such as sarcoidosis, amyloidosis, endomyocardial fibrosis, or eosinophilia.

6. Cardiac ^{18}F-fluorodeoxyglucose positron emission tomography (FDG-PET) may be useful in the diagnosis and assessment of treatment response in sarcoidosis.

Diagnostic Criteria

RCM is diagnosed on the basis of imaging studies and in some cases on the basis of histologic examination of cardiac biopsy specimens.

Differential Diagnosis

RCM should be mainly differentiated from constrictive pericarditis. This usually requires a specialized cardiology assessment and may involve invasive testing.

→ TREATMENT

1. Symptomatic treatment: As in chronic heart failure.

2. Long-term anticoagulation is used in patients with atrial fibrillation.

3. Heart transplantation is used in end-stage heart failure not responding to treatment.

4. Treatment of the underlying condition is used in patients with potentially reversible causes.

→ SPECIAL CONSIDERATIONS

1. Cardiomyopathy associated with hemochromatosis may lead to heart failure but frequently causes only minor symptoms. Treatment is with phlebotomy.

2. Cardiomyopathy associated with amyloidosis develops in 50% of patients with AL amyloidosis, 10% of patients with AA amyloidosis, and rarely in those with familial disease. Amyloid deposits lead to significant cardiac dysfunction and wall thickening, causing features of restriction and diastolic LV dysfunction, as well as to reduced right ventricular function. Amyloidosis also leads to arrhythmia, conduction disease, and a tendency to orthostatic hypotension. It must be suspected in the case of RCM developing in a person with proteinuria, hepatomegaly, anemia, or a chronic inflammatory condition. Echocardiographic features include marked hypertrophy of the ventricles, diastolic dysfunction with or without LV systolic dysfunction, biatrial enlargement, interatrial hypertrophy, and pericardial effusion. Diagnosis may be confirmed with biopsy of the abdominal fat pad, gingiva, rectum, or affected organ. Chemotherapy is available for patients with AL amyloidosis associated cardiomyopathy. Caution is noted with angiotensin-converting enzyme inhibitors, angiotensin receptor blockers, digoxin, β-blockers, and calcium channel blockers, given their predisposition to cause hypotension in patients with this disease. β-Blockers can be used, however, in the context of atrial fibrillation to improve diastolic filling time. Otherwise, careful use of diuretics is the pharmacotherapy of choice.

6.5. Unclassified Cardiomyopathies

1. Stress-induced (takotsubo) cardiomyopathy is a nonfamilial cardiomyopathy characterized by acute left ventricular (LV) dysfunction after emotional or physiologic stress. It is a form of myocardial stunning that is associated with hyperkinesis of the basal LV segments, akinesis of mid LV segments, and dyskinesis of the apical LV segments.

Clinically takotsubo cardiomyopathy can present with ST-segment elevations followed by inverted T waves associated with chest pain and elevations in serum troponin levels. As such, this is a diagnosis of exclusion after acute coronary syndrome has been ruled out. LV contractility normalizes within days, and electrocardiography changes resolve much later, within weeks or months. The prognosis is often good.

2. LV noncompaction is a congenital cardiomyopathy characterized by prominent trabeculation in the LV myocardium due to failure of compaction of the trabeculae during gestation. Clinical features include systolic dysfunction with heart failure, thromboembolic complications, arrhythmias, and sudden cardiac death. Diagnosis is made based on characteristic features found on echocardiography, magnetic resonance imaging, or LV ventriculography.

7. Congenital Heart Disease in Adults

7.1. Atrial Septal Defect

➔ DEFINITION, ETIOLOGY, PATHOGENESIS

Atrial septal defects are the most common congenital heart disease diagnosed in adults, accounting for >30% of all defects seen in adults.

Types of atrial septal defect (ASD):

1) **Ostium secundum ASD** (~70%).
2) **Ostium primum ASD** (partial atrioventricular septal defect) (~15%).
3) **Sinus venosus ASD** (~7%).
4) **Coronary sinus ASD** (<1%).

A common feature of all types of ASD is an atrial level shunt and its consequences, while differences include location of the defect and other coexisting heart defects. Approximately 30% of all ASDs are associated with other cardiac malformations, most common of which are anomalous pulmonary venous drainage (seen in all patients with superior sinus venosus defects), ventricular septal defects, and patent ductus arteriosus. All patients with ostium primum defects have abnormality of the mitral valve (a cleft anterior leaflet) with a varying degree of regurgitation.

➔ CLINICAL FEATURES AND NATURAL HISTORY

1. Symptoms: The most common symptom is dyspnea on exertion with progressive reduction of exercise tolerance and palpitations, which are initially paroxysmal (usually caused by atrial fibrillation [AF] or atrial flutter). For many women with undiagnosed defects, the initial symptoms are noticed during pregnancy. Rarely initial symptoms may be related to paradoxical embolization.

2. Signs: Typically, physical examination findings are quite subtle and can be missed. The jugular venous pulse may appear normal. However, an *a* wave dominance may be noticed, and in the presence of severe tricuspid regurgitation (TR), a *cv* wave will be clearly visible. A right ventricular lift is present in patients with significant right ventricular enlargement. A classic finding of an ASD on auscultation is a fixed splitting of the second heart sound. Special attention should be paid to the intensity of the pulmonic component. A loud pulmonic valve component of the second heart sound would indicate the presence of significant pulmonary hypertension. Many patients with an ASD will also have a systolic outflow murmur audible over the main pulmonary artery, which is related to increased flow across the right ventricular outflow tract. In individuals with very large shunts, a soft mid-diastolic rumble in the fourth left intercostal space may be heard, indicative of a significant increase in flow across the tricuspid valve. Patients may also have a holosystolic murmur caused by secondary TR. In the case of significant TR, its symptoms may be dominant, sometimes including central cyanosis (when the regurgitant jet is directed through the ASD to the left atrium).

3. Natural history: There is a direct link between the size of the defect and associated morbidity. Furthermore, the presence of additional cardiac defects will influence treatment and mortality. Patients with ostium secundum ASD have a relatively benign course and can remain asymptomatic for decades. Symptoms usually appear in the third to fourth decades of life and are generally progressive. The overall survival of patients is close to that of the normal population, but the quality of life is impaired due to progressive heart failure, sustained AF or atrial flutter, and dyspnea.

→ DIAGNOSIS

The final diagnosis is based on echocardiography, less commonly on magnetic resonance imaging (MRI) or computed tomography (CT). Suspected increased pulmonary vascular resistance is an indication for cardiac catheterization prior to referral for surgical or interventional closure.

Diagnostic Tests

1. Electrocardiography (ECG):

1) **Ostium secundum ASD**: Incomplete right bundle branch block (RBBB), in 90% of cases with rsR' pattern, right axis deviation or rightward axis, wide P waves, features of right ventricular overload (prominent R in V_1 and V_2), and supraventricular arrhythmias (frequently AF and atrial flutter).

2) **Ostium primum ASD**: First-degree atrioventricular block in some patients, incomplete RBBB, features of right ventricular overload (prominent R in V_1 and V_2) and left axis deviation. Evidence of left atrium enlargement in those with significant mitral regurgitation.

3) **Sinus venosus defect**: Incomplete RBBB, right axis deviation or rightward axis, abnormal P-wave axis with negative P waves in leads II, III, and aVF.

2. Chest radiographs: Increased pulmonary perfusion (shunt vascularity), dilated right ventricle and main pulmonary artery, narrow aorta.

3. Echocardiography: Transthoracic echocardiography (TTE) allows visualization of the defect and cardiac remodeling secondary to the shunt as well as visualization of the shunt using color Doppler imaging. In some individuals, calculation of the pulmonary (Qp) to systemic (Qs) flow ratio is possible with good accuracy (shunt is significant in patients with Qp:Qs ≥1.5). Furthermore, calculation of the right ventricular systolic pressure, which in those without right ventricular outflow tract obstruction equals the pulmonary artery systolic pressure, is an important component of echocardiographic evaluation.

Additionally, detection of associated heart defects is possible. In equivocal cases, transesophageal echocardiography (TEE) is conclusive; this is necessary when transcatheter closure of the defect is considered (in ostium secundum ASDs only). Sinus venosus defects are very difficult to visualize on TTE and are routinely missed. Hence, unexplained right heart enlargement on TTE should raise the suspicion of a sinus venosus defect, anomalous pulmonary venous drainage, or both and requires TEE examination.

4. Cardiac catheterization: Although there is no role for routine cardiac catheterization in patients with ASDs, it is performed in patients being considered for ASD closure who:

1) Have established coronary artery disease.

2) Are >40 years.

3) Have a significant risk factor profile for coronary artery disease.

4) Have significant pulmonary hypertension (to assess pulmonary vascular reactivity).

5. Cardiac MRI: Cardiac MRI provides a robust noninvasive way of assessing not only cardiac anatomical anomalies such as ASDs and anomalous pulmonary venous connections, but can also provide accurate measures of the shunt ratio (Qp:Qs) as well as ventricular volumes and function. In many centers, this modality has become a routine part of assessment of patients with shunt lesions.

➡ TREATMENT

1. Patients with minor shunts, normal right heart size, and normal pulmonary pressures require neither treatment nor specific recommendations. However, there is a small risk of paradoxical embolization; such risk is especially important in patients requiring intracardiac device therapy, such as permanent pacemakers or implantable defibrillators. This is due to the development of microthrombi on intracardiac leads, which can then embolize paradoxically to the central nervous system. In these patients, percutaneous closure of the defect (ostium secundum ASDs only) should be considered prior to device implantation.

2. Patients with significant left-to-right shunts (with right ventricular volume overload) require invasive treatment; pharmacotherapy with diuretics can only provide symptomatic relief. Invasive treatment should also be considered in the case of paradoxical embolism (after other causes have been excluded). Closure of the defect is contraindicated in patients with severe pulmonary hypertension (pulmonary artery systolic pressure >2/3 systolic blood pressure) or Eisenmenger syndrome. Transcatheter (percutaneous) closure is only suitable for ostium secundum ASDs and may be used in eligible patients (depending on the size of the defect/defects); following the procedure, both dual antiplatelet therapy (acetylsalicylic acid [ASA] 75-100 mg/d and clopidogrel 75 mg/d or ticlopidine 250 mg bid; treatment regimens may be slightly different in various centers) and infective endocarditis prophylaxis should be administered for a total of 6 months. After a successful closure of the defect, many patients have a significant reduction in the right heart size. Requirements for ongoing follow-up depend on the size of the defect and associated abnormalities, presence and degree of pulmonary hypertension (more than mild) prior to closure, and age (closed in adulthood) of the patient at closure.

3. Severe TR: In patients with ostium secundum ASDs and severe TR, surgical treatment of the ASD with concomitant repair of the tricuspid valve is necessary.

4. Ostium primum ASDs: All patients with ostium primum ASDs have associated cardiac defects, which include a cleft anterior mitral valve leaflet leading to a variable degree of mitral regurgitation, and in many patients inlet ventricular septum defects. All patients with hemodynamically significant shunts will require surgical intervention with closure of the defect or defects and repair of the mitral valve. It is recommended that surgeons with expertise in congenital heart disease perform the operation.

5. Sinus venosus defects: All patients with superior sinus venosus defects (a majority of patients belong to this category) have associated anomalous pulmonary venous drainage and/or connection and require surgical intervention for closure of the defect and rerouting the anomalous vein to the left atrium. Surgery should be performed by surgeons with expertise in congenital heart disease.

→ COMPLICATIONS AND PROGNOSIS

The prognosis is directly related to the size of the defect, degree of pulmonary hypertension (prior to closure), and age at closure. Supraventricular arrhythmias, rarely sick sinus syndrome or complete heart block (sometimes as a consequence of surgery), Eisenmenger syndrome, and paradoxical embolism (during intraventricular pacing) are some of the complications of untreated ASDs. Patients without significant pulmonary hypertension and Eisenmenger syndrome have a favorable prognosis.

7.2. Coarctation of the Aorta

→ DEFINITION, ETIOLOGY, PATHOGENESIS

Coarctation of the aorta refers to a narrowing of the aorta, most frequently at the level of the aortic isthmus, that is, distal to the origin of the left subclavian artery, opposite to the ligamentum arteriosum. Usually collateral circulation develops via the internal thoracic arteries and intercostal arteries. The most common association is the presence of a bicuspid aortic valve. Intracranial aneurysms of the circle of Willis (the most common extracardiac anomaly) occur in 3% to 5% of patients. Turner syndrome is a commonly associated chromosomal abnormality.

→ CLINICAL FEATURES

1. Symptoms usually develop in the second or third decade of life and are associated with prestenotic hypertension in the aorta. However, there is an inverse relationship between the severity of stenosis and age at which symptoms develop. Other factors that determine severity and age at which symptoms occur are the presence and quality of collateral circulation and presence (or absence) of additional defects. Symptoms include headaches, epistaxis, and disturbances of vision.

2. Signs involve hypertension (blood pressures measured on the upper extremities are >10 mm Hg higher than those measured on the popliteal artery); different blood pressures on both brachial arteries in patients with stenosis including the origin of the left subclavian artery; weak or absent pulse on the femoral arteries; and rarely, intermittent claudication (usually collateral circulation is well developed). A continuous murmur caused by blood flow in the narrowed aorta is audible in the left interscapular area as well as posteriorly. Precordial murmurs caused by a coexisting aortic valve disease (a bicuspid aortic valve) may also be present. The presence of a systolic ejection click with or without a systolic murmur should make one suspect the presence of an associated bicuspid aortic valve. A sustained apical impulse and a fourth heart sound are found in many patients due to the underlying left ventricular (LV) hypertrophy.

3. Complications (may be fatal): Heart failure, aortic rupture or dissection, infection of the aortic wall, intracranial hemorrhage, and complications of rapidly developing coronary artery disease.

→ DIAGNOSIS

Coarctation of the aorta is usually diagnosed in the course of a workup of secondary hypertension or headache and is confirmed by imaging studies.

Diagnostic Tests

1. Electrocardiography (ECG): Features of LV hypertrophy. Atrial arrhythmias such as atrial fibrillation can be seen.

2. Chest radiographs: A characteristic indentation of the outline of the aorta (the so-called figure-3 configuration) and erosions (notching) of the lower edges of the ribs by well-developed collateral circulation, dilatation of the left subclavian artery and the ascending aorta.

3. Transthoracic echocardiography is useful in assessing functional consequences, prestenotic and poststenotic pressure differences, and the nature of flow in the abdominal aorta. Frequently, stenosis is not immediately apparent. Assessment of the degree of LV hypertrophy as well as of the systolic and diastolic function are important components of the evaluation. The presence of a congenitally abnormal aortic valve and associated aortic dilatation are also assessed on echocardiography.

4. Traditional aortography or magnetic resonance angiography (MRA): Direct assessment of aortic stenosis, especially when qualifying the patient for surgery. MRA with hemodynamic assessment can be performed in many sites and has replaced conventional cardiac catheterization. Computed tomography angiography (CTA) can also provide anatomic evaluation of the presence and severity of coarctation. Catheterization is performed for evaluation of coronary arteries (preoperatively), in individuals with discrepant data from noninvasive assessment, as well as in those in whom percutaneous therapy is being considered.

→ TREATMENT

Invasive treatment (surgical or percutaneous) in patients with a pressure gradient >20 mm Hg between the right upper extremity and the right lower extremity and blood pressure >140/90 mm Hg, significant LV hypertrophy, or a pathologic blood pressure response to exercise. Systemic hypertension frequently persists after surgery. Annual follow-up visits are recommended to detect possible restenosis as well as local site complications (such as pseudoaneurysms). In patients with an associated bicuspid aortic valve continued surveillance of the valve is recommended.

7.3. Ebstein Anomaly

→ DEFINITION AND CLINICAL FEATURES

Ebstein anomaly is a congenital malformation of the tricuspid valve resulting in failure of delamination during cardiac development. This congenital anomaly may remain undiagnosed until adulthood. It includes a wide range of lesions, which depend on the degree of displacement of the septal tricuspid leaflet into the right ventricle, "atrialization" of the right ventricle, severity of functional changes (regurgitation or stenosis of the tricuspid valve), coexisting interatrial shunt (patent foramen ovale and atrial septal defects in 50%-75% of patients), accessory conduction pathways (usually right-sided, may be multiple), and other coexisting congenital malformations. Although mild forms of Ebstein anomaly may be asymptomatic, severe forms may cause a significant reduction in exercise tolerance.

Symptoms: Palpitations, dyspnea, reduced exercise tolerance, often mild cyanosis. Patients with mild defects are usually asymptomatic until a late age; in others, symptoms develop in the second and third decades of life.

Signs: On auscultation, midsystolic heart sounds (clicks, often multiple), a holosystolic murmur that intensifies during inspiration (this is caused by tricuspid regurgitation), wide splitting of the first and second heart sounds, and a right ventricular third heart sound.

→ DIAGNOSIS

Diagnosis is usually based on echocardiography with evidence of apical displacement of septal and posterior leaflets of the tricuspid valve.

Diagnostic Tests

1. Electrocardiography (ECG): Right atrial enlargement and right bundle branch block are typically seen. ECG should be inspected for the presence of preexcitation.

2. Chest radiographs may be nearly normal in mild cases and show severe enlargement (globular) of the right atrium in severe cases. The lungs and pulmonary vasculature appear normal.

3. Echocardiography: Apical displacement of septal and posterior leaflets of the tricuspid valve (for septal leaflets, ≥ 0.8 cm/m^2). There are varying degrees of tricuspid regurgitation. The presence of an atrial-level shunt should be documented; this is usually best achieved with intravenous bubble contrast injection during echocardiography.

4. Magnetic resonance imaging (MRI): Preoperative evaluation may be warranted to provide a complete anatomical assessment. Accurate volumetric evaluation of the right ventricle can be obtained with MRI.

→ TREATMENT

Surgery is indicated in patients with New York Heart Association class III or higher, cyanosis, right ventricular heart failure, or paradoxical embolism. Relative indications include recurrent supraventricular arrhythmias resistant to treatment (including ineffective ablation) and significant asymptomatic heart enlargement. Surgery should be performed by surgeons with special expertise in operating in adults with congenital heart disease as well as special expertise in different techniques used in surgical repairs in patients with Ebstein anomaly. Surgical treatment improves prognosis. Continuing periodic follow-up in specialized clinics postoperatively is recommended.

7.4. Eisenmenger Syndrome

→ DEFINITION, ETIOLOGY, PATHOGENESIS

Eisenmenger syndrome (pulmonary vascular disease) is a result of an untreated large left-to-right shunt (interatrial, interventricular, or aortopulmonary) and increased pulmonary perfusion, leading to severe irreversible pulmonary hypertension and shunt reversal (ie, a right-to-left shunt). It is a complication of simple or complex defects associated with large shunts. Eisenmenger syndrome frequently develops in childhood; in adults, the diagnosis is made mainly in patients with an atrioventricular septal defect, interatrial shunt, nonrestrictive ventricular septal defect, or patent ductus arteriosus (PDA).

→ CLINICAL FEATURES

1. Symptoms: Significant reduction in exercise tolerance, resting dyspnea exacerbated with exercise, palpitations, and chest pain. Patients with high hematocrit levels develop symptoms of hyperviscosity and hemoptysis. Syncope may occur in patients with advanced disease. Cyanosis and symptoms are often exacerbated in conditions associated with decreased systemic vascular resistance. This typically happens during fever.

2. Signs: Central cyanosis, clubbing of the nail beds, evidence of right ventricular lift, and a palpable second heart sound. Auscultation often reveals accentuation of the second heart sound; a right ventricular third heart sound and fourth heart sound may be present in patients with right ventricular hypertrophy. Disappearance of the murmurs caused by the underlying defect, for instance, the continuous murmur caused by PDA or the systolic murmur caused by a ventricular septal defect, should raise the suspicion of development of Eisenmenger physiology. Frequently, a soft systolic murmur at the left sternal border is audible, which is probably due to the dilation of the main pulmonary artery. In patients with pulmonary regurgitation, a relatively low-grade proto--meso-diastolic murmur, resulting from a high pulmonary vascular resistance (Graham Steell murmur), may be audible. In individuals with Eisenmenger PDA differential cyanosis is seen (cyanosis and clubbing in the lower extremities only).

3. Natural history: Patients with Eisenmenger syndrome and simple defects (shunts) have an average life expectancy >40 years, while in those with complex defects, the survival is shorter. The most common causes of death are heart failure, sudden cardiac death, and massive hemoptysis. The risk factors for severe complications or death include pregnancy, general anesthesia, dehydration, hemorrhage, surgical procedures (noncardiac), diuretics overuse, certain oral contraceptives, anemia (usually after unnecessary phlebotomies), cardiac catheterization, intravenous therapy, and pulmonary infections.

→ DIAGNOSIS

Diagnosis is based on the presence of a high pulmonary vascular resistance that does not respond to vasodilators (oxygen, nitric oxide) in a patient with a congenital heart disease with a shunt. Invasive diagnostic methods are indicated when noninvasive assessment suggests feasibility of surgical repair of the defect.

Diagnostic Tests

1. Laboratory tests reveal abnormalities that are secondary to hypoxemia; hemoglobin oxygen saturation (SaO_2) is usually <90% (measured at rest for at least 5 minutes). Complete blood count (CBC), hematocrit, renal function assessment, clotting profile, and serum uric acid levels should be measured regularly. Further testing with additional tests to assess iron indices, serum brain natriuretic peptide, folic acid, and vitamin B_{12} can be done.

2. Electrocardiography (ECG): Features of right atrial enlargement (if in sinus rhythm) and features of right ventricular hypertrophy (often with strain pattern) and overload are the dominant features of ECG.

3. Chest radiographs: The size of the heart may vary depending on the primary defect and severity of Eisenmenger syndrome. Pulmonary perfusion is clearly reduced, with a pruning pattern of the arteries; the hilar vessels are dilated.

4. Echocardiography: Right ventricular hypertrophy with color and spectral Doppler evidence of bidirectional flow through the shunt, and severe elevation in right ventricular systolic pressures. Often, there is an associated significant dilation of pulmonary arteries. Other abnormalities such as mitral or tricuspid regurgitation can be present and depend on the severity of Eisenmenger syndrome. Transesophageal echocardiography, magnetic resonance imaging (MRI), or computed tomography (CT) may detect proximal pulmonary artery thrombosis.

5. Exercise capacity should be assessed with the 6-minute walk test.

→ TREATMENT

1. General measures:
1) Administration of influenza vaccine every year, and pneumococcal vaccine every 5 years.

2) Monitoring for the signs and symptoms of bleeding.

3) Aggressive and prompt treatment of upper respiratory tract infections.

4) Avoidance of dehydration, excessive physical exercise, and staying at high altitudes. Smoking is prohibited.

5) Patients should be followed in specialized centers with expertise in care of adults with congenital heart disease and pulmonary hypertension.

6) Contraceptive advice: Pregnancy is a contraindication in women with Eisenmenger syndrome. Given the high failure rates, the use of single--barrier methods is not recommended. Estrogen-containing contraceptives should be avoided in these patients.

2. Treatment of hyperviscosity should only be performed in patients with hematocrit >65% who have moderate to severe symptoms of hyperviscosity and in whom iron deficiency and dehydration have been excluded. Perform therapeutic phlebotomy of 250 to 500 mL of blood with isovolumic fluid replacement. An air filter is recommended for all intravenous lines to avoid air embolism.

3. Iron supplementation should be performed in all patients with iron deficiency anemia related to repeated phlebotomies.

4. Treatment of arrhythmias: Sinus rhythm should be maintained with individualization of antiarrhythmic therapy. Transvenous leads must be avoided due to the increased risk of paradoxical embolization.

5. Treatment of hemoptysis is usually not necessary; however, an initial assessment with chest radiography followed by CT imaging of the chest if an infiltrate is present is recommended. Life-threatening events (rupture of an aortopulmonary collateral artery, pulmonary artery, or arteriole) are an indication for percutaneous embolization or surgery. Bronchoscopy should be avoided in patients with Eisenmenger syndrome and hemoptysis.

6. Targeted treatment of pulmonary hypertension: In patients with World Health Organization functional class III symptoms, the endothelin--receptor antagonist (ERA) bosentan should be initiated.◐◯ Other ERAs, phosphodiesterase inhibitors (eg, sildenafil, tadalafil), and prostacyclins can also be considered in patients with class III symptoms. In selected patients combination therapy may be considered. Also →Chapter 13.15. Initiation of therapy and follow-up is recommended to take place in conjunction with specialized pulmonary hypertension clinics.

7. Single-lung or total heart-lung transplantation may be used in patients with severe hypoxemia or heart failure and no contraindications to surgery in whom the risk of death within 1 year is >50%. Single-lung transplantation is performed in conjunction with repair of the cardiac defect (eg, ventricular septal defect) in selected cases.

8. Treatment of hyperuricemia: Asymptomatic hyperuricemia does not need treatment. In patients with acute gout, treatment with colchicine and anti--inflammatory drugs should be instituted with attention to the increased risk of renal function deterioration and increased risk of bleeding. Also →Chapter 14.8.

9. Noncardiac surgery: This should only be performed when absolutely necessary and unavoidable due to the high mortality associated with Eisenmenger syndrome. An experienced cardiac anesthesiologist with a clear understanding of Eisenmenger physiology should be requested to administer anesthesia. An air filter should be used on all intravenous lines. Preoperative phlebotomy (with isovolumic fluid replacement) can be considered in patients with hematocrit >65% (in absence of hyperviscosity symptoms). The blood withdrawn can be used for autologous transfusion if needed.

10. Endocarditis prophylaxis is indicated in all patients with cyanotic congenital heart disease.◐◯

11. Routine anticoagulation: Although patients with Eisenmenger syndrome are at risk of thrombosis (especially in the dilated pulmonary arteries), currently available data do not support the routine use of anticoagulation in these patients due to the inherent increased risk of bleeding as well as difficulty with the routine monitoring of anticoagulation.

7.5. Patent Ductus Arteriosus

→ DEFINITION

In fetal circulation the ductus arteriosus connects the proximal left pulmonary artery to the aortic arch immediately distal to the origin of the left subclavian artery, allowing nutrient-rich blood from the mother to bypass the developing lungs. If it fails to close after birth, the patent ductus arteriosus (PDA) causes a left-to-right shunt at the level of pulmonary artery. In adults, this is usually an isolated defect.

→ CLINICAL FEATURES AND DIAGNOSIS

The clinical significance of PDA depends on its size and hence volume of the left-to-right shunt:

1) **Small shunt**: Usually discovered incidentally by echocardiography, it is asymptomatic and associated with normal pulmonary pressures and normal left atrial and ventricular volumes.

2) **Moderate shunt**: Exertional dyspnea, reduced exercise tolerance, and palpitations; a continuous murmur in the second left intercostal space, enlargement of the left atrium and left ventricle; pulmonary hypertension may develop, but this is usually reversible after surgery.

3) **Large shunt**: Rare in adults; adult patients with large shunts usually present at the stage of Eisenmenger syndrome (such patients have no continuous murmur but develop differential cyanosis and clubbing, affecting the lower parts of the body and occasionally the left arm depending on whether the PDA joins the aorta before or after the left subclavian artery).

Diagnosis is based on the physical findings and results of echocardiographic evaluation (with magnetic resonance imaging [MRI] and computed tomography [CT] in equivocal cases). However, PDAs can be missed on echocardiography if the pulmonary arteries are not well visualized.

→ TREATMENT

1. PDA with a continuous murmur: These defects should be closed, preferably using the percutaneous approach. Percutaneous closure is the method of choice and can be performed safely in the vast majority of adults. After invasive treatment, patients without residual hemodynamic disturbances do not need a specialized follow-up. Endocarditis prophylaxis is required in the first 6 months after device closure and in patients in whom there may be residual shunting adjacent to the device, thus not allowing for complete endothelialization.

2. Patients with Eisenmenger syndrome: Medical treatment geared towards complications of Eisenmenger syndrome. Selective pulmonary vasodilators can be used.

7.6. Patent Foramen Ovale

→ DEFINITION, ETIOLOGY, PATHOGENESIS

In fetal circulation the foramen ovale provides the necessary anatomic and functional communication between the right and left atria. The foramen ovale closes after birth in ~75% of people due to increased left atrial pressures; in others it remains patent and is considered a normal anatomic variant.

A patent foramen ovale (PFO) can cause interatrial, mainly right-to-left shunting, which can predispose to paradoxical embolization, orthodeoxia-platypnea syndrome (dyspnea and arterial desaturation in the upright position with improvement in the supine position) in susceptible patients, and decompression sickness in divers. The role of PFOs in pathophysiology of migraines is not well established, however its association has been implicated in a number of retrospective studies.

→ CLINICAL FEATURES AND DIAGNOSIS

The presenting feature may be stroke or a transient ischemic attack, usually in young persons. There is occasional imaging evidence of cerebral embolization without the presence of symptoms. PFOs can be diagnosed using transthoracic echocardiography (with Doppler imaging); the sensitivity of detection can be increased using agitated bubble contrast injection with imaging at rest and with the release phase of the Valsalva maneuver. However, the gold standard for detection of a PFO remains transesophageal echocardiography with bubble contrast injection at rest and with the release phase of the Valsalva maneuver. Transcranial Doppler (TCD) ultrasonography can also be used as a noninvasive alternative for diagnosis. However, TCD can only detect presence of right-to-left shunting and not the location of this shunt.

→ TREATMENT

1. In the event of **recurrent central nervous system embolism** in younger individuals (≤60 years of age) and in the absence of other etiologies after a comprehensive evaluation that should include assessment of thrombophilias, the patient can be referred for percutaneous PFO closure, particularly in the case of a coexisting atrial septal aneurysm or large right-to-left shunting observed on transesophageal echocardiography.⊘◔

2. Antiplatelet treatment and prevention of infective endocarditis is necessary **for up to 6 months after device closure of a PFO**.

7.7. Tetralogy of Fallot

→ DEFINITION AND INITIAL MANAGEMENT

Tetralogy of Fallot is the most common form of cyanotic congenital heart defect, accounting roughly for ~10% of all congenital heart diseases. The defect is due to the antero-cephalad deviation of the outlet septum, leading to the four features of a nonrestrictive ventricular septal defect (VSD), an overriding aorta, right ventricular outflow tract obstruction (usually infundibular and valvular), and right ventricular hypertrophy. There is a slight male predominance.

Initial Palliative Shunts

Most of the patients who had the initial systemic-to-pulmonary palliative procedures performed had these reversed or closed at the time of definitive repair later in childhood.

Types of palliative shunts:

1) **Blalock-Taussig shunt** (classic or modified): Anastomosis between the subclavian artery and the pulmonary artery.
2) **Waterston shunt**: The ascending aorta and the right pulmonary artery are anastomosed.
3) **Potts shunt**: This is an anastomosis of the descending aorta and the left pulmonary artery.

Surgical Repair in Infancy

Surgical repair is performed in infancy and involves patch closure of the VSD, relief of the right ventricular outflow tract obstruction involving resection of the infundibular muscle, insertion of a transannular patch to augment the outflow, and closure or ligation of the previous palliative shunt.

In individuals who have had transannular patch repair there is usually severe pulmonary regurgitation present in patients with transannular patch repair. Although well tolerated for many years, it can lead to significant right ventricular dilation and dysfunction. There might also be residual obstruction to the right ventricular outflow tract at multiple levels. Many patients will also develop supraventricular arrhythmias (atrial flutter and fibrillation) as a result of the increased right atrial pressures. Of more concern is the development of sustained ventricular tachycardia, the electrical focus of which is usually at the site of infundibulectomy or the VSD patch. Some patients have aortic root and/or ascending aortic dilation with associated significant aortic regurgitation.

Contemporary surgical techniques do not use transannular patch augmentation and try to maintain some integrity of the pulmonary valve to avoid the sequelae of long-term severe pulmonary regurgitation. In patients whose anatomy is not suitable for direct repair (eg, due to an anomalous coronary artery course across the right ventricular outflow tract) an alternative surgical repair such as Rastelli repair (VSD closure and right ventricle to pulmonary artery valved conduit placement) is undertaken. The main issue with these patients in long--term follow-up is conduit stenosis/regurgitation and requirements for periodic interventions in the conduit.

→ CLINICAL FEATURES

Symptoms: In adulthood, many patients are relatively asymptomatic; however, many of these patients have limited their daily activities (subconsciously) and hence may not have significant symptoms. Most adult patients will demonstrate significant abnormalities in objective tests of functional capacity. When patients have symptoms, these will be of dyspnea on exertion and decrease in exercise tolerance. Particular attention should be paid to symptoms of palpitations, presyncope, and syncope, as these might be related to ventricular tachycardia.

Signs: Patients after repair have a previous midline sternotomy scar; those with initial palliation have additional left or right lateral thoracotomy scars. Individuals with previous Blalock-Taussig shunts have an absent (or very faint) radial and/or brachial pulse on the side of the shunt. Blood pressure should be measured in the arm with the normal pulse. Palpation of the precordium usually reveals a right parasternal lift associated with right ventricular enlargement. If a thrill is felt, it may indicate the presence of a VSD patch leak. Auscultation usually reveals a normal first heart sound and often a widely split second heart sound (presence of right bundle branch block [RBBB]). In cases where a transannular patch has been used to augment the right ventricular outflow tract, there usually is very little pulmonary valve tissue present, which is reflected by a single second heart sound (the aortic valve component of the second heart sound only). A right-sided fourth heart sound and third heart sound may be present depending on the function of the right ventricle. A systolic ejection murmur is heard in almost all patients and reflects the flow across the right ventricular outflow tract even in the absence of obstruction. There is also a low-pitched diastolic murmur from pulmonary regurgitation heard along the sternal border.

→ DIAGNOSIS

Diagnostic Tests

1. Electrocardiography (ECG): In the majority of patients, the rhythm is sinus; however, atrial flutter and fibrillation may be seen. RBBB is present in virtually all patients. Particular attention should be paid to the QRS complex duration, as there is a strong correlation between a QRS complex duration >180 milliseconds and the risk of sudden death from arrhythmia. Signs of right ventricular hypertrophy are present, and there may be evidence of right atrium enlargement.

2. Chest radiographs reveal evidence of previous sternotomy. The right ventricle is usually enlarged.

3. Echocardiography can assess the size and function of the right ventricle as well as the presence and degree of pulmonary regurgitation and right ventricular outflow tract obstruction. The VSD patch can also be assessed for the presence of patch leaks. In patients after Rastelli repair, evaluation for conduit stenosis and regurgitation can be challenging on echocardiography due to the location of the conduit; often alternative imaging modalities are used for to evaluate the severity of conduit dysfunction.

4. Cardiac magnetic resonance imaging (MRI): Serial assessment (quantitative) of right ventricular volumes, ejection fraction, and pulmonary regurgitation fraction is performed with cardiac MRI, which is considered the gold standard for evaluating the right ventricle. In individuals with intracardiac devices that are not MRI compatible, **gated computed tomography (CT)** imaging can provide right ventricular volumetric evaluations. Both MRI and CT should be performed in centers with expertise in congenital heart disease imaging.

➔ TREATMENT

Current recommendations for surgical reintervention (after the initial repair) are aortic valve replacement for severe aortic regurgitation with signs or symptoms of left ventricular dysfunction, pulmonary valve replacement in severe symptomatic pulmonary regurgitation, and severe or symptomatic right ventricular outflow tract obstruction. Pulmonary valve replacement can be considered in patients with asymptomatic but severe pulmonary regurgitation associated with decreased exercise capacity on objective testing; progressive right ventricular dilation, dysfunction, or both; and sustained ventricular tachycardia.

➔ FOLLOW-UP AND PROGNOSIS

Annual follow-up (clinical evaluation and imaging) in specialized centers is recommended for all patients with tetralogy of Fallot.

The prognosis in patients with repaired tetralogy of Fallot depends on several factors including type of corrective surgery (eg, using transannular patch), associated defects, and age at initial surgery, to name a few. For most adult patients with repaired tetralogy of Fallot, the most important factor that influences prognosis is the degree of pulmonary regurgitation and resultant right ventricular dilatation. Tachyarrhythmias (both atrial and ventricular) have significant impact on morbidity and mortality. In many patients the development of arrhythmias is directly linked to worsening hemodynamics. For this reason, early evaluation of these patients is key.

7.8. Transposition of Great Arteries

➔ DEFINITION AND CLINICAL FEATURES

Two different conditions are classified under the transposition complexes: complete transposition of great arteries (or d-TGA) and so-called congenitally corrected transposition of great arteries (CCTGA or l-TGA).

1. In patients with complete TGA, there is atrioventricular concordance and ventriculoarterial discordance. Obviously, this situation is not compatible with life, unless adequate mixing of the venous and arterial blood takes place. Newborns become progressively cyanotic with the physiologic closure of the ductus arteriosus and survival is dependent on mixing of blood, either through existing communications (such as a ventricular septal defect [VSD], atrial septal defect [ASD], and patent ductus arteriosus [PDA]) or by catheter or surgical interventions to create shunting (at the atrial level). Unoperated patients have >90% mortality in the first year of life; hence, almost all adult patients have had a surgery, usually early in childhood (atrial switch operation, arterial switch operation, or Rastelli repair).

2. In patients with congenitally corrected TGA, there is both atrioventricular and ventriculoarterial discordance. The majority of the patients (>95%) have associated cardiac abnormalities including VSDs, systemic tricuspid valve abnormalities, and pulmonary or subpulmonary stenosis. There is also a significant risk of development of complete heart block with a rate of ~2% per year.

3. Symptoms: The majority of patients have had previous operations. Rarely, a patient with previously unrecognized isolated congenitally corrected TGA is seen with presyncope or syncope. Patients may develop progressive dyspnea, fatigue, and decreased exercise tolerance as the function of the systemic ventricle deteriorates. Most patients with a previous atrial switch operation develop atrial arrhythmias and may present with palpitations and presyncope. Patients who have had the arterial switch operation may present with signs or symptoms of ischemia related to the coronary artery stenosis.

4. Signs (details on surgical interventions: →Treatment, below):

1) **Patients after the atrial switch**: Previous sternotomy is present. A right parasternal lift is felt. Auscultation usually reveals a normal first heart sound and a single loud second heart sound. There may be a pansystolic murmur related to systemic tricuspid regurgitation (note that in these patients the anatomic right ventricle supports systemic circulation: it is subaortic and the atrioventricular valve that allows inflow into this ventricle is a tricuspid valve).

2) **Patients after the arterial switch**: Usually these patients have relatively normal examination findings with the exception of the previous sternotomy. However, particular attention should be paid to the presence of a diastolic murmur associated with neoaortic regurgitation. A systolic ejection murmur may also be heard, which is associated with right ventricular outflow tract obstruction.

3) **Patients after the Rastelli operation**: Usually there is a systolic thrill associated with the flow through the conduit. Auscultation reveals a loud systolic murmur from the conduit. The duration of time in systole occupied by the murmur is helpful in detecting significant conduit obstruction. This may be associated with a systolic thrill. A diastolic murmur may be heard due to conduit regurgitation.

4) **Patients with congenitally corrected TGA**: The majority of these patients have undergone the classic repair and have a previous sternotomy scar. The jugular venous pressure is usually normal except in patients with complete heart block, where an intermittent cannon a wave is seen. Usually a right parasternal lift is present. Auscultation reveals a normal first heart sound with a single loud second heart sound. A third heart sound or a fourth heart sound may be present depending on the function of the systemic ventricle. There may be a holosystolic murmur, which is related to systemic atrioventricular valve regurgitation.

→ DIAGNOSIS

Diagnostic Tests

1. Electrocardiography (ECG): In patients with complete transposition after the atrial switch operation, ECG may show junctional rhythm at varying rates. Signs of right ventricular hypertrophy and right atrial overload are present. In patients after the arterial switch operation, ECG is usually normal. However, special attention should be paid to signs of ventricular hypertrophy (both left and right) and evidence of ischemia and infarction. In patients with CCTGA, there may be complete heart block present. Typically, there are Q waves present in leads V_1 to V_2 and absent in leads V_5 to V_6. This reflects the initial right-to-left septal depolarization in patients with ventricular inversion (this should not be mistaken for previous anteroseptal myocardial infarction).

2. Chest radiographs: In patients with complete transposition after the atrial switch operation, radiographs shows a narrow vascular pedicle with a cardiac silhouette that is somewhat oblong. Following the arterial switch, radiographs are usually normal (with the exception of evidence of previous sternotomy). In patients with CCTGA, radiographs usually show evidence of cardiomegaly. There is an abnormal contour to the left heart border, which reflects the left--sided ascending aorta.

3. Echocardiography: In patients after the atrial switch operation, echocardiography is used to assess the size and function of the systemic right ventricle as well as the degree of systemic atrioventricular valve regurgitation. Baffle obstruction or leak can be assessed by echocardiography with or without the use of IV agitated bubble contrast. In patients after the arterial switch operation, echocardiography may be entirely normal. However, the assessment of aortic stenosis or regurgitation as well as aortic dimensions are important. Similarly, the degree of pulmonary stenosis and pulmonary regurgitation should be documented. In patients after Rastelli operation, the main echocardiographic index is the degree and progression of conduit stenosis or regurgitation. In patients with CCTGA, echocardiography provides the size and function of the systemic ventricle; these patients will have more important degrees of systemic atrioventricular valve regurgitation and echocardiography can provide information with regards to its severity and progression when compared with previous studies.

→ TREATMENT

Surgical Intervention

1. Complete TGA: There are 3 major operative procedures for patients with complete transposition:

1) **Atrial switch operation**: Two similar operations (Mustard and Senning procedures). The goal of both operations is to redirect blood at the atrial level to provide physiologic correction. Hence, the systemic venous return is directed via the atrial baffle through the mitral valve to the subpulmonic left ventricle, and the pulmonary venous flow is redirected through the tricuspid valve to the systemic right ventricle.

2) **Arterial switch operation (Jatene procedure)**: This provides both anatomic and physiologic correction, as the great arteries are switched. The arterial switch operation has been in widespread use since the late 1970s and for the most parts has replaced the atrial switch operations.

3) **Rastelli operation**: This is reserved for patients with VSD and pulmonary or subpulmonary stenosis. In this operation blood is redirected through the VSD to the aorta via an artificial tunnel, while a valved conduit connects the right ventricle to the pulmonary artery. In these patients, the morphologic left ventricle supports the systemic circulation.

2. Congenitally corrected TGA: These patients usually have undergone a classic repair in childhood, where the VSD is closed with left ventricle to pulmonary artery valved conduit placement (in those with subpulmonary or pulmonary stenosis).

→ FOLLOW-UP

Many patients with transposition of great arteries have complex issues and should be seen regularly by a specialist with expertise in adult congenital heart disease. In general, these patients need a serial follow-up of systemic right ventricular function as well as the assessment of baffle patency (patients with complete transposition after the atrial switch operation and those with CCTGA) with different imaging modalities (echocardiography, radionuclide angiography, or magnetic resonance imaging [MRI]).

7.9. Ventricular Outflow Tract Obstruction

7.9.1. Left Ventricular Outflow Tract Obstruction

▶**DEFINITION, CLINICAL FEATURES, NATURAL HISTORY**

Left ventricular outflow tract obstruction may develop as a result of defects of the aortic valve, defects of the adjacent parts of the left ventricle (LV), and defects of the ascending aorta that cause obstruction of the outflow of blood from the LV.

1. Classification:
1) **Valvular obstruction**: The most common type, usually associated with a bicuspid aortic valve.
2) **Subvalvular obstruction**: In the form of membranous stenosis or a fibro-muscular tunnel.
3) **Supravalvular obstruction**: Usually in the form of an hourglass (with fibrosis of the aortic intima); it may involve a large part of the ascending aorta. Etiology: Williams-Beuren syndrome, congenital rubella syndrome.

2. Symptoms depend on the severity of stenosis and do not differ significantly from those found in patients with acquired valvular aortic stenosis.

3. Signs: In subvalvular stenosis, a loud ejection murmur with a systolic thrill along the left sternal border (in severe stenosis) and diastolic murmur of aortic regurgitation (AR) (common) are present. Similar auscultatory signs are seen in supravalvular stenosis, but usually without the diastolic murmur. Other features include increased accentuation of the second heart sound (resulting from increased aortic pressures proximal to the stenosis), very distinct radiation of the murmur and the thrill to the carotid arteries, and a late systolic or holosystolic murmur caused by stenosis of the peripheral pulmonary arteries. In people with significant stenosis, a fourth heart sound is often present. In those with a congenitally abnormal aortic valve an ejection click is audible. In individuals with supravalvular aortic stenosis, the systolic blood pressure in the right arm is higher than the left arm.

4. Natural history: Congenital valvular stenosis progresses with time to significant stenosis (particularly when valve calcifications occur, usually in patients aged <60 years) and regurgitation with dilation of the aorta (with increased risk of dissection), which require surgery. Subvalvular membranous stenosis can be progressive and often leads to significant aortic regurgitation. Tunnel stenosis is usually severe and requires surgery. The condition is associated with an increased risk of infective endocarditis.

▶**DIAGNOSIS**

Diagnosis is mainly based on echocardiography. Differential diagnosis includes the individual morphologic forms of the disease. Cardiac magnetic resonance imaging (MRI) or computed tomography (CT) should be performed in individuals with supravalvular aortic stenosis and those with multilevel stenosis to delineate the locations of stenosis and identify additional lesions in the aorta and the peripheral vessels (such as renal arteries). Coronary angiography should be performed in all patient with supravalvular aortic stenosis undergoing surgical correction (CT coronary angiography may be performed).

▶**TREATMENT**

Symptomatic patients with a mean gradient ≥50 mm Hg on Doppler echocardiography require surgery. Asymptomatic patients with severe defects require individual assessment; in asymptomatic patients, surgery may be performed in the presence of LV systolic dysfunction (ejection fraction <50%), with the development of symptoms during exercise stress testing, and in the presence of severe AR and LV dilatation. Surgery may be considered in patients with subvalvular stenosis and progressive AR (on serial assessment) in order to prevent further progression of AR. An independent indication for surgery is a dilation of the ascending aorta >50 to 55 mm. After surgery annual follow--up visits are required.

7.9.2. Right Ventricular Outflow Tract Obstruction

➔ DEFINITION, CLINICAL FEATURES, NATURAL HISTORY

Right ventricular outflow tract obstruction may be caused by defects of the pulmonary valve, adjacent parts of the right ventricle, and main pulmonary artery that cause obstruction of the outflow of blood from the right ventricle.

1. Classification:

1) **Valvular obstruction**: The most common type; usually involves an isolated defect, often as a feature of congenital rubella syndrome, component of the tetralogy of Fallot, Noonan syndrome, or Alagille syndrome. Acquired pulmonary stenosis can occur in the setting of carcinoid syndrome.

2) **Subvalvular obstruction**: Usually a part of complex defects, most commonly associated with ventricular septal defect, tetralogy of Fallot, and subvalvular aortic stenosis.

3) **Supravalvular obstruction**: Rarely an isolated defect, it may be a part of the tetralogy of Fallot, Noonan syndrome, Williams syndrome, and Alagille syndrome.

2. Symptoms: In moderate and severe stenosis, fatigue, dyspnea, chest pain, and syncope are the common presenting features. Patients can also present with palpitations related to underlying atrial arrhythmias.

3. Signs: In cases of severe stenosis, the jugular venous pressure reveals an augmented a wave. A prominent right ventricular impulse is often palpable in individuals with significant right ventricular outflow tract obstruction. On auscultation, there is an ejection murmur best audible in the second intercostal space at the left sternal border and accompanied by a thrill in many patients with hemodynamically important stenosis. There is a normal first heart sound, wide-splitting (not fixed) of the second heart sound with a soft pulmonary component (in severe stenosis), and systolic ejection click that fades during inspiration (in patients with thin and mobile valve leaflets; rarely in supravalvular or subvalvular stenosis). A right-sided S_4 sound is audible in patients with a noncompliant right ventricle who are in sinus rhythm. In individuals with associated atrial septal defect or ventricular septal defect and severe stenosis there may be cyanosis and clubbing present related to right-to-left shunting.

4. Natural history: Moderate or severe pulmonary stenosis is usually progressive; in milder forms, progression is rare in adults. Subvalvular or supravalvular stenosis causes right ventricular hypertrophy and increasing pressure gradients.

➔ DIAGNOSIS

Diagnosis is mainly based on echocardiography, while differential diagnosis includes the individual morphologic forms of the disease. Echocardiography can also provide the level of obstruction(s) and presence of associated congenital defects. A measure of the severity of stenosis is the peak pressure gradient between the right ventricle and the main pulmonary artery:

1) Mild: <36 mm Hg.

2) Moderate: 36 to 64 mm Hg.

3) Severe: >64 mm Hg.

→ **TREATMENT**

Right ventricular outflow tract obstruction at any level requires invasive treatment if the peak pressure gradient on Doppler imaging is >64 mm Hg (peak flow velocity >4 m/s) and the right ventricular function is normal. In valvular stenosis, percutaneous pulmonary balloon valvotomy is the procedure of choice. In subvalvular and supravalvular stenosis as well as in stenosis with calcified or dysplastic valve, surgical repair is indicated. In general, long-term survival rates in patients undergoing valvular stenosis repair are similar to those of the general population. However, individuals with significant pulmonary regurgitation after valvotomy develop symptoms related to progressive right ventricular enlargement.

7.10. Ventricular Septal Defect

Ventricular septal defects (VSDs) are the most common congenital heart disease seen at birth (excluding bicuspid aortic valves), accounting for 30% to 40% of all defects.

Classification of VSDs based on their location:

1) **Perimembranous VSD** (most common, accounting for ~80% of all cases): Located in the membranous septum.

2) **Muscular/trabecular VSD** (up to 15%-20% of cases): Completely surrounded by muscle. These could be multiple ("Swiss cheese" defects).

3) **Outlet VSDs** (~5% of cases): Located underneath the semilunar valves.

4) **Inlet/atrioventricular canal**: Directly inferior to the atrioventricular valves. A component of the atrioventricular septal defect.

→ **CLINICAL FEATURES AND NATURAL HISTORY**

1. Symptoms: Small VSDs are asymptomatic. Symptoms of a larger VSD include exertional dyspnea, reduced exercise tolerance, and palpitations. The development of pulmonary vascular disease (which eventually leads to shunt reversal and Eisenmenger syndrome) causes a significant limitation of the patient's activity.

2. Signs: In patients with small VSDs, the apical impulse is normal in location and size; however, in those with large VSDs, the apical impulse is located inferiorly and laterally. This is also the case in patients with hemodynamically important aortic regurgitation (associated with aortic cusp prolapse) or significant mitral regurgitation (associated with inlet-type VSDs). A loud holosystolic murmur in the fourth left intercostal space with a systolic thrill is the predominant sound heard during auscultation (the smaller the defect, the louder the murmur and the more pronounced the presence of the associated thrill). Muscular VSDs often have murmurs that are not holosystolic due to the systolic compression of the defect. In patients with large-volume shunts, there may be a diastolic apical rumble. With the development of Eisenmenger syndrome, the systolic murmur disappears, the second heart sound becomes distinctly accentuated, and a diastolic murmur of pulmonary regurgitation (a Graham Steell murmur) may appear. A low-frequency diastolic decrescendo murmur along the sternal border should make one suspect the presence of aortic regurgitation, which can be related to aortic cusp prolapse.

3. Natural history: Moderate left-to-right shunts lead to left ventricle (LV) volume overload, congestive heart failure, and subsequently to the development of Eisenmenger syndrome and shunt reversal. The defect may close spontaneously at any age, although this rarely occurs in adults (<10%) and applies to perimembranous and muscular defects only.

→ DIAGNOSIS

Diagnosis is largely made on the basis of echocardiography. However, muscular VSDs located at the apex, even when multiple, may be missed on routine echocardiographic evaluation. Differential diagnosis includes other lesions that lead to holosystolic murmurs, such as mitral regurgitation or tricuspid regurgitation.

Diagnostic Tests

1. Electrocardiography (ECG): In a large VSD, the features of LV and left atrial hypertrophy are observed. When severe pulmonary vascular disease develops (→Chapter 3.7.4), there is evidence of right ventricular hypertrophy and right atrial enlargement.

2. Chest radiographs: In patients with a significant VSD, there are features of increased pulmonary perfusion (shunt vascularity), and there could also be evidence of LV and left atrial enlargement. With the development of pulmonary hypertension, varying degrees of pulmonary artery enlargement are seen.

3. Echocardiography: Echocardiography can identify the location and size of VSD(s) as well as assess cardiac remodeling caused by the shunt. Furthermore, calculation of the pulmonary (Qp) to systemic (Qs) flow ratio can be performed in individuals with good imaging windows. An important component of an echocardiographic evaluation is the assessment of pulmonary artery systolic pressures as well as evaluation for possible coexisting defects.

4. Cardiac catheterization: Although not routinely performed, in some patients it may be necessary to assess the hemodynamic significance of the VSD (shunt ratio calculation), main pulmonary artery pressures, as well as pulmonary vascular resistance. In individuals with significantly elevated pulmonary artery pressures on noninvasive imaging, preoperative cardiac catheterization is necessary to evaluate pulmonary vascular reactivity. Furthermore, in patients being forwarded for surgical closure of the defect who are at risk of coronary artery disease, assessment of coronary arteries is performed via cardiac catheterization.

→ TREATMENT

1. Patients with normal pulmonary artery pressures and a small shunt (with less than moderate aortic regurgitation): No treatment is necessary. Current guidelines do not recommend routine endocarditis prophylaxis in these patients.

2. Surgical treatment is recommended in patients who are:
1) Symptomatic but do not have Eisenmenger syndrome.
2) Asymptomatic but have LV volume overload (more than mild LV dilation) that is not related to other etiologies.

3. Surgical treatment may also be considered in patients with:
1) A history of infective endocarditis.
2) Progressive aortic regurgitation due to aortic cusp prolapse.
3) Pulmonary hypertension, if the Qp:Qs ratio is >1.5 and pulmonary artery pressures or pulmonary vascular resistance are <2/3 of the respective systemic values (in baseline conditions, after the administration of a pulmonary artery vasodilator, or following targeted treatment for pulmonary hypertension).

→ FOLLOW-UP

Patients after surgery with no residual hemodynamic disturbances and with cardiovascular symptoms only require a periodic specialist follow-up (a 5-year interval is adequate). However, patients with LV dysfunction, pulmonary hypertension, residual shunt, aortic regurgitation, right ventricular outflow obstruction, or LV outflow obstruction require a more regular (annual) evaluation in specialized clinics.

→ **COMPLICATIONS**

Infective endocarditis (reported up to 2 in 1000 patient-years), aortic regurgitation requiring surgery, paradoxical embolism (during intraventricular pacing), and complete heart block (rare).

8. Heart Failure

→ **DEFINITION AND CLASSIFICATION**

Heart failure (HF) is a condition in which an abnormal heart structure or function causes a reduction in cardiac output relative to metabolic requirements or in which cardiac output is maintained with an increase in filling pressures. Clinically, HF is a syndrome in which patients have symptoms (eg, shortness of breath, ankle and/or abdominal swelling, fatigue) and signs (eg, elevated jugular venous pressure, pulmonary crackles) of volume or pressure overload.

Heart failure can be classified as:

1) **New-onset HF**: Occurring for the first time, regardless of the dynamics of symptoms.

2) **Acute decompensated HF**: A rapid onset of or increase in symptoms and signs of HF.

3) **Chronic HF**, which can be further classified as **stable**, **progressive**, or **advanced**. Advanced HF represents a subset of chronic HF and is characterized by refractory, "end-stage" symptoms and circulatory compromise despite evidence-informed treatment.

For therapeutic and prognostic purposes, heart failure is also classified according to left ventricular ejection fraction (LVEF), which is defined as stroke volume (end-diastolic minus end-systolic volume) divided by the end-diastolic volume.

1) **HF with reduced ejection fraction (HFrEF)** is typically defined as clinical HF with ejection fraction (EF) $\leq 40\%$.

2) **HF with preserved ejection fraction (HFpEF)** is typically defined as clinical HF with EF $\geq 50\%$ and evidence of diastolic dysfunction or elevated LV filling pressure.

The LVEF threshold for the diagnosis of HFrEF and HFpEF has varied across clinical trials and clinical practice guidelines. LVEF between 41% to 49% is considered to be in the gray zone, recently referred to as midrange EF (HFmrEF).

Clinically, HF may also be classified as **left ventricular**, **right ventricular**, or **biventricular failure**, depending on whether the predominant symptoms of congestion are pulmonary, systemic, or both.

High-output HF refers to clinical HF occurring due to increased cardiac output and hyperdynamic states, which may not always be associated with an underlying structural heart disease.

8.1. Acute Heart Failure

→ **ETIOLOGY AND PATHOGENESIS**

Acute heart failure (AHF) may develop de novo, that is, in a person without prior documented heart dysfunction, or as acute decompensation of prior heart failure (HF).

Causes of AHF: Acute coronary syndrome (ACS), mechanical complications of myocardial infarction (MI), acute valvular regurgitation, markedly elevated blood pressure (BP), arrhythmia or conduction disturbances, peripartum cardiomyopathy, cardiac surgical complications, infections (including myocarditis and infective endocarditis), endocrinopathy, high cardiac output states (severe infection [particularly sepsis], thyroid storm, anemia, arteriovenous fistula, Paget disease), nonadherence to medications.

Ischemic heart disease and long-standing poorly controlled hypertension are the most common causes of AHF, especially in the elderly. Predominant etiologies in young patients include dilated cardiomyopathy, arrhythmia, congenital heart disease, valvular heart disease, and myocarditis.

→ CLINICAL FEATURES AND NATURAL HISTORY

Signs and symptoms:

1) Features of low cardiac output (hypoperfusion) if cardiogenic shock is present: Fatigue; weakness; confusion; drowsiness; pale, cool, and moist extremities, occasionally with peripheral cyanosis; thready pulse; hypotension; oliguria.

2) Congestion:

   a) In systemic circulation (right ventricular failure): Peripheral edema (ankle or sacral pitting edema; this may be absent in early AHF); jugular vein distention; epigastric tenderness (caused by liver enlargement); sometimes ascites and pleural and/or pericardial effusions.

   b) In pulmonary circulation (left ventricular [LV] failure, which may lead to pulmonary edema): Dyspnea, tachypnea and orthopnea, crackles over lungs.

3) Features of the underlying condition causing AHF.

Based on the features of peripheral hypoperfusion, the patient may be classified as "**cold**" (with hypoperfusion) or "**warm**" (without hypoperfusion), and based on the features of pulmonary congestion, as "**wet**" (with congestion) or "**dry**" (without congestion).

→ DIAGNOSIS

Diagnosis is made on the basis of signs and symptoms as well as results of diagnostic tests.

Diagnostic Tests

1. Electrocardiography (ECG) usually reveals abnormalities corresponding to the underlying condition, which most frequently are features of myocardial ischemia, arrhythmia, or conduction abnormalities.

2. Chest radiographs: In addition to features of the underlying condition, they may reveal pulmonary congestion, pleural effusions, and cardiac enlargement.

3. Echocardiography reveals cardiac abnormalities, which may be functional (systolic or diastolic myocardial dysfunction, valvular dysfunction) or anatomical (eg, mechanical complications of MI).

4. Laboratory tests: The basic set of tests includes complete blood count; serum levels of creatinine, urea/blood urea nitrogen, sodium, potassium, glucose, cardiac troponin, and liver enzymes; arterial blood gas levels (in patients with mild dyspnea, pulse oximetry may be used, with the exception of patients with shock causing very low cardiac output and peripheral vasoconstriction). Natriuretic peptide levels (B-type natriuretic peptide [BNP]/N-terminal pro–B-type natriuretic peptide [NT-proBNP]) can be useful in differentiating between cardiogenic (higher levels) and noncardiogenic causes of dyspnea.

5. Endomyocardial biopsy: Indications: →Chapter 3.8.2.

Differential Diagnosis

Other causes of dyspnea and edema. Consider also causes of noncardiogenic pulmonary edema (features facilitating differentiation between noncardiogenic

Table 8-1. Initial differentiation between cardiogenic and noncardiogenic pulmonary edema

Clinical features	Pulmonary edema	
	Cardiogenic	Noncardiogenic
Skin	Cold	Usually warm
Gallop	Present	Usually absent
Electrocardiography	Features of myocardial ischemia or myocardial infarction	Usually normal
Chest radiographs	Hilar pulmonary venous congestion and edema	Initially peripheral pulmonary venous congestion and edema
Blood levels of cardiac troponins	May be increased	Usually normal

and cardiogenic pulmonary edema: →Table 8-1), acute respiratory failure, and (acute) interstitial lung disease.

→ TREATMENT

General Considerations

1. Short-term treatment goals: Control of symptoms (primarily of dyspnea) and hemodynamic stabilization of the patient.

2. Treatment of the underlying condition is mandatory in every case.

3. Close monitoring of respiratory rate, heart rate, ECG, and BP. Measure these parameters regularly (eg, every 5-10 minutes) or continuously (in unstable patients) until the patient's condition is stable and drug doses need no further adjustment. Noninvasive automated BP monitors are reliable as long as there is no severe vasoconstriction or significant tachycardia. Rhythm and ST-segment monitoring is mandatory in AHF, particularly when caused by ACS or arrhythmia. In patients treated with oxygen, monitor hemoglobin oxygen saturation in arterial blood (SaO_2) using a pulse oximeter regularly (eg, every hour) or continuously (preferable approach).

Occasionally invasive hemodynamic monitoring is necessary, particularly in patients with concomitant congestion, hypoperfusion, and a poor response to pharmacotherapy. It may be helpful in selecting an appropriate therapy. Note that the influence of these devices on survival is unclear. In selected scenarios, the following devices may be considered:

1) A Swan-Ganz catheter placed in the main pulmonary artery allows measurement of pressures in the superior vena cava, right atrium, right ventricle, main pulmonary artery, as well as pulmonary capillary wedge pressure, cardiac output (→Chapter 3.16), and oxygen saturation of mixed venous blood; the use is limited.

2) A central venous catheter is used to measure central venous pressure and oxygen saturation of the venous blood (SvO_2) in the superior vena cava or in the right atrium.

3) A peripheral arterial catheter (usually placed in the radial artery) is used for continuous BP monitoring.

4. Treatment of specific types of AHF:

1) **Worsening or decompensation of HF**: Use vasodilators in combination with loop diuretics (in patients with impaired kidney function or those already receiving long-term diuretic treatment, consider using higher doses

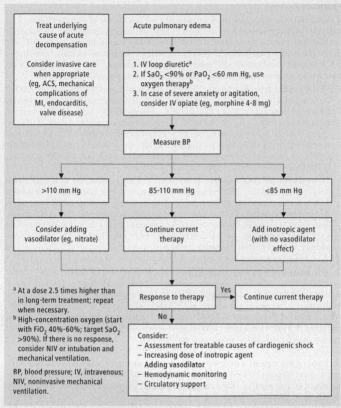

Figure 8-1. Management algorithm in patients with acute pulmonary edema. *Based on Eur J Heart Fail. 2016;18(8):891-975.*

of diuretics). Use inotropic agents in patients with hypotension and features of organ hypoperfusion.

2) **Pulmonary edema**: →Figure 8-1.

3) **AHF with high BP**: Vasodilators (close monitoring is necessary). Use low-dose diuretics in patients with volume overload or pulmonary edema.

4) **Cardiogenic shock**.

5) **Isolated right ventricular AHF**: Maintain right ventricular preload. If possible, avoid vasodilators (opiates, nitrates, angiotensin-converting enzyme inhibitors [ACEIs], angiotensin receptor blockers [ARBs]) and diuretics. Cautious administration of intravenous fluids may be effective (with careful hemodynamic monitoring). Low-dose dopamine is sometimes used.

6) **AHF in the course of ACS**. Perform echocardiography to determine the cause of AHF. In patients with ST-segment elevation MI or non–ST-segment elevation MI, perform coronary angiography and revascularization. In patients with mechanical complications of acute MI, urgent surgical treatment is necessary.

Pharmacotherapy

1. Vasodilators may be used in patients with features of hypoperfusion and congestion but without hypotension. They are generally avoided in patients with systolic blood pressure (SBP) <110 mm Hg. Vasodilators lower SBP, LV, and right ventricular filling pressures as well as peripheral vascular resistance while improving dyspnea. BP monitoring is mandatory. Use vasodilators with particular caution in patients with mitral or aortic stenosis.

1) IV **nitroglycerin**: Start with 10 to 20 µg/min and increase the dose as needed by 5 to 10 µg/min every 3 to 5 minutes up to the maximal hemodynamically tolerated dose (maximum, 200 µg/min); alternatively, nitroglycerin may be administered orally or in the form of translingual spray at a dose of 400 µg every 5 to 10 minutes. Because tolerance develops after 24 to 48 hours of treatment with high-dose nitroglycerin, the drug should be used intermittently. In case of BP dropping <90 mm Hg, reduce the dose of nitroglycerin. If BP continues to fall, discontinue the infusion.

2) IV **sodium nitroprusside**: Start with 0.3 µg/kg/min, up to a maximum dose of 5 µg/kg/min. Nitroprusside is recommended in patients with severe AHF in the course of hypertension and in patients with AHF caused by mitral insufficiency. Do not use nitroprusside in patients with AHF in the course of ACS, as it may cause a coronary steal effect. In patients receiving long-term treatment with nitroprusside, particularly patients with severe kidney or liver failure, toxicity caused by its metabolites—thiocyanate and cyanide—may occur (abdominal pain, confusion, seizures).

2. Diuretics are mainly used in patients with AHF and features of volume overload, that is, pulmonary congestion or peripheral edema. High doses of diuretics may cause a transient deterioration in kidney function. Algorithm of diuretic treatment in patients with AHF: →Figure 8-2. In patients treated with diuretics, monitor urine output (catheterization may be necessary); adjust the dose of diuretics to the clinical response; restrict sodium intake; monitor serum creatinine, potassium, and sodium levels every 1 to 2 days, depending on the urine output; and correct for potassium and magnesium loss.

3. Inotropic agents may be used in patients with AHF associated with peripheral hypoperfusion and hypotension (SBP <85 mm Hg). Monitor ECG because of the risk of tachycardia, myocardial ischemia, and arrhythmia. Agents and dosage: →Table 8-2.

4. Vasoconstrictors are considered in patients with persistent hypotension and hypoperfusion despite appropriate volume status. Agents and dosage: →Table 8-2.

5. Other agents:

1) **Amiodarone** is the only antiarrhythmic agent with no negative inotropic effects that is effective in most types of supraventricular and ventricular arrhythmia.

2) In patients with HF receiving long-term treatment with **β-blockers** who are hospitalized due to HF exacerbation, the β-blockers generally should not be discontinued unless it is necessary to use inotropic agents. In patients with bradycardia or an SBP decreased to <100 mm Hg, reduce the dose of the β-blocker. If the β-blocker has been discontinued, resume the treatment once the patient is hemodynamically stable.

3) In patients receiving long-term **ACEI/ARB** treatment, these agents should not be discontinued unless it is unavoidable (eg, in a patient with shock). Caution is advised when starting ACEIs/ARBs in patients with HF in the acute setting. If ACEI/ARB are indicated and no contraindications exist, start the treatment before discharge.

4) **Antithrombotic prophylaxis** with heparin or other anticoagulants should be used (→Chapter 3.19.2)

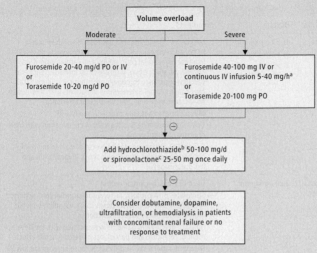

Figure 8-2. Algorithm of diuretic therapy in patients with acute heart failure. *Based on Eur J Heart Fail 2016;18(8):891-975*.

5) Once the patient is stable, add an **aldosterone antagonist** in patients with ACS, ejection fraction ≤40%, and no contraindications. Assess kidney function and serum potassium levels before starting the treatment.

Supportive Treatment

1. Ventilatory support: Consider this in patients with persistent SaO_2 <90% despite maintained airway and oxygen treatment. Generally start with non-invasive support, but invasive support may also be considered if patients are tiring out due to work of breathing or severe pulmonary edema causing hypoxia.

2. Circulatory support, such as extracorporeal membrane oxygenation (ECMO), may be considered in patients with AHF resistant to pharmacologic treatment (except for those with increased cardiac output) if improvement in cardiac function is expected or as a bridging therapy before heart transplantation or another intervention that may restore cardiac function.

Surgical Treatment

Indications:

1) Multivessel ischemic heart disease causing severe myocardial ischemia.
2) Acute mechanical complications of MI.
3) Acute mitral or aortic regurgitation caused by endocarditis, trauma, or aortic dissection (in the case of aortic insufficiency).
4) Some complications of percutaneous coronary intervention.

Table 8-2. Use of intravenous inotropic agents in patients with acute heart failure

Agents	Dosage	Comments
Dopamine	1) <3 µg/kg/min 2) 3-5 µg/kg/min 3) >5µg/kg/min(max, 30 µg/kg/min)	– Low doses (1) mainly cause vasodilation of the visceral, renal, and coronary vascular beds; intermediate doses (2) increase myocardial contractility and cardiac output via adrenergic stimulation; high doses (3) increase peripheral vascular resistance through α-adrenergic stimulation (this may cause clinical deterioration in patients with AHF due to an increase in LV and right ventricular afterloads) – May be used in patients with AHF and low BP – Low-dose dopamine is often used in combination with higher doses of dobutamine – Survival on dopamine may be worse compared to norepinephrine in case of cardiogenic shock (hypotension and hypoperfusion)⊖
Dobutamine	2-20 µg/kg/min	– Used to increase cardiac output – Stimulates β_1-receptors, increases myocardial contractility, increases heart rate; lower doses cause vasodilation while higher doses cause vasoconstriction – Infusion over >24 to 48 hours is associated with the development of tolerance and partial loss of hemodynamic effects – Discontinuation may be difficult because of recurrent low BP, congestion, or kidney failure, which is why the infusion rates should be reduced gradually (by 2 µq/kq/min per day) and used together with optimized vasodilator therapy (eg, oral ACEIs) – May cause ventricular or supraventricular arrhythmia and chest pain in patients with IHD
Milrinone	Bolus 25-75 µg/kg over 10-20 min followed by infusion of 0.375--0.75 µg/kg/min	– Phosphodiesterase inhibitor (inhibits cAMP degradation); has positive inotropic effects and facilitates myocardial relaxation and vasodilation – Indicated in patients with peripheral hypoperfusion and normal BP with or without pulmonary congestion in whom diuretic and vasodilator treatment was ineffective – May be used instead of dopamine in patients treated with β-blockers in the case of inadequate response to dobutamine – May have proarrhythmic effects and should be used with caution in patients with IHD
Norepinephrine	0.2-2 µg/kg/min	– Use (with caution!) only in patients with cardiogenic shock and BP <90 mm Hg when organ perfusion is inadequate in spite of other interventions – May be indicated in shock patients with AHF and sepsis – May be combined with each of the above inotropic agents (use with caution in combination with dopamine)
Epinephrine	1 mg every 3-5 min (only during CPR); 0.05-0.5 µg/kg/min	Use only during CPR in patients with cardiac arrest or in the case of dobutamine resistance and persistent hypotension
Digoxin	Loading dose 0.5--1 mg, followed by 0.125-0.375 mg/d (monitor serum drug levels)	Effective in patients with AHF caused by tachyarrhythmia (eg, AF); not recommended in patients with AHF after acute MI because of its proarrhythmic effects

ACEI, angiotensin-converting enzyme inhibitor; AF, atrial fibrillation; AHF, acute heart failure; BP, blood pressure; cAMP, cyclic adenosine monophosphate; CPR, cardiopulmonary resuscitation; IHD, ischemic heart disease; LV, left ventricle; MI, myocardial infarction.

→ **SPECIAL CONSIDERATIONS**

1. Prosthetic valve thrombosis is often fatal. If this is suspected, perform echocardiography immediately.

1) In patients with a **thrombosed prosthetic pulmonary or tricuspid valve or at high surgical risk**, use **fibrinolytic agents**: alteplase (10 mg IV bolus followed by an IV infusion of 90 mg over 90 minutes) or streptokinase (250,000-500,000 IU IV over 20 minutes followed by an IV infusion of 1-1.5 million IU over 10 hours and then by unfractionated heparin treatment).

2) In patients with a **thrombosed prosthetic mitral or aortic valve**, the preferred treatment is valve replacement.

2. Acute kidney injury in the course of AHF leads to nonrespiratory acidosis and electrolyte disturbances that may cause arrhythmia, reduce effectiveness of treatment, and affect the prognosis. Moderate to severe renal failure (serum creatinine levels >190 µmol/L [2.5 mg/dL]) is associated with an impaired response to diuretics. In patients with persistent volume overload despite appropriate pharmacotherapy, consider continuous venous hemofiltration with ultrafiltration.

3. In the case of **bronchoconstriction** in a patient with AHF, administer nebulized **salbutamol** 0.5 mL of a 0.5% solution (2.5 mg) in 2.5 mL of 0.9% saline over 20 minutes. Administer subsequent doses every hour for the first few hours, then continue as needed.

8.2. Chronic Heart Failure

→ **DEFINITION**

Definition and classification of heart failure: →Chapter 3.8.

→ **EPIDEMIOLOGY, ETIOLOGY, PATHOPHYSIOLOGY**

Heart failure with reduced ejection fraction (HFrEF) is better understood than heart failure with preserved ejection fraction (HFpEF) and represents approximately half of all heart failure (HF) cases. The most common etiology of HFrEF is coronary artery disease (CAD) and arterial hypertension. Other causes include viral infection, alcohol abuse, valvular heart disease, chemotherapy (eg, doxorubicin or trastuzumab), peripartum cardiomyopathy, "idiopathic" dilated cardiomyopathy, and genetic cardiomyopathies.

In HFrEF, maladaptive changes after myocardial injury lead to pathologic remodeling of the ventricle with dilatation and impaired contractility. This is mediated by:

1) Maladaptive left ventricle (LV) hypertrophy associated with the reexpression of fetal isoforms of contractile proteins and progressive loss of cardiomyocytes via apoptosis or necrosis.

2) Abnormal calcium homeostasis and depressed β-receptor density in cardiomyocytes.

3) Myocardial fibrosis.

4) Progression of mitral insufficiency and pulmonary hypertension.

5) Neurohormonal activation involving the renin-angiotensin-aldosterone system, the sympathetic nervous system, and enhanced vasopressin secretion accompanied by impaired vasodilatory and renal responses to natriuretic peptides, which increases preload and afterload. These systemic neurohormonal responses are triggered by cardiac output lowering, have detrimental long-term effects on the heart and systemic vasculature, and create a vicious cycle of further myocardial injury and remodeling, which in turn exacerbates neurohormonal activation.

Additionally, the following systemic abnormalities both underlie HF symptoms and contribute to HF progression: depressed sensitivity of baroreceptors, enhanced reactivity of chemoreceptors and muscular ergoreceptors, vascular endothelial dysfunction and impaired vasodilatory reserve, renal dysfunction, skeletal muscle dysfunction, functional or absolute iron deficiency with or without anemia, chronic inflammatory activation, and neuroendocrine dysfunction favoring catabolic pathways.

HFpEF is less understood and is increasing in prevalence. Patients are more likely to be older, female, and obese, and have a better prognosis than those with HFrEF. They are less likely to have coronary heart disease and more likely to have hypertension, atrial fibrillation, and sleep apnea. Pathophysiology involves heterogeneous factors, such as impaired LV relaxation due to excessive afterload (owing to elevated blood pressure, aortic stenosis, increased arterial stiffness, and impaired peripheral vasodilatory reserve), decreased passive LV compliance (mediated by changes in the extracellular matrix associated with concentric LV hypertrophy), chronotropic incompetence, microvascular coronary dysfunction, and accompanying myocardial oxidative stress with consequent stimulation of proinflammatory and profibrotic pathways.

Causes of high-output HF include conditions associated with hyperdynamic circulation: severe anemia, thyrotoxicosis, large systemic arteriovenous fistulas, advanced cirrhosis, polycythemia or secondary erythrocytosis, Paget disease, beriberi, carcinoid syndrome, or pregnancy. HF usually develops in patients with hyperdynamic circulation superimposed on an underlying heart disease, although it can occur in absence of structural heart disease.

Cardiomyopathies (abnormalities in cardiac myocytes that result in impaired function) are a predisposing condition for clinical HF but may not always be associated with clinical HF. The World Health Organization categorizes the etiology of HF based on the type of underlying cardiomyopathy, which is defined as pathologic myocardial processes and dysfunction that are a direct consequence of cardiovascular abnormalities other than valvular heart disease, systemic hypertension, congenital heart disease, and atherosclerotic coronary artery disease. The European Society of Cardiology classification scheme helps with identifying etiology based on cardiac structure:

1) Dilated cardiomyopathy: Dilatation of ventricle or ventricles with impaired ability to contract leading to eccentric hypertrophy. Etiologies may include toxins (eg, alcohol, cocaine, and chemotherapeutic agents such as anthracyclines, fluorouracil, and trastuzumab), myocarditis, Chagas disease, peripartum cardiomyopathy, and familial cardiomyopathies (eg, Becker or Duchenne muscular dystrophy), among others.

2) Hypertrophic cardiomyopathy: Concentric hypertrophy of the ventricle or its segments, with resulting diastolic dysfunction.

3) Restrictive cardiomyopathy: Impaired ventricular filling with no or minimal dilatation or hypertrophy, although ventricular thickening may occur.

4) Arrhythmogenic right ventricular cardiomyopathy: Fatty and fibrous replacement of the normal myocardium, usually affecting the right ventricular free wall.

5) Unclassified cardiomyopathies: Cardiomyopathies that do not fit the above types. Takotsubo and noncompaction are examples of unclassified cardiomyopathies.

Causes of HF exacerbations: Patients with chronic heart failure may develop exacerbations due to the following reasons:

1) Acute coronary syndrome.

2) Poorly controlled hypertension.

3) Tachyarrhythmia (most commonly atrial fibrillation) or bradyarrhythmia.

4) Pulmonary embolism.

Table 8-3. New York Heart Association (NYHA) classification of heart failure	
Class	Functional capacity
I	No limitation of physical activity. Ordinary physical activity does not cause undue fatigue, dyspnea, or palpitation
II	Slight limitation of physical activity. The patient is comfortable at rest, but ordinary physical activity results in fatigue, palpitation, or dyspnea
III	Marked limitation of physical activity. The patient is comfortable at rest, but less than ordinary activity causes fatigue, palpitation, or dyspnea
IV	Any physical activity causes discomfort. Symptoms of heart failure may be present even at rest. Discomfort increases with any physical activity

Based on: The Criteria Committee of the New York Heart Association. Nomenclature and Criteria for Diagnosis of Diseases of the Heart and Great Vessels. 9th ed. Boston, Mass: Little, Brown & Co; 1994:253-256.

5) Endocarditis, myocarditis.
6) Conditions associated with hyperdynamic circulation.
7) Infections (particularly pneumonia).
8) Renal dysfunction.
9) Dietary indiscretion (high sodium intake).
10) Nonadherence to prescribed medications.
11) Iatrogenic: Intravenous fluids, use of medications with negative chronotropic or inotropic effects (eg, verapamil, diltiazem, or inappropriate doses of β-blockers), cardiotoxic agents (eg, anthracyclines), drugs causing sodium and/or water retention (eg, glucocorticoids, estrogens, nonsteroidal anti--inflammatory drugs [NSAIDs]).
12) Abnormalities in thyroid function (eg, caused by amiodarone).
13) Alcohol abuse, cocaine use.
14) Untreated sleep apnea.

→ CLINICAL FEATURES

Symptoms of HF are a combination of pulmonary and/or systemic congestion with or without low output. The New York Heart Association (NYHA) classification of the severity of HF (functional status) is based on the assessment of fatigue, dyspnea, and palpitations, which are caused by physical activity (→Table 8-3). A validated scale, such as that by the NYHA, is commonly used to document functional capacity.

1. Clinical manifestations of LV failure (pulmonary congestion):

1) **Symptoms**: Dyspnea (at rest or on exertion); orthopnea (occurs 1-2 minutes after lying down and resolves within a few minutes of sitting or standing up); paroxysmal nocturnal dyspnea, which unlike orthopnea occurs much later after lying down, wakes the patient up, and takes much more time (usually ≥30 minutes) to resolve; cough (an equivalent of exertional dyspnea or orthopnea), generally dry, occasionally producing pink sputum (usually in patients with pulmonary edema); fatigue.

2) **Signs**: Dilated LV or displaced apex with a third heart sound; crackles over the lung fields (typically audible in the basal regions, although they may extend up to the apical regions), which may be accompanied by wheezing and rhonchi (caused in part by edema of the bronchial mucosa).

2. Clinical manifestations of right ventricular failure (systemic congestion):

1) **Symptoms**: Peripheral dependent edema (most commonly affecting the feet and ankles, or the sacral area in bedridden patients), abdominal pain or discomfort caused by liver congestion, or nocturia. The symptoms may also include anorexia, nausea, and constipation caused by venous congestion of the gastric and intestinal mucosa and by reduced cardiac output, which in some cases may lead to malabsorption and subsequent malnutrition or even cachexia in patients with advanced HF.

2) **Signs**: Exudates, including pleural effusions (usually bilateral; when unilateral, they occur more frequently on the right) or ascites; right ventricular heave or a right ventricle that is palpable in the subxiphoid region; an enlarged and tender liver (tenderness is due to stretching of the hepatic capsule and occurs when congestion develops rapidly); a firm and atrophic liver may be observed in a long-standing (several years-long) HF. Other signs include mild jaundice, jugular vein distention with or without sustained elevation, and in some patients Kussmaul sign (increased jugular venous pressure during inspiration, similar to that observed in constrictive pericarditis).

3. Manifestations common to right and left ventricular failure (including manifestations of low cardiac output):

1) **Symptoms**: Impaired exercise tolerance, oliguria (in advanced HF).

2) **Signs**: Pale and cool skin of the extremities, diaphoresis, rarely acrocyanosis (features of sympathetic stimulation); tachycardia, third heart sound (often audible in patients with systolic LV dysfunction) or fourth heart sound (more suggestive of isolated diastolic HF), an accentuated pulmonary component of the second heart sound; occasionally murmurs associated with valvular heart disease, which is a cause of HF or is secondary to ventricular dilatation; low pulse pressure, mild elevation of diastolic blood pressure; Cheyne-Stokes respiration; symptoms of abnormal cerebral perfusion, especially in the elderly.

4. Symptoms and signs of HF with an increased cardiac output caused by hyperdynamic circulation: High pulse pressure (reduction in diastolic blood pressure); increased precordial pulsation; pulsus altus et celer, capillary pulsation (Quincke pulse); tachycardia; abnormal features on auscultation (hyperdynamic heart sounds, sometimes a third or fourth heart sound, midsystolic ejection murmur audible along the left sternal border, sometimes midsystolic murmur over the mitral or tricuspid valve and constant venous hum, carotid bruit); warming and erythema of the skin (not present in patients with ischemia; it may be local, eg, in patients with Paget disease or arteriovenous fistulas). In patients with arteriovenous fistulas, applying pressure on a fistula causes a decrease in heart rate.

5. Clinical features of HFpEF are similar to those of HFrEF and include exertional dyspnea and other symptoms of pulmonary congestion, while the features of peripheral hypoperfusion are usually absent.

→ DIAGNOSIS

Diagnostic Tests

A thorough history and physical examination are essential to screen for conditions that cause or precipitate HF.

Basic laboratory investigations are used to establish the cause of HF, detect associated complications, or ascertain prognosis. Chest radiographs and echocardiography play a key role in diagnosing HF.

1. Laboratory investigations:

1) Hyponatremia caused by volume overload may be observed in patients with advanced HF or those who are treated with thiazide diuretics.

2) Hypokalemia or hyperkalemia and increased serum creatinine levels may be caused by diuresis, kidney injury, and/or adverse effects of drugs (→below).

3) Elevated serum aminotransferase, lactate dehydrogenase, and bilirubin levels are observed in patients with hepatic congestion.

4) Anemia (worsening or triggering HF) or high hematocrit values (eg, in chronic obstructive pulmonary disease and congenital heart disease with right-to-left shunt).

5) Serum levels of the natriuretic peptides can be measured to diagnose patients with a clinical suspicion of HF (especially in case of diagnostic uncertainty and unavailability of bedside echocardiography, which is increasingly being used in clinical practice). Due to a high negative but limited positive predictive value, natriuretic peptides are recommended to exclude HF but not to establish HF diagnosis. Exclusionary cut-off points for natriuretic peptides are higher in the acute than in the nonacute setting:

a) HF is unlikely in patients with no acute worsening of the symptoms (ie, in the nonacute setting), B-type natriuretic peptide (BNP) levels <35 pg/mL, N-terminal pro–B-type natriuretic peptide (NT-proBNP) levels <125 pg/mL, and normal ECG.

b) In patients with rapidly worsening symptoms (ie, in the acute setting), the cut-points are as follows: BNP <100 pg/mL, NT-proBNP <300 pg/mL, midregional proatrial natriuretic peptide (MR-proANP) <120 pmol/L.

c) BNP/NT-proBNP can be used for prognostic stratification in patients with known HF. In ambulatory patients aged <75 years and with low EF, BNP/NT-proBNP can be used to guide management.⊘●

It should be noted that (1) because natriuretic peptides tend to be lower in HFpEF than in HFrEF, the BNP/NT-proBNP threshold for diagnosis of HF in HFpEF is lower than in HFrEF; (2) BNP, but not NT-proBNP, is a substrate of neprilysin. Thus, BNP levels cannot be used to assess HF severity or treatment response in patients on angiotensin receptor neprilysin inhibitors (ARNIs); NT-proBNP, however, can be used for these purposes in patients on ARNIs.

2. ECG can reveal clues about the underlying etiology: ischemic heart disease, arrhythmia, conduction disturbances, or ventricular hypertrophy.

3. Chest radiographs usually reveal an enlarged cardiac silhouette (except for the majority of patients with hyperdynamic circulation or HFpEF) and features of pulmonary congestion. They help identify pulmonary edema while excluding other lung diseases that may be contributing.

4. Echocardiography is a key diagnostic study in HF and is usually performed in patients with suspected HF as it allows assessment of:

1) LV systolic function through the analysis of global and segmental LV contractility and measurements of LVEF.

2) LV diastolic function through the analysis of tissue Doppler indices, left atrial volume, estimated pulmonary pressure, and presence of predisposing conditions.

3) Structural heart disease: Ventricular and/or atrial hypertrophy or dilatation, valvular heart disease, congenital heart disease, pericardial effusion.

In some cases (eg, a poor acoustic window in transthoracic echocardiography, significant native or prosthetic valve dysfunction, suspected thrombus in the left atrial appendage in patients with atrial fibrillation, diagnosis of bacterial endocarditis or congenital heart disease), transesophageal echocardiography may be indicated.

Dobutamine stress echocardiography is useful in the diagnosis of coronary artery disease and can be considered in patients with intermediate pretest probability or for assessment of reversible ischemia prior to proceeding to coronary angiography and revascularization.

5. Coronary angiography is indicated in patients with suspected ischemic heart disease, a history of unexplained cardiac arrest, severe ventricular arrhythmias if myocardial ischemia is suspected as a cause, HF that is treatment resistant or of unknown etiology, or prior to an elective cardiac surgery.

6. Exercise stress test may be useful in patients with a discrepancy between the severity of symptoms and signs of the disease, in patients qualified for heart transplantation, and to differentiate between cardiac and pulmonary causes of dyspnea.

7. Multislice CT (MSCT) and cardiac MRI may be used in determining the etiology of HF and in differential diagnosis when other methods (especially echocardiography and coronary angiography) are not sufficient to make a diagnosis. MSCT and MRI are particularly useful when differentiating between various forms of cardiomyopathy, cardiac tumors, pericardial disease, and congenital heart disease.

8. Endomyocardial biopsy has utility in selected patients with HF of unexplained etiology and with a suspected disease requiring specific treatment, including myocarditis (giant cell or eosinophilic), infiltrative or storage diseases (amyloidosis, sarcoidosis, hemochromatosis, or Fabry disease), and in diagnostics of transplant rejection.

Diagnostic Criteria

HF is diagnosed in patients with typical signs and symptoms accompanied by objective features of systolic or significant diastolic LV dysfunction at rest, usually observed in echocardiography. Chest radiography criteria include interstitial or pulmonary edema. Another important indicator of the dysfunction is an increase in serum levels of natriuretic peptides (→above) and clinical improvement in response to standard HF pharmacotherapy. The Boston criteria offer objective scoring to facilitate the diagnosis of heart failure.

Differential Diagnosis

Differential diagnosis includes other causes of dyspnea, edema, and jugular vein distension.

→ TREATMENT

Treatment of HF includes:

1) Definitive treatment of the underlying condition (eg, coronary revascularization, valvular surgery).
2) Long-term treatment of HF (→below).
3) Treatment of exacerbations of HF (→Chapter 3.8.1).

Nonpharmacologic Management

1. In patients with symptoms of sodium and fluid retention, **sodium restriction** to 2 to 3 g/d is usually recommended (<2 g/d if the symptoms persist, especially if they are resistant to diuretic treatment). In patients with hyponatremia and severe symptoms (NYHA classes III-IV), add **fluid restriction** to 1.5 to 2 L/d.

2. Regular body weight monitoring:

1) Monitor the patient's body weight; an increase >2 kg in body weight over 3 days may indicate fluid retention caused by HF.
2) Reduce body weight in obese patients, especially those with a body mass index (BMI) >35 kg/m^2.
3) Improve nutrition in patients with features of malnutrition (BMI <22 kg/m^2, <90% of ideal body weight).

3. Reduction in alcohol consumption to ≤10 to 12 g/d in women and ≤20 to 25 g/d in men. Abstinence is necessary in patients with suspected alcohol cardiomyopathy.

4. Smoking cessation.

5. In patients with HF who have recently been hospitalized for an acute HF exacerbation, nurse home visits, nurse case management, and outpatient disease management/heart failure clinics should be considered, as they reduce all-cause mortality and readmissions.⊘●

6. Avoidance of the following drugs (if possible):

1) NSAIDs, including cyclooxygenase-2 (COX-2) inhibitors (these increase fluid retention; reduce the effectiveness of diuretics, angiotensin-converting enzyme inhibitors [ACEIs], angiotensin receptor blockers [ARBs], and aldosterone antagonists; and increase the risk of adverse effects of these classes of drugs).

2) Glucocorticoids (these increase fluid retention and the risk of hypokalemia).

3) Class I antiarrhythmic drugs (particularly class Ia and Ic agents) and class III sotalol and ibutilide (→Table 4-1).

4) Tricyclic antidepressants (these have proarrhythmic effects and are associated with a risk of hypotension and HF exacerbation; selective serotonin reuptake inhibitors are relatively safe).

5) Dronedarone is contraindicated in patients with HF, as it increases cardiovascular mortality and risk of HF exacerbation.⊗●

6) Verapamil and diltiazem (except in patients with HFpEF; high doses of verapamil are routinely used in patients with hypertrophic cardiomyopathy); dihydropyridine calcium-channel blockers (in patients with coexisting hypertension or angina, only long-acting agents [amlodipine and felodipine] may be used). Nondihydropyridine calcium-channel blockers are usually avoided in patients with HFrEF, given their negative inotropic effect.

7) α_1-Blockers (these cause fluid retention and increase the risk of hypotension; in the case of voiding problems caused by symptomatic prostatic hyperplasia, switch to 5α-reductase inhibitors).

8) Moxonidine (increases the risk of death).

9) Metformin should be avoided in the patients with contraindications (risk of lactic acidosis in patients with acute HF or severe respiratory, liver, or renal failure; it is commonly used and considered the first-line antidiabetic drug in patients with stable HF).

10) Thiazolidinediones (rosiglitazone, pioglitazone; these increase fluid retention and are absolutely contraindicated in NYHA class III or IV).⊗●

11) Anthracyclines (in the case of life-saving therapy, consider using liposomal doxorubicin or pretreatment with dexrazoxane; closely monitor LV function).

7. Annual influenza and pneumococcal vaccination.

8. Regular moderate physical activity: 30 minutes of aerobic exercise at least 3 times a week (clinically stable HF patients).

9. Caution is advised when **traveling to altitudes >1500 meters above sea level or to hot and humid climates**. In the case of long-distance journeys, air travel is preferred over land travel to **avoid prolonged periods of immobilization**.

10. Diagnosis and treatment of clinically significant depression (→Chapter 12.5).

11. In the case of **concomitant central sleep apnea**, consider continuous positive airway pressure (→Chapter 13.11).

Pharmacotherapy

Pharmacotherapy of HFrEF: →Figure 8-3.

General recommendations: Start with low doses of drugs and titrate them up to a target dose that has been proven effective in clinical trials or up to the maximum tolerated dose.

In hospitalized patients, start treatment with low-dose β-blockers (after HF is stabilized), ACEIs, ARBs, or aldosterone antagonists before discharge, if possible. The pattern of use of ARBs + ARNIs is evolving rapidly.

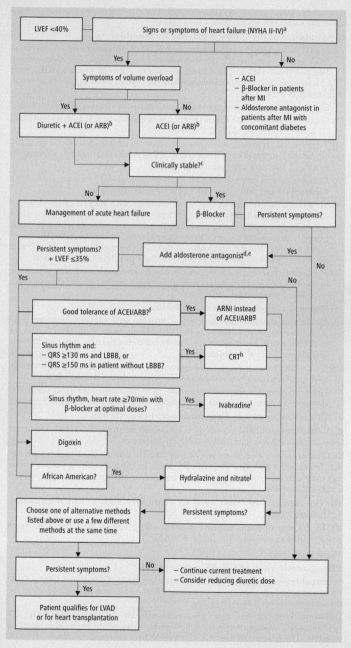

Note: ICD is indicated at any management stage if:
1) LVEF ≤35% persists ≥3 months despite optimal therapy, or
2) Patient has a history of ventricular fibrillation, sustained ventricular tachycardia, or unexplained syncope.

[a] In patients with atrial fibrillation and rapid ventricular rhythm in case of hemodynamic instability use electrical cardioversion (if arrhythmia cannot be quickly controlled with pharmacotherapy). If this is not feasible or is contraindicated, use IV amiodarone (alternatively IV digoxin for rate control after excluding an accessory conduction pathway). If there are no features of acute hemodynamic decompensation, control heart rate using a β-blocker (add digoxin if necessary).

[b] In patients with intolerance of or contraindications to ACEIs (persistent cough or angioedema).

[c] Patients without significant symptoms of volume overload, symptomatic hypotension, or hypoperfusion who have not required nondigitalis inotropic agents in the past few days.

[d] In patients with an LVEF ≤35% receiving a β-blocker and an ACEI (or an ARB) at optimal doses. Use particular caution in patients with serum potassium >5 mmol/L and serum creatinine >220 μmol/L (2.5 mg/dL).

[e] In patients hospitalized in the past 6 months, if BNP is >250 pg/mL, or if NT-proBNP is >500 pg/mL in men or >750 pg/mL in women.

[f] In a dose equivalent to enalapril 10 mg twice a day.

[g] Provided that serum BNP is ≥150 pg/mL or NT-proBNP is ≥600 pg/mL; in the case of patients hospitalized in the past 12 months, BNP ≥100 pg/mL or NT-proBNP ≥400 pg/mL.

[h] In patients with sinus rhythm and QRS morphology other than LBBB, consider CRT in the case of QRS ≥150 ms; this may be also considered in those with QRS 130-149 ms. In patients with atrial fibrillation, consider CRT in case of QRS ≥130 ms provided that dual chamber pacing is used.

[i] In patients hospitalized due to heart failure in the past year; this may be also considered if β-blockers are contraindicated or not tolerated.

[j] Consider also in the case of intolerance of or contraindications to both ACEIs and ARBs.

ACEI, angiotensin-converting enzyme inhibitor; ARB, angiotensin receptor blocker; ARNI, angiotensin receptor neprilysin inhibitor; BNP, B-type natriuretic peptide; CRT, cardiac resynchronization therapy; ICD, implantable cardioverter-defibrillator; LBBB, left bundle branch block; LVAD, left ventricular assist device; LVEF, left ventricular ejection fraction; MI, myocardial infarction; NT-proBNP, N-terminal pro-B-type natriuretic peptide; NYHA, New York Heart Association.

Figure 8-3. Suggested management of chronic heart failure. *Based on Eur J Heart Fail. 2016;18(8):891-975.*

1. Diuretics (loop with or without potassium-sparing diuretics) are used in patients with symptoms of volume overload and then continued at the lowest dose that prevents water retention. Agents and dosage: →Table 8-4.

General recommendations:

1) Loop diuretics are generally the first-line agents in managing volume overload, particularly in symptomatic HF.

2) Adjust doses to the patient's needs. Closely monitor the clinical status as well as serum levels of potassium, sodium, and creatinine.

3) Increase doses of diuretics until the signs and symptoms of volume overload improve (a recommended rate of body weight reduction is 0.5 to 1 kg/d). Adjust doses of diuretics (particularly when the desired dry body weight has been achieved) to avoid kidney injury and dehydration.

4) Encourage patients or caregivers to self-adjust the doses of diuretics based on the daily measurements of body weight and signs and symptoms of fluid retention.

5) In the case of resistance to diuretics, assess the patient's adherence to the treatment regimen; make sure that the patient does not use NSAIDs, COX--2 inhibitors, glucocorticoids, cyclosporine (INN ciclosporin), or estrogens; assess the patient's sodium/fluid intake; and then increase the dose of diuretics. If this is not effective, consider replacing furosemide with another loop diuretic (eg, bumetanide). At this point, administer the loop diuretic

Table 8-4. Dosage of oral diuretics in patients with chronic heart failure

Agent	Starting dose (mg/d)	Usual dose (mg/d)
Loop diuretics		
Furosemide[a]	20-40	40-240
Torasemide	5-10	10-20
Thiazide and thiazide-like diuretics		
Chlorthalidone	12.5-25	25-100
Hydrochlorothiazide	25	12.5-100
Indapamide	2.5 (1.5 mg when using controlled-release formulations)	2.5-5
Potassium-sparing diuretics[b]		
Amiloride (available only in a fixed combination with hydrochlorothiazide)	2.5 (5)	5-10 (10-20)
Eplerenone	25 (50)	50 (100)
Spironolactone	12.5-25 (50)	50 (100-200)

[a] The diuretic effect starts within 30 to 60 minutes, peaks in 1 to 2 hours, and ends after 6 to 8 hours.

[b] Doses used in patients who are not treated with an angiotensin-converting enzyme inhibitor or an angiotensin receptor blocker are given in parenthesis.

bid or when fasting, and finally consider a short-term intravenous infusion of a loop diuretic.

6) Ensure optimal afterload reduction, use of an aldosterone antagonist, and use of other guideline-recommended medical therapy.

Management of adverse effects:

1) In patients with **hypokalemia/hypomagnesemia**, start potassium or magnesium supplementation. Consider increasing the dose of the ACEI/ARB or aldosterone antagonist for long-term prevention of hypokalemia/hypomagnesemia.

2) **Hyperkalemia** may occur in patients treated with ACEIs or ARBs in combination with potassium-sparing diuretics, including aldosterone antagonists. Do not use potassium-sparing diuretics other than aldosterone antagonists.

3) In patients with **hyponatremia**, restrict fluid intake, discontinue the thiazide diuretic and substitute it (if possible) with a loop diuretic, and reduce the dose of or discontinue (if possible) the loop diuretic.

4) In patients with **hyperuricemia and gout**, avoid NSAIDs.

5) In patients with possible **hypovolemia**, determine the volume status and consider reducing doses of diuretics.

6) In patients with renal failure, exclude hypovolemia and concomitant use of other nephrotoxic agents (eg, NSAIDs), then discontinue aldosterone antagonists and thiazides (in patients treated with loop diuretics in combination with thiazides) and consider reduction of the dose of the ACEI/ARB.

7) High-dose loop diuretics may be **ototoxic**.

2. β-Blockers: Evidence supporting β-blockers is drug-specific to bisoprolol, carvedilol, and metoprolol. They should be used in patients with NYHA

Table 8-5. Dosage of evidence-informed β-blockers in patients with chronic heart failure

β-Blocker	Starting dose (mg)[a]	Subsequent doses up to target dose (mg)
Bisoprolol	1.25	2.5 to 3.75 to 5 to 7.5 to 10
Carvedilol	3.125	6.25 to 12.5 to 25 to 50
Metoprolol succinate controlled-release	12.5 or 25	25 to 50 to 100 to 200

[a] Carvedilol is administered 2 times a day, while other listed β-blockers are administered once daily. The table lists single doses of the agents.

classes II to IV and LVEF ≤40% or in patients with asymptomatic systolic LV dysfunction after myocardial infarction (MI) who have already been receiving an optimal ACEI or ARB dose and are clinically stable.◉● Treatment with a β-blocker may be started with caution in patients with a recent history of HF decompensation as long as their condition has improved as a result of other treatments or the use of ongoing intravenous inotropic agents is not required. Agents and doses: →Table 8-5.

General recommendations: During dose titration follow-up visits should be scheduled every 2 to 4 weeks and the dose should be doubled at each visit as tolerated. Do not increase the dose in case of symptoms of HF exacerbation, symptomatic hypotension (eg, dizziness), or bradycardia <50 beats/min.

Management of adverse effects:

1) **Symptomatic hypotension** frequently resolves spontaneously with time. Consider reducing doses of other antihypertensive agents (except for ACEIs and ARBs), for instance, diuretics or nitrates.

2) **HF exacerbation**: Increase the dose of diuretics (frequently a temporary increase is sufficient) and continue the β-blocker treatment (frequently at a lower dose), if possible. In case of cardiogenic shock/hypoperfusion, discontinue the β-blocker and use an intravenous inotropic agent such as milrinone or dobutamine (→Table 8-2).

3) **Excessive bradycardia**: Perform ECG (or Holter ECG) to exclude a heart block. Consider discontinuation of digoxin if the patient is treated with this agent. Dose reduction or discontinuation of the β-blocker may be necessary.

3. ACEIs: ACEIs should be initiated in patients with LVEF ≤40%, regardless of symptoms.◉● Once target or maximal tolerated doses are achieved, consideration should be given for persistently symptomatic patients to be switched to the equivalent dose of ARNIs (→below). Doses: →Table 8-6.

General recommendations:

1) Avoid excessive diuretic treatment before starting ACEIs (you may reduce the doses of diuretics 24 hours before the start of ACEI treatment).

2) Consider increasing the dose after 2 to 4 weeks of ACEI treatment. Do not increase the dose in patients with significant deterioration in renal function or with hyperkalemia. In hospitalized or closely monitored patients who tolerate the drug, the dose may be uptitrated more rapidly.

3) Monitor renal function and serum electrolyte levels at baseline; within 1 to 2 weeks of starting ACEI treatment; 1 and 4 weeks after the dose increase; 1, 3, and 6 months after reaching the target maintenance dose; and subsequently every 6 months.

Management of adverse effects (suggestions):

1) **Kidney function impairment**: Serum blood urea nitrogen and creatinine levels may increase after the initiation of ACEI treatment; this is not clinically relevant unless rapid and severe. Exclude hypovolemia, dehydration,

Table 8-6. Recommended dosage of ACEIs, ARBs, and ARNIs in patients with chronic heart failure

Agent	Dose	
	Starting	Target
ACEIs		
Enalapril	2.5 mg bid	10-20 mg bid
Captopril	6.25 mg tid	50 mg tid
Lisinopril	2.5-5 mg once daily	20-35 mg once daily
Ramipril	2.5 mg once daily	5 mg bid
Trandolapril	0.5 mg once daily	4 mg once daily
ARBs		
Candesartan	4 mg or 8 mg once daily	32 mg once daily
Valsartan	40 mg bid	160 mg bid
Losartan[a]	50 mg once daily	150 mg once daily
ARB + ARNI		
Valsartan/sacubitril[b]	24/26 mg bid	97/103 mg bid

Contraindications: →Table 9-4.

[a] Losartan is mentioned in the 2012 European Society of Cardiology guidelines but it has been stressed in the text that the benefits of using the agent may be lower.

[b] Valsartan component in the valsartan/neprilysin combination pill Entresto is more potent than valsartan monotherapy pills available on the market. Therefore, caution must be exercised not to equate valsartan dosage found in current monotherapy with the dose found in Entresto, as it will lead to prescribing a higher than the intended dose.

ACEI, angiotensin-converting enzyme inhibitors; ARB, angiotensin receptor blockers; ARNI, angiotensin receptor neprilysin inhibitor; bid, 2 times a day; tid, 3 times a day.

other medications (eg, NSAIDs, COX-2 inhibitors, cyclosporine, excessive doses of diuretics). The patient should be closely monitored.

a) An increase in serum creatinine levels ≤50% is acceptable unless it exceeds 265 µmol/L (~3 mg/dL).

b) In patients with a serum creatinine increase of 50% to 100% or >265 µmol/L but ≤310 µmol/L (~3.5 mg/dL), reduce the ACEI dose by half.

c) In patients with a serum creatinine increase >100% or >310 µmol/L, discontinue the ACEI immediately.

2) **Hyperkalemia**: Check for other agents that may be the cause (eg, potassium supplements, potassium-sparing diuretics) and discontinue them.

a) In patients with serum potassium levels >5.5 mmol/L, reduce the ACEI dose by half.

b) In patients with serum potassium levels >6.0 mmol/L, discontinue the ACEI immediately and admit for cardiac monitoring and treating hyperkalemia.

3) **Symptomatic hypotension** (eg, dizziness) often resolves spontaneously even if the ACEI dose is not changed. Consider reducing the dose of diuretics and other hypotensive agents (except for ARBs, β-blockers, and aldosterone antagonists).

4) **Cough** (in ~10% patients): Independent of the ACEI dose, cough usually appears within 1 week of ACEI treatment but may also occur after up to several months. It generally resolves within 3 to 5 days after discontinuation of ACEIs but may persist for up to a month or in rare cases even for several months. It usually recurs with the use of a different ACEI. If the cough is persistent and troublesome, switch to an ARB, if needed.

5) **Angioedema** (<1% patients): Switch to an ARB (although on very rare occasions angioedema may also occur after ARBs).

4. ARNIs: Use these preferentially over ACEIs in patients with HFrEF (LVEF <40%) who remain symptomatic (NYHA classes II-IV) and have elevated levels of BNP or NT-proBNP despite treatment with optimal medical therapy, including maximally tolerated ACEIs (ARBs), β-blockers, and mineralocorticoid-receptor antagonists.◐◔ Patients on ACEIs should be converted to the equivalent dose of ARNIs after a washout period of 36 hours (→above). Patients who do not tolerate ARNIs may be switched back to ACEIs after a 36-hour washout period. The role of ARNIs is rapidly evolving, and long-term data on this class of medications are unavailable at this time.

ARNIs are contraindicated in patients with hypotension (systolic blood pressure ≤95 mm Hg), significant renal impairment (glomerular filtration rate ≤30 mL/min), hyperkalemia (K^+ ≥5.2 mmol/L), or severe hepatic disease (liver enzymes >2×upper limit of normal).

Closely monitor serum levels of K^+ (≤5.2 mmol/L) and creatinine (estimated glomerular filtration rate ≥30 mL/min).

Ensure that patients are not concomitantly on an ACEI (a 36-hour washout period from ACEIs is required to reduce the risk of angioedema).

Agents and dosage: →Table 8-6. Doses can be uptitrated every 2 to 4 weeks.

5. ARBs: ARBs are used in NYHA classes II to IV patients with LVEF ≤40% who do not tolerate ACEIs or ARNIs because of persistent cough or angioedema.◐◔ Do not use a combination of an ACEI and an ARB due to the risk of adverse events.

General recommendations and management of adverse effects are the same as in ACEIs except for cough. Agents and dosage: →Table 8-6.

6. Aldosterone antagonists (eplerenone, spironolactone) should be used in patients with◐◔:

1) LVEF ≤35% and NYHA classes II to IV.

2) LVEF ≤40%, recent MI, and HF symptoms or diabetes mellitus.

In both cases, patients should have been already treated with an ACEI or an ARB (but not both!) and a β-blocker, all in optimal doses. Agents and dosage: →Table 8-4.

General recommendations:

1) Consider increasing the dose 4 to 8 weeks after starting the treatment. Do not increase the dose in case of significant deterioration of kidney function or hyperkalemia.

2) Monitor kidney function and serum electrolyte levels 1 and 4 weeks after starting the treatment and after increasing the dose; then at 2, 3, 6, 9, and 12 months; and subsequently every 4 months.

3) Do not use aldosterone antagonists in pregnant patients.

Management of adverse effects:

1) In patients with **deterioration of kidney function**, close monitoring is necessary (suggestions below):

   a) In patients with serum creatinine levels >220 µmol/L (~2.5 mg/dL), reduce the dose by half (eg, 25 mg every other day).

   b) In patients with serum creatinine levels >310 µmol/L (~3.5 mg/dL), immediately discontinue aldosterone antagonists.

2) In patients with **hyperkalemia**, close monitoring is necessary:

   a) In patients with serum potassium levels >5.5 mmol/L, reduce the dose by half.

   b) In patients with serum potassium levels >6.0 mmol/L, immediately discontinue aldosterone antagonists.

3) In patients with **breast tenderness and/or enlargement**, switch from spironolactone to eplerenone.

7. Consider **ivabradine**,⊘◯ which reduces the heart rate by having selective effects on the sinus node, in patients with:

1) LVEF ≤35%, preserved sinus rhythm ≥70 beats/min, and NYHA classes II to IV despite the use of an ACEI (or an ARB), an aldosterone antagonist, and a β-blocker at optimal doses.

2) Contraindications to or intolerance of β-blockers.

General recommendations: Start with 5 mg bid and after 2 weeks increase the dose to 7.5 mg bid, provided the patient continues to be in sinus rhythm with a rate of >60 beats/min (treatment with ivabradine cannot be the reason for reducing the dose of a β-blocker without a strong justification, as the benefit of ivabradine is in reducing readmissions [no effect on mortality]).

Management of adverse effects:

1) **Asymptomatic sinus bradycardia <50 beats/min or symptomatic bradycardia**: Reduce the dose to 2.5 mg bid. If the symptoms persist, discontinue ivabradine.

2) **Bradycardia associated with hemodynamic instability**: Discontinue ivabradine. Consider administration of a β-agonist (eg, isoproterenol [INN isoprenaline]) or temporary pacing, if necessary.

3) **Vision disturbances** (transient sensation of bright light in a portion of the visual field, which may interfere with the ability to drive) usually occur in the first 2 months of treatment and generally resolve spontaneously. However, discontinuation of treatment must be considered in case of a sudden vision impairment.

Note: Occurrence of atrial fibrillation (AF) or atrial flutter during treatment with ivabradine increases the risk of rapid ventricular rate if the patient does not receive concomitant β-blockers or low-dose β-blockers. Ivabradine should be discontinued ≥24 hours before an elective cardioversion.

8. Digoxin reduces hospitalization with no survival benefit. It may be considered in HF patients with LVEF ≤40% who remain symptomatic (NYHA classes II-IV) despite receiving treatment with an ARNI or ACEI (or an ARB in patients intolerant to either ARNIs or ACEIs), a β-blocker, and an aldosterone antagonist at optimal doses.⊘◯

Once the clinical status is stabilized, digoxin is preferably used in combination with a β-blocker. Digoxin may be used in stable patients in whom β-blockers are not tolerated, ineffective, or contraindicated. If the effects of the combined treatment with digoxin and a β-blocker are insufficient for rate control in AF, you may switch from digoxin to amiodarone. Avoid the combination of digoxin, a β-blocker, and amiodarone.

Contraindications: Hypertrophic cardiomyopathy with LV outflow tract obstruction, preexcitation syndromes, hypokalemia, hypercalcemia, life-threatening ventricular arrhythmia, cardiac amyloidosis (digoxin binds to amyloid), multifocal atrial tachycardia, patients prior to planned electric cardioversion, bradycardia, second-degree and third-degree atrioventricular blocks, sick sinus syndrome (unless the patient has an implanted pacemaker).

General recommendations:

1) Boluses of 0.25 to 0.5 mg IV (loading dose up to 1 mg over 8-24 hours) may be used to slow down rapid ventricular rate in digoxin-naive patients with HF and AF in an acute setting followed by 0.125 to 0.25 mg/d. Loading doses are

not recommended in hemodynamically stable patients with AF and in patients with preserved sinus rhythm. With routine maintenance doses (0.125-0.25 mg orally per day), steady state serum drug levels are achieved within ~7 days.

2) In elderly patients and in patients with impaired renal function, hypothyroidism, or low body weight, the maintenance doses are 0.0625 or 0.125 mg/d orally. Exercise caution with the loading dose in this population.

3) It has not been proven that regular serum digoxin level measurements are associated with improved outcomes (therapeutic range is 0.6-1.2 ng/mL).

4) Serum digoxin levels may be increased by amiodarone, diltiazem, verapamil, certain antibiotics (macrolides, tetracyclines), proton pump inhibitors, H_2--blockers, and quinidine.

Management of adverse effects: →Chapter 15.6.

9. A fixed-dose combination of **hydralazine** (or dihydralazine) and **isosorbide dinitrate**: In patients with LVEF ≤35% (or LVEF ≤45% and LV dilation), this may be considered an alternative to the ACEI/ARNI/ARB if none of these agents are tolerated due to renal dysfunction (in such cases, use it in combination with a β-blocker and an aldosterone antagonist). Adding the combination to treatment may also be considered in patients who have persistent symptoms of HF when receiving treatment with an ACEI/ARNI/ARB, a β-blocker, and an aldosterone antagonist and is recommended in HF patients self-described as African Americans who remain symptomatic despite treatment with an ACEI, a β-blocker, and an aldosterone antagonist.

Adverse effects: Symptomatic hypotension, tachycardia, arthralgia, myalgia, drug-induced lupus-like syndrome.

10. ω-3 Polyunsaturated fatty acids: 1 g/d may be considered.

11. Antithrombotic treatment should be used in patients with additional indications, that is, paroxysmal or persistent AF or atrial flutter, intracardiac thrombus, or a history of peripheral embolism.

Treatment of HFpEF

There is no convincing data to date for treatments that reduce morbidity or mortality in patients with HF and preserved EF. Nonetheless, the current standard of practice includes:

1) **Optimal treatment of the underlying condition**: This may involve rate control in the setting of AF, treatment of sleep apnea with continuous positive airway pressure, strict control of hypertension (preferably using agents that reduce LV remodeling [ACEIs and ARBs]), revascularization in CAD.

2) **Restriction of sodium and of fluid intake if the patient is hyponatremic**: As in HFrEF.

3) **β-Blockers** are used to improve LV filling by extending diastole (target resting heart rates 60-70 beats/min, or 55-60 beats/min in patients with angina), particularly in patients after MI or with angina, either with sinus rhythm or with AF. Digoxin may be used in patients with AF and rapid ventricular rhythm or in patients with AF not responding to monotherapy with a β-blocker, verapamil, or diltiazem (digoxin reduces mainly the resting heart rate, while β-blockers reduce heart rates on exertion). Assess the feasibility of restoring sinus rhythm.

4) **Diuretics** are used in patients with symptoms of fluid retention. Use these with caution to avoid excessive reduction in cardiac output and subsequent hypotension (measure supine and standing BP) as well as impairment of kidney function.

Invasive Treatment

Consider referral to a specialized center.

1. Cardiac resynchronization therapy (CRT) involves placement of 2 electrodes to stimulate the right and left ventricles, and an additional electrode the right atrium to synchronize the stimulation of the ventricles with the intrinsic atrial rhythm. CRT improves exercise tolerance, reduces the incidence of hospitalization caused by symptom exacerbation, and in patients with preserved sinus rhythm also reduces the risk of death.

Consider referral to a specialized center in patients who are clinically stable, have life expectancy >1 year with reasonable functional status, and (1) are symptomatic with EF ≤35%, and QRS ≥130 milliseconds in the case of left bundle branch block (LBBB); or (2) have QRS ≥150 milliseconds in the case of non-LBBB QRS morphology.

Note: Patients with a decreased EF may be candidates for CRT-D (CRT defibrillator; CRT + ICD placement). Therefore, when qualifying patients for CRT, we typically assess LVEF and the NYHA class after ≥3 months of optimal pharmacotherapy; in patients with ischemic heart disease, after >40 days post-MI; and after >3 months post–percutaneous coronary intervention.

2. Implantable cardioverter-defibrillator (ICD): These devices have been shown to reduce sudden cardiac death (SCD) and are typically considered in patients receiving optimal pharmacotherapy for ≥3 months, after revascularization (where indicated), and with >1-year life expectancy of good functional status. Consider referral to a specialized cardiac center for assessment in the following cases:

1) **Primary prevention**:
   a) Post-MI systolic LV dysfunction (LVEF ≤35% measured >40 days after MI and >3 months after coronary revascularization, whenever performed) in patients with NYHA classes II to III.
   b) NYHA classes II to III systolic LV dysfunction (LVEF ≤35%) of a nonischemic etiology (primary prevention of SCD).

2) **Secondary prevention**: History of ventricular fibrillation or ventricular tachycardia causing a loss of consciousness or hemodynamic instability regardless of LVEF, as long these were not due to a transient or reversible condition, for instance, in the first 48 hours of MI.

   In patients who meet the above criteria and have concomitant indications for CRT, implantation of a device with both CRT and ICD functions (CRT-D) is preferred.

3. Coronary revascularization is usually done in patients with HF caused by ischemic heart disease, particularly with symptoms of angina. In the absence of angina, establish indications for revascularization on the basis of documented ischemia of a viable myocardium supplied by an artery suitable for revascularization.

4. In patients refractory to medical, invasive, and device treatments, consider referral to a specialized center for **heart transplantation assessment**. **Left ventricular assist devices** (LVADs) may be used when waiting for the transplant in patients with HFrEF.

➔ REHABILITATION

Participation in interval or continuous training programs is recommended in HF regardless of LVEF values as long as the patient is clinically stable and physical activity does not lead to exhaustion or trigger new HF symptoms.◐◑ Isometric exercise is not recommended.

➔ PROGNOSIS

SCD accounts for up to 50% of all deaths among patients with HF. An improved prognosis in HF has been documented in:

1) Patients treated with ACEIs or ARBs or ARNIs, β-blockers, aldosterone antagonists, and hydralazine/isosorbide (the last one in African Americans

on contemporary treatments with other drugs). Diuretics in monothera
have no effect on prognosis.

2) Certain subgroups of patients treated with CRT or ICD as well as patients
after coronary revascularization.

Chronic heart failure is marked by periods of stability interspersed with exacerbations requiring hospitalization. Epidemiologic data from Medicare beneficiaries hospitalized for HF suggested a 30-day readmission risk of 25% and a 1-year mortality risk of 37%. Advanced HF is characterized by frequent exacerbations, intolerance of preventive therapies, metabolic perturbations, and overall deterioration that culminates in death. In the current era of ICD use, SCD has been replaced by pump failure as a common mechanism of death.

Overall, patients with HFpEF may have a better prognosis than those with HFrEF. A meta-analysis of published trials in HF patients found the 3-year all-cause mortality rate to be 32% in HFrEF (adjusted for prognostic risk factors) versus 24% in HFpEF.

Patients with HFpEF are typically older, more often female, less likely to have ischemic heart disease, and more likely to have a history of hypertension than patients with HFrEF patients.

9. Hypertension

→ INTRODUCTION

Hypertension is defined as a **systolic blood pressure (SBP) ≥140 mm Hg and/or diastolic blood pressure (DBP) ≥90 mm Hg**. Clinical classification based on blood pressure values: →Table 9-1. Target blood pressure values: →Chapter 3.9.1.

Depending on etiology, **hypertension is classified as**:

1) **Essential hypertension** (>90% of cases).

2) **Secondary hypertension**.

Causes of secondary hypertension:

1) Kidney diseases:
   a) Renal parenchymal diseases (→Chapter 3.9.3).
   b) Renovascular diseases (→Chapter 3.9.4).
   c) Renin-secreting tumors originating from the renal juxtaglomerular apparatus.
   d) Primary sodium retention syndromes: Liddle syndrome, Gordon syndrome.

2) Endocrine diseases: Primary aldosteronism, Cushing syndrome, pheochromocytoma, thyrotoxicosis, hypothyroidism, hyperparathyroidism, carcinoid syndrome, acromegaly.

3) Coarctation of the aorta.

4) Preeclampsia or eclampsia.

5) Acute stress: Burns, alcohol withdrawal syndrome, psychogenic hyperventilation, hypoglycemia, major surgery.

6) Obstructive sleep apnea.

7) Increased intravascular fluid volume.

8) Diseases of the nervous system: Increased intracranial pressure, Guillain-Barré syndrome, quadriplegia, familial dysautonomia.

9) Drugs: Sympathomimetic agents, glucocorticoids, erythropoietin, nonsteroidal anti-inflammatory drugs, calcineurin inhibitors (cyclosporine

Table 9-1. Definitions and classification of blood pressure levels (mm Hg)[a]

Category	Systolic blood pressure		Diastolic blood pressure
Optimal	<120	And	<80
Normal	120-129	And/or	80-84
High-normal	130-139	And/or	85-89
Grade 1 hypertension	140-159	And/or	90-99
Grade 2 hypertension	160-179	And/or	100-109
Grade 3 hypertension	≥180	And/or	≥110
Isolated systolic hypertension	≥140	And	<90

Patients with systolic and diastolic blood pressures falling into different categories are classified into the higher category.

Isolated systolic hypertension should also be classified by grades (1, 2, and 3) based on systolic blood pressure levels.

[a] Based on office measurements of blood pressure.

Based on Eur Heart J. 2018;39(33):3021-3104.

[INN ciclosporin], tacrolimus), monoamine oxidase inhibitors, oral contraceptives, herbal drugs (eg, ginseng, yohimbine).

10) Toxic substances: Amphetamines, cocaine, heavy metals, alcohol, nicotine.

Causes of isolated systolic hypertension:

1) Increased stiffness of the aorta, most often in the elderly.
2) Conditions causing increased cardiac output: Aortic regurgitation, anemia, thyrotoxicosis, Paget disease, arteriovenous fistulas.

9.1. Essential Hypertension

→ ETIOLOGY AND PATHOGENESIS

Essential (or primary) hypertension is caused by a variety of genetic and environmental factors that interfere with the functioning of one or more of the systems involved in the regulation of blood pressure (BP) and thus lead to increased BP. The following factors play an important role in the development of hypertension: the renin-angiotensin-aldosterone (RAA) system, sympathetic nervous system, natriuretic peptides, and substances produced by the vascular endothelium (prostacyclin, nitric oxide, endothelins). Family history increases one's risk of developing essential hypertension; it is likely that genetic contributions to hypertension risk are mediated through many or all of the factors enumerated above. The lifetime risk of developing hypertension approaches 80% in those aged 80 years or older.● The risk and/or severity of hypertension are increased by excessive sodium intake, physical inactivity, obesity (especially abdominal), and stress (increased sympathetic activation).

→ CLINICAL FEATURES AND NATURAL HISTORY

Clinical classification (grading) based on BP values: →Table 9-1.

Hypertension is usually asymptomatic. Headache, sleep disturbance easy fatigability may occur. Other signs and symptoms appear with velopment of target organ complications of hypertension. In the major patients with uncomplicated essential hypertension, physical examina reveals no significant abnormalities aside from an increase in BP. Over ti. ranging from months to decades, hypertension may lead to pathophysiolog changes, including the accelerated development of atherosclerosis, arteria. stiffness, and left ventricular (LV) hypertrophy. The clinical manifestations of these changes lead to an increased risk of:

1) Coronary artery disease, including myocardial infarction and angina.

2) Stroke (ischemic and hemorrhagic).

3) Congestive heart failure.

4) Peripheral vascular disease.

5) Premature death from cardiovascular causes.

6) Persistent kidney injury (a urinary albumin-to-creatinine ratio [ACR] elevated ≥3 mg/mmol [30 mg/g] and/or decline in estimated glomerular filtration rate [eGFR] usually develops slowly; in mild to moderate hypertension the development of end-stage renal disease is rare and usually appears after many years of hypertension).

7) Aortic dissection.

8) Visual impairment.

→ DIAGNOSIS

Diagnostic workup includes:

1) Confirmation of the diagnosis of hypertension.

2) If appropriate, search for causes of secondary hypertension.

3) Assessment of cardiovascular risk factors, target organ complications, and comorbidities.

Diagnostic Tests

1. BP measurements: To determine the BP, perform traditional measurements (office measurements using either the manual auscultatory method or automated oscillometric blood pressure; the latter allows a sufficient rest period with the health-care provider out of the room, is typically 5-10 mm Hg [or more] lower, and is **preferred**), and make use of the self-measurements performed by the patient (→below) as well as, in some cases, also of the results of ambulatory BP monitoring (ABPM).

2. Laboratory tests that are suggested include:

1) Serum levels of sodium, potassium, glucose (fasting) and/or serum glycated hemoglobin (HbA$_{1c}$), creatinine (with calculation of eGFR using the CKD-EPI formula; →Chapter 9.2), uric acid, total cholesterol, high-density (HDL-C) and low-density (LDL-C) lipoprotein cholesterols, and triglycerides.

2) Urinalysis: Urine dipstick test for blood and protein.

3. 12-lead electrocardiography (ECG) is suggested in all patients.

4. Additional studies are suggested as guided by the clinical assessment and routine laboratory tests:

1) Quantitative assessment of urinary albumin and urine microscopy (in patients with positive results of the dipstick test).

2) Measurements of daily urinary sodium excretion to evaluate sodium intake.

3) ABPM and/or home BP measurements.

4) Echocardiography with the assessment of LV hypertrophy and cardiovascular risk in patients where it is unclear if pharmacologic therapy should be initiated or in those with suspected LV dysfunction.

ening for obstructive sleep apnea if clinically suspected (consider using
Epworth Sleepiness Scale [→Chapter 13.11] or the STOP-Bang ques-
onnaire [stopbang.ca]).

**Suggested studies based on suspected etiology of secondary hyper-
nsion** (frequently performed in referred/specialized care):

.) Renal parenchymal etiology if suggested by history (urinary tract infection
or obstruction, hematuria, analgesic abuse; family history of polycystic
kidney disease [PKD]), laboratory tests (protein and red blood cells in
urine, decreased eGFR), or physical examination showing renal masses
(PKD): Consider renal ultrasonography as a first-line additional test. If
needed, follow with referral and more specialized tests (→Chapter 9.2).

2) Renal vascular etiology if suggested by history (difficult to control hypertension, especially with early onset [fibromuscular dysplasia] or rapid onset
[atherosclerosis]), physical examination (abdominal bruit) or tests (difference in kidney size on ultrasonography, rapid worsening of eGFR either
spontaneously or after exposure to RAA system inhibitors (angiotensin-
-converting enzyme inhibitors [ACEIs] or angiotensin receptor blockers
[ARBs]): Investigations: →Chapter 3.9.4.

3) Primary hyperaldosteronism if suggested by history (early onset, cardiovascular events at an age <40 years), physical examination (arrhythmia secondary
to low potassium), or laboratory tests (hypokalemia, either spontaneous or
diuretic-induced): Investigations: →Chapter 5.1.4.

4) Cushing syndrome if suggested by history (rapid weight gain, polyuria
and polydipsia), physical examination showing typical body habitus, and
laboratory tests showing hyperglycemia: Investigations: →Chapter 5.1.2.

5) Pheochromocytoma may be suggested by history (paroxysmal hypertension
or crisis in the course of sustained hypertension; headache, sweating, palpitations, and pallor; family history of pheochromocytoma), physical examination (cutaneous neurofibromatosis (café au lait spots or neurofibromas), and
laboratory tests (adrenal mass), with further investigations for the presence
of excessive urinary catecholamines or their metabolites (metanephrines).

6. BP self-measurement may be indicated:

1) As part of diagnostic workup.

2) When starting or intensifying antihypertensive treatment.

3) As part of long-term monitoring of patients.

Diagnostic Criteria

The diagnosis is made on the basis of BP values obtained from ≥2 measurements
performed on ≥2 visits. Essential hypertension (common) is considered probable if the history and/or initial testing do not suggest underlying secondary
hypertension (rare).

Perform screening BP measurement in all adults periodically (frequency is
based on underlying risk factors, including age and previous BP patterns).

Differential Diagnosis

1. Secondary hypertension: Clinical indications and diagnostics of secondary
hypertension: →above.

2. White coat hypertension: Increase in BP in some patients during measurement performed by a physician or nurse; in such patients use ABPM.
If the office BP levels are consistent with hypertension while the results of
repeated home measurements or ABPM are normal, the diagnosis of white
coat hypertension is made.

3. Masked hypertension: Conversely, if the patient has normal office BP levels
and elevated results of home and ABPM measurements, the diagnosis of masked
hypertension is established. This may be due to smoking, exercise-induced

Table 9-2. Treatment of hypertensive emergencies

Clinical presentation	Target BP	Recommended drugs
Accelerated (malignant) hypertension	MAP reduced by 20%-25%	– First choice: Labetalol or nicardipine[a] – Second choice: Nitroprusside or urapidil[a]
Hypertensive encephalopathy	MAP reduced by 20%-25%	– First choice: Labetalol or nicardipine[a] – Second choice: Nitroprusside
Acute coronary event	SBP <140 mm Hg	– First choice: Nitroglycerine or labetalol – Second choice: Urapidil[a]
Acute cardiogenic pulmonary edema	SBP <140 mm Hg	– First choice: Nitroglycerine or nitroprusside (with loop diuretic) – Second choice: Urapidil[a] (with loop diuretic)
Acute aortic dissection	SBP <120, HR <60 beats/min	– First choice: β-Blocker (esmolol, propranolol); add nitroglycerine, nitroprusside, or nicardipine[a] if needed – Second choice: Labetalol or metoprolol
Eclampsia and severe preeclampsia/HELLP	SBP <160 mm Hg, DBP <105 mm Hg	– Magnesium sulfate plus one or more of labetalol, nicardipine,[a] or oral nifedipine – Consider immediate delivery

Notes:

1) Treatment in the ICU or an equivalent setting is mandatory.

2) Drugs are usually delivered IV.

3) BP reduction should occur immediately (or within several hours in case of accelerated/ malignant hypertension).

[a] Not available in Canada.

Adapted from Eur Heart J. 2018;39(33):3021-3104.

BP, blood pressure; DBP, diastolic blood pressure; HELLP, hemolysis, elevated liver enzymes, and low platelets; IV, intravenous; MAP, mean arterial pressure; SBP, systolic blood pressure.

hypertension, anxiety, job stress, or other factors and is not only difficult to detect but also associated with an increased cardiovascular risk.

4. Pseudohypertension: In the elderly the results of BP measurements using auscultation may be significantly elevated due to increased arterial stiffness (sclerosis), which causes the early appearance and disappearance of pulse. This may be observed if the pulse remains palpable even after filling the cuff above the systolic blood pressure (SBP) level (the stiffened artery cannot be sufficiently compressed by the cuff). Another feature suggestive of pseudohypertension is the absence of target organ damage caused by hypertension. In patients with suspected pseudohypertension, measure the BP using oscillometric devices and not auscultation.

→ TREATMENT

Acute and Urgent Treatment

The management procedure is determined by the BP values, type of target organ complications, patient's age, and comorbidities (→Table 9-2). In emergencies, such as pulmonary edema, hypertensive encephalopathy, or aortic dissection, immediately lower the BP using parenteral antihypertensive drugs (→Table 9-3),

Table 9-3. Parenteral drugs for treatment of hypertensive emergencies

Drug	Dose	Onset/duration of action	Contraindications	Adverse effects[a]	Special indications
Vasodilators					
Enalaprilat	0.625-1.25 mg IV bolus	5-15 min/4-6 h	History of angioedema		Acute LV failure; avoid in acute MI
Fenoldopam	0.1-0.3 µg/kg/min as IV infusion	<5 min/30 min		Tachycardia, headache, nausea, flushing	In most hypertensive emergencies; use with caution in patients with glaucoma
Hydralazine	10-20 mg IV	10-20 min/1-4 h		Tachycardia, flushing, headache, vomiting, worsening of angina pectoris	Eclampsia
Nicardipine	5-15 mg/h IV infusion, starting dose 5 mg/h, increase every 15-30 min by 2.5 mg until target BP is achieved, then decrease to 3 mg/h	5-15 min/30-40 min	Liver failure	Headache, reflex tachycardia	In most hypertensive emergencies except for acute heart failure; use with caution in patients with coronary ischemia
Nitroglycerin	5-100 µg/min as IV infusion	2-5 min/5-10 min		Headache, vomiting, methemoglobinemia, development of tolerance with prolonged use	Myocardial ischemia, heart failure
Sodium nitroprusside	0.25-10 µg/kg/min as IV infusion (max dose may be administered only for 10 min)	Immediate/1-2 min	Liver/kidney failure (relative)	Nausea, vomiting, muscle cramps, sweating, cyanide and thiocyanate poisoning	In most hypertensive emergencies; use with caution in patients with high intracranial pressure or CKD

Adrenergic inhibitors			
Esmolol	250-500 µg/kg/min IV bolus followed by 50-100 µg/kg/min as IV infusion; bolus may be repeated after 5 min or infusion rate increased to 300 µg/min	1-2 min/10-30 min	Second- or third-degree AV block, systolic heart failure, asthma, bradycardia	Nausea, AV block	Aortic dissection, perioperative emergencies
Labetalol	20-80 mg IV bolus every 10 min or 0.5-2 mg/min as IV infusion	5-10 min/3-6 h	Second- or third-degree AV block, systolic heart failure, asthma, bradycardia	Vomiting, scalp tingling, burning sensation in throat, dizziness, AV block	In most hypertensive emergencies except for acute heart failure
Phentol-amine	5-15 mg IV	1-2 min/10-30 min		Tachycardia, headache, flushing	Catecholamine excess (eg, pheochromocytoma)
Urapidil (not available in Canada)	10-50 mg IV bolus then repeat once; or as IV infusion starting with 2 mg/min, then continued at average rate of 9 mg/h	1-5 min/1-2 h		Dizziness, headache, nausea, vomiting, dyspnea, palpitations, tachycardia or bradycardia, chest discomfort, arrhythmia	In most hypertensive emergencies

[a] Each of these drugs may cause hypotension.

Based on JAMA. 2014;311(5):507-20 and Eur Heart J. 2018;39(33):3021-3104.

AV, atrioventricular; CKD, chronic kidney disease; IV, intravenous; LV, left ventricle; MI, myocardial infarction.

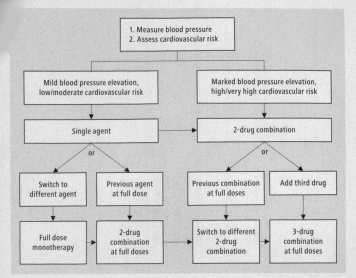

Figure 9-1. Decision algorithm for monotherapy vs combination treatment strategies in hypertension. Treatment should be intensified whenever target BP values are not achieved. *Adapted from guidelines by the European Society of Hypertension, European Society of Cardiology, and Hypertension Canada.*

preferably in a continuous IV infusion. We suggest that in such cases the mean arterial pressure should be reduced by <25% of BP reduction during the first hours and cautiously thereafter. In the case of acute stroke, BP should be reduced more gradually, if at all.

Long-Term Treatment

General Considerations

Comprehensive lifestyle optimization strategies have been shown to lower SBP and diastolic blood pressure (DBP) among patients with hypertension by 14.2 mm Hg and 7.4 mm Hg on average, respectively.◔ The evidence to date indicates that although some patients may not have hypertension as currently defined (ie, BP >140/90 mm Hg), they may nevertheless benefit from BP-lowering therapy, particularly if they have a higher baseline cardiovascular risk. One must therefore consider the current BP (and not just whether the patient has hypertension), the BP target based on the patient's characteristics as outlined below, past tolerability of treatment, and personal preferences. With increasing evidence that targets vary among different patient groups, the utility of grading hypertension may ultimately be limited to guiding the rapidity at which to initiate pharmacologic therapy, the number of pharmacologic agents that will likely be required, and consideration of secondary causes. We have recommended a target BP in each case as a range of 10 mm Hg and suggested that treatment be initiated when the measured BP is persistently at or above the upper limit of that range.

1. Long-term treatment of hypertension includes:

1) Lifestyle optimization.
2) Treatment with antihypertensive drugs (→Figure 9-1).
3) Optimization of other cardiovascular risk factors.

2. Decisions on the choice of treatment modalities depend on the patient's BP levels and overall cardiovascular risk:

1) In patients with grade 3 hypertension (SBP ≥180 mm Hg and/or DBP ≥110 mm Hg), promptly start pharmacotherapy combined with lifestyle optimization regardless of the cardiovascular risk.

2) In patients with grade 2 hypertension (SBP 160-179 mm Hg and/or DBP 100-109 mm Hg), start treatment simultaneously with lifestyle modifications, especially in those with >2 cardiovascular risk factors or any one of the following: target organ damage, diabetes mellitus, cardiovascular disease, or chronic kidney disease. In patients not fulfilling these criteria it may be acceptable to delay treatment for a few weeks to observe the effects of lifestyle modifications.

3) In patients with grade 1 hypertension (SBP 140-159 mm Hg and/or DBP 90-99 mm Hg), start pharmacotherapy if the response to lifestyle optimization is inadequate.

3. Target BP levels: Note that these targets are guides and that in many cases the achieved BP will be higher due to treatment and patient factors, including undue adverse effects. The BP target may be 5 to 10 mm Hg higher if measured using methods different than automated oscillometric BP measurements, as described above. It is also worth noticing that different expert bodies, using similar data, have reached different conclusions regarding exact targets◐:

1) **SBP <140 mm Hg** in all patients with hypertension, with the following exceptions:

a) In noninstitutionalized patients without dementia, diabetes mellitus, symptomatic heart failure, or prior stroke and (i) who are aged >50 years and have either clinically evident cardiovascular disease, an eGFR <60 mL/min/1.73m^2, or a 10-year risk score >15% (which corresponds to ≥13 points for men and ≥16 points for women; →Table 15-1), or (ii) who are ≥75 years of age, the target SBP is **<120 mm Hg (if measured using automated oscillometric BP measurement)**. Patients with ≥1 of these indications should participate in discussion about benefits and risks of more intensive therapy and give their consent.◉◐ Examples of risk calculators: Framingham Coronary Heart Disease Risk Score at mdcalc.com; ACC/AHA 2013 Cardiovascular Risk Assessment at medscape.com.

b) Patients with diabetes mellitus: →Special Considerations, below.

2) DBP <90 mm Hg in all patients.

Lifestyle Modifications

1. Reduction of weight in overweight patients and maintenance of a normal body weight (waist circumference ≤88 cm in women, ≤102 cm in men; body mass index <25 kg/m^2).

2. A diet that emphasizes fruits and vegetables, low-fat dairy products, whole grains, and protein from plant sources that is reduced in saturated fat and cholesterol, including nuts, seeds, and legumes (the DASH [Dietary Approaches to Stop Hypertension] diet).

3. Reduction of sodium intake to ≤5 to 6 g of salt.

4. Limitation of daily alcohol consumption to a maximum of 20 to 30 g of ethanol in men and 10 to 20 g in women and individuals with a low body weight.

5. Appropriate physical activity: Regular aerobic exercise, such as brisk walking for 30 to 45 minutes daily.

6. Smoking cessation.

Antihypertensive Treatment

1. The **major classes of antihypertensive agents** are diuretics (mainly thiazide and thiazide-like diuretics), β-blockers, calcium channel blockers, ACEIs, and ARBs. Their BP-lowering efficacy is similar. β-Blockers have been shown to be inferior to the other agents in their efficacy to reduce cardiovascular events● and are generally not recommended as first-line therapy in North American guidelines anymore. Specific indications and contraindications: →Table 9-4. Agents and dosage: →Table 9-5.

2. Additional antihypertensive drugs: Renin inhibitors (aliskiren), angiotensin receptor blocker/neprilysin inhibitor combinations, α_1-blockers (doxazosin, terazosin, prazosin), centrally acting sympathetic inhibitors (methyldopa, clonidine), direct vasodilators (hydralazine, minoxidil), nonthiazide or thiazide-like diuretics. These agents are used in combination treatment and in special situations. Agents, dosage, specific indications and contraindications: →Table 9-6.

3. Principles of pharmacotherapy: Depending on the cardiovascular risk as well as the baseline and target BP levels, start with 1 drug at a low dose (any agent of the main antihypertensive classes may be used, unless specific indications for or contraindications to any particular class exist), or 2 drugs at low doses (in patients with BP elevated by >20/10 mm Hg [ie, grade 2 or 3 hypertension] or at high cardiovascular risk). Most agents produce the full antihypertensive effect after a few weeks of treatment, so their effectiveness should be assessed after 2 to 4 weeks.

In patients in whom treatment with 1 drug at a low dose does not provide BP control (in a significant majority of patients treatment with ≥2 antihypertensive agents is necessary), you may:

1) Add a second drug (the preferred strategy).

2) Change to another drug (only if no hypotensive effects have been achieved or if adverse reactions occurred).

3) Increase the dose of the currently used drug (this increases the risk of adverse effects).

In patients in whom treatment with 2 drugs at low doses (either from the beginning or at a subsequent phase of treatment) is not effective, you may:

1) Increase the doses of the currently used drugs; or

2) Add a third drug at a low dose.

Usually 2 or 3 antihypertensive agents are used; less commonly more drugs are necessary. The main benefits of a combination therapy are higher efficacy and fewer adverse effects (drug doses used in combinations are lower than those used in monotherapy). Preferred combinations include:

1) A thiazide/thiazide-like diuretic + an ACEI.

2) A thiazide/thiazide-like diuretic + an ARB.

3) A thiazide/thiazide-like diuretic + a calcium channel blocker.

4) A calcium channel blocker + an ACEI.

5) A calcium channel blocker + an ARB.

The most rational triple-drug combination includes a drug acting on the RAA system (an ACEI or an ARB) + a calcium channel blocker + a thiazide/thiazide-like diuretic.

→ FOLLOW-UP

The frequency of follow-up visits depends on the overall cardiovascular risk, BP level, and patient's compliance (eg, regarding BP self-measurements at home). Once the target BP has been achieved and other risk factors have been adequately controlled, the frequency of visits can be significantly reduced. It may be of value to ask patients to record their resting BP, when possible, on several occasions prior to their follow-up visit.

Suggested schedule of follow-up visits in patients with hypertension:

1) After 2 to 4 weeks of starting antihypertensive treatment.

2) After 4 weeks of introducing a change in the treatment regimen.

3) Every 3 months after achieving the target BP.

Table 9-4. Preferred indications and contraindications for the use of key classes of antihypertensive drugs

Drug class	Preferred indications	Contraindications
Diuretics		
Thiazide and thiazide-like diuretics	Isolated systolic hypertension (in the elderly), HF, hypertension in black patients	Gout, pregnancy,[a] hypercalcemia,[a] hyponatremia, hypokalemia[a]
Aldosterone antagonists	HF, prior MI, prevention of AF (may be considered)	Hyperkalemia
β-Blockers	Angina pectoris, prior MI, HF, aortic aneurysm, pregnancy, prevention of AF (may be considered), ventricular rate control in AF	Asthma, second-degree/third-degree AV block, peripheral artery disease,[a] metabolic syndrome,[a] IGT,[a] COPD (except for β-blockers with vasodilation effects),[a] athletes or physically active patients
Calcium channel blockers		
Dihydropyridines	LV hypertrophy, asymptomatic atherosclerosis, angina pectoris, peripheral artery disease, isolated systolic hypertension (in the elderly), pregnancy, hypertension in black patients	Tachyarrhythmia,[a] HF[a]
Verapamil and diltiazem	Ventricular rate control in AF, LV hypertrophy, asymptomatic atherosclerosis, angina pectoris, peripheral artery disease, isolated systolic hypertension (in the elderly), metabolic syndrome, pregnancy, hypertension in black patients	Second-degree/third-degree AV block, severe LV dysfunction, HF
ACEIs	LV hypertrophy, asymptomatic atherosclerosis, microalbuminuria, renal dysfunction, prior MI, HF, prevention of AF (may be considered), end-stage renal failure/proteinuria, peripheral artery disease, metabolic syndrome, DM	Pregnancy, angioedema, hyperkalemia, bilateral renal artery stenosis, renal artery stenosis of a solitary functioning kidney
ARBs	LV hypertrophy, microalbuminuria, renal dysfunction, previous MI, HF, prevention of AF (may be considered), end-stage renal failure/proteinuria, metabolic syndrome, DM	Pregnancy, hyperkalemia, bilateral renal artery stenosis, renal artery stenosis of a solitary functioning kidney

[a] Relative contraindications.

Adapted from Can J Cardiol. 2018;34(5):506-525, Eur Heart J. 2018; 29(33):3021-3104, and Eur Heart J. 2013;34(28):2159-219.

ACEI, angiotensin-converting enzyme inhibitor; AF, atrial fibrillation; ARB, angiotensin receptor blocker; AV, atrioventricular; COPD, chronic obstructive pulmonary disease; DM, diabetes mellitus; HF, heart failure; IGT, impaired glucose tolerance; LV, left ventricle; MI, myocardial infarction.

Table 9-5. Typical dosage of oral antihypertensive agents

Agents and formulations	Dosage
β-Blockers	
Acebutolol	400 mg once daily or 200 mg bid
Atenolol	25-100 mg once daily
Betaxolol	5-20 mg once daily
Bisoprolol	2.5-10 mg once daily (max 20 mg/d)
Celiprolol[a]	100-400 mg once daily
Carvedilol	6.25-25 mg once daily or bid
Metoprolol	
Standard release	25-100 mg bid
Controlled release	50-100 mg once daily (up to 200 mg once daily)
Nebivolol	5 mg once daily
Pindolol	5-10 mg/d bid (doses up to 20 mg/d may be administered once daily; max 60 mg/d)
Propranolol	40-80 mg bid to qid
Calcium channel blockers	
Amlodipine	2.5-10 mg once daily
Diltiazem	
Standard release	30-60 mg tid
Controlled release	90-480 mg once daily or 90-240 mg bid
Felodipine	5-10 mg once daily
Isradipine[a]	2.5-10 mg once daily or 5 mg bid
Lacidipine[a]	4-6 mg once daily
Lercanidipine[a]	10-20 mg once daily
Nitrendipine[a]	10-20 mg once daily (max 20 mg bid)
Verapamil	
Standard release	40-120 mg tid to qid
Extended release	120-240 mg once daily to bid
Diuretics	
Amiloride in a fixed-dose combination with hydrochlorothiazide	2.5-5 mg once daily to bid
Chlorthalidone (INN chlortalidone)	12.5-50 mg once daily or 50 mg every other day
Furosemide	20-40 mg daily to bid (typically bid when used as an anti-hypertensive)

Agents and formulations	Dosage
Hydrochlorothiazide	12.5-50 mg once daily
Indapamide	
Standard release	1.25-2.5 mg once daily
Extended release	1.5 mg once daily
Clopamide[a]	5-20 mg once daily
Spironolactone	25-50 mg once daily to bid
Torasemide[a]	2.5-10 mg once daily
Angiotensin-converting enzyme inhibitors	
Benazepril	5-20 mg once daily to bid
Quinapril	5-40 mg once daily to bid
Cilazapril	2.5-5 mg once daily
Enalapril	2.5-20 mg once daily to bid (bid preferred)
Imidapril[a]	5-20 mg once daily
Captopril	25-50 mg bid to tid
Fosinopril	10-40 mg daily
Lisinopril	10-40 mg once daily
Perindopril	4(5)-8(10) mg once daily
Ramipril	2.5-5 mg once daily (max 10 mg)
Trandolapril	2-4 mg once daily
Zofenopril[a]	30 mg once daily (max 60 mg once daily or in 2 divided doses)
Angiotensin receptor blockers	
Eprosartan	600 mg once daily
Irbesartan	150-300 mg once daily
Candesartan	8-32 mg once daily
Losartan	25-100 mg once daily or in 2 divided doses
Telmisartan	20-80 mg once daily
Valsartan	80-320 mg once daily

[a] Not available in Canada.

bid, 2 times a day; INN, international nonproprietary name; qid, 4 times a day; tid, 3 times a day.

Table 9-6. Additional antihypertensive drugs

Drugs	Dosage	Specific indications	Contraindications
Aliskiren	150-300 mg once daily		As in ARBs (→Table 9-4)
Sacubitril/ valsartan	24/26-97/103 mg bid	Congestive heart failure	As in ARBs (→Table 9-4)
Doxazosin	1-16 mg once daily	Prostatic hypertrophy	Orthostatic hypotension, heart failure
Terazosin	1-20 mg once daily		
Methyldopa	0.25-1 g bid	Hypertension in pregnancy; use in combination with a diuretic	Liver failure, pheochromocytoma, hemolytic anemia, depression, sexual dysfunction
Clonidine	0.05-0.2 mg bid to tid	Use in combination with a diuretic	Renal or liver failure, depression, sick sinus syndrome, bradyarrhythmia
Moxonidine[a]	0.2-0.6 mg/d	Mild and moderate hypertension, especially in young patients with symptoms of sympathetic activation	Severe depression, severe renal failure
Rilmenidine[a]	1 mg once daily to bid		
Hydralazine	75-200 mg/d in 3-4 divided doses	Use in exceptional cases in combination with a diuretic and a β-blocker	Tachycardia, cerebrovascular disease, mitral stenosis, aortic aneurysm, hypertrophic cardiomyopathy, ischemic heart disease, liver and kidney dysfunction, porphyria

[a] Not available in Canada.

ARB, angiotensin receptor blocker; bid, 2 times a day; tid, 3 times a day.

→ SPECIAL CONSIDERATIONS

Elderly Patients

1. In elderly patients (>65 years of age) the most common form of hypertension is isolated systolic hypertension. Additionally, orthostatic hypotension is frequent (**BP must also be measured in the upright position**).

2. General principles of antihypertensive treatment in the elderly:

1) Lower BP gradually, initially using low doses of drugs.

2) Note that interactions with other drugs may occur.

3) For many, a target SBP <140 mm Hg will be reasonable. In those who have been identified as potentially benefiting from an SBP target <120 mm Hg (→above), consider cautiously lowering SBP further while monitoring for adverse effects including orthostatic hypotension.

3. You can start treatment with a drug from any major antihypertensive class; however, in patients with isolated systolic hypertension start with a diuretic (thiazide or thiazide-like) or a calcium channel blocker. As comorbidities are frequent in patients with hypertension, these should be taken into consideration when choosing antihypertensive agents.

4. In a significant proportion of patients, it is necessary to use ≥2 antihypertensive drugs to achieve the target BP levels.

Patients With Diabetes Mellitus

1. There is currently some uncertainty as to the BP target, as demons
by differences in the most key clinical practice guidelines. SBP targets r
between 130 and 140 mm Hg and DBP between 80 and 90 mm Hg. We sug
a BP target <130/80 mm Hg, particularly in those with diabetic nephropat
if it can be achieved without undue treatment burden (→Chapter 5.2).

2. All the major classes of antihypertensive drugs have beneficial effects in
this group of patients.

3. ACEIs and ARBs have renal protective effects, significantly reduce proteinuria, and are the preferred option in patients with albuminuria.

4. In a significant proportion of patients, the target BP values can only be
achieved with ≥3 appropriately selected antihypertensive drugs.

5. BP should also be measured in the upright position due to the increased
risk of orthostatic hypotension.

6. Intensive lifestyle modifications are of particular importance (→Lifestyle
Modifications, above).

White Coat Hypertension

In patients with no additional cardiovascular risk factors, consider limiting
the intervention to lifestyle changes, as long as careful follow-up is continued.
In patients with a higher cardiovascular risk due to metabolic disturbances or
asymptomatic target organ damage, you may consider adding antihypertensive
pharmacotherapy.

Masked Hypertension

Consider introducing both lifestyle changes and antihypertensive drugs, as
this category of hypertension is associated with a cardiovascular risk similar
to that of hypertension observed in both office and home measurements.

Resistant Hypertension

Hypertension is defined as resistant if target BP values cannot be achieved
despite the use of ≥3 antihypertensive drugs (including a diuretic) at optimal
doses and in appropriate combinations.

Causes:

1) Noncompliance with the antihypertensive drug regimen and with lifestyle
   modifications (alcohol abuse, tobacco smoking, excessive sodium intake,
   persistent obesity).

2) Inappropriate drug combinations (failure to include a diuretic in treatment,
   using a diuretic at inadequate doses, or failure to adapt the type of the
   diuretic to the patient's renal function).

3) Pseudoresistance to treatment (BP measurement errors, white coat hypertension [→above]).

4) Pseudohypertension (→Differential Diagnosis, above).

5) Obstructive sleep apnea.

6) Drug interactions reducing the efficacy of antihypertensive drugs (nonsteroidal anti-inflammatory drugs [NSAIDs]).

7) Treatment with drugs that increase BP.

8) Metabolic syndrome (insulin resistance).

9) Chronic kidney disease.

10) Unrecognized secondary hypertension.

Management:

1) **Resistance to treatment is confirmed** in patients in whom target office
   BP levels are not achieved despite treatment with ≥3 antihypertensive drugs
   at optimal doses, including a diuretic.

2) **Exclude pseudoresistance**: Determine whether the patient is compliant
   with the recommended treatment and exclude white coat hypertension

he patient has abnormal office BP levels with normal BP levels in self-
asurement or ABPM, pseudoresistance to treatment is confirmed).

Identify and attempt to modify adverse lifestyle factors, such as
obesity, excessive alcohol consumption, or high sodium intake.

**Eliminate or minimize the effect of substances that increase blood
pressure**, such as NSAIDs, sympathomimetic agents (appetite suppressants,
decongestants), stimulants, and oral contraceptives.

5) **Search for causes of secondary hypertension**.

6) **Modify pharmacotherapy**: Maximize diuretic treatment (consider adding
an aldosterone antagonist or amiloride, use loop diuretics in patients with
renal failure), use drugs with different mechanisms of action.

7) **Refer the patient to a specialist** in the case of a confirmed or suspected
secondary hypertension, or if hypertension remains uncontrolled despite
a sufficient duration of treatment.

Accelerated Hypertension

The most severe form of hypertension, characterized by a DBP >120 to
140 mm Hg, rapid progression of target organ complications, and particularly
by the development of heart failure, renal failure, and severe lesions in the retinal vessels (transudates, ecchymoses, papilledema). This type of hypertension
may develop in the course of hypertension of various etiologies, both essential
and secondary, and is most common in patients with renal artery stenosis or
glomerulonephritis. The term "malignant hypertension" was used in the past
to indicate the very poor prognosis in such patients.

Symptoms are often present and can include weakness, headache, dizziness,
dyspnea, chest pain, and less commonly abdominal pain (caused by abnormalities of intestinal vessels). Symptoms of rapidly progressive renal failure
as well as central nervous system symptoms of varying severity, up to severe
encephalopathy, may predominate. The patients are at increased risk of stroke
and heart failure, often in the form of pulmonary edema.

Diagnosis is based on the clinical and laboratory manifestations.

9.2. Pregnancy-Related Hypertension

→ ETIOLOGY AND PATHOGENESIS

During pregnancy the maternal cardiovascular system undergoes several major
physiologic changes. As early as 8 weeks' gestation, peripheral vasodilatation
can lead to a fall in systemic vascular resistance. To mitigate this effect, maternal cardiac output steadily increases, reaching upwards of 50% above the
prepregnancy levels by weeks 20 to 24. As there is usually a lag in compensation,
maternal blood pressure often falls by 10 to 15 mm Hg of systolic blood pressure
(SBP), reaching a nadir around 20 to 22 weeks' gestation before slowly rising
back up to prepregnancy levels by term. After delivery, blood pressure may
transiently decrease before peaking after 3 to 5 days.

Despite these physiologic changes, hypertension is one of the most common medical problems encountered in pregnancy. Complicating 5% to 10% of all pregnancies,
certain etiologies are associated with significant maternal and fetal morbidity
and mortality, requiring prompt identification, intervention, and management.

→ CLASSIFICATION

Classification of hypertension in pregnancy:

1) **Preexisting hypertension**: Chronic hypertension diagnosed before pregnancy or hypertension occurring before 20 weeks' gestation. It may also present
as persistent hypertension >3 to 6 months into the postpartum period.

a) **Essential hypertension**: No secondary cause identified.

b) **Secondary hypertension (hypertension with an identifiab**
Consider endocrine, renal, cardiac, or vascular abnormalities, de
on the clinical presentation.

2) **Gestational hypertension**: Hypertension identified after 20 weeks'
tion without other features of preeclampsia; it may evolve into preeclam

3) **Preeclampsia**: Hypertension occurring after 20 weeks' gestation w
proteinuria and/or end-organ dysfunction.

   a) **De novo preeclampsia**: New-onset hypertension and proteinuria or
   end-organ dysfunction.

   b) **Preexisting hypertension with superimposed preeclampsia**:
   Worsening hypertension with new or worsening proteinuria or end-organ
   dysfunction.

   c) **Preexisting proteinuria with superimposed preeclampsia**: New
   or worsening hypertension with worsening proteinuria or end-organ
   dysfunction; this is often due to chronic kidney disease, and the diagnosis
   of superimposed preeclampsia is complex. Involvement of a specialist in
   renal disease in pregnancy is advisable.

→ DIAGNOSIS

Blood pressure should be taken in a sitting rather than a supine position, as the
gravid uterus may decrease venous return to the heart and produce abnormal
increases or decreases in blood pressure. Measurements should be taken with
a manual sphygmomanometer. Ensure the cuff size is appropriate for the patient so as not to overestimate the measurement (such as can occur with a cuff
size too small). Phase V (disappearance) rather than phase IV (muffling) of
Korotkoff sounds should be used.

The diagnosis of hypertension in pregnancy is made when the patient has **at
least 2 readings >140/90 mm Hg**, taken in the office or hospital, measured **at
least** 15 minutes apart. The severity of hypertension is based on BP readings
and evidence of end-organ damage. Nonsevere hypertension is considered any
BP between 140 to 159 mm Hg SBP and 90 to 109 mm Hg diastolic BP (DBP).
Severe hypertension is defined as a BP ≥160/110 mm Hg.

Isolated office (white coat) hypertension may be revealed by home blood-pressure
measurement. If there is any conflict between home and office readings,
a 24-hour ambulatory blood-pressure monitor can be considered.

All patients with hypertension diagnosed before or during pregnancy should
be followed closely by an obstetrician. Baseline blood tests to look for causes of
secondary hypertension and exclude end-organ involvement should be ordered
at the first visit at which hypertension is diagnosed.

The issue of when to search for a possible cause of secondary hypertension
(→Chapter 3.9.1) is not always clear. The need for other tests may be prompted
by the clinical features or clinical course. At a minimum, electrolytes, creatinine
(estimated glomerular filtration rate), and urinalysis should be ordered. It is
our practice to also obtain a complete blood count and liver function tests to
use as a baseline or, in the case of patients at >20 weeks' gestation, to exclude
end-organ involvement from preeclampsia. Further information may be taken
into account when judging the need for additional investigations (→Table 9-7).

→ MANAGEMENT AND TREATMENT

General Approach

Regardless of the etiology of hypertension (preeclampsia, preexisting, gestational), the pharmacologic treatment of hypertension in pregnancy is approached in
a similar manner. However, unlike the management of nonpregnant patients,
the decision to treat hypertension must consider the risks and benefits to both

. Screening for secondary causes of hypertension at initial assessment	
	Red flags
First-order testing	
Creatinine	Evidence of renal impairment
Electrolytes (potassium)	Hypokalemia suggesting potential mineralocorticoid excess
Midstream urine	Evidence of proteinuria or hematuria suggesting a renal etiology
Urine PCR or 24-hour urine collection for protein	If midstream urine is positive for proteinuria, recommend for baseline and quantitative assessment
Second-order testing[a]	
Renal ultrasonography with Doppler	If sudden-onset or worsening hypertension, presence of abdominal bruit, resistance to ≥3 drugs, increase in serum creatinine ≥30% after using ACEI/ARB, significant asymmetry (>1.5 cm) in kidney size, recurrent pulmonary edema, significant atherosclerosis, family history of fibromuscular dysplasia, or personal history in another vascular territory
Sleep study	If evidence of sleep apnea in history (headache, nocturnal choking and gasping, early morning fatigue, snoring)
Plasma renin and aldosterone	If evidence of spontaneous hypokalemia (K <3.5 mmol/L) or hypokalemia with diuretics, resistance to ≥3 drugs, incidental adrenal adenoma
24-h urine metanephrines	If severe ≥180/110 mm Hg refractory hypertension, symptoms of catecholamine excess (headaches, palpitations, sweating, panic attacks, orthostatic syncope), hypertension triggered by β-blockers, history of multiple endocrine neoplasia 2A or 2b, or incidental adrenal mass
Thyroid-stimulating hormone	If evidence of hypothyroidism or hyperthyroidism on clinical assessment

[a] Only undertaken if signs and symptoms present (→Chapter 3.9.1).

ACEI, angiotensin-converting enzyme inhibitor; ARB, angiotensin receptor blocker; PCR, protein-to-creatinine ratio.

mother and fetus. For this reason, the initiation of antihypertensive therapy should always be undertaken in consultation with an obstetrician. It is also vital to determine the etiology of the hypertension (primary, secondary, pregnancy-related) so that the clinical course and prognosis may be appropriately predicted.

1. General recommendations: Blood pressure levels, gestational age, and the presence of maternal and fetal comorbidities and complications must be taken into consideration.

1) Advise avoiding the supine position when lying down, as it may increase vasoconstriction.
2) Recommend maintaining a normal diet without salt restriction.
3) Normal physical activity need not be limited. Bed rest, unless in the setting of severely uncontrolled hypertension and/or severe preeclampsia, is not indicated.

2. Target blood pressure and levels at which to start antihypertensive treatment are controversial. On the one hand, maternal risk of cerebral

Table 9-8. Oral drugs for the management of hypertension in pregnancy

Drug	Starting dose	Maximum dose	Onset of action	Adverse effects	Special indications and notes
Labetalol	100 mg bid	500 mg qid	20-40 min	Headache; avoid in uncontrolled asthma	Often requires tid or qid dosing in pregnancy; safe for breastfeeding
Nifedipine (slow release)	20 mg bid	60 mg bid	20-40 min	Peripheral edema	Safe for breastfeeding
Methyldopa	250 mg bid	1 g qid	1-3 h	Fatigue; avoid in uncontrolled depression	Safe for breastfeeding

bid, 2 times a day; qid, 4 times a day; tid, 3 times a day.

hemorrhage increases with blood pressures >160/110 mm Hg; on the other, aggressive lowering of blood pressure may run the risk of compromising the uteroplacental blood supply due to reduced perfusion pressure into this largely passive vascular bed. Most clinicians will **initiate treatment at levels >140 to 150 mm Hg SBP and >90 to 100 mm Hg DBP**. A target DBP between 85 and 100 mm Hg in women with preexisting or pregnancy-induced hypertension (without preeclampsia) can be considered a safe zone for both mother and fetus. We suggest **a target between 130 and 150 mm Hg SBP and 85 and 100 mm Hg DBP**, recognizing that women with blood pressures closer to 150/100 mm Hg run an increased risk of developing severe hypertension and that slightly lower targets may also be reasonable.☺☺

3. Treatment of nonsevere hypertension in pregnancy: First-line antihypertensive therapies include slow-release **nifedipine**, **labetalol**, or **methyldopa** (→Table 9-8). These agents can be used alone or in combination as required. Second-line therapies (a fourth agent is rarely necessary) can include metoprolol, clonidine, hydralazine, or thiazide diuretics. Hydrochlorothiazide should be avoided if there is concern regarding a low amniotic fluid volume or in the setting of preeclampsia. Angiotensin-converting enzyme inhibitors (ACEIs) and angiotensin receptor blockers are contraindicated.

4. Treatment of severe hypertension in pregnancy: Although there is a divergence in opinion regarding the optimal blood pressure cutoff at which to initiate medications and target treatment, **a blood pressure of 160 mm Hg SBP or 110 DBP should always be treated**. In such cases, both maternal and fetal well-being must be assessed and hospital admission considered. Medications including intravenous labetalol, oral short-acting nifedipine, or intravenous hydralazine can be used. Our preference is to use short-acting nifedipine, as it has been found to be as effective and safe as intravenous labetalol and does not require a parenteral route.☺☺ We prefer not to use hydralazine if other options are available. With all these drugs, small doses repeated every 30 to 40 minutes until the target blood pressure is reached are the safest regimen; this allows the full effect of each incremental dose to be seen and avoids overdose and an inappropriate reduction in perfusion pressure (all 3 of these drugs have an onset within 20 minutes and a peak effect within 40 minutes, whether given orally or intravenously). Medication doses: →Table 9-9.

5. Postpartum management: After delivery, maternal blood pressure often declines before **rising once more between days 3 to 5 postpartum, sometimes to levels higher than in pregnancy**. Although this will often return to prepregnancy values within the following weeks, women who have had a pregnancy complicated by hypertension may be particularly vulnerable

Table 9-9. Drugs for the treatment of hypertensive emergencies in pregnancy

Drug	Dose	Onset/duration of action	Adverse effects	Special indications
Labetalol	20-40 mg IV bolus every 20+ min	10-20 min/3-6 h	Vomiting, scalp tingling, burning sensation in the throat, dizziness, AV block	In most hypertensive emergencies except for acute heart failure
Nifedipine (short acting)	10 mg PO every 20+ min	10-20 min/3-6 h	Headache, facial flushing	
Nitroglycerin	5-100 μg/min as IV infusion	2-5 min/5-10 min	Headache, vomiting, methemoglobinemia, developing tolerance with prolonged use	Myocardial ischemia or pulmonary edema
Hydralazine	10 mg IV bolus every 20+ min	10-20 min/1-4 h	Tachycardia, flushing, headache, vomiting, worsening of angina pectoris	Eclampsia
AV, atrioventricular; IV, intravenous; PO, oral.				

to this postpartum surge, requiring an adjustment or addition of medication to prevent severe hypertension. All women with hypertension during pregnancy must be followed closely in the postpartum period. The use of nonsteroidal anti-inflammatory drugs for analgesia should be avoided, as it may aggravate hypertension. Women with new or sudden worsening of hypertension with any associated signs and symptoms of end-organ dysfunction should be carefully assessed for postpartum preeclampsia.

Antihypertensives used in pregnancy may be continued, as labetalol, slow-release nifedipine, and methyldopa are all considered safe in breastfeeding. However, ACEIs—particularly enalapril and quinapril—are both effective and safe and have the particular advantage that they have been shown not to cross into breast milk in an active form. Transition to prepregnancy medications may also be considered in the postpartum period.

9.2.1. Eclampsia

→ **DEFINITION**

Eclampsia is defined as the occurrence of a generalized seizure during pregnancy or the postpartum period usually in association with a diagnosis of preeclampsia. While eclampsia develops in 2% of women with severe preeclampsia, it is important to recognize that in >20% of cases, prior hypertension may be absent. In at least a third of patients, eclampsia occurs for the first time postpartum, usually within the first 5 days, but it can develop up to several weeks after. In these late cases, alternative etiologies are more likely.

→ **TREATMENT**

1. Place the mother in a lateral decubitus position, ensure her airway is patent, and administer oxygen at a rate of 8 to 10 L/min. Ensure she is moved to a monitored setting such, as a labor and delivery or an intensive care unit, where mental status, blood pressure, and oximetry can be continuously monitored.

2. Start anticonvulsant treatment: **magnesium sulfate**✓● 4 g IV over 20 minutes followed by 1 to 2 g/h in a continuous IV infusion for 24 hours after delivery or after the last seizure. Magnesium is cleared entirely through the kidney; therefore, if there is any evidence of renal impairment (creatinin >100 µmol/L or urine output <25 mL/h), the infusion rate of magnesium m need to be reduced to avoid toxicity, which can occur at levels >3.5 mmol/. (>3.5-5 mmol/L, loss of deep tendon reflexes; 5-6.5 mmol/L, respiratory pa ralysis; >7.5 mmol/L, cardiac conduction abnormalities). Magnesium levels should ideally be monitored in this situation to guide adjustment. If magnesium sulfate is ineffective (repeated seizures occur in about 10% of patients), our practice is to give one repeat bolus of magnesium 2 g IV **before administering diazepam or midazolam** 5 to 10 mg IV.

3. Maintain blood pressure at 140 to 160/90 to 110 mm Hg, for instance, using **labetalol** up to 20 to 40 mg IV every 20 minutes or as infusion if required (→Table 9-9). Use diuretics only if pulmonary edema is present. Oral agents can be used once the mother has recovered consciousness.

4. In the case of signs of fetal distress, urgent cesarean section may be necessary once the mother has been stabilized. However, the baby may also recover in utero as the maternal condition improves. In other cases, eclampsia is not an indication for cesarean section and vaginal delivery is possible (induced when necessary). The timing and mode of delivery is a decision for the obstetrician.

➔ PROPHYLAXIS

The choice for both primary and secondary seizure prophylaxis in preeclamp-sia is **magnesium sulfate**.◐◑ It is thought to act as a neurostabilizer and cerebral vasodilator. In its use as primary prophylaxis, magnesium is given as a loading dose of 4 g IV over 20 to 40 minutes, then in a maintenance infusion of 1 g/hour for 24 hours after delivery. Magnesium must be given in a monitored setting where adverse effects and urine output can be watched closely. Many obstetrical units have a protocol that includes frequent evaluation for signs of magnesium toxicity. These can include loss of deep tendon reflexes, double vision, respiratory depression, or signs of hypocalcemia. Magnesium levels are not usually monitored unless the serum creatinine level is increased or oliguria is present (→above).

Potential indications for primary magnesium sulfate prophylaxis include preeclampsia with any signs of neurologic involvement (vision change, irritability, severe headache, marked hyperreflexia and/or clonus); prophylaxis may also be given in patients with preeclampsia and severe features mandating urgent delivery. A decision to initiate magnesium as primary prophylaxis should always be undertaken in consultation with the treating obstetrician.

➔ FOLLOW-UP

Women should be followed clinically for resolution of hypertension, proteinuria, and end-organ dysfunction. Hypertension and/or proteinuria persisting for >6 months postpartum requires evaluation for causes unrelated to pregnancy.

Long-term cardiovascular risk: There is increasing recognition that pre-eclampsia is a risk factor for the development of both short-term and long-term cardiovascular events. Women with a history of a hypertensive disorder of pregnancy have increased risk of developing chronic hypertension, diabetes mellitus, early-onset coronary artery disease, and stroke, at a rate of roughly 2 to 4 times their baseline risk. The optimal timing and method of screening after the index pregnancy is still be determined. However, we recommend exercise (150 minutes per week of aerobic activity), aggressive cardiovascular risk factor modification, and regular screening for the development of risk factors in addition to the usual age-appropriate preventative screening.◐○

Recurrence risk: The risk of recurrence in a subsequent pregnancy is ~20%; however, the actual number is subject to some variation dependent on individual factors (→Chapter 3.9.2.2). Acetylsalicylic acid (ASA) is thought to improve development of placental vascularization around the time of placentation, thereby reducing the risk of subsequent early onset preeclampsia by up to 20%. All women who have had a pregnancy complicated by preeclampsia should be advised to start receiving ASA◉◉ 81 to 160 mg daily (the dose is not entirely clear but likely >100 mg) during subsequent pregnancies initiated by 8 to 10 weeks' and no later than 16 weeks' gestation as well as supplemental calcium if their daily intake is <600 mg/d (target daily calcium of 1.2-2.5 g/d).◉◉

9.2.2. Preeclampsia

→ ETIOLOGY AND PATHOGENESIS

Preeclampsia is a pregnancy-specific syndrome characterized by new-onset or worsening hypertension after 20 weeks' gestation associated with new or increasing proteinuria and/or evidence of end-organ involvement. Fetal manifestations may occur with, precede, or occur in the absence of maternal manifestations.

While the pathophysiology of preeclampsia is still incompletely understood, it is **likely related to abnormal placentation occurring in the first trimester**. Failure of the spiral arteries in the placental bed to undergo remodeling may cause uteroplacental ischemia and abnormal perfusion, leading to local and systemic inflammation. The fact that the majority of preeclampsia resolves rapidly after delivery of the placenta is a testament to the causal role of the placenta.

Risk factors for preeclampsia: Preeclampsia likely involves a genetic predisposition. Women with a family history (mother or sister) of preeclampsia are at a heightened risk. Other risk factors include a previous history of preeclampsia, obesity (body mass index >30), age >40 years, multiple pregnancy, autoimmune disease, preexisting kidney disease, chronic hypertension, diabetes mellitus, assisted reproduction, and antiphospholipid antibodies. Some other factors include first pregnancy, black populations, age >35 years, >10-year pregnancy interval, family history, new partner, and a previous adverse pregnancy outcome. Women felt to be at risk for preeclampsia should be started on acetylsalicylic acid (ASA) (→Chapter 3.9.2.1).

The maternal syndrome of preeclampsia is a systemic syndrome associated with endothelial injury resulting in vasoconstriction, capillary leak, and activation of the coagulation system. The effect on maternal organ systems can be quite variable (→below).

The fetal syndrome can be characterized by intrauterine growth restriction (IUGR), oligohydramnios, asymmetric growth, or abnormalities in the uterine and umbilical arteries on ultrasonography. All women with suspected preeclampsia should have a fetal and placental assessment by an obstetrician.

→ CLINICAL FEATURES AND DIAGNOSIS

A diagnosis of preeclampsia requires the following:

1) Systolic blood pressure (SBP) ≥140 mm Hg or diastolic blood pressure (DBP) ≥90 mm Hg on 2 occasions at least 4 hours apart after 20 weeks' gestation, or one-time SBP ≥160 mm Hg or DBP ≥110 mm Hg, **and**

2) At least one of the following:
   a) Proteinuria >0.3 g/d in a 24-hour urine collection, protein-to-creatinine ratio >30 mg/mmol in a spot urine sample, or, if not available, urine analysis with >1+ protein.
   b) Evidence of end-organ dysfunction (→below).

Note that not all patients with these clinical features have preeclampsia (eg, patients with diabetic nephropathy or other underlying renal disease).

In these cases, consultation with a specialist with considerable experience ~
preeclampsia is often warranted.

In patients without proteinuria, the diagnosis of preeclampsia requires at least
one of the following **criteria for end-organ dysfunction**:

1) **Neurologic**:
   a) Symptoms and signs: Headache and vision changes, marked hyperreflexia.
   b) Severe manifestations: Irritability, cortical blindness (rare), altered
   mental status (Glasgow Coma Scale <13), sustained ankle clonus, stroke,
   eclampsia.
   c) Investigations: Radiologic evidence of intracerebral hemorrhage, posterior
   reversible encephalopathy syndrome, or reversible cerebral vasoconstriction syndrome (however, imaging is frequently normal).

2) **Hematologic**:
   a) Symptoms and signs: Bleeding or bruising, platelets count $<100 \times 10^9$/L.
   b) Severe manifestations: Platelet count $<50 \times 10^9$/L, transfusion of any blood
   product.
   c) Investigations: Thrombocytopenia, hemolysis (elevated lactate dehydrogenase or indirect bilirubin, decreased haptoglobin).

3) **Renal**:
   a) Symptoms and signs: Decreased urine output.
   b) Severe manifestations: Acute kidney injury with creatinine >150 µmol/L,
   decreased urine output or oliguria despite 500 mL trial of fluids, new
   indication for dialysis.
   c) Investigations: Acute kidney injury (serum creatinine levels >100 µmol/L
   or a 2-fold increase compared with the baseline value indicates severe
   disease), acutely elevated uric acid levels.

4) **Hepatic**:
   a) Symptoms and signs: Epigastric and/or right upper quadrant pain, nausea
   or vomiting.
   b) Severe manifestations: Hepatic hematoma or rupture.
   c) Investigations: Liver cell damage (serum aminotransferase levels $\geq 2 \times$ upper limit of normal).

5) **Respiratory**:
   a) Symptoms and signs: Shortness of breath, cough.
   b) Severe manifestations: Oxygen saturation <90%, intubation, pulmonary
   edema.
   c) Investigations: Pulmonary edema on radiologic imaging.

6) **Cardiac**:
   a) Symptoms and signs: Angina-like chest pain, dyspnea, elevated jugular
   venous pressure.
   b) Severe manifestations: Uncontrolled severe hypertension (inability to
   control after >12 hours or requiring 3 antihypertensive drugs).
   c) Investigations: Heart failure (reduced left ventricular ejection fraction,
   diastolic dysfunction), elevated troponin levels.

7) **Fetal**:
   a) Fetal manifestations: Intrauterine growth restriction (IUGR), abnormal
   fetal heart rate, oligohydramnios, stillbirth.
   b) Uterine artery manifestations: Absent or reversed end-diastolic flow,
   uterine artery nicking.
   c) Investigations: Fetal ultrasonography and uterine artery ultrasonography.

Biochemical markers in the prediction and diagnosis of preeclampsia:
Specific angiogenic factors implicated in the pathogenesis of preeclampsia can
be measured but are not yet widely available in North America. These include

Table 9-10. Investigations for evidence of end-organ dysfunction

Diagnostic test	Red flags
Complete blood count	Anemia if hemolysis is present, thrombocytopenia
AST, ALT	Elevation of transaminases can occur in both preeclampsia and other causes of HELLP syndrome
Creatinine, uric acid	Baseline creatinine values in pregnancy are decreased. Elevations may be reported as "normal"; therefore, it is helpful to have a pre-pregnancy/early pregnancy value
LDH, bilirubin	Elevated if hemolysis is present
INR	Any increase suggests coagulation factor deficit. INR >1.3 suggests serious liver disease (consider acute fatty liver of pregnancy)
Placental growth factor	Not currently available in Canada
Midstream urine	Evidence of proteinuria or hematuria
Urine PCR or 24-h urine collection for protein	24-h urine >0.3 g/d or protein-to-creatinine ratio >30 mg/mmol
ECG, chest radiography, troponin	Warranted if chest pain, shortness of breath, or other clinical signs suggestive of ischemia, edema, or ventricular depression are present. Consider in the case of a first presentation of hypertension to investigate for evidence of chronicity or underlying structural heart disease
Fetal and uterine artery ultrasonography	Fetal growth restriction, abnormal heart rate, stillbirth; abnormal uterine artery flow

ALT, alanine aminotransferase; AST, aspartate aminotransferase; ECG, electrocardiography; HELLP, hemolysis, elevated liver enzymes, low platelets; INR, international normalized ratio; LDH, lactate dehydrogenase; PCR, protein-to-creatinine ratio.

the antiangiogenic soluble fms-like tyrosine kinase-1 (sFlt-1) and angiogenic placental growth factor (PlGF). Normal levels of circulating PlGF have been found to have a high negative predictive value in excluding suspected preeclampsia between 20 to 35 weeks' gestation and the role of these assays as an adjunct to usual clinical practice is currently under investigation.

The syndrome of HELLP (**h**emolysis, **e**levated **l**iver enzymes, **l**ow **p**latelets) is most often seen in preeclampsia but can occur in other situations, for example, in placental abruption, amniotic fluid embolism, or septicemia. The exact pathophysiology of HELLP is unclear, but it is considered a subtype of severe preeclampsia. The majority of women have hypertension with proteinuria, but some may have hypertension or proteinuria or, rarely, neither. The management of the HELLP syndrome is the same as in preeclampsia.

Key diagnostic studies to look for evidence of end-organ dysfunction: →Table 9-10.

→ MANAGEMENT

Preeclampsia is a progressive disease that will resolve only with delivery of the placenta. However, if this syndrome occurs before term, the risk of continued pregnancy to the mother must be weighed against the risk to the baby from preterm delivery. For this reason, the management of preeclampsia should not be undertaken without close partnership with an obstetrician, as it is the obstetrician who is usually best equipped to weigh the risks and benefits of expediting delivery versus expectant management. Before 37 weeks' gestation,

this is a complex decision that is outside the scope of this chapter. In gene~
however, women who are likely to deliver prior to 34 weeks' gestation will recer
betamethasone for fetal lung maturation. After 37 weeks' gestation, treatmen
is almost always delivery of the baby. The diagnosis of preeclampsia is not ar
indication for cesarean section if not otherwise required for obstetric indications.

Urgent delivery, regardless of gestational age, is often indicated in the presence of preeclampsia with any of the following severe manifestations: eclampsia,
severe fetal compromise (severe IUGR, reversed diastolic umbilical artery
flow), cortical blindness, stroke, platelets <50,000 µmol/L, acute kidney injury
(creatinine >110 µmol/L with no prior disease), inability to control hypertension
after >12 hours on >3 antihypertensive agents.

Supportive management is directed towards mitigating the effects of vasoconstriction, capillary leak, and activation of clotting. The priorities for
management are therefore:

1) Vasodilation (vasodilators and fluid).

2) Restoration of intravascular volume.

3) Clotting factor replacement when depleted.

Increased blood pressure needs to be reduced to safe levels (usually <160 mm Hg
SBP and 110 mm Hg DBP). Treatment should be initiated promptly but then
titrated to produce a steady rather than precipitous decrease to target levels
(→Table 9-9). Blood pressure lowering will be augmented by volume expansion
(→below), magnesium sulfate, and epidural or spinal anesthesia, so antihypertensive therapy needs to be adjusted with these factors taken into consideration.

The goal of treatment of severe hypertension is to reduce the maternal risk of
stroke. Treatment does not alter the course of preeclampsia.

Women with preeclampsia almost always have intravascular hypovolemia
when they present. This aggravates vasoconstriction, increases hypertension
and organ ischemia, and increases the risk of acute kidney injury. Volume expansion can reduce the overall systemic vascular resistance, improving blood
pressure control and ischemia, but may result in fluid overload. The optimum
management remains controversial. Usually at least 500 mL to 1 L of normal
saline or Ringer solution can be given quickly; however, the administration of
fluids should be associated with meticulous input/output documentation, so
as to avoid inadvertent volume overload. Clinical assessment of the jugular
venous pressure is an important guide to intravascular volume. In severe cases,
colloid replacement could be considered, especially if the serum albumin level
is very low (<20 g/L). A urine output >30 mL/h usually indicates adequate
intravascular volume, but not if the woman is receiving magnesium (osmotic
diuretic effect). The volume management of patients with preeclampsia that
is associated with pulmonary capillary leak (causing pulmonary edema) can
be extremely difficult. In such situations, we would recommend consultation
and transfer of the patient to a high acuity care ward (an intensive care or
a step-down unit) before the administration of fluids is considered.

The use of vasodilators (primarily to lower blood pressure) and volume expansion
is important also to reduce multiorgan ischemia.

Otherwise, supportive management is directed at the affected organ systems:

1) **Neurologic**: Prevention or treatment of seizures: Anticonvulsant treatment
   (usually magnesium sulfate) is indicated for seizures and also for signs
   of cerebral irritability (agitation, visual scotomata, clonus). Treatment:
   →Chapter 3.9.2.1.

   Red flags: Confusion and obtundation (except in the immediate postictal
   phase) and fixed neurologic deficits are rarely seen; these should be investigated with imaging of the brain.

2) **Hematologic**:

   a) Thrombocytopenia, even severe (platelets $<25 \times 10^9$/L), is not usually
      associated with a major risk of hemorrhage. As platelet transfusion

is a consumptive process, the life-span of transfused platelets is very short (minutes), so this measure should be reserved for situations when treatment of active bleeding is required (eg, after the baby is delivered by cesarean section). **Red flag**: The platelet count will usually begin to rise by 48 hours following delivery of the placenta. If not, thrombotic thrombocytopenic purpura or hemolytic-uremic syndrome (HUS) need to be considered.

b) Hemolysis: This rarely requires transfusion. While hemolysis is microangiopathic, the associated disseminated intravascular coagulation (DIC) is of greater concern.

c) Coagulation: A small decrease in fibrinogen and increase in the international normalized ratio (INR) may be seen in patients with severe preeclampsia and DIC. Close monitoring for progression is vital. **Red flag**: Fibrinogen <1.5 g/L implies serious defibrination. A prolonged INR (>1.3) is rare in preeclampsia and usually indicates severe liver dysfunction (acute fatty liver of pregnancy needs to be considered). Prompt clotting factor replacement in these situations may be life-saving.

3) **Renal**: Correcting the intravascular volume deficit is a priority to mitigate acute kidney injury.

Red flag #1: Oliguria (urine output <25 mL/h) should be treated with volume expansion unless or until there are definite signs of left ventricular failure. Furosemide is not appropriate in such cases and may in fact worsen oliguria.

Red flag #2: Serum creatinine may increase up until 48 hours postpartum before stabilizing and decreasing. An increase after this period is of serious concern, warranting consideration of an alternative renal diagnosis (eg, complement-mediated HUS).

Red flag #3: Polyuria (>3 L/d) may simply be due to clearance of excess extravascular water as the woman recovers from preeclampsia. However, it may be due to renal tubular dysfunction (acute tubular necrosis) and may precipitate secondary severe hypovolemia a few days after delivery. Monitoring jugular venous pressure and serum creatinine levels is helpful.

4) **Hepatic**: Serum transaminases may be markedly elevated (10-20 times the upper limit of normal) due to ischemic liver cell injury. This usually begins to resolve promptly as perfusion is improved (vasodilators and volume expansion).

Red flag #1: Jaundice is relatively uncommon and usually associated with the combination of severe hemolysis, DIC, and often liver dysfunction.

Red flag #2: The INR is usually normal or only slightly raised in preeclampsia. An INR >1.3 suggests significant liver dysfunction (such as can occur with acute fatty liver of pregnancy). The coagulation defect is the greatest threat and requires prompt treatment.

5) **Respiratory**: Pulmonary edema is primarily due to capillary leak and possible diastolic dysfunction; it may be aggravated by reduced plasma oncotic pressure due to reduced serum albumin levels. Left ventricular failure or fluid overload is rarely a factor. Management is aimed at maintaining adequate oxygenation, adding positive airway pressure if necessary. Volume restriction and diuretics are usually unhelpful in such situations and indicated only for pulmonary edema not responding to oxygen or positive airway pressure.

6) **Cardiac**: Myocardial cell injury (increased troponin and cardiac enzymes) is not uncommon as a consequence of preeclampsia-induced ischemia. This usually resolves quickly with improved perfusion/vasodilation. Coronary arteriography is rarely indicated.

Red flag: Heart failure is rare but can occur as a consequence of "stunned myocardium" and/or diastolic dysfunction. Cardiac ultrasonography is invaluable in identifying left ventricular failure (reduced ejection fraction) and wall motion abnormalities. Diuretics are indicated if heart failure is demonstrated.

→ **FOLLOW-UP**

Follow-up is the same as in eclampsia.

→ **SPECIAL CONSIDERATIONS**

Postpartum Preeclampsia

Although delivery of the placenta usually results in the resolution of preeclampsia, there is a subset of women who will go on to develop delayed preeclampsia in the postpartum period. Clinical symptoms may be more atypical and, in many cases, without antecedent hypertension. It is for this reason that all women should be instructed on the signs and symptoms of preeclampsia prior to discharge from the hospital and, ideally, have blood pressure taken between days 3 and 6 postpartum. Treatment is similar to that of antepartum preeclampsia, with the exception that delivery has already occurred. Angiotensin-converting enzyme inhibitors may be preferred in the treatment of ongoing hypertension.

9.3. Renal Parenchymal Hypertension

→ **DEFINITION, ETIOLOGY, PATHOGENESIS**

Renal parenchymal hypertension is a form of secondary hypertension caused by kidney disease. It may occur in the course of glomerulonephritis, diabetic nephropathy (diabetic kidney disease), kidney damage in the course of systemic connective tissue diseases (systemic lupus erythematosus, systemic sclerosis, systemic vasculitis), tubulointerstitial nephritis, obstructive nephropathy, polycystic kidney disease, large solitary kidney cysts (rare), postirradiation nephropathy, hypoplastic kidney, renal tuberculosis (rare).

The **main mechanisms** leading to hypertension in chronic kidney disease (CKD) include impaired urinary sodium and water excretion (impaired pressure natriuresis); excessive kidney release of vasoconstrictors (angiotensin II and endothelin 1); vasodilator deficiency (eg, nitric oxide); sympathetic activation; endocrine and metabolic disturbances (including calcium/phosphate metabolism). The accelerated development of atherosclerosis and calcification of the vascular wall leads to an increased stiffness of the walls of large arteries. Sodium and water retention with subsequent volume overload increase with progression of kidney disease. An increase in venous return and cardiac output causes sympathetic activation, which results in increased vasoconstriction of the resistance vessels and an increase in peripheral vascular resistance.

→ **CLINICAL FEATURES AND NATURAL HISTORY**

Hypertension often develops at an early stage of kidney disease, when the glomerular filtration rate (GFR) is only slightly reduced (it may be the presenting feature). Symptoms of the underlying kidney disease are usually the predominant clinical feature. Sodium and water retention manifest as peripheral edema only in some patients. Untreated hypertension accelerates the progression of kidney disease and may itself be a cause of (hypertensive) nephropathy. Kidney diseases are the most common causes of treatment--resistant and malignant hypertension.

→ **DIAGNOSIS**

Perform the same diagnostic tests as in all patients with hypertension (→Chapter 3.9.1) as well as studies necessary for the diagnosis of the kidney disease responsible for the hypertension. Note that there may be other contributors to hypertension in patients with renal parenchymal disease, cluding renovascular disease and drug therapy (eg, erythropoietin-stimulating agents, calcineurin inhibitors). Consider also unrecognized nonsteroidal anti-inflammatory drug (NSAID) use as a potential contributor to both hypertension and CKD.

➔ TREATMENT

General Considerations

1. Treatment of renal parenchymal hypertension involves treating the underlying kidney disease and hypertension.

2. Target blood pressure: <130 to 140/90 mm Hg in all patients (exceptions: →Chapter 3.9.1) and <140/90 mm Hg in patients treated with renal replacement therapy (RRT). General principles: →Chapter 3.9.1.

Nonpharmacologic Management

1. Restriction of salt intake (sodium chloride) to 5 to 6 g/d.

2. Monitoring fluid balance to maintain normal volume status (this is of particular importance in patients on dialysis).

Pharmacotherapy

1. Drug selection: Angiotensin-converting enzyme inhibitors (ACEIs) and angiotensin receptor blockers (ARBs) are preferred in patients with CKD and proteinuria, but these two classes should not be used in combination. As in other patients treated with these agents, the risk of acute kidney injury is increased with dehydration, generalized atherosclerosis, and heart failure.

Diuretics are a key component of blood pressure control in patients with renal parenchymal disease. Use thiazide diuretics in patients with a GFR $\geq$30 mL/min/1.73 m^2 and loop diuretics in patients with a GFR <30 mL/min/1.73 m^2 and/or with severe proteinuria and edema. Potassium-sparing diuretics should be used cautiously, if at all, due to the risk of hyperkalemia. Further agents that can be used include calcium channel blockers and cardioselective β-blockers. Other agents, including α-blockers, centrally acting α-agonists, or vasodilators, are typically reserved for adjunctive therapy when alternative drugs are insufficient to control blood pressure and/or are not tolerated. With advancing CKD, attention to the route of excretion of the various agents should be reviewed.

Starting treatment with an ACEI or ARB:

1) In patients who have not been previously treated with antihypertensive agents, start with an intermediate dose of an ACEI or ARB and titrate it up every 4 to 8 weeks, checking the serum estimated glomerular filtration rate (eGFR) and potassium levels prior to the initiation and 2 to 4 weeks following the initiation or dose escalation.

2) In patients who are already treated with antihypertensive drugs, add an ACEI or ARB at a low dose and titrate it up while reducing the dose of the previously used antihypertensive agent(s) at the same time.

2. Monitoring of treatment with ACEIs/ARBs: In patients with a reduced GFR in whom treatment with an ACEI or ARB has been started or the dose of the agent has been increased, monitor the following parameters at time intervals dependent on their baseline values (→Table 9-11):

1) **eGFR**: In patients with a substantial decrease in the GFR (eg, >10%), closer monitoring is recommended, as this is associated with an increased risk of adverse cardiovascular and renal events and our practice is not to escalate the doses of the ACEI/ARB in such situations. In patients with a GFR decrease >30% from baseline, consider a dose reduction or switch to an antihypertensive agent from another class. In patients who are on a diuretic and may be volume depleted, consider reducing the diuretic dose and rechallenging with the ACEI/ARB at a reduced dose.

Table 9-11. Monitoring of serum creatinine (GFR) and serum potassium levels during treatment with an ACEI or ARB in patients with chronic kidney disease

GFR (mL/min/1.73 m^2)	Serum potassium level (mmol/L)	After treatment initiation or dose change	In a stable patient[a,b]
≥60	≤4.5	In 2-4 weeks	Every 6-12 months
30-59	4.6-5	In 2-4 weeks	Every 3-6 months
<30	5.1-5.5	In 2 weeks	Every 2-4 months

[a] After determining dosage and stabilizing blood pressure, GFR, and serum potassium level.

[b] In patients with a decrease in the GFR ≥15% during ACEI or ARB treatment, measure serum creatinine levels (GFR) every 1 to 2 months.

ACEI, angiotensin-converting enzyme inhibitor; ARB, angiotensin receptor blocker; GFR, glomerular filtration rate.

2) **Serum potassium levels**:

  a) 5.1 to 5.5 mmol/L: Recommend restricted consumption of potassium-rich foods (renalnetwork.on.ca) and reduce the doses or discontinue other drugs that may increase potassium levels if the potassium level does not fall into an acceptable range.

  b) 5.6 to 5.9 mmol/L: Recommend restricted consumption of potassium-rich foods, reduce the dose of the ACEI/ARB by 50% or add a diuretic, and measure serum potassium levels approximately every week until they return to an acceptable range. If this does not occur within 4 weeks, either discontinue the ACEI/ARB and use an antihypertensive drug from another class, or potassium-binding therapy (eg, sodium polystyrene sulfonate, sodium zirconium cyclosilicate, patiromer sorbitex calcium).

  c) >5.9 mmol/L: Consider the need for a more urgent evaluation, discontinue the ACEI/ARB, recommend restricted consumption of potassium-rich foods, and reduce the doses or discontinue other drugs that may increase potassium levels. Consider reinitiation of the ACEI/ARB at a reduced dose if the serum potassium level normalizes.

After establishing dose(s) of the drug(s) and achieving stable blood pressure, GFR, and potassium levels, serum creatinine and potassium levels are monitored less frequently (→Table 9-11).

In patients with an eGFR falling to <15 mL/min/1.73 m^2, discontinuation of ACEIs/ARBs in some cases may improve the GFR and delay the need to start RRT.

9.4. Renovascular Hypertension

→ DEFINITION, ETIOLOGY, PATHOGENESIS

Renovascular hypertension is a secondary cause of hypertension due to renal ischemia and subsequent hypersecretion of renin. **Ischemic nephropathy** is a reduction in the glomerular filtration rate (GFR) and impairment of other kidney functions due to hemodynamically significant renal artery stenosis.

Causes of renal artery stenosis: The most common causes are atherosclerosis (usual risk factors apply) and fibromuscular dysplasia. Other causes include atherosclerotic renal-artery stenosis, fibromuscular dysplasia, renal artery aneurysm, arterial embolus, arteriovenous fistula (congenital/traumatic), segmental arterial occlusion (posttraumatic), extrinsic compression of renal artery (eg, pheochromocytoma), renal compression (eg, metastatic tumor), stenosis to a solitary functioning kidney, aortic coarctation, systemic vasculitis (eg, Takayasu, polyarteritis), atheroembolic disease, vascular occlusion due to an endovascular aortic stent graft.

A hemodynamically significant stenosis (ie, >60%-70% of the artery diameter) of the renal artery or arteries results in hypoperfusion of the kidney as well as an increase in the activity of the renin-angiotensin-aldosterone (RAA) system and its subsequent effects.

→ CLINICAL FEATURES AND NATURAL HISTORY

1. Clinical features of renovascular hypertension:

1) A sudden onset of hypertension, development of hypertension before the age of 30 years.

2) Development of severe hypertension after the age of 50 years.

3) Treatment-resistant or malignant hypertension.

4) Deterioration of renal function (eg, >30%) after the administration of an angiotensin-converting enzyme inhibitor (ACEI) or an angiotensin receptor blocker (ARB).

5) Unexplained renal atrophy or a difference >1.5 cm in the kidney size.

6) Unexplained progressive deterioration in kidney function.

7) Unexplained flash pulmonary edema.

8) Fibromuscular dysplasia of other vascular beds.

9) An epigastric or abdominal bruit.

2. Natural history: Over time significant renal artery stenosis—particularly when bilateral—may lead to the development of ischemic nephropathy and progressive chronic kidney disease (CKD). Fibromuscular dysplasia is also progressive and is associated with the development of new stenoses and arterial lesions (aneurysms and dissections).

→ DIAGNOSIS

Diagnostic and management algorithm: →Figure 9-2.

General Principles

Most patients with atherosclerotic renal artery stenosis should be managed medically.◐◑ Investigation for renal artery stenosis should therefore be reserved for those with compelling indications to proceed with interventional approaches if renal artery stenosis is identified (→below).

Diagnostic Tests

1. Laboratory tests may reveal hypokalemia and albuminuria, although the latter is usually mild. An increase in serum creatinine levels and decrease in the GFR are frequently observed. Plasma renin activity (PRA) and aldosterone levels are often increased.

2. Imaging studies:

1) **Intra-arterial digital subtraction angiography (DSA)** is the most accurate method of imaging renal vasculature and is considered the gold standard. It is indicated in patients in whom the final diagnosis cannot be established using less invasive studies and there is an intent to proceed with an intervention if renal artery stenosis is confirmed.

2) **Duplex ultrasonography, computed tomography angiography (CTA),** and **magnetic resonance angiography (MRA)** are reasonable initial noninvasive imaging modalities. Duplex ultrasonography may provide better functional versus anatomical information but is often limited due to the length of the procedure and lack of expertise. Limitations have been identified in the use of all noninvasive modalities, although many of the studies predate more recent advances in imaging quality. Ultimately, the choice of the initial test should be decided based on availability and local

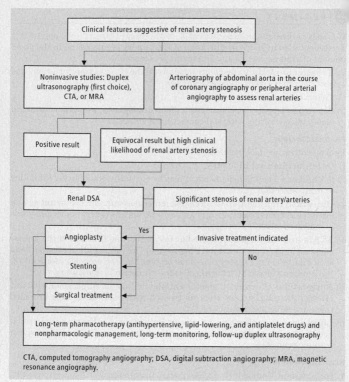

CTA, computed tomography angiography; DSA, digital subtraction angiography; MRA, magnetic resonance angiography.

Figure 9-2. Management algorithm in patients with hypertension and renal artery stenosis. *Adapted from Eur Heart J. 2018;39(9):763-816.*

expertise, recognizing that most patients do not require imaging and can be managed medically. As a general rule, a positive test is more helpful than a negative one. CTA and MRA may miss lesions of fibromuscular dysplasia that are subsequently detected on DSA.

3) The advantages of **captopril renal scintigraphy** are its noninvasive nature and the absence of nephrotoxic effects of radiopharmaceuticals (unlike in the case of radiographic contrast media). However, this test has fallen out of favor due to high false-positive and false-negative rates and limitations in those with preexisting CKD or bilateral renovascular disease.

3. Renal vein catheterization may be useful in determining indications for nephrectomy but is used infrequently. It allows for measuring PRA in the venous blood.

Diagnostic Criteria
Diagnosis is based on the results of the imaging studies.

Differential Diagnosis
Focus on:
1) Primary and secondary hyperaldosteronism (hypokalemia).
2) Renal parenchymal disease (renal failure).

→ TREATMENT

1. Goals of treatment: Achievement of blood pressure targets (→Chapter 3.9.1). Treatment also includes modification of the factors predisposing to the development of atherosclerosis and treatment of comorbidities.

2. Treatment modalities (choice depends on the clinical manifestations and severity of renal artery stenosis [→below]):

1) Pharmacotherapy.
2) Revascularization: Percutaneous balloon angioplasty, percutaneous angioplasty with stenting, surgical correction of stenosis.

Pharmacotherapy

Pharmacotherapy may include:

1) **Calcium channel blockers**.
2) **β-Blockers**: Their beneficial effect may be partially related to the inhibition of renin secretion.
3) **Diuretics**: Thiazide diuretics and/or a mineralocorticoid receptor antagonist are often effective. Monitoring of kidney function and serum potassium levels is indicated when initiating.
4) **ACEIs and ARBs** are effective but may affect the function of the kidney supplied by the stenotic artery. These agents are contraindicated in patients with bilateral renal artery stenosis or renal artery stenosis of a solitary functioning kidney. Monitoring of kidney function is mandatory.
5) **Antiplatelet therapy**: Consider antiplatelet agents in patients with atherosclerotic renal artery stenosis treated with medical therapy provided there are no contraindications.✓○
6) **Lipid-lowering therapy (statins)**: Patients with atherosclerotic renal artery stenosis warrant treatment with statins provided there are no contraindications.✓�🌑

Revascularization

1. Indications: Consider revascularization in patients with hemodynamically significant renal artery stenosis (stenosis of 80%-99% of the artery diameter, or of 60%-79% with a systolic pressure gradient across the stenosis ≥20 mm Hg; the latter is only measurable if the patient has already had intra-arterial angiography) and one of the following:

1) Coexisting uncontrolled hypertension despite maximal medical therapy.
2) Rapidly declining kidney function.
3) The etiology of the renal artery stenosis is fibromuscular dysplasia.

2. Techniques of revascularization:

1) **Percutaneous renal angioplasty** is the method of choice in most patients with renal artery stenosis caused by fibromuscular dysplasia. It is also effective in individuals with inflammatory stenosis (eg, Takayasu disease). The procedure may be performed only in patients in remission. Stenting is very rarely necessary and could impede the ability to proceed with surgical revascularization, when required.
2) **Percutaneous renal angioplasty with stenting**: In atherosclerotic renal artery stenosis, stenting is preferred over balloon angioplasty alone. In patients with stenosis caused by fibromuscular dysplasia, stenting is performed only in case of complications of angioplasty (arterial dissection).
3) **Surgical renal revascularization** is currently rarely performed and usually involves an aortorenal bypass graft. Occasionally surgical revascularization is required in lesions secondary to fibromuscular dysplasia, when angioplasty is not possible or ineffective.

3. Management of patients after percutaneous renal angioplasty:

1) Assess kidney function 24 hours after the procedure and then after 2 to 3 days. Carefully monitor blood pressure on the first day after the procedure because of the risk of hypotension.

2) Extrapolating from the interventional cardiology literature, the pattern of practice is to administer acetylsalicylic acid (ASA) 75 to 325 mg/d for lifetime; for the first 4 weeks after stent implantation, add clopidogrel 75 mg/d (in patients with implanted drug-eluting stents, consider extending clopidogrel therapy to 12 months).

3) To assess long-term effects of the procedure, continue to monitor blood pressure and renal function, initially more often and periodically thereafter.

→ SPECIAL CONSIDERATIONS

Fibromuscular Dysplasia

1. Definition: A segmental, nonatherosclerotic, and noninflammatory disease of unknown etiology typically affecting the muscular layer of blood vessels, which causes stenosis of small and medium arteries. Fibromuscular dysplasia often presents with hypertension at a young age and is more common in women (a female to male ratio of ~4:1). The classical appearance on angiography is a "string-of-beads."

2. Diagnosis: Indications for diagnostic workup of fibromuscular dysplasia: →Clinical Features, above. If first-degree relatives of a patient with fibromuscular dysplasia develop hypertension at a young age or have dissection of any artery, an aneurysm, or cerebral bleeding, they should be evaluated for fibromuscular dysplasia.

Diagnostic tests:

1) Duplex ultrasonography (a potentially useful screening test with the same caveats as raised previously [→General Principles, above]).

2) MRA or CTA (the latter is preferred) to confirm the diagnosis or as a first--line study (in patients in whom duplex ultrasonography is presumed to be suboptimal [eg, obese patients]; these diagnostic methods are also used in the case of a very strong suspicion of fibromuscular dysplasia and/or serious clinical implications of the diagnosis [patients who are very young; patients with malignant hypertension or complications of hypertension, including complications affecting other vascular beds; patients with elevated serum creatinine levels]).

3) Intra-arterial DSA in patients with a strong suspicion of fibromuscular dysplasia in whom after performing all the above studies diagnosis is still equivocal or in patients with fibromuscular dysplasia confirmed by CTA or MRA in whom revascularization is indicated.

4) **Differential diagnosis**: Consider other rare diagnoses, including renal artery spasm; arteritis; and genetic diseases, such as type 1 neurofibromatosis, tuberous sclerosis, pseudoxanthoma elasticum, Ehlers-Danlos syndrome, Alagille syndrome, Williams syndrome, and Turner syndrome.

3. Treatment: Revascularization should be considered in most patients with hypertension and renal artery stenosis caused by fibromuscular dysplasia. Advancing age and longer duration of hypertension are negatively associated with improved outcomes after revascularization.⊘○ Other scenarios in patients with fibromuscular dysplasia when revascularization should be considered include:

1) A recent onset of hypertension (this is the treatment of choice to normalize blood pressure).

2) Treatment-resistant hypertension or intolerance of antihypertensive drugs.

3) Renal failure or deteriorating renal function, particularly after the administration of an ACEI or ARB.

Preferred modalities of revascularization: →Revascularization, above.

In **patients in whom revascularization is not performed**:

1) Measure blood pressure monthly until target values are achieved.

2) Our pattern of practice is to measure serum creatinine (estimated glomerular filtration rate [eGFR]) levels and perform ultrasonography on a yearly basis to assess the kidney size.

In **patients after revascularization**:

1) Measure blood pressure and calculate the eGFR 1 month after the procedure.

2) Our pattern of practice is to perform renal imaging studies 6 months after the procedure, or earlier in case of elevated blood pressure or serum creatinine levels.

10. Infective Endocarditis

→ DEFINITION, ETIOLOGY, PATHOGENESIS

Infective endocarditis (IE) is an infection of the endocardium involving the valves (most frequently), ventricles, atria, or endothelium of vessels (eg, in patients with coarctation of the aorta) or systemic infection of cardiac implantable electronic devices extending to the electrode leads, valves, or endocardial surface. Most frequently IE affects the mitral and aortic valves; less frequently the tricuspid valve may be involved. IE can involve >1 valve and the proportion of these patients varies in reported literature. IE is preceded by bacteremia, which can last from <2 weeks (80% of patients) to several months (in particular in patients with IE involving a prosthetic valve).

Etiologic agents:

1) Bacteria (>90% of cases). Most frequent pathogens:

   a) Staphylococci (an increasingly more common cause of IE; *Staphylococcus aureus*, *Staphylococcus epidermidis*, coagulase-negative staphylococci).

   b) Streptococci (viridans-group streptococci; until recently the most frequent cause of native valve infections).

   c) Enterococci.

   d) Gram-negative bacteria, including the HACEK group (*Haemophilus* spp, *Aggregatibacter* [formerly *Actinobacillus*] spp, *Cardiobacterium hominis*, *Eikenella corrodens*, and *Kingella* spp).

   e) Mixed bacterial etiology is frequently found among IV drug abusers.

2) Fungi (<1%).

3) Rare: Chlamydia, rickettsia, or mycoplasma.

Depending on criteria definitions for IE, etiology cannot be established in 5% to 20% of patients.

Etiologic agents in patients with negative blood cultures: Culture-negative IE may be seen in the context of antimicrobial use prior to blood cultures being drawn or infections caused by fastidious organisms. These organisms include:

1) Nutritionally variant streptococci.

2) *Coxiella burnetii*.

3) *Bartonella* spp.

4) *Mycoplasma pneumoniae*.

5) *Brucella* spp.

6) *Legionella pneumophila*.

7) Fungi (eg, *Aspergillus* spp).

8) *Tropheryma whipplei*.

Diseases and conditions predisposing to native valve endocarditis (NVE): Certain heart diseases predisposing to IE are indications for antibiotic prophylaxis (→Prevention, below). Other risk factors include history of rheumatic disease, mitral valve prolapse with regurgitation, hypertrophic cardiomyopathy, valvular or congenital heart disease (particularly affecting the aortic valve, eg, bicuspid aortic valve, coarctation of the aorta), degenerative cardiac lesions, prolonged maintenance of indwelling central venous catheters, foreign bodies in the heart (eg, intracardiac electrodes, vascular patches), chronic hemodialysis, and IV drug use (IVDU) (associated with involvement of right-sided heart valves).

Prosthetic valve endocarditis (PVE) accounts for 10% to 30% of all cases of IE. It most frequently develops within 5 to 6 weeks of surgery. IE occurring within 12 months of surgery is considered a postoperative complication. In the first 2 months after surgery, PVE is most frequently caused by *S aureus* followed by coagulase-negative staphylococci (mainly methicillin-resistant strains) and *Candida* spp. In PVE developing >1 year after surgery, etiologic agents are similar to those seen in NVE.

Cardiac device–related infective endocarditis (CDRIE) is most frequently caused by coagulase-negative staphylococci and *S aureus*.

→ CLINICAL FEATURES

IE presentation is highly variable and differential diagnosis is often broad, sometimes leading to delay in establishing diagnosis. IE is manifested mainly by nonspecific symptoms, including high-grade fever with chills or prolonged low-grade fever (the most frequent feature), malaise, weakness, arthralgia, myalgia, loss of appetite, weight loss, headache, and nausea.

1. Left-sided endocarditis may also cause symptoms associated with:

1) Regurgitation murmur over the affected valve.

2) Features of heart failure, including pulmonary edema in patients with no prior history of valvular disease.

3) Conduction abnormalities.

4) Rarely large vegetations leading to functional mitral stenosis.

5) Embolic phenomena (most frequently associated with *S aureus*), including:

   a) Central nervous system (CNS) symptoms (30%-40% of patients; hemiparesis, aphasia; behavioral changes in those with microembolism).

   b) Rarely intracranial hemorrhage due to ruptured mycotic aneurysm.

   c) Renal, splenic, or mesenteric embolism, which may lead to adynamic ileus resulting in abdominal pain or back pain.

   d) Coronary artery embolism (rare) manifesting as chest pain.

   e) Ocular disturbances associated with retinal artery embolism.

   f) Peripheral vascular and inflammation symptoms (petechiae on skin and under nail plates, Osler nodes [painful red nodules located mainly on fingers and toes due to deposition of immune complexes], Janeway lesions [painless hemorrhagic lesions on palms and soles], Roth spots [retinal hemorrhages with pale centers]).

   g) Splenomegaly and hepatomegaly (more frequent in patients with long--standing IE).

2. Right-sided endocarditis may also cause symptoms associated with:

1) Pulmonary embolism, with associated cough and pleuritic chest pain (caused by septic pulmonary emboli): This is the most common manifestation.

2) Murmur caused by tricuspid or pulmonary regurgitation: This is often absent or seen in advanced disease.

3) Features of right ventricular failure in patients with long-standing IE.

4) Often recurrent right-sided IE in the case of IVDU, frequently in the absence of other predisposing heart conditions.

Note: IE must always be excluded in patients with embolism and fever.

→ DIAGNOSIS

Diagnostic Workup

The following studies should be performed in every patient with suspected IE.

1. Blood cultures (before starting antimicrobial treatment): Obtain ≥3 blood culture sets at 30-minute intervals, regardless of body temperature. Each sample should contain 10 mL of blood collected to an aerobic tube and another 10 mL collected to an anaerobic tube. Mark the order form as suspected IE. In all patients undergoing cardiac surgery, and particularly those with negative results of previous cultures, perform specimen cultures and pathologic examination and, if needed, use molecular identification methods, to identify the etiologic agent.

2. Serologic studies: Perform these in the case of suspected infection with *C burnetii*, *Bartonella* spp, *Brucella* spp, *Histoplasma capsulatum*, *Legionella* spp, or *Chlamydia* spp.

3. Echocardiography: In suspected endocarditis it is important to evaluate for vegetations (mobile echogenic structures attached to the endocardium or intracardiac prosthetic material), valvular damage (regurgitation of the infected valve due to vegetations, leaflet perforation, or rupture of chordae tendineae), and perivalvular complications (abscess, pseudoaneurysm, intracardiac fistula).

In all patients without prosthetic valves with IE suspected on the basis of clinical criteria, transthoracic echocardiography (TTE) should be performed.✅● In those with a low clinical probability of IE and a negative TTE result (provided that good-quality images are obtained), IE is unlikely and another diagnosis should be considered. If good-quality TTE images cannot be obtained, transesophageal echocardiography (TEE) should be performed. TEE should be also performed in:

1) Patients with a high clinical probability of IE and a negative TTE result.

2) Patients with suspected IE and a prosthetic valve or intracardiac device.

3) Patients with suspected IE affecting the aortic valve.

4) Patients with IE and significant valvular regurgitation.

5) Patients with a TTE result suggestive of IE (except for those with IE affecting right-sided native heart valves and unequivocal TTE findings). In the case of a negative TEE result and reasonable suspicion of IE, repeat TEE after 5 to 7 days.

Although the mainstay for diagnosis of IE, echocardiography has limitations (it cannot reliably differentiate between active and healed IE, and TTE and TEE sensitivity and specificity are both not 100%). As such, results must be interpreted in the context of clinical presentation.

4. Laboratory tests: There are no biochemical parameters that have been proven to be sensitive or specific for the diagnosis of IE. IE has been associated with elevated erythrocyte sedimentation rate (ESR), increased levels of C-reactive protein (CRP) and fibrinogen, leukocytosis with neutrophilia (most frequent in acute IE), anemia (usually normocytic and normochromic), hematuria, and minor proteinuria.

5. Electrocardiography: Nonspecific findings and conduction abnormalities.

6. Chest radiography: Nonspecific findings, which may include congestive heart failure findings and signs of pulmonary complications.

7. Multislice computed tomography (CT) and magnetic resonance imaging (MRI): CT provides a valuable addition to echocardiography in the diagnosis of perivalvular lesions: abscesses, pseudoaneurysms, and fistulas. It may be also used in patients with prosthetic valves. Multislice CT is useful in the anatomical assessment of the aortic valve (eg, leaflet perforation) and aorta and in the diagnosis of pulmonary embolism in patients with right-side IE, metastatic abscesses (eg, in the spleen), and CNS-related emboli. CT has lower sensitivity than MRI but is more available.

Diagnostic Criteria

The diagnosis of IE can be made in a patient with sepsis or generalized infection and objective features of endocardial involvement. Relevant diagnostic terminology includes:

1) **Definite IE**: →Table 10-1.

2) **Possible IE**: →Table 10-1.

3) **Active IE**:

   a) Positive blood cultures or positive intraoperative specimens.

   b) Intraoperative confirmation of features of endocarditis.

   c) Unfinished course of antimicrobial treatment for IE.

4) **Relapse**: IE caused by the same microorganism within <6 months of a confirmed episode of IE.

5) **Reinfection**: IE caused by the same microorganism after >6 months of a previous episode of IE or caused by a different microorganism.

6) **CDRIE**: CDRIE is difficult to differentiate from local infection of the device. It should be suspected in the case of fever of unknown origin in a patient with a cardiac implantable electronic device. The key diagnostic procedures are echocardiography (TEE has superior sensitivity and specificity but TTE should be performed first) and blood cultures.

Differential Diagnosis

Other causes of fever (→Chapter 1.10), systemic connective tissue disease, malignancy, rheumatic fever.

Causes of false-positive echocardiography results: Sterile intracardiac thrombus or tumor resembling vegetations, sterile valvular vegetations (eg, in Libman-Sacks endocarditis in the course of systemic lupus erythematosus, or less frequently in Behçet syndrome, carcinoid, or acute rheumatic fever).

→TREATMENT

IE requires initial therapy and stabilization of the patient in the hospital. Outpatient parenteral therapy can be considered once this is achieved. Intravenous treatment may vary in duration from 2 weeks (in a highly selective population meeting predefined criteria) up to 4 to 6 weeks (most commonly) or longer.

Treatment of PVE lasts ≥6 weeks. Intravenous treatment is currently recommended, although this may change in the future.

Pharmacologic Treatment

1. Intravenous antibiotics: In acutely ill patients with suspected IE, start empiric treatment immediately after obtaining blood cultures (→Figure 10-1). The choice of empiric treatment should take into consideration the most likely pathogens. Treatment may be tailored to blood culture results (identified pathogens) and sensitivities once these become available; for instance, streptococcal IE: →Figure 10-2; staphylococcal IE: →Figure 10-3; or IE caused by other pathogens (including those causing IE with negative blood cultures): →Table 10-2.

2. Antithrombotic treatment: Data to guide the use of antithrombotic therapy in the setting of IE are limited, and decisions should be made on a case-by-case basis with consideration given to risks and benefits. IE by itself is not an indication for antithrombotic treatment, but such therapy is

---

Table 10-1. The Duke criteria for diagnosis of infective endocarditis modified by the European Society of Cardiology (2015)

Pathologic criteria

1) Microorganisms demonstrated by culture or on histologic examination of a vegetation, a vegetation that has embolized, or an intracardiac abscess specimen; or

2) Pathologic lesions; vegetation or intracardiac abscess confirmed by histologic examination showing active endocarditis.

Clinical criteria

Major criteria

1) Blood cultures positive for IE:

   a) Typical microorganisms consistent with IE from 2 separate blood cultures: Viridans-group streptococci, *Streptococcus gallolyticus* (formerly *bovis*), HACEK group, *Staphylococcus aureus*; or community-acquired enterococci in the absence of a primary focus; or

   b) Microorganisms consistent with IE from persistently positive blood cultures: ≥2 positive blood cultures of samples drawn >12 h apart or all of 3 or a majority of ≥4 separate cultures of blood (with first and last samples drawn ≥1 h apart); or

   c) Single positive blood culture for *Coxiella burnetii* or phase I IgG antibody titer >1:800.

2) Imaging studies positive for IE:

   a) Echocardiography positive for IE: Vegetation; abscess, pseudoaneurysm, intracardiac fistula; valvular perforation or aneurysm; new partial dehiscence of a prosthetic valve.

   b) Abnormal activity around the site of prosthetic valve implantation detected by ^{18}F-FDG PET/CT (only if the prosthesis was implanted for >3 months) or radiolabeled leukocyte SPECT/CT.

   c) Definite paravalvular lesions on cardiac CT.

Minor criteria

1) Predisposition, such as predisposing heart condition or injection drug use.

2) Fever defined as temperature >38°C.

3) Vascular phenomena (including those detected by imaging only): Major arterial emboli, septic pulmonary infarcts, infectious (mycotic) aneurysm, intracranial hemorrhage, conjunctival hemorrhages, and Janeway lesions.

4) Immunologic phenomena: Glomerulonephritis, Osler nodes, Roth spots, and rheumatoid factor.

5) Microbiological evidence: Positive blood culture but not meeting a major criterion as noted above or serologic evidence of active infection with an organism consistent with IE.

Definite IE: 2 major criteria; 1 major criterion and 3 minor criteria; or 5 minor criteria.

Possible IE: 1 major criterion and 1 minor criterion; or 3 minor criteria.

Rejected IE:

1) Firm alternative diagnosis; or

2) Resolution of symptoms suggesting IE with antibiotic therapy for ≤4 days; or

3) No pathologic evidence of IE at surgery or autopsy with antibiotic therapy for ≤4 days; or

4) Not fulfilling the criteria for possible IE, as defined above.

Based on Eur Heart J. 2015;36(44):3075-3128.

---

^{18}F-FDG PET/CT, ^{18}F-fluorodeoxyglucose positron emission tomography/computed tomography; CT, computed tomography; HACEK, *Haemophilus* spp, *Aggregatibacter* spp, *Cardiobacterium hominis*, *Eikenella corrodens*, *Kingella* spp; IE, infective endocarditis; SPECT, single-photon emission computed tomography.

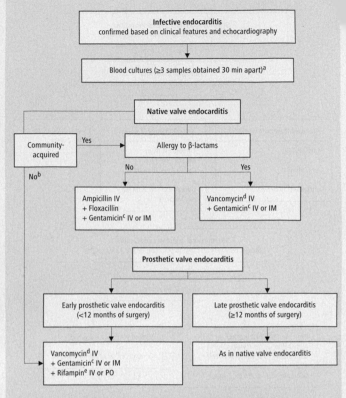

Infective endocarditis
confirmed based on clinical features and echocardiography

Blood cultures (≥3 samples obtained 30 min apart)[a]

Native valve endocarditis

Community-acquired

No[b]

Yes → Allergy to β-lactams

No / Yes

Ampicillin IV
+ Floxacillin
+ Gentamicin[c] IV or IM

Vancomycin[d] IV
+ Gentamicin[c] IV or IM

Prosthetic valve endocarditis

Early prosthetic valve endocarditis
(<12 months of surgery)

Late prosthetic valve endocarditis
(≥12 months of surgery)

Vancomycin[d] IV
+ Gentamicin[c] IV or IM
+ Rifampin[e] IV or PO

As in native valve endocarditis

Dosage: Ampicillin and floxacillin 12 g/d in 4-6 divided doses. **Gentamicin** 3 mg/kg/d in 1 dose.
Rifampin 900-1200 mg/d in 2-3 divided doses. **Vancomycin** 30-60 mg/kg/d in 2-3 divided doses.[f]

[a] Once the pathogen has been identified (usually within 48 h), modify treatment according to results of susceptibility testing. If blood cultures are negative and there is no clinical response to treatment, consider adding antimicrobial agents with activity against pathogens causing blood culture–negative infective endocarditis (doxycycline, fluoroquinolones) and maybe surgery for molecular diagnosis and treatment.

[b] In health-care–associated native valve endocarditis in settings with high prevalence (>5%) of *S aureus* infections some experts recommend a combination of cloxacillin and vancomycin until *S aureus* infection is confirmed.

[c] Renal function and serum levels of gentamicin should be monitored closely to prevent the development of renal injury. In patients receiving the drug once a day, the trough level should be <1 mg/L and level 1 hour after an IV dose should be 10-12 mg/L.

[d] Serum vancomycin concentrations should be 10-15 mg/L at the predose level and 30-45 mg/L 1 hour after completing IV infusion of the drug.

[e] Rifampin is used only in case of prosthetic valve endocarditis. According to some experts it should be started after 3-5 days of using vancomycin and gentamicin.

[f] In native valve endocarditis or late prosthetic valve endocarditis; 30 mg/kg/d in 2 divided doses in early prosthetic valve endocarditis.

IM, intramuscular; IV, intravenous; PO, oral.

Figure 10-1. Empiric antibiotic treatment for infective endocarditis before pathogen identification and in the case of negative cultures. *Based on Eur Heart J. 2015;36(44):3075-3128.*

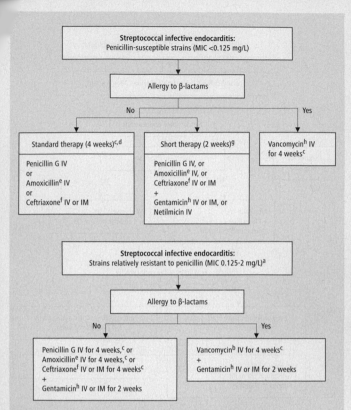

Dosage: Amoxicillin 100-200 mg/kg/d in 4-6 divided doses; in patients with relative or complete resistance, 200 mg/kg/d in 4-6 divided doses. **Ceftriaxone** 2 g once daily. **Gentamicin** 3 mg/kg once daily. **Netilmicin** 4-5 mg/kg once daily. **Penicillin G** 12-18 million IU/d (in patients with relative resistance 24 million IU/d) in 4-6 divided doses or continuous infusion. **Vancomycin** 30 mg/kg/d in 2 divided doses.[i]

[a] In case of complete resistance (MIC >2 mg/L) use treatment as in enterococcal endocarditis (see Infective Endocarditis).

[b] Serum vancomycin concentrations should be 10-15 mg/L at the predose (trough) level and 30-45 mg/L 1 hour after completing IV infusion of the drug.

[c] 6 weeks in patients with prosthetic valve endocarditis.

[d] Preferred in patients aged >65 years or with impaired renal or VIII (vestibulocochlear) cranial nerve function.

[e] Or an equivalent dose of ampicillin.

[f] Preferred in outpatients.

[g] Only in patients with uncomplicated native valve endocarditis and normal renal function.

[h] Monitor renal function and serum levels of gentamicin closely. In patients receiving the drug once daily, trough levels should be <1 mg/L and the level 1 hour postdose should be ~10-12 mg/L.

[i] According to some experts up to 45-60 mg/kg/d in 2-3 divided doses to achieve serum drug levels 15-20 mg/L.

IM, intramuscular; IV, intravenous; MIC, minimal inhibitory concentration.

Figure 10-2. Infective endocarditis caused by oral streptococci or *Streptococcus gallolyticus* group: targeted antibiotic treatment. *Based on Eur Heart J. 2015;36(44):3075-3128.*

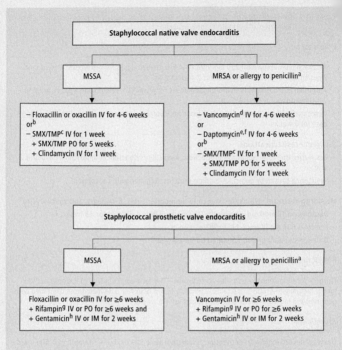

Staphylococcal native valve endocarditis

MSSA
− Floxacillin or oxacillin IV for 4-6 weeks
or[b]
− SMX/TMP[c] IV for 1 week
  + SMX/TMP PO for 5 weeks
  + Clindamycin IV for 1 week

MRSA or allergy to penicillin[a]
− Vancomycin[d] IV for 4-6 weeks
or
− Daptomycin[e,f] IV for 4-6 weeks
or[b]
− SMX/TMP[c] IV for 1 week
  + SMX/TMP PO for 5 weeks
  + Clindamycin IV for 1 week

Staphylococcal prosthetic valve endocarditis

MSSA
Floxacillin or oxacillin IV for ≥6 weeks
 + Rifampin[g] IV or PO for ≥6 weeks and
 + Gentamicin[h] IV or IM for 2 weeks

MRSA or allergy to penicillin[a]
Vancomycin IV for ≥6 weeks
 + Rifampin[g] IV or PO for ≥6 weeks
 + Gentamicin[h] IV or IM for 2 weeks

Dosage: Floxacillin or oxacillin 12 g/d in 4-6 divided doses. **Gentamicin** 3 mg/kg/d in 1-2 divided doses. **Rifampin** 900-1200 mg/d in 2-3 divided doses. **Vancomycin** 30-60 mg/kg/d in 2-3 divided doses. **SMX/TMP** 4800 mg/d + 960 mg/d in 4-6 doses (if IV). **Clindamycin** 1800 mg/d in 3 divided doses. **Daptomycin** 10 mg/kg once a day.

[a] In case of methicillin-susceptible staphylococci in patients with penicillin allergy and nonanaphylactic reactions use cephalosporins (cefazolin 6 g/d or cefotaxime 6 g/d IV in 3 divided doses).

[b] Alternative therapy for *S aureus* (this regimen may be considered [weak recommendation]).

[c] Renal function and SMX/TMP blood concentrations should be monitored once a week (twice a week in patients with renal failure).

[d] Trough serum levels of vancomycin should be ≥20 mg/L.

[e] Superior to vancomycin with vancomycin MIC >1 mg/L.

[f] Monitor creatine kinase levels once a week. Some experts recommend adding cloxacillin (12 g/d in 6 divided doses) or fosfomycin (8 g/d in 4 divided doses) to daptomycin.

[g] Rifampin increases hepatic metabolism of warfarin and other drugs. The agent is believed to be of particular importance in patients with prosthetic valve endocarditis, as it helps to eradicate bacteria on foreign material. Rifampin should be used in combination with another antistaphylococcal agent to minimize the risk of emergence of resistant strains. It is suggested to start rifampin 3-5 days later than gentamicin and vancomycin.

[h] Serum gentamicin levels and renal function should be monitored closely to prevent renal injury.

IM, intramuscular; IV, intravenous; MIC, minimum inhibitory concentration; MRSA, methicillin-resistant *Staphylococcus aureus*; MSSA, methicillin-susceptible *Staphylococcus aureus*; PO, oral; SMX/TMP, sulfamethoxazole/trimethoprim.

Figure 10-3. Infective endocarditis caused by staphylococci: targeted antibiotic treatment. *Based on Eur Heart J. 2015;36(44):3075-3128.*

Table 10-2. Antibiotic treatment for infective endocarditis caused by microorganisms other than streptococci and staphylococci

Enterococci

– Amoxicillin (or ampicillin) 200 mg/kg/d IV in 4-6 divided doses for 4-6 weeks[a] + gentamicin[b] 3 mg/kg/d IV or IM as single dose for 2-6 weeks; or

– Ampicillin 200 mg/kg/d IV in 4-6 divided doses for 6 weeks + ceftriaxone 4 g/d IV or IM in 2 divided doses for 6 weeks[c]; or

– Vancomycin 30 mg/kg/d in 2 divided doses for 6 weeks + gentamicin[b] 3 mg/kg IV as single dose for 6 weeks

β-Lactam–resistant strains

– Resistance due to β-lactamase production: Ampicillin/sulbactam or amoxicillin/clavulanic acid

– Resistance caused by penicillin-binding proteins: Regimen with vancomycin

Multidrug-resistant strains (resistance to aminoglycosides, β-lactams, and vancomycin)[d]

– Daptomycin 10 mg/kg/d + ampicillin 200 mg/kg/d IV in 4-6 doses for ≥8 weeks; or

– Linezolid 600 mg IV or po bid for ≥8 weeks; or

– Quinupristin/dalfopristin 7.5 mg/kg tid for ≥8 weeks

HACEK group

Third-generation cephalosporin (eg, ceftriaxone 2 g/d for 4 weeks in NVE or 6 weeks in PVE); non-β-lactamase–producing strains: ampicillin 12 g/d IV in 4 or 6 divided doses combined with gentamicin 3 mg/kg/d in 2 or 3 divided doses for 4-6 weeks

Brucella spp

Doxycycline 200 mg/d + trimethoprim/sulfamethoxazole 960 mg bid + rifampin 300-600 mg/d for ≥3-6 months po; in the first few weeks you may add streptomycin 15 mg/kg/d in 2 divided doses

Coxiella burnetii

Doxycycline 200 mg/d + hydroxychloroquine 200-600 mg/d PO (regimen preferred over doxycycline alone) for >18 months

Bartonella spp

Doxycycline 100 mg PO bid for 4 weeks + gentamicin 3 mg/kg/d IV for 2 weeks

Legionella spp

Levofloxacin 500 mg IV or PO bid for ≥6 weeks or clarithromycin 500 mg bid IV for 2 weeks, then PO for 4 weeks + rifampin 300-1200 mg for 6 weeks

Mycoplasma spp

Levofloxacin 500 mg IV or PO bid for ≥6 months

Tropheryma whipplei

Doxycycline 200 mg/d + hydroxychloroquine[d] 200-600 mg/d PO (regimen preferred over doxycycline alone) for ≥18 months a Six-week treatment is recommended in patients with symptoms persisting for >3 months and in those with a prosthetic valve.

b Monitor renal function and serum levels of gentamicin closely. The trough level should be <1 mg/L and level 1 hour after IV dose should be 10-12 mg/L.

c Regimen recommended in *Enterococcus faecalis* infection. It is the treatment of choice for aminoglycoside-resistant *E faecalis* species. Ineffective for *Enterococcus faecium*.

d Cooperation with an infectious disease specialist is essential.

Based on Eur Heart J. 2015;36(44):3075-3128.

bid, 2 times a day; HACEK, *Haemophilus* spp, *Aggregatibacter* spp, *Cardiobacterium hominis*, *Eikenella corrodens*, *Kingella* spp; IM, intramuscular; IV, intravenous; NVE, native valve endocarditis; PO, oral; PVE, prosthetic valve endocarditis; tid, 3 times a day.

generally continued if started previously for other indications in the absence of contraindications. In patients who may need to be qualified for urgent surgery or with international normalized ratio (INR) values showing wide variations, anticoagulation is often switched to unfractionated heparin (UFH). In cases of ischemic or hemorrhagic stroke, all anticoagulants and antiplatelet drugs should be stopped for a minimum of 2 weeks. The optimal length of time for discontinuation is unknown and based on limited evidence. In patients with a prosthetic heart valve and intracerebral hemorrhage, antithrombotic treatment (using UFH) should be resumed as soon as it is safe to do so. In the event of serious hemorrhagic complications, antithrombotic treatment should be stopped, and neurology and hematology service consultations are prudent.

Invasive Treatment

Need for and optimal timing of surgical treatment are among the most difficult therapeutic decisions in the treatment of IE. Surgical intervention may be prompted by hemodynamic instability despite antimicrobial therapy. Decisions regarding surgery should be made by an experienced clinical team with cardiac surgery service and infectious disease consultations and should consider individual risks and benefits.

Indications for emergency surgery (within the first 24 hours): Refractory pulmonary edema or cardiogenic shock caused by severe acute mitral or aortic regurgitation, obstruction, or fistula.🗹⬤

Indications for urgent surgery in active IE:

1) Symptoms of heart failure or echocardiographic signs of poor hemodynamic tolerance caused by severe regurgitation or obstruction of a native or prosthetic valve.

2) Locally uncontrolled infection with involvement of perivalvular structures (annular or aortic abscess, fistula, leaflet rupture, conduction disturbances).

3) Persistent infection despite appropriate antibiotic treatment: This is defined as persisting bacteremia and fever after 3 to 7 days of antibiotic treatment and exclusion of other causes of persistent positive blood cultures (according to the European Society of Cardiology) or persistent bacteremia or fever for 5 to 7 days in patients in whom other sites of infection have been excluded (according to the American Heart Association).

4) Infection with difficult-to-treat organisms (fungi or multidrug-resistant organisms).

5) PVE endocarditis caused by staphylococci or non-HACEK gram-negative bacteria.

6) Persistent aortic or mitral vegetations >10 mm after ≥1 embolic episode despite appropriate antibiotic treatment (particularly during the first 2 weeks of treatment).

7) Aortic or mitral NVE vegetations >10 mm, associated with severe valve stenosis or regurgitation, and low operative risk.

8) Aortic or mitral NVE and PVE with isolated large vegetations (>15 mm) and no other indications for surgery.

9) Aortic or mitral NVE and PVE with isolated very large vegetations (>30 mm).

Decision for surgery in patients with large vegetations (>15 mm) can be difficult and requires a careful individual approach.

Surgical treatment may also be considered after CNS embolism (including transient ischemic attack or asymptomatic embolism) as long as intracranial hemorrhage has been excluded, the patient is not in a comatose state, stroke has not caused very severe CNS damage, and no other contraindications to surgery are present. The risk of an embolic event is highest before the start of antimicrobial therapy and in the early days of treatment and decreases significantly after 2 weeks of therapy. Head CT or MRI should be conducted in every patient with neurologic complications. Indications for surgery in such patients include severe heart failure, uncontrolled sepsis, infection not responding to antimicrobial therapy, presence of an abscess, or persistence of a high embolic risk. Surgery using a cardiopulmonary bypass within the first 30 days of stroke is associated with a high risk of complications.

Treatment of CDRIE: Prolonged antimicrobial treatment (initially empiric treatment, optimally using an antistaphylococcal agent [vancomycin, given the high resistance rates], followed by targeted treatment based on susceptibility testing) and complete hardware removal is generally recommended.⊘○ A center capable of performing percutaneous removal of the implanted device including leads should be involved in such cases. In patients with vegetations >20 mm, surgical treatment should be considered. Given the risk of reinfection, indications for reimplantation of devices should be evaluated. If the patient is clinically stable, blood cultures should be negative for a minimum of 72 hours while antimicrobial therapy is continued. If the patient is dependent on the device, a temporary electrode should be implanted contralaterally. In case of evidence of remaining valvular infection, implantation should be delayed for 14 days.

Treatment of IE in IV drug abusers: Valve replacement is rarely recommended because substance dependence results in frequent recurrences of IE in this group of patients. Surgery may be considered in those with bacteremia persisting >7 days in spite of adequate antimicrobial treatment, fungal infections, right ventricular heart failure refractory to treatment, or those with persisting large (>20 mm) vegetations with recurrent pulmonary embolism.

Duration of therapy varies based on operative tissue cultures when surgery is pursued. In patients with negative operative tissue cultures, the first day of negative blood cultures on antimicrobial treatment is the first day of targeted therapy. In patients with positive valve tissue cultures, a new postoperative complete course of antimicrobial treatment using agents to which the isolated organisms are susceptible is recommended (with the operative day considered as day 0).

→ FOLLOW-UP

The patient should be carefully monitored for cardiac and extracardiac complications, especially for embolic events. In particular, the following parameters should be monitored: temperature (febrile or afebrile), white blood cell counts, and biochemical markers associated with any potential drug toxicities (eg, renal function). Repeat blood cultures after 48 to 72 hours should be collected to evaluate treatment response. Serial physical examinations should also be conducted to evaluate for endocarditis-related complications and sequelae. In patients undergoing antimicrobial treatment, the severity of valvular disease and any indications for surgery should be evaluated. After completing treatment, perform follow-up TTE for functional and morphologic evaluation.

Regular clinical follow-up is recommended following the completion of initial therapy.

→ COMPLICATIONS

→Clinical Features, above.

→ PREVENTION

1. General preventative measures, such as maintenance of general oral and skin hygiene, avoiding body piercings and tattoos, and minimizing unnecessary IV catheterization and invasive procedures, are important.

2. Indications for antimicrobial prophylaxis: Indications for prophylaxis of IE have been narrowed over time. Prophylaxis is currently indicated **only before dental procedures** involving gingival or periapical instrumentation or perforation of the oral mucosa (dental extraction, periodontal procedures, root canal treatment, scaling, dental implants)☺☻ and **only in the following specific circumstances**:

1) Prosthetic valve (including transcatheter valve replacement) or history of valve repair using prosthetic materials.

2) History of IE.

3) Congenital heart disease (cyanotic; up to 6 months after complete surgical or percutaneous repair of congenital heart disease using prosthetic materials; residual regurgitation or leak in the area of surgical or transcatheter implantation of prosthetic material).

4) Cardiac transplant patients with a structurally abnormal valve (as per the American Heart Association/American Society of Cardiology recommendations).

3. Recommended antimicrobial agents (a single dose 30-60 minutes before the procedure):

1) **Patients with no allergy to penicillin**: Oral or IV amoxicillin or ampicillin 2 g in adults or 50 mg/kg in children. Alternative agents are IV cefazolin or ceftriaxone 1 g in adults or 50 mg/kg in children.

2) **Patients with allergy to penicillin**: Oral or IV clindamycin 600 mg in adults or 20 mg/kg in children.

11. Ischemic Heart Disease

Ischemic heart disease (IHD) comprises all types of myocardial ischemia (ie, reduced blood supply or imbalance), regardless of the pathologic mechanism. **Coronary artery disease (CAD)** is IHD due to atherosclerosis of a coronary artery.

→ CLASSIFICATION

1. Classification of CAD:
1) Stable CAD:
   a) Stable angina pectoris.
   b) Vasospastic angina (Prinzmetal variant angina).
   c) Microvascular angina (syndrome X).
   d) Angina associated with myocardial bridging of coronary arteries.
2) Acute coronary syndromes (ACSs).

2. ACS classification based on initial electrocardiographic (ECG) findings:

1) Non–ST-segment elevation ACS.

2) ST-segment elevation ACS.

3. Classification of ACS based on clinical manifestations, biochemical markers of myocardial necrosis, and ECG:

1) Unstable angina (UA).

2) Non–ST-segment elevation myocardial infarction (NSTEMI).

3) ST-segment elevation myocardial infarction (STEMI).

4) Unspecified myocardial infarction (MI). ECG abnormalities that do not allow an unequivocal diagnosis of ST-segment elevation: left bundle branch block (acute or preexisting), pacemaker rhythm, or infarction diagnosed on the basis of clinical and biochemical criteria, with ECG performed >24 hours after the onset of symptoms.

5) Sudden cardiac death.

4. Classification of MI based on the evolution of ECG features:

1) Q-wave MI.

2) Non–Q-wave MI.

→ ETIOLOGY AND PATHOGENESIS

---

1. Etiology of IHD:

1) Most commonly IHD is due to coronary atherosclerosis.

2) Less commonly IHD is due to coronary artery spasm (Prinzmetal variant angina, illicit drug use [eg, cocaine], or discontinuation of nitrates), coronary artery embolism, vasculitis of the coronary arteries, metabolic disorders affecting the coronary arteries, anatomic defects of the coronary arteries, coronary artery injury, arterial thrombosis due to disorders of hemostasis, reduced oxygen supply in relation to demand (aortic stenosis or regurgitation, hypertrophic cardiomyopathy, carbon monoxide poisoning, decompensated thyrotoxicosis, long-standing hypotension [shock]), anemia, myocardial bridging), or aortic dissection.

3. Etiology of ACS: A sudden imbalance between the myocardial oxygen demand and supply, most frequently due to a sudden occlusion of a coronary artery by a thrombus formed on a ruptured atherosclerotic plaque.

1) **UA** most frequently results from rupture of an eccentric plaque. The resulting thrombus reduces coronary blood flow but occlusion is not complete.

2) **NSTEMI** is the result of a process similar to UA and is associated with elevation of troponin levels.

3) In **STEMI** the thrombus usually causes a complete and sudden occlusion of a coronary artery. Necrosis starts to develop within 15 to 30 minutes of the cessation of blood flow and spreads from the subendocardium to the epicardium. The rate at which necrosis develops depends on diameter of the occluded artery and collateral circulation.

4. Myocardial injury versus MI: Myocardial injury is defined as elevation of cardiac troponin values >99th percentile. In some situations myocardial injury is associated with MI (→Table 11-1).

11.1. Acute Coronary Syndromes

Acute coronary syndrome (ACS) is a clinical syndrome of acute chest pain related to acute myocardial ischemia. ACS is classified based on electrocardiography (ECG) results into ST-segment elevation ACS and non–ST-segment elevation ACS. This approach has important practical implications because patients presenting with ST-segment elevation ACS require immediate reperfusion therapy.

Table 11-1. Types of MI based on the fourth universal definition of MI

Criteria for types 1 and 2 MI[a]

Type 1	MI caused by atherothrombotic event precipitated by plaque erosion or plaque rupture with thrombus formation
Type 2	Ischemic myocardial injury, usually in the setting of coronary atherosclerosis, from oxygen supply-demand mismatch without plaque erosion or rupture (eg, sudden anemia, prolonged tachyarrhythmia, coronary artery spasm or dissection, shock)

Criteria for type 3 MI

Sudden cardiac death with new ischemic ECG changes or ventricular fibrillation with symptoms suggestive of myocardial ischemia; death occurs before blood biomarkers can be obtained or before increases in biomarkers are identified

Criteria for types 4 and 5 MI (procedure-related MI within 48 hours after index procedure)[b]

Type 4a	PCI-related MI
Type 4b	In-stent thrombosis documented angiographically or by the same criteria as type 1 MI
Type 4c	In-stent restenosis or restenosis after balloon angioplasty documented angiographically or by the same criteria as type 1 MI
Type 5	CABG-related MI

[a] Rise and fall of cardiac troponins with ≥1 troponin value >99th percentile of URL along with either new ischemic ECG changes, development of pathologic Q waves, symptoms of acute myocardial ischemia, imaging evidence of new wall motion abnormality or loss of viable myocardium, or angiographic identification of coronary thrombus

[b] Further specific criteria: Coronary procedure–related MI ≤48 hours after the index procedure with an elevation in cardiac troponin values >5 × >99th percentile of URL for type 4a MI, >10 × for type 5 MI in patients with normal values at baseline. Patients with elevated but stable or declining baseline values must meet the criterion of >5-fold or >10-fold increase as well as have a change ≥20% from the baseline value. Patients must also have one of the following: new ischemic changes (type 4a MI only), new pathologic Q waves, imaging evidence of loss of viable myocardium, or angiographic findings of a procedure-related flow-limiting complication.

Adapted from Circulation. 2018;138(20):e618-e651.

CABG, coronary artery bypass graft; ECG, electrocardiography; MI, myocardial infarction; PCI, percutaneous coronary intervention; URL, upper reference limit.

→ DEFINITION

Classification of ACS: →Chapter 3.11.

Definition of myocardial infarction: →Table 11-1.

1. Non–ST-segment elevation ACSs (unstable angina [UA]/non–ST--segment elevation myocardial infarction [NSTEMI]) are caused by acute myocardial ischemia that in some patients leads to myocardial necrosis manifested by elevated serum markers of myocardial necrosis without an acute ST-segment elevation seen on ECG. Patients with UA/NSTEMI constitute a heterogeneous group due to the complex pathogenesis, which includes atherosclerotic plaque rupture with superimposed thrombosis, progressive obstruction of a coronary artery, arterial constriction, inadequate oxygen supply relative to myocardial demand, or spontaneous coronary dissection.

2. ST-segment elevation myocardial infarction (STEMI) is a clinical syndrome usually caused by the cessation of blood flow through a coronary artery due to its occlusion, which results in transmural ischemia leading to ST-segment elevation and typically myocardial necrosis manifested by increased blood levels of specific biomarkers.

11.1.1. Non–ST-Segment Elevation Myocardial Infarction (NSTEMI) and Unstable Angina (UA)

➡ CLINICAL FEATURES AND NATURAL HISTORY

1. Symptoms: Chest pain or equivalent ischemic discomfort (features: →Chapter 3.11.2.2). Unlike in stable coronary artery disease (CAD), the pain is not relieved within 5 minutes of removing the precipitating factors or administering sublingual nitrate, but it lasts longer and may occur at rest.

2. Classification of pain in unstable angina (UA)/non–ST-segment elevation myocardial infarction (NSTEMI):

1) **Angina occurring at rest**, lasting >20 minutes.
2) **New-onset angina** within the prior month, Canadian Cardiovascular Society (CCS) class III (→Table 11-9).
3) **Angina with a crescendo pattern**: Angina that is becoming more frequent, is caused by less intense physical exertion than previously, lasts longer, has increased by at least one CCS class, and is at least CCS class III.

➡ DIAGNOSIS

Clinicians should assess the likelihood that signs and symptoms represent an acute coronary syndrome (ACS). This is an important step in the assessment of patients with a possible ACS, as it helps to avoid unnecessary invasive procedures in patients with a low likelihood of ACS. Patients with a history of obstructive CAD have a higher likelihood of presenting symptoms related to ACS.

The second step is to assess the risk of adverse events. Standardized risk scores are available, for instance, Global Registry of Acute Coronary Events (GRACE) score (→Table 11-2) or Thrombolysis in Myocardial Infarction (TIMI) NSTEMI score (available at www.timi.org).

Definition of myocardial infarction: →Table 11-1.

Diagnostic Tests

1. Resting electrocardiography (ECG): Abnormalities may be observed in ≥2 contiguous leads (groups of contiguous leads include: V_1-V_6, anterior leads; II, III, aVF, inferior leads; I, aVL, lateral/apical leads; V_3R, V_4R, supplemental leads covering the free wall of the right ventricle).

1) **ST-segment depression (less commonly, transient ST-segment elevation)**: Abnormalities of diagnostic value are new horizontal or downsloping ST-segment depressions ≥0.05 mV.
2) **T-wave inversion** (>0.1 mV; inversions ≥0.2 mV are associated with higher risk) or reversal of a prior T-wave inversion. T-wave flattening is relatively nonspecific.
3) ECG is normal in 30% to 50% of patients.

2. Blood tests: Patients may have elevated blood levels of markers of myocardial necrosis (the markers may also be elevated in UA, but in such cases they do not exceed the acute MI cutoff values):

1) **Cardiac-specific troponin T (cTnT)**, troponin I (cTnI), or high-sensitivity troponin I or T.
2) **Creatine kinase MB subunit (CK-MB) concentration** (CK-MB_{mass}) >510 µg/L (depending on the assay); this is used only when cardiac-specific troponin measurements are not available.

Table 11-2. Global Registry of Acute Coronary Events (GRACE) acute coronary syndrome risk model

Risk factor	Score
Age	The GRACE risk model calculator for the calculation of risk scores is available at www.gracescore.org (risk factors are scored separately at admission and at discharge)
Resting heart rate	
Systolic blood pressure	
Serum creatinine	
Congestive heart failure, Killip class	
Cardiac arrest at admission	
ST-segment deviation	
Elevated enzymes/markers of myocardial ischemia	
Inhospital PCI[a]	
Inhospital CABG[a]	
Past history of MI[a]	

Probability of death in hospital according to the score on admission		
Score	Risk (%)	Risk group
≤108	<1%	Low
109-140	1%-3%	Intermediate
>140	>3%	High

Probability of death within 6 months according to the score at discharge		
≤88	<3%	Low
89-118	3%-8%	Intermediate
>118	>8%	High

[a] Risk factor assessed at discharge only.

CABG, coronary artery bypass graft; MI, myocardial infarction; PCI, percutaneous coronary intervention.

CK-MB activity and myoglobin concentrations are no longer used in the diagnostic workup of MI.

3. Chest radiographs may reveal signs of other diseases that may have caused angina or features of heart failure.

4. Resting echocardiography may reveal regional wall motion abnormalities or other etiologies of chest pain, such as valvular heart disease, including aortic stenosis or hypertrophic cardiomyopathy.

5. Coronary angiography reveals lesions located in the coronary arteries that are responsible for UA/NSTEMI or STEMI (usually arterial occlusion) and determine the optimal form of revascularization. Routine coronary angiography has been shown to be beneficial in moderate- to high-risk patients and should be performed.

Differential Diagnosis

In patients presenting with acute chest pain, differential diagnosis includes but is not limited to aortic dissection, pulmonary embolism, myopericarditis, and musculoskeletal chest pain.

Other Diagnostic Considerations

The term "myocardial infarction" does not include the death of cardiomyocytes due to mechanical injury (eg, in the course of coronary artery bypass graft [CABG]), renal failure, heart failure, cardioversion, ablation, sepsis, myocarditis, cardiac toxins, or malignancy.

Criteria for the diagnosis of periprocedural MI:

1) **Percutaneous coronary intervention (PCI)-related MI**: Elevation in troponin values (>5×99th percentile of the upper reference limit [URL]) in patients with normal baseline values (≤99th percentile of URL) or a rise in troponin values >20% (if the baseline values are elevated and are stable or falling) plus signs of myocardial ischemia or evidence of ischemia found on ECG, angiography, or imaging.

2) **MI associated with CABG**: Elevation in troponin values (>10×99th percentile of URL) in patients with normal baseline troponin values (≤99th percentile of URL), plus new pathologic Q waves or new left bundle branch block, an angiographically documented new graft or a new native coronary artery occlusion, or imaging evidence of a new loss of viable myocardium.

⟶ T R E A T M E N T

General Considerations

Treatment of high-risk patients in an intensive cardiac care or coronary care unit or equivalent; high-risk patients can be transferred to a nonintensive care ward after 24 hours of being free of the symptoms of myocardial ischemia, significant arrhythmias, and hemodynamic instability.

1. Monitoring: Continuous ECG monitoring for 24 hours after admission and further monitoring depending on clinical status and ongoing ischemia.

2. Assess the risk of death or MI using **risk scores**, for instance, **GRACE** (→Table 11-2) or **TIMI** (visit www.timi.org). Treatment is tailored to the patient's risk of adverse events (→Figure 11-1):

1) **High-risk patients** (GRACE score >140, a defined increase in troponin levels, or dynamic ST-segment or T-wave changes) and **intermediate-risk patients** (recurrent symptoms or additional high-risk factors) without contraindications for invasive procedures benefit from a routine coronary angiography, which is recommended.◯● High-risk patients (GRACE score >140) should have an early invasive approach (ie, within 24 hours if possible).◯● Patients with refractory or recurrent angina accompanied by ST-segment depression (≥2 mm) or deep T waves, heart failure, hemodynamic instability (shock), or life-threatening arrhythmias (ventricular fibrillation or ventricular tachycardia) should undergo an early invasive approach as well.

2) **Low-risk patients** are those with no recurrent chest pain, without symptoms of heart failure, without abnormal ECG findings, and with normal cardiac troponin (or any other appropriate marker of myocardial necrosis) levels. The determination should be made whether these symptoms are related to ACS or a noncardiac cause. Low-risk patients may have a noninvasive assessment, and if it is normal or low risk, they may be treated medically. Low-risk patients with the classical description of low-threshold angina should undergo an invasive assessment.

3. Oxygen should be administered to each patient with hypoxia (arterial saturation <90%). Monitor saturation using pulse oximetry and assess blood gases in patients with abnormal results. The use of oxygen in patients without hypoxia may be detrimental.◯

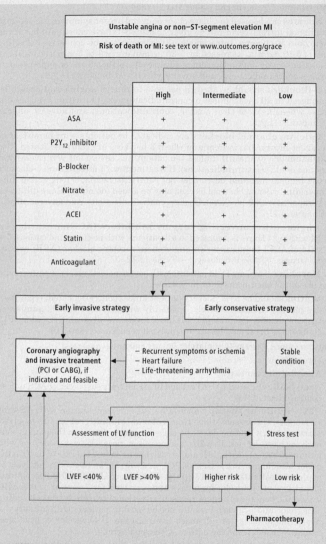

	High	Intermediate	Low
ASA	+	+	+
P2Y$_{12}$ inhibitor	+	+	+
β-Blocker	+	+	+
Nitrate	+	+	+
ACEI	+	+	+
Statin	+	+	+
Anticoagulant	+	+	±

Unstable angina or non–ST-segment elevation MI

Risk of death or MI: see text or www.outcomes.org/grace

Early invasive strategy

Early conservative strategy

Coronary angiography and invasive treatment (PCI or CABG), if indicated and feasible

– Recurrent symptoms or ischemia
– Heart failure
– Life-threatening arrhythmia

Stable condition

Assessment of LV function

Stress test

LVEF <40%

LVEF >40%

Higher risk

Low risk

Pharmacotherapy

ACEI, angiotensin-converting enzyme inhibitor; ASA, acetylsalicylic acid; CABG, coronary artery bypass graft; LV, left ventricle; LVEF, left ventricular ejection fraction; MI, myocardial infarction; PCI, percutaneous coronary intervention.

Figure 11-1. Management algorithm of unstable angina or non–ST-segment elevation myocardial infarction.

Anti-Ischemic Treatment and Plaque Stabilization

1. Nitrates can be used to relieve chest pain and are for symptomatic use only. Sublingual nitroglycerin can be given to acutely relieve chest pain but if the chest pain is ongoing, intravenous nitroglycerin can be considered (loading dose of 5-10 µg/min, increased by 5-20 µg/min every 3 to 5 minutes until the resolution of pain or development of adverse effects [headache or hypotension]). Dosage, contraindications, and adverse effects: →Chapter 3.11.2.2.

2. β-Blockers should be used in patients to relieve angina and should be considered in all cases unless a contraindication exists (resting bradycardia, active wheezing).◉● Oral dosage, contraindications, and adverse effects: →Chapter 3.11.2.2.

3. Calcium channel blockers are indicated in patients with persistent or recurrent myocardial ischemia in whom β-blockers are contraindicated. Use **diltiazem** or **verapamil** (unless the patient has severe left ventricular dysfunction or other contraindications). If treatment with nitrates and β-blockers at the highest tolerated doses does not control ischemia, a long-acting dihydropyridine calcium channel blocker may be added (do not combine diltiazem or verapamil with β-blockers). Dosage, contraindications, and adverse effects: →Chapter 3.11.2.2.

4. Angiotensin-converting enzyme inhibitors (ACEIs): Starting an ACEI within 24 hours is indicated in all patients with no contraindications.◉● In case of ACEI intolerance, an angiotensin receptor blocker (ARB) may be used. Drugs: →Table 9-5; dosage: →Table 11-12.

5. Morphine: 3 to 5 mg IV in patients with severe persistent chest pain despite the use of the treatments described above.

6. Statins should be used in every patient unless contraindicated, regardless of the plasma cholesterol levels, optimally within 1 to 4 days of admission. Target low-density lipoprotein cholesterol levels are <1.8 mmol/L (70 mg/dL). High-dose statins should be used to prevent recurrent events.◉●

Antithrombotic Therapy (Antiplatelet Agents and Anticoagulants)

Agents and dosage: →Table 11-3.

1. Antiplatelet therapy:

1) **Acetylsalicylic acid (ASA)** is used in all patients suspected of ACS unless contraindicated.◉●

2) **$P2Y_{12}$ inhibitor therapy** should be used in combination with ASA for 12 months. On presentation, **ticagrelor** or **clopidogrel** should be given, starting with a loading dose; the decision may be based on the patient's underlying bleeding risk. In a direct comparison, ticagrelor was associated with a reduced rate of death, MI, and stroke but an increased rate of non-CABG major bleeding.◕ At the time of PCI, **prasugrel** can be used in addition to aspirin in patients without an increased risk of bleeding.◉● Discontinue clopidogrel or ticagrelor for 5 days and prasugrel for 7 days prior to CABG unless the benefits of urgent revascularization outweigh the risks bleeding. Ticagrelor and prasugrel should not be used in patients with a history of hemorrhagic stroke or advanced liver disease. If ticagrelor or prasugrel cannot be used, treat the patient with clopidogrel.

2. Anticoagulant therapy should be used in every patient with a documented ACS. Options for anticoagulant therapy include **fondaparinux** (2.5 mg subcutaneously daily),◉● **enoxaparin** (1 mg/kg subcutaneously bid),◉● or intravenous **unfractionated heparin (UFH)**.◉◕ In a direct comparison, fondaparinux was associated with a reduced major bleeding risk compared to enoxaparin.◕ Anticoagulant therapy is usually discontinued after PCI unless there are additional indications, such as increased risk of thromboembolism. In patients receiving conservative treatment, anticoagulant therapy may be continued until discharge or to a maximum of 8 days, whichever comes first.

Table 11-3. Dosage of anticoagulants in patients with non–ST-segment elevation acute coronary syndrome

Agent	Dosage
Oral antiplatelet agents	
ASA	Loading dose (only in patients not receiving prior ASA) 150-300 mg (preferably chewing an uncoated tablet), then lifelong treatment 75-100 mg/d
Clopidogrel	Loading dose 600 mg, followed by 75 mg/d or 150 mg/d (after PCI for 7 days), followed by 75 mg/d
Prasugrel	Loading dose 60 mg followed by 10 mg once daily
Ticagrelor	Loading dose 180 mg followed by 90 mg bid
Anticoagulants[a]	
Fondaparinux	2.5 mg SC every 24 h
Enoxaparin	1 mg/kg SC every 12 h[b]
Dalteparin	120 IU/kg SC every 12 h
Nadroparin	86 IU/kg SC every 12 h
Unfractionated heparin	60-70 IU/kg (up to 5000 IU) in IV injection, followed by 12 IU/kg/h (up to 1000 IU/h) as infusion; maintain aPTT 1.5-2.5 × ULN
Bivalirudin	In urgent invasive strategy 0.75 mg/kg IV injection followed by 1.75 mg/kg/h IV infusion; in other cases, 0.1 mg/kg IV injection and 0.25 mg/kg/h IV infusion until PCI; administer additional 0.5 mg/kg injection and increase infusion rate to 1.75 mg/kg/h prior to PCI
GP IIb/IIIa receptor antagonists (used in some high-risk patients at the discretion of the invasive cardiologist)[c]	
Abciximab	0.25 mg/kg IV injection followed by 0.125 µg/kg/min (up to 10 µg/min) IV infusion for 12 h
Eptifibatide	180 µg/kg IV injection repeated after 10 min and followed by 2 µg/kg/min IV infusion for 18 h
Tirofiban	25 µg/kg IV injection over 3 min followed by 0.15 µg/kg/min infusion for 18 h

[a] In patients with renal failure, use unfractionated heparin.

[b] Patients with renal failure require dose adjustment.

[c] Consider dose reduction in elderly patients and patients with moderate renal insufficiency.

aPTT, activated partial thromboplastin; ASA, acetylsalicylic acid; bid, two times a day; IV, intravenous; PCI, percutaneous coronary intervention; SC, subcutaneous; ULN, upper limit of normal.

Management After The Acute Phase

In patients with **ongoing angina after medical treatment**, perform coronary angiography with no prior noninvasive studies.

→ FOLLOW-UP

Long-term follow-up as in patients with stable angina (→Chapter 3.11.2.2).

Table 11-4. Long-term postdischarge pharmacotherapy as secondary prevention in patients with acute coronary syndrome

Agent and dosage	Indications
ASA 70-100 mg/d	Lifelong in all patients unless contraindicated
Clopidogrel 75 mg once daily	– Lifelong in patients with ASA contraindications or intolerance – Combined with ASA for 12 months after ACS
or Ticagrelor 90 mg bid	– Combined with ASA for 12 months after ACS
or Prasugrel 10 mg once daily	– Combined with ASA for 12 months after ACS
β-Blocker	– All patients after UA/NSTEMI with LV dysfunction unless contraindicated – All patients after STEMI unless contraindicated
ACEI	– Patients after UA/NSTEMI with heart failure, LV dysfunction (LVEF <40%), hypertension, diabetes mellitus, or chronic kidney disease. Consider in all other patients as prevention of further ischemic events – All patients after STEMI
Statin	All patients (unless contraindicated) regardless of baseline cholesterol levels. Target LDL-C <1.8 mmol/L (70 mg/dL)
ARB	All patients who do not tolerate ACEI, and particularly those with heart failure and LV dysfunction (LVEF <40%)
Aldosterone antagonist	Patients after MI treated with β-blockers and ACEI with LVEF <40% and with diabetes mellitus or heart failure but without significant renal dysfunction or hyperkalemia

Based on Eur Heart J. 2016;37(3):267-315 and Eur Heart J. 2018;39(2):119-177.

ACEI, angiotensin-converting enzyme inhibitor; ACS, acute coronary syndrome; ARB, angiotensin-receptor blocker; ASA, acetylsalicylic acid; bid, 2 times a day; LDL-C, low-density lipoprotein cholesterol; LV, left ventricle; LVEF, left ventricular ejection fraction; MI, myocardial infarction; NSTEMI, non–ST-segment elevation myocardial infarction; STEMI, ST-segment elevation myocardial infarction; UA, unstable angina.

→ **SECONDARY PREVENTION**

1. Control of risk factors of atherosclerosis (→Chapter 3.15).

2. Cardiac rehabilitation.

3. Pharmacotherapy (specific indications, including antiplatelet agents [ASA and/or clopidogrel or prasugrel or ticagrelor], β-blockers, ACEIs [or ARBs], aldosterone antagonists, statins: →Table 11-4).

4. Anticoagulant treatment is recommended after coronary stenting in patients with atrial fibrillation and a moderate to high risk of thromboembolic complications. Treatment with a direct oral anticoagulant (DOAC) is preferred according to the 2018 CCS antiplatelet guidelines. Dual therapy with clopidogrel + DOAC without acetylsalicylic acid (ASA) for 1 year has been shown to be associated with reduced bleeding compared with triple therapy and should generally be considered.⊘◓

11.1.2. ST-Segment Elevation Myocardial Infarction (STEMI)

→ CLINICAL FEATURES AND NATURAL HISTORY

ST-segment elevation myocardial infarction (STEMI) most often occurs in the early morning hours (→Table 11-1). Some patients die before reaching hospital, mainly due to ventricular fibrillation (VF). In ~10% of cases symptoms are minor and the diagnosis is established only after a few days, weeks, or even months, on the basis of electrocardiography (ECG) and imaging studies.

1. Symptoms: Chest pain, epigastric pain, nausea, vomiting, dyspnea, syncope, or palpitations.

2. Signs:

1) Skin pallor and sweating are usually associated with severe pain. Peripheral cyanosis is present in patients developing cardiogenic shock.

2) Tachycardia (most frequently >100 beats/min; heart rates decrease with relief of pain), arrhythmia (most frequently premature ventricular complexes), bradycardia (in 10% of patients, frequent in inferior wall myocardial infarction [MI]).

3) Abnormal heart sounds: Gallop sounds, frequently a transient systolic murmur caused by a dysfunctional ischemic papillary muscle (more frequently in inferior wall MI) or left ventricular (LV) dilatation. A sudden-onset, loud apical systolic murmur accompanied by a thrill, most frequently caused by papillary muscle rupture (usually accompanied by symptoms of shock); a similar murmur, although most prominent along the left sternal border, occurs in ventricular septal rupture. Pericardial friction rub in large MI (usually on day 2 or 3).

4) Rales are audible over the lungs in patients with LV failure.

5) Symptoms of right ventricular failure, including hypotension and jugular venous distention, in right ventricular MI (it may accompany inferior wall MI).

→ DIAGNOSIS

Diagnostic Tests

1. ECG:

1) **Diagnostic ECG criteria for STEMI**: A persistent ST-segment elevation at the J point in 2 contiguous leads with the following cutoff points:

   a) >0.1 mV in all leads other than leads V_2 to V_3.

   b) For leads V_2 to V_3, the following cutoff points apply: ≥ 0.2 mV in men aged ≥ 40 years, ≥ 0.25 mV in men aged <40 years, or ≥ 0.15 mV in women.

2) **New-onset left bundle branch block (LBBB)** on its own is no longer considered specific for STEMI. Acute MI is suggested in patients with LBBB and an ST-segment elevation ≥ 1 mm that is in the same direction (concordant) as the QRS complex in any lead or an ST-segment depression of ≥ 1 mm in any lead from V_1 to V_3, or an ST-segment elevation ≥ 5 mm that is discordant with the QRS complex; MI may be also suspected if there is a QS complex in leads V_1 to V_4 and a Q wave in leads V_5 and V_6.

3) Typical **evolution of ECG changes** lasts several hours to several days. The initial appearance of tall peaked T waves is followed by a convex or horizontal ST-segment elevation. Then pathologic Q waves with reduced R waves appear (Q waves may be absent in patients with a small MI or those undergoing reperfusion therapy), the ST segment returns to the isoelectric line, and the amplitudes of R waves decrease further. Q waves become deeper, and inverse T waves appear. The probable location of MI based on ECG changes: →Table 11-5.

Table 11-5. Probable location of myocardial infarction based on ECG findings

ECG leads	Location of MI
V_1-V_4	LV anterior wall, ventricular septum, apex
I, aVL, V_5-V_6	LV lateral wall, apex
II, III, aVF	LV inferior wall
V_1-V_3 (tall R waves), V_7-V_9 (ST-segment elevation ≥0.05 mV[a] and Q waves)	LV posterior wall
V_{r4}-V_{r6} (ST-segment elevation ≥0.05 mV)[b]	Right ventricle

[a] ≥0.1 mV in male patients aged <40 years.

[b] ≥0.1 mV in male patients aged <30 years.

In 50%-70% of cases of inferior wall ST-segment elevation myocardial infarction, so-called mirror ST-segment depressions are found in the anterior or lateral leads; this is also true for 40%-60% of anterior wall MIs with mirror elevation in the inferior leads. This finding is associated with more extensive infarction and a worse prognosis. ST-segment depression in anterior leads may also represent posterior MI.

ECG, electrocardiography; LV, left ventricle; MI, myocardial infarction.

2. Blood tests should not be used for the acute diagnosis of STEMI because this would delay acute reperfusion. In acute MI elevated blood levels of markers of myocardial necrosis can be seen:

1) **Cardiac-specific troponin T (cTnT) levels** 10 to 14 ng/L (depending on assay), **cardiac-specific troponin I (cTnI) levels** 9 to 70 ng/L (depending on assay).

2) **Creatine kinase MB (CK-MB) concentration (CK-MBmass)** >5 to 10 µg/L (depending on assay); this is used only when cTn measurements are not available.

3) CK-MB activity and myoglobin concentrations are no longer used in the diagnostic workup of MI.

3. Chest radiographs may reveal signs of other diseases that may have caused angina, or features of heart failure.

4. Resting echocardiography may reveal regional wall-motion abnormalities or other etiologies of chest pain, such as valvular heart disease including aortic stenosis or hypertrophic cardiomyopathy.

5. Rapid coronary angiography reveals lesions located in the coronary arteries that are responsible for STEMI (usually arterial occlusion) and allows reperfusion (percutaneous coronary intervention [PCI]).🗹🔴

Differential Diagnosis

In patients presenting with acute chest pain, the differential diagnosis includes—but is not limited to—aortic dissection, pulmonary embolism, myopericarditis, or musculoskeletal chest pain (→Chapter 1.1). The presence of certain characteristics markedly increases the probability of ACS as opposed to other causes: features similar to current symptoms documented before as related to CAD; known history of MI; transient hypotension, diaphoresis, pulmonary congestion, or mitral regurgitation murmur; presumably new dynamic changes of ST-segment deviation (≥1 mm) or T-wave inversion in multiple precordial leads; elevated cardiac markers.

The probability is intermediate with a new type of chest pain (not documented before as CAD-related) and presence of only nonspecific ECG changes (ST-segment depression <0.5-1 mm, T-wave inversion >1 mm, or nonspecific fixed Q waves)

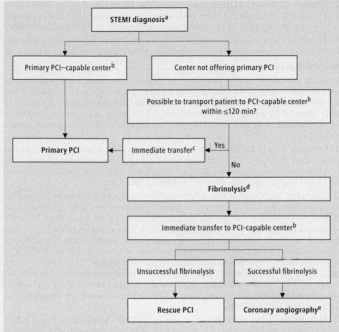

^a Based on symptoms and ECG, ideally within 10 minutes.
^b A PCI laboratory open 24 hours a day, 7 days a week. PCI should ideally be performed within
≤60 minutes.
^c PCI should ideally be performed within ≤90 minutes (≤60 minutes in patients presenting within
120 minutes of symptom onset).
^d Ideally ≤10 minutes.
^e Within 2-24 hours.

Note: Time frames for interventions are from the first medical contact.
ECG, electrocardiography; PCI, percutaneous coronary intervention; STEMI, ST-segment elevation
myocardial infarction.

Figure 11-2. Management algorithm for patients with acute myocardial infarction with ST-segment
elevation presenting within 24 hours of the first medical contact. *Based on Eur Heart J. 2018;39(2):119-
-177 and Eur Heart J. 2019;40(2):87-165.*

but increased particularly in older patients with a history of diabetes mellitus
and vascular disease in other areas. In the absence of above features (specifically
no elevation in cardiac markers and no relevant ECG changes) the probability of
CAD is low, especially if the chest pain may be reproduced by palpation.

→ **TREATMENT**

Management algorithm: →Figure 11-2.

Prehospital Management

1. Acetylsalicylic acid (ASA) 160 mg to chew should be administered by
emergency personnel to every patient with suspected MI, unless there are
contraindications or the patient has previously taken ASA on their own.

2. Prehospital ECG: If the prehospital ECG confirms the diagnosis of STEMI, when possible and practical these patients should be brought to a center capable of primary PCI as long as the time from contact to PCI is <120 minutes.⊘●

3. In areas where timely primary PCI is not available, **prehospital fibrinolysis** should be considered if possible within the existing systems of care.⊘●

Hospital Management

Patients should be treated at a coronary care unit or an equivalent monitored unit for ≥24 hours. Then patients may be moved to a step-down monitored bed for subsequent 24 to 48 hours. Patients may be transferred to a regular ward only after 12 to 24 hours of clinical stability, that is, no signs or symptoms of myocardial ischemia, heart failure, or arrhythmias with hemodynamic consequences.

1. Oxygen should be administered to every patient with hypoxia (arterial saturation [SpO_2] <90%) and monitored using pulse oximetry. Routine administration of supplemental oxygen for patients with SpO_2 possibly as low as ≥90% and certainly >94% should be avoided.⊘○

2. Nitrates: Sublingual nitroglycerin (0.4 mg every 5 minutes as long as the pain persists and as long as no significant adverse effects develop, up to a total of 3 doses), subsequently continued via an IV route (dosage: Non–ST--Segment Elevation Myocardial Infarction) in patients with persistent symptoms of myocardial ischemia (particularly pain), heart failure, significantly elevated blood pressures (do not use routinely in the early phase of STEMI). Contraindications to the use of nitrates in patients with STEMI: systolic blood pressure (SBP) <90 mm Hg, tachycardia >100 beats/min (in patients without heart failure), suspected right ventricular MI, administration of a phosphodiesterase inhibitor within the prior 24 hours (for sildenafil or vardenafil) or 48 hours (for tadalafil).⊗○

3. Morphine is the analgesic of choice in STEMI. Administer 4 to 8 mg IV with subsequent injections of 2 mg every 5 to 15 minutes until the resolution of pain (in some patients the total dose required to control the pain is as high as 2 mg/kg and is well tolerated). Adverse effects include nausea and vomiting, hypotension with bradycardia, and respiratory depression. There is recent evidence that morphine may reduce absorption and effects of oral $P2Y_{12}$ inhibitors.

4. Antiplatelet agents: ASA, administered immediately with the first medical contact, whether in the field with the emergency medical service or in the emergency department, and $P2Y_{12}$ inhibitors should be used:

1) Prasugrel or ticagrelor (rather than clopidogrel) in patients undergoing primary PCI;⊘● for ticagrelor, use a loading dose of 180 mg and then 90 mg bid, and for prasugrel, use a loading dose of 60 mg and then 10 mg daily. Prasugrel should not be used in patients with a history of stroke or transient ischemic attack (TIA).❷●

2) Clopidogrel in patients undergoing primary PCI (if prasugrel and ticagrelor are not available) or if at higher bleeding risk. In patients treated with fibrinolysis, for clopidogrel use a loading dose of 300 mg in patients aged ≤75 years and 75 mg for those aged >75 years.⊘●

3) Ticagrelor may be administered in patients who have received fibrinolysis,⊘○ with the understanding that this was a strategy tested in patients <75 years of age within 24 hours of the beginning of symptoms and an approximate median time from fibrinolysis of 8 to 10 hours.

5. β-Blockers should be used in patients without contraindications, such as bradycardia, Killip class II or greater heart failure, or active bronchospasm.⊘● In patients in whom β-blockers are contraindicated and in whom suppression of heart rate is necessary because of atrial fibrillation (AF), atrial flutter, or persistent myocardial ischemia, a calcium channel blocker (diltiazem and verapamil) may be used unless LV systolic dysfunction or atrioventricular (AV) block is present (calcium channel blockers should not be used routinely in patients with STEMI). Patients with baseline contraindications to β-blockers should be monitored for possible resolution of the contraindications in the course of hospital treatment, as this may allow the start of long-term β-blocker treatment. Dosage of oral agents, contraindications, and adverse effects: →Chapter 3.11.2.2.

6. Anticoagulants: The choice and dosage depend on the treatment method of STEMI: PCI, coronary artery bypass graft (CABG), fibrinolysis, or no reperfusion treatment (→below).

7. Angiotensin-converting enzyme inhibitors (ACEIs): Start as early as day 1 of MI unless contraindicated, particularly in patients with left ventricular ejection fraction (LVEF) ≤40% or symptoms of heart failure in the early phase of STEMI.◐◉ Start with low doses and then titrate up, depending on tolerance. In the case of ACEI intolerance (cough), switch to an angiotensin--receptor blocker (ARB). Dosage: →Table 11-12.

8. Statins are used in every patient regardless of plasma cholesterol levels, unless contraindicated, preferably within 1 to 4 days of admission. The target low-density lipoprotein cholesterol (LDL-C) levels are <1.8 mmol/L (70 mg/dL).

Invasive Reperfusion Therapy

1. Primary PCI is indicated if the time from the first medical contact to PCI is <120 minutes;◐◉ otherwise administer fibrinolysis unless contraindicated.◐◉ Primary PCI is indicated in the case of:

1) All patients with an indication for reperfusion therapy: chest pain or discomfort lasting <12 hours and persistent ST-segment elevation.
2) Patients with shock or contraindications to thrombolytic therapy (→below), regardless of the time since the onset of MI.
3) Evidence of ongoing myocardial ischemia even if symptoms of MI appeared >12 hours earlier or if the pain and ECG changes have been stuttering.◐◉

2. Rescue PCI is indicated after failed fibrinolysis, that is, when clinical symptoms and ST-segment elevations have not resolved (<50% reduction in the ST-segment elevation) within 60 to 90 minutes of the initiation of fibrinolysis; PCI should be considered as soon as possible.

3. A pharmacoinvasive approach should be used in patients without contraindications, with coronary angiography and/or PCI performed within 3 to 24 hours of successful fibrinolysis.◐◉

4. Indications for CABG:

1) Coronary anatomy best treated with CABG and Thrombolysis in Myocardial Infarction (TIMI)-3 flow of the infarct vessel.
2) Cardiogenic shock in a patient with left main or multivessel CAD.
3) Mechanical complications of MI.

5. Anticoagulant therapy in patients treated with primary PCI: There are alternatives and, at the discretion of the person performing the procedure, the choice and combination of which to use depends on the perceived bleeding risk as compared with the thrombotic risk and concomitant use of glycoprotein IIb/IIIa receptor antagonists.◐◉

1) Unfractionated heparin (UFH) in an IV injection at a standard dose of 70 to 100 IU/kg (or 50-60 IU/kg in patients treated with glycoprotein IIb/IIIa receptor antagonists).
2) Bivalirudin in an IV injection 0.75 mg/kg, followed by an IV infusion 1.75 mg/kg/h (regardless of the activated clotting time [ACT]) for the duration of the procedure.
3) Enoxaparin in an IV injection 0.5 mg/kg. Do not use fondaparinux during primary PCI.

Table 11-6. Fibrinolysis in patients with STEMI

Fibrinolytic agent	Dosage	Anticoagulant therapy[a]
tPA	IV bolus 15 mg, then 0.75 mg/kg over 30 min, then 0.5 mg/kg over 60 min (up to a total of ≤100 mg)	**UFH:** 60 IU/kg in IV bolus (up to 4000 IU), then 12 IU/kg/h in IV infusion (up to 1000 IU/h) for 24-48 hours. Target aPTT, 50-70 s; check aPTT after 3, 6, 12, and 24 h **Enoxaparin:** – Patients <75 years: 30 mg IV bolus, then after 15 min 1 mg/kg SC every 12 h. The 2 initial SC doses should be ≤100 mg – Patients >75 years: No IV bolus; start with 0.75 mg/kg SC every 12 h. The 2 initial SC doses should be ≤75 mg – Patients with creatinine clearance <30 mL/min, regardless of age: SC injections every 24 h **Fondaparinux:** 2.5 mg IV, then 2.5 mg SC every 24 h
TNK tPA	Single IV injection at a dose based on body weight: <60 kg: 30 mg 60-70 kg: 35 mg 70-80 kg: 40 mg 80-90 kg: 45 mg >90 kg: 50 mg	
SK	1.5 million IU in 100 mL of 5% glucose (dextrose) or 0.9% saline, IV infusion over 30-60 min	**Fondaparinux:** 2.5 mg SC, then 2.5 mg/d SC every 24 h

[a] Administer until discharge but no longer than for 8 days. In patients with severe renal failure (creatinine clearance <20 mL/min), use unfractionated heparin rather than other anticoagulants.

aPTT, activated partial thromboplastin time; IV, intravenous; SC, subcutaneous; SK, streptokinase; STEMI, ST-segment elevation myocardial infarction; TNK tPA, tenecteplase; tPA, alteplase; UFH, unfractionated heparin.

Fibrinolysis

1. Indications: Patients in whom primary PCI cannot be performed within the recommended timeframe (time from the first medical contact to PCI >120 minutes).

2. Contraindications: Absolute contraindications to fibrinolysis: history of intracranial hemorrhage or stroke of unknown origin; ischemic stroke in the last 6 months; central nervous system injury or cancer (primary or metastatic); recent major trauma, surgery, or head injury in the last 3 weeks; prior gastrointestinal bleeding in the last month; known bleeding disorder; aortic dissection; noncompressible punctures in the past 24 hours (eg, liver biopsy, lumbar puncture). Relative contraindications: transient ischemic attack in the last 6 months; oral anticoagulant therapy; pregnancy; first week postpartum; traumatic cardiopulmonary resuscitation; treatment-refractory hypertension (SBP >180 mm Hg and/or diastolic blood pressure >110 mm Hg); advanced liver disease; infective endocarditis; active peptic ulcer.

3. Fibrinolytic agents and concomitant anticoagulants: →Table 11-6. Fibrinolytic agents should be started within 30 minutes of the arrival of emergency medical services or of the moment the patient arrived at the hospital. Fibrin-specific agents (alteplase, tenecteplase) are preferred; never administer streptokinase to a patient who has been previously treated with streptokinase or anistreplase due to its immunogenic properties and risk of reactions including anaphylaxis.

Patients who receive fibrin-specific agents should be treated with fondaparinux, ●● concomitant UFH, or low-molecular-weight heparin (LMWH).●● Patients receiving streptokinase should not receive UFH●● and should be treated with fondaparinux. Fondaparinux is associated with reduced bleeding compared to enoxaparin. Every patient should also receive antiplatelet therapy: ASA and clopidogrel (→above).

4. Complications of fibrinolysis most frequently include bleeding; in the case of streptokinase, allergic reactions may also develop. If you suspect intracranial bleeding, discontinue all fibrinolytic, anticoagulant, and antiplatelet agents immediately. Then perform imaging studies (eg, computed tomography [CT] or magnetic resonance imaging [MRI] of the head) and laboratory tests (hematocrit, hemoglobin, prothrombin time [PT], activated partial thromboplastin time [aPTT], platelet count, fibrinogen and D-dimer levels; repeat these studies as needed) and request an urgent neurosurgical consultation. Give 2 units of fresh frozen plasma every 6 hours for 24 hours plus platelet concentrate when necessary, as well as protamine in patients who have received UFH (dosage: →Chapter 3.1.1.3).

5. Indications for coronary angiography in patients receiving fibrinolytic treatment:

1) Lack of reperfusion (<50% resolution of ST-segment elevation at 60-90 minutes), then emergency rescue PCI.◐◕

2) Within 3 to 24 hours of the beginning of successful fibrinolysis (as evidenced by ST-segment resolution by >50% at 60-90 minutes, typical reperfusion arrhythmia, or disappearance of chest pain) in high-risk patients (anterior MI or high-risk inferior MI).◐◕

3) In patients with low-risk STEMI (inferior MI without high-risk features), consider coronary angiography.

Management of Patients Who Have Not Received Reperfusion Therapy

1. In addition to the drugs indicated in all patients with STEMI (→above), including the antiplatelet agents (ASA and clopidogrel), administer an anticoagulant: **fondaparinux**; if fondaparinux is not available, use **enoxaparin** or **UFH** (dosage: →Table 11-6).

2. Coronary angiography should be performed immediately in hemodynamically unstable patients. In stable patients it may be considered before discharge. Administer IV UFH in a bolus of 60 IU/kg (up to a maximum of 4000 IU) prior to PCI.

⇥ COMPLICATIONS

Complications of MI:

1. Acute heart failure due to extensive myocardial necrosis and ischemia, arrhythmias/conduction disturbances, or mechanical complications of MI. Symptoms and treatment: →Chapter 3.8.1.

2. Recurrent ischemia or MI:

1) In patients with recurrent ST-segment elevation, perform emergency coronary angiography.

2) In patients with recurrent chest pain after reperfusion therapy, intensify medical treatment with nitrates and β-blockers. Administer heparin (unless already started earlier).

3) Patients with signs of hemodynamic instability should be urgently referred for cardiac catheterization.

3. Free wall rupture usually develops within 5 days of anterior wall MI; it rarely occurs in patients with LV hypertrophy or well-developed collateral circulation. **Signs** of acute rupture include cardiac tamponade and cardiac arrest, usually with fatal outcome; symptoms of slowly progressing rupture: gradually developing cardiac tamponade and symptoms of shock. Diagnosis is based on echocardiography. **Treatment**: Urgent surgical intervention.

4. Ventricular septal rupture (VSR) usually develops on days 3 to 5 of MI. **Signs**: A new-onset holosystolic murmur heard along the left sternal border (it may be poorly audible in patients with large ruptures) and rapidly worsening symptoms of left and right ventricular failure. Diagnosis is based on echocardiography. **Treatment**: Management of shock, including intra-aortic balloon counterpulsation and invasive hemodynamic monitoring; surgery must be performed as soon as possible (this usually involves resection of the necrotic tissues and closing the defect with a prosthetic patch).

5. Papillary muscle rupture develops on days 2 to 10 of MI; it is most frequently associated with inferior wall MI and affects the posterior LV papillary muscle, causing acute mitral regurgitation. **Signs**: Acute heart failure; a typical loud holosystolic apical murmur that may have widespread radiation; in many patients, there is absence of murmur or only a soft murmur. Diagnosis is based on clinical features confirmed by echocardiography. **Treatment**: Surgery, usually mitral valve replacement. Mitral regurgitation may also occur as a result of dilatation of the mitral annulus and ischemic dysfunction of the subvalvular apparatus without mechanical damage; in such cases, PCI may be the treatment of choice.

6. Arrhythmias and conduction disturbances: In addition to specific treatment (→below), correct electrolyte disturbances (target potassium levels >4 mmol/L and magnesium levels >0.8 mmol/L) and acid-base disturbances, if present.

1) **Ventricular premature beats (VPBs)** are very common on day 1 of MI; they generally do not require antiarrhythmic treatment unless they cause hemodynamic deterioration. A routine prophylactic use of antiarrhythmic drugs (eg, lidocaine) is not recommended.

2) **Accelerated idioventricular rhythm (AIVR)** (<120 beats/min) is relatively common on day 1 of MI; it usually does not require the administration of antiarrhythmic drugs. AIVR is not associated with an increased risk of ventricular fibrillation. It may be a sign of successful reperfusion.

3) **Nonsustained ventricular tachycardia (VT)** does not usually have hemodynamic consequences and does not require specific treatment. In the later phases of MI, particularly in patients with reduced LVEF, it may indicate an increased risk of cardiac arrest and may require pharmacologic treatment and diagnostic workup as in sustained ventricular tachycardia.

4) **Sustained VT**:
   a) **Polymorphic VT**: Prompt defibrillation (as in VF). In the event of bradycardia or QT prolongation as the cause of polymorphic VT, use temporary pacing.
   b) **Monomorphic VT**: Cardioversion. In patients who tolerate VT well (SBP >90 mm Hg, no angina or pulmonary edema), pharmacotherapy with intravenous β-blockers (drugs of choice) may be attempted before cardioversion, but such treatment rarely leads to the resolution of tachycardia. Alternatives include amiodarone 150 mg (or 5 mg/kg) in an IV infusion over 10 minutes, and repeat every 10 to 15 minutes when necessary (alternatively, 360 mg over 6 hours [1 mg/min], followed by 540 mg over the subsequent 18 hours [0.5 mg/min]; total dose ≤1.2 g/d); lidocaine 1 mg/kg in an IV injection, followed by 0.5 mg/kg every 8 to 10 minutes, up to a maximum of 4 mg/kg; alternatively, 1 to 3 mg/min in an IV infusion.

5) **VF**: Defibrillation. Primary VF (within 4 hours of hospitalization) is not associated with a poorer long-term prognosis in patients surviving the hospital phase of MI. In patients with sustained VT or VF occurring after the first 48 hours of hospitalization, consider a consultation with an electrophysiologist regarding an implantable defibrillator (ICD) (indications for ICD implantation after MI: →Chapter 3.4.3.6).

6) **AF** is more frequent in the elderly, in patients with anterior MI, extensive myocardial necrosis, heart failure, other arrhythmias, and conduction disturbances or post-MI pericarditis. It is an adverse prognostic factor.

a) **Persistent AF causing hemodynamic consequences or symptoms of myocardial ischemia**: Cardioversion. If cardioversion is ineffective, use antiarrhythmic agents controlling ventricular rate (IV amiodarone or IV digoxin in patients with heart failure).

b) **Persistent AF with no hemodynamic consequences or symptoms of myocardial ischemia**: Antiarrhythmic agents controlling ventricular rate. Consider the indications for anticoagulant therapy.

7) **Bradyarrhythmias**:

a) **Symptomatic sinus bradycardia, sinus pauses >3 seconds, or sinus bradycardia <40 beats/min with hypotension and symptoms of hemodynamic impairment**: IV atropine 0.5 to 1 mg (up to a maximum dose of 2 mg). In patients with persistent disturbances, temporary cardiac pacing.

b) **First-degree AV block** (→Chapter 3.4.2.2.1): No treatment.

c) **Second-degree AV block (Wenckebach type) with hemodynamic disturbances**: Atropine; if ineffective, temporal cardiac pacing.

d) **Mobitz type II second-degree AV block or third-degree AV block**: Temporary cardiac pacing is usually indicated; it may be avoided in patients with ventricular rates >50 beats/min, narrow QRS complexes, and no signs of hemodynamic instability.

Usually heart block is transient after MI and typically does not require permanent pacing. Indications for permanent cardiac pacing: →Chapter 3.2.1.

7. Stroke usually occurs after 48 hours of hospitalization. Predisposing factors include a prior stroke or TIA, CABG, advanced age, low LVEF, AF, and hypertension. If the stroke is caused by emboli originating from the heart (AF, intracardiac thrombi, akinetic LV segments), start a vitamin K antagonist (VKA) combined with heparin to achieve a target international normalized ratio (INR) of 2.0 to 3.0 (principles of treatment: →Chapter 3.1.1.4). A neurologist should be involved in the decision of when to start heparin due to the risk of hemorrhagic conversion.

→REHABILITATION

Patients with STEMI should be referred to an outpatient cardiac rehabilitation program where feasible. This may include an exercise program, dietary advice, and smoking cessation programs.

→PROGNOSIS

Discharge Planning: Risk Stratification, Prognosis, Management

Mortality of patients with uncomplicated STEMI who have undergone primary PCI is between 2% and 5%. The TIMI risk score (→Table 11-7) or the Zwolle risk score (→Table 11-8) can be used to determine the risk and timing of discharge. The probability of 30-day and 1-year mortality ranges from about 2% and 4%, respectively, for Zwolle scores 0 to 3; 4% and 7% for scores 4 to 6; 10% and 20% for scores 7 to 9; and 30% and 40% for a score >10. In low-risk patients (a Zwolle risk score ≤3), early discharge at 48 to 72 hours is feasible.

For the purpose of assessing prognosis, TIMI flow 0 means no perfusion, TIMI 1 means only faint flow with incomplete filling of the distal arteries, TIMI 2 means complete filling but with sluggish flow, and TIMI 3 means normal flow. For Killip class, Killip class IV means cardiogenic shock, Killip class III means acute pulmonary edema, Killip class II means signs of heart failure, and Killip class I stands for no heart failure.

In patients not treated with coronary revascularization procedures, the risk of death or MI should be assessed in the context of indications for coronary angiography and subsequent invasive treatment.

Table 11-7. TIMI risk score for STEMI

Risk factor	Score
Age	Individual risk factors receive varying numbers of points. Total points correspond to odds of death at 30 days
Diabetes mellitus/hypertension or angina	
Systolic blood pressure	
Heart rate	
Killip class II-IV	
Weight	
Anterior ST-elevation or left bundle branch block	
Time to treatment	

Original data and tool can be found in Circulation. 2000;102(17):2031-7.

STEMI, ST-segment elevation myocardial infarction; TIMI, thrombolysis in myocardial infarction.

Table 11-8. Zwolle risk score for STEMI

Killip class	
Killip class II	4
Killip class III	9
Killip class IV	9
TIMI flow	
TIMI flow 0	2
TIMI flow 1	2
TIMI flow 2	1
Age	
Age ≥60 years	2
3-vessel disease	
3-vessel disease present	1
Myocardial infarction	
History of anterior myocardial infarction	1
Ischemia time	
Ischemia time >4 hours	1
Total score	

Based on Circulation. 2004;109(22):2737-43.

STEMI, ST-segment elevation myocardial infarction; TIMI, thrombolysis in myocardial infarction.

1. Prior to discharge, assess the risk of death or recurrent MI. As indicated above, one of the tools for early risk assessment is the TIMI STEMI score (→Table 11-7; also available at mdcalc.com).

2. Indications for coronary angiography without prior stress testing:

1) Symptoms of myocardial ischemia that develop spontaneously or with minimal effort in the post-MI recovery period, or persistent hemodynamic instability.

2) Before radical treatment of mechanical complications of STEMI in patients with acceptable hemodynamic stability.

3. Do not perform the stress test:

1) Within 2 to 3 days of the onset of STEMI in patients who did not undergo successful reperfusion therapy.

2) In patients with unstable post-MI angina, symptomatic heart failure, or life-threatening arrhythmias.

4. Do not perform coronary angiography in patients who are not candidates for revascularization because of specific contraindications or lack of consent.

→ FOLLOW-UP

Long-term follow-up as in patients with stable angina (→Chapter 3.11.2.2).

→ SECONDARY PREVENTION

1. Control of risk factors of atherosclerosis (→Chapter 3.15).

2. Regular exercise: ≥30 minutes of moderate aerobic exercise (the intensity is determined on the basis of the stress test) ≥5 times a week or supervised rehabilitation programs in high-risk patients.

3. Pharmacotherapy (specific indications: →Table 11-4): Antiplatelet agents (ASA and/or clopidogrel, prasugrel, or ticagrelor), β-blockers, ACEIs (or ARBs), aldosterone antagonists, statins.

4. Anticoagulant treatment is recommended after coronary stenting in patients with atrial fibrillation and a moderate to high risk of thromboembolic complications. Treatment with a direct oral anticoagulant [DOAC] is indicated according to the Canadian Cardiovascular Society antiplatelet guidelines.

11.2. Stable Coronary Artery Disease

11.2.1. Microvascular Angina

→ DEFINITION AND CLINICAL FEATURES

Microvascular angina refers to angina pectoris with accompanying ST-segment depression on the electrocardiography (ECG) stress test (resting ECG is usually normal) and normal coronary angiography (without epicardial coronary artery spasm on ergonovine or acetylcholine challenge). Microvascular angina was formerly termed cardiac syndrome X.

Symptoms: Chest pain is often atypical; it may be very severe and usually develops on exertion but may also occur at rest. The pain usually lasts >10 minutes (up to >30 minutes after the end of exertion); it responds poorly to nitroglycerin. Symptoms of anxiety disorders may occur. Acute coronary syndrome may occur despite the absence of significant epicardial artery occlusion on angiography.

→ DIAGNOSIS

Diagnosis is based on the exclusion of significant (or dominant) coronary artery disease and other diseases that may cause chest pain (→Chapter 1.1).

→ TREATMENT

Acetylsalicylic acid (ASA) and statins are recommended in all patients; treatment of chest pain using β-blockers (first-line agents), nitrates, or calcium channel blockers: →Table 11-13, →Table 11-14. In patients not responding to these agents, used either alone or in combination, administer imipramine 50 mg once daily. Some studies have reported beneficial effects of angiotensin--converting enzyme inhibitors (ACEIs), sildenafil, ranolazine, L-arginine, and metformin. Behavioral interventions and physical exercise also may be beneficial.

→ PROGNOSIS

Prognosis is good with respect to survival and maintaining good left ventricular systolic function, but chronic symptoms affect the quality of life.

11.2.2. Stable Angina Pectoris

This chapter addresses symptomatic stable coronary artery disease (CAD).

→ DEFINITION, ETIOLOGY, PATHOGENESIS

Angina pectoris is a clinical syndrome characterized by chest pain (or its equivalent) due to myocardial ischemia, usually developing on exertion or caused by stress and not associated with necrosis of cardiomyocytes. In some patients the pain may be spontaneous. Angina reflects an inadequate oxygen supply in relation to myocardial demand. Stable angina pectoris is diagnosed in patients with symptoms of angina and no worsening over the prior 2 months. Etiology and pathogenesis: →Chapter 3.11.

→ CLINICAL FEATURES AND NATURAL HISTORY

1. Symptoms: The clinical diagnosis of angina is based on history. Therefore, a detailed characterization of the symptom complex is critical to the patient assessment.

Anginal chest pain is typically retrosternal in location and may radiate to the neck, jaw, left shoulder, and/or left arm (and usually further along the ulnar nerve to the wrist and fingers), to the epigastrium, or rarely to the interscapular region. The pain is caused by exertion (threshold may vary from patient to patient) and emotional stress; it usually lasts a few minutes and is relieved by rest or sometimes decreases in the course of continued exercise. The pain is frequently more severe in the morning and may be exacerbated by cold air or a heavy meal. Pain intensity is not related to body position or phase of the respiratory cycle; it usually resolves within 1 to 3 minutes of sublingual administration of nitroglycerin (if it resolves after 5-10 minutes, it is probably not related to myocardial ischemia and may be caused, eg, by esophageal disease). The pain may be absent in patients with an anginal "equivalent," particularly exertional dyspnea; however, it may be challenging to distinguish the anginal equivalent from a pulmonary cause.

Typical angina (1) is substernal and referred in a typical way; (2) is caused by exertion or emotional stress; (3) resolves at rest or after sublingual administration of a nitrate. Atypical angina fulfills 2 of these criteria. Nonanginal pain meets only 1 criterion.

2. Grading of angina based on its severity (→Table 11-9): Grading the severity of angina is helpful in monitoring the course of symptoms and provides a basis for therapeutic decisions. In a significant proportion of patients, the symptoms of angina remain stable for many years. Long-term spontaneous remissions may occur (these are sometimes only apparent and related to reduction of physical activity).

Table 11-9. Grading of angina pectoris based on its severity according to the Canadian Cardiovascular Society (CCS)

Grade I: Ordinary physical activity (such as walking and climbing stairs) does not cause angina. Angina occurs with strenuous, rapid, or prolonged exertion at work or recreation

Grade II: A slight limitation of ordinary activity. Angina occurs when:
- Walking or climbing stairs rapidly
- Walking uphill
- Walking or climbing stairs after meals, in cold, or in wind, or when under emotional stress, or only during the few hours after awakening
- Walking >200 meters or climbing more than 1 flight of stairs at a normal pace and in normal conditions

Grade III: Marked limitation of ordinary physical activity. Angina occurs when walking 100--200 meters or climbing 1 flight of stairs at a normal pace in normal conditions

Grade IV: Inability to carry on any physical activity without discomfort; anginal syndrome may be present at rest

Source: Canadian Cardiovascular Society. Angina pectoris, a CSS Grading Scale. www.ccs.ca/images/Guidelines/Guidelines_POS_Library/Ang_Gui_1976.pdf. Accessed September 5, 2019.

---

3. Signs: No signs are specific for angina. Signs of atherosclerosis of other arteries (eg, carotid bruit, ankle-brachial index <0.9 or >1.15) increase the risk of coronary artery disease.

→ DIAGNOSIS

Diagnostic Tests

1. Laboratory tests may reveal risk factors for atherosclerosis and disorders that may trigger angina. Baseline tests in a patient with stable coronary disease include:

1) Fasting lipid profile (total cholesterol [TC], low-density lipoprotein cholesterol [LDL-C], high-density lipoprotein cholesterol [HDL-C], and triglycerides [TG]).
2) Fasting blood glucose and glycated hemoglobin (HbA_{1c}) (and oral glucose tolerance test, when indicated [→Chapter 5.2]).
3) Complete blood count (CBC).
4) Serum creatinine level and estimated glomerular filtration rate.

Moreover, in patients with clinical indications perform:

1) Measurement of cardiac troponin levels (in the case of suspected acute coronary syndrome).
2) Thyroid function tests.
3) Liver function tests (after starting statin therapy).
4) Measurement of creatine kinase levels (in patients with features of myopathy).
5) B-type natriuretic peptide (BNP)/N-terminal pro–B-type natriuretic peptide (NT-proBNP) (in the case of suspected heart failure).

2. Resting electrocardiography (ECG) should be performed in every patient with suspected angina. Although the results are normal in the majority of patients, some patients may have significant Q waves, indicating prior myocardial infarction (MI) (even in the absence of a clinical history suggestive of prior MI) or ECG features of myocardial ischemia, mainly ST-segment depression or T-wave inversion.

3. Resting echocardiography is indicated in all patients to detect other diseases that may cause angina, assess impaired myocardial contractility and

Table 11-10. Pretest probability of coronary artery disease in patients with stable chest pain depending on age, sex, and type of pain

Type of pain	30-39 years		40-49 years		50-59 years		60-69 years		70-79 years		≥80 years	
	M	F	M	F	M	F	M	F	M	F	M	F
Typical chest pain									■		■	
Atypical chest pain												
Nonanginal chest pain												

PTP of CAD <15% (white boxes) indicates no need for further diagnostics.

In patients with PTP of CAD 15%-65% (grey boxes), ECG stress test may be performed as the first-line test. If well-conducted noninvasive imaging stress testing is available, this is the preferred method because of higher diagnostic yield. In young patients, irradiation must be taken into consideration.

In patients with PTP of CAD 66%-85% (light red boxes), CAD should be confirmed using noninvasive imaging stress test, not by ECG stress test.

In patients with PTP of CAD >85% (dark red boxes), CAD is diagnosed and the risk of complications should be assessed.

Based on Eur Heart J. 2011;32(11):1316-30.

CAD, coronary artery disease; ECG, electrocardiography; F, female patients; M, male patients; PTP, pretest probability.

diastolic function, and measure left ventricular (LV) ejection fraction (LVEF), which is necessary for risk stratification.

4. ECG Holter monitoring rarely provides significant diagnostic information and therefore should not be performed routinely. It can be considered in the case of suspected arrhythmia or vasospastic angina (Prinzmetal variant angina).

Noninvasive Imaging Diagnostic Tests for CAD

The choice of diagnostic tests depends on the clinical probability of CAD. The probability can be estimated by considering the age and sex of the patient and the nature of discomfort. Clinically useful classification is divided into a low (~15%), intermediate (~15%-85%), and high (~>85%) probability (→Table 11-10).

In patients with a high pretest probability (PTP), noninvasive testing is performed to assess the risk of cardiovascular events. However, invasive coronary angiography may be an alternative in many such patients (→below). In patients with a low PTP, a search for other causes should be considered, and noninvasive testing has limited usefulness. In patients with an intermediate PTP, noninvasive testing should be performed to confirm the diagnosis and assess prognosis. There are several noninvasive strategies commonly used in practice (→Figure 11-3).

1. ECG stress testing is used in patients with an intermediate PTP who are able to exercise and have interpretable ECG. The test has only modest sensitivity but very high specificity. It should be considered in patients with a PTP of 15% to 65%. Due to its limited sensitivity, the test is of less value for diagnostic purposes in patients with a PTP of 66% to 85%. The study is also of limited diagnostic value in patients in whom the baseline ECG features make it impossible to interpret the recordings during exercise (left bundle branch block [LBBB], preexcitation syndromes, pacemaker rhythms).

2. ECG stress testing with imaging: The addition of imaging to stress testing improves sensitivity, specificity, and prognostic information. Stress imaging is especially useful in assessing patients with a PTP of 66% to 85% with LVEF <50% and in those who have uninterpretable ECG. The 2 common types of imaging are single-photon emission computed tomography (SPECT) with sestamibi or thallium isotopes and stress echocardiography. Imaging can be performed with pharmacologic stress (dipyridamol [trade name Persantine] or dobutamine) in individuals who are not able to exercise. However, exercise is always preferred whenever possible for the additional prognostic information that it provides.

3. Coronary computed tomography angiography (CCTA) is used in patients with a PTP of 15% to 85% and in intermediate-risk patients in whom stress testing yields equivocal results or is not feasible (due to limited exercise capacity or uninterpretable ECG). CCTA has a very high negative predictive value, which allows for the exclusion of CAD in lower-risk patients. Specificity and diagnostic accuracy are reduced in the setting of extensive coronary calcification and fast or irregular heart rates.

4. Cardiac magnetic resonance imaging (MRI) and **positron emission tomography (PET)** are the emerging modalities for cardiac imaging. They have value for the assessment of myocardial viability and ventricular function; however, they are not widely used as stress testing modalities.

In patients with an intermediate PTP, clinical outcomes were similar whether an initial strategy with stress testing or CCTA was compared.⊘● However, when CCTA was used in addition to stress testing compared with stress testing alone, the use of CCTA was associated with lower rates of death and MI as well as increased diagnostic certainty and performance of fewer invasive angiographies without subsequent revascularization. The radiation dose with CCTA is lower than with nuclear imaging but higher than with stress echocardiography or stress ECG, where no radiation is administered. Although either stress testing or CCTA are usually recommended in patients with an intermediate PTP, recent national guidelines from the United Kingdom recommend a strategy of CCTA first in eligible patients.⊘●

Coronary angiography is the gold standard for demonstrating coronary anatomy, establishing prognosis, and assessing the feasibility of invasive treatment. Coronary angiography should be considered for the diagnosis of CAD in the following situations:

1) A high PTP of CAD in patients with severe symptoms or clinical features suggestive of high risk of cardiovascular events. In such cases it is justified to proceed to early coronary angiography without prior noninvasive imaging with the intention of revascularization.

2) Coexistence of typical angina and systolic LV dysfunction (LVEF <50%).

3) Equivocal diagnosis made on the basis of noninvasive tests or conflicting results of various noninvasive tests (this is an indication for coronary angiography with measurement of functional flow reserve [FFR], if necessary).

4) Unavailability of imaging stress testing, special legal requirements associated with certain professions (eg, aircraft pilots).

Risk Stratification Based on Clinical Data and Noninvasive Imaging

Estimating the subsequent risk of cardiovascular events uses data from the clinical evaluation, ventricular function, and results of stress testing or CCTA. **Markers of increased risk**:

1) **Clinical**: Increased age, history of diabetes mellitus, current smoker status, hypertension, elevated cholesterol, peripheral vascular disease, and chronic kidney disease (CKD). Evidence of clinical heart failure and ECG abnormalities are additional risk markers.

2) **LV function**: Ventricular function is the strongest long-term predictor of survival. An LVEF <50% indicates elevated risk; the risk continues to increase with a lower LVEF.

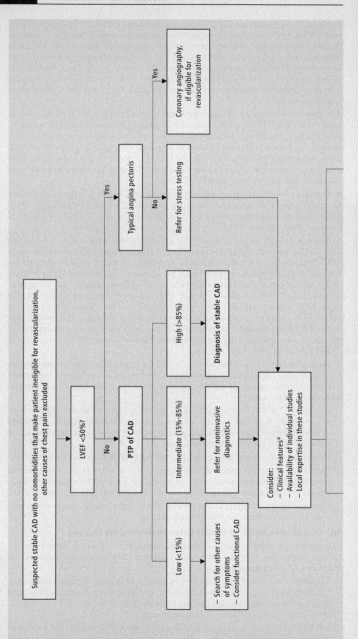

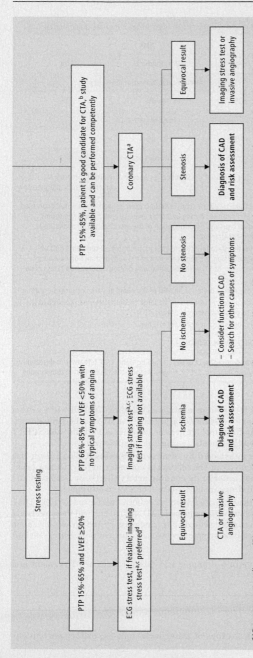

CAD, coronary artery disease; CTA, computed tomography angiography; ECG, electrocardiography; FFR, fractional flow reserve; LVEF, left ventricular ejection fraction; PTP, pretest probability.

a Consider the patient's age and radiation exposure.

b The patient is able to hold his/her breath, does not have severe obesity, has an appropriate coronary calcium score (<400 Agatston units) and distribution of calcifications, has sinus rhythm ≤65 beats/min (preferred ≤60 beats/min; if necessary use a short-acting β-blocker or another rate-control agent). In patients with severe disseminated or focal calcifications, the result is classified as equivocal.

c Echocardiography, single photon emission computed tomography, stress positron emission tomography (exercise or pharmacologic if the patient is unable to exercise), or stress magnetic resonance imaging (only pharmacologic).

d If available and can be performed competently.

Figure 11-3. Proposed diagnostic algorithm in patients with suspected stable coronary artery disease.

Study	Risk		
	High	**Intermediate**	**Low**
ECG stress test[a]	**Annual cardiovascular mortality**		
	>3%	1%-3%	<1%
Imaging studies	**Area of ischemia**		
	>10%[b]	1%-10%[c]	–
Coronary CTA	**Coronary lesions**		
	Significant stenosis[d]	Significant stenosis[e]	Normal coronary arteries or atherosclerotic plaques only

Table 11-11. Definitions of risk of cardiovascular events in various diagnostic studies

[a] Risk assessment using the Duke treadmill score including exercise workload in time expressed in metabolic equivalents, ST-T changes during and after exercise, and clinical symptoms (no angina, angina, or angina causing discontinuation of the test). Calculator available at www.cardiology.org/tools/medcalc/duke.

[b] >10% in SPECT; the quantitative data for MRI are limited: probably ≥2 segments (out of 16) with new areas of hypoperfusion; ≥3 segments (out of 17) with dysfunction caused by dobutamine; or ≥3 segments (out of 17) with abnormal wall motion observed on stress echocardiography.

[c] Or any ischemia rated as lower than high-risk on MRI of the heart or stress echocardiography.

[d] That is 3-vessel disease with proximal stenosis of the large coronary arteries, stenosis of the left main coronary artery, or proximal stenosis of the LAD.

[e] Non–high-risk stenosis of proximal large coronary arteries.

Adapted from Eur Heart J. 2013;34(38):2949-3003.

CTA, computed tomography angiography; ECG, electrocardiography; LAD, left anterior descending artery; MRI, magnetic resonance imaging; SPECT, single-photon emission computed tomography.

3) **Noninvasive tests for ischemia**: High-risk findings include >10% area of ischemia on SPECT or >3 dysfunctional segments on stress echocardiography. Intermediate-risk findings include area of ischemia of 1% to 10% on SPECT or 1 to 2 dysfunctional segments on stress echocardiography.

4) **Coronary anatomy assessed by noninvasive tests** (CCTA): High-risk findings include stenosis in the left main coronary artery, in the proximal section of the left anterior descending artery (LAD), or 3-vessel CAD. Intermediate-risk findings include 1-vessel or 2-vessel disease.

Management based on the estimated risk of a cardiovascular event: →Table 11-11, →Figure 11-4. In all patients with confirmed CAD optimal medical therapy should be started. The decision to proceed to coronary angiography and revascularization depends on the estimated risk, symptom control, and patient preference (→below).

Differential Diagnosis

Other causes of chest pain (→Chapter 1.1). Other causes of ST-segment and T-wave abnormalities.

→TREATMENT

General Considerations

1. Control of the risk factors of atherosclerosis (secondary prevention): →Chapter 3.15.

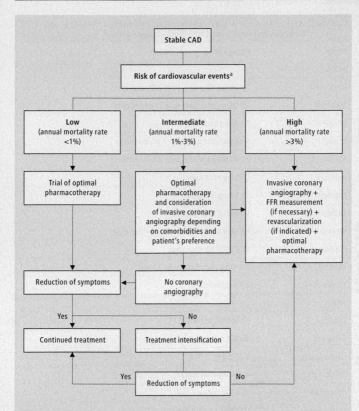

^a In patients with 15%-85% PTP of CAD, a stress test has already been performed and can be the basis for risk assessment. If PTP of CAD is >85%, additional studies to assess the risk must be performed only in those patients who have minor symptoms when receiving pharmacotherapy but nevertheless made an informed decision to undergo revascularization in case of a high risk of cardiovascular events.

CAD, coronary artery disease; FFR, fractional flow reserve; PTP, pretest probability.

Figure 11-4. Management algorithm in patients with confirmed stable coronary artery disease depending on the risk of cardiovascular events. *Adapted from Eur Heart J. 2013;34(38):2949-3003.*

2. Treatment of diseases worsening angina, such as anemia, hyperthyroidism, or tachyarrhythmias.

3. Increasing physical activity (below the threshold of angina): 30 minutes daily ≥3 days a week.

4. Influenza vaccination: Annually.

5. Optimal medical therapy to improve prognosis and control the symptoms of angina.

6. Invasive treatment (percutaneous coronary intervention [PCI], coronary artery bypass grafting [CABG]): In eligible patients.

Table 11-12. Typical dosage of angiotensin-converting enzyme inhibitors (ACEIs) and angiotensin-receptor blockers (ARBs) in angina pectoris

Agent	Dosage (PO)
ACEIs	
Benazepril	10-40 mg once daily or in 2 divided doses
Quinapril	10-80 mg once daily or in 2 divided doses
Cilazapril	2.5-5 mg once daily
Enalapril	5-40 mg once daily or in 2 divided doses
Fosinopril	20-40 mg once daily or in 2 divided doses
Imidapril	5-20 mg once daily
Captopril	25-50 mg bid to tid
Lisinopril	10-40 mg once daily
Moexipril	7.5-30 mg once daily or in 2 divided doses
Perindopril	4(5)-8(10) mg once daily
Ramipril	2.5-5 mg once daily (max, 10 mg)
Trandolapril	2-4 mg once daily
ARBs	
Losartan	50-100 mg once daily
Valsartan	80-320 mg once daily
Candesartan	8-32 mg once daily
Telmisartan	40-80 mg once daily
Irbesartan	150-300 mg once daily
Eprosartan	600-800 mg once daily
Olmesartan	20-40 mg once daily
bid, 2 times a day; PO, oral; tid; 3 times a day.	

Optimal Medical Therapy: Treatment to Improve Prognosis

In every patient the following oral agents should be administered on a lifelong basis:

1) **Antiplatelet agents**: Acetylsalicylic acid (ASA) 75 mg once daily; in the case of adverse gastrointestinal effects, add an antacid (→Chapter 6.1.2.4). In patients with contraindications to ASA (allergy, aspirin-induced asthma), use clopidogrel 75 mg once daily (dosage: →Table 11-3); a combination therapy with ASA and clopidogrel is not recommended in stable patients except after stenting (→below).🗙⬤

2) **Low-dose oral anticoagulants**: ASA in addition to a low-dose oral anticoagulant (rivaroxaban 2.5 mg bid) may be considered as an added risk-reduction strategy in patients who are at elevated risk of future coronary events compared with bleeding events.⊘⬤

3) **Statins** (→Table 12-2): Make attempts to lower LDL-C levels ≤2.0 mmol/L, and if this cannot be achieved, to reduce them by >50% compared with baseline levels.⊘⬤ In cases of poor tolerance or ineffectiveness of statins,

Table 11-13. Typical dosage of nitrates in angina pectoris

Agent	Preparations	Dosage[a]	Duration of action
Nitroglycerin (INN glyceryl trinitrate)	Aerosol	0.4 mg	1.5-7 min
	Transdermal patch	5-20 mg/24 h (patch should be detached for the night)	
	Prolonged-release tablets	6.5-15 mg bid	4-8 h
Isosorbide dinitrate	Tablets	5-10 mg	Up to 60 min
Isosorbide mononitrate	Tablets	10-40 mg bid	Up to 8 h
	Prolonged-release tablets	50-100 mg once daily	12-24 h
	Prolonged-release capsules	40-120 mg once daily	

[a] In a long-term bid administration, the second dose should be administered within 8 h of the first dose (eg, 7:00 and 15:00), and the nitroglycerin patches should be detached for 10 h.

bid, 2 times a day; INN, international nonproprietary name.

the use of ezetimibe or proprotein convertase subtilisin/kexin type 9 (PCSK9) inhibitors can be considered.

4) **Angiotensin-converting enzyme inhibitors (ACEIs)** (or angiotensin--receptor blockers [ARBs]) are indicated in patients with coexisting hypertension, diabetes mellitus, heart failure, or LV systolic dysfunction (dosage: →Table 11-12).◐●

Optimal Medical Therapy: Treatment to Control Symptoms

1. Acute symptom control and prevention prior to planned exercise: Use a short-acting nitrate: nitroglycerin aerosol (→Table 11-13). Patients should be instructed to use nitroglycerin 3 times at 5-minute intervals. If no relief is achieved, the patient should call an ambulance and should be assessed by the medical personnel for acute chest pain. Relative contraindications include hypertrophic cardiomyopathy with outflow tract obstruction, severe aortic stenosis, use of phosphodiesterase-5 (PDE-5) inhibitors (eg, sildenafil). Other drug interactions include α-blockers (in male patients with benign prostatic hyperplasia, the combined use of nitrates and a selective α-blocker [tamsulosin] is allowed). Adverse effects: headache, facial flushing, dizziness, syncope.

2. Prevention of angina and increasing exercise tolerance:

1) β-Blockers reduce heart rate, contractility, and atrioventricular (AV) conduction. They are the first-line agents for treatment of angina. Physicians should titrate the dose on the basis of heart rate and blood pressure with a goal to achieve the maximum recommended dose. Typical dosage: →Table 11-14. A β-blocker may be considered in asymptomatic patients with extensive ischemia (>10% of LV). Absolute contraindications: symptomatic bradycardia, symptomatic hypotension, second-degree or third-degree AV block, sick sinus syndrome, severe decompensated heart failure. Adverse effects: bradycardia, AV block, bronchospasm, peripheral artery spasm, and peripheral hypoperfusion in patients with severe peripheral artery disease; sexual dysfunction and loss of libido; and particularly in the case of propranolol, fatigue, headache, sleep disturbances, insomnia, vivid dreams, depression. Caution should be exercised in combining β-blockers with verapamil and diltiazem due to their additive effects on AV conduction and heart rate.

Table 11-14. Typical dosage of β-blockers and calcium channel blockers in angina pectoris

Agent	Dosage (PO)
β-Blockers	
Acebutolol	200-600 mg bid
Atenolol	50-200 mg once daily
Betaxolol	10-20 mg once daily
Bisoprolol	5-10 mg once daily
Carvedilol	12.5-25 mg bid
Metoprolol	
Immediate-release formulations	25-100 mg bid
Extended-release formulations	25-200 mg once daily
Pindolol	2.5-10 mg bid or tid
Propranolol	10-80 mg bid or tid
Dihydropyridine calcium channel blockers	
Amlodipine	5-10 mg once daily
Felodipine	5-10 mg once daily
Nondihydropyridine calcium channel blockers	
Diltiazem	
Immediate-release formulations	30-90 mg tid
Extended-release formulations	120-480 mg once daily (or in 2 divided doses)
Verapamil	
Immediate release formulations	40-160 mg tid
Extended-release formulations	120-480 mg once daily
bid, 2 times a day; tid, 3 times a day; PO, oral.	

2) **Calcium channel blockers** are smooth muscle vasodilators; they have
   a negative inotropic effect. They can be used in patients who cannot take
   β-blockers or do not respond to monotherapy with a β-blocker. Typical dosage:
   →Table 11-14.
   a) **Diltiazem and verapamil** lower the heart rate. They are of value in patients
      with contraindications to or intolerance of β-blockers. Contraindications:
      heart failure, bradycardia, AV conduction disturbances, hypotension.
      Adverse effects: constipation, bradycardia, AV block, hypotension.
   b) **Dihydropyridines** are vasodilators. Their mechanism of action is com-
      plementary to β-blockers. They can be used in combination with a β-blocker
      in patients not responding to a β-blocker alone. Adverse effects: facial
      flushing, headache, peripheral edema.
3) **Long-acting nitrates** are arterial and venous vasodilators; they reduce
   preload. **Isosorbide dinitrate**, **isosorbide mononitrate**, or **nitroglycerin**

are recommended as second-line agents; typical dosage: →Table 11-13. When administered bid, ensure ~10-hour intervals between the doses. The onset of action of nitroglycerin patches occurs a few minutes after they are attached; their antianginal effect is maintained for 3 to 5 hours.

3. Other agents, such as ivabradine, molsidomine, nicorandil, ranolazine, and trimetazidine, are used for their antianginal properties in some countries around the world.

Invasive Angiography and Revascularization

In patients with a diagnosis of stable angina based on noninvasive testing, invasive angiography is indicated for high-risk patients or those with severe or refractory symptoms to assess the potential for revascularization:

1) Invasive coronary angiography (with assessment by FFR measurement, when necessary) is recommended:

   a) For risk stratification in patients with severe stable angina or with a high risk of cardiovascular events, especially if symptoms do not improve with medical therapy.

   b) For patients with mild or no symptoms if noninvasive risk stratification suggests a high risk of cardiovascular events and revascularization has the potential to improve prognosis.

2) Invasive coronary angiography (with FFR measurement) should be considered in patients with inconclusive or conflicting noninvasive test results to obtain a definitive diagnosis and inform prognosis.

Findings of invasive angiography (extent and complexity of CAD, LV dysfunction) as well as clinical factors (age, comorbidities, history of diabetes mellitus) dictate the decision to perform revascularization and the choice of the revascularization strategy. In patients with multivessel disease, the angiographic extent and complexity of CAD can be quantified using the SYNTAX score (www.syntaxscore.com). Decisions about the revascularization strategy are usually taken by an interventional cardiologist in consultation with a cardiovascular surgeon as part of the heart team approach.

Choice of PCI vs CABG

1. PCI is the preferred treatment in patients with:

1) One-vessel disease (including the proximal section of the LAD) or 2-vessel disease that does not involve the proximal LAD.

2) Anatomic features of a low-risk lesion.

3) Comorbidities increasing the risk of cardiac surgery.

2. CABG is preferred in patients with:

1) Three-vessel disease and a SYNTAX score >22 or reduced LV function.

2) Patients with diabetes mellitus and multivessel disease.

3) Left main coronary artery stenosis combined with 2-vessel or 3-vessel disease in patients with a SYNTAX score >32.

3. Anatomic subsets where either PCI or CABG may be considered include patients with 2-vessel disease involving the proximal LAD, 3-vessel disease with a low SYNTAX score (<22), or left main coronary artery stenosis with limited CAD at other sites.

4. Patients after prior revascularization: In patients with prior CABG or with prior PCI presenting with in-stent restenosis, PCI is the preferred treatment option, unless angiographic complexity or the extent of the disease favors bypass surgery.

5. Patients with diabetes mellitus: Patients with diabetes mellitus are at increased risk of disease progression and cardiovascular events. Patients with diabetes mellitus and multivessel disease have a survival advantage with bypass surgery. PCI with drug-eluting stents (DESs) should be considered in patients with 1-vessel disease.○○●

6. Patients with CKD: In patients with nonsevere CKD in whom CABG is indicated because of the extent of CAD, surgical risk is acceptable, and life expectancy justifies the procedure, consider CABG rather than PCI.

7. Intracoronary assessment: For patients without diagnostic noninvasive evidence of ischemia, FFR measurement with administration of IV or intracoronary adenosine may be used to guide revascularization decisions, especially in uncertain clinical situations, such as an angiographically moderate coronary stenosis or atypical symptoms. Revascularization is recommended in patients with angina, a positive stress test result, or with an FFR value <0.80, but it should be deferred in those with FFR >0.80.

Choice of Stents and Management After Stent Insertion

1. Choice of stents and antiplatelet therapy in patients undergoing elective PCI: Second-generation DESs with thinner struts and biodegradable or more biocompatible polymers have shown superior outcomes compared with first-generation DESs and BMSs. Dual antiplatelet therapy should be used for 6 months in all patients undergoing elective PCI with DESs and continued for up to 3 years in patients in whom the risk of ischemic versus bleeding outcomes is favorable.⊘● BMSs require only 1 month of dual antiplatelet therapy and may be chosen in patients who are not candidates for a longer-duration combined therapy. Dual antiplatelet therapy is recommended with aspirin and clopidogrel for patients undergoing stenting for chronic coronary disease. Ticagrelor or prasugrel should be chosen in combination with aspirin for patients presenting with acute coronary syndromes, stent thrombosis, or in other high-risk situations.

2. Antithrombotic treatment is recommended after stenting in patients with atrial fibrillation and a moderate or high risk of thromboembolism in whom the use of vitamin K antagonists or direct oral anticoagulants is necessary. The duration of dual antiplatelet therapy and/or triple therapy should be individualized based on the balance of risks of thrombosis and bleeding. Bleeding is minimized in regimens that limit the duration of triple therapy. Clopidogrel and an anticoagulant for long-term treatment combined with the use of ASA during the time of stent implantation and shortly afterwards may be preferred as compared with an extended course of triple therapy because of the elevated risk of bleeding with this approach.⊘●

→ FOLLOW-UP

Regular monitoring of modifiable risk factors: →Chapter 3.15. The frequency of follow-up visits depends on the severity of risk factors and angina: usually every 3 to 4 months in the first year of treatment, and then (in stable patients) every 6 months to 1 year.

→ PROGNOSIS

The annual mortality rate is 1.2% to 3.8%, risk of cardiac death is 0.6% to 1.4%, and risk of nonfatal MI is 0.6% to 2.7%. Adverse prognostic factors include advanced age, more severe angina pectoris (→Table 11-9), poor performance status, resting ECG abnormalities, silent myocardial ischemia, LV systolic dysfunction, extensive ischemia documented by noninvasive stress tests, advanced lesions observed in coronary angiography, diabetes mellitus, renal failure, LV hypertrophy, and resting heart rate >70 beats/min.

11.2.3. Vasospastic Angina (Prinzmetal Variant Angina)

→ DEFINITION AND CLINICAL FEATURES

Vasospastic angina (Prinzmetal variant angina) is a type of angina in which chest pain is caused by transient ischemia secondary to spontaneous coronary artery spasm. Chest pain generally occurs at rest and usually in the absence of flow-limiting coronary stenoses.

Symptoms include chest pain occurring at rest, commonly in the late night or early morning hours, which is frequently transient and lasts between 5 and 15 minutes (pain characteristics: →Chapter 3.11.2.2). On occasion, it may also develop on exertion, although this is less common. Other associated symptoms may include nausea, diaphoresis, palpitations, dyspnea, and lightheadedness.

→ DIAGNOSIS

Diagnosis is based on the occurrence of unprovoked chest pain at rest with accompanying ST-segment elevation (less commonly depression) on electrocardiography (ECG) and absence of significant coronary artery stenosis on coronary angiography. If an episode occurs during coronary angiography, coronary spasm may be directly observed during the procedure. Interventionalists can provoke coronary spasm via medications such as acetylcholine, ergonovine, or via hyperventilation, but this is not done commonly and only performed when the diagnosis is unclear.

In patients with recurrent pain, Holter monitoring may reveal ST-segment changes with pain. Whether ST-segment elevation or ST-segment depression is seen depends on the severity of spasms: full occlusion causes ST-segment elevation, while a less severe spasm may cause ST-segment depression. Rises in the levels of biomarkers of ischemia depend on the duration of the spasm. While most times the spasm is transient, a prolonged spasm may lead to actual infarction and arrhythmia in up to 25% of patients.

→ TREATMENT

Medical Treatment

1. Modification of risk factors, particularly smoking cessation.

2. Low-dose acetylsalicylic acid (ASA).

3. High-dose oral calcium channel blockers: Diltiazem 120 to 360 mg/d, verapamil 240 to 480 mg/d (→Table 11-14). If treatment with 1 calcium channel blocker is not effective, add another calcium channel blocker of a different group or a long-acting nitrate (→Table 11-13).

4. Nonselective β-blockers are contraindicated as they may exacerbate vasospasm.

Invasive Treatment

Percutaneous intervention is not recommended as the first-line therapy for patients with coronary vasospasm and nonobstructive coronary disease. Consideration may be given to percutaneous coronary intervention (PCI) if a significant plaque (≥70%) is present and if the plaque is thought to be a trigger for localized vasospasm with the patient developing pain at rest. Further, PCI of a vasospastic segment may be of benefit in patients who are refractory to medical therapy if the vasospastic segment is clearly visualized on the diagnostic catheterization. Outcomes overall are variable as vasospasm may occur in a different section of the artery, and thus medical therapy is considered the first-line treatment. Vasospasm-associated severe arrhythmias may require treatment with a pacemaker or implantable cardioverter-defibrillator (ICD).

→ PROGNOSIS

Among patients with vasospastic angina, 95% survive 5 years from diagnosis. Prognosis is worse in patients with concurrent atherosclerotic plaque and in those with vasospasm-induced ventricular fibrillation.

12. Lipid Disorders

→ DEFINITION

Dyslipidemias are conditions in which plasma concentrations of lipids, lipoproteins, or triglycerides are considered elevated based on the patient's total cardiovascular disease risk.

Total cholesterol, high-density cholesterol, and triglycerides used to be measured in the fasting state after 12 to 14 hours since the last meal. New guidelines suggest that lipid measurement could be done in a nonfasting state for the purpose of risk assessment and screening, but fasting measurements should be taken while assessing the efficacy of treatment, especially in patients with elevated triglyceride levels.

Low-density lipoprotein levels are usually calculated using the Friedewald formula:

$$LDL\text{-}C = TC - HDL\text{-}C - (TG/5 \text{ [mg/dL]} \text{ or } TG/2.2 \text{ [mmol/L]})$$

Where: LDL-C, low-density lipoprotein cholesterol; TC, total cholesterol; HDL-C, high-density lipoprotein cholesterol; TG, triglyceride.

The calculations are unreliable in patients with a triglyceride level >4.6 mmol/L (400 mg/dL).

12.1. Atherogenic Dyslipidemia

→ DEFINITION, ETIOLOGY, PATHOGENESIS

A combination of:

1) High triglyceride (TG) levels: **≥1.7 to 5.6 mmol/L (150-500 mg/dL)**.
2) Low high-density lipoprotein cholesterol (HDL-C) levels: **<1 mmol/L (40 mg/dL)** in men, **<1.2 mmol/L (45 mg/dL)** in women (or <1.3 mmol/L [50 mg/dL] in the case of coexisting metabolic syndrome).
3) Abnormal (small, dense) low-density lipoprotein cholesterol (LDL-C) particles (not typically measured in practice).

Insulin resistance plays a major role in the development of atherogenic dyslipidemia in metabolic syndrome and type 2 diabetes mellitus.

→ CLINICAL FEATURES AND DIAGNOSIS

There are no typical symptoms. Overweight/obesity or type 2 diabetes mellitus may coexist. Diagnosis is based on TG and HDL-C levels. LDL-C levels are moderately increased; patients with significantly increased LDL-C are diagnosed with mixed (familial) hyperlipidemia.

→ TREATMENT

General Principles

1. Aim at normalization of the LDL-C level.

2. Currently there are no specific target concentrations for TG and HDL-C (lack of clinical trials). A desirable TG concentration of <1.7 mmol/L (150 mg/dL) is suggested. Pharmacotherapy is recommended in patients at high risk for cardiovascular disease if TG levels are >2.3 mmol/L (200 mg/dL) despite nonpharmacologic treatment.

Nonpharmacologic Management

1. Reduction of body weight by appropriate diet and exercise.

2. Dietary modification is aimed at reducing TG and increasing HDL-C levels. This also includes restricted intake of carbohydrates (particularly simple carbohydrates).

3. Increased physical activity.

4. Limit alcohol consumption to reduce TG levels. Abstinence is recommended in patients with a TG level ≥5.6 mmol/L (500 mg/dL).

Pharmacotherapy

Agents and dosage: →Table 12-1.

1. Statins:

1) In patients with high LDL-C, high TG, and low HDL-C levels, start with a statin.

2) In patients who have achieved the target LDL-C level but continue to have TG ≥1.7 mmol/L (150 mg/dL), HDL-C <1 mmol/L (40 mg/dL), or both, exclude secondary dyslipidemia (→Chapter 3.12.2) and evaluate compliance. If this does not result in adequate improvements, you may try adding a fibrate or nicotinic acid.

2. Fibrates should be used in patients with high TG or low HDL-C levels and LDL-C at the target level. In patients with a TG concentration ≥5.6 mmol/L (500 mg/dL), start with a fibrate (prevention of pancreatitis) and then add a statin when necessary.

Contraindications: Severe chronic kidney disease (do not use fenofibrate in patients with a glomerular filtration rate [GFR] <50 mL/min/1.73 m^2 or gemfibrozil in patients with a GFR <15 mL/min/1.73 m^2), liver failure, cholelithiasis, pregnancy, and breastfeeding.

Major adverse effects: Increased serum alanine aminotransferase (ALT); myopathy; gastrointestinal complaints such as dyspepsia, abdominal pain, diarrhea, bloating. If the ALT or aspartate aminotransferase (AST) level is > 3×upper limit of normal (ULN), discontinue the fibrate. The risk of serious complications, especially myopathy, is increased in the case of combination treatment with a fibrate and a statin (not as increased with fenofibrate). When using such treatment, be especially cautious and warn the patient about muscle complaints; if such complaints occur, measure the creatine kinase (CK) level (an increase in CK > 4×ULN is an indication for treatment discontinuation). Do not combine gemfibrozil (not used in many countries) with a statin because of the risk of adverse effects.

3. Nicotinic acid is rarely used because of disturbing adverse effects, which include flushing, pruritus, paresthesias, and nausea (these are less frequent with sustained-release formulations used alone).

Contraindications: Gout, active liver disease, acute myocardial infarction, peptic ulcer disease, pregnancy, breastfeeding, diabetes mellitus (only for crystalline nicotinic acid).

12.2. Hypercholesterolemia

→ DEFINITION, ETIOLOGY, PATHOGENESIS

In healthy individuals a plasma/serum **low-density lipoprotein cholesterol (LDL-C) level ≥3.0 mmol/L (115 mg/dL)** may be considered abnormal. Current guidelines are not specific on abnormal levels but rather correlate the LDL-C concentration with a risk category and recommend lifestyle changes or pharmacotherapy on this basis.

Table 12-1. Selected lipid-lowering agents	
Agent	Dosage
Statins	
Atorvastatin	10-80 mg once daily
Fluvastatin	20-80 mg once daily
Lovastatin	20-80 mg once daily
Rosuvastatin	5-40 mg once daily
Simvastatin	5-80 mg[a] once daily
Bile acid sequestrants (resins)	
Cholestyramine	Start from 4 g once daily to bid, then titrate up to 4 g/d (max, 24 g/d in divided doses)
Colesevelam	Monotherapy 1.875 g bid or 3.75 g once daily (max, 4.375 g/d) Combination treatment 2.5-3.75 g/d (max, 3.75 g/d)
Fibrates	
Ciprofibrate	100 mg once daily
Fenofibrate	
Nonmicronized	Start from 100 mg tid; maintenance dose 200 mg/d
Micronized	145, 160, 200, 215, or 267 mg once daily
Other	
Ezetimibe	10 mg once daily
PCSK9 inhibitors	
Evolocumab	140 mg SC every 2 weeks or 420 mg once monthly
Alirocumab	75 mg SC every other week, then dose may be increased to 150 mg every 2 weeks or 300 mg every 4 weeks

[a] Note: The US Food and Drug Administration does not recommend the use of simvastatin at a dose of 80 mg/d because of increased incidence of myopathy.

SC, subcutaneous.

Classification:

1) **Primary hypercholesterolemia**:
   a) Polygenic hypercholesterolemia (most common) involving environmental factors, such as diet.
   b) Familial (monogenic) hypercholesterolemia (FH): Most often heterozygous familial hypercholesterolemia (HeFH) caused by a mutation affecting the LDL receptor, apolipoprotein B, or proprotein convertase subtilisin/kexin type 9 (PCSK9) protease.

2) **Secondary hypercholesterolemia**: Hypercholesterolemia caused by medical conditions, including hypothyroidism, nephrotic syndrome, chronic kidney disease, liver disease with cholestasis, Cushing syndrome, anorexia nervosa, or drug induced (secondary to progestogens, glucocorticoids, protease inhibitors).

→ CLINICAL FEATURES

Clinical signs in patients with FH: Tendon xanthomas (of the Achilles tendon and tendon of the extensor digitorum muscle), corneal arcus.

→ SCREENING

Consider screening patients with the following:

1) Men aged ≥40 years; women ≥40 years or after menopause.
2) Ethnic groups at increased risk (eg, South Asian, First Nations).
3) Diabetes mellitus.
4) Aortic aneurysm.
5) Chronic obstructive pulmonary disease.
6) Hypertension.
7) Family history of early cardiovascular disease (men <55 years, women <65 years).
8) Chronic kidney disease (CKD).
9) HIV.
10) Erectile dysfunction.
11) Clinical features of atherosclerosis.
12) Obesity.
13) Chronic inflammatory disease.
14) Active smokers.
15) Hypertensive disease in pregnancy.

→ DIAGNOSIS

Diagnostic Criteria

Indirect evidence is provided by LDL-C levels >4.9 mmol/L (190 mg/dL) or signs of premature atherosclerosis (these can occur in childhood in homozygous patients) and first-degree relatives with FH. Detection of a mutation causing hypercholesterolemia confirms the diagnosis of FH but has no impact on the clinical management.

Differential Diagnosis

1. Familial combined hyperlipidemia (lower total cholesterol [TC] and higher triglyceride [TG] levels).

2. Polygenic hypercholesterolemia (lower TC levels, no family history of high TC levels, no xanthomas).

Note that in most countries <1% of patients with heterozygous FH are diagnosed.◕

→ TREATMENT

General Considerations

Target LDL-C levels and indications (→Table 12-2) depend on the patient's total cardiovascular risk rather than on the absolute lipid level. In North America the risk of cardiovascular disease (CVD) is assessed using the Framingham risk score (→Table 15-1). The Framingham Heart Study website provides numerous ways of calculating the 10-year CVD risk. Canadian guidelines consider a probability of cardiovascular complications over 10 years that is >20% as **high risk** and a probability between 10% and 19% as **intermediate risk**. Cardiovascular complications include coronary death, myocardial infarction, coronary insufficiency, angina, ischemic stroke, hemorrhagic stroke, transient ischemic attack, peripheral artery disease, and heart failure.

Table 12-2. Management targets for dyslipidemia

Risk category (10-year CVD risk)[a]	Serum target
High risk (FRS ≥20%)	LDL-C <2.0 mmol/L or reduce by >50%[c]
Intermediate risk (FRS 10%-19%) and ≥1 of: 1) LDL-C ≥3.5 mmol/L 2) Non–HDL-C ≥4.3 mmol/L 3) Apolipoprotein B >1.2 g/L 4) Men >50 years, women >60 years (only with +1 additional CVD risk factor)[b]	or Apolipoprotein B <0.8 g/L or Non–HDL-C <2.6 mmol/L
LDL-C >5.0 mmol/L	>50% reduction in LDL-C

[a] →Table 15-1.
[b] Low HDL-C, impaired fasting glucose, high waist circumference, active smoker, hypertension.
[c] LDL-C <1.8 mmol/L in patients with acute coronary syndrome in the last 3 months.

Based on Can J Cardiol. 2016;32(11):1263-1282.

CVD, cardiovascular disease; FRS, Framingham risk score; HDL-C, high-density lipoprotein cholesterol; LDL-C, low-density lipoprotein cholesterol.

According to Canadian guidelines, indications for statins include high and intermediate risk categories and are also based on the presence of certain clinical conditions (→Chapter 3.15). Treatment targets are similar with the exception of lower LDL-C in patients with acute coronary syndrome in the last 3 months (→Table 12-2).

Lifestyle Modifications

1. The Mediterranean diet, characterized by a high consumption of vegetables and olive oil with a moderate consumption of protein (including nuts), can reduce the risk of cardiovascular events.○ Suggestions include replacement of saturated fats with polyunsaturated fats; restriction of fatty acids to <7% of caloric requirements (<15 g/d with a caloric intake of 2000 kcal/d) by partial substitution with polyunsaturated fatty acids or complex carbohydrates (optimally high-fiber products); restricted intake of trans-unsaturated fatty acids (hard margarines, ready-made pastries, instant soups); limiting cholesterol to <300 mg/d.

2. Exercise reduces individual risk factors. However, its effect on cumulative risk factors remains unclear.

3. Smoking cessation may improve the lipid profile.○

4. There is no evidence that improved sleep hygiene has beneficial effects.○

Pharmacotherapy

Agents and dosage: →Table 12-1.

1. Statins are the first-line agents to lower LDL-C levels and have a moderate effect on TG and high-density lipoprotein cholesterol (HDL-C) concentrations.

Contraindications: Pregnancy, breastfeeding, active liver disease (alanine aminotransferase [ALT] or aspartate aminotransferase [AST] levels >3×upper limit of normal [ULN]; a smaller increase is not an absolute contraindication but requires close monitoring and control after 4-6 weeks). Certain liver conditions are not absolute contraindications: chronic liver disease or stable cirrhosis, nonalcoholic fatty liver, liver transplantation, autoimmune (nonchronic) hepatitis.

Significant adverse effects:

1) Patients at increased risk of adverse events include those with any of the following: >80 years of age, renal failure, hypothyroidism, inflammatory diseases of the muscles, and those in a perioperative period.

2) Increased serum ALT or AST levels occur in 0.5% to 2% of patients, are dose-dependent, and usually return to baseline values after reducing the statin dose. An increase in AST or ALT may not have clinical implications and further liver assessment may be of value (albumin, international normalized ratio [INR], bilirubin). Measure serum transaminase levels within the first 3 months. In patients with ALT >3×ULN, discontinue statins and measure the ALT level again after 4 to 6 weeks. Restarting statins in lower doses may be considered after the ALT concentration returns to normal.

3) Muscle discomfort may be present in up to 10% to 15% of patients.

4) Myopathy develops in <0.2% of patients. It manifests with pain, muscle weakness or tenderness (or both), and increased serum creatine kinase (CK) levels. Very rarely, myopathy may lead to rhabdomyolysis; this may occur at any time of statin therapy. Measurement of CK is advised prior to treatment initiation. Subsequent monitoring in patients with no muscle pain is not necessary. However, CK must be measured in all patients who develop muscle pain, tenderness, weakness, or brownish urine (all patients should be advised to report such symptoms immediately).

In patients with CK levels >4×ULN, discontinue statins immediately and measure CK (if >10×ULN, measure CK and creatinine every 2 weeks). Remember to review drugs for interactions (eg, fibrates [particularly gemfibrozil], azole antifungal agents [fluconazole, itraconazole, ketoconazole], macrolide antibiotics, other drugs inhibiting the metabolism of statins). If there is an attempt to restart statins, you can try to use atorvastatin or rosuvastatin in a low dose every other day or 1 to 2 days per week in combination with ezetimibe; in patients at very high cardiovascular risk who have not reached the target LDL-C level, subsequently consider a PCSK9 inhibitor as the third drug. If the patient does not tolerate statins even at a low dose, use ezetimibe and, if justified by the risk, possibly a PCSK9 inhibitor.

In patients with a CK level <4×ULN, monitor CK and symptoms every 6 weeks. If the discomfort persists, stop the statin. If symptoms resolve after 2 to 4 weeks, you can try another statin while monitoring muscle aches and CK activity.

If CK measurement is performed in a patient with no muscle symptoms and the level is ≥4×ULN (and <10×ULN), you can continue statin treatment if the CK concentration is monitored.

2. Ezetimibe should be used primarily in combination with a statin in patients with significant hypercholesterolemia to achieve target LDL-C levels. Ezetimibe may be useful as monotherapy in patients with intolerance of statins, but it has lower effectiveness.

3. Bile acid sequestrants (resins): Cholestyramine, colestipol, colesevelam; these are used as monotherapy in patients with contraindications to or intolerance of statins and in combination treatment when the efficacy of statins is suboptimal. Colesevelam is used in pregnant women.

Contraindications: High serum TG levels (>5.6 mmol/L [500 mg/dL] or, according to some experts, >3.4 mmol/L [300 mg/dL]).

Adverse effects: Troublesome gastrointestinal symptoms, including constipation, eructation (belching), abdominal pain, flatulence (except for colesevelam); malabsorption of fat-soluble vitamins and other drugs, such as β-blockers, thiazide diuretics, thyroxine, digoxin, and oral anticoagulants. All other drugs should be administered 1 hour before or 4 hours after a bile acid sequestrant.

4. Inhibitors of PCSK9: Evolocumab and alirocumab (subcutaneous injection once every 2-4 weeks). Generally the absolute benefit is proportional to cholesterol lowering◉; the major limitation is high cost of medications. Indications include:

1) Homozygous FH or heterozygous FH with high LDL-C levels despite using a statin at the maximum tolerated dose.

2) Very high cardiovascular risk in patients who have not reached the target LDL-C level despite using a statin at the maximum tolerated dose in combination with ezetimibe. Threshold serum LDL-C concentrations in qualifying for the initiation of a PCSK9 inhibitor:

   a) In patients with atherosclerotic CVD without additional risk factors: >3.6 mmol/L (140 mg/dL).

   b) In patients with atherosclerotic CVD with additional risk factors: >2.6 mmol/L (100 mg/dL).

   c) In patients with FH without additional risk factors: >4.5 mmol/L (180 mg/dL).

   d) In patients with FH with additional risk factors: >3.6 mmol/L (140 mg/dL).

5. Lomitapide (inhibitor of the microsomal TG transfer protein in hepatocytes): Usually authorized for reimbursement for homozygous FH treatment, which is very rare. Treatment should be conducted in specialized centers.

Other Approaches

LDL-C apheresis (extracorporeal removal of LDL-C) in homozygotic FH (TC usually 18-31 mmol/L) or severe heterozygotic FH in patients with CVD. The procedure is repeated every 2 weeks and the patient should be also treated with high-dose potent statins (eg, atorvastatin 80 mg/d or rosuvastatin 40 mg/d). It is a rare treatment conducted in specialized centers only.

12.3. Severe Hypertriglyceridemia

➡ ETIOLOGY AND PATHOGENESIS

Classification and etiology of severe hypertriglyceridemia:

1) **Type V hyperlipoproteinemia**: A combination of genetic, demographic, and clinical factors. Causes include obesity, diabetes mellitus, untreated hypothyroidism, HIV infection, lipodystrophy, anorexia, Cushing syndrome, sarcoidosis, systemic lupus erythematosus, alcohol consumption, and certain drugs (oral estrogen, glucocorticoids, protease inhibitors, hydrochlorothiazide, nonselective β-blockers, retinoic acid, tamoxifen, raloxifene, cyclosporine [INN ciclosporin], sirolimus).

2) **Familial chylomicronemia syndrome**: Genetic (type I hyperlipoproteinemia according to the Fredrickson classification).

Type V hyperlipoproteinemia includes fasting chylomicronemia and high very low-density lipoprotein (VLDL) levels. The very rare type I hyperlipoproteinemia does not predispose to atherosclerosis, as chylomicrons are too large to penetrate the arterial wall. Nevertheless, there is still an increased risk of cardiovascular disease.

➡ CLINICAL FEATURES AND DIAGNOSIS

Clinical symptoms of severe hypertriglyceridemia with the presence of chylomicrons: Abdominal pain, acute pancreatitis.

Lipid profile: High TG levels, usually >11.3 mmol/L (1000 mg/dL). Low-density lipoprotein cholesterol (LDL-C) levels are low, whereas total cholesterol may be high, depending on the cholesterol content of chylomicrons and in type V hyperlipoproteinemia also of VLDL.

Chylomicronemia is usually an incidental diagnosis, which is prompted either by the occurrence of acute pancreatitis or by finding turbid plasma in a fasting patient or high serum TG levels in routine laboratory tests. The diagnosis is confirmed by identifying **flotation of chylomicrons** in the patient's serum left overnight at 4°C. If chylomicrons are present, a creamy supernatant of varying thickness (depending on the concentration of chylomicrons) is observed. Under the fatty supernatant, the serum is transparent in patients with type I hyperlipoproteinemia and turbid in patients with type V hyperlipoproteinemia.

→ TREATMENT

The main goal of treatment is prevention of acute pancreatitis.

1. A very low-fat diet (<10% of daily caloric requirements covered by fats), including both saturated and unsaturated fats. Additionally, reduce the intake of carbohydrates, particularly simple carbohydrates.

2. Abstinence from alcohol.

3. Fibrates (→Chapter 3.12.1).

4. Statins are used after lowering TG levels if the LDL-C target level is not reached.

13. Myocarditis

→ DEFINITION, ETIOLOGY, PATHOGENESIS

Myocarditis is an inflammatory process involving cardiomyocytes, connective tissue, blood vessels, and sometimes also the pericardium. In the majority of cases etiologic agents cannot be identified. Apart from de novo infection, myocarditis can also be caused by reactivation of a latent infection.

Causes:

1) Viral infection (the most frequent cause; etiologic factors include parvovirus B19 [the most common etiologic factor of acute myocarditis with features similar to acute coronary syndrome, including diffuse ST-segment elevations], human herpesvirus type 6, coxsackievirus B, adenoviruses, other herpesviruses); bacteria (*Borrelia burgdorferi*, *Mycobacterium tuberculosis*, pneumococci, staphylococci, *Haemophilus* spp, *Salmonella* spp, *Legionella* spp), rickettsiae, mycoplasma, chlamydia, fungi (eg, *Candida* spp); protozoa (eg, *Toxoplasma gondii*, *Entamoeba histolytica*); parasites (eg, *Trichinella spiralis*).

2) Factors causing autoimmune reactions to allergens (tetanus toxin, vaccines, drugs), allogenic antigens (rejection of a heart transplant), autoantigens (systemic connective tissue diseases, eg, systemic lupus erythematosus; celiac disease).

3) Drugs and toxins: Antibiotics, antimycobacterial agents, antiepileptic agents, nonsteroidal anti-inflammatory drugs (NSAIDs), diuretics, sulfonylureas, methyldopa, amitriptyline, clozapine, heavy metals, cocaine, excess catecholamines (pheochromocytoma), ionizing radiation, sodium azide, insect and snake venoms.

→ CLINICAL FEATURES AND NATURAL HISTORY

1. Symptoms: Dyspnea caused by heart failure, chest pain caused by myocardial ischemia or coexistent pericarditis, palpitations.

2. Signs: Features of heart failure, pericarditis, peripheral embolism (this may be the presenting symptom).

3. Manifestations characteristic for specific types of myocarditis:

1) **Acute myocarditis:** History of a recent viral infection. Prodromal symptoms characteristic of the infection (involving the upper respiratory or gastrointestinal tract) precede cardiac symptoms by several days or weeks. Myocarditis may mimic acute coronary syndrome with elevated troponin levels and normal results of coronary angiography; it is usually caused by adenovirus or parvovirus B19.

2) **Eosinophilic myocarditis:** Rash and peripheral eosinophilia. The most severe type (acute necrotizing eosinophilic myocarditis) can cause fulminant heart failure.

3) **Giant cell myocarditis:** Most frequently features of heart failure, including fulminant heart failure and cardiogenic shock. Arrhythmias, including ventricular tachyarrhythmias, as well as heart block are also commonly noted.

4. Classification of myocarditis based on its course:

1) **Fulminant myocarditis:** A sudden and clearly defined onset of the disease with rapidly developing heart failure, which may even progress to cardiogenic shock. Myocardial dysfunction resolves spontaneously or (less frequently) leads to death.

2) **Acute myocarditis:** A less clearly defined onset. In some patients left ventricular (LV) dysfunction may progress to dilated cardiomyopathy.

3) **Subacute or chronic myocarditis:** Progressive heart failure as in dilated cardiomyopathy.

→ DIAGNOSIS

Diagnostic Tests

1. Laboratory tests: Increased erythrocyte sedimentation rate (ESR) (in 70% of patients); leukocytosis with neutrophilia (in 50% of patients); severe eosinophilia in the majority of patients with myocarditis in the course of parasitic infections, systemic vasculitides, or hypereosinophilic syndrome; elevated serum creatine kinase MB subunit (CK-MB) and cardiac troponin levels. Elevated CK levels are usually found in patients with acute or fulminant myocarditis or patients with acute exacerbation of myocarditis.

2. Electrocardiography (ECG) is usually abnormal; however, ECG features are typically nonspecific. Most frequent findings include diffuse ST-T changes, ventricular and supraventricular arrhythmias, and atrioventricular conduction abnormalities, as well as Q waves, which are less frequent than in the case of myocardial infarction (MI).

3. Echocardiography is useful in the identification of patients with fulminant myocarditis, who usually have a nondilated LV with increased thickness and severe global hypokinesis. Other features in myocarditis can include regional wall motion abnormalities and preserved ejection fraction with diastolic dysfunction. The progression of heart failure is associated with features similar to dilated cardiomyopathy.

4. Magnetic resonance imaging (MRI) reveals myocardial edema and a pattern of late gadolinium enhancement characteristic for myocarditis. MRI may also be helpful to exclude inflammatory and infiltrative etiologies, such as sarcoidosis, which has a characteristic pattern of patchy infiltration.

5. Endomyocardial biopsy is usually reserved for patients with life-threatening presentations, including cardiogenic shock with recurrent ventricular arrhythmias. In these situations biopsy may differentiate between specific etiologies of myocarditis, such as giant cell, lymphocytic, or eosinophilic myocarditis. If a diagnosis of giant cell or eosinophilic myocarditis is made, it helps guide immunosuppressive therapy to possibly reverse the underlying etiology.

Diagnostic Criteria

Acute myocarditis should be suspected in young individuals with a sudden onset of heart failure, persistent arrhythmia or conduction disturbances, or with clinical features of MI accompanied by normal results of coronary angiography. In patients with symptoms of congestive heart failure and unclear onset of the disease, other causes of dilated cardiomyopathy must be excluded. The diagnosis of myocarditis is usually made based on a combination of the clinical presentation, laboratory testing, ECG, imaging studies (echocardiography, cardiac catheterization, and MRI), and, in some instances, endomyocardial biopsy.

Criteria for the clinical diagnosis of myocarditis (based on the 2013 European Society of Cardiology position statement):

1) Clinical presentations:
   a) Acute chest pain, pericarditic or pseudoischemic.
   b) New-onset (≤3 months) or worsening of dyspnea at rest or with exercise, and/or fatigue.
   c) Subacute or chronic (>3 months) dyspnea at rest or with exercise, and/or fatigue.
   d) Palpitation, and/or unexplained arrhythmia, and/or syncope, and/or aborted sudden cardiac death.
   e) Unexplained cardiogenic shock.

2) Diagnostic test criteria:
   a) Newly abnormal ECG (atrioventricular block or fascicular block, ST-segment elevation, T-wave inversion, ventricular tachycardia or fibrillation, asystole, atrial fibrillation, reduced R-wave height, intraventricular conduction delay [widened QRS], abnormal Q waves, low voltage, frequent premature beats, supraventricular tachycardia).
   b) Elevated levels of troponin T or troponin I.
   c) Functional and structural abnormalities on cardiac imaging (echocardiography, angiography, or cardiac MRI): New, otherwise unexplained LV and/or right ventricular structure and function abnormalities (including an incidental finding in apparently asymptomatic patients): regional wall motion or global systolic or diastolic function abnormality.
   d) Tissue characterization by cardiac MRI: Edema or late gadolinium enhancement typical for myocarditis.

Myocarditis is clinically suspected if ≥1 clinical presentations and ≥1 diagnostic test criteria are found in a patient with excluded coronary artery disease or excluded other conditions that may cause similar symptoms (such as valve disease, congenital heart disease, hyperthyroidism). The higher the number of fulfilled criteria, the stronger the suspicion. In asymptomatic patients not fulfilling any clinical criteria, the presence of ≥2 diagnostic criteria is required (criteria 2a-2d) for the diagnosis of myocarditis.

Differential Diagnosis

Acute MI, sepsis, acute mitral regurgitation, tachycardia-induced cardiomyopathy and other causes of dilated cardiomyopathy, other causes of heart failure.

➡ TREATMENT

Symptomatic Treatment

1. General measures:

1) **Restricted physical activity**, especially in the case of fever and other symptoms of systemic infection or features of heart failure.
2) **Restricted alcohol intake**.
3) **Avoidance of NSAIDs** (these may worsen myocarditis, particularly during the first 2 weeks of viral infection).

2. In patients with chest pain and generalized ST-T changes suggestive of ischemia, you may use **β-blockers** or **amlodipine** in low doses (to avoid lowering systemic blood pressure) as antianginals. In patients with mild systolic LV dysfunction, use **angiotensin-converting enzyme inhibitors (ACEIs)**.

3. Treatment of severe ventricular arrhythmia: β-Blockers and antiarrhythmic agents may be used. However, short-acting β-blockers (eg, esmolol) are preferred over longer-acting β-blockers in the case of refractory ventricular arrhythmias because of the concern for worsening end-organ perfusion from their negative inotropic effect during a low-output shock state. In patients with **bradyarrhythmias** temporary cardiac pacing may be justified.

4. Treatment of heart failure: Standard management (→Chapter 3.8). In patients with fulminant myocarditis, restriction of physical activity, extracorporeal membrane oxygenation, and in some cases ventricular assist devices are used; the patients should be urgently transferred to a center capable of mechanical circulatory support.

5. Heart transplantation in patients in whom all other treatment modalities have been ineffective or patients with severe heart failure.

Treatment of the Underlying Condition

1. Antimicrobial treatment is feasible in some viral infections, for instance, with herpes simplex virus, and in infections caused by other pathogens (eg, *Borrelia* spp).

2. Immunosuppressive treatment is effective in patients with myocarditis caused by systemic connective tissue diseases, sarcoidosis, hypereosinophilic syndrome, or in giant cell myocarditis.

3. Discontinuation of the offending drug with or without concomitant glucocorticoid treatment in patients with myocarditis caused by drug hypersensitivity.

➡ PROGNOSIS

The majority of patients with acute or fulminant myocarditis recover completely. In a small proportion of cases, a subclinical inflammatory process persists, leading to the development of dilated cardiomyopathy. The prognosis is poor in patients with subacute myocarditis; it is better in patients with a higher baseline LV ejection fraction and shorter duration of the disease. Adverse prognostic factors include New York Heart Association (NYHA) class III/IV heart failure at diagnosis and focal late gadolinium enhancement on MRI.

14. Pericarditis

➡ DEFINITION, ETIOLOGY, PATHOGENESIS

Pericardial syndromes refer to diseases that involve the pericardium. These include pericarditis, pericardial effusion, cardiac tamponade, pericardial masses, and constrictive pericarditis.

Pericarditis is the most common pericardial syndrome worldwide. It refers to an inflammatory process involving the pericardial sac.

Causes:

1) **Infectious:**

a) **Viral**: Parvovirus B19, Ebstein-Barr Virus, echovirus, coxsackievirus, cytomegalovirus, adenovirus.

Table 14-1. Course of acute pericarditis

	Viral	Bacterial	Tuberculous	Autoimmune
Spontaneous remission	Frequent	Never	Never	Rare
Relapse rates	30%-50%	Rare	Frequent	Frequent (>25%)
Mortality rates in untreated disease	Depends on type of virus and occurrence of cardiac tamponade	100%	85%	Death in case of untreated cardiac tamponade
Constriction	Rare	Frequent	Frequent	Rare

b) **Bacterial**: *Mycobacterium tuberculosis*, *Coxiella burnetii*, *Borrelia burgdorferi*. Other bacterial causes are rare.

c) **Fungal**: *Histoplasma* spp, *Aspergillus* spp, *Blastomyces* spp, *Candida* spp. Fungal causes are rarely seen in immunocompetent patients.

2) **Noninfectious**:

a) **Inflammatory**: Post–myocardial infarction (MI) pericarditis (early after MI), postpericardiotomy syndrome after cardiac surgery.

b) **Autoimmune diseases**: Dressler syndrome (post–cardiac injury syndrome weeks after MI), systemic lupus erythematosus, rheumatoid arthritis, scleroderma, sarcoidosis, Sjögren syndrome, Behçet syndrome, other systemic vasculitides. Rarely pericarditis can be seen in familial Mediterranean fever and tumor necrosis factor receptor–associated periodic syndrome.

c) **Neoplastic**: Primary tumors (rare; most frequently pericardial mesothelioma) or secondary tumors (common; most frequently lung cancer, breast cancer, lymphoma, melanoma).

d) **Metabolic**: Uremia, hypothyroidism (myxedema), anorexia nervosa, hypoadrenalism.

e) **Traumatic and iatrogenic**: Direct injury (penetrating thoracic injury, esophageal perforation); indirect injury (nonpenetrating thoracic injury, radiation injury); and other iatrogenic injury due to complications related to coronary percutaneous intervention, pacemaker lead insertion, or radiofrequency ablation.

f) **Drug-related** (rare): Procainamide, hydralazine, phenytoin, antineoplastic drugs (eg, doxorubicin, daunorubicin, cytarabine, fluorouracil, cyclophosphamide), penicillins, streptokinase, para-aminosalicylic acid, amiodarone, cyclosporine (INN ciclosporin), thiazide diuretics, granulocyte and macrophage colony-stimulating factors, tumor necrosis factor α inhibitors.

The mechanism for pericardial fluid accumulation in malignancy may be related to pericardial inflammation caused directly by cancer cells in the pericardium or as a consequence of treatment (ie, certain chemotherapies or radiation) or obstruction of lymphatic drainage of pericardial fluid by malignant deposits.

→ **CLINICAL FEATURES AND NATURAL HISTORY**

Natural history of acute pericarditis depends on etiology (→Table 14-1). Pericarditis can be **acute**, **incessant** (>4-6 weeks but <3 months with no remission), **chronic** (>3 months), or **recurrent** (recurring after an episode of acute pericarditis and following an asymptomatic period lasting ≥4-6 weeks; recurrence usually takes place within 18-24 months).

Adverse prognostic factors:

1) **Major**: Fever >38°C, subacute onset, large pericardial effusion, cardiac tamponade, lack of response to high-dose acetylsalicylic acid (ASA) or non-steroidal anti-inflammatory drugs (NSAIDs) for ≥1 week.

2) **Minor**: Myopericarditis, immunosuppression, trauma, oral anticoagulant therapy.

Patients with ≥1 of the above adverse prognostic factors, either major or minor, are considered to be at **high risk** of complications. Patients at **moderate risk** have no risk factors but their response to NSAIDs is incomplete. Patients at **low risk** have no risk factors and a good response to anti-inflammatory treatment.

1. Symptoms: In acute pericarditis symptoms include pleuritic and positional chest pain that is worse with inspiration and recumbency (the key symptom; →Chapter 1.1). This may be accompanied by dry cough and dyspnea and preceded by low-grade or high-grade fever (usually <39°C), malaise, arthralgia, and myalgia. Chronic pericarditis is characterized by chest pain, palpitations, loss of appetite, and sometimes weight loss.

2. Signs: Pericardial friction rub (transient, not always present; most easily audible during held expiration with the patient seated and leaning slightly forward). Cardiac tamponade may occur in patients with acute pericarditis. Features of myocarditis may be present in patients with infectious causes of pericarditis.

→ DIAGNOSIS

Diagnostic Tests

1. Laboratory tests: Elevations in erythrocyte sedimentation rate (ESR) and C-reactive protein (CRP) levels, less frequently leukocytosis (in patients with bacterial pericarditis), and sometimes elevated levels of cardiac troponins if associated with myocarditis (perimyocarditis).

2. Electrocardiography (ECG): Generalized/diffuse upsloping ST-segment elevations and PR-segment depressions (except for lead aVR, where ST-segment depression and PR-segment elevation is seen in acute pericarditis). The evolution of pericarditis on ECG follows 4 stages: diffuse ST-elevation (stage 1); normalization of the ST segment over a few days (stage 2); T-wave inversions (stage 3); return to normal baseline ECG (stage 4). No pathologic Q-wave formation or precordial lead R-wave disappearance is observed.

3. Chest radiographs: In patients with pericardial effusions >250 mL, the cardiac silhouette may be enlarged ("water bottle" configuration).

4. Echocardiography: Images may be normal. A pericardial effusion may be present. Transthoracic echocardiography is recommended in all patients with suspected acute pericarditis to assess for the presence of pericardial effusion and echocardiographic features of increased intrapericardial pressures or overt pericardial tamponade.

5. Computed tomography (CT): CT may be useful to detect pericardial calcification or thickening. Nongated CT scans generally overestimate the size of pericardial effusion (it is normally measured at end diastole but nongated CT obtains pictures throughout cardiac cycle).

6. Analysis of pericardial fluid: Evaluation of pericardial fluid requires pericardiocentesis.

7. Pericardial biopsy: Histologic examination of biopsy specimens is helpful in the diagnosis of pericarditis caused by neoplastic or inflammatory processes.

Diagnostic Criteria

Diagnosis is based on clinical features and results of diagnostic tests, particularly echocardiography.

Acute pericarditis is diagnosed in patients fulfilling ≥2 out of 4 criteria:

1) Chest pain with features typical of pericarditis (ie, pleuritic, worse when lying flat).

2) Pericardial friction rub on auscultation.

3) New-onset widespread/diffuse ST-segment elevation, PR-segment depression on ECG (except for lead aVR, which is opposite, ie, ST depression and PR elevation), or both.

4) Pericardial effusion on echocardiography (new-onset or worsening).

Further supportive findings of acute pericarditis include elevation of inflammatory markers (ESR or CRP) or imaging features suggestive of pericardial inflammation shown on CT or magnetic resonance imaging (MRI).

To confirm viral etiology (rarely needed), consider studies (histologic, cytologic, immunohistologic, molecular) of pericardial fluid and pericardial/epicardial biopsy. If diagnosis is uncertain, use the term "presumed viral pericarditis." Routine viral serologic studies are not recommended except if HIV or hepatitis C virus is suspected to be the cause.

Malignancy as a cause of pericarditis or pericardial effusion is confirmed on the basis of cytology studies of pericardial fluid, histologic examination of pericardial specimens, elevated levels of tumor markers in pericardial fluid (high concentrations of carcinoembryonic antigen with low adenosine deaminase levels are typical for malignant effusions compared with those caused by tuberculosis [TB]), and identification of the primary tumor in the case of metastatic disease.

⇨ TREATMENT

1. Patients at high or moderate risk of complications (→Clinical Features and Natural History, above) are sometimes hospitalized to establish the etiology and monitor the course of disease. Low-risk patients may be treated on an outpatient basis with evaluation of response to anti-inflammatory treatment after approximately 1 week.

2. Management algorithm: →Figure 14-1.

General Measures

1. First-line agents in acute pericarditis:

1) **ASA** or **NSAIDs** with concomitant gastric protection (proton pump inhibitors). Dosage: →Table 14-2.

2) Oral **colchicine** 0.5 to 0.6 mg (European tablets are 0.5 mg, North American tablets are 0.6 mg) bid for 3 months usually in combination with a shorter course of ASA or an NSAID. The dose may be given once daily in patients weighing <70 kg or with gastrointestinal intolerance. Compared with placebo, colchicine reduces the risk of recurrence, improves remission rates, and decreases hospitalization rates.⊘●

2. Glucocorticoids: Low doses are used. Dosage: →Table 14-2. Glucocorticoids are indicated when treatment with ASA or NSAIDs is contraindicated or ineffective and in situations where infection has been excluded (or is very unlikely). They are also used in patients who have specific indications for glucocorticoid treatment (eg, those with autoimmune disease, some postpericardiotomy syndrome patients, pregnant women). If infection cannot be excluded, particularly of bacterial etiology (including TB), do not use glucocorticoids. Colchicine is usually added to glucocorticoids.

3. Restriction of strenuous physical activity: In patients with acute pericarditis, strenuous physical activity should be restricted until symptoms, ECG findings, and elevated inflammatory markers (ESR or CRP) resolve. If there is evidence of concomitant myocarditis, at least 6 months of strenuous exercise restriction is advised, based on expert recommendations.

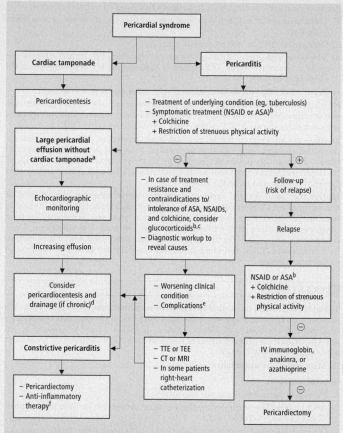

⊕ Symptoms resolving. ⊖ Symptoms persisting.

a Markers of inflammation not elevated, cause unknown. If markers of inflammation are elevated, treat as in pericarditis.

b Consider low-dose glucocorticoids in case of steroid-responsive diseases or in case of contraindications to or intolerance of ASA, NSAIDs, or colchicine.

c After an infectious cause has been excluded.

d Persisting >3 months.

e Hemodynamic instability, obstructive shock leading to signs of right-sided heart failure or volume overload, or unexplained cardiovascular symptoms.

f In patients with features of inflammation.

ASA, acetylsalicylic acid; CT, computed tomography; IV, intravenous; MRI, magnetic resonance imaging; NSAID, nonsteroidal anti-inflammatory drug; TEE, transesophageal echocardiography, TTE, transthoracic echocardiography.

Figure 14-1. Management algorithm in pericarditis. *Based on the 2015 European Society of Cardiology guidelines.*

Table 14-2. Typical dosage of anti-inflammatory agents in acute and recurrent pericarditis

Agent	Dosage	
	Acute pericarditis	Recurrent pericarditis
ASA	650-1000 mg every 6-8 h[a,b]	500-1000 mg every 6-8 h (1.5-4 g/d)[b,c]
Ibuprofen	600-800 mg every 8 h[a,d]	600 mg every 8 h (1200-2400 mg)[b,c]
Colchicine	0.5-0.6 mg (once daily[e] or bid[f])[g,h]	0.5-0.6 mg (bid[f] or once daily[e,i])[h,j]
Indomethacin	–	25-50 mg every 8 h[c,k,l]
Glucocorticoids	Doses depend on agents used[m,n]	

[a] For 1-2 weeks.

[b] Decrease the dose by 250-500 mg every 1-2 weeks. In case of recurrent pericarditis in patients showing more resistance to treatment, you may consider more gradual and longer tapering of doses down to discontinuation.

[c] For weeks or months.

[d] Decrease the dose by 200-400 mg every 1-2 weeks. In case of recurrent pericarditis in patients showing more resistance to treatment, you may consider more gradual and longer tapering of doses down to discontinuation.

[e] In patients <70 kg.

[f] In patients ≥70 kg.

[g] For 3 months. Note that in North America colchicine is only available in 0.6 mg tablets, whereas the 0.5 mg dose is available in Europe.

[h] Tapering down is not necessary; however, you may decrease the dose by 0.5 mg every other day in patients <70 kg or by 0.5 mg once a day in the last weeks of treatment in patients ≥70 kg.

[i] In patients who do not tolerate higher doses.

[j] For ≥6 months.

[k] Start from low doses and titrate them up to avoid headache and dizziness.

[l] Decrease the dose by 25 mg every 1-2 weeks. In patients resistant to treatment, you may consider more gradual and longer tapering of doses down to discontinuation.

[m] The starting dose of prednisone is 0.25-0.5 mg/kg/d. A dose of 25 mg of prednisone is equivalent to 20 mg of methylprednisolone. Higher doses should be avoided except for selected patients (higher doses are then used over a few days and rapidly tapered down to 25 mg/d).

[n] Prednisone dose may be tapered down (particularly <25 mg/d) when symptoms have resolved and CRP normalized.

Based on Eur Heart J. 2015;36(42):2921-64.

ASA, acetylsalicylic acid; bid, twice a day; CRP, C-reactive protein.

Treatment of Specific Types of Pericarditis

1. Purulent pericarditis: Open pericardial drainage through the substernal pericardiotomy approach with 0.9% saline irrigation and appropriate IV antimicrobial treatment. Consider intrapericardial administration of fibrinolytic agents and pericardiectomy in patients with significant adhesions, loculated or thick purulent effusion, recurrent cardiac tamponade, persistent infection, or disease progressing to constrictive pericarditis.

2. Tuberculous pericarditis: Administration of 4 anti-TB drugs is necessary (→Chapter 13.18.2). In patients not residing in endemic areas, empiric anti-TB treatment is not recommended if the diagnosis of TB pericarditis has not been confirmed. Empiric anti-TB treatment is recommended in residents of endemic areas with confirmed exudative pericardial effusion once other causes have been excluded. Some authors recommend addition of glucocorticoids: prednisone 1 to 2 mg/kg/d for 5 to 7 days with the dose gradually tapered down to discontinuation over 6 to 8 weeks.

3. Uremic pericarditis: Increasing the frequency of dialysis usually leads to resolution of symptoms within 1 to 2 weeks. In patients with persistent symptoms, use NSAIDs (with caution in patients with severe renal injury) and glucocorticoids. In patients with large pericardial effusions not responding to adequate treatment, use intrapericardial glucocorticoids. Colchicine is contraindicated in patients with severe renal failure.

4. Pericarditis in patients with systemic connective tissue disease or sarcoidosis resolves with adequate treatment of the underlying condition. Intrapericardial glucocorticoids are not routinely recommended but may be considered in selected cases.

5. Post-MI pericarditis: ASA 650 mg every 4 hours for 2 to 5 days or ibuprofen (dosage: →Table 14-2). Usually ASA is preferred, as these patients will require antiplatelet therapy following MI.

6. Postpericardiotomy syndrome: NSAIDs or ASA in the same doses as in presumed viral pericarditis with colchicine for several weeks or months (even after resolution of pericardial effusion). If ineffective, perform pericardiocentesis combined with intrapericardial administration of glucocorticoids and oral glucocorticoids for 3 to 6 months.

7. Neoplastic pericarditis: In patients with chemosensitive cancer use systemic chemotherapy. In patients with large effusions who are symptomatic, pericardiocentesis may be necessary. In patients with recurrent effusions, consider administering an intrapericardial sclerosing agent (eg, tetracycline, bleomycin) or a nonsclerosing cytotoxic agent (eg, cisplatin; this is particularly effective in pericarditis caused by non–small cell lung cancer). Pericardial irradiation controls neoplastic effusions in >90% of cases of radiation-sensitive cancers (eg, lymphoma, leukemia) but it may by itself cause myocarditis, pericarditis, or both. Palliative treatment options include pericardiotomy or creation of a pericardial window.

8. Radiation pericarditis: Glucocorticoids. Dosage: →Table 14-2.

9. Pericarditis in patients with hypothyroidism: Treatment of the underlying condition.

10. Recurrent pericarditis: First-line agents are (1) **ASA or NSAIDs** until complete resolution of symptoms, and (2) **colchicine** for 6 months in combination. Alternatively, low-dose **glucocorticoids** may be used as in acute pericarditis (→above). Dosage: →Table 14-2. The use of glucocorticoids is only recommended in patients who are refractory to NSAIDs or ASA and colchicine therapy. Sometimes colchicine treatment should be prolonged, depending on clinical response. Regularly perform follow-up measurements of serum CRP levels to establish the duration of therapy and response to treatment. When CRP levels normalize, gradually taper down the dose of anti-inflammatory medications while monitoring symptoms and CRP levels. Do not discontinue all agents at the same time. If symptoms of pericarditis recur in the period of tapering treatment, do not increase the dose of glucocorticoids and use maximal doses of ASA or NSAIDs instead (usually in divided doses every 8 hours) in addition to colchicine. Use analgesics for pain control. In glucocorticoid-dependent recurrent pericarditis in patients not responding to colchicine, consider IV immunoglobulins, anakinra, or azathioprine (this requires specialist consultation).

→ FOLLOW-UP

In patients with recurrent or chronic pericarditis, as well as in patients after surgical procedures on the pericardium, echocardiographic monitoring is indicated for early detection of cardiac tamponade or constrictive pericarditis.

→ COMPLICATIONS

1. Cardiac tamponade.

2. Constrictive pericarditis: A rare but serious complication of chronic pericarditis (particularly frequent in patients with bacterial or TB pericarditis), which is characterized by loss of elasticity of the pericardium.

Symptoms: Progressive weakness, chest pain, palpitations; signs of chronic systemic venous congestion (jugular vein distension, absence of jugular vein collapse during inspiration [Kussmaul sign], ascites, hepatic enlargement and pulsation, peripheral edema); early diastolic heart sound (pericardial knock); hypotension with low pulse pressure.

Diagnosis: Diagnosis is based on imaging studies: chest radiographs (revealing pericardial calcifications, atrial enlargement, pleural effusion), CT, MRI, and echocardiography. Intracardiac pressure measurements may also be performed. ECG may reveal low-amplitude QRS complexes, generalized T-wave inversions or T-wave flattening, widening of P waves, sometimes atrial fibrillation, atrioventricular conduction disturbances, or intraventricular conduction disturbances. However, ECG may also be normal.

Differential diagnosis: Restrictive cardiomyopathy. Differentiation is based on echocardiography (including tissue Doppler echocardiography), CT, MRI, and cardiac catheterization.

Treatment: Pericardiectomy.

15. Prevention of Cardiovascular Diseases

→ DEFINITION

Cardiovascular disease (CVD) prevention is based on the assessment or identification and modification or elimination of cardiovascular risk factors.

Modifiable cardiovascular risk factors:

1) Atherogenic diet.
2) Smoking.
3) Physical inactivity.
4) High blood pressure.
5) Dyslipidemia: Elevated serum low-density lipoprotein cholesterol (LDL-C) levels, low high-density lipoprotein cholesterol (HDL-C) levels, elevated triglyceride (TG) levels.
6) Impaired glucose tolerance or diabetes mellitus.
7) High body mass index (BMI).

Nonmodifiable cardiovascular risk factors:

1) Age (men ≥45 years, women ≥55 years).
2) Family history of early (<55 years in men and <65 years in women) ischemic heart disease (IHD) or atherosclerosis of other arteries.
3) Chronic kidney disease (CKD).
4) Chronic inflammatory disease (eg, systemic lupus erythematosus, rheumatoid arthritis).
5) Ethnicity (eg, South Asian).
6) Menopause at an age <40 years.
7) History of preeclampsia.

Table 15-1. Framingham risk score: estimation of the 10-year risk of cardiovascular disease

Risk factor	Risk points			
	Men		Women	
Age				
35-39	2		2	
40-44	5		4	
45-49	7		5	
50-54	8		7	
55-59	10		8	
60-64	11		9	
65-69	12		10	
70-74	14		11	
≥75	15		12	
HDL-C (mmol/L)				
>1.60	−2			
1.30-1.60	−1			
1.20-1.29	0			
0.90-1.19	1			
<0.90	2			
Total cholesterol (mmol/L)				
4.10-5.19	1		1	
5.20-6.19	2		3	
6.20-7.20	3		4	
>7.20	4		5	
Systolic blood pressure (mm Hg)				
	Untreated	Treated	Untreated	Treated
<120	−2	0	−3	−1
120-129	0	2	0	2
130-139	1	3	1	3
140-149	2	4	2	5
150-159	2	4	2	5
>160	3	5	5	7
Smoking status				
Smoker	4		3	

Interpretation
10-year risk of CVD is assumed to be:
High if risk is ≥20%;
Intermediate if risk is 10%-19%;
Low if risk is <10%.
For women:
High risk: ≥18 points
Intermediate risk: 13-17 points
For men:
High risk: ≥15 points
Intermediate risk: 11-14 points
Based on Circulation. 1998;97(18):1837-47 and Can J Cardiol. 2016;32(11):1263-1282.
CVD, cardiovascular disease; HDL-C, high-density lipoprotein cholesterol.

➔ RISK ASSESSMENT

The frequency of cardiovascular risk assessment should depend on the degree of risk and presence of borderline indications for treatment. It should be performed at least every 5 years.

In persons with no additional risk factors (such as CVD, diabetes mellitus, CKD, or a markedly expressed individual risk factor), the 10-year CVD risk assessment can be calculated using the Framingham risk score, which takes into account age, sex, systolic blood pressure (treated or untreated), HDL-C, and smoking status (→Table 15-1). Of note, there are many modifications of this risk score, some taking into account BMI or diabetes; see the official website of the Framingham Heart Study.

➔ PREVENTION

Prevention goals based on the Canadian Cardiovascular Society guidelines:

1) **Nonsmoking status**.
2) **Healthy diet** (minimizing intake of processed food, refined carbohydrates, trans fats, and unsaturated fats).
3) **Physical activity** reduces individual risk factors for cardiovascular disease; however, the absolute effect of physical activity on reducing the risk of developing CVD remains unclear.
4) **Body weight reduction**: Optimally maintain BMI within 20 to 25 kg/m^2 and waist circumference <94 cm in men and <80 cm in women. Recommend weight loss if waist circumference is >102 cm in men and >88 cm in women.
5) **Blood pressure <140/90 mm Hg** for all patients, possibly <130 mm Hg in those who tolerate treatment well. In patients with diabetes a target systolic blood pressure <130 and diastolic blood pressure <80 mm Hg is currently provided in clinical practice guidelines, including Hypertension Canada guidelines.
6) **LDL-C levels** depending on the risk category (→Table 12-2).
7) **Glycated hemoglobin (HbA$_{1c}$)** <7% in patients with type 2 diabetes. A less strict target can be used in frail patients and those at higher risk for developing hypoglycemia. A target of <6.5% has been recommended for patients with diabetic microvascular complications.
8) **Secondary prevention**: Note that similar treatment goals occur in the presence of certain clinical conditions (secondary prevention): atherosclerosis;

abdominal aortic aneurysm; diabetes mellitus at an age >40 years (type 1 diabetes at an age >30 years), of >15 years' duration, or with microvascular disease; CKD at an age >50 years (estimated glomerular filtration rate [eGFR] <60 mL/min/1.73 m^2 or albumin-to-creatinine ratio [ACR] >3 mg/mmol), LDL-C >5.0 mmol/L. Atherosclerosis is defined as acute coronary syndrome, stable angina, angiographically documented CAD, stroke, transient ischemic attack, or carotid or peripheral vascular disease. Patients with acute coronary syndrome within the last 3 months have lower treatment targets for LCD-C (1.8 mmol/L; →Table 12-2).

16. Shock

→ DEFINITION, ETIOLOGY, PATHOGENESIS

Shock is a life-threatening generalized form of acute circulatory failure associated with inadequate oxygen utilization by cells. In this state circulation is unable to deliver enough oxygen to meet the demands of tissues. As a result, the patient develops cellular dysoxia that is associated with a transition to anaerobic metabolism and subsequent lactate production. Although it is frequently accompanied by hypotension (reduction of blood pressure), in the early stages of shock—referred to as **compensated shock**—blood pressure may be normal or even elevated.

Etiology and Pathomechanisms

Shock is due to one or more often a combination of the following pathophysiologic mechanisms.

1. A decrease in the total blood volume (absolute hypovolemia), referred to as **hypovolemic shock**, which may result from:

1) **Loss of whole blood** due to an internal or external hemorrhage. This leads to **hemorrhagic shock**.

2) A **decrease in the plasma (effective circulating) volume** due to:

   a) Leakage of plasma to damaged tissues (trauma) or exudation from the skin surface (eg, burns, Lyell syndrome, Stevens-Johnson syndrome, exfoliative dermatitis).

   b) Reduction of the extracellular fluid volume (dehydration) because of reduced water intake (most frequently in the elderly [with hypodipsia] or incapacitated persons) or an increased loss of water and electrolytes via the gastrointestinal (GI) tract (diarrhea and vomiting), kidneys (osmotic diuresis in diabetic ketoacidosis or hyperglycemic hyperosmolar state, polyuria and excessive excretion of sodium in glucocorticoid and mineralocorticoid deficiencies, central or nephrogenic diabetes insipidus), or skin (fever, hyperthermia).

   c) Shifting of fluids into the third space, such as the intestinal lumen (ileus or intestinal obstruction) or less commonly to the serous cavities (eg, the peritoneum; this may lead to ascites).

   d) Increased vascular permeability in anaphylactic shock or septic shock.

2. Increased volume of the vascular bed, maldistribution of flow, or both, leading to relative hypovolemia with a potentially hyperkinetic state—**distributive shock**—due to vasodilation or peripheral shunting and reduction in the effective tissue blood flow. The main etiologies of distributive shock:

1) **Septic shock**.

2) **Anaphylactic shock**.

3) **Neurogenic shock**: Secondary to spinal cord injury, traumatic brain injury, stroke, brain edema, orthostatic hypotension (long-standing), or vasodilation caused by pain.

4) **Hormone-induced shock**: Secondary to acute adrenal insufficiency, thyroid storm, myxedema coma.

3. Cardiac dysfunction (usually secondary to acute myocardial dysfunction, arrhythmia, or valvular dysfunction) that causes decreased cardiac output due to loss of contractility or significant rhythm change. This leads to **cardiogenic shock**.

4. Impaired left ventricular (LV) filling due to compression of the heart secondary to cardiac tamponade, severely reduced venous return (eg, tension pneumothorax, abdominal compartment syndrome), intracardiac impairment of ventricular filling caused by heart tumors or intracardiac thrombi, or a sudden increase in cardiovascular resistance (pulmonary embolism, acute pulmonary hypertension in the course of acute respiratory failure). This leads to **obstructive shock**.

Consequences

1. Compensatory responses by the body in an attempt to maintain homeostasis. Importantly, their effectiveness usually declines with time.

1) Compensatory autonomic response and adrenaline release from the adrenal glands, which causes tachycardia and attempts to maintain central perfusion (this leads to constriction of precapillaries and veins in less essential organ vascular beds [first in the skin, then in muscles, later in visceral and renal circulation] and instead maintains perfusion to the vital organs, such as the heart and brain). In hypovolemic shock the deficient plasma volume is replaced by transudation of the intracellular fluid to the capillaries. In some cases of noncardiogenic shock, myocardial contractility (and sometimes also cardiac output) may increase. Hyperventilation and hyperglycemia can also occur as a result of increased sympathetic stimulation.

2) Stimulation of the renin-angiotensin-aldosterone system as well as secretion of antidiuretic hormone (ADH) and glucocorticoids, which all contribute to maintaining central perfusion and cause sodium and water retention.

3) Increased tissue oxygen uptake in response to low oxygen supply, which leads to increased deoxygenation of hemoglobin and decreased venous hemoglobin oxygen saturation (SvO_2).

2. Metabolic and electrolyte disturbances due to hypoxia:

1) Increased anaerobic metabolism and lactate production, leading to metabolic acidosis ($\rightarrow$Chapter 4.1.1).

2) Release of potassium, phosphate, and some intracellular proteins (lactate dehydrogenase [LDH], creatine kinase [CK], aspartate aminotransferase [AST], alanine aminotransferase [ALT]) to the extracellular fluid, increased sodium influx into the cells (due to impaired adenosine triphosphate synthesis). Both of these processes may lead to hyponatremia, hyperkalemia, and hyperphosphatemia.

3. Consequences of organ ischemia: Multiple organ dysfunction syndrome including acute kidney injury (prerenal azotemia), altered mental status (which may progress to coma), acute respiratory insufficiency (potentially leading to acute respiratory distress syndrome), acute liver failure, disseminated intravascular coagulation (DIC), GI bleeding (due to acute and erosive hemorrhagic gastropathy), gastric or duodenal stress ulcers, ischemic colitis, adynamic ileus, and penetration of microorganisms from the GI tract to the bloodstream.

→ CLINICAL FEATURES

1. Cardiovascular symptoms:

1) Tachycardia (in rare cases bradycardia may be seen, usually in the terminal phase before cardiac arrest).

2) Hypotension. This is traditionally defined as a drop in systolic blood pressure (SBP) <90 mm Hg, significant decrease in SBP (eg, by >40 mm Hg), or drop

in mean arterial pressure (MAP) <65-70 mm Hg. Decreased diastolic blood pressure (DBP) and resulting decreased MAP may precede a drop in SBP. (MAP is defined as approximately 1/3 of SBP plus 2/3 of DBP.) The early phases of shock may be accompanied by orthostatic hypotension alone or no hypotension at all.

3) A low-amplitude and slow-rising pulse (at SBP <60 mm Hg radial pulse is usually not palpable).

4) Reduced jugular vein filling (although this may be increased with comorbid cardiac tamponade, pulmonary embolism, or tension pneumothorax).

5) Chest pain.

6) Cardiac arrest (special attention is needed not to overlook pulseless electrical activity, which is undetected by electrocardiographic [ECG] monitoring alone).

2. Symptoms of organ hypoperfusion:

1) Skin: Usually pale, mottled, and cold, may be sweaty (in septic shock the skin is usually dry and warm; in dehydration, dry and hypoelastic); delayed capillary refill (after releasing pressure on a nail plate or peripheral soft tissue pallor disappears only after >2 seconds); cyanosis.

2) Central nervous system: Anxiety, restlessness, confusion, psychomotor agitation, somnolence, stupor, coma, focal neurologic deficits.

3) Kidneys: Oliguria or anuria and other symptoms of acute kidney injury.

4) Muscles: Weakness.

5) GI tract: Nausea, vomiting, flatulence, weak or no peristaltic sounds, bleeding.

6) Liver: Jaundice (a rare symptom, may occur late or after recovery from shock).

7) Respiratory system: Variable breathing patterns are possible. Initially, breaths may be shallow and rapid (in metabolic acidosis respiration may be slower but deeper, or even fast and deep [Kussmaul respirations]); subsequently, the respiratory rate may decrease and the patient may develop apnea. Acute respiratory failure with hypoxia (type I), inappropriate hypercapnia (type II), or both may occur.

3. Symptoms and signs of the underlying condition: Dehydration, bleeding, anaphylaxis, infection (sepsis), cardiovascular diseases, pulmonary embolism, tension pneumothorax, ileus, and other conditions.

The classically described triad of shock (hypotension, tachycardia, oliguria) may not be present in all patients.

→ DIAGNOSIS

The clinical diagnosis of shock based on signs, symptoms, and results of biochemical tests is usually straightforward, but establishing the cause of shock may be more difficult; sometimes this is possible on the basis of history (eg, fluid or blood loss, symptoms of infection or anaphylaxis) or physical examination (eg, signs of bleeding, dehydration, cardiac tamponade, or tension pneumothorax). When evaluating the possible etiologies of shock, it is also important to consider other causes of reduced oxygen supply and tissue hypoxia (anemia, respiratory insufficiency, poisonings with substances that inhibit blood oxygen transport and cellular oxygen utilization).

Diagnostic Tests

1. Cardiovascular investigations:

1) **Blood pressure measurements** (including use of invasive methods, eg, arterial cannulation).

2) **12-lead ECG** and continuous ECG monitoring looking for signs of arrhythmias, myocardial ischemia or infarction, or other heart diseases.

3) **Echocardiography** may be helpful in determining the cause of cardiogenic or obstructive shock (myocardial dysfunction, valvular dysfunction, cardiac tamponade; focused ultrasonography allows for the assessment of LV pressure and volume through direct and indirect measures). When hemodynamic assessment is needed, echocardiography may be preferable, given its noninvasive approach.

4) **Cardiac output (CO)** and **pulmonary capillary wedge pressure (PCWP)**: Measurements of CO and PCWP are sometimes performed in case of diagnostic uncertainties and treatment difficulties. Measurements of PCWP using a Swan-Ganz (pulmonary artery) catheter may be useful in the assessment of volume status and preload (LV filling), which is essential for differential diagnosis and ultimately for the therapeutic plan. PCWP reflects left atrial pressures and is an indirect indicator of LV end-systolic pressure; PCWP values of ~15 to 18 mm Hg indicate optimal LV filling. The Swan-Ganz catheter allows for the measurement of CO using the thermodilution method (other methods of CO measurements are also available). CO is reduced in cardiogenic and obstructive shock and usually increased in the initial phases of hypovolemic shock as well as in septic or anaphylactic shock. Of note, the evidence for efficacy of any invasive CO-measuring devices in terms of improving patient-important outcomes is lacking and therefore the use of Swan-Ganz catheters is usually reserved for complex patients who are not otherwise responding to initial therapy.

5) **Dynamic measures of volume status**: Measures of volume status such as pulse pressure variation (PPV), systolic pressure variation (SPV), stroke volume variation (SVV), passive leg raise, and inferior vena cava (IVC) collapsibility attempt to predict fluid responsiveness in patients with shock to guide fluid resuscitation. PPV, SPV, SVV, and IVC collapsibility reflect changes in hemodynamic measurements that accompany respiration-related fluctuations in intrathoracic pressure. Patients who are volume-responsive tend to have larger degrees of variation in hemodynamic measures during the respiratory cycle. These measurements have not gained widespread acceptance, possibly due to limitations such as lack of applicability; they are only useful in patients receiving full mechanical ventilation (no spontaneous breathing activity) and with no arrhythmias. Another limitation is that the sensitivity of the test is affected when tidal volumes <8 mL/kg of ideal body weight are used.

2. Laboratory tests of venous blood:

1) **Serum biochemical tests**:

a) Assessment of the effects of shock: Elevated levels of lactate, electrolyte disturbances (sodium and potassium levels); elevated levels of creatinine, urea/blood urea nitrogen (BUN), bilirubin, and glucose; elevated AST, ALT, CK, or LDH levels. We recommend measuring serum lactate levels in all patients with suspected shock and using the trend in lactate to guide, monitor, and assess the ongoing management of shock.◐◔

b) Elevated levels of cardiac troponins, creatine kinase MB subunit (CK-MB), or myoglobin may indicate acute myocardial infarction.

c) Elevated levels of natriuretic peptides (B-type natriuretic peptide [BNP] or N-terminal pro–B-type natriuretic peptide [NT-proBNP]) may indicate heart failure being either a cause or a consequence of shock.

2) **Complete blood count (CBC)**:

a) Hematocrit, hemoglobin concentration, and red blood cell count: These are reduced in hemorrhagic shock (except for the initial phase) and usually increased in other forms of hypovolemic shock.

b) White blood cell count: Neutrophilic leukocytosis or leukopenia in septic shock. Leukocytosis and increase in neutrophil counts may also be observed in other forms of shock (eg, hypovolemic). Eosinophilia may be present in some cases of anaphylaxis.

c) Platelet count: Thrombocytopenia is usually the first sign of DIC (most frequently developing in septic shock or after a major trauma), but it may also be a result of massive bleeding and packed red blood cells transfusions.

3) **Coagulation tests**: Prolonged prothrombin time (PT) and activated partial thromboplastin time (aPTT) as well as low fibrinogen levels may suggest DIC or result from posthemorrhagic or posttransfusion coagulopathy; sometimes prolonged PT and prolonged aPTT are manifestations of liver failure (either acute or chronic). Elevated D-dimer levels are not specific to pulmonary embolism, as they may also occur in DIC and other conditions.

3. Pulse oximetry: Monitor for a possible fall in hemoglobin oxygen saturation (SaO_2).

4. Arterial blood gases: Metabolic or mixed acidosis. Respiratory alkalosis may sometimes be present in the early stages of shock due to hyperventilation; possible hypoxemia ($\rightarrow$Chapter 4.1).

5. Imaging studies: Chest radiographs: Look for the signs of heart failure (cardiac enlargement, pulmonary congestion, pulmonary edema) and causes of respiratory insufficiency or sepsis. **Chest computed tomography (CT) scans** are indicated in patients with suspected pulmonary embolism (computed tomography angiography [CTA]), aortic dissection, or aortic aneurysm rupture. **Plain abdominal radiographs** are performed in the case of suspected GI perforation or mechanical intestinal obstruction. **Abdominal ultrasonography or CT** is used to search for the source of infection in sepsis. **Venous ultrasonography and pulmonary CTA (pulmonary embolism protocol)** is indicated in the case of suspected deep vein thrombosis or pulmonary embolism. **Head CT scans** are indicated in the case of suspected stroke, brain edema, or posttraumatic lesions.

6. Blood group is to be determined in each patient either directly or on the basis of medical records.

7. Other studies: Venous blood hemoglobin oxygen saturation (preferably in the superior vena cava [$SvcO_2$] or pulmonary trunk [mixed venous blood, or $SvmO_2$]) and venous blood gases from those central areas ($SvcO_2$ <70% or $SvmO_2$ <65% indicates compromised oxygen delivery to tissues and a compensatory increase in oxygen extraction from the blood), microbiology (in septic shock), hormonal tests (thyroid-stimulating hormone and free thyroxine in case of suspected myxedema coma or thyroid storm, cortisol in case of suspected adrenal crisis), toxicology (suspected poisoning), allergy tests (IgE and allergic skin tests after recovery from an anaphylactic shock).

→ TREATMENT

1. Maintain the airway ($\rightarrow$Chapter 3.3), intubate the patient, and start mechanical ventilation as deemed necessary. Note that introducing positive-pressure ventilation in addition to patient sedation and effects of drugs used during intubation may all lead to hypotension. Be prepared to take appropriate action to treat worsening hypotension if needed (rapid volume replacement, vasoconstrictors).

2. Position the patient with elevated lower extremities (Trendelenburg position): This may be transiently helpful in hypovolemic hypotension, particularly when no medical equipment is available, but it may impair ventilation as well as cardiac function in patients with cardiogenic shock and pulmonary congestion.

3. Insert intravascular catheters:

1) Two large-bore catheters in peripheral veins (preferably ≥1.8 mm [≤16 gauge]) to allow for effective fluid resuscitation ($\rightarrow$below).

2) Central venous catheter in patients in whom administration of multiple drugs (including catecholamines; $\rightarrow$below) is necessary. Although central access

may be necessary in some cases, measurement of central venous pressure (CVP) to guide fluid resuscitation in patients with shock has not been shown to be beneficial. We suggest that central venous catheter insertion is not essential in all shock patients and suggest against CVP monitoring.⊘⊖

3) Arterial catheter (usually in the radial artery) to allow for invasive blood pressure monitoring (not essential in shock easily responding to therapy). Central venous and arterial line placement should not delay appropriate treatment.

4. Treat causes of shock (→below) **while maintaining cardiovascular function and tissue oxygen supply:**

1) Discontinue all antihypertensive drugs that may have been used by the patient.

2) In most types of shock **IV fluid resuscitation** is essential; an exception is cardiogenic shock with signs of pulmonary congestion. In theory, colloids restore the intravascular volume by remaining almost entirely in the circulation (plasma substitutes, eg, gelatin, 4%-5% albumin solution) or by remaining in blood vessels and causing transfer of water from the extravascular to the intravascular space; crystalloid solutions compensate for the deficit of the entire extracellular fluid (both extravascular and intravascular). Glucose (dextrose) solutions increase total body water (both extracellular and intracellular fluid). Of the colloid solutions, gelatin, dextran, and starches have been associated with harm and should not be used. Albumin solutions have not been associated with clear benefit and in comparison with crystalloid solutions (Ringer solution or 0.9% NaCl) and are more costly. The 2016 Surviving Sepsis guidelines recommend to start fluid resuscitation using crystalloids, either normal saline or a more physiologic balanced crystalloid (Ringer lactate solution, Ringer acetate solution, Hartmann solution, Plasma-Lyte). Usually the initial management involves the administration of 500 mL of a crystalloid over 30 minutes, and then the infusion is repeated, depending on the effects on blood pressure, CVP, urine output, or other dynamic measures of volume status, as well as adverse effects (symptoms of volume overload). Balanced crystalloids may be preferred compared with normal saline; however, ongoing studies will further address this question. In the case of intensive fluid resuscitation, some may choose to administer 5% albumin solutions after 3 or 4 L of a crystalloid, although this practice has not been studied in proper randomized controlled trials. Do not use hypotonic fluids (eg, 5% glucose) for fluid resuscitation in shock even in patients with hypernatremia, as this fluid will not remain in the intravascular space.

3) In the case of persistent hypotension despite fluid resuscitation, a continuous IV infusion of catecholamines should be started (optimally via a central venous catheter). For almost all etiologies of shock, we recommend starting with **norepinephrine**, usually 1 to 20 μg/min (up to 1-2 μg/kg/min).⊘⊕ However, **epinephrine** 0.05 to 0.5 μg/kg/min may be considered. We suggest to use vasopressin as a second-line vasopressor, which can be administered at a rate of 2 IU/h. In anaphylactic shock start with an IM injection of 0.3 to 0.5 mg epinephrine to the lateral thigh.

4) In patients with evidence of low CO despite adequate hydration (or volume overload), **dobutamine** in a continuous IV infusion (2-20 μg/kg/min) may be beneficial (this requires careful consideration in the presence of arrhythmia, including sinus tachycardia, as dobutamine may worsen the arrhythmia). In the case of concomitant hypotension, you may simultaneously administer vasoconstrictors.

5) At the same time administer **oxygen therapy** (maintaining an oxygen saturation [SaO_2] >92%).

6) In patients with signs of hypoperfusion and hematocrit <30% despite the above treatment, consider transfusion of packed red blood cells.

5. The basis of management in patients with lactic acidosis is **treatment of the underlying condition and maintaining cardiovascular function.**

Consider IV administration of **NaHCO$_3$** in patients with a pH <7.15 (7.20) and bicarbonate levels <14 mmol/L, although beneficial effects of this intervention have not been proven.

6. Monitor vital parameters (blood pressure [initially in most circumstances the target MAP is ≥65 mm Hg; exceptions: →Chapter 3.16.2.1], pulse rate, respiratory rate), level of consciousness, ECG, SaO$_2$, blood lactate levels (aim to normalize), blood gases, sodium and potassium levels, renal and liver function tests, CVP, as well as CO, PCWP, or dynamic measures of volume status, when necessary.

7. Protect the patient from hypothermia and ensure a quiet environment.

8. In the case of persistent shock and the need for ongoing intensive care:

1) **Prevent GI bleeding and thromboembolic complications** (do not use anticoagulants in patients with active bleeding or at high risk of bleeding; in such cases use mechanical methods only): →Chapter 3.19.2.

2) **Treat hyperglycemia** (in patients with glucose levels >10-11.1 mmol/L [180-200 mg/dL], possibly with a continuous IV infusion of a short-acting insulin, but avoid hypoglycemia. Make attempts to maintain blood glucose levels from between 6.7 and 7.8 mmol/L (120-140 mg/dL) to between 10 and 11.1 mmol/L (180-200 mg/dL).

16.1. Cardiogenic Shock

➡ DEFINITION, ETIOLOGY, PATHOGENESIS

Cardiogenic shock is shock due to dysfunction of the heart (→Chapter 3.8.1) that leads to reduced cardiac output. **Causes:**

1) **Myocardial injury:** Acute systolic heart failure caused by acute coronary syndrome (ACS) (most commonly myocardial infarction [MI], usually ST-elevation myocardial infarction with a left ventricular [LV] function decrease >40%) and its complications (acute mitral insufficiency, free wall rupture, ventricular septal defect), myocarditis, cardiac injury (trauma), cardiomyopathies, exacerbation of or end-stage chronic heart failure.

2) **Cardiac arrhythmias:** Bradycardia, tachyarrhythmias (particularly ventricular tachycardia and atrial fibrillation).

3) **Acute valvular heart disease** (acute mitral or aortic regurgitation), **prosthetic valve dysfunction.**

Traditionally, the term "cardiogenic shock" has denoted a shock caused by impaired cardiac contractility (pump function).

➡ CLINICAL FEATURES AND DIAGNOSIS

Symptoms of shock and of the underlying disease are seen.

Diagnostic Tests
→Chapter 3.16; →Chapter 3.8.1.

➡ TREATMENT

Use of the following methods of treatment depends on the specific underlying pathophysiology.

1. Discontinue β-blockers, angiotensin-converting enzyme inhibitors, and other drugs that may lower blood pressure unless used specifically to counteract the mechanism of shock (eg, a β-blocker in a patient with mitral stenosis and very rapid atrial fibrillation).

2. In case of **ventricular tachycardia, atrial fibrillation, or atrial flutter** (or other supraventricular tachycardia causing shock), perform **cardioversion**. Consider subsequent administration of medications to prevent or treat arrhythmia recurrence (→Chapter 3.4).

3. In patients with **bradycardia**, consider **atropine**, chronotropic agents (such as epinephrine 2-10 µg/min in a continuous IV infusion; alternatively isoproterenol [INN isoprenaline] 5 µg/min or dopamine), or **cardiac pacing** (→Chapter 3.3).

4. In patients **without symptoms of volume overload and pulmonary congestion**, initiate **fluid resuscitation** to achieve optimal LV filling (this is particularly important in right ventricular dysfunction). Start with 250 mL of a crystalloid over 10 to 15 minutes, continue fluid resuscitation, and make adjustments based on response to treatment and appearance of volume overload. In patients with volume overload (pulmonary congestion) and patients without volume overload who do not respond to fluid therapy, consider one of treatment interventions discussed below.

5. In patients with documented myocardial dysfunction, an inotropic agent may be beneficial. For most patients, starting with **norepinephrine** is reasonable ⊘ ⊖ as its pharmacologic effects include not only vasoconstriction but also some inotropy (via β_2 stimulation). In patients with ongoing signs of shock despite initial therapy, **dopamine** or **dobutamine** can be administered via a continuous IV infusion. In case of unsatisfactory response or issues with significant arrhythmias, consider milrinone, enoximone, or levosimendan (all of these drugs may have serious adverse effects and their use is controversial).

6. In patients with **pulmonary congestion** in whom blood pressure has been raised to a physiologically adequate level (usually at least 90 mm Hg) without catecholamine support, you may consider a **loop diuretic** (→Chapter 3.8.1). In patients in whom diuretic treatment is ineffective, consider ultrafiltration. In patients with renal failure consider hemodialysis.

7. In patients with **pulmonary congestion** and systolic blood pressure >110 mm Hg, consider a vasodilator, usually **nitroglycerin or nitroprusside** (dosage: →Chapter 3.8.1; these should not be used in isolated right ventricular failure).

8. Treatment of the underlying condition. In the case of ACS, refer the patient for urgent invasive revascularization (→Chapter 3.11.1). In the case of mechanical complications of MI, acute valvular disease, or prosthetic valve dysfunction, refer the patient for cardiac surgery.

9. In patients with **refractory cardiogenic shock** (persisting despite medical support), specialized centers may consider intra-aortic counterpulsation (after excluding contraindications: aortic regurgitation and aortic dissection) or short-term mechanical circulatory support, depending on the patient's age, comorbidities, and neurologic function.

10. Other management steps (including oxygen therapy): As in other forms of shock.

16.2. Hypovolemic Shock

➔ CLINICAL FEATURES AND DIAGNOSIS

The signs and symptoms of shock may be accompanied or preceded by signs and symptoms of dehydration: dry mucous membranes, dry and hypoelastic skin, and increased thirst (except for elderly patients with hypodipsia). Altered mental status may develop before hypotension (particularly in the elderly). Tachycardia and orthostatic hypotension usually occur before the drop in blood pressure that may be observed in a patient when they are sitting or supine. History and results of physical examination indicative of the cause of shock are helpful in establishing the diagnosis. Also →Chapter 4.3.1. Acid-base (eg, contraction alkalosis or metabolic acidosis) or electrolyte disturbances (eg, hyponatremia or hypernatremia, hypokalemia or hyperkalemia) can be also considered as warnings of hypovolemic conditions.

→ TREATMENT

1. IV infusion of crystalloid, colloid, or blood product solutions (→Chapter 3.16). In patients with persistent hypotension and hypoperfusion despite a rapid administration of ~1500 to 2000 mL of a crystalloid (or ~1000 mL of a colloid), administer norepinephrine or epinephrine (or dopamine) in a continuous IV infusion (→Chapter 3.16) while continuing fluid resuscitation. The basis of treatment of hypovolemic shock is volume resuscitation, not catecholamines; nevertheless, catecholamines may be helpful in maintaining vital organ perfusion. Subsequent to the initial volume resuscitation, smaller boluses of fluids in the form of fluid challenge can be used to titrate the overall fluid loading. When applicable, dynamic indices of preload (→Chapter 3.16) can be useful for predicting the response to fluids.

2. Simultaneously **treat the underlying causes of shock**, for instance, treat the disease that causes vomiting, diarrhea, intestinal obstruction, polyuria, or fluid loss via the skin.

3. Other management procedures: →Chapter 3.16.

16.2.1. Hemorrhagic Shock

→ CLINICAL FEATURES AND DIAGNOSIS

Local symptoms of bleeding (hemorrhage) depend on its location and are not always overt. Locations include, among other sites, the gastrointestinal (GI) tract (→Chapter 6.1.3.4) and wounds due to trauma. The sites of potential major bleeding in a hemodynamically unstable trauma patient are the long bones, chest, abdomen, retroperitoneum, and external sites. Blood pressure may not drop until 750 to 1500 mL of blood is lost. In the early stages of bleeding it is sometimes important to compare the blood pressures and heart rates measured in supine and standing positions. An orthostatic drop in blood pressure ≥10 mm Hg and increase in pulse rate ≥20 beats/min suggests hypovolemia. A blood loss up to 1500 mL is usually accompanied by subtle changes in mental status, while losing half of the blood volume (2000-2500 mL) is associated with a significantly altered mental status (usually loss of consciousness). A decrease in hematocrit, hemoglobin levels, and red blood cell counts usually occurs ≥1 to 3 (4) hours after the blood loss.

→ TREATMENT

1. Stop the bleeding, if possible. When necessary, refer the patient for a specialist minimally invasive surgery (eg, endoscopy in the case of GI bleeding) or radiologic assessment for embolization.

2. Continue fluid resuscitation with crystalloids (eg, ~3 mL for every 1 mL blood lost) or colloids (eg, ~1 mL for every 1 mL of blood lost) only until packed red blood cells (PRBCs) are available for transfusion (→Chapter 3.16). Once blood products are available, they are the best resuscitative fluid to use in hemorrhagic shock. We suggest a target systolic blood pressure of 80 to 90 mm Hg (mean arterial pressure, 40 mm Hg) until major bleeding has been stopped in the initial phase following trauma without brain injury.⊘⊖ A mean arterial pressure ≥80 mm Hg should be maintained in patients with combined hemorrhagic shock and severe traumatic brain injury (Glasgow Coma Scale ≤8 [→Chapter 10.3, Table 3-2]) in order to maintain cerebral perfusion pressures.

3. Collect blood samples for cross-matching. Request blood group typing if the group cannot be quickly and reliably established on the basis of medical records. Order and transfuse PRBCs. In patients with massive hemorrhages, do not wait for the results of the cross-matching and transfuse O Rh− blood before compatible blood arrives. If shock persists, do not allow for a hematocrit fall <30%. In patients with severe blood loss, supplement the PRBC transfusions with the administration of fresh frozen plasma (FFP) and consider platelet transfusion as well as administration of cryoprecipitate (as a reasonable example, supplement transfusion of >2 units of PRBCs with 1 unit of FFP for every 2 units of PRBCs and 1 unit of platelets for 5 units of PRBCs; in massive bleeding it is advised to supplement transfusions of PRBCs with FFP or fibrinogen from the beginning of treatment). In case of coagulopathy, consider FFP, cryoprecipitate, and platelet transfusions. In massive bleeding that cannot be controlled by surgical procedures, blood transfusion, or tranexamic acid (→below), consider administration of recombinant factor VIIa concentrate as rescue treatment.

4. Prevent and treat complications of massive bleeding and transfusion, including hypothermia, acidosis, and hypocalcemia (these impair blood coagulation).

5. In patients receiving anticoagulants, discontinue treatment and neutralize the effects of the drugs, if possible (→Chapter 3.1.1.1; →Chapter 3.1.1.4).

6. In patients with a severe hemorrhage following trauma, we recommend the administration of IV tranexamic acid (loading dose 1 g over 10 minutes, then 1 g over 8 hours).✓●

7. Other management procedures: →Chapter 3.16.

For rapid fluid resuscitation and blood transfusions, use large-bore peripheral venous catheters (preferably ≥1.8 mm [≤16 gauge]; establish 2 separate IV lines) as these allow for higher infusion rates compared with central lines. If peripheral access is not possible, a large-bore central line (such as employed for renal replacement therapy or angiography/pacing [vascular sheaths]) should be used.

16.3. Obstructive Shock

➔ DEFINITION, ETIOLOGY, PATHOGENESIS

→Chapter 3.16.

➔ CLINICAL FEATURES AND DIAGNOSIS

Symptoms of shock (usually rapidly evolving) and of the underlying disease are seen.

Diagnostic Tests

Imaging studies are crucial: **Chest radiographs** may show pneumothorax. **Computed tomography (CT) angiography** may confirm pulmonary embolism. **Ultrasonography** may detect or suggest cardiac tamponade, heart tumors, intracardiac thrombosis, pneumothorax, and venous thrombosis associated with pulmonary embolism.

Also →Chapter 3.16.

➔ TREATMENT

Manage the underlying condition as soon as possible. In patients with cardiac tamponade, perform pericardiocentesis. In case of tension pneumothorax, perform decompression. In patients with pulmonary embolism, consider administration of thrombolysis and start anticoagulation therapy if feasible (→Chapter 3.19.3). In case of a heart tumor, intracardiac thrombosis, or cardiac tamponade related to aortic dissection or heart wall rupture, refer the patient for cardiac surgery.

17. Valvular Heart Disease

17.1. Aortic Valve Disease

17.1.1. Aortic Regurgitation

→ **DEFINITION, ETIOLOGY, PATHOGENESIS**

Aortic regurgitation (AR) is a reversal of blood flow from the aorta into the left ventricle (LV) due to incomplete closure of the aortic valve leaflets. **Primary regurgitation** is caused by damage to or a congenital abnormality of the leaflets, with subsequent dilation of the left ventricular outflow tract, aortic annulus, and ascending aorta. **Secondary regurgitation** is caused by dilation of the aortic annulus and the ascending aorta (secondarily causing malcoaptation of the aortic valve leaflets) in the absence of significant aortic valve leaflet pathology.

Etiology:

1) **Primary**: Congenital (bicuspid aortic valve, quadricuspid aortic valve, valve damage in subaortic stenosis); degenerative (calcifications, fibrosis); infective endocarditis (active or healed); rheumatic; drug-induced (fenfluramine, phentermine) damage of the leaflets.

2) **Secondary**: Idiopathic aortic dilation; hypertensive aortic dilation; systemic connective tissue diseases (rheumatic disease, rheumatoid arthritis, aortic stenosis); dilation or dissection of the ascending aorta (hypertension, Marfan or Marfan-like syndrome, atherosclerosis, inflammation, trauma, myxomatous degeneration); aortopathy associated with bicuspid aortic valve; syphilitic aortic disease.

→ **CLINICAL FEATURES AND NATURAL HISTORY**

1. Symptoms: In acute AR, a sudden-onset tachycardia and increasing dyspnea (in AR caused by aortic dissection, symptoms of the underlying condition predominate). Chronic AR may be asymptomatic for years, and even in severe AR, the symptoms are at times mild, often involving fatigue.

2. Signs: A wide (high) pulse pressure (with elevated systolic blood pressure and low, at times undetectable diastolic blood pressure), rapidly rising and rapidly collapsing pulse (so-called water hammer pulse or Corrigan pulse); sometimes a bisferiens pulse (more easily recognized on the brachial or femoral arteries than on the carotid arteries). The first heart sound is usually normal (although it may be silent in acute AR due to mitral valve preclosure). The aortic component of the second heart sound may be accentuated (in the case of aortic pathology) or soft (in the case of pathology of the leaflets). A holodiastolic decrescendo murmur is audible, frequently most prominent at the left sternal border (in the case of pathology of the ascending aorta, it is frequently better audible at the right sternal border); the Austin Flint murmur—a diastolic rumble due to relative mitral stenosis from preclosure of the mitral valve—may also be present. Frequently, a systolic ejection murmur is audible over the aortic valve (due to increased stroke volume, resulting in increased transaortic valve gradients).

3. Natural history of acute AR depends on the underlying condition. Chronic AR is usually asymptomatic for several years; in patients with a normal left ventricular ejection fraction (LVEF), the sudden cardiac death risk is <0.2% per year. The prevalence of cardiovascular events is ~5% per year in patients with severe AR and preserved LV function, and 25% per year in patients with New York Heart Association (NYHA) class III/IV symptoms. Some patients with asymptomatic severe AR may develop irreversible LV dysfunction; thus, early detection and appropriate treatment of severe AR is paramount.

Table 17-1. Classification of aortic regurgitation

	Regurgitation		
	Mild	Moderate	Severe
Vena contracta width (mm)	<3	4-6	≥7
Effective regurgitant orifice area (cm^2)	<0.10	0.1-0.29	≥0.30
Regurgitant volume (mL)	<30	30-59	≥60
Regurgitant fraction (%)	<30	30-49	≥50
Based on Circulation. 2014;129(23):e521-643.			

➔ DIAGNOSIS

Diagnosis is based on typical clinical features and echocardiography.

Diagnostic Tests

1. Electrocardiography (ECG): Features of LV hypertrophy and strain pattern; features of left atrial enlargement (P mitrale). Ventricular arrhythmias can occur.

2. Chest radiographs: LV hypertrophy, dilation of the ascending aorta and the aortic arch. In acute AR, pulmonary congestion with a normal cardiac silhouette is observed.

3. Doppler echocardiography allows for detection of a regurgitation jet and its quantitative and qualitative assessment (→Table 17-1).

4. Gated computed tomography (CT) is best for aortic dilation measurement using the inner-edge-to-inner-edge technique.

Differential Diagnosis

Echocardiography combined with clinical manifestations has very high accuracy in the diagnosis of AR. Consideration of the differential diagnosis of the causes of AR (primary valve damage and/or secondary to dilation of the aortic root or ascending aorta) is necessary to guide therapy.

➔ TREATMENT

General Considerations

1. Mild or moderate chronic AR: Asymptomatic patients with normal systolic LV function require no treatment.

2. Chronic severe AR: In general, medical or surgical management may be considered with surgical opinion for potential aortic valve replacement (AVR) recommended in the presence of any of the following:

1) Symptoms attributable to AR (dyspnea, chest pain, orthopnea, paroxysmal nocturnal dyspnea).
2) No symptoms and severe AR with normal LV systolic function (LVEF ≥50%) but with severe LV dilation (LV end-systolic diameter >50 mm or 25 mm/m^2 for patients with small body habitus).
3) LV systolic dysfunction (LVEF <50%).

3. Acute symptomatic AR: Typically due to endocarditis or aortic dissection. Urgent surgery is required: AVR with the implantation of a mechanical or bioprosthetic valve, or an aortic homograft (details of invasive treatment: →below). Prior to surgery, vasodilators can be used. Aortic balloon counterpulsation is contraindicated.

Table 17-2. Echocardiographic follow-up of patients with asymptomatic aortic regurgitation

Severity of regurgitation	Left ventricular function	Follow-up
Mild or moderate	Normal LVEF and LVESD	Every 2 years
Severe	LVEDD 60-65 mm	Every year[a]
	LVEDD >65 mm	Every 6 months
Aortic dilation <50 mm		Every year[b]

[a] The first follow-up visit within 6 months of the diagnosis.

[b] Increases >3 mm should be confirmed on CT.

CT, computed tomography; LVEDD, left ventricular end-diastolic diameter; LVEF, left ventricular ejection fraction; LVESD, left ventricular end-systolic diameter.

Invasive Treatment

AVR (mechanical vs bioprosthetic valve, depending on the patient's age and ability to take warfarin [the latter necessary for mechanical prosthesis]) is the mainstay of surgical therapy in chronic severe AR and in acute symptomatic AR. In cases of AR caused by aortic root dilation where the aortic valve is structurally normal, surgical aortic root replacement may be performed with preservation of the native aortic valve leaflets. In cases of both aortic root enlargement and abnormal aortic valves, concomitant AVR and aortic root replacement (Bentall procedure) may be performed.

Medical Treatment

1. Vasodilators (agents: →Table 9-5), for instance, enalapril 10 to 20 mg bid, quinapril 10 to 20 mg/d, or losartan 50 to 100 mg bid (but also other angiotensin--converting enzyme inhibitors and angiotensin-receptor blockers)◐◔ may be used in:

1) Patients with hypertension.

2) Patients with severe AR who have symptoms and/or LV dysfunction (stages C2 and D) when surgery is not performed because of comorbidities.

2. Prevention of infective endocarditis: →Chapter 3.10.

→ FOLLOW-UP

Follow-up: →Table 17-2.

→ PROGNOSIS

In symptomatic patients receiving medical treatment, 5-year survival rates are 30% for NYHA class III/IV patients and 70% for NYHA class II patients.

17.1.2. Aortic Stenosis

→ DEFINITION, ETIOLOGY, PATHOGENESIS

Aortic stenosis (AS) results from thickened or calcified valve leaflets leading to restricted leaflet motion, reduced aortic valve area (AVA), and transvalvular flow obstruction. AS is most frequently an acquired disease (age-related degenerative valve disease, with rheumatic disease rarely seen) but may also be congenital (most frequently a bicuspid aortic valve).

Table 17-3. Classification of aortic stenosis

	Aortic stenosis		
	Mild	Moderate	Severe
AVA (cm²)	>1.5	1.0-1.5	<1.0 (0.6 cm²/m² BSA)
Mean gradient (mm Hg)	<25	25-39	≥40
Jet velocity (m/s)	<3	3-3.9	≥4

Based on Circulation. 2014;129(23):e521-643.

AVA, aortic valve area; BSA, body surface area.

→ CLINICAL FEATURES AND NATURAL HISTORY

1. Symptoms: AS remains asymptomatic for a long time. It may cause angina, palpitations, dizziness, presyncope or syncope, dyspnea, and in more advanced disease, resting dyspnea. Classification of severity: →Table 17-3.

2. Signs: Cardiac impulse is diffuse, sustained, and displaced laterally and inferiorly. A systolic thrill may be palpable at the base of the heart and transmitted to the carotid arteries (in patients with severe stenosis). An ejection systolic murmur is present, although its intensity may not reflect the severity of stenosis; the murmur radiates to the carotid arteries and the later the murmur peaks, the more severe the stenosis. An aortic ejection click is audible in patients with elastic leaflets (commonly bicuspid valves). The aortic component of the second heart sound is soft, reverse split, or absent (in severe stenosis); sometimes a fourth heart sound is audible. The pulse is low-amplitude and slow-rising—"parvus and tardus" (in elderly patients these pulse features may be absent due to systemic arteriosclerosis). Patients may have a brachial--radial delay.

3. Natural history: The rate of progression of AS is highly variable. In asymptomatic patients the risk of sudden cardiac death is low but rapidly increases with the onset of the 3 cardinal symptoms: syncope, angina, and heart failure. The average survival of untreated patients with such symptoms is 2 to 3 years.

→ DIAGNOSIS

Diagnosis is based on typical clinical features and echocardiography results.

Diagnostic Tests

1. Electrocardiography (ECG) is usually normal in mild to moderate AS. In severe AS, features of left ventricular (LV) hypertrophy with strain pattern are commonly present.

2. Chest radiography remains normal for many years. In severe AS, LV hypertrophy and poststenotic dilation of the ascending aorta are observed. Calcifications of the aortic valve may be seen.

3. Doppler echocardiography is used to confirm the diagnosis of AS, assess its severity, evaluate LV structure and function, assess valve morphology, aortic root, and ascending aorta, and monitor the course of the disease. A thickened, calcified aortic valve with reduced leaflet excursion is seen. Doppler echocardiography allows for determination of the severity of stenosis by measuring the aortic jet velocity, peak and mean transvalvular pressure gradients, and AVA (→Table 17-3). In patients with low-flow low-gradient AS (AVA <1 cm², but a mean aortic valve gradient <40 mm Hg and/or peak aortic valve velocity

<4.0 cm/s), the most common cause is depressed left ventricular ejection fraction (LVEF) (ejection fraction <40%) resulting in low transvalvular flow; in such cases, dobutamine stress echocardiography can be performed to distinguish true severe AS from "pseudosevere AS" and to help predict perioperative mortality (expert input usually required).◗

4. Noncontrast gated cardiac computed tomography (CT): Aortic valve calcium scoring can provide a morphologic estimation of the severity of AS and risk of adverse outcomes with medical therapy. Severe AS is unlikely with calcium scores <800 in women and <1600 in men but likely with calcium scores >1200 in women and >2000 in men.

5. Cardiac catheterization may be considered in cases of inconsistent clinical and echocardiographic findings, and to exclude significant coronary artery stenosis before aortic valve surgery. Coronary angiography is recommended before surgical treatment of AS in patients with severe valvular heart disease and one of the following:

1) A history of coronary artery disease (CAD).

2) Suspected myocardial ischemia (chest pain, abnormal results of noninvasive investigations).

3) LV systolic dysfunction.

4) Men >40 years of age, postmenopausal women.

4) ≥1 cardiovascular risk factor (in patients at low risk of atherosclerosis, the diagnosis of CAD may be excluded using coronary CT angiography.

Differential Diagnosis

Differential diagnosis should include supravalvular AS and membranous subvalvular stenosis, both of which can be readily identified by echocardiography. Dynamic LV outflow tract obstruction can cause flow acceleration and high transvalvular gradients; however, the carotid upstroke is rapid (not delayed as in AS), while on echocardiography, the aortic valve is not restricted in motion and the shape of the Doppler spectral tracing is "dagger-shaped," not parabolic as in AS.

→ TREATMENT

General Considerations

1. Mild or moderate AS: Medical treatment and follow-up visits (every 1-2 years in mild AS and every year in moderate AS) with echocardiography (every 3-5 years in mild AS and every 1-2 years in moderate AS).

2. Severe AS: In general, an opinion regarding valve replacement from a multidisciplinary team should be obtained; further details: →below.

Invasive Treatment

1. Aortic valve replacement (AVR) is the key method of treatment in the case of severe AS. AVR is recommended in:

1) Patients with severe AS and symptoms related to AS (syncope, angina, or heart failure); in such cases, urgent surgery is indicated.

2) Asymptomatic patients with severe AS in any of the following cases:

   a) LVEF <50% due to AS.

   b) Abnormal exercise test results showing symptoms on exercise clearly related to AS (valve replacement may be considered if exercise leads to a drop in blood pressure below baseline).

   c) Other indications for cardiac surgery including severe coronary disease, aortopathy, and nonaortic valve disease.

2. Modality of AVR: Surgical aortic valve replacement (SAVR) and transcatheter aortic valve replacement (TAVR) are options for treatment of aortic stenosis.

Table 17-4. Factors influencing transcatheter versus surgical valve replacement for aortic stenosis

Factors favoring TAVR	Factors favoring SAVR
– Isolated symptomatic severe aortic stenosis with acceptable aortic and vascular anatomy for transcatheter replacement – Noncardiac comorbidities that increase operative risks and reduce ability to recover from sternotomy	– Young patients benefiting from durability of mechanical valves – Multilevel obstruction (eg, involving left ventricular outflow tract) – Surgical intervention required for coronary disease, aortopathy, nonaortic valve disease, or endocarditis – Presence of left ventricular thrombus – Inadequate vascular access (vessel size, calcification, tortuosity) or factors that increase technical difficulty of TAVR

SAVR, surgical aortic valve replacement; TAVR, transcatheter aortic valve replacement.

Choice among treatment modalities is best made by an interdisciplinary valve team. Specific treatment options include:

1) **SAVR with a bioprosthetic valve**: SAVR with a bioprosthetic valve is preferred in older patients (usually >65 years of age) as durability is superior compared with younger patients and the need for long-term anticoagulation is avoided.

2) **SAVR with a mechanical valve**: SAVR with a mechanical valve is used in younger patients because of their durability. Lifelong anticoagulation with warfarin is required in these patients.

3) **SAVR with pulmonary homograft (Ross procedure)**: SAVR with transplantation of the pulmonary valve to the aortic position is a desirable but more technically complex approach in younger patients.

4) **TAVR with balloon-expandable or self-expanding valve**: TAVR involves implantation of a bioprosthetic valve via transarterial access (usually transfemoral). Balloon-expandable and self-expanding technologies are used.

Among patients eligible for both SAVR and TAVR, TAVR is associated with reduced rates of mortality and stroke, kidney injury, new-onset atrial fibrillation, and major bleeding but with increased rates of vascular complications, need for permanent pacemaker implantation (depending on valve type), and paravalvular leak.⊚⊖ Patients with other indications for cardiac surgery should undergo SAVR. TAVR should be considered in those ineligible for surgery.⊚⊖ TAVR is an acceptable (and may be the preferred) option in patients at both low⊚⊖ and high surgical risk⊚⊖ (→Table 17-4).

Patients with implanted prosthetic mechanical valves require lifelong oral anticoagulant therapy (with international normalized ratio [INR] dependent on thrombogenicity of the artificial valve: →Table 17-5). In patients considered to have acceptable risk of bleeding, especially those with coexisting CAD, low-dose acetylsalicylic acid (ASA) could be added.⊚⊖ In the case of relative contraindications to oral anticoagulants (eg, athletes or women planning to become pregnant), consider other modalities of surgical treatment: valvuloplasty, implantation of a heterograft (bioprosthetic valve) or a homograft, the Ross procedure (using the patient's own pulmonary valve to replace the diseased aortic valve, with implantation of a homograft to replace the pulmonary valve).

Patients with implanted bioprosthetic or TAVR valves are typically prescribed lifelong low-dose ASA for thromboprophylaxis. Dual antiplatelet therapy is continued after TAVR in patients already receiving therapy for coronary stents.⊖ Anticoagulation is commonly prescribed for the first 3 to 6 months following bioprosthetic SAVR.

Table 17-5. Antithrombotic treatment in patients with mechanical prosthetic valves

Risk of thrombosis associated with the prosthesis	Examples of mechanical valves	Target international normalized ratio depending on the number of risk factors[a]	
		0	≥1
Low	– Carbomedics (aortic) – Medtronic Hall – St. Jude Medical – On-X	2.5	3.0
Medium	Other bileaflet valves	3.0	3.5
High	– Lillehei-Kaster – Omniscience – Starr-Edwards – Björk-Shiley – Other tilting disc valves	3.5	4.0

[a] Risk factors: replacement of the mitral or tricuspid valve; prior thromboembolic event, atrial fibrillation, mitral stenosis of any severity, left ventricular ejection fraction <35%.

Adapted from Eur Heart J. 2012;33(19):2451-96.

Medical Treatment

1. To reduce or control symptoms:

1) **Hypertension**: Control hypertension with β-blockers or angiotensin-
-converting enzyme inhibitors (ACEIs) (care should be taken to avoid over-
medication and resultant hypotension). With ACEIs, start with a low dose
and slowly titrate. In patients who have symptomatic AS, try to avoid
preload- and afterload-reducing agents that may produce hypotension.

2) **Pulmonary congestion**: Diuretics and ACEIs (use with caution, as a too
rapid preload reduction decreases cardiac output and blood pressure), β-blockers (in patients with LV hypertrophy and LV systolic dysfunction, or with
atrial fibrillation).

3) **Atrial fibrillation**: Electrical cardioversion (not to be performed prior to
surgical treatment of AS in patients with severe AS who are hemodynamically
stable). In the case of persistent atrial fibrillation, administer β-blockers
(the preferred agents) or calcium channel blockers (diltiazem or verapamil)
to control the ventricular rate, although such calcium channel blockers are
contraindicated in patients with depressed LVEF (<50%). Digoxin can be
added to β-blockers or calcium channel blockers to augment ventricular rate
control. Amiodarone can be used in selected cases alone or with β-blockers or
calcium channel blockers, but it should be avoided if the patient is receiving
digoxin.

4) **Angina**: β-Blockers, nitrates (use with caution).

2. Prevention of infective endocarditis: →Chapter 3.10.

▶ COMPLICATIONS

Sudden cardiac death, peripheral embolism, infective endocarditis (more frequent in younger patients with minor valvular lesions), coagulopathy (acquired
von Willebrand syndrome), aortic dissection (most often in patients with a bicuspid aortic valve and aortopathy), right ventricular failure (rare).

→ PROGNOSIS

The prognosis is favorable in asymptomatic patients. The onset of symptoms is associated with a worse prognosis, as the average survival time is 2 years from the onset of heart failure, 3 years from the onset of syncope, and 5 years from the onset of angina. Surgical treatment improves prognosis.

17.1.3. Mixed Aortic Stenosis and Regurgitation

→ DEFINITION, ETIOLOGY, CLINICAL FEATURES

Mixed aortic stenosis (AS) and aortic regurgitation (AR) refers to concomitant stenosis and regurgitation of the aortic valve.

Etiology: Congenital (most commonly a bicuspid aortic valve), degenerative, rheumatic disease, prior balloon valvuloplasty for AS in childhood, or prior mediastinal irradiation.

Clinical features are similar to other types of acquired aortic valve disease and depend on the dominant lesion (AS vs AR). The coexisting AR causes a louder systolic murmur by increasing transvalvular flow across the stenotic valve.

→ TREATMENT

1. Surgery: The decision is made on an individual basis, taking into consideration the symptoms, transvalvular gradient, aortic valve area, and left ventricular size and function.

Indications: In patients with dominant stenosis, even if the symptoms are mild; in patients with dominant regurgitation in the case of severe symptoms or reduced left ventricular ejection fraction. In patients with postradiation disease, the most common indication for surgery is concomitant coronary artery disease.

2. Pharmacotherapy: Depends on the dominant lesion. Note that vasodilators used for AR may increase the transvalvular gradient of AS; agents that slow the heart rate (β-blockers) may increase regurgitant volumes in AR.

3. Prevention of infective endocarditis: →Chapter 3.10.

17.2. Mitral Valve Disease

17.2.1. Mitral Regurgitation

→ DEFINITION, ETIOLOGY, PATHOGENESIS

Mitral regurgitation (MR) is a backward blood flow from the left ventricle (LV) to the left atrium due to an incomplete closure of the mitral valve leaflets. In 10% to 40% of people in whom Doppler echocardiography is performed results show a mild regurgitant jet with no evident abnormalities of the valve apparatus (so-called physiologic regurgitation).

Primary (organic) MR is due to a primary damage of the valve apparatus (leaflets, chordae tendineae, or both). **Secondary (functional) MR** is due to changes in LV size and function (eg, in ischemic or dilated cardiomyopathy) in the presence of structurally normal leaflets.

Etiology of chronic MR:

1) Primary: Degenerative lesions of the valve apparatus (myxomatous mitral valve disease, idiopathic rupture of the chordae tendineae, Marfan syndrome, Ehlers-Danlos syndrome, calcification of the mitral annulus, degenerative lesions of the leaflets), infective endocarditis of an initially normal or damaged valve, systemic connective tissue diseases (systemic lupus erythematosus, antiphospholipid syndrome, scleroderma), rheumatic disease, iatrogenic

Table 17-6. Classification of mitral regurgitation

	Regurgitation		
	Mild	Moderate	Severe
Effective regurgitant orifice area (cm²)	<0.20	0.2-0.39	≥0.40
Regurgitant volume (mL)	<30	30-59	≥60
Regurgitant fraction (%)	<30	30-49	≥50
PASP (mm Hg)	<30	30-50	>50

Based on Circulation. 2014;129(23):e521-643.

MVA, mitral valve area; MVG, mitral valve gradient; PASP, pulmonary artery systolic pressure.

(ergotamines, appetite suppressants [eg, fenfluramine; currently withdrawn]), congenital (mitral valve clefts).

2) Secondary: Diseases of the myocardium (ischemic heart disease, dilated cardiomyopathy, hypertrophic cardiomyopathy), storage and infiltrative diseases (amyloidosis, idiopathic eosinophilia, carcinoid syndrome, endomyocardial fibrosis).

Etiology of acute MR:

1) Primary (organic): Lesions of the valve leaflets (infective endocarditis, leaflet trauma, eg, during balloon valvotomy), rupture of the chordae tendineae (idiopathic, myxomatous degeneration, infective endocarditis, acute rheumatic fever, leaflet trauma, eg, during balloon valvotomy), diseases of the annulus (infective endocarditis [periannular abscess]).

2) Secondary (functional): Papillary muscle diseases (acute myocardial infarction [MI] complicated by papillary muscle rupture or LV dysfunction; acute LV dilation, eg, acute myocarditis; amyloidosis or sarcoidosis), left atrial myxoma.

→ CLINICAL FEATURES AND NATURAL HISTORY

1. Symptoms: Mild or moderate chronic MR is usually asymptomatic (in the case of slow progression of regurgitation—even if it is severe—the symptoms may be minor). With time, patients develop symptoms related to changes in LV diastolic function, left atrial compliance, LV filling pressure, pulmonary artery pressure, and right ventricular function, as well as dyspnea and palpitations (in the case of atrial fibrillation [AF]). In acute MR, sudden dyspnea and hypotension or cardiogenic shock may occur. Classification of severity: →Table 17-6.

2. Signs: A holosystolic murmur, whose loudness is usually correlated with the size of the regurgitant volume (except for ischemic regurgitation); a short diastolic rumble (in severe MR); a late systolic murmur (preceded by a systolic click; usually associated with mitral valve prolapse or papillary muscle dysfunction); a diminished first heart sound (in clinically significant MR); splitting of the second heart sound; mid or late systolic click (with prolapsing valves); third heart sound (correlating with the regurgitant volume and with LV enlargement); laterally displaced apex. Pulmonary crepitations may occur. In patients with severe MR and pulmonary hypertension, symptoms of right ventricular failure (→Chapter 3.8.2) may be present.

3. Natural history: In functional MR, disease progression is related to the underlying condition (LV disease). Acute MR is rapidly progressive and usually fatal when left without surgical treatment: 25% of patients with moderate or severe MR related to acute MI die within 30 days, and 50% die within one year. In the case of papillary muscle rupture in the course of acute MI, 95% of patients die within two weeks. Chronic MR may remain asymptomatic for over a decade. The regurgitant volume is of a significant prognostic value in asymptomatic patients. Severe MR may lead to irreversible asymptomatic LV dysfunction.

→ DIAGNOSIS

Diagnosis is based on clinical features (if present) and echocardiography.

Diagnostic Tests

1. Electrocardiography (ECG) is usually normal; the most frequent abnormalities include AF and atrial flutter. Patients with preserved sinus rhythm may have features of left atrial enlargement (or enlargement of both atria in patients with coexisting tricuspid regurgitation). Signs of LV hypertrophy and overload may be present in chronic severe MR.

2. Chest radiographs: Significant LV and left atrial enlargement; right ventricular and right atrial enlargement in patients with coexisting tricuspid regurgitation and pulmonary hypertension. Patients with acute MR have features of pulmonary congestion with a normal cardiac silhouette. Calcifications of the mitral annulus may be present.

3. Doppler echocardiography is used to detect a regurgitant jet, allowing quantitative and qualitative assessment. A specific cause of MR (primary or secondary) and effects on LV and left atrium can be elucidated. The pulmonary artery pressure can often be measured. In the case of equivocal results of transthoracic imaging, transesophageal echocardiography is helpful.

4. Exercise stress testing is helpful for objective evaluation of exercise tolerance. Echocardiographic stress test is used for noninvasive assessment of exertional increase in pulmonary artery systolic pressures.

5. Cardiac catheterization and coronary angiography are rarely performed in MR, except to assess for concomitant coronary artery disease in patients referred for mitral valve surgery in whom coronary disease is a clinical concern (>40 years of age, coronary disease risk factors).

6. Magnetic resonance imaging (MRI) is more reliable than echocardiography in the determination of the end-diastolic and end-systolic LV volume, as well as of the LV mass; however, echocardiography with Doppler remains the gold standard for assessment of the mitral valve apparatus and MR severity.

Differential Diagnosis

On physical examination, differential diagnosis includes aortic stenosis and tricuspid regurgitation. On echocardiography, there is usually little doubt as to whether hemodynamically significant (moderate or severe) MR is present or not.

→ TREATMENT

Treatment of Acute Mitral Regurgitation

1. Vasodilators (nitroglycerin or sodium nitroprusside). In the case of shock, these are used in combination with catecholamines and intra-aortic balloon counterpulsation (the latter is contraindicated in patients with coexisting significant aortic regurgitation). Agents and dosage: →Table 9-3.

2. Surgical treatment is necessary in all patients with severe acute MR who are surgical candidates; emergency surgery is necessary in the case of hemodynamic instability. Depending on the anatomy, this includes either mitral valvuloplasty (eg, partial leaflet resection, annuloplasty using a prosthetic ring) or mitral valve replacement (bioprosthetic or mechanical).

Table 17-7. Echocardiographic monitoring of mitral regurgitation

Severity of regurgitation	Follow-up
Mild	Every 5 years
Moderate	Every 1 to 2 years
Severe	Every year

Treatment of Chronic Mitral Regurgitation

Management of severe chronic primary MR: In general, medical therapy, surgical therapy, or both may be used, depending mainly on the presence of symptoms, LV function and size, and need for coronary revascularization:

1) **Primary MR** (due to an organic leaflet abnormality, eg, mitral valve prolapse): In general, mitral valve repair is preferred to replacement, and is indicated in patients with severe MR who have left ventricular ejection fraction (LVEF) ≤60% or have significant LV dilation (LV end-systolic diameter ≥40 mm). Ideally, it is recommended that mitral valve surgery should be performed before these thresholds are reached. In patients with very poor LV function (LVEF <30%), surgery can be considered in experienced hands, with the option of percutaneous mitral valve repair (a mitral valve clip) in patients with prohibitive surgical risk. In asymptomatic patients with severe organic MR and LVEF ≥60% without significant LV dilation (LV end-systolic diameter ≤40 mm), surgery can be considered in centers with significant MV repair experience and a high chance of repair success (as opposed to replacement).

2) **Secondary MR** (due to LV dilation with structurally normal leaflets): Patients with severe secondary MR should receive optimal medical therapy for heart failure with reduced ejection fraction including angiotensin--converting enzyme inhibitors (ACEIs) (or angiotensin receptor neprilysin inhibitors [ARNIs]), β-blockers, aldosterone antagonists, and diuretics as needed. Cardiac resynchronization can reduce MR in those qualifying based on LVEF and QRS duration.⊘⊖ Patients with persistent symptomatic severe MR despite therapy for LV dysfunction should be referred to an interdisciplinary heart team to consider percutaneous or surgical intervention. Among patients who are undergoing coronary artery bypass graft (CABG), surgery for mitral valve is indicated in patients with severe MR and LVEF >30% and could be considered (but is rarely done) in symptomatic patients with severe MR and LVEF <30%. Surgical mitral valve replacement rather than surgical repair is associated with less recurrent MR.⊘⊖ Surgery is not routinely indicated in patients with moderate MR who undergo CABG.⊗⊖ For patients without other indications for sternotomy, percutaneous mitral valve repair with mitral valve clip(s) is an option in experienced centers.⊘⊖

Vasodilators (carvedilol, isosorbide mononitrate, ACEIs, angiotensin-receptor blockers): These are most effective in patients with contraindications to surgery who have LV enlargement, significant systolic LV dysfunction, and severe symptoms.⊘⊖ In asymptomatic patients with minor LV enlargement, vasodilators offer little or no benefit. Agents and dosage: →Table 9-5.

➡ FOLLOW-UP

Follow-up: →Table 17-7.

➡ COMPLICATIONS

AF, heart failure and pulmonary edema, pulmonary hypertension, sudden cardiac death (in patients with a flail leaflet).

The annual mortality rate in severe chronic structural MR without surgical treatment is 5%.

17.2.2. Mitral Stenosis

→ **DEFINITION, ETIOLOGY, PATHOGENESIS**

Mitral stenosis (MS) is a reduction of the mitral valve orifice area causing obstruction of blood flow from the left atrium to the left ventricle (LV). **Classification based on etiology**:

1) **Structural MS**: Limited mobility of the leaflets and chordae tendineae due to organic lesions. Etiology: rheumatic (most frequently, especially if more than mild), degenerative (due to severe mitral annular calcification, increasingly common in aging populations), infective endocarditis; rarely, systemic lupus erythematosus, rheumatoid arthritis, carcinoid syndrome, or storage diseases.

2) **Functional MS**: Inhibited opening of structurally normal valve leaflets. Etiology: aortic regurgitation, left atrial thrombus, tumor (usually left atrial myxoma).

→ **CLINICAL FEATURES AND NATURAL HISTORY**

1. Symptoms: Impaired exercise tolerance, fatigue, exertional dyspnea, sometimes cough with expectoration of frothy sputum, hemoptysis, recurrent respiratory tract infections, palpitations, right upper abdominal quadrant discomfort, rarely hoarseness (due to compression of the left recurrent laryngeal nerve by an enlarged left atrium [Ortner syndrome]), chest pain (in 15% of patients due to high right ventricular pressures or coexisting coronary artery disease).

2. Signs: An accentuated first heart sound, opening snap of the mitral valve, a low-pitched decrescendo diastolic rumble with presystolic accentuation (the rumble can occur in patients with preserved sinus rhythm). A Graham Steell murmur caused by pulmonary regurgitation in patients with severe pulmonary hypertension and dilation of the main pulmonary artery. In advanced MS, pinkish-purple patches on the cheeks, peripheral cyanosis, systolic pulsation in the epigastrium, displacement of the apical impulse to the left, symptoms of right ventricular failure (→Chapter 3.8.2).

3. Natural history: The severity of MS gradually increases. The first symptoms usually develop approximately 15 to 20 years after an episode of rheumatic fever. The usual presenting symptoms are exertional dyspnea; supraventricular arrhythmias (particularly atrial fibrillation [AF]; the risk increases with age and with progressive left atrial enlargement); and thromboembolic events (up to 6/100 patients/y; risk factors: age, AF, small mitral valve orifice area, spontaneous left atrial contrast on echocardiography).

→ **DIAGNOSIS**

Diagnosis is based on typical clinical features and echocardiography results.

Diagnostic Tests

1. Electrocardiography (ECG): Features of left atrial enlargement, often P mitrale, frequently atrial arrhythmias, particularly AF. In patients with pulmonary hypertension, right axis deviation, incomplete right bundle branch block (less frequently other features of right ventricular hypertrophy and overload), P mitrale that may evolve into P cardiale or P pulmonale.

Table 17-8. Classification of mitral stenosis			
	Stenosis		
	Mild	Moderate	Severe
Mean MVG (mm Hg)	<5	5-10	>10
PASP (mm Hg)	<30	30-50	>50
MVA (cm²)	>2.0	1.5-2.0	<1.5 (<1.0: very severe)

Based on Circulation. 2014;129(23):e521-643.

MVA, mitral valve area; MVG, mitral valve gradient; PASP, pulmonary artery systolic pressure.

2. Chest radiographs: Left atrial enlargement, dilation of the upper lobe pulmonary veins, dilation of the main pulmonary artery, pulmonary alveolar edema, pulmonary interstitial edema, right ventricular enlargement, calcifications of the mitral valve (rare).

3. Echocardiography is used to evaluate the anatomic features of the valve (heavily calcified valves are generally not amenable to percutaneous procedures; this is important for the percutaneous vs surgical approach), detect left atrial thrombi (transesophageal echocardiography is useful as most thrombi occur in the left atrial appendage, which is not well-visualized on transthoracic echocardiography), measure the mean transvalvular gradient, calculate the mitral valve area (MVA), estimate the pulmonary artery pressure, and classify the severity of MS (→Table 17-8).

4. Exercise stress testing is used to assess exercise tolerance and the increase in pulmonary artery pressures (especially important for management of patients with moderate MS at rest and exertional symptoms).

5. Cardiac catheterization and coronary angiography are used in cases that are equivocal by clinical and echocardiographic criteria to confirm the severity of MS and to measure pulmonary artery pressures. Coronary angiography is recommended in patients >40 years of age who are undergoing intervention for MS (→below), or in younger patients with LV dysfunction or suspected coronary artery disease.

⇨ TREATMENT

General Considerations

1. Mild asymptomatic MS: Pharmacologic treatment.

2. Moderate or severe MS: Management depends primarily on the presence of symptoms and the anatomy of the valve. Specialist referral is usually required; however, in general, the following factors increase the potential benefits of invasive therapy: severe MS; presence of symptoms; and favorable valve morphology (to consider percutaneous options). More details: below.

Invasive Treatment

1. Percutaneous mitral commissurotomy (PMC), also referred to as **percutaneous balloon mitral valvuloplasty (PBMV)**: Separation or tearing apart of the fused commissures with a balloon inserted via the atrial septum using a catheter. Owing to high efficacy and low risk of complications (death, cardiac tamponade, peripheral embolism), it is the first therapeutic choice for appropriate MS cases.◉◯

Indications: Patients with severe MS (MVA <1.5 cm²), symptoms attributable to MS (or asymptomatic patients with new-onset AF), mild or mild to moderate mitral regurgitation, and valve anatomy amenable to PMC (generally, the less calcified and mobile valves are amenable to PMC, whereas heavily calcified, immobile valves require surgical treatment).

Contraindications: MVA >1.5 cm^2; left atrial thrombus; concomitant moderate or greater mitral regurgitation; nonrheumatic etiology of MS; poorly mobile valves; severe leaflet or bicommissural calcification; absence of commissural fusion; severe concomitant aortic valve disease, or severe combined tricuspid stenosis and regurgitation; concomitant coronary artery disease requiring bypass surgery.

2. Surgical valve repair:

1) Open (direct vision) mitral commissurotomy using cardiopulmonary bypass.
2) Closed mitral commissurotomy using a transatrial approach (this is rarely if ever used).

3. Mitral valve replacement (MVR) is indicated in patients with New York Heart Association class III/IV heart failure and severe abnormalities of the valvular apparatus when balloon and surgical commissurotomy are not possible. MVR is associated with higher hospital and long-term mortality rates as well as more frequent complications than PMC (this may be confounded by patient selection, ie, candidates not amenable to PMC [higher risk, with more severe valvular calcification] are referred for surgery). In patients with mechanical valves, lifetime oral anticoagulant treatment is necessary (target international normalized ratio [INR] values: →Table 17-5).

Medical Treatment

1. Patients not eligible for or refusing consent to invasive treatment: Diuretics (in the case of symptoms of pulmonary congestion), **β-blockers** with or without **digoxin** (particularly in the case of AF with a fast ventricular rhythm), and **angiotensin-converting enzyme inhibitors (ACEIs)** (in the case of coexisting LV dysfunction).

2. Anticoagulant treatment (INR, 2.0-3.0): In patients with AF, after embolic events, or with a documented left atrial thrombus, anticoagulation is definitely indicated. In patients with an enlarged left atrium (>55 mm), spontaneous left atrial contrast on echocardiography, and/or coexisting systolic LV failure, anticoagulation may be considered but is not supported by evidence. There is no current evidence supporting novel oral anticoagulants for patients with MS and indication for anticoagulation.

3. Electrical cardioversion: In patients with AF and hemodynamic instability. Electrical cardioversion may be considered in the case of the first AF occurrence in patients with mild to moderate MS, and after successful invasive treatment of MS in patients with a short episode of AF and minor left atrial enlargement. If medical therapy fails and AF is producing heart failure, clinical instability, or both, electrical cardioversion can be considered in patients with MS who are therapeutically anticoagulated; transesophageal echocardiography may also be helpful in such patients to exclude left atrial and left atrial appendage thrombi prior to cardioversion, particularly those with severe MS and marked left atrial enlargement. Pharmacologic cardioversion (usually with amiodarone) is generally less effective than electrical.

4. Prevention of infective endocarditis and of recurrent rheumatic fever.

→ FOLLOW-UP

The frequency of follow-up visits in patients receiving noninvasive treatment depends on the severity of MS. Patients with mild asymptomatic MS: follow-up visits every 2 to 3 years. Asymptomatic patients with significant MS and patients after successful PMC: clinical and echocardiographic examination every year; in symptomatic patients, every 6 months.

→ PROGNOSIS

In asymptomatic patients, the 10-year survival rates are >80% and 20-year survival rates are ~40%. The prognosis is affected by the onset of even minor symptoms and significantly improved by PMC or MVR in patients with severe MS, symptoms attributable to MS, or both. The causes of death are heart failure and thromboembolic events.

17.2.3. Mitral Valve Prolapse

→ DEFINITION, ETIOLOGY, PATHOGENESIS

Mitral valve prolapse (MVP) is displacement of a part of one or more mitral leaflets into the left atrium during left ventricular contraction, which may or may not be associated with mitral regurgitation.

MVP syndrome (formerly termed the "floppy valve" or Barlow syndrome) is a group of symptoms, including chest pain, palpitations, arrhythmias, dizziness, and syncope, which occur in patients with MVP.

Primary MVP results from myxomatous degeneration of the leaflets and chordae tendineae; it may be familial or associated with other conditions, for instance, Marfan syndrome. **Secondary MVP** occurs in patients with connective tissue diseases, acute endocarditis (due to rupture of chordae tendineae), as well as ischemic heart disease (eg, due to rupture of a papillary muscle in patients with myocardial infarction). Rupture of chordae tendineae may present as a flail leaflet. MVP may be accompanied by tricuspid valve prolapse (in 10%-20% of cases), aortic or pulmonary valve prolapse (2%-10%), and sometimes by an aneurysm or atrial septal defect.

→ CLINICAL FEATURES AND NATURAL HISTORY

1. Symptoms: Chest pain, palpitations, dizziness, collapse, and syncope.

2. Signs: Typically a mid- or late-systolic click, late-systolic or holosystolic murmur (abnormal heart sounds are more pronounced with standing; absence of these symptoms argues against MVP).

3. Natural history varies from mild, asymptomatic cases to patients at high risk of death.

→ DIAGNOSIS

Diagnosis is based on clinical features (if present) and echocardiography results.

Diagnostic Tests

1. Electrocardiography (ECG) is normal in the majority of patients; in some symptomatic patients, nonspecific ST-segment changes in leads II, III, and aVF (rarely in V_4-V_6) and arrhythmia may be observed.

2. Chest radiographs are usually normal, except for severe chronic or acute mitral regurgitation (MR).

3. Echocardiography is performed to diagnose MVP in asymptomatic patients with typical findings on auscultation, and to rule out MVP in patients with suspected MVP who have no typical findings on auscultation.

→ TREATMENT

1. Asymptomatic patients or patients with mild symptoms and favorable echocardiographic findings: Reassure the patient of a good prognosis; recommend normal lifestyle, regular exercise, and follow-up every 3 to 5 years (unless there is significant MR).

2. Patients with paroxysmal palpitations accompanied by anxiety, chest pain, and fatigue: β-Blockers may be beneficial.

3. Patients after a transient ischemic attack: Start acetylsalicylic acid (ASA) 75 to 325 mg/d, unless the patient otherwise qualifies for systemic anticoagulation.

4. Patient with a history of stroke and MR, atrial fibrillation, or left atrial thrombus: Start long-term anticoagulant treatment with a vitamin K antagonist (international normalized ratio [INR] ~2.5).

5. Surgical treatment should be considered in **patients with myxomatous valves and severe MR**, even in the absence of symptoms, if the mitral valve has a high chance of repair in experienced surgical hands.⊘◯ In cases where mitral valve repair is not possible or fails, mitral valve replacement must be performed.

6. Percutaneous mitral valve repair using the edge-to-edge procedure (a mitral valve clip) is a new method of percutaneous treatment in selected patients who are ineligible for surgery because of high perioperative risk (commonly severe left ventricular dysfunction).

→ PROGNOSIS

Prognosis is generally favorable. Factors associated with an increased risk of death include severe and possibly moderate MR, left ventricular ejection fraction <50%, unfavorable echocardiographic findings (severe thickening or elongation of a leaflet, or both), and presence of pulmonary hypertension. Patients with MVP and ≥1 of the following conditions should not engage in competitive sports: history of loss of consciousness of unexplained cause, family history of sudden cardiac death in persons with MVP, paroxysmal supraventricular arrhythmias or complex ventricular arrhythmias (particularly occurring or worsening during exercise), severe MR, left ventricular dysfunction, Marfan syndrome, long QT syndrome.

17.2.4. Mixed Mitral Valve Disease

→ DEFINITION, ETIOLOGY, CLINICAL FEATURES

Mixed mitral valve disease refers to coexisting mitral stenosis (MS) and mitral regurgitation (MR).

Etiology: Rheumatic disease, less frequently degenerative or endocarditic lesions.

Clinical features are similar to that of MS and MR, and depend on which of these hemodynamic lesions is dominant (→Chapter 3.17.2.2; →Chapter 3.17.2.1). Most frequently the systolic murmur typical of MR is prominent and may mask the soft rumble typical of MS. The first heart sound may be increased in intensity.

→ DIAGNOSIS

Diagnostic Tests

In patients with hemodynamically significant combined MS and MR, **chest radiographs** reveal enlargement of the left atrium and ventricle (also the right ventricle if the valve disease is severe and chronic) and features of pulmonary congestion, less frequently pulmonary hypertension. In patients with dominant MS the size of LV may be normal.

→ TREATMENT

1. Pharmacologic treatment of heart failure.

2. Antithrombotic treatment in patients with atrial fibrillation.

3. Prevention of infective endocarditis and of recurrent rheumatic disease (→Chapter 8.12).

4. Invasive treatment: Patients with coexisting moderate or severe MR are ineligible for percutaneous valvuloplasty; usually, treatment involves mitral valve replacement.

17.3. Multivalvular Disease

→ DEFINITION, ETIOLOGY, PATHOGENESIS

Multivalvular disease affects ≥2 venous or arterial valves; in general order of descending frequency in the contemporary European or North American practice:

1) Mitral regurgitation (MR) and tricuspid regurgitation (TR).

2) Aortic stenosis (AS) and MR.

3) Aortic regurgitation (AR) and MR.

4) AS and TR.

5) Mitral stenosis (MS) and AR.

6) MS and AS.

Previously multivalvular disease with secondary effects on the left ventricle and the left atrium used to be mainly caused by rheumatic heart disease (eg, MS and AS); however, with ageing populations (and increased use of antibiotics in childhood and youth), degenerative or functional MR with secondary TR as well as degenerative AS with secondary MR or TR are increasingly common.

→ CLINICAL FEATURES AND DIAGNOSIS

In general, the predominant clinical features are caused by the hemodynamically more severe lesion; however, assuming similar degrees of valvular severity, symptoms are related to the disease of the more proximal (upstream) valvular lesion (eg, AS in combined AS/MR). The primary valve lesion can create secondary ("back pressure") effects on the secondary valve lesion (eg, chronic severe MR [or AS] leading to right ventricular dilation, secondary functional TR, and pulmonary hypertension). In advanced multivalvular disease, symptoms of heart failure are often present, and are accompanied by secondary hemodynamic effects on the cardiac chambers (eg, chronic severe AR leading to left ventricular and left atrial dilation and secondary functional MR). Features of various types of multivalvular disease: →Table 17-9.

The diagnostic workup of multivalvular heart disease is not significantly different from that of individual valvular lesions.

→ TREATMENT

To establish indications for surgical treatment, the clinical and hemodynamic significance of the components of multivalvular heart disease must be assessed. Any defect assessed separately may not be severe enough to warrant surgical treatment; however, when combined, these may have significant hemodynamic consequences that require surgery. In some cases it may not be necessary to replace all the affected valves (eg, surgical treatment of severe AS may, by relieving afterload challenge to the left ventricle, relieve secondary functional MR). Double-valve replacement is generally associated with higher perioperative and long-term risks, owing to a more complex surgical technique and longer cardiopulmonary bypass times, compared to single valve repair or replacement (with or without coronary artery bypass graft); thus, whenever feasible, repair is often preferred (eg, mitral valve repair for severe myxomatous mitral regurgitation with concomitant tricuspid valve annuloplasty for secondary TR). It is important to recognize that management of multivalve disease is essentially

Table 17-9. Characteristics of multivalvular disease

Multi-valvular disease	Pathophysiology	Auscultation	Surgical treatment	Comments
MR + TR	Chronic MR causes pulmonary hypertension, leading to RV dilation and secondary TR	Apical systolic murmur caused by MR and lower sternal border murmur of TR	Mitral repair or replacement with tricuspid valve repair or annuloplasty	MR most commonly the dominant lesion; at times relief of MR alone may result in decrease in TR
AS + MR	AS leads to LV afterload challenge or strain and secondary MR; impaired aortic valve outflow can further aggravate MR	Ejection murmur radiating to carotid arteries and murmur caused by MR radiating to axilla	Simultaneous aortic valve replacement and mitral repair or replacement	MR may be reduced after aortic valve replacement (or TAVI) without specific mitral valve intervention
AR + MR	AR leads to LV dilation and secondary MR	Apical systolic murmur caused by MR and diastolic murmur caused by AR	Simultaneous aortic valve repair or replacement and mitral repair or replacement	AR frequently dominant; in such cases it is difficult to distinguish primary from secondary MR due to LV enlargement; at times treatment of AR alone may relieve significant MR due to LV dilation caused by chronic AR
MS + TR	MS leads to pulmonary hypertension and secondary regurgitation of anatomically normal tricuspid valve; in some patients tricuspid valve also affected by rheumatic fever	Typical signs of MS and holosystolic murmur (more prominent during inspiration) caused by TR	Mitral valve replacement (or mitral valvuloplasty) and tricuspid annuloplasty	Hemodynamically significant TR may improve following mitral valve valvuloplasty (or surgery) without specific surgical treatment of the tricuspid valve
MS + AS	MS restricts blood inflow to LV and aggravates the drop of cardiac output caused by AS	Typical signs of MS and murmur caused by AS (less prominent than in isolated AS)	Simultaneous replacement of both valves	Percutaneous balloon mitral valvuloplasty in patients with significant AS may result in pulmonary edema
MS + AR	Impaired LV filling from left atrium is compensated by reverse blood flow through aortic valve	Typical signs of MS and diastolic murmur along left sternal border	Before surgical treatment of aortic valve percutaneous balloon mitral valvuloplasty should be considered	MS reduces LV volume overload and can mask AR

AR, aortic regurgitation; AS, aortic stenosis; LV, left ventricle; MR, mitral regurgitation; MS, mitral stenosis; RV, right ventricle; TAVI, transcatheter aortic valve implantation; TR, tricuspid regurgitation.

an "evidence-free zone," and thus recommendations in the most current 2014 American College of Cardiology and American Heart Association guidelines are brief and consensus-based.

17.4. Tricuspid Valve Disease

17.4.1. Tricuspid Regurgitation

→ DEFINITION, ETIOLOGY, PATHOGENESIS

Tricuspid regurgitation (TR) is a reversal of blood flow from the right ventricle to the right atrium due to an incomplete closure of tricuspid valve leaflets. Patients with isolated TR (without tricuspid stenosis) usually have functional TR related to pulmonary hypertension (secondary or primary) or coexisting mitral valve disease, particularly stenosis.

Etiology:

1) **Structural (organic) TR**: Rheumatic fever, infective endocarditis, carcinoid syndrome, Marfan syndrome, Fabry disease, Whipple disease, tricuspid valve prolapse, rheumatoid arthritis, systemic lupus erythematosus, congenital heart disease (Ebstein anomaly and other conditions), papillary muscle dysfunction, drugs (methysergide, fenfluramine).

2) **Functional TR** (most frequent in patients with acquired valvular disease): Dilation of the tricuspid annulus of an anatomically normal valve secondary to the altered right ventricular geometry most commonly caused by pulmonary hypertension, mitral valve disease, right ventricular myocardial infarction, or congenital heart disease (eg, right ventricular outflow obstruction).

3) **TR associated with intracardiac devices**: Pacemaker and defibrillator leads can interfere with function of the tricuspid valve and lead to varying degrees of regurgitation, which may be progressive.

→ CLINICAL FEATURES

Clinical features are usually dominated by symptoms of the coexisting pulmonary hypertension or mitral valve disease.

1. Symptoms: Reduced exercise tolerance, weakness, peripheral edema, right upper abdominal discomfort and distension.

2. Signs: Pulsation of significantly distended neck veins, a positive hepatojugular reflux; in patients with severe TR, pulsations of the vessels of the neck and head, less commonly pulsations of the eyes; right ventricular impulse; pulsations of the liver; in advanced TR, generalized subcutaneous edema, ascites, and cyanotic-yellowish color of the skin; a holosystolic murmur intensified during deep inspiration and diastolic rumble (in severe TR).

→ DIAGNOSIS

Diagnostic Tests

1. Electrocardiography (ECG): P pulmonale, features of right ventricular hypertrophy, frequently incomplete right bundle branch block. Atrial fibrillation and atrial flutter are usually seen.

2. Chest radiographs: In functional TR, the heart is significantly enlarged and includes a prominent right atrium; pleural effusion and distension of the azygos vein may be seen. Right ventricular enlargement in severe TR.

3. Echocardiography is used to assess the morphology of the tricuspid valve and severity of TR, as well as right ventricular systolic pressures (pressures >55 mm Hg suggest secondary TR). Significant TR with a normal tricuspid valve morphology may develop in patients with main pulmonary artery systolic pressures ≥55 mm Hg. TR in patients with pulmonary artery systolic pressures <40 mm Hg suggests structural valve abnormalities. In many healthy individuals, clinically irrelevant TR is seen.

→ TREATMENT

1. Medical therapy: Diuretics play a major role in symptomatic relief in patients with TR.

2. TR combined with mitral valve disease:

1) Surgical treatment of mitral stenosis alone may significantly reduce the severity of functional TR.

2) Surgical tricuspid valvuloplasty is indicated in patients with severe TR or dilation of the annulus ($\geq$40 mm or >21 mm/m^2) accompanied by mitral valve disease requiring surgery.

3) After left-sided valve surgery, tricuspid valve surgery may be considered in symptomatic patients with severe TR who have progressive right ventricular dilation or dysfunction in the absence of left-sided valve dysfunction, severe right or left ventricular dysfunction, and severe pulmonary vascular disease.

3. Severe symptomatic isolated primary TR without severe right ventricular dysfunction: Tricuspid valve repair; if not possible, tricuspid valve replacement is indicated.

4. Severe asymptomatic or mildly symptomatic isolated primary TR with progressive right ventricular dilation or deterioration of right ventricular function: Surgery should be considered.

5. TR with coexisting conduction disturbances: Implantation of an epicardial pacemaker during valve replacement surgery.

Recently developed transcatheter techniques have provided an alternative for patients with severe symptoms and prohibitive surgical risks. These patients should be evaluated in heart valve centers by a multidisciplinary team including surgeons, imaging specialists, and interventional cardiologists for eligibility.

→ PROGNOSIS

Regardless of the underlying condition, severe TR is associated with a poor long-term prognosis due to the progressive right ventricular dysfunction and systemic venous congestion.

17.4.2. Tricuspid Stenosis

→ DEFINITION, ETIOLOGY, PATHOGENESIS

Tricuspid stenosis (TS) is a reduction of the tricuspid valve orifice area, which causes impaired right ventricular filling.

Etiology: Rheumatic fever; other, very rare etiologies include carcinoid syndrome. Right atrial myxoma or other tumors of the right atrium, tricuspid valve vegetations, and right atrial thrombus can cause tricuspid inflow stenosis not related to the valve but with similar physiologic consequences. Tricuspid atresia is a rare congenital anomaly affecting the tricuspid valve with other associated lesions. Patients with previous tricuspid valve replacement can develop prosthetic valve stenosis. The majority of patients have mixed TS and tricuspid regurgitation (TR), such as those with carcinoid syndrome.

→ CLINICAL FEATURES

1. Symptoms: Progressive fatigue, loss of appetite, mild dyspnea. Palpitations related to atrial arrhythmias are common.

2. Signs: A tricuspid opening snap, presystolic murmur (in patients with sinus rhythm), an early- and mid-diastolic murmur (rarely holodiastolic), most prominent during inspiration; signs of right ventricular failure ($\rightarrow$Chapter 3.8.2), pulsations of the liver (presystolic pulsation is typical).

➔ DIAGNOSIS

Diagnostic Tests

1. Electrocardiography (ECG): P pulmonale; frequently atrial fibrillation or atrial flutter. There may be features of enlargement of both atria (due to the frequent coexisting mitral valve disease). The amplitude of the QRS complex may be low in V_1 due to right atrial enlargement.

2. Chest radiographs: Right atrial enlargement and dilation of the superior vena cava. Pulmonary perfusion may be reduced.

3. Echocardiography: Evaluation of the valve morphology and severity of the defect. A mean transvalvular gradient of ≥5 mm Hg at a normal heart rate is considered indicative of clinically significant TS. Given the association with rheumatic heart disease, the left-sided valve should be fully assessed. In cases of suspected carcinoid syndrome, there is often pulmonary valve involvement with combined stenosis and regurgitation.

➔ TREATMENT

1. Medical treatment: Diuretics (agents: →Table 9-5) and fluid and sodium restriction.

2. Invasive treatment should be considered in patients with severe TS who are (1) symptomatic; or (2) undergoing intervention on other left heart valves (percutaneous valvotomy may be attempted in patients eligible for percutaneous mitral commissurotomy). In patients with isolated severe TS, consider percutaneous tricuspid balloon valvotomy; in patients with coexisting mitral valve disease, surgical treatment is indicated. Valve morphology can provide clues as to the underlying etiology.

18. Peripheral Vascular Diseases

18.1. Aortic Diseases

18.1.1. Aortic Aneurysms

➔ DEFINITION, ETIOLOGY, PATHOGENESIS

Aortic aneurysm is a local dilation of the aorta by >50% of its normal diameter. Normal aortic dimensions in adults: →Table 18-1.

Anatomy of the aorta: →Figure 18-1.

Classifications of aortic aneurysms:

1) Based on etiology: **Atherosclerotic aneurysm (most common by far)**, **degenerative aneurysm** (Marfan syndrome, Ehlers-Danlos syndrome type IV, cystic degeneration of the aorta), **postinflammatory aneurysm** (Takayasu disease, giant cell arteritis, inflammation in the course of systemic diseases, syphilis, infective endocarditis, sepsis), **posttraumatic aneurysm**.

2) Based on shape: **Fusiform aneurysm** (much more frequent), **saccular aneurysm** (→Figure 18-2).

3) Based on wall structure: **True aneurysm**, **pseudoaneurysm** (or "false aneurysm"; after disruption of the intima and media, the aneurysm wall is formed by the adventitia together with surrounding tissues; this type is often posttraumatic; →Figure 18-2).

Table 18-1. Normal aortic dimensions in adults measured from the outer wall

Aortic segment	Diameter (mm)	Imaging study
Aortic annulus	F: 23 ± 2 M: 26 ± 3	Transthoracic US
Sinus of Valsalva	F: 30 ± 3 M: 34 ± 3	Transthoracic US
Aortic root	<37	Transthoracic US
Proximal ascending aorta	F: 26 ± 3 M: 29 ± 3	Transesophageal US
Ascending aorta	$14-21/m^2$ BSA	Transesophageal US
	25-38	CT
Descending aorta	$10-16/m^2$ BSA	Transesophageal US
	17-28	CT
Abdominal aorta	14-21	B-mode US

BSA, body surface area; CT, computed tomography; F, female patients; M, male patients; US, ultrasonography.

4) Based on location: **Thoracic aneurysm** (usually of the ascending aorta but also can be seen in the aortic arch or descending thoracic aorta), **abdominal aneurysm** (located below the diaphragm; infrarenal aneurysms constitute ~90% of aortic aneurysms), **thoracoabdominal aneurysm** (more extensive, involving both the thoracic and abdominal aorta).

5) Based on clinical presentation: **Asymptomatic**, **symptomatic**, **dissecting** (→Figure 18-2), **ruptured**.

→ CLINICAL FEATURES AND NATURAL HISTORY

What follows below pertains to an aneurysm that is either asymptomatic or causing symptoms related to the space it occupies. It does not correspond to acute medical emergency of aortic dissection or aneurysm rupture (→Complications, below).

The majority of aortic aneurysms, regardless of location, are asymptomatic and most commonly identified as an incidental finding on imaging. The first manifestation of an aortic aneurysm may be a thromboembolic incident, such as stroke, lower limb ischemia, intestinal ischemia, renal infarction, or blue toe syndrome (acute ischemia [sometimes necrosis] of the toes caused by small emboli originating from the aneurysm cavity).

1. Symptoms and signs of a thoracic aortic aneurysm: Chest pain and back pain (in 25% of patients without dissection; usually persistent, stabbing, often severe), dysphagia (rare), hoarseness, cough, dyspnea (sometimes dependent on body position), hemoptysis, recurrent pneumonia, and Horner syndrome. Aneurysms of the ascending aorta or aortic arch may cause symptoms of aortic regurgitation (often with manifestations of heart failure) or symptoms of superior vena cava syndrome.

2. Symptoms and signs of an abdominal aortic aneurysm: Symptoms are usually absent. The most frequent manifestation is a constant dull pain that may be abdominal, hypogastric, or lumbar and mimics radicular pain

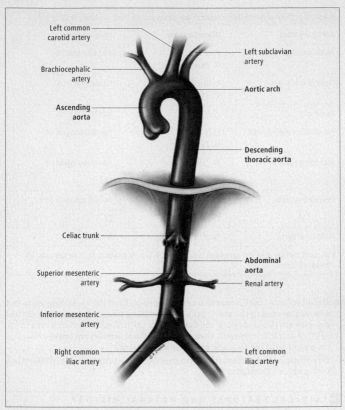

Figure 18-1. Anatomy of the aorta. *Illustration courtesy of Dr Shannon Zhang.*

(movement has no effect on pain intensity; may be less severe in the supine position with bent knees). Aneurysms ≥5 cm in diameter may be palpable if examined for. They are frequently tender, especially when expanding rapidly. Murmurs may be audible over the abdominal aorta.

3. Natural history: Aneurysms have a tendency to expand and rupture (→Complications, below). The 5-year risk of rupture of an abdominal aortic aneurysm is 2% for aneurysms <40 mm in diameter, 20% for aneurysms >50 mm in diameter, and 40% for aneurysms >60 mm in diameter. An increase in aneurysm diameter by 5 mm over 6 months is associated with a 2-fold increase in the risk of rupture.

Ascending thoracic aortic aneurysms expand by an average of 0.1 cm per year (aneurysms of the descending aorta, large aneurysms, and those associated with Marfan syndrome grow faster; in patients with Loeys-Dietz syndrome they may expand >1 cm per year). The 1-year risk of rupture is 7% for aneurysms >60 mm in diameter and 2% for aneurysms <50 mm in diameter.

Aortic aneurysms may undergo dissection, although this happens rarely, as preexisting aneurysms generally do not dissect but rather expand, rupture, or embolize.

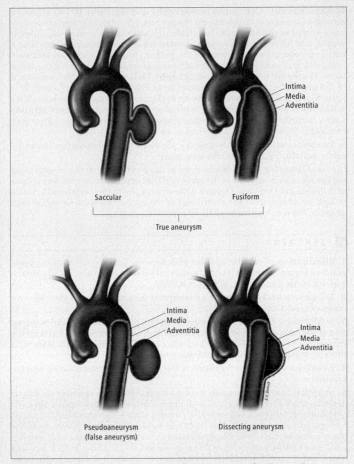

Saccular

Fusiform

Intima
Media
Adventitia

True aneurysm

Pseudoaneurysm
(false aneurysm)

Intima
Media
Adventitia

Dissecting aneurysm

Intima
Media
Adventitia

Figure 18-2. Different types of aortic aneurysm. *Illustration courtesy of Dr Shannon Zhang.*

→ DIAGNOSIS

Aortic aneurysms are usually detected incidentally on imaging studies performed for unrelated indications.

1. Chest radiographs reveal dilation of the aorta (a normal aortic silhouette does not exclude an aneurysm of the ascending aorta).

2. Transthoracic echocardiography (TTE) is a useful screening test of the ascending aorta; visualization of the aortic arch and descending aorta is more difficult. **Transesophageal echocardiography (TEE)** allows for assessment of the entire thoracic aorta except for the short distal segment of the ascending aorta.

3. Ultrasonography is a key technique for diagnosing abdominal aortic aneurysms.

4. Angiography: Computed tomography angiography (CTA) allows for accurate assessment of the size (to the nearest 0.2 cm) and extent of an aneurysm as well as the anatomical relationships between the aneurysm, adjacent organs, and arteries branching off from the aorta (sometimes this is sufficient for the preoperative assessment of the patient); it is also used to detect coexisting aortic dissection, aortic intramural hematoma, and penetrating aortic ulcer. **Magnetic resonance angiography (MRA)** is useful for assessment of the size and extent of an aneurysm when CTA cannot be performed. It is particularly justified in serial periodic evaluations in younger patients. MRA is less useful in acute disease and does not reveal calcifications. **Aortography** with a calibrated catheter is sometimes used intraoperatively to confirm measurements prior to the final selection of an endovascular stent.

5. Intravascular ultrasonography allows for optimal visualization of the aortic wall during endovascular treatment.

In case of detecting an aortic aneurysm at any level of the aorta, consider imaging the remaining sections of the aorta and iliac arteries to exclude aneurysms in different locations and Doppler ultrasonography of the peripheral arteries to look for aneurysms. For aneurysms of the ascending aorta or aortic arch, examine the aortic valve (usually by echocardiography).

➡ TREATMENT

1. Elimination of cardiovascular risk factors, particularly smoking cessation and normalization of blood pressure (at least <140/90 mm Hg in patients without aortic dissection [→Chapter 3.9.1]).

2. Diagnosis and treatment of ischemic heart disease before elective invasive treatment of aneurysm.

3. β-Blockers: Long-term treatment with oral β-blockers slows down expansion of abdominal aortic aneurysms >4 cm in diameter but has no effect on the frequency of ruptures. Beta-blockers are also recommended in patients with thoracic aortic aneurysms and Marfan syndrome.

4. Losartan slows down expansion of the aortic root in patients with Marfan syndrome.

5. Surgical treatment usually involves implantation of a vascular prosthetic graft in place of an aneurysm. Indications include asymptomatic thoracic aortic aneurysms (in acceptable-risk patients with a life expectancy ≥2 years) >55 mm in diameter (ascending aorta and aortic arch) or >60 mm in diameter (descending aorta; if possible, endovascular treatment is preferred); smaller aneurysms in patients with Marfan syndrome and in those with a bicuspid aortic valve and risk factors; asymptomatic abdominal aortic aneurysms >55 mm in diameter (or smaller if located below or at the level of ostia of the renal arteries and larger if located above), rapidly expanding aneurysms (≥5 mm in 6 months or ≥7 mm in a year); and all symptomatic or ruptured aneurysms. Lower threshold values for invasive treatment may be used in patients with small body weight, with rapidly expanding aneurysms, with aortic regurgitation, those planning to become pregnant, or those with a borderline aorta diameter who prefer earlier invasive treatment. The recommended follow-up after surgery is duplex ultrasonography or computed tomography (CT) performed every 5 years.

6. Endovascular stenting has become the preferred treatment in most centers for patients with favorable anatomy, in particular of the descending thoracic aorta and infrarenal abdominal aorta (for patients at both low and high risk for open surgical repair). Patients with more complicated anatomy, such as with aneurysm involvement of the aortic arch, visceral vessels, or both, may be offered traditional surgery (if low risk) or custom-designed "fenestrated" or "branched" endovascular grafts if they are felt to be at higher risk of perioperative complications. Indications for endovascular repair (size, expansion, symptoms) are similar to those for open surgical treatment. The decision to proceed with endovascular repair over surgical repair is made after a discussion with the patient about considerations such as recovery time, durability of repair, feasibility, and risk, as noted earlier. Endovascular stents are increasingly being used in urgent and emergent circumstances in addition to their longstanding use in elective (planned) repairs.

→ FOLLOW-UP

1. Screening for abdominal aortic aneurysms: Perform abdominal ultrasonography in all male patients >65 years (this may be also considered in female patients >65 years) and consider it in first-degree relatives of patients with an abdominal aortic aneurysm. In patients with an aortic diameter of 26 to 29 mm, a subsequent imaging study is recommended after 4 years.

2. Asymptomatic thoracic aortic aneurysms: Perform CTA or MRA 6 months after detecting an aneurysm. Subsequent studies—using the same method at the same facility—are performed once every 12 months if the aneurysm is not expanding or every 6 months if the aneurysm expands significantly on subsequent studies.

3. Abdominal aortic aneurysms: Investigations may depend on the speed of development and expansion. Suggestions include follow-up ultrasonography or CT:

1) In patients with aneurysms 30 to 39 mm in diameter, every 3 years.

2) In patients with aneurysms 40 to 44 mm in diameter, every 2 years.

3) In patients with aneurysms >45 mm in diameter, every year.

4. In **patients after surgery**, perform follow-up duplex ultrasonography or CT every 5 years.

5. In **patients after endovascular surgery**, imaging and regular surveillance are required to ensure that the stent graft remains in good position and there are no endoleaks (persisting blood flow in the aneurysm sac) that result in elevated pressure in the aneurysm sac and its expansion. For abdominal endovascular grafts, CT is performed at 1 month following implantation to assess graft position and check for endoleaks. Subsequent imaging with duplex ultrasonography or CT is performed for surveillance, with the choice of modality and interval for imaging depending on the results or stability of the repair and surgeon preference. Thoracic endovascular grafts cannot be adequately visualized with duplex ultrasonography and generally require CTA for follow-up, with the interval also determined by the results and surgeon preference.

→ COMPLICATIONS

1. Aneurysm rupture manifests as a severe constant pain in the chest or abdomen with rapidly developing hypovolemic shock. Thoracic aortic aneurysms may rupture into the pleural cavity (usually on the left), mediastinum, pericardium (leading to rapidly developing cardiac tamponade), or esophagus (rare; this causes life-threatening hematemesis). Abdominal aortic aneurysms may rupture into the retroperitoneal space (producing a characteristic group of symptoms: sudden severe pain in the abdomen and lumbosacral region, hypovolemic shock, perineal and scrotal hematoma); peritoneal cavity (abdominal pain, symptoms of shock, and abdominal distention); duodenum (rare; massive gastrointestinal bleeding); inferior vena cava or renal or iliac vein (rare; symptoms of rapidly progressing heart failure with increased cardiac output).

2. Aortic dissection.

18.1.1.1. Aortic Pseudoaneurysm

→ DEFINITION, ETIOLOGY, PATHOGENESIS

Aortic pseudoaneurysm refers to disruption of all aortic wall layers that does not lead to fatal exsanguination thanks to periaortic connective tissue.

Causes:

1) Blunt thoracic trauma in motor vehicle accidents (impact of safety belts, motor bike crashes), falls, sports injuries.
2) Iatrogenic: Aortic surgery, percutaneous catheter-based interventions.
3) Rarely, due to aortic infection or penetrating aortic ulcer.

→ NATURAL HISTORY

An increase in blood pressure may cause an aortic pseudoaneurysm to rupture and result in fatal hemorrhage. In some patients aortic pseudoaneurysms may be an incidental finding.

→ TREATMENT

Invasive treatment (endovascular or surgical), regardless of the size of the pseudoaneurysm.

→ COMPLICATIONS

Pseudoaneurysm rupture; fistula and compression of the surrounding structures, which leads to their destruction.

18.1.1.2. Contained Rupture of Aortic Aneurysm

→ DEFINITION, ETIOLOGY, PATHOGENESIS

Contained rupture of aortic aneurysm refers to disruption of the aortic wall (sometimes also involving formation of a pseudoaneurysm) associated with the development of perivascular hematoma that is sealed off by periaortic structures: the pleura, pericardium, retroperitoneal space, or adjacent organs.

→ CLINICAL FEATURES AND NATURAL HISTORY

Symptoms:

1) A sudden-onset acute pain in the chest or back (or both). In patients with a thoracoabdominal aortic aneurysm, abdominal pain may be present.
2) Acute respiratory failure due to aortic rupture into the left hemithorax.
3) Rarely, bleeding from the respiratory tract or from the upper gastrointestinal tract.

The closer the location of rupture to the aortic valve, the higher the risk of death. Over 75% of patients die within 24 hours.

→ DIAGNOSIS

Suspected aortic rupture is an indication for urgent computed tomography angiography (CTA) without contrast enhancement to detect possible intramural hematomas and subsequently for contrast-enhanced CTA to locate the rupture.

→ TREATMENT

Invasive treatment (endovascular treatment is superior), regardless of the size of the aneurysm.

18.1.2. Acute Aortic Syndrome

Acute aortic syndrome refers to emergency aortic conditions that produce similar clinical manifestations.

Acute aortic syndrome includes:

1) **Acute aortic dissection**.
2) **Intramural hematoma**.
3) **Penetrating aortic ulcer**.

18.1.2.1. Aortic Dissection

→ DEFINITION, ETIOLOGY, PATHOGENESIS

Aortic dissection is caused by a tear of the intima with blood penetrating into the media. This results in the separation of the intima from the media and adventitia and creates a false lumen of the aorta.

Aortic dissections may be divided according to the **Stanford classification** into **type A and type B**. **Type A aortic dissections** refer to dissections involving the ascending aorta, aortic arch, or both regardless of the site of origin (70%). These may extend down into the descending thoracic or thoracoabdominal aorta. **Type B aortic dissections** involve the thoracic or thoracoabdominal aorta. These arise distal to the left subclavian artery and do not involve the ascending aorta.

The **DeBakey classification** for aortic dissections is also commonly used. **DeBakey type I dissections** involve the ascending aorta, arch, and descending thoracic aorta and may extend into the abdominal aorta. **DeBakey type II dissections** are limited to the ascending aorta. **DeBakey type III dissections** (like Stanford type B) arise distal to the left subclavian artery.

Risk factors for aortic dissection include hypertension (usually poorly controlled), bicuspid aortic valve and coarctation of the aorta (including patients after surgical correction of these malformations), history of aortic disease (eg, aortic aneurysm) or aortic valve disease, positive family history of aortic disease, congenital connective tissue diseases (Marfan syndrome, Ehlers-Danlos syndrome), cystic medial degeneration (in patients >50 years of age), aortitis, trauma (traffic accidents, iatrogenic), hemodynamic and hormonal factors during pregnancy (50% of aortic dissections in patients aged <40 years occur in pregnant women), Turner syndrome, cardiovascular surgery, professional weightlifting, tobacco smoking, and IV use of cocaine or amphetamines.

→ CLINICAL FEATURES

Aortic dissection usually manifests as severe chest pain (features: →Chapter 1.1, Table 1-1) that often leads to syncope and does not respond to sublingual or oral nitrates. It may be accompanied by symptoms of shock, neurologic symptoms (cerebral ischemia, less commonly paraplegia, upper or lower limb ischemic neuropathy, Horner syndrome, hoarseness), myocardial infarction (if dissection involves the coronary artery ostia), heart failure (in the case of severe aortic regurgitation) and cardiac tamponade, pleural effusion, acute kidney injury (involvement of the ostia of renal arteries), abdominal pain (involvement of the ostia of mesenteric arteries), features of acute limb ischemia, and limb paralysis due to spinal cord ischemia. Physical findings may include high blood pressure (BP) (50% of patients) or hypotension, diastolic murmur audible over the aortic valve caused by severe aortic regurgitation, and pulse deficit in one extremity (in ~30% of patients with dissection of the ascending aorta, aortic arch, or both). The presenting feature may also be syncope without pain and neurologic symptoms.

Symptoms indicative of the severity of the patient's condition: Very severe pain, tachycardia, tachypnea, hypotension, cyanosis, shock.

> **Table 18-2. Factors increasing the probability of acute aortic syndrome**
>
> **Conditions**
> Marfan syndrome (or other connective tissue disease)
> Family history of aortic disease
> Known aortic valve disease
> Known thoracic aortic aneurysm
> Previous aortic manipulation (including cardiac surgery)
>
> **Pain features**
> Chest, back, or abdominal pain characterized by any of:
> – Abrupt onset
> – Severe intensity
> – Ripping or tearing
>
> **Examination features**
> Evidence of perfusion deficit:
> – Pulse deficit
> – Systolic blood pressure difference in upper limbs
> – Focal neurologic deficit (in conjunction with pain)
> Aortic diastolic murmur (new and with pain)
> Hypotension or shock
>
> The presence of features from one of the groups amounts to 1 point; from 2 groups, 2 points; and from 3 groups, 3 points. The higher the score on a scale from 0 to 3, the higher the risk of acute aortic syndrome before additional diagnostic tests are performed.
>
> *Based on Circulation. 2010 Apr 6;121(13):e266-369.*

→ DIAGNOSIS

Diagnosis should be established immediately (do not prolong diagnostics in a center not capable of providing invasive treatment). Assess the clinical risk of dissection (→Table 18-2). Aortic dissection should be differentiated from other causes of chest pain. Diagnosis must be confirmed with an imaging study (preferably computed tomography angiography [CTA]; in unstable patients transesophageal echocardiography is equivalent). Chest radiographs may reveal enlargement of the cardiac silhouette, rarely of the upper mediastinum; in the case of rupture into the pleural cavity, radiographs reveal pleural effusion. Normal results of imaging studies do not exclude aortic dissection. In case of sustained suspicion of aortic dissection despite normal baseline imaging study results, repeated imaging study using CTA or magnetic resonance angiography (MRA) is recommended. Proposed diagnostic algorithm: →Figure 18-3.

→ TREATMENT

Secure peripheral venous access and—if this does not interfere with the rapidity of the diagnostic process—central venous access. Monitor urine output, heart rate, BP, electrocardiography (ECG), and arterial oxygen saturation (SaO$_2$); continue monitoring while transporting the patient to a specialist center.

1. Medical treatment: Medical treatment is used in the initial treatment and stabilization of patients with all types of aortic dissections and may be the sole treatment for uncomplicated type B dissections. (All type A and complicated type B dissections should be considered for immediate surgery [type A] or endovascular repair [type B].)

1) Administer IV **morphine** for pain control.

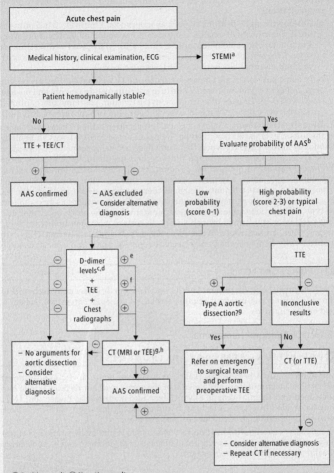

⊕ Positive result. ⊖ Negative result.

ª In rare cases STEMI can be associated with AAS.
ᵇ See text.
ᶜ Preferably point-of-care, otherwise classical.
ᵈ Also troponin levels to detect non–ST-segment elevation myocardial infarction.
ᵉ Features of aortic dissection.
ᶠ Enlargement of the mediastinum.
ᵍ Proof of type A aortic dissection by the presence of flap, aortic regurgitation, and/or pericardial effusion.
ʰ Depending on the local availability, patient's characteristics, and physician's experience.

AAS, acute aortic syndrome; CT, computed tomography; MRI, magnetic resonance imaging; STEMI, ST-segment elevation myocardial infarction; TEE, transesophageal echocardiography; TTE, transthoracic echocardiography.

Figure 18-3. Diagnosis of suspected acute aortic syndrome. *Based on Eur Heart J. 2014;35(41).2873-926.*

2) Quickly lower BP (systolic BP to 100-120 mm Hg after excluding severe aortic regurgitation):

   a) Administer an IV **β-blocker**, such as propranolol 1 mg every 3 to 5 minutes until the target BP is achieved (up to a maximum of 10 mg) then every 4 to 6 hours; or esmolol (dosage: →Table 9-3). In patients with asthma or severe chronic obstructive pulmonary disease, replace β-blockers with calcium channel blockers (or short-acting esmolol).

   b) In some patients it may be necessary to add IV **nitroglycerin**, and if this is ineffective, you may use IV **sodium nitroprusside** (agents and dosage: →Table 9-3). In case of refractory hypertension, you may add enalapril (start from 0.625-1.25 mg IV every 6 hours [up to a maximum of 5 mg]).

2. Invasive treatment: Urgent surgical intervention is the treatment of choice in the majority of patients with type A dissection (perform CT only in hemodynamically stable patients when the study does not delay transfer to a cardiac surgery center). Complicated type B dissections are those defined as ≥1 of the following: end-organ malperfusion (bowel, renal, spinal cord, lower extremity ischemia), rapid aortic expansion, refractory chest or back pain, uncontrolled hypertension despite adequate pharmacotherapy, signs of rupture (hemothorax, expanding periaortic or mediastinal hematoma). Treatment options for complicated type B dissections include endovascular stenting of the aortic entry tear and fenestration or stenting of branch vessels to restore perfusion in any ischemic organs. Open surgical repair of complicated type B dissections is increasingly rare and generally happens when endovascular repair is unavailable or not feasible.

→ COMPLICATIONS

Aortic regurgitation (in patients with ascending aortic dissection), ischemia of the extremities and internal organs, stroke, paraplegia, intestinal ischemia, and aortic rupture.

18.1.2.2. Intramural Hematoma

→ DEFINITION, ETIOLOGY, PATHOGENESIS

Aortic intramural hematoma (IMH) is a type of acute aortic syndrome in which blood accumulates in the media of the aortic wall but no false lumen has developed and intimal tear is absent. Just like acute aortic dissection, IMH may be divided into type A or type B and generally presents as chest or back pain without evidence of rupture or malperfusion.

The greatest concern with intramural hematomas is that most clinicians believe they are part of the same spectrum of disease as dissections and as such carry similar risks in case of progression.

→ NATURAL HISTORY

In 30% to 40% of patients with IMH type A, aortic dissection occurs (the risk is highest within 8 days of symptom onset).

→ DIAGNOSIS

Computed tomography (CT) and magnetic resonance imaging (MRI) are the key diagnostic studies used to diagnose and classify IMH.

→ TREATMENT

1. Medical treatment: Control of pain and blood pressure. Repeat imaging studies.

2. Invasive treatment:

1) In IMH type A coexisting with a pericardial effusion, periaortic hematoma, or large aneurysm, start **emergency surgical treatment**.

2) In other cases of IMH type A, **urgent surgical treatment** is necessary (within <24 hours of diagnosis), although in many elderly patients and those with significant comorbidities initial medical treatment may be justified (provided the aortic diameter is ≤50 mm and thickness of the intramural hematoma is <11 mm).

3) In IMH type B, medical management is the primary treatment but invasive treatment (usually endovascular stenting) is indicated in case of complications.

→ COMPLICATIONS

Recurrent pain, hematoma expansion, periaortic hematoma, or disruption of the intima.

Risk factors for complications of IMH: Persistent or recurrent pain despite aggressive medical treatment, difficult blood pressure control, ascending aortic involvement, maximum aortic diameter ≥50 mm, progressive maximum aortic wall thickness (>11 mm), enlarging aortic diameter, recurrent pleural effusion, unstable atherosclerotic plaque (penetrating ulcer or ulcer-like projection) secondary to localized dissections in the involved segment, organ ischemia (brain, myocardium, bowels, kidneys).

18.1.2.3. Penetrating Aortic Ulcer

→ DEFINITION, ETIOLOGY, PATHOGENESIS

Penetrating aortic ulcer (PAU) refers to ulceration of an aortic atherosclerotic plaque that penetrates through the internal elastic lamina into the media. In the acute phase, penetrating aortic ulcers may present and are managed in a similar fashion to acute aortic dissections and intramural hematomas.

→ CLINICAL FEATURES AND NATURAL HISTORY

PAU may result in intramural hematoma, pseudoaneurysm, aortic dissection, or aortic rupture. Clinical features usually found in patients with PAU include advanced age, male sex, tobacco smoking, hypertension, coronary artery disease, chronic obstructive pulmonary disease, and abdominal aneurysm. Clinical manifestations may be similar to those in aortic dissection but signs of organ hypoperfusion are rarely seen. PAUs are associated with progressive enlargement of the aorta and development of aneurysms.

→ DIAGNOSIS

Contrast-enhanced computed tomography angiography (CTA) is the study of choice.

→ TREATMENT

1. Medical treatment: Control of pain and blood pressure.

2. Invasive treatment: Consider surgery in patients with a PAU in the ascending aorta. Indications for invasive treatment in the descending thoracic aorta (preferably endovascular) include recurrent or refractory pain as well as signs of contained rupture (a rapidly growing aortic ulcer with periaortic hematoma or pleural effusion).

18.2. Carotid and Vertebral Artery Stenosis

→ ETIOLOGY, PATHOGENESIS, CLINICAL FEATURES

Atherosclerosis is the cause of >90% of all cases of stenosis or occlusion of the carotid arteries and most cases of stenosis of the vertebral arteries; rare causes include postradiotherapy stenosis, systemic vasculitis, spontaneous or traumatic artery dissection, and fibromuscular dysplasia. Carotid or vertebral artery stenosis may be symptomatic or asymptomatic.

1. Symptomatic carotid artery stenosis is defined as a transient ischemic attack (TIA) or stroke that has occurred within the prior 6 months in the vascular territory of the stenotic carotid artery. Neurologic symptoms may include:

1) Motor or sensory disturbances contralateral to the stenosis.
2) Speech disorder in the case of stenosis of the artery supplying the dominant hemisphere.
3) Inattention or neglect in the case of stenosis of the artery supplying the nondominant hemisphere.
3) Monocular visual disturbances ipsilateral to the stenosis (amaurosis fugax).

2. Symptomatic vertebral artery stenosis is defined as a TIA or stroke that has occurred in the vascular territory of the vertebrobasilar or posterior cerebral arteries. Neurologic symptoms may include:

1) Motor or sensory disturbances with cranial nerve involvement.
2) Crossed motor or sensory disturbances (face ipsilateral, arm and leg contralateral).
3) Gait ataxia especially if associated with limb ataxia or the symptoms and signs listed above.

→ DIAGNOSIS

Auscultation for a carotid bruit is not sufficient to confirm or exclude carotid stenosis and should not be used for this purpose.❸⊖

Diagnostic Tests

Computed tomography (CT) or **magnetic resonance imaging** (MRI) of the brain should be done to identify cerebral infarction and to exclude hemorrhage. MRI is more sensitive for detecting ischemia than CT, especially in the posterior fossa. **Color Doppler ultrasonography** can accurately locate the atherosclerotic plaque, assess its morphology, and determine the severity of stenosis in carotid artery disease but not vertebral disease or intracranial disease. **Magnetic resonance angiography** (MRA) or **computed tomography angiography** (CTA) should be done to confirm the degree of stenosis and assess for vertebral or intracranial stenosis.❷⊖ Because of the risk of complications, **arteriography** is reserved for situations when the severity or cause of stenosis cannot be assessed using other modalities.

→ TREATMENT

Recommended treatment of carotid artery stenosis: →Table 18-3.

Medical Treatment

1. Management of risk factors for atherosclerosis: →Chapter 3.15. Use a statin in all patients, including those with asymptomatic stenosis. Make attempts to control diabetes mellitus. Smoking should be strongly discouraged.

2. Antiplatelet treatment: All patients should receive lifelong treatment with acetylsalicylic acid (ASA) 75 to 325 mg/d. If ASA is contraindicated, use

Table 18-3. Recommended treatment of carotid artery stenosis

Degree of stenosis	Treatment
Patients with recent (<6 months) stroke or TIA[a]	
<50%	Pharmacotherapy
50%-69%	– Consider revascularization[a,b,d] – Pharmacotherapy
70%-99%	– Revascularization[a,b,c] – Pharmacotherapy
Occluded or near-occluded	Pharmacotherapy
Patients without recent (<6 months) stroke or TIA	
<60%	Pharmacotherapy
60%-99%	– Pharmacotherapy – Consider revascularization[b,d] in patients with life expectancy >5 years, favorable anatomy, and ≥1 feature suggesting higher risk of stroke with pharmacotherapy[e]
Occluded or near-occluded	Pharmacotherapy

[a] Revascularization should be performed as soon as possible (<14 days).

[b] After a multidisciplinary discussion including neurologists.

[c] CEA is preferred. Consider CAS in patients at high risk for CEA (age >80 years, clinically significant cardiac disease, severe pulmonary disease, contralateral internal carotid artery occlusion, contralateral recurrent laryngeal nerve palsy, previous radical neck surgery or radiotherapy, recurrent stenosis after CEA).

[d] Consider CEA. CAS may be considered as a second choice.

[e] Contralateral TIA/stroke; ipsilateral silent infarction on cerebral imaging; ultrasonographic features: stenosis progression >20%, spontaneous embolization on transcranial Doppler, impaired cerebral vascular reserve, large (>40 mm²) or echolucent plaques, increased juxtaluminal hypoechogenic area; MRA features: intraplaque hemorrhage, lipid-rich necrotic core.

Adapted from Eur Heart J. 2018;39(9):763-816.

CAS, carotid artery stenting; CEA, carotid endarterectomy; CTA, computed tomography angiography; MRA, magnetic resonance angiography; TIA, transient ischemic attack.

clopidogrel 75 mg/d. For symptomatic intracranial disease, administer 2 antiplatelet agents for 90 days.◐◔ Antiplatelet treatment is recommended over anticoagulation in patients with symptomatic intracranial disease.◐◔ Add clopidogrel 300 to 600 mg as a loading dose followed by 75 mg/d to ASA 50 to 325 mg for 30 days in patients with a recent TIA or minor stroke and extracranial carotid disease◐◔ (→Chapter 10.7). After endovascular angioplasty and stenting, our practice—acknowledging the lack of high-quality evidence to determine the duration of treatments—is to administer 2 antiplatelet agents for at least 30 days and ASA indefinitely.

Invasive Treatment

1. Carotid artery stenosis: Surgical removal of the atherosclerotic plaques that cause the stenosis (endarterectomy) or endovascular angioplasty with stent implantation. Treatment should be started as soon as possible after the symptomatic event to reduce the risk of recurrent stroke.◐◔ Endarterectomy is preferred over carotid artery stenting in older patients (eg, >75 years) to reduce the risk of periprocedural stroke.⊘● Either treatment could be considered in younger patients. Endovascular treatment is, however, the treatment of choice for high-risk patients with any of the following⊘●:

1) Stenosis eligible for invasive treatment in a patient with general contraindications to surgery.

2) Severe cardiac or pulmonary disease.

3) Contralateral carotid occlusion.

4) Stenosis that is inaccessible to the surgeon for anatomical reasons.

5) Restenosis of the internal carotid artery after endarterectomy.

6) Postradiotherapy stenosis.

Medical management is usually preferred over a surgical or endovascular intervention for patients with asymptomatic carotid stenosis.⊘⊘

2. Vertebral or basilar artery stenosis: In patients with symptomatic or asymptomatic vertebral or basilar artery stenosis, dual antiplatelet treatment for 90 days after a neurologic event and single antiplatelet treatment indefinitely is recommended over invasive treatment.⊘● Antiplatelet treatment is recommended over anticoagulation in patients with symptomatic or asymptomatic vertebral or basilar stenosis.⊘●

18.3. Lower Limb Ischemia

18.3.1. Acute Lower Limb Ischemia

➡ **DEFINITION, ETIOLOGY, PATHOGENESIS**

Acute lower limb ischemia refers to any sudden deterioration of limb perfusion that carries a risk of amputation.

Causes:

1) Embolism of cardiac origin (80% of cases; most often associated with atrial fibrillation) or originating from the aorta or large arteries (from aneurysms or atherosclerotic plaques). It usually leads to occlusion at branch points, such as the aortic bifurcation/proximal common iliac artery, common femoral artery bifurcating into superficial femoral and profunda arteries, and distal popliteal artery/proximal tibial arteries.

2) Thrombosis:

   a) Primary thrombosis (usually a complication of atherosclerotic stenosis or aneurysm).

   b) Thrombosis at the site of previous revascularization (bypass, endarterectomy, stent).

   c) Thrombosis due to hypercoagulable states.

3) Arterial trauma or dissection (including iatrogenic trauma from catheters and arterial punctures).

4) Compartment syndrome.

➡ **CLINICAL FEATURES AND NATURAL HISTORY**

Manifestations: Arterial occlusion, which initially manifests as lack of pulse and pale cold skin. The subsequent timeline can vary depending on etiology and preexisting disease; times presented here serve only as approximation: after 15 minutes, pain in the limb develops. After 2 hours, hypoesthesia and paresthesia are present. After 6 hours, mottled cyanosis and anesthesia occur. After 8 hours, motor paralysis and muscle rigidity develop. After 10 hours, the patient develops blisters, local hemostasis disturbances, and

Table 18-4. Clinical classification and treatment of acute limb ischemia (based on the Rutherford classification)

Grade/category	Prognosis	Clinical features		Treatment
		Sensory loss	Motor deficit	
I. Viable	Not immediately threatened	None	None	Thrombolysis or surgery
II. Threatened				
IIa. Marginally	Salvageable if promptly treated	None or minimal (toes)	None	Thrombolysis or surgery
IIb. Immediately	Salvageable if promptly revascularized	More than toes	Mild or moderate	Surgery, may be combined with thrombolysis
III. Irreversible	Inevitable high-level amputation or permanent nerve damage	Profound, anesthetic	Profound, paralysis (rigor)	Primary amputation

Adapted from J Vasc Surg. 1997;26(3):517-38 and Eur Heart J. 2011;32(22):2851-906.

necrosis. The dynamics and severity of symptoms depend on the location and extent of occlusion. Arterial thrombosis usually has a less dynamic course than arterial embolism. Preexisting chronic limb ischemia reduces the dynamics and severity of symptoms because of the previously developed collateral circulation.

Clinical classification: →Table 18-4.

→ DIAGNOSIS

Diagnosis should be established on the basis of clinical manifestations by the physician who examines the patient first and who should immediately refer the patient to a specialist vascular surgery center. Arterial duplex ultrasonography is used to reveal the absence of blood flow in limb arteries and to locate the occlusion (this is particularly helpful in the assessment of patency of bypass grafts). Computed tomography (CT) arteriography reveals the site of occlusion, provides information on the etiology of acute ischemia, and enables planning for revascularization. Conventional (catheter) arteriography can be both diagnostic and allow for immediate intervention if the underlying pathology is amenable to endovascular treatment.

→ TREATMENT

Invasive Treatment

1. Indications: Surgery or endovascular treatment in patients with acute lower limb ischemia are potentially limb-saving procedures to which no contraindications exist. Urgently refer the patient to a surgical center.

2. Preoperative management:

1) As early as possible administer **unfractionated heparin (UFH)** 5000 to 10,000 IU followed by a continuous IV infusion (dosage: →Table 19-3).

2) Analgesics (**opioid analgesics**).

3) **Protect the limb** against heat loss, pain, and potential trauma.

Table 18-5. Classification of peripheral artery disease

Fontaine classification stage	Symptoms		Rutherford classification stage
I	Asymptomatic		0
IIa	Claudication >200 meters	Mild claudication	1
IIb	Claudication <200 meters	Moderate claudication	2
		Severe claudication	3
III	Rest pain		4
IV	Ischemic necrosis or ulceration	Minor tissue damage[a]	5
		Major tissue damage[b]	6

[a] Nonhealing ulceration, focal gangrene with diffuse pedal ischemia.

[b] Extending above the transmetatarsal level, functional foot no longer salvageable.

Adapted from Helv Chir Acta. 1954;21(5-6):499-533 and J Vasc Surg. 1997;26(3):517-38.

3. Methods:

1) **Surgery**: Prompt revascularization surgery is indicated in patients with Rutherford stage IIb and early stage III ischemia (→Table 18-5). Most often this involves thromboembolectomy, which should be performed within 6 to 8 hours of the onset of symptoms of ischemia. An arterial repair, stent, or bypass may be required in addition to or instead of thromboembolectomy, particularly if there is preexisting arterial occlusive disease or dissection.

2) **Endovascular treatment**: Intra-arterial thrombolysis administered via a catheter with the catheter tip placed (embedded) in the thrombus; this involves a continuous infusion of low-dose streptokinase and alteplase. **Thrombolytic therapy** may be considered in patients with no contraindications and recent (<14 days) thrombosis or embolism. It may be the method of choice in patients with Rutherford stage I and IIa ischemia (where there is time to allow for thrombolysis to work) and may eliminate the need for or reduce the extent of surgical treatment. Any deterioration in perfusion during thrombolysis indicates a need to stop the infusion and perform immediate surgery. After restoring arterial patency, percutaneous angioplasty or reconstructive surgery may be performed to ensure sustained patency. Percutaneous aspiration thrombectomy or percutaneous mechanical thrombectomy may also be performed in place of or together with thrombolysis.

After thrombolysis, use an anticoagulant (→Chapter 3.1) for ≥3 months (or lifelong in patients with thromboembolism associated with atrial fibrillation or a prosthetic valve).

18.3.2. Lower Extremity Peripheral Artery Disease

→ DEFINITION, ETIOLOGY, PATHOGENESIS

Lower extremity peripheral artery disease (PAD) is a condition in which the supply of oxygen to tissues of the lower extremities is inadequate due to chronically impaired arterial blood flow. In >97% of patients this is caused by atherosclerosis of the lower extremities. Other causes of chronic lower extremity ischemia: →Differential Diagnosis, below.

→ CLINICAL FEATURES

The staging of PAD is based on the severity of symptoms: →Table 18-5.

PAD is often accompanied by features of atherosclerosis of other arteries: coronary, cranial, or renal. Sometimes patients have a coexisting abdominal aortic aneurysm.

1. Symptoms: Early PAD is asymptomatic. With time, patients develop easy fatigability of the limbs, increased sensitivity to cold, and paresthesia. They usually seek medical attention because of intermittent claudication, that is, pain occurring relatively regularly after defined physical exercise (eg, walking a certain distance). The pain, sometimes described as muscle numbness or stiffness, involves muscles below the level of artery stenosis/occlusion, is not referred, forces the patient to stop walking, and resolves spontaneously after several seconds or minutes of rest. Claudication pain usually involves large muscle groups of the lower extremity, such as the buttocks, thighs, and most frequently the calf. Claudication of the foot (deep pain in the middle of the foot [short flexor muscles of the foot]) occurs rarely and results from narrowing or occlusion of the more distal arteries in the lower leg (tibial arteries) or foot. It can be seen in conditions such as thromboangiitis obliterans (Buerger disease) and diabetes mellitus. Severe narrowing or occlusion of the aorta, iliac arteries, or both may present as Leriche syndrome, which is defined as intermittent claudication, absent femoral pulses, and erectile dysfunction.

In advanced stages patients complain of foot pain, leg pain, or both occurring at night (often hanging the limb over the side of a bed to keep it in the lowest possible position and allow gravity to improve blood flow) or pain at rest throughout the day and night.

2. Signs: The skin of the feet is pale or cyanotic (especially when standing) and cold. In advanced PAD trophic lesions (discoloration, hair loss, ulcers, necrosis) may be present. Patients also have muscle atrophy and a weak, absent, or asymmetric pulse over the arteries below the stenosis/occlusion, sometimes with a vascular bruit over the large arteries of the extremities. On the lower extremities, pulse is assessed on the following arteries: the dorsalis pedis artery (on the dorsum of the foot between the first and second metatarsal bone; not palpable in 8% of healthy persons), posterior tibial artery (behind the medial malleolus), popliteal artery (in the popliteal fossa), and femoral artery (in the groin, just below the inguinal ligament).

→ DIAGNOSIS

Diagnostic Tests

1. Ankle-brachial index (ABI) (→Figure 18-4): A ratio of the systolic blood pressure (SBP) measured using continuous wave Doppler ultrasonography in the ankle to the SBP measured in the arm (if pressures vary between the arms, consider the higher value). A normal value is from 0.9 to 1.15; an ABI <0.9 indicates the presence of stenosis (in critical ischemia usually <0.5), while an ABI >1.3 is suggestive of abnormal arterial stiffness (eg, in patients with diabetes mellitus).

If tibial arteries cannot be compressed due to their stiffness, use the

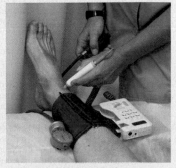

Figure 18-4. Ankle-brachial index.

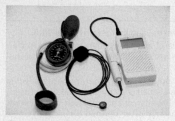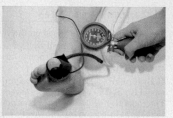

Figure 18-5. Toe-brachial index.

toe-brachial index (TBI) (→Figure 18-5). The measuring principle is the same as in the ABI, but SBP is measured in the toe; the pressure measured in the toe should be ~10 mm Hg lower than the pressure measured at the level of the ankle. A normal TBI is >0.7; lower values indicate the possibility of lower limb ischemia.

2. Stress testing on a treadmill is performed in case of diagnostic doubts, particularly in patients with borderline ABI values, as well as to objectively assess the claudication distance. The ABI is calculated before and at the peak of exercise. If pain forcing the patient to interrupt testing is caused by ischemia, the ankle pressure after exercise will be significantly lower than before exercise (often <50 mm Hg).

3. Imaging studies: Arterial duplex **ultrasonography of the arteries** (including B-mode imaging [ultrasonography] and Doppler spectral waveform analysis) is the key method used in the initial diagnostics and for surveillance of patients with PAD, in particular those who have undergone surgical treatment (patency of prosthesis and bypasses) or endovascular interventions. The study should always be preceded by a thorough physical examination and ABI measurement. **Computed tomography angiography (CTA)** and **magnetic resonance angiography (MRA)** allow for the assessment of the entire vascular system and type of lesions in the vascular walls as well as qualification or planning of the patient for an appropriate invasive procedure; these studies should not be used for screening. **Arteriography** is performed in the case of diagnostic doubts or more commonly in the course of therapeutic endovascular procedures such as angioplasty (with or without stenting).

Diagnostic Criteria

The diagnosis of PAD is made on the basis of symptoms, signs, and ABI (or the walking test). If arteries at the ankle cannot be compressed or if the ABI is >1.40, use alternative methods (eg, TBI or Doppler). **Critical limb ischemia** is diagnosed in a patient with chronic ischemia with pain at rest, necrosis, or ulceration (Fontaine classification stages III-IV or Rutherford stages 4-6).

Differential Diagnosis

1. Causes of chronic lower limb ischemia other than atherosclerosis: There are multiple other nonatherosclerotic causes of lower extremity arterial narrowing or occlusion that can present as chronic lower limb ischemia. Peripheral emboli from the heart (arrhythmias, valvular heart disease) or proximal arteries (plaque or aneurysms) may more typically present as acute ischemia but can also cause chronic symptoms. Inflammatory changes as well as thickening and narrowing of the artery wall and lumen can occur with large-vessel vasculitis, thromboangiitis obliterans (Buerger disease), and radiation injury (especially in iliac arteries following pelvic irradiation). Trauma can narrow arteries with dissection or chronic repetitive injury including external iliac artery endofibrosis (cyclist hip pain). The popliteal artery in particular can be extrinsically narrowed by muscles and tendons (popliteal artery entrapment)

be performed 1, 3, and 6 months after intervention and then every 6 months, but such a rigid schedule may need adjustment to surgical observations and stability of the graft.

18.4. Microcirculation Disorders

18.4.1. Erythromelalgia

→ DEFINITION, ETIOLOGY, CLINICAL FEATURES

Erythromelalgia is a vasomotor disorder associated with acute (and sometimes followed by chronic) episodic dilation of the arterioles and arteriovenous connections. It manifests as sudden erythema and warmth of the extremities, particularly fingers and toes, that involves the feet more often than the hands and is accompanied by severe burning pain. The features are usually symmetric and sometimes also occur on the ears and face. Each episode can last for hours to years.

Causes: Secondary erythromelalgia develops in the course of myeloproliferative neoplasms (particularly essential thrombocythemia and polycythemia vera), systemic connective tissue diseases, type 1 or type 2 diabetes mellitus, multiple sclerosis, neuropathy of various etiologies, infectious diseases (eg, AIDS), and peripheral embolism (especially cholesterol emboli). It may also be caused by certain drugs (bromocriptine, nifedipine) or trauma.

→ TREATMENT

Symptoms of erythromelalgia may be improved by cooling and elevating the affected extremity and by avoiding high temperatures and strenuous exercise. In some patients sedatives and pharmacologic nerve blockade may be helpful. Treatment, particularly in the case of secondary erythromelalgia, involves acetylsalicylic acid (ASA) up to 100 mg/d, indomethacin, propranolol, serotonin reuptake inhibitors (eg, sertraline), and clonazepam. In case of severe pain, you may consider IV infusion of sodium nitroprusside, lidocaine, or prostaglandin E_1.

18.4.2. Livedo Reticularis

→ DEFINITION AND ETIOLOGY

Livedo reticularis is a vasomotor disorder involving the skin of the extremities or less commonly the trunk. It leads to persistent unevenly disseminated vasoconstriction affecting the arterioles and concomitant congestion and dilation of venules filled with deoxygenated blood, which results in a mottled reddish or blue discoloration of the skin (→Figure 18-6). It is most frequently a cosmetic

Figure 18-6. A, livedo reticularis. **B**, livedo racemosa.

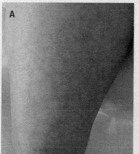
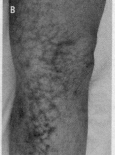

Table 18-7. Causes of secondary Raynaud phenomenon

Systemic connective tissue diseases	– Eosinophilic fasciitis – Mixed connective tissue disease – Juvenile idiopathic arthritis – Primary biliary cirrhosis – Rheumatoid arthritis – Systemic lupus erythematosus – Scleroderma – Antiphospholipid syndrome – Sjögren syndrome – Polymyositis – Dermatomyositis
Vasculitides	– Behçet disease – Buerger disease – Takayasu disease – Polyarteritis nodosa – Other systemic vasculitides – Atherosclerosis (rare) – Diabetic microangiopathy – Microembolization – Giant cell arteritis – Granulomatosis with polyangiitis (Wegener)
Occupational exposure	– Vibration and repetitive mechanical finger injuries – Exposure to cold
Intoxication and chemical agents	– Vinyl chloride poisoning – Cocaine – Heavy metal poisoning (lead, thallium) – Nicotine – Acrylic artificial nails
Blood disorders	– Leukemia and lymphoma – Cold agglutinin disease – Polycythemia vera – Monoclonal and polyclonal cryoglobulinemia – Cryofibrinogenemia – Essential thrombocythemia – Multiple myeloma – Disseminated intravascular coagulation
Central nervous system disorders	– Syringomyelia – Tabes dorsalis
Compression syndromes	– Thoracic outlet syndrome – Carpal tunnel syndrome – Compression syndrome following use of forearm crutches
Drugs	– Ergot derivatives – β-Blockers – Oral contraceptives – Vincristine – Bleomycin – Cyclosporine – Interferon α – Interferon γ

Infectious diseases	– Leprosy
	– Cytomegalovirus infection
	– Parvovirus infection
	– *Mycoplasma pneumoniae* infection
	– *Helicobacter pylori* infection
	– Hepatitis B
	– Hepatitis C
Other disorders	– Anorexia nervosa
	– Cancer
	– Frostbite
	– Primary or secondary pulmonary hypertension
	– Arteriovenous shunts (including those related to dialysis)
	– Familial cold urticaria
	– Carney complex

defect rather than a disease, but a similar process may accompany variety of systemic diseases (livedo racemosa).

Etiologic classification:

1) Livedo reticularis without other symptoms or association with other diseases: Physiologic (mainly on the lower extremities, resolves completely after warming up the limb); primary (independent of ambient temperature); idiopathic (does not decrease with warming; most frequently affects women aged 20-60 years).

2) Livedo reticularis in the course of other diseases (livedo racemosa), including antiphospholipid syndrome (most frequently), cryoglobulinemia, Sneddon syndrome, polycythemia vera, cold agglutinin disease, systemic connective tissue diseases (especially systemic lupus erythematosus), peripheral embolism (cholesterol [eg, after endovascular intervention] or bacterial embolism), or diabetes mellitus.

→DIAGNOSIS

Diagnosis is based on history and physical examination. In some cases (eg, in patients with a history of venous or arterial thrombosis) determine the presence of lupus anticoagulant and anticardiolipin antibodies to exclude antiphospholipid syndrome.

→TREATMENT

Treatment is not necessary unless there is an underlying condition that needs therapy. Exposure to cold should be avoided.

18.4.3. Raynaud Phenomenon

→DEFINITION AND ETIOLOGY

Raynaud phenomenon is an acute reversing blanching of the fingers and toes, rarely also of the nose and ears, in response to cold, emotional stressors, or without an obvious cause. The following types of Raynaud phenomenon are distinguished:

1) **Primary Raynaud phenomenon**, found in ~80% of patients.

2) **Secondary Raynaud phenomenon**, which may develop as a result of various diseases and conditions (→Table 18-7).

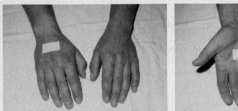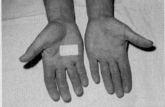

Figure 18-7. Raynaud phenomenon. Cyanosis affecting fingers of both hands.

→ CLINICAL FEATURES

Phases of Raynaud phenomenon:

1) **Ischemic phase**: Whitening or blanching of the fingers or toes, rarely of entire hands or feet; sharply demarcated pallor of the affected body parts with accompanying numbness (→Figure 18-7).

2) **Cyanotic phase**: Blue or purple discoloration accompanied by a feeling of numbness and pain.

3) **Hyperemic phase**: Reddening, mild edema, cutaneous sensation of burning and heat.

In patients with secondary Raynaud phenomenon the vasomotor symptoms are usually more pronounced than in patients with primary Raynaud phenomenon; the cyanotic phase is often dominant and ulcerations and necrosis of the fingertips develop more frequently. The thumb is not usually involved in primary Raynaud phenomenon.

→ DIAGNOSIS

Diagnostic Criteria

Primary Raynaud phenomenon is diagnosed when there are no features of an underlying condition in history, physical examination, or results of specific investigations suggestive of etiology, making an idiopathic cause likely.

Secondary Raynaud phenomenon is diagnosed after identifying an underlying condition that may be causative. Secondary causes should be established through history, physical examination, and any relevant laboratory investigations. The adequacy of cancer screening should be reviewed, particularly in men and in patients with the onset of Raynaud phenomenon >30 years of age.

Differential Diagnosis

Differential diagnosis should include benign cold sensitivity, peripheral neuropathy, acrocyanosis, Buerger disease, vascular disease (atherosclerosis), vasculitis, toxins, cryoglobulinemia, and erythromelalgia.

→ TREATMENT

1. Nonpharmacologic treatment: Avoidance of exposure to cold, smoking cessation, avoidance of caffeinated beverages, avoidance of oral contraceptives and vasoconstrictive drugs.

2. Pharmacologic treatment: In severe primary and secondary Raynaud phenomenon, treat the underlying condition (where applicable) and use a long--acting oral **dihydropyridine calcium channel blocker** (eg, amlodipine, nifedipine). Start at low doses and titrate upwards based on the efficacy of treatment and adverse effects. Additional therapeutic options include topical nitrates, angiotensin receptor blockers, phosphodiesterase-5 inhibitors (eg, sildenafil, tadalafil), selective serotonin reuptake inhibitors (eg, fluoxetine), or endothelin-1 receptor antagonists (eg, bosentan, macitentan). In patients with severe digital ischemia or development of necrotic lesions, urgent treatment with warming and calcium channel blockers should be initiated; prostaglandin infusion (eg, iloprost) can limit the damage and can be considered in case of secondary Raynaud phenomenon.☺◯ Antithrombotic agents, acetylsalicylic acid, or therapeutic doses of low-molecular-weight heparin are used to treat potential thrombotic events after considering contraindications (eg, gastric antral vascular ectasia or severe gastritis, both of which are seen in systemic sclerosis).

3. Surgical treatment: In selected patients not responding to pharmacologic treatment, in particular those at high risk for necrosis of the fingers, digital sympathectomy may be considered.

18.5. Venous Diseases

18.5.1. Chronic Venous Insufficiency

▶ DEFINITION, ETIOLOGY, PATHOGENESIS

Chronic venous insufficiency is venous stasis due to a retrograde flow of blood, stenosis, or occlusion of the veins. Chronic venous insufficiency may be caused by **varicose veins** (persistent dilation of a superficial vein ≥3 mm in diameter measured in a standing position), **postthrombotic syndrome**, **primary venous valve incompetence**, and **venous compression syndromes** (eg, popliteal entrapment syndrome).

Risk factors: Age >40 years, female sex, genetic factors causing weakness of the vein walls and valves (causing so-called primary varicose veins), pregnancy, working in sitting or standing positions, obesity. Regardless of the cause, the primary factor leading to the development of chronic venous insufficiency is venous hypertension, which may result from agenesia, hypoplasia, incompetence, or damage of the venous valves, as well as from venous occlusion or stenosis caused by thrombosis (and lack of or incomplete recanalization following a thrombotic event) or by compression of the veins.

In some cases, venous ulcers are accompanied by **stasis dermatitis**, which may be caused by trauma, microtrauma, bacterial infection, or contact allergy.

▶ CLINICAL FEATURES

1. Symptoms: Patients with early venous insufficiency complain of a feeling of "heaviness" and "fullness" in the lower extremities, which usually worsens in the evening and improves after resting with elevated legs. Other symptoms include blue-colored, dilated superficial veins, painful muscle cramps in the calf (particularly at night), as well as restless leg syndrome. In the more advanced stages, patients usually develop dull pain that worsens during the day; pain while walking (called venous claudication), which is rarely observed in patients with venous insufficiency, indicates occlusion of deep veins of the lower leg.

2. Signs:
1) Telangiectasias (→Figure 18-8) (dilated intradermal venules <1 mm in diameter, small spider veins, reticular varicose veins) that with time progress to wide, tortuous varicose veins of the long (great) saphenous vein (→Figure 18-9) and short (small) saphenous vein.
2) Edema (in early disease this is pitting, reversible, and resolves after an overnight rest; later it becomes hard, nonpitting and irreversible).

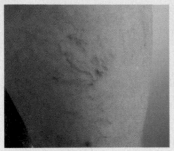

Figure 18-8. Telangiectasias.

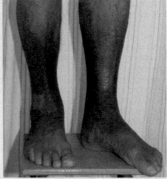

Figure 18-10. Rusty-brown discoloration of the skin in chronic venous insufficiency.

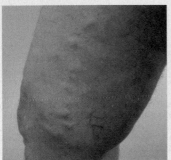

Figure 18-9. Varicose veins of the great saphenous vein.

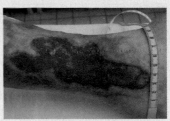

Figure 18-11. Venous ulcerations.

3) Rusty-brown discoloration of the skin of the lower leg (→Figure 18-10).

4) Venous ulcers (→Figure 18-11) (typically above the medial malleolus; advanced ulcers involve the entire circumference of the lower leg).

5) Dry or oozing eczema of varying severity and persistent cellulitis (frequent in patients with advanced chronic venous insufficiency).

6) Lipodermatosclerosis.

7) Secondary lymphedema.

3. Signs and symptoms of **stasis dermatitis** include severe erythema and inflammatory lesions on one or both lower extremities, in some cases with a generalized hematogenous reaction (associated with erythematous or fine papular rash that frequently includes the skin of the head, trunk, and upper extremities) and severe pruritus. Bacterial superinfections of the cutaneous lesions are frequent.

→ DIAGNOSIS

Diagnosis is based primarily on the clinical manifestations and, secondarily, on the results of **color Doppler ultrasonography** of the veins in the lower extremity.

Differential Diagnosis

Bilateral or unilateral edema of the lower extremities (→Chapter 1.9).

Table 18-8. Classes of compression stockings and indications for their use

Class	Pressure[a]	Indications
I	20-30	Prevention of venous thrombosis, prophylaxis of thrombosis and varicose veins in pregnant patients, small varicose veins during pregnancy, complaints of heavy and tired legs, small varicose veins with no visible edema, postsurgical treatment of varicose veins
II	30-40	Large varicose veins during pregnancy, varicose veins with mild edema, history of superficial vein phlebitis, prior sclerotherapy of varicose veins, healed small ulcers
III	40-50	Very large varicose veins with significant edema, successfully healed large ulcers, posttraumatic edema, reversible lymphedema
IV	50-60	Severe postthrombotic syndrome, irreversible lymphedema

[a] Pressure at ankle level (mm Hg).

→TREATMENT

Medical Treatment

1. General recommendations: Avoidance of exposure to high temperatures and intense sunlight, avoidance of prolonged standing or prolonged sitting with the knee and hip joints flexed at right angles; maintaining an ergonomic workplace, including a chair with reclining backrest and a footstool; several minutes of walking or limb exercises after longer periods of sitting; regular recreational exercise (walking, jogging, cycling, swimming); frequent rests with the lower extremities raised above the heart level, supported along the entire length of the lower leg (not by a few isolated support points).

2. Compression therapy is the only method that can slow down the development of chronic venous insufficiency; it may also be used prophylactically in patients with early manifestations of venous insufficiency. The therapy involves the use of compression bandages (in patients with venous ulcerations), compression stockings (selected on an individual basis to fit the limb after edema has improved or resolved: →Table 18-8), and intermittent pneumatic compression (→Chapter 3.19.1).

Contraindications: acute cellulitis, exudative skin diseases, Fontaine class III/IV arterial ischemia (ankle-brachial index [ABI] <0.6; before applying any type of compression, always examine the pulse in the lower extremities and measure the ABI), limb deformities or severe arthritis that make it impossible to precisely apply the appropriate pressure.

3. Pharmacologic treatment is an addition to but never a replacement of compression therapy. Natural or synthetic flavonoids (rutoside and its derivatives, hesperidin, diosmin), saponins (aescin), calcium dobesilate, and grape seed or citrus extracts may improve quality of life and alleviate symptoms in some patients, but they do not prevent the progression of the disease. The best evidence of efficacy exists for saponins.○

Treatment of Venous Ulcers

1. Elevation of the limbs while sitting or lying down.

2. Compression therapy: Multilayer compression using special bandages or commercial multilayer compression systems for treatment of ulcers (recommended pressures are 40 mm Hg at ankle level and 17-20 mm Hg at popliteal level; maximum pressures in patients with mixed arteriovenous ulcers and patients with an ABI 0.6-0.9 are 17-25 mm Hg).

3. Removal of necrotic tissues, wound debridement, transplantation of cutaneous and/or musculocutaneous flaps.

4. Treatment of infection: Topical disinfectants containing octenidine, dressings with 7% to 10% iodinated povidone or with ethacridine solution, and systemic (not topical!) antibiotics.

5. Treatment of pain is particularly important during debridement and when changing the dressings.

6. Treatment of stasis dermatitis: Oral antihistamines, topical glucocorticoids, and compresses of 1% tannin and 0.1% silver nitrate.

7. Correction of possible protein malnutrition impairing the healing process (assessment of the patient's nutritional status is necessary before starting treatment of venous ulcers).

8. Patients with ulcers that have not healed for >3 months despite appropriate treatment should be referred for a specialist consultation. Malignant lesions within the ulcer must be excluded.

Invasive Treatment

1. Indications: Severe symptoms of chronic venous insufficiency, complications of varicose veins (inflammation, rupture, bleeding, trophic skin lesions, venous ulcers), cosmetic reasons. Do not refer patients with occlusion of the deep veins for surgical treatment.

2. Methods: Stripping of varicose veins, open surgical treatment of incompetent perforators (Linton method), minimally invasive surgery (microphlebectomy, cryosurgery, laser surgery), sclerotherapy (obliteration of the veins by injecting sclerotic agents). Recurrences of varicose veins after surgery are frequent (affecting up to 50% of patients). Good long-term effects of the surgery largely depend on the continued use of compression treatment.

18.5.2. Superficial Thrombophlebitis

→ DEFINITION, ETIOLOGY, PATHOGENESIS

Superficial thrombophlebitis refers to inflammation of the veins located above the fascial layer that is usually accompanied by thrombosis of varying severity.

Thrombophlebitis of varicose veins accounts for ~90% of all cases of superficial thrombophlebitis, more frequently affecting the medial greater (long) saphenous vein, less often the lateral lesser (short) saphenous vein. The mechanism of thrombophlebitis includes stasis in the varicose veins and abnormalities of the venous wall, which lead to thrombosis and subsequent inflammation of the venous wall.

Idiopathic superficial thrombophlebitis usually affects the lesser saphenous vein or the greater saphenous vein but may develop in any superficial vein.

Recurrent superficial thrombophlebitis usually occurs in the same area of the affected leg. Migratory superficial thrombophlebitis may precede or coexist with thromboangiitis obliterans (Buerger disease), Behçet disease (→Chapter 14.23.2), or with adenocarcinomas (Trousseau sign), most frequently pancreatic cancer. The risk of concomitant deep vein thrombosis (DVT) is low (~5%).

Catheter-related superficial thrombophlebitis (excluding catheters inserted directly into the central vein) most frequently affects the superficial veins of the upper extremities, less frequently the superficial veins of the lower extremities. It is caused by the insertion and long-term use of peripheral venous catheters. Factors contributing to the development of thrombophlebitis include large-bore catheters, central venous catheters inserted via a peripheral vein (eg, antecubital vein), infection, hypercoagulability, hormone treatment, and irritants (eg, drugs or potassium chloride administered via the catheter).

Purulent superficial thrombophlebitis may develop in patients with bacteremia persisting for >72 hours despite an appropriate antimicrobial therapy, particularly in patients with indwelling venous catheters. The most frequent etiologic factors include *Staphylococcus aureus*, streptococci, and gram-negative rods.

→ CLINICAL FEATURES AND NATURAL HISTORY

Signs of superficial thrombophlebitis include painful localized edema and erythema of the skin. In the case of **superficial thrombophlebitis of the varicose veins**, they can be easily palpated as a nodular or cordlike thickening. In patients with **catheter-related superficial thrombophlebitis**, the signs are observed in the area of the affected vein. Drawing blood from the catheter is impossible if a thrombus is blocking its entry. In some patients (5%-13%) the condition may be asymptomatic. Patients with **purulent superficial thrombophlebitis** additionally develop fever, severe erythema, pain, and purulent exudate in the area of the affected vein.

Untreated superficial thrombophlebitis usually resolves spontaneously after several days or weeks, but can progress to deep vein thrombosis or pulmonary embolism in 1% to 2% of patients. Patients with thrombophlebitis of the greater saphenous vein, especially if the thrombus is in close proximity to the adductor canal, are likely at higher risk of DVT. Within several months, the varicose veins usually undergo at least partial recanalization.

→ DIAGNOSIS

Diagnosis is based on the clinical manifestations. In the case of **catheter--related superficial thrombophlebitis**, cultures may reveal the etiologic agent (the specimen is usually the tip of the removed catheter). Diagnostic tests are not necessary in localized superficial thrombophlebitis, particularly when it is catheter-related or caused by irritants. In patients with **superficial thrombophlebitis of the varicose veins of the lower extremities**, perform ultrasonography to localize the head of the thrombus and determine its distance from the deep venous system, because thrombophlebitis of the greater (long) saphenous that is in close proximity to the saphenofemoral junction may extend to the deep venous system. In patients with **migratory thrombophlebitis without an apparent cause**, perform a thorough diagnostic workup to exclude malignancy. In patients with **thrombophlebitis of previously normal (nonvaricose) veins**, consider underlying causes such as oral contraceptive use, vasculitis (eg, Behçet disease), or thrombophilia.

→ TREATMENT

1. Catheter-related superficial thrombophlebitis: In patients with a short peripheral catheter, stop using the catheter and remove it. In cases of mild to moderate pain, use **nonsteroidal anti-inflammatory drugs (NSAIDs)** (oral or topical; agents: →Chapter 14.11, Table 11-2) or **heparin** (topical gel) until the resolution of symptoms, but no longer than for 2 weeks.

The use of heparin at therapeutic doses for DVT (eg, enoxaparin 1 mg/kg bid) is not recommended. Low-dose antithrombotic treatment (eg, fondaparinux 2.5 mg once daily or enoxaparin 40 mg once daily) could be considered if symptoms from superficial thrombophlebitis persist despite the removal of the catheter. The duration of treatment should be 4 weeks, but can be decreased if symptoms resolve promptly and if the catheter is removed.

Assess the site of the catheter for signs of inflammation or an abscess.

Superficial vein thrombosis is not an indication for a routine removal of the peripherally inserted central venous catheter, particularly if it is functioning and required for medically necessary treatments (eg, administration of antibiotics).

2. Purulent superficial thrombophlebitis: Remove the source of infection (eg, a catheter) and use antimicrobial treatment, which should optimally be targeted; if ineffective, consider drainage or resection of the affected segment of the vein.

3. Superficial thrombophlebitis affecting a segment of a vein of a lower extremity ≥5 cm: Subcutaneous **fondaparinux** 2.5 mg/d, **low-molecular--weight heparin** at a prophylactic dose (→Table 19-10) for ≥4 weeks. In selected patients with severe, extensive superficial thrombophlebitis, typically involving the entire length of the greater saphenous vein, consider a therapeutic-dose anticoagulation as done for the treatment of DVT (eg, a vitamin K antagonist [acenocoumarol or warfarin] at a dose adjusted to maintain the international normalized ratio [INR] in the range of 2.0-3.0, in combination with heparin for 5 days, and continued as monotherapy for ≥4 weeks). Additional indications for anticoagulation treatment (in patients with thrombophlebitis affecting a segment <5 cm) include thrombophlebitis in the area of the saphenofemoral junction, severe clinical manifestations, history of venous thromboembolism or superficial vein thrombosis, active malignancy, recent surgery. Once acute inflammation and edema have subsided, consider using appropriate compression stockings.

Localized superficial vein thrombosis (thrombus involving a short vein segment [<5 cm] located far from the saphenofemoral junction) probably requires no anticoagulation therapy. Use NSAIDs (oral or topical) to alleviate the symptoms.

18.5.3. Superior Vena Cava Syndrome

→ **DEFINITION, ETIOLOGY, PATHOGENESIS**

Superior vena cava syndrome (SVCS) is caused by the impairment of blood flow from the superior vena cava (SVC) to the right atrium.

Causes:

1) Cancer (compression or infiltration of the SVC): Lung cancer (50%-80% of all cases, most frequently non–small cell lung cancer), lymphoma, metastatic disease (mainly breast cancer), primary mediastinal tumors (thymoma and other).

2) Nonneoplastic causes: Compression by a thoracic aortic aneurysm, chronic mediastinitis, catheter-related central venous thrombosis, right atrial tumor.

→ **CLINICAL FEATURES AND NATURAL HISTORY**

Typical signs and symptoms include edema and erythema or cyanosis of the face and neck, conjunctival congestion, edema of the upper extremities, persistent jugular vein distention, headache, dizziness, visual disturbances (the symptoms result from venous congestion distal to the obstruction). Dilated superficial veins of the chest are a visible sign of collateral circulation (these are observed in patients in whom SVCS develops slowly). Severe venous drainage impairment is associated with dysphagia, dyspnea, hoarseness, and stridor (often due to compression of the esophagus, trachea, or the recurrent laryngeal nerve). Pleural effusion is observed in approximately one quarter of patients.

→ **DIAGNOSIS**

Imaging studies (chest radiographs, computed tomography [CT], and/or magnetic resonance imaging [MRI]) show a widening of the mediastinum caused by a paratracheal, hilar, or mediastinal tumor. MRI may also provide information on the cause of SVCS in the case of thrombosis, although CT is usually easier to obtain and highly accurate.

→ TREATMENT

The goal of treatment is to improve venous drainage from the regions distal to the obstruction.

1. Treatment of the underlying condition: Promptly determine the cause (including tumor histology) to start targeted therapy as soon as possible (if available). In patients with cancer:

1) Urgent mediastinal irradiation is the treatment of choice for most cancers; this leads to a symptomatic improvement within 2 weeks in ~70% of patients.

2) In patients with small cell lung carcinoma and germinal tumors, chemotherapy should be considered as the initial treatment modality; in patients with lymphoma, radiation, chemotherapy, or both should be considered.

3) Other treatment modalities: Stenting of the SVC; in the case of thrombosis, consider thrombolysis followed by anticoagulant treatment.

2. Symptomatic treatment:

1) **Symptomatic treatment of dyspnea** (oxygen therapy in patients with decreased SaO_2; for palliative management, low-dose opioids [eg, oral or subcutaneous morphine 1-2.5 mg every 4-6 hours] or benzodiazepines [eg, sublingual lorazepam 0.5-2 mg every 8-12 hours] may help to alleviate symptoms).

2) **Dexamethasone** 16 to 32 mg/d IV for 7 days, then taper down the dose (this is used for malignant compression of steroid-responsive tumors, such as non-Hodgkin lymphoma, and for symptomatic management to lessen tumor-associated edema).

3) In some cases administer a loop diuretic IV.

19. Venous Thromboembolism (VTE)

19.1. Deep Vein Thrombosis (DVT)

→ DEFINITION, ETIOLOGY, PATHOGENESIS

Deep vein thrombosis (DVT) refers to the development of a thrombus in the deep venous system (below the deep fascia) of the lower extremities or, less commonly, the upper extremities. Thrombosis of other deep veins (eg, the portal vein) is considered a separate disease entity. Formation of a thrombus in the vein depends on the presence of one or more factors referred to as the **Virchow triad**, which includes the following:

1) Impaired blood flow (eg, due to immobilization of the limb or compression of the veins).

2) Procoagulant activity prevailing over the effects of coagulation inhibitors and fibrinolytic factors (congenital or acquired thrombophilia).

3) A damaged vascular wall (eg, as a result of injury during surgical procedures on a limb).

Risk factors:

1) **Patient-related factors and clinical conditions**: Age >40 (the risk increases with age), obesity (body mass index >30 kg/m^2), prior episodes of venous thromboembolism (VTE), trauma (particularly multiorgan trauma or fractures of the pelvis, proximal femur, and other long bones of the lower extremities), prolonged immobilization of the lower limb (eg, due to paresis, immobilization of 2 adjacent joints in a cast, general anesthesia [in particular involving muscle relaxants]), stroke that resulted in lower limb

paresis, cancer (particularly pancreatic, brain, lung, ovarian, and kidney), family history of VTE, congenital or acquired thrombophilia (particularly antithrombin deficiency and antiphospholipid syndrome), sepsis, medical treatment of a severe debilitating disease (eg, severe pneumonia), New York Heart Association class III or IV heart failure, respiratory failure, autoimmune diseases (eg, Crohn disease, ulcerative colitis, systemic lupus erythematosus), nephrotic syndrome, myeloproliferative neoplasms, paroxysmal nocturnal hemoglobinuria, venous compression (eg, due to a tumor, hematoma, arterial malformation), pregnancy and postpartum, a long flight (>6 hours, particularly when sleeping in a sitting position), varicose veins of the lower extremities, severe infection.

2) **Diagnostic, therapeutic, and prophylactic interventions**: Major surgery, particularly involving the lower extremities, pelvis, and abdomen; an indwelling catheter in the large veins (particularly in the femoral vein); cancer treatment (chemotherapy, hormone therapy, and particularly the use of angiogenesis inhibitors); use of oral contraceptives, hormone replacement therapy, or selective estrogen receptor modulators; use of erythropoietin-stimulating agents.

Some risk factors are transient (surgery, trauma, temporary immobilization in a cast), while others are permanent (such as congenital thrombophilia).

Causes of upper extremity DVT: An indwelling central venous catheter (the most frequent cause); compression of the subclavian or axillary vein by enlarged lymph nodes; a malignant infiltrate; a fractured clavicle; compression of the veins by the scalene muscles between the clavicle and the tendon of the subclavius muscle or the residual tendon band in the axillary fossa associated with strenuous physical activity or bodybuilding (Paget-Schrötter syndrome).

→ CLINICAL FEATURES AND NATURAL HISTORY

1. Lower extremity DVT. Types:

1) **Distal DVT** involves one of the calf veins (peroneal, anterior tibial, posterior tibial). It is often asymptomatic, typically resolves spontaneously, and is associated with a low risk of clinically significant pulmonary embolism (PE), but it can progress to proximal vein thrombosis, typically in patients with ongoing VTE risk factors.

2) **Proximal DVT** involves one or more of the popliteal, femoral, and iliac veins, and rarely extends into the inferior vena cava. It is usually symptomatic and carries a high risk of PE if untreated. **Extensive DVT** is an anatomic distinction that refers to DVT involving iliofemoral vein segments, and may warrant a different treatment approach than less extensive DVT. **Massive DVT** is a clinical distinction that refers to DVT manifesting with phlegmasia and is limb-threatening; most cases of massive DVT are extensive anatomically, that is, they involve the iliofemoral veins. **Submassive DVT** is seen most commonly (>90% of cases) and is not limb-threatening.

3) **Phlegmasia dolens**: An acute form of DVT involving the majority of the veins of the limb, accompanied by pain and massive edema.

   a) **Phlegmasia alba dolens**: Severe edema, spasm of the arterioles in the skin, impaired capillary flow.

   b) **Phlegmasia cerulea dolens**: The most severe form of DVT associated with an increased risk of amputation or death. Patients develop occlusion of nearly all veins in the limb, which leads to a significant increase in venous pressure and impairment of blood flow in the congested vascular bed, thus resulting in tissue hypoxia.

Signs and symptoms: DVT is often asymptomatic or manifests as minor symptoms only. The patient may complain of calf pain while walking. Edema of the lower leg or the entire limb may be seen, sometimes perceived as a thickening, in which case it is necessary to compare the circumferences of the limbs (in unilateral thrombosis the difference is ≥2 cm); 70% of cases of unilateral edema of the lower limb are caused by DVT. Bilateral edema may be caused by bilateral DVT, thrombosis of the inferior vena cava, or conditions unrelated to thrombosis. Tenderness or pain on palpation may be present, with some patients complaining of limb pain at rest and in rare cases developing the Homans sign (calf pain that occurs with passive dorsal flexion of the foot). The limb may be warm and dilation of the superficial veins may persist with the limb elevated at a 45 degrees angle. Low-grade or sometimes high-grade fever may be seen (due to inflammation of the tissues adjacent to the thrombotic vein). In patients with phlegmasia alba dolens, the skin of the limb is pale. Phlegmasia cerulea dolens causes massive edema and severe pain at rest; the limb (usually the foot) initially turns cyanotic and subsequently, with the development of necrosis, its color changes to black.

2. Upper extremity DVT usually involves the axillary and subclavian veins. Limb edema and pain are the predominant symptoms.

3. Complications of DVT: Deep venous thrombi may undergo fragmentation, thus becoming embolic material that is carried into the pulmonary circulation.

1) A newly formed deep venous thrombus may detach from the vascular wall or undergo fragmentation and subsequently be carried to the lungs and cause **PE**. A massive PE may block pulmonary blood flow and cause cardiac arrest, which may be the initial manifestation of DVT. Undiagnosed and untreated DVT can be complicated by recurrent PE caused by small fragments of the thrombi that embolize and frequently is misdiagnosed as pneumonia or asthma.

2) **Rarely DVT may cause stroke or systemic embolism** as a result of a paradoxical embolism in patients with a functional right-to-left cardiac shunt (eg, a patent foramen ovale).

3) Long-term complications of DVT include **postthrombotic syndrome** (chronic venous insufficiency) as well as **pulmonary hypertension** as a complication of PE. In approximately two-thirds of patients treated for DVT, the thrombus undergoes organization and the affected vein is partially recanalized (a total dissolution of the thrombus occurs only in a third of patients). This leads to chronic venous insufficiency and postthrombotic syndrome: organization of the thrombus results in damage to the venous valves, a retrograde flow of venous blood, and eventually in venous hypertension.

→ DIAGNOSIS

Due to the subtle and nonspecific clinical manifestations of VTE, it should be considered in patients with suggestive clinical features, especially when an alternative diagnosis is unlikely or has been excluded. Whenever in doubt, attempt to confirm or exclude the diagnosis of DVT, because the disease is associated with a high risk of complications (including death) if left untreated. A prompt diagnosis of VTE allows initiation of anticoagulant therapy, which is highly effective at preventing VTE-related sequelae.

Diagnostic Tests

1. Measurement of plasma D-dimer levels: The test performed to exclude DVT and PE (the reference range and cutoff values depend on the assay; most frequently thrombosis is unlikely in patients with D-dimer levels <500 µg/L). The diagnosis of VTE cannot be made on the basis of an increase in D-dimer levels alone, because an elevated D-dimer level is nonspecific and can occur in the elderly and in patients with other conditions not associated with thrombosis (eg, cancer, infection, inflammation). However, in patients with a low to intermediate clinical suspicion for DVT (assessed using a validated clinical

Table 19-1. Assessment of the clinical probability of deep vein thrombosis using the Wells score

Clinical feature	Score
Cancer (treated or diagnosed within the prior 6 months)	1
Paralysis, paresis, or recent lower limb immobilization in a cast	1
Recently bedridden for >3 days or major surgery within the prior 4 weeks	1
Localized tenderness along distribution of the deep veins of the lower extremity[a]	1
Edema of the entire leg[a]	1
Calf swelling >3 cm compared to the asymptomatic leg (measured 10 cm below the tibial tuberosity)[a]	1
Pitting edema (more prominent on the symptomatic leg)[a]	1
Visible collateral superficial veins (nonvaricose)[a]	1
Other diagnosis as likely or more likely than deep vein thrombosis	−2

Interpretation
  Low clinical probability: Total score ≤0
  Intermediate clinical probability: Total score 1-2
  High clinical probability: Total score ≥3

[a] If symptoms occur in both lower limbs, the limb in which symptoms are more severe should be assessed.

Adapted from Lancet. 1997;350(9094):1795-8 and N Engl J Med. 2003;349(13):1227-35.

prediction guide such as the Wells score), a normal D-dimer value when using a high-sensitivity D-dimer assay (eg, enzyme-linked immunosorbent assay--based) is associated with a low likelihood for DVT (≤2%).

2. Compression ultrasonography (CUS) is the key method of confirming proximal vein thrombosis. A positive result means that a vein filled with thrombi does not collapse when compressed by the transducer. Ultrasonography of the entire deep vein system of the limb allows for the detection of distal thrombosis. In patients who have below-knee CUS for detection of distal thrombosis, this should be done by an experienced vascular laboratory, since below-knee CUS may produce a high proportion of false-positive and false-negative results.

Diagnostic Criteria

In the case of suspected DVT always attempt to confirm or exclude the diagnosis to allow a prompt initiation of anticoagulant therapy (if confirmed) and avoidance of anticoagulation and associated bleeding risk (if excluded).

The diagnosis is based on a combination of the **assessment of the clinical probability of thrombosis** (eg, using the Wells score: →Table 19-1), measurements of D-dimer levels, and/or CUS. If the diagnosis based on ultrasonography is doubtful, repeat the study; in exceptional cases, consider magnetic resonance venography or computed tomography (CT) venography.

1. Outpatients:

1) A **low clinical probability of DVT**: Measure **D-dimer levels** using a high-sensitivity (~95%) or moderate-sensitivity (~85%) assay. A negative D-dimer result is sufficient to exclude DVT.◐ ● In patients with a positive result, perform CUS; if the CUS is negative, no further testing is needed.◐ ●

2) An **intermediate clinical probability of DVT**: Measure **D-dimer levels** using a high-sensitivity (~95%) assay. A negative D-dimer result is sufficient to exclude thrombosis.☑ ⬤ In patients with a positive result, perform CUS; if the CUS is negative, repeat it after 5 to 7 days.☑ ⬤

3) A **high clinical probability of DVT** or **intermediate probability of DVT without the possibility to measure D-dimer levels** using a high-sensitivity (~95%) assay: Perform **CUS**, and if the result of the study is negative, repeat it after 5 to 7 days.☑ ⬤

2. Hospitalized patients: It is necessary to perform **CUS** due to the low specificity and predictive value of positive D-dimer test results (the level is increased in many hospitalized patients, for instance due to major trauma, surgery, cancer, or inflammation), and sometimes also a reduced sensitivity of the assay (due to the use of anticoagulants or the assay being performed a few days after the onset of clinical manifestations). In patients with a negative CUS result and a high probability of DVT, repeat CUS after 5 to 7 days. In patients with a lower probability of DVT, measure the D-dimer level, and if positive, repeat CUS.

Differential Diagnosis

Limb injury (most frequent), chronic venous insufficiency (dysfunction of the venous valves, venous muscle pump, and plantar venous pump), superficial vein thrombosis, a Baker cyst (the posterior protrusion of the popliteal bursa [eg, due to trauma or in association with rheumatoid arthritis], which may rupture or compress the popliteal vein; this condition may cause thrombosis upon severe compression or as a result of local inflammation), cellulitis or lymphangitis, drug-induced edema (particularly in patients treated with calcium-channel blockers; edema is usually bilateral), lymphedema (in a third of patients with severe chronic venous insufficiency), hematomas of the lower leg muscles, plantaris muscle tendon rupture, myositis, tendinitis (particularly involving the Achilles tendon), or arthritis.

➡ TREATMENT

General Considerations

1. Treatment of symptomatic and asymptomatic DVT is the same. Management algorithm: →Figure 19-1.

2. Conventional anticoagulant therapy is used for patients with **clinically submassive DVT**, whereas thrombolytic therapy is considered for patients with **massive DVT**. Submassive DVT is characterized by proximal vein thrombosis, which may extend into the iliofemoral vein segment, but does not produce severe symptoms and signs. Massive DVT, which typically involves the iliofemoral veins, is characterized by severe symptoms and signs that include extensive entire leg swelling, phlegmasia cerulea dolens, and limb ischemia.

3. A patient with **acute submassive DVT** does not have to be hospitalized and the treatment can be started at home (using low-molecular-weight heparin [LMWH]), provided the following conditions are fulfilled:

1) The patient is clinically stable with normal vital signs.
2) There are no severe symptoms (severe pain and major edema of the lower limbs).
3) The risk of bleeding is low.
4) The patient has a creatinine clearance >30 mL/min.
5) An appropriate follow-up care is provided.

4. Early mobilization (this applies to the majority of patients): The patient should remain in bed with the limb elevated (with the lower leg in a horizontal position, the thigh directed at an angle towards the pelvis, and the limb supported along its whole length) only on the day the diagnosis of DVT is made and heparin treatment started.

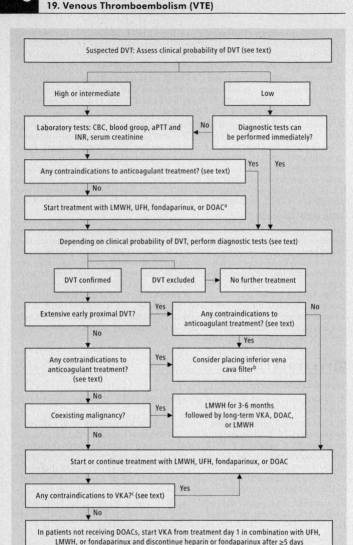

Figure 19-1. Management algorithm of lower extremity deep venous thrombosis.

5. Treatment with graduated compression: Elastic compression stockings (pantyhose, stockings, or knee-high socks are available; in most cases knee-high socks are sufficient) should not be routinely used in all patients with DVT but should be considered in patients with edema or other swelling. Typically, elastic compression stockings are initiated during the first week after diagnosis when the associated pain and inflammation have subsided enough to allow the patient to comfortably wear the stockings. The patient should wear a knee-high sock or stocking (or bandage) throughout the day and walk as much as possible; at night it should be taken off, and the bed mattress in the region of the leg should be elevated by 10 to 15 cm. **Contraindications** to compression treatment include phlegmasia cerulea dolens, concomitant limb ischemia due to arterial disease (measure the ankle-brachial index [ABI] or at least make sure that the pulse assessed on the dorsalis pedis artery and posterior tibial artery is present and symmetric on both lower extremities), and severe peripheral neuropathy.

6. Anticoagulant treatment: →below; this treatment modality is of key importance.

7. Placement of inferior vena caval filters should be considered in patients with acute proximal DVT of the lower extremities in whom the use of anticoagulants at therapeutic doses is contraindicated (because of the risk of bleeding or need for a major surgical procedure that cannot be postponed) or ineffective (recurrent PE or a significant enlargement of the thrombus despite an adequate anticoagulant treatment). Retrievable filters, which are typically removed after 1 to 3 weeks, are preferred. Anticoagulant treatment should be started or resumed once the risk of bleeding has decreased.

8. Thrombolysis: Consider systemic thrombolysis for patients with clinically massive DVT that may be accompanied by phlegmasia cerulea dolens, and only if local infusion of a thrombolytic agent via a catheter is not feasible. Local thrombolysis may be beneficial in the following groups of patients:

1) Patients with clinically massive DVT (eg, iliofemoral DVT with severe edema and pain), <14 days from the onset of symptoms, who are in good general condition (a low risk of bleeding).

2) Patients with early upper extremity DVT (<14 days from the onset of symptoms) or at risk of amputation.

Thrombolytic agents are administered locally via a catheter inserted into the thrombus; this is preferably combined with mechanical fragmentation of the thrombus and aspiration of its fragments. Following a successful thrombolysis, use the same anticoagulant treatment as in similar patients receiving medical treatment only.

Initial Anticoagulant Treatment

1. General principles of anticoagulant treatment in VTE: →Figure 19-2.

2. In patients with a **high or intermediate clinical probability of DVT** or with **confirmed DVT**, start anticoagulant treatment immediately once contraindications have been excluded, even if the results of diagnostic tests are not yet available. If the tests cannot be performed promptly and the probability of DVT is at least intermediate, start treatment before the diagnosis is established.

In **nonhospitalized patients with acute isolated distal lower extremity DVT** (veins of the lower leg [peroneal vein; anterior and posterior tibial veins]), it is suggested to start anticoagulant therapy if there are severe symptoms or risk factors for thrombus extension (eg, positive D-dimer test results, active cancer, immobility, thrombus in close proximity to the proximal veins, thrombus >5 cm in length). In patients who have mild to moderate symptoms and do not have risk factors for thrombus extension, it is suggested to withhold anticoagulant therapy and undertake serial compression ultrasonography over 2 weeks. If there is worsening of symptoms or evidence of thrombus extension

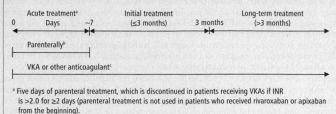

Figure 19-2. General principles of anticoagulant treatment in patients with venous thromboembolism. *Based on the 2012 Polish guidelines.*

Table 19-2. Dosage of low-molecular-weight heparin in the initial treatment of venous thromboembolism

Low-molecular-weight heparin	Dosage	
	Twice daily	Once daily
Dalteparin	100 IU/kg every 12 h	200 IU/kg every 24 h (a single dose cannot exceed 18,000 IU)
Enoxaparin	1 mg/kg every 12 h	1.5 mg/kg every 24 h (a single dose cannot exceed 180 mg)
Nadroparin	85 IU/kg every 12 h	170 IU/kg every 24 h

into the proximal veins on ultrasonography testing, it is suggested to start anticoagulant therapy.⊘○

3. LMWH, unfractionated heparin (UFH), fondaparinux, rivaroxaban, apixaban, edoxaban, or dabigatran: LMWH or fondaparinux are preferred over UFH due to the convenient dosage and no need for laboratory monitoring of the anticoagulant effects. In patients treated with a vitamin K antagonist (VKA) who have developed acute lower extremity DVT, start parenteral anticoagulant treatment (LMWH, fondaparinux, or UFH). In patients with kidney failure (creatinine clearance <30 mL/min), UFH is preferred (you may also reduce the dose of LMWH by 50% or monitor plasma anti-Xa levels). In certain clinical situations (eg, patients at risk of hemorrhagic complications, patients in whom thrombolytic therapy is considered or urgent surgery is likely) starting the therapy with UFH is preferred because of its shorter duration of action and the possibility of easy neutralization of anticoagulant effects with protamine, when necessary. In patients at risk of heparin-induced thrombocytopenia (HIT), use fondaparinux (→Chapter 3.1.1.3). **Dosage**:

1) Subcutaneous **LMWH** at a therapeutic dose every 12 hours (initial treatment) or every 24 hours (in long-term and outpatient treatment) (→Table 19-2). If the clinical efficacy of LMWH is questionable (eg, thrombus progression is seen), measure the anti-Xa level (preferably 4 hours after the last LMWH administration; the target anti-Xa levels are 0.6-1.0 IU/mL in patients receiving LMWH every 12 hours and 1-1.3 IU/mL in those receiving LMWH

Table 19-3. Protocol of IV unfractionated heparin dose adjustment based on aPTT

aPTT (s)[a]	IV bolus	Continuous IV infusion
First dose	80 IU/kg	18 IU/kg/h
<35 (<1.2 × control)	80 IU/kg	Increase by 4 IU/kg/h
35-45 (1.2-1.5 × control)	40 IU/kg	Increase by 2 IU/kg/h
46-70 (1.5-2.5 × control)[b]	Without IV injection	No change
71-90 (2.5-3 × control)	Without IV injection	Reduce by 2 IU/kg/h
>90 (>3 × control)	Without IV injection	Stop the infusion for 1 h, then reduce by 3 IU/kg/h

[a] Sample numerical values expressed in seconds may vary depending on the reference (control) values in a given laboratory.

[b] The therapeutic aPTT range of 46-70 seconds should correspond to the anti-Xa activity of 0.3-0.7 IU/mL. Note: Repeat aPTT and adjust the unfractionated heparin dose after 6 hours.

aPTT, activated partial thromboplastin time; IV, intravenous.

once daily). If anti-Xa measurement is not feasible, administer IV UFH and monitor the activated partial thromboplastin time (aPTT).

2) **UFH**:
   a) **IV administration**: Inject 80 IU/kg (or up to 5000 IU) as an IV bolus followed by a continuous IV infusion at the rate of 18 IU/kg/h (or up to 1300 IU/h). Assess aPTT after 6 hours. If the aPTT value is within the therapeutic range (1.5-fold to 2.5-fold prolongation compared with the reference value; usually aPTT in the course of treatment should be 60--90 seconds), continue the infusion at the same dose (the average maintenance dose is 25,000-35,000 IU/d); otherwise increase or decrease the dose of UFH accordingly (→Table 19-3).
   b) **Subcutaneous administration**: If the anticoagulant effect is being monitored, use a concentrated formulation of 25,000 IU/mL, initially 80 IU/kg IV followed by 250 IU/kg subcutaneously every 12 hours, and adjust the doses so that 6 hours after the injection of the drug aPTT remains in the therapeutic range (the average maintenance dose is 17,500 IU every 12 hours). If the anticoagulant effect is not being monitored, start with 333 IU/kg subcutaneously, followed after 12 hours by 250 IU/kg subcutaneously every 12 hours.

In patients who fail to achieve the target aPTT values despite the use of high-dose UFH, adjust the dose on the basis of the anti-Xa levels.

3) **Fondaparinux**: Administer 7.5 mg subcutaneously every 24 hours. In patients with a body weight >100 kg, you may increase the dose to 10 mg every 24 hours.

4) **Rivaroxaban**: Administer 15 mg orally bid for 3 weeks, followed by 20 mg once daily (15 mg if GFR is <50 mL/min; do not use if GFR is <30 mL/min).

5) **Apixaban**: Administer 10 mg orally bid for the first 7 days, then 5 mg bid. In long-term treatment (>3 months), use 2.5 mg bid.

6) **Dabigatran**: Switch from LMWH or UFH to dabigatran after 5 to 7 days of LMWH or UFH treatment; administer dabigatran 150 mg orally bid (110 mg bid is suggested in patients at high risk of bleeding).

7) **Edoxaban**: Switch from LMWH or UFH to edoxaban after 5 to 7 days of LMWH or UFH treatment; administer edoxaban 60 mg orally once daily

(30 mg once daily is suggested in patients with moderate renal insufficiency [creatinine clearance 30-50 mL/min], body weight <60 kg, concomitant use of potent p-glycoprotein inhibitors).

4. Duration of heparin and fondaparinux treatment:

1) In the majority of patients in whom VKA use is planned, these agents should be administered from the first day of treatment. Discontinue heparin and fondaparinux if the international normalized ratio (INR) is ≥2.0 for 2 consecutive days of combination treatment with VKAs, but not earlier than after 5 days of the administration of heparin or fondaparinux. Do not discontinue heparin/fondaparinux on the day of starting the VKA, because in the first days the anticoagulant effect of VKAs is incomplete, and therefore the concomitant administration of heparin/fondaparinux is necessary.

2) In patients with extensive iliofemoral DVT causing severe edema and limb pain, use heparin or LMWH for 7 to 10 days (or longer, until symptom relief) and consider deferring the start of VKA administration.

3) In patients in whom VKAs are contraindicated or not recommended, continue LMWH. This pertains in particular to the following situations:

   a) Pregnant women with VTE, since VKAs cross the placenta and may be harmful to the developing fetus.

   b) Patients with cancer, as LMWHs are more effective and safer than VKAs; the agents should be used at least during the first 3 to 6 months of treatment. An alternative to VKAs for patients with cancer and VTE are selected direct oral anticoagulants (DOACs) (edoxaban, rivaroxaban), which are administered in the same manner as in patients without cancer.

   c) When regular and accurate INR monitoring cannot be performed.

   d) If the current episode of VTE occurred despite the administration of appropriate doses of a VKA.

5. Treatment with VKAs:

1) Start the administration of **acenocoumarol** or **warfarin** simultaneously with heparin or fondaparinux, usually on the first day of treatment. If you plan to use heparin for >7 days (→above), you may delay the administration of a VKA.

2) In the first 2 days, use 6 mg of acenocoumarol or 10 mg of warfarin; do not use >6 mg of acenocoumarol or >10 mg of warfarin. In the elderly, debilitated, or malnourished patients, as well as in patients with heart failure, liver disease, those receiving drugs that enhance the effects of VKAs, or those at increased risk of bleeding, start treatment with 4 mg of acenocoumarol or 5 mg of warfarin.

3) Assess the INR on day 3 and adjust the dose on the basis of the results.

4) In patients with an INR ≥2.0 for 2 consecutive days, discontinue heparin/fondaparinux and continue treatment with a VKA alone for a time dependent on the risk of relapse (≥3 months; →Table 19-4) at doses adjusted to maintain the INR within the range of 2.0 to 3.0.

5) Principles of safe VKA treatment (contraindications, monitoring, dose adjustment, management of complications): →Chapter 3.1.1.4.

6. Treatment with rivaroxaban or apixaban:

1) Rivaroxaban or apixaban may be used from the beginning of DVT treatment.

2) Unlike with VKAs, it is not necessary to start treatment with the concomitant administration of heparin.

3) As the cost of rivaroxaban treatment is higher than that of VKA treatment, consider whether the patient will be able to continue the therapy for several months. Note that due to its shorter duration of action, skipping a dose of rivaroxaban may have more serious consequences than in the case of VKAs.

7. Treatment with dabigatran:

Table 19-4. Duration of venous thromboembolism treatment depending on the clinical setting

3 months

– Proximal lower extremity DVT or pulmonary embolism caused by surgery or other transient risk factor
– Upper extremity DVT associated with a central venous catheter that has already been removed in patients with or without cancer
– Upper extremity DVT unrelated to a central venous catheter or to cancer
– First episode of VTE in the form of idiopathic proximal lower extremity DVT or idiopathic pulmonary embolism in patients at high risk of bleeding[a]
– First episode of isolated distal lower-extremity DVT
– Second episode of idiopathic VTE in patients at high risk of bleeding[a]

>3 months[b]

– Upper extremity DVT associated with a central venous catheter that has not yet been removed (anticoagulant treatment should be administered as long as the catheter remains in the central vein or for 3 months if the catheter is removed)
– Lower extremity DVT and active cancer (metastatic or treated within the prior 6 months)
– First episode of VTE in the form of idiopathic proximal lower extremity DVT in patients at low or moderate risk of bleeding[a]
– Second episode of idiopathic VTE in patients at low or moderate risk of bleeding[a]

[a] Risk factors for bleeding: →Table 19-5.
[b] The need for continued treatment should be assessed periodically (eg, once a year).

DVT, deep vein thrombosis; VTE, venous thromboembolism.

1) Dabigatran is used only after 5 to 7 days of LMWH treatment.
2) Bearing in mind that the cost of dabigatran treatment is higher than that of VKA treatment, consider whether the patient will be able to continue the therapy for several months. Note that due to its shorter duration of action, skipping a dose of dabigatran may have more serious consequences than in the case of VKAs.

8. Treatment with edoxaban:
1) Edoxaban is used only after 5 to 7 days of LMWH treatment.
2) Bearing in mind that the cost of edoxaban treatment is higher than that of VKA treatment, consider whether the patient will be able to continue the therapy for several months. Note that due to its shorter duration of action, skipping a dose of edoxaban may have more serious consequences than in the case of VKAs.

Duration of Treatment

1. Patients with VTE require long-term anticoagulant treatment if there is a **high risk of recurrent thrombosis** and their **risk for bleeding is not high**. The risk is higher in the case of cancer, severe thrombophilia (eg, antithrombin deficiency, antiphospholipid antibody syndrome), elevated plasma D-dimer levels after anticoagulation, male sex, or a history of recurrent VTE.

2. Methods of preventing recurrence of VTE after upper or lower extremity DVT and after PE are similar. In the majority of patients, best results are obtained with long-term administration of VKAs at a dose that maintains the INR in the range of 2.0 to 3.0. LMWHs are recommended in patients with cancer. The recommended duration of anticoagulant treatment depends on the clinical condition (→Table 19-4) and the risk of bleeding (→Table 19-5).

Table 19-5. Risk of bleeding during anticoagulant therapy
Factors associated with bleeding during anticoagulant therapy: – Older age (>65 years and particularly >75 years)[a] – Previous bleeding (particularly if the cause was not correctable) – Cancer (particularly if metastatic or highly vascular) – Renal insufficiency – Liver failure – Diabetes mellitus – Previous stroke – Thrombocytopenia – Anemia – Concomitant antiplatelet therapy – Recent surgery – Frequent falls – Alcohol abuse – Reduced functional capacity – Poor control of VKA therapy
With an increase in the severity of individual factors and with an increase in the number of factors present, the risk of bleeding is expected to increase (both at baseline and while on anticoagulants).
[a] Young (eg, <65 years) healthy patients with good VKA control will have a low risk of major bleeding (≤1% per patient-year), those with less severe factors have an intermediate risk, and elderly patients with severe or multiple factors are at high risk for major bleeding (>4% per patient-year).
Based on Blood. 2014;123(12):1794-801.
VKA, vitamin K antagonist.

3. In patients with **recurrent VTE despite maintaining the INR in the range of 2.0 to 3.0**, consider the use of VKAs at a dose that maintains INR in the range of 2.5 to 3.5. This therapeutic range may be also more adequate for patients with antiphospholipid antibodies (APLAs) and additional VTE risk factors or with a thromboembolic event despite maintaining the INR in the range of 2.0 to 3.0, as well as in patients with an elevated baseline INR due to the presence APLAs.

4. If **VKAs cannot be used** (eg, if regular monitoring of anticoagulant effects is contraindicated or not feasible), administer a DOAC or LMWH subcutaneously.

5. To **prevent recurrent VTE in the course of long-term treatment**, you may consider switching from a VKA to rivaroxaban 20 mg once daily or to dabigatran 150 mg bid (consider using lower doses in patients at high risk of bleeding).

6. Periodically evaluate the benefits and risks of the anticoagulant treatment, as it reduces the risk of VTE recurrence but at the same time increases the risk of bleeding.

7. Compression therapy: Use class II compression elastic stockings (→Table 18-8) in patients with persistent edema or other leg swelling. In most cases, knee-length socks are the best option when fitted to the size of the limb in accordance with the manufacturer's recommendations.

Treatment of Deep Vein Thrombosis in Pregnant Women

1. Drugs (options, dosage: →Table 19-6):

1) **Subcutaneous LMWHs** (the preferred treatment) at doses adjusted to the body weight before pregnancy, administered until the end of the pregnancy.

Table 19-6. Selected heparin dosage in pregnant patients with venous thromboembolism

	Adjusted dose
Unfractionated heparin	Dose to maintain aPTT within therapeutic range, SC administration every 12 h
Dalteparin	100 IU/kg SC every 12 h or 200 IU/kg SC every 24 h
Enoxaparin	1 mg/kg SC every 12 h or 1.5 mg/kg SC every 24 h
Nadroparin	85 IU/kg SC every 12 h or 190 IU/kg SC every 24 h

aPTT, activated partial thromboplastin time; SC, subcutaneous.

Monitoring of anti-Xa levels every 1 to 3 months in the course of treatment is recommended (if available). Measure the anti-Xa level ~4 hours after the last injection of LMWH; the target levels are 0.6-1.0 IU/mL in patients receiving LMWHs every 12 hours and 1-1.3 IU/mL in those receiving LMWHs every 24 hours.

2) **UFH** (if LMWHs are not available);

a) **IV administration** (as initial treatment and in certain situations: →below): Inject 80 IU/kg (or up to 5000 IU) as an IV bolus followed by a continuous IV infusion at a dose that maintains the aPTT in the therapeutic range for 5 days (1.5-fold to 2.5-fold prolongation compared with the reference value; usually in the course of treatment aPTT should be 60-90 seconds), then treat the patient with subcutaneous LMWHs or UFH until the end of pregnancy.

b) **Subcutaneous administration** at an individually adjusted dose until the end of pregnancy: Start with the subcutaneous administration of 333 IU/kg followed after 12 hours by 250 IU/kg every 12 hours, and adjust the dose to maintain the aPTT within the therapeutic range 6 hours after the injection (the average maintenance dose is 17,500 IU every 12 hours).

2. Use **heparin** at an individually adjusted dose for ≥3 months. Subsequently, you can reduce the dose by 25% to 50% without a loss of efficacy, especially in women at an increased risk of bleeding or osteoporosis.

3. Management at delivery: The delivery should be planned. In patients with VTE there is no preference for either cesarean section or induced vaginal delivery.

1) Before the planned induction of vaginal delivery or cesarean section, discontinue subcutaneous LMWH/UFH 24 hours prior to the scheduled time of delivery.

2) Before the planned induction of vaginal delivery or cesarean section in patients at a very high risk of VTE recurrence (eg, proximal lower extremity DVT within 4 prior weeks), switch from subcutaneous LMWH/UFH to a full therapeutic dose of IV UFH and then discontinue heparin 4 to 6 hours before the scheduled time of delivery. You may consider placing a retrievable inferior vena caval filter before the delivery and removing it afterwards (this may be used in special situations only, eg, VTE within 4 weeks, as sometimes the filter cannot be retrieved).

3) Spontaneous labor: In women receiving subcutaneous UFH, closely monitor the aPTT. If it is significantly prolonged at labor, consider the administration of protamine (dosage: →Chapter 3.1.1.3).

4) Spinal or epidural anesthesia can be administered as long as the last dose of LMWH was 24 hours ago, the last dose of subcutaneous UFH was 12 hours ago, or IV UFH was stopped 4 to 6 hours ago.

4. Postdelivery management: For 6 weeks (or longer, so that the entire duration of anticoagulant treatment is ≥6 months) use VKAs at a dose that maintains the INR in the range of 2.0 to 3.0, initially in combination with LMWHs or UFH until an INR ≥2.0 is achieved on 2 consecutive days.

→ PREVENTION

1. →Chapter 3.19.2.

2. Prevention of recurrent VTE by appropriate treatment of a VTE episode: →Duration of Treatment, above.

19.2. Primary Prevention of Venous Thromboembolism

→ METHODS OF PREVENTION

The **choice of the method** depends on the patient's characteristics (risk of venous thromboembolism [VTE], of bleeding, and of other complications) as well as the feasibility of the method (availability, cost, ability to monitor the anticoagulant effect).

1. Early mobilization.

2. Mechanical treatment:

1) **Graduated compression stockings** (or appropriately applied short-stretch bandages).

2) An **intermittent pneumatic compression device**, which facilitates outflow of venous blood from the lower extremities. The device consists of a cuff applied to the lower or upper extremity and an electrical pneumatic pump, which periodically fills segments of the cuff with compressed air.

3. Anticoagulant terminology (contraindications and complications: →Chapter 3.1):

1) Heparins: **Unfractionated heparin (UFH) and low-molecular-weight heparins (LMWHs)**.

2) Selective factor Xa inhibitors: **Fondaparinux, rivaroxaban, apixaban, edoxaban, betrixaban** (in the United States).

3) Direct thrombin inhibitors: **Dabigatran** (oral; the other are parenteral), **bivalirudin, argatroban, desirudin**.

3) Vitamin K antagonists (VKAs): **Acenocoumarol, warfarin**.

4) Direct oral anticoagulants (DOACs): **Apixaban, edoxaban, rivaroxaban, dabigatran**.

→ PATIENTS AFTER SURGERY OR TRAUMA

Prevention of VTE is usually started before the surgery or within 24 hours afterwards and is continued until the patient is completely mobilized; in the case of major orthopedic surgery, prevention continues for ≥10 to 14 days.◐◐

Because of high incidence of VTE after discharge from the hospital, it is suggested to continue the VTE prophylaxis, typically with a LMWH, for up to 35 days in patients after major orthopedic surgery◐◐ and it is recommended to continue prophylaxis up to 4 weeks in high-risk patients (eg, with prolonged immobilization) after abdominal or pelvic cancer surgery, as long as these patients are not at high risk of bleeding.◐◐ The choice of the prevention method depends on the individual risk of thrombosis (→Table 19-7).

After elective hip or knee replacement surgery, prophylaxis with a DOAC can be considered, with apixaban 2.5 mg bid, dabigatran 150 mg to 220 mg daily, or rivaroxaban 10 mg daily. An alternative option involves a hybrid approach comprising 5 days of rivaroxaban 10 mg daily followed by 14 to 28 days of acetylsalicylic acid (ASA) 75 to 100 mg daily.

Also →Chapter 3.1.3.

→ MEDICAL PATIENTS

Risk factors: →Table 19-8.

Principles of prevention: →Table 19-9.

Drug dosage: →Table 19-10.

→ PATIENTS WITH CANCER

1. The **risk of VTE** in patients with cancer is approximately 6-fold higher than in patients without cancer; this concerns in particular patients with malignant brain tumors and adenocarcinomas of the ovary, pancreas, colon, stomach, lung, prostate, or kidney, as well as with hematologic malignancies. It is further increased by immobilization, hospitalization, treatment with angiogenesis inhibitors (thalidomide, lenalidomide, bevacizumab), erythropoietin, darbepoetin, chemotherapy (particularly with platinum analogues), and surgical procedures. VTE in patients with cancer can be asymptomatic (so-called incidental VTE) and it is diagnosed as a result of imaging performed for the staging of cancer or evaluation of the effects of cancer therapy. Both incidental and symptomatic thrombosis are independent risk factors for recurrent VTE and reduced survival of the patients. Risk score: →Table 19-11.

2. Recommended prevention of VTE in outpatients with solid tumors: VTE prophylaxis can be considered in selected high-risk outpatients with solid tumors who are receiving chemotherapy. Treatment options include LMWH or selected DOACs:

1) Consider a prophylactic-dose anticoagulant in the following patients:

   a) Patients with additional risk factors of VTE (→above) or risk factors included in the Khorana score (→Table 19-11), and at low risk of bleeding (do not use prophylactic anticoagulant treatment in patients with none of these features).

   b) Patients receiving chemotherapy for pancreatic cancer or lung cancer who are at low risk of bleeding (such prophylactic treatment is ineffective in patients with metastatic breast cancer, and it increases the risk of intracranial hemorrhage in patients with brain tumors).

   c) Patients treated with angiogenesis inhibitors combined with glucocorticoids or doxorubicin (other therapeutic options in this group of patients include low-dose ASA (eg, 80-100 mg/d) or a VKA at a low dose or at a dose maintaining the international normalized ratio [INR] in the range of 2.0-3.0).

2) Do not use routine prophylactic anticoagulant treatment to prevent central venous catheter-associated thrombosis in patients with no additional risk factors for VTE.

3. Recommended prevention of VTE in hospitalized medical patients: →Table 19-9.

→ LONG-DISTANCE TRAVEL

Overall, there is only low-quality evidence regarding the use of intervention to prevent VTE during long distance travel (>6 hours) and all statements below represent suggestions.

1. For long-distance air travelers, suggest wearing loose-fitting clothing that does not compress the lower extremities or the waist, drinking plenty of nonalcoholic beverages, avoiding alcohol and caffeinated beverages, frequent

Table 19-7. A modified Caprini risk assessment score	
Risk factor	**Score**
Age	
41-60 years	1
61-74 years	2
≥75 years	3
BMI >25 kg/m^2	1
Women	
Oral contraceptives or HRT	1
Pregnancy or postpartum	1
History of unexplained or recurrent miscarriage/stillborn infant	1
Thrombophilia	
Elevated serum homocysteine	3
Positive factor V Leiden	3
Positive prothrombin 20210A	3
Positive lupus anticoagulant	3
Positive anticardiolipin antibodies	3
Positive anti−β_2-GPI antibodies	3
HIT	3
Other congenital or acquired thrombophilia	3
Venous disease	
Lower limb edema	1
Varicose veins of lower limb	1
History of VTE	3
Family history of VTE	3
Immobilization	
Medical patient currently at bed rest	1
Patient confined to bed (>72 h)	2
Limb immobilized in plaster cast	2
Surgery	
Minor surgery planned	1
Arthroscopic surgery	2
Major surgery (>45 min)	2
Laparoscopic surgery (>45 min)	2
Elective arthroplasty	5
Hip, pelvis, or leg fracture	5

Risk factor	Score
Other	
Sepsis (<1 month)	1
Serious lung disease, including pneumonia (<1 month)	1
Abnormal pulmonary function	1
Acute myocardial infarction	1
Onset or exacerbation of heart failure (<1 month)	1
History of inflammatory bowel disease	1
Central venous access	2
Malignancy	2
Stroke (<1 month)	5
Acute spinal cord injury (<1 month)	5
Interpretation of risk level:	
Score 0: Very low risk	
Score 1-2: Low risk	
Score 3-4: Moderate risk	
Score ≥5: High risk	

Adapted from Chest. 2012;141(2 Suppl):e227S-e277S.

Anti−β$_2$-GPI, anti−β$_2$-glycoprotein I; BMI, body mass index; HIT, heparin-induced thrombocytopenia; HRT, hormone replacement therapy; VTE, venous thromboembolism.

tightening of the muscles of the calf during the flight, flexing the toes or standing on tiptoes, and avoiding sleeping in a sitting position.

2. For long-distance air travelers at increased risk for VTE, suggest frequent ambulation, calf muscle exercises, or sitting in an aisle seat, if feasible. The use of knee-high graduated compression socks with 15 to 30 mm Hg compression at the ankle level is suggested in the following groups: individuals with a history of VTE, recent (<6 weeks) trauma, or surgery; patients with cancer; women who are pregnant or receive estrogens; elderly persons; physically handicapped or obese persons; patients with thrombophilia. A single prophylactic dose of a LMWH before departure can be used in selected patients at increased risk for VTE (eg, VTE within the past year). The prophylactic use of antiplatelet agents is not recommended.

3. For long-distance travel by car, bus, or train, in addition to the above-mentioned propositions we suggest periodic ambulation during car stops or while travelling.

▸ PREGNANCY

1. Appropriate prevention of VTE in pregnant patients is very important. In developed countries, PE is the most common cause of death in women during pregnancy and the postpartum period.

2. Recommended methods of prevention in pregnant women at increased risk of VTE: →Table 19-12.

3. LMWHs are the drugs of choice (agents and dosage: →Table 19-10), but UFH may also be used (5000 IU administered subcutaneously every 12 hours),

Table 19-8. Risk factors for venous thromboembolism in hospitalized patients: the Padua risk assessment score

Baseline features	Score
Active cancer (patients with regional lymph node involvement or distant metastases who received chemotherapy or radiotherapy in the prior 6 months)	3
A history of VTE (except for superficial vein thrombosis)	3
Immobilization (bed rest with bathroom privileges, either due to patient's limitations or physician order, for at least 3 days)	3
Previous diagnosis of thrombophilia (deficiencies of antithrombin, protein C, protein S, or factor V Leiden, prothrombin gene G20210A mutation, or antiphospholipid syndrome)	3
Recent (≤1 month) trauma or surgery	2
≥70 years of age	1
Heart failure or respiratory failure	1
Acute myocardial infarction or ischemic stroke	1
Acute infection or rheumatologic disorder	1
Obesity (BMI ≥30 kg/m^2)	1
Hormonal therapy	1
Interpretation: Score ≥4: High risk of VTE	
Adapted from J Thromb Haemost. 2010;8(11):2450-7.	
BMI, body mass index; VTE, venous thromboembolism.	

because—unlike VKAs—heparins do not cross the placenta and do not cause fetal malformations or bleeding. New oral anticoagulants (factor Xa inhibitors and thrombin inhibitors) have not been studied in pregnant women and thus are not recommended.

4. The use of LMWHs, UFH, or VKAs by a mother is not a contraindication to breastfeeding; however, fondaparinux, oral factor Xa inhibitors, and thrombin inhibitors should not be administered during lactation.

5. In women receiving long-term VKA treatment who plan to become pregnant, frequent pregnancy testing is recommended. Once the patient becomes pregnant, she should be switched from VKAs to UFH or LMWHs. An alternative approach is to switch from a VKA to an LMWH before attempting to become pregnant. This does not apply to women with implanted mechanical heart valves, who should be referred to a specialist center.

6. DOACs should be avoided during pregnancy because they cross the placenta and their effects on the developing fetus are uncertain.

19.3. Pulmonary Embolism

→ DEFINITION, ETIOLOGY, PATHOGENESIS

Pulmonary embolism (PE) refers to the occlusion of the pulmonary artery or some of its branches by an embolus. The embolus may be formed by thrombi (the most frequent cause of PE; these usually originate from deep veins of the

Table 19-9. Prevention of venous thromboembolism in medical patients

Clinical condition	Recommended prevention
Ischemic stroke with impaired mobility[a]	Options: – Adequate prophylactic dose of LMWH[b] (preferred); – SC UFH 5000 IU every 12 hours; – IPC and/or graduated compression elastic stockings in patients with contraindications to anticoagulant treatment. **Note:** You can safely use a prophylactic dose of heparin in combination with ASA. Do not use heparin in the first 24 hours after thrombolytic treatment of stroke.
Hemorrhagic stroke[a]	– Use IPC in early treatment; – In clinically stable patients at very high risk of VTE you may use LMWH at an adequate prophylactic dose[b] (preferred dose) or SC UFH 5000 IU every 12 h starting on day 2-4 after the bleeding if considered safe (documented cessation of bleeding). **Note:** The time for starting heparin administration depends on the evaluation of the risk of thrombosis and the risk of recurrent bleeding in the patient.
Hospitalized acutely ill medical patients at high risk of VTE (Padua Score ≥4)[c]	Options: – Adequate prophylactic dose of LMWH[b]; – SC UFH 5000 IU every 12 h; – SC fondaparinux 2.5 mg[d] SC every 24 h; – In the case of bleeding or high risk of bleeding[e] use IPC and/or graduated compression elastic stockings at least in early treatment until the risk of bleeding is reduced. Use pharmacologic prophylaxis during the patient's immobilization or hospitalization.
Long-term immobilized patients remaining at home or in an institution	Do not use VTE prevention routinely.

[a] Recommendations for the management of patients with stroke apply to VTE prophylaxis only, and not to the anticoagulant and thrombolytic treatment of stroke.

[b] Agents: →Chapter 3.19.1. Dosage: →Table 19-10.

[c] →Table 19-8.

[d] 1.5 mg in patients with a creatinine clearance <50 mL/min.

[e] The risk of bleeding is highest in patients with active gastric or duodenal ulcers, a history of severe bleeding within the prior 3 months, platelet counts of $<50 \times 10^9$/L, or liver failure (INR >1.5). Other risk factors of bleeding: ≥85 years of age (vs <40 years), severe renal failure (GFR <30 mL/min/1.73 m^2), admission to an intensive care unit or coronary care unit, insertion of a central venous catheter, chronic arthritis, cancer, male sex. The coexistence of several of these factors indicates a significant increase in the risk of bleeding. Moreover, these factors often increase the risk of VTE. Hence the decision to start anticoagulant treatment should be based on a joint evaluation of all these risks.

ASA, acetylsalicylic acid; GFR, glomerular filtration rate; INR, international normalized ratio; IPC, intermittent pneumatic compression; LMWH, low-molecular-weight heparin; SC, subcutaneous; UFH, unfractionated heparin; VTE, venous thromboembolism.

Table 19-10. Prophylactic doses of low-molecular-weight heparin in medical patients and pregnant women

Low-molecular-weight heparin	Prophylactic doses	
	Medical patients	**Pregnant women**
Dalteparin	5000 IU every 24 h	5000 IU SC every 24 h
Enoxaparin	40 mg every 24 h	40 mg SC every 24 h[a]
Nadroparin	2850 IU every 24 h	3800 IU SC every 24 h

[a] Dose adjustment may be necessary in the case of extremely low or extremely high body weight.

SC, subcutaneous.

Table 19-11. Risk assessment score for venous thromboembolism in outpatients with cancer treated with chemotherapy (Khorana score)

Clinical features	Score
Type of cancer	
Stomach, pancreas (very high risk)	2
Lung, lymphoma, gynecologic, genitourinary (high risk)	1
Platelet count before chemotherapy $\geq 350 \times 10^9$/L	1
White blood cell count before chemotherapy $>11 \times 10^9$/L	1
Hemoglobin level before chemotherapy <100 g/L and/or planned use of erythropoiesis stimulating agents	1
Body mass index ≥ 35 kg/m^2	1

Interpretation:
    Score 0: Low risk
    Score 1-2: Intermediate risk
    Score ≥ 3: High risk	

Adapted from Blood. 2008;111(10):4902-7.

lower extremities or the pelvis, less commonly from veins of the upper parts of the body; this type of PE is a clinical manifestation of deep vein thrombosis [DVT]), or occasionally by amniotic fluid, air (during insertion or removal of a central venous catheter), fat (after a long bone fracture), tumor cells (eg, renal cancer), or a foreign body (eg, material used for embolization procedures).

Risk factors for PE are the same as in the case of DVT (→Chapter 3.19.1). In approximately a half of all cases no risk factors are identified (idiopathic PE).

Complications of PE (their severity depends on the size of the embolus and individual cardiovascular reserve):

1) Ventilation-perfusion mismatch leading to impairment of gas exchange and subsequent hypoxemia (it may be aggravated by a shunt of poorly oxygenated blood from the right to the left atrium via a patent foramen ovale).

2) An increase in pulmonary vascular resistance (aggravated by vasoconstriction due to hypoxemia) results in increased right ventricular afterload, right

Table 19-12. Prevention of venous thromboembolism in high-risk pregnant women

Clinical setting	Recommended prevention	
	During pregnancy	Postpartum
History of 1 VTE episode associated with a transient risk factor (except pregnancy and estrogen use)	Careful monitoring[a]	LMWH[b] or VKA[c]
History of 1 VTE episode associated with pregnancy or estrogen use	LMWH[d]/UFH[d]	LMWH[b] or VKA[c]
History of 1 idiopathic VTE episode (in a patient without thrombophilia and currently not receiving long-term anticoagulant treatment)	LMWH[d]/UFH[d] or careful monitoring[a]	LMWH[b] or VKA[c]
History of 1 VTE episode in a patient with low-risk thrombophilia[e] (currently not receiving long-term anticoagulant treatment)	LMWH[d]/UFH[d] or careful monitoring[a]	LMWH[b] or VKA[c]
History of 1 VTE episode in a patient with high-risk thrombophilia[f] (currently not receiving long-term anticoagulant treatment)	LMWH[g]/UFH[g]	LMWH[b] or VKA[c] or LMWH/UFH[h]
Negative history of VTE in a patient with low-risk thrombophilia	Careful monitoring[a]	Careful monitoring[a] or anticoagulant treatment if positive family history of VTE (LMWH[b] or VKA[c])[i]
Negative history of VTE in a patient with high-risk thrombophilia[g]	LMWH[d]/UFH[d]	LMWH[b] or VKA[c]
History of ≥2 VTE episodes in a patient receiving long-term anticoagulant treatment	LMWH[j]/UFH[j]	Continuation of long-term treatment used before pregnancy
History of ≥2 VTE episodes (currently not receiving long-term anticoagulant treatment)	LMWH[g]/UFH[g]	LMWH[b] or VKA[c] or LMWH/UFH[h]

[a] Plus prompt diagnostic workup in patients with suspected DVT/PE.

[b] At a prophylactic dose (→Table 19-10) for 4-6 weeks. Do not reduce the dose of LMWH used during pregnancy.

[c] For 4-6 weeks, INR 2.0-3.0 (initially together with LMWH/UFH until the INR is ≥2.0 for 2 consecutive days).

[d] At a prophylactic dose.

[e] Heterozygotes for factor V Leiden, heterozygotes for the prothrombin G20210A gene, deficiency of protein C or protein S.

[f] Antithrombin deficiency, double heterozygotes for the prothrombin G20210A gene and factor V Leiden, homozygotes for factor V Leiden or homozygotes for the prothrombin G20210A gene.

[g] Adjusted or prophylactic dose.

[h] Adjusted dose for 6 weeks.

[i] If additional risk factors are present (a first-degree relative with an episode of VTE before 50 years of age or other major risk factors for thrombosis, eg, obesity, prolonged immobilization).

[j] Adjusted dose.

Note: In patients with a history of DVT, use adequately fitted graduated compression stockings during pregnancy, labor, and postpartum.

DVT, deep vein thrombosis; INR, international normalized ratio; LMWH, low-molecular-weight heparin; PE, pulmonary embolism; UFH, unfractionated heparin; VKA, vitamin K antagonist; VTE, venous thromboembolism.

ventricular dilation, a decrease in left ventricular filling, a reduction in cardiac output, hypotension/shock, and impaired coronary blood flow, eventually leading to acute ischemia and injury to the overloaded right ventricle. Impairment of coronary blood flow may cause myocardial injury or even a transmural myocardial infarction with normal coronary arteries, and irreversible progressive right ventricular failure is one of the major causes of death. In patients with heart failure, occlusion of even a small proportion of the pulmonary artery branches may result in shock, whereas in young and otherwise healthy individuals, a substantial occlusion of the pulmonary vascular bed may cause only minor clinical symptoms. Emboli in the peripheral branches of the pulmonary arteries may lead to lung infarcts and focal atelectasis. An increase in right atrial pressure may cause opening of the foramen ovale (this is anatomically patent in approximately a third of the healthy population), thus allowing a venous thrombus to pass and embolize into the systemic circulation (paradoxical embolism). After hemodynamic stabilization, a gradual recanalization of the pulmonary arteries takes place; in rare cases, the emboli do not dissolve despite adequate treatment and slowly undergo organization, which may lead to the development of chronic pulmonary hypertension.

→ CLINICAL FEATURES AND NATURAL HISTORY

1. Symptoms often have a sudden onset and include dyspnea (in ~80% of patients), chest pain (~50%; usually with features of pleural pain, less commonly resembling coronary pain [10%]), cough (20%, usually dry), less frequently collapse or syncope and hemoptysis.

2. Signs: More than half of patients develop tachypnea and tachycardia. In the case of right ventricular dysfunction, the signs include dilation of the jugular veins, a loud pulmonary component of the second heart sound, sometimes a tricuspid regurgitation murmur, hypotension, and signs of shock.

3. Natural history: Symptoms of DVT occur in an approximately one-fourth of patients. Mortality in untreated PE depends on the clinical severity of the disease (→Diagnostic Workup, below) and is up to 30%.

→ DIAGNOSIS

Diagnostic Tests

1. Blood tests: Increased serum D-dimer levels; in the majority of patients with high-risk or intermediate-risk PE, elevated levels of cardiac troponins and/or natriuretic peptides (B-type natriuretic peptide [BNP] or N-terminal pro–B-type natriuretic peptide [NT-proBNP]) are seen, which are indicative of right ventricular overload.

2. Electrocardiography (ECG): Tachycardia; supraventricular arrhythmias as well as nonspecific ST-segment and T-wave changes (typically inverted T waves in leads III and V_1-V_2) may also occur. Rare features include $S_IQ_{III}T_{III}$ syndrome, right axis deviation, and incomplete or complete right bundle branch block. In patients with PE causing hemodynamic instability, negative T waves in leads V_2 to V_4 and sometimes up to lead V_6 are often observed.

3. Chest radiographs may reveal enlargement of the cardiac silhouette, pleural effusion, elevated hemidiaphragm, dilation of the pulmonary artery, atelectasis, and parenchymal opacification.

4. Computed tomography angiography (CTA) allows for an accurate assessment of the pulmonary arteries from the pulmonary trunk to the segmental arteries. Multislice CT (MSCT) also includes the subsegmental arteries (the clinical significance of isolated thrombi in these arteries is controversial). Additionally, CTA reveals interstitial pulmonary lesions.

5. Echocardiography: In patients with high-risk or intermediate-risk PE, this may reveal right ventricular dilation and thinning of the interventricular septum. A characteristic finding is a hypokinetic right ventricular free wall with preserved apical contractility, as well as dilation of the inferior vena cava due to right ventricular failure and right atrial hypertension. Transesophageal echocardiography allows for the visualization of the pulmonary arteries up to the proximal parts of the lobar arteries and thus detects emboli more effectively than transthoracic echocardiography.

6. Ultrasonography of the deep veins of the lower extremities: Compression ultrasonography (CUS) and/or ultrasonography of the entire venous system of the limb may reveal thrombosis.

7. Other studies: Pulmonary ventilation-perfusion (V/Q) scintigraphy is performed less often because of its limited availability and the advantages of CT angiography. However, V/Q scintigraphy provides less radiation exposure than CT angiography and is a first-line test during pregnancy; moreover, it should be considered in women of child-bearing age or other patients who do not have concomitant lung pathology (which can lead to indeterminate test results). Pulmonary angiography is used rarely because of its invasiveness.

Diagnostic Workup

A patient with suspected PE requires a rapid diagnostic workup. The management strategy depends on the patient's condition and the availability of diagnostic studies.

1. Evaluate the risk of early death:

1) **High-risk PE: Symptoms of shock or hypotension** (systolic blood pressure [SBP] <90 mm Hg or SBP fall by ≥40 mm Hg lasting >15 minutes, if not caused by arrhythmia, hypovolemia, or sepsis).

2) **Non–high-risk PE**: No manifestations of shock or hypotension.

   a) **Intermediate-risk PE**: Features of right ventricular dysfunction (observed on echocardiography or CTA; elevated BNP/NT-proBNP levels) or positive markers of myocardial damage (increased levels of troponin T or I). The risk is additionally increased if the features of right ventricular dysfunction and myocardial damage occur simultaneously.

   b) **Low-risk PE**: Absence of the above-mentioned features of right ventricular dysfunction and markers of myocardial damage.

2. Evaluate the clinical probability of PE (eg, using the **Wells score** [→Table 19-13] or the **modified Geneva score** [→Table 19-14]) in a patient with non–high-risk PE. In patients with suspected high-risk PE, the clinical probability of PE is usually high. Diagnostic tests can also be used to consider an alternative diagnosis, for instance, ECG may be used to assess for an acute coronary syndrome or acute pericarditis and a chest radiograph may be used to assess for pneumonia or pneumothorax. The exclusion of alternative diagnoses can increase the clinical probability for PE, which requires specific diagnostic testing.

3. Diagnostic tests in patients at high risk with suspected PE: →Figure 19-3. To confirm the diagnosis, perform an urgent **CTA** or a **V/Q lung scan**. If CTA or a V/Q scan is unavailable, or if CTA cannot be performed due to the patient's condition, bedside echocardiography may be helpful in providing indirect evidence for PE (eg, dilated right ventricle, increased pulmonary artery pressure).

4. Diagnostic tests in patients not at high risk with suspected PE: →Figure 19-4.

1) Patients with a **low clinical probability of PE**: Measure the **D-dimer level** using a high-sensitivity (~95%) or moderate-sensitivity (~85%) assay. A normal D-dimer level is sufficient to exclude PE and further investigations and treatment are not necessary. If the D-dimer level is elevated, perform **CTA**; a negative CTA result excludes PE and allows for the safe discontinuation of anticoagulant treatment.

Table 19-13. Assessment of the clinical probability of pulmonary embolism using the original and simplified Wells score

Parameter	Score (original)	Score (simplified)
Predisposing factors		
History of DVT or PE	1.5	1
Recent surgery or immobilization	1.5	1
Cancer	1	1
Symptoms: Hemoptysis	1	1
Signs		
Heart rate >100 beats/min	1.5	1
Signs and symptoms of DVT	3	1
Clinical assessment: Alternative diagnosis less likely than PE	3	1
Interpretation		
Clinical probability (3 levels; original score) Low clinical probability: Total score 0-1 Intermediate clinical probability: Total score 2-6 High clinical probability: Total score ≥7 **Clinical probability (2 levels; original score)** PE not likely: Total score 0-4 PE likely: Total score >4 **Clinical probability (2 levels; simplified score)** PE not likely: Total score 0-1 PE likely: Total score ≥2		

Adapted from Thromb Haemost. 2000;83(3):416-20 and Thromb Haemost. 2008;99(1):229-34.

DVT, deep vein thrombosis; PE, pulmonary embolism.

2) Patients with an **intermediate clinical probability of PE**: Measure the **D-dimer** level using a high-sensitivity (~95%) assay. A normal D-dimer level is sufficient to exclude PE and further investigations and treatment are not necessary. If the D-dimer level is elevated, perform **CTA**; a negative CTA result excludes PE and allows for the safe discontinuation of anticoagulant treatment.

3) Patients with a **high clinical probability of PE**: Measurement of D-dimer levels is not recommended and **CTA** should be performed. In patients with an indeterminate CTA result, consider a V/Q scan or bilateral CUS to assess for DVT.

The **diagnosis of PE in non–high-risk patients** is confirmed by a thrombus observed in CTA and extending to the level of the segmental arteries. If the embolism is limited to a single subsegmental artery and there is no evidence of thrombosis elsewhere (eg, lower limb DVT), anticoagulant therapy may not be warranted.

5. Diagnosis of PE in pregnancy: The measurement of D-dimer levels is of limited value because these may be elevated due to pregnancy, particularly in the second half of pregnancy. If the D-dimer is negative, there

Table 19-14. Assessment of the clinical probability of pulmonary embolism using the original and simplified revised Geneva score

Parameter	Score (original)	Score (simplified)
Predisposing factors		
Age >65 years	1	1
Previous deep vein thrombosis or pulmonary embolism	3	1
Surgery or fracture in the past month	2	1
Active malignant condition	2	1
Symptoms		
Unilateral lower limb pain	3	1
Hemoptysis	2	1
Signs		
Heart rate 75-94 beats/min	3	1
Heart rate ≥95 beats/min	5	2
Pain on deep venous palpation of the lower limb and unilateral edema	4	1
Interpretation		

Clinical probability (3 levels; original score)
 Low clinical probability: Total score 0-3
 Intermediate clinical probability: Total score 4-10
 High clinical probability: Total score ≥11
Clinical probability (3 levels; simplified score)
 Low clinical probability: Total score 0-1 points
 Intermediate clinical probability: Total score 2-4 points
 High clinical probability: Total score ≥5 points
Clinical probability (2 levels; original score)
 Pulmonary embolism unlikely: Total score 0-5 points
 Pulmonary embolism likely: Total score ≥6 points
Clinical probability (2 levels; simplified score)
 Pulmonary embolism unlikely: Total score 0-2 points
 Pulmonary embolism likely: Total score ≥3 points

Adapted from Arch Intern Med. 2008;168(19):2131-6 and Ann Intern Med. 2006;144(3):165-71.

is insufficient evidence that it can be used to exclude DVT without further diagnostic imaging. The initial diagnostic test is lower extremity venous ultrasonography, because the diagnosis of DVT is sufficient to start antico-agulant therapy without further diagnostic testing for PE. Diagnostic tests involving ionizing radiation should only be performed in pregnant women with normal bilateral lower limb venous ultrasonography. A V/Q scan and CTA can be done during pregnancy, but V/Q scanning is suggested as an initial test because it has been better studied and there is more radiation exposure to the mother with CTA.

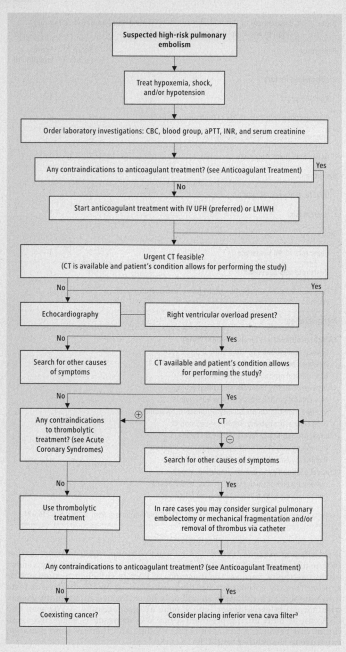

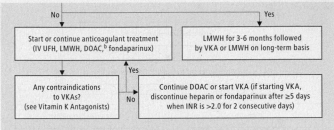

^a Applies in particular to patients at high risk for VTE recurrence, eg, immediately after neurosurgery or other major surgical procedure and in pregnant women with acute extensive proximal thrombosis a few weeks before delivery.

^b Dabigatran and edoxaban are used only after 5-7 days of parenteral medication.

aPTT, activated partial thromboplastin time; CBC, complete blood count; CT, computed tomography; DOAC, direct oral anticoagulant; INR, international normalized ratio; IV, intravenous; LMWH, low-molecular-weight heparin; UFH, unfractionated heparin; VKA, vitamin K antagonist.

⊕ Positive result. ⊖ Negative result.

Figure 19-3. Management algorithm in patients with high-risk pulmonary embolism.

Differential Diagnosis

Pneumonia and pleurisy, asthma, chronic obstructive pulmonary disease, pneumothorax, acute respiratory distress syndrome, heart failure, acute coronary syndrome (eg, in the case of ST-T changes in a patient with chest pain), intercostal neuralgia and other causes of chest pain; and in the case of high-risk PE, also cardiogenic shock, cardiac tamponade, and aortic dissection.

Severe heart failure and exacerbation of COPD are risk factors for VTE and may coexist with PE.

→ TREATMENT

Treatment of High-Risk Pulmonary Embolism

Treatment of high-risk PE: →Figure 19-3.

1. Start symptomatic treatment:

1) Treat hypotension/shock as in patients with right ventricular failure (→Chapter 3.8.1). **Note** that intensive fluid resuscitation may have harmful effects due to an increase in right ventricular overload.

2) Depending on the presence and severity of respiratory failure, administer oxygen and consider indications for mechanical ventilation.

2. IV unfractionated heparin (UFH): Administer UFH immediately at a loading dose of 80 IU/kg (up to 5000 IU) as an IV bolus provided that anticoagulant treatment is not contraindicated (→Chapter 3.1.1.3).

3. Thrombolytic therapy: Thrombolytic therapy is suggested if not contraindicated ⊕⊖ (→Chapter 3.11.1.2) (most contraindications are relative in the case of life-threatening PE, particularly when immediate embolectomy is not possible). Early confirmation of PE using imaging studies is indicated, but in critically ill patients the decision to use thrombolysis can be made solely on the basis of the clinical features suggestive of PE. In some patients, bedside cardiac echocardiography may provide indirect evidence to support a diagnosis of massive PE (right ventricular dilation, elevated pulmonary artery pressure, paradoxical septal motion). In patients with cardiac arrest, the immediate administration of 50 mg of IV alteplase and starting cardiopulmonary resuscitation may be life-saving. Thrombolytic therapy is most effective when administered

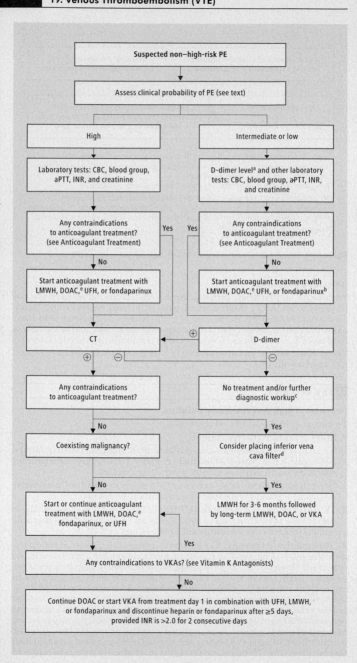

[a] D-dimer levels in hospitalized patients are of limited use. In this population starting diagnostic workup from a CT scan may be justified also in those with low or intermediate probability of PE. The same approach can be used in patients with moderate probability of PE when a high-sensitivity D-dimer assay is not available.

[b] In patients with low probability of PE, anticoagulant treatment should be started after obtaining test results (if available within 24 hours).

[c] Further studies (eg, compression ultrasonography) in case of a negative single-slice CT result regardless of the clinical probability of PE and in case of a negative multislice CT result in patients with high clinical probability of PE.

[d] Applies in particular to patients at high risk of VTE recurrence, eg, immediately after neurosurgery or other major surgical procedure and in pregnant women with acute extensive proximal thrombosis a few weeks before delivery.

[e] Dabigatran and edoxaban are used only after 5-7 days of parenteral medication.

aPTT, activated partial thromboplastin time; CBC, complete blood count; CT, computed tomography; DOAC, direct oral anticoagulant; INR, international normalized ratio; LMWH, low-molecular-weight heparin; PE, pulmonary embolism; UFH, unfractionated heparin; VKA, vitamin K antagonist; VTE, venous thromboembolism.

⊕ Positive result. ⊖ Negative result.

Figure 19-4. Management algorithm of non–high-risk pulmonary embolism.

within 48 hours of the onset of PE symptoms, but may have beneficial effects even after 6 to 14 days.

Dosage of thrombolytic agents:

1) **Streptokinase**:

  a) Accelerated regimen (preferred): 1.5 million IU IV over 2 hours.

  b) Standard regimen: 250,000 IU IV over 30 minutes followed by 100,000 IU/h.

2) **Recombinant tissue plasminogen activator (rtPA) (alteplase)**:

  a) Standard regimen: 100 mg IV over 2 hours.

  b) Accelerated regimen: 0.6 mg/kg (maximum, 50 mg) over 15 minutes.

4. If the patient has not received heparin prior to the administration of the thrombolytic agent, administer IV **UFH** 80 IU/kg (up to 5000 IU) and then start a continuous infusion of UFH at a rate of 18 IU/kg/h (up to 1300 IU/h) while monitoring the activated partial thromboplastin time (aPTT). If a loading dose of UFH has been used before the thrombolytic agent, you may continue the UFH infusion together with an infusion of the thrombolytic agent or start UFH after the discontinuation of the agent. Evidence is lacking in regards to whether UFH should be continued during the concurrent administration of thrombolytic therapy; it is suggested that UFH not be coadministered during thrombolytic therapy.

5. Once thrombolytic treatment has been discontinued, with the patient stabilized while still receiving heparin, start long-term anticoagulation with a **VKA or direct oral anticoagulants (DOACs)** following the same principles as in DVT (→Chapter 3.19.1).

6. In the case of contraindications to anticoagulant treatment in patients at high risk of PE recurrence, ie, with extensive proximal DVT, consider placement of an **inferior vena caval filter**. The filter is inserted via the femoral vein or the internal jugular vein and placed in the inferior vena cava, below the ostia of the renal veins. This treatment is sometimes also indicated in selected patients with severe pulmonary hypertension (to protect against even a minor PE episode, which in this situation could be life-threatening) or after pulmonary embolectomy. If the risk of bleeding has decreased, start anticoagulant treatment and remove the filter. Do not place the inferior vena caval filter in patients receiving anticoagulant treatment.

7. If thrombolytic therapy is contraindicated or has been ineffective (hypotension or shock persist), as well as in the case of a **mobile thrombus**

in the right ventricle or right atrium (particularly passing through the foramen ovale), consider **pulmonary embolectomy** (surgical removal of the thrombus from the pulmonary arteries, performed using extracorporeal circulation). In the case of a thrombus located proximally in the pulmonary arteries, you can also consider **percutaneous embolectomy or fragmentation of the thrombus using a catheter**. Such interventions should only be considered in experienced specialized centers.

Treatment of Low-Risk Pulmonary Embolism

1. In all patients with suspected PE, start anticoagulant treatment while still waiting to perform diagnostic tests if the results cannot be obtained within 24 hours. In patients with a high or intermediate clinical probability of PE, start anticoagulant treatment immediately, without waiting for the results of diagnostic tests.

2. Anticoagulant treatment regimen: →Chapter 3.19.1.

Treatment of Intermediate-Risk Pulmonary Embolism

The treatment is the same as in patients with low-risk PE, but in patients with right ventricular overload and myocardial dysfunction it should be started in a clinical setting with continuous monitoring of heart rate and blood pressure. In case of clinical deterioration, start "rescue" thrombolytic treatment, and if this is contraindicated, perform embolectomy or percutaneous intervention, depending on the clinical setting and availability.

Treatment of Pulmonary Embolism in Pregnancy

1. Non–high-risk PE: →Chapter 3.19.1.

2. High-risk PE: If this is life-threatening for the pregnant patient, consider thrombolytic therapy (it may cause bleeding into the placenta and lead to miscarriage). Pulmonary embolectomy is also associated with a high risk for both the child and the mother.

3. Do not use DOACs in pregnancy.

Duration of Treatment

→Chapter 3.19.1. While continuing treatment with heparin, consider switching from UFH to LMWH or fondaparinux.

➡ PREVENTION

1. →Chapter 3.19.2.

2. Prevention of recurrent VTE: →Chapter 3.19.1.

1. Acid-Base Disorders

→ **OVERVIEW OF ACID-BASE HOMEOSTASIS**

Under physiologic conditions, blood concentration of hydrogen ions [H^+] ranges from 35 to 45 nmol/L. The constant [H^+] in the body fluids is the basis for normal enzymatic reactions, particularly those associated with the formation of high-energy compounds. It is largely maintained by the lungs (elimination of CO_2) and kidneys (excretion of H^+ in the form of ammonium and titratable acids). This is described by the Henderson-Hasselbalch equation:

$$\text{Blood pH} = \frac{6.1 + \log [HCO_3^-]}{0.03 \times PaCO_2}$$

Where: [HCO_3^-], bicarbonate level in mmol/L; $PaCO_2$, blood level of CO_2 in mm Hg. The equation can be rearranged in the following way:

$$[H^+] \text{ (in nmol/L)} = \frac{24 \times PaCO_2 \text{ (in mm Hg)}}{[HCO_3^-] \text{ (in mmol/L)}}$$

Blood pH depends on the respiratory component (partial pressure of carbon dioxide in arterial blood [$PaCO_2$]) and on the metabolic (renal) component. Consequently, blood pH may be normal despite considerable changes in $PaCO_2$ and bicarbonate concentration [HCO_3^-].

Under physiologic conditions, blood pH is 7.35 to 7.45 and $PaCO_2$ is 35 to 45 mm Hg (4.65-6.00 kPa).

Key factors involved in the maintenance of a constant pH of blood and body fluids:

1) **Blood and tissue buffers**, which consist of bicarbonate, phosphate, proteinate, and hemoglobin buffers. They are characterized by the following: (a) addition of an acid or a base to the buffer results in only minor changes in buffer pH; (b) the buffer binds or releases hydrogen ions, depending on the conditions.

2) **Lungs**: Blood pH depends on $PaCO_2$, which in turn depends mostly on alveolar ventilation. Respiratory disturbances of acid-base homeostasis are mainly caused by abnormal alveolar ventilation, with hypoventilation leading to respiratory acidosis and hyperventilation leading to respiratory alkalosis.

3) **Kidneys**: The main role of kidneys in pH regulation involves the reabsorption of filtered HCO_3^-, excretion of H^+ in the form of titratable acid (mainly phosphoric acid) and ammonium, and formation of HCO_3^-. Impaired renal function with respect to these processes results in metabolic acidosis. Kidneys are the most important organ involved in compensatory responses to primary respiratory acid-base disturbances.

→ **PARAMETERS OF ACID-BASE HOMEOSTASIS**

The following 3 parameters are required to accurately describe the acid-base equilibrium. Values of these parameters are obtained from blood gas analysis (parameters: →Table 1-1; interpretation: →Table 1-2).

1) **pH** is measured in arterial or arterialized capillary blood. A normal blood pH does not exclude very serious metabolic or respiratory (nonmetabolic) disturbances. Venous blood pH is usually 0.01 to 0.03 lower than arterial blood pH.

Table 1-1. Parameters of arterial blood gas analysis[a]

Symbol	Definition	Normal range
pH	Negative logarithm of hydrogen ion concentration	7.35 to 7.45
$PaCO_2$	Arterial level of carbon dioxide	32 to 45 mm Hg (4.27-6.00 kPa)
HCO_{3curr}^-	Current plasma bicarbonate level	21 to 27 mmol/L
HCO_{3std}^-	Standard plasma bicarbonate level	24 (21-25) mmol/L
BE	Base excess in blood	−2.3 to +2.3 mEq/L
PaO_2	Arterial oxygen level	75 to 100 mm Hg[b] (10.00-13.33 kPa)
$ctCO_2$	Total plasma content of carbon dioxide	22 to 28 mmol/L 47.0% to 60.5% (volume)
SaO_2	Oxygen saturation of hemoglobin in arterial blood	95% to 98%[b]

[a] Blood drawn without contact with air.

[b] When interpreting PaO_2 and SaO_2, always record the fraction of inspired oxygen (FiO_2). The normal ranges given here are for respiration with atmospheric air at sea level (an oxygen concentration of 20.9%, which corresponds to an FiO_2 of 0.209). When a healthy individual is breathing 100% oxygen ($FiO_2 = 1.0$), PaO_2 may be as high as ~600 mm Hg and SaO_2 may reach 100%.

2) $[HCO_3^-]$, expressed in mmol/L, is a parameter of the metabolic component. It reflects the current plasma $[HCO_3^-]$ measured in blood drawn without contact with air. Venous blood $[HCO_3^-]$ is usually 1 to 3 mmol higher than arterial blood $[HCO_3^-]$.

3) **Partial pressure of carbon dioxide** is a parameter of the respiratory component. Partial pressure of CO_2 in venous blood is usually 1 to 3 mm Hg higher than partial pressure of CO_2 in arterial blood ($PaCO_2$).

If 2 of the above 3 parameters are measured, the remaining one can be calculated using the Henderson-Hasselbalch equation (→above).

Other useful parameters:

1) **Buffer base (BB)** is the sum of levels of bicarbonate, plasma proteins, phosphate, and hemoglobin (in mEq/L). It is rarely used clinically.

2) **Base excess (BE)** is the amount of titratable acid or alkali obtained when titrating a solution to a pH of 7.40 at a $PaCO_2$ of 40 mm Hg and a temperature of 37°C. If BE is negative, the solution contains an excess of nonvolatile acids or a deficit of bases.

3) **Anion gap (AG)** is the difference between $[Na^+]$ and the sum of $[Cl^-]$ and $[HCO_3^-]$. Under physiologic conditions, AG is from 8 to 12 mEq/L (note reference values in your laboratory). On the basis of AG, acidosis can be subdivided into non-AG acidosis (≤12 mEq/L), also termed hyperchloremic acidosis and caused mainly by loss of bases, and high-AG acidosis with normal serum chloride levels, caused by exogenous or endogenous nonvolatile acids (eg, lactic acidosis or ketoacidosis), decreased bicarbonate regeneration, toxins (eg, methanol, ethylene glycol, acetylsalicylic acid) or decreased H^+ excretion.

→ **CLASSIFICATION OF ACID-BASE DISORDERS**

Classification of acid-base disorders: →Table 1-2.

1. Changes in $[H^+]$ due to primary changes in $PaCO_2$ levels:

1) **Respiratory acidosis** caused by an increase in $PaCO_2$ and $[H^+]$ and a decrease in blood pH.

Table 1-2. Diagnosis of acid-base disorders based on blood gas analysis

Diagnosis	pH	PaCO$_2$	HCO$_3^-$
Simple acid-base disorders			
Respiratory acidosis			
Uncompensated[a]	↓	↑	N
Partially compensated[a]	↓	↑	↑
Completely compensated respiratory acidosis or completely compensated metabolic alkalosis[b]	N	↑	↑
Metabolic acidosis			
Uncompensated	↓	N	↓
Partially compensated	↓	↓	↓
Completely compensated metabolic acidosis or completely compensated respiratory alkalosis[b]	N	↓	↓
Respiratory alkalosis			
Uncompensated[a]	↑	↓	N
Partially compensated[a]	↑	↓	↓
Metabolic alkalosis			
Uncompensated	↑	N	↑
Partially compensated	↑	↑	↑
Mixed acid-base disorders[c]			
Metabolic and respiratory acidosis	↓	↑	↓
Metabolic and respiratory alkalosis	↑	↓	↑

[a] In patients with respiratory disturbances, changes in pH and in PaCO$_2$ develop in opposite directions.

[b] These entities may be differentiated only on the basis of a complete clinical presentation.

[c] In mixed acid-base disorders, changes in PaCO$_2$ and in [HCO$_3^-$] develop in opposite directions.

↑, increased; ↓, decreased; N, normal; PaCO$_2$, partial pressure of carbon dioxide in arterial blood.

2) **Respiratory alkalosis** caused by a decrease in PaCO$_2$ and [H$^+$] and an increase in blood pH.

2. Changes in [H$^+$] due to primary changes in [HCO$_3^-$]:

1) **Metabolic acidosis** caused by an increase in [H$^+$] and a decrease in blood pH and [HCO$_3^-$].

2) **Metabolic alkalosis** caused by a decrease in [H$^+$] and an increase in [HCO$_3^-$] and blood pH.

3. Changes in [H$^+$] due to changes in both PaCO$_2$ and [HCO$_3^-$] cause **mixed acid-base disorders**.

1.1. Metabolic Acidosis

→ **DEFINITION, ETIOLOGY, PATHOGENESIS**

Metabolic acidosis is defined as a decrease in blood pH to <7.35 (an increase in $[H^+]$ >45 nmol/L) due to a primary decrease in bicarbonate concentration $[HCO_3^-]$.

Causes (more than one mechanism may be present):

1) Excessive intake or excessive endogenous production of nonvolatile acids: Diabetic ketoacidosis, lactic acidosis, acidosis caused by intake of acid precursors (eg, poisoning with ethanol, methanol, ethylene glycol, or salicylates).

2) Impaired renal regeneration of bicarbonate (acidosis in acute or chronic renal failure) or impaired excretion of H^+ by the distal tubule (distal renal tubular acidosis).

3) Loss of bases: Renal loss (proximal renal tubular acidosis), gastrointestinal loss (diarrhea; external biliary, pancreatic, or intestinal fistulas, due to a high $[HCO_3^-]$ in bile, pancreatic juice, and intestinal juices).

Acidosis may be compensated by respiratory mechanisms, that is, by hyperventilation, which results in a decrease in the partial pressure of carbon dioxide in arterial blood ($PaCO_2$) and a complete or near-complete normalization of blood pH (resulting in complete or partial compensation of acidosis).

→ **CLINICAL FEATURES AND DIAGNOSIS**

Manifestations of metabolic acidosis depend on the underlying condition. Compensatory hyperventilation in patients with severe acute metabolic acidosis is manifested by an increased depth and frequency of breathing.

Diagnostic criteria of metabolic acidosis include a decrease in pH, a decrease in $[HCO_3^-]$, and often hypocapnia as a manifestation of the respiratory compensation of acidosis. The anion gap (AG) may be normal or increased, depending on the pathogenesis of acidosis.

→ **TREATMENT**

1. Treatment of the underlying condition.

2. Symptomatic treatment: The use of bicarbonate treatment is controversial and frequently not based on studies considering patient-important outcomes. When used, an IV $NaHCO_3$ infusion may have a target of 15 to 18 mmol/L (rather than 20-24 mmol/L). Start by calculating the bicarbonate space using the following formula:

$$\text{Bicarbonate space (L)} = \frac{0.4 + 2.6}{[HCO_3^-]_{current}} \times \text{body weight (kg)}$$

Then calculate the $[HCO_3^-]$ deficit using the following formula:

$$[HCO_3^-] \text{ deficit} = \text{bicarbonate space} \times ([HCO_3^-]_{current} - [HCO_3^-]_{target})$$

The rate of $NaHCO_3$ administration depends on the severity of acidosis, rate at which it developed, and cardiovascular function. Uncontrolled administration of $NaHCO_3$ may lead to hypernatremia and acute left-ventricular heart failure. When $NaHCO_3$ is used, our pattern of practice is to avoid boluses and rather infuse at a rate of 5 to 25 mmol/h.

1.2. Metabolic Alkalosis

→ **DEFINITION, ETIOLOGY, PATHOGENESIS**

Metabolic alkalosis is defined as an increase in blood pH to >7.45 due to a primary increase in the concentration of bicarbonate [HCO_3^-] or other bases, or due to loss of H^+.

Causes:

1) Excessive loss of H^+ or Cl^- through the gastrointestinal tract (vomiting, gastric suction, congenital chloride diarrhea), with urine (diuretics), and through the skin (cystic fibrosis).

2) Excessive intake of bases or potential bases: $NaHCO_3$, sodium citrate or lactate, or calcium carbonate; posthypercapnic alkalosis.

3) Severe hypokalemia.

Metabolic alkalosis may result from the primary loss of H^+, Cl^-, or K^+, or from a shift of K^+ from the extracellular to the intracellular compartment, which leads to hypokalemia.

→ **CLINICAL FEATURES AND DIAGNOSIS**

Clinical manifestations depend on the underlying condition. Hypokalemia, depending on its severity, may manifest as muscle weakness and arrhythmia, while alkalosis may manifest as signs and symptoms of tetany or its equivalents (→Chapter 4.2.1.2).

Diagnostic criteria of metabolic alkalosis include pH >7.45, increase in [HCO_3^-], increase in the partial pressure of carbon dioxide in arterial blood ($PaCO_2$) (as a compensatory mechanism), and often hypokalemia.

Differential diagnosis of compensated metabolic alkalosis (with a normal pH) should include compensated respiratory acidosis (features of respiratory failure are present).

→ **TREATMENT**

1. Treatment of the underlying condition is the mainstay of the management of metabolic alkalosis.

2. In patients with hypokalemia, correct potassium deficiency using KCl (→Chapter 4.2.4.2).

1.3. Respiratory Acidosis

→ **DEFINITION, ETIOLOGY, PATHOGENESIS**

Respiratory acidosis is defined as a decrease in blood pH to <7.35 due to hypercapnia.

Causes of abnormal ventilation: →Chapter 13.16.

Hypoventilation leads to CO_2 retention, hypercapnia, and respiratory acidosis. Respiratory acidosis may be acute or chronic. Physiologic mechanisms that counteract respiratory acidosis include the binding of H^+ by intracellular buffers and increased renal production of bicarbonate HCO_3^- in the process of ammonia production.

→ **CLINICAL FEATURES AND DIAGNOSIS**

Manifestations of respiratory acidosis include features of acute or chronic respiratory failure. Blood pH may be normal or decreased and variable increases in blood [HCO_3^-] may be seen as a compensatory mechanism.

Treatment of respiratory acidosis depends on the underlying condition.

1.4. Respiratory Alkalosis

Respiratory alkalosis is defined as an increase in blood pH to >7.45 due to primary hypocapnia (caused by hyperventilation).

Hypocapnia due to hyperventilation may be caused by stimulation of the respiratory center (eg, due to pain, excitement, cold), hypoxia (causes of hypoxemia and hypoxia: →Chapter 13.16), organic central nervous system changes (cerebrovascular disease in >90% of cases), or psychiatric disorders.

Renal compensation for respiratory alkalosis involves an increase in the urinary excretion of bicarbonate and a decrease in bicarbonate production. Maximal renal compensation of respiratory alkalosis takes several days.

Clinical manifestations depend on the underlying condition. Hypocapnia is manifested by altered mental status, features of cerebral ischemia, paresthesia, and pyramidal symptoms. Alkalosis may precipitate tetany or its equivalents (→Chapter 4.2.1.2).

Diagnostic criteria for respiratory alkalosis include permanent or episodic hyperventilation, pH >7.45, low partial pressure of carbon dioxide in arterial blood ($PaCO_2$), and normal or low bicarbonate concentration [HCO_3^-]. In patients with compensated respiratory alkalosis, pH is (close to) normal, $PaCO_2$ is low, and [HCO_3^-] is decreased.

1. Treatment of the underlying condition.

2. Symptomatic treatment (rarely; only in patients without hypoxia):

1) Instruct the patient to breathe into a plastic bag (to increase the respiratory dead space) in case of symptomatic respiratory alkalosis, usually acute.
2) Short-term use of sedatives or drugs that have depressive effects on the respiratory center (benzodiazepines, barbiturates) may play a limited role in anxiety-induced hyperventilation, leading to symptomatic chronic respiratory alkalosis.

2. Electrolyte Disturbances

1. Electroneutrality of body fluids: Body fluids are electrically neutral in all body water compartments, which means that in each body fluid the sum of anions (negative charges) equals the sum of cations (positive charges). In the extracellular fluid (ECF), the key cation is Na^+, while the key anions are Cl^- and HCO_3^-. In the intracellular fluid (ICF), the key cation is K^+, while the key anions are proteinates and phosphates.

2. Isomolality (iso-osmolality) of body fluids: The osmotic pressure of body fluids in all water compartments is equal. An increase or a decrease in the concentration of effective osmolytes (osmotically active substances that do not readily pass through cell membranes) in one water compartment causes a shift of water between the compartments and stabilization of the osmotic pressure at a new level. Fluids with effective osmolality below the physiologic level are called **hypotonic**, while those with effective osmolality above the physiologic level are called **hypertonic**. The normal osmolality of body fluids ranges from 280 to 290 mmol/kg H_2O. The osmolality of serum can be calculated on the basis of sodium, glucose, and urea levels (all in mmol/L) using the following formula:

Serum osmolality = $2 \times [Na^+] + [glucose] + [urea]$

Osmolar gap is a difference between measured serum osmolality and osmolality calculated using the formula above. Under physiologic conditions, the osmolar gap is ≤10. An osmolar gap >15 suggests the presence of substances that are effective osmolytes in serum, such as ethanol, methanol, isopropanol, ethylene glycol, propylene glycol, or acetone.

2.1. Calcium Disturbances

→ PHYSIOLOGIC BACKGROUND

Total body calcium content is 20 to 25 g/kg lean body weight, which accounts for ~1.4% to 1.6% of total body weight. The normal range of serum $[Ca^{2+}]$ is 2.25 to 2.75 mmol/L (9-11 mg/dL).

In the body, 98% of calcium is located in bones. The remaining 1% to 2% can undergo rapid mobilization; half of this is ionized (biologically active) calcium, and the rest is protein-bound (mainly albumin-bound). Alkalosis increases binding of calcium to proteins, thus decreasing the levels of ionized calcium; acidosis has the opposite effect.

Daily dietary calcium intake is ~1 g; ~30% of this is absorbed. The gastrointestinal absorption of calcium is increased by $1,25(OH)_2D_3$ and parathyroid hormone—mediated by $1,25(OH)_2D_3$—and decreased by oxalate, phosphate, and fatty acids as a result of binding in the intestinal lumen. From 98% to 99% of calcium filtrated in the glomeruli undergoes reabsorption in the renal tubules. Daily urinary calcium excretion is 3 to 5 mmol.

Intracellular and extracellular calcium are important in many enzymatic reactions and play a regulatory role in vital body functions (eg, blood coagulation, signal transmission in the nervous system, muscle contraction).

2.1.1. Hypercalcemia

→ DEFINITION, ETIOLOGY, PATHOGENESIS

Hypercalcemia is defined as a **serum $[Ca^{2+}]$ >2.75 mmol/L (>11 mg/dL)**.
Causes:

1) **Hypercalcemia with high parathyroid hormone (PTH) levels** (PTH--dependent hypercalcemia) due to primary hyperparathyroidism (sporadic, induced by lithium salts); multiple endocrine neoplasia syndromes type 1, 2A, and 4; inactivating mutations of the calcium-sensing receptor gene (familial hypocalciuric hypercalcemia); antibodies to the calcium-sensing receptor; or PTH secretion by neoplasms.

2) **Hypercalcemia with low PTH levels** (PTH-independent hypercalcemia) due to cancer (oversecretion of parathyroid hormone–related peptide [PTHrP] and other substances), thyrotoxicosis (increased osteolysis), overdose of vitamin D or its metabolites, production of $1,25(OH)_2D_3$ by granulomas (sarcoidosis) or lymphomas, vitamin A overdose (increased osteolysis), milk-alkali syndrome, long-term immobilization (mobilization of calcium from bone),

thiazide diuretics, theophylline (decreased urinary calcium excretion), or Williams syndrome.

3) **Hypercalcemia with normal PTH levels**: Jansen syndrome (activating mutations of the PTH-PTHrP receptor gene).

The most common causes (90%) of hypercalcemia are hyperparathyroidism and malignancy.

→ CLINICAL FEATURES

Mild hypercalcemia (<3 mmol/L) may be asymptomatic or manifested by signs and symptoms of the underlying condition.

In moderate to severe or rapidly developing hypercalcemia, clinical manifestations of **hypercalcemic syndrome** are present: renal dysfunction (polyuria, hypercalciuria, nephrocalcinosis, and nephrolithiasis), gastrointestinal (GI) tract dysfunction (loss of appetite, nausea, vomiting, constipation, peptic ulcer disease, pancreatitis, cholelithiasis), cardiovascular dysfunction (hypertension, tachycardia, arrhythmia, increased susceptibility to digitalis), neuromuscular manifestations (muscle weakness, hyperreflexia, transient facial muscle paresis), cerebral manifestations (headache, depression, confusion, somnolence, coma), and dehydration. **Hypercalcemic crisis** is caused by severe hypercalcemia (usually >3.75 mmol/L) and manifests as altered mental status, nausea, vomiting, abdominal pain, arrhythmia, polyuria, and dehydration. Features of the underlying condition are often present.

Electrocardiography (ECG) features of hypercalcemia may include a long PR interval and a short QT interval.

→ DIAGNOSIS

The diagnosis of hypercalcemia is based on measurement of serum $[Ca^{2+}]$ (>2.75 mmol/L [>11 mg/dL]).

In patients with hypoalbuminemia or hyperalbuminemia, adjust serum $[Ca^{2+}]$ (→Chapter 4.2.1.2). Ionized calcium levels are a more accurate indicator of the severity of hypercalcemia. In all patients with hypercalcemia, measure serum levels of creatinine, chloride, phosphate, magnesium, potassium, PTH, thyroid-stimulating hormone (TSH), and alkaline phosphatase, and consider performing blood gas analysis. The majority of cases of hypercalcemia with normal or increased PTH levels are caused by hyperparathyroidism.

In patients with low PTH levels perform diagnostic workup for malignancy, unless the available data indicate another cause of PTH-independent hypercalcemia. Malignancies that most frequently cause hypercalcemia include breast cancer, lung cancer, kidney cancer, multiple myeloma, lymphoma, and leukemia.

In patients with suspected excess of exogenous or endogenous vitamin D, measure blood levels of vitamin D metabolites. PTHrP levels can be measured.

→ TREATMENT

1. Treatment of the underlying condition is the mainstay of the management of hypercalcemia.

2. Reduce total body calcium content:

1) Increase renal calcium excretion by intensive administration of fluids (up to ~5 L of 0.9% NaCl on the first day) combined with IV **furosemide** 20 to 40 mg after assessment of renal function. Carefully monitor urine output and electrolyte levels.

2) Decrease calcium mobilization from bone. The available options include IV **calcitonin** 100 IU bid to qid, **pamidronate disodium** (INN pamidronic acid) 60 to 90 mg in 200 mL of 0.9% NaCl as an IV infusion over 2 hours, or

IV **zoledronate disodium** (INN zoledronic acid) 4 mg in 50 mL of 0.9% NaCl over 15 minutes. Zoledronate is preferred over pamidronate in malignancy--related hypercalcemia.🔵⚫ In patients with hypercalcemia associated with malignancy and resistant to bisphosphonates, use subcutaneous denosumab 120 mg every 7 days for 3 weeks and then every 4 weeks. In patients with advanced chronic kidney disease, denosumab should be used with caution and requires close monitoring of calcium levels because of the risk of severe symptomatic hypocalcemia.

3) Inhibit GI absorption of calcium using IV **hydrocortisone** 100 mg every 6 hours.

3. In patients with renal failure and symptomatic or refractory hypercalcemia, elimination of calcium using **hemodialysis** may be necessary.

2.1.2. Hypocalcemia

➡️ DEFINITION, ETIOLOGY, PATHOGENESIS

Hypocalcemia is defined as a **serum [Ca^{2+}] <2.25 mmol/L (<9 mg/dL)**.
Causes:

1) Insufficient dietary calcium intake.
2) Impaired absorption of calcium from the gastrointestinal (GI) tract due to malabsorption syndromes or vitamin D deficiency.
3) Excessive deposition of calcium in soft tissues or bone due to acute pancreatitis, so-called hungry bone syndrome after parathyroidectomy, hyperphosphatemia, bisphosphonates, fluoride poisoning, or foscarnet.
4) Excessive urinary excretion of calcium due to treatment with loop diuretics, deficiency of or resistance to parathyroid hormone (PTH), or tubular acidosis.
5) Absolute or relative vitamin D deficiency due to impaired 25-hydroxylation of vitamin D in patients with liver disease, impaired 1-α-hydroxylation of 25(OH)D$_3$ in patients with acute or chronic renal failure, inadequate absorption of vitamin D from the GI tract (celiac disease, cholestatic jaundice, pancreatic enzyme deficiency), increased vitamin D inactivation in patients treated with certain antiepileptic drugs (hydantoin derivatives and barbiturates), hyperphosphatemia, or tumor lysis syndrome.
6) PTH deficiency: Hypoparathyroidism.
7) Tissue resistance to PTH: Pseudohypoparathyroidism.

Pseudohypocalcemia is falsely low serum calcium levels caused by the presence of a gadolinium-containing contrast agent in blood.

➡️ CLINICAL FEATURES

Clinical manifestations of hypocalcemia result from the deficiency of ionized (biologically active) calcium and are mainly a consequence of nervous system and neuromuscular dysfunctions.

Hypocalcemia is manifested as tetany or its equivalents. An **episode of tetany** is characterized by numbness and symmetric tonic spasms of the muscles of the hand ("obstetrician's hand"), which then extend to the muscles of forearms and arms, face (blepharospasm, "carp mouth"), chest, and lower limbs (equinovarus positioning), with preserved consciousness. Latent tetany may be demonstrated by the **Chvostek sign** (twitching of the facial muscles after tapping the facial nerve ~2 cm anterior to the earlobe, just below the zygomatic process; →Chapter 5.5, Figure 5-3), the **Trousseau sign** (carpal spasm causing the "obstetrician's hand" induced by inflating a blood pressure cuff on the patient's arm to a pressure 20 mm Hg above systolic blood pressure for 3 minutes; →Chapter 5.5, Figure 5-4), or by triggering an episode of tetany through hyperventilation.

Other manifestations of hypocalcemia include seizures, hypotension, and papilledema. Electrocardiography (ECG) may reveal a long QT interval (due to the long ST interval). Chronic hypocalcemia is often asymptomatic, as ionized calcium levels are normal or near-normal.

→ DIAGNOSIS

The diagnosis of hypocalcemia is based on measurement of serum $[Ca^{2+}]$ (<2.25 mmol/L [<9 mg/dL]). In patients with hypoalbuminemia and a normal pH level, add 0.2 mmol/L (0.8 mg/dL) for every 10 g/L of reduction in the plasma albumin level below 40 g/L (the **corrected calcium level**). A low ionized calcium level confirms deficiency of the biologically active form of calcium.

Tests performed to establish the underlying cause of hypocalcemia may include serum levels of creatinine, phosphate, magnesium, potassium, alkaline phosphatase, PTH, and vitamin D; 24-hour urinary calcium excretion; and imaging studies (to detect skeletal abnormalities, abnormal lymph nodes, and cancer).

→ TREATMENT

1. Treatment of the underlying condition is the mainstay of the management of hypocalcemia.

2. In patients with **symptomatic hypocalcemia (tetany)**, administer 20 mL of 10% **calcium gluconate** IV; repeat the injection if symptoms recur. Measure serum $[Ca^{2+}]$ every 4 to 6 hours (in patients with hypoalbuminemia measure ionized calcium levels). At the same time, start oral administration of calcium and vitamin D, usually in the form of active metabolites—alfacalcidol or calcitriol—in a dose of 0.5 to 2 µg/d. Refractory symptomatic hypocalcemia may be due to hypomagnesemia.

3. In patients with **chronic hypocalcemia where the underlying cause cannot be resolved**, administer oral calcium 1000 to 2000 mg/d in the form of **calcium carbonate** (1 g of calcium carbonate contains 400 mg of calcium) or **calcium acetate** (1 g of calcium acetate contains 253 mg of calcium) combined with vitamin D, usually also in the form of active metabolites. Periodically measure serum or urine $[Ca^{2+}]$ (hypercalciuria is the first sign of overtreatment).

4. In patients with hypocalcemia due to excessive urinary calcium loss, administer thiazide diuretics, for example, oral **hydrochlorothiazide** 25 to 50 mg/d as accessory treatment (to reduce urinary calcium excretion).

2.2. Magnesium Disturbances

→ PHYSIOLOGIC BACKGROUND

Total body magnesium content in an adult person weighing 70 kg is 1000 mmol. The daily magnesium requirement is 0.15 to 0.20 mmol/kg, and the average dietary magnesium intake is 20 mmol/d. The normal range of plasma magnesium levels is 0.65 to 1.20 mmol/L, out of which 30% is bound to albumin. Kidneys are the key regulator of magnesium homeostasis.

Mg^{2+} is a catalyst for glycolytic enzymes, respiratory enzymes, and enzymes responsible for nucleic acid synthesis. It is involved in contraction of cardiac myocytes and platelet stabilization (preventing platelet activation).

2.2.1. Hypermagnesemia

→ DEFINITION, ETIOLOGY, PATHOGENESIS

Hypermagnesemia is defined as a **total serum $[Mg^{2+}]$ >1.2 mmol/L**.
Causes:
1) Excessive intake of magnesium due to the use of magnesium oxide preparations (eg, as treatment for peptic ulcer disease or hypomagnesemia).

2) Excessive absorption of magnesium from the gastrointestinal tract due to gastric or intestinal inflammatory conditions.

3) Impaired renal excretion of magnesium due to acute or chronic renal failure, adrenal insufficiency, hypothyroidism (deficiency of cortisol, aldosterone, and thyroid hormones impairs renal excretion of magnesium), or treatment with lithium salts.

→ CLINICAL FEATURES

Hypermagnesemia impairs neuromuscular transmission.

Clinical manifestations of hypermagnesemia include hyporeflexia; facial paresthesia; symptoms of smooth muscle paralysis (constipation, urinary retention); hypotension; and muscle weakness, particularly affecting the respiratory muscles. Electrocardiography (ECG) reveals a long PR interval, and in severe hypermagnesemia also atrioventricular and intraventricular conduction abnormalities (in extreme hypermagnesemia a heart block or even asystole may develop). Signs and symptoms of hypocalcemia may also be present (because of parathyroid hormone suppression).

→ DIAGNOSIS

The diagnosis of hypermagnesemia is based on measurement of serum $[Mg^{2+}]$ (>1.2 mmol/L). In all patients measure serum levels of other ions and creatinine.

→ TREATMENT

1. Try to **control the cause** of hypermagnesemia.

2. In case of emergency (arrhythmia, ventilation abnormalities) administer Ca^{2+} in the form of 10 to 20 mL of 10% **calcium gluconate** IV. You may increase the renal magnesium excretion by IV administration of 1000 to 2000 mL of **0.9% NaCl** and **furosemide** 20 to 40 mg. In patients with life-threatening hypermagnesemia, serum $[Mg^{2+}]$ may be decreased rapidly by hemodialysis using magnesium-free or low-magnesium dialysate.

2.2.2. Hypomagnesemia

→ DEFINITION, ETIOLOGY, PATHOGENESIS

Hypomagnesemia is defined as a **total serum $[Mg^{2+}]$ <0.65 mmol/L**.
Causes:

1) Inadequate intake due to a low-magnesium diet or long-term parenteral nutrition using products with inadequate magnesium content.

2) Impaired magnesium absorption in the gastrointestinal (GI) tract due to chronic malabsorption syndromes (particularly involving the small intestine).

3) Increased magnesium loss:
   a) Through the kidneys due to tubulopathies, which may be congenital (Gitelman syndrome; Bartter syndrome; isolated hypomagnesemia with hypocalciuria or normal urinary calcium excretion; familial hypomagnesemia with hypercalciuria, nephrocalcinosis, or both; hypomagnesemia with secondary hypocalcemia; activating mutation of the gene encoding the calcium receptor) or acquired (primary aldosteronism, chronic alcohol abuse, hypercalcemia, hypokalemia, diuretics, aminoglycosides, cisplatin, amphotericin B, cyclosporine [INN cyclosporin], polyuria in the course of acute tubular necrosis or after relief of urinary tract obstruction).
   b) With body fluids (fistulas).

4) A magnesium shift from the extracellular compartment during intensive treatment of diabetic ketoacidosis, in so-called hungry bone syndrome after surgical treatment of hyperparathyroidism, in refeeding syndrome, during sympathetic stimulation, in chronic alcohol abuse, or in acute pancreatitis (saponification at the sites of fat necrosis).

Although hypomagnesemia is most frequently associated with reduced total body magnesium content, it may occur in patients with normal or even increased magnesium stores. Normal magnesium levels do not exclude magnesium deficiency.

→CLINICAL FEATURES

Clinical features of hypomagnesemia are nonspecific. The most frequent manifestations are metabolic disturbances (hypocalcemia and hypokalemia resistant to supplementation, hypophosphatemia), arrhythmia (premature supraventricular and ventricular beats, tachycardia, atrial fibrillation, ventricular fibrillation), neuromuscular symptoms (hand and tongue tremor; symptomatic or latent tetany; muscle weakness, especially affecting respiratory muscles). Electrocardiography (ECG) may reveal a long QT interval, flat T waves, and the presence of U waves. Chronic mild hypomagnesemia is more frequent in patients with hypertension and ischemic heart disease.

→DIAGNOSIS

The diagnosis of hypomagnesemia is based on measurement of serum $[Mg^{2+}]$ (<0.65 mmol/L). In severe hypoalbuminemia, the value should be corrected by adding 0.05 mmol/L for each 1 g/dL (10 g/L) of reduction in the plasma albumin level below 4 g/dL (40 g/L). In all patients measure serum levels of other ions and creatinine. Blood gas analysis may be of use in more complex situations.

A baseline daily urinary magnesium excretion >1 mmol in a patient with hypomagnesemia is suggestive of renal magnesium loss, while values <1 mmol suggest other causes.

In the case of suspected magnesium deficiency in a patient with normal serum $[Mg^{2+}]$, you may perform a magnesium loading test that involves IV administration of 4 g of $MgSO_4$ dissolved in 500 mL of a 5% glucose (dextrose) solution over 8 hours. A urinary magnesium excretion <15 mmol/d on the day of administration of the loading dose indicates magnesium deficiency.

→TREATMENT

1. Try to **control the cause** of hypomagnesemia.

2. Correct magnesium deficiency (suggested doses):

1) In patients with **symptomatic hypomagnesemia** (arrhythmia, tetany, seizures), administer IV **magnesium sulfate** 1 to 2 g over 10 to 15 minutes (to achieve a serum increase in $[Mg^{2+}]$ by ≥0.4 mmol/L as quickly as possible) followed by 5 g in 500 mL of 5% glucose over 5 hours as a slow IV infusion (≤2 g/h); in patients with torsades de pointes, administer the initial dose over 30 to 60 seconds and repeat if necessary after 5 to 15 minutes. If serum $[Mg^{2+}]$ is <0.25 mmol/L, magnesium deficiency is estimated to be 0.5 to 1.0 mmol/kg. The rate of correction follows local patterns and may include a rapid IV infusion (over a few hours) of $MgSO_4$ 1 to 4 g in 250 to 1000 mL of 5% glucose followed by more doses as needed.

2) In patients with asymptomatic hypomagnesemia, administer oral magnesium such as magnesium oxide (in patients with normal GI magnesium absorption). All oral magnesium formulations cause diarrhea (extended-release formulations least commonly), which may worsen magnesium deficiency.

3. Simultaneously correct coexisting hypokalemia, hypocalcemia, and hypophosphatemia, as these cause treatment-resistant hypomagnesemia.

4. Perform frequent serum magnesium measurements, depending on the severity of deficiency and doses used, and monitor the patient's clinical status to avoid hypermagnesemia caused by magnesium overdose.

2.3. Phosphate Disturbances

→ **PHYSIOLOGIC BACKGROUND**

Total body phosphorus content is 11 to 14 g/kg lean body mass, which accounts for ~1% of total body mass. The normal range of serum phosphate levels is 0.9 to 1.6 mmol/L (2.8-5 mg/dL). The daily dietary phosphate intake is 19.4 to 29.0 mmol (600-900 mg) and depends on the quantity of dietary protein.

Gastrointestinal absorption of phosphate is increased by $1,25(OH)_2D_3$ and parathyroid hormone (PTH)—mediated by $1,25(OH)_2D_3$—and decreased by high quantities of dietary calcium and magnesium and by intake of substances that bind inorganic phosphate. A total of 90% to 95% of phosphate filtrated in the glomeruli undergoes reabsorption in the renal tubules. Urinary excretion of phosphate is increased by PTH, phosphatonins, nonrespiratory acidosis, and glucocorticoids, and decreased by PTH deficiency and physiologic concentrations of $1,25(OH)_2D_3$.

Phosphorus-rich foods include fresh and canned fish, milk, cheese, cold meats, offal (brain, liver, kidney), dry fruit, chicken eggs, porridge, cereal, and bran.

2.3.1. Hyperphosphatemia

→ **DEFINITION, ETIOLOGY, PATHOGENESIS**

Hyperphosphatemia is defined as a **serum inorganic phosphate [Pi] >1.6 mmol/L (>5 mg/dL)**.
Causes:

1) Impaired renal Pi excretion due to acute or chronic renal failure (the most frequent cause), hypoparathyroidism, parathyroid hormone (PTH) resistance, excess growth hormone, severe hypomagnesemia, bisphosphonates, or activating mutations of the gene encoding the sodium/phosphate cotransporter type 2a or 2c.
2) Excessive Pi release from cells due to rhabdomyolysis, tumor lysis syndrome, hemolysis, severe acidosis, malignant hyperthermia, or strenuous exercise.
3) Excessive Pi intake due to milk-alkali syndrome, laxatives containing Pi, or parenteral use of Pi.
4) Excessive absorption of Pi from the gastrointestinal (GI) tract due to vitamin D overdose.

Hyperphosphatemia leads to hypocalcemia (as a result of calcium binding and calcium deposition in the soft tissues, a factor markedly accelerating the development of atherosclerosis) and inhibits the synthesis of $1,25(OH)_2D_3$, which subsequently leads to secondary hyperparathyroidism.

→ **CLINICAL FEATURES**

No signs or symptoms are specific for hyperphosphatemia. Clinical presentation depends on the underlying condition.

→ **DIAGNOSIS**

The diagnosis of hyperphosphatemia is based on measurement of serum [Pi] (>1.6 mmol/L [>5 mg/dL]).

Signs and symptoms may indicate the underlying cause of hyperphosphatemia. Studies useful in establishing the cause of hyperphosphatemia include serum levels of creatinine, calcium, magnesium, PTH, and vitamin D, and urinary Pi excretion.

→TREATMENT

1. Treatment of the underlying condition is the mainstay of the management of hypophosphatemia.

2. Reduce total body phosphate content:

1) Recommend dietary restriction of high-phosphate foods (→Chapter 4.2.3).

2) Use substances that bind Pi in the lumen of the GI tract: **calcium carbonate** or **calcium acetate** 3 to 6 g/d, **sevelamer** 1.5 to 6 g/d, **lanthanum carbonate** 200 to 1200 mg/d. These drugs are to be taken usually in divided doses during or immediately before meals.

3) In patients with normal renal function and acute hyperphosphatemia, induce forced diuresis with a loop diuretic to increase renal Pi excretion.

4) In patients with end-stage kidney disease, use intensive hemodialysis (this is the only way to remove excess Pi).

3. Also →Chapter 9.1.1.

2.3.2. Hypophosphatemia

→DEFINITION, ETIOLOGY, PATHOGENESIS

Hypophosphatemia is defined as a **serum inorganic phosphate [Pi] <0.9 mmol/L (<2.8 mg/dL)**.

Causes:

1) Insufficient dietary Pi intake due to chronic protein malnutrition.

2) Impaired gastrointestinal (GI) absorption of Pi due to ingestion of substances that bind Pi (most frequently antacids), vitamin D deficiency, or malabsorption syndromes.

3) Excessive renal Pi loss due to hyperparathyroidism, excess of phosphatonins (secreted by certain cancers), vitamin D deficiency, glucocorticoids, or congenital or acquired renal tubulopathies.

4) A shift of Pi from the extracellular to the intracellular compartment caused by respiratory alkalosis, refeeding syndrome, the blood glucose normalization phase during treatment of diabetic ketoacidosis, so-called hungry bone syndrome after parathyroidectomy, or the anabolic phase after severe trauma.

The most common clinical situations in which hypophosphatemia should be expected include respiratory alkalosis, intensive treatment of diabetic ketoacidosis, long-term use of antacids, and nutritional treatment of malnourished patients. Phosphate deficiency leads to decreased synthesis of adenosine triphosphate (ATP) and other high-energy phosphate compounds, which considerably impairs functioning of all cells in the body and leads to osteomalacia.

→CLINICAL FEATURES

Clinical manifestations of hypophosphatemia depend on the severity of phosphate depletion and on the rate at which it developed. Chronic mild and moderate hypophosphatemia may be asymptomatic for a long time or manifest as bone pain and muscle weakness. Severe acute hypophosphatemia may manifest as muscle weakness including respiratory compromise paralysis or even rhabdomyolysis, intention tremor, seizures or even coma, hemolysis, bleeding due to platelet disorders, features of liver injury, and severe infections.

→ **DIAGNOSIS**

The diagnosis of hypophosphatemia is based on measurement of serum [Pi] (<0.9 mmol/L [<2.8 mg/dL]).

History may suggest the pathogenesis of hypophosphatemia. Studies useful in establishing the cause of hypophosphatemia include serum levels of calcium, potassium, magnesium, parathyroid hormone (PTH), and vitamin D; blood gas analysis; urinalysis; and measurement of urinary Pi excretion.

→ **TREATMENT**

1. Treatment of the underlying condition is the mainstay of the management of hypophosphatemia.

2. Correct body phosphate deficiency:

1) Recommend a high-phosphate diet (→Chapter 4.2.3).

2) Administer oral repletion: 30 to 80 mmol of phosphate per day in divided doses over a 24-hour period. Commonly used oral supplements include sodium phosphate or potassium phosphate (a 250 mg tablet contains 8 mmol Pi). Serum [Pi] should be rechecked 2 to 6 hours after the last dose to determine if additional doses are required.

3) In patients with hypophosphatemia and serious symptoms and in those unable to take oral medication, administer an IV sodium or potassium phosphate solution at a dose of 15 to 30 mmol over 2 to 6 hours. Remeasure serum [Pi] and calcium levels.

2.4. Potassium Disturbances

→ **PHYSIOLOGIC BACKGROUND**

Total body potassium content in an adult person weighing 70 kg is ~3500 mmol (~50 mmol/kg). A total of 90% of body potassium is intracellular.

The most important factors that determine blood potassium concentration are potassium intake, renal regulation of potassium excretion, and shifts of potassium between the extracellular and the intracellular compartments.

Daily dietary intake of potassium is typically from 20 to 100 mmol. Of the absorbed potassium, 90% is excreted in urine and 10% in stool. The percentage of potassium excreted in stool may increase to 30% to 40% in adults with chronic renal failure. Potassium is excreted into urine mainly by cells of the collecting ducts. Daily renal excretion of potassium in individuals with normal renal function may reach 300 to 400 mmol.

2.4.1. Hyperkalemia

→ **DEFINITION, ETIOLOGY, PATHOGENESIS**

Hyperkalemia is defined as a **serum [K$^+$] >5.5 mmol/L**.

Causes:

1) Excessive potassium intake in patients with impaired renal function or with impaired transport of potassium into cells.

2) Impaired renal excretion of potassium due to acute or chronic renal failure, aldosterone or glucocorticoid deficiency (congenital or acquired), hyporeninemic hypoaldosteronism (in patients with diabetic, lupus, analgesic-induced, or HIV-associated nephropathy), or resistance of renal tubules to aldosterone (pseudohypoaldosteronism type I, II, or III).

3) Drug-induced hyperkalemia due to angiotensin-converting enzyme inhibitors (ACEIs), angiotensin receptor blockers (ARBs), aldosterone receptor antagonists (spironolactone, eplerenone), renin inhibitors, potassium supplements, nonsteroidal anti-inflammatory drugs (NSAIDs), amiloride, triamterene, trimethoprim, cyclosporine (INN ciclosporin), tacrolimus, heparin, or digoxin.

4) Impaired transport of potassium into cells due to nonrespiratory acidosis, β_2-adrenergic receptor blockade, insulin deficiency, aldosterone deficiency, or blockade of the renin-angiotensin-aldosterone (RAA) system.

5) Excessive release of potassium from cells due to rhabdomyolysis, tumor lysis syndrome, nonrespiratory acidosis, sepsis, hyperkalemic periodic paralysis, too rapid correction of hypothermia, or malignant hyperthermia.

Common causes of hyperkalemia include drugs such as ACEIs, ARBs, or aldosterone receptor antagonists and acute or chronic renal failure.

Pseudohyperkalemia is a laboratory artifact caused by the release of potassium from blood cells in a blood sample due to hemolysis, thrombocytosis ($>900 \times 10^9$/L), or leukocytosis ($>70 \times 10^9$/L).

➡ CLINICAL FEATURES

The presence and severity of clinical manifestations are not consistently correlated with the severity of hyperkalemia. Patients with slowly increasing serum $[K^+]$ are usually asymptomatic despite severe hyperkalemia (>7.0 mmol/L).

Hyperkalemia decreases the resting potential of cell membranes and therefore impairs the generation and propagation of stimuli. Dysfunction of myocytes and neurons is manifested by skeletal muscle weakness or paralysis, hyporeflexia, cardiac arrhythmias (bradycardia, asystole, ventricular fibrillation), decreased stroke volume, electrocardiography (ECG) changes, paresthesia, and altered mental status (confusion).

The clinical presentation of hyperkalemia may be dominated by features of the underlying condition.

➡ DIAGNOSIS

The diagnosis of hyperkalemia is based on measurement of serum $[K^+]$ (>5.5 mmol/L; exclude pseudohyperkalemia). History may indicate the underlying condition. Take a thorough history of medications, including over-the-counter drugs and herbal remedies. Assess renal function and acid-base homeostasis. While previously in common use, the transtubular potassium gradient (TTKG) has been demonstrated to be invalid and should not be used for diagnosis of hyperkalemia.❸〇

➡ TREATMENT

1. **Try to control the cause of hyperkalemia.**

2. **Restrict potassium intake** (fruit, fruit juices, plant products).

3. Monitor ECG and vital signs, especially if $[K^+]$ is >6.3 mmol/L.

4. If the patient develops ECG features of hyperkalemia or arrhythmia, immediately administer 10 to 20 mL of 10% **calcium gluconate** IV or calcium chloride (use with particular caution in patients treated with digitalis) and 25 to 50 mL of 50% glucose (dextrose) IV and 5 to 10 units of short-acting insulin. If acidosis is present, add 50 mL of 8.4% $NaHCO_3$. A temporary shift of potassium into cells may be achieved by administering a β_2-agonist, for instance, nebulized salbutamol 2.5 mg every 15 minutes even up to a dose of 10 to 20 mg, or 0.5 mg IV. A smaller dose may be delivered through multiple inhalations of salbutamol using a metered-dose inhaler (MDI). Watch for tachycardia and limit the dose as required.

5. At the same time, start treatment to remove excess potassium from the body:

1) A loop diuretic in patients with normal urine output, for instance, IV **furosemide** 20 to 40 mg, which may be repeated after 6 to 8 hours. Loss of fluids due to increased urine output should be corrected with 0.9% NaCl infusion.

2) Oral or rectal **polystyrene sulfonate** 30 g in 150 mL water or 10% glucose (dextrose). This acts as an ion-exchanger in the gastrointestinal tract and causes a decrease of 0.5 to 1.0 mmol/L in serum potassium levels within 4 to 6 hours.

3) **Hemodialysis** (rarely peritoneal dialysis) in life-threatening hyperkalemia refractory to medical management and in patients with severe renal failure.

6. In patients with diabetes mellitus and hyporeninemic hypoaldosteronism, start by discontinuing drugs known to increase serum potassium levels (β-blockers, ACEIs, ARBs, mineralocorticoid receptor antagonists, NSAIDs). If serum [K$^+$] continues to be >6.5 mmol/L, administer oral **fludrocortisone** 0.5 mg/d. Maintain the target serum [K$^+$] in a range <5.5 mmol/L.

7. In patients with suspected adrenal insufficiency, start IV glucocorticoids (→Chapter 5.1.1.2).

2.4.2. Hypokalemia

→ DEFINITION, ETIOLOGY, PATHOGENESIS

Hypokalemia is usually defined as a **serum [K$^+$] <3.5 mmol/L**.

Causes:

1) Inadequate potassium intake: Anorexia nervosa; protein-energy malnutrition; normal intake of potassium in patients losing potassium through the kidneys, gastrointestinal (GI) tract, or skin.

2) Increased influx of potassium into cells (transmineralization): Alkalosis, β$_2$-adrenergic receptor stimulation (β$_2$-agonists, increased sympathetic activity, thyrotoxicosis), phosphodiesterase inhibitors (theophylline, caffeine), insulin, aldosterone, refeeding syndrome, hypokalemic periodic paralysis.

3) Renal potassium loss (urinary potassium excretion >20 mmol/d in a patient with hypokalemia): Primary aldosteronism, secondary aldosteronism (renovascular hypertension, cancer, reninoma), glucocorticoid-remediable hyperaldosteronism, Bartter syndrome, Gitelman syndrome, apparent mineralocorticoid excess, Liddle syndrome, congenital adrenal hyperplasia (11-β-hydroxylase or 17-α-hydroxylase deficiency), Cushing syndrome, hypokalemia-associated types of proximal or distal tubular acidosis, hypomagnesemia, drugs and toxins (loop and thiazide diuretics, acetazolamide, glucocorticoids, mineralocorticoids, amphotericin B, cisplatin, aminoglycosides, sirolimus, Chinese herbs, toluene).

4) Potassium loss via the GI tract: Vomiting, diarrhea, VIPoma (WDHA syndrome: watery diarrhea, hypokalemia, achlorhydria), fistulas, laxatives.

5) Loss of potassium via the skin: Excessive sweating, burns.

Common causes of hypokalemia include loop/thiazide diuretics, laxatives/diarrhea, and primary aldosteronism.

In some patients **pseudohypokalemia** is found; it is a laboratory artifact caused by storage of uncentrifuged blood samples with white blood cell counts >100 × 10^9/L (young granulocytes consume potassium), obtaining blood samples within 20 to 30 minutes of insulin administration, or prolonged storage of uncentrifuged blood samples at 25°C to 28°C.

→ CLINICAL FEATURES

Clinical manifestations of hypokalemia result from its influence on the resting potential of myocytes and neurons (increased resting potential that may completely block action potentials), renal excretion of water (impaired urinary concentration leading to polyuria), and increased generation of ammonia (resulting in metabolic alkalosis). Manifestations depend on the severity of hypokalemia and rate at which it developed. Rapidly developing hypokalemia, even if moderate, may have a dramatic clinical course and manifest as dangerous arrhythmia (eg, torsades de pointes), muscle weakness, constipation up to adynamic ileus, urinary retention, and neurologic abnormalities (paresthesia, agitation, or apathy). Severe hypokalemia may be fatal due to arrhythmia or serious complications of rhabdomyolysis.

→ **DIAGNOSIS**

The diagnosis of hypokalemia is based on measurement of serum [K^+] (<3.5 mmol/L). History may suggest the underlying condition. Because hypokalemia may be accompanied by other electrolyte or acid-base disturbances (most frequently by metabolic alkalosis), serum magnesium, calcium, and phosphate levels should be measured and blood gas analysis may be considered. Determining the cause of hypokalemia may require measurements of plasma renin activity, serum aldosterone and cortisone levels, and urinary potassium excretion. While previously in common use, the transtubular potassium gradient (TTKG) has been demonstrated to be invalid and should not be used for diagnosis of hypokalemia.🔾○

→ **TREATMENT**

1. Administer potassium (usually as KCl; in exceptional cases, in patients with metabolic acidosis, as potassium carbonate or citrate).

2. The method for potassium supplementation depends on the severity and symptoms of hypokalemia:

1) In **asymptomatic patients with [K^+] ≥2.5 mmol/L**, administer 20 to 30 mmol of K^+ (up to 40 mmol per dose) orally bid to qid.

2) In **patients with [K^+] <2.5 mmol/L or symptomatic hypokalemia**, start from an IV infusion of up to 20 mmol K^+/h (usually solutions containing ≥40 mmol K^+/L should be administered via central venous access).

3. A decrease of 1 mmol/L in serum [K^+] represents a potassium deficit of approximately 100 to 200 mmol. The existing potassium loss should be added to this deficit. Serum [K^+] should be usually remeasured after supplementing 60 to 80 mmol.

4. Correct concomitant water and electrolyte disturbances.

5. In patients who are able to take oral medications, you may use an **aldosterone receptor antagonist** (spironolactone, eplerenone), or possibly an angiotensin-converting enzyme inhibitor or angiotensin receptor blocker if there are other indications for using these drugs as well.

6. Patients with hypokalemia may fail to respond to treatment because of coexisting hypomagnesemia.

2.5. Sodium Disturbances

→ **PHYSIOLOGIC BACKGROUND**

The body of an average adult weighing 70 kg contains ~4200 mmol (~60 mmol/kg) of sodium. A total of 91% of the body sodium is in the extracellular fluid (ECF) and the remainder is the intracellular fluid (ICF).

Dietary sodium intake is 80 to 160 mmol/d. In individuals with a normal sodium balance, 95% of dietary sodium is filtered into the renal tubule, 4.5%

with feces, and 0.5% through the skin. Less than 1% of sodium filtered into the renal tubule is excreted with urine, while the remaining sodium is reabsorbed.

2.5.1. Hypernatremia

→ **DEFINITION, ETIOLOGY, PATHOGENESIS**

Hypernatremia is usually defined as a **serum [Na$^+$] >145 mmol/L**. It is classified as chronic when persisting >48 hours.

Hypernatremia is most frequently caused by loss of water or hypotonic fluids, insufficient water intake (in such cases total body sodium content is unchanged or decreased), or less frequently by excessive sodium intake (in such cases total body sodium content is increased).

Causes:

1) Loss of water: Fever, hypercatabolic conditions (thyrotoxicosis, sepsis).

2) Loss of hypotonic fluids via the skin (excessive sweating), gastrointestinal tract (vomiting, diarrhea), kidneys (central or nephrogenic diabetes insipidus; osmotic diuresis caused by hyperglycemia, mannitol, or urea).

3) Insufficient water intake in patients unable to drink fluids unassisted (unconscious patients, young children, residents of long-term care facilities) or due to impaired thirst.

4) Excessive sodium intake: Administration of excessive doses of NaHCO$_3$ in patients with lactic acidosis or undergoing cardiopulmonary resuscitation, feeding infants high-salt foods (salt poisoning), drinking of seawater by marine accident survivors, use of dialysis solutions containing excessively high sodium levels in patients undergoing hemodialysis or peritoneal dialysis.

Extracellular fluid (ECF) volume may be reduced (hypovolemia), normal (euvolemia), or increased (hypervolemia).

In the early phase of hypernatremia, water is shifted from the intracellular fluid (ICF) to the ECF (cellular dehydration). With time, osmolytes are generated in cells and an influx of Na$^+$, K$^+$, and Cl$^-$ ions into the cells occurs, which causes a decrease in the osmotic gradient between the ICF and the ECF. For this reason, in patients with chronic hypernatremia manifestations of central nervous system (CNS) dehydration may be absent. In physiologic conditions, kidneys respond to hypernatremia by achieving the maximum urine concentration (because of increased effective plasma osmolality).

→ **CLINICAL FEATURES**

Manifestations of hypernatremia depend on the rate of serum [Na$^+$] increase, severity of hypernatremia, and coexisting blood volume changes. Signs and symptoms of the underlying condition causing hypernatremia are frequently seen.

Early manifestations of developing hypernatremia include loss of appetite as well as nausea and vomiting. In later stages patients develop impaired mental status and agitation or somnolence, which may progress to coma. Increased muscle tone and hyperreflexia may be present.

In patients with hypernatremia caused by hypotonic fluid loss or insufficient water intake, manifestations of hypovolemia may be present, urine volume is usually low, and urine is highly concentrated. Urine output is high in patients with diabetes insipidus (with low urine specific gravity) or osmotic diuresis.

Patients with chronic hypernatremia are often asymptomatic. A too rapid correction of chronic hypernatremia may result in cerebral edema, which is manifested by the onset of neurologic signs and symptoms in a previously asymptomatic patient.

→ **DIAGNOSIS**

Hypernatremia is usually defined as a serum $[Na^+]$ >145 mmol/L.

In every patient consider total body water status to establish the cause of hypernatremia. **Hypernatremia with hypovolemia** suggests extrarenal or renal fluid loss or insufficient water intake. **Hypernatremia with hypervolemia** suggests excessive sodium intake (as dietary sodium or as solutions used for treatment of hyponatremia or acidosis). **Hypernatremia with euvolemia** occurs in the case of moderate extrarenal or renal fluid loss. In patients with renal water loss in whom osmotic diuresis has been excluded, establish the type and cause of diabetes insipidus.

→ **TREATMENT**

General Measures

1. Try to control the cause of hypernatremia and correct serum $[Na^+]$ by administering fluids without effective osmolytes.

2. Correction of hypernatremia should correspond to the rate at which hypernatremia developed. The rate of the serum $[Na^+]$ decrease during the first 24 hours should not be >1 mmol/L/h in acute hypernatremia and >0.5 mmol/L/h in chronic hypernatremia.◉○

Pharmacotherapy

1. Select infusion fluid based on volume status:

1) In patients with **hypovolemia**, administer a balanced crystalloid until blood pressure is normalized, then use a 1:1 mixture of 0.45% NaCl and 5% glucose (dextrose) solutions.

2) In patients with **euvolemia or hypervolemia**, administer a 5% glucose solution. In patients with hypervolemia, add oral or IV furosemide; repeat the dose every 6 to 8 hours if necessary.

2. Estimate the serum $[Na^+]$ change after the administration of 1 L of the solution, using the same formula as for hyponatremia. The resulting value will be negative (meaning that serum $[Na^+]$ is decreasing). Using the same method, calculate the volume of the solution to be infused over 1 hour to achieve the target reduction of serum $[Na^+]$. Measure serum $[Na^+]$ frequently (initially every 1-2 hours) and adjust the management accordingly.

3. Another approach involves initial calculation of the water deficit using the following formula:

$$\Delta H_2O = \frac{([Na^+]_{ser} - [Na^+]_{target}) \times BM \times 0.6}{[Na^+]_{target}}$$

Where: $[Na^+]_{ser}$, current serum $[Na^+]$; $[Na^+]_{target}$, target serum $[Na^+]$; BM, body mass expressed in kilograms; BM×0.6, total body water in liters.

Add the volume of the current water loss to the calculated water deficit and administer the resulting volume over 72 hours (half of the volume over the first 24 hours). Frequently measure serum $[Na^+]$.

4. In conscious patients with mild hypernatremia, water deficit may be corrected by the oral route.

5. In patients with extreme hypernatremia, you can consider removing sodium and water excess using dialysis.

→ **PROGNOSIS**

Mortality rates in patients with severe hypernatremia are >50%, but death is most frequently caused by the underlying condition.

2.5.2. Hyponatremia

→ **DEFINITION, ETIOLOGY, PATHOGENESIS**

Hyponatremia is defined as a **serum [Na$^+$] <135 mmol/L**.

In the majority of cases, hyponatremia is a consequence of water disturbances that result in a relative excess of body water compared with the body sodium content. The most frequent cause is impaired renal free water excretion due to inappropriate antidiuretic hormone (ADH) hypersecretion caused by nonosmotic factors. Less frequently, the relative excess of body water may be due to excessive free water intake, which exceeds renal capacity for free water excretion.

Severity of hyponatremia:

1) Mild ([Na$^+$], 130-134 mmol/L).

2) Moderate ([Na$^+$], 125-129 mmol/L).

3) Severe ([Na$^+$] <125 mmol/L).

Classification of hyponatremia based on its duration:

1) **Acute hyponatremia** is that of a documented duration <48 hours.

2) **Chronic hyponatremia** is that of a documented duration ≥48 hours, or any case of hyponatremia of undocumented duration unless clinical features and history indicate acute hyponatremia.

Classification of hyponatremia based on plasma osmolality (measured, not calculated!), and volume status:

1) **Hypotonic hyponatremia**: Sodium ions are the key extracellular osmolyte. Low serum [Na$^+$] is most commonly associated with a hypotonic extracellular fluid (ECF) and a shift of water from the ECF to the intracellular fluid (ICF), which leads to cellular swelling. The most frequent cause of hypotonic hyponatremia is water retention due to syndrome of inappropriate antidiuretic hormone secretion (SIADH).

   a) **Hypotonic hyponatremia with hypovolemia** is caused by sodium and water loss that is partially replaced with fluids containing no electrolytes. Water and sodium may be lost via the skin (excessive sweating), gastrointestinal (GI) tract (vomiting, diarrhea, GI fistulas), kidneys (mainly loss of sodium due to diuretic use; mineralocorticoid deficiency; osmotic diuresis caused by hyperglycemia, urea, or mannitol; salt-losing nephritis; or congenital or acquired tubulopathy), or a shift of fluids into the "third space."

   b) **Hypotonic hyponatremia with euvolemia**, the most frequent type of hyponatremia, is caused by SIADH (→above), glucocorticoid deficiency, use of thiazide diuretics, prolonged strenuous exercise, primary polydipsia, long-term use of a low-sodium diet, hypothyroidism, increased sensitivity to ADH, or mutations of genes encoding V$_2$ or aquaporin 2 receptors.

   c) **Hypotonic hyponatremia with hypervolemia** is caused by increased ADH secretion in patients with a relative decrease in effective intravascular volume (chronic heart failure, cirrhosis with ascites, nephrotic syndrome with edema) or by excessive intake of fluids containing no electrolytes in patients with impaired free water excretion (acute kidney injury, advanced chronic kidney disease).

2) **Nonhypotonic (isotonic or hypertonic) hyponatremia**, also called translocational hyponatremia, is caused by an increase in plasma concentrations of effective osmolytes leading to a shift of water from the ICF to the ECF and subsequent hyponatremia due to dilution. Depending on plasma concentrations of osmolytes, plasma osmolality may be normal or increased. The most frequent cause is severe hyperglycemia (an increase in the blood glucose level by each 5.5 mmol/L causes a decrease in the serum sodium level by ~2.0 mmol/L). Less frequent causes include IV infusions of mannitol; administration of high doses of hyperosmolal contrast media; or leakage of

isotonic mannitol, sorbitol, or glycine to blood during transurethral prostate resection.

Pseudohyponatremia is a falsely low serum [Na⁺] caused by high plasma lipid or paraprotein levels. Plasma osmolality is normal.

→ CLINICAL FEATURES

Clinical manifestations depend on the severity and rate of plasma sodium level decrease, effective plasma osmolality, and direction and magnitude of blood volume changes.

In the majority of patients with slowly developing mild to moderate hyponatremia, no serious central nervous system (CNS) symptoms are seen, but impaired concentration, impaired cognitive functions, and dizziness may occur. Neurologic manifestations of hyponatremia depend on the severity and rate of plasma sodium level decrease and the resulting changes in plasma osmolality. They may be:

1) Moderate, including nausea (without vomiting), confusion, and headache.
2) Severe, including vomiting, somnolence, seizures, and coma (Glasgow coma score ≤8).

Note: These manifestations are nonspecific and may have other causes.

Acute hyponatremia is suspected in the following clinical situations (in patients with undocumented duration of hyponatremia): postoperative period, polydipsia, after or during strenuous exercise, recently started treatment with thiazide diuretics, preparation to colonoscopy, treatment with IV cyclophosphamide, amphetamine use, recently started treatment with ADH analogues.

Clinical features suggestive of dehydration and hypovolemia include dry mucous membranes, reduced skin turgor, orthostatic or constant hypotension, tachycardia, and decreased urine output.

→ DIAGNOSIS

Diagnostic algorithm in hyponatremia: →Figure 2-1.

Hyponatremia is diagnosed in patients with serum [Na⁺] <135 mmol/L after pseudohyponatremia has been excluded (→below).

1. At the beginning of workup, **exclude hyperglycemia and measure plasma osmolality** to establish whether the patient has hypotonic or nonhypotonic (isotonic or hypertonic) hyponatremia. Nonhypotonic hyponatremia may be due to only a few known causes (most frequently severe hyperglycemia) and is not associated with a risk of neurologic complications (cerebral edema, osmotic demyelination syndrome [ODS]).

2. In patients with isotonic hyponatremia, **exclude pseudohyponatremia**. Determination of [Na⁺] in a nondiluted serum sample using ion-selective electrodes provides accurate values. If this technique is not available, measure serum triglyceride, cholesterol, and total protein levels.

3. In patients with hypotonic hyponatremia, **measure urine osmolality (U$_{osm}$) and urine sodium level (U$_{Na}$)** in the same urine sample or in separate urine samples collected at the same time.

In patients with **U$_{osm}$ ≤100 mmol/kg H$_2$O**, hyponatremia is caused by a relative excess of water resulting from polydipsia, long-term use of a low-solute diet (eg, in patients with anorexia or those following a diet based on biscuits and tea or beer), or excessive intake of fluids containing no electrolytes (particularly in patients with impaired kidney function).

In patients with **U$_{osm}$ >100 mmol/kg H$_2$O**, measure U$_{Na}$:

1) In patients with **U$_{Na}$ ≤30 mmol/L**, hyponatremia may be caused by low effective intravascular volume. Estimate water content in the ECF based on clinical data.

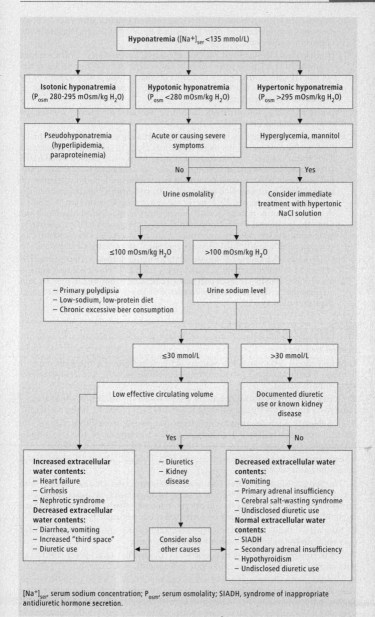

Figure 2-1. Diagnostic algorithm in hyponatremia. *Adapted from Eur J Endocrinol. 2014;170(3):G1-47.*

[Na+]$_{ser}$, serum sodium concentration; P$_{osm}$, serum osmolality; SIADH, syndrome of inappropriate antidiuretic hormone secretion.

a) In patients with increased ECF water content (edema, effusions to body cavities), hyponatremia may be caused by heart failure, cirrhosis, or nephrotic syndrome.

b) In patients with decreased ECF water content (features of dehydration and hypovolemia), hyponatremia may be caused by loss of water and sodium via the GI tract, skin, or due to a shift of water to the "third space"; or by diuretic treatment (with information about treatment either lacking or concealed by the patient).

2) Patients with U_{Na}>30 mmol/L should be assessed for kidney disease or diuretic treatment (or both).

a) In patients who have no kidney disease and do not use diuretics, estimate ECF water content on the basis of clinical data. In patients with normal ECF water content, hyponatremia is most frequently caused by SIADH. Other possible causes include glucocorticoid deficiency (secondary adrenal insufficiency), diuretic treatment (with information about treatment either lacking or concealed by the patient), and severe hypothyroidism. In patients with decreased ECF water content, hyponatremia may be caused by vomiting, mineralocorticoid deficiency (primary adrenal insufficiency), diuretic treatment (with information about treatment either lacking or concealed by the patient), or renal sodium loss (salt-losing nephritis, congenital or acquired tubulopathy, cerebral salt-wasting syndrome).

b) In patients with kidney disease and those using diuretics, determination of the cause of hyponatremia based on U_{Na} and ECF water content may be unreliable. Because in such patients all causes of hypotonic hyponatremia are possible, differential diagnosis should be based on the available clinical data and history.

⇨ TREATMENT

General Measures

1. Management depends on the severity of hyponatremia, its duration, clinical features (cerebral edema, abnormalities of volume status), and risk of neurologic complications.

2. Symptomatic hyponatremia (ie, associated with cerebral edema) always requires immediate treatment, even if serum [Na⁺] is 125 to 129 mmol/L.

3. In **patients with asymptomatic hyponatremia**, start by identifying the cause. Treatment is aimed at achieving a slow increase in serum [Na⁺] up to 130 mmol/L (→below), with a maximum rise of 8 mmol/L per day.◐○

4. Subsequent measurements of serum [Na⁺] should always be performed using the same assay.

5. The longer hyponatremia has been developing, the slower it should be corrected. Chronic hyponatremia that is asymptomatic or associated with minor neurologic symptoms should be corrected very slowly. Documented acute hyponatremia (<48 hours) may be corrected relatively rapidly.

6. Stop all IV fluids unless they are essential and discontinue all drugs that may contribute to the development of hyponatremia.

7. Try to control the cause of hyponatremia (if possible) and correct coexisting potassium disturbances (hypokalemia is frequent).

8. Patients with chronic hyponatremia and serum [Na⁺] ≤120 mmol/L are at risk of ODS if sodium levels are increased too quickly. In such cases, the rate of serum sodium increase should be 4 to 8 mmol/L/d and should not be >10 mmol/L over any 24-hour period. In patients with risk factors for ODS (hyponatremia ≤105 mmol/L, coexisting hypokalemia, alcohol abuse, malnutrition, female sex, advanced liver disease), the rate of serum sodium increase should be 4 to 6 mmol/L/d and should not be >8 mmol/L over 24 hours.

9. Special caution is necessary when correcting hyponatremia ([Na$^+$] <120 mmol/L) caused by a transient impairment of renal free water excretion (SIADH; hyponatremia with hypovolemia, particularly caused by thiazide diuretics; aldosterone or cortisol deficiency). In such patients resolution of the cause of hyponatremia may lead to a rapid increase in free water clearance (with a decrease in urine specific gravity <1.009) and a dangerously rapid increase in serum sodium levels. Monitor urine output; values >100 mL/h indicate an increase in renal free water excretion. If the serum sodium level reaches the recommended safe range (→above), discontinue treatment aimed at increasing sodium concentration and correct water loss or administer IV desmopressin 2 to 4 µg. In the case of a too rapid increase in serum sodium levels (exceeding the recommended safe range), reduce serum [Na$^+$] using a 5% glucose (dextrose) infusion at a rate of, for example, 10 mL/kg over 1 hour or 3 mL/kg/h until a safe serum sodium level is achieved. To prevent further water loss, administer IV desmopressin 2 to 4 µg every 8 hours.⊘◯

Pharmacotherapy

1. The target serum [Na$^+$] during pharmacotherapy is 130 mmol/L. After reaching the target value, try to normalize serum sodium levels using water restriction and a diet with normal sodium and protein contents.

2. NaCl solutions: Usually 0.9% or 3%.

To estimate the change in serum [Na$^+$] after infusion of 1 L of NaCl solution, use the following formula:

$$\Delta[\text{Na}^+] = \frac{[\text{Na}^+]_{\text{inf}} - [\text{Na}^+]_{\text{ser}}}{\text{TBW} + 1}$$

Where: $\Delta[\text{Na}^+]$, change in sodium concentration (mmol/L); $[\text{Na}^+]_{\text{inf}}$, sodium concentration in administered solution (mmol/L) (eg, 513 mmol/L in a 3% NaCl solution); $[\text{Na}^+]_{\text{ser}}$, current serum [Na$^+$] (mmol/L); TBW, estimated total body water volume expressed in liters (in adults assumed to be 0.6 [men] or 0.5 [women] of body weight; in individuals aged ≥65 years, 0.5 and 0.45, respectively).

Note: This is an expected serum [Na$^+$] increase from baseline after the administration of 1 L of NaCl solution. If the calculated increase is 10 mmol/L and the target increase rate is 1 mmol/L/h, administer 100 mL of the (hypertonic) solution over 1 hour. Measure serum [Na$^+$] and calculate the change in serum [Na$^+$] again (using the current serum [Na$^+$]!) to avoid a too rapid correction of hyponatremia. Note that in many cases the actual increase in serum sodium levels is higher than values estimated using the formula.

In the case of simultaneous correction of hyponatremia and hypokalemia, one may use the following modified formula that takes into account the amount of administered potassium, which also contributes to the increase in serum [Na$^+$]:

$$\Delta[\text{Na}^+] = \frac{([\text{Na}^+]_{\text{inf}} + [\text{K}^+]_{\text{inf}}) - [\text{Na}^+]_{\text{ser}}}{\text{TBW} + 1}$$

Where: $\Delta[\text{Na}^+]$, change in sodium concentration (mmol/L); $[\text{Na}^+]_{\text{inf}}$, sodium concentration in the administered solution (mmol/L); $[\text{K}^+]_{\text{inf}}$, potassium concentration in the infused solution (mmol/L); $[\text{Na}^+]_{\text{ser}}$, current serum [Na$^+$] (mmol/L); TBW, estimated total body water volume expressed in liters (→above).

3. Oral solutes: Oral NaCl tablets, in addition to free water restriction, can be administered to promote free water diuresis and increase in serum sodium levels in patients with SIADH. The usual dose is 2 to 6 g (split into bid dosing). Oral urea can also be used in this situation by giving 15 to 60 g/d (0.25-0.5 g/kg/d) in several divided doses. The unpleasant bitter taste of urea can be improved by adding sweeteners.

4. Vasopressin receptor antagonists (vaptans): Blockade of the V_2 receptor will produce a selective free water diuresis and thus correct hyponatremia. This approach can be considered in patients with increased or normal ECF water content but should be avoided in patients with decreased ECF water content because of the risk of further volume depletion. Use should also be avoided in patients with liver disease owing to the risk of liver injury.⊘●

Special Clinical Situations

1. Chronic or acute hyponatremia with severe symptoms of cerebral edema (vomiting, somnolence, seizures, coma): The goal of treatment is a rapid increase in serum [Na^+] by ~5 mmol/L. In the first hour of treatment you may administer, for example, 150 mL of 3% NaCl IV over 20 minutes; the dose may be repeated twice if necessary. After the administration of each dose, measure serum [Na^+]. If symptoms of cerebral edema have resolved following an increase in serum [Na^+] by 5 mmol/L over 1 hour, discontinue 3% NaCl and start treatment of the underlying condition, trying to at least maintain the achieved sodium level and prevent a further serum [Na^+] increase from exceeding safe daily ranges (→above). In case of no improvement of symptoms after an increase in serum [Na^+] by 5 mmol/L over 1 hour, continue the administration of 3% NaCl. The goal of treatment is an increase in serum [Na^+] by 1 mmol/L during every subsequent hour. Calculate the volumes of subsequent doses using the formula above. Discontinue 3% NaCl in case of clinical improvement, an increase in serum [Na^+] by 10 mmol/L compared with baseline, or upon reaching serum [Na^+] of 130 mmol/L.

Neurologic symptoms persisting after an increase in serum [Na^+] by 10 mmol/L compared with baseline or after reaching a serum [Na^+] of 130 mmol/L indicate causes other than cerebral edema due to hyponatremia.

If 3% NaCl is unavailable, a rescue treatment that may be effective in patients with hyponatremia and features of cerebral edema is the administration of 100 to 200 mL of 20% mannitol IV.

2. Chronic or acute hyponatremia with moderate symptoms of cerebral edema (nausea without vomiting, confusion, headache): Immediately administer 150 mL of 3% NaCl IV over 20 minutes followed by NaCl solution to increase serum [Na^+] by 5 to 10 mmol/L over 24 hours. Start treatment of the underlying condition and administer NaCl solution to achieve a serum [Na^+] of 130 mmol/L while maintaining the serum sodium increase in the safe daily range (→above).

3. Acute hyponatremia without symptoms of cerebral edema: If possible, discontinue the administration of fluids and drugs that may contribute to hyponatremia, identify the cause of hyponatremia, and start treatment of the underlying condition. In patients with a serum sodium decrease >10 mmol/L, you may administer a single dose of 150 mL of 3% NaCl IV over 20 minutes to prevent a further decrease in serum [Na^+] and reduce the risk of cerebral edema.

4. Chronic hyponatremia without symptoms of cerebral edema: Treat hyponatremia according to the general rules (→General Measures, above). Before starting treatment, assess volume status.

1) In patients with **hypovolemia**, administer a balanced crystalloid solution (eg, lactate Ringer solution) 0.5 to 1 mL/kg/h as IV infusion until hypovolemia is corrected. If serum [Na^+] remains <130 mmol/L, manage the patient according to the general rules of hyponatremia treatment. Note that there is a risk of a rapid increase in free water clearance and a dangerous rapid increase in serum [Na^+] once hypovolemia has been corrected.

2) In patients with **hypervolemia**, do not start treatment aimed only at correcting hyponatremia if it is mild to moderate. Treatment of the underlying condition (eg, heart failure, cirrhosis, nephrotic syndrome, polydipsia) is of key importance. Fluid restriction may prevent a further increase in ECF volume.

3) In patients with **euvolemia**, treat the underlying condition. Manage patients with moderate to severe hyponatremia according to the general rules. Note that there is a risk of a rapid increase in free water clearance and a dangerous rapid increase in serum $[Na^+]$ after the resolution of the cause of hyponatremia (eg, treatment with glucocorticoids or mineralocorticoids, resolution of the cause of SIADH).

Management of Hyponatremia of Known Etiology

Always follow the general rules of hyponatremia treatment ($\rightarrow$General Measures, above).

1. SIADH: $\rightarrow$Chapter 5.3.3.

2. Heart failure causes chronic hyponatremia. Treatment includes fluid restriction and use of a loop diuretic in case of water overload.

3. Hyponatremia caused by thiazide diuretics is almost always chronic. Discontinuation of the thiazide diuretic and normalization of volume status may lead to a rapid increase in free water clearance and a rapid increase in serum $[Na^+]$. It is important to avoid a too rapid increase in serum $[Na^+]$ ($\rightarrow$General Measures, above).

4. Hyponatremia caused by mineralocorticoid deficiency, glucocorticoid deficiency, or both: These conditions usually cause chronic hyponatremia with hypovolemia (aldosterone deficiency) or with euvolemia (cortisol deficiency). Correction of hypovolemia or starting hormone replacement therapy may lead to rapid increases in free water clearance and in serum $[Na^+]$. It is important to avoid a too rapid increase in serum $[Na^+]$ ($\rightarrow$General Measures, above).

5. Hyponatremia in patients with cirrhosis is usually chronic. Increasing serum $[Na^+]$ requires restriction of water intake to a volume lower than the daily urine output (usually <750 mL/d). Urine output is most effectively increased by using a loop diuretic in combination with spironolactone; watch for the effect on renal function.

6. Hyponatremia caused by prolonged strenuous exercise is acute and associated with neurologic features of cerebral edema that usually develop after ending the exercise. It is a specific type of transient SIADH. Patients with neurologic symptoms should be managed as in the case of cerebral edema (administer 150 mL of 3% NaCl IV over 20 minutes; this may be repeated twice when necessary). Water diuresis that starts after the exercise leads to a rapid normalization of serum $[Na^+]$. Prevention of this type of hyponatremia is based on drinking fluids during exercise only in case of thirst and in volumes ≤400 to 800 mL/h.

7. Cerebral salt-wasting syndrome is a rare condition that develops in patients with intracranial pathology (eg, subarachnoid hemorrhage). Typical features include hypotonic hyponatremia, very high urine sodium levels, low serum uric acid levels, orthostatic hypotension, and low central venous pressure. Urine output is high. Treat hyponatremia according to the general rules and correct sodium and water deficits.

→ COMPLICATIONS

ODS is a potentially life-threatening complication that may occur in the course of treatment of chronic hyponatremia. Clinical manifestations develop over several days and include rapidly developing tetraplegia, pseudobulbar palsy, seizures, and coma. The condition may be fatal.

→ PROGNOSIS

The prognosis in patients with severe hyponatremia causing cerebral edema and with ODS is uncertain; these conditions may cause permanent brain damage. In other patients, the prognosis depends on the underlying condition.

3. Fluid Disturbances

3.1. Dehydration

3.1.1. Isotonic Dehydration

→ **DEFINITION, ETIOLOGY, PATHOGENESIS**

Isotonic dehydration is loss of water with preserved normal effective osmolality of body fluids.

Causes include loss of isotonic fluids via the gastrointestinal tract, kidneys, or skin (burns); loss of blood; or as a result of fluid sequestration in the "third space" (eg, the peritoneum).

→ **CLINICAL FEATURES**

Manifestations include features of hypovolemia (decreased blood pressure and central venous pressure, tachycardia), features of central nervous system ischemia, oliguria (prerenal acute kidney injury), dry mucous membranes, dry skin, and reduced skin turgor. In case of extremely severe dehydration, the patient develops hypovolemic shock.

→ **DIAGNOSIS**

Diagnosis is based on a positive history of current or prior loss of body fluids as well as the presence of clinical features of dehydration and hypovolemia, and in some cases prerenal azotemia (→Chapter 9.1). Differential diagnosis includes all conditions associated with hypotension, such as cardiovascular or central nervous system diseases, poisonings, or other disorders.

→ **TREATMENT**

1. Volume resuscitation using balanced crystalloid fluids, unless there are specific indications for blood or plasma, to compensate for the prior and current volume loss.◐◉

2. Intensive treatment of causes of dehydration.

3.1.2. Hypertonic Dehydration

→ **DEFINITION, ETIOLOGY, PATHOGENESIS**

Hypertonic dehydration is loss of water associated with increased effective osmolality of body fluids.

Causes include inadequate water intake (most frequently in unconscious patients); loss of water via the lungs (hyperventilation); or loss of hypotonic fluids via the skin, gastrointestinal tract, or kidneys (diabetes insipidus, osmotic diuresis caused by glycosuria). An increased osmotic pressure of the extracellular fluid (ECF) results in a shift of water from the intracellular fluid (ICF) to the ECF, which reduces the volume of the intracellular compartment (cellular dehydration).

→ **CLINICAL FEATURES**

Manifestations depend on the severity of dehydration of central nervous system (CNS) cells and the severity of hypovolemia. The key factor is the time over which dehydration developed; CNS manifestations are less severe when hypertonic dehydration develops slowly. The patient has symptoms of dehydration (dry mucous membranes and skin, hypotension, tachycardia, oliguria), features of hypertonicity (extreme thirst), and CNS symptoms (confusion, hallucinations, hyperthermia).

➔ DIAGNOSIS

Diagnosis is based on a positive history of current or prior loss of body fluids as well as the presence of clinical manifestations of dehydration, hypovolemia, hypernatremia, and increased serum osmolality.

➔ TREATMENT

Administer hypotonic fluids:

1) **Oral administration** of glucose-free fluids, such as unsweetened tea or water.
2) Slow **IV administration** of hypotonic fluids (except for patients with hypotension, in whom isotonic fluids should be administered until hypotension is corrected) to achieve a simultaneous decrease in the hyperosmolality of the ECF and the ICF (excessively rapid correction of ECF hyperosmolality is associated with a risk of cerebral edema).

Also →Chapter 4.2.5.1.

3.1.3. Hypotonic Dehydration

➔ DEFINITION, ETIOLOGY, PATHOGENESIS

Hypotonic dehydration is loss of water associated with decreased effective osmolality of body fluids.

Causes include loss of isotonic fluids via the kidneys or gastrointestinal tract that has been partially compensated by drinking hypotonic fluids (eg, unsweetened tea). This results in a shift of water from the extracellular fluid (ECF) to the intracellular fluid (ICF), which leads to cellular edema (particularly affecting the central nervous system) and a further reduction of the extracellular compartment (worsening of hypovolemia).

➔ CLINICAL FEATURES

Manifestations are a consequence of hypovolemia and, if present, of cerebral edema. Thirst is usually absent.

➔ DIAGNOSIS

Diagnosis is based on the presence of symptoms of dehydration, hypovolemia, hyponatremia, and on decreased serum osmolality.

➔ TREATMENT

The management is similar to **hyponatremia with hypovolemia**. The rate of correction of hyponatremia must be carefully controlled.

3.2. Water Overload

3.2.1. Hypertonic Water Overload

➔ DEFINITION, ETIOLOGY, PATHOGENESIS

Hypertonic water overload is an increase in body water content associated with increased effective osmolality of body fluids.

Causes most frequently include excessive intake of hypertonic sodium solutions (drinking of seawater by marine accident survivors, enteral nutrition via a nasogastric tube) or excessive intake of isotonic solutions by patients with impaired renal function. A hypertonic extracellular fluid (ECF) results in cellular dehydration, reduction of the intracellular compartment, and expansion of the extracellular compartment.

→ CLINICAL FEATURES

Manifestations of hypervolemia (peripheral edema, pulmonary edema, hypertension) and central nervous system symptoms (impaired consciousness, hyperthermia).

→ DIAGNOSIS

Diagnosis is based on history, the presence of hypernatremia, and symptoms of hypervolemia.

→ TREATMENT

Treatment may be difficult, as both excess sodium and excess water need to be removed.
1. Use a **sodium-free diet** (the rice diet). Principles of hypernatremia management: →Chapter 4.2.5.1.
2. Use **loop diuretics** to remove excess water.
3. In particularly severe cases that involve impairment in kidney function, hemodialysis may be necessary.

3.2.2. Hypotonic Water Overload (Water Intoxication)

→ DEFINITION, ETIOLOGY, PATHOGENESIS

Hypotonic water overload is an increase in body water content relative to body sodium content, which leads to hyponatremia and reduced effective osmolality of body fluids.

The **most frequent causes** are impaired renal excretion of free water due to renal failure (acute kidney injury or chronic kidney disease) or increased antidiuretic hormone (ADH) secretion caused by nonosmotic factors (this leads to hypotonic hyponatremia with hypervolemia). The most frequent precipitating factor is the administration of electrolyte-free fluids in patients with renal failure. A rare cause of hypotonic water overload is excessive water intake by a person with normal renal function (primary polydipsia).

→ CLINICAL FEATURES

Manifestations are a result of excess body water (peripheral edema, effusions into body cavities) and possibly cerebral edema (as a consequence of the hypotonicity of the extracellular fluid).

→ DIAGNOSIS

Diagnosis is based on the presence of clinical features of water overload accompanied by hyponatremia and serum hypo-osmolality, which are most frequently present in patients with conditions predisposing to this type of water overload.

→**TREATMENT**

The management is similar to **hyponatremia with hypervolemia**. The rate of correction of chronic hyponatremia must be carefully controlled.◑○

3.2.3. Isotonic Water Overload

→**DEFINITION, ETIOLOGY, PATHOGENESIS**

Isotonic water overload is characterized by an increase in the extracellular fluid (ECF), which manifests as edema. It is caused by increased sodium content in the body in the form of an isotonic solution. Sodium and water retention is mediated by hormonal factors (activation of the renin-angiotensin-aldosterone system; relative deficiency of natriuretic hormones, such as atrial natriuretic peptide) and nervous system factors (sympathetic activation).

Causes include heart failure, cirrhosis, nephrotic syndrome, and renal failure.

→**CLINICAL FEATURES AND DIAGNOSIS**

Signs, symptoms, and abnormalities in diagnostic studies depend on the underlying condition. Differential diagnosis of edema: →Chapter 1.9.

→**TREATMENT**

1. Intensive treatment of the underlying condition.
2. Sodium and water restriction, administration of diuretics.◑◔

1. Adrenal Gland Diseases

1.1. Adrenal Insufficiency

1.1.1. Acute Adrenal Insufficiency (Adrenal Crisis)

▶ DEFINITION, ETIOLOGY, PATHOGENESIS

Adrenal crisis is a life-threatening clinical syndrome caused by acute severe cortisol deficiency. It may occur in:

1) Patients with chronic adrenal insufficiency in case of stress without administration of an appropriate additional dose of hydrocortisone (the most frequent cause). Adrenal crisis may be the presenting manifestation of previously undiagnosed adrenal insufficiency.

2) Patients with adrenal injury caused by trauma, hemorrhage in the course of disseminated intravascular coagulation (DIC) (eg, in sepsis), anticoagulant treatment, or eclampsia, as well as in the case of sudden discontinuation of long-term treatment with glucocorticoids (secondary adrenal insufficiency).

3) Critically ill patients with severe diseases due to dysregulation of the hypothalamic-pituitary-adrenal (HPA) axis with concomitant tissue insensitivity to glucocorticoids and a severe inflammatory reaction.

▶ CLINICAL FEATURES AND NATURAL HISTORY

Prodromal symptoms: Loss of appetite, nausea, muscle pain, and malaise.

Symptoms of impending crisis: Increasing weakness, influenza-like muscle pain, abdominal pain, nausea, gradual blood pressure decrease. These may be accompanied by elevated body temperature caused by cytokines released in cortisol deficit.

Symptoms of crisis: Severe weakness, altered mental status, vomiting, diarrhea; blood pressure decrease and tachycardia; shock.

In patients with **adrenal crisis caused by DIC in the course of sepsis**, particularly of meningococcal etiology, the symptoms of acute adrenal insufficiency are accompanied by extensive cutaneous hemorrhages (Waterhouse-Friderichsen syndrome). In critically ill patients with severe diseases, the key symptom is a blood pressure drop not responding to fluid resuscitation and vasopressor drugs. It may be accompanied by symptoms of sepsis or acute respiratory failure.

Diagnostic Tests

1. Laboratory tests:

1) **Biochemical tests** may reveal hyperkalemia, hyponatremia, and hypoglycemia.

2) **Hormone tests** reveal low basal serum cortisol levels (<138 nmol/L [5 µg/dL]). There is no need for stimulation tests as the adrenal crisis is a stimulation per se.

2. Imaging studies depend on the suspected cause of adrenal crisis.

▶ TREATMENT

The goal of treatment is to correct the deficits of cortisol, fluids, and glucose; correct electrolyte disturbances; and control the infection or other underlying condition that may have precipitated the crisis.

1. Treatment of acute adrenal insufficiency after collection of blood samples for key biochemical (glucose, sodium, potassium, creatinine) and hormonal (cortisol, adrenocorticotropic hormone [ACTH]) tests, as well as for microbiological studies where appropriate:

1) **Hydrocortisone**: Immediately administer 100 mg IV followed by 200 mg over 24 hours as an IV infusion or 50 mg IV every 4 to 6 hours. When blood pressure and heart rate return to normal, administer 50 mg IV or IM every 6 hours. Treatment of patients with septic shock: →**Chapter 8.14**.

2) **Volume expansion** with crystalloids or colloids to treat hypovolemia (including glucose solutions in case of low serum glucose levels). A reasonable starting point is a 1-L bolus with further doses according to the precipitating condition and individual patient requirements.

3) **Treatment of hyponatremia**: Monitor the patient closely. The type and volume of administered fluids depend on the fluid balance, severity of electrolyte disturbances, cardiovascular and renal status, and body weight. Also →Chapter 4.2.5.2.

2. Treatment of impending adrenal crisis: Early administration of IV hydrocortisone 100 mg can halt the development of adrenal crisis. Ensure appropriate hydrocortisone replacement, correct for possible electrolyte disturbances, and treat the underlying condition.

→ PROGNOSIS

Appropriate treatment of adrenal crisis is life-saving but the prognosis may be affected by underlying conditions that precipitated the crisis.

1.1.2. Primary Adrenal Insufficiency (Addison Disease)

→ DEFINITION, ETIOLOGY, PATHOGENESIS

Primary adrenal insufficiency (Addison disease) is a clinical syndrome caused by a long-term deficit of hormones of the adrenal cortex, primarily cortisol, due to a direct injury to the adrenal gland. Symptoms of adrenal insufficiency develop only in the case of major bilateral involvement of the adrenal glands. **Causes**:

1) Autoimmune disorders (most common).◕ The autoantigens are enzymes of the steroid pathway—most frequently 21-hydroxylase, 17-hydroxylase, and 20-22-lyase. Other autoimmune diseases may coexist, most often thyroid disease (autoimmune polyglandular syndromes). In the early stages adrenal glands may be enlarged (due to lymphocytic infiltrates), while in later stages they become small (due to atrophy).

2) Tuberculosis and other infectious diseases (histoplasmosis, cryptococcosis, blastomycosis, coccidioidomycosis; AIDS-related infections, most commonly cytomegalovirus). Symptoms of Addison disease develop when ~90% of the adrenal cortex is destroyed (this is preceded by subclinical Addison disease). Tuberculous and fungal granulomas may calcify (lesions are visible on chest radiographs and computed tomography [CT]).

3) Malignancy (lymphoma; metastatic lesions, eg, renal or lung carcinoma, and rarely bilateral adrenocortical carcinoma).

4) Metabolic disorders, including amyloidosis, adrenoleukodystrophy, and hemochromatosis.

5) Hereditary disorders, including hereditary adrenal hypertrophy or adrenocorticotropic hormone (ACTH) insensitivity.

6) A drug-induced reduction in the secretion of adrenal hormones. The reduction is usually transient and resolves after discontinuation of the offending drug (eg, mitotane, aminoglutethimide, ketoconazole, metyrapone, etomidate). Adrenal insufficiency may persist longer after discontinuation of mitotane.

7) An increase in cortisol metabolism by enzyme inducers such as rifampin (INN rifampicin).

8) Bilateral adrenal gland hemorrhage (Waterhouse-Friderichsen syndrome [*Neisseria meningitidis*] or anticoagulant agents).

→ CLINICAL FEATURES AND NATURAL HISTORY

1. Symptoms: Weakness, syncope (due to orthostatic hypotension or hypoglycemia), poor exercise tolerance, weight loss, appetite loss, sometimes nausea (less frequently vomiting), craving for salty foods, oligomenorrhea, loose stools, muscle and joint pain, abdominal pain. Symptoms are often associated with stress, such as infection or major trauma. In subclinical Addison disease episodes of weakness, loss of appetite, and muscle pain are only transient and caused by stress, particularly related to strenuous exercise.

2. Signs: Skin hyperpigmentation, which is particularly evident in areas exposed to sunlight or pressure, with brown discoloration of elbows, palmar and dorsal hand creases, nipple areolae, and scars; some patients also have brown spots on the oral mucosa that are caused by excess ACTH and melanotropin (melanocyte-stimulating hormone [MSH]), whose secretion is inadequately inhibited by cortisol feedback. Low blood pressure and orthostatic hypotension may also be present.

3. Coexisting autoimmune disorders affecting organs other than adrenal glands may change the clinical features and course of Addison disease. Concomitant secondary adrenal deficiency leads to resolution of skin hyperpigmentation. Cutaneous depigmentation may also occur in patients with diffuse vitiligo.

→ DIAGNOSIS

Diagnostic Tests

1. Basic blood tests:

1) **Complete blood count (CBC)** may reveal neutropenia, lymphocytosis, monocytosis, and eosinophilia.

2) **Serum biochemical tests** may reveal hyperkalemia, hyponatremia, sometimes hypoglycemia (especially during longer periods between meals and after strenuous exercise), rarely hypercalcemia, sometimes elevated serum urea and creatinine levels (due to decreased glomerular filtration rate).

2. Hormone tests: If these are performed to confirm diagnosis, discontinue hydrocortisone 24 hours before a test.

1) Low levels of **serum cortisol** (<138 nmol/L [5 µg/dL]) and high levels of **serum ACTH** (2×upper limit of normal) in morning blood samples collected at the same time are the key feature of Addison disease. Serum ACTH levels become elevated first (if serum cortisol is normal, subclinical Addison disease is diagnosed).

2) The **short stimulation test with 250 µg synthetic ACTH** can be performed in an outpatient setting to exclude primary adrenal insufficiency. The test involves the administration of synthetic human ACTH (cosyntropin [INN tetracosactide] 0.25 mg IV or IM) with measurements of serum cortisol levels at baseline, 30 minutes, and 60 minutes. An increase in the cortisol level >497 nmol/L (18 µg/dL) in any of the measurements excludes primary adrenal insufficiency; results close to this value may suggest a reduced adrenal reserve. A trend to use lower-dose ACTH stimuli in the recent years may suggest that 1 µg could also be used as a provocative dose with reported higher sensitivity in detecting secondary adrenal dysfunction.

3) The **insulin-induced hypoglycemia test** (performed rarely, only in specialized centers): Rapid IV insulin (0.05-0.15 IU/kg) is given to achieve adequate hypoglycemia (<40 mg/dL [2.2 mmol/L)]; measurements of glucose and cortisol are obtained at −30, 0, 30, 60, and 120 minutes. Cortisol levels <500 to 550 nmol/L (18-20 µg/dL) are considered diagnostic for adrenal

insufficiency. The test is contraindicated in patients with seizures or cardiac disease. It is rarely performed, with the exception of recent suspected ACTH deficiency or concomitant growth hormone deficiency (eg, suspected secondary adrenal insufficiency).

4) The **adrenal reserve test** (performed rarely, only in specialized centers): Performed to differentiate between primary and secondary adrenal insufficiency. The test involves the administration of long-acting IM cosyntropin (synthetic ACTH) 0.5 mg every 12 hours for 2 days and daily measurements of urinary excretion of free cortisol or 17-hydroxycorticosteroids (17-OHCS) on both test days.

Interpretation of the test is made by comparing the increase in excretion of free cortisol or 17-OHCS with baseline values: A ≥4-fold increase is consistent with normal adrenal response; in the case of a 2- to 4-fold increase and ACTH in the normal range, the diagnosis of secondary adrenal insufficiency is made; a <2-fold increase is consistent with primary adrenal insufficiency (Addison disease). Currently, the adrenal reserve test has become less important, as the results of ACTH and cortisol level measurements and the short ACTH stimulation test are considered sufficient for diagnosis.

5) Other results include low dehydroepiandrosterone sulfate (DHEAS), androstenedione, and aldosterone levels and a high plasma renin activity (PRA) or renin level (an early manifestation).

3. Immunologic studies: Most frequently specific adrenal antibodies are measured (antibodies to 21-hydroxylase, less often to desmolase or to 17-hydroxylase). Antibody levels decrease over time with the disappearance of autoantigens. In autoimmune polyglandular syndromes antibodies to the thyroid gland or other organs are present.

4. Electrocardiography (ECG) may reveal features of hyperkalemia or rarely hypercalcemia.

5. Imaging studies: Abdominal radiography, CT, and ultrasonography may reveal adrenal calcifications caused by prior adrenal tuberculosis or fungal infection. In the late stages of autoimmune Addison disease, abdominal CT or magnetic resonance imaging (MRI) reveals adrenal atrophy. Bilateral adrenal tumors most frequently indicate metastatic lesions or lymphoma.

Diagnostic Criteria

Criteria of overt adrenal insufficiency: A high serum ACTH level and low serum cortisol level at baseline. Clinical manifestations: →Clinical Features and Natural History, above.

→ TREATMENT

Hormone Replacement Therapy

Ongoing replacement therapy should be augmented in periods of increased hormone requirements. Advise the patient how to modify hydrocortisone dosage to adjust to stress (eg, infection, trauma, minor procedures such as tooth extraction; →below). The patient should receive and always carry a drug dosage handout. Schedule follow-up studies. In patients with adrenocortical insufficiency, replacement of glucocorticoids, mineralocorticoids, and androgens may be necessary.

1. Glucocorticoid replacement aims to reproduce the diurnal rhythm of cortisol secretion, which equals 8 to 12 mg/m^2 (with the highest dose administered in the morning). Assess the effects of hormone replacement doses on the basis of symptoms, physical performance, and serum sodium and potassium levels. Consider the duration of action of each dose (4-8 hours), body weight, height, and increased requirement in case of stress. In patients with diabetes mellitus, an additional dose of 5 mg administered in the evening may prevent nocturnal hypoglycemia. Use **hydrocortisone** 15 to 30 mg/d in 2 divided doses, for instance, in the morning and at approximately 15:00 (15 mg + 5 mg or 20 mg + 10 mg); alternatively, you may use a 3-dose regimen: in the morning, at approximately 13:00, and at approximately 18:00 (15 mg + 10 mg + 5 mg).⊘⊖ Sustained-release hydrocortisone in the forms of 5-mg and 20-mg tablets provides more stable blood levels of hydrocortisone and may be administered once daily. The patient should receive a dosage handout and should be advised to carry it at all times. Although prednisone, dexamethasone, and other long--acting synthetic analogues of cortisol are usually not recommended as the first option (they do not mimic the normal diurnal rhythm), they represent a valid alternative and may be unavoidable when hydrocortisone is not available.

Guidance on hydrocortisone dosage:

1) In case of moderate stress, the patient should increase the dose by 10 to 30 mg/d.

2) Before major physical exercise, the patient should take an additional dose of 5 to 10 mg.

3) In case of infection with fever (>39°C), for instance, of the upper respiratory tract, the dose should be increased 2- to 3-fold. If after 3 days symptoms of infection worsen or the patient is unable to return to the previous doses, medical attention should be sought.

4) In case of vomiting or diarrhea, the patient should seek medical attention. In such situations, administer IM or IV hydrocortisone 50 mg every 8 to 12 hours. In special cases (eg, in patients with hypertension or edema), hydrocortisone may be replaced with prednisolone at equivalent doses (20 mg hydrocortisone equals 5 mg prednisolone).

2. Mineralocorticoid replacement: Fludrocortisone 0.025 to 0.2 mg/d in the morning (starting dose, 0.025-0.1 mg/d; in hot weather use the upper range of the dose). Individual dose adjustment is necessary. Reduce the dose or consider discontinuation in case of hypertension or edema, especially in the elderly. Note that hydrocortisone has a weak mineralocorticoid effect. When using a well-adjusted mineralocorticoid dose, orthostatic hypotension should not occur. In patients with essential hypertension, add an appropriately selected antihypertensive agent without changing the replacement treatment; however, do not use diuretics, as these may cause a sudden blood pressure decrease associated with hypovolemia.

3. Adrenal androgen replacement: Dehydroepiandrosterone (DHEA): In women, use 5 to 50 mg after breakfast, most frequently 10 mg/d; consider using 25 mg/d, particularly in women with depressive symptoms, low libido, or low energy levels. In men, use 10 to 25 mg/d. Using higher doses in women may cause symptoms of androgen excess; determining serum DHEAS levels is useful if such excess is suspected. In patients after surgery with impaired wound healing, DHEA 50 mg/d may be beneficial.

→ FOLLOW-UP

The key goals of treatment are reduction of symptoms, normalization of blood pressure and electrolyte levels, and general improvement of the patient's condition. Use the lowest effective doses of hydrocortisone and fludrocortisone. Serum ACTH measurements are of little use as they can be above the upper limit of normal; morning values within or below the lower limit of normal indicate excess hydrocortisone, in which case the dose should be reduced.

→ SPECIAL CONSIDERATIONS

Pregnancy

A common approach is to increase hydrocortisone dose by 20% to 40% during the third trimester, especially in case of worsening of symptoms (particularly weakness). In patients with hypertension reduce the dose of fludrocortisone.

Administration of hydrocortisone during and after delivery in women with adrenal insufficiency: **At the beginning of delivery**, our approach is to administer hydrocortisone 100 mg IV followed by 50 mg IV or IM every 6 to 8 hours or by a continuous infusion of 200 mg over 24 hours; in case of a blood pressure decrease, add 100 mg as an IV infusion in 500 mL of 0.9% saline. **On days 1 and 2 after delivery**, administer 50 mg IM or IV every 6 to 8 hours. **On days 3 and 4 after delivery**, administer 60 mg/d orally in 3 divided doses (eg, in the morning, at approximately 13:00, and at approximately 18:00; 30 mg + 20 mg + 10 mg). **On days 5 and 6 after delivery**, administer 40 mg/d orally in 2 to 3 divided doses (eg, in the morning, at approximately 13:00, and at approximately 18:00; 25 mg + 10 mg + 5 mg). **On day 7 after delivery**, administer 30 mg/d orally (eg, in the morning and approximately at 15:00; 20 mg + 10 mg).

Surgery

Administration of hydrocortisone during major surgery in patients with adrenal insufficiency◯: **On the day before surgery**, our approach is to administer 40 mg/d orally. **On the day of surgery**, administer 100 mg as an IV infusion during surgery followed by 100 mg IV every 8 hours or by an IV infusion of 200 mg over 24 hours. **On day 1 after surgery**, administer 100 mg IV every 8 hours. **On day 2 after surgery**, administer 50 mg IM or IV every 6 hours, and in case of a blood pressure decrease, add 100 mg as an IV infusion. This management should be continued until the patient is able to tolerate food and drink, and then it should be followed by oral hydrocortisone. Administer oral hydrocortisone for 2 days at a dose twice as high as before surgery and taper it down, so that at the end of the first week the dose is the same as the baseline dose administered before surgery. This dosage is based on our pattern of practice; slightly lower or slightly higher doses may be equally reasonable.

Administration of hydrocortisone during minor surgery in patients with adrenal insufficiency: Our approach is to administer 100 mg as an IV infusion before anesthesia, followed by oral hydrocortisone over the next 24 hours at a dose twice as high as the previous oral dose. Before **tooth extraction**, use additional 20 mg of oral hydrocortisone 1 hour prior to surgery. The subsequent dose administered on that day should be doubled.

Administration of hydrocortisone during colonoscopy in patients with adrenal insufficiency: The patient may need to be hospitalized. In the evening, administer IM or IV hydrocortisone 100 mg and IV fluids to ensure adequate volume status. Immediately before colonoscopy, administer another dose of IM hydrocortisone 100 mg.

→ PROGNOSIS

In patients who receive appropriate hormone replacement treatment, Addison disease does not affect life expectancy; however, untreated disease is always fatal. In patients with adrenal insufficiency caused by tuberculosis, the prognosis depends on the extent of infection. In patients with bilateral adrenal metastases or lymphoma, the prognosis is poor.

1.1.3. Secondary Adrenal Insufficiency

→ DEFINITION, ETIOLOGY, PATHOGENESIS

Secondary adrenal insufficiency is a clinical syndrome caused by a long-term deficit of adrenal cortex hormones due to adrenocorticotropic hormone (ACTH) deficiency.

Most frequent causes: Inhibition of ACTH secretion by long-term glucocorticoid therapy, large tumors of the pituitary and craniopharyngiomas, neurosurgical treatment of pituitary and parasellar tumors, autoimmunization.

Less frequent causes: Pituitary infarction, postpartum pituitary necrosis (Sheehan syndrome: →Chapter 5.3.2), infiltrative and posttraumatic lesions.

▶ CLINICAL FEATURES

Symptoms are as in Addison disease but usually develop much more slowly and are less severe. The key difference is reduced skin pigmentation, especially of the nipple areolae, due to ACTH and melanocyte-stimulating hormone (MSH) deficits. Electrolyte disturbances (particularly hyperkalemia) are not frequent (secretion of mineralocorticoids is usually not impaired, as it depends to a greater degree on the renin-angiotensin system than on ACTH). Hypoglycemia is more common and hyponatremia may develop due to cortisol deficiency. Symptoms of an underlying condition are present.

▶ DIAGNOSIS

Diagnostic Tests

1. Hormone tests:

1) Low **cortisol levels** (<138 nmol/L [5 µg/dL]) and low **ACTH levels** (<2.2 pmol/L [10 pg/mL]) in blood samples collected simultaneously in the morning (the key feature); low cortisol levels in the evening (an early manifestation). The tests listed below are usually performed in specialized settings:

2) **24-hour urinary excretion of free cortisol or 17-hydroxycorticosteroids (17-OHCS)** is usually decreased.

3) Low serum dehydroepiandrosterone sulfate (DHEAS) levels.

4) Serum gonadotropin and prolactin levels are normal in isolated secondary adrenal insufficiency and decreased in hypopituitarism.

5) The **short stimulation test with 250 µg of synthetic ACTH** involves the administration of synthetic human ACTH (cosyntropin [INN tetracosactide] 0.25 mg IV or IM) and measurements of serum cortisol levels at baseline, 30 minutes, and 60 minutes to reveal a delayed increase in cortisol levels in secondary adrenal insufficiency. Adrenal reserve test, if done (stimulation with long-acting synthetic ACTH; →Chapter 5.1.1.2), reveals a gradual 2- to 4-fold increase in free cortisol or 17-OHCS levels in 24-hour urine and confirms secondary adrenal insufficiency.

6) The **corticotropin-releasing hormone (CRH) stimulation test** (stimulation of ACTH and cortisol secretion using CRH): Administer 100 µg (or 1 µg/kg) of synthetic CRH IV. Measure serum ACTH levels before CRH administration and at 15, 30, 60, and 90 minutes after the administration; measure serum cortisol levels at baseline and at 30, 60, 90, and 120 minutes after the administration. Under normal conditions, serum ACTH levels increase 2 to 4 times and serum cortisol levels increase by >552 nmol/L (20 µg/dL) (or >276 nmol/L [10 µg/dL] above the baseline value). Absence of response confirms secondary (pituitary) adrenal insufficiency.

2. Imaging studies: Magnetic resonance imaging (MRI) or **computed tomography (CT)** may reveal an empty or partially empty sella resulting from prior lymphocytic pituitary hypophysitis or a tumor of the hypothalamus--pituitary region.

▶ TREATMENT

1. High-sodium diet.

2. Glucocorticoid replacement: Hydrocortisone, usually at doses lower than in Addison disease (5-20 mg/d orally), most frequently in 2 or 3 divided doses (aim at reproducing the circadian cortisol secretion rhythm).☺☻

3. Mineralocorticoid replacement: In many cases this is not necessary, because aldosterone secretion is regulated by the renin-angiotensin-aldosterone system. In patients with long-standing disease lasting many years, the mineralocorticoid requirement may be similar as in primary adrenal insufficiency due to degenerative changes in the adrenal glands.

4. Adrenal androgen replacement: Consider oral dehydroepiandrosterone (DHEA) at a dose of 5 to 10 mg/d in the morning in women and 25 to 50 mg/d in men (evaluate the prostate before treatment).

→ SPECIAL CONSIDERATIONS

Surgery

Indications for hydrocortisone during surgery○: Prior glucocorticoid therapy (in our practice we use an approximate threshold for oral glucocorticoids of prednisone or equivalent ≥7.5 mg for >2-3 weeks in the past year); prior surgical resection of a hormonally functioning adrenal tumor (secondary adrenal insufficiency develops in the contralateral adrenal gland due to chronic inhibition of ACTH secretion); secondary adrenal insufficiency of another origin.

On the day of surgery, our approach is to administer hydrocortisone 100 mg as an IV infusion during surgery followed by 50 mg IM or IV every 8 hours or a continuous infusion of 200 mg over 24 hours. **On day 1 after surgery**, administer 50 mg IM or IV every 8 to 12 hours, and in case of a blood pressure decrease add 100 mg as an IV infusion. **On day 2 after surgery**, administer 50 mg IM or IV in the morning, and in case of a blood pressure decrease add 100 mg as an IV infusion. **Starting from day 3 after surgery** (or earlier if the patient tolerates fluids well), switch to oral hydrocortisone. In case of surgical complications, such as infection, maintain a higher hydrocortisone dose (eg, 50 mg IV tid to qid) and delay switching to oral treatment.

→ PROGNOSIS

Adrenal insufficiency caused by glucocorticoid treatment may be reversible. Appropriately treated isolated secondary adrenal insufficiency is not life--threatening and does not affect life expectancy. In patients with overt hypopituitarism, the prognosis depends on disturbances caused by deficiencies of other pituitary hormones (→Chapter 5.3.2).

1.2. Cushing Syndrome

→ DEFINITION, ETIOLOGY, PATHOGENESIS

Cushing syndrome is a clinical syndrome composed of signs and symptoms resulting from longstanding exposure of tissues to excess glucocorticoids.

Subclinical Cushing syndrome refers to a minor excess of glucocorticoids due to increased cortisol secretion by an adrenal tumor that results in inhibition of glucocorticoid secretion by the contralateral adrenal gland, milder clinical presentation, and absence of signs common to overt Cushing syndrome (eg, supraclavicular fullness caused by fat pads).

Cushing syndrome is classified based on etiology.

1. Exogenous Cushing syndrome is caused by administration of glucocorticoids at doses exceeding their physiologic levels. This is the most common cause of excess glucocorticoids.

2. Endogenous Cushing syndrome results from adrenal overproduction of glucocorticoids.

1) **Adrenocorticotropic hormone (ACTH)-independent Cushing syndrome** (primary adrenal overproduction of glucocorticoids):

a) **Autonomous adrenal tumors**: Usually a solitary tumor, less frequently multiple adenomas; adrenal carcinoma. Tumors originating from the zona fasciculata cause selective cortisol overproduction, whereas other tumors (arising from the zona reticularis or mixed tumors) additionally secrete androgens. Excess cortisol inhibits corticotropin-releasing hormone (CRH) and ACTH secretion, causing atrophy of the adrenal cortex located outside the tumor capsule and atrophy of the contralateral adrenal gland.

b) **Macronodular adrenal hyperplasia** is caused by ectopic receptors in the adrenal cortex, which are activated by atypical stimuli; most commonly, they are activated by the gastric inhibitory peptide (GIP)—currently called the glucose-dependent insulinotropic peptide—which is secreted postprandially in the gastrointestinal tract. Other stimulating factors include catecholamines, antidiuretic hormone, thyroid-stimulating hormone, luteinizing hormone, human chorionic gonadotropin, follicle-stimulating hormone, high levels of estrogens, prolactin, and interleukin 1.

c) **Micronodular adrenal hyperplasia (primary pigmented nodular adrenal disease [PPNAD])** is a familial genetic disease. It may either be part of Carney complex, which includes various other abnormalities (cutaneous, cardiac, or breast myxoma; light-brown cutaneous nevi; testicular tumors; less commonly other endocrine abnormalities, such as acromegaly), or it may be the sporadic type, where immunoglobulins stimulating hyperplasia of the adrenal cortex may play a role. Like in other ACTH-independent types of Cushing syndrome, the adrenal tissue between the nodules may be atrophic.

2) **ACTH-dependent Cushing syndrome** (secondary adrenal overproduction of glucocorticoids) may be caused by ACTH overproduction in the pituitary (Cushing disease, the most common cause of endogenous Cushing syndrome), ectopic ACTH secretion by an extrapituitary tumor (much less frequent), or ectopic CRH secretion (least frequent).

→ CLINICAL FEATURES AND NATURAL HISTORY

Signs and symptoms are unspecific but some are more distinctive than others.

1. Symptoms: Muscle weakness and poor exercise tolerance, skin prone to injury with poorly healing ulcers and easy bruising; excessive thirst and polyuria (measure blood glucose levels); excessive appetite; headache and dizziness (measure blood pressure); emotional instability, depressive tendencies, memory impairment, rarely psychotic conditions; bone pain (in the case of osteoporosis look for pathologic fractures of vertebral bodies, ribs, pubic rami, and the ischium); frequent infections, especially opportunistic (eg, fungal), often with a severe clinical course; symptoms of coronary artery disease or peptic ulcer disease (particularly in patients treated with nonsteroidal anti-inflammatory drug [NSAIDs]); erectile dysfunction in men, oligomenorrhea or secondary amenorrhea in women; acne and hirsutism in patients with androgen-secreting tumors.

2. Signs: Presence of purple striae, facial plethora (due to polycythemia and thinned skin) and dilated vessels, facial fullness ("moon face"), dorsocervical fat pad ("buffalo hump"), supraclavicular fullness caused by fat pads, thin extremities, thin skin, easy bruising, sometimes spontaneous cutaneous hemorrhages or purpura. Other consequences of cortisol excess can be present, but these are also common in the general population (eg, obesity, depression, diabetes mellitus, hypertension, hyperandrogenism). The presence of thin skin (<2 mm) markedly increases the probability of Cushing syndrome; similarly, patients who have ≥3 nontraumatic ecchymoses that are >1 cm in diameter are a few times more likely to have Cushing syndrome than patients without such findings.

3. Natural history: Overt Cushing syndrome is diagnosed only in the advanced stage of a chronic disease. Significantly more often, just some of the

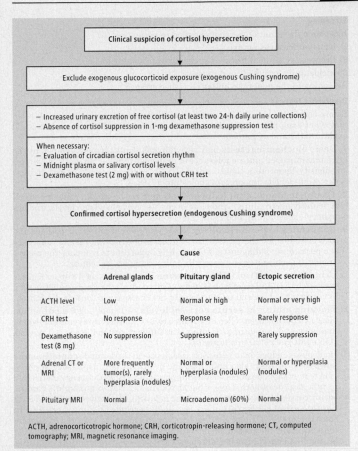

Figure 1-1. Diagnostic algorithm in Cushing syndrome.

manifestations are present, such as impaired glucose tolerance or diabetes, dyslipidemia, hypertension, and rapid body weight gain (obesity), which constitute metabolic syndrome. The risk of osteoporosis is also increased. For these reasons, screening hormone tests for Cushing syndrome should be considered in patients, especially young, who have been unsuccessfully treated for metabolic syndrome or its components (eg, hypertension).

In **subclinical Cushing syndrome**, even if it is long-standing, the typical clinical manifestations may be absent. Because the risk of progression to overt Cushing syndrome is low, subclinical Cushing syndrome should not be regarded as an early stage of Cushing syndrome.

→ DIAGNOSIS

Diagnostic algorithm: →**Figure 1-1**. Always exclude prior use of glucocorticoids (exogenous Cushing syndrome).

Screening

Biochemical evaluation is recommended in patients with:

1) Unusual features for age.

2) Progressive clinical features suggestive of Cushing disease.

3) Incidentally found adrenal masses.

Screening in the general population is discouraged.

Diagnostic Tests

Before beginning biochemical evaluation for hypercortisolism, take a detailed history of drug use to exclude exogenous glucocorticoid exposure that could explain signs and symptoms.

1. Basic biochemical tests may reveal hypokalemia; hypercalciuria; hyperglycemia (impaired glucose tolerance or diabetes); high serum total cholesterol, low-density lipoprotein cholesterol (LDL-C), and triglyceride levels; and low serum high-density lipoprotein cholesterol (HDL-C) levels.

2. Complete blood count (CBC) reveals high red blood cell, white blood cell (particularly neutrophilia), and platelet counts; low hemoglobin levels; and low lymphocyte, eosinophil, and monocyte counts.

3. Confirming hypercortisolism: Note that different collection methods and assays available for the measurement of cortisol exist and results may vary. When performing a diagnostic workup, it is important to evaluate the assays available at each center and carefully collect samples for testing.

1) **Urinary free cortisol (UFC) excretion** increased to 3 or 4×upper limit of normal (ULN) (330 nmol/24 h [120 µg/24 h]) confirms the diagnosis of Cushing syndrome; ≥2 abnormal measurements are necessary to confirm diagnosis.

2) **Elevated midnight serum cortisol levels** >50 nmol/L (1.8 µg/dL) if the blood sample has been collected within 5 to 10 minutes of awakening or, where available and standardized, late-night salivary cortisol levels (>4 nmol/L [145 ng/dL] at 23:00 to midnight).

3) Inadequate reduction in serum cortisol levels in the **1-mg dexamethasone suppression test** (also known as the overnight dexamethasone suppression test or short dexamethasone suppression test): Patients are instructed to take oral dexamethasone 1 mg at bedtime (23:00 to midnight). Fasting serum cortisol levels are measured the following day between 8:00 and 9:00. Serum cortisol levels <50 nmol/L (1.8 µg/dL) exclude Cushing syndrome. In some centers the ULN of 138 nmol/L (5 µg/dL) has been accepted in relation to incidentally diagnosed adrenal tumors. Recently, a modified criterion of 83 nmol/L (3 µg/dL) has been proposed and proved more practical. Note that a single abnormal result of the dexamethasone test cannot be the basis for the decision on surgical treatment.

4) Loss of the **normal circadian cortisol secretion rhythm** (the late afternoon serum cortisol level, usually lower, is >50% of the morning level).

5) Elevated **serum cortisol levels** >690 nmol/L (25 µg/dL).

6) Inadequate reduction in urinary free cortisol excretion in the **2-mg dexamethasone suppression test**: Instruct the patient to take oral dexamethasone 0.5 mg every 6 hours for 2 days. The response is considered normal when free cortisol excretion on day 2 decreases to <27 nmol/24 h (10 µg/24 h).

4. Diagnostics of causes of high serum cortisol levels: Once hypercortisolism is documented, the next diagnostic step is to determine if it is ACTH-dependent (ACTH-secreting tumor) or ACTH-independent (adrenal). This is done by measuring serum ACTH levels.

1) Serum ACTH levels <1.1 pmol/L (5 ng/L) in a patient with a high serum cortisol level indicate ACTH-independent Cushing syndrome, whereas serum ACTH levels >4.4 pmol/L (20 ng/L) indicate ACTH-dependent Cushing syndrome. In patients with serum ACTH levels 1.1 to 4.4 pmol/L (5-20 ng/L), the CRH stimulation test (→below) may be useful to distinguish the cause.

2) The **CRH stimulation test** involves stimulation of ACTH secretion and indirect stimulation of cortisol secretion with CRH. In Cushing disease (which is ACTH-dependent) a characteristic several-fold elevation in ACTH levels is seen after the administration of CRH, but in the case of markedly increased baseline values, an increase in ACTH level by $\geq 35\%$ to 50% and cortisol by $\geq 14\%$ to 20% is considered significant. In ACTH-independent Cushing syndrome usually no response to CRH is seen or it is minor only.

3) The **8-mg dexamethasone suppression test** (2 mg every 6 hours for 2 days) is considered unreliable and is now rarely used; it played a role in the differentiation between Cushing disease (ACTH-dependent pituitary disease) and autonomous adrenal cortisol hypersecretion (functioning adrenal tumor, ectopic ACTH secretion, or nodular adrenal hypertrophy). In patients with Cushing disease urinary excretion of cortisol and its metabolites usually decreases by $\geq 50\%$, whereas in patients with autonomous cortisol secretion no suppression is seen. The test result is not reliable in patients with tumors causing ectopic ACTH secretion.

4) The **adrenal response to atypical stimuli** could be assessed in patients with suspected macronodular adrenal hyperplasia; this is performed in specialized centers. Measure serum cortisol levels at baseline and at 30, 60, 90, and 120 minutes after breakfast or oral intake of 75 g of glucose; after standing up; after oral administration of 10 mg of metoclopramide, or after IV administration of 100 µg of gonadotropin-releasing hormone (GnRH) or 200 µg of thyrotropin-releasing hormone (TRH). The diagnosis is supported by an increase in serum cortisol levels.

5. Imaging studies: Computed tomography (CT) is the first choice for the evaluation of the adrenal gland in Cushing syndrome. CT helps distinguish between tumors and hyperplasia and in most cases can differentiate between adrenal adenomas and carcinomas. **Magnetic resonance imaging (MRI)** is a good option when CT is contraindicated or unavailable. **Skeletal radiographs** may reveal features of osteoporosis and pathologic fractures; delayed bone age is frequently seen in children and adolescents. **Dual-energy x-ray absorptiometry (DXA)** may reveal features of osteopenia or osteoporosis, particularly in the lumbar spine and proximal femur. **Receptor scintigraphy** with somatostatin analogues is used in specialized settings to detect neuroendocrine neoplasms causing ectopic ACTH secretion and to diagnose asymmetric hormone functioning of bilateral adrenal tumors.

CT and MRI of the adrenal glands reveal findings dependent on the cause of Cushing syndrome (→Figure 1-1):

1) **Autonomous adrenal cortex tumor or tumors**: CT reveals a unilateral adrenal tumor with features of adenoma, atrophy of the contralateral adrenal gland, and less frequently bilateral multiple adenomas of the adrenal cortex. MRI reveals significant fat content and rapid contrast washout.

2) **Macronodular adrenal hyperplasia**: CT reveals symmetric adrenal glands that are usually enlarged and often polycyclic; their density is typical for adenomas. MRI reveals high fat content in the adrenal glands.

3) **Micronodular adrenal hyperplasia**: CT and MRI reveal symmetric adrenal glands that are small or of normal size. Diagnosis is established during surgery (characteristic yellow-black color of the nodules caused by lipofuscin deposition).

Diagnostic Criteria

Diagnostic algorithm: →Figure 1-1. Elevated serum cortisol levels must be found on ≥ 2 separate test results. The diagnostic process is usually conducted in a specialized setting.

1. Features of overt Cushing syndrome: Signs and symptoms of Cushing syndrome; high serum cortisol levels with low serum ACTH levels (in ACTH-independent Cushing syndrome) or with high serum ACTH levels (in ACTH-dependent Cushing syndrome caused by pituitary adenoma or ectopic ACTH or CRH secretion);

CRH test results dependent on the cause of elevated cortisol levels; absence of cortisol secretion suppression (in adrenal tumors) or suppression of cortisol secretion only with high-dose (8 mg) dexamethasone (in pituitary adenoma); sometimes elevated androgen levels. CT and MRI may reveal adrenal tumor or tumors, MRI may reveal pituitary tumors, and much less frequently receptor scintigraphy may reveal ectopic ACTH or CRH secretion.

2. Subclinical Cushing syndrome: The earliest and longest-lasting abnormality is inadequate suppression of late-night cortisol levels. Suppression with dexamethasone is impaired, while morning blood and salivary cortisol levels and UFC excretion may approach or slightly exceed the ULN. The most important diagnostic findings are considered to be the reduction of morning plasma ACTH levels below the lower limit of normal (LLN) and inadequate suppression of cortisol secretion by dexamethasone (serum cortisol levels >83 nmol/L [3 μg/dL] in the overnight suppression test with dexamethasone 1 mg). This type of Cushing syndrome is diagnosed in a small proportion of incidentally detected, usually unilateral autonomous tumors of the adrenal cortex. A small group of patients who undergo unilateral adrenalectomy for an apparently nonfunctioning adrenal tumor are retrospectively diagnosed with subclinical Cushing syndrome based on secondary adrenal insufficiency of the remaining adrenal gland in the postoperative period.

Differential Diagnosis

Differential diagnosis of ACTH-dependent and ACTH-independent Cushing syndrome: →Figure 1-1.

Other conditions associated with elevated glucocorticoid levels:

1) Glucocorticoid resistance: A syndrome of partially impaired response of the glucocorticoid receptor (a rare genetic condition). It is associated with high serum ACTH, cortisol, androgen, and aldosterone levels without symptoms of excess cortisol, with features of androgenization and aldosteronism in women. The circadian rhythm of cortisol secretion as well as pituitary and adrenal response to CRH are preserved. Treatment: Dexamethasone 1 to 1.5 mg/d to suppress ACTH secretion.

2) Functional syndromes (pseudo–Cushing syndrome), with high serum cortisol levels resulting not from organic lesions in the pituitary-adrenal system but rather from other abnormalities (high serum cortisol levels require no treatment).

   a) **Depression**: High serum cortisol levels and impaired dexamethasone suppression with a preserved circadian rhythm of cortisol secretion and normal serum ACTH levels.

   b) **Pregnancy**: High blood levels of transcortin (corticosteroid-binding globulin) and, consequently, also high cortisol levels. Placental CRH secretion increases in the third trimester of pregnancy. UFC excretion is increased and the circadian rhythm of cortisol secretion is preserved.

   c) **Alcohol dependence**: Few patients have clinical features of Cushing syndrome (because of altered cortisol metabolism in the liver and effects of alcohol on the central nervous system). Abstinence results in resolution of symptoms.

   d) **Anorexia nervosa**: Elevated cortisol levels, mainly as a result of decreased renal clearance of cortisol. An increase in ACTH secretion may also occur. Impaired dexamethasone suppression caused by acquired glucocorticoid-receptor resistance is present, which explains the lack of any features of adrenal overproduction of glucocorticoids.

⇥ TREATMENT

Symptomatic Treatment

Treatment of complications of Cushing syndrome, which may include hypertension, diabetes mellitus, dyslipidemia, osteoporosis, and psychological disturbances. Some complications resolve after successful treatment of the underlying conditions that have caused Cushing syndrome.

Treatment of Cortisol Hypersecretion

This depends on the etiology of Cushing syndrome.

1. Autonomous tumors of the adrenal cortex: The treatment of choice is usually **surgical resection of the adrenal tumor**.◐○ Medical therapy is recommended as second-line treatment, as primary treatment in metastatic ectopic ACTH syndrome, and as adjuvant therapy in reducing cortisol levels in adrenocortical carcinoma.◐○ Use ketoconazole 400 to 800 mg/d in 3 divided doses (rarely up to 1200 mg/d) or less frequently aminoglutethimide 500 to 750 mg/d or mitotane in an average dose of ~3 g/d. Care should be taken to avoid precipitating glucocorticoid deficit and features of impending adrenal crisis. Clinical improvement is seen at ~3 weeks of treatment, provided the dose is appropriately selected. Perioperative administration of glucocorticoids is the same as in perioperative management of patients with adrenal insufficiency. After surgical tumor resection, use hydrocortisone replacement (typical starting dose, 30 mg/d) as functioning of the contralateral adrenal gland is usually impaired. Over the course of the following weeks, taper the dose of hydrocortisone down to discontinuation. For the following 2 years, hydrocortisone treatment may be occasionally necessary in the event of severe stress (eg, surgery). In rare cases discontinuation of hydrocortisone is not possible.

Patients with subclinical Cushing syndrome after adrenal tumor resection develop secondary adrenal insufficiency of the contralateral adrenal gland. This requires hydrocortisone replacement with subsequent dose tapering (typical starting dose, 20 mg/d).

2. Macronodular or micronodular adrenal hyperplasia: The treatment of choice is resection of both adrenal glands. Administer hydrocortisone as in patients after resection of an adenoma.

3. Management of **pituitary adenoma**.

→ PROGNOSIS

Regardless of etiology, patients with long-standing Cushing syndrome may develop vascular complications of hypertension.

1. Resection of adrenal adenoma or adenomas results in complete resolution of Cushing syndrome. Periodic replacement therapy may be needed.

2. Bilateral adrenalectomy in patients with micronodular and macronodular adrenal hyperplasia results in resolution of symptoms of Cushing syndrome, but lifelong glucocorticoid replacement therapy is necessary. In patients with Carney complex, the prognosis depends on coexisting abnormalities.

3. In patients with adrenocortical carcinoma, the prognosis depends on the stage of cancer and extent of surgery. Patients after bilateral adrenalectomy require lifelong replacement therapy.

1.3. Hypoaldosteronism

→ ETIOLOGY, PATHOGENESIS

Hypoaldosteronism can be caused by defective stimulation of aldosterone secretion, primary defects in adrenal synthesis or secretion of aldosterone, and aldosterone resistance. The major clinical manifestations are hyperkalemia and mild hyperchloremic metabolic acidosis. When hyponatremia is present, primary adrenal insufficiency should be suspected. **Most frequent causes include**:

1) **Primary aldosterone deficiency** should be suspected in persons who have hyperkalemia despite normal renal function and lack of potassium

Table 1-1. Differential diagnosis of different causes of hypoaldosteronism

Etiology	Plasma renin activity	Serum aldosterone	Serum cortisol
Hyporeninemic hypoaldosteronism	↓	↓	Normal
Primary adrenal insufficiency	↑	↓	↓
Adrenal enzyme deficiency	↑	↓	Normal
↑, increased; ↓, decreased.			

supplementation or treatment with potassium-sparing diuretics; this may be caused by primary adrenal insufficiency, bilateral adrenalectomy, 21-hydroxylase deficiency (leading to hypersecretion of adrenal androgens with reduced production of cortisol and aldosterone), or aldosterone synthase deficiency (leading to isolated hypoaldosteronism). Causes of hyperkalemia other than endocrine disorders should also be considered, including drugs inhibiting adrenal steroid synthesis (eg, ketoconazole) and, although infrequently, heparin, which reduces the number of angiotensin II receptors in the zona glomerulosa of the adrenal cortex and results in suppression of aldosterone synthesis and hyperkalemia.

2) **Renin-angiotensin-aldosterone system suppression**: Hyporeninemic hypoaldosteronism (diabetic nephropathy, advanced age), drugs inhibiting renin secretion (nonsteroidal anti-inflammatory drugs, β-blockers, ciclosporin [INN cyclosporine]), angiotensin-converting enzyme inhibitors, angiotensin receptor blockers.

3) **Aldosterone resistance**: Type I and type II pseudohypoaldosteronism, potassium-sparing diuretics that compete for the aldosterone receptor (eg, spironolactone and eplerenone) or that close the sodium channels in the luminal membrane (eg, amiloride and triamterene), and certain antibiotics that inhibit the collecting tubule sodium channel (trimethoprim and pentamidine).

→ DIAGNOSIS

Diagnosis is based on clinical history, focusing primarily on the use of medications or presence of diseases that could interfere with aldosterone metabolism and on laboratory findings. The different causes of hypoaldosteronism can be differentiated by measurement of plasma renin activity (PRA), serum aldosterone levels, and serum cortisol concentrations (→Table 1-1).

→ TREATMENT

Treatment depends on etiology:

1) **Primary hypoaldosteronism**: →Chapter 5.1.1.2.

2) **Hyporeninemic hypoaldosteronism**: Potassium restriction, fludrocortisone 0.2 to 1 mg/d. In case of hypertension or edema, consider furosemide or a thiazide diuretic. Monitor serum potassium levels.

3) **Drug-induced hypoaldosteronism**: Attempt to discontinue or reduce the dose of the offending drug. Correct electrolyte abnormalities.

1.4. Primary Aldosteronism

➔ DEFINITION, ETIOLOGY, PATHOGENESIS

Primary aldosteronism is caused by aldosterone hypersecretion that is relatively independent from regulators of its secretion (renin-angiotensin system, intravascular volume, and potassium concentration) and is not suppressed by sodium administration. Aldosterone acts in the distal renal tubule, increasing $[Na^+]$ concentration and water reabsorption as well as excretion of K^+ and H^+. Excess aldosterone classically leads to the development of hypertension and hypokalemia.

Causes and types of primary aldosteronism:

1) The most common causes and types:

   a) **Unilateral aldosterone-producing adenoma** (30%-40% of patients), which develops as a result of monoclonal hyperplasia. Aldosterone production is independent from angiotensin II and shows a correlation with circadian fluctuations in plasma adrenocorticotropic hormone (ACTH) levels.

   b) **Bilateral idiopathic hyperaldosteronism** or idiopathic hyperplasia (60-70% of patients).

2) Infrequent causes and types:

   a) **Unilateral adrenal hyperplasia** (micronodular or macronodular).

   b) **Familial aldosteronism**: **Type I** is caused by a mutation in the *CYP11B2* gene, encoding aldosterone synthase, and in the *CYP11B1* gene, encoding 11-β-hydroxylase. The mutation results in the formation of a chimeric gene, which causes aldosterone synthesis in the ACTH-dependent zona fasciculata of the adrenal cortex. In such patients, administration of dexamethasone (reducing ACTH levels) suppresses aldosterone hypersecretion, which is why this type is also called glucocorticoid-remediable aldosteronism. **Type II** refers to familial aldosterone-producing adenoma, bilateral idiopathic hyperplasia, or both; aldosteronism is not ACTH--dependent and the underlying genetic defect has not been yet identified, but it most likely involves the *CYP11B2* gene. **Type III** is caused by a germline mutation of the potassium channel *KCNJ5* gene and is associated with severe adrenal hyperplasia and severe manifestations of aldosteronism.

   c) Aldosterone-secreting **adrenocortical carcinoma**.

   d) **Ectopic aldosterone-producing tumors** (eg, ovarian tumors or renal cancers).

In ~50% of patients with aldosterone-secreting adrenal adenoma, somatic mutations of the *KCNJ5* gene have been found, which make the potassium channels less selective and allow the flow of sodium ions followed by calcium ions into the cells of the zona glomerulosa of the adrenal cortex. This leads to increased aldosterone synthesis. Patients with adrenal adenoma and confirmed *KCNJ5* mutations have particularly severe symptoms of aldosteronism.

➔ CLINICAL FEATURES AND NATURAL HISTORY

The major clinical finding is hypertension, although most patients are asymptomatic.

The inappropriate production of aldosterone causes hypertension, sodium retention, hypervolemia, and increased hydrogen and potassium excretion, leading to symptoms of hypokalemia. This has been described as the triad of hypertension, hypokalemia, and metabolic alkalosis. However, nowadays only a minority of patients (10%-40%) are reported to have hypokalemia at the time of diagnosis (probably because of diagnosis made earlier in the natural course of the disease).

Currently it is also rare to see treatment-resistant hypertension, which often could be severe and accompanied by other symptoms, including muscle weakness, hypomagnesemia, polyuria, excessive thirst, paresthesia, cramps, and tetany (symptoms of a significant potassium deficit and alkalosis). Blood volume is normal. (At early stages blood volume is increased due to sodium and water retention; this is followed by spontaneous diuresis and normalization of the extracellular fluid volume, called an "aldosterone escape," which is probably associated with increased secretion of atrial natriuretic peptide [ANP].) Excess aldosterone, acting synergistically with angiotensin II, causes necrosis, fibrosis, and proliferation of myocytes; myocardial hypertrophy; vascular remodeling and fibrosis; and impaired endothelial function; in the kidney this results in damage to small and intermediate arteries and the development of nephropathy (particularly in the case of increased sodium intake). As a result, there is an increase in the risk of cardiovascular morbidity and mortality in such patients when compared with patients with the same blood pressure (BP) and primary hypertension. In addition, metabolic syndrome and type 2 diabetes mellitus are more prevalent in patients with primary aldosteronism, which further increases their cardiovascular risk. Finally, aldosterone may increase glomerular filtration rate, albumin excretion, and renal perfusion pressure independent of systemic pressure.

→ DIAGNOSIS

Perform studies to detect primary aldosteronism in:

1) Patients with moderate (>160-179/100-109 mm Hg) or severe (>180/110 mm Hg) hypertension.
2) Patients with refractory hypertension (>140/90 mm Hg despite treatment with a maximum dose of 3 antihypertensive drugs including a diuretic).
3) Patients with hypertension and idiopathic or spontaneous low-dose diuretic--induced hypokalemia.
4) Patients with hypertension and incidentally diagnosed adrenal tumor (incidentaloma).
5) Patients with hypertension and first-degree relatives diagnosed with primary aldosteronism or with a family history of early-onset hypertension or cerebrovascular hemorrhage at a young age (<40 years).

Diagnostic Tests

1. Basic biochemical tests may reveal:

1) Hypokalemia (may be absent in bilateral adrenal hyperplasia, more often found in patients with adenoma). Serum potassium levels should be measured after discontinuation of drugs that affect sodium-potassium metabolism and renin-angiotensin-aldosterone (RAA) system activity (→below) and during periods of normal dietary sodium and potassium intake; the higher the sodium intake, the greater the likelihood of hypokalemia. In some patients hypokalemia appears during antihypertensive treatment with low-dose diuretics.
2) Increased urinary excretion of potassium in patients with hypokalemia (>30 mmol/d).
3) Normal serum sodium levels approaching the upper limit of normal (ULN) or mild hypernatremia (<150 mEq/L).
4) Mild metabolic alkalosis.

2. Hormone tests (initial tests): Blood samples for measurements of plasma renin activity (PRA) and plasma aldosterone concentration (PAC) should be collected in the morning (8:00). Correction of potassium deficit before performing the RAA system hormone studies is recommended. It was traditionally thought that any drugs affecting sodium-potassium metabolism and the RAA system should be discontinued; it is now recommended to continue most of them with the exception of mineralocorticoid receptor antagonists (eg, eplerenone and spironolactone), which should be discontinued for 4 to 6 weeks unless there is hypokalemia, as this indicates that the system is not completely blocked. Tests may be done while patients are treated with angiotensin-converting enzyme inhibitors (ACEIs), angiotensin receptor blockers (ARBs) and direct renin inhibitors, which usually increase PRA and decrease the PAC/PRA ratio (consequently, a negative result would not exclude the diagnosis of primary aldosteronism). However, low PRA and a high PAC/PRA ratio despite pharmacotherapy is a strong predictor of aldosteronism. When making the decision about testing, it is important to take into account that discontinuing drugs and changing treatment regimens can worsen hypertension and increase the risk of adverse events such as arrhythmias, heart failure, and hypertensive crisis. If the patient requires treatment with other antihypertensive drugs because of high BP, this must be taken into consideration when interpreting test results.

1) **Low baseline (resting) PRA and high baseline (resting) serum aldosterone levels**:

   a) **PRA** <0.77 nmol/L/h (1.0 ng/mL/h).

   b) **PAC** >416 pmol/L (15 ng/dL).

   c) **Aldosterone-renin ratio (ARR)** (aldosterone in ng/dL to PRA in ng/mL/h) >20 to 40 (depending on assay).

2) **PRA and serum aldosterone levels in dynamic conditions** (confirmatory tests, done in specialized settings only):

   a) No increase in PRA and aldosterone levels after stimulating the RAA system using a **3-day low-sodium diet** (up to 20-30 mmol/d; eg, a rice and fruit diet) followed by 3 to 4 hours in a standing position, or alternatively **20 to 40 mg furosemide followed by 2 to 3 hours in a standing position**. Under normal conditions, the increase in PRA and aldosterone levels after 2 to 3 hours in a standing position is 2- or 3-fold, whereas a sodium-restricted diet or administration of furosemide results in a multiple-fold increase.

   b) Aldosterone levels are not reduced when the RAA system is suppressed by a **3-day sodium-rich diet** (confirmed by urinary sodium excretion >200 mmol/24 h; primary aldosteronism confirmed by urinary aldosterone excretion >39 nmol/24 h [12-14 µg/24 h]); the **captopril test** (25 mg orally after remaining in a standing position for ≥1 hour; primary aldosteronism confirmed by no decrease [>30%] in serum aldosterone after 2 hours in a sitting position); or the **0.9% saline suppression test** using 0.9% saline as a 4-hour IV infusion at a rate of 500 mL/h (monitor BP and serum potassium; a high sodium load may be dangerous as it can precipitate hypertensive crisis in patients with hypertension and severe hypokalemia in patients with primary aldosteronism; primary aldosteronism is confirmed by serum aldosterone levels >277 pmol/L [10 ng/dL]).

   After confirming the diagnosis of primary aldosteronism, it is critical to distinguish a unilateral aldosterone-producing adenoma from bilateral idiopathic hyperplasia, as treatment options differ. This is usually done in specialized settings. Adenomas usually have higher aldosterone secretion rates resulting in higher levels of hypertension, hypokalemia (<3.2 mEq/L), aldosterone >25 ng/dL, and PAC/PRA ratios >30.

3. Imaging studies: Computed tomography (CT) allows the visualization of adrenal tumors >8 to 10 mm in diameter; enlargement of one segment of an adrenal gland >6 to 7 mm or of the whole adrenal gland >10 mm is considered abnormal. A result <10 Hounsfield units and assessment of the rate of washout of IV contrast allows for differentiating adrenal adenoma (rapid washout) from adrenal carcinoma (usually >4 cm), metastatic lesions, and pheochromocytoma. However, it should be noted that in some studies CT was accurate in only half of the cases (eg, patients with clearly visualized adenoma

Table 1-2. Causes of mineralocorticoid-dependent hypertension (aldosterone-related and non–aldosterone-related)

Cause of hypertension	Mineralocorticoid	Key clinical[a] and hormonal features
Primary aldosteronism	Aldosterone	Hypokalemia ↓↓ PRA ↑↑ Aldosterone
Congenital adrenal hyperplasia: 17-α-hydroxylase deficit	DOC	Hypogonadism ↓↓ PRA ↓ Aldosterone ↓ Cortisol
Congenital adrenal hyperplasia: 11-β-hydroxylase deficit	DOC	Virilization ↓ PRA ↓ Aldosterone
DOC-secreting adrenal tumors	DOC	Adrenal tumor ↓↓ PRA ↓ Aldosterone
Apparent mineralocorticoid excess 11-β-HSD2 deficit	Cortisol	Excessive thirst Polyuria ↓↓ PRA ↓↓ Aldosterone ↑ Cortisol or cortisone metabolites

[a] Apart from hypertension.

↓, decrease; ↑, increase; 11-β-HSD2, 11-β-hydroxysteroid dehydrogenase isozyme 2; DOC, 11-deoxycorticosterone; PRA, plasma renin activity

may still have bilateral idiopathic hyperplasia and absence of a mass does not exclude an adenoma). **Magnetic resonance imaging (MRI)** has similar sensitivity and specificity to CT and is useful in differentiating aldosterone--secreting adenomas from nonfunctioning tumors. Adrenal **scintigraphy** using a ^{131}I-labeled cholesterol analogue is helpful in detecting aldosterone-secreting tumors >1.5 cm in diameter.

4. Adrenal vein catheterization with aldosterone sampling: The limitations of imaging studies dictate the need for further localization of excess aldosterone production, especially if the treatment of choice is surgery and the patient is >35 years (in younger patients the probability of adrenal incidentalomas is low; in such cases biochemical tests and CT are sufficient). Aldosterone levels on the side of the tumor are 4 to 5 times higher than contralaterally. This study is performed in specialized centers only.

Diagnostic Criteria

Diagnosis is based on results of diagnostic tests (→above).

Familial aldosteronism should be suspected in patients who developed hypertension and aldosteronism in early childhood, or in the case of a family history of aldosteronism in relatives who suffered cerebrovascular accidents at a young age. In familial aldosteronism type I, administration of dexamethasone causes suppression of aldosterone secretion.

Differential Diagnosis

1. Other causes of mineralocorticoid-related hypertension (aldosterone and nonaldosterone mineralocorticoids): →Table 1-2.

2. Other causes of hypokalemia.

3. Secondary aldosteronism caused by long-term activation of the RAA system (high PRA and high serum angiotensin II levels), which stimulates the zona glomerulosa of the adrenal cortex to hypersecrete aldosterone. The most frequent causes include sodium loss, hypovolemia, treatment with high doses of laxatives or diuretics, cirrhosis with ascites, heart failure, myocardial infarction, nephrotic syndrome, renal artery stenosis, renin-secreting tumors, malignant hypertension (regardless of etiology), and estrogen use (as replacement therapy or oral contraceptives; these increase angiotensinogen synthesis).

4. Activating mutation of the mineralocorticoid receptor that becomes apparent during pregnancy (the receptor is stimulated by progesterone).

→ TREATMENT

1. Treatment goals: Prevent adverse outcomes associated with excess aldosterone. Include normalization of BP and serum potassium levels and prevention of cardiovascular damage.

2. Recommend maintaining an appropriate body weight, moderate physical exercise, and sodium-restricted diet (<100 mmol/d; the same applies to patients planned for surgical resection of adenoma).

Surgical Treatment

Unilateral laparoscopic adrenalectomy is the treatment of choice in aldosterone--producing adenomas.

Pharmacotherapy

1. Mineralocorticoid receptor blockers are indicated before resection of an aldosterone-secreting adenoma; they are also used in patients with contraindications to surgery and in bilateral adrenal hyperplasia (idiopathic or familial).

1) **Spironolactone** is administered with meals. Start from 12.5 to 50 mg bid, and when necessary titrate up to 100 mg bid (use a dose that ensures normal serum potassium levels without the need for supplementation; after several months the dose may be reduced even to 25 mg bid). Adverse effects include gynecomastia (at doses >150 mg/d), erectile dysfunction, menstrual disorders caused by inhibition of androgens and progestagens, nausea, vomiting, and diarrhea.

2) **Eplerenone** 25 mg bid (dose may be increased to 100 mg/d); this causes fewer adverse effects than spironolactone. After a few months of treatment, you may try to taper down the dose provided that good BP control is maintained.

2. Other potassium-sparing diuretics: In case of spironolactone intolerance and unavailability of eplerenone, use **amiloride** 5 mg bid, up to 20 mg/d.

3. ACEIs are used in patients with bilateral adrenal hyperplasia when BP normalization cannot be achieved using mineralocorticoid receptor blockers.

4. Glucocorticoids are used in patients with familial aldosteronism type I. The most frequently used agent is dexamethasone 0.5 to 0.75 mg/d.

→ PROGNOSIS

Surgical resection of aldosterone-secreting adenoma leads to complete resolution of signs and symptoms in 35% to 70% of patients. If the disease is undiagnosed or inappropriately treated, the excess aldosterone, especially with a concomitant high salt intake, not only causes hypokalemia and hypertension but also has direct adverse cardiovascular effects and may lead to nephropathy.

2. Diabetes Mellitus

→ DEFINITION, ETIOLOGY, PATHOGENESIS

Diabetes mellitus (DM) is a group of metabolic disorders where various genetic and environmental factors result in the progressive loss of β-cell mass or function (or both) that manifests clinically as hyperglycemia. Chronic hyperglycemia in the course of DM is associated with damage, dysfunction, and failure of multiple organs, particularly the eyes, kidneys, peripheral nerves, heart, and blood vessels.

1. Type 1 DM is caused by the destruction of pancreatic β cells due to an autoimmune process (type 1A, associated with β-cell autoantibodies) or due to unknown mechanisms (idiopathic or type 1B) that typically results in absolute insulin deficiency. Type 1A DM (5%-10% of all patients with diabetes) develops more frequently in children, adolescents, and younger adults, but it can occur at any age. The disease occurs in genetically susceptible individuals with particular gene polymorphisms (human leukocyte antigen [HLA] associations, with linkage to *DQA* and *DQB* genes) and in many cases appears to be triggered by environmental factors (eg, perinatal events, viral infections, ingestion of cow's milk). The autoantibodies (islet cell autoantibodies and autoantibodies to GAD65, insulin, tyrosine phosphatases IA-2 and IA-2β, and ZnT8) may appear several years before symptoms of DM are observed. Their persistence is almost a certain predictor of clinical hyperglycemia and DM. Age at the first detection of an antibody, number of antibodies, antibody specificity, and antibody titers are the main factors that predict the rate of progression to DM. After disease onset, the process of destruction of β cells continues for some time until their total destruction.

There are 3 staging phases of type 1 DM that have been described:

1) Stage 1 is characterized by the presence of autoimmunity but with normal glucose levels and absence of symptoms.
2) Stage 2 is associated with glucose levels in the range of impaired fasting glucose (5.6-6.9 mmol/L [100-125 mg/dL]) and/or impaired glucose tolerance (2-hour plasma glucose of 7.8-11 mmol/L [140-199 mg/dL]) with glycated hemoglobin (HbA$_{1c}$) between 5.7% and 6.4% (or an increase ≥10% in HbA$_{1c}$).
3) Stage 3 is characterized by the onset of symptoms with glucose levels that meet the criteria for the diagnosis of DM.

In some cases autoimmune destruction of β cells leads to the onset of DM in older adults (latent autoimmune diabetes in adults [LADA]; →Table 2-1). These patients initially appear to have type 2 DM but have positive circulating β-cell autoantibodies and progress to insulin dependence after a few months or years. LADA includes a heterogeneous group of patients, with some having high titers of β-cell autoantibodies and progressing to insulin dependence faster. The disappearance of serum C-peptide (→Diagnostic Tests, below) indicates a total destruction of β cells.

2. Type 2 DM is the most common form of DM (~90% of patients). It is characterized by varying degrees of insulin resistance coexisting with progressive impairment of insulin secretion in the absence of autoimmune destruction of β cells. Hyperglycemia occurs when insulin secretory capacity is inadequate to overcome peripheral insulin resistance. Both genetic (polygenic inheritance) and environmental factors (obesity, particularly abdominal, and low physical activity) play a strong role in the occurrence of insulin resistance. The hereditary component results in significant differences in the prevalence of type 2 DM among ethnic groups (eg, type 2 DM is common in Pima Indians and North American Indians). The pathophysiologic pathways leading to insulin resistance and deficient insulin secretion are not completely understood, but it appears that an excessive release of free fatty acids by visceral adipose tissue,

Table 2-1. Differential diagnosis and treatment of latent autoimmune diabetes in adults and type 2 diabetes mellitus

Differential features	LADA	Type 2 diabetes mellitus
Body mass index	As in general population	Obese or overweight
Hypertension	No	Yes
Family history of diabetes	No	Yes
Past or family history of autoimmune diseases	Yes	No
Anti-GAD or other islet cell antibodies	Yes	No
C-peptide (glucagon test)	Low level	Normal or initially increased
Treatment of choice	Insulin	Initial treatment with PO antidiabetic agents

GAD, glutamic acid decarboxylase; LADA, latent autoimmune diabetes in adults; PO, oral.

lipotoxicity caused by these free fatty acids, effects of several adipokines, metabolic stress, and chronic inflammation associated with obesity all play a role in the development of DM and also contribute to the cardiovascular complications of this disease. The risk of developing DM is increased with advancing age, obesity, and lack of physical activity, as well as in patients with hypertension, dyslipidemia, women with prior gestational DM (GDM), and in certain ethnic groups.

Prediabetes is diagnosed when glucose levels and/or HbA_{1c} does not meet the criteria for DM but is higher than what is considered normal. Its presence is associated with an increased risk of overt DM: the 5-year incidence is from 9% to 25% for HbA_{1c} in the range of 5.5% to 6%; the incidence rises to 25% to 50% with HbA_{1c} in the range of 6% to 6.5%. Of note, the threshold at which experts suggest diagnoses of prediabetes and DM change with time and geography (similarly to lipid levels or blood pressure thresholds).

3. Other specific types of DM may be caused by genetic defects of pancreatic β-cell function (eg, maturity-onset diabetes of the youth [MODY]: a group of autosomal dominant monogenic defects of insulin secretion that lead to DM diagnosed at a young age and with negative β-cell autoantibodies [→Table 2-2]), genetic defects of insulin action, pancreatic exocrine disorders and cystic fibrosis–related diabetes, endocrinopathies (eg, Cushing syndrome; acromegaly; catecholamine-producing tumors, including pheochromocytomas, glucagonomas, somatostatinomas), drug-induced DM (eg, glucocorticoids and posttransplantation DM), viral infections (eg, congenital rubella), rare immune-mediated DM (eg, stiff man syndrome), and other genetic syndromes associated with DM (eg, Down syndrome, Klinefelter syndrome, Turner syndrome, Wolfram syndrome, and maternally inherited DM and deafness).

4. GDM (→Chapter 5.2.2.2) is defined by the presence of DM that is first diagnosed in the second or third trimester of pregnancy in women without preexisting DM. Women diagnosed with DM (standard diagnostic criteria) during the first trimester should be classified as having preexisting pregestational diabetes. GDM develops due to pregnancy-related elevation of hormones antagonistic to insulin, leading to insulin resistance, increased insulin requirements, and increased glucose availability for the developing fetus. These mechanisms result in increased risk of abnormal glucose metabolism in otherwise healthy women.

Table 2-2. Differential diagnosis and treatment of maturity-onset diabetes of youth (MODY) and type 1 diabetes mellitus

Differential features	MODY	Type 1 diabetes mellitus
Congenital malformations (most frequently affecting the kidneys and urogenital system)	Possible	No
≥3 generations of family history of diabetes mellitus	Yes	No
Past or family history of autoimmune diseases	No	Yes
Islet cell antibodies	No	Yes
C-peptide (glucagon test)	Initially normal	Low level
Treatment of choice	Initial treatment with oral antidiabetic agents	Insulin
Onset	Slow	Usually acute

→ CLINICAL FEATURES AND NATURAL HISTORY

1. The natural history of DM depends on the rate and extent of β-cell dysfunction and destruction caused by the combination of genetic and environmental factors. In type 1 DM the progression seems to depend on expression of antibodies (age of detection, their number and levels). The mechanism of type 2 DM is through a state of insulin resistance and β-cell dysfunction. Initially type 2 DM can be underdiagnosed because of the lack of typical clinical symptoms. As the disease progresses, patients typically go from a stage of mild hyperglycemia (eg, prediabetes) to overt type 2 DM. Signs and symptoms are nonspecific and variable; they are associated with the type of DM and dynamics of disease progression, which tend to be much more abrupt in type 1 than in type 2. This may result in hyperglycemic crisis such as ketoacidosis or coma. Because of difficulties in achieving complete DM control, the development of chronic complications cannot be fully prevented (→Chapter 5.2.1.2).

2. Signs and symptoms of DM: Nonspecific and variable, including polyuria (osmotic diuresis caused by glucosuria when serum glucose rises >10 mmol/L [180 mg/dL]), nocturia (urinating during the night), polydipsia (increased thirst), polyphagia (increased hunger), blurred vision, weight loss, weakness, and signs of hypovolemia (eg, decreased skin turgor, dry skin and mucous membranes, hypotension). Hyperglycemia may become particularly evident during a concurrent illness (eg, infection, myocardial infarction).

1) **Type 1 DM**: The sudden loss of β-cell reserve leads to an acute onset of the disease with marked insulinopenia and hyperglycemia; in fact, in many patients with type 1 DM the degree of insulinopenia is significant enough to cause ketoacidosis at presentation.

2) **Type 2 DM**: In contrast, >50% of patients with type 2 DM are asymptomatic when the diagnosis is made (disease is frequently detected incidentally or on screening glucose measurements). The majority of patients with type 2 DM are obese, most commonly showing abdominal-type obesity, and frequently have a cluster of comorbidities that includes hypertension, nonalcoholic fatty liver disease, and dyslipidemia (with low serum high-density lipoprotein cholesterol [HDL-C] and high triglyceride concentrations). Insulin resistance is a key feature in type 2 DM, although it is not a pathognomonic finding of this type of DM (eg, obese patients with type 1 DM may have varying degrees of insulin resistance).

→ **DIAGNOSIS**

Diagnostic Tests

Laboratory tests:

1) **Blood glucose**: Fasting plasma glucose (FPG) in venous blood (reference range, 3.9-5.5 mmol/L [70-99 mg/dL]) is used as a diagnostic test for DM and for monitoring glycemic control, whereas glucose levels in capillary full blood (measured using a glucometer) are used only for monitoring DM treatment.

2) **HbA$_{1c}$** reflects mean glycemia over the 3 months preceding the test. It is used both for the diagnosis of DM and for evaluation of metabolic control of the disease. The advantage of this test is that it can be measured at any time during the day and it is not affected by acute blood glucose level changes. When interpreting the results, consider other conditions that may affect its accuracy; if a condition results in a shorter life-span and greater proportion of younger erythrocytes (eg, hemolytic anemias), falsely low HbA$_{1c}$ values are likely. Red blood cell transfusion can also decrease HbA$_{1c}$ levels in patients with DM. In contrast, a longer erythrocyte life-span is associated with longer exposure to elevated blood glucose, hence falsely increasing HbA$_{1c}$ levels (eg, iron or vitamin B$_{12}$ deficiency anemias). To avoid misdiagnosis of DM, HbA$_{1c}$ should be measured using a method certified by the NGSP and standardized to the Diabetes Control and Complications Trial (DCCT) assay.

3) A **75-g oral glucose tolerance test (OGTT)** can be used for the screening or diagnosis of DM. In this test a patient without acute illness is instructed to eat a diet with normal carbohydrate content in the days before the test. The OGTT is performed in the morning after 8 to 12 hours of fasting and includes measurement of FPG. Plasma glucose measurement is obtained 2 hours after the ingestion of 75 g of glucose in the form of a solution. Normal plasma glucose levels at 2 hours are <7.8 mmol/L (140 mg/dL). A modified version of this test is used to diagnose GDM.

4) **Urine glucose**: Glucosuria is typically seen in patients with DM when the blood glucose level rises >10 mmol/L (180 mg/dL). In patients without DM, this can result from defects in renal tubular function (eg, proximal renal tubular acidosis). Measurement of urine glucose is not useful for the screening, diagnosis, or treatment monitoring of DM. However, finding glucosuria is an indication for blood glucose tests.

5) **Fructosamine**: This rarely used test demonstrates mean glycemia over the preceding 2 weeks (the half-life of albumin). Fructosamine levels are mainly measured in patients in whom HbA$_{1c}$ is unreliable or in whom it is necessary to evaluate short-term blood glucose control (eg, pregnant women).

6) **Islet cell antibodies** can be used to confirm the autoimmune etiology of DM. At least 1 antibody is present in >90% of patients with type 1 DM, and the presence of antibodies defines patients with LADA. These antibodies may be detectable before the clinical onset of DM:

   a) Antibodies to glutamate decarboxylase 65 (**anti-GAD65**).

   b) Antibodies against tyrosine phosphatase–related proteins (**IA-2, IA-2 β**).

   c) Insulin autoantibodies (**IAAs**).

   d) β-Cell-specific zinc transporter antibody (**ZnT-8**).

7) **Serum C-peptide level** reflects endogenous insulin levels. It is decreased or undetectable in type 1 DM, elevated in early type 2 DM (when insulin resistance is a dominant mechanism and insulin secretion increases), and decreased in type 2 DM after the deterioration of β-cell secretory capacity. Measurements of C-peptide levels are not required in most cases of DM.

Screening

Screening for type 1 DM is not recommended, because this condition is rare and there are no interventions to prevent the progression of subclinical disease.

In contrast, type 2 DM is common, develops slowly, can be asymptomatic for a relatively long time, and can be treated at an early stage to prevent or delay its complications.

As an example, in the case of asymptomatic individuals the American Diabetes Association (ADA) recommends to screen for type 2 DM in adults of any age who have a body mass index (BMI) ≥25 kg/m^2 (or Asian Americans with a BMI ≥23 kg/m^2) and have ≥1 additional risk factors for DM:

1) Physical inactivity.

2) A first-degree relative with DM.

3) A high-risk race/ethnicity (eg, African American, Latino, Native American, Asian American, Pacific Islander).

4) Delivery of a baby weighing >4.08 kg or confirmed diagnosis of GDM.

5) Hypertension (≥140/90 mm Hg or being treated for hypertension).

6) An HDL-C level <0.90 mmol/L (35 mg/dL) and/or triglyceride level >2.82 mmol/L (250 mg/dL).

7) Polycystic ovary syndrome (PCOS).

8) HbA$_{1c}$ ≥5.7% (39 mmol/mol), impaired glucose tolerance (IGT), or impaired fasting glucose (IFG) on previous testing.

9) Other clinical conditions associated with insulin resistance (eg, severe obesity, acanthosis nigricans).

10) A history of cardiovascular disease (CVD).

In the absence of the above criteria, testing for DM should begin at the age of 45 years. FPG, HbA$_{1c}$, and a 75-g OGTT are appropriate tests for screening. If results are negative, the ADA recommends repeating testing at least at 3-year intervals, with consideration of more frequent testing depending on the initial results and presence of risk factors. Other organizations issued similar suggestions, noting that the quality of evidence supporting the type of screening and its overall benefit is at most moderate.

Diabetes mellitus screening tests in pregnant women: →Chapter 5.2.2.2.

Diagnostic Criteria

Diagnostic workup in patients with hyperglycemia should not be performed during acute phases of other diseases (eg, infection or acute coronary syndrome), immediately following trauma or surgery, or during treatment with drugs that may cause elevated blood glucose levels (eg, glucocorticoids, thiazide diuretics, certain β-blockers).

According to the ADA, the **diagnosis of DM** is established when either of these criteria is met:

1) There are **typical signs and symptoms of hyperglycemia** (eg, increased thirst, polyuria, weight loss, blurry vision, weakness) or **hyperglycemic crisis** and a **random plasma glucose level ≥11.1 mmol/L** (200 mg/dL).

2) **HbA$_{1c}$ ≥6.5%** (48 mmol/mol) (using a certified method), **FPG ≥7.0 mmol/L** (126 mg/dL) (fasting is defined as no caloric intake for ≥8 hours), or **2-hour plasma glucose ≥11.1 mmol/L** (200 mg/dL) during a 75-g OGTT. In the absence of unequivocal signs and symptoms of hyperglycemia, one abnormal test result should be confirmed by repeating the same test on a subsequent day. If 2 different tests are available (eg, FPG and HbA$_{1c}$) and both are consistent with DM, additional testing is not needed. If results of different tests are discordant, the test that is diagnostic for DM should be repeated.

According to the ADA, the category of **increased risk for DM** (prediabetes) is defined by the presence of any of the following:

1) HbA$_{1c}$ between 5.7% and 6.4% (39-46 mmol/mol).

2) IFG (FPG between 5.6-6.9 mmol/L [100-125 mg/dL]).

3) IGT (2-hour plasma glucose after a 75-g OGTT between 7.8-11.0 mmol/L [140-199 mg/dL]).

Differential Diagnosis

1. Other causes of clinical signs and symptoms, such as polyuria (diabetes insipidus).

2. Other causes of hyperglycemia: Stress-induced hyperglycemia, which refers to transient hyperglycemia and may occur during acute illness or significant stress in patients without DM (eg, sepsis, acute coronary syndrome, immediately following trauma or major surgery).

➡ TREATMENT

General Considerations

The management of DM includes:

1) **Patient education**, which is indispensable for treatment success.

2) Nonpharmacologic management: **Nutrition, weight loss, and exercise**.

3) **Glucose-lowering treatment**: Oral and injectable antidiabetic agents, insulin.

4) Management of other cardiovascular risk factors, particularly **hypertension** (→Chapter 3.9.1) and **dyslipidemia** (→Chapter 3.12.2).

5) Prevention and management of **chronic diabetic complications**.

1. In type 2 DM **lifestyle modification and weight loss** are the fundamental aspects of care. An intensive behavioral lifestyle intervention program should be suggested to all patients with type 2 DM, including those with prediabetes, in order to induce and maintain a loss of ~7% of initial body weight and to increase moderate-intensity physical activity to at least 150 min/wk. In patients with prediabetes this program has been shown to reduce the incidence of type 2 DM by 58% over 3 years. Of note, patients' willingness and ability to conform to recommendations concerning lifestyle modifications vary widely and cannot be assumed or even expected.

2. Insulin therapy:

1) In **type 1 DM** insulin therapy is mandatory once the diagnosis of DM is established.

2) In **type 2 DM** insulin therapy is indicated in patients not achieving appropriate glycemic control with other medications. Insulin should also be started in patients with type 2 DM and marked hyperglycemia at the time of diagnosis (eg, HbA_{1c} >11% [97 mmol/mol]) and in patients with hyperglycemic crisis (ie, diabetic ketoacidosis [DKA], hyperosmolar hyperglycemic state [HHS]). If insulin treatment is used early in the course of DM because of β-cell glucotoxicity, recovery of β-cell function after achieving adequate control of hyperglycemia may allow for de-escalation of insulin therapy and often switching to oral antidiabetic medications. As type 2 DM is a progressive disease with gradual deterioration of the secretory capacity of pancreatic β cells, many patients with type 2 DM eventually need insulin therapy.

3. In type 2 DM **metformin** is typically the first medication used. Because type 2 DM is a progressive disease, second-line and third-line agents are frequently required for appropriate glycemic control. Different glucose-lowering medications are currently available, including insulin secretagogues (eg, sulfonylureas, meglitinides, dipeptidyl peptidase-4 [DPP-4] inhibitors, glucagon-like peptide-1 [GLP-1] receptor agonists), insulin sensitizers (eg, metformin, thiazolidinediones [TZDs]), α-glucosidase inhibitors (eg, acarbose), and sodium-glucose cotransporter 2 (SGLT-2) inhibitors (eg, canagliflozin or empagliflozin).

4. If the type of DM is unclear (ie, type 1 versus type 2) in a patient presenting with **hyperglycemic crisis**, the final diagnosis and appropriate long-term treatment can be established after control of metabolic abnormalities is achieved with insulin therapy. If autoimmune etiology of DM is excluded, patients can be sometimes successfully switched to oral glucose-lowering medications.

5. Target HbA$_{1c}$ levels should be achieved gradually (ie, over several months) because a rapid reduction of plasma glucose levels carries a risk of hypoglycemia (particularly in type 1 DM), and in patients with advanced microangiopathy (primarily retinopathy) it may accelerate progression of this complication; in type 2 DM it may additionally increase the cardiovascular risk. In patients who do not achieve target HbA$_{1c}$ levels despite maintaining target FPG, make attempts to reduce postprandial glucose levels.

6. Criteria of DM control: Glycemic goal: The intensity of glucose-lowering treatment, determined by target blood glucose and HbA$_{1c}$ values, should be individualized based on the patient's cooperation and motivation, risk of hypoglycemia, disease duration, life expectancy, comorbidities, cardiovascular complications, as well as financial resources and support available. Higher glucose levels may be acceptable in patients achieving target HbA$_{1c}$ levels. The criteria of DM control may be less stringent in the elderly, in patients with comorbidities, and in those with frequent episodes of hypoglycemia. If target values cannot be achieved, attempts should be made to achieve results as close as practically possible. Of note, **different professional societies recommend different targets**, from 6.5% (American Association of Clinical Endocrinologists) through 7% (ADA) to between 7% and 8% (American College of Physicians). This may make clinicians less anxious about rigid adherence to specific values.◐ The ADA suggests:

1) Target **HbA$_{1c}$** levels <7.0% (53 mmol/mol) and **preprandial capillary blood glucose levels** between 3.9 and 7.2 mmol/L (70-130 mg/dL) in most nonpregnant adults with DM. To achieve this in young patients with type 1 DM, a multiple daily injection insulin therapy is usually required. ADA experts acknowledge that individual patients' goals may be slightly lower or slightly higher. We consider the recommendation to achieve this target as strong in type 1 DM◐◐ and weak in type 2 DM.◯◐

2) **HbA$_{1c}$** levels <6.5% (48 mmol/mol) are suggested for selected patients with a short duration of DM, long life expectancy, and no significant CVD, as long as treatment does not induce significant hypoglycemia.

3) In contrast, the criteria of DM control may be less stringent (HbA$_{1c}$ <8.0% [64 mmol/mol]) in the elderly, in patients with significant comorbidities, advanced microvascular or macrovascular complications, limited life expectancy, and in patients who developed hypoglycemia unawareness or those with severe or frequent episodes of hypoglycemia.

4) Considering the lack of clear benefits on the major outcomes, risk of hypoglycemia, and potential burden and higher costs of more intensive treatment, a strong recommendation against intensive glycemic control (eg, HbA$_{1c}$ ≤6.5% [48 mmol/mol]) can be made for older patients with long-standing type 2 DM and risk for CVD.◐◯

5) The role of postprandial blood glucose targets is unclear because outcome studies relied mostly on HbA$_{1c}$ and preprandial glucose levels for assessing the glycemic effect of evaluated interventions. According to the ADA, postprandial testing aiming for blood glucose values <10 mmol/L (180 mg/dL) 1 to 2 hours after the beginning of a meal is a reasonable strategy in patients with high HbA$_{1c}$ and preprandial glucose levels within target values.

6) According to the Fifth International Workshop-Conference on Gestational Diabetes Mellitus, the following target values should be used for capillary glucose concentrations in pregnant patients: preprandial, ≤5.3 mmol/L (95 mg/dL); and 1-hour postprandial level ≤7.8 mmol/L (140 mg/dL) and/or 2-hour postprandial level ≤6.7 mmol/L (120 mg/dL). For patients with preexisting type 1 or type 2 DM who become pregnant, the optimal recommended glycemic goals are as follows, provided they can be achieved without excessive hypoglycemia: (i) preprandial, bedtime, and overnight glucose: 3.3 to 5.4 mmol/L (60-99 mg/dL); (ii) peak postprandial glucose: 5.4 to 7.1 mmol/L (100-129 mg/dL); (iii) HbA$_{1c}$: <6.0% (42 mmol/mol).

7. Principles of lipid control:

1) The ADA recommends to intensify lifestyle therapy and optimize glycemic control for patients with triglyceride levels ≥1.7 mmol/L (150 mg/dL) and/or HDL-C levels <1.0 mmol/L (40 mg/dL) for men or <1.3 mmol/L (50 mg/dL) for women.

2) For patients with triglyceride levels ≥5.7 mmol/L (500 mg/dL), medical therapy (eg, fibrates) should be considered to reduce the risk of pancreatitis.

3) For patients with DM of all ages and overt CVD, high-intensity statin therapy should be added to lifestyle therapy.

4) For patients aged 40 to 75 years with additional cardiovascular risk factors, consider using high-intensity statin therapy added to lifestyle therapy.

5) For patients aged <40 years or >75 years with additional cardiovascular risk factors, consider using moderate or high-intensity statin therapy added to lifestyle therapy.

6) For patients aged >40 years without additional cardiovascular risk factors, consider using moderate-intensity statin therapy added to lifestyle therapy.

8. Principles and criteria of blood pressure control:

1) General criteria: <140/90 mm Hg.

2) Less than 130/80 mm Hg (but not <120/70 mm Hg) in patients with diabetic nephropathy and in patients with recently diagnosed hypertension and no target organ damage if these targets can be achieved without undue treatment burden.

3) Angiotensin-converting enzyme inhibitors (ACEIs) or angiotensin-receptor blockers (ARBs) are suggested as first-line antihypertensive agents, particularly among patients with evidence of diabetic nephropathy.⊘◐

Education

1. Patient education is an important component of DM management, together with nutrition therapy, exercise, and pharmacotherapy, and it should be offered to all patients.⊘◐

2. Patient education aims to improve knowledge, skills, and confidence in DM management and to promote the patient's cooperation with a multidisciplinary therapeutic team. The reinforcement for diabetes self-management education must be addressed at diagnosis, annually, in case of appearance of new complicating factors, and when transitions in care occur.

3. Education programs typically cover aspects of the pathophysiology of DM, lifestyle modification, glucose self-monitoring, insulin dose-adjustment, management of hypoglycemia, prevention and detection of acute and chronic DM complications, and foot care. Additionally, health status and quality of life evaluation is also included.

4. Educational sessions should be patient-centered and repeated and their effects should be evaluated, including not only the patients' knowledge but also their capability of coping with the disease and empowerment to make informed self--management decisions. The inclusion of patient-centered care must be respectful of and responsive to individual patient preferences, needs, and values. Structured education programs that promote intensive basal-bolus insulin therapy and teach the principles of dose-adjustment have been associated with improvements in glycemic control and quality of life in patients with type 1 DM. In patients with type 2 DM education should include teaching about the likely progressive nature of the disease and the necessary gradual modifications of treatment.

5. Patient education can be optimally conducted both in individual and group settings.

Self-Monitoring of Blood Glucose

All patients with DM who use insulin or take other glucose-lowering medications that can cause hypoglycemia (eg, sulfonylureas) should learn how to check their finger-stick capillary blood glucose with a glucose meter. The recommended frequency of self-monitoring of blood glucose (SMBG) depends on the type of antidiabetic therapy and long-term stability of clinical status. SMBG is a fundamental aspect of management in type 1 DM and is also important in patients with type 2 DM treated with complex insulin regimens. The ADA suggests that patients treated with multiple-dose insulin or insulin pump therapy should consider SMBG prior to meals and snacks, occasionally postprandially, at bedtime, prior to exercise, when hypoglycemia is suspected, after treating hypoglycemia, and prior to critical tasks such as driving. For some patients it may mean 6 or more measurements per day. Patients with type 2 DM treated with oral agents that can cause hypoglycemia also likely benefit from SMBG, particularly during uptitration of these medications (eg, testing once to twice per day before breakfast and before the evening meal).

In contrast, the benefit of SMBG in patients with type 2 DM only on diet or who are treated with medications not associated with hypoglycemia is controversial. The ADA suggests that SMBG results may be helpful to guide treatment decisions in patients treated with noninsulin therapies. In this context a reasonable frequency of measurements will depend on the patient's preference. Motivated patients with type 2 DM could take action to modify diet or exercise patterns based on SMBG readings and therefore improve their HbA_{1c} values.

Medical Nutrition Therapy: General Considerations

The ADA recommends nutrition therapy for all patients with type 1 and type 2 DM. Nutrition therapy consists of the development of eating patterns designed to achieve and maintain an ideal body weight, improve glycemic control, lower blood pressure, improve lipid profile, reduce cardiovascular risk, and reduce the overall risk for both acute and long-term complications of DM while preserving the pleasure of eating. Nutrition therapy should aim for a beneficial effect in the overall health of patients while taking into consideration their personal and cultural preferences as well as their individual nutritional needs and their ability to sustain recommendations in the plan.

1) Adequate caloric intake should ensure maintaining an ideal body weight or gradual reduction of body weight in obese or overweight patients. A weight loss of ≥5% in patients with type 2 DM is needed in order to produce beneficial outcomes in glycemic control, lipids, and blood pressure.

2) An optimal body weight is usually a BMI between 18.5 and 24.9 kg/m^2. Healthy weight-loss diets typically aim to achieve an energy deficit of 500 to 750 kcal/d or reduce daily energy intake to 1200 to 1500 calories in women and 1500 to 1800 calories in men, depending on the initial weight (eg, in women >135 kg start with 1600 calories per day, in men >135 kg start with 1800 calories per day). Diets <1200 calories per day for women or <1500 calories per day in men are not generally recommended because they may be deficient in nutrients. Furthermore, very low-calorie diets have not been found to produce greater long-term weight losses than conventional low-calorie diets. The Mediterranean diet, structured low-calorie meal plan, low-fat eating plan, plant-based diet, or Dietary Approaches to Stop Hypertension (DASH) meal plan are the ones most suggested for patients with prediabetes and DM. Low-carbohydrate diets have been shown to improve hyperglycemia, reduce HbA_{1c}, and reduce the need for antihyperglycemic medications in some patients with type 2 DM. Overall, lifestyle modifications, which include dietary changes, are strongly recommended.◉◔

3) The optimal distribution of calories from carbohydrates, protein, and fat to facilitate weight loss is unknown and likely not absolute. Macronutrient distribution should be based on an individual assessment of current eating patterns, preferences, and metabolic goals.

4) Carbohydrate intake is the most important determinant of postprandial glucose levels in patients with DM. The ADA suggests choosing nutrient--dense carbohydrates containing vitamins, minerals, and fiber (eg, vegetables,

whole grains, legumes, or fruit) over processed carbohydrates high in calories, sugar, sodium, and fat. Avoiding sugar-sweetened beverages and processed "low-fat" or "nonfat" food products with high amounts of refined grains and added sugars is also recommended. In patients with type 2 DM taking insulin secretagogues (eg, sulfonylureas) or insulin, meals should include carbohydrates to reduce the risk of hypoglycemia.

5) Protein intake recommendations are the same as for the general population (1-1.5 g/kg of body weight per day or 15%-20% of total calories). It can be increased to 20% to 30% of total calories to increase satiety in some patients, based on an individual approach. A reduction to 0.8 g/kg of body weight per day should be achieved in patients with diabetic kidney disease.

6) Fat quality is more important than quantity for reducing the risk for CVD. An acceptable macronutrient distribution for total fat is generally 20% to 35% of total calorie intake. The ADA suggests limiting the intake of saturated fat to 10% of calories, limiting the intake of cholesterol to <300 mg/d, and avoiding trans-fat as much as possible. These recommendations apply to the general population. It is also suggested to limit sodium intake to <2300 mg/d.

7) In patients treated with metformin, periodic testing of vitamin B_{12} levels should be recommended, especially in those with anemia and peripheral neuropathy. There is lack of evidence with regards to efficacy of routine supplementation with antioxidants (vitamins E and C, carotene), herbals, and micronutrients (cinnamon, curcumin, vitamin D, chromium). Therefore, their use should not be recommended, except for special populations (pregnant or lactating women, older adults, vegetarians, and people with very low-calorie or low-carbohydrate diets).

Dietary Considerations in Patients on Insulin Therapy

1. For patients with type 2 DM (or type 1 DM) treated with fixed doses of short-acting and intermediate-acting insulin (frequently premixed), day-to-day consistency in the time of insulin administration, mealtimes, and amount of carbohydrate intake is an important consideration in order to avoid variable and unpredictable blood glucose levels and hypoglycemia. These patients should not skip meals.

2. For patients with type 1 DM (or type 2 DM) following a multiple daily injection program treated with a long-acting insulin and fixed doses of a rapid-acting prandial insulin, it is important to eat similar amounts of carbohydrates during each meal to match the prandial insulin doses. This program gives more flexibility regarding the time when meals can be consumed. Different meal planning strategies can be used to quantify carbohydrate intake (eg, sample menus, the exchange system [list of servings in 6 categories that may be exchanged for one another, as they contain a similar amount of main nutrients], or carbohydrate counting). The ADA recommends the carbohydrate-counting approach for patients with type 1 DM on a flexible multiple daily injection program. Patients using insulin pumps also need to learn carbohydrate counting.

Physical Activity

1. The ADA and the American Heart Association (AHA) recommend performing ≥150 minutes of moderate-intensity aerobic physical activity (eg, brisk walking) per week. Physical activity should be distributed over ≥3 days per week, with no more than 2 consecutive days without activity, and should be supplemented by increase in daily lifestyle activities (eg, gardening, household work). The exercise regimen should also include resistance training. At least 90 minutes of vigorous aerobic exercise per week is an alternative. For long-term maintenance of a major weight loss, the ADA and AHA recommend a larger amount of exercise (eg, 7 hours of moderate or vigorous aerobic physical activity per week). Special considerations should be addressed in patients with CVD, uncontrolled retinopathy or nephropathy, and severe neuropathy.

2. Exercise can improve glycemic control, assist with weight loss and maintenance, and affect positively different cardiovascular risk factors, including hypertension and dyslipidemia. Resistance training (eg, exercise with elastic bands or weight machines) may confer additional benefits, as it has the potential to enhance skeletal muscle mass and improve muscle strength and insulin sensitivity.

3. Patients with significant hyperglycemia (eg, blood glucose ≥13.9 mmol/L [250 mg/dL]) should avoid vigorous exercise because they may experience worsening of hyperglycemia and ketosis. Other occasional complications associated with strenuous physical activity include foot-stress fractures, retinal bleeding in patients with proliferative retinopathy (particularly during resistance training), and acute coronary events.

4. Although many individuals with DM do not need exercise stress testing before undertaking exercise more intense than brisk walking, pre-exercise evaluation and exercise stress testing should be considered in those at high risk for CVD (eg, multiple cardiovascular risk factors, known coronary artery disease, cerebrovascular disease, or peripheral artery disease), advanced nephropathy with renal failure, or cardiovascular autonomic neuropathy.

5. Patients receiving insulin treatment should measure their blood glucose before, during, and after exercise to identify glycemic patterns that can be used to develop strategies to avoid hypoglycemia. Ideally, exercise should be performed at similar times and in a consistent relation to meals and insulin injections. Some strategies to prevent hypoglycemia include consuming extra carbohydrates before exercise and then at 30-minute intervals during exercise (eg, 15-30 g of quickly absorbed carbohydrates) as well as after the end of exercise if it was prolonged; this is particularly important in type 1 DM. In type 2 DM the risk of hypoglycemia is lower; obese patients do not usually need extra carbohydrates during exercise.

6. Avoid insulin injections in the body areas that are especially active during a particular activity (eg, thigh) and reduce the dose of insulin that affects the time when exercise will be performed (eg, by 30%-50%), depending on exercise intensity and glucose levels.

Pharmacotherapy: Insulin

Of note, the term human insulin denotes genetically human insulin produced by *Escherichia coli* (examples: Humulin; neutral protamine Hagedorn [NPH] insulin, also known as isophane insulin). For a major proportion of patients treated with insulin, the advantages of using insulin analogues (modified human insulin) over human insulin are far from clear or obvious despite the cost of modified insulins being 2 to 10 times higher.◒

1. Indications for insulin therapy:

1) **Type 1 DM**: All patients with type 1 DM should be treated with insulin from the moment of diagnosis (LADA may be an exception). These patients should not stop their basal insulin administration, even during fasting.

2) **Type 2 DM**:

    a) Patients presenting with an acute DM complication or with significant hyperglycemia at the time of diagnosis (eg, DKA, HHS, FPG >16.7 mmol/L [300 mg/dL], HbA_{1c} >11% [97 mmol/mol], or signs of increased catabolism such as weight loss, polyuria, and polydipsia). The requirement for insulin may be temporal.

    b) Failure of noninsulin antidiabetic treatment despite the intensification of pharmacotherapy as well as lifestyle and behavioral interventions. In these patients insulin therapy should not be delayed. Insulin regimens can be combined with other noninsulin antidiabetic medications. Combined GLP-1 and insulin can be considered if HbA_{1c} is >10% (86 mmol/mol) and/or >2% (23 mmol/mol) above the glycemic goal.

    c) Hospitalized patients, as it allows greater flexibility in the management of hyperglycemia during acute illness.

Table 2-3. Insulin pharmacokinetics (effective duration may differ markedly)				
Insulin preparations		**Time of action**		
		Onset	Peak	Effective duration
Rapid-acting insulin analogues	Aspart	5-20 min	40-75 min	3-5 h
	Glulisine	5-20 min	40-75 min	3-5 h
	Lispro	5-20 min	40-75 min	3-5 h
Short-acting insulins	Regular	30 min	2-4 h	5-8 h
Intermediate-acting insulins	NPH (isophane)	2 h	4-12 h	10-18 h
Long-acting insulin analogues	Detemir	2 h	3-9 h	8-24 h
	Glargine	2 h	No peak	20 to >24 h
	Degludec	2 h	No peak	>40 h
NPH, neutral protamine Hagedorn.				

2. Types of insulin: →Table 2-3. The selection of insulin preparations and insulin regimen should be individualized to the patient's lifestyle, usual mealtimes, and preferences.

1) **Basal insulin preparations**:
   a) **Intermediate-acting human insulin** (insulin isophane [NPH]) is administered subcutaneously once or twice daily (typically in the morning before breakfast and before the evening meal or at bedtime). It is frequently given in combination with a short-acting insulin.
   b) **Long-acting insulin analogues** are usually administered subcutaneously once daily, in the morning or evening, at a fixed time. However, the effect of insulin detemir can last <24 hours, and therefore bid administration is frequently required with this basal insulin (in the morning and evening). In occasional situations insulin glargine also requires twice-daily dosing (eg, early morning hyperglycemia in patients taking insulin glargine before breakfast who also experience hypoglycemia while fasting during the day, patients susceptible to hypoglycemia while on very low total daily doses of insulin, or patients using very high basal insulin doses). Long-acting analogues are frequently used in combination with rapid-acting insulin analogues as part of an intensive insulin therapy regimen (→Figure 2-1).

2) **Prandial insulin preparations**:
   a) **Rapid-acting insulin analogues** are administered subcutaneously immediately (within 0-15 minutes) before a meal, although they may also be administered during and immediately after mealtime, usually 3 times a day.
   b) **Short-acting human insulin** (regular insulin) is administered subcutaneously within 45 minutes before meals, usually 3 times a day. It is commonly used together with an intermediate-acting insulin (→Figure 2-2).

3) **Premixed insulin preparations** (insulin combinations, biphasic insulins):
   a) **Premixed human insulins**: A short-acting human insulin combined with an intermediate-acting insulin.
   b) **Premixed insulin analogues**: A rapid-acting insulin analogue combined with a long-acting protamine suspension of this analogue.

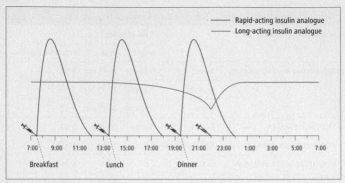

Figure 2-1. Intensive insulin therapy regimen with 4 insulin injections a day: a rapid-acting insulin analogue combined with a long-acting insulin analogue.

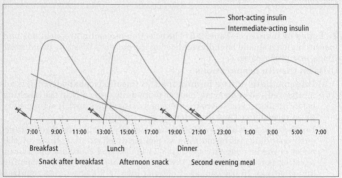

Figure 2-2. Intensive insulin therapy regimen with 4 insulin injections a day: a short-acting insulin combined with an intermediate-acting insulin (neutral protamine Hagedorn).

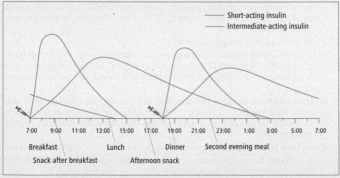

Figure 2-3. Treatment regimen with a premixed human insulin (short-acting insulin plus intermediate--acting insulin) administered twice a day.

Table 2-4. Premixed insulins (insulin combinations, biphasic insulins)

Types of insulins in the combination	Brand names
Premixed human insulin (longer/shorter)	Humulin® 20/80; Humulin® 70/30; Novolin® ge 30/70; Novolin® ge 40/60; Novolin® ge 50/50
Aspart plus aspart protamine suspension (30% longer)	NovoMix® 30
Lispro plus lispro protamine suspension (25% longer)	Humalog® Mix 25

With premixed insulin preparations the proportion of short-acting to long-acting insulin is fixed. Depending on preparation, 50% to 80% of the insulin dose is given as an intermediate-acting or long-acting form of insulin (→Table 2-4). Each of insulin preparations in a combination product achieves its peak activity at a different time. The peaks associated with the effect of rapid-acting insulin or short-acting insulin are higher and their duration is shorter than those associated with intermediate-acting or long-acting insulins. These premixed insulin preparations are typically administered as 2 daily doses, before breakfast and before the evening meal (→Figure 2-3). Patients must consume a meal after each injection and should follow a diet consistent in carbohydrates from day to day with meals consumed at similar times of the day. Because of the fixed ratios of insulins, individual basal and prandial dose adjustments cannot be made. Premixed insulin preparations should ideally be used after basal insulin requirements have been first established.

3. Initial insulin doses: Most patients with type 1 DM are sensitive to insulin. It is recommended to start with a dose of 0.5 IU/kg/d. However, patients with type 1 DM may require a total daily insulin dose that ranges from 0.4 to 1.0 IU/kg/d. In type 1 DM insulin regimens typically try to mimic the physiologic release of insulin by administering a basal form of insulin (eg, glargine or detemir) and mealtime (prandial) boluses of short-acting or rapid-acting insulin. As an initial strategy, half of the total daily insulin dose can be administered as basal (eg, 0.25 IU/kg) and half as the daily prandial dose (eg, 0.25 IU/kg divided into 3 doses given with each main meal).

In contrast, in type 2 DM it should be considered if significant hyperglycemia requires full doses of insulin (eg, 0.3-0.6 IU/kg/d) or if appropriate glycemic control can be achieved with low doses of intermediate-acting or long-acting insulin added to other glucose-lowering medications (10 U or 0.1-0.2 IU/kg/d of a long-acting or intermediate-acting insulin). When full doses of insulin are required (0.3-0.6 IU/kg/d), patients who are sensitive to insulin or predisposed to complications of hypoglycemia (eg, thin, elderly, those with adrenal insufficiency, advanced kidney disease, cirrhosis, unstable coronary disease, active intracranial pathology, terminal illness) require lower starting insulin doses than those who are more insulin-resistant (eg, obese, receiving supraphysiologic glucocorticoid treatment).

4. Insulin regimens: It is important to note that there is no uniformly accepted "best available" way of prescribing insulin and monitoring its effects. In general, in type 2 DM all insulin regimens should be combined with metformin, if not contraindicated. Insulin therapy should not be unduly delayed, because persistent hyperglycemia and elevated proinsulin levels accelerate the progression of the complications of DM.

1) **Single-dose insulin program**: Typically used in patients with type 2 DM when combined treatment with 2 or 3 oral antidiabetic agents (with or without a GLP-1 agonist) is ineffective and who are transitioning to insulin therapy. One injection of intermediate-acting insulin (NPH) or a long--acting insulin analogue (eg, glargine, detemir, or degludec) is given once

a day at about the same time. Patients with high FPG levels are commonly advised to administer insulin at bedtime, while patients with normal FPG levels and daytime hyperglycemia are advised to administer insulin in the morning before breakfast. Preprandial glucose targets are individualized (eg, glucose levels between 4.4 and 6.7 mmol/L [80-130 mg/dL] in younger patients without major comorbidities or between 5.6 and 7.8 mmol/L [100- -140 mg/dL] in elderly patients with long-standing DM). At least 4 hours should elapse between a meal and subsequent preprandial measurement. In patients with persistently elevated HbA$_{1c}$ levels despite a single-dose insulin program or doses > 0.5 IU/kg/d, a more complex insulin regimen is frequently needed. Once prandial insulin is added, oral insulin secretagogues should be discontinued.

Patients using a single dose of NPH insulin are instructed to monitor their capillary glucose levels before breakfast and before the evening meal. If blood glucose levels are consistently (eg, for 3 consecutive days) above the individualized target range before breakfast and before the evening meal, the insulin dose should be increased by 10% to 20%. If blood glucose levels are consistently below the individualized target range before breakfast and before the evening meal, the insulin dose should be decreased by 10% to 20%. If unexplained symptomatic hypoglycemia occurs at any time (despite consuming adequate meals), the insulin dose may be too high and therefore should be decreased by 10% to 20%. If blood glucose levels are consistently within the individualized target range at one time of the day but consistently outside the individualized target range at another, the single-dose insulin program likely needs to be changed.

2) **Split-dose intermediate-acting insulin program**: A split-dose intermediate-acting insulin program with NPH insulin twice a day is used by some patients with type 2 DM. Patients following this program take one NPH insulin injection 30 minutes before breakfast and one NPH insulin injection 30 minutes before the evening meal or at bedtime (depending on the patient's sleep habits, early morning hyperglycemia between 2:00 and 8:00—the "dawn phenomenon"—may be better controlled with NPH insulin given at bedtime because to the timing of its peak effect). Capillary blood glucose measurements before breakfast and before the evening meal are required to estimate if the insulin doses are appropriate. For the morning dose adjustments, blood glucose measurements before the evening meal are evaluated. For the evening dose adjustments, blood glucose measurements before breakfast of the following day are evaluated. The insulin doses can be adjusted by 10% to 20% based on personalized preprandial glycemic targets. Patients following this program need a diet that has a consistent amount of carbohydrates and have to eat their meals at about the same time every day.

3) **Split mixed-dose insulin program**: A split mixed-dose insulin program with intermediate-acting insulin (NPH) plus either short-acting insulin (regular) or rapid-acting insulin (aspart, lispro, or glulisine) administered each with breakfast and the evening meal is occasionally used. Before breakfast, patients on this program take an injection of NPH insulin plus an injection of either rapid-acting insulin or short-acting insulin. Before the evening meal, they also get an injection of NPH insulin plus an injection of one of the prandial insulin preparations. Patients are instructed to check their capillary glucose levels before breakfast, before the noon meal, before the evening meal, and at bedtime. They need to follow a diet that has a consistent amount of carbohydrates and eat their main meals at about the same time every day. Glucose measurements before breakfast indicate the effectiveness of the evening-meal NPH insulin administered the previous day. Glucose measurements before the noon meal indicate the effectiveness of the breakfast rapid-acting insulin (or short-acting insulin). Glucose measurements before the evening meal indicate the effectiveness

of the breakfast NPH insulin dose. Glucose measurements before bedtime indicate the effectiveness of the evening-meal prandial insulin. The insulin doses are changed by 10% to 20% during each dose adjustment.

4) **Premixed split-dose insulin program**: In a premixed split-dose insulin program one of the premixed insulin preparations (→Table 2-4) is administered twice a day, before breakfast and before the evening meal. A common practice is to initially give about 60% of the total daily insulin doses in the morning and about 40% in the evening. Patients are instructed to check their capillary blood glucose levels before breakfast, before the noon meal, before the evening meal, and at bedtime. Patients need to follow a diet that has a consistent amount of carbohydrates and eat their main meals at about the same time every day. Hypoglycemia could be the consequence, for example, of skipping or delaying a meal, eating fewer carbohydrates than usual, or doing an unusual amount of physical activity. In this program glucose measurements before the noon meal and before the evening meal indicate the effectiveness of the morning premixed insulin dose. Glucose measurements before bedtime and before breakfast the next day indicate the effectiveness of the evening premixed insulin dose.

If blood glucose values before the noon meal and before the evening meal are both consistently (eg, for 3 consecutive days) above or below the individualized target range, the breakfast premixed insulin dose should be increased or decreased by 10% to 20%. If blood glucose levels are within the goal range either before the noon meal or before the evening meal but outside the goal range at the other time (before the evening meal or before the noon meal), then the premixed split-dose insulin program may need to be changed. If blood glucose values at bedtime and before breakfast the next day are both consistently above or below the individualized target range, the evening-meal premixed insulin dose should be increased or decreased by 10% to 20%. If blood glucose levels are within the goal range either at bedtime or before breakfast the next day but outside the goal range at the other time (before breakfast the next day or at bedtime), then the premixed split-dose insulin program may need to be changed.

5) **Multiple daily injection insulin program**: This is the principal method of treatment of type 1 DM, which is also recommended in patients with type 2 DM who require full insulin replacement and insulin injections 4 times a day. Typically the program consists of a combination of long-acting basal insulin (eg, glargine, detemir, or degludec) given once daily in the morning or evening and rapid-acting insulin (aspart, lispro, or glulisine) with meals 3 times a day. A starting dose in type 2 DM is recommended as either 4 IU or 10% of basal dose at each meal; titration depends on capillary glucose measurements and Hb_{A1c}. This basal-bolus regimen is supplemented by correction scales that add or subtract units to the rapid-acting insulin prandial doses. Patients are instructed to check their capillary blood glucose levels before breakfast, before the noon meal, before the evening meal, and at bedtime. When the dose of a long-acting insulin analogue is appropriate, overnight blood glucose levels (difference between glucose readings at bedtime and before breakfast) should remain stable (eg, not increasing or decreasing >2.2 mmol/L [40 mg/dL]). Postprandial glycemic excursions (high glucose levels that are transitory during a period of time during the day), different levels of physical activity, and effects of prandial insulin are not present overnight; therefore, this period is optimal to assess the basal insulin requirements. If blood glucose levels consistently drop overnight (eg, >2.2 mmol/L [40 mg/dL] between bedtime and breakfast), the dose of the long-acting insulin should be decreased by 10% to 20%. If blood glucose levels consistently rise overnight (eg, >2.2 mmol/L [40 mg/dL] between bedtime and breakfast), the dose of the long-acting insulin should be increased by 10% to 20%.

To adjust the prandial insulin doses, the blood glucose values before the next meal (or at bedtime) should be assessed. Glucose measurements before the noon meal indicate the effectiveness of the breakfast rapid-acting insulin. Glucose measurements before the evening meal indicate the effectiveness of the noon-meal rapid-acting insulin. Glucose measurements before bedtime indicate the effectiveness of the evening-meal rapid-acting insulin. The objective is to keep the preprandial glucose values (typically 80-130 mg/dL) and bedtime glucose values within the individualized glycemic target. Another way to adjust the prandial insulin doses is to check the postprandial glucose levels (1-2 hours after the beginning of a meal) targeting levels <180 mg/dL. However, this approach adds burden to the program by requiring more capillary glucose measurements and is not necessary in the majority of cases. The prandial insulin doses depend on how many carbohydrates are present in diet. Two strategies can be followed when planning the prandial insulin therapy: (a) fixed meal insulin doses following a diet consistent in carbohydrates on consecutive days; (b) carbohydrate counting. For the purpose of carbohydrate counting, the ratio of insulin to grams of carbohydrate (number of grams of carbohydrate covered by 1 IU of rapid-acting insulin) is calculated for each meal. Usually the ratio will be started with 1 IU of insulin for every 15 g of carbohydrate and the scale will be readjusted individually.

6) **Continuous subcutaneous insulin infusion (CSII) or insulin pump therapy**: Insulin pumps are devices designed to administer short-acting or rapid-acting insulin analogues in a subcutaneous infusion, providing both a continuous basal infusion (40%-60% of total daily insulin dose) and mealtime boluses. Insulin pumps allow for programming delivery for multiple basal rates. The dose of prandial boluses is based on the estimated meal carbohydrate content and capillary blood glucose level immediately before each meal. Insulin pumps also have features that allow adjustments for the "residual insulin" action from previous boluses, potentially reducing the risk of hypoglycemia from frequent administration of boluses.

The advantages of insulin pump therapy include fewer injections, possibility of giving very low doses of insulin (doses as low as 0.05 IU can be accurately delivered, a feature particularly useful in small children), possibility of delivering >1 basal rate (useful, eg, for treating the dawn phenomenon or for patients with different basal requirements during periods of intense physical activity), and lifestyle flexibility with respect to eating schedules. There is also evidence indicating that in motivated patients properly trained on pump management skills, CSII can provide better glycemic control and lower risk of severe hypoglycemia. Insulin pump therapy is not recommended for patients who are unwilling or unable to perform a minimum of 4 blood glucose tests per day. CSII requires patient training in the fundamental aspects of intensive insulin therapy, carbohydrate counting, and manipulation of insulin pump settings. Potential risks associated with insulin pump therapy include blockage or leakage of the system (leading to rapid hyperglycemia and potentially DKA in patients with type 1 DM), infections at the site of infusion, and hypoglycemia (eg, if the basal insulin dose is too high and the patient skips a meal). Another disadvantage is the high cost of the pump and supplies.

Continuous glucose monitoring (CGM) systems measure the interstitial fluid glucose level, which is generally within 15% to 20% of the capillary glucose concentration, and provide semicontinuous real-time information about glucose levels that identifies fluctuations difficult to assess with conventional capillary blood glucose self-monitoring. These systems are now commonly used in conjunction with CSII (a sensor-augmented insulin pump) to provide more detailed information about the patients' glycemic patterns (eg, average glucose, percentage of hypoglycemic and target ranges). CGM systems can play a valuable role in the management of patients with hypoglycemia unawareness and hyperglycemic excursions and are highly recommended in children and adolescents with type 1 DM. There are also other devices that allow measuring of the glucose levels intermittently but they lack alarms and glucose measurements are only obtained on demand. Some sensor-augmented pumps can be programmed to interrupt insulin delivery for up to 2 hours at a preset sensor glucose value (the threshold-suspend feature). This feature can reduce the frequency of nocturnal hypoglycemia and severe hypoglycemia without increasing HbA_{1c} values or causing DKA. Patients considering using a CGM device should be willing to perform frequent capillary blood glucose measurements and to calibrate the system daily.

Overall, CSII (particularly sensor-augmented insulin pumps with threshold-suspend feature) should be offered to individuals with type 1 DM in whom there is concern about hypoglycemia unawareness or high risk for severe hypoglycemia, ✓⊖ to patients requiring very low doses of insulin that cannot be given by syringes or pens, or to those who wish a tighter glycemic control with more flexible eating schedules.⊘⊖ All such patients should be willing and able to learn the complexities of CSII therapy and follow closely their glycemic patterns.

Pharmacotherapy: Oral Antidiabetic Agents

1. When choosing an antidiabetic medication for patients with type 2 DM, the glucose-lowering efficacy, safety profile, tolerability, convenience, patient preferences, comorbidities, concurrently used drugs, adverse effects, and costs of available agents should be considered. The effect on weight and the risk of causing hypoglycemia are also important to review. As demonstrated by the most recent evidence, the reduction in mortality, CVD, heart failure, and progression of kidney disease are additional factors that should be considered in the initial selection of treatment.

2. A patient-centered approach with shared decision-making is recommended. Although there are uncertainties regarding the best choice and sequence of therapy, the general consensus is that metformin should be used as the initial drug for treatment of type 2 DM if there are no contraindications (eg, advanced renal failure).⊘⊖ Metformin has a relatively strong glucose-lowering effect, possible cardiovascular benefits, proven long-term safety, and is widely available at a low cost.

3. In patients with type 2 DM progression or in whom metformin alone is contraindicated or has failed to meet the individualized glycemic targets, a stepwise therapy with the addition of other oral or injectable medications (including insulin) is frequently needed. Treatment should be individualized on a case-by-case basis rather than by applying one possible algorithm rigidly. The benefits and downsides of each medication should be evaluated in the specific context of each patient. Dosage, mechanism of action, advantages, and disadvantages of available antidiabetic agents: →Table 2-5.

4. In patients with established CVD, ≥2 cardiovascular risk factors, and/or diabetic kidney disease, the use of an SGLT-2 inhibitor or GLP-1 receptor agonist with proven cardiovascular benefits and reduction of kidney disease progression should be considered as part of the therapeutic plan. SGLT-2 inhibitors should be specifically recommended in the setting of atherosclerotic CVD and heart failure. The renal outcome benefit is most pronounced with the use of SGLT-2 inhibitors.

5. Shared decision-making tools have been developed and can be used as aids that enable conversations resulting in DM treatment regimens consistent with patients' preferences and values.

6. Do not delay insulin therapy in patients in whom it is indicated.

7. Always adjust doses of oral antidiabetic agents to achieve glycemic targets. Dose adjustment is also recommended to avoid hyperglycemia when adding a new agent to a regimen containing insulin, sulfonylurea or glinide therapy, particularly in patients at or near glycemic goals (→Follow-Up, below).

Table 2-5. Antidiabetic agents

Biguanides

Drug and dosage	**Metformin**: Initially 500 or 850 mg PO once daily taken with largest meal. Dose increased by 500 mg/wk up to the usual dose of 1000 mg bid or 850 mg tid (with meals). Max dose 2550 mg/d
Comments[a]	**Mechanism of action**: ↓ liver production of glucose **Efficacy**[b]: HbA$_{1c}$ ↓ 1%-2% **Contraindications**: Renal failure with GFR <30 mL/min (or serum creatinine ≥132.6 µmol/L [1.5 mg/dL] in men or ≥123.8 µmol/L [1.4 mg/dL] in women according to manufacturer), severe hepatic dysfunction, decompensated or advanced HF, acidosis, hypoxia, shock, history of severe hypersensitivity to metformin **Frequent adverse effects**: Diarrhea, nausea, vomiting, bloating, abdominal cramping, metallic taste **Rare adverse effects**: Lactic acidosis **Risk of hypoglycemia**: No if monotherapy **Effect on weight**: Neutral or modest weight loss **Miscellaneous advantages**: Extensive experience, low cost **Miscellaneous disadvantages**: Can cause vitamin B$_{12}$ deficiency. Manufacturer recommends temporarily discontinuing metformin in patients undergoing radiologic studies where intravascular iodinated contrast media are used **Other comments**: GI adverse effects more frequent early in the course of treatment. Extended-release metformin may be better tolerated in patients with GI adverse effects. Elderly patients should not be titrated to max dose. Careful use in patients ≥80 years (normal renal function has to be established)

Sulfonylureas

Drug and dosage	**Glipizide**: 2.5-20 mg PO once daily. Doses >15 mg/d should be administered in 2 divided doses. Immediate-release tablets should be administered 30 min before meals (typically before breakfast if once daily); extended-release tablets should be given with breakfast. Titrate in 2.5-5 mg increments. Max recommended dose 20 mg/d **Glimepiride**: 1-8 mg PO once daily. Administer once daily with breakfast or first main meal of the day. Titrate in 1-2 mg increments. Max recommended dose 8 mg/d **Glyburide (INN glibenclamide)**: 1.25-20 mg PO once daily. Patients receiving >10 mg daily may have more satisfactory response with bid dosing. Administer with meals (typically before breakfast or first main meal of the day if once daily). Titrate in 1.25-2.5 mg increments. Max recommended dose 20 mg/d **Micronized glyburide** (greater bioavailability): 0.75-12 mg PO once daily. Patients receiving >6 mg daily may have more satisfactory response with bid dosing. Administer with meals (typically before breakfast or first main meal of the day if once daily). Titrate in 0.75-1.5 mg increments. Max recommended dose 12 mg/d **Gliclazide**: 80-320 mg/d in 2 divided doses, 30 min before meals. Modified-release tablets 30 mg once daily (with breakfast). Increase dose (by 30 mg every 2 weeks) up to max of 120 mg/d
Comments[a]	**Mechanism of action**: Closes KATP channels on β-cell plasma membranes. ↑ insulin secretion **Efficacy**[b]: HbA$_{1c}$ ↓ 1%-2% **Contraindications**: History of severe hypersensitivity reactions **Frequent adverse effects**: Lack of energy and strength **Rare adverse effects**: Diarrhea, nausea, constipation, flatulence, dizziness, headaches **Risk of hypoglycemia**: Present, particularly in the elderly, with strenuous exercise, or due to interactions with other drugs (eg, sulfonamides, alcohol) **Effect on weight**: Modest gain

Miscellaneous advantages: Extensive experience, low cost

Miscellaneous disadvantages: Failure rate may exceed other drugs (this is attributed to exacerbation of islet dysfunction)

Other comments: Reduces postprandial glucose excursions. Usually start with lowest dose and increase every 1-2 weeks based on blood glucose. Patients with decreased caloric intake or fasting may need doses held to avoid hypoglycemia. Long-acting sulfonylureas (eg, glyburide) may be associated with higher risk of hypoglycemia than short-acting sulfonylureas (eg, glipizide, glimepiride)

Meglitinides (glinides)

Drug and dosage	**Repaglinide:** 0.5-4 mg PO 1-30 min before each meal 2, 3, or 4 times/d based on meal pattern. Titrate in 1-2 mg increments weekly. Max recommended dose 16 mg/d **Nateglinide:** 60-120 mg PO 1-30 min before each meal 2, 3, or 4 times/d based on meal pattern
Comments[a]	**Mechanism of action:** Closes KATP channels on β-cell plasma membranes. ↑ insulin secretion **Efficacy[b]:** HbA$_{1c}$ ↓ 1%-2% **Contraindications:** History of severe hypersensitivity reactions **Frequent adverse effects:** Headaches **Rare adverse effects:** Diarrhea, arthralgias **Risk of hypoglycemia:** Present (possibly smaller than with sulfonylureas) **Effect on weight:** Modest gain **Miscellaneous advantages:** Both can be used in patients allergic to sulfonylureas. Short duration of action allows dosing flexibility **Miscellaneous disadvantages:** Tid dosing, expensive **Other comments:** Reduces postprandial glucose excursions. Repaglinide is more effective at lowering HbA$_{1c}$ than nateglinide. Repaglinide is principally metabolized by liver with <10% excreted by kidneys (dose adjustments not typically required in patients with renal insufficiency). Nateglinide has active metabolites excreted by kidneys and should be used with caution in renal insufficiency. If patient misses a meal, glinides should not be administered to avoid hypoglycemia

α-Glucosidase inhibitors

Drug and dosage	**Acarbose:** Initially 25 mg PO tid immediately before main meals (some patients benefit from starting with 25 mg once daily with gradual titration to 25 mg tid to reduce GI adverse effects). Dose may be increased every 2-4 weeks. Max dose 50 mg tid (≤60 kg) or 100 mg tid (>60 kg)
Comments[a]	**Mechanism of action:** Inhibits intestinal α-glucosidase and slows down the final enzymatic stage of intestinal digestion of polysaccharides, oligosaccharides, and some disaccharides (maltose and sucrose) **Efficacy[b]:** HbA$_{1c}$ ↓ 0.5%-1% (mainly ↓ postprandial glucose levels) **Contraindications:** History of severe hypersensitivity reactions, IBD, colonic ulceration, conditions that may deteriorate due to increased intestinal gas formation, predisposition to intestinal obstruction, partial intestinal obstruction, cirrhosis, renal impairment (serum creatinine >2 mg/dL) **Frequent adverse effects:** Flatulence, diarrhea, abdominal pain **Rare adverse effects:** Ileus, hepatotoxicity **Risk of hypoglycemia:** No if monotherapy **Effect on weight:** Neutral **Miscellaneous advantages:** No systemic effects **Miscellaneous disadvantages:** Frequent GI adverse effects; frequent dosing; expensive **Other comments:** Reduces postprandial glucose excursions. In case of hypoglycemia (eg, concomitant use of sulfonylureas), glucose (dextrose) recommended for treatment. GI adverse effects may be decreased by restricting dietary sucrose (table sugar)

Thiazolidinediones (TZD)

Drug and dosage	**Pioglitazone:** 15-30 mg PO once daily, administered without regard to meals. Dose can be increased in 15 mg increments with careful monitoring of adverse effects (eg, weight gain, edema, symptoms of heart failure). Max dose 45 mg once daily
	Rosiglitazone: 4 mg PO once daily or in divided doses bid, administered without regard to meals. Dose can be increased up to 8 mg daily, as a single daily dose or in divided doses bid. Max dose 8 mg/d
Comments[a]	**Mechanism of action:** Activates the nuclear transcription factor PPAR-γ, ↑ insulin sensitivity
	Efficacy[b]: HbA$_{1c}$ ↓ 0.5%-1.5%
	Contraindications: History of severe hypersensitivity reactions, HF, serious hepatic impairment, active bladder cancer, history of bladder cancer; uninvestigated macroscopic hematuria, pregnancy
	Frequent adverse effects: Edema, headaches
	Rare adverse effects: HF exacerbation, bone fractures, anemia, possibly ischemic heart disease (rosiglitazone), possibly bladder cancer (pioglitazone)
	Risk of hypoglycemia: No if monotherapy
	Effect on weight: Modest gain
	Miscellaneous advantages: Effectiveness may be more durable than sulfonylureas and metformin. ↑ HDL-C, ↓ triglycerides
	Miscellaneous disadvantages: Rosiglitazone may ↑ LDL-C and is expensive
	Other comments: Limit max dose of pioglitazone to 15 mg/d—and consider dose reduction of rosiglitazone—when used in combination with strong CYP2C8 inhibitors (eg, gemfibrozil)

Dipeptidyl peptidase-4 (DPP-4) inhibitors (gliptins)

Drug and dosage	**Sitagliptin:** 100 mg PO once daily. Administer with or without food. If eGFR 30-50 mL/min, dose 50 mg once daily; if eGFR is <30 mL/min, dose 25 mg once daily
	Linagliptin: 5 mg PO once daily. Administer with or without food. No dosage adjustment necessary for renal impairment
	Saxagliptin: 2.5-5 mg PO once daily. Administer with or without food. If eGFR is ≤50 mL/min, dose 2.5 mg once daily. If concomitant use of strong CYP3A4/5 inhibitors, dose 2.5 mg once daily
	Alogliptin: 25 mg PO once daily. Administer with or without food. If eGFR is 30-60 mL/min, dose 12.5 mg once daily. If eGFR is <30 mL/min, dose 6.25 mg once daily
Comments[a]	**Mechanism of action:** Inhibition of DPP-4 activity leads to ↑ endogenous incretins (GLP-1 and GIP) after meals, ↑ glucose-dependent insulin secretion
	Efficacy[b]: HbA$_{1c}$ ↓ 0.5%-0.8%
	Contraindications: History of severe hypersensitivity reactions
	Frequent adverse effects: Generally well tolerated
	Rare adverse effects: Headaches, nausea, possibly pancreatitis
	Risk of hypoglycemia: No if monotherapy
	Effect on weight: Neutral
	Miscellaneous advantages: Can be used in patients with advance renal disease
	Miscellaneous disadvantages: Modest glucose-lowering efficacy, expensive
	Other comments: Limited long-term safety data. Saxagliptin may increase risk of HF

Glucagon-like peptide 1 (GLP-1) agonists

Drug and dosage

Exenatide: Immediate release: Initial dose 5 µg SC bid within 60 min prior to 2 main meals (≥6 h apart). After 1 month dose may be increased to 10 µg bid. Extended release: 2 mg once weekly without regard to meals or time of day. Rotate injection sites weekly

Liraglutide: Initial dose 0.6 mg SC once daily for 1 week (dose intended to reduce GI symptoms but ineffective for glycemic control), then increase to 1.2 mg once daily. Dose may be increased to 1.8 mg once daily. Administer without regard to meals or time of day

Albiglutide: 30 mg SC once weekly. Dose may be increased to 50 mg once weekly. Administer without regard to meals or time of day. Rotate injection sites weekly

Dulaglutide: 0.75 mg SC once weekly. Dose may be increased to 1.5 mg once weekly. Administer without regard to meals or time of day. Rotate injection sites weekly

Lixisenatide: Initial dose 10 µg once daily for 14 days; on day15 increase to 20 µg once daily. Maintenance dose 20 µg once daily. If dose is missed, administer within an hour of next meal

Semaglutide: Initial dose 0.25 mg once weekly for 4 weeks. Increase to 0.5 mg once weekly for ≥4 weeks. If further glycemic control necessary, increase to max 1 mg once weekly

Comments[a]

Mechanism of action: Stimulation of GLP-1 receptors leads to ↑ glucose-dependent insulin secretion; ↓ glucagon secretion; slow gastric emptying; ↑ satiety

Efficacy[b]: HbA_{1c} ↓ 0.5%-1.5%

Proven CV benefit: Only liraglutide; semaglutide may be considered as it was shown to reduce MACE but at expense of stroke reduction rather than CV death. No CV benefit demonstrated with exenatide or lixisenatide

Reduction of CKD progression: Liraglutide and semaglutide

Contraindications: History of severe hypersensitivity reactions, history of pancreatitis, severe GI disease (eg, gastroparesis), history or family history of medullary thyroid carcinoma or MEN syndrome type 2; caution with severe renal impairment (exenatide contraindicated if eGFR <30 mL/min)

Frequent adverse effects: Nausea, vomiting, diarrhea, injection site reactions (eg, pruritus, swelling), headaches, dizziness, nervousness

Rare adverse effects: Possibly pancreatitis, possibly pancreatic cancer

Risk of hypoglycemia: No if monotherapy

Effect on weight: Modest to significant weight loss

Miscellaneous advantages: Once-weekly preparations can reduce treatment burden

Miscellaneous disadvantages: Injectable medications, expensive

Other comments: GI adverse effects more frequent early in the course of treatment. Administer SC injections in upper arm, thigh, or abdomen. Some patients develop high titers of antibodies that may ↓ glycemic response. Limited long-term safety data

Sodium-glucose cotransporter 2 (SGLT-2) inhibitors (flozins)

Drug and dosage

Canagliflozin: 100 mg PO once daily before first meal of day. Dose may be increased to 300 mg once daily. If eGFR is 45-59 mL/min, dose 100 mg once daily. Has also inhibitory effect on SGLT-1

Dapagliflozin: 5 mg PO once daily. Administer in the morning with or without food. Dose may be increased to 10 mg once daily

Empagliflozin: 10 mg PO once daily, may be increased to 25 mg

Sotagliflozin: Currently an investigational drug, under regulatory review by EMA and FDA for treatment of both type 1 and 2 DM. Has also inhibitory effect on SGLT-1

Comments[a] **Mechanism of action:** Promote renal excretion of glucose

Efficacy[b]: HbA$_{1c}$ ↓ 0.5%-0.8%

Proven CV benefit: Empagliflozin, canagliflozin, and dapagliflozin; empagliflozin has modestly stronger benefit

Reduction of CKD progression: Canagliflozin, dapagliflozin, and empagliflozin

Contraindications: History of severe hypersensitivity reactions, severe renal impairment (canagliflozin, GFR <45 mL/min, dapagliflozin, GFR <30 mL/min), severe hepatic impairment, active bladder cancer

Frequent adverse effects: Vulvovaginal candidiasis, urinary frequency, polyuria

Rare adverse effects: Urinary tract infections, symptomatic hypotension (particularly in the elderly), hyperkalemia

Risk of hypoglycemia: No if monotherapy

Effect on weight: Modest weight loss

Miscellaneous advantages: Can decrease blood pressure. Empagliflozin has been shown to reduce mortality among patients with type 2 DM at high risk of CV events

Miscellaneous disadvantages: Uncertain long-term effect of chronic glycosuria, modest glucose-lowering efficacy, expensive, LDL-C levels may increase, careful use in conditions associated with risk of dehydration

Other comments: Correct volume depletion prior to administration. Limited long-term safety data. May reduce postprandial hyperglycemia by delaying intestinal glucose absorption

Warning: Recent FDA review applied to all sodium-glucose cotransporter-2 inhibitors pointed to risk of ketoacidosis and serious urinary tract infections (fewer than 100 cases reported over >1 year)

---

[a] Adapted from the American Diabetes Association and the European Association for the Study of Diabetes 2012 position statement.

[b] Predicted reduction of HbA$_{1c}$ levels with monotherapy (expressed in percentage points).

↑, increase; ↓, decrease; bid, 2 times a day; CKD, chronic kidney disease; CV, cardiovascular; DM, diabetes mellitus; eGFR, estimated glomerular filtration rate; EMA, European Medicines Agency; FDA, US Food and Drug Administration; GFR, glomerular filtration rate; GI, gastrointestinal; GIP, glucose-dependent insulinotropic polypeptide; GLP-1, glucagon-like peptide-1; HbA$_{1c}$, hemoglobin A1c; HDL-C, high-density lipoprotein cholesterol; HF, heart failure; IBD, inflammatory bowel disease; INN, international nonproprietary name; LDL-C, low-density lipoprotein cholesterol; MACE, major adverse cardiovascular events; MEN, multiple endocrine neoplasia; PO, oral administration; PPAR-γ, peroxisome proliferator-activated receptor γ; tid, 3 times a day.

Management of Hypoglycemia

Hypoglycemia is defined by blood glucose levels <3.9 mmol/L (70 mg/dL). Its severity is further classified as **level 1** (≥3.0 mmol/L [54 mg/dL]), **level 2** (<3.0 mmol/L [54 mg/dL]; sufficiently low to indicate serious, clinically important hypoglycemia), and **level 3** (altered mental and/or physical status requiring assistance of a third party for recovery; →Chapter 5.2.1.1.2). Patients with DM should learn to recognize the symptoms of hypoglycemia (eg, sweating, tremors, weakness, hunger) and learn how to treat it. The "rule of 15" can be used to treat conscious patients with level 1 or level 2 hypoglycemia:

1) Check the capillary glucose level immediately when there are symptoms of hypoglycemia.

2) If the patient is awake and able to swallow, treat with 15 g of carbohydrates (eg, 4 glucose tablets [4 g each], 100 to 125 mL of fruit juice, 1 tablespoon of sugar or syrup).

3) Wait 15 minutes and recheck the blood glucose level.

4) If the capillary blood glucose level remains low or if there are still symptoms of hypoglycemia, treat the patient again with 15 g of carbohydrates and

continue to recheck the capillary glucose levels until the target glucose levels are reached and symptoms resolve.

In patients with level 3 hypoglycemia and those who are unwilling or unable to swallow, treatment with IV glucose and/or a glucagon injection should be provided immediately.

Patients with DM receiving insulin therapy with a history of level 2 hypoglycemia should have a glucagon injection available (→Chapter 5.2.1.1.2).

Serious Intercurrent Illness and Sick-Day Guidelines

Acute illnesses frequently lead to worsening of hyperglycemia and increased insulin requirements. Patients with type 1 or type 2 DM following a multiple daily injection insulin program likely benefit from learning management strategies that can be applied during acute sickness ("sick-day guidelines"). These strategies include monitoring blood glucose levels more frequently, keeping good hydration, avoiding exercise as it may worsen hyperglycemia, checking for urine ketones if there is severe and persistent hyperglycemia, using extra doses of rapid-acting insulin to temporarily correct hyperglycemia—"insulin supplements"—and knowledge of when to contact health-care providers.

Alternative Treatment Methods

1. Whole pancreas transplantation is most frequently used in patients with renal failure in whom pancreas transplantation is combined with kidney transplantation.

2. Pancreatic islet transplantation is associated with lower risk than whole pancreas transplantation and allows for the normalization of blood glucose levels. Its use is limited by poor graft survival.

→ FOLLOW-UP

1. Glycemic control: The ADA recommends checking HbA_{1c} levels based on clinical situation. For patients with well-controlled DM, testing twice per year is appropriate. For unstable or highly intensively managed patients, testing every 3 months is appropriate.

2. Screening for hypertension: The ADA advises to measure blood pressure at every routine medical visit. Elevated values should be confirmed on a separate day.

3. Screening for dyslipidemia: The ADA recommends to measure the fasting lipid profile at least annually in most adult patients with DM but suggests postponing lipid assessment for 2 years in adults with low-risk lipid values (low-density lipoprotein cholesterol [LDL-C] <2.6 mmol/L [100 mg/dL], HDL-C >2.8 mmol/L [50 mg/dL], and triglycerides <8.3 mmol/L [150 mg/dL]).

4. Screening for chronic complications of DM:

1) **Nephropathy**: The ADA advises performing an annual test to quantitate urine albumin excretion in patients with type 1 DM lasting ≥5 years, and in all patients with type 2 DM since the time of diagnosis. Serum creatinine with estimated glomerular filtration rate should also be measured at least annually.

2) **Retinopathy**: The ADA recommends that patients with type 1 DM should have an initial dilated and comprehensive eye examination by an ophthalmologist or optometrist within 5 years after the onset of DM. In patients with type 2 DM this should be done shortly after the diagnosis of DM. If there is no evidence of retinopathy for ≥1 eye examination, then examinations every 2 years may be considered. If diabetic retinopathy is present, subsequent examinations should be repeated at least annually or more frequently as per ophthalmologic recommendations.

3) **Diabetic foot complications**: The International Working Group on Diabetic Foot Editorial Board and the ADA recommend that all patients with DM

should have a thorough foot examination at least once annually, and more frequently if high-risk foot conditions (eg, diabetic peripheral neuropathy, foot deformities, or peripheral artery disease) are identified. The ADA also advises that visual inspection of the feet should be performed at every health-care visit.

→ PREVENTION

1. Type 1 DM: There are no effective methods of prevention.

2. Type 2 DM: Effective preventive measures include a healthy diet and increased physical activity to reduce excessive weight and maintain appropriate body weight. Metformin can reduce the risk of progression of prediabetes to DM and therefore could be considered in this situation.

2.1. Complications of Diabetes Mellitus

2.1.1. Acute Complications of Diabetes Mellitus

2.1.1.1. Diabetic Ketoacidosis

→ DEFINITION, ETIOLOGY, PATHOGENESIS

Diabetic ketoacidosis (DKA) is an acute life-threatening syndrome of metabolic disturbances involving carbohydrate, fat, and protein metabolism as well as the water-electrolyte and acid-base balances that result from an acute severe insulin deficiency or insulin resistance and an elevation in the levels of counterregulatory hormones, such as glucagon, catecholamines, cortisol, and growth hormone; in particular, glucagon is elevated due to the absence of the normal suppressive effect of insulin. A typical feature is the triad of hyperglycemia, elevated anion gap metabolic acidosis, and serum and urine ketone bodies (eg, acetoacetic acid, acetone, and β-hydroxybutyric acid). DKA has been characteristically described as a feature of type 1 diabetes mellitus (many times in new-onset diabetes); however, patients with type 2 diabetes and any other type of diabetes may develop DKA.

Regarding DKA pathogenesis, insulin deficiency or severe resistance results in excessive glucose production through hepatic gluconeogenesis and increased lipolysis, which leads to the production of ketone bodies. This in turn causes hyperglycemia, urinary glucose loss, osmotic diuresis, dehydration, electrolyte disturbances (particularly hyperkalemia with coexisting intracellular potassium deficiency), and elevated anion gap metabolic acidosis. DKA is also considered a proinflammatory state in which tumor necrosis factor α, interleukin (IL) 1, IL-6, IL-8, and reactive oxygen species are generated.

Precipitating factors include interruption of insulin therapy (eg, due to a gastrointestinal disease resulting in fasting) or inappropriate insulin use (most common cause in type 1 diabetes mellitus), infections (bacterial, viral, or fungal; most common cause in type 2 diabetes), acute cardiovascular events (myocardial infarction, stroke), delayed diagnosis of type 1 diabetes, acute pancreatitis, alcohol abuse, drugs (glucocorticoids, high-dose thiazide diuretics), and any conditions causing a sudden increase in insulin requirements (eg, sepsis, surgery).

→ CLINICAL FEATURES

1. Symptoms: Excessive thirst (polydipsia), dry mouth, polyuria, polyphagia, weakness, fatigue and somnolence, altered mental status to coma, vertigo, headache, nausea, vomiting, abdominal and/or chest pain (the latter usually associated with DKA severity).

Table 2-6. Diagnostic criteria of diabetic ketoacidosis

	Mild	Moderate	Severe
Blood glucose level in mmol/L (mg/dL)	>13.9 (>250)	>13.9 (>250)	>13.9 (>250)
Arterial blood pH	7.25-7.30	7.00-7.24	<7.0
Serum bicarbonate level (mmol/L)	15-18	10-15	<10
Urine and serum ketones	Present	Present	Present
Anion gap (mmol/L)	>10	>12	>12
Altered mental status	Alert	Alert/drowsy	Stupor/coma

2. Signs: Hypotension, tachycardia, rapid and deep and then shallow breathing (Kussmaul breathing), features of dehydration (weight loss, reduced skin turgor), hyporeflexia, odor of acetone on patient's breath, facial redness, reduced eyeball turgor, abdominal guarding (similar to peritonitis).

An important feature of DKA is that all symptoms evolve rapidly (usually within 24 hours).

→ DIAGNOSIS

Initial evaluation:

1) Airway, breathing, circulation status (volume status), and mental status.
2) Fingerstick glucose levels (later confirmed with a plasma glucose test).
3) Arterial blood gases (usually including bicarbonate and lactate levels).
4) Electrocardiogram.
5) Complete blood count with differential count, serum electrolytes (sodium, potassium, and chlorine), blood urine nitrogen, and creatinine.
6) Serum and urine ketones.
7) Urinalysis.
8) Effective plasma osmolality calculated as:

Effective $P_{osm} = (2 \times Na\,[mEq/L]) + (glucose\,[mmol/L\ or\ \{mg/dL \div 18\}])$

Additional tests, such as chest and/or abdominal radiographs; amylase/lipase; computed tomography of the head; and cultures of urine, sputum, and blood may be evaluated, depending on the particular case.

The diagnosis of DKA and assessment of its severity are based on laboratory test results (→Table 2-6).

Differential Diagnosis

Starvation ketosis (hyperglycemia is absent), alcoholic ketoacidosis (blood glucose levels are rarely >13.9 mmol/L [250 mg/dL], bicarbonate levels ≥18 mmol/L), lactic acidosis (blood glucose levels are not severely increased, symptoms of shock are the dominant features; elevated serum lactate levels [some moderate lactate elevation may be observed in DKA]), coma (uremic, hepatic, and cerebral coma; these may sometimes be accompanied by elevated blood glucose levels), nonrespiratory acidosis with a high anion gap >20 mEq/L (poisonings with ethylene glycol, methyl alcohol, paraldehyde, or salicylates).

With the development of new antihyperglycemic drugs, such as sodium glucose cotransporter-2 (SGLT-2) inhibitors, one of differential diagnoses to be considered is euglycemic DKA. This condition has been reported in patients with type 1 and type 2 diabetes mellitus, being more prevalent in type 1 diabetes.

The risk factors for the development of euglycemic DKA include reduction or discontinuation of insulin, major surgery, alcohol consumption, and low--carbohydrate diet. Although this is a potential risk with the use of SLGT-2 inhibitors, the 2016 position statement from the American Association of Clinical Endocrinologists and American College of Endocrinology remarks that the risk-benefit ratio is in favor of continued use.

→ TREATMENT

1. Fluid replacement: Large volumes of isotonic IV fluids is the mainstay therapy. The exact amount may depend on the resolution of metabolic abnormalities (particularly the anion gap) and severity of dehydration.

The fluid administered initially in most cases is 0.9% saline but balanced solutions or 0.45% saline may also be used. The choice may depend on the progression and resolution of electrolyte abnormalities, especially hyperchloremia. The aggressiveness of fluid replacement therapy will depend on the patient's hemodynamics: state of hydration, serum electrolyte levels, and urinary output. One of the reasonable regimens, initiated while monitoring volume status and metabolic parameters, may start in the following way (following fluid balance may be more important than absolute infusion rates, as urine output may exceed the infusion rate):

1) Administer 1000 mL of 0.9% saline IV over the first hour, or at a rate of 15 to 20 mL/kg/h.

2) Administer 500 mL/h of 0.9% saline IV (or a balanced solution) over the following 4 to 6 hours.

3) Then administer 0.9% saline (or a balanced solution) as an IV infusion at a rate of 250 mL/h until the normalization of acid-base homeostasis.

4) When the blood glucose level decreases <11.1 mmol/L (200 mg/dL), add an IV infusion of 5% glucose (dextrose) to maintain serum glucose between 8.3 and 11.1 mmol/L (150-200 mg/dL) until ketoacidosis resolves.

5) After adding the glucose infusion, reduce the rate of the 0.9% saline and 5% glucose IV infusion to 150 mL/h.

6) Once the serum sodium results are available, in patients with normal to high corrected serum sodium levels, a 0.45% saline infusion can be used until hypernatremia is controlled (the actual serum sodium level may be calculated by adding 1.6 mEq/L to the measured serum sodium level for every 5.6 mmol/L [100 mg/dL] of blood glucose over 5.6 mmol/L [100 mg/dL]); more recent studies suggest that the correction factor is closer to 2.4 mEq/L. If 0.45% saline is not available, you can connect 2 infusion sets to one IV catheter: one with 0.9% saline and another with hyponatremic solution (2/3/1/3; sterile water) for IV infusion and administer both fluids at the same rate. Another option is to take away 500 mL of the 0.9% infusion and add 500 mL of sterile water to the remaining 500 mL of the 0.9% saline infusion. In patients with low corrected serum sodium levels, use 0.9% saline.

2. Reduce hyperglycemia: Start IV insulin (use a short-acting insulin):

1) Start from an IV bolus injection of 0.1 IU/kg and immediately follow with a continuous IV infusion at a rate of ~ 0.1 IU/kg/h (usually 4-8 IU/h) and monitor blood glucose levels frequently (as often as hourly).⊘◯

2) Alternatively, start directly (without the bolus) with an IV continuous insulin infusion at a rate of ~0.14 IU/kg/h.

3) Adjust the insulin dose to maintain a constant rate of blood glucose reduction by 2.7 to 4.1 mmol/L/h (50-75 mg/dL/h, or 10% per hour) not exceeding 5.6 mmol/L/h (100 mg/dL/h). If the expected reduction in the blood glucose level is not achieved within 1 hour, give an insulin bolus of 0.14 IU/kg and return to the previous rate of insulin infusion. Then reassess the treatment effect hourly and adjust the insulin dose as appropriate.

4) Once the serum glucose level reaches 11.1 mmol/L (200 mg/dL), reduce the infusion rate of IV insulin to 0.02 to 0.05 IU/kg/h and maintain serum glucose between 8.3 and 11.1 mmol/L (150-200 mg/dL) until DKA resolves.

5) To switch from the IV infusion to a subcutaneous insulin regimen, you may start the latter in insulin-naive patients with a dose of 0.5 to 0.8 IU/kg/d of human insulin (two-thirds of insulin isophane [NPH] and one-third of regular insulin), maintaining the insulin infusion for 1 to 2 hours after the subcutaneous regimen begins and the patient has eaten. In patients previously treated with insulin, a prior insulin regimen can be restarted.

3. Correct potassium deficit (approximate doses of replacements may differ markedly in individual patients, especially in those with impaired renal function). The treatment goal is to maintain potassium levels within 4.0 to 5.0 mEq/L:

1) In patients with serum potassium levels between 3.3 and 5.2 mEq/L, give 20 to 30 mEq per each liter of IV fluid to keep serum potassium levels in the range of 4.0 to 5.0 mEq/L.

2) In patients with serum potassium levels <3.3 mEq/L, you may decrease the insulin infusion and administer 20 to 30 mEq/h until the serum potassium level is >3.3 mEq/L.

3) In patients with serum potassium levels >5.2 mEq/L, do not administer potassium but check the serum potassium level every 2 hours. Note that potassium deficit becomes apparent with continued insulin therapy and worsens with an increase in pH (remember about potassium administration once acidosis is controlled, particularly if sodium bicarbonate is used).

4. Control acidosis:

1) Mild and moderate acidosis is gradually controlled with fluid replacement, insulin administration, and correction of water-electrolyte abnormalities.

2) Severe metabolic acidosis (with a pH level <6.9) may lead to impaired myocardial contractility, cerebral vasodilatation and coma, and several gastrointestinal complications; therefore, administration of IV sodium bicarbonate in this situation may be considered.⊘⊙ Sodium bicarbonate use is open to debate and some (including some reviewers of this chapter) suggest not to use it at all. Our pattern is to administer it only in patients with an arterial blood pH <6.9. In these patients, 100 mmol of bicarbonate is infused in 400 mL of sterile water with 20 mEq of potassium chloride at an infusion rate of 200 mL/h every 2 hours until pH is >7.0. Monitor potassium levels every 2 hours, as they can decrease dangerously with the infusion.

5. Monitor and correct hypophosphatemia, especially if severe (<0.5 mmol/L). As with potassium, correction of acidosis may lead to rapid unmasking of hypophosphatemia.

6. Look for an underlying condition and start appropriate treatment (eg, antimicrobial therapy in case of infection; usually suspected with leukocytosis with cell counts >25,000 mm^3).

⇥ FOLLOW-UP

The following points present our suggested pattern of practice.

1) If feasible, **as often as every 1 hour** monitor blood pressure, pulse rate, respiratory rate, mental status, capillary blood or plasma glucose levels, and fluid balance.

2) **Every 2 to 4 hours** monitor the serum potassium level and arterial blood gases. **Every 4 hours** monitor serum sodium, chloride, and (less importantly) ketone levels (β-hydroxybutyrate), as well as phosphate and calcium levels (these may be monitored less often if the values are within the reference range or normalizing).

3) Monitor body weight and temperature as needed.

4) **When the patient has voided**, urinary ketone and glucose levels may be assessed (however, if judged important, the most accurate method of monitoring DKA is the quantitative determination of blood β-hydroxybutyrate levels).

→ COMPLICATIONS

In the course of treatment of DKA and coma, the following **adverse events** may occur:

1) Sudden hypokalemia.

2) Hypernatremia that may contribute to lung edema with respiratory failure and to brain edema (brain edema may be caused by an excessively rapid reduction of blood glucose levels).

3) Hyperglycemia due to premature discontinuation of insulin infusion.

4) Hypoglycemia (most common complication).

5) Hyperchloremic metabolic acidosis (with a normal anion gap) caused by an excessive saline intake.

6) Hypophosphatemia.

7) Renal failure.

8) Thromboembolic complications.

2.1.1.2. Drug-Induced Hypoglycemia

→ DEFINITION AND ETIOLOGY

Drug-induced hypoglycemia is a **plasma glucose level <3.9 mmol/L (70 mg/dL)** regardless of symptoms of hypoglycemia. Symptoms may first appear in patients with lower blood glucose levels (eg, in those with long-standing well-controlled type 1 diabetes mellitus [hypoglycemia unawareness]) or in patients with blood glucose levels still >5.6 mmol/L (100 mg/dL) when the level has rapidly decreased.

Hypoglycemia is an important treatment-related complication of diabetes mellitus to take into account. Repeated episodes of hypoglycemia increase the risk of cardiovascular and all-cause mortality, both in patients with type 1 and type 2 diabetes.

Causes:

1) An excessively high dose of antidiabetic drugs (insulin or sulfonylureas) in relation to food intake and physical activity levels.

2) Impaired physiologic mechanisms preventing hypoglycemia recognition, such as autonomic failure or as in patients with renal impairment.

3) Decreased endogenous glucose production (eg, after alcohol intake).

4) Increased insulin sensitivity (eg, after a decrease in body weight, as a delayed effect of exercise, or as a result of improved diabetes control).

Caution: The risk of hypoglycemia is increased in patients in whom intensive insulin therapy is used to achieve normalization of blood glucose levels and glycated hemoglobin levels (HbA$_{1c}$) <7.0%. Episodes of hypoglycemia are less frequent in patients with type 2 diabetes mellitus, even in those receiving intensive insulin therapy.

Hypoglycemia classification:

1) **Level 1**: Blood glucose levels <3.9 mmol/L (70 mg/dL) and ≥3.0 mmol/L (54 mg/dL).

2) **Level 2**: Blood glucose levels <3.0 mmol/L (54 mg/dL), sufficiently low to indicate serious, clinically important hypoglycemia.

3) **Level 3** (defined by symptoms): A severe event characterized by altered mental and/or physical status requiring assistance of a third party for recovery. Repeated level 3 hypoglycemia may cause cognitive impairment in the long term.

→ CLINICAL FEATURES AND DIAGNOSIS

1. Clinical features:

1) General signs and symptoms: Dizziness, blurred vision, pallor, nausea, and light-headedness.

2) Neurogenic symptoms such as perspiration, palpitations, tremor, hunger, anxiety, and profuse perspiration are caused by sympathetic stimulation. These develop in patients with blood glucose levels of ~3.0 mmol/L (54 mg/dL).

3) Confusion, somnolence, dysarthria, abnormal coordination, atypical behavior, visual disturbances, migrant paresthesia, seizures, loss of consciousness, coma, and death are **manifestations of neuroglycopenia** (glucose deficit in the central nervous system), which may develop in patients with blood glucose levels <2.8 mmol/L (50 mg/dL). These symptoms are usually seen in patients with level 3 hypoglycemia.

2. In some patients symptoms and signs of hypoglycemia may be absent despite very low glucose levels. This is referred to as **hypoglycemia unawareness**. Causes:

1) Autonomous nervous system dysfunction in patients with long-standing diabetes mellitus causes a loss of warning signs related to adrenergic stimulation. This leads to features of neuroglycopenia appearing without warning symptoms.

2) Dysregulation of mechanisms that prevent hypoglycemia, which may occur after previous episodes of severe hypoglycemia and may require temporary adoption of less stringent criteria of glycemic control.

Differential Diagnosis

1. Hypoglycemia caused by other factors: Insulinoma and other conditions.

2. Loss of consciousness caused by other conditions: Coma in the course of diabetes mellitus (→Chapter 5.2.1.1.1), syncope, epilepsy.

→ TREATMENT

Acute Treatment

1. Level 1 and 2 hypoglycemia (conscious patients): Intake of fast--acting carbohydrates should be recommended at a blood glucose alert value of 3.9 mmol/L (70 mg/dL). Glucose (10-15 g) is the preferred treatment, although any foods or fluids that contain glucose (fruit juice, hard bar candy) will raise blood glucose levels; this may be repeated as necessary. Ingestion of fatty foods may delay and then prolong acute glycemic response. Subsequently, the patient should consume a meal or snack with complex (long-lasting) carbohydrates and added fat to prevent recurrent hypoglycemia (eg, bread, potatoes, cereal, nuts, peanuts). All patients, and particularly patients using insulin pumps or treated with insulin analogues as part of an intensive insulin therapy regimen, should consume 15 g of glucose and measure their blood glucose level after 15 minutes (the 15/15 rule; →Chapter 5.2); this should be repeated in case of persistent hypoglycemia. Glucagon should be prescribed for all individuals with level 2 hypoglycemia to have it available if needed.

2. Level 3 hypoglycemia (unconscious or impaired patients): In patients with altered mental status or those unable or unwilling to consume carbohydrates by mouth, administer 20% glucose (dextrose) IV solution (0.2 g of glucose/kg, even up to 80-100 mL of the solution; in Canada up to 50 mL of a 50% glucose solution is used), followed by an IV infusion of a 10% glucose solution until the mental status improves and the patient is able to tolerate oral carbohydrates.

In case of level 3 hypoglycemia in patients with type 1 diabetes mellitus in whom it is difficult to establish IV access, administer glucagon 0.5 to 1 mg as an IM or subcutaneous injection; if there is no improvement, repeat the injection after 10 minutes. Glucagon should be used with caution in patients with type 2 diabetes. Do not use glucagon in patients with hypoglycemia caused by sulfonylureas (as it may paradoxically stimulate the secretion of endogenous insulin and worsen the hypoglycemic episode). Glucagon is also contraindicated in patients with recent alcohol use.

Further Management

1. Assess the risk of recurrence: Hypoglycemia caused by long-acting sulfonylureas, intermediate-acting insulins, or long-acting insulin analogues may recur even after 16 to 20 hours (particularly in patients with impaired renal function). When using premixed insulins, note that they have 2 peaks of action (one after 2-4 hours and another after 8-12 hours).

2. Assess the frequency and time of occurrence of hypoglycemia and adjust treatment of diabetes mellitus appropriately:

1) Hypoglycemia occurring **at a specified time**: Adjust nutrition management and insulin doses.

2) Hypoglycemia occurring **at irregular intervals**: Identify and address the causes, including irregular meals, inappropriate insulin injection techniques, variable intensity of exercise, alcohol use, gastric motility disorders, and variable rates of carbohydrate absorption from the gastrointestinal tract.

3) **Hypoglycemia unawareness**: Adjust treatment to reduce the incidence of episodes of hypoglycemia. Educate patients and their caregivers or family members on how to recognize the less typical prodromal symptoms of hypoglycemia. Consider the use of a continuous glucose monitoring system. Consider the risk of hypoglycemia unawareness at work or when driving. Patients with hypoglycemia unawareness and level 2 hypoglycemia should be advised to raise their glycemic targets for several weeks. This may prevent hypoglycemia and partially reverse hypoglycemia unawareness. Hypoglycemia unawareness or repeated level 3 hypoglycemia should prompt reevaluation of the patient's treatment regimen.

3. Assess chronic sequelae of hypoglycemia, such as cognitive impairment.

2.1.1.3. Hyperglycemic Hyperosmolar State

→ **DEFINITION, ETIOLOGY, PATHOGENESIS**

Hyperglycemic hyperosmolar state (HHS) is characterized by severe hyperglycemia, increased plasma osmolality, dehydration, and often prerenal azotemia (water loss is significantly higher than in diabetic ketoacidosis [DKA]). Despite the very high blood glucose levels, no ketosis or acidosis is observed, which is explained by residual insulin secretion that does not protect against hyperglycemia but is sufficient to inhibit ketone production; in addition, hyperosmolality inhibits lipolysis.

HHS develops mainly in patients with type 2 diabetes mellitus, most frequently as a result of its delayed diagnosis or inappropriate treatment, especially in the elderly. However, it may also develop in patients with type 1 diabetes. The risk of HHS increases with the presence of precipitating factors, including severe infections (the most common precipitating factor, especially with dehydration), acute cardiovascular conditions (myocardial infarction, stroke), alcohol poisoning, use of diuretics or psychotropic drugs, and renal failure. The prognosis in HHS, in comparison with DKA, is markedly worse.

Table 2-7. Diagnostic criteria for hyperglycemic hyperosmolar state (HHS)	
Parameters	Values typical for HHS
Blood glucose level in mmol/L (mg/dL)	≥33.3 (≥600)
pH	>7.30
Serum bicarbonate level	>15 mmol/L
Urine ketone bodies/serum ketone bodies	Low
Effective serum osmolality	>320 mOsm/kg H_2O[a]
Altered mental status	Altered level of consciousness to lack of response (coma)
Anion gap	Variable
[a] Reference range: 280 to 290 mOsm/kg H_2O.	

→ CLINICAL FEATURES

Signs and symptoms of HHS are very similar to DKA. However, the clinical course of HHS is characterized by an onset of days before hospital admission and altered mental status is almost always present (≥90% of patients). In addition, compared with DKA, patients with HHS are usually more dehydrated and do not develop a rapid and deep breathing pattern (Kussmaul) or abdominal pain.

Symptoms including manifestations of the underlying condition from altered mental status to coma.

Signs including tachycardia, tachypnea, shallow or deep respirations, features of extreme dehydration (reduced skin turgor, dry mucous membranes, and reduced eyeball turgor), facial redness, and hypotension. Neurologic signs, such as abnormal movements, seizures, hemiparesis and hemianopia, may occur.

→ DIAGNOSIS

The initial evaluation is the same as in DKA.

Diagnostic Criteria

Diagnosis is based on laboratory test results (→Table 2-7).

Differential Diagnosis

1. DKA with concomitant hyperosmolality.

2. Coma due to a primary neurologic condition (hyperosmolality is not a constant feature).

3. Hepatic or uremic coma (no severe hyperglycemia is seen; patients with hepatic coma may even have hypoglycemia).

4. Poisoning or intoxication.

5. Dehydration secondary to other causes (diabetes insipidus, excessive use of diuretics, polyuria).

→ TREATMENT

1. Fluid replacement: Similarly to DKA, in HHS, due to the severe dehydration, fluid replacement therapy is considered the most critical part of treatment. The rate of infusion and type of saline solution (0.45% vs 0.9% vs balanced crystalloid solutions) depend on serum sodium and chloride levels, plasma osmolality, and cardiac function. The rate of correction of plasma osmolality should not be >3 mOsm/kg H_2O/h. Use 0.45% saline until normal plasma osmolality is restored. The starting point for a reasonable regimen of fluid resuscitation may be as follows:

1) Administer 1000 mL of 0.9% saline IV over the first hour in severe hypovolemia.

2) Administer 500 mL of 0.45% or 0.9% saline IV per hour for the subsequent 4 to 6 hours.

3) Administer 250 mL 0.45% or 0.9% saline per hour until the correction of water deficit is achieved.

4) When serum glucose reaches ≤16.6 mmol/L (300 mg/dL), change to 5% glucose (dextrose) with 0.45% NaCl at a rate of 150 to 250 mL/h.

5) In patients with heart failure it may be necessary to reduce the infusion rates.

6) In case of hypotension use 0.9% saline or a balanced isotonic solution.

2. Reduce hyperglycemia: Start insulin IV (use a short-acting insulin)⊘◯:

1) Start with approximately 0.1 IU/kg (usually 4-8 IU) in an IV injection bolus and start a continuous insulin infusion at a rate of ~0.14 IU/kg/h as a follow-up to bolus or as a direct step, without the bolus.

2) Adjust the dose as required to achieve a serum glucose level ≤16.6 mmol/L (300 mg/dL).

3) Once serum glucose reaches 16.6 mmol/L (300 mg/dL), reduce the infusion rate of IV insulin to between 0.02 and 0.05 IU/kg/h, maintain the serum glucose level between 11.1 and 16.6 mmol/L (200-300 mg/dL), then switch from the IV infusion to a subcutaneous insulin regimen. In insulin-naive patients, start with 0.5 to 0.8 IU/kg/d of human insulin (our pattern of practice is to use two-thirds of insulin isophane and one-third of regular insulin), maintaining the insulin infusion for 1 to 2 hours after the subcutaneous regimen begins and the patient has eaten. In patients previously treated with insulin, a prior insulin regimen can be restarted.

3. Correct potassium deficit as in DKA.

4. Search for the precipitating cause and treat appropriately.

→ FOLLOW-UP

Follow-up is similar to DKA.

The criteria of resolution are normal osmolality and normal mental status. There is no need to monitor serum phosphate, calcium, or ketone levels. In patients in whom acidosis has been excluded, arterial blood gas analysis may be done only as otherwise indicated.

→ COMPLICATIONS AND PROGNOSIS

Rhabdomyolysis resulting from severe hyperosmolality, gastroparesis, and venous thromboembolism (common; thromboprophylaxis with subcutaneous heparin is recommended: →Chapter 3.19.2).

The estimated mortality rate in HHS is ~20% and is 10 times higher than in DKA. Prognosis depends on the presence of comorbidities, age, and severity of dehydration, with infants and elderly being the most affected.

2.1.1.4. Lactic Acidosis

→ DEFINITION, ETIOLOGY, PATHOGENESIS

Lactic acidosis is a metabolic acidosis with a high anion gap characterized by serum lactate levels >5 mmol/L (4 mEq/L). It is caused by increased anaerobic glucose metabolism and consequent lactate accumulation in the bloodstream. Lactic acidosis is not a disease-specific complication of diabetes mellitus; it is triggered by precipitating factors and is most frequently and nonspecifically seen in patients with shock. Metformin-associated lactic acidosis is more specific to diabetes, with an estimated incidence of 4.3 cases per 100,000 person-years in patients treated with metformin. Lactic acidosis is less frequent than other complications in patients with diabetes that may lead to coma, but when present, the mortality rate may be as high as 50%. It develops more often in patients with type 2 diabetes, especially when associated with conditions that can precipitate drug accumulation (eg, renal insufficiency or failure) and/or decrease in lactate clearance (eg, liver impairment). In patients with type 1 diabetes, advanced microangiopathy (especially in patients with renal failure) can be a risk factor for lactic acidosis.

Types of lactic acidosis associated with diabetes:

1) **Type A lactic acidosis (anaerobic)** develops in the case of tissue hypoxia or hyperperfusion (sepsis, shock, heart failure, respiratory failure, and severe trauma).

2) **Type B lactic acidosis (aerobic)** is caused by factors other than hypoxia. In patients with diabetes mellitus, it accompanies severe complications of diabetes (eg, diabetic ketoacidosis [DKA]), renal failure, liver failure, and malignancy. Type B lactic acidosis is also caused by inappropriate use of metformin (a condition known as metformin-associated lactic acidosis [MALA]), precipitated by an imbalance between lactate production, drug accumulation, and lactate clearance (contraindications: →Table 2-5). Ingestion of high doses of salicylates, methyl alcohol, ethyl alcohol, propylene glycol, and certain drugs like antiretroviral agents and propofol that impair oxidative phosphorylation can also cause type B lactic acidosis. Malignancy, high alcohol consumption, and HIV infection have also been associated with this kind of acidosis.

→ CLINICAL FEATURES AND DIAGNOSIS

Symptoms include severe weakness, nausea, vomiting, and abdominal pain. Patients may have a history of ingestion of a toxic substance, alcohol, or treatment with metformin despite contraindications.

Signs include hyperpnea (Kussmaul respiration), altered mental status with hallucinations and coma, moderate dehydration, oliguria, hypothermia, hypotension, and shock.

→ DIAGNOSIS

Diagnostic Criteria

Diagnosis is based on lactate levels ≥5 mmol/L (4 mEq/L), even in the absence of overt acidemia. Minor hyperglycemia (or sometimes normal glucose levels), serum lactate levels usually >7 mmol/L (increasing with deteriorating renal function and resulting in elevated mortality with higher levels), low blood pH <7.35, serum bicarbonate levels <10 mmol/L, anion gap >16 mEq/L, usually hyperkalemia (except in grand mal seizures, which present with normokalemia), and normal serum sodium levels (these may be low in patients abusing alcohol) are also typically found.

Measurement of metformin plasma concentration is important to confirm involvement of this drug in patients with suspected MALA. The mean plasma concentrations of metformin in healthy patients fluctuate between about 0.5 and 1 mg/L while fasting and 1 to 2 mg/L after a meal.

Differential Diagnosis

Differential diagnosis includes DKA (higher levels of glucose and ketone bodies without signs and symptoms of shock, lactate usually not as high), hyperglycemic hyperosmolar state (HHS) (significant hyperosmolality; serum lactate levels and blood pH within reference ranges), alcohol poisoning (no significant decrease in blood pH, normal blood glucose levels, no features of shock, serum lactate levels <5 mmol/L), other types of coma (hepatic, uremic), and other causes of shock.

⇒ TREATMENT

1. Prevention and treatment of shock:

1) Use fluid resuscitation to increase intravascular volume as in DKA or HHS. Crystalloid and colloid solutions are both effective.

2) In patients with hypotension, IV administration of catecholamines may be ineffective (as in other instances of severe acidosis).

3) High doses of catecholamines can aggravate hyperlactatemia by reducing tissue perfusion or overstimulating β2-adrenergic receptors; therefore, the dose should be adjusted carefully.

2. Improvement of blood oxygenation and treatment of hypoxia: Administer oxygen as needed. Invasive ventilation may also be required to prevent hypercapnia, particularly if acidemia persists or worsens (note that achieving levels of hyperventilation required to mimic spontaneous hyperventilation may be difficult or impossible).

3. Reduction of hyperglycemia:

1) Administer insulin infusion as in the treatment of HHS.

2) When blood glucose levels decrease <11.1 mmol/L (200 mg/dL), administer a 5% glucose (dextrose) infusion. Once blood glucose levels have normalized, administer a 10% glucose infusion and continue the insulin infusion.

4. Treatment of acidosis: Administer IV sodium bicarbonate (this remains a controversial intervention; it is usually done with a pH <7.2; associated with some benefits in other instances of lactic acidosis)⊘ ● (→Chapter 4.1.1).

5. Hemodialysis: Renal replacement therapy may be needed.

6. Treatment of the underlying condition.

7. Measurement of the blood lactate level remains the cornerstone of monitoring for lactic acidosis. Lactate can be measured in arterial or venous blood. Although a single elevated blood lactate level often predicts an adverse outcome, sustained hyperlactatemia is associated with even worse prognoses. An interval of 2 to 6 hours has been suggested for repeat lactate measurements.

⇒ PREVENTION

Consider risk factors. MALA develops when there is an imbalance between increased lactate production and impaired metabolism/reduced clearance. This is observed in individuals with poor renal function (reduced metformin clearance), impaired hepatic metabolism (reduced lactate clearance), and/or in the presence of increased lactate production (eg, sepsis, reduced tissue perfusion, anoxia). Other conditions that may increase the risk of lactic acidosis include severe dehydration, shock, alcohol use, and advanced age.

2.1.2. Chronic Complications of Diabetes Mellitus

⇒ INTRODUCTION

Diabetes mellitus is a worldwide public health problem that affects >420 million people of all ages, genders, and racial and ethnic groups. One of the paramount aspects of treating patients with diabetes mellitus is the association of the disease with chronic complications, which represent a burden not only to public health-care systems but predominantly to individuals who cope with them on a day-to-day basis.

While the exact pathophysiologic mechanisms behind both microvascular and macrovascular diabetes complications remain uncertain, oxidative stress appears to play a determining role in their development. An increased mitochondrial superoxide production is the first event that leads to activation of other pathways involved in the pathogenesis of chronic diabetes complications (eg, formation of advanced glycation end products, activation of protein kinase C isoforms, increased polyol pathway flux). Those changes may lead to defective formation of new vessels in response to ischemia and activation of inflammatory processes that may persist after relative normalization of glucose metabolism. Endothelial dysfunction also plays a critical role in diabetes-related complications and represents an imbalance in the production of vasodilator factors.

The duration of diabetes mellitus along with glycemic, blood pressure, and lipid control are common risk factors for the development of complications. Criteria for recognizing these conditions are well established, but other causes must be excluded to confirm diagnosis.

Chronic complications of diabetes mellitus:

1) **Microvascular complications**:
   a) **Diabetic nephropathy**.
   b) **Diabetic retinopathy**.
   c) **Diabetic neuropathy**.
2) **Macrovascular complications** are mainly related to the accelerated development of atherosclerosis (diabetes mellitus is an independent risk factor for atherosclerosis). It is characterized by early onset, disseminated lesions in smaller arteries, impaired development of collateral circulation due to microvascular complications, and a painless course of atherosclerosis--related conditions (eg, myocardial infarction, stroke, death). Macrovascular complications are the leading cause of morbidity and mortality in individuals with diabetes.
3) **Diabetic foot syndrome**, which is caused by microvascular and macrovascular lesions and neuropathy.
4) **Other complications**: Skeletal (eg, Dupuytren contracture), joint (eg, Charcot foot), visual impairment (eg, subcapsular cataracts), and cutaneous (eg, necrobiosis lipoidica).

2.1.2.1. Diabetic Foot Syndrome

→ DEFINITION, ETIOLOGY, PATHOGENESIS

Diabetic foot syndrome is defined as infection, ulceration, or destruction of deep tissues of the foot (including bones) in a patient with diabetes mellitus. It affects nearly 6% of individuals with diabetes. Around 0.5% to 1.5% of patients with diabetic foot syndrome require amputation. Most amputations start with ulcerations and can be prevented with good foot care and screening to assess the risk of foot complications. Diabetic foot syndrome is associated with neurologic abnormalities and peripheral arterial disease of the lower limbs of varied severity.

Neuropathy and vascular abnormalities both play a role in the development of diabetic foot syndrome (→Table 2-8). Motor neuropathy results in atrophy of the muscles of the foot, thus disturbing the flexor-extensor balance and leading to contractures. Sensory neuropathy (abnormal sensation of pain, temperature, and touch) exposes the patient to repeated uncontrolled injuries, increasing the risk of ulcerations. Autonomic neuropathy results in the formation of arteriovenous fistulae and trophic changes. Atherosclerosis of the lower extremities results in foot ischemia. All these changes are associated with the development of local osteoporosis and may also lead to osteomyelitis, avascular necrosis, fractures, dislocations, and significant disfigurement of the foot (Charcot foot arthropathy).

Table 2-8. Pathogenesis of diabetic foot syndrome	
Causative factors	**Contributory factors**
– Peripheral neuropathy: Present in 50% of patients with diabetes aged >60 years. Increases the risk of foot ulceration 7-fold – Excessive plantar pressure: Related to limited joint mobility and foot deformities – Repetitive trauma	– Atherosclerotic peripheral vascular disease affecting femoropopliteal and smaller vessels below the knee – Several intrinsic wound-healing disturbances: Impaired collagen cross-linking and metalloproteinase function, immunologic perturbations, higher rates of onychomycosis and toe-web tinea infections – Obesity and poor vision leading to impaired self-care

Stages of Charcot foot arthropathy:

1) Stage 1: Warmth, redness, and edema of the foot, with features suggestive of tissue inflammation.
2) Stage 2: Bone fractures and joint dislocations.
3) Stage 3: Foot deformation, joint destruction.
4) Stage 4: Ulcerations of the foot arch (bottom foot).

Classification based on pathogenesis includes neuropathic foot, ischemic foot, and neuropathic-ischemic foot. Differentiation of the neuropathic and the ischemic foot is of great importance, as their treatment differs significantly (→Table 2-9).

→ CLINICAL FEATURES AND DIAGNOSIS

Inquire about factors known to be associated with foot ulcers: previous foot ulceration, prior lower extremity amputation, Charcot foot arthropathy, long history of diabetes (>10 years), poor glycemic control (glycated hemoglobin [HbA_{1c}] >9.0%), angioplasty or vascular surgery, cigarette smoking, peripheral neuropathy, visual impairment, and chronic kidney disease (especially in patients treated with dialysis). Perform a **complete foot examination**, which should include inspection of the skin, assessment of muscular deformities, and neurologic and vascular evaluations. The neurologic examination performed as part of foot examination is designed to identify loss of protective sensation (LOPS) rather than early neuropathy. The 10-g monofilament is the most useful test to diagnose LOPS. Ideally, it should be performed with at least one other assessment (pinprick, temperature or vibration sensation using a 128--Hz tuning fork, or ankle reflexes). Absent monofilament sensation suggests LOPS, while at ≥2 normal test results (and no abnormal results) exclude LOPS. Initial screening for peripheral arterial disease (PAD) should include history of decreased walking speed, leg fatigue, claudication, and assessment of pedal pulses. Ankle-brachial index (ABI) testing should be performed in patients with symptoms or signs of PAD (→Table 2-10).

The **Perfusion, Extent, Depth, Infection, and Sensation (PEDIS) classification** of the diabetic foot includes assessment of perfusion, size, and depth of ulceration, severity of infection, and presence of sensory neuropathy; this classification is reflected in the Infectious Diseases Society of America (IDSA) classification of diabetic foot infection (→Table 2-11).

Clinical diagnostic criteria for infection of the soft tissues of the foot: Acute ulceration with classic inflammation signs (redness, pain, warming, swelling, lymphangitis, phlegmon, purulent discharge or abscess), fluctuance, increased discharge, friable or discolored granulation tissue, undermining of wound edges, and foul odor. Deep ulceration reaching the bone (visible or confirmed at clinical examination using a sterile probe) indicates a risk of

Table 2-9. Differential diagnosis of neuropathic and ischemic foot

Feature	Foot ischemia	Neuropathic foot
Pain on movement	++	–
Pain at rest	+++	±
Sensory abnormalities	–	++
Pulse on the lower extremity	Absent	Present
Skin	Cold	Warm
Bone structure	Normal	Damaged
Lesion type	Gangrene	Ulceration
Lesion location	Depends on location of arterial lesions	Depends on internal and external pressure areas
Pain	Increases with physical activity	Increases with rest, usually appears at night

Table 2-10. Tools for identification of the at-risk foot

Symptoms	Identifying tool	Description
Loss of protective sensation	Monofilament	Performed using 10-g (5.07 Semmens-Weinstein) monofilament. Inspect 8-10 anatomic sites and 4 plantar sites
	Biothesiometer	Used to assess vibration perception thresholds. Reading >25 V has sensitivity of 83%, specificity of 63%, positive LR of 2.2, and negative LR of 0.27 for predicting foot ulceration over 4 years
	Tuning fork	Performed using 128 Hz tuning fork. Abnormal response occurs when patient loses vibratory sensation while it is still perceived by examiner
Peripheral vascular disease	Clinical features	History of decreased walking speed, leg fatigue, claudication; assessment of pedal pulses
	ABI (→Chapter 3.18.3.2)	>1.30 — Arterial calcification 0.90-1.30 — Normal 0.60-0.89 — Mild arterial obstruction 0.40-0.59 — Moderate obstruction <0.40 — Severe obstruction
	Arterial oxygen supply	Transcutaneous oximetry >30 mm Hg correlates with high likelihood of wound healing

ABI, ankle-brachial index; LR, likelihood ratio.

bone infection; in such cases perform magnetic resonance imaging (MRI) or histologic examination of bone samples.

Microbiological examination of soft tissues is not used to confirm the diagnosis of infection but to establish its etiology and provide treatment guidance. Specimens for culture should be obtained prior to starting empiric antibiotic therapy, if possible. Make sure the samples are collected in an appropriate

Table 2-11. Classification of diabetic foot infection according to the Infectious Diseases Society of America (IDSA) and International Working Group on the Diabetic Foot (2012)

Clinical manifestation of infection	PEDIS grade	IDSA infection severity
No symptoms or signs of infection[a]	1	Uninfected
Local infection involving only skin and subcutaneous tissue (no involvement of deeper tissues or systemic signs described below); if erythema is present, it must be >0.5 cm to ≤2 cm around the ulcer Exclude other causes of an inflammatory skin response (eg, trauma, gout, acute Charcot arthropathy, fracture, thrombosis, venous stasis)	2	Mild
Local infection (as above) with erythema >2 cm or involving structures deeper than skin and subcutaneous tissues (eg, abscess, osteomyelitis, septic arthritis, fasciitis) and no systemic inflammatory response signs (→below)	3	Moderate
Local infection (as above) with signs of SIRS[b]	4	Severe[c]

[a] Infection defined as the presence of ≥2 of the following: local swelling or induration; erythema; local tenderness or pain; local warmth; purulent discharge (thick, opaque to white or sanguineous secretion)

[b] At least 2 of the following: temperature >38°C or <36°C; heart rate >90 beats/min; respiratory rate >20 breaths/min or $PaCO_2$ <32 mm Hg; white blood cell count >12 × 10⁹/L or <4 × 10⁹/L or ≥10% immature (band) forms

[c] Ischemia may increase the severity of any infection, and the presence of critical ischemia often makes the infection severe. Systemic infection may sometimes manifest with other clinical findings, such as hypotension, confusion, vomiting, or evidence of metabolic disturbances, such as acidosis, severe hyperglycemia, and new-onset azotemia

Adapted from Clin Infect Dis. 2012;54(12):e132-73.

IDSA, Infectious Diseases Society of America; $PaCO_2$, partial pressure of arterial carbon dioxide; PEDIS, perfusion, extent, depth, infection, and sensation; SIRS, systemic inflammatory response syndrome.

way; optimally, they should be obtained from deeper parts of the wound during tissue biopsy or curettage after the wound has been cleansed and debrided. Superficial smears are insufficient, as they reveal the colonizing flora and are of little diagnostic value. Mild (superficial and limited) infection is generally caused by staphylococci and streptococci, while chronic and severe infections are often polymicrobial and involve aerobic gram-negative rods and anaerobes.

→ PREVENTION

1. Examine or inspect the feet at every visit (usually every 3 months) for structural abnormalities (eg, calluses, hammer or claw toes, flat feet, bunions), reduced joint mobility, dry or fissured skin, tinea or onychomycosis, loss of protective sensation, diminished arterial supply, and improper footwear. Determine the risk of diabetic foot syndrome during the annual complete foot examination and schedule further control foot examinations at intervals depending on the presence of abnormalities found. Assess the ABI (→Chapter 3.18.3.2) every 2 years starting from 35 years of age.

2. Instruct the patient with diabetic neuropathy, foot deformities, exostosis, peripheral ischemia, or prior ulcers to do the following:

1) Inspect the feet daily, including interdigital spaces (if the patient is not capable of self-inspection, they should ask for assistance).

2) Wash the feet regularly with water (<37°C) and dry them thoroughly, paying special attention to the interdigital spaces.

3) Avoid walking barefoot or using footwear without socks. Change socks daily. Wear socks and stockings with seams turned inside out, or optimally use seamless hosiery. Perform daily visual and manual inspection of the inner surfaces of footwear.

4) Clip toenails straight. Visually impaired patients should not clip toenails by themselves.

5) Avoid cutting hard skin and calluses by the patients themselves (including the use of chemical preparations and patches).

6) Seek medical attention immediately in case of blisters, cuts, scratches, or ulcerations.

→ TREATMENT

1. Good control of diabetes mellitus is of key importance.

2. Treatment aimed at optimizing cardiovascular function: →Chapter 3.18.3.2.

3. Management of an uninfected foot: Ensure appropriate foot care procedures, patient education, and avoidance of weight-bearing of the foot. Do not use antimicrobial treatment. Perform repeated foot assessments including effects of treatment and perfusion and search for features of infection. Hyperbaric oxygen therapy (HBOT) in patients with diabetic foot ulcerations has mixed and nondefinitive evidence supporting its use as adjunctive treatment to enhance wound healing and prevent amputation.○ With the high cost and burden of therapy, HBOT should be a topic of shared decision-making before treatment is considered for selected patients with diabetic foot ulcerations.

4. Treatment of an infected foot:

1) In patients who are not treated with insulin, start **insulin therapy**.

2) **Reduce weight-bearing on the foot**, for instance, by using molded footwear inserts, crutches, or casts.

3) **Ensure restoration of skin perfusion**. Implement measures focused on cardiovascular risk reduction: cessation of smoking, treatment of hypertension and dyslipidemia, use of acetylsalicylic acid. Consider revascularization in patients with an ABI <0.6 (→Chapter 3.18.3.2), toe pressures <50 mm Hg, or transcutaneous partial pressure of oxygen <30 mm Hg.

4) Consider **hospitalization** in all patients with severe infection, selected patients with moderate infection and complicating features (eg, severe peripheral arterial disease or lack of home support), and any patient unable to comply with the required outpatient treatment regimen for psychological or social reasons.

5) **Antimicrobial treatment**: The guidelines specific for diabetic wound infections (IDSA 2012) recommend that clinically uninfected wounds do not get treated with antibiotics; if the wounds are infected, antibiotic treatment should be supported by debridement as needed and wound care. In patients with cellulitis surrounding a wound that is mild in severity, start empiric treatment by targeting *Staphylococcus aureus* and group A streptococcus by using dicloxacillin, a first-generation cephalosporin (eg, cephalexin [INN cefalexin] 500 mg qid), or amoxicillin/clavulanate 875/125 mg bid. Other options are clindamycin, levofloxacin, and doxycycline or trimethoprim/sulfamethoxazole for potential or confirmed methicillin-resistant *S aureus* (MRSA) infections.

Broader coverage is indicated in patients with moderate to severe deep wound infection, where polymicrobial infection is more likely. Therapy could include ceftriaxone (1 g IM bid) and metronidazole (500 mg orally or IV every 12 hours), ampicillin/sulbactam (1.5 g IM every 6 hours), and piperacillin/tazobactam (4.5 g qid). Other options include clindamycin/ciprofloxacin (600 mg orally tid/500 mg bid), levofloxacin (750 mg orally once daily), or a carbapenem (eg, meropenem 500 mg IV tid); however, these should be used judiciously to avoid contributing to fluoroquinolone and carbapenem resistance. If there has been a recent known exposure to MRSA or in centers where exposure is likely (eg, local MRSA incidence >10%), consider adding vancomycin for empiric therapy. If results of susceptibility testing are available, use targeted antimicrobial treatment (eg, in patients with laboratory-confirmed MRSA infection, use vancomycin [1 g IV bid]).

The duration of antibiotic treatment can be variable and depends on a number of factors, with the evidence base for duration being very poor. Patients with complicated infections should be seen by an infectious disease specialist who would determine treatment duration. As a rough approximation, the **usual duration of antimicrobial treatment** in patients with a PEDIS grade 2 infection (→Table 2-11) is 1 to 2 weeks, and in patients with PEDIS grade 3 or 4 infection, 2 to 4 weeks, until the infection resolves; do not continue treatment until ulceration is healed. In patients with infection of bones and joints, the duration of treatment is usually as follows: in patients after amputation (indications: →below) with no residual infection, 5 days; in patients with bone infections without a residual sequestrum, 4 to 6 weeks; in patients with bone infection and residual sequestrum after surgical treatment, >3 months.

6) **Drainage, incision, and debridement of necrotic tissues or surrounding callus**: Debridement should be aimed at removing debris, eschar, and surrounding callus. Urgent surgical intervention should be offered to patients with foot infections accompanied by gas in the deeper tissues, abscess, or necrotic fasciitis.

7) **Dressings**: Adjust the type of dressing to the stage of wound healing. The choice of dressing should be based on the size, depth, and nature of the ulcer (eg, dry, exudative, purulent).

8) **Intravascular and surgical procedures** may be used in patients with clinical or imaging evidence of significant ischemia in the infected limb.

9) **Amputation**: An absolute indication for amputation is life-threatening extensive necrosis with inflammation. Relative indications include distal phalangeal osteomyelitis of the foot and liquefactive necrosis. Additional signs of a possibly imminently limb-threatening infection include evidence of a systemic inflammatory response, rapid progression of infection, extensive necrosis or gangrene, crepitus on examination, tissue gas on imaging, extensive ecchymoses or petechiae, new-onset wound anesthesia, pain out of proportion to clinical findings, recent loss of neurologic function, critical limb ischemia, extensive soft tissue loss, extensive bony destruction, or failure of infection to improve with appropriate therapy. In patients with coagulative necrosis, watchful waiting for spontaneous amputation is recommended.

5. Treatment of acute Charcot arthropathy: Avoiding weight-bearing of the affected foot until resolution of the acute phase of arthropathy (cast or orthesis). Consider bisphosphonates combined with vitamin D and calcium supplements (long-term treatment, not always effective).

6. Long-term treatment to reduce the risk of ulcerations: Educate the patients and their family or caregivers on appropriate foot hygiene, necessity of daily foot inspections, and avoidance of foot injury. Use special orthopedic footwear with appropriate inserts allowing correction of deformities and reducing excessive load-bearing in the foot.

2.1.2.2. Diabetic Kidney Disease

➡ ETIOLOGY, PATHOGENESIS, CLASSIFICATION

The development of diabetic kidney disease (DKD) depends on the duration of diabetes mellitus (DM), severity of metabolic disturbances, coexisting hypertension, and genetic factors. DKD is present in up to 25% to 40% of patients with DM, and some of them develop end-stage kidney disease requiring renal replacement therapy. It is caused by changes in the basal membrane, which lead to a decrease in its negative charge and increase in the pore size. Concurrently, high blood glucose levels and blood pressure increase the intraglomerular pressure. As a result, albumin filtration is increased, initially in the form of albuminuria of 30 to 300 mg/24 hours or equivalent 30 to 300 mg/g creatinine in a random urine sample (albumin-to-creatinine ratio [ACR], 3-30 mg/mmol) and then overt proteinuria >300 mg/24 hours or >300 mg/g creatinine (ACR >30 mg/mmol). Over time, this leads to glomerular hyalinosis, fibrosis of the interstitial tissue, and development of renal failure. Moreover, the presence of renal failure in patients with DM has been related to increases in cardiovascular risk and health-care costs.

According to the current Kidney Disease: Improving Global Outcomes (KDIGO) guidelines, the use of the term "microalbuminuria," corresponding to an ACR between 3 and 30 mg/g, has been discouraged. Additionally, DKD is preferred over diabetic nephropathy because DM studies are often observational and lack biopsy data to prove involvement of lesions.

Major **risk factors** for the development of DKD include ethnicity, male sex, family history, gestational DM, hypertension, dyslipidemia, obesity, and insulin resistance, as well as elevated glycated hemoglobin (HbA_{1c}) level, elevated systolic blood pressure, inflammation, hypovitaminosis D, proteinuria, and smoking.

The **clinical classification** of DKD includes 4 key stages:

1) **Asymptomatic nephropathy** (corresponding to stages 1 and 2 of the Mogensen classification, also referred to as the classification of the natural history of diabetic nephropathy; →Table 2-12).

2) **Albuminuria** (30-300 mg/24 h; corresponding to stage 3 of the Mogensen classification).

3) **Overt proteinuria** (urinary albumin excretion >300 mg/24 h or >300 mg/g creatinine in a random urine sample; corresponding to stage 4 of the Mogensen classification).

4) **Renal failure** (corresponding to stage 5 of the Mogensen classification). The dynamics of renal failure does not always correspond to the rate of worsening of proteinuria.

Other urinary system disorders that are more frequent in patients with DM include recurrent urinary tract infections (neurogenic bladder is a risk factor), acute renal cortical necrosis, and tubulopathies.

➡ DIAGNOSIS

Chronic kidney disease (CKD) is defined as abnormalities of kidney structure or function present for >3 months with implications for health (→Table 2-13). DKD is diagnosed when albuminuria, reduced estimated glomerular filtration rate (eGFR), or other manifestations of CKD are detected in patients with DM in the absence of other primary causes of renal failure.

Diagnostic Tests

All patients should have eGFR and albuminuria measurement for staging and to guide treatment decisions. In patients without overt proteinuria, the key screening test is the **measurement of 24-hour urinary albumin excretion**

Table 2-12. Mogensen classification of diabetic nephropathy and its course

Diabetes duration	Stage	Clinical features	Prognosis
Since disease onset	1: Increased GFR, renal hypertrophy	GFR increased to 160 mL/min/1.73 m^2, kidney enlargement (20%) and increase in renal plasma flow (10%-15%), no albuminuria or hypertension	Potentially reversible
2-5 years	2: Onset of histologic changes, altered structure and function of basement membrane	Thickening and altered electrical charge of basement membrane, mesangial proliferation, normal GFR, no albuminuria, no clinical symptoms	May be partially reversible
5-10 (15) years	3: Early clinical nephropathy	Albuminuria 30-300 mg/24 h, GFR reduced from 160 to 130 mL/min/1.73 m^2, ± HTN	Lesion progression may be stopped, sometimes reversible
10 (15)-25 years	4: Overt nephropathy	Persistent and irreversible proteinuria, GFR <60 mL/min/1.73 m^2 and sustained HTN, edema, dyslipidemia	Lesion progression may be slowed and sometimes stopped
>15 years	5: Renal failure	End-stage kidney disease with GFR <15 mL/min/1.73 m^2, HTN	Irreversible progression to end-stage renal failure

Based on Diabetes. 1983;32 Suppl 2:64-78.

GFR, glomerular filtration rate; HTN, hypertension.

or its equivalent ACR (→Table 2-14). Two of 3 specimens used for the urinary ACR collected within 3 to 6 months should yield abnormal results before the patient is considered to have albuminuria. **Serum creatinine should be used to calculate eGFR** using the Chronic Kidney Disease Epidemiology Collaboration (CKD-EPI) equation (→Chapter 9.2).

Screening for kidney damage can be most easily performed by measuring the urinary ACR using a random spot urine collection. Measurement of a spot urine sample for albumin alone without simultaneously measuring urine creatinine is less expensive but susceptible to false-negative and false-positive determinations as a result of variations in urine concentration due to hydration. Some factors that may elevate the urinary ACR ratio (independently of kidney damage) include infection, marked hyperglycemia, congestive heart failure, exercise within 24 hours, fever, menstruation, and marked hypertension.

Perform the screening test for albuminuria and eGFR in patients with **type 1 DM within 5 years** of establishing the diagnosis, in all patients with **type 2 DM at the time of diagnosis**, and in all patients with **comorbid hypertension**. Repeat follow-up tests for albuminuria and serum creatinine measurements annually (or earlier if needed) to enable a timely diagnosis of CKD, monitor the progression of CKD, detect superimposed kidney diseases, assess the risk of CKD complications, dose drugs appropriately, and determine whether nephrology referral is needed. All patients with CKD stages 3 to 5 should undergo evaluation for renal failure complications.

Table 2-13. CKD stages in diabetic nephropathy

Stage	eGFR (mL/min/1.73m^2)	Evidence of kidney damage
No clinical evidence of CKD	≥60	–
1	≥90	+
2	60-89	+
3	30-59	+/–
4	15-29	+/–
5	<15	+/–

CKD stages 1-2 are defined by evidence of kidney damage (+), while CKD stages 3-5 are defined by reduced eGFR with or without evidence of kidney damage (+/–). Kidney damage is most often manifest as albuminuria (UACR >30 mg/g) but can also include glomerular hematuria, other abnormalities of urinary sediment, radiographic abnormalities, and other presentations. Focus on kidney-related care: diagnose the cause of kidney injury in stages 1-3, evaluate and treat risk factors for CKD progression in stages 1-4, evaluate and treat CKD complications in stages 3-5, and prepare for RRT in stages 4-5. At any stage of CKD, the degree of albuminuria, observed history of eGFR loss, and cause of kidney damage (including possible causes other than diabetes mellitus) may also be used to characterize CKD, evaluate prognosis, and guide treatment decisions.

Adapted from Diabetes Care. 2019;42(Suppl 1):S124-S138.

CKD, chronic kidney disease; eGFR, estimated glomerular filtration rate; RRT, renal replacement therapy; UACR, urine albumin-to-creatinine ratio.

→ PREVENTION AND TREATMENT

1. Careful individualized targets of glycemic control, medication prescription, patient education, therapeutic planning, and vigilance for hypoglycemia are all important in the management of patients with DKD. For both type 1 and type 2 DM **optimize glucose levels** to achieve and maintain DM control according to appropriate criteria (→Chapter 5.2); this is of key importance for reducing the risk and delaying the development of nephropathy and may even result in reversal of its early stages. Target levels of HbA$_{1c}$ are <7.0% (53 mmol/mol) for primary prevention, especially in patients with type 1 DM. Aim at an HbA$_{1c}$ <8.0% when eGFR is <60 mL/min/1.73m^2 because of the increased risk of hypoglycemia with more intensive treatment. Doses of insulin and other injectable and oral glucose-lowering medications often need to be reduced or suspended at these eGFR levels. In the presence of established CKD, consider the use of a sodium-glucose cotransporter 2 (SGLT-2) inhibitor or glucagon-like peptide 1 (GLP-1) receptor agonist with proven efficacy in reducing the risk of CKD progression or cardiovascular events.

2. In patients with **hypertension and albuminuria, overt proteinuria, and/or an eGFR <60 mL/min/1.73 m^2**, use an angiotensin-converting enzyme inhibitor (ACEI) or angiotensin-receptor blocker (ARB), aiming to maintain a target blood pressure level <140/90 mm Hg◐◑ (do not combine these two drug classes). Lower blood pressure targets (<130/80 mm Hg) may be considered for patients based on individual anticipated benefits and risks, such as those with stroke or progressive kidney disease. In patients who tolerate these agents poorly, hypertension may be treated with other drugs, for example, nondihydropyridine calcium channel blockers or thiazide-type diuretics. Serum creatinine and potassium levels must be monitored periodically for the development of increased creatinine or hyperkalemia when ACEIs, ARBs, or diuretics are used.

Table 2-14. Albuminuria categories according to the 2012 Kidney Disease: Improving Global Outcomes (KDIGO) guidelines

Parameter	Category		
	Normal to mildly increased	Moderately increased	Severely increased[a]
Albumin-to-creatinine ratio[b]			
mg/g	<30	30-300	>300
mg/mmol	<3	3-30	>30
Urinary albumin excretion rate (mg/24 h)[c]	<30	30-300	>300
Protein-to-creatinine ratio[b]			
mg/g	<150	150-500	>500
mg/mmol	<15	15-50	>50
Urinary protein excretion rate (mg/24 h)[c]	<150	150-500	>500
Urine dipstick test for protein[d]	Negative or trace	Trace or +	+ or more

[a] Nephrotic proteinuria is diagnosed in patients with an albumin-to-creatinine ratio >2200 mg/g (>2200 mg/24 h) or a protein-to-creatinine ratio >3000 mg/g (>3000 mg/24 h).

[b] In the first morning urine sample or a random urine sample. The assumed average urinary creatinine excretion rate is 1 g/24 h or 10 mmol/24 h.

[c] In 24-hour urine.

[d] The results of the dipstick test depend on urine specific gravity.

Based on: Kidney Disease: Improving Global Outcomes (KDIGO) Acute Kidney Injury Work Group. KDIGO Clinical Practice Guideline for Acute Kidney Injury. Kidney Inter., Suppl. 2012; 2: 1-138.

3. Treat **dyslipidemia** using a statin. There are no specific target goals for low-density lipoprotein cholesterol (LDL-C). Consider measuring lipids to assess adherence to the drug regimen. A reduced statin dose is recommended in patients with an eGFR <60 mL/min/1.73 m^2 (→Chapter 9.2). The initiation of statin therapy has not been shown to be beneficial in patients undergoing chronic dialysis treatment. The use of antiplatelet and antithrombotic agents in patients with DKD for the prevention of CKD remains controversial.

4. For patients with non–dialysis-dependent DKD, the suggested **dietary protein intake** is the same as in the general population—approximately 0.8 g/kg of body weight per day (usual recommended daily allowance)—and **sodium intake** could be restricted to 50 to 100 mmol/d. Reducing the amount of dietary protein below the recommended daily allowance of 0.8 g/kg/d is not recommended because it does not alter glycemic control, cardiovascular risk, or glomerular filtration rate (GFR) decline. Of note, considering some uncertainty regarding the effects of dietary protein intake, any restriction below normal intake should be limited to highly motivated, well-nourished patients with access to a wide variety of foods and expert dietary supervision following a discussion of the uncertain effectiveness of this intervention.

5. Educate the patient about the need to **avoid nephrotoxic substances, smoking cessation, and maintaining a recommended body weight**.

6. When diagnosing renal failure (GFR <60 mL/min/1.73 m^2), our pattern of practice is to **refer the patient to a nephrologist** for the evaluation and management of potential complications of CKD. A suspicion of alternative or additional causes of nephropathy should also be the reason for referral. Other, more conservative criteria for referral and principles of CKD treatment: →Chapter 9.2.

2.1.2.3. Diabetic Neuropathy

→ ETIOLOGY, PATHOGENESIS, CLINICAL FEATURES

Diabetic neuropathy is the most frequent chronic complication of diabetes mellitus (DM), present in 20% of patients with type 1 DM after 20 years of disease duration and in 10% to 15% of newly diagnosed patients with type 2 DM (50% after 10 years of disease duration). Metabolic abnormalities and changes in blood vessels supplying the nerves result in segmental demyelination, axonal atrophy and degeneration, and atrophy of neurons of the anterior horns and intervertebral ganglia; they may be accompanied by features of neuronal regeneration and changes in blood vessels supplying the nerves. Causative factors include persistent hyperglycemia, microvascular insufficiency, oxidative and nitrosative stress, defective neurotropism, and autoimmune-mediated nerve destruction.

Diabetic neuropathy is a diagnosis of exclusion. The most important differential diagnoses include neuropathies caused by alcohol abuse, uremia, hypothyroidism, vitamin B_{12} deficiency, peripheral arterial disease, cancer, inflammatory and infectious diseases, and neurotoxic drugs. Nondiabetic neuropathies may be present in patients with DM and may be treatable.

Diabetic neuropathy is classified as peripheral or autonomic.

1. Diabetic peripheral neuropathy: The most frequent type of diabetic neuropathy. Up to 50% of patients may be asymptomatic. The most common symptoms include paresthesia and dysesthesia of the hands and feet, neuropathic pain (burning, lancinating, tingling, or shooting), painful muscle cramps and acute pain attacks, superficial and deep sensory deficits (hyperalgesia or allodynia), muscle weakness, hyporeflexia or areflexia, trophic changes, and autonomic disturbances. The symptoms are chronic, not related to exercise, and usually worsen at night. The loss of protective sensation indicates the presence of distal sensorimotor polyneuropathy, which is considered a risk factor for diabetic foot ulceration. If this is not recognized and if preventive foot care is not implemented, patients are at risk for injuries to their insensate feet. Diabetic peripheral neuropathy has also been strongly associated with falls and fractures.

Classification of diabetic peripheral neuropathy:

1) **Distal symmetric polyneuropathy**: Accounting for 75% cases of diabetic neuropathies. It is defined by the presence of distal symmetric symptoms and/or signs of peripheral nerve dysfunction in patients with DM after other causes have been excluded. It is classified as primarily small-fiber, primarily large-fiber, and mixed small-fiber and large-fiber neuropathy. Tests for assessing the involvement of small and large fibers:

   a) Small-fiber function: Pinprick and temperature sensation.

   b) Large-fiber function: Vibration perception, ankle reflex, and proprioceptive sensation.

2) **Mononeuropathy**: Isolated cranial or peripheral (cranial neuropathies, carpal tunnel syndrome, and ulnar, femoral, or peroneal entrapment) and mononeuritis multiplex. These are more prevalent in the older population, have an acute onset with localized pain, and a self-limiting course with resolution in 6 to 8 weeks.

3) **Radiculopathy or polyradiculopathy**: Radiculoplexus neuropathy (lumbosacral polyradiculopathy, proximal motor amyotrophy) and thoracic radiculopathy. Proximal motor amyotrophy primarily affects the elderly, has an acute or gradual onset, and usually manifests with severe pain in the thighs, hips, and buttocks followed by significant weakness of the proximal muscles of the lower limbs and inability to rise from the sitting position.

Nondiabetic neuropathies common in DM include pressure palsies, chronic inflammatory demyelinating polyneuropathy, radiculoplexus neuropathy, and treatment-induced acute painful small-fiber neuropathies.

Assessment of peripheral neuropathy should be performed at diagnosis of type 2 DM and 5 years after diagnosis of type 1 DM. Follow-up should be done every 6 to 12 months. Diagnostic studies include assessment of the sense of touch (plantar) using a 10-g monofilament (eg, Semmes-Weinstein 5.07 monofilament applied at selected locations on the foot for ~1.5 second using a force that causes bending of the monofilament), testing the sense of vibration with a tuning fork (128 Hz, applied at the lateral malleolus and medial malleolus, superior portion of the tibia, and bases of the big toe and fifth toe), and testing the sense of temperature using a double-tipped metal or plastic probe. When previous tests are inconclusive and another type of neuropathy is suspected, nerve conduction studies and electromyography may be performed. Atypical features include motor greater than sensory neuropathy, rapid onset, or asymmetric presentation.

2. Diabetic autonomic neuropathy: Major clinical manifestations include hypoglycemia unawareness, resting tachycardia, orthostatic hypotension, gastroparesis, constipation, diarrhea, neurogenic bladder, and sudomotor dysfunction with either increased or decreased sweating.

1) **Involving the cardiovascular system**: Associated with cardiovascular mortality, arrhythmia, silent ischemia, myocardial dysfunction, and any major cardiovascular event independently of other cardiovascular risk factors. The key features are orthostatic hypotension (a fall in systolic blood pressure by >20 mm Hg or in diastolic blood pressure >10 mm Hg upon standing without an appropriate increase in heart rate), syncope, resting tachycardia (>100 beats/min), and sudden death (malignant arrhythmia). The diagnostic study performed is the Ewing cardiovascular test battery, which detects absence of heart rate variability on deep respiration, getting up, and Valsalva maneuver, as well as orthostatic hypotension when standing up, or absence of blood pressure increase on squeezing a dynamometer.

2) **Involving the gastrointestinal system**: This usually manifests as delayed gastric emptying, esophageal dysmotility, gastroparesis, constipation, diarrhea, and/or fecal incontinence. Diagnostic studies include contrast barium studies, gastric ultrasonography, gastrointestinal manometry, electrogastrography, and radionuclide studies (to assess retention of gastric contents). Exclude organic causes of gastric outlet obstruction or peptic ulcer disease before considering specialized testing for gastroparesis.

3) **Involving the genitourinary system**: One of the most frequent causes of erectile dysfunction and/or retrograde ejaculation, which is seen in ~50% of men with DM. In women it may result in vaginal dryness (increased pain during intercourse, decreased sexual arousal, inadequate lubrication) and loss of libido. Consider hormonal evaluation to exclude hypogonadism. Urogenital neuropathy also causes urinary retention (this is assessed using ultrasonography performed after voiding), urinary incontinence, and bladder dysfunction (nocturia, frequent urination, urination urgency, weak urinary stream). All patients with recurrent urinary tract infections, pyelonephritis, incontinence, or a palpable bladder should be assessed for the presence of neuropathy.

4) **Other**, which may involve the eyes (including abnormal pupil reactions to light) as well as sudomotor dysfunction (distal hypohidrosis/anhidrosis, abnormal perspiration, and gustatory sweating).

Assessment of autonomic neuropathy should be done in all patients with microvascular and neuropathic complications. Recognition and treatment of autonomic neuropathy may improve symptoms, reduce sequelae, and improve quality of life.

▶ **TREATMENT**

1. Good DM control and lifestyle modifications (exercise and healthy dietary plan) are of key importance. Glucose control has been shown to prevent diabetic peripheral neuropathy and cardiac autonomic neuropathy in type 1 DM and to modestly slow their progression in type 2 DM without reversal of neuronal loss. Avoid hypoglycemia, particularly for primary prevention. Consider using an angiotensin-converting enzyme inhibitor (ACEI) only when blood pressure does not meet the target level (140/90 mm Hg). Evaluate the risk of falls by assessing gait and balance, cognitive function, concomitantly used drugs, and presence of neuropathic pain.

2. Symptomatic treatment of painful polyneuropathy:

1) **Treatment of neuropathic pain**: →Chapter 1.20. Pregabalin (300--600 mg/d) and duloxetine (60-120 mg/d) are both approved by the US Food and Drug Administration (FDA), Health Canada, and the European Medicines Agency for the treatment of neuropathic pain in DM. Other therapies include antiepileptic drugs (gabapentin 900-3600 mg/d), tricyclic antidepressants (amitriptyline 25-100 mg/d, imipramine 25-150 mg/d, nortriptyline 50-150 mg/d, desipramine 25-150 mg/d), opioids (tramadol, tapentadol), venlafaxine (75-225 mg/d), carbamazepine, and topical capsaicin.⊘◯ Nonsteroidal anti-inflammatory drugs (eg, oral ibuprofen 400-800 mg tid, oral naproxen 500 mg bid) or acetaminophen (INN paracetamol) (1 g orally tid) are short-term alternatives if pain is too intense.

2) **α-Lipoic acid** (INN thioctic acid) 600 mg/d IV for the first 2 to 4 weeks followed by oral administration may be tried as an alternative. It may be useful in reduction of oxidative stress-induced nerve damage exacerbated by chronic hyperglycemia.

3. Symptomatic treatment of autonomic neuropathy:

1) **Syncope**: →Chapter 10.4.2.

2) **Orthostatic hypotension**: Nonpharmacologic and pharmacologic measures are used. Patients should ensure adequate fluid and salt intake and avoid medications that aggravate hypotension. Compressive garments over the legs and abdomen may be used. Therapeutic options include midodrine and droxidopa. Low-dose fludrocortisone may be of benefit in some patients.

3) **Gastroparesis**: Nutritional management (a low-fiber low-fat eating plan with frequent small-volume meals and foods with small particle size; in severe cases a semiliquid or liquid diet), prokinetic drugs (eg, domperidone, metoclopramide), erythromycin, and proton pump inhibitors (→Chapter 6.1.2.4). Prokinetic agents should be used at the lowest doses and for the shortest duration possible, generally not exceeding 3 months. Avoid drugs with adverse effects on gastrointestinal motility (opioids, anticholinergics, tricyclic antidepressants, glucagon-like peptide-1 [GLP-1] receptor agonists, pramlintide, and dipeptidyl peptidase-4 [DPP-4] inhibitors). In patients with severe gastroparesis surgical treatment and stimulation of gastric bioelectrical activity can be considered.

4) **Abnormal intestinal motility**: Nutritional management (eg, gluten-free diet, lactose restriction), cholestyramine, clonidine, octreotide, antidiarrheal drugs (loperamide), pancreatic enzymes, antibiotics; each may be tried if other interventions fail despite the lack of convincing evidence of efficacy.

5) **Atonic bladder**: Avoidance of urine retention, parasympathomimetic drugs (eg, bethanechol), catheterization (an intermittent or indwelling catheter).

6) **Erectile dysfunction**: Phosphodiesterase-5 (PDE-5) inhibitors (avanafil, sildenafil, tadalafil, vardenafil). Consider intracorporeal or intraurethral prostaglandins, vacuum devices, or penile prostheses in advanced cases. Note the interactions with nitrates in patients with coronary heart disease.

7) **Sudomotor dysfunction**: Botulinum toxin, vasodilator drugs, moisturizing creams, and topical antimuscarinic agents (glycopyrrolate).

3. Symptomatic treatment of atypical neuropathies:

1) **Mononeuropathies**: Cranial neuropathies usually resolve spontaneously over several months. Nerve entrapments may require surgical decompression.

In both cases anti-inflammatory medications and glucocorticoid injections may be needed in selected patients.

2) **Diabetic radiculoplexus neuropathy**: Usually self-limiting, with improvement in symptoms with medical management and physical therapy.

2.1.2.4. Diabetic Retinopathy

→ ETIOLOGY, PATHOGENESIS, CLASSIFICATION

Diabetic retinopathy is present in most patients with diabetes mellitus (DM) (after 20 years from diagnosis in almost all patients with type 1 DM and in more than half of patients with type 2 DM). It is the most frequent cause of new cases of blindness and visual impairment among adults aged 20 to 74 years in developed countries and is a frequent cause of glaucoma, cataracts, and other disorders in the eye at early ages. The key factors in the pathogenesis and progression of diabetic retinopathy are DM duration, baseline retinopathy at the diagnosis of DM, chronic hyperglycemia, nephropathy, dyslipidemia, and hypertension.

Retinopathy usually progresses from mild nonproliferative abnormalities (microaneurysm formation and intraretinal hemorrhages) to retinal capillary nonperfusion, cotton wool spots, increased numbers of hemorrhages, venous abnormalities, and intraretinal microvascular abnormalities. Eventually this leads to increased vascular permeability, vascular occlusion, and neovascularization on the disc, retina, iris, and in the filtration angle, resulting in traction retinal detachments and neovascular glaucoma. All these changes can be accelerated by the presence of pregnancy and puberty.

The American Academy of Ophthalmology established the International Classification of Diabetic Retinopathy and Diabetic Macular Edema, which describes **5 clinical levels of diabetic retinopathy**:

1) No apparent retinopathy and no abnormalities.
2) Mild nonproliferative diabetes retinopathy (NPDR) with microaneurysms only.
3) Moderate NPDR with microaneurysms and other abnormalities but less than severe NPDR.
4) Severe NPDR with any of the following: $\geq$20 intraretinal hemorrhages in each of the 4 retinal quadrants, definite venous beading in $\geq$2 retinal quadrants, prominent intraretinal microvascular abnormalities in $\geq$1 retinal quadrants, and no proliferative diabetic retinopathy (PDR).
5) PDR with $\geq$1 of the following: Retinal neovascularization, vitreous hemorrhage, or preretinal hemorrhage. Neovascular glaucoma can result from new vessels growing in the iris and anterior chamber angle structures.

Diabetic macular edema (DME) can be present with any level of diabetic retinopathy. It develops as a consequence of increased retinal vascular permeability that results in retinal thickening and lipid deposits (hard exudates). The DME classification is based on the ophthalmic findings (retinal thickening or hard exudates in the posterior pole):

1) Mild DME: Some retinal thickening or hard exudates in the posterior pole but distant from the center of the macula.
2) Moderate DME: Findings approaching but not involving the center of the macula.
3) Severe DME: Findings involving the center of the macula.

Clinically significant DME is considered, for example, when retinal edema or hard exudates are located at or within 500 μm of the center of the macula.

Vision loss due to diabetic retinopathy develops when the retinal neurons are damaged as a result of macular edema, capillary nonperfusion, retinal detachment, neovascularization, and/or in the preretinal or vitreous hemorrhage.

→ DIAGNOSIS AND FOLLOW-UP

The **first ophthalmologic examination** should be performed within 5 years of establishing the diagnosis of type 1 DM and at the moment of diagnosis of type 2 DM. Perform **follow-up** examinations every 1 to 2 years in patients with no retinopathy, every 6 to 12 months in those with early stages of NPDR, every 3 months in patients with more advanced retinopathy, and within 3 to 4 months in patients with non–clinically significant DME. In women with **preexisting DM who are planning pregnancy**, eye examinations should take place before pregnancy or in the first trimester and then should be followed up every trimester and for 1 year postpartum, as dictated by the degree of retinopathy. Follow-up should be done every 1 to 3 months in case of severe NPDR or worse. No eye examinations are required during pregnancy in patients who develop gestational DM.

Eye examinations should be performed by an ophthalmologist or optometrist who is knowledgeable and experienced in diagnosing diabetic retinopathy. Examination must include visual acuity and color vision, dilated slit-lamp biomicroscopy with a hand-held lens, intraocular pressure, gonioscopy, pupillary assessment for optic nerve dysfunction, stereoscopic examination of the posterior pole, and examination of the peripheral retina and vitreous. Rarely **specialized studies** such as optical coherence tomography and **fluorescein angiography** of the fundus are indicated. These can be useful in patients with very early retinopathy (undetectable by ophthalmoscopy), macular edema, and NPDR, as well as for the assessment of the effects of laser therapy. **Retinal photography with remote reading** can be a useful screening tool in areas where qualified eye-care professionals are not available; however, it should not be a substitute for a comprehensive eye examination, at least initially.

→ PREVENTION AND TREATMENT

1. The goal of treatment in patients with no apparent retinopathy and mild and moderate NPDR is to optimize medical therapy. **Early detection and optimal control of DM** can reduce the risk or slow down the progression of diabetic retinopathy: a 10% reduction in glycated hemoglobin (HbA_{1c}) reduces the risk of retinopathy progression by 43% in patients with type 1 DM, and every percentage-point decrease in HbA_{1c} is associated with a 35% reduction in the risk of microvascular complications in patients with type 2 DM. Target levels of preprandial glucose are 4.4 to 7.2 mmol/L (80-130 mg/dL) and target levels of postprandial glucose are ≤10.0 mmol/L (180 mg/dL), with HbA_{1c} ≤7.0% in the general population.

2. Effective treatment of **hypertension and dyslipidemia** is of key importance. Angiotensin-converting enzyme inhibitors (ACEIs) and angiotensin receptor blockers (ARBs) are both effective treatments in diabetic retinopathy. The addition of fenofibrate has shown to slow down the progression of retinopathy in patients with dyslipidemia and preexisting diabetic retinopathy. The presence of retinopathy is not a contraindication to acetylsalicylic acid (ASA) therapy for prevention of cardiovascular disease.

3. The mainstay of treatment aimed at inhibiting the progression of vascular lesions is grid, focal, or panretinal **laser photocoagulation therapy**, which is used in patients with DME, advanced NPDR, and early proliferative retinopathy to reduce the risk of severe vision loss. Advanced proliferative retinopathy (vitreous hemorrhages, connective tissue proliferation) is an indication for **vitrectomy**.

4. In patients with severe central-involved DME, injections of intravitreal **anti–vascular endothelial growth factor (anti-VEGF)** preparations (bevacizumab, ranibizumab, and aflibercept) have replaced the need for laser photocoagulation, although the cost of treatment and need for frequent follow-up visits may limit their use.⊘⊖ Anti-VEGF preparations can also be used as an alternative or adjunct to laser photocoagulation in patients with DPR, as rapid regression of retinal neovascularization has been observed in several studies. Ranibizumab, a selective monoclonal antibody to VEGF, is the first-line agent in all patients with DME with central foveal involvement. Aflibercept is another agent indicated for the treatment of visual impairment due to DME, especially in patients with lower levels of acuity (20/50 or worse). The therapeutic regimen is based on near-monthly administrations during the first 12 months with fewer injections administered as needed in subsequent years as maintenance therapy.

5. Other treatments such as intravitreal glucocorticoids, topical nonsteroidal anti-inflammatory drugs, antioxidants, inflammatory molecule inhibitors, renin-angiotensin-aldosterone system blockers, and natural anti-inflammatory therapies can be considered, in a specialized settings, as adjunct therapies to reduce the rate of administration of anti-VEGF agents or in cases where anti--VEGF agents are contraindicated.

2.2. Diabetes Mellitus in Pregnant Patients

In general terms, we distinguish between **diabetes mellitus in pregnancy** (usually preexisting or diagnosed in the first half of pregnancy) and **gestational diabetes** (usually developed and diagnosed in the second half of pregnancy).

Details of treatment are presented in respective chapters. Generally speaking, most oral drugs are not proven to be safe during pregnancy with the exception of metformin and glyburide. Women with type 1 diabetes mellitus require insulin, and most women with type 2 diabetes mellitus will need some insulin as well. For gestational diabetes, the majority of patients are controlled with diet. In terms of pharmacotherapy, insulin but also metformin or glyburide can be the first choice, depending on patient preferences and individual patient circumstances.

2.2.1. Diabetes Mellitus in Pregnancy

▶ DEFINITION AND NATURAL HISTORY

Diabetes mellitus in a pregnant woman is any type of diabetes that has been diagnosed before pregnancy or early in pregnancy on the basis of standard diabetes criteria for nonpregnant patients (→Chapter 5.2).

1. The effect of pregnancy on the course of diabetes: In pregnancy, mainly due to placental secretion, the levels of insulin antagonist hormones (placental lactogen, placental growth hormone [growth hormone isoform V], insulin-like growth factor 1 [IGF-1], estrogen, progesterone, prolactin, and cortisol), as well as binding proteins (IGF-binding proteins, cortisol-binding globulin) are significantly increased, which results in insulin resistance and increased β-cell activity demand. In patients with diabetes this leads to hyperglycemia, increased insulin requirements, as well as difficult-to-control diabetes and accelerated development of diabetes-specific microvascular complications (retinopathy, nephropathy).

2. The effect of diabetes on the course of pregnancy: Unlike insulin, glucose crosses the placental barrier—facilitated by glucose transporter proteins, predominantly glucose transporter 1, independently from insulin—and thus hyperglycemia in the mother results in elevated fetal blood glucose levels, stimulation and hypertrophy of fetal pancreatic islets, and insulin hypersecretion. This leads to anabolic effects, causing fetal macrosomia, and to fetal immaturity, which together increase the risk of obstetric complications associated with more frequent deliveries by cesarean sections, birth weight ≥4000 g, shoulder dystocia, perinatal injury, polyhydramnios, preeclampsia, and low Apgar scores.

Significant hyperglycemia may also result in miscarriage, growth restriction, preterm delivery, intrauterine death, or congenital malformations, most commonly neural tube defects and congenital heart malformations.

→ **TREATMENT**

1. When planning pregnancy:

1) Preconception management and counseling is important for good pregnancy outcomes. Counseling is mandatory to start in patients with diabetes at puberty. Contraception should be offered and encouraged until a woman is planning to become pregnant. Counseling should address the importance of maintaining glycemic control close to normal.

2) Try to maintain a fasting blood glucose level ≤5.5 mmol/L (100 mg/dL) and glycated hemoglobin level (HbA_{1c}) <6.5%, if safely achieved.⊙◯ Monitor for infections and treat them as required. Diagnose and treat chronic complications and intensify patient education.

3) Fundoscopic eye examination should be performed before pregnancy or in the first trimester of pregnancy and repeated each trimester until 1 year postpartum (treatment may be provided if needed).

4) Folic acid in a dose 400 μg daily is recommended at least 3 months before the planned pregnancy.

5) Statins should be withheld during pregnancy as they have been associated with congenital malformations.

6) Angiotensin-converting enzyme inhibitors and angiotensin receptor blockers should be stopped and β-blockers or calcium channel blockers should be considered as needed.

7) Thyroid-stimulating hormone is recommended to be checked before pregnancy, particularly in patients with type 1 diabetes, as subclinical hypothyroidism has been associated with preterm delivery, preeclampsia, and pregnancy loss.

2. During pregnancy: Strict control of diabetes is suggested throughout the entire duration of pregnancy (HbA_{1c} <6.0% if achieved without hypoglycemia; otherwise <7.0%). This is especially important during the first trimester of pregnancy,⊙◯ because the risk of congenital malformations is higher in this period. The goals of treatment are to maintain normoglycemia with the minimum risk of hypoglycemia and to maintain fetal well-being and maternal health during pregnancy. This can be achieved through nutritional and pharmacologic therapy. Low-dose acetylsalicylic acid (60-120 mg) may be recommended for women who are at high risk of preeclampsia from the end of the first trimester until delivery (→Chapter 3.9.2.2.). In patients with preexisting hypertension, blood pressure targets of 120 to 140 systolic blood pressure and 80 to 90 mm Hg diastolic blood pressure are suggested.

3. Postpartum care: Insulin sensitivity increases dramatically after delivery of the placenta. Insulin requirements are usually 1/3 lower than during pregnancy and return to their prepregnancy baseline within several days. Attention should be paid to avoid hypoglycemia in the setting of breastfeeding and erratic sleep schedules. In the immediate postpartum period it is suggested to review contraception options to prevent unplanned pregnancy.

Monitoring and Target Blood Glucose Values

As indicated above, the **suggested HbA_{1c} target level is <6.0% if it can be safely achieved or otherwise <7.0% to prevent hypoglycemia**; we suggest measuring the level every 6 weeks.⊙◯ **Target blood glucose levels** (based on glucometer measurements) may slightly differ from the values specified below as long as they allow the target HbA_{1c} levels to be maintained.

Fasting blood glucose and glucose levels:

1) Fasting or before meals: <5.3 mmol/L (95 mg/dL).

2) 1 hour after meals: < 7.8 mmol/L (140 mg/dL).

3) 2 hours after meals: <6.7 mmol/L (120 mg/dL).

4) At night between 2:00 and 4:00: >3.3 mmol/L (60 mg/dL).

It is important to avoid hypoglycemic episodes, as they have been closely associated with an increased maternal and fetal morbidity. The most accurate assessment of 24-hour blood glucose levels is obtained using continuous blood glucose monitoring systems. The target mean 24-hour glucose level is ≤5.3 mmol/L (95 mg/dL). Pregnant women can self-monitor glucose levels 8 to 10 times a day (to meet all the goals), although this is often not needed. In our experience, measurements performed 3 to 4 times a day, alternating times between days, are sufficient in most cases.

Nutritional Therapy

No specific diet regimen is recommended to improve maternal or fetal outcomes.⊘◌ The goals of nutritional therapy are to prevent ketone formation and promote adequate maternal weight gain and fetal growth. The suggested caloric intake is per current weight and prepregnancy body mass index (BMI) calculation:

1) Underweight: 40 kcal/kg/d.

2) Normal weight: 30 kcal/kg/d.

3) Overweight: 20 to 25 kcal/kg/d.

4) Morbid obesity (BMI ≥40): 12 to 14 kcal/kg/d.

The Dietary Reference Intakes (DRI) recommend a minimum of 175 g of carbohydrate, 71 g of protein, and 28 g of dietary fiber intake for all pregnant women.

Pharmacologic Therapy

In most cases, if insulin therapy has not been used before, it is suggested to start it immediately and continue throughout pregnancy (using a basal-bolus regimen or an insulin pump). Intermediate-acting human insulin (insulin isophane [NPH]) and rapid-acting insulin are the preferred choices. However, in patients using long-acting insulin (glargine or detemir) who were well controlled before pregnancy, these agents can be continued. Consider the possibility of increased (as much as 2-fold) insulin requirements particularly during the second and third trimesters.

Systematic reviews have found oral medications could be safely used in pregnancy.⊘◌ Accordingly, oral medications such as metformin and glyburide may be used in type 2 diabetes and other types of diabetes, such as maturity-onset diabetes of the youth (MODY), during pregnancy (→Table 2-15). Although metformin crosses the placenta, its use during pregnancy has been tested and is considered to be safe. Some of the advantages of metformin are the low risk of hypoglycemia, reduced maternal weight gain, and a reduction in perinatal morbidity, particularly in obese women or those using concomitantly high doses of insulin. Glyburide also crosses the placental barrier, and some studies have shown an increased rate of neonatal hypoglycemia and birth weight ≥4000 g. Therefore, our pattern is to use metformin or glyburide (especially if such treatment was received before pregnancy), and if the patient remains well controlled, the agents may be continued. If glycemic targets are not met, insulin therapy may be added to the oral medication; in most cases, during the second and third trimesters some insulin will be required to achieve glycemic targets (→Table 2-15).

1. During delivery (either vaginal or cesarean): Administer continuous intravenous insulin infusion (continuous subcutaneous infusion using an insulin pump is acceptable) at doses corresponding to daily requirements and ensure appropriate caloric intake (800-1200 kcal) by intravenous glucose (dextrose) infusion. Blood glucose levels should be within the range of 5.6 to 10.0 mmol/L (100-180 mg/dL). Insulin administration should not be discontinued at this point, especially in type 1 diabetes, since there is an increased risk for developing diabetic ketoacidosis.

Table 2-15. Medical management of diabetes during pregnancy

	Duration	Onset	Time to peak	Peak effect	Pregnancy risk factor
Oral agents					
Biguanides: Metformin					B
Immediate-release	4-9 h	–	2-3 h	–	
Extended-release		–	7 h	–	
Sulfonylureas					
Glyburide	<24 h	–	2-4 h	–	B/C
Insulin					
Short-acting					
Lispro	–	15-30 min	–	0.5-3 h	B
Aspart	–	12-30 min	–	1-2 h	B
Regular	–	15-30 min	–	2.5-5 h	B
Intermediate-acting					
NPH	–	1-2 h	–	4-12 h	B
Long-acting					
Detemir	–	3-4 h	–	3-9 h	B
Glargine	–	3-4 h	–	No peak	C

B: Animal reproduction studies have failed to demonstrate a risk to the fetus and there are no adequate and well-controlled studies in pregnant women.

C: Animal reproduction studies have shown an adverse effect on the fetus and there are no adequate and well-controlled studies in humans, but potential benefits may warrant use of the drug in pregnant women despite potential risks.

NPH, insulin isophane (intermediate-acting human insulin).

2. After delivery: Insulin requirements may decrease to 50% or even as little as 30% of the predelivery levels. In patients with type 1 diabetes, hypoglycemia is very common during the first 24 to 48 hours. After delivery, for patients with type 2 diabetes, our pattern of practice is to stop insulin infusion, monitor glucose levels every 4 to 6 hours, and prescribe the insulin sliding scale therapy. Standard diabetes therapy can be restarted by reducing the total insulin dose used before delivery by 50%. In patients who have been treated with oral antidiabetic drugs, these agents may be restarted. Metformin has been usually considered the first-line therapy. The evidence regarding oral glucose-lowering agents is scarce but, in general, those agents are considered safe (entering milk in minimal amounts), particularly metformin and glyburide. The risk of infant hypoglycemia is minimal with these drugs.

2.2.2. Gestational Diabetes Mellitus

→ DEFINITION, ETIOLOGY, PATHOGENESIS

Gestational diabetes mellitus (GDM) describes diabetes mellitus (DM) diagnosed in the second or third trimester of pregnancy in patients who meet ≥1 of the appropriate diagnostic criteria without clear diagnosis of overt diabetes prior to that time. Experts differ slightly in their views on optimal strategies for the diagnosis of GDM (→Table 2-16).

Risk factors include multiparity, age >35 years, previous delivery of a child >4000 g of birth weight, delivery of a child with malformations, intrauterine death, hypertension or a body mass index (BMI) >30 kg/m^2 before pregnancy, high-risk ethnic groups (eg, Hispanics, African American), family history of type 2 DM, or history of GDM (in ~30% of patients GDM develops again in a subsequent pregnancy).

→ DIAGNOSIS

The American Diabetes Association (ADA) suggests measuring fasting plasma glucose (FPG) levels and glycated hemoglobin (HbA$_{1c}$) in every pregnant woman at the first office visit to diagnose previously unrecognized type 2 DM. If FPG and HbA$_{1c}$ are within the reference range (<100 mg/dL and <6%, respectively) at the first visit, preferably in the first trimester, in all pregnant women within 24 to 28 weeks of pregnancy the ADA suggests to perform:

1) One-step diagnostic oral glucose tolerance test (OGTT) (fasting, with the administration of 75 g of glucose); or

2) Two-step OGTT, which starts with a nonfasting 50-g OGTT. If the result is ≥7.8 mmol/L (140 mg/dL) at 1 hour, then a fasting 100-g 3-hour OGTT is required.

GDM is diagnosed in patients with ≥1 abnormal glucose level found in the 1-step 75-g OGTT and 2 abnormal glucose levels in the 100-g OGTT (→Table 2-16).

In patients in whom blood glucose levels fail to normalize after delivery (6-12 weeks), testing for DM using standard diabetes criteria is recommended (→Chapter 5.2).

Diagnostic Criteria
→Table 2-16.

→ TREATMENT

1. Start with **nutritional therapy**. There is a paucity of evidence that one diet compared to others improves maternal or fetal outcomes.⊘◯ However, ~80% of pregnant patients with GDM can be controlled solely with an adequate diet. The daily caloric intake depends on the prepregnancy BMI, physical activity, and term of pregnancy:

1) Underweight: 40 kcal/kg/d.

2) Normal weight: 30 kcal/kg/d.

3) Overweight and obesity: 20 to 25 kcal/kg/d.

4) Morbid obesity (BMI ≥40): 12 to 14 kcal/kg/d.

The suggested diet may include 35% to 45% of carbohydrates (mainly complex carbohydrates), 25% to 35% of fats (with equal proportions of saturated and unsaturated fats), and 20% of protein (1.3 g/kg/d). It is recommended to substitute a percentage of animal protein by nonanimal protein (eg, broccoli, mushrooms). A high fiber (≥20 g/1000 kcal) daily intake is suggested. It is also recommended to consume 3 moderate-sized meals in addition to 2 to 4 snacks, including an evening snack.

Table 2-16. Diagnostic criteria for gestational diabetes mellitus

	75-g OGTT			100-g OGTT		
	WHO[a]	EASD[a]	IADPSG[a,d]	O'Sullivan and Mahan[b]	NDDG[b,c]	Carpenter and Coustan[b,c,d]
Sample	Venous plasma	Venous plasma	Venous plasma	Venous whole blood	Venous plasma	Venous plasma
Fasting glucose levels	5.1-6.9 mmol/L (92-125 mg/dL)	≥6.0 mmol/L (108 mg/dL)	≥5.1 mmol/L (92 mg/dL)	≥5.0 mmol/L (9C mg/dL)	≥5.8 mmol/L (105 mg/dL)	≥5.3 mmol/L (95 mg/dL)
1 h	≥10.0 mmol/L (180 mg/dL)	–	≥10.0 mmol/L (180 mg/dL)	>9.1 mmol/L (164 mg/dL)	≥10.6 mmol/L (190 mg/dL)	≥10.0 mmol/L (180 mg/dL)
2 h	8.5-11.0 mmol/L (153-199 mg/dL)	≥9.0 mmol/L (162 mg/dL)	≥8.5 mmol/L (153 mg/dL)	>8.0 mmol/L (144 mg/dL)	≥9.2 mmol/L (165 mg/dL)	≥8.6 mmol/L (155 mg/dL)
3 h	–	–	–	>6.9 mmol/L (124 mg/dL)	≥8.0 mmol/L (145 mg/dL)	≥7.8 mmol/L (140 mg/dL)

[a] Diagnosis is defined by one abnormal glucose value at any time point.
[b] Diagnosis is defined by two or more abnormal values at different time points.
[c] Diagnostic thresholds recommended by the American College of Obstetricians and Gynecologists.
[d] Diagnostic thresholds recommended by the American Diabetes Association.

EASD, European Association for the Study of Diabetes; IADPSG, International Association of Diabetes and Pregnancy Study Group; NDDG, National Diabetes Data Group; OGTT, oral glucose tolerance test; WHO, World Health Organization.

The Dietary Reference Intake (DRI) suggests a minimal consumption of 175 g of carbohydrate, 71 g of protein, and 24 g of fiber. The design of nutritional therapy has to be individualized in each patient and it is highly recommended that the assessment is done by a dietitian with expertise in GDM. The goal of this treatment is to have an adequate balance in caloric intake that benefits both the offspring and the mother and to achieve adequate glycemic control.

2. Pharmacologic therapy: In patients who have been compliant with appropriate nutritional therapy for 5 to 7 days and have not achieved normal blood glucose levels (criteria for glycemic control: →Chapter 5.2.2.1) or those with an initial highly elevated glucose level, insulin is suggested as the first-line therapy. **Intensive insulin therapy** (a multiple daily injection regimen) using subcutaneous injections of short-acting human insulin or a rapid-acting insulin analogue and intermediate-acting human insulin (insulin isophane [NPH]) can be started. There is not enough data from randomized trials to prove the safety of long-acting insulin analogues (glargine and detemir) and NPH is preferred. Oral glucose-lowering drugs were previously considered to be contraindicated; however, metformin and glyburide (alone or in combination with insulin) have been proven effective and safe in patients with GDM and can be also used as a first-choice or add-on therapy. Metformin, compared with other therapeutic options like insulin or sulfonylureas, has been associated with smaller weight gain and lower prevalence of pregnancy-induced hypertension and neonatal hypoglycemia despite the fact that metformin crosses the placental barrier. Glyburide can also be used during pregnancy, but it has been associated with increased prevalence of neonatal hypoglycemia (fetal hyperinsulinism) and birth weights ≥4000 g.⊘◔

3. Management during delivery: In patients treated with insulin, the management is the same as in preexisting DM (→Chapter 5.2.2.1). In women who have achieved satisfactory blood glucose control with diet alone, insulin should be administered during delivery only if blood glucose levels are >7.2 mmol/L (130 mg/dL).

4. Any type of therapy should be discontinued immediately after delivery unless there is a high suspicion for type 1 DM. Since patients with GDM are at increased risk of developing type 2 DM, a 2-hour 75-g OGTT is recommended 6 to 12 weeks after delivery. Patients meeting the criteria for prediabetes should be counseled about their increased risk of DM and should consider lifestyle modification strategies (nutritional therapy, metformin and exercise). In patients with a diagnosis of DM, start lifestyle changes and oral medications as in any other patient with a recent diagnosis of type 2 DM.

3. Hypothalamus and Pituitary Diseases

3.1. Diabetes Insipidus

→ DEFINITION, ETIOLOGY, PATHOGENESIS

Diabetes insipidus (DI) is a condition characterized by increased water loss (polyuria) and excessive thirst (polydipsia) due to:

1) **Central DI** (neurohypophyseal): Arginine vasopressin (antidiuretic hormone) (ADH) deficiency. This may result from:

   a) Damage to the vasopressin-secreting neurons located in the supraoptic and paraventricular nuclei in the hypothalamus or to the pituitary stalk or posterior pituitary gland (vasopressin transport and storage sites, respectively). The most common cause of central DI is idiopathic (autoimmune process) followed by tumors (germinoma, metastatic lesions, craniopharyngioma), infiltrative diseases (sarcoidosis, Langerhans cell histiocytosis), hypoxic encephalopathy, and head trauma.

b) Genetic defects, such as familial central DI (autosomal dominant gene defect encoding ADH), Wolfram syndrome (DIDMOAD syndrome [**d**iabetes **i**nsipidus, **d**iabetes **m**ellitus, **o**ptic **a**trophy, and **d**eafness]), congenital hypopituitarism, and septo-optic dysplasia.

2) **Nephrogenic DI**: Loss of sensitivity of the renal tubules to ADH (ADH resistance), which may result from a genetic defect of the renal vasopressin receptors (aquaporin-2 water channels). Nephrogenic DI may also occur in hypercalcemia (eg, hyperparathyroidism), hypokalemia (eg, primary hyperaldosteronism), renal diseases (eg, bilaterally urinary tract obstruction, polycystic kidney disease, renal amyloidosis), and drugs (eg, lithium [most common], amphotericin B, cidofovir, and foscarnet).

→ CLINICAL FEATURES

DI manifests as excessive thirst (polydipsia) and polyuria (>3 L/24 h). Patients characteristically report nocturia (sometimes voiding several times throughout the night) and night thirst. Signs and symptoms due to hypernatremia or an underlying hypothalamic-pituitary tumor may also be present.

Onset of polyuria:

1) Children: Familiar central DI and hereditary nephrogenic DI manifest with severe polyuria in the first week of life.

2) Adults: Central DI manifests in an abrupt manner. Nephrogenic DI has a gradual onset.

→ DIAGNOSIS

Diagnostic Tests

1. Laboratory studies:

1) Urine specific gravity ≤**1.005**.

2) Plasma sodium concentration: High-normal (≥142 mmol/L).

3) Urine osmolality: Low and characteristically lower than plasma osmolality.

4) Urinary sodium: Usually <20 mmol/L.

5) **Water restriction test** (combined with the desmopressin stimulation test): In patients with suspected DI before performing this test it is important to confirm hypotonic polyuria (suggested values: →Table 3-1). The test is performed usually in an inpatient setting only after diabetic polyuria has been excluded. The patient should stop drinking water in the morning before arriving to the clinic (avoid nocturnal water restriction) and have urine volume, urine osmolality, plasma sodium concentration, plasma osmolality, and body weight measured at baseline. Urine specific gravity or osmolality is measured in each consecutive urine sample (with frequency depending on the clinical situation, even hourly if needed) along with plasma osmolality, serum sodium levels, and body weight; serum ADH level may be determined at the end of the test. Terminate the test when: (1) body weight decreases ≥3%; (2) urine osmolality is stable (difference <10%) in 2 or 3 samples despite rising plasma osmolality; (3) serum sodium levels are above the upper limit of normal (≥145 mmol/L) with plasma osmolality >295-300 mOsm/kg (in patients with DI, this usually occurs within a few hours); or (4) urine osmolality reaches a normal value (500-600 mOsm/kg). If the criteria for termination of the test are not met, it should be continued for 18 hours to exclude DI. Interpretation of test results: →Table 3-1.

6) **Desmopressin stimulation test** (second phase of the water restriction test) is performed to differentiate central DI from nephrogenic DI. Administer

Table 3-1. Differential diagnosis of psychogenic, central, and nephrogenic DI using water restriction and desmopressin stimulation

	Psychogenic polydipsia (psychogenic DI)	Central (neurohypophyseal) DI	Nephrogenic DI
Water restriction test (fluid deprivation test)			
Urine specific gravity	>1.005	<1.005	<1.005
Urine osmolality	>500-600 mOsm/kg	<250 mOsm/kg	<250 mOsm/kg
Plasma ADH level	Initially low, then increasing	Low	High
Desmopressin stimulation test (desmopressin 0.2 mg PO, 10-20 µg intranasally, or 2-4 µg SC or IV)			
Urine specific gravity	No indication for the test[a]	Increased by ≥50%	Low, not increasing
Urine osmolality	No indication for the test[a]	Increase by 100% in complete central DI and 15% to 50% in partial central DI	No elevation

[a] As the results of the fluid deprivation test are normal.

ADH, antidiuretic hormone; DI, diabetes insipidus; IV, intravenous; PO, oral; SC, subcutaneous.

desmopressin 0.2 mg orally, 10 to 20 µg intranasally, or 2 to 4 µg subcutaneously or IV at the end of the fluid deprivation test. Measure the volume, specific gravity, and osmolality every 30 minutes for the next 2 hours. Interpretation of test results: →Table 3-1.

2. Imaging studies: A confirmed diagnosis of central DI is an absolute indication for magnetic resonance imaging (MRI) of the hypothalamic-pituitary area. The absence of T1 hyperintensity in the posterior pituitary lobe is seen in most patients with central DI.

Diagnostic Criteria and Differential Diagnosis
→Table 3-1.

➜ TREATMENT

1. Central DI: Replacement therapy with a long-acting ADH analogue desmopressin. Usually desmopressin is administered intranasally 10 to 20 µg once a day or bid, orally 0.05 to 0.2 mg in 1 or 2 doses or, where available, sublingually up to 60 to 120 µg tid. In patients with altered mental status, an IV or subcutaneous injection (2-4 µg daily) may be used. Adjust the dosage individually on the basis of resolution of clinical symptoms and normalization of plasma osmolality and serum sodium levels.

2. Nephrogenic DI: Management depends on the causative factor:

1) **Acquired renal injury**: Symptomatic treatment involving appropriate fluid replacement and management of the underlying condition.

2) **Electrolyte disturbances**: Signs and symptoms of DI improve with normalization of electrolyte levels.

3) **Genetic defects of ADH receptors**: Low-sodium diet plus a thiazide diuretic. Consider high-dose desmopressin in patients with a partial ADH-receptor response.

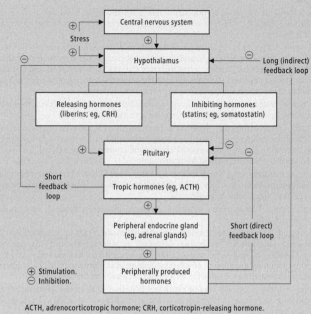

ACTH, adrenocorticotropic hormone; CRH, corticotropin-releasing hormone.

Figure 3-1. Stimulation and feedback loops in the endocrine system.

→ **PROGNOSIS**

Prognosis depends on the cause of central DI (tumor, trauma, metastases, inflammation, idiopathic). If the patient maintains appropriate fluid intake, untreated DI is not life-threatening. Special attention (fluid balance!) is warranted in the case of unconscious trauma patients, patients after central nervous system surgery, and patients with an altered sense of thirst due to the damaged hypothalamic thirst center. Advise the patients to carry information about their DI at all times. Patients with DI treated with hormone replacement may lead normal lives. Desmopressin overdose may cause syndrome of inappropriate antidiuretic hormone secretion (SIADH) (water retention and hyponatremia).

3.2. Hypopituitarism

→ **DEFINITION, ETIOLOGY, PATHOGENESIS**

Hypopituitarism refers to a syndrome caused by deficiency of one or more pituitary hormones, which can result from pituitary or hypothalamic disease (deficiency of pituitary hormone–releasing hormones). Deficiency of all pituitary hormones is known as panhypopituitarism. The resulting changes in hormonal levels and in the choice of diagnostic tests are related to the presence of several short and long feedback loops among different parts of the hypothalamic-pituitary-peripheral gland system (→Figure 3-1).

Causes:

1) **Congenital:** Familial hypopituitarism with multiple hormone deficiencies (*PROP1, HESX1, PIT1*) or developmental abnormalities (pituitary hypoplasia or aplasia).

2) **Tumors:** Pituitary tumors (functioning and nonfunctioning pituitary adenomas, Rathke or arachnoid cysts), posterior pituitary tumors (ganglioneuroma, astrocytoma), hypothalamic tumors (astrocytoma, germinoma), craniopharyngioma, tumors of the optic chiasm (meningioma, glioma), and metastases (most frequently breast and lung cancer).

3) **Cranial trauma and iatrogenic:** Severe head trauma, surgery (most frequently transsphenoidal), and pituitary/sellar irradiation.

4) **Vascular:** Postpartum pituitary infarction (due to postpartum hemorrhage [Sheehan syndrome]), pituitary apoplexy (sudden hemorrhage into the pituitary gland), internal carotid artery aneurysm (compression), and stroke (ischemic or subarachnoid hemorrhage).

5) **Inflammatory and infiltrative lesions:** Sarcoidosis, hemochromatosis, Langerhans cell histiocytosis, granulomatosis with polyangiitis, lymphocytic (autoimmune) hypophysitis.

6) **Infectious:** Tuberculosis, syphilis, mycoses, pituitary abscess, encephalitis, or meningitis.

7) **Isolated hormone deficiencies:** Growth hormone (GH) or gonadotropin deficiency (Kallmann syndrome: defective gonadotropin-releasing hormone synthesis [causing hypogonadotropic hypogonadism] associated with hyposmia). Isolated deficiency of adrenocorticotropic hormone (ACTH), thyroid--stimulating hormone (TSH), or prolactin is very rare.

In general, the acquired loss of pituitary function follows the sequence of GH, luteinizing hormone (LH)/follicle-stimulating hormone (FSH), TSH, ACTH, and prolactin.

⮕ CLINICAL FEATURES AND NATURAL HISTORY

Clinical manifestations can present suddenly or gradually, can be mild or severe, and can affect one, several, or all of the pituitary hormones. Consequently, the clinical presentation varies depending on the age of onset, severity of the hormonal deficiency, velocity (chronic or acute) at which the disease affects the pituitary gland, and number of cell lines affected (→Table 3-2). Additional specific situations are described below.

In patients with **pituitary apoplexy** (sudden hemorrhage into the pituitary gland), the presentation depends on the severity of hemorrhage and may include sudden-onset headache, nausea, vomiting, and confusion, which result from elevated intracranial pressure; visual disturbances resulting from compression of the optic chiasm and oculomotor nerves; and paralysis of extraocular muscles caused by a hemorrhage to the cavernous sinus. The most serious signs and symptoms of acute hypopituitarism are due to ACTH deficiency, which can result in life-threatening hypotension (refractory shock) and severe neurologic signs and symptoms in the case of a subarachnoid or intraventricular hemorrhage. On the other hand, hemorrhagic apoplexy of a pituitary adenoma may result in spontaneous healing and subsequent resolution of symptoms of hormone hypersecretion.

Acute ACTH deficiency may occur when the pituitary gland is damaged in the course of pituitary apoplexy, stroke, head trauma, or neurosurgical procedures. It is a life-threatening condition (adrenal crisis: →Chapter 5.1.1.1). **Chronic ACTH deficiency** (→Chapter 5.1.1.3) may become symptomatic and potentially lead to adrenal crisis after a sudden increase in the glucocorticoid requirements, especially in the setting of acute stress or infection.

Signs and symptoms of **posttraumatic hypopituitarism** usually develop gradually, becoming clinically overt within ~1 year after the event. In ~30%

Table 3-2. Signs and symptoms of anterior pituitary insufficiency according to deficiencies of individual pituitary hormones

Deficiency	Signs and symptoms
GH	Growth retardation (in children), decreased muscle mass, increased body fat (primarily visceral fat), decreased bone mineral density, hypoglycemia, hyperlipidemia (in adult-onset deficiency, signs and symptoms are nonspecific)
ACTH	Orthostatic hypotension, syncope, nausea and vomiting, anorexia, weight loss, elevated body temperature, decreased skin pigmentation, tendency to hypoglycemia (particularly in patients with coexisting GH deficiency)
TSH	Secondary hypothyroidism (signs and symptoms are less pronounced than in primary hypothyroidism, goiter is absent)
LH and FSH	Amenorrhea, male sexual dysfunction, decreased libido, disappearance or lack of tertiary sexual characteristics (pubic hair)
PRL	No lactation after childbirth

ACTH, adrenocorticotropic hormone; FSH, follicle-stimulating hormone; GH, growth hormone; LH, luteinizing hormone; PRL, prolactin; TSH, thyroid-stimulating hormone.

of patients severe head trauma may also cause damage to the hypothalamic supraoptic nucleus or the posterior pituitary lobe, resulting in antidiuretic hormone deficiency and the development of central diabetes insipidus.

→ DIAGNOSIS

Diagnosis entails a clinical examination looking for clinical manifestations of hormone deficiency (→Table 3-2) and requires the documentation of subnormal secretion of pituitary hormones in basal and/or stimulated tests exploring stimulation and feedback loops in the endocrine system (→Figure 3-1). Each pituitary hormone must be tested separately.

Diagnostic Tests

1. Laboratory studies:

1) Basal cortisol (8:00) levels.

2) TSH and free thyroxin levels.

3) Men: LH and basal testosterone (8:00). Women: In patients with normal menses, no tests are needed; if menses are abnormal, measure levels of FSH, LH, and estradiol.

4) Insulin-like growth factor 1 (IGF-1) (also called somatomedin C; its production is stimulated by GH).

5) Prolactin.

2. Magnetic resonance imaging (MRI) of the parasellar region should be performed in every case of hypopituitarism to determine its cause.

3. Visual fields should be assessed in patients with suspected pathologic lesions in the area of the optic chiasm.

Diagnostic Criteria

1. Hypothalamic-pituitary-adrenal axis:

1) Basal cortisol value (8:00):

   a) ≤3 mg/dL (82.7 nmol/L): Repeat the test. If the results are consistent, this is a strong evidence of adrenal insufficiency (of any cause).

   b) 3 to 18 mg/dL (83.7-496.6 nmol/L): This is an indication for evaluating the ACTH reserve (→below).

   c) ≥18 mg/dL (496.6 nmol/L): ACTH secretion is sufficient.

2) ACTH:

    a) Measure ACTH only if the cortisol level is ≤3 mg/dL. Low or normal ACTH values in this setting are consistent with central (pituitary/secondary or hypothalamic/tertiary) adrenal insufficiency. The corticotropin-releasing hormone stimulation test may be used to discriminate between pituitary and hypothalamic localizations of central adrenal insufficiency.

    b) ACTH reserve (applying physiological stimuli to enhance ACTH secretion): The gold standard is the insulin-induced hypoglycemia test (careful monitoring and physician attendance required). The test used most frequently is the metyrapone stimulation test.

2. Thyroid function: TSH and free thyroxine: Low free thyroxine levels with TSH in the normal range are most frequent seen. Low or slightly elevated TSH levels (usually <10 mIU/L) are consistent with central hypothyroidism (in other words, with a clear decrease in thyroid hormones one expects a marked elevation in TSH, usually >20 mIU/L).

3. Gonadotropins:

1) Men: Total testosterone measured at 8:00 and LH levels. A low testosterone level with a normal or low LH level is consistent with hypogonadotrophic hypogonadism.

2) Women: In patients with normal menses, no tests are needed. In patients with abnormal menses, measure the levels of FSH, LH, and estradiol. Low estradiol concentrations with normal or low FSH and LH levels are consistent with hypogonadotrophic hypogonadism.

4. GH:

1) IGF-1: A concentration lower than the age-specific lower limit of a normal range in a patient with pituitary disease confirms GH deficiency (IGF-1 production is stimulated by GH).

2) Provocative tests: Insulin-induced hypoglycemia or the arginine with growth hormone–releasing hormone (GHRH) stimulation test. Subnormal increases of GH ≤5 ng/mL are consistent with GH deficiency.

5. Prolactin:

1) Patients with low prolactin concentrations usually have no manifestations. An exception are women in the postpartum period, who may not be able to nurse.

2) 20-100 ng/dL: Prolactin levels are usually elevated due to stalk compression or secondary hypothyroidism. If pituitary adenoma is the etiology, dilute prolactin to exclude the "hook effect" (spuriously low prolactin levels due a very high concentration of prolactin saturating the antibodies used in the prolactin assay).

3) ≥100 ng/dL: Consider the diagnosis of prolactinoma.

6. Antidiuretic hormone deficiency: Consider testing (water restriction test [→Chapter 5.3.1]) if history is consistent with diabetes insipidus.

Differential Diagnosis

Differential diagnosis depends on the signs and symptoms and will vary, depending on the pituitary deficiencies, but may include primary adrenal insufficiency, primary hypothyroidism, or hypogonadism. Nevertheless, measurements of biochemical hormone levels, basal and/or stimulated, will confirm a definite diagnosis.

▶ TREATMENT

Hormone Replacement Therapy

Management of hormone deficiencies in secondary (pituitary) and tertiary (hypothalamic) insufficiency is similar and involves the administration of appropriate target hormones.

1. Secondary adrenocortical insufficiency: Hydrocortisone (→Chapter 5.1.1.3).

2. Secondary hypothyroidism: L-thyroxin in individually adjusted doses (first correct the adrenocortical insufficiency). Increase the dose gradually, for instance, starting with 25 µg and titrating the dose up to 75 to 100 µg/d, based not on TSH levels but on the patient's clinical condition and free thyroxin levels.

3. Secondary hypogonadism:

1) Male patients:

   a) Not interested in fertility: **Testosterone** (IM **testosterone enanthate** 100 mg weekly or 200 mg every 2 weeks) or short-acting testosterone (topical gel 50 mg/d).

   b) Interested in fertility: Gonadotropins (LH and FSH) or gonadotropin--releasing hormone therapy.

   Note that testosterone replacement should not be given to patients with prostate cancer, uncontrolled heart failure, and erythrocytosis (hematocrit ≥54%).🗹 ◯

2) Female patients (<50 years of age): Sequential low-dose estrogens combined with progesterone. In patients with no uterus, use low-dose estrogen replacement therapy without progestin.

4. Growth retardation in children: Recombinant human GH. The GH replacement therapy is also suggested in adults with severe GH deficiency.◔ ◖

Treatment of Underlying Conditions

1. Tumors in the pituitary:

1) **Surgical resection** (transsphenoidal) is the treatment of choice for all pituitary adenomas (except for prolactinoma [→below]), tumors derived from Rathke pouch, and other parasellar tumors (except for germinomas).

2) **Pharmacotherapy**: Dopamine agonists for prolactinoma (cabergoline and bromocriptine). In TSH-secreting pituitary adenomas, long-acting somatostatin analogues are used to restore euthyroidism prior to the definitive treatment with transsphenoidal surgery. In the case of GH-secreting tumors, the routine use of pharmacotherapy (somatostatin analogues) as pretreatment before the neurosurgical resection is not recommended except in patients with pharyngeal thickness, sleep apnea, or high-output heart failure.

3) **Radiotherapy** is indicated for germinoma and should be considered for other unresectable tumors, either primary or recurring after radical neurosurgical treatment. Modern radiotherapy (stereotactic) approaches are associated with a lower risk of complications.

4) **Chemotherapy** is used in the case of metastatic tumors of the pituitary or as an adjuvant treatment in patients with central nervous system tumors sensitive to chemotherapy.

2. Hemorrhagic pituitary apoplexy:

1) **IV glucocorticoids**: Hydrocortisone 100 mg qid or dexamethasone ~4 mg bid at the early stages of pituitary apoplexy to correct the possible ACTH deficiency and reduce edema.

2) **Surgical decompression**: The decision to proceed to surgery usually should be made within 1 week from hemorrhagic apoplexy in patients whose neurologic status does not improve despite the administration of glucocorticoids.

→ PROGNOSIS

Adequate hormone replacement therapy allows maintaining a good overall clinical status. However, the mortality rates are higher compared to the general population, regardless of the cause of pituitary insufficiency. The prognosis is less favorable in patients with malignant central nervous system tumors causing pituitary insufficiency and depends on the type and stage of the tumor.

3.3. Syndrome of Inappropriate Antidiuretic Hormone Secretion (SIADH)

➡ DEFINITION, ETIOLOGY, PATHOGENESIS

Syndrome of inappropriate antidiuretic hormone secretion (SIADH) is caused by excessive blood levels of antidiuretic hormone (ADH) in relation to the osmolality of plasma in patients with clinical euvolemia. The excess of ADH causes water retention with normal sodium excretion, which results in euvolemic hyponatremia, plasma hypo-osmolality (<280 mOsm/kg), urine hyperosmolality (≥100 mOsm/kg), and urine sodium concentration usually >40 mmol/L.

Causes: Central nervous system pathology (trauma, tumor, surgery, inflammation, psychosis), pulmonary diseases (pneumonia, tuberculosis, pleural empyema, asthma), cancer (lung, renal, gastrointestinal, prostate, thymoma, carcinoid), right ventricular failure, HIV infection, surgery, drugs (analgesic, psychotropic, diuretic, cytotoxic), and substance abuse.

The **pathogenesis** of SIADH is complex. For instance, cancers may cause ectopic secretion of ADH, while in nonneoplastic conditions, such as pulmonary diseases, the secretion of ADH is stimulated by hypoxia. This results in concentrated urine, reduced urine volumes, water retention, and transitory extracellular volume expansion with a consequent increase in urinary sodium excretion.

➡ CLINICAL FEATURES AND NATURAL HISTORY

The two most important determinants of the clinical presentation of SIADH are the severity and rapidity with which hyponatremia develops. Signs and symptoms may include headache, apathy, fatigue, nausea, vomiting, muscle cramps, altered mental status, and in severe cases, coma, seizures, and respiratory arrest, which may be fatal (with the serum sodium level usually ~100 mmol/L or less). If hyponatremia develops rapidly, life-threatening signs and symptoms of cerebral edema may occur even with sodium levels of 120 mmol/L. Despite high ADH levels, neither peripheral edema nor arterial hypertension is observed (the "vasopressin escape" phenomenon, in which blood volume is normal and fluids are evenly distributed between body compartments).

➡ DIAGNOSIS

Determine serum sodium level, urinary sodium excretion, urine osmolality, and plasma osmolality. Exclude renal failure, adrenal insufficiency, and hypothyroidism by measuring serum creatinine, morning cortisol, and thyroid-stimulating hormone (TSH) levels. Once these etiologies and related drugs have been excluded, perform diagnostic tests to identify an organic cause of SIADH.

Diagnostic Criteria

Hyponatremia (<135 mmol/L), low plasma osmolality (<280 mOsm/kg), and urinary sodium excretion >40 mmol/L along with a normal sodium intake and normal renal, adrenal, and thyroid function test results. The diagnosis of SIADH is established in the context of euvolemia (neither hypovolemia nor hypervolemia can be present).

Differential Diagnosis

Chronic hypovolemia caused by thiazide diuretics, diarrhea or vomiting (SIADH is suggested by elevated urinary sodium excretion in the absence of features of dehydration), acute or chronic renal failure, hypopituitarism, adrenal insufficiency, hypothyroidism, pseudohyponatremia (apparently low serum sodium levels in patients with severe hyperlipidemia or hyperproteinemia).

Table 3-3. Selected drugs associated with syndrome of inappropriate antidiuretic hormone secretion

Drug class	Drug
Anticonvulsants	– Carbamazepine – Oxcarbazepine – Valproic acid
Antineoplastics	– Vincristine – Vinblastine – Cyclophosphamide – Ifosfamide – Melphalan – Cisplatin
Antidiabetics	– Chlorpropamide – Tolbutamide
Psychotropics	– Sertraline – Fluoxetine – Amitriptyline – Haloperidol
Others	– Vasopressin/desmopressin – Ciprofloxacin – Bromocriptine – Imatinib – Methotrexate – Amiodarone – Ecstasy (3,4-methylenedioxymethamphetamine)

→ **TREATMENT**

Use the same general treatment principles as in patients with hypotonic hyponatremia (→Chapter 4.2.5.2), particularly in terms of the rate of hyponatremia correction.

Drugs used in SIADH: →Table 3-3.

1. Whenever possible, **eliminate or treat the underlying disease causing SIADH**.

2. Fluid restriction is the mainstay of therapy, with a suggested goal intake of 500 to 1000 mL/d, including liquid in foods. The fluid intake should be 500 mL less than the daily urine output. The restriction may not yield satisfactory results in patients with high urine osmolality (>500 mmol/kg H_2O), combined urine sodium and potassium levels exceeding serum sodium levels, daily urine output <1500 mL, or in the setting of a serum sodium increase <2 mmol/L/d after a 48-hour restriction of fluid intake (<1 L/d).

3. In mild to severe hyponatremia where fluid restriction has proven to be ineffective or in a patient who is unable/unwilling to comply, **increase oral sodium intake** (3-9 g/d), **administer a low-dose loop diuretic** (furosemide 20-40 mg/d), or consider oral urea 0.25-0.5 g/kg of body weight/d. Note that an excessively rapid increase in serum sodium concentration (>8--10 mmol/L in a 24-hour period) may cause osmotic demyelination syndrome (→Chapter 4.2.5.2).

4. In **severe, life-threatening hyponatremia** (altered mental status, seizures, or coma) in which serum sodium levels usually fall <120 mmol/L in <48 hours, the administration of hypertonic saline (3% saline) is warranted until neurologic symptoms are reverted.

5. Vasopressin V_2-receptor and $V_{1a/2}$-receptor antagonists (tolvaptan, conivaptan) are not used routinely in treatment of SIADH-associated hyponatremia except in severe unresponsive hyponatremia (intravenous conivaptan). This is in accordance with the current European guidelines; however, some experts consider SIADH with coexisting hyponatremia to be an indication for the use of the antagonists.

4. Metabolic Syndrome

➔ DEFINITION AND PATHOGENESIS

The co-occurrence of cardiovascular risk factors including central obesity, elevated blood pressure, dyslipidemia (high triglyceride and low high-density lipoprotein cholesterol [HDL-C] levels), and hyperglycemia is known as the metabolic syndrome. The pathophysiology behind the metabolic syndrome has been traditionally ascribed to insulin resistance; however, genetic predisposition and our contemporary "obesogenic" environment (ie, nutrient composition, high-calorie diets, decreased energy expenditure) are also major determinants in its development.

➔ DIAGNOSIS

According to the 2009 joint statement of International Diabetes Federation; National Heart, Lung, and Blood Institute; American Heart Association; World Heart Federation; International Atherosclerosis Society; and International Association for the Study of Obesity, the diagnosis of metabolic syndrome is made in patients who fulfill any 3 of the following 5 criteria:

1) **Increased waist circumference/abdominal obesity** (depending on the country of origin and ethnicity):

   a) European, Middle East, Mediterranean, and sub-Saharan African population: ≥80 cm in women and ≥94 cm in men.

   b) South Asian, Chinese, and ethnic Central and South American population: ≥80 cm in women and ≥90 cm in men.

   c) Japanese population: ≥90 cm in women and ≥85 cm in men.

   d) United States and Canada population: ≥102 cm in men and ≥88 cm in women.

2) Serum **triglyceride levels** >1.7 mmol/L (150 mg/dL) or current treatment for this type of dyslipidemia.

3) Serum **HDL-C levels** <1.0 mmol/L (40 mg/dL) in men and <1.3 mmol/L (50 mg/dL) in women or current treatment for this type of dyslipidemia.

4) **Systolic blood pressure** ≥130 mm Hg and/or **diastolic blood pressure** ≥85 mm Hg, or current antihypertensive treatment.

5) **Fasting plasma glucose levels** ≥5.6 mmol/L (100 mg/dL) or pharmacotherapy for elevated blood glucose levels.

The dominant feature of the metabolic syndrome is abdominal obesity with visceral fat deposition. The second most frequent feature is hypertension (patients with early metabolic syndrome may only have an altered circadian blood pressure rhythm with no blood pressure drop at night). Untreated metabolic syndrome leads to overt type 2 diabetes mellitus (if not present already) and premature atherosclerosis.

➔ TREATMENT

Reduction of cardiovascular risk is the rationale behind treatment of the metabolic syndrome. Consequently, the cornerstone treatment for any component of the metabolic syndrome is lifestyle modification (diet [low-calorie, low glycemic index/load, high-fiber, DASH, Mediterranean] and exercise) including weight reduction.◕◔ Treatment of any of the individual components is no different from treatment related to the metabolic syndrome.

5. Parathyroid Gland Diseases

➔ PHYSIOLOGICAL BACKGROUND

In ~95% of the general population 4 parathyroid glands (parathyroids) are present; the number of glands in the remaining 5% of the population may be higher—up to 8 glands—or lower. The glands are usually located adjacent to the thyroid gland, near to its upper and lower poles; in ~10% of people one or more parathyroid glands are located ectopically, for instance, within the thyroid gland, in the thymus, upper neck, or mediastinum. Anatomy of the parathyroid gland: →Figure 5-1.

Parathyroid glands secrete parathyroid hormone (PTH), which is an amino acid polypeptide that undergoes cleavage necessary for transport, release, and final biologic activity. The predominant form of the hormone present in the serum is dependent on the serum calcium level. PTH 1-84 is the biologically active form of the hormone. Currently, the universally adopted method for measurement of PTH is the determination of the so-called intact PTH (iPTH), which includes both PTH 1-84 and large terminal PTH fragments (normal range, 1.1-6.7 pmol/L or 10-60 pg/mL). The most recent assays measure the so-called bio-intact PTH (bio-iPTH), which is believed to measure only PTH 1-84 (normal range, 6-37 pg/mL).

The key factor regulating the secretion of PTH is the serum ionized calcium level (→Figure 5-2). The secretion of PTH is stimulated by hypocalcemia and inhibited by hypercalcemia. PTH increases the synthesis of 1,25-dihydroxycholecalciferol ($1,25(OH)_2D_3$, the active form of vitamin D_3) in the kidney, increases the reabsorption of calcium in the distal renal tubules, and inhibits the renal reabsorption of phosphate. It also increases the intestinal absorption of calcium and phosphate mediated by $1,25(OH)_2D_3$. At physiological levels, PTH has substantial effects on bone formation and remodeling, as it increases serum calcium levels and urinary excretion of phosphate, thus reducing serum phosphate levels. Excess PTH has osteolytic effects.

Regulation of the plasma phosphate concentration is determined mainly by the renal threshold for phosphate reabsorption in the proximal tubule, in addition to bone release and gut absorption. Hyperphosphatemia can lead to a reduction in calcium levels, inhibition of $1,25(OH)_2D_3$ synthesis and stimulation of PTH secretion irrespectively of hypocalcemia and $1,25(OH)_2D_3$ deficiency. A decreased level of inorganic phosphate stimulates the synthesis of $1,25(OH)_2D_3$ even in the absence of PTH. New, currently researched metabolic links in the regulation of calcium and phosphate metabolism are phosphatonins, which appear to have mostly a phosphaturic effect (eg, fibroblast growth factor 23), and the Klotho protein; they act by suppressing the expression of the sodium-dependent phosphate cotransporters in the renal proximal tubules. In addition, a vitamin D

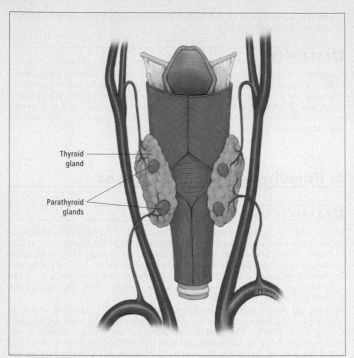

Figure 5-1. Anatomy of the parathyroid gland (posterior view). *Illustration courtesy of Dr Shannon Zhang.*

counterregulatory effect has also been described, acting through the inhibition of the synthesis of $1,25(OH)_2D_3$, and the stimulation of 24-hydroxylation of both 25-OH-D and $1,25(OH)_2D_3$, rendering the hormones inactive.

5.1. Hyperparathyroidism

5.1.1. Primary Hyperparathyroidism

→ DEFINITION, ETIOLOGY, PATHOGENESIS

Primary hyperparathyroidism (PHPT) results from an excessive parathyroid hormone (PTH) secretion caused by a defect in the parathyroid cells that makes them resistant or hyposensitive to the suppressive effects of hypercalcemia. It is the most common cause of hypercalcemia and should be considered in the differential diagnosis of any person with an elevated serum calcium level.

Causes of PHPT include **sporadic causes**: single adenomas (80%-85% of patients; double adenomas can be found in 5%), glandular hyperplasia (10%-15%; all 4 glands affected), and only rarely parathyroid carcinoma (<1%). In ~5% of patients PHPT can be part of **hereditary syndromes**, such as multiple endocrine neoplasia (type 1 or type 2A), hyperparathyroidism-jaw tumor syndrome (HPT-JT), or very rarely familial isolated hyperparathyroidism, which results from an inactivating mutation of the gene encoding the calcium-sensing receptor.

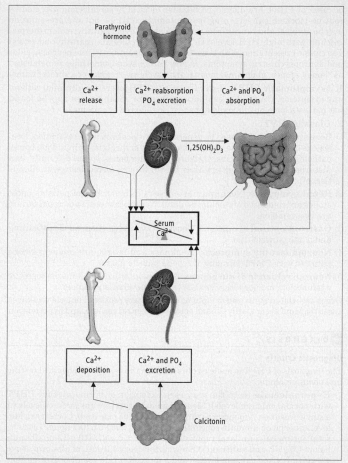

Figure 5-2. Physiological control of calcium metabolism by parathyroid hormone and its thyroid--produced counter, calcitonin. *Illustration courtesy of Dr Shannon Zhang.*

Increased PTH levels cause increased osteolysis (bone resorption), increased gastrointestinal absorption of calcium (due to the increased production of calcitriol), decreased urinary calcium excretion, and increased urinary phosphate excretion; all of these cause elevations in total and ionized calcium levels.

→ CLINICAL FEATURES AND NATURAL HISTORY

Women are affected 2 to 3 times more frequently than men, with the peak incidence occurring in the sixth decade of life. Clinical features of hyperparathyroidism are directly related to the degree of hypercalcemia and PTH elevation, and less so to the duration of the disease, as PHPT may remain asymptomatic for many years or even decades. As a result, the vast majority of cases of PHPT are diagnosed because of mild hypercalcemia detected by routine biochemical screening (asymptomatic PHPT), but the presentation may be atypical and ranges from normocalcemic hyperparathyroidism (normal calcium with high PTH levels) to severe hypercalcemia (parathyroid crisis). The classic presentation, with bone disease, nephrolithiasis, and neuromuscular and neuropsychiatric symptoms, is now rarely seen (sometimes remembered as "bones, stones, abdominal moans, and psychotic groans," or a similar name).

1. Asymptomatic PHPT: High calcium and PTH levels (usually mild) without any symptoms. On further evaluation a bone or renal disease may be found, but patients have no clinically apparent or referred symptoms.

2. Classic PHPT:

1) Bone symptoms are caused by generalized or localized bone resorption, local lesions of osteitis fibrosa cystica (back pain; arthralgia; pain in long bones; pathologic fractures of ribs, vertebrae, or other bones; spinal deformity; gait disturbances [waddling]; epulis or brown tumors [osteoclasts with fibrous tissue]).

2) **Renal symptoms**: Nephrolithiasis occurs in 5% to 15% of patients (most stones are composed of calcium oxalate). Nephrocalcinosis and renal failure are less common.

3) **Gastrointestinal symptoms**: Constipation, indigestion, nausea/vomiting, and acute pancreatitis.

4) **Neuromuscular symptoms**: Weakness and fatigue are common among patients with PHPT (atrophy of type II muscle fibers).

5) **Neuropsychiatric disturbances**: Depression, lethargy, confusion, cognitive dysfunction, memory loss, anxiety, and/or psychosis/paranoia.

Other associated signs and symptoms of PHPT are proximal muscle weakness, keratitis, band keratopathy (a band across the central cornea), and hypertension.

→ DIAGNOSIS

Diagnostic Criteria

The diagnosis of PHPT is made **exclusively** on the basis of biochemical testing and should include:

1) **Hypercalcemia** (with the very rare exception of normocalcemic PHPT with normal calcium levels): Measurement of total serum calcium levels (if a single elevation is found, measurement should be repeated). Correct calcium levels depend on albumin concentration; **add** 0.8 mg/dL (0.2 mmol/L) to the total serum calcium level reported for every 1.0 g/dL (10 g/L) of albumin below 4.0 g/dL and **subtract** 0.8 mg/dL for every 1.0 g/dL of albumin above 4.0 g/dL. Ionized calcium levels yield a more accurate result providing that the test is done in a laboratory known to measure the levels reliably; it is suggested mainly in cases of known or suspected hypoalbuminemia or hyperalbuminemia.

2) **Elevated PTH**: Intact (second-generation) or third-generation PTH assays (in 90% of patients PTH levels are ≥65 pg/mL [7.15 pmol/L]). According to the diagnostic algorithm of hypercalcemia once an elevated serum calcium level is confirmed, the next **obligatory step in all patients** should be the measurement of serum PTH.

3) Exclusion of other causes: Vitamin D deficiency, secondary hyperparathyroidism, lithium and thiazide use, familial hypocalciuric hypercalcemia (FHH).

Diagnostic Tests

1. Blood tests: Serum creatinine concentration should be measured in all cases, as hypercalcemia can diminish renal function and hypocalcemia due to kidney diseases (usually resulting in low vitamin D levels) is the main cause of secondary hyperparathyroidism. Ionized calcium (measured in a reliable laboratory) should be used when protein abnormalities are suspected. Alkaline phosphatase concentration is sometimes high, serum phosphate is usually normal-low (≤3.5 mg/dL [1.13 mmol/L]) or low (≤2.5 mg/dL [0.81 mmol/L]), and mild hyperchloremic metabolic acidosis may be observed.

2. Urine tests: Low urine specific gravity; increased urinary excretion of calcium (>250 mg/d [6 mmol/d]) and phosphate; minor proteinuria (in the presence of interstitial nephritis); microscopic hematuria (in the presence of nephrolithiasis).

3. Electrocardiography (ECG): Features of hypercalcemia may be present (→Chapter 4.2.1.1).

4. Bone mineral density (dual-energy x-ray absorptiometry [DXA]): Features of osteopenia (T-score ≤−1.0 to −2.4 standard deviation) or osteoporosis (T-score ≤−2.5 standard deviation).

5. Vertebral fracture assessment (VFA) can be assessed with plain radiographs or with VFA by DXA (used only when patients do not have osteoporosis in DXA).

6. Imaging studies: Localization studies (eg, ultrasonography, technetium--99m sestamibi, computed tomography [CT], magnetic resonance imaging [MRI]) **should not be used** to establish the diagnosis. Rather, they should be done when the decision to perform surgery has been made.

1) Neck **ultrasonography** detects enlarged parathyroid glands with a sensitivity of 70% to 90% (in experienced hands) and has the advantages of being noninvasive and inexpensive. It cannot always distinguish abnormal parathyroids from abnormal thyroid tissue or abnormal lymph nodes and cannot detect mediastinal adenomas.

2) **Radionuclide scans** using ^{99m}Tc-labeled sestamibi detect 60% to 80% of adenomas when performed in high-volume centers.

3) **Spiral CT** is done either with timed flow (4-dimensional, or 4D CT) or in conjunction with both contrast and noncontrast imaging. This last technique appears to be far superior to any of the other methods used to detect abnormal parathyroids, since it can identify additional adenomas, can often detect multiglandular disease when all 4 parathyroid glands are only minimally enlarged, accurately demonstrates the anatomy of the neck and the upper mediastinum, and is useful in evaluating abnormalities of the thyroid and the adjacent anatomy.

4) **MRI** has a sensitivity of 85% to 95%, is noninvasive, and is not associated with exposure to ionizing radiation. It is usually used for reoperative surgery.

5) **Bone radiographs** are rarely indicated. When performed in advanced PHPT, they may reveal generalized osteoporosis, subperiosteal resorption (most prominent in phalanges), bone cysts in very advanced disease (located in the jaw, ribs, and long bones), osteolysis (calcaneus, pubic bone, distal clavicle, alveolar lamina dura, cranial vault bones ["salt and pepper" appearance on radiographs]), thinning of the cortex of long bones, and pathologic fractures. **Plain abdominal radiographs**, if done for other reasons, may show urolithiasis, nephrocalcinosis, or calcifications in the pancreas. **Other radiographs** may reveal calcifications in muscles or in other soft tissues.

6) **Venography with PTH sampling** from the veins in the neck and the mediastinum is used only when all other methods of localizing have failed, following a previous negative exploration.

7) **Positron emission tomography (PET)** using either ^{18}F-fluorodeoxyglucose (FDG) or ^{11}C-labeled methionine is performed rarely, in complicated cases.

7. Ophthalmology examination may sometimes reveal calcium deposits in the cornea (band keratopathy).

Diagnostic Difficulties

1. Patients with elevated serum PTH and normal calcium levels usually have vitamin D deficiency rather than PHPT. Vitamin D deficiency is exceedingly common, and in most patients in this situation the PTH concentration will decrease to a normal range over time with correction of the low vitamin D level. Only a small number of these individuals subsequently develop hypercalcemia with a persistent elevation of PTH levels.

2. Patients with normal or slightly elevated serum PTH levels and hypercalcemia usually do have PHPT, with elevated serum calcium levels partially inhibiting PTH secretion. In most of these patients, serial ionized calcium and PTH concentrations show a gradual increase over time.

3. "Undetectable" PTH and hypophosphatemic hypercalcemia are observed in hyperparathyroidism caused by secretion of a PTH-related peptide (PTHrP) (secreted by malignant cells); the molecule is biologically active but cannot be detected by the antibodies used in PTH assays.

Differential Diagnosis

Distinguishing between:

1) **PHPT and FHH**: Measure 24-hour urine calcium excretion. In PHPT, calcium urinary excretion is usually >200 mg/d (5 mmol/d) or 4 mg/kg/d (0.1 mmol/kg/d). In FHH, calcium excretion is usually <50 mg/d (1.25 mmol/d) and the calcium/creatinine (Ca/Cr) clearance ratio is usually <0.01.

   Ca/Cr clearance ratio = (24-hour urine Ca × serum Cr) / (serum Ca × 24-hour urine Cr) [with all units either in mg or molar amount or concentration]

2) **PHPT and thiazide/lithium adverse effects**: In the case of drug use, there are usually mildly elevated/normal calcium and PTH (with lithium use) concentrations; otherwise, the two scenarios are indistinguishable. These should be excluded on the basis of clinical history.

3) **PHPT and secondary hyperparathyroidism**: Measure creatinine and serum 25-hydroxyvitamin D (25(OH)D) concentrations; it is recommended to measure 25(OH)D levels in all suspected cases of PHPT. If the concentration of 25(OH)D is ≤20 ng/mL (50 nmol/L), repletion with vitamin D_3 or D_2 is warranted before making any management decisions.

Differential diagnosis should also include other diseases associated with hypercalcemia, osteopenia, osteoporosis or osteomalacia, primary and metastatic bone tumors, multiple myeloma, and Paget disease. Differential diagnosis may prove difficult in familial hypocalciuric hypercalcemia (calciuria <5 mmol/d [200 mg/d]); in parathyroid adenoma in patients with hypercalcemia caused by malignancy (elevated serum PTH and PTHrP levels); and in paraneoplastic endocrinopathy (secretion of PTH and other osteolytic factors by cancers of nonparathyroid origin).

→ TREATMENT

Surgical Treatment

Surgery for PHPT is rarely required urgently. Even patients with markedly elevated calcium levels seldom have significant symptoms. Those rare patients who present to the emergency department obtunded usually respond promptly to basic medical treatment (→Chapter 4.2.1.1). The urgency of surgery depends on the severity of symptoms and serum calcium levels. The procedure involves a total removal of adenoma or carcinoma, and in the case of parathyroid hyperplasia, removal of 3.5 parathyroid glands with preservation of 50% of one gland (**subtotal parathyroidectomy**), or removal of all parathyroid glands (**total parathyroidectomy**) with transplantation of a small portion of one of the removed glands into an adjacent muscle in the neck (usually the sternocleidomastoid muscle or a muscle of the upper extremity). A portion of the remaining glands can be frozen and stored so that they may be transplanted in case of postoperative hypoparathyroidism. The effectiveness of parathyroidectomy may be evaluated by intraoperative measurements of PTH levels in blood samples collected 5 to 10 minutes following the removal of the gland (after a successful surgery, levels are <50% of baseline).

Minimally invasive surgical removal of solitary adenomas has been increasingly popular. More surgical details: →Chapter 5.5.1.1.

Recommended criteria for surgery (according to the Fourth International Workshop on the Management of Asymptomatic Primary Hyperparathyroidism):

1) **Classic or symptomatic PHPT**: Surgery is warranted in all patients.

2) **Asymptomatic PHPT**: One or more of the following criteria:

   a) Age <50 years.

   b) Serum calcium ≥1 mg/dL above the upper limit of normal.

   c) DXA T-score ≤−2.5 standard deviation in the lumbar spine, total hip, femoral neck, or distal 1/3 radius, or vertebral fracture confirmed by radiography, CT, MRI, or VFA.

   d) Creatinine clearance ≤60 mg/dL/min, 24-hour urinary calcium >400 mg/d, or presence of nephrolithiasis.

In specialized centers the success rates of surgical treatment are >90%. After parathyroidectomy, significant hypocalcemia and hypophosphatemia may occur (hungry bone syndrome) but it is rare.

In patients with primary hyperparathyroidism and a genetic syndrome (MEN 1, MEN 2, or HPT-JT), the results of genetic testing are important in the choice of adequate treatment and, in confirmed cases, subtotal or total parathyroidectomy with transplant is almost always required.

Pharmacotherapy

1. Treatment of hypercalcemia (→Chapter 4.2.1.1).

2. Calcimimetics in patients with contraindications to surgery (these agents inhibit PTH secretion but hypercalcemia recurs upon drug discontinuation): cinacalcet 30 mg bid; the dose may be titrated up every 2 to 4 weeks to 90 mg bid (maximum dose, 90 mg qid).

3. Bisphosphonates inhibit bone resorption by osteoclasts; they may also be used to control hungry bone syndrome (→above) prior to parathyroidectomy.

4. Correction of hypocalcemia and hypophosphatemia following parathyroidectomy.

→ FOLLOW-UP

In patients with asymptomatic PHPT and no indications for surgery, monitor serum calcium and creatinine levels every 12 months and perform DXA of 3 skeletal locations every 1 to 2 years. The calcium-phosphate metabolism parameters and serum PTH levels should be measured after the confirmation of a normal 25(OH)D concentration (20-50 ng/mL [50-125 nmol/L]).

→ PROGNOSIS

In patients with mild to moderate bone and renal abnormalities and in those with general symptoms in whom surgical treatment has been successful, the prognosis is excellent with usual marked improvement. Untreated classical PHPT is associated with increased mortality due to cardiovascular disease (20%-100% risk increase). In asymptomatic PHPT patients, data are limited but appear to be the same when compared to healthy individuals. In parathyroid carcinoma, a complete cure is achieved in 30% to 50% of patients, 30% of individuals can have a prolonged course with recurrence that is still treatable with surgery or radiation, and 20% have rapidly progressive disease.

5.1.2. Secondary Hyperparathyroidism

→ DEFINITION, ETIOLOGY, PATHOGENESIS

Secondary hyperparathyroidism refers to parathyroid hormone (PTH) hypersecretion by hypertrophic parathyroid glands, mainly due to reduced influx of calcium ions to parathyroid cells. It is usually accompanied by low or normal calcium level. On occasions, long-standing chronic kidney disease (CKD), the most common cause of secondary hyperparathyroidism, leads to persistent parathyroid stimulation, PTH hypersecretion, and parathyroid gland hypertrophy and hyperplasia accompanied by elevation of serum calcium and worsening symptoms requiring treatment. Over time, the function of the hypertrophic parathyroid glands may become autonomous and could be defined as advanced secondary hyperparathyroidism. We choose this label over the more traditionally used tertiary hyperparathyroidism, as this situation represents a continuum of the pathophysiologic process. It is also distinct from a situation which evolves after causes of secondary hyperparathyroidism are removed but hypersecretion of PTH persists (→Chapter 5.5.1.3).

Causes: CKD (the most frequent cause; hyperparathyroidism develops at a glomerular filtration rate [GFR] ≤45 mL/min/1.73 m^2), acute kidney injury, diseases associated with chronic hypocalcemia, vitamin D deficiency (hereditary or acquired), gastrointestinal malabsorption syndromes, malnutrition, and hypermagnesemia.

→ CLINICAL FEATURES AND NATURAL HISTORY

Signs and symptoms depend on the underlying condition that causes chronic hypocalcemia, its duration, and prior treatment. Advanced secondary hyperparathyroidism in patients with CKD leads to the development of renal osteodystrophy associated with high bone turnover (→Chapter 9.2). These patients have significant bone pain, which is most noticeable in the legs, and marked weakness. They can develop severe osteodystrophy, soft tissue calcification, persistent pruritus and, in extreme cases, calciphylaxis or spontaneous rupture of tendons.

→ DIAGNOSIS

Diagnostic Tests

1. Biochemical tests: High serum PTH levels, frequently with hypocalcemia or serum calcium levels in the lower range of the normal limits. With progression to advanced secondary hyperparathyroidism and autonomous parathyroid functioning, calcium level becomes high-normal or elevated. Other abnormalities are related to the underlying condition (most frequently elevated serum creatinine and phosphate levels in patients with CKD), usually low 25(OH)D levels, and diminished 1-25(OH)$_2$D$_3$ levels.

2. Imaging studies may reveal enlarged parathyroid glands (best seen on computed tomography [CT] scans) and various bone lesions similar to those found in primary hyperparathyroidism.

Diagnostic Criteria

Elevated serum PTH levels and hypocalcemia or, more commonly, normal serum calcium levels in a patient with an underlying disease known to cause secondary hyperparathyroidism (eg, CKD or low 25(OH)D levels). Hypercalcemia may develop gradually with progression to autonomously functioning parathyroid glands (advanced secondary hyperparathyroidism).

→ TREATMENT

Treatment of the underlying condition. If this is not feasible, use symptomatic treatment, which involves:

1) Correction of hyperphosphatemia (→Chapter 4.2.3.1).

2) Correction of hypocalcemia (→Chapter 4.2.1.2).

3) Active vitamin D metabolites (calcitriol), precursors that require no renal hydroxylation (alfacalcidol), or analogues (eg, IV paricalcitol administered via a central venous catheter during hemodialysis at doses calculated on the basis of serum PTH levels).

4) If the above treatment is ineffective in lowering PTH, use a calcimimetic: cinacalcet 30 to 90 mg/d (unless the patient has hypocalcemia).

5) Surgical treatment of secondary hyperparathyroidism may be required when failure of the above measures results in persistent elevation of PTH and ongoing or worsening symptoms. Despite advances in medical treatment, 10% of patients with end-stage renal disease will require parathyroid surgery that is tailored to renal disease and the likelihood of renal transplant: subtotal parathyroidectomy is preferred in patients in whom renal transplant is anticipated, and total parathyroidectomy with parathyroid transplant in those with no immediate plan for renal transplantation.

Management of secondary hyperparathyroidism in patients with CKD: →Chapter 9.2.

5.1.3. Tertiary Hyperparathyroidism

→ DEFINITION, ETIOLOGY, PATHOGENESIS

Tertiary hyperparathyroidism is best described as the persistence of increasingly autonomously functioning hypertrophied parathyroid glands with parathyroid hormone (PTH) hypersecretion and hypercalcemia in a patient after correction of causes of secondary hyperparathyroidism. Tertiary hyperparathyroidism is most commonly observed in patients with a history of chronic kidney disease (CKD) previously treated with chronic hemodialysis or peritoneal dialysis who received a functioning renal transplant but in whom the parathyroid glands fail to involute. Approximately 10% to 20% of these patients require subsequent subtotal or total parathyroidectomy (→Chapter 5.5.1.1).

Of note, the traditional concept of tertiary hyperparathyroidism also includes a combination of progressively increasing hyperplasia, hypertrophy, and autonomy of the parathyroid glands accompanied by hypercalcemia—a process that we describe as advanced secondary hyperparathyroidism (→Chapter 5.5.1.2).

→ CLINICAL FEATURES AND NATURAL HISTORY

Since renal transplantation removes many of the symptoms of CKD, including weakness and tiredness, symptoms of tertiary hyperparathyroidism are considerably less severe than that of advanced secondary hyperparathyroidism and the need for surgery depends on careful evaluation of blood calcium and PTH levels and frequent reassessment of symptoms that persist. In 80% to 90% of such patients hyperparathyroidism resolves spontaneously within several months of transplantation, as measured by decreasing calcium and PTH levels. In a small group of patients, when this involution of the parathyroid glands does not occur, surgery needs to be considered, because the persistent elevation of PTH and calcium levels may lead to damage to the new kidney.

→ DIAGNOSIS

Diagnostic Tests

1. Biochemical tests: Hypercalcemia, high serum PTH levels (>10 × the upper limit of normal), hyperphosphatemia (in patients with CKD), elevated levels of bone turnover markers (markers of osteolysis and of osteogenesis).

2. Imaging studies may reveal enlarged parathyroid glands and various bone lesions similar to those found in primary hyperparathyroidism.

Diagnostic Criteria

Hypercalcemia and elevated PTH in a patient with treated secondary hyperparathyroidism in whom other causes of hypercalcemia have been excluded.

→**TREATMENT**

Pharmacotherapy

As in secondary hyperparathyroidism.

Surgical Treatment

Total or subtotal parathyroidectomy in patients with serum PTH levels >1000 pg/mL despite medical treatment; hypercalcemia >3 mmol/L; persistent pruritus, bone pain, extraskeletal calcifications (lungs, muscles, skin), or severe myopathy. A complication of total parathyroidectomy may be adynamic bone disease (low-turnover bone disease). Discussion on the choice of surgery: →Chapter 5.5.1.3.

5.2. Hypoparathyroidism

→**DEFINITION, ETIOLOGY, PATHOGENESIS**

Hypoparathyroidism is a relatively uncommon condition associated with hypocalcemia and hyperphosphatemia in the presence of low or inappropriately normal parathyroid hormone (PTH) levels. It is associated with significant symptoms of hypocalcemia as well as long-term complications of inadequate PTH levels, hypocalcemia, and hyperphosphatemia.

Causes:

1) Neck surgery is the most common cause of primary hypoparathyroidism, accounting for 75% of all cases. During neck surgery the parathyroid glands may be damaged or deprived of their blood supply. Patients with transient hypoparathyroidism after surgery may recover; however, if the serum calcium level remains low for ≥6 months, the diagnosis of chronic hypoparathyroidism is confirmed.

2) Nonsurgical causes of hypoparathyroidism account for 25% of cases:

   a) Autoimmune hypoparathyroidism is the most common cause of nonsurgical primary hypoparathyroidism. It may occur in isolation or as part of autoimmune polyendocrine syndrome type 1 (APS-1). APS-1 is caused by mutations in the *AIRE* (autoimmune regulator) gene. Among such patients, 80% have only hypoparathyroidism; other major features of APS-1 are adrenal insufficiency and oral or vaginal candidal infections. Individuals with APS-1 should be followed up to ensure that other major or minor features of APS do not develop.

   b) Infiltrative causes include destruction of the parathyroid glands secondary to granulomatous infiltration (eg, Riedel thyroiditis, amyloidosis, sarcoidosis).

   c) Metastatic cancer can be a rare cause of hypoparathyroidism, with the most common tumors being tumors of the breast, skin, or lung, as well as leukemia, lymphomas, and sarcomas.

   d) Radiation destruction can also be a cause, although high doses of ionizing radiation exposure have been rarely associated with hypoparathyroidism.

   e) Mineral deposition can result in hypoparathyroidism with iron overload in hemochromatosis or with repeat blood transfusions and can also develop in individuals with thalassemia. Wilson disease with copper deposition in the parathyroid glands has been reported to cause hypoparathyroidism.

   f) Transient hypoparathyroidism can be seen in the presence of severe burn injuries and acute illness.

Table 5-1. Causes of abnormal serum magnesium levels	
Low serum magnesium	
Decreased intake or absorption	– Decreased intake, – Malabsorption (short bowel syndrome, steatorrhea, diarrhea, vomiting)
Drugs	– Diuretics (especially thiazides) – Proton pump inhibitors – Foscarnet, amphotericin B, aminoglycosides, pentamidine, rapamycin – Anticancer drugs (cisplatin, carboplatin) – Immunosuppressants (calcineurin inhibitors: tacrolimus, cyclosporine A) – EGRF inhibitors (cetuximab)
Rare genetic disorders	– Familial hypomagnesemia with secondary hypocalcemia (*TRPM6* gene mutation) – Autosomal dominant hypocalcemia (activating mutation in the *CASR* gene) – Familial hypomagnesemia with hypercalciuria and nephrocalcinosis
High serum magnesium	
– Magnesium administration for eclampsia or preeclampsia – Intake in laxatives or cathartics – Metabolic syndromes (familial hypocalciuric hypercalcemia) – Chronic kidney disease	
EGFR, epidermal growth factor receptor.	

g) Functional hypoparathyroidism is caused by hypomagnesemia as well as hypermagnesemia, both of which impair parathyroid function (→Table 5-1).

h) Maternal hyperparathyroidism can result in suppressed parathyroid function in infants exposed to hypercalcemia in utero.

i) Idiopathic hypoparathyroidism is confirmed if the cause of hypoparathyroidism is not identified after laboratory and clinical evaluation.

j) Two additional clinical states have traditionally carried "hypoparathyroidism" as part of their name but are either distinct or not a disease entity. **Pseudohypoparathyroidism (PHP)** is defined as target organ resistance to PTH. PHP is characterized by elevated PTH levels in association with low serum calcium and high phosphate levels. **Secondary hypoparathyroidism** is not a disease state but a physiologic response where PTH levels are low in response to a primary process that has caused hypercalcemia (→Chapter 4.2.1.1).

→ CLINICAL FEATURES AND NATURAL HISTORY

1. Symptoms of hypocalcemia include muscle cramping; twitching; numbness and tingling in the face, hands, or feet; depression or irritability; seizures; bradyarrhythmias; wheezing; and laryngospasm (→Table 5-2). On physical examination the Chvostek sign (→Figure 5-3) and Trousseau sign (→Figure 5-4) can be somewhat helpful, but they are not sensitive or specific enough for diagnosis and are mostly of historical interest.

2. Target organ damage: In patients with chronic hypoparathyroidism prolonged hypercalciuria and hyperphosphatemia can result in the development of nephrocalcinosis, nephrolithiasis, and renal insufficiency. Renal function and urine calcium losses should be closely monitored with 24-hour urine calcium

Table 5-2. Symptoms associated with abnormal calcium levels	
Hypocalcemia	– Numbness, tingling in face, hands and feet – Muscle spasms or cramps, laryngospasm – Bradyarrhythmia, heart failure – Wheezing – Depression, confusion, seizures
Hypercalcemia	– Nausea, vomiting, anorexia – Polyuria, polydipsia – Constipation – Weakness – Confusion – Headaches

measurements as well as assessments of renal function. Nephrocalcinosis or nephrolithiasis can be identified using renal imaging such as ultrasonography. The risk for developing renal stones and renal insufficiency in individuals with postsurgical hypoparathyroidism was found to be increased 4.8 times and 3.1 times, respectively, as compared with control populations.�🖝

Patients with hypoparathyroidism are at risk of developing cataracts, which occur in ~50% of cases.

Intracranial calcification with calcification of the basal ganglia has also been observed in individuals with hypoparathyroidism. This has been associated with elevations in serum phosphate levels and was noted to

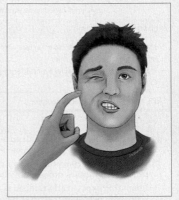

Figure 5-3. Chvostek sign. *Illustration courtesy of Dr Shannon Zhang.*

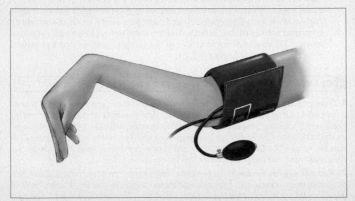

Figure 5-4. Trousseau sign. *Illustration courtesy of Dr Shannon Zhang.*

occur in the presence of a normal calcium phosphate product by the Canadian National Hypoparathyroidism Registry. Intracranial calcification has also been associated with dystonias and parkinsonism. Brain imaging and electroencephalography are helpful tools in evaluating neurocognitive decline, movement disorders, or seizures in individuals with hypocalcemia.

The standards of care for hypoparathyroidism advise lowering urine calcium losses and maintaining serum phosphate levels in the normal reference range to reduce the risk of extra skeletal calcification as well as the risk of renal, neurologic, and ocular complications associated with hypoparathyroidism. The calcium phosphate product should be maintained in the normal reference range; however, renal complications have been observed even in the presence of a normal calcium phosphate product.

3. Quality of life: Hypoparathyroidism is associated with diminished quality of life. Complaints of "brain fog," myalgias, numbness, paresthesias, fatigue, weakness, anxiety, and depression all contribute to a lower quality of life. Studies assessing the quality of life in patients with hypoparathyroidism using standardized measurements show that patients with hypoparathyroidism have a lower quality of life relative to control populations irrespective of disease duration, etiology, and treatment with activated vitamin D and calcium supplements. Loss of PTH may have significant effects on cognition and overall well-being; this is an area of active research.

→ DIAGNOSIS

For patients with nonsurgical hypoparathyroidism, a detailed family history is required including the presence of consanguinity. Clinical evaluation is used to determine if other features associated with genetic or autoimmune causes of hypoparathyroidism are present. Currently genetic testing is available, enabling a molecular diagnosis of the cause of hypoparathyroidism.

Diagnostic Tests
Low serum calcium levels (corrected for low albumin levels if needed) or low ionized calcium levels should be confirmed on ≥2 separate occasions prior to confirming the diagnosis of hypocalcemia. Low PTH levels should also be confirmed on ≥2 occasions. If PTH levels are not clearly elevated in the presence of hypocalcemia, this confirms the diagnosis of hypoparathyroidism, as it indicates an impaired parathyroid response to the low serum calcium levels.

After parathyroid surgery hypoparathyroidism can be acute and transient (present for <6 months after surgery) or chronic and permanent (present for >6 months after surgery). The diagnosis of permanent surgical hypoparathyroidism is confirmed by the presence of hypocalcemia (ionized calcium or low total serum calcium levels corrected for albumin) for ≥6 months after surgery (in the presence or absence of clinical symptoms) and in the presence of low or inappropriately normal PTH levels on 2 separate occasions.

→ TREATMENT

Management requires close monitoring of the biochemical profile and drug therapy in order to minimize symptoms of hypocalcemia while avoiding overtreatment with the development of hypercalcemia. Prevention of long-term complications requires avoidance of hypercalciuria and hyperphosphatemia. Conventional therapy includes calcium and active vitamin D supplementation. PTH replacement therapy is of value in those in whom conventional therapy has failed.

Acute Hypocalcemia in Hypoparathyroidism
Acute hypocalcemia may require **IV calcium**, depending on the rate of onset, clinical symptoms, and biochemical severity of hypocalcemia. Symptomatic hypocalcemia requires IV administration of calcium, with the preferred

preparation being calcium gluconate. If the total serum calcium level corrected for albumin is <1.75 mmol/L, our advice is that IV calcium should be administered even if the patient is asymptomatic to avoid serious complications of hypocalcemia, including laryngospasm, seizures, or cardiac arrythmias.

A bolus of IV calcium transiently elevates serum calcium for ~2 to 3 hours and a continuous infusion is required to prevent subsequent decreases in serum levels. **Calcium gluconate** is preferred to avoid local venous irritation, which can be seen with calcium chloride infusions. Electrocardiographic (ECG) monitoring is required for early detection of any cardiac arrythmias that may occur with calcium infusion.

In the presence of acidosis the ionized calcium level is higher, as calcium ions are displaced from binding to albumin by hydrogen ions. It is important to correct serum calcium levels prior to correcting acidosis to prevent significant declines in serum calcium concentration.

Avoid infusing sodium bicarbonate or phosphate in the same IV administration line as calcium to prevent precipitation of calcium carbonate or calcium phosphate.

Following the administration of the initial bolus of IV calcium gluconate, a calcium infusion is initiated. A calcium bolus is given over 10 minutes and consists of a 1-g of calcium gluconate in 10 mL of a 10% solution or 90 mg of elemental calcium. Following the bolus, a calcium infusion is started, with 10 ampoules of calcium gluconate containing 900 mg of elemental calcium in 1 L of 5% glucose (dextrose) or 0.9% saline (1 mg/mL solution). The infusion is started at 50 mL/h and is titrated to normal serum calcium concentration. To elevate serum calcium levels by 0.5 to 0.75 mmol/L, ~15 mg/kg of elemental calcium IV must be administered over 4 to 6 h.

If the patient is able to take oral calcium supplements, these are also started at the same time as the calcium infusion. Oral **calcium salts** can be given in the form of calcium carbonate, which contains 40% elemental calcium and is easier to comply with as fewer tablets are required orally. **Calcium citrate** contains 21% elemental calcium and can be useful in the presence of proton pump inhibitors or achlorhydria, as an acidic pH is not required for absorption of calcium citrate (this is a requirement for the absorption of calcium carbonate). Calcium supplements are initiated in doses of 500 mg to 1000 mg taken with food bid to tid. Patients may require up to 9 g daily. **Calcitriol supplementation** is of great value as it replaces the deficient $1,25(OH)_2D$, which is also low in the absence of PTH. Calcitriol is started at a dose of 0.25 µg once daily or bid and gradually titrated upwards to a maximum of 2 µg daily. Calcitriol has a rapid onset of action with a peak occurring at 3 to 6 hours of administration and a half-life of 4 to 6 hours. Vitamin D stores must also be replenished with cholecalciferol or ergocalciferol and hypomagnesemia (→Chapter 4.2.2.2) must be corrected.

Chronic Hypocalcemia in Hypoparathyroidism

Treatment goals of chronic management are to reduce symptoms of hypocalcemia and the risk of long-term complications of hypercalciuria and hyperphosphatemia. Conventional therapy includes calcium supplementation, active vitamin D and its analogues, as well as hydrochlorothiazide, which is helpful in enhancing renal calcium reabsorption. Serum magnesium and potassium levels should be closely monitored as renal losses leading to hypomagnesemia and hypokalemia are common with thiazide use. Begin hydrochlorothiazide with low doses of 12.5 mg daily and gradually titrate upwards. Magnesium supplementation is used as necessary to normalize magnesium levels.

Hyperphosphatemia

Hyperphosphatemia can be controlled by using phosphate binders and by following a low-phosphate diet. Calcium is an ideal phosphate binder and all patients are advised to take calcium supplements with food, as it binds phosphate in the meal and enables loss of phosphate in the stool. A low-salt diet will also lower urinary calcium losses.

Failure of conventional therapy is confirmed in the presence of poor control of serum calcium, complications of hypoparathyroidism, or poor quality of life; in such cases patients can be offered PTH therapy (→below).

PTH Peptides in the Management of Chronic Hypoparathyroidism

Conventional therapy with calcium and active vitamin D supplementation has been associated with worsening hypercalciuria, renal stones, ectopic calcifications, impaired renal function, and nephrocalcinosis. PTH therapy enhances renal calcium reabsorption and contributes to improved renal phosphate clearance.

Recombinant human PTH (rhPTH) (1-84) therapy has been approved as an adjunct to conventional treatments in Europe and in the United States. PTH(1-84) has been shown to lower urinary calcium losses and serum phosphate levels and allows the patient to decrease the dose of calcium and calcitriol required to maintain target serum calcium concentration. It also makes it possible to achieve normal serum phosphate and urine calcium levels. The majority of patients are able to stop or lower the dose of calcium and calcitriol supplementation required to maintain serum calcium concentration in the low-normal reference range.

PTH(1-34) in doses of 20 μg bid resulted in reductions in the dose of calcium and calcitriol required daily and increased serum calcium while lowering serum phosphate.

Replacement therapy with PTH(1-84) resulted in maintenance of serum calcium and phosphate levels in the appropriate range with reduced daily doses of calcium and active vitamin D metabolites.

PTH therapy is well tolerated and has mild and/or transient adverse events. Long-term data is limited, with no long-term studies evaluating the potential benefits and risks of PTH(1-84) therapy. The US Food and Drug Administration (FDA) has approved PTH(1-84) for the treatment of hypoparathyroidism with a "black box" warning due to a potential increased risk of osteosarcoma observed in rats treated with high doses of PTH(1-34). PTH therapy can be considered in the presence of:

1) Poorly controlled serum calcium levels with calcium and calcitriol therapy.

2) Requirements of high doses of oral calcium or vitamin D metabolites (>2.5 g of calcium or >1.5 μg of calcitriol per day).

3) Hypercalciuria, renal stones, nephrocalcinosis, reduced creatinine clearance, or reduced estimated glomerular filtration rate (eGFR) (<60 mL/min/1.73 m^2).

4) Hyperphosphatemia and/or calcium-phosphate product >55 mg^2/dL^2 (4.4 mmol^2/L^2).

→ FOLLOW-UP

Recommendations from the standards of care for hypoparathyroidism (the 2018 Canadian and international consensus):

1) Corrected serum calcium levels (albumin-corrected or ionized calcium), phosphorus, magnesium, urea nitrogen, and creatinine should be monitored every 3 to 6 months. If changes are made in the dose of calcium or calcitriol, or if symptoms of hypocalcemia or hypercalcemia occur, serum calcium and phosphate may require weekly evaluation.

2) Annual monitoring of urinary calcium excretion, creatinine, and sodium (either by 24-hour urine collection or random urine collection), and 25(OH)D levels is currently advised.

3) Renal imaging by ultrasonography for the presence of nephrocalcinosis or nephrolithiasis is recommended at baseline and is of particular importance in individuals with persistent hypercalciuria, history of renal stones, abnormal urinalysis, or a decline in eGFR.

4) Signs and symptoms of hypercalcemia and hypocalcemia should be evaluated every 6 months, depending on the stability of hypoparathyroidism.

5) The general health of the patient should also be assessed, as many symptoms of hypoparathyroidism are nonspecific and include brain fog and low energy.

6) Basal ganglia calcification can be assessed with brain computed tomography (CT) or susceptibility-weighted magnetic resonance imaging (MRI).

7) An eye examination is of value to determine if cataracts are present.

8) Bone mineral density (BMD) is usually higher than expected for age and gender as evaluated by dual x-ray absorptiometry (DXA). Spinal radiographs may be completed with exclusion of vertebral fractures in the presence of significant height loss, back pain, or spinal deformity. At this time there is very limited data on the effects of hypoparathyroidism on fracture risk.

6. Thyroid Gland Diseases

6.1. Hypothyroidism

→ DEFINITION, ETIOLOGY, PATHOGENESIS

The clinical manifestations of hypothyroidism are caused by deficiency of thyroxine (T_4) and the resulting insufficient cellular effects of triiodothyronine (T_3), leading to a general slowing down of metabolic processes and development of interstitial edema due to deposition of fibronectin and hydrophilic glycosaminoglycans in the subcutaneous tissue, muscles, and other tissues.

The following types of hypothyroidism may be distinguished:

1) **Primary hypothyroidism**, which results from damage to the thyroid gland. It may be caused by:

   a) Chronic autoimmune thyroiditis (most frequently Hashimoto thyroiditis), other types of thyroiditis.

   b) Total or subtotal thyroidectomy (with a possible autoimmune process leading to the damage of the remaining thyroid parenchyma).

   c) Treatment with ^{131}I (radioiodine).

   d) Irradiation of the neck.

   e) Excessive intake of iodides, including the administration of amiodarone and iodine contrast media (by inhibiting iodide organification and T_4 and T_3 synthesis—known as the Wolff-Chaikoff effect—which could be transient or result in permanent hypothyroidism in cases of failure to escape the acute effect).

   f) Overdose of antithyroid drugs (transient and reversible hypothyroidism, improves upon discontinuation of the drug).

   g) Administration of lithium salts (inhibition of T_4 and T_3 secretion), sodium nitroprusside, phenytoin, some tyrosine kinase inhibitors (eg, sunitinib, sorafenib), interferon α, or interleukin 2.

   h) Significant environmental iodine deficiency and chronic exposure to goitrogens, that is, substances that inhibit the accumulation of iodides by the thyroid gland (eg, perchlorates, thiocyanates, nitrates).

   i) Infiltrative diseases (eg, hemochromatosis, sarcoidosis).

   j) Congenital hypothyroidism (eg, thyroid agenesis, dysgenesis, or defects in hormone synthesis).

2) **Secondary hypothyroidism**, which results from a decrease in or lack of thyroid-stimulating hormone (TSH) secretion due to hypopituitarism caused by:

   a) Parasellar neoplasia.

   b) Inflammatory or infiltrative conditions.

    c) Vascular, traumatic, or iatrogenic injury (irradiation, neurosurgery procedures).

    d) Hemorrhagic necrosis (Sheehan syndrome).

3) **Tertiary hypothyroidism**, resulting from a decrease in or lack of secretion of thyrotropin-releasing hormone (TRH), which is caused by damage to the hypothalamus (malignancy, sarcoidosis) or by a disrupted pituitary stalk.

→ CLINICAL FEATURES AND NATURAL HISTORY

In secondary and tertiary hypothyroidism the signs and symptoms are usually less pronounced than in primary hypothyroidism, but there may be coexisting features of other endocrine deficiencies (look for the features of adrenal insufficiency, diabetes insipidus, or other symptoms directly related to hypopituitarism). Hypothyroidism can also be a part of polyglandular autoimmune syndromes.

Subclinical Hypothyroidism

In patients with subclinical hypothyroidism typical signs and symptoms of hypothyroidism are absent. Mood disorders and depression may be present along with abnormal laboratory test results, such as elevated serum total and low--density lipoprotein cholesterol (LDL-C) levels. The risk of developing clinically overt hypothyroidism increases 2-fold if an elevated TSH level is accompanied by high titers of thyroperoxidase (TPO) antibodies. The nonspecific symptoms of both subclinical and overt hypothyroidism may make the distinction difficult.

Overt Hypothyroidism

1. General signs and symptoms: Weight gain, fatigue, weakness and poor exercise tolerance, somnolence, general slowing down (affecting both psychomotor functions and speech), feeling cold, cold intolerance.

2. Cutaneous manifestations: Dry, cold, pale, and/or slightly yellowish skin; reduced perspiration, excessive epidermal keratosis, for instance, on the elbows; subcutaneous edema (so-called myxedema) with coarse facial features, typical edema of the eyelids and hands; coarse, brittle hair; loss of hair, sometimes including the eyebrows.

3. Cardiovascular manifestations: Bradycardia, hypokinetic pulse, distant heart sounds; enlarged cardiac silhouette; hypotension or, less commonly, hypertension (diastolic).

4. Respiratory manifestations: Hoarse and mellow voice (due to thickened vocal cords and an enlarged tongue); shallow breathing and a low respiratory rate; chronic signs and symptoms of upper respiratory tract congestion; in severe cases symptoms of respiratory failure.

5. Gastrointestinal manifestations: Chronic constipation; ileus (in severe cases); ascites (in advanced disease; usually accompanied by pericardial and pleural effusion).

6. Urinary manifestations: Impaired water excretion (decreased renal filtration is important because of the risk of volume overload). In the absence of clinically overt edema the abnormalities are probably insignificant.

7. Nervous system manifestations: Cognitive dysfunction, nerve entrapment syndromes (eg, carpal tunnel syndrome), paresthesias, hyporeflexia, a delayed relaxation phase of the deep tendon reflexes. Some patients may have hearing impairment.

8. Musculoskeletal manifestations: Muscle weakness and fatigue, loss of energy, lethargy, muscle cramps, myalgia; joint edema, particularly affecting the knees (due to synovial hypertrophy and effusion).

9. Reproductive system manifestations: In women, menstrual dysfunction (reduced cycle duration, menorrhagia), infertility, miscarriage, and galactorrhea; in men, loss of libido, sometimes also erectile dysfunction.

10. Psychiatric manifestations: Impaired concentration and memory, subclinical or overt depression, mood lability, sometimes symptoms of bipolar disorder or paranoid psychosis. In extremely severe cases dementia and coma.

Myxedema Coma

Myxedema coma is a life-threatening condition that develops in extremely severe untreated hypothyroidism; it may be triggered by comorbidity, for instance, by sepsis. Symptoms include hypothermia (body temperature <30°C, but it may be as low as 23°C), significant bradycardia, hypotension, hypoxemia and hypercapnia (caused by hypoventilation), hypoglycemia, hyponatremia with symptoms of volume overload, edema, cognitive dysfunction, coma, and shock. Patients may have reduced muscle tone (although they may develop seizures) and hyporeflexia. Signs and symptoms of comorbidities may be observed, for instance, pneumonia or other infections, acute myocardial infarction, or gastrointestinal bleeding.

→ DIAGNOSIS

Diagnostic Tests

1. Hormone tests:

1) Serum TSH concentrations: Elevated in primary hypothyroidism (the key diagnostic criterion), low or not appropriately elevated in secondary and tertiary hypothyroidism.

2) Low serum free thyroxine (FT_4) levels.

3) Serum free triiodothyronine (FT_3) levels may often be normal, or sometimes low.

4) Serum TSH levels in the thyrotropin-releasing hormone test (now rarely used): In primary hypothyroidism there is TSH hypersecretion. In secondary hypothyroidism, no significant TSH increase. In tertiary hypothyroidism, delayed and moderate elevation of TSH levels.

2. Other laboratory tests:

1) Elevated antithyroid antibody levels (primarily TPO antibodies) in autoimmune thyroid disease.

2) Elevated levels of total cholesterol, LDL-C, and triglycerides.

3) Anemia.

4) Hyponatremia and mild hypercalcemia may be seen in some patients.

3. Imaging studies:

1) **Thyroid ultrasonography**: Features are variable and depend on the cause of hypothyroidism (the thyroid gland may be small, normal, or enlarged with heterogeneous appearance; foci of altered echogenicity may be seen).

2) **Abdominal ultrasonography**: Ascites in advanced disease.

3) **Chest radiography**: In advanced disease, pleural effusion, an enlarged cardiac silhouette.

4) **Echocardiography**: In advanced disease, pericardial effusion, left ventricular enlargement, reduced ejection fraction (due to impaired myocardial contractility).

5) **Radionuclide thyroid imaging**: Radioactive iodine uptake may be low or normal.

4. Electrocardiography (ECG): Sinus bradycardia, low amplitudes of ECG waveforms, particularly the QRS complex; flat or inverted T waves, a prolonged PR interval; rarely third-degree atrioventricular block, a prolonged QT interval.

Diagnostic Criteria

1. Primary hypothyroidism:

1) **Overt**: Low serum FT_4 and elevated serum TSH levels.

2) **Subclinical**: Normal serum FT_4 (often close to the lower limit of normal) with normal serum FT_3 and mildly elevated serum TSH levels (typically <10 mIU/L).

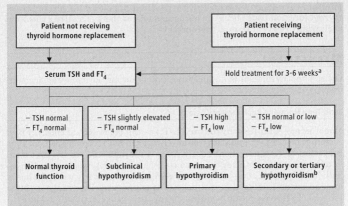

a If the diagnosis of hypothyroidism is questionable.
b A thyrotropin-releasing hormone test is sometimes useful in differentiating these conditions from primary hypothyroidism.

FT$_4$, free thyroxine; TSH, thyroid-stimulating hormone.

Figure 6-1. Diagnostic algorithm of hypothyroidism based on TSH and FT$_4$ levels.

2. Secondary and tertiary hypothyroidism: Low serum FT$_4$ with normal or low serum TSH levels.

3. Myxedema coma: Low serum FT$_4$ and usually markedly elevated serum TSH. The diagnosis depends primarily on clinical manifestations and exclusion of other causes of coma.

Differential Diagnosis

Differential diagnostic algorithm for hypothyroidism: →Figure 6-1. When considering the differential diagnosis of primary hypothyroidism, look for a family history of thyroid diseases, exposure to iodine or chemical goitrogens, recent childbirth, treatment with antithyroid drugs, previous thyroid surgery, ^{131}I therapy, or neck irradiation (including treatment completed several years earlier). Autoimmune hypothyroidism may be accompanied by insufficiency of other endocrine glands. In the case of secondary hypothyroidism look for coexisting adrenal insufficiency before initiating hormone replacement therapy. Edema, effusions in body cavities, hypercholesterolemia, and anemia must be differentiated from nephrotic syndrome, pernicious anemia, and heart failure.

In patients hospitalized in an intensive care unit (ICU) or recovering from a severe disease not related to the thyroid gland, the TSH level may be above the reference range but still remain <20 mIU/L. Certain medications used in the acute setting (eg, dopamine, dobutamine, glucocorticoids) decrease serum TSH levels. Predominantly as a result of impaired synthesis, the levels of thyroid hormone-binding proteins decrease in nonthyroidal illness, which leads to low serum total T$_3$ and T$_4$ levels. FT$_4$ levels may also be found to be low, although methods for assessing FT$_4$ are unreliable during severe illness. Reverse T$_3$ (rT$_3$) levels increase; the measurement of rT$_3$ levels can be useful in distinguishing between nonthyroidal illness and central hypothyroidism (rT$_3$ levels are low in central hypothyroidism) but is not commonly ordered; the term **euthyroid sick syndrome** is used to describe these laboratory abnormalities. Despite such abnormal findings, patients usually do not warrant thyroid hormone replacement therapy. In view of the abnormal results of hormone tests of the pituitary-thyroid axis observed in hospitalized patients with severe illness, thyroid function tests should be performed only if there is a strong suspicion of clinically relevant thyroid dysfunction.

→ TREATMENT

Overt hypothyroidism is an absolute indication for hormone replacement therapy, usually lifelong.

Long-Term Hormone Replacement Therapy

Monotherapy with **levothyroxine (L-T$_4$)** is the treatment of choice. Fixed combinations of L-T$_4$ and liothyronine (L-T$_3$) are not recommended, as T$_4$ is converted to T$_3$. Dosage: once daily, 30 to 60 minutes before the first meal or at bedtime 4 hours after the last meal. The daily dose is estimated on an individual basis: in adults usually ~1.7 µg/kg/d; in the elderly use lower doses, even as low as 1 µg/kg/d. In the majority of patients the dose range is 100 to 150 µg/d (TSH levels should be within the reference range, optimally 2-3 mIU/L). In young healthy adults initiating treatment with full replacement doses is suggested.☉☻ For patients >50 to 60 years without evidence of coronary heart disease, you may consider a low dose (50 µg/d) when initiating therapy, whereas among those with evidence of coronary heart disease the usual starting dose is 12.5 to 25 µg/d. Dose adjustments are guided by measuring the TSH level 4 to 8 weeks following the initiation of L-T$_4$. Once the therapeutic dose has been established, reevaluate TSH levels after 6 months, and later after 1 year and in the event new clinical manifestations are observed. Note that some drugs may reduce the absorption or metabolism of L-T$_4$ (eg, calcium or iron supplements, bisphosphonates, sulfonylureas). Measure TSH levels within 4 to 8 weeks of introducing a new therapy. In regions with adequate iodine intake, iodine products should not be used in the treatment of hypothyroidism, except in pregnant women.

In patients with low levels of thyroid hormones, serum cortisol half-life is prolonged and normalizes during L-T$_4$ therapy; in the case of **coexisting adrenal insufficiency** this may trigger symptoms of acute adrenal crisis. Therefore, in patients with coexisting hypothyroidism and adrenal insufficiency, always start cortisol replacement first (→Chapter 5.1.1.2).

In **subclinical hypothyroidism** L-T$_4$ treatment is suggested in patients with serum TSH levels >10 mIU/L.☉☻ If TSH levels are 5 to 10 mIU/L, treatment should likely be considered in patients with TPO antibodies, ischemic heart disease, heart failure, or risk factors for these conditions.

Treatment monitoring: Assess serum TSH levels no sooner than 3 weeks after the last L-T$_4$ dose adjustment. In patients with secondary and tertiary hypothyroidism, measure the FT$_4$ level (TSH is not useful in such cases).

Increasing the previously established hormone replacement dose (under TSH level monitoring) may be necessary in the following cases:

1) Oral L-T$_4$ malabsorption (eg, in patients with inflammatory bowel diseases).

2) In patients requiring concomitant administration of drugs that cause L-T$_4$ malabsorption (eg, cholestyramine, aluminum hydroxide, calcium and iron supplements), maintain a several-hour interval between the administration of L-T$_4$ and these agents.

3) Starting estrogen products (eg, oral contraceptives).

Treatment of Myxedema Coma

Myxedema coma is an endocrine emergency associated with a high mortality risk (>20%) that should be treated aggressively.

Management in the ICU

1. L-T$_4$. On day 1 administer 200 to 400 µg IV in a single infusion or using an infusion pump (to correct L-T$_4$ deficiency; this may result in evident clinical improvement within several hours), and on subsequent days administer 50 to 100 µg IV once daily in a rapid infusion or using an infusion pump (take special care in patients with coronary heart disease due to the high risk of triggering angina, heart failure, or arrhythmia). When improvement is seen, switch to oral administration, usually 1.7 µg/kg/d or 100 to 150 µg/d (it is not necessary to start with a low dose of L-T$_4$ and titrate it up). Alternatively, IV **L-T$_4$ and L-T$_3$** may be used: on day 1 administer 200 to 300 µg of IV L-T$_4$ (4 µg/kg lean body weight) plus a separate T$_3$ preparation (5-20 µg IV infusion); on subsequent days administer L-T$_4$ 50 to 100 µg/d IV plus L-T$_3$ 2.5 to 10 µg tid IV (use lower doses in the elderly and in patients at high risk of cardiovascular complications; continue IV L-T$_3$ until clinical improvement is seen and the patient's clinical condition is stable). If IV preparations are not available, oral combinations containing 20 µg of L-T$_3$ and 100 µg of L-T$_4$ may be used: on day 1 administer 3 to 4 tablets once daily via a nasogastric tube; on subsequent days, 1 or 2 tablets via a nasogastric tube. When the patient's condition improves, administer 1 tablet once daily or L-T$_4$ 100 to 150 µg/d. Note that oral treatment is less reliable than the IV route due to the possibility of malabsorption.

2. Ensure good ventilation: Intubation and ventilatory support are usually required.

3. Correct any electrolyte disturbances and hypoglycemia using IV fluids; do not use hypotonic fluids due to the risk of water intoxication. In case of severe dilutional hyponatremia and hypovolemia, consider a hypertonic NaCl infusion (→Chapter 4.2.5.2). In euvolemic patients with hyponatremia treatment is the same as in patients with syndrome of inappropriate antidiuretic hormone secretion (→Chapter 5.3.3).

4. Aggressively treat concomitant diseases, such as heart failure or infection (administer empiric antibiotic therapy until culture and susceptibility results are available).

5. Until the possibility of concomitant adrenal insufficiency is excluded, use **glucocorticoids** in stress doses (eg, IV hydrocortisone 50-100 mg every 6 hours); they may be discontinued immediately after a normal serum cortisol level is confirmed in a sample collected before the administration of hydrocortisone.

6. Do not actively rewarm a hypothermic patient as this may cause vascular dilation and shock (a warm blanket is sufficient to prevent further heat loss).

➔ SPECIAL CONSIDERATIONS

Pregnancy

1. According to the 2012 Endocrine Society guidelines, screening for thyroid disorders before planned pregnancy is indicated in women at high risk of thyroid diseases, which includes patients with thyroid disorders, after thyroidectomy, with a history of postpartum thyroiditis, with a family history of thyroid disease, with a goiter, with elevated plasma levels of thyroid antibodies, with signs or symptoms suggestive of thyroid disorders, with type 1 diabetes mellitus or other autoimmune disorders, with infertility, with a history of miscarriage or preterm delivery, and with prior therapeutic head or neck irradiation.

2. In pregnant women the TSH level is usually measured in weeks 4 to 8 of pregnancy, during the first obstetric visit. According to the American Thyroid Association, if a population-specific and trimester-specific reference range for serum TSH is not available, an upper reference limit of ~4 mIU/L may be used. For most assays this limit represents a reduction in the upper reference limit for TSH in nonpregnant patients by ~0.5 mIU/L.

3. Measure TPO antibody levels in:

1) Patients with a coexisting autoimmune disease (in particular type 1 diabetes mellitus) or a family history of such disorders.

2) Patients with a TSH level >2.5 mIU/L.

3) Patients in whom ultrasonography of the thyroid gland suggests autoimmune disease.

4) Patients with a positive history of postpartum thyroiditis.

5) Patients who are treated for infertility or have a history of miscarriage or preterm delivery. Significant correlations between elevated TPO antibodies and miscarriage, preterm delivery, and neonatal respiratory failure have been identified.

4. Supplementation with potassium iodide is not recommended in North America, although it is used in some geographic areas where access to iodine is of concern.

5. In pregnant patients with overt hypothyroidism start L-T_4 at a dose that covers the daily requirement. In patients diagnosed with hypothyroidism before pregnancy, increase the dose of L-T_4 by 30% to 50%, usually in weeks 4 to 6 of pregnancy. In the majority of patients the dose has to be reduced after delivery. In pregnant women with subclinical hypothyroidism, L-T_4 is recommended for TPO-positive women if TSH is greater than the pregnancy-specific reference range (or, if the range is unavailable, >4 mIU/L) and suggested for TPO-positive women if TSH is >2.5 mIU/L or for TPO-negative women if TSH is from 4 to 10 mIU/L.⊘○ In the first half of pregnancy monitor TSH levels (as well as T_4 and FT_4) every 4 weeks and measure TSH levels at least once between weeks 26 and 32. Measuring FT_4 levels does not always allow for an accurate evaluation of thyroid status during pregnancy. In the second and third trimesters the reference ranges are adapted by multiplying the total T_4 (TT_4) levels from before pregnancy by 1.5. However, due to the changing levels of T_4-binding globulin, TT_4 levels may be considered less accurate than FT_4 levels.

6.2. Nontoxic Multinodular Goiter

→ DEFINITION AND ETIOLOGY

Nontoxic multinodular goiter (MNG) is a disease of the thyroid gland characterized by the presence of thyroid nodules (dominant focal structural lesions) without biochemical abnormalities of the thyroid gland. The etiology of nontoxic MNG is multifactorial, with the important factors including, among others, iodine deficiency (initially manifesting as a simple goiter), genetic predisposition, goitrogens, exposure to ionizing radiation, and history of thyroiditis.

A **goiter** is defined as an enlarged thyroid gland. A precise cutoff value for the size on physical examination or the volume measured by ultrasonography is controversial and difficult to provide given the expected differences due to age, sex, and presence of iodine deficiency in patients from different populations.

A **simple goiter** refers to an enlarged thyroid gland with no structural echographic abnormalities, which most frequently develops as a result of iodine deficiency in children and adolescents. It is a risk factor for the development of MNG in adults. A **substernal goiter** is an enlarged thyroid gland with more than one-third of the thyroid volume located below the upper margin of the jugular notch. It may remain undiagnosed until compression symptoms develop.

A **nontoxic goiter** is a goiter in a euthyroid patient. **Euthyroid status** refers to normal function of the thyroid gland with no abnormal findings in history and on clinical examination, which has been confirmed by normal results of thyroid hormone tests.

An **incidental thyroid nodule** is a nodule not suspected clinically that is identified during an imaging study performed for other clinical reasons.

→ CLINICAL FEATURES AND NATURAL HISTORY

Nontoxic goiter develops slowly and often remains undiagnosed for years; it is not accompanied by biochemical abnormalities of the thyroid gland. The enlarged thyroid gland with nodular hypertrophy may be evident through an increased neck circumference and its visible asymmetry. In rare cases it may present with dyspnea, cough, or dysphagia resulting from the compression of adjacent tissues by a large or retrosternal goiter.

→ DIAGNOSIS

Diagnostic Tests

1. Laboratory tests: Serum thyroid-stimulating hormone (TSH) levels are usually obtained to rule out biochemical thyroid abnormalities; normal results usually exclude abnormal thyroid function without the need for the determination of free thyroid hormone levels.

2. Imaging studies: Thyroid ultrasonography is used for the evaluation and monitoring of the thyroid size and nodules, including their location, size (3-dimensional), echogenicity (iso-, hyper-, or hypoechogenic solid nodules; nonechogenic cysts), internal structure (homogeneous or heterogeneous), borders (clearly demarcated or fuzzy and irregular), calcifications (microcalcifications or macrocalcifications), blood supply (vascularity) of the whole parenchyma and nodules (color Doppler or power Doppler). Ultrasonography cannot reliably differentiate nonmalignant from malignant nodules, but it may detect an increased risk of malignancy (→below). Thyroid ultrasonography is recommended in all patients with suspected thyroid nodules and for the initial evaluation of thyroid nodules discovered through other modalities.◐◐ **Radionuclide thyroid imaging** has limited use in the diagnosis of nontoxic goiter and should not be routinely used for this purpose (however, it is useful in the evaluation of patients with hyperthyroidism, as it can help distinguish between toxic multinodular goiter and Graves disease).

3. Fine-needle aspiration biopsy (FNB) and cytologic examination is an extremely useful technique in the evaluation of thyroid nodules. It helps guide clinical management and evaluate the need for surgery. One of the most commonly used cytology-reporting classifications is the Bethesda classification; it has 6 diagnostic categories (→Table 6-1). FNB allows the cytologic diagnosis of papillary thyroid cancer but does not differentiate benign lesions (hyperplastic nodule, thyroiditis, or follicular adenoma [nonmalignant neoplasm]) from malignant follicular carcinoma, where only histologic examination of surgical specimens is conclusive. Therefore, the diagnosis of "follicular neoplasm" has been replaced with "suspicious for follicular neoplasm" and the respective oxyphilic variant. Molecular testing of the aspirate, if available, allows better classification and risk prediction.

Indications for FNB of a thyroid nodule include (but are not limited to):
1) A nodule of any size with the presence of suspicious cervical lymphadenopathy assessed clinically or with imaging studies.
2) A nodule >1 cm with ultrasound features associated with a high risk of malignancy.
3) A nodule with ^{18}F-fluorodeoxyglucose positron emission tomography (FDG-PET) avidity.

Features of a thyroid nodule associated with a high risk of malignancy:
1) **Clinical**: Worrisome clinical lymphadenopathy, rapidly increasing nodule size, hoarseness (due to laryngeal nerve palsy), metastases from an unknown primary lesion, previous neck or chest irradiation, family history of thyroid cancer, age <18 years.
2) **Ultrasonography**: Internal microcalcifications, hypoechogenicity, increased central blood flow, infiltrative margins, taller than wider nodules, features

Table 6-1. Diagnostic categories in cytology of the thyroid gland

Diagnostic category	Risk of thyroid cancer	Most common histologic diagnoses	Indications for repeated FNB	Commonly recommended management[a]
I: Nondiagnostic biopsy	5%-10%[c,d]	Any diagnosis possible	Repeated FNB with US guidance, usually in 3-12 months, depending on risk; in case of clinical suspicion of anaplastic cancer, further diagnostics must be continued immediately	Indications for surgery depend on clinical risk of malignancy; nondiagnostic biopsy likely in patients with cysts or thyroiditis
II: Benign	0%-3%[c,d]	Multinodular goiter, including hyperplastic nodules and colloid nodules; thyroiditis	No (except in cases of new US risk factors of suspicious lymphadenopathy)	Follow-up (clinical and US)
III: AUS or FLUS	6%-18%[c] (10%-30%)[d]	Category used only if accurate cytologic diagnosis not possible	Yes (in 3-12 months, depending on risk)	Possible options: (1) molecular testing (if available); (2) active surveillance; (3) surgery
IV: Suspicious for follicular neoplasm[a]	10%-40%[b,c] (25%-40%)[d]	May reflect nonneoplastic lesion or benign tumor, which cannot be differentiated from malignancy by cytology alone	No but if surgery is planned diagnosis must be confirmed by another cytologist	Possible options: (1) molecular testing (if available); (2) active surveillance; (3) surgery
V: Suspicious for malignancy	45%-60%[c] (50%-75%)[d]	Suspected thyroid cancer	No but diagnosis must be confirmed by another cytologist	Surgery
VI: Malignant	94%-96%[c] (97%-99%)[d]	Papillary thyroid cancer; medullary thyroid cancer; anaplastic thyroid cancer; other malignancy	No but diagnosis must be confirmed by another cytologist	Surgery

[a] Actual management also depends on other clinical and US risk factors.

[b] The diagnosis of nodules "suspicious for follicular neoplasm" includes those "suspicious for oxyphil neoplasm," which is more frequently an unequivocal indication for surgery.

[c] Risk of malignancy if NIFTP is excluded because it is benign; previously classified as noninvasive follicular variant of papillary thyroid carcinoma.

[d] Risk of malignancy if NIFTP is included.

Based on Thyroid. 2017 Nov; 27: 1341-1346 and Endokrynol Pol. 2018;69(1):34-74.

↑, increase; ↓, decrease; FT_3, free triiodothyronine; FT_4, free thyroxine; TSH, thyroid-stimulating hormone.

Table 6-2. Treatment of nontoxic multinodular goiter: advantages and disadvantages of various therapeutic options

Treatment method	Disadvantages	Advantages
Surgery (nodules suspicious for malignancy, tracheal compression)	Surgical complications; hospitalization required	Total removal of nodule; complete resolution of symptoms; histologic diagnosis
Radioiodine therapy (age >40-60 years, goiter volume >60 mL, contraindications to surgery; not commonly used)	Slow reduction in the goiter volume; hypothyroidism (10% in 5 years); radiation-induced thyroiditis (1%-2%); effective contraception required	Minor side effects; 40% reduction in goiter volume in 2 years
Percutaneous ethanol injections (subtoxic nodules, simple cysts; not commonly used)	Difficult evaluation of subsequent cytology; repeated injections necessary; ineffective in large nodules; painful procedure; transient dysphonia (1%-2%)	Does not cause hypothyroidism

suggestive of lymph node metastases, features of infiltration of the thyroid capsule or adjacent tissues. Suspicious cervical adenopathy (microcalcifications, loss of the hilum, and a round shape) strongly suggests the presence of a metastatic disease. FDG-PET–avid thyroid nodules are more likely to be malignant than FDG-PET–negative thyroid nodules (the study is usually performed for other reasons).

Diagnostic Criteria

Diagnostic criteria for nontoxic MNG:

1) At least 1 clinically evident thyroid nodule (regardless of the total volume of the thyroid gland) or an enlarged thyroid gland on ultrasonography with focal abnormalities of the echogenic structure lesions >1 cm in diameter.

2) Normal serum TSH levels.

Follow-Up Investigations to Exclude Thyroid Cancer

FNB should be considered in every case of MNG. The criteria for selection of nodules to perform FNB are based on clinical and ultrasound features (→above). In patients with multiple nodules, each nodule should be assessed independently.

1. If the initial FNB yields no features of malignancy of the examined nodules ("benign" nodule; →Table 6-1) and the study is reliable, the biopsy does not need to be repeated and a follow-up ultrasonography of the thyroid gland is sufficient. If the clinical suspicion is high and follow-up imaging reveals findings suspicious of malignancy, repeat FNB should be performed.◉◯ Of note, the initial clinical suspicion appears more relevant than, for example, the rate of growth.

2. If the initial FNB result indicates a "follicular lesion of undetermined significance," repeat the FNB at 3 to 12 months depending on the degree of clinical suspicion of malignancy.

⇥ T R E A T M E N T

Advantages and disadvantages of individual treatment modalities: →Table 6-2.

Surgical Treatment

A surgical approach for thyroid nodules is recommended as a treatment modality in cases where the clinical evaluation (ultrasound features, FNB) demonstrates a high risk of malignancy. In addition, surgery might be recommended as both a diagnostic and treatment modality in cases where the clinical evaluation is suggestive of malignancy. In cases of benign nodules surgery can be performed in the setting of compressive symptoms or for cosmetic concerns.

Indications:

1) Cytologic diagnosis of a "malignant" or "suspicious for malignancy" nodule (→Table 6-1) denoting suspicion of thyroid cancer or insufficient data for its exclusion (an absolute indication). The diagnosis of "suspicious for oxyphilic neoplasm" is associated with a 15% to 20% risk of cancer and can be an important indication for surgery. The diagnosis of "suspicious for follicular neoplasm" is a relative indication for surgery, as the risk of cancer is ~5% (the decision is taken on a case-by-case basis, depending on the size of the nodule and presence of risk factors; surgery is mandatory in nodules >4 cm in diameter).

2) A large goiter causing airway compression.

3) A retrosternal goiter (regardless of airway compression).

Nonsurgical Treatment

Nonsurgical treatment may be considered in cases where both the FNB findings and clinical features do not suggest thyroid cancer (→Table 6-2).

→ P R O G N O S I S

If the FNB is correctly performed and interpreted, the risk of overlooking a malignant thyroid nodule ranges between <1% and 10%, according to center. A benign nodule may increase in size and cause compression symptoms during follow-up; there is also some risk of gradual development of hyperthyroidism (→Chapter 5.6.4, →Figure 6-9).

6.3. Thyroiditis

1. Clinical classification of thyroiditis:

1) Acute.

2) Subacute.

3) Chronic (most frequent).

2. Histologic classification of thyroiditis:

1) Bacterial thyroiditis (acute suppurative thyroiditis).

2) Other (nonbacterial) acute thyroiditis: Radiation-induced thyroiditis; palpation-induced or trauma-induced thyroiditis; drug-induced thyroiditis (interferon α, interleukin 2, amiodarone, or lithium).

3) Subacute granulomatous thyroiditis (synonyms: subacute thyroiditis, granulocytic thyroiditis, giant cell thyroiditis, de Quervain thyroiditis).

4) Subacute lymphocytic thyroiditis (painless thyroiditis; postpartum thyroiditis).

5) Chronic lymphocytic thyroiditis (also called chronic autoimmune thyroiditis and Hashimoto thyroiditis; most common).

6) Chronic infiltrative fibrosing thyroiditis (Riedel thyroiditis).

3. Classification of thyroiditis based on thyroid function:

1) **Destructive thyroiditis** with periodic or continuous thyrotoxicosis caused by the destruction of thyroid follicles and release of variable (sometimes very high) amounts of thyroid hormones to the circulation. This class includes many types of thyroiditis with different etiologies; most frequently, they are acute or subacute, but chronic thyroiditis may also occur. Pain or tenderness are not always present and are not required for the diagnosis. The clinical spectrum includes numerous types of thyroiditis:

   a) Subacute painful granulomatous thyroiditis (de Quervain thyroiditis).

   b) Viral painless granulomatous thyroiditis.

   c) Subacute painless lymphocytic thyroiditis (silent thyroiditis).

  d) Painful lymphocytic thyroiditis.
  e) Posttraumatic thyroiditis (including palpation-induced thyroiditis).
  f) Radiation-induced thyroiditis.
  g) Infectious thyroiditis.
  h) Drug-induced thyroiditis, for instance, caused by amiodarone, interferon α, interleukin 2, or lithium, and recently tyrosine kinase inhibitors.
2) **Nondestructive thyroiditis**: All the other conditions that do not cause thyrotoxicosis.

6.3.1. Acute Thyroiditis

1. Acute bacterial (suppurative) thyroiditis is rare. Infection spreads by the hematogenous route or by continuity from adjacent tissues.

Etiology: Streptococci (*Streptococcus pyogenes*), staphylococci (*Staphylococcus aureus*), less frequently *Escherichia coli* and *Salmonella typhimurium*; in recurrent infections, anaerobic bacteria. The disease initially manifests as a painful swelling of the thyroid gland with fever and rigors. Formation of an abscess is accompanied by painful regional lymphadenopathy. Thyroid function is usually normal.

Ultrasonography shows decreased heterogeneous echogenicity of the abscess. On **radionuclide imaging** the abscess is "cold" and shows no radionuclide uptake. Cytology shows only purulent contents (send a sample for culture and antibiotic susceptibility). White blood cell counts are high and erythrocyte sedimentation rate is markedly elevated.

The **treatment of choice** is inpatient antibiotic therapy and surgical drainage of the abscess or a total or partial surgical resection of the affected thyroid gland. Immediately after collecting samples for microbiology start empiric antibiotic therapy based on risk factors, severity of infection, previous history of allergic reactions to antibiotics, and recently used antimicrobial treatment.

2. Radiation-induced thyroiditis develops after radioiodine treatment. Following the acute inflammatory phase, patients can develop hypothyroidism. The disease may also occur after external beam irradiation used in oncology; in such cases it appears late, has no acute phase, and is termed "radiation--induced hypothyroidism."

3. Thyroiditis caused by trauma (including vigorous palpation) of the thyroid gland.

4. Drug-induced thyroiditis: Some drugs, such as, lithium, interferon α, interleukin 2, amiodarone, and tyrosine kinase inhibitors, may cause symptoms of acute thyroiditis. Amiodarone-induced thyroiditis: →Chapter 5.6.3.3.

6.3.2. Chronic Autoimmune Thyroiditis (Hashimoto Thyroiditis)

➔ DEFINITION, ETIOLOGY, PATHOGENESIS

Chronic autoimmune (lymphocytic) thyroiditis (Hashimoto thyroiditis) is a painless thyroiditis associated with antibodies against thyroid peroxidase (TPO) and, in some cases, against thyroglobulin (Tg), presenting with thyroid lymphocytic infiltrates and slow-onset hypothyroidism. Pathogenesis is primarily attributed to the activity of cytotoxic T cells, which are responsible for the destruction of the follicular thyroid cells.

➔ CLINICAL FEATURES AND NATURAL HISTORY

The disease may take one of two clinical forms: with a normal thyroid volume (atrophic form) or with a goiter (painless enlargement and increased density of the thyroid gland). Both forms may present with normal thyroid levels and subclinical or overt hypothyroidism. The course of the disease is chronic, indolent, and in some cases results in permanent hypothyroidism. Exacerbations with sudden enlargement and tenderness of the thyroid gland and general features of inflammation (elevated C-reactive protein [CRP] levels and erythrocyte sedimentation rate [ESR], rarely with fever) are very rare; they may be accompanied by clinical features of thyrotoxicosis (hashitoxicosis, hyperthyroiditis) caused by excessive release of thyroid hormones from the affected gland. These symptoms resolve spontaneously and are followed by the development of hypothyroidism.

→ DIAGNOSIS

Diagnostic Tests

1. Laboratory tests:

1) Increased titers of **antibodies to TPO and, in some cases, to Tg**.

2) Elevated serum **thyroid-stimulating hormone (TSH)** levels (they may be decreased in the rarely observed hyperthyroid phase).

3) Decreased serum **free thyroxine (FT_4)** levels (in subclinical hypothyroidism FT_4 levels are normal, whereas in the rare hyperthyroid phase the levels of free thyroid hormones may be elevated).

2. Imaging studies: Results of ultrasonography and ^{131}I radionuclide thyroid imaging are frequently not conclusive and not needed. Ultrasonography shows a heterogeneous hypodense parenchyma both in patients with a goiter and with thyroid atrophy; if nodular lesions are found, consider the indications for fine-needle biopsy (FNB) (→Chapter 5.6.2).

3. FNB and morphology studies: Cytologic findings may vary from mild fibrosis to massive lymphocytic and plasmacytic infiltrates with the formation of lymphoid follicles and oncocytic metaplasia of the follicular epithelium.

Diagnostic Criteria

The key diagnostic criterion is an elevated level of TPO antibodies in a patient who presents with a goiter, reduced size of the thyroid gland (atrophic thyroid), or hypothyroidism. The diagnostic importance of Tg antibodies is considerably lower than that of TPO antibodies due to their lower specificity. In patients with concomitant hypothyroidism and elevated levels of TPO antibodies, FNB should not be performed to confirm diagnosis.⊘⊜

Differential Diagnosis

1. Other thyroid diseases causing hypothyroidism: History, different morphologic features.

2. Differentiation of hashitoxicosis from other causes of hyperthyroidism: History, elevated TPO antibody levels, negative thyrotropin-stimulating hormone receptor (TSH-R) antibodies, and different morphologic features.

→ TREATMENT

There are no effective methods of treating the cause of the disease. Patients with overt hypothyroidism should receive levothyroxine ($L-T_4$) replacement therapy (→Chapter 5.6.1). In subclinical hypothyroidism, $L-T_4$ replacement is suggested when TSH levels are >10 mIU/L⊘⊜ or in pregnancy. Uncertainty exists regarding the management of patients with subclinical hypothyroidism and TSH levels between 5 and 10 mIU/L; thus the decision of treatment with $L-T_4$ replacement is based on the presence of symptoms suggestive of hypothyroidism and age of the patient (TSH values between 5 and 10 mIU/L may be normal in elderly people). In the rare cases of hashitoxicosis use of antithyroid drugs is not mandatory and usually accelerates the development of hypothyroidism.

→ PROGNOSIS

The disease may lead to permanent hypothyroidism, which requires lifelong hormone replacement therapy (with adequate treatment, the disease causes no sequelae). The risk of developing overt hypothyroidism in patients with subclinical hypothyroidism increases with age. Very rarely thyroiditis may progress to primary lymphoma of the thyroid gland; transformation of Hashimoto thyroiditis into Graves disease is also rare and caused by the development of TSH-R antibodies early in the course of the disease along with subsequent overstimulation of the thyroid gland.

6.3.3. Other Types of Chronic Thyroiditis

1. Painless (silent) thyroiditis (subacute lymphocytic thyroiditis): Autoimmune, painless, chronic thyroiditis, which is considered to be a variant of Hashimoto thyroiditis. It is characterized by a 4-phase course that includes a transient phase of thyrotoxicosis with low iodine uptake (phase 1) followed by a transient euthyroid phase (phase 2), a hypothyroid phase (phase 3), and subsequent return to the euthyroid status (phase 4). A small painless goiter is observed; the course is otherwise similar to that of subacute thyroiditis (→below). The disease occurs spontaneously or within 1 year of childbirth (or miscarriage); in the latter case, it is referred to as **postpartum thyroiditis** (develops in ~50% of women with elevated thyroperoxidase [TPO] antibody levels during pregnancy, may recur after subsequent pregnancies, and is associated with a slightly elevated risk of permanent hypothyroidism). In the thyrotoxicosis phase administer a β-blocker or, in severe cases, a glucocorticoid. In patients who develop permanent hypothyroidism start levothyroxine (L-T$_4$) replacement therapy (→Chapter 5.6.1).

2. Riedel thyroiditis: Very rare fibrosing thyroiditis, which gradually involves the whole thyroid gland and other tissues of the neck (the thyroid gland is very hard on palpation). Patients may develop dyspnea, recurrent laryngeal nerve palsy, Horner syndrome, or hypoparathyroidism. Fine-needle biopsy (FNB) does not yield diagnostic samples. Total thyroidectomy is practically impossible; the tracheal compression can be reduced by wedge resection of the thyroid isthmus. Treatment with glucocorticoids is sometimes effective.

3. Chronic interferon α–induced thyroiditis: In persons with a genetic predisposition interferon α induces the production of autoantibodies, including antithyroid antibodies, thus increasing the risk of developing subacute lymphocytic thyroiditis, chronic autoimmune thyroiditis, or (rarely) Graves disease. Thyroiditis is not fully reversible.

4. Chronic amiodarone-induced thyroiditis: The drug causes **hypothyroidism** or (less frequently) **thyrotoxicosis** (amiodarone-induced thyrotoxicosis [AIT]). **Type 1 AIT** is caused by excess iodine, coming from the amiodarone molecule, which is used as a substrate for the synthesis of thyroid hormones (increased production of thyroid hormones in patients with subclinical disorders or in genetically predisposed persons). **Type 2 AIT** is a chronic thyroiditis causing destruction of the previously structurally intact thyroid gland and release of excess thyroid hormones to the circulation (the production of thyroid hormones is not increased).

Diagnosis: Signs and symptoms of hyperthyroidism may be subtle; exacerbation of preexisting arrhythmia may be the only sign (in such patients it is necessary to assess thyroid-stimulating hormone levels).

Differential diagnosis and treatment: →Table 6-4. **In patients with mixed features of type 1 and type 2 AIT**, combined treatment is recommended: start therapy with an antithyroid drug and prednisone in patients in whom thyrotoxicosis-related symptoms do not improve. When amiodarone is used for non–life-threatening arrhythmias, cardiology consultation is suggested to consider the possibility of drug discontinuation.

Table 6-3. Clinical phases of subacute thyroiditis (de Quervain thyroiditis)

	Hormone levels	Iodine uptake	Clinical features
Phase 1	↑FT_4, ↑FT_3, ↓TSH	Low	Thyrotoxicosis
Phase 2	Normal	Low	Euthyroidism
Phase 3	↓FT_4, ↓FT_3, ↑TSH	High	Hypothyroidism
Phase 4	Normal	Normal	Euthyroidism

↑, increase; ↓, decrease; FT_3, free triiodothyronine; FT_4, free thyroxine; TSH, thyroid-stimulating hormone.

6.3.4. Subacute Thyroiditis (de Quervain Thyroiditis)

→ DEFINITION, ETIOLOGY, PATHOGENESIS

Subacute thyroiditis (de Quervain thyroiditis, granulocytic thyroiditis, granulomatous thyroiditis, giant cell thyroiditis) is probably of viral origin and follows a 4-phase course. There is a strong correlation of subacute thyroiditis with the presence of certain human leukocyte antigens (HLAs). The disease is usually preceded (2-8 weeks earlier) by an upper respiratory tract infection.

→ CLINICAL FEATURES AND NATURAL HISTORY

The disease can be divided into 4 distinct phases (→Table 6-3). Initially the dominant features are painful swelling of the thyroid gland and fever; pain is referred to the ears, mandibular angle, and upper chest. Thyrotoxicosis (lasting 3-8 weeks) results from destruction of the glandular parenchyma and release of thyroid hormones; usually it is not associated with prominent clinical features but it may be accompanied by malaise and muscle pain. The pain and fever subside spontaneously and hormone levels normalize after 8 to 16 weeks. Phase 3 (hypothyroidism) is not always present. Permanent hypothyroidism is extremely rare and recovery is almost always complete (phase 4). A rapidly growing nodule, requiring cytologic assessment to exclude malignancy, may actually be an inflammatory infiltrate in the course of subacute thyroiditis. In ~2% of patients the disease may recur after a long remission (up to 20 years).

→ DIAGNOSIS

Diagnostic Tests

1. Laboratory tests:

1) Extremely elevated erythrocyte sedimentation rate (ESR) (accompanied by exquisite tenderness of the thyroid gland).
2) Thyroid-stimulating hormone (TSH) and thyroid hormones: →Table 6-3.
3) Antithyroid antibodies (present only in 10%-20% of patients; thyroglobulin [Tg] antibodies are more frequent than thyroperoxidase [TPO] antibodies).

2. Imaging studies: Thyroid ultrasonography reveals diffuse or focal hypoechogenicity of the thyroid gland. **Radionuclide thyroid imaging** shows a very low iodine uptake (in the early phase of the disease).

3. Cytology: The dominant cells are neutrophils, giant cells (characteristic polynuclear macrophages), and epithelioid cells (mononuclear macrophages).

Diagnostic Criteria

The key diagnostic criteria are a painful or tender goiter, elevated ESR, transient thyrotoxicosis, and significantly decreased iodine uptake.

Differential Diagnosis

Other rare types of granulomatous thyroiditis: tuberculous thyroiditis, fungal thyroiditis (*Aspergillus*, *Candida*, *Cryptococcus*); *Pneumocystis jiroveci* thyroiditis in immunodeficient patients. If pain is not a dominant feature, differential diagnosis should include silent thyroiditis (markedly elevated ESR and association with a prior viral infection suggest de Quervain thyroiditis).

→TREATMENT

The hyperthyroid phase requires no antithyroid treatment (propranolol may be used in patients with bothersome symptoms of hyperthyroidism). Administer acetylsalicylic acid 2 to 4 g/d or nonsteroidal anti-inflammatory drugs to control pain and inflammation; if pain is severe, consider prednisone 40 to 60 mg/d for the first week, then taper the dose down to discontinue treatment in ≤4 weeks. In the hypothyroid phase consider levothyroxine (L-T$_4$) replacement therapy (to prevent exacerbation of the disease); note that hypothyroidism is transient and therapy should not be continued indefinitely. There is no indication for surgery, as the disease is self-limiting and does not cause permanent thyroid damage.

6.4. Thyrotoxicosis and Hyperthyroidism

→DEFINITION, ETIOLOGY, PATHOGENESIS

Subclinical (occult) thyrotoxicosis is a usually asymptomatic mild elevation in tissue levels of thyroid hormones with low or suppressed thyroid-stimulating hormone (TSH) levels and free thyroxine (FT$_4$) and free triiodothyronine (FT$_3$) levels within normal limits.

Clinically overt thyrotoxicosis refers to suppressed TSH with high FT$_4$ and FT$_3$ levels.

Thyrotoxicosis is a clinical state that results from any condition leading to high thyroid hormone action in tissues.

Hyperthyroidism is a form of thyrotoxicosis caused by high synthesis and secretion of thyroid hormone by the thyroid gland.

Thyrotoxic crisis (thyroid storm) is a life-threatening, sudden, and rapid collapse of homeostasis, developing as a result of undiagnosed or inadequately treated hyperthyroidism and involving altered mental status that may progress to coma, multiorgan failure, shock, and death. Causes of thyrotoxicosis: →Figure 6-2.

→CLINICAL FEATURES AND NATURAL HISTORY

Thyrotoxicosis usually develops over the course of several months. It may also appear suddenly (eg, when associated with exposure to iodinated contrast media), develop over several years (autonomously functioning nodule, toxic multinodular goiter), or be transient and resolve spontaneously (subacute or postpartum thyroiditis). Various causes of thyrotoxicosis coexist rarely; for instance, a hyperfunctioning thyroid nodule in a patient with Graves disease may produce an unusual clinical course without periods of remission typical of Graves disease.

Subclinical Thyrotoxicosis

Subclinical thyrotoxicosis is the asymptomatic or occult phase of thyrotoxicosis regardless of its cause. In ~50% of cases serum TSH levels spontaneously normalize and the estimated risk of progression to overt thyrotoxicosis is ~5% per year (the progression may be triggered by exposure to iodine). Subclinical thyrotoxicosis may include subtle signs and symptoms of hypersecretion of thyroid hormones such as tachycardia, supraventricular arrhythmias (atrial fibrillation,

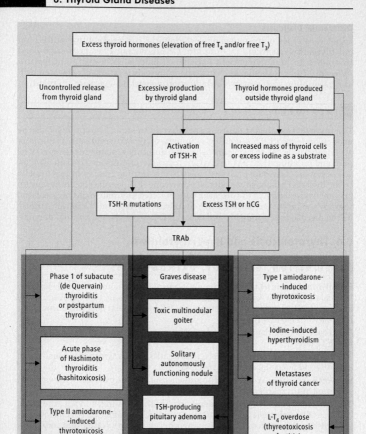

Figure 6-2. Causes of thyrotoxicosis.

premature supraventricular contraction), and (rarely) ventricular arrhythmias. If long-standing and untreated, subclinical thyrotoxicosis leads to decreased bone mineral density, and in elderly patients with TSH levels <0.1 mIU/L it may be associated with elevated risk of cardiovascular complications.

Overt Thyrotoxicosis

1. General symptoms: Loss of weight despite normal or good appetite (elderly people may present with weight loss and low appetite), weakness, and heat intolerance.

2. Neuropsychiatric symptoms: Anxiety, irritability, hyperactivity (hyperkinetic behavior), concentration problems, insomnia; rarely psychotic symptoms (suggestive of schizophrenia or bipolar disorder); fine tremor and hyperreflexia.

3. Ocular symptoms:

1) Eyelid retraction (staring appearance) resulting from sympathetic overactivity.
2) Graefe sign (more sclera exposed over the upper border of the iris when the patient looks downward [upper lid lag over the globe]).
3 Kocher sign (a similar sign observed in a patient looking up).
4) Möbius sign (deviation of one eye on convergent gaze).
5) Stellwag sign (infrequent blinking).
6) Signs and symptoms of Graves orbitopathy: Eye pain, tearing, diplopia, periorbital edema, and conjunctival injection.

4. Cutaneous symptoms: Hyperhidrosis and skin hyperemia (warm, pink, moist, and excessively smooth skin); rarely hyperpigmentation (not including mucosal surfaces) or urticaria; hair loss, thinning, and breaking; thin and fragile nails, which may separate from nail beds (onycholysis); thyroid dermopathy (pretibial myxedema) (→Figure 6-3) and acropachy (→Figure 6-4) may be present in Graves disease.

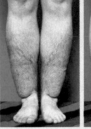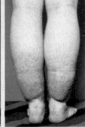

Figure 6-3. Thyroid dermopathy (pretibial myxedema) in Graves disease.

5. Musculoskeletal symptoms: Decrease of muscle mass and strength (in more severe thyrotoxicosis); in severe cases, thyrotoxic myopathy involving muscles of the face and distal limbs. Involvement of extraocular muscles may mimic myasthenia gravis.

6. Abnormalities of the neck: In some patients increased neck circumference and sensation of pressure are observed. On physical examination the thyroid gland is of normal size or, more frequently, enlarged (in overt thyrotoxicosis this is indicative of a toxic goiter). Finding a thrill or bruit on physical examination of the thyroid gland is indicative of a vascular goiter

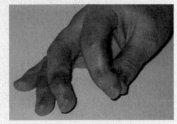

Figure 6-4. Thyroid acropachy.

(typical of Graves disease) and if ≥1 nodule is present, it is necessary to consider toxic nodular goiter in the differential diagnosis (the presence of nodules does not exclude Graves disease).

7. Respiratory symptoms: Dyspnea caused by tracheal compression due to an enlarged thyroid gland is rare.

8. Cardiovascular symptoms: Palpitations, hyperkinetic circulation (tachycardia, systolic hypertension, widened pulse pressure, loud heart sounds); frequently arrhythmia with premature ventricular contractions or atrial fibrillation, systolic murmurs (due to mitral prolapse or regurgitation), sometimes end-diastolic murmurs; symptoms of heart failure, particularly in patients with preexisting heart disease.

9. Gastrointestinal symptoms: Increased stool frequency or diarrhea. In severe thyrotoxicosis hepatomegaly and jaundice may develop due to liver damage.

10. Abnormalities of the reproductive system and breast: Sometimes decreased libido, oligomenorrhea (generally with ovulation); in exceptional cases, amenorrhea, erectile dysfunction, or gynecomastia.

Thyrotoxic Crisis (Thyroid Storm)

Thyrotoxic crisis due to a sudden and large excess of thyroid hormones may develop in a patient with hyperthyroidism as a result of stress, infection, trauma, or other serious condition, or if the patient undergoes thyroid surgery without appropriate pretreatment with antithyroid drugs. In case of a sudden deterioration in the status of a patient with hyperthyroidism, always consider the possibility of impending or overt thyrotoxic crisis. The predominant signs and symptoms may be those related to the underlying disease that precipitated thyrotoxic crisis.

1. Precedent symptoms: Agitation, insomnia (hallucinations and other psychotic symptoms may occur at night), significant weight loss, worsening of tremor, fever, nausea, and vomiting.

2. Overt thyrotoxic crisis: Fever; extreme agitation and worsening of psychotic symptoms; sometimes somnolence, apathy, or even coma; in some cases status epilepticus; sudden worsening of cardiovascular symptoms (severe tachycardia, atrial fibrillation, symptoms of heart failure, sometimes shock) and gastrointestinal symptoms of thyrotoxicosis (nausea, diarrhea, and hepatic dysfunction); signs and symptoms of dehydration (often following a period of hyperhidrosis).

→ DIAGNOSIS

Always inquire about a family history of thyroid disorders, exposure to high doses of iodine (certain disinfecting agents [eg, iodine tincture] or expectorants; amiodarone; iodinated contrast media), and previous treatment of thyroid diseases and autoimmune diseases of other organs. Simultaneously assess thyroid function and morphology and aim at identifying the causative factors. Always make sure that serum TSH and free thyroid hormone levels are consistent and correspond with the presenting signs and symptoms. General diagnostic algorithm: →Figure 6-5.

Diagnostic Tests

In patients suspected of thyrotoxicosis evaluate serum TSH levels and FT_4 levels (in patients with low TSH and normal FT_4 levels measure serum total T_3 levels) and examine the thyroid gland for enlargement and presence of nodules in the parenchyma (palpable nodules or nodules detected on ultrasonography may fulfill the criteria for fine-needle biopsy [FNB]; →Chapter 5.6.2). Antibodies to TSH receptors allow for a reliable differential diagnosis of autoimmune and nonautoimmune causes of thyrotoxicosis.

1. Hormone tests:

1) Serum **TSH** concentrations are the most sensitive marker of activity of thyroid hormones. They are decreased in primary thyrotoxicosis (both overt and subclinical) and increased in secondary thyrotoxicosis (very rare TSH-producing pituitary adenoma). Circadian fluctuations of serum TSH levels are of no significance for routine diagnostics.

2) Serum FT_4 **and** FT_3 concentrations are increased in overt thyrotoxicosis (more commonly FT_4 or both FT_4 and FT_3 are affected; isolated FT_3 elevation is rare but confirms thyrotoxicosis if TSH level is low and FT_4 level is normal) and normal (often close to the upper limit of normal [ULN]) in subclinical thyrotoxicosis.

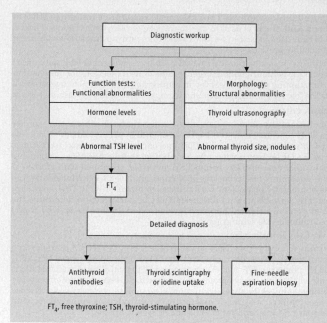

FT$_4$, free thyroxine; TSH, thyroid-stimulating hormone.

Figure 6-5. General diagnostic algorithm for disorders of the thyroid gland.

2. Other laboratory tests:

1) Serum **antibodies to TSH receptor (TRAb)**: Measurement of TRAb antibodies is suggested to differentiate autoimmune causes of thyrotoxicosis (eg, Graves disease) from nonautoimmune causes.☺◯

2) Serum **antibodies to thyroperoxidase (TPO Ab)**, and **antibodies to thyroglobulin (Tg Ab)**; least specific: Measurement of TPO Ab and Tg Ab is not suggested for the workup of patients with low TSH values,⊗◯ as they do not definitely indicate etiology (may also be present in healthy individuals and patients with nonautoimmune thyroid diseases, most frequently in subacute thyroiditis) and can lead to unnecessary tests.

3) Serum Tg levels are useful only for excluding thyrotoxicosis caused by exogenous thyroid hormone excess (low levels of Tg).

3. Imaging studies: Ultrasonography of the thyroid gland is used to measure thyroid size and diagnose goiter, visualize thyroid nodules, select areas for biopsy, and monitor the position of the needle during FNB. Ultrasonography of the thyroid gland can be used in patients with suppressed TSH and palpable thyroid nodules but it is usually not helpful in the differential diagnosis of thyrotoxicosis. In **thyroid radionuclide scintigraphy** technetium scans are used to differentiate an autonomously functioning thyroid gland or nodules (hot) from subacute thyroiditis (cold); radioiodine scans are used to estimate iodine uptake when planning radioiodine treatment for hyperthyroidism. To prepare a patient for scintigraphy, discontinue all antithyroid drugs >5 days before the study. Inquire about any iodine-containing drugs, as they reduce iodine uptake by the thyroid gland. For radioiodine scans the patient should be fasting. **Radiographs of the chest or neck** are used to assess tracheal compression and/or dislocation by a large nodular goiter or to diagnose a retrosternal goiter.

Computed tomography (CT) or magnetic resonance imaging (MRI) of the neck and chest is used to assess the size of retrosternal goiter. Orbital CT or MRI is used in patients with Graves orbitopathy to diagnose involvement of extraocular muscles.

4. Cytology is used to classify thyroid nodules as malignant (thyroid cancer), suspicious, or nonmalignant in order to determine indications for surgery. For hyperfunctioning nodules observed in scintigraphy, FNB is not suggested⊗○ due to the low risk of malignancy and increased risk of indeterminate results.

Diagnostic Criteria

1. Subclinical thyrotoxicosis is diagnosed on the basis of hormone tests: low serum TSH concentrations (<0.1 mIU/L; in mild hyperthyroidism TSH levels may be in the range of 0.1-0.4 mIU/L) accompanied by normal (sometimes close to the ULN) serum concentrations of free thyroid hormones in patients in whom other causes of low serum TSH levels (eg, treatment with glucocorticoids or dopamine, first trimester of pregnancy) have been excluded and who are asymptomatic or present with minor symptoms only. If TSH levels are persistently low, differential diagnosis must be performed to determine the cause of excessive thyroid hormone levels (serum antibodies to TSH-R and thyroid radionuclide scintigraphy).

2. Overt thyrotoxicosis:

1) **Primary**: Low serum TSH concentrations (<0.05 mIU/L) and elevated (above the ULN) serum concentrations of free thyroid hormones (FT_4; FT_4 and FT_3; or rarely FT_3 alone) accompanied by typical clinical manifestations or atypical signs and symptoms (**thyrocardiac disease**: thyrotoxicosis presenting mainly with atrial fibrillation, symptomatic coronary heart disease, or heart failure; very rarely **apathetic thyrotoxicosis** in the elderly, with dominant fatigue, apathy, depression, or even confusion).

2) **Secondary**: Elevated serum FT_4 and FT_3 concentrations with normal or elevated serum TSH levels.

3. Thyrotoxic crisis (thyroid storm) should be suspected in every case of sudden deterioration in a patient with known thyrotoxicosis (serum TSH levels <0.05 mIU/L; FT_4 and FT_3 levels may not be markedly elevated). **Assess the risk of thyrotoxic crisis using the Burch-Wartofsky criteria**:

1) **Temperature**:
   a) 38°C to 38.5°C: 5 points.
   b) 38.6°C to 39°C: 10 points.
   c) 39.1°C to 39.5°C: 15 points.
   d) 39.6°C to 40°C: 20 points.
   e) 40.1°C to 40.6°C: 25 points.
   f) >40.6°C: 30 points.

2) **Central nervous system disturbance**:
   a) Absent: 0 points.
   b) Mild (agitation): 10 points.
   c) Moderate (delirium, psychosis, extreme lethargy): 20 points.
   d) Severe (seizure, coma): 30 points.

3) **Gastrointestinal-hepatic dysfunction**:
   a) Absent: 0 points.
   b) Moderate (diarrhea, abdominal pain, nausea/vomiting): 10 points.
   c) Severe (jaundice): 20 points.

4) **Cardiovascular dysfunction**:
   a) Tachycardia (beats/min):
   – <90/minute: 0 points.
   – 90 to 109/minute: 5 points.

		TSH concentration (mIU/L)				
		Very low <0.05	Slightly decreased 0.05-0.4	Normal 0.4-4.0	Slightly elevated 4.0-10.0	High >10.0
FT$_4$ concentration[a]	Very high	Primary thyrotoxicosis	Borderline	Differentiate between TSH-producing adenoma and resistance to thyroid hormones (take special care to exclude laboratory error or positive anti-T$_4$ or TRAb antibodies)		
	Slightly elevated			Probably euthyroid[b]		
	Normal	Subclinical thyrotoxicosis		Confirmed euthyroid	Subclinical hypothyroidism	
	Low	Secondary and tertiary hypothyroidism[c] (rare)		Secondary and tertiary hypothyroidism[d]	Primary hypothyroidism	

[a] FT$_4$ concentration ranges depend on the assay and its particular reference range; usually the normal FT$_4$ levels are 10-25 pmol/L (8-20 ng/L).
[b] Is the patient treated with L-T$_4$?
[c] TSH may even be normal.
[d] After exclusion of euthyroid sick syndrome, as a result of severe disease.

FT$_4$, free thyroxine; L-T$_4$, levothyroxine; TRAb, thyroid-stimulating hormone receptor antibody; TSH, thyroid-stimulating hormone.

Figure 6-6. Differential diagnosis of thyroid disorders based on serum TSH and FT$_4$ concentrations.

- 110 to 119/minute: 10 points.
- 120 to 129/minute: 15 points.
- 130 to 139/minute: 20 points.
- ≥140/minute: 25 points.

b) Congestive heart failure:
- Absent: 0 points.
- Mild (pedal edema): 5 points.
- Moderate (bibasilar rales): 10 points.
- Severe (pulmonary edema): 15 points.

c) Atrial fibrillation:
- Absent: 0 points.
- Present: 10 points.

5) A **precipitating event** in patients with untreated or inappropriately treated hyperthyroidism: acute infection, trauma, surgery, childbirth, ketoacidosis, myocardial infarction, stroke or transient ischemic attack, radioiodine treatment (rarely), or administration of iodinated contrast media:

a) Absent: 0 points.

b) Present: 10 points.

Score interpretation: <25 points, unlikely to represent thyrotoxic crisis; 25 to 44 points, suggestive of impending crisis; ≥45 points, highly suggestive of thyrotoxic crisis.

Differential Diagnosis

Thyroid function disturbances are differentiated on the basis of serum TSH and FT$_4$ levels (→Figure 6-6) and other test results (→Table 6-5). Note other causes of thyrotoxicosis: hashitoxicosis, subacute thyroiditis or postpartum thyroiditis, trophoblastic disease, TSH-secreting pituitary adenoma, iodine-induced or amiodarone-induced hyperthyroidism (→Chapter 5.6.3.3;

Table 6-4. Differential diagnosis and treatment[a] of type I and type II amiodarone-induced thyrotoxicosis

	Type I	Type II
Previous history of thyroid disease	Multinodular goiter or Graves disease (usually undiagnosed)	None
Pathomechanism	Excess iodine causing increased synthesis of thyroid hormones	Toxic effect of amiodarone (inflammation) causing damage of thyroid cells and release of thyroid hormones
Iodine uptake	>5%	<2%
Thyroid ultrasonography + Doppler	Thyroid gland frequently enlarged, nodules may be present; increased blood flow	Normal appearance of thyroid gland; decreased blood flow
TRAb	Increased in Graves disease	Negative
Pharmacologic treatment[a]	Eg, methimazole 40-60 mg/d + sodium perchlorate (<4 weeks) 200-250 mg qid (inhibits iodine accumulation in thyroid gland); consider radical treatment	For instance, prednisone 40-60 mg/d for 1-3 months, then taper off the dose over another 2 months

[a] When differential diagnosis of these types is impossible and thyroid status from before amiodarone use is unknown, combined treatment can be used: start with methimazole and sodium perchlorate; add glucocorticoids if there is no improvement.

qid, 4 times a day; TRAb, thyroid-stimulating hormone receptor antibody.

→Table 6-4), levothyroxine (L-T_4) overdose, functioning metastases of thyroid cancer, struma ovarii. In the differential diagnosis of TSH-secreting pituitary adenoma, consider conditions associated with elevated serum FT_4 levels: high T_4 syndrome and thyroid hormone resistance syndrome.

➡ TREATMENT

General Principles of Hyperthyroidism Treatment

The choice of treatment depends on the causes of thyrotoxicosis (→Table 6-6; →Chapter 5.6.4.1; →Chapter 5.6.2; →Chapter 5.6.4.3), its course, and the patient's decisions.

In subclinical thyrotoxicosis with serum TSH levels <0.1 mIU/L, treatment is unequivocally indicated in patients >65 years of age and in younger individuals with coexisting comorbidities (cardiovascular disease, osteoporosis, postmenopause) and/or symptoms of thyrotoxicosis; in the remaining cases, watchful waiting is acceptable. Treatment may sometimes be considered in mild subclinical hyperthyroidism with TSH levels 0.4 to 0.1 mIU/L in patients >65 years of age, and in younger individuals only in the case of coexisting serious heart disease or symptomatic hyperthyroidism.

Management of L-T_4–induced subclinical thyrotoxicosis depends on indications for the use of this drug. In patients with thyroid cancer on TSH suppression therapy, consider L-T_4 dose reduction. In subclinical thyrotoxicosis in a patient treated for hypothyroidism or a nontoxic goiter, reduce the dose of L-T_4 immediately.

Treatment Options

Pharmacotherapy

Pharmacotherapy can be used as the primary treatment of hyperthyroidism or as pretreatment before radical therapy (radioiodine or surgery).

1. Antithyroid drugs: **Thionamides**: The effects develop after 1 to 3 weeks of treatment (these agents inhibit synthesis of thyroid hormones but do not inhibit secretion of hormones that were synthesized earlier). Minor granulocytopenia may be a result of hyperthyroidism and is not a contraindication to the use of thionamides. If the patient has a history of agranulocytosis or liver disease, thionamides are contraindicated.

1) **Methimazole** (INN thiamazole): The drug of choice. Initially administer 20 to 40 mg/d orally (in 2 divided doses); the dose should be reduced, usually after 3 to 6 weeks (euthyroidism is achieved in up to 6 weeks). The maintenance dose is 2.5 to 10 mg/d orally and is usually administered once daily. In severe hyperthyroidism use up to 60 mg/d orally in 2 to 3 divided doses (in outpatient setting), and in impending thyrotoxic crisis, up to 120 mg/d orally or IV (in hospitalized patients). Currently methimazole is recommended instead of propylthiouracil in the second and third trimester of pregnancy due to the lower risk of adverse effects (initial dose 10-15 mg/d orally; the drug crosses the placenta, so the lowest effective doses should be used).

2) **Propylthiouracil** is a second-line drug (it should be used only in exceptional cases due to reports of serious liver injury and deaths); some authors consider it the drug of choice in the first trimester of pregnancy. It is also used in exceptional cases of patients allergic to methimazole in whom antithyroid treatment is required (in 50% of cases there is no cross-reactivity). The initial dose is 100 to 150 mg every 8 hours (in pregnant women 100 mg/d); the dose should be reduced after 4 to 8 weeks (euthyroidism is achieved after a longer time than with methimazole, in up to 10-17 weeks), and the maintenance dose is 50 to 150 mg/d. In pregnant women the dose should be reduced as soon as FT_4 approaches the ULN (eg, 10% above the ULN). When switching antithyroid medications, 100 to 150 mg of propylthiouracil is equivalent to 10 mg of methimazole.

Monitoring treatment:

1) Evaluate improvement in clinical manifestations of hyperthyroidism. A rapid improvement may indicate a need for earlier reduction of doses of the antithyroid drug.

2) Measure serum TSH and FT_4 concentrations at 3 to 6 weeks of treatment; if symptoms of thyrotoxicosis have improved and serum FT_4 levels are in the lower range or below the normal limit, reduce the dose of the antithyroid drug (serum TSH levels may still be low). Normalization of serum TSH levels indicates a need for a rapid dose reduction.

3) The subsequent follow-up studies should be performed after another 3 to 6 weeks. If hyperthyroidism was not long-standing, only TSH concentrations should be measured; in patients in whom the blockade of TSH secretion was longer, this test may not be useful and management should be guided by FT_4 levels.

No regular monitoring of white blood cell (WBC) differential counts is recommended during antithyroid treatment; however, it is necessary in patients with suspected granulocytopenia or agranulocytosis. If granulocyte counts during treatment are $1.5 \times 10^9/L$ to $1 \times 10^9/L$, more frequent follow-up is necessary and reduction of antithyroid drug dose should be considered. If granulocyte counts are $1 \times 10^9/L$ to $0.5 \times 10^9/L$, the dose of antithyroid drugs should be reduced and their discontinuation considered. If granulocyte counts are $<0.5 \times 10^9/L$, discontinuation of the antithyroid drug is mandatory (treatment with granulocyte colony-stimulating factor may be effective). Inform the patient about the possible adverse effects of treatment; if fever and sore throat appear (usually the first symptoms of agranulocytosis), the patient should discontinue the thionamide and promptly seek medical attention. Check WBC and differential counts.

Adverse effects:

1) Rare but warranting discontinuation of thionamide treatment: Agranulocytosis, aplastic anemia; acute hepatitis (propylthiouracil), obstructive jaundice (methimazole); vasculitis with antineutrophil cytoplasmic antibodies, lupus-like syndrome.

2) Not requiring immediate discontinuation of thionamides: Pruritus, rash, urticaria, sometimes very intense skin symptoms (administer antihistamines, reduce thionamide dose, or switch to another thionamide); muscle or joint pain (in case of arthritis consider discontinuation of the antithyroid drug); fever (do not use salicylates; advise the patient to seek prompt medical attention and obtain a CBC in every case of fever with sore throat; if the WBC count is normal, antithyroid treatment may be continued); taste disturbances, nausea and vomiting (reduce thionamide dose and administer the drug in divided doses); minor increases in serum aminotransferase levels (use the lowest effective dose and schedule follow-up tests; discontinue the drug if alanine aminotransferase [ALT] levels increase to $>3 \times$ ULN); transient granulocytopenia or thrombocytopenia (reduce thionamide dose and schedule follow-up studies).

2. Other drugs lowering thyroid hormone levels should not be routinely administered due to adverse effects. They should only be used for limited periods of time and in specific situations: in patients with contraindications to thionamides (eg, due to agranulocytosis); for treatment of thyrotoxic crisis (→below); in cases when rapid control of hyperthyroidism is required.

1) **Iodine (inorganic) in the form of potassium iodide** administered as Lugol solution (1 drop contains 8 mg of iodine) or saturated solution of potassium iodide (SSKI) (1 drop contains 50 mg of iodine). Potassium iodide inhibits the synthesis and secretion of thyroid hormones; it is used in treatment of thyrotoxic crisis and sometimes in the preoperative treatment of patients with Graves disease, a coexisting vascular goiter, and no thyroid nodules. It is contraindicated in iodine-induced hyperthyroidism and in patients in whom radioiodine treatment is planned (it causes reduced iodine uptake for ≥6 months). A longer use (eg, >6 weeks) of iodine for treatment of thyrotoxicosis could lead to a paradoxical increase in the synthesis and secretion of thyroid hormones.

2) **Iodinated contrast media** (organic iodine; IV iohexol and oral sodium ipodate) inhibit T_4 to T_3 conversion and the inorganic iodine they release inhibits the synthesis and secretion of thyroid hormones; they are rarely used in treatment of thyrotoxic crisis.

3) **Lithium carbonate** has questionable efficacy. It decreases the secretion of thyroid hormones by inhibiting proteolysis of Tg. Oral lithium carbonate may be used in doses of 750 to 900 mg/d in treatment of thyrotoxic crisis or sometimes in severe hyperthyroidism (particularly in patients with contraindications to thionamides), although the drug is only approved for use in psychiatric indications. Monitoring of serum drug levels is required.

4) **Sodium perchlorate or potassium perchlorate** inhibits transport of iodine to the thyroid gland and may be used in treatment of iodine-induced hyperthyroidism. It should be used for a limited period only (<4 weeks) due to adverse effects (the most serious adverse effect is bone marrow suppression) at a dose ≤1 g/d.

5) **Glucocorticoids** have questionable efficacy. They inhibit the conversion of T_4 to T_3. For instance, oral dexamethasone 8 mg/d can be used in 2 to

3 divided doses in patients in whom rapid correction of thyroid hormone levels is required (when used in combination with thionamide and inorganic iodine glucocorticoids allow for significant reduction or normalization of FT_3 levels within 24-48 hours).

3. β-Blockers: Indications include tachycardia and supraventricular arrhythmias, eyelid retraction, tremor, and hyperhidrosis. If antithyroid drugs alone are effective, β-blockers are not required. Usually oral **propranolol** is used at doses of 10 to 40 mg tid; larger doses may be used in treatment of thyrotoxic crisis. Less frequently $β_1$-selective drugs are used: atenolol, metoprolol, or bisoprolol.

Radioiodine (^{131}I) Treatment

1. Effects and risks: Radioiodine (radioactive iodine, ^{131}I) emits radiation limited to the thyroid gland. A portion of the administered ^{131}I that has not been taken up by the thyroid gland is rapidly excreted with urine. Radiation exposure of sensitive organs (bone marrow, gonads) is low.

2. Contraindications: Pregnancy and breastfeeding; confirmed or suspected thyroid malignancy in a patient with hyperthyroidism; patients unable to follow the recommended safety precautions, including contraception.

3. Safety precautions: Before starting treatment, make sure that female patients are not pregnant; because of radiation emitted by ^{131}I taken up by the thyroid gland, the patient must avoid any contact with young children and pregnant women for 1 to 2 weeks, depending on the dose given, to avoid causing their exposure to ionizing radiation. After completing the treatment, female patients should not become pregnant for 6 months (4-6 months according to the American Thyroid Association); the recommended 6-month contraception also applies to male patients treated with ^{131}I. There is no risk of permanent fertility impairment or congenital malformations in children; therefore, reproductive age is not a contraindication to radioiodine treatment. If radioiodine treatment is used in patients with active thyroid-associated orbitopathy, concomitant prophylactic glucocorticoid therapy should be used (→below).

4. Preparation for radioiodine treatment:

1) Discontinue methimazole or propylthiouracil 5 to 7 days before planned radioiodine treatment.

2) Check iodine uptake (to plan required ^{131}I activity; thyroid radiation sensitivity differs in patients with Graves disease and other types of hyperthyroidism).

3) Exclude pregnancy immediately before the administration of ^{131}I (a negative pregnancy test result).

4) Advise the patient on the requirement of overnight fasting before the administration of radioiodine (^{131}I is administered orally) and on subsequent management (including precautions and other radiation safety measures).

5. Management after radioiodine therapy: Euthyroidism is achieved within 6 weeks to 6 months after ^{131}I administration. Some patients require continued antithyroid treatment throughout this time.

6. Indications for repeated radioiodine therapy: Persistent hyperthyroidism 6 months after therapy or recurrence of hyperthyroidism. A final evaluation of treatment efficacy is performed at 1 year.

7. Monitoring of thyroid function is required for early detection and treatment of hypothyroidism (which may develop as a consequence of radioiodine therapy; the risk is lowest in Graves disease and highest in solitary autonomously functioning nodules). Measure serum TSH concentrations at 6 weeks; at 3, 6, and 12 months; and then every year. Prevention of overt hypothyroidism with early detection can avoid or decrease symptoms of Graves ophthalmopathy.

Surgical Treatment (Thyroidectomy)

1. Indications:

1) **Absolute**: Confirmed or suspected thyroid cancer in a patient with hyperthyroidism.

2) **Relative**: An alternative to radioiodine therapy (surgery is indicated in patients with large nodular goiters causing compression of adjacent structures, large nonfunctioning nodules, or retrosternal goiters).

2. Preparation for surgery:

1) **Elective surgery**: In patients with previously untreated hyperthyroidism, administer methimazole at full doses for ≥4 to 6 weeks to achieve clinical remission of thyrotoxicosis and normalization of serum free thyroid hormone concentrations. Elevated serum TSH levels are not a contraindication to surgery (they result from previous potent inhibition of pituitary function by excess thyroid hormones). In patients with vascular goiters administration of Lugol solution may facilitate surgery by reducing goiter size and vascularity: give 3 to 7 drops of Lugol solution tid for 7 to 10 days before surgery. In patients with large goiters titrate the dose up to 10 to 15 drops tid; 1 to 2 drops of SSKI tid can be given instead of Lugol solution.

2) **Urgent surgery** may require administration of high doses of iodine and glucocorticoids, as in treatment of thyrotoxic crisis (→below).

3. Extent of surgery: Near-total thyroidectomy (leaving <1 mL of thyroid parenchyma) or total thyroidectomy are recommended for patients with Graves disease who opted for surgical options.◐◕ Less extensive procedures carry a high risk of recurrence.

4. Complications following surgery: Permanent complications (lasting >12 months) are rare (they are more frequently associated with total or repeated thyroidectomy). Temporary complications, usually lasting several weeks to months, are more common and include hypoparathyroidism (→Chapter 5.5.2) and iatrogenic injury of the recurrent laryngeal nerve with resulting vocal cord paralysis (most commonly unilateral and causing hoarseness; very rarely bilateral paralysis with serious respiratory compromise, which may require emergency tracheotomy).

5. Postoperative L-T$_4$ replacement therapy should be started immediately after surgery (calculated dose 1.6 µg/kg/d). Start from a low dose of L-T$_4$, for instance, 50 µg/d, or 25 µg/d in the elderly (in the initial period of treatment patients may have increased sensitivity to thyroxine), and titrate up slowly based on TSH values.

Treatment of Thyrotoxic Crisis (Thyroid Storm)

Start treatment immediately, without waiting for confirmation by laboratory tests. Continue treatment at an intensive care unit.

1. Drugs:

1) To reduce serum thyroid hormone levels:

    a) **Methimazole** 20 to 30 mg orally qid or propylthiouracil (PTU) 200 mg orally every 4 to 6 hours (PTU for acute phase only; either drug via a nasogastric tube if needed). Both drugs may be specially prepared for rectal or IV use.

    b) Give **iodine** as soon as possible (unless thyrotoxic crisis is induced by iodine exposure but ≥1 hour after the first dose of methimazole (to avoid utilization of iodine for synthesis of new thyroid hormones): oral SSKI 800 to 1000 mg/d in 4 divided doses (4-5 drops qid) or Lugol solution (10-30 drops bid to qid). Alternatively use IV iohexol 0.6 g (2 mL) bid.

2) **β-Blockers**, for instance, IV propranolol 2 mg over 2 minutes (the dose may be repeated after a few minutes), then 2 mg every 4 hours; alternatively 40 to 80 mg orally tid to qid (this also causes minor inhibition of T$_4$ to T$_3$ conversion).

3) **Hydrocortisone** 50 to 100 mg IV qid (it has an antishock effect and inhibits T_4 to T_3 conversion).

4) **Antibiotics** if there is a suspicion of infection (continue empiric antibiotic therapy until culture and sensitivity results are available).

5) **Sedative or anticonvulsive drugs** if necessary.

2. Administer oxygen 2 L/min via a nasal tube. Increase oxygen flow if necessary.

3. Correct water-electrolyte disturbances while monitoring volume status and assess serum electrolyte levels every 12 hours.

4. Treat hyperthermia: Use noninvasive external cooling and acetaminophen (INN paracetamol) or, less preferably, nonsteroidal anti-inflammatory drugs (salicylates are contraindicated because they block binding of T_4 to its carrier protein: thyroxine-binding globulin).

5. Aggressively treat the precipitating condition, such as infection, ketoacidosis, pulmonary embolism, or other conditions.

6. Use thromboprophylaxis (→Chapter 3.19.2) if indicated, for instance, in atrial fibrillation, severe heart failure, or immobilization.

7. Plasmapheresis may be considered if there is no effect of treatment after 24 to 48 hours.

Mortality rates in thyrotoxic crisis are 30% to 50%. Therefore, efforts should be made to prevent it with early and effective therapy of thyrotoxicosis.

COMPLICATIONS

Indirect (eg, stroke in a patient with atrial fibrillation caused by hyperthyroidism) or direct and acute (thyrotoxic crisis—a life-threatening complication) or chronic (atrial fibrillation, osteoporotic fractures) consequences of the excess of thyroid hormones. The risk of persistent atrial fibrillation in hyperthyroidism is increased ~3-fold and attempts to restore normal sinus rhythm are unsuccessful until the resolution of thyrotoxicosis is achieved. Increased cardiovascular morbidity and mortality results from elevated risk of arrhythmias, thromboembolic complications associated with atrial fibrillation, and worsening of coronary heart disease or heart failure.

6.4.1. Graves Disease

DEFINITION, ETIOLOGY, PATHOGENESIS

Graves disease (GD) is an autoimmune disease in which the thyroid--stimulating hormone (TSH) receptor (TSH-R) is the autoantigen. Stimulation of this receptor in the thyroid gland by TSH-R antibodies (TRAb) results in increased secretion of thyroid hormones, development of signs and symptoms of hyperthyroidism, thyroid hypertrophy, and vascular proliferation. The activation of cellular immune-response mechanisms against the same antigen present in orbital and skin fibroblasts results in the development of clinical symptoms that are not directly related to the thyroid gland.

Thyroid-associated orbitopathy (Graves orbitopathy [GO]) is a condition associated with ocular symptoms caused by autoimmune inflammation of the soft tissues of the orbit in the course of GD, leading to a temporary or permanent damage to the eye. Patients may develop a severe form of progressive ophthalmopathy with infiltrates and edema, which is associated with particularly high risk of permanent complications.

CLINICAL FEATURES

1. Clinically overt or moderately symptomatic hyperthyroidism (→Chapter 5.6.4); in the elderly cardiac symptoms may be the only manifestation of the condition. Usually GD presents with a vascular goiter associated with a typical vascular bruit; exophthalmos may be seen (→Figure 6-7; but overt orbitopathy is not a necessary diagnostic criterion for GD). Less commonly there are signs and symptoms of autoimmune dermatitis, including pretibial myxedema (thyroid dermopathy, a pathognomonic but rare sign) and thyroid acropathy (clubbing [very rare]).

2. GO develops simultaneously with hyperthyroidism or within 24 months from its onset. It may precede other symptoms of hyperthyroidism and rarely is the only symptom of GD. In exceptional cases it may be associated with hypothyroidism. Patients with GO complain of eye pain and burning,

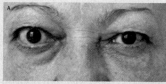
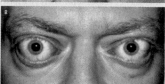

Figure 6-7. Thyroid-associated orbitopathy. **A,** mild orbitopathy (eyelid retraction, mild right eye proptosis without other symptoms affecting soft tissues). **B,** overt orbitopathy.

tearing, reduced visual acuity, sensation of grittiness, photophobia, and diplopia. The findings on clinical examination include exophthalmos, palpebral and periorbital swelling, conjunctival injection, and impaired ocular movement. The risk of sight loss is related to corneal ulcerations caused by incomplete eyelid closure and to possible optic nerve compression (with an early symptom of impaired color vision).

⮞ DIAGNOSIS

GD may manifest as overt or subclinical primary hyperthyroidism (→Chapter 5.6.4) accompanied by features of autoimmune inflammation, either clinically overt or limited to laboratory test results only.

Diagnostic Tests

1. Laboratory tests:

1) Low serum **TSH** concentrations and high (less commonly normal) serum free thyroid hormone concentrations (usually **free thyroxine [FT$_4$]** levels are sufficient for diagnosis; in patients with normal FT$_4$ levels serum **free [FT$_3$] or total triiodothyronine** concentrations should be assessed). In patients in remission the hormone test results are normal.

2) Elevated **TRAb** levels confirm the diagnosis of GD (they should be assessed before starting antithyroid therapy or within the first 3 months of treatment). Normalization of TRAb levels indicates immunologic remission of the disease.

3) Other laboratory test results are as in hyperthyroidism (→Chapter 5.6.4).

2. Imaging studies: Thyroid ultrasonography is not needed to confirm GD; however, when done, it reveals hypoechogenic thyroid parenchyma. The thyroid gland is usually enlarged. Presence of nodules does not exclude GD. **Thyroid scintigraphy** with radioactive iodine shows elevated and diffuse thyroid uptake of iodine; normal uptake of iodine in the setting of suppressed TSH values is also considered abnormal and suggestive of GD. **Computed tomography (CT) imaging of the orbits** (contrast enhancement is not necessary) in patients with active and severe ophthalmopathy allows for the evaluation of the soft tissues of the orbit, its bone walls (important for planning surgical decompression), and thickening of the extraocular muscles. **Magnetic resonance imaging (MRI) of the orbits** allows for the assessment of edema or fibrosis of the extraocular muscles.

Diagnostic Criteria for Graves Disease

The **diagnosis of GD is confirmed** in patients with:

1) Overt or subclinical hyperthyroidism and elevated TRAb levels.
2) Hyperthyroidism with concomitant thyroid-associated orbitopathy and evident involvement of the orbital soft tissues (→Figure 6-7) or with thyroid dermopathy (→Figure 6-3).
3) Hyperthyroidism with increased radioactive iodine uptake in thyroid scintigraphy if TRAb levels cannot be measured.
4) Isolated thyroid-associated orbitopathy with elevated TRAb levels.

Isolated elevation of TRAb levels is not sufficient for the diagnosis of GD (it may occur in relatives of patients with GD who do not develop the disease themselves).

Diagnostic Criteria for Graves Orbitopathy

It is important not only to recognize inflammation of the orbital soft tissues and establish the diagnosis of GO but to determine whether the severity of symptoms warrants initiating treatment (this requires a complete ophthalmologic examination and in many cases also CT imaging of the orbits).

A **classification of GO** with respect to the activity of autoimmune inflammation (according to the 2008 consensus statement of the European Group on Graves' Orbitopathy [EUGOGO]):

1) **Sight-threatening orbitopathy**: Optic neuropathy and/or corneal breakdown.
2) **Moderate to severe orbitopathy** (→Figure 6-7): Eyelid retraction ≥2 mm, moderate or severe involvement of the orbital soft tissues, exophthalmos ≥3 mm, constant or intermittent diplopia.
3) **Mild orbitopathy** (→Figure 6-7): Minor eyelid retraction <2 mm, mild involvement of the orbital soft tissues, exophthalmos <3 mm, transient or no diplopia, corneal exposure responsive to lubricants.

Evaluation of the activity of GO based on features of inflammation: Clinical Activity Score (CAS) corresponds to the total number of symptoms (symptom present, score 1; symptom absent, score 0):

1) Spontaneous retrobulbar pain.
2) Pain on attempted up or down gaze.
3) Redness of the eyelids.
4) Redness of the conjunctiva.
5) Swelling of the eyelids.
6) Inflammation of the caruncle, plica, or both.
7) Conjunctival edema.

CAS scores ≥3 on a scale of 1 to 7 indicate active orbitopathy.

Differential Diagnosis of Hyperthyroidism

Differential diagnosis of GD and other causes of thyrotoxicosis: →Figure 6-2; →Table 6-5. Elevated TRAb levels confirm an active autoimmune process in GD.

Differential Diagnosis of Graves Orbitopathy

Ocular signs and symptoms accompanying nonautoimmune hyperthyroidism (TRAb levels are the key parameter). If proptosis is unilateral, differentiate with orbital lymphoma, metastasis, or granuloma (pseudotumor of the orbit).

→ TREATMENT

There is no effective treatment for the causes of GD. Treatment focuses on controlling the symptoms of hyperthyroidism and orbitopathy (→Figure 6-8).

Treatment of Hyperthyroidism

The primary goal is to achieve euthyroidism as soon as possible, and then a joint decision should be taken with the patient to plan the subsequent treatment

Table 6-5. Differential diagnosis of autoimmune and nonautoimmune hyperthyroidism

Criteria	Graves disease	Nonautoimmune hyperthyroidism (toxic MNG, solitary autonomously functioning nodule)
History	Recurrent hyperthyroidism; family history of autoimmune thyroid disease or other autoimmune diseases	Previous nontoxic MNG
Signs and symptoms of thyrotoxicosis	No differential features	
Goiter[a]	Features of vascular goiter[b]	MNG or solitary nodule
Ocular signs and symptoms	Features of orbitopathy (immunologic inflammation), overt orbitopathy in 20%-30% of patients, severe form of progressive ophthalmopathy with infiltrates and edema in 2%-3% of patients	Ocular signs and symptoms of sympathetic hyperactivity (eg, Graefe sign) do not preclude the diagnosis
Pretibial myxedema	1%-3% of patients	None
Laboratory thyroid function tests	↓ TSH and ↑ FT$_4$ (less commonly ↑ FT$_3$), no differential features	
TRAb	95% of patients	Absent
↑ Anti-TPO[c]	70% of patients	15% of patients (elderly)
Thyroid ultrasonography	Diffuse hypoechogenicity of thyroid parenchyma[b]	Nodules
Thyroid radionuclide scintigraphy	No evident nodules, frequently slightly heterogeneous marker uptake	Autonomously functioning nodules and nonfunctioning areas

[a] Lack of goiter is not a differential feature.
[b] Nodules may be present in one-fourth of patients.

↑, increased level; ↓, decreased level; anti-TPO, anti-thyroperoxidase; FT$_3$, free triiodothyronine; FT$_4$, free thyroxine; MNG, multinodular goiter; TRAb, thyroid-stimulating hormone receptor antibody; TSH, thyroid-stimulating hormone.

strategy. If pharmacotherapy is the principal treatment modality, try to achieve and maintain immunologic remission. Normalization of TRAb levels is a good prognostic factor. Similarly, reduction of goiter size and resolution of features of a vascular goiter (due to the reduction of the stimulating effect of TRAb and resolution of lymphocytic infiltrates) are good prognostic factors as indirect signs of immunologic remission. Recurrence of hyperthyroidism is usually an indication for radical treatment with radioiodine or surgery.

Pharmacotherapy

Principles of hyperthyroidism treatment: →Chapter 5.6.4.

The optimal duration of pharmacologic treatment is 18 months and ≥12 months are necessary to achieve a durable immunologic remission. Patients can also receive long-term therapy with methimazole if GD remission has not been achieved in 18 months.

1. Regimens of antithyroid treatment in GD: Treatment with methimazole (dosage: →Chapter 5.6.4) should be continued until the patient is euthyroid (~3-6 months); the dose is usually 20 mg/d, and then it is gradually tapered

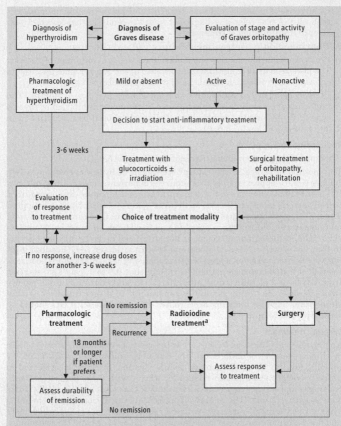

Figure 6-8. Algorithm of treatment of Graves disease.

to the maintenance dose (→above; to be continued for ~18 months or longer).
Propylthiouracil may only be used in patients with allergy to methimazole in
whom this treatment is indispensable (dosage: →Chapter 5.6.4). The time to
achieving euthyroidism is usually longer.

2. Features suggestive of the need for long-term pharmacotherapy:

1) Lack of hormonal remission: Despite antithyroid treatment levels of thyroid
   hormones do not normalize or increase again on attempts of dose reduction.
2) Lack of initial immunologic remission: Persistent TRAb levels >10 IU/L
   after 6 months of drug therapy (resolution of clinical signs and symptoms
   of hyperthyroidism does not guarantee immunologic remission).
3) Lack of durable immunologic remission: Elevated TRAb levels after 12 months
   of treatment indicate a high risk of recurrence (75%-90%) despite euthyroidism.

4) Recurrence of hyperthyroidism after achieving hormonal and immunologic remission. A true relapse is diagnosed when the remission has lasted ≥1 year after discontinuation of treatment.

3. Pharmacologic pretreatment before radical therapy:

1) Pretreatment before surgery should last 4 to 6 weeks (a minimum of 2 weeks). The preferred drug is methimazole because of the shorter time required to achieve euthyroidism; it should be discontinued after surgery.
2) Pretreatment before radioiodine therapy should last 1 to 3 months. The preferred drug is methimazole because of the lower inhibition of thyroid sensitivity to ionizing radiation (methimazole should be discontinued in due course [→Chapter 5.6.4]).

Radioiodine Therapy (^{131}I)

Principles of hyperthyroidism treatment: →Chapter 5.6.4.

The method of choice in the radical treatment of hyperthyroidism in GD: →Table 6-6. In approximately three-fourths of patients one administration of ^{131}I is sufficient, whereas in the remaining cases a repeated dose is required, usually after 6 months. Patients with large goiters causing tracheal compression and airway compromise may need to be treated in the hospital (a transient increase in thyroid volume is possible due to edema). In severe or moderate active GO, radioiodine treatment is not suggested as a therapy for GD due to the risk of worsening GO symptoms.⊗◒ In mild active GO concomitant glucocorticoid therapy is suggested to accompany ^{131}I treatment (because of the risk of transient exacerbation)⊘◯: prednisone 0.3 to 0.5 mg/kg/d starting from day 1 to 3 of radioiodine administration and continued for 1 month; then the dose should be gradually tapered off to discontinuation within ≤3 months. Because smoking exacerbates GO, patients with GO should be recommended to quit.

Surgical Treatment

An unequivocal indication for surgery is the presence of a nodule with cytologic or clinical features of malignancy (the risk of thyroid cancer in GD is 2%-7% lifelong, similar to other forms of nodular goiter). Surgery is preferred in patients with concomitant severe orbitopathy or with large goiters (>80 mL) causing compression symptoms, particularly if the goiter contains large areas with no iodine uptake. The volume of fragments of the thyroid gland remaining after surgery strongly correlates with the risk of recurrence of GD, which more and more often is a rationale for performing total or near-total thyroidectomy; however, due to a higher risk of long-term complications, this approach is not universally accepted. An unavoidable sequela of the surgery is hypothyroidism (at least subclinical), requiring hormone replacement therapy.

Treatment of Thyroid-Associated Orbitopathy

Durable effects cannot be achieved without effective treatment of hyperthyroidism. Achieving remission of hyperthyroidism alone may result in improvement or remission of GO within 2 to 3 months. Anti-inflammatory treatment with glucocorticoids should be started early when the patient is still in the active inflammatory phase. An indication may be a rapid development of symptomatic GO. Management depends on the severity of orbitopathy:

1) Sight-threatening orbitopathy: Start IV glucocorticoids immediately, consider orbital decompression surgery.
2) Moderate to severe orbitopathy: Start immunosuppressive treatment with glucocorticoids (in active disease; CAS ≥3/7) or consider surgery (if the disease is not active).
3) Mild orbitopathy: Symptoms do not affect daily activities and do not warrant immunosuppression or surgery. Use symptomatic treatment only.

Table 6-6. Methods of treatment of thyrotoxicosis

Cause of thyrotoxicosis		BB	T	131I	Op
Graves disease	First episode				
	Recurrence				
	Overt thyroid-associated orbitopathy			a	
	Severe thyroid-associated orbitopathy (progressive ophthalmopathy with infiltrates and edema)				
	Plus confirmed or suspected malignant nodule			b	
	Recurrence of Graves disease after surgery				
Toxic multinodular goiter	Small goiter without airway compression, nonmalignant				
	Large goiter, previous biopsy of nodules: nonmalignant				
	Goiter with confirmed or suspected malignant nodule			b	
Solitary autonomously functioning nodule	FNB: nonmalignant nodule or suspected follicular thyroid cancer with no evidence of clinical and ultrasound risk factors of malignancy			c	
	Confirmed thyroid cancer (very rare)			b	
Iodine-induced hyperthyroidism	Amiodarone-induced hyperthyroidism		d		
	Other cases				
Thyroiditis	Subacute				
	Silent or postpartum				
	Early Hashimoto thyroiditis				
Thyrotoxicosis in pregnancy[e]			f		
Subclinical thyrotoxicosis					g

□ No indication ■ Optional method ■ Method in use ■ Preferred method
■ Contraindicated method

[a] Oral glucocorticoids are administered to prevent exacerbation of orbitopathy.

[b] After surgical treatment of cancer radioiodine treatment is usually necessary.

[c] Radioiodine treatment is also acceptable in patients with suspected follicular thyroid cancer based on FNB results if no clinical features suggestive of malignancy are present. The risk of cancer in a true solitary autonomously functioning nodule is 2% (it should be differentiated from an isolated autonomously hyperfunctioning area in toxic MNG).

[d] Depending on type. In type I sodium perchlorate is often indicated. In type II glucocorticoids are preferred.

[e] Differentiate from thyrotoxicosis of pregnancy, which rarely requires any treatment.

[f] At markedly lower doses; in the first trimester of pregnancy propylthiouracil can be used.

[g] Only if the indications for surgery are clinical symptoms of compression or malignancy.

BB, β-blocker; FNB, fine-needle biopsy; 131I, radioiodine therapy; MNG, multinodular goiter; Op, surgery; T, thionamides (methimazole is the drug of choice).

Glucocorticoids

Glucocorticoids are the first-line drugs in moderate to severe GO and should be started after careful evaluation and confirmation of disease activity. IV pulse glucocorticoids are more effective and better tolerated than oral glucocorticoids in moderate to severe GO; thus, IV pulses of glucocorticoids are recommended as the treatment of choice.◐◐ Methylprednisolone pulses are given IV in a cumulative dose of 4.5 to 8 g (eg, 1 g every week for 6 weeks or 0.5 g twice weekly for 1-4 weeks, then 0.25-0.5 g/wk for up to 8-12 weeks); when IV glucocorticoids are contraindicated, oral prednisone is given 1 mg/kg/d for 6 to 8 weeks, then the dose is tapered off to discontinuation at 3 months.

Orbital Irradiation

An optional method. The combination of glucocorticoids and radiotherapy yields better and longer-lasting effects than either method used alone. Diabetic retinopathy is the only contraindication.

Surgical Treatment

The only method of treatment of long-term sequelae of orbitopathy after resolution of active disease. It is frequently a multistep procedure including orbital decompression, treatment of strabismus resulting from fibrosis of the extraocular muscles, and surgical procedures on the eyelids. Urgent orbital decompression surgery should be considered in patients with symptoms of optic nerve compression and when 1-week to 2-week intensive immunosuppressive treatment is ineffective.

▶ PROGNOSIS

1. Hyperthyroidism: Sometimes spontaneous remissions are observed in patients with untreated hyperthyroidism, but life-threatening complications may develop earlier (→Chapter 5.6.4). Pharmacologic treatment alleviates symptoms of thyrotoxicosis and accelerates remission but recurrence rates are ~50%. In the majority of patients TRAb levels normalize after ~6 months of treatment, but this does not guarantee a durable remission. The risk of recurrence is higher in male patients and in patients <20 years of age, as well as in patients with large goiters and high baseline FT_3 and/or FT_4 values. Hypothyroidism is always observed after surgery and is very frequent after effective radioiodine therapy; it may also develop after long-term pharmacologic treatment of GD.

2. GO: Spontaneous remissions with no long-term sequelae may be observed in untreated patients, particularly with mild orbitopathy. Nevertheless, in patients with severe active GO the risk of permanent damage to the orbital structures (disturbances of eye movements and visual impairment or even loss of vision) is high, particularly in the severe form of progressive ophthalmopathy with infiltrates and edema. If treatment is started early (in active disease), serious sequelae can often be avoided. If exophthalmos is advanced and significant involvement of the soft tissues and extraocular muscles is present, or in cases of corneal involvement or optic nerve compression, the risk of permanent damage to the eye and alteration of the patient's appearance is high. Strabismus and exophthalmos are surgically corrected after remission of active disease is achieved.

6.4.2. Toxic Multinodular Goiter

▶ DEFINITION, ETIOLOGY, PATHOGENESIS

A toxic multinodular goiter (MNG) (MNG with functional autonomy) is the end stage of the development of MNG, often caused by iodine deficiency (→Figure 6-9), in which nodules show autonomous secretion of thyroid hormones independent from thyroid-stimulating hormone (TSH) due to somatic mutations in the TSH receptor.

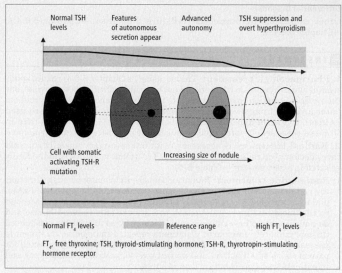

Figure 6-9. Development of an autonomously functioning thyroid nodule.

➡ CLINICAL FEATURES AND NATURAL HISTORY

Hyperthyroidism usually develops very slowly (presentation of overt disease is preceded by a subtoxic MNG with subclinical hyperthyroidism [→Chapter 5.6.4]), but it may also occur suddenly after exposure to large doses of iodine, for instance, in the contrast media or drugs (amiodarone or certain disinfectants). Enlargement of the goiter or appearance of a nodule is frequently unnoticed by the patient. If the goiter is large, a sensation of neck compression may occur with dyspnea or much less commonly with dysphagia and cough.

➡ DIAGNOSIS

Diagnostic Tests

1. Hormone tests: Significantly decreased **TSH** secretion and significant elevation of serum concentrations of free thyroxine (FT_4) and free triiodothyronine (FT_3) (or FT_3 only).

2. Imaging studies: Thyroid ultrasonography is used to measure goiter size and accurately assess the nodules. **Thyroid radionuclide imaging** is helpful in an accurate evaluation of the uptake of radioactive markers and identification of autonomously functioning nodules, which are the basis for the decision to start radioiodine therapy.

3. Cytology: For autonomously hyperfunctioning nodules observed on thyroid radionuclide imaging, fine-needle biopsy is not suggested due to the low risk of malignancy and increased risk of indeterminate results (→Chapter 5.6.4). For nonfunctioning nodules the indications for fine-needle biopsy are the same as in nontoxic MNG (→Chapter 5.6.2).

Diagnostic Criteria

A visible or palpable multinodular goiter of varying size (the key feature is the presence of >2 nodules >1 cm in diameter found on clinical examination or on ultrasonography) with concomitant hyperthyroidism.

Differential Diagnosis

Other causes of thyrotoxicosis (→Figure 6-2). Also →Chapter 5.6.4.1; →Chapter 5.6.4.3.

➡ TREATMENT

1. Pharmacologic treatment: Thionamides (→Chapter 5.6.4) reduce symptoms of hyperthyroidism (they should not be combined with levothyroxine), but their discontinuation invariably results in the recurrence of hyperthyroidism (after a period from several days to several months). **β-Blockers** are used as in other cases of hyperthyroidism, but in toxic MNG higher doses than in Graves disease are often required because of the more severe cardiac symptoms.

2. Radical treatment is necessary, with either surgery (usually subtotal thyroidectomy) or radioiodine treatment. Treatment modality is individually selected in every patient (→Table 6-6).

1) **Radioiodine treatment**: Radiation sensitivity of autonomously functioning nodules is lower than in Graves disease (this must be considered when planning radioiodine treatment). Nonfunctioning nodules do not respond to treatment and most functioning nodules are only reduced in size and do not disappear; nevertheless, remission of hyperthyroidism is achieved (in approximately one-fourth of patients repeated radioiodine treatment is necessary after 6 months). Radioiodine treatment is usually selected for patients with small goiters and no features suggestive of malignancy and in patients with contraindications to surgery.

2) **Surgical treatment** is required in patients with nodules revealing cytologic or clinical features suggestive of malignancy. It should also be considered in patients with large goiters causing compression symptoms, particularly if nonfunctioning nodules are present.

➡ PROGNOSIS

Untreated toxic MNG increases the risk of arrhythmias, other cardiovascular complications, and thyrotoxic crisis (→Chapter 5.6.4). The risk of malignancy is the same as in other forms of nodular goiter.

6.4.3. Toxic Thyroid Nodule

➡ DEFINITION, ETIOLOGY, PATHOGENESIS

A toxic thyroid nodule is an adenoma (toxic adenoma) or hyperplastic nodule observed on radionuclide scintigraphy that usually (but not always) causes hyperthyroidism. It develops most commonly as a result of a somatic mutation of the thyrotropin-stimulating hormone receptor or stimulatory G protein α subunit (Gs α). Unlike multinodular goiter, it is not related to iodine deficiency.

➡ CLINICAL FEATURES

Symptoms of hyperthyroidism are similar to those caused by toxic multinodular goiter, and the typical pattern of development is from a compensated autonomously functioning nodule to overt hyperthyroidism: →Figure 6-9.

➡ DIAGNOSIS

Diagnosis is based on radionuclide thyroid scintigraphy. Clinical examination and ultrasonography reveal a solitary nodule. TSH secretion can be decreased (but still within normal limits) or suppressed (subclinical or overt hyperthyroidism [→Chapter 5.6.4]).

→ TREATMENT

The treatment of choice is radioiodine therapy (→Table 6-6). Due to low serum TSH levels, iodine uptake of the thyroid parenchyma is inhibited (therefore, the risk of developing posttreatment hypothyroidism is low). Radioiodine therapy should be started after discontinuation of thionamides and when serum TSH levels are <0.1 mIU/L. In patients with indications for fine-needle biopsy (→Chapter 5.6.2), the biopsy should not be performed within 1 to 2 weeks before radioiodine therapy, as it may cause transient inhibition of iodine uptake by the nodule. Serum TSH levels should be monitored and follow-up ultrasonography performed to evaluate the size of the nodule every 6 to 12 months. In some centers ethanol injections into the nodule are used with satisfactory outcomes.

→ PROGNOSIS

The 6-year risk of developing overt hyperthyroidism in patients with a compensated or subtoxic nodule (ie, with subclinical thyrotoxicosis) is 2% to 5%. With appropriately conducted radioiodine therapy a complete resolution of hyperthyroidism may be achieved. The risk of malignancy is ~2%.

1. Gastrointestinal Diseases

1.1. Esophageal Diseases

1.1.1. Eosinophilic Esophagitis

▶ **DEFINITION, ETIOLOGY, PATHOGENESIS**

Eosinophilic esophagitis (EoE) is a chronic immune-mediated esophageal disease affecting up to 1 in 2000 people in Europe and North America and, nowadays, the second most common esophageal disease, after gastroesophageal reflux disease (GERD). It occurs in all age groups but is more prevalent in white males from childhood to midlife. Clinically, EoE is characterized by symptoms of esophageal dysfunction and histologically, by eosinophil-predominant esophageal inflammation. EoE is distinct from other systemic and local causes of esophageal eosinophilia and from GERD, although EoE and GERD may coexist.

In many patients EoE is associated with concomitant atopic diseases, such as asthma, allergic rhinitis, and atopic dermatitis. In EoE food and environmental antigens stimulate a Th2 inflammatory response, which leads to the production of eotaxin-3, a potent chemokine that recruits eosinophils to the esophageal mucosa. Activated eosinophils secrete proinflammatory and profibrotic mediators, causing tissue damage and with time also fibrosis and remodeling that may ultimately progress to esophageal dysmotility and stricture.

Although EoE is considered to be an immune-mediated disease, the underlying pathogenetic mechanisms remain unclear. Whilst the therapeutic response to glucocorticoids and elimination diets in many patients is consistent with EoE being an immune-mediated disease, the improvement produced by proton pump inhibitors (PPIs) suggests that there may be other, non–immune-mediated mechanisms at play in some patients who have esophageal eosinophilia. When PPI-responsive esophageal eosinophilia (PPI-REE) was first reported, it was thought to be different from EoE. Now it appears that this condition is comparable to EoE and distinct from GERD with respect to clinical, pathologic, and genetic features of EoE. As a result, PPI-REE is no longer considered to be a separate diagnostic entity, distinct from EoE.

▶ **CLINICAL FEATURES**

There are no specific symptoms diagnostic of EoE. In young children, the most common symptoms are vomiting, abdominal pain, feeding difficulties, refusal of food, and failure to thrive. In older children and adults, dysphagia, food impaction, GERD-like symptoms, and chest pain predominate; in this age group, EoE is now the most common cause of dysphagia and food bolus impaction. Assessment of symptom severity is hampered by patients' attempts to minimize symptoms by avoiding foods that are difficult to swallow, chewing their food for prolonged periods, and drinking more fluids when eating.

▶ **DIAGNOSIS**

Diagnostic Tests

In patients with clinical features consistent with EoE, diagnosis is based on upper endoscopy and esophageal biopsies confirming esophageal eosinophilia. Currently, there are no noninvasive tests that are sufficiently accurate to diagnose EoE or evaluate response to therapy. Absolute serum eosinophil counts correlate with the degree of esophageal eosinophilia at baseline and after glucocorticoid therapy but their diagnostic accuracy is insufficient for use in clinical practice. Similarly, other biomarkers associated with EoE pathogenesis have proved inadequate, alone or in combination, for diagnosis or disease monitoring.

1. Endoscopy: The 5 key endoscopic features of EoE are highlighted in the endoscopic reference score, a standardized tool which uses the acronym EREFS to grade the severity of **e**xudates (whitish plaques), **r**ings (trachealization), **e**dema (loss of vascular pattern), **f**urrows (longitudinal markings), and **s**trictures. However, these features have only modest accuracy for the diagnosis of EoE and the esophageal mucosa may be normal in ~10% of adult patients. A diagnosis of EoE must therefore be confirmed by histology; because inflammation is variable, ≥6 biopsies should be taken from 2 different sites in the esophagus and, in particular, from areas that are endoscopically abnormal. Gastric and duodenal biopsies should also be taken at the initial diagnostic endoscopy to exclude eosinophilic gastroenteritis and other conditions.

2. Histology: Histologic assessment, using hematoxylin-eosin (HE) staining, identifies typical EoE features including eosinophils in the epithelium and other layers of the esophageal wall, eosinophilic clusters (microabscesses), dilated intercellular spaces, basal cell hyperplasia, expansion of the papillae, and fibrosis of the lamina propria. However, apart from esophageal eosinophilia and microabscesses, the other histologic features are not specific for EoE; furthermore, low-grade esophageal eosinophilia also occurs in GERD (usually <5 eosinophils per high power field [HPF]). The histologic diagnostic criterion is the finding of >15 eosinophils per HPF (~60 eosinophils/mm^2), which has a sensitivity of 100% and a specificity of 96% for the diagnosis of EoE.

3. Contrast radiography: Barium esophagography may occasionally be helpful to evaluate dysphagia, because EoE strictures, when present, tend to be longer and more tapered than the localized distal strictures associated with GERD (as such, they can be missed at endoscopy).

4. Allergy testing: Skin prick tests to evaluate mast cell–bound IgE in the context of immediate allergic reactions and atopy patch tests to evaluate non-IgE cell-mediated reactions to potential food triggers of EoE have shown consistently low utility in adults and variable utility in children, with a poor positive predictive value (on average <50%) and only moderate to good negative predictive value (40%-90%). Elimination diets based on skin allergy testing lead to histologic remission in less than a third of adult EoE patients. Skin allergy tests are therefore not sufficiently accurate for use in clinical practice to determine food elimination or reintroduction strategies for EoE patients.

Diagnostic Criteria

The most recent consensus publication states that a diagnosis of EoE requires all 3 of:

1) Symptoms of esophageal dysfunction.
2) Esophageal biopsy findings of >15 eosinophils per HPF (~60 eosinophils/mm^2).
3) Exclusion of non-EoE disorders associated with esophageal eosinophilia (causes of esophageal eosinophilia other than EoE and GERD; →below).

The efficacy of PPIs in reducing esophageal eosinophilia and EoE symptoms, limited correlation between esophageal acid exposure and PPI response, clinical and pathophysiologic similarities between PPI-responders and nonresponders, and coexistence of EoE and GERD as distinct conditions in the same patient have all recently led to the consensus recommendation that a trial of PPI therapy is no longer required to fulfill the diagnosis of EoE and recognition that a diagnosis of EoE cannot be excluded definitively in patients by normal biopsy results if they are taking PPIs at their initial endoscopy.

Differential Diagnosis

There are many diagnoses that should be considered in a patient with features of EoE, the most common being GERD. There are several epidemiologic and clinicopathologic features that differ between EoE and GERD (→Table 1-1), but

Table 1-1. Features differentiating EoE and GERD

Characteristic features	EoE	GERD
Coexisting atopic diseases	Common	As in general population
Food hypersensitivity	Common	As in general population
Sex	M > F	M = F
Dysphagia (particularly with allergenic foods)	Common	Uncommon
pH-metry	Normal in most	Abnormal
Endoscopy	Frequent lesions, characteristic appearance	Normal in 40%-60%
Histology		
Distal esophagus	Lesions present	Lesions present
Proximal esophagus	Lesions present	Normal findings
Epithelial hyperplasia	Significant	Mild
Mucosal eosinophilia	>15 per HPF	0-7 per HPF
Treatment		
H$_2$ blockers	Useful in some	Useful in some
PPIs	Useful in some	Useful
Glucocorticoids	Useful	No effect
Elimination diet	Useful	No effect

EoE, eosinophilic esophagitis; F, female; GERD, gastroesophageal reflux disease; HPF, high-power field; M, male; PPI, proton pump inhibitor.

currently there is no single test that can reliably distinguish between these two conditions. A definitive diagnosis may be difficult, as EoE and GERD may occur concurrently in the same patient.

The differential diagnosis for EoE includes other causes of symptoms, such as dysphagia and chest pain, and other causes of esophageal eosinophilia (→Table 1-2).

→ TREATMENT

The mainstays of treatment are elimination diets, PPIs, or topical glucocorticoids (→Table 1-3). In general, the choice of therapy is guided by the nature and severity of symptoms, comparative evaluation of the potential harms and benefits of each therapy, and patient preferences, with PPIs recommended as early or initial treatment by recent practice guidelines. There are limited data comparing these different therapies individually,⊜ and there are no data on the use of 2 or more treatments in combination, either for those who have not responded to initial therapy or those who have concurrent GERD and EoE.

The goals of therapy are alleviation of symptoms and histologic remission (<15 eosinophils/HPF) in the short term, maintenance of remission and prevention of recurrent food bolus impaction in the medium and long term, and prevention of progressive fibrosis and strictures in the very long term.

Table 1-2. Conditions associated with esophageal eosinophilia (other than EoE or GERD)

Associated conditions	Comment
Eosinophilic gastritis, gastroenteritis, or colitis	With esophageal involvement
Crohn disease	With esophageal involvement
Esophageal motor disorders	– Achalasia of cardia – Esophagogastric outlet obstruction – Esophageal body dysmotility
Infections	Viral, fungal, bacterial
Medications	– Drug hypersensitivity reactions – Pill esophagitis
Autoimmune disorders	– Connective tissue disorders – Vasculitides
Dermatologic conditions	– With esophageal involvement – Pemphigus vulgaris
Graft-versus-host disease	
Mendelian disorders	– Marfan syndrome type II – Hyper-IgE syndrome – PTEN hamartoma tumor syndrome – Netherton syndrome – Severe atopy metabolic wasting syndrome
HES	– Primary (neoplastic) HES – Secondary (reactive) HES – Idiopathic HES
Hypermobility syndromes	Ehlers-Danlos syndrome

EoE, eosinophilic esophagitis; GERD, gastroesophageal reflux disease; HES, hypereosinophilic syndrome; PTEN, phosphatase and tensin homolog.

Regardless of treatment, it is recommended that the effect of any therapeutic change should be evaluated by endoscopy and biopsy (usually after 6-12 weeks of treatment), because of the poor correlation between symptoms and histologic features. However, it should be recognized that this may be considered a significant burden by the patient and the payer.

Nutritional Management

Dietary therapy to prevent exposure to foods that trigger the immune response and inflammation is a common initial approach, particularly in children. Adults are usually less motivated to follow a precise, very restricted diet, which may have a substantial detrimental effect on the patient's social life, nutritional status, financial commitments, and quality of life. Prolonged avoidance of food triggers may lead to sustained drug-free remission, but symptoms and inflammation commonly recur after diet discontinuation.

Elimination diets:

1) Hypoallergenic elimination diets involve the elimination of up to 6 most frequent sources of food allergens: milk, egg, fish/shellfish, nuts/peanuts, soy, and wheat (→Table 1-3). An empiric six-food elimination diet (SFED)

Table 1-3. Medical treatment for eosinophilic esophagitis

Treatment	Comments
Acid suppression	
PPI: – Dexlansoprazole – Esomeprazole – Lansoprazole – Omeprazole – Pantoprazole – Rabeprazole	Standard-dose PPI: – Once daily or bid – 8-12 weeks
Glucocorticoids (topical)	
Fluticasone propionate: – Metered-dose inhaler – Spray (swallowed)	Infants: 44 µg inhaler 2 puffs bid Children: 110 µg inhaler 2 puffs bid Adults: 220 µg inhaler 2 puffs bid
Budesonide: – Nebulizer solution – Swallowed as solution or in viscous sucralose slurry	Children: 0.25-0.5 mg bid Adults: 1-2 mg bid
Dietary therapy	
Elemental diet	– Amino acid–based formula (antigen-free) – Oral intake: Poor adherence due to taste
6-food elimination diet	– Eliminate eggs, milk, nuts, seafood, soy, and wheat for 6 weeks – If effective, reintroduce food groups individually every 6-8 weeks; repeat endoscopy and biopsy to evaluate response
4-food elimination diet	– Eliminate eggs, milk, soy, and wheat for 6 weeks – If effective, reintroduce food groups individually every 6-8 weeks; repeat endoscopy and biopsy to evaluate response
2-food elimination diet	– Eliminate milk and wheat for 6 weeks – If effective, reintroduce food groups individually every 6-8 weeks; repeat endoscopy and biopsy to evaluate response

bid, 2 times a day; PPI, proton pump inhibitor.

leads to histologic remission in about three-quarters of patients; stepwise food reintroduction may then identify the specific food triggers. Four-food (FFED) and two-food (TFED) elimination diets lead to histologic remission in about a half and one-third of EoE patients, respectively, but they are also less restrictive.

2) The targeted elimination diet is individually tailored to the patient on the basis of history, results of skin prick tests, and elimination and provocation tests. It leads to histologic remission in less than one-third of adult EoE patients.

3) The elemental diet is a particular type of commercial diet. Although it is well balanced and free of allergens, some patients cannot tolerate its taste. After 4 to 6 weeks of following the diet and achieving remission, individual foods are reintroduced one by one. The elemental diet is recommended only in case other elimination diets and pharmacotherapy have failed. In adults, the elemental diet should usually be supplemented with pharmacologic treatment.

Pharmacotherapy

1. PPIs: Currently there is limited information suggesting that PPIs (mostly esomeprazole) are comparable in efficacy to topical glucocorticoids.☉ However, there is a large body of observational evidence that PPIs relieve symptoms and reduce esophageal eosinophilia in EoE and this—along with the low cost, convenience, and good safety profile of PPIs—supports their use for initial treatment.

A standard-dose PPI, taken bid for 8 weeks, results in clinical remission in 60% of patients and histologic remission in 50% of patients. Maintenance treatment used for ≥1 year extends remission in 75% of patients who responded to treatment. In case of recurrence, in some patients the dose of the PPI may be increased.

2. Topical glucocorticoids: No agents are specifically designed for use in patients with EoE. Oral administration of inhaled glucocorticoid formulations is used: budesonide (2-4 mg/d, usually in divided doses; oral solution is prepared using nebulization suspension [0.5 mg/mL] mixed with sucralose 5 mg to increase viscosity) or fluticasone (880-1760 µg bid via metered-dose inhaler; instruct the patient to activate the inhaler while holding their breath to deposit the drug in the mouth, and then to swallow the medication, which minimizes the amount of the drug delivered to the lungs). After administering these agents, the patient should not eat or drink for 30 to 60 minutes. Esophageal candidiasis is a possible adverse effect. Systemic glucocorticoids should not be used, as they are no more effective than topical therapy but are associated with more adverse events.

3. Nonglucocorticoid immunosuppressive drugs: There are case reports that azathioprine and 6-mercaptopurine may induce and maintain remission in a few patients but other medications, including disodium cromoglicate, antihistamines, montelukast, anti-interleukin (IL)-5 antibody, anti-IL-13 antibody, anti–tumor necrosis factor (TNF) antibody, and anti-IgE antibody, have all been ineffective.

Endoscopic Treatment

EoE patients who have an esophageal stricture that affects swallowing and do not respond to medical therapy should be offered endoscopic esophageal dilation. This is a generally safe procedure with a risk of perforation <1% and a mean duration of response typically >1 year.

→ PROGNOSIS

EoE is a chronic disease that usually responds to therapy in the short term, but if treatment is stopped, most patients experience recurrent symptoms leading to reduced quality of life and possibly esophageal strictures. Long-term maintenance therapy seems appropriate for those with persistent symptoms, although there are very scarce data on long-term outcomes in EoE patients in the presence or absence of long-term therapy.

1.1.2. Esophageal Motility Disorders

→ CLASSIFICATION

Classification of esophageal motility disorders:

1) **Primary**: Achalasia; major disorders of esophageal peristalsis including distal esophageal spasm (formerly diffuse esophageal spasm) and hypercontractile (jackhammer) esophagus (previously nutcracker esophagus); other nonspecific abnormal motility patterns.

2) **Secondary**: In the course of scleroderma, diabetes mellitus, alcohol abuse, psychiatric disorders, Chagas disease, and associated with aging.

1.1.2.1. Achalasia

→ DEFINITION, ETIOLOGY, PATHOGENESIS

Achalasia is the most common (>70% of cases) primary esophageal motility disorder of unclear etiology characterized by impairment of lower esophageal sphincter (LES) relaxation and lack of a primary peristaltic wave in the esophageal body. An increase in resting LES pressure may also be present. Impairment of LES relaxation is probably caused by damage to and decrease in the number of postganglionic inhibitory neurons of the esophageal myenteric plexus (Auerbach plexus), which are responsible for relaxation of the LES. As the disease progresses, an esophageal stricture develops, which in turn leads to dilation of the esophageal lumen and marked thinning of the esophageal wall above the hypertrophic LES.

→ CLINICAL FEATURES AND NATURAL HISTORY

The most typical feature is dysphagia, which is initially limited to solid foods and later includes liquids. It may be accompanied by regurgitation, chest pain, heartburn, chronic cough, and aspiration. Dysphagia leads to weight loss and malnutrition, while regurgitation may cause aspiration pneumonia and lung abscess. Other complications include esophagitis, development of diverticula of distal parts of the esophagus, and bleeding (rare). After 15 to 25 years the risk of developing squamous cell carcinoma of the esophagus is ~30 times higher than in the general population.

→ DIAGNOSIS

Diagnostic Tests

1. Barium esophagography reveals a beak-like appearance of the distal esophagus with smooth outlines of the walls that sharply taper downwards to the closed LES.

2. Endoscopy is necessary to exclude other causes of the stricture, particularly esophageal cancer, which may have similar symptoms (eg, dysphagia and weight loss). It also helps to exclude hiatal hernia, which may present as dysphagia but requires different treatment. In advanced achalasia the esophagus is atonic, dilated, and tortuous, and its mucosa is damaged due to chronic irritation by residual food (erythema, fragility, ulcerations, candidiasis). The LES keeps closed and does not open with insufflation of air into the distal esophagus, although passage of the endoscope to the stomach is possible with slight resistance. Marked resistance to passage of the endoscope and stiffening of the cardia suggest other causes (postinflammatory stricture, cancer).

3. Esophageal manometry reveals impaired LES relaxation with elevated LES integrated relaxation pressure and 100% failed peristalsis (absence of peristalsis; no contractions) or spastic contractions in the esophageal body. The LES may show normal or increased resting pressure.

Diagnostic Criteria

Diagnosis is based on barium esophagography and endoscopy. Esophageal manometry is performed to confirm diagnosis. Increased resting pressure of the LES is not a prerequisite for diagnosis.

Differential Diagnosis

Other causes of dysphagia. History and endoscopy are the basis of differential diagnosis.

→ TREATMENT

General Measures

1. Avoidance of foods that are difficult to swallow; in some patients soft (blended, minced, or pureed) foods may be recommended. Hot water (50°C) may help to relax the LES.

2. Lifestyle modifications such as elevated bedhead to prevent aspiration with food retained in the esophagus.

Pharmacotherapy

Drugs relaxing the smooth muscle of the LES and esophageal body supplement surgical or endoscopic treatment. **Isosorbide dinitrate** 5 to 20 mg or **nifedipine** 10 to 30 mg administered sublingually 10 to 30 minutes before a meal (duration of action, ~1.5 hours) are used. The benefit is not durable.

Endoscopic Treatment

1. Pneumatic balloon dilation of the LES weakens the LES by circumferential stretching or tearing of its muscle fibers. It should be performed by an experienced endoscopist. The efficacy may last 12 to 24 months and retreatment is required for symptom recurrence in >50% of patients over a 5-year period. Complications include esophageal perforation, upper gastrointestinal bleeding, reflux esophagitis, intramural hematomas, esophageal mucosal tears, aspiration pneumonia, and diverticula at the gastric cardia. Postprocedural fever and postprocedural chest pain can be self-limiting.

2. Intrasphincteric injection of botulinum toxin during endoscopy paralyses the LES by poisoning the excitatory (acetylcholine-releasing) neurons that increase the LES smooth muscle tone, thereby reducing LES resting pressure.

3. Peroral endoscopic myotomy (POEM) is a longitudinal cut of the esophageal muscle with a special knife inserted through the gastroscope. The procedure is performed under general anesthesia with endotracheal intubation. Myotomy is performed inside the esophagus with subsequent closure of the esophageal mucosa. Leakage of air and esophageal fluid may complicate the procedure.

Surgical Treatment

Cardiomyotomy (Heller myotomy) has been the primary alternative to pneumatic dilation for achalasia. It is a longitudinal incision of the muscle fibers of the LES and cardia. Heller myotomy is usually performed laparoscopically and is frequently combined with partial fundoplication to reduce the risk of symptomatic gastroesophageal reflux. The advantages of surgical myotomy are high initial success rates and, compared with pneumatic dilation, lower rates of symptom recurrence. Indications include stricture of the cardia that blocks passage of the endoscope to the stomach and age <30 years; the procedure is also indicated in situations when multiple sessions of esophageal dilation will probably be necessary. The main complication is gastroesophageal reflux. In certain cases (eg, severe esophageal dilation) esophageal resection may be indicated.

→ PROGNOSIS

The majority of patients require multiple endoscopic procedures (dilation, injection of botulinum toxin) or myotomy (endoscopic or surgical), which are often only partially effective. Even after successful treatment the risk of developing esophageal cancer is probably increased, which is why some authors advise periodic endoscopic follow-up.

1.1.2.2. Major Disorders of Esophageal Peristalsis: Distal Esophageal Spasm, Hypercontractile (Jackhammer) Esophagus

→ ETIOLOGY AND CLINICAL FEATURES

The etiology of distal esophageal spasm (DES) and hypercontractile (jackhammer) esophagus is unknown. They may occur at any age but usually develop in patients aged >40 years.

Clinical manifestations include noncardiac chest pain, usually retrosternal, and dysphagia to solid foods and liquids in the majority of patients. The pain may occur immediately after a meal but sometimes is independent of food intake. Dysphagia may be severe and may lead to malnutrition.

➔ DIAGNOSIS

Diagnosis is based on high-resolution esophageal manometry after other esophageal disorders have been excluded on the basis of upper gastrointestinal endoscopy with biopsy or barium esophagram. DES is characterized by increased simultaneous or premature contractions in the distal esophagus. Hypercontractile esophagus is characterized by high pressure but normally sequential contractions in the smooth muscles of the esophagus.

➔ TREATMENT

The most effective treatment of DES and jackhammer esophagus in not well defined. Pharmacologic treatment includes calcium channel blockers (nifedipine and diltiazem) or nitrates (nitroglycerin, isosorbide dinitrate) if patients have no gastroesophageal reflux disease or if it is well controlled. Many patients require antisecretory therapy with proton pump inhibitors. The advantages of surgical over medical treatment have not been proven.

1.1.3. Gastroesophageal Reflux Disease (GERD)

➔ DEFINITION, ETIOLOGY, PATHOGENESIS

Gastroesophageal reflux disease (GERD) is defined as the occurrence of troublesome symptoms or complications caused by the reflux of gastric contents, including acid and pepsin, into the esophagus. It is an increasingly common gastrointestinal (GI) disorder with a prevalence of 10% to 20% in the Western world. The incidence and prevalence of GERD appear to be rising. The reason for this is unclear, but it may be associated with obesity and diet.

The pathogenesis of GERD is multifactorial and one or more causative factors, alone or in combination, may lead to reflux-related symptoms or injury. However, it is important to recognize that gastroesophageal reflux is a normal occurrence and that disease (GERD) occurs only if there are adverse consequences. Factors associated with the development of GERD may be categorized according to the underlying mechanisms:

1) **Greater reflux into the esophagus**:
   a) Impaired antireflux mechanisms: Inappropriate transient lower esophageal relaxations (TLESRs), hypotensive lower esophageal sphincter (LES), hiatus hernia, supine position, medication (ethanol, oral contraceptives, nitrates, calcium channel blockers, β-blockers, anticholinergics).
   b) Increased intragastric pressure: Obesity, pregnancy.
   c) Increased gastric contents: Impaired gastric emptying (idiopathic gastroparesis, diabetic gastroparesis); large calorically dense meals.
2) **Greater toxicity of reflux**:
   a) Greater acidity (Zollinger-Ellison syndrome).
   b) Increased bile acids and pancreatic secretions (duodenogastric reflux).
3) **Decreased clearance of reflux from the esophagus**:
   a) Hiatus hernia.
   b) Failed peristalsis (scleroderma, esophageal dysmotility, chronic graft--versus-host disease).
4) **Greater sensitivity of the esophagus to reflux**:
   a) Esophageal epithelial hypersensitivity.
   b) Central mechanisms (hyperalgesia, stress).

5) **Decreased neutralization of reflux**:

a) Sjögren syndrome.

b) Salivary gland dysfunction (radiotherapy).

GERD-like symptoms or injury may also be related to other nonreflux mechanisms, including ingested irritants (antibiotics, potassium supplements, bisphosphonates, caustic agents and lyes, alcoholic spirits, acidic or spicy foods and drinks), inflammation (eosinophilic esophagitis), or functional heartburn.

Classification

GERD may be further subclassified into esophageal and extraesophageal syndromes.

1. Esophageal syndromes:

1) Symptomatic syndromes:

a) Typical reflux syndrome: 40% to 60% of symptomatic patients have nonerosive reflux disease (NERD) with no mucosal injury.

b) Reflux chest pain syndrome.

2) Syndromes with esophageal injury:

a) Reflux esophagitis: Distal esophageal injury ("mucosal breaks," encompassing erosions and ulcers) on endoscopy in patients who may or may not have typical GERD symptoms.

b) Reflux stricture.

c) Barrett esophagus.

d) Esophageal adenocarcinoma.

2. Extraesophageal syndromes:

1) Established associations (symptoms associated with GERD in some patients, although GERD is usually one of several etiologic factors and reflux therapy is usually effective only in patients who have typical reflux symptoms):

a) Reflux cough syndrome.

b) Reflux laryngitis syndrome.

c) Reflux asthma syndrome.

d) Reflux dental erosion syndrome.

2) Proposed associations (symptoms occurring concurrently with GERD; there is no high-quality evidence to support a causal relationship between reflux and the reported extraesophageal symptoms):

a) Pharyngitis.

b) Sinusitis.

c) Idiopathic pulmonary fibrosis.

d) Recurrent otitis media.

> ### → CLINICAL FEATURES AND NATURAL HISTORY

Typical symptoms: Heartburn (a retrosternal burning sensation), regurgitation, and water brash (hypersalivation) are the cardinal symptoms of GERD. They may be worsened in a supine position, on bending, and while straining (especially after a large or fatty meal) and may be temporarily relieved by antacids.

Atypical symptoms: Nausea, eructation (belching), slow digestion, early satiety, epigastric pain, bloating, vomiting, and chest pain are the atypical esophageal or upper GI symptoms attributed most commonly to GERD. Extraesophageal symptoms including dry cough, wheeze, chronic rhinosinusitis, hoarseness, pharyngeal pain, and globus, as well as early awakening, nocturnal awakening, and nightmares.

Alarming symptoms: Dysphagia (difficulty swallowing), odynophagia (pain on swallowing), unintentional weight loss, anemia, and suspected upper GI bleeding (overt or occult) warrant prompt investigation, usually beginning with urgent endoscopy.

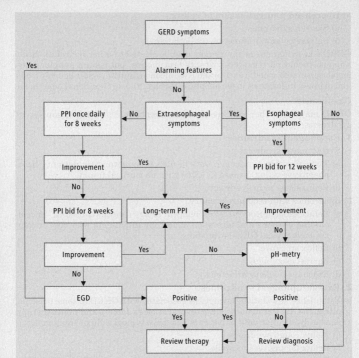

bid, 2 times a day; EGD, esophagogastroduodenoscopy; GERD, gastroesophageal reflux disease;
PPI, proton pump inhibitor.

Figure 1-1. Initial diagnostic management algorithm for gastroesophageal reflux disease.

GERD syndromes with esophageal injury may be asymptomatic and discovered incidentally on endoscopy performed for indications other than typical GERD symptoms. The course of GERD is associated with exacerbations and remissions. In most patients exacerbations do not lead to significant adverse outcomes. Untreated severe GERD may lead to bleeding, strictures, Barrett esophagus and, rarely, esophageal adenocarcinoma.

→ **DIAGNOSIS**

Diagnostic Criteria

The presence of typical GERD symptoms ≥2 times a week and the absence of alarming features is suggestive of GERD and warrants an empiric trial of a proton pump inhibitor (PPI) once daily for 8 weeks. If symptoms persist, the dosage may be increased to bid for another 8 weeks without further investigation.

Diagnostic algorithm for suspected GERD: →Figure 1-1.

Alarming Features

Features suggestive of complicated GERD (syndromes with esophageal injury; →Classification, above) or GI malignancy include the recent onset of symptoms in a patient >60 years, iron deficiency anemia or evidence of GI bleeding, anorexia, unintended weight loss, dysphagia, odynophagia, recurrent unexplained vomiting, or a family history of GI tract malignancy.

Differential Diagnosis

Symptoms consistent with GERD may be caused by other types of esophagitis (fungal, viral, drug-induced, eosinophilic esophagitis), diseases of the stomach and duodenum (*Helicobacter pylori*, peptic ulcer disease), esophageal motility disorders (achalasia of the cardia, distal esophageal spasm), esophageal cancer, ischemic heart disease, and functional heartburn.

Diagnostic Tests

1. Endoscopy is the initial investigation for patients who have alarming features and those who have persistent symptoms despite appropriate escalated therapy with a PPI to assess for the presence and severity of erosive esophagitis (Los Angeles grade A and B, mild; Los Angeles grade C and D, severe), hiatus hernia, and Barrett esophagus, as well as other potential causes of persistent or atypical symptoms. Esophageal biopsy is not required to confirm GERD in the presence of erosive esophagitis but is indicated for suspected Barrett esophagus, eosinophilic esophagitis, malignancy, or other diagnoses. Repeat endoscopy is appropriate to confirm healing in severe esophagitis, to evaluate and (if needed) dilate strictures, and to monitor for progression of Barrett esophagus. Endoscopic follow-up is not needed for NERD or mild erosive esophagitis.

2. Ambulatory 24-hour esophageal pH monitoring (esophageal pH-metry) measures esophageal luminal acidity 5 cm above the gastroesophageal junction to determine whether there is excessive esophageal exposure to acid and a temporal relationship between the patient's symptoms and the occurrence of an acid reflux episode. Concurrent esophageal impedance monitoring allows for the additional detection of weakly acid or nonacid reflux episodes that might cause symptoms despite PPI therapy sufficient to reduce esophageal acid exposure to normal levels. While esophageal pH-impedance monitoring is the gold standard for detecting and quantifying reflux, it has only moderate sensitivity and specificity for the diagnosis of GERD and should generally be reserved for patients who had an unsatisfactory response to adequate PPI therapy. Esophageal reflux monitoring may be performed after the patient has stopped PPI therapy for ≥1 week if the goal is to determine whether there is abnormal reflux; alternatively, it may be performed while the patient continues PPI therapy to determine whether adequate acid suppression has been achieved.

3. High-resolution esophageal manometry measures esophageal contraction pressures at multiple points along the esophagus to assess the function of the upper esophageal sphincter (UES), esophageal body, and LES. It cannot be used directly to make a diagnosis of GERD but is often performed to allow accurate placement of the pH electrode for esophageal pH-metry. Additionally, it can identify risk factors for GERD, including hiatus hernia, impaired LES function, and impaired esophageal motility, as well as achalasia of the cardia, which can induce GERD-like symptoms by impairing clearance of esophageal contents.

4. Barium swallow radiography has limited usefulness and should not be performed routinely to diagnose GERD. In rare circumstances, in patients with concurrent dysphagia it may reveal a hiatus hernia or GERD complications, such as esophageal stricture or features of achalasia, which can mimic GERD symptoms.

→ TREATMENT

Symptoms of GERD differ in severity and frequency between patients and result in varying intensity of treatment. Generally, a stepwise approach is recommended, starting with lifestyle modifications and over-the-counter antacids. In patients with more frequent symptoms (≥2 times per week), empiric treatment with drugs that inhibit gastric acid secretion (→below) is warranted. Because GERD is a chronic disease, to control the symptoms and prevent complications patients should receive continual treatment (that will frequently be lifelong).

General Measures

There is little if any evidence that lifestyle measures, detailed below, will lead to healing of erosive esophagitis, but these nonpharmacologic approaches may reduce GERD symptoms:

1) Avoiding eating for 2 to 3 hours before going to bed.
2) Raising the head of the bed by 15 to 20 cm using blocks or foam wedges.
3) Quitting smoking.
4) Limiting dietary fats, alcohol, and coffee.
5) Reducing weight (in obese patients).
6) Avoiding drugs that may reduce LES pressure (eg, methylxanthines, nitrates, calcium channel blockers, β_2-agonists, and anticholinergics).

Pharmacotherapy

1. Gastric acid suppression therapy with a PPI or a histamine type 2 (H_2) receptor antagonist (H_2-RA) is the mainstay of treatment, with PPIs being more effective. For short-term treatment, PPIs are more effective than H_2-RAs for symptom relief in patients with GERD symptoms (PPIs effective in up to three-fourths of symptomatic GERD patients, H_2-RAs in about a half; for every 4 patients treated, one more will achieve remission with PPIs [number needed to treat, or NNT, of 4]) and in those with NERD (PPIs effective in about a half of patients, with H_2-RA slightly less effective, resulting in NNT of ~8). PPIs are usually administered once daily 30 to 60 minutes before the first meal of the day at standard doses (dexlansoprazole 30 mg, esomeprazole 40 mg, lansoprazole 30 mg, omeprazole 20 mg, pantoprazole 40 mg, rabeprazole 20 mg) for 8 weeks. If GERD symptoms persist, PPIs may be given bid for a further 8 weeks before considering investigation or symptom reevaluation (→Figure 1-1). The addition of a standard-dose H_2-RA at bedtime may be considered but any benefit may be transient due to tachyphylaxis (pharmacologic tolerance).

Many GERD patients require long-term treatment to prevent or minimize recurrent symptoms and injury, including bleeding, stricture formation, and progression to Barrett esophagus and esophageal adenocarcinoma. In the majority of patients the lowest dose of a PPI that effectively controls the symptoms should be used—daily or as needed—although bid PPI therapy⊘⊖ with acetylsalicylic acid (ASA) 325 mg daily⊘⊖ reduces patient-important outcomes, including mortality, in patients with Barrett esophagus. For maintenance therapy of reflux esophagitis, PPI therapy is the most effective; H_2-RAs (eg, famotidine 20-40 mg bid, ranitidine 150 mg bid) may be effective in less severe GERD but tachyphylaxis has been demonstrated after as little as 2 weeks of therapy, potentially rendering H_2-RAs less useful for maintenance therapy.

2. Antacids and gastric mucosal protectants containing magnesium or aluminum, alginic acid, sucralfate, or hyaluronic acid/chondroitin sulfate are effective in patients with less severe or less frequent GERD symptoms and may be used as needed. The combination of mucosal protection (hyaluronic acid/ chondroitin sulfate) with acid suppression (PPIs) may be indicated in symptom control of NERD, particularly in cases of partial or unsatisfactory response to PPIs alone. In **pregnant women** preparations of alginic acid or sucralfate are preferred, and when these are ineffective, ranitidine may be used for as short a time as possible and at the lowest effective dose.

3. Prokinetic drugs, such as domperidone or metoclopramide, or LES modifiers, such as baclofen, are not recommended for first-line use in GERD patients. There is little evidence to support their use, either alone or in combination with acid suppression, and their use is associated with appreciable adverse effects.

Surgical Treatment

Antireflux surgery is now generally performed as a laparoscopic Nissen fundoplication procedure in which the gastric fundus is mobilized and then "wrapped" around the distal esophagus as a "collar" to reduce the likelihood that gastric contents will reflux into the esophagus. Long-term PPI therapy and laparoscopic antireflux surgery achieve comparable 5-year remission rates of 92% and 85%, respectively. Open fundoplication is usually restricted to patients with technical challenges, often related to prior antireflux surgery; there is no good evidence that endoscopic antireflux procedures or antireflux implants provide comparable symptom relief or long-term benefits.

Surgical therapy may be considered for patients who are unwilling or unable to take long-term medical therapy and those who do not achieve complete or sustained benefit with medical therapy; this applies in particular to patients who have large-volume reflux due to a large hiatal hernia or significant LES dysfunction and an increased risk of aspiration and respiratory symptoms. However, it is important to confirm the presence of pathologic reflux or reflux-induced disease before considering surgery in patients who report no benefit from medical therapy.

→ COMPLICATIONS

1. Barrett esophagus is defined as the presence of ≥1 cm of metaplastic columnar epithelium replacing the normal stratified squamous epithelium of the distal esophagus, proximal to the uppermost limit of the gastric folds. Risk factors include a long-standing history of GERD, male sex, age >50 years, white populations, hiatal hernia, increased body mass index, and abdominal-type obesity. Barrett esophagus develops in about 10% to 15% of patients with symptomatic GERD but may also occur in those who have no reflux symptoms.

Treatment: Until recently, there have been no high-quality studies of the effect of PPI therapy on long-term outcomes for Barrett esophagus. Therefore, current guidelines recommend that pharmacotherapy should use the lowest doses of PPIs needed to achieve freedom from reflux symptoms, as in uncomplicated GERD. However, a recent study has reported that a high-dose PPI (esomeprazole 40 mg bid) with ASA (300 or 325 mg daily) in patients with Barrett esophagus was associated with a significantly longer time to all-cause mortality, esophageal adenocarcinoma, and high-grade dysplasia at 9 years, with an NNT of 34 for PPIs and an NNT of 43 for ASA. There is no evidence that surgical antireflux therapy reduces the risk of progression to malignancy.

Barrett esophagus is associated with increased risk of esophageal adenocarcinoma. Endoscopic surveillance to identify areas of epithelial irregularity supplemented by 4-quadrant biopsies of the Barrett epithelium every 1 to 2 cm is mandatory, at intervals determined by the grade of dysplasia:

1) No dysplasia: Endoscopy every 3 to 5 years.
2) Indefinite for dysplasia: Repeat endoscopy in 6 months (if indefinite for dysplasia again, the surveillance strategy should follow recommendations for no dysplasia).
3) Low-grade dysplasia: Endoscopy every 6 to 12 months (initially repeat endoscopy at 6 months, later the surveillance interval can be extended to 12 months).
4) High-grade dysplasia: Endoscopy every 3 months, pending resection or ablation therapy.

Dysplasia, particularly low-grade, may regress. In patients with high-grade dysplasia or persistently low-grade dysplasia, the preferred treatment methods are endoscopic mucosal resection (EMR) or mucosal ablation (radiofrequency ablation [RFA], cryotherapy, or photodynamic therapy). Ablation combined with intensive acid suppression may lead to partial or total replacement of metaplastic columnar epithelium with squamous epithelium. In patients with high-grade dysplasia, esophageal resection may also be considered. To date, none of the above methods has been proven to improve survival.

2. Esophageal strictures result from more severe esophagitis (Los Angeles grade D) and ulceration. Diagnosis is based on history (dysphagia) and endoscopy (including biopsy to exclude malignancy). Treatment consists of endoscopic dilation and long-term PPI therapy, often bid, to prevent recurrent injury and scarring.

3. GI bleeding.

4. Esophageal adenocarcinoma.

→ PROGNOSIS

GERD is a chronic condition and recurrent symptoms are common, often requiring long-term medical therapy. Most patients have NERD or mild erosive esophagitis and although these can lead to impaired quality of life, progression to more severe erosive esophagitis, stricturing, Barrett esophagus, and esophageal adenocarcinoma is uncommon. Most patients can be managed with long-term medical therapy without any requirement for additional investigations, which are generally indicated only in the presence of alarming features or symptoms unresponsive to adequately titrated PPI therapy.

1.2. Gastric Diseases

1.2.1. Gastric Cancer

→ DEFINITION, ETIOLOGY, PATHOGENESIS

A precancerous stage of gastric cancer is **intraepithelial neoplasia** (formerly called cancer in situ, preinvasive cancer, or high-grade dysplasia). It is diagnosed microscopically. **Early cancer** is an invasive cancer involving mucosa or submucosa, regardless of involvement of regional lymph nodes.

Epidemiology

Although it is one of the most common types of cancer in the world, the overall incidence of gastric cancer has decreased over the last few decades. The frequency is highest in countries like Japan and South Korea but much lower in North America, except for the first generation of immigrants from high-prevalence countries.

Risk Factors

For **intestinal-type gastric cancer**, precancerous lesions include atrophic gastritis (3-fold to 18-fold risk increase), intestinal metaplasia (6-fold risk increase), and dysplasia (10-fold risk increase). For **diffuse-type gastric cancer**, no precancerous pathology has been identified and it could be difficult to diagnose with ordinary investigations.

Factors increasing the risk of gastric cancer include male sex, atrophic gastritis, partial gastrectomy, Ménétrier disease, dietary factors (salt or salt-preserved food; food with high nitrite levels; diet low in fruits, vegetables, or folate), lifestyle factors (smoking and obesity), infection with *Helicobacter pylori*, and genetic factors.● Two hereditary types of gastric cancer are known:

1) Hereditary diffuse gastric cancer (HDGC), which is due to an autosomal dominant mutation in *CDH1* gene regulating E-cadherin. Most affected patients require early preventive total gastrectomy.

2) Familial intestinal gastric cancer, which is also an autosomal dominant disease.

Gastric cancer has been associated with group A blood type. It can also be linked to other hereditary cancer syndromes (Lynch syndrome, juvenile polyposis syndrome, Peutz-Jeghers syndrome, familial adenomatous polyposis [FAP]).

→ CLINICAL FEATURES AND NATURAL HISTORY

1. Symptoms of early cancer: Epigastric discomfort or vague pain, early satiety, nausea, belching. The disease is rarely asymptomatic.

2. Typical and late clinical manifestations of gastric cancer: Loss of appetite, weight loss and malnutrition, vomiting, dysphagia/odynophagia, constant epigastric pain, sometimes a palpable epigastric tumor; these features develop very late and indicate advanced cancer. Specific symptoms of gastric cancer spread include metastases to the liver (palpable liver mass, jaundice), peritoneum (ascites), left supraclavicular lymph nodes (Virchow node), enlarged ovary (Krukenberg tumor), metastatic umbilical nodule (Sister Mary Joseph nodule), a shelf-like tumor of the anterior rectal wall palpable on rectal examination (Blumer shelf).

→ DIAGNOSIS

Diagnostic Tests

1. Endoscopy: The accuracy of endoscopy in detecting early gastric cancer has been reported to be >95%; however, the lesions may be difficult to detect, flat, or erosion-like (indigo carmine stain or magnifying endoscopy may be helpful). Advanced cancer presents as a tumor (frequently irregularly ulcerated), a fairly uniform infiltrate with impaired gastric distention on insufflation of air (in the case of diffuse-type gastric cancer or linitis plastica), or both. Mapping biopsy defined as taking ≥2 biopsy specimens from each of the antrum, incisura, and body of the stomach is often recommended to check for precancerous lesions while performing gastroscopy in people at higher risk of gastric cancer. All patients with gastric ulcers should undergo follow-up endoscopy to verify healing. Multiple (6-8) biopsy specimens should be obtained from suspicious lesions for histologic examination and particularly from the edge of any unhealed ulceration, even in patients with known peptic ulcer disease (in 10% of chronic peptic ulcers gastric cancer tissue is found).

2. Endoscopic resection: Endoscopic mucosal resection (EMR) or endoscopic submucosal dissection (ESD) of early gastric cancer will provide an accurate T stage of the tumor.

3. Imaging studies: Endoscopic ultrasonography (EUS), computed tomography (CT), and positron emission tomography (PET) are used to assess the extent and depth of local cancer infiltration before surgery and to detect metastases to regional lymph nodes (mainly endosonography) as well as distant metastases. CT is superior to EUS in detecting distant metastases, but EUS is significantly more sensitive and specific in detecting the depth of invasion and lymph node involvement with a possibility of fine-needle aspiration (FNA). EUS is also very accurate in detecting early gastric cancer and determining the criteria for endoscopic resectability. PET is more sensitive than CT in identifying distant metastases.

4. Histology: Adenocarcinoma in 95% of patients.

5. Serology: Currently available serologic markers do not provide reasonable sensitivity or specificity in detecting gastric cancer.

Diagnostic Criteria

Diagnosis is based on histologic examination of gastric mucosa specimens obtained during endoscopy.

Staging

Gastric cancer is staged based on the American Joint Committee on Cancer (AJCC) and the Union for International Cancer Control (UICC) recommendations. Initial staging should include physical examination, blood tests (blood count, liver and renal function tests), endoscopy, pathology, and imaging studies including CT (of the thorax, abdomen, and possibly pelvis) and EUS with or without FNA of suspected lymph nodes. Staging laparoscopy may be required for accurate results. The AJCC recommends evaluating a minimum of 16 and preferably 30 lymph nodes for the purpose of staging. Early stages are considered curable but more advanced stages are usually palliative.

Screening

The rationale for screening depends on the baseline risk, which differs between countries and depends on additional personal risk factors. At present, in North America screening of the general population is not recommended. Screening with endoscopy every 2 to 3 years is currently implemented in some high-risk areas (eg, Japan and South Korea). In Western countries screening is considered controversial and if done, it is reserved for individuals with conditions that are supposed to be precancerous, such as gastric intestinal metaplasia, gastric adenoma, pernicious anemia, FAP, Lynch syndrome, Peutz-Jeghers syndrome, or juvenile polyposis syndrome. It might be reasonable to screen patients with a strong family history of gastric cancer as the risk is increased 2-fold to 3-fold.⊘○

→ TREATMENT AND PROGNOSIS

Formerly gastric cancers were thought to be insensitive to radiotherapy and to show poor response to chemotherapy. Recently there have been attempts to use preoperative (neoadjuvant) chemoradiotherapy, with some success. The criteria for unresectability in gastric cancer are distant metastases and involvement of major vessels.

1. Early cancer: In patients with suspicion of cancer based on endoscopic findings, endoscopic resection (EMR or ESD) may be performed. If histologic examination of the removed lesion reveals advanced cancer, gastrectomy should be done. The overall 5-year survival rates after resection of early gastric cancer are >90%. *H pylori* infection should be treated if present.

2. Advanced cancer: A multidisciplinary approach in a specialized center is required. Patients with resectable cancers at stage T2 or higher and any N stage may benefit from perioperative chemotherapy or chemoradiation, with trastuzumab for human epidermal growth factor receptor 2 (HER2)-overexpressing metastatic carcinoma. Total or subtotal gastrectomy with regional lymphadenectomy should include as many lymph nodes as possible (D1 dissection: limited to perigastric nodes; D2 dissection: extended to include nodes along the main branches of the celiac axis). The overall postoperative 5-year survival rates differ between countries but are usually >20%. The prognosis in patients undergoing this radical surgery depends on dimensions of the resected tumor, depth of infiltration, and number of lymph nodes with metastases.

→ FOLLOW-UP

Postoperative Follow-Up

A reasonable approach may involve follow-up visits every 3 to 6 months for the first 1 to 2 years and then every 6 to 12 months for the next 3 to 5 years (clinical evaluation, complete blood count, and liver function tests). Imaging studies (chest CT, CT of the abdomen and pelvis) should be performed every 12 months.

In patients with early cancer, particularly after EMR, reasonable follow-up includes endoscopic evaluation with the collection of mucosal specimens 3 to 6 months after surgery, then every 6 to 12 months for 3 to 5 years, and annually thereafter.

After subtotal gastrectomy endoscopy should be performed every year for 4 to 5 years after the surgery and later based on clinical manifestations. The follow-up schedule in patients after total gastrectomy is less certain.

1.2.2. Gastric Mucosa-Associated Lymphoid Tissue (MALT) Lymphoma

→ DEFINITION, ETIOLOGY, PATHOGENESIS

Low-grade B-cell lymphoma or extranodal marginal zone lymphoma of mucosa-
-associated lymphoid tissue (MALT) is a non-Hodgkin lymphoma presumably
originating from the post–germinal center memory B cells. There are common
chromosomal translocations associated with this type of lymphoma, the most
frequent ones being t(11;18)(q21;q21) and t(14;18)(q32;q21).

Epidemiology

Stomach is the most common site of gastrointestinal (GI) extranodal lymphomas,
accounting for two-thirds of cases. MALT lymphoma and diffuse large B-cell
lymphoma (DLBCL) are the two most common types found in the stomach.
MALT lymphoma is more frequent in middle-aged patients and accounts for
a half of all cases of gastric lymphoma. The overall incidence is estimated to
be ~4 in 1,000,000 and involves both men and women equally.

Risk Factors

1. *Helicobacter pylori* (the most common risk factor).

2. Autoimmune disorders (most commonly Sjögren syndrome and systemic
lupus erythematosus).

3. Immune deficiency or immunosuppressive therapy.

4. Celiac disease.

5. Inflammatory bowel disease.

6. Nodular lymphoid hyperplasia.

→ CLINICAL FEATURES

In most people MALT lymphoma is an incidental finding. The symptoms are
very nonspecific and include epigastric pain, weight loss, anorexia, nausea
and vomiting, early satiety, or GI bleeding. Occasionally anemia or elevated
erythrocyte sedimentation rate may be detected.

→ DIAGNOSIS

Diagnostic Tests

1. Upper endoscopy: Endoscopic assessment with biopsy is the most important
diagnostic tool. Findings may include erythema, mass, ulcer, nodularity, and
thickened gastric folds. Biopsies should be taken from any abnormal-appearing
mucosa as well as the duodenum, gastric antrum, gastric body, and gastroesophageal junction. Endoscopic ultrasonography (EUS) can also play a role
in determining the depth of invasion and can be used to obtain core specimens
from surrounding enlarged lymph nodes.

The need for confirmation or exclusion of *H pylori* infection dictates the use of
the most sensitive diagnostic strategy. Apart from having a diagnostic value for
MALT lymphoma itself, biopsies should be obtained from the normal stomach
and examined for the presence of *H pylori*.

2. Alternative tests, such as the urea breath test, should be used if biopsies are
negative for *H pylori* (effectively performing 2 tests, each with high sensitivity).
Genetic testing for t(11;18) identifies tumors that are less likely to transform to
high-grade lymphoma or less likely to respond to *H pylori* eradication therapy.
It is important to obtain chest, abdominal, and pelvic computed tomography
(CT) scans to exclude distant metastasis.

Differential Diagnosis

DLBCL is the second most common type of lymphoma in the stomach and, given
its prognosis, it should always be excluded. The less common types include
mantle cell lymphoma, follicular lymphoma, and peripheral T-cell lymphoma.

Staging

The Lugano staging system is used to stage MALT lymphoma and accounts for distant nodal involvement. Stage I and II disease include a single primary lesion or multiple noncontiguous lesions confined to the GI tract that may have nodal involvement. Stage IV (advanced) disease is associated with widespread extranodal involvement or simultaneous supradiaphragmatic nodal involvement.

Screening

At this time there are no defined strategies recommended to screen the general population for MALT lymphoma.

→ TREATMENT

Treatment depends on the stage of MALT lymphoma. In nonadvanced disease, which is the most common clinical scenario, **eradication of *H pylori*** is the mainstay of treatment. Local guidelines should be applied in choosing the best therapeutic regimen to treat *H pylori*. It is essential to confirm eradication of *H pylori* at least 4 weeks after completion of an eradication regimen. It is also key to avoid proton pump inhibitors for ≥1 week (or 2 weeks if well tolerated by the patient) before the confirmation test to prevent false-negative results, as the use of PPIs decreases test sensitivity (sensitivity difference of 3%-4% between 1 and 2 weeks of PPI abstinence).◔ It is not uncommon for *H pylori* to require a second or third line of treatment to achieve eradication. The preferred test for confirming eradication is the urea breath test or endoscopic biopsy. Serology should not be used for this purpose. Also →Chapter 6.1.2.4.

If eradication is confirmed, surveillance endoscopies are required to monitor tumor response. It is crucial to exclude more advanced lymphomas, such as DLBCL. If the disease persists despite *H pylori* eradication, localized radiotherapy is the next universally accepted therapeutic option. Those with stage IV MALT lymphoma may require rituximab or chemotherapy.

Patients without *H pylori* infection do not require eradication treatment and should receive localized radiotherapy as the first line of treatment.

→ PROGNOSIS

Prognosis is generally good, with the 5-year survival rate >90%.

1.2.3. Gastritis and Gastropathy

Gastritis refers to the histologic presence of mucosal inflammation in the gastric tract. It encompasses a number of different entities, including *Helicobacter pylori*–related gastritis, erosive gastropathy secondary to substance use or biliary reflux, stress-related gastritis, autoimmune gastritis, and phlegmonous gastritis.

Gastritis is differentiated from gastropathy, which is a term that refers to gastric mucosal damage with minimal to no active inflammation. Gastritis is primarily driven by active mucosal inflammation. The distinction may require histologic examination.

1.2.3.1. Acute Hemorrhagic/Erosive and Stress-Related Gastropathy

→ DEFINITION, ETIOLOGY, PATHOGENESIS

Acute hemorrhagic (erosive) gastropathy is reactive noninflammatory damage to the gastric mucosa caused by various exogenous and/or endogenous irritants or hypoxia. It manifests as bleeding from multiple superficial mucosal erosions. Acute erosive gastropathy may be caused by one of the following:

1) **Nonsteroidal anti-inflammatory drugs (NSAIDs)**: Chronic NSAID use is associated with both acute and chronic reactive gastritis and ulceration

due to inhibited prostaglandin production, decreased mucosal blood flow, and degradation of the protective mucosal barrier.

2) **Alcohol**: Chronic or excessive use is associated with decreased mucosal blood flow, degradation of the protective mucosal barrier, and depletion of mucosal sulfhydryl compounds.

3) **Bile exposure**: Reflux of biliary salts into the stomach due to pyloric sphincteric incompetence, such as may be seen in the context of gastric surgery.

4) **Other**: Exposure to oral preparations of iron salts, bisphosphonates, sodium phosphate; exposure to endogenous toxins (eg, in uremia).

Gastritis may also be seen in the setting of critical illness with stress-induced gastrointestinal (GI) bleeding. Mechanical ventilation for ≥2 days, coagulopathy, and likely sepsis are associated with increased risk of clinically significant hemorrhage related to stress-induced gastritis. Other causes of mucosal ischemia that may lead to gastritis—including trauma, burns (Curling ulcers), shock of any origin, severe central nervous system injury (Cushing ulcers), hypovolemia, and cocaine use—may also be associated with similar stress-induced gastritis.

Glucocorticoids likely do not cause gastritis or gastropathy but may worsen NSAID-induced lesions.

Bacterial invasion of the gastric wall (with organisms other than *Helicobacter pylori*) may also be associated with infection-driven gastritis.

→ CLINICAL FEATURES AND NATURAL HISTORY

Patients may present with dyspepsia, nausea, emesis, or loss of appetite. Some patients may experience upper GI bleeding, which may be associated with no other signs or symptoms or may be accompanied by dyspepsia. Deep ulcers may develop, complicated by hemorrhage or perforation. Patients with gastritis may also be asymptomatic.

→ DIAGNOSIS

A detailed **medical history** should include:

1) Recent NSAID use (dose, frequency, duration).
2) Concurrent anticoagulant or glucocorticoid use.
3) Recent or history of alcohol misuse.
4) Prior peptic ulcers or GI bleeding.
5) Age (age >60 years is associated with increased risk).
6) Previous gastric or abdominal surgery (including biliary surgery).
7) History of gastroesophageal reflux disease (GERD).
8) Critical illness or mechanical ventilation exposure and associated duration of hospitalization, intensive care unit (ICU) admission, and invasive therapy.
9) History of coagulopathies or thrombocytopenia.
10) Symptoms: Dyspepsia, abdominal pain, fever, nausea, emesis; signs and symptoms of critical illness, infection, sepsis, or other concurrent medical conditions.

Diagnostic Tests

Endoscopy allows to directly evaluate the gastric mucosa for gastritis or other abnormalities. In patients with suspected erosive gastritis mucosal biopsy may not be necessary, although it is often obtained for histopathologic examination and to exclude alternative etiologies, such as *H pylori* infection.

Endoscopy is recommended for patients aged ≥60 years with dyspepsia and for patients <60 years with alarming symptoms (anemia, weight loss, dysphagia, emesis). Patients with a family history of esophageal or GI cancer, lymphadenopathy, suspected or known abdominal mass, or treatment-refractory symptoms should undergo endoscopy.

Endoscopic evaluation may reveal mucosal edema and erythema, petechiae, hemorrhage, erosions, or ulcerations (in severe cases). Curling ulcers are usually located in the gastric fundus (or may also involve the gastric body). Lesions caused by NSAID or alcohol use most often cover the entire stomach; these erosions are usually smaller and heal more rapidly than those associated with ischemic gastritis and gastropathy.

The diagnosis of bile reflux–related gastritis is based on gross endoscopic examination showing severe erythema of the gastric mucosa (fiercely red discoloration) and incrustation of the mucosa with bile crystals (note that the presence of bile in the stomach does not warrant by itself the diagnosis of bile reflux gastropathy).

NSAID-induced gastritis and alcohol-induced gastritis are primarily diagnosed based on clinical suspicion. Patients with prior ulceration, age >60 years, high NSAID use, or concurrent anticoagulant or glucocorticoid use are at especially high risk of NSAID-related complications.

Differential Diagnosis

Differential diagnosis includes gastric lymphoma or carcinoma, dyspepsia not associated with ulcers, GERD, and peptic ulcer disease (PUD) (although this is often related to gastritis).

→TREATMENT

Treatment of gastritis is focused on discontinuation of the offending agent and therapy aimed at preventing further mucosal injury. The goals of treatment are reduction of gastric inflammation, symptomatic relief, and resolution of the underlying cause.

1. Discontinuation of the offending agent: When NSAID-induced or alcohol-induced erosive gastritis is suspected, reduction or discontinuation of the offending agent is recommended. When the cause of hemorrhagic gastropathy is removed, it generally resolves without further treatment.

2. Acid suppression (dosage: →Chapter 6.1.1.3): Therapy with either H_2 antagonists or proton pump inhibitors (PPIs) is effective in the suppression of acid secretion and associated with both symptomatic relief and mucosal healing.

3. Patients with biliary reflux–associated gastritis: Therapy with a PPI or sucralfate may be indicated.⊙⊙ Antacid drugs may be added.

→PREVENTION

1. Prevention of NSAID-induced gastritis and gastropathy: →Chapter 6.1.2.4.

2. Prevention of stress ulcers in seriously ill patients: H_2 antagonists or PPIs have traditionally been recommended for stress ulcer prophylaxis in the setting of critical illness. Recently their benefit has been questioned and new clinical studies are being conducted. The strongest risk factors are mechanical ventilation >48 hours and coagulopathy (platelet counts $<50 \times 10^9$/L or international normalized ratio [INR] >1.5).

1.2.3.2. Autoimmune Gastritis

→DEFINITION, ETIOLOGY, PATHOGENESIS

Autoimmune gastritis (autoimmune metaplastic atrophic gastritis [AMAG]) is a chronic inflammation of the gastric mucosa leading to irreversible atrophy. It is associated with circulating antibodies against parietal cells (90% of patients) and against intrinsic factor, which are responsible for vitamin B_{12} deficiency; this leads to the development of pernicious anemia in some patients. Associated autoimmune diseases such as thyroiditis, Addison disease, Sjögren syndrome, type 1 diabetes mellitus, hypoparathyroidism, or rheumatoid arthritis may coexist and are associated with elevated risk of gastritis. Patients of North European or Scandinavian ancestry are also at increased risk of autoimmune gastritis.

CLINICAL FEATURES AND NATURAL HISTORY

Clinical features associated with autoimmune gastritis are nonspecific. Patients may be asymptomatic or may develop symptoms related to pernicious anemia, such as neurologic abnormalities, cognitive impairment, angular cheilitis, and atrophic glossitis. Even individuals with total mucosal atrophy and intestinal metaplasia may remain asymptomatic, which suggests that endoscopic findings may not completely correlate with clinical presentation.

There is a small increased risk for the development of gastric adenocarcinoma and gastric carcinoid.

DIAGNOSIS

Routine blood tests may be helpful in identifying megaloblastic anemia as the first sign of a potential autoimmune etiology and low vitamin B_{12} levels (→Chapter 7.7.1). Serum vitamin B_{12} and autoantibody studies should be completed in the setting of suspected autoimmune gastritis. Antibodies to intrinsic factor and parietal cell are highly sensitive for pernicious anemia. Patients with confirmed pernicious anemia should usually undergo endoscopy to evaluate for the presence of potential gastric malignancy (the risk is a few times higher compared with the general population). In early disease numerous pseudopolyps may be observed in the gastric body and fundus. At later stages gastric fold flattening or absence and atrophic mucosa with vascular abnormalities may be seen.

TREATMENT

Vitamin B_{12} supplementation (→Chapter 7.7.1). Patients should be monitored to confirm their response to supplementation.

1.2.3.3. Gastritis Due to *Helicobacter pylori* Infection

DEFINITION, ETIOLOGY, PATHOGENESIS

The prevalence of *Helicobacter pylori* is highest in developing countries, with Africa having the highest pooled prevalence globally (70.1%) and Oceania having the lowest (24.4%). Approximately 4.4 billion individuals were estimated to be infected globally as of 2015. The prevalence of *H pylori* infection is also determined by geography, age, strain virulence, environmental factors, and socioeconomic status.

H pylori infection is associated with gastric mucin degradation, epithelial cytotoxicity, and increased mucosal permeability. It causes inflammatory reactions and increased gastric acid secretion by stimulating gastrin-secreting G cells.

Acute gastritis may progress to a chronic phase, leading to mucosal atrophy and hypochlorhydria or achlorhydria. Early *H pylori* infection and uncomplicated chronic gastritis are usually asymptomatic. Complications and long-term sequelae include peptic ulcer disease (PUD), gastric cancer, gastric mucosa-associated lymphoid tissue (MALT) lymphoma, immune thrombocytopenia, iron deficiency anemia, and in very rare cases bacterial overgrowth secondary to achlorhydria. Chronic *H pylori* infection predisposes affected individuals to atrophic and autoimmune gastritis.

→ **CLINICAL FEATURES AND NATURAL HISTORY**

Clinical features associated with *H pylori*–related gastritis are similar to that of gastritis due to other causes (→Chapter 6.1.2.3.1).

→ **DIAGNOSIS**

Endoscopy is used for gastric mucosal assessment and biopsy for histopathologic and *H pylori* testing (biopsies should include the prepyloric region). It is recommended for patients with dyspepsia aged >60 years, and for those <60 years with alarming symptoms (anemia, weight loss, dysphagia, emesis). Mucosal biopsies can be tested using the rapid urease test and with direct culture and molecular studies.

The endoscopic features of acute gastritis usually include enlarged and stiffened folds as well as erosions and erythema of the mucosa. In chronic gastritis the antral mucosa is nodular and has a "cobblestone" appearance (due to "follicular" inflammation of the gastric mucosa), and areas of intestinal metaplasia, either multifocal or limited to the prepyloric region, are observed. Histologic examination of gastric mucosa specimens is necessary to assess the severity of chronic gastritis and to diagnose potential epithelial dysplasia. Details of the diagnosis of *H pylori* infection: →Chapter 6.1.2.4.

The **urea breath test and fecal antigen test** are 2 noninvasive tests for active infection that may be also used to monitor treatment response. Because proton pump inhibitor (PPI) therapy may interfere with test results, if possible it should be withheld for 1 to 2 weeks after treatment when confirming *H pylori* eradication.

→ **TREATMENT**

1. Eradication therapy: →Chapter 6.1.2.4. Eradication testing is now recommended following completion of treatment using urea breath test, fecal antigen test, or biopsy-based confirmatory testing. Eradication failure has been associated with medication nonadherence, smoking, and alcohol use, among other variables. Eradication of *H pylori* leads to regression of inflammatory infiltrates, but regression of intestinal metaplasia and reduction of the risk of gastric cancer have not been proven.

2. Nonsteroidal anti-inflammatory drug (NSAID) discontinuation is generally recommended.

Prognosis is usually very good with appropriate therapy.

1.2.4. Peptic Ulcer Disease

→ **DEFINITION, ETIOLOGY, PATHOGENESIS**

Peptic ulcer disease (PUD) is a recurring formation of gastric and/or duodenal peptic ulcers. A **peptic ulcer** is a demarcated mucosal defect extending through the muscularis mucosa with associated inflammatory infiltrates and coagulative necrosis. Peptic ulcers are most frequently located in the duodenal bulb or stomach or less commonly in the lower part of the esophagus or duodenal loop.

Etiology: Frequently *Helicobacter pylori* infection or nonsteroidal anti-inflammatory drugs (NSAIDs). Rarely critical illness, Zollinger-Ellison syndrome, glucocorticoids in combination with NSAIDs, or other drugs (potassium chloride, bisphosphonates, mycophenolate mofetil).

H pylori **infection** is responsible for >50% of duodenal and gastric ulcers. *H pylori* is able to survive in the gastric environment thanks to the production of urease, which degrades urea, thus releasing ammonia that neutralizes gastric acid and creates a less acidic microenvironment within the gastric mucus layer. Initially *H pylori* causes acute gastritis in the prepyloric region, which after several weeks progresses to chronic gastritis; *H pylori* also induces hypergastrinemia, leading to an increased secretion of hydrochloric acid, which plays an important role in the pathogenesis of duodenal ulcers. All **NSAIDs**, including acetylsalicylic acid (ASA) (even at the low doses used for cardiovascular indications), damage the gastrointestinal (GI) mucosa, primarily by reducing the production of prostaglandins as a result of inhibition of cyclooxygenase-1 (COX-1), and are associated with ulcer generation. The extent to which NSAIDs damage the mucosa depends on the type of NSAID, but all increase the risk of peptic ulceration; moreover, they inhibit platelet activity and, to a various degree, increase the risk of bleeding from those ulcers. The risk of serious upper GI events (including bleeding) is doubled with selective cyclooxygenase-2 (COX-2) inhibitors (coxibs) or diclofenac and quadrupled with naproxen or ibuprofen.⊜ Clopidogrel, an antiplatelet drug, is unlikely to be ulcerogenic per se for the upper GI tract, but it significantly increases the risk of bleeding of gastric erosions and ulcers caused by other drugs or *H pylori* infection. The use of this drug should be taken into account when assessing the risk of bleeding from peptic ulcers.

Risk factors for mucosal damage by NSAIDs include history of peptic ulcers or bleeding ulcers, *H pylori* infection, age ≥60 years, concomitant administration of several NSAIDs, treatment with high-dose NSAIDs, and NSAIDs combined with glucocorticoids (induction of peptic ulcers by glucocorticoid monotherapy has not been proven) or anticoagulants.

→ CLINICAL FEATURES AND NATURAL HISTORY

The leading symptom is epigastric pain or epigastric discomfort. In patients with duodenal ulcers the pain typically occurs in the fasting state (often at night or early in the morning) and resolves after consuming food or taking antacids. Epigastric pain is not specific for peptic ulcers; in ~50% of cases it may be caused by other conditions, most frequently by functional dyspepsia. Nausea and vomiting may occur. However, the course of PUD is often asymptomatic, especially in patients receiving NSAIDs who may develop bleeding or perforation as the first presentation. Possible complications: →Complications, below.

→ DIAGNOSIS

Diagnostic Tests

1. Endoscopy: A gastric ulcer is a sharply demarcated circular mucosal defect or an irregular cavity with infiltrated edges, most often located at the lesser curvature or in the prepyloric region. It is usually isolated, although ulcers caused by NSAIDs may be multiple. Duodenal ulcers are most frequently found in the anterior wall of the bulb. Mucosal defects smaller than an arbitrary size of 5 mm in diameter are called erosions. Upper GI bleeding warrants urgent endoscopy (→Chapter 6.1.3.4).

2. Tests for detection of *H pylori* (proton pump inhibitors [PPIs] decrease the sensitivity of all tests except serology and therefore should be discontinued 2 weeks before the tests, if possible; testing for *H pylori* should be avoided, if possible, within 4 weeks from administration of bismuth or antibiotics):

1) **Invasive methods (requiring endoscopy and mucosal biopsy)**:

   a) **Urease test** (most commonly used): A specimen of the gastric mucosa is placed on a plate containing urea and a color indicator. The degradation of urea to ammonia by bacterial urease alkalinizes the medium, causing a change in its color. Sensitivity is 90% and specificity is 95%.

   b) **Histology of a mucosal specimen** obtained from the antrum (an additional sample from the gastric body increases sensitivity). Sensitivity and specificity are ~95%.

c) **Bacterial culture of a mucosal specimen**: This allows the determination of antimicrobial sensitivity. Specificity is 100% but sensitivity is poor.

2) **Noninvasive methods**:

a) **Urea breath test**: A solution containing portions of ^{13}C-labeled or ^{14}C-labeled urea are consumed by the patient. The urea is hydrolyzed by bacterial urease to labeled CO_2, which is measured in the expired air after 30 minutes. This test can either be performed in the office (the vials of expired air are then mailed to a central laboratory) or in a laboratory. Both sensitivity and specificity are >95%.

b) **H pylori stool antigen test**: A laboratory test using the enzyme-linked immunosorbent assay (ELISA) and monoclonal antibodies (not the office-rapid test kits); the test is almost as accurate as the breath test.

c) **Serology**: Serologic assays are useful in epidemiologic research but less so in clinical practice. This is because a positive result does not indicate an ongoing infection, since antibodies are still detectable for 1 or more years after treatment. Laboratory-based ELISAs are better validated than whole blood office-based kits and can be used in clinical practice in special situations, such as patients who cannot safely withhold PPI treatment for 2 weeks and in whom other tests were negative while receiving PPIs.

Overall, invasive tests (urease test or histology) are used when endoscopy is required for another reason. Rarely endoscopy may be indicated solely for obtaining mucosal samples for culture and antimicrobial sensitivity in refractory *H pylori* infection. In most clinical scenarios the urea breath test is the preferred test both pretreatment and posttreatment.

Diagnostic Criteria

The diagnosis of ulcer is based on endoscopy.

Differential Diagnosis

Other causes of dyspepsia, nausea and vomiting, and epigastric pain. To assess the nature of the gastric ulcer (benign or malignant), it is customary to perform a histologic evaluation of ≥6 specimens taken from the edges and the floor of the ulcers. In duodenal ulcers biopsy is only indicated when an etiology different from *H pylori* infection or NSAIDs is suspected.

➡ TREATMENT

General Considerations

1. Diet: Although patients often identify specific foods that cause or worsen the symptoms, there is no evidence that any specific diet, restriction of coffee, or moderate alcohol consumption helps in the healing of peptic ulcers.

2. Avoidance of smoking is recommended. Tobacco smoking is a risk factor for peptic ulcers, which also delays their healing and increases the risk of their recurrence.◐○

3. Avoidance of NSAIDs or, if NSAIDs cannot be avoided, use of **gastro-protective treatment** (→below).

Treatment of Patients With *H Pylori* Infection

H pylori should be eradicated in patients with PUD.◐●

Further eradication indications: →Table 1-4.

1. In regions where >15% of *H pylori* strains are resistant to clarithromycin, the preferred regimen is **bismuth-containing quadruple therapy or concomitant therapy**:

1) Bismuth-containing quadruple therapy includes 14-day treatment with a **PPI** (esomeprazole 20 mg bid, lansoprazole 30 mg bid, omeprazole 20 mg bid, pantoprazole 40 mg bid, or rabeprazole 20 mg bid), **bismuth subsalicylate**

Table 1-4. Indications for treatment of *Helicobacter pylori* infection, where present, according to the Maastricht IV/Florence Consensus Conference

1. Gastric and/or duodenal ulcer (active or healed, as well as complications of ulcer disease)
2. Gastric MALT lymphoma
3. First-degree relatives of patients with gastric cancer
4. Prior endoscopic or subtotal gastric resection in the treatment of gastric neoplasia (MALT lymphoma, gastric adenoma, gastric cancer)
5. Severe pangastritis, corpus-predominant gastritis, or severe atrophy
6. Chronic gastric acid inhibition for >1 year
7. Strong environmental risk factors for gastric cancer (heavy smoking, high exposure to dust, coal, quartz, cement, and/or work in quarries)
8. At the patient's request in case of fear of gastric cancer
9. Dyspepsia not associated with peptic ulcer
10. Undiagnosed dyspepsia (test-and-treat strategy)[a]
11. Prevention of development of ulcers and their complications before or during a long-term NSAID treatment[b]
12. Unexplained iron deficiency anemia
13. Primary immune thrombocytopenic purpura
14. Vitamin B_{12} deficiency

[a] In regions with a low prevalence of *Helicobacter pylori* infection, the effectiveness of this strategy is low and empiric acid inhibition is an equivalent option.

[b] In patients who are already receiving long-term NSAID treatment, it is recommended to combine eradication with PPI administration.

MALT, mucosa-associated lymphoid tissue; NSAID, nonsteroidal anti-inflammatory drug; PPI, proton pump inhibitor.

525 mg qid, **metronidazole** 250 mg qid, and **tetracycline** 500 mg qid. Alternatively, a combined preparation containing **bismuth subcitrate potassium** 140 mg, **metronidazole** 125 mg, and **tetracycline** 125 mg in 1 capsule can be used in a dose of 3 capsules qid with a PPI bid.

2) Concomitant therapy includes 14-day treatment with a PPI, clarithromycin 500 mg, metronidazole 500 mg, and amoxycillin 1 g, all bid.

2. In regions where *H pylori* strains resistant to clarithromycin are rare (ie, <15%) or regions with proven high local eradication rates (> 85%) of clarithromycin-based triple therapies, **clarithromycin** can still be used as a first-line agent within the conventional triple therapy: 14-day treatment with a **PPI** (dosage as above) + **clarithromycin** 500 mg bid + either **amoxicillin** 1 g bid or **metronidazole** 500 mg bid. Increasing the duration of triple therapy increases eradication rates: 7-day regimens should not be used, while 14-day regimens are more effective than 10-day regimens. Therefore, the recommended duration of triple therapy is 14 days.◐◔

3. Patients should be tested to prove eradication at least 1 month after completion of antibiotic therapy:

1) Patients with duodenal ulcers should be tested with noninvasive methods. There is no need to repeat endoscopy for these patients unless severe symptoms persist or reoccur. Similarly, there is no need for PPI treatment after the 14-day eradication regimen unless severe symptoms persist or reoccur or unless there is still a clear indication for PPI gastroprotective treatment (→below) despite *H pylori* eradication.

2) Patients with gastric ulcers at endoscopy require PPI treatment (standard doses once daily; →above) for 1 to 2 months and should have repeat endoscopy to confirm complete healing of ulcers at the end of treatment. During repeat

endoscopy biopsies from nonulcerated mucosa can be obtained to test for *H pylori* infection (with the caveat that sensitivity is reduced if PPIs had been taken in the 2 weeks prior to endoscopy; →above), and if the ulcers have not healed completely, additional mucosal samples should be obtained from the base and edges of ulcers (to exclude malignancy) and repeat endoscopy scheduled after a repeat course of PPI treatment.

4. Second-line empiric regimens in case of eradication failure:

1) Failure of bismuth-containing quadruple therapy: Use **levofloxacin** 500 mg bid + **amoxicillin** 1 g bid + **PPI** bid (doses as above).

2) Failure of clarithromycin-containing regimens: Use **bismuth-containing quadruple therapy** or **levofloxacin-containing regimen** (→above).

Patients with second-line treatment failure must be treated according to the actual antibiotic resistance of the *H pylori* strain as determined by culture and sensitivity assessment.

5. Bleeding peptic ulcer: Extended treatment with a PPI aimed at achieving an increased speed and rate of ulcer healing.

Treatment of Patients Without *H Pylori* Infection

1. A PPI or H_2-blocker for 1 to 2 months is usually effective:

1) A **PPI** once daily, in the morning, 20 to 30 minutes before a meal. Dosage: **esomeprazole** and **pantoprazole** 40 mg daily, **lansoprazole** 30 mg daily, **omeprazole** and **rabeprazole** 20 mg daily.

2) H_2 **blockers** inhibit the secretion of hydrochloric acid stimulated by histamine. These agents are less effective than PPIs and their repeated dosing leads to tolerance (reduced pharmacodynamic effect); therefore, we prefer not to use those.⊗� However, H_2 blockers could be used in patients who do not tolerate PPIs because of suspected adverse effects. Dosage, when used: **famotidine** 40 mg once daily at bedtime, **ranitidine** 150 mg bid or 300 mg once daily at bedtime.

2. There is no need to repeat endoscopy for duodenal ulcers unless severe symptoms persist. If the ulcer was initially associated with NSAIDs with or without *H pylori* infection and neither of these 2 risk factors is present any longer, treatment need not be prolonged for more than 1 to 2 months, provided that the patient is asymptomatic.

Similarly to *H pylori*-positive ulcers, endoscopy should be repeated in patients with gastric ulcers 1 to 2 months after the initial endoscopy. If the ulcers have not healed completely, repeat biopsy samples from ulcerations should be obtained to exclude undiagnosed malignancy.

3. Causes of treatment failure: Use of NSAIDs by the patient, false-negative *H pylori* test results, noncompliance, or other causes of ulcers.

Surgical Treatment

Surgical treatment does not eliminate the risk of ulcer recurrence and is associated with late complications.

Main potential indications: Ineffectiveness of pharmacotherapy (failure to heal the ulcer, frequent [≥2 times a year] and early [<3 months after treatment] recurrence of ulcers after exclusion of other causes of ulcers including Zollinger-Ellison syndrome), ulcer complications (perforation, hemorrhage, pyloric stenosis) not responding to pharmacotherapy.

Surgical approach:

1) **Duodenal ulcers**: Usually highly selective vagotomy or truncal vagotomy with antrectomy. In the case of pyloric stenosis, truncal vagotomy with pyloroplasty or vagotomy with antrectomy.

2) **Gastric ulcers**: The type of surgery depends on ulcer location. The usual procedure consists of:

a) For ulcers in the gastric body, partial gastrectomy with gastroduodenal anastomosis without vagotomy.

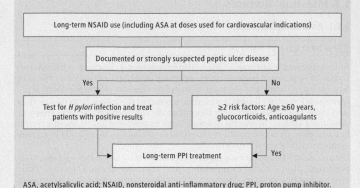

Figure 1-2. Limiting the risk of ulcer complications associated with the use of nonsteroidal anti-inflammatory drugs. *Based on Circulation. 2008;118(18):1894-1909.*

b) For ulcers in the prepyloric region or gastric ulcers plus duodenal ulcers, vagotomy with antrectomy.

c) For ulcers in the subcardial region, partial gastrectomy including the pyloric region.

COMPLICATIONS

1. Upper GI bleeding manifests as bloody or coffee-ground emesis and/or bloody or tarry stools. Treatment: →Chapter 6.1.3.4.

2. Perforation manifests as a sudden, severe, piercing epigastric pain followed by rapidly developing symptoms of diffuse peritonitis. In >50% of patients there are no preceding dyspeptic symptoms. This complication often requires surgical intervention.

3. Pyloric stenosis results from permanent scarring or edema and inflammation associated with an ulcer located in the pylorus or duodenal bulb. It manifests as gastric retention, nausea, and profuse vomiting; some patients develop hypokalemia and alkalosis. In the course of antiulcer treatment the inflammation and edema subside and patency of the pylorus may improve. Endoscopic dilation or surgical treatment may be indicated in patients with persistent stenosis.

PREVENTION

In patients at risk of ulcer recurrence or complications due to the use of NSAIDs in whom these drugs cannot be discontinued or replaced with less harmful agents (eg, acetaminophen [INN paracetamol]), use full antiulcer doses of a PPI as an adjunct to NSAIDs (→Figure 1-2). The use of film-coated (releasing active substance in the small intestine) or buffered preparations of ASA does not reduce the risk of complications. Do not replace ASA with clopidogrel to reduce the risk of recurrent ulcer bleeding in high-risk patients; this approach is inferior in terms of bleeding risk to the use of ASA in combination with a PPI. Before a planned long-term treatment with NSAIDs, particularly in patients with a history of ulcer disease, test for *H pylori* infection and administer eradication treatment if the result is positive.

1.3. Intestinal Diseases

1.3.1. Anorectal Diseases

→ **INTRODUCTION**

Anorectal complaints may be due to benign anorectal disorders or malignancy. Common symptoms include pain, swelling, discharge, and rectal bleeding. Systemic symptoms and changes in bowel movements may also occur.

One useful way of classifying benign anorectal disorders is to divide them into those that cause pain and those that do not. Common painful anorectal conditions include anorectal abscess, anal fissure, and thrombosed external hemorrhoids. Common painless anorectal conditions include fistula in ano and symptomatic internal hemorrhoids.

Diagnostic studies to investigate anorectal disorders include assessment of the perineum, digital rectal examination, and anoscopy or sigmoidoscopy. Other studies that are sometimes necessary include transrectal/endoanal ultrasonography (evaluation of the structure of and defects in the anal sphincter), anal manometry (evaluation of anal sphincter function), and magnetic resonance imaging (MRI).

1.3.1.1. Anal Fissures

→ **DEFINITION, ETIOLOGY, PATHOGENESIS**

An anal fissure is a tear in the epithelial lining of the distal anal canal.

The exact cause of anal fissures is not known. An initiating event, such as passage of a hard stool or trauma, causes a tear in the epithelial lining. High resting anal canal pressure and reduced blood flow prevents healing and results in mucosal ischemia and fissure formation. Some risk factors that may contribute are diets lacking in fiber, previous anal surgery, childbirth, and laxative abuse.

The most common location is the posterior midline (up to 90% of cases). Anterior midline fissures are less frequent and are more common in women than in men. However, the most common location in women are posterior midline fissures. Lateral fissures are the least common.

Atypical fissures that are lateral, nonhealing, or nonsolitary should raise suspicion of diseases such as Crohn disease, tuberculosis, syphilis, HIV/AIDS, other dermatologic conditions (eg, psoriasis), leukemia, or anal carcinoma.

→ **CLINICAL FEATURES AND NATURAL HISTORY**

The main symptoms are sharp or burning pain on defecation that can last for hours after defecation and mild rectal bleeding (eg, bright red blood on toilet paper).

The most important physical examination is inspection of the perianal area by gentle effacement of the anus by separation of the buttocks. Chronic fissures (symptoms persisting for >6-8 weeks) also have associated features, such as an external sentinel anal tag and hypertrophied anal papilla internally. Digital rectal examination is often deferred due to severe pain and increased anal sphincter tone that makes the examination difficult.

→ **DIAGNOSIS**

Diagnosis is usually made on the basis of history and physical examination. Endoscopic examination may be delayed until pain resolution after treatment. Biopsies should be done if the fissure is atypical or nonhealing to exclude other diagnoses.

→ TREATMENT

The goal of treatment is to achieve internal sphincter relaxation to allow healing without fecal incontinence. Special attention should be paid to treatment of atypical fissures, such as in Crohn disease; expert opinion should be sought.

1. Conservative management includes dietary modification for prevention of constipation, fiber supplementation, stool softeners if necessary, and warm sitz baths.

2. Medical treatment involves the use of topical medications that produce reversible chemical sphincterotomy as an initial treatment for acute fissures.◐◒ Topical calcium channel blockers such as diltiazem (2%) or nifedipine ointment may be used. Topical nitroglycerin (0.2% or 0.4%) is another option; however, adverse effects are more common than with calcium channel blockers. Medical treatment has marginally better healing rates than placebo.

3. Botulinum toxin injections into the internal sphincter can be performed in medically refractory chronic fissures.◐◒ Healing rates are no different from medical treatment but there is significant variability in dose, site, and frequency of injections that may affect the results.

4. Surgical treatment is reserved for severe chronic medically refractory fissures. In such situations lateral internal sphincterotomy is the treatment of choice with the highest healing rates, although the risk of incontinence exists.◐●

1.3.1.2. Anorectal Abscess and Fistula in Ano

→ DEFINITION, ETIOLOGY, CLASSIFICATION

Anal canal anatomy and anorectal spaces: →Figure 1-3.

Anorectal abscess and fistula in ano are entities along a spectrum of disease with the same underlying pathogenesis.

Anorectal abscesses are infections that usually develop as a result of obstruction of anal crypts causing stasis in ducts (also described as of cryptoglandular origin). Less common causes are inflammatory bowel disease, trauma, and malignancy. Anorectal abscesses occur in patients aged 20 to 40 years and are more frequent in men than in women.

A **fistula in ano** is an abnormal communication between the anal canal (usually at the level of the dentate line) and the skin. It develops due to chronic infection and epithelialization of an abscess drainage tract. Fistula in ano is found in 30% to 70% of patients presenting with an anorectal abscess. About a third of patients that do not have a concomitant fistula will develop a fistula after drainage of the abscess.

Abscesses are classified based on the anatomic location in which they develop as perianal, ischiorectal, intersphincteric, or supralevator (→Figure 1-4). Horseshoe abscesses are those that track to the contralateral side via the deep postanal space. Perianal and ischiorectal abscesses compose about 80% of anorectal abscesses.

Fistulas may be classified based on their relationship to the external anal sphincter (under voluntary control; →Figure 1-5). Intersphincteric fistulas penetrate only through the internal anal sphincter (under involuntary control). Transsphincteric fistulas penetrate through both internal and external sphincters. Suprasphincteric fistula tracts loop over the external sphincter and perforate the levator ani. Extrasphincteric fistulas are completely external to the sphincter complex. Intersphincteric and transsphincteric fistulas are most common.

Fistulas can also be classified as **simple** versus **complex fistulas**. Simple fistulas are intersphincteric or transsphincteric fistulas that do not involve a significant portion of the external sphincter (<30%). The following are

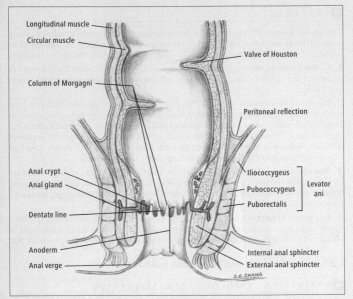

Figure 1-3. Anal canal anatomy. *Illustration courtesy of Dr Shannon Zhang.*

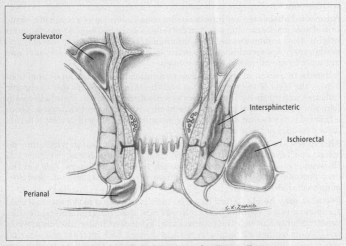

Figure 1-4. Location of abscesses. *Illustration courtesy of Dr Shannon Zhang.*

classified as complex fistulas: transsphincteric fistulas involving a significant amount of the external sphincter; anterior fistulas in women; suprasphincteric fistulas; extrasphincteric fistulas; horseshoe fistulas; and fistulas associated with inflammatory bowel disease, radiation, or malignancy.

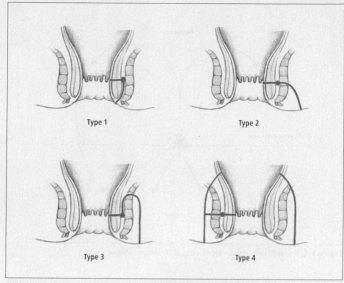

Figure 1-5. Types of fistula in ano. **Type 1**, intersphincteric fistula. **Type 2**, transsphincteric fistula. **Type 3**, suprasphincteric fistula. **Type 4**, extrasphincteric fistula. *Illustration courtesy of Dr Shannon Zhang.*

→ CLINICAL FEATURES

The most common symptoms of anorectal abscesses are acute perianal pain and swelling. Patients may report spontaneous drainage. Less commonly fever and malaise develop. Supralevator abscesses may present with referred pain in the lower back and buttocks.

The most common history suggestive of a fistula is intermittent perianal pain and swelling with constant or occasional drainage from the external opening of the fistula. Exacerbation of the inflammatory process is often observed following a spontaneous closure of the external opening (ie, increased pain and swelling after drainage stops).

It is important to elicit information about sphincter function, prior anorectal surgery, and any associated gastrointestinal, urologic, or gynecologic history.

Physical examination starts with inspection of the perineum. Erythema, signs of perianal Crohn disease, spontaneous drainage, or external openings of fistula in ano are noted. External perianal and digital rectal examination (DRE) are done to identify areas of induration, fluctuance, and tenderness. An intersphincteric abscess should be suspected if there is exquisite tenderness and fluctuance on DRE with a relatively unremarkable external examination. Careful examination of the contralateral side should also be performed to exclude a horseshoe abscess. Physical examination is not very helpful in supralevator abscesses.

→ DIAGNOSIS

Clinical examination is usually sufficient for diagnosis. However, if there is uncertainty or physical examination cannot be performed due to pain, the patient may require imaging or examination under anesthesia with anoscopy.

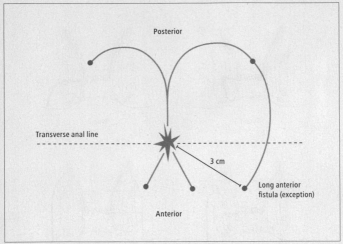

Figure 1-6. Goodsall rule. *Illustration courtesy of Dr Shannon Zhang.*

Imaging studies may be helpful in occult or complicated anorectal abscesses and Crohn disease. Computed tomography (CT) or magnetic resonance imaging (MRI) may identify and characterize abscesses and fistulas. MRI is more helpful in identifying and delineating fistulas.

→ TREATMENT

1. Abscess: Prompt **incision and drainage** of the abscess is required. Incision should be large enough for adequate drainage and as close as possible to the anal verge to minimize the length of the potential fistula.

Antibiotic therapy is usually not necessary. It may be considered in patients with significant cellulitis, systemic signs, or underlying immunosuppression.⊘○

2. Fistula: The first step in treatment is an **examination under anesthesia**, which is performed to confirm diagnosis, identify the internal opening(s), and characterize the fistula tract(s). Goodsall rule is helpful in locating the internal opening of the fistula (→Figure 1-6). To apply the rule, an imaginary line is drawn transversely across the buttocks, through the anus. If the external opening of a fistula is anterior to this line, the tract will likely be a straight radial tract with the internal opening at the end of this straight tract. If the external opening is posterior to this line, the tract will likely be curved, with the internal opening in the posterior midline location. An exception is a long anterior fistula with an external opening anterior to this line but further away from the anus (>3 cm) that has a curved tract with a posterior internal opening.

Surgical treatment may require multiple stages, depending on the characteristics of the fistula. Surgical treatment for a simple fistula with normal sphincter function is a fistulotomy.⊘⊖ In patients with complex fistulas, when continence and/or wound healing may be compromised with surgical treatment, it is necessary to place a seton (drain) to ensure drainage. Other surgical treatments that are effective include ligation of the intersphincteric fistula tract (LIFT) and endoanal advancement flaps. Fistula plugs and fibrin glue are relatively ineffective.

1.3.1.3. Hemorrhoids

➔ **DEFINITION, ETIOLOGY, PATHOGENESIS**

Hemorrhoids are vascular cushions in the anal canal, formed by the submucosa containing blood vessels, smooth muscle, and connective tissue. Three main vascular cushions are located in the left lateral, right anterior, and right posterior positions. Hemorrhoids are a part of normal anatomy with the potential to become symptomatic.

Hemorrhoids are classified as **internal** or **external hemorrhoids** depending on their location relative to the dentate line (above or below the dentate line, respectively). **Mixed hemorrhoids** have both components.

➔ **CLINICAL FEATURES**

A common symptom is rectal bleeding (bright red blood on toilet paper or in the toilet bowl). It is rare to have significant bleeding that causes anemia. Prolapse is another common symptom.

Classification of internal hemorrhoids based on degree of prolapse is as follows:

1) Grade I: Enlargement of hemorrhoids without prolapse.
2) Grade II: Prolapse of hemorrhoids with spontaneous reduction.
3) Grade III: Prolapse of hemorrhoids requiring manual reduction.
4) Grade IV: Irreducible prolapse of hemorrhoids.

Sometimes patients complain of perianal pruritus. Sudden-onset pain is usually associated with thrombosed external hemorrhoids; it is rare in symptomatic internal hemorrhoids.

It is important to elicit information on bowel habits and any recent changes as well as family history.

Physical examination includes inspection of the perianal region, digital rectal examination, and anoscopy. Careful examination should be done to exclude other pathology (eg, fissure, abscess, fistula in ano, dermatitis, condyloma, inflammatory bowel disease, malignancy).

➔ **DIAGNOSIS**

Physical examination and anoscopy/sigmoidoscopy is usually sufficient for diagnosis.

Colonoscopy should be performed in patients with rectal bleeding that is not typical for hemorrhoids (eg, blood is mixed with feces, anemia) or if indicated for other clinical reasons (eg, family history of colorectal cancer).

➔ **TREATMENT**

Treatment includes:

1) **Conservative management**:
   a) **Dietary and lifestyle changes**: Dietary modification to achieve a high--fiber diet with fiber supplementation and increased water intake is the first-line conservative management for symptomatic hemorrhoids.◐◯ Lifestyle modifications such as minimizing the time spent on the toilet and straining should be adopted to decrease symptoms.
   b) **Treatment of local symptoms** (pruritus, burning sensation, pain) using warm sitz baths may be helpful. Suppositories/ointments containing ingredients such as local anesthetics and hydrocortisone have little science to support their use; however, some patients report relief.
2) **Office-based procedures**: In patients with **grade I, II, and III hemorrhoids** in whom medical treatment is ineffective, obliteration of hemorrhoidal

tissue is performed in an outpatient setting. Available techniques include sclerotherapy, bipolar diathermy, infrared coagulation, and rubber band ligation. Rubber band ligation is the most common and effective method of office-based procedures but it still requires multiple repeat treatments.

3) **Surgery**: Surgery is reserved for symptomatic hemorrhoids that have failed conservative and office-based procedures, grade IV hemorrhoids, or mixed hemorrhoids with a significant external component. Acutely incarcerated (nonreducible) or strangulated (vascular compromise) internal hemorrhoids require emergency excisional hemorrhoidectomy. Hemorrhoidectomy is the most effective treatment; however, it is associated with significant pain and potential serious complications.

Thrombosed external hemorrhoids may require incision and evacuation of thrombus in patients who present within 72 hours of the onset of symptoms. Patients presenting later should be followed up without intervention because the pain associated with thrombosis usually resolves spontaneously within 7 to 10 days. Most patients do not require any intervention.

1.3.2. Bacterial Overgrowth Syndrome

→ **DEFINITION, ETIOLOGY, PATHOGENESIS**

Small intestinal bacterial overgrowth (SIBO) is a condition in which the small bowel is colonized by excessive numbers of aerobic and anaerobic microbes that normally colonize the colon.

The prevalence of SIBO in the general population is unknown. It is often associated to other disorders and therefore frequently underdiagnosed.

Etiology and pathogenesis: There are several mechanisms that prevent bacterial colonization of the small intestine, such as low gastric pH, gastrointestinal (GI) motility, enzymes in pancreatic and biliary secretions, integrity of the intestinal mucosa, direct effects of commensal bacteria, decreased secretion of IgA, and the ileocecal valve. When any of these mechanisms is altered, the risk for SIBO increases:

1) Alteration of the GI tract: Duodenal or jejunal diverticulosis, fistulas, strictures, inflammatory bowel disease, gastric resection or bypass, blind loop syndrome, resection of ileocecal valve.

2) Decreased gastric acid: Hypochlorhydria or achlorhydria, gastrectomy, vagotomy, inhibitors of acid secretion or acid blockers.

3) Altered GI motility: Gastroparesis, pseudo-obstruction, connective tissue diseases (scleroderma, polymyositis, lupus), medications (opiates, anticholinergics, tricyclic antidepressants), radiation enteropathy, muscular dystrophy, amyloidosis.

4) Decreased pancreatic enzymes or biliary secretion: Chronic pancreatitis, cirrhosis.

Intestinal motility disorders and chronic pancreatitis are estimated to account for approximately 90% of cases of SIBO.

Consequences: Bacterial overgrowth leads to:

1) Deconjugation of bile salts and impaired digestion of fats, with consequent steatorrhea and malabsorption of fat-soluble vitamins (specifically vitamins A, D, and E, but not vitamin K, as it is produced by luminal bacteria).

2) Depletion of vitamin B_{12}, leading to megaloblastic anemia. Vitamin B_{12} is used by anaerobic bacteria to produce inactive cobamides, which in turn decrease vitamin B_{12} absorption in the ileum by competing for its binding sites.

3) Protein malabsorption.

4) Damage to the enterocytes of the intestinal villi and disturbance of disaccharide digestion with lactose intolerance, which contributes to diarrhea.

5) Increased absorption of bacterial antigens into the bloodstream.

→ CLINICAL FEATURES AND NATURAL HISTORY

SIBO can be asymptomatic or can present with nonspecific symptoms, such as bloating, flatulence, diarrhea, abdominal discomfort, or abdominal pain. These symptoms may mimic irritable bowel syndrome (IBS). In fact, a recent meta-analysis showed that one-third of patients with IBS may test positive for SIBO.◯

Patients with SIBO may develop chronic fatty diarrhea and megaloblastic anemia as well as weight loss and malnutrition. They may have symptoms of vitamin A and D deficiencies (osteomalacia and osteoporosis, tetany, trophic epithelial lesions, night blindness), symptoms of vitamin B_{12} deficiency (ataxia and peripheral neuropathy), erythema nodosum, and maculopapular rash.

Patients with SIBO may also present glomerulonephritis, hepatitis or hepatic steatosis, and arthritis.

→ DIAGNOSIS

Although there is no perfect test for the diagnosis of SIBO, the current gold standard involves measurement of bacterial concentrations and culture of jejunal aspirate samples taken endoscopically. Because this test is invasive, hydrogen breath testing (HBT) with substrates such as glucose or lactulose has become a widely accepted alternative.

If available, HBT using glucose as the substrate should be considered, with additional measurement of methane concentration to improve the sensitivity of the test. If HBT is not available, culture of small bowel aspirate should be attempted. If clinical suspicion is high and no test is available, empiric antibiotic therapy seems appropriate.

1. Microbiology of intestinal contents: Quantitative and qualitative microbiological examination of samples collected via a nasogastric tube or during endoscopy from jejunal aspirate. This is considered the gold standard for the diagnosis of bacterial overgrowth syndrome; however, the examination is invasive, expensive, and flawed by false-positive results due to contamination with oral and esophageal flora as well as false-negative results due to inability to reach the middle and distal sections of the small bowel. There is a lack of consensus regarding the definition of a positive test. While some studies suggest $>10^3$ colony-forming units (CFU)/mL are required to define SIBO, for others $>10^7$ CFU/mL are needed. However, most experts have accepted a bacterial count of $>10^3$ CFU/mL for the diagnosis of SIBO.

2. HBT: Hydrogen and methane are gas productions from colonic anaerobic bacterial fermentation of carbohydrates used in this test as the substrate for fermentation (eg, glucose or lactulose). These gases can then be measured in exhaled breath using gas chromatography. In patients with SIBO bacteria present in the small intestine produce a premature rise in the concentration of hydrogen, methane, or both following the intake of glucose or lactulose.

Breath testing to measure hydrogen and methane concentrations after the intake of glucose or lactulose as substrates is a noninvasive and relatively inexpensive tool to diagnose SIBO. There is, however, a lack of standardization regarding indications and methodology for testing as well as interpretation of results. A recent North American consensus has proposed a rise ≥20 ppm from baseline in hydrogen concentration and ≥10 ppm in methane concentration using a glucose or lactulose substrate for the diagnosis of SIBO, although the characteristics of these tests are unclear and likely poor.◯ The sensitivity and specificity of HBT is variable, with studies reporting a sensitivity range from 31% to 68% and a specificity range from 44% to 100%. When using glucose as a substrate, HBT is more specific but not as sensitive, as glucose is absorbed mainly in the proximal bowel and can therefore miss distal SIBO. On the other hand, the lactulose breath test is more sensitive than specific, but lactulose is an osmotic laxative, which accelerates transit and may lead to false-positive results and overtreatment.

3. Laboratory tests: There is no specific laboratory test to diagnose SIBO. Indirect findings may be macrocytic anemia, hypoalbuminemia, and other abnormalities depending on clinical manifestations and target organ damage.

4. Radiography of the GI tract: Radiographs may reveal impaired intestinal passage or anatomical defects (eg, diverticulum, duplication, "blind loop," intestinal stricture).

5. Stool fat analysis: Microscopic examination of a freshly prepared stool specimen stained with a 1% solution of Sudan III may reveal an increased number of fat droplets in the stool.

Differential Diagnosis

Other causes of chronic diarrhea (→Chapter 1.5).

SIBO often presents with other concomitant conditions, such as celiac disease or IBS, or after a GI surgery. Concomitant celiac disease and SIBO commonly manifest as a lack of an adequate response to a gluten-free diet. In patients with other underlying diseases, like Crohn disease or pancreatitis, SIBO may present as unexplained clinical deterioration.

→ TREATMENT

1. Treatment of the underlying diseases or correcting factors promoting bacterial overgrowth: This is the most important part of SIBO treatment. However, because it is not always possible to completely control the underlying condition, the risk of recurrence remains high.

2. Nutritional management:

1) Formulas containing medium-chain triglycerides (MCTs) may facilitate the absorption of fats.

2) In the case of disaccharide intolerance, dietary lactose restriction may contribute to better symptom control.

3) Supplementation of vitamins A, D, E, and, B_{12} in patients with deficiencies.

4) A diet low in fermentable oligosaccharides, disaccharides, monosaccharides, and polyols (FODMAPs) may improve clinical symptoms.

3. Antimicrobial treatment: Wide-spectrum antimicrobial drugs against gram-negative aerobic and anaerobic bacteria may be used. The most commonly used antibiotics and doses:

1) Amoxicillin/clavulanate 500/125 mg tid.

2) Ciprofloxacin 250 to 500 mg bid.

3) Doxycycline 100 mg bid.

4) Metronidazole 250 mg bid or tid.

5) Neomycin 500 mg bid.

6) Norfloxacin 400 mg bid.

7) Rifaximin 550 mg bid or tid.

8) Tetracycline 250 to 500 mg bid or qid.

9) Sulfamethoxazole/trimethoprim 800/160 mg bid.

Most guidelines recommend administering treatment for 7 to 10 days as a single treatment course or as a cyclic therapy.

Rifaximin is the most studied antimicrobial drug for SIBO. It has been preferred over other antibiotics because of its limited absorption and systemic effects. Furthermore, it is probably the only antibiotic capable of achieving a long-term favorable clinical effect in patients with IBS and SIBO.○ However, the drug is expensive and not widely available.

4. Probiotics for SIBO: Different probiotic strains have shown benefits in reducing abdominal pain as well as decreasing hydrogen concentration and may help to restore microbial balance in patients with SIBO. However, they do not seem effective in preventing SIBO.○

→ PROGNOSIS

SIBO is considered a relapsing condition, with up to 44% of patients having a recurrence of symptoms at 9 months after initial successful antibiotic treatment. Therefore, multiple cycles of antibiotics may be needed. The role of retesting after a course of an antibiotic is currently unknown.

1.3.3. Celiac Disease

→ DEFINITION, ETIOLOGY, PATHOGENESIS

Celiac disease (CD) is an autoimmune enteropathy triggered by gluten and developing in patients that carry the HLA-DQ2 or HLA-DQ8 haplotype.

Gluten is the collective name for a group of proteins found in wheat (gliadins and glutenins), rye (secalin), and barley (hordein). Gluten proteins have a high concentration of the amino acids proline and glutamine, rendering them resistant to enzymatic degradation by digestive enzymes. As a result, large and potentially immunogenic peptides may reach the mucosa of the small intestine and initiate an immune response. The high proline and glutamine content in gluten peptides also renders them excellent substrates for tissue transglutaminase type 2 (tTG2). tTG2 is a ubiquitous intracellular enzyme that is released extracellularly and activated during inflammation. tTG2 deamidates gluten peptides, which converts glutamine to negatively charged glutamic acid residues, increasing their binding affinity to HLA-DQ2 and HLA-DQ8 molecules on antigen-presenting cells. Gluten-specific T cells from patients with CD preferentially recognize deamidated gluten peptides and produce the type 1 helper T cell (Th1) cytokines interferon γ and interleukin 21. Gluten-specific Th1 cells also provide help for the activation of B cells to form antigluten and anti-tTG2–producing plasma cells. The presence of antibodies to tTG2 (anti-tTG2 IgA) or endomysial antibodies (EmAs) and/or IgA or IgG antibodies against deamidated forms of gliadin peptides (DGPs) is a valuable tool for diagnosing CD. In clinical practice IgA antibodies to tTG2 along with total IgA levels to exclude IgA deficiency are the primary serologic diagnostic tests used. Duodenal biopsies to assess the presence of enteropathy are encouraged to confirm diagnosis.

Contrary to what was previously thought, the onset of CD occurs at any age, and today the disease is more often diagnosed in adulthood. Although ~30% of the world population carries the HLA-DQ2 or HLA-DQ8 genes, only 1% will develop the disease. This together with the rising prevalence of CD in the past 40 years suggests that unknown environmental factors may also play a role in disease pathogenesis.

→ CLINICAL FEATURES AND NATURAL HISTORY

1. Signs and symptoms: CD is frequently asymptomatic and diagnosis often follows a screening test. However, it may present with different gastrointestinal and extraintestinal manifestations, with extraintestinal symptoms usually predominating in adults:

1) **Gastrointestinal**: Chronic diarrhea, abdominal pain, bloating, constipation, recurrent aphthous stomatitis, vomiting, reflux, micronutrient deficiencies, steatohepatitis, and weight loss (rare).

2) Extraintestinal:

a) **Cutaneous**: Dermatitis herpetiformis (Duhring disease: →Figure 1-7; ~15%-25% of patients), urticaria, atopic dermatitis, psoriasis (~4%).

b) **Hematologic**: Iron deficiency anemia (~50% of patients at diagnosis), thrombocytosis, IgA deficiency, leukopenia, neutropenia.

c) **Gynecologic**: Delayed puberty (including delayed menarche), infertility, recurrent abortions.

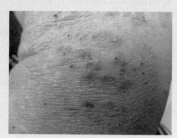

Figure 1-7. Dermatitis herpetiformis (Duhring disease).

d) **Neurologic**: Central nervous system: seizures, migraine, ataxia; peripheral neuropathy.

e) **Psychological**: Anxiety, depression.

f) **Bones**: Osteopenia, osteoporosis, bone fractures.

g) **Other**: Muscle weakness, tetany, short stature, dental enamel defects.

2. Clinical classification of CD: →Table 1-5.

3. Natural history: Undiagnosed or untreated CD may lead to complications, some of them serious (eg, increased risk of certain types of cancers). The **clinical course of CD** depends on compliance with a gluten-free diet (GFD). Poor compliance is associated with increased risk of complications and mortality. The most common complications associated with CD:

1) **Gastrointestinal**: Pharyngeal or esophageal cancer, lymphoma or cancer of the small intestine, refractory CD (symptoms persisting despite compliance with a GFD).

2) **Hematopoietic**: Non-Hodgkin lymphoma.

3) **Urogenital**: Infertility, recurrent miscarriage, premature birth, premature menopause.

4) **Musculoskeletal**: Osteoporosis and increased risk of bone fractures.

→ DIAGNOSIS

CD may be suspected in:

1) Symptomatic patients with:

a) Gastrointestinal symptoms and signs: Diarrhea, weight loss, gas/bloating, constipation (more commonly in children), elevated aminotransferase levels.

b) Extraintestinal symptoms and signs: Iron deficiency anemia, dermatitis herpetiformis, osteoporosis, neuropsychiatric conditions (eg, neuropathy, ataxia).

2) Patients with associated conditions: Autoimmune thyroiditis, type 1 diabetes mellitus, Down syndrome, other autoimmune conditions.

3) First-degree family members of patients with CD.

Diagnostic tests should be performed in patients consuming a gluten containing diet (≥6 weeks of daily intake of ≥1 meal containing gluten).

Diagnostic Tests

1. General laboratory tests:

1) Hemoglobin to investigate for anemia (a frequent abnormality in adults); most likely iron deficiency anemia, rarely megaloblastic anemia.

2) Micronutrients: Reduced serum levels of iron, folic acid, calcium, vitamins D, B_6, B_{12}, zinc, copper, selenium.

Table 1-5. Clinical classification of different forms of celiac disease based on the Oslo consensus

Descriptors of CD	Characteristics
Classical CD	Symptoms and signs of malabsorption including diarrhea, steatorrhea, weight loss; in children growth failure is required
Nonclassical CD	CD presenting without symptoms of malabsorption
Symptomatic CD	Clinically evident GI and/or extraintestinal symptoms attributable to gluten intake
Asymptomatic CD	Lack of GI or extraintestinal symptoms at diagnosis
CD autoimmunity	Increased antibodies to tTG2 or EMAs on ≥2 occasions (if biopsy is negative, it is "potential CD"; if positive, it is CD)
Subclinical CD	CD below threshold for clinical detection without symptoms or signs sufficient to trigger CD-testing in routine practice
Potential CD	Positive CD serology with normal small intestinal mucosa
Genetically at risk for CD	Family members of patients with CD who test positive for HLA-DQ2 and/or HLA-DQ8
Refractory CD	Persistent villous atrophy and malabsorptive symptoms and signs despite strict gluten-free diet for >12 months

CD, celiac disease; EMA, endomysial antibody; GI, gastrointestinal; tTG2, tissue transglutaminase type 2.

3) Hypoalbuminemia (due to protein loss into the gastrointestinal tract).

4) Liver enzymes (transient elevation of liver aminotransferases is seen in active CD).

2. Specific serology: IgA antibodies to tissue transglutaminase (tTG) (total IgA levels must also be measured to exclude IgA deficiency), EmA IgA, and DGPs are used for the diagnosis of CD. tTG IgA antibody is the preferred single test for detection of CD in individuals aged >2 years.◎● Because of their low sensitivity and specificity, the use of antigliadin antibodies (IgA and IgG) for the diagnosis of CD is discouraged. In patients with IgA deficiency IgG antibodies to tTG2 or DGPs need to be measured. Alternatively, DGP IgG can be added to tTG IgA to increase sensitivity.

Sensitivity and specificity differ depending on the type of antibodies and substrate. The most sensitive and specific test is tTG IgA, which is considered the first-line choice for the diagnosis of CD. The new DGP IgA or IgG have lower sensitivity compared with tTG IgA but may detect CD in some patients who are falsely negative for tTG. DGP IgG is also useful as a first-line test in addition to tTG IgA, especially in those with IgA deficiency. EmA IgA is the most specific test for the diagnosis of CD, but it requires immunofluorescence and is operator-dependent. EmA IgG has lower sensitivity compared with EmA IgA.

Indications for serologic studies:

1) Case finding in patients with suspected CD.

2) Screening in high-risk groups (eg, family members of patients with diagnosed CD; patients with related autoimmune diseases, such as type 1 diabetes mellitus or hypothyroidism).

3) Monitoring of compliance with a GFD. In compliant patients results of serologic tests normalize in the first year after diagnosis.

3. Endoscopy: Grooved or scalloped margins of duodenal folds, reduction in the number of folds (which are flattened or atrophic), a mosaic pattern of the mucosal surface, and prominent submucosal blood vessels (normally not visible).

4. Histologic examination of samples of the small intestinal mucosa is key for the diagnosis of CD, particularly in adult patients. The European Society for Paediatric Gastroenterology Hepatology and Nutrition (ESPGHAN) criteria propose specific clinical situations where biopsy could be avoided in the diagnosis of CD in children. Tissue samples (≥4 biopsy specimens collected from the second and third portion of the duodenum and 1-2 specimens from the duodenal bulb) are usually obtained by esophagogastroduodenoscopy (EGD). A typical histologic finding is villous atrophy accompanied by high intraepithelial lymphocyte counts and hyperplasia of intestinal crypts (villous atrophy). The Marsh classification includes types 0 to 2 with increasing intraepithelial lymphocyte counts and increasing degree of hyperplasia and type 3 with villous atrophy (3a, mild; 3b, moderate; 3c, severe).

5. Genetic testing: The great majority (95%-99%) of patients with CD carry the HLA-DQ2 haplotype and the remaining patients (5%-10%) carry HLA--DQ8. In rare cases (<1%) patients not carrying these heterodimers express the other half of the DQ2.5 heterodimer (DQ7.5). Therefore, the absence of HLA-DQ2 or HLA-DQ8 molecules practically excludes the diagnosis of CD. However, ~30% of the general population carries HLA-DQ2 and HLA-DQ8 in the absence of CD; therefore, HLA-DQ2 and HLA-DQ8 should not be used for the diagnosis of CD.◐◒ HLA-DQ2/DQ8 testing is indicated to exclude CD in the following situations:

1) Marsh type 1 or 2 histology in patients with negative CD serology.

2) Assessment of the risk for CD in patients on a GFD not previously investigated for CD.

3) Discrepancy between CD-specific serology and histology results.◐◒

Diagnostic Criteria

Positive serologic study results and typical histologic findings. General diagnostic algorithm: →Figure 1-8.

Differential Diagnosis

Differential diagnosis should include other causes of enteropathy (villous atrophy): chronic giardiasis, tropical sprue, protein malnutrition, anorexia nervosa, food hypersensitivity (lesions are usually focal), viral infection (including HIV), bacterial infection (eg, tuberculosis), bacterial overgrowth syndrome, Whipple disease, postirradiation complications, immunodeficiency (eg, hypogammaglobulinemia, common variable immunodeficiency), Crohn disease, ulcerative colitis, and lymphoma of the small intestine.

→ **TREATMENT**

The only currently available treatment for CD is adherence to a strict GFD. Very small amounts of gluten (50 mg or a breadcrumb) can induce changes ranging from villous to crypt abnormalities in patients with CD.

1. GFD: Lifelong elimination of all wheat, rye, and barley products.

Products allowed: Dairy products (liquid and powdered milk, hard cheese, cottage cheese, cream, eggs); all meats and meat products (note: diced bread and semolina may be added to certain meat products such as sausages, pates, liverwurst), offal (liver, lungs, kidneys), fish; all fruits and vegetables; nuts; rice, corn, soybeans, tapioca, buckwheat; all fats; sugar, honey; spices, salt, and pepper; coffee, tea, cocoa; gluten-free breads, cakes, and desserts. All gluten--free products are labeled with a crossed-grain symbol.

Products not allowed: Wheat, rye, barley, and noncertified gluten-free oat products (as they are often contaminated with gluten); bread rolls, white

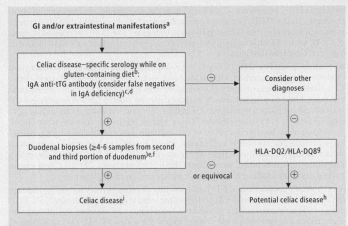

⊕ Positive. ⊖ Negative.

a Screening for celiac disease in high-risk asymptomatic populations is controversial due to the lack of knowledge of natural history and benefit of screening in such groups.

b If the patient self-started a gluten-free diet, consider testing after a challenge with >3 g of gluten per day (equivalent to 1-2 slices of bread per day) for ≥2 weeks.

c The addition of total IgA may be useful to detect IgA deficiency.

d An alternative approach is to include both IgA-based and IgG-based testing, such as IgG deamidated gliadin peptides.

e There are scarce data evaluating the diagnosis of celiac disease in the adult population based on serology alone. Therefore, the combined use of biopsy and serologic analyses for the diagnosis of celiac disease is recommended.

f Current guidelines recommend 1-2 biopsies from the bulb in addition to ≥4 biopsies from the distal duodenum. However, the advantages (increased sensitivity) and disadvantages (reduced specificity) of bulb biopsies are under scrutiny.

g HLA-DQ2/HLA-DQ8 negative results exclude celiac disease in the majority of cases.

h Other reasons for discrepant serology and biopsy results include reduced gluten in diet, inadequate biopsy sampling, and lack of expert histopathology reporting.

i The diagnosis is confirmed after clinical or histologic improvement (or both) after following a gluten-free diet.

tTG, tissue transglutaminase.

Figure 1-8. Approach to the diagnosis of celiac disease in the adult population. *Adapted with permission from the Society for the Study of Celiac Disease.*

bread, whole-grain bread, crispbread; pasta; semolina, barley; other products containing gluten, such as cakes, biscuits, confectionery.

Supplementation of iron, folic acid, calcium, and sometimes vitamin B_{12} may be indicated (in case of deficiency). Repeated monitoring of the effectiveness of treatment includes evaluation of diet and nutritional status of the patient. Undetectable levels of tTG, DGP, or EMA are an indirect confirmation of compliance with a GFD.

2. Immunosuppressive drugs (eg, glucocorticoids, azathioprine, cyclosporine [INN ciclosporin]) may be used in refractory CD not responding to dietary restrictions.

3. Treatment difficulties and future pharmacologic therapies: A strict GFD is difficult to achieve and follow in the long term. Without proper monitoring, following a GFD can lead to nutritional deficiencies. The diet is also expensive. Therefore, noncompliance, either voluntary or through inadvertent contamination, is common. This highlights the need for development of adjuvant therapies to the GFD. Several approaches are being pursued, but so far none is clinically applicable. These potential therapies are to be used as adjuvants of GFD, with the idea to help the patient tolerate minimal amounts of gluten (eg, cross-contamination).

4. Nonresponsive CD: Patients with symptoms and sings of malabsorption (abdominal pain, diarrhea, weight loss) and histologic or serologic abnormalities that persist or recur despite their best efforts to follow a GFD for ≥6 months are considered nonresponsive. The most common reason for nonresponsive CD is inadvertent gluten exposure. Therefore, the first approach is an exhaustive assessment of GFD compliance. Once gluten exposure has been excluded, symptoms may be attributed to other common associated conditions, including exocrine pancreatic insufficiency, small intestinal bacterial overgrowth, inflammatory bowel diseases, microscopic colitis, or functional disorders including irritable bowel syndrome (IBS). Patients with CD may develop an eating disorder leading to persistent symptoms in the follow-up.

A very small proportion of CD patients may develop refractory celiac disease (RCD) (1% of patients with CD or 10% of patients with nonresponsive CD). RCD patients are recognized for persistent symptoms and signs of malabsorption and villous atrophy despite 1 year of following a strict GFD. tTG or CD serology is often negative, supporting the strict compliance with a GFD. There are 2 types of RCD, based on the evidence of aberrant patterns of intraepithelial lymphocytes (IELs). RCD type 1 has a typical pattern of IELs (CD3$^+$ and CD8$^+$) and is associated with better prognosis compared with RCD type 2 (aberrant pattern of IELs: CD3$^-$ and CD8$^-$), which is associated with mortality and risk of lymphoma of 50% at 5 years. Management of RCD patients is complex and they are usually followed up in specialized centers.

→ FOLLOW-UP

Regular follow-up is recommended after the diagnosis of CD is made.

1. In the first year follow-up visits need to be more frequent to improve dietary adherence, provide psychological support, and optimally motivate the patient to adapt to changes. Even though the evidence on the frequency of visits and type of tests that should be performed is low, guidelines recommend follow-up visits with the physician and ideally a dietitian at 4 to 6 months and 12 months in the first year. The objectives are to symptom assessment, dietary review, CD serologic testing (tTG or DGPs). Nutrients should be monitored at this stage only if they were low at diagnosis. Follow-up endoscopy is not necessary in asymptomatic patients, as mucosal healing is seen only in 30% of individuals in the first year of a strict GFD.

2. After one year or when results of serologic testing become negative, annual visits are recommended to monitor GFD adherence, CD serology (tTG or DGPs), and nutrients (iron, copper, zinc, selenium, folate, vitamin B$_{12}$). Bone density measurements may be repeated at 1 to 2 years if the results were abnormal at diagnosis. If osteopenia or osteoporosis are present, in addition to a strict GFD it is prudent to ensure adequate calcium and vitamin D intake for all patients. Follow-up endoscopy is reasonable after 1 to 2 years of starting a GFD to assess for mucosal healing, especially in patients with severe initial presentation.

3. It is advisable to screen first-degree family members for CD.

4. Assessment by a skilled dietitian is the gold standard for evaluating GFD adherence, but it is time-consuming (each visit takes 45 minutes to 1 hour). New tools for detecting gluten immunogenic peptides in stool or urine by enzyme-linked immunosorbent assay (ELISA) (currently available in research settings) or as point-of-care testing may be useful to identify inadvertent gluten consumption. The tests are highly sensitive (98%) and specific (100%) for detecting gluten consumption within 4 to 5 days (stool) or 1 to 2 days (urine). Gluten can be detected in food by a similar method, using a point-of-care sensor.

1.3.4. Gastrointestinal Bleeding

→ DEFINITION, ETIOLOGY, PATHOGENESIS

Gastrointestinal (GI) bleeding may be divided into:

1) **Upper gastrointestinal (GI) bleeding** (from a source located above the ligament of Treitz), which occurs in ~80% of patients hospitalized due to GI bleeding. The most common **causes** include gastric or duodenal ulcers, acute hemorrhagic (erosive) gastropathy, esophageal varices, Mallory-Weiss syndrome, and esophagitis; less common causes include Dieulafoy lesions, duodenitis, neoplasms, esophageal ulcers, and vascular malformations. Acute upper GI bleeding may be precipitated by shock, systemic inflammatory response syndrome, sepsis, multiple trauma, acute respiratory failure, multiorgan failure, severe burns, and other acute and severe diseases.

2) **Lower GI bleeding** (from a source located below the ligament of Treitz), which occurs in ~20% of patients hospitalized due to GI bleeding. The most common **causes** of severe lower GI bleeding in adults are colonic diverticula and vascular malformations, while the less common causes include inflammatory bowel disease (IBD), hemorrhoidal disease, and neoplasms. In children and adolescents the causes may include intussusception (secondary to polyps), IBD, Meckel diverticular bleed, and small intestinal or colonic polyps.

Bleeding may be exacerbated by coagulopathy.

GI bleeding can be also divided into:

1) **Overt GI bleeding**: Bleeding that is visible, such as hematemesis (bloody or coffee-ground emesis), hematochezia (presence of blood and blood clots in feces), or melena (black tarry stools). It may be overt-obscure if investigations do not establish the exact source.

2) **Occult GI bleeding**: Bleeding which is not overt (eg, detected through occult blood testing or confirmed only after investigations for iron-deficiency anemia). It may also be occult-obscure.

→ CLINICAL FEATURES

1. Acute bleeding:

1) **Upper GI bleeding**: The most common presentation is melena (tarry, black, foul-smelling stools). If the bleeding is brisk, hematochezia or maroon stools may be observed. Sometimes the presenting symptom is hematemesis or coffee-ground emesis. Epigastric or diffuse abdominal pain may be present (chest pain mimicking coronary disease occurs in some patients) as well as symptoms of hypovolemia (shock).

2) **Lower GI bleeding**: Hematochezia is the most common presentation but ~10% of lower GI bleeding presents with melena. Symptoms of hypovolemia may occur (shock).

2. Chronic bleeding: Iron deficiency anemia, fecal occult blood. These patients often have obscure GI bleeding.

→ DIAGNOSIS

History may indicate the source of bleeding, but usually diagnosis can only be established on the basis of endoscopy or, in the case of a massive hemorrhage, during radiologic intervention or surgery.

Diagnostic Tests

1. Laboratory tests:

1) **Complete blood count (CBC)**: A decrease in hematocrit, hemoglobin levels, and red blood cell (RBC) counts may not be evident until blood becomes diluted by the transition of the intercellular fluid into the intravascular space, which may take hours, or by infused fluids that contain no blood cells (eg, 0.9% NaCl).

2) **International normalized ratio (INR) and other coagulation tests**: These are particularly important in patients treated with anticoagulants, such as warfarin, especially because information concerning such treatment sometimes cannot be obtained from individuals with altered mental status. Coagulopathy may be also indicative of liver dysfunction or depletion of coagulation factors.

2. Endoscopy of the upper GI tract is the key diagnostic and often therapeutic modality for suspected upper GI bleeding. The most common lesion identified on upper endoscopy is peptic ulcer.

Ulcers are generally characterized by the **Forrest classification**, which reliably predicts the likelihood of rebleeding:

– Class I: Active spurting bleeding (Ia) or active oozing bleeding (Ib).
– Class IIa: Visible nonbleeding vessel.
– Class IIb: Adherent clot at the ulcer base.
– Class IIc: Flat pigmented spot at the ulcer base.
– Class III: Clean (white) ulcer base.

Classes Ia, Ib, and IIa are associated with high risk for rebleeding and are usually treated endoscopically in combination with injection therapy, coagulation, or clips. Class IIb lesions warrant targeted irrigation to attempt to dislodge the clot and then treat the underlying lesion. Classes IIc and III usually do not require endoscopic therapy, as they are associated with low risk for rebleeding.

If urgent endoscopy is not feasible, introduce a nasogastric tube (after securing the airway if needed). The presence of bile without blood in the gastric aspirate suggests a lower GI source of bleeding.

3. Colonoscopy is the initial diagnostic procedure for patients with lower GI bleeding. It should be performed after adequate bowel preparation ideally within 24 hours of presentation. Of note, urgent upper GI endoscopy may be indicated in patients who are unstable with hematochezia, as it is prudent to exclude a briskly bleeding upper GI source.

4. Computed tomography angiography (CTA) may be helpful in locating and potentially treating the source of active bleeding, using subsequently an interventional radiologic procedure.

5. Some patients with obscure GI bleeding (usually after repeat endoscopy and/or colonoscopy) may require small bowel evaluations with **push enteroscopy**, **double balloon enteroscopy**, and **wireless capsule endoscopy**; each may be combined with CT enterography.

➔ TREATMENT

Management algorithm for bleeding ulcers: →Figure 1-9.
Management algorithm for bleeding varices: →Figure 1-10.

1. Patients should be treated in an acute setting and then transferred to a general ward or monitored setting depending on the severity of their condition. In patients with significant blood loss and impaired mental status, **maintain the airway** and intubate if necessary.

2. Measure **blood pressure**. If it is normal, perform the measurement in a standing position. A decrease in systolic blood pressure >20 mm Hg, decrease

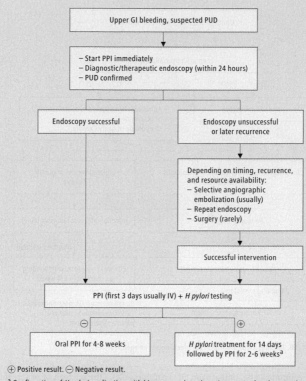

Figure 1-9. Management algorithm for bleeding ulcers.

in diastolic blood pressure >10 mm Hg, or increase in heart rate >30 beats/min indicates significant volume depletion. Check for signs of hypoperfusion, such as delayed capillary refill and other symptoms of shock. If the above signs are present, **start treatment of shock** (→Chapter 3.16).

3. Correct blood volume for the blood lost due to the bleeding: Insert 2 large--bore peripheral vein catheters or a central venous catheter. Crystalloid is usually administered first as it is readily available. Packed RBCs should be administered as soon as possible in patients with signs of hemodynamic instability or shock.

4. Perform **urgent endoscopy and make attempts to stop the bleeding** using local injections of vasoconstrictors (such as epinephrine) or saline, electrocoagulation, argon coagulation, hemostatic clips, and ligation of esophageal varices.

5. Start pharmacologic treatment:

1) In patients with **high-risk bleeding gastric or duodenal ulcers or acute hemorrhagic gastropathy**, administer an IV proton pump inhibitor (PPI)

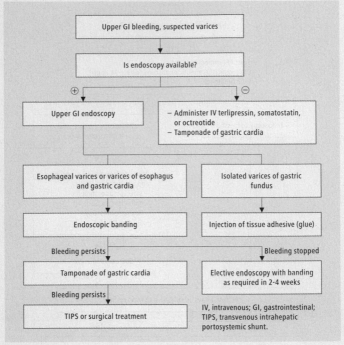

Figure 1-10. Management algorithm for bleeding esophageal varices.

(eg, esomeprazole, omeprazole, or pantoprazole). Our pattern of practice is to administer a bolus injection followed by a continuous infusion for 3 days (this also includes patients in whom bleeding was successfully stopped using endoscopy). If no further bleeding has occurred after 3 days of monitoring, the patient can be switched to an oral PPI. Low-risk lesions can be managed with initial oral PPI therapy. Of note, there is insufficient evidence to reach a firm conclusion about the superiority or noninferiority of PPI regimens for acute ulcer bleeding based on route (oral vs IV) and dose (high vs medium or low) of PPIs. ○ All patients with peptic ulcers should be tested and, if positive, treated for *Helicobacter pylori* infection. Nonsteroidal anti-inflammatory drugs (NSAIDs) should be avoided if possible with the exception of acetyl-salicylic acid (ASA), which should be continued if there is a good indication for cardiovascular protection.

2) In patients with **bleeding esophageal varices**, administer one of the following IV agents lowering portal pressure:

a) **Terlipressin**, a synthetic analogue of vasopressin with fewer adverse effects: 5 to 20 µg/min in a 20- to 40-minute infusion; if necessary, repeat the infusion every 8 hours for a maximum of 5 days. Alternatively injections of 1 to 2 mg every 4 to 6 hours may be used.

b) **Somatostatin**: 250 µg injection followed by a continuous infusion of 250 µg/h for 5 days.

c) **Octreotide**: 50 µg injection followed by a continuous infusion of 50 µg/h for 5 days.

3) **Patients with cirrhosis and GI bleeding** should receive antibiotics (eg, ceftriaxone for 1 week; switch to oral ciprofloxacin is possible if the patient is discharged earlier), as this is associated with a mortality benefit.◐◔

4) In **patients treated with anticoagulants**, neutralize the anticoagulant effects (vitamin K antagonists: →Chapter 3.1, Table 1-4; heparin: →Chapter 3.1.1.3; fibrinolytic agents: →Chapter 3.11.1.2). However, this should not delay endoscopy once needed. Hematology consultation may be required in case of use of direct oral anticoagulants. Also →Chapter 3.1.3.

6. In patients with bleeding esophageal varices in whom endoscopic attempts to stop the bleeding have failed, you can introduce a **Sengstaken-Blakemore tube** into the esophagus and stomach or another type of tube (eg, Linton-Nachlas) allowing for balloon compression of the varices; the tubes should be removed within 24 hours.

7. If endoscopic and pharmacologic treatment is ineffective, proceed with **visceral angiography and selective embolization** of the bleeding vessel or administration of terlipressin into the visceral vessels.

8. Since patients may require emergency surgery, involve a surgeon in the management at early stages of treatment. **Indications for consideration of surgery include** uncontrolled massive bleeding (ie, causing uncontrolled hemodynamic instability), also after an endoscopic or angiographic attempt to stop the bleeding; recurrent bleeding (following 2 endoscopic procedures); prolonged bleeding combined with an estimated blood loss >50% of circulating volume; and repeated hospitalizations due to a bleeding ulcer. The following surgical procedures are used:

1) **Bleeding duodenal ulcer**: Usually pyloroplasty or antrectomy are performed, both with oversewing of the bleeding ulcer. Vagotomy was historically performed as well, but it is now generally avoided as effective pharmacologic suppression of gastric acid is available.

2) **Bleeding gastric ulcer or gastric erosions**: Various types of resection, depending on the clinical situation and patient's condition.

3) **Bleeding esophageal varices unresponsive to pharmacotherapy and insertion of tubes compressing varices**: Transvenous intrahepatic portosystemic shunt (TIPS) is a minimally invasive method. If this is ineffective, perform portosystemic anastomosis or revascularization and transection (dissection and suturing) of the esophagus as well as splenectomy.

4) **Lower GI bleeding**: Colonoscopy performed during surgery and guided by the operating surgeon sometimes enables localization of the source of bleeding. If this is successful, segmental intestinal resection with anastomosis is performed; if the source of bleeding in the colon cannot be located, partial colectomy with ileorectal anastomosis is performed.

1.3.5. Gastrointestinal Infections and Parasitic Diseases

1.3.5.1. Acute Appendicitis

⇒ETIOLOGY AND PATHOGENESIS

Acute appendicitis is one of the most common causes of abdominal pain and peritonitis. It most frequently results from obstruction of the appendiceal lumen by a fecalith. The obstruction allows bacterial stasis and overgrowth while also causing intramural and intraluminal fluid accumulation and edema. The resultant increase in local pressure may compromise vascular flow, leading to appendiceal ischemia and possibly necrosis and/or perforation. Bacteria may be able to translocate through an inflamed/ischemic appendiceal wall or may freely enter the peritoneal cavity through a perforation. If the infectious process is able to be contained by the body's immune or inflammatory response, a localized phenomenon such as abscess or phlegmon may develop. However, if free perforation occurs, diffuse peritonitis may result.

→ CLINICAL FEATURES

1. Symptoms:

1) Abdominal pain is the most common presenting symptom. In early appendicitis the patient typically has poorly localized discomfort in the periumbilical region. As peritonitis develops, the pain may localize, most frequently to the right iliac fossa. In advanced pregnancy the pain may be located in the right upper quadrant due to superior displacement of the abdominal viscera by the gravid uterus. In patients with an extraperitoneal or retrocecal appendix, the pain may also occur elsewhere.

2) Anorexia is a frequent symptom. Nausea and vomiting may also occur.

2. Signs: Common vital sign abnormalities include tachycardia and fever. Local abdominal guarding (on palpation or percussion), local pain when attempting to cough, and rebound tenderness may be observed. Special signs that have been described in appendicitis include McBurney point tenderness (a point two-thirds of the distance from the umbilicus to the anterior superior iliac spine), Rovsing sign (tenderness in the right lower quadrant elicited by palpation in the left lower quadrant), obturator sign (pain when the right hip is internally rotated passively with the hip and knee flexed), and psoas sign (pain when the right hip is actively flexed with the knee extended). Pain on coughing and rebound tenderness are indicative of the development of peritonitis, which may be localized or generalized. Digital rectal examination most often shows no specific abnormalities but should be performed, as it may reveal other causes of pain.

→ DIAGNOSIS

The diagnosis of appendicitis should be considered in all patients with abdominal pain and should be established promptly to minimize the risk of progression to perforation. In the setting of clinical uncertainty it may be appropriate to admit the patient for observation and monitoring with serial assessments.

Diagnostic Tests

1. Blood tests: In 80% to 85% of cases elevated white blood cell (WBC) and neutrophil counts are observed. Other blood tests such as liver function tests and creatinine should be considered to evaluate for a different underlying cause.

2. Urinalysis: Results may be suggestive of another underlying cause of symptoms. However, microscopic hematuria and pyuria may accompany appendicitis adjacent to the ureter or bladder, and these findings should not be used to discredit the diagnosis of appendicitis.

3. Imaging studies: Computed tomography (CT) is considered the study of choice for the diagnosis of appendicitis, given its high accuracy and low rate of nondiagnostic studies. However, **ultrasonography** is often used as the initial diagnostic modality because of its availability and lack of radiation exposure or use of IV contrast. Compression ultrasonography (CUS) confirms diagnosis with high specificity if results reveal a tubular structure >6 mm in diameter that cannot be compressed, shows no peristalsis, and is surrounded by a layer of fluid (a normal appendix is often not visualized by ultrasonography). A fecalith may also be visualized on ultrasonography. Only positive results of the study are of diagnostic value. This is the preferred test in pregnant women and children. **Magnetic resonance imaging (MRI)** may also have a role in diagnosis, particularly in patients in whom radiation exposure is problematic (such as pregnant women), but its use is limited by accessibility and timeliness.

4. Diagnostic laparoscopy: In the setting of clinical uncertainty diagnostic laparoscopy may be undertaken to evaluate for evidence of appendicitis versus alternative pathology.

5. Clinical scores: The Modified Alvarado Scoring System may help in quantifying the probability of confirmed acute appendicitis.◌ It gives 2 points for the presence of right lower quadrant tenderness and elevated WBC counts and 1 point each for anorexia, nausea and vomiting, migratory pain in the right inguinal fossa, rebound tenderness in the same area, elevated temperature, and a left shift on WBC evaluation.

→ **TREATMENT**

1. The standard treatment method is **surgical appendectomy** via either laparoscopy or laparotomy. Several trials and subsequent meta-analyses have now been conducted comparing surgical therapy to nonsurgical therapy with antibiotics alone in acute uncomplicated appendicitis where no fecalith is evident. Although initial success has been reported with antibiotics alone in the majority of patients, a meaningful number of patients either fail initial medical management (~10%), or have recurrent symptoms that later require surgery (~30% within 1 year). Therefore, appendectomy remains the standard of care, with conservative treatment being a less commonly chosen option.⊘○ There is no justification to avoid analgesics before surgery for fear of obscuring symptoms or signs. To minimize the risk of surgical site infection, prior to surgery broad--spectrum IV **antibiotics** are administered, for instance, **ceftriaxone** 1 to 2 g/24 hours (50-75 mg/kg/d in children) and **metronidazole** 500 mg/12 hours (in children 15-30 mg/kg/d and a maximum of 2 g/d). If no perforation has occurred, antibiotics are not necessary after surgery. In case of perforation antibiotics are typically continued for 4 to 7 days after source control is achieved.

2. Periappendiceal abscesses should be drained. In Canada, this is most commonly done by interventional radiologists.

3. Periappendiceal phlegmons are treated with IV antibiotics in a hospital setting until general symptoms have resolved and significant reduction in the abdominal guarding in the right iliac region is observed. Oral antibiotic therapy is continued at home. Selective interval appendectomy may be performed after 8 weeks. There is accumulating data suggesting a meaningful rate of underlying malignancy in adults with perforated appendicitis and some advocate routine interval appendectomy for this reason.

1.3.5.2. Acute Infectious Diarrhea: General Considerations

→ **DEFINITION, ETIOLOGY, PATHOGENESIS**

Definition, criteria, and classification of diarrhea: →Chapter 1.5.

1. Etiologic agents: Viruses (noroviruses and other caliciviruses; rotaviruses, astroviruses, adenoviruses); bacteria (most commonly *Salmonella* spp and *Campylobacter* spp; *Escherichia coli*, *Clostridium difficile*, *Yersinia* spp, rarely *Shigella* spp; *Listeria monocytogenes*); rarely parasites (*Giardia lamblia*, *Cryptosporidium parvum*, *Cystoisospora belli* [formerly *Isospora belli*]; microsporidia).

2. Transmission: Oral route (contaminated hands, food, or water). Typically the source of infection is a sick individual or carrier.

3. Risk factors: Contact with a sick person or carrier; poor hand hygiene; consumption of food and drinking water of dubious origin (potentially contaminated); consumption of raw eggs, mayonnaise, raw or undercooked meat (*Salmonella* spp), poultry or dairy products (*Campylobacter* spp, *Salmonella* spp), seafood (noroviruses), cold meats and aged cheese (*L monocytogenes*); antibiotic treatment (*C difficile*); traveling to endemic areas (cholera) and developing countries (traveler's diarrhea); achlorhydria or gastric mucosal damage (eg, drug-induced); immunodeficiency.

4. Incubation and contagious period: The incubation period lasts a few hours or days. Shedding of the pathogen in feces may continue from a few days to a few months (eg, in the case of *Salmonella* spp carriers).

→ **CLINICAL FEATURES AND NATURAL HISTORY**

1. Classification of infectious diarrhea based on pathogenesis:
1) Type I: Enterotoxin-related (eg, enterotoxigenic *E coli* [ETEC]).
2) Type II: Inflammatory (eg, *C difficile*).
3) Type III: Invasive (eg, *Salmonella* spp, *Shigella* spp, *L monocytogenes*).

2. Clinical manifestations: Various syndromes may occasionally overlap:
1) **Acute gastroenteritis** (the most frequent manifestation): Starts with vomiting, which is followed by the development of nonbloody diarrhea without pus and mucus. Patients are at risk of significant dehydration.
2) **Bloody diarrhea (dysentery):** The dominant clinical features are diarrhea with fresh blood in stools and abdominal cramping. It may be caused by *Shigella* spp or *Salmonella* spp, enteroinvasive *E coli* (EIEC), or amebiasis.
3) **Dysentery syndrome:** Frequent small-volume bowel movements containing fresh blood or pus and large quantities of mucus, painful and unproductive urge to defecate, and severe abdominal cramping.
4) **Typhoid syndrome (enteric fever):** The dominant features are high-grade fever (39°C-40°C), headache, abdominal pain, and relative bradycardia (pulse <100 beats/min with a fever >39°C), which may be accompanied by diarrhea or constipation.

3. Other signs and symptoms: Abdominal pain, nausea and vomiting, fever, signs and symptoms of dehydration (the most important and most common complication of acute diarrhea), abdominal tenderness, altered mental status (caused by infection [eg, with *Salmonella* spp] or dehydration).

4. Natural history: In the majority of patients the disease has a mild course and resolves spontaneously after a few days. A chronic (>1 year) carrier status develops in <1% patients with *Salmonella* spp infection (rates are higher in patients treated with antibiotics).

→ **DIAGNOSIS**

Diagnosis and treatment of infectious diarrhea: →Figure 1-11. Diagnostic tests are not necessary in the majority of cases, particularly in individuals treated on an outpatient basis. Assess the severity of dehydration in each patient (→Chapter 1.5).

Diagnostic Tests

1. Laboratory tests:
1) **Biochemical tests** (performed in severely ill or significantly dehydrated patients treated with intravenous fluids) may reveal hypernatremia or hyponatremia (isotonic dehydration is most frequent), hypokalemia, hypocalcemia, hypomagnesemia, metabolic acidosis, and increased levels of urea/blood urea nitrogen (prerenal acute kidney injury).
2) **Fecal leukocyte test** (a smear of a freshly collected stool specimen stained with 0.5% methylene blue): The presence of ≥5 leukocytes in a high-power field indicates inflammatory or invasive diarrhea (in the case of amebiasis despite dysentery no neutrophils are found in stool but erythrocytes are present). The test should be performed on a fresh stool sample.
3) **Fecal lactoferrin:** A positive result is suggestive of inflammatory or invasive diarrhea of a bacterial etiology (there is no need for urgent shipment of the stool samples to the laboratory as lactoferrin is released by disintegrating neutrophils).

2. Stool microbiology: Bacterial cultures (may be repeated a few times because pathogen shedding is not continuous), in justified cases followed by parasitology and virology studies. Indications for microbiological stool testing

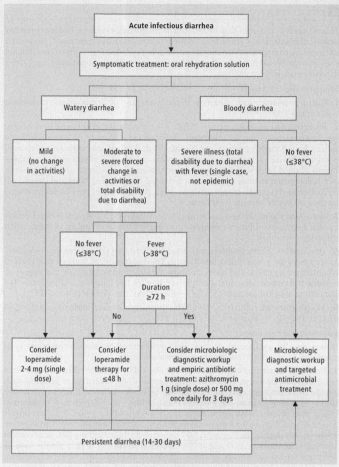

Figure 1-11. Management algorithm in patients with infectious diarrhea.

include dysentery, high numbers of neutrophils in stools or positive test results for fecal lactoferrin, severe diarrhea with severe dehydration and fever, suspected nosocomial diarrhea, diarrhea persisting for >2 weeks, extraintestinal signs and symptoms (eg, arthritis in *Salmonella* spp, *Campylobacter* spp, *Shigella* spp, or *Yersinia* spp infections), epidemiologic reasons (eg, epidemiologic investigation; suspicion of cholera, typhoid fever, or type A, B, or C paratyphoid fever; testing for the possible carrier status in carriers and convalescents with a history of cholera, typhoid fever, paratyphoid fever, salmonellosis, or shigellosis, as well as in individuals who may be at risk of infecting others due to their occupation).

Differential Diagnosis

Other causes of acute diarrhea (→Chapter 1.5).

→ TREATMENT

The majority of patients may be treated on an outpatient basis. **Indications for hospitalization** may include need for intravenous fluid treatment, suspected bacteremia, complications of infectious diarrhea, enteric fever syndrome (typhoid fever; paratyphoid fever A, B, or C), immunocompromised patients, and stays in areas endemic for cholera.

Symptomatic Treatment

1. Fluid replacement therapy is the mainstay of symptomatic treatment (→Chapter 1.5).

2. Nutritional management: After a successful fluid therapy (3-4 hours) resume oral nutrition as tolerated. A potential diet may be based on foods rich in boiled starch (rice, pasta, potatoes) and on groats, with an addition of crackers, bananas, natural yoghurt, soups, and boiled meats and vegetables. Spices should be avoided if they are not tolerated. Patients should consume meals according to their preferences but avoid heavy, fried foods and sweetened milk. Frequent smaller meals are beneficial. A regular diet may be reintroduced as soon as stools become well formed.

3. Antidiarrheal drugs: Loperamide (→Chapter 1.5). Antidiarrheal drugs should be reserved for the second-line therapy and avoided in patients with infectious diarrhea.

4. Probiotics: Some probiotics (*Lactobacillus casei* GG, *Saccharomyces boulardii*) may be a beneficial addition to the treatment of watery diarrhea of a confirmed or suspected viral etiology. Oral administration of one sachet or capsule bid reduces the duration of diarrhea by 1 to 2 days.◔◕ Probiotics are not effective in inflammatory and invasive diarrhea (types II and III).

5. Management of other disturbances (metabolic acidosis, electrolyte disturbances): →Chapter 4.

Antimicrobial Treatment

Indications for antimicrobial treatment are limited because in the majority of cases infectious diarrhea resolves spontaneously.

1. Empiric antimicrobial treatment should be considered in patients with traveler's diarrhea and while awaiting results of stool cultures in patients with severe inflammatory diarrhea (associated with fever, painful urge to defecate, blood or leukocytes in stools, positive results of fecal lactoferrin test, ie, features typical for infection with *Salmonella* spp, *Campylobacter jejuni*, *Yersinia* spp, or *Shigella* spp). Use an oral **quinolone** for 3 to 5 days (ciprofloxacin 750 mg once daily or 500 mg bid, norfloxacin 800 mg once daily or 400 mg bid, or ofloxacin 400 mg once daily or 200 mg bid) or **azithromycin** (1 g in a single dose or 500 mg/d for 3 days). Do not use these agents in afebrile patients with dysentery, as it may have been caused by enterohemorrhagic *E coli* (EHEC) (→below).

2. Targeted antimicrobial treatment:

1) *Salmonella* spp (other than *Salmonella typhi*): Treatment is not indicated in patients with asymptomatic or mild infection; however, it should be started in patients with severe disease, sepsis, or risk factors for extraintestinal infection (→Complications, below). Use oral ciprofloxacin (dosage as above) for 5 to 7 days; alternatively use azithromycin 1 g followed by 500 mg once daily for 6 days or a third-generation cephalosporin (eg, ceftriaxone 1-2 g/d).

2) *S typhi*: Use a fluoroquinolone for 10 to 14 days (ciprofloxacin as above, norfloxacin 400 mg bid); alternatively use azithromycin 1 g followed by 500 mg once daily for 6 days or a third-generation cephalosporin (eg, ceftriaxone 1-2 g/d). Rise in quinolone resistance and multiresistant isolates from South East Asia and Africa must be taken into account based on the patient's travel history.

3) *C jejuni*: Use azithromycin (1 g in a single dose or 500 mg once daily for 3 days) or a fluoroquinolone for 5 days (eg, ciprofloxacin, norfloxacin as above).

4) *Shigella* spp: Use a fluoroquinolone bid for 3 days (ciprofloxacin 500 mg, ofloxacin 300 mg, or norfloxacin 400 mg); alternatively use azithromycin 500 mg in a single dose followed by 250 mg once daily for 4 days or a third--generation cephalosporin (eg, ceftriaxone 1-2 g/d).

5) *E coli*:

   a) ETEC, enteropathogenic *E coli* (EPEC), and EIEC, as well as *Aeromonas* spp and *Plesiomonas* spp: Use sulfamethoxazole/trimethoprim 960 mg or a fluoroquinolone bid for 3 days (eg, ofloxacin 300 mg, ciprofloxacin 500 mg, norfloxacin 400 mg).

   b) Enteroaggregative *E coli* strains (EAggEC): Generally antimicrobial treatment is not recommended as the effects are unknown.

   c) EHEC: Avoid drugs that may inhibit peristalsis and antibiotics because of their undetermined role in the treatment and a risk of hemolytic-uremic syndrome.

6) *Yersinia* spp: Antibiotics are usually not necessary. In patients with severe infection or bacteremia, use doxycycline combined with an aminoglycoside, sulfamethoxazole/trimethoprim, or a third-generation cephalosporin.

7) *Vibrio cholerae* strains O1 or O139: Ciprofloxacin 1 g once daily, alternatively doxycycline 300 mg once daily or sulfamethoxazole/trimethoprim (160 mg trimethoprim) bid for 3 days.

8) *L monocytogenes*: Usually no treatment is required as the infection is self-limiting. If it persists or in the case of an immunocompromised host, use oral amoxicillin 500 mg tid or sulfamethoxazole/trimethoprim (160 mg trimethoprim) bid for 7 days.

9) *Giardia lamblia*: Acceptable options include oral metronidazole 250 mg tid for 5 to 7 days, oral tinidazole as a single dose of 2 g, or nitazoxanide 500 mg bid for 3 days. In pregnant patients use oral paromomycin 10 mg/kg tid for 5 to 10 days.

10) *Cryptosporidium* spp: In patients with severe infection, use paromomycin 500 mg tid for 7 days.

11) *Cystoisospora (Isospora)* spp, *Cyclospora* spp: Use sulfamethoxazole/trimethoprim (160 mg trimethoprim) bid for 7 to 10 days; this is not recommended in patients with microsporidia infections.

→ COMPLICATIONS

Complications depend on etiology and include:

1) Hemorrhagic colitis (EHEC, *Shigella* spp, *Vibrio parahaemolyticus*, *Campylobacter* spp, *Salmonella* spp).

2) Toxic megacolon, intestinal perforation (EHEC, *Shigella* spp, *C difficile*, *Campylobacter* spp, *Salmonella* spp, *Yersinia* spp).

3) Hemolytic-uremic syndrome (EHEC serotype O157:H7 and *Shigella* spp, rarely *Campylobacter* spp).

4) Reactive arthritis (*Shigella* spp, *Salmonella* spp, *Campylobacter* spp, *Yersinia* spp).

5) Postinfectious irritable bowel syndrome (*Campylobacter* spp, *Shigella* spp, *Salmonella* spp).

6) Distant localized extraintestinal infections (meningitis, encephalitis, osteitis, arthritis, wound infection, cholecystitis, abscesses in various organs) or sepsis (*Salmonella* spp, *Yersinia* spp, rarely *Campylobacter* spp or *Shigella* spp). Risk factors are age <6 months or >50 years, prosthetic implants, congenital or acquired heart disease, severe atherosclerosis, malignancy, uremia,

immunodeficiency, diabetes mellitus, and iron overload (increased risk of severe infection with certain pathogens, including *Yersinia* spp, *Listeria monocytogenes*, *Vibrio cholera*, *E coli*).

7) Malnutrition and cachexia (various pathogens).

8) Guillain-Barré syndrome (*C jejuni*).

▶ PROGNOSIS

In the majority of patients the prognosis is good. However, elderly patients are at risk of severe disease and death.

▶ PREVENTION

The key prevention measures include:

1) Good hand hygiene: Thorough hand washing with soap and water after defecation, after changing soiled diapers, after any contact with toilet/washroom facilities, before meal preparation and consumption, after handling raw meat and eggs.

2) Regular sanitary inspections, adherence to food and water safety guidelines (concerning both production and distribution).

3) Mandatory notification of local public health authorities for reportable pathogens (may vary among jurisdictions), epidemiologic vigilance, identification of sources of infection (epidemiologic investigations).

4) Carrier status testing in carriers if applicable based on public health regulations.

1.3.5.3. Antibiotic-Associated Diarrhea

▶ DEFINITION, ETIOLOGY, PATHOGENESIS

Antibiotic-associated diarrhea develops in the course of antimicrobial treatment or within 2 months of its discontinuation.

1. Etiologic agents: Antibiotic treatment has a direct influence on the gastrointestinal tract and induces quantitative and qualitative changes in the intestinal flora, which lead to impaired digestion and metabolism of some nutrients (this is nonspecific antibiotic-associated diarrhea, accounting for 70%-80% of cases). The disease may also be caused by selection of antibiotic-resistant bacterial strains, predominantly *Clostridium difficile* strains producing toxin B (15%-25% of cases, associated with the most severe disease) or rarely other bacteria (~3% of cases: *Klebsiella oxytoca*, enterotoxic strains of *Staphylococcus aureus*, *Clostridium perfringens* type A).

2. Epidemiology: The disease occurs in up to 30% of patients receiving antibiotics. Regarding **risk factors**, the risk of antibiotic-associated diarrhea is higher in patients treated with cephalosporins, amoxicillin/clavulanic acid, ampicillin and other semisynthetic broad-spectrum penicillins, clindamycin, fluoroquinolones, patients receiving long-term treatment (>4 weeks), and patients with multiple comorbidities. The route of antibiotic administration (oral vs parenteral) does not influence the risk. Risk factors for *C difficile* infection: →Chapter 6.1.3.5.5.

▶ CLINICAL FEATURES AND TREATMENT

Most commonly a nonspecific mild diarrhea that resolves after discontinuation of the antimicrobial agent. In some patients the disease is more severe, requiring IV fluid therapy and discontinuation of the antimicrobial agent or agents.

Severe colitis (including pseudomembranous colitis caused by *C difficile*) may develop. Diagnosis and treatment: →Chapter 6.1.3.5.5.

→**PREVENTION**

1. Judicious use of antimicrobial agents is of crucial importance.

2. Probiotics: Consider administration of probiotics in children and adults aged <65 years throughout the entire duration of antimicrobial treatment (usually 7-10 days).⊘⊖ In pediatric population the available data suggest the use of *Saccharomyces boulardii* and *Lactobacillus rhamnosus* may be an appropriate strategy.

1.3.5.4. Bacterial Food Poisoning

→**DEFINITION, ETIOLOGY, PATHOGENESIS**

Food poisoning refers to signs and symptoms caused by consumption of food contaminated with bacteria or bacterial toxins. It may be also due to certain parasites and chemicals.

1. Etiologic agents: Predominantly *Salmonella* spp and *Campylobacter* spp or bacterial exotoxins (produced by *Staphylococcus aureus*, rarely by *Clostridium perfringens*, *Bacillus cereus*, *Clostridium botulinum* [→Chapter 8.3.1]).

2. Risk factors: Consumption of boiled and fried rice, boiled beef, grilled chicken (*B cereus*); creams (*S aureus*, *B cereus*); pastries and cakes (including ice cream and cakes filled with cream), milk and dairy products (*S aureus*, *Salmonella* spp, *Yersinia enterocolitica*, *Escherichia coli*, *Listeria monocytogenes*, *Campylobacter* spp, *Shigella* spp); chocolate (*Y enterocolitica*); pork, ham (*S aureus*, *Y enterocolitica*, *Salmonella* spp); raw or undercooked beef (*E coli* [particularly strain O157:H7], *Campylobacter* spp, *L monocytogenes*, *C perfringens*); turkey, chicken (*Salmonella* spp, *Campylobacter* spp, *L monocytogenes*, *C perfringens*); raw vegetables (*L monocytogenes*); salads (*E coli*, *Shigella* spp); raw eggs, raw or undercooked meat (*Salmonella* spp).

3. Incubation period ranges from a few hours (eg, *S aureus*, *B cereus*, *L monocytogenes*, *E coli*) to a few days (eg, *Campylobacter* spp, *Yersinia* spp).

→**CLINICAL FEATURES**

Signs and symptoms have a sudden onset and include nausea, vomiting, and diarrhea (usually of moderate intensity, may contain blood). Other symptoms may include asthenia, abdominal cramping, fever, and malaise. The patient's history indicates consumption of contaminated food, attendance of a social event with catering, or cases of diarrhea among other individuals who consumed the same foods. The diarrhea is usually short-lasting, resolves spontaneously, and in the majority of cases is associated with good prognosis. Also →Chapter 8.3.1.

→**DIAGNOSIS**

Diagnosis is confirmed upon isolating a pathogen from a stool sample or a toxin from a suspected food sample (→Chapter 8.3.1).

→**TREATMENT AND PREVENTION**

Treatment and prevention are the same as in acute infectious diarrhea. Notification of appropriate epidemiologic authorities and securing samples of the suspicious food for testing may be mandatory.

1.3.5.5. *Clostridium (Clostridioides) difficile* Infection

→ **DEFINITION, ETIOLOGY, PATHOGENESIS**

The clinical presentation of *Clostridium* (now *Clostridioides*) *difficile* infection (CDI) ranges from mild diarrheal disease to fulminant colitis with septic shock. Asymptomatic carriers may be a reservoir of the disease.

Pseudomembranous colitis is an acute diarrhea with typical yellow-grey plaques (pseudomembranes) developing on the surface of the mucosa of the large intestine (one of the more severe forms of antibiotic-associated diarrhea).

1. Etiologic agents: Toxin A and toxin B produced by *C difficile*, a spore- -forming, anaerobic, gram-positive bacilli.

2. Reservoir and transmission: Soil, environment (especially hospitals, long-term medical care institutions, daycare facilities), and individuals with *C difficile* carriage (5% of adults, more often the elderly; up to 50% of newborns and infants) are an important reservoir for environmental contamination, with or without an underlying clinical infection. Transmission occurs via the fecal-oral route by ingesting the spore form of the organisms.

3. Risk factors: The most significant risk factor for CDI is current or recent (up to 2 months prior to disease onset) antibiotic treatment, especially with clindamycin, cephalosporins, broad-spectrum penicillins, or fluoroquinolones. Additional identified risk factors are recent hospitalization, advanced age, and serious comorbidities. Some other risk factors include gastrointestinal surgery, chemotherapy, inflammatory bowel disease (IBD), and gastric acid suppression (proton pump inhibitors [PPIs] and H_2-receptor antagonists).

4. Recurrence of infection: Recurrence is defined as complete resolution of CDI symptoms followed by the subsequent development of CDI symptoms within 8 weeks after the onset of a previous episode. Up to 25% of patients have recurrent CDI within 30 days of treatment. After ≥2 recurrences the risk for further recurrences is >60%.

→ **CLINICAL FEATURES AND NATURAL HISTORY**

The **dominant clinical feature** is diarrhea of varying intensity, ranging from 3 loose stools up to 30 watery stools over 24 hours; fresh blood may be occasionally present in stools. Lower abdominal cramping and fever may also be present. In more severe cases patients may develop dehydration, ileus, and shock. Approximately 15% of patients with a milder form of CDI recover spontaneously, particularly when the causative antibiotic is discontinued. Patients with severe CDI may develop ileus of the colon or toxic megacolon (→Chapter 6.1.3.7.2) with minimal to no diarrhea.

Severe complicated CDI (defined as CDI leading to intensive care unit [ICU] admission), colectomy, or death occurs in 3% to 20% of patients. Some indicators of a more severe disease include high fever (38.5°C), markedly increased white blood cell count (>15,000), low albumin levels (<30 g/L), increased creatinine levels (a 50% increase from the premorbid level or levels ≥133 µmol/L), and advanced age (≥65 years).

→ **DIAGNOSIS**

Diagnostic Tests

1. Laboratory assays: Establishing the diagnosis of CDI **requires the presence of toxins or a toxigenic strain of *C difficile*** in a liquid stool sample shown using enzyme immunoassay (EIA) testing or polymerase chain reaction (PCR). Stool samples from symptomatic patients only should be sent for laboratory testing, as the currently available laboratory assays cannot

Table 1-6. Characteristics of laboratory tests used in the diagnosis of *Clostridium* (*Clostridioides*) *difficile* infection

Test	Target	Sensitivity	Specificity	NPV	PPV	Turnaround time
EIA	Toxins A + B	60%	98%	Low	High	20-90 min
GDH	Common antigen	90%	50%	High	Low	20-90 min
NAAT (PCR, LAMP)	Toxin B gene	90%	65%	High	Low	90-200 min

GDH, glutamate dehydrogenase; LAMP, loop-mediated isothermal amplification; NAAT, nucleic acid amplification test; NPV, negative predictive value; PCR, polymerase chain reaction; PPV, positive predictive value.

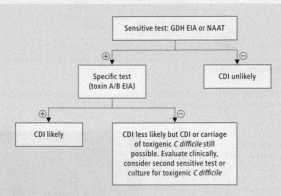

⊕ Positive result. ⊖ Negative result.

CDI, *Clostridium difficile* infection; EIA, enzyme immunoassay; GDH, glutamate dehydrogenase; NAAT, nucleic acid amplification test.

Figure 1-12. Testing for *Clostridium* (*Clostridioides*) *difficile* infection: glutamate dehydrogenase or nucleic acid amplification test. *Adapted from Clin Microbiol Infect. 2016;22 Suppl 4:S63-81.*

distinguish between infection and asymptomatic carriage of *C difficile*. Given that no single test has sufficiently high negative and positive predictive values, results of the laboratory tests must be interpreted only when the clinical context is consistent with CDI. Approximate characteristics of currently available tests: →Table 1-6.

One approach is to use an algorithm of screening the stool sample with a sensitive test (eg, EIA for the detection of the common antigen glutamate dehydrogenase [GDH]) or a nucleic amplification test (NAAT) and, if positive, proceed to test the sample with more specific EIA testing to detect toxins directly (→Figure 1-12). The other possibility is to perform both sensitive and specific tests simultaneously (eg, GDH and EIA for toxins) and if results are discrepant, do another sensitive test (NAAT; →Figure 1-13). Of note, clinical context and judgment are always needed, especially with discrepant test results, as mild CDI or carriage of toxigenic *C difficile* is possible. Toxigenic culture of the stool sample may provide additional information.

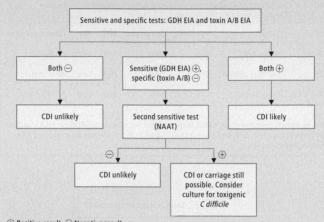

⊕ Positive result. ⊖ Negative result.

CDI, *Clostridium difficile* infection; EIA, enzyme immunoassay; GDH, glutamate dehydrogenase; NAAT, nucleic acid amplification test.

Figure 1-13. Testing for *Clostridium* (*Clostridioides*) *difficile* infection: glutamate dehydrogenase and toxin A/B. *Adapted from Clin Microbiol Infect. 2016;22 Suppl 4:S63-81.*

2. Colonoscopy reveals pseudo-membranes, which are characteristic whitish-yellow, yellowish-golden, or honey-colored plaques ranging from a few millimeters to 1 to 2 centimeters in diameter (→Figure 1-14). They are relatively evenly distributed over the mucosa of the rectum and distal sigmoid colon; in ~30% of patients the lesions develop exclusively in the ascending colon. Pseudomembranes may not be apparent in patients with immunodeficiency or IBD.

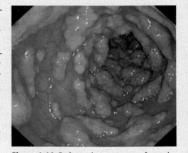

Figure 1-14. Endoscopic appearance of pseudomembranous colitis.

Diagnostic Criteria

The diagnosis of CDI consists of a combination of symptoms and one of the following:

1) Colonoscopic or histopathologic evidence of pseudomembranous colitis.
2) A stool sample positive for toxins or toxigenic *C difficile*, including the toxin gene detected by the NAAT.

Differential Diagnosis

Diarrhea of another etiology (→Chapter 1.5); this diagnosis can be confirmed by medical history and microbiology results. Ulcerative colitis may be differentiated from pseudomembranous colitis caused by CDI based on the persistent presence of fresh blood in stools, lack of laboratory evidence of CDI, and (predominantly) distinct microscopic appearance of mucosal lesions. Other causes of pseudomembranous colitis are collagenous colitis and infections due to *Campylobacter*, *Salmonella*, *Strongyloides*, and cytomegalovirus.

→ TREATMENT

Nonpharmacologic Management

1. Mild CDI: If possible, discontinuation of the implicated antimicrobial agent causing diarrhea. If continued treatment of the primary infection is necessary, switch to an alternative antibiotic that is not as strongly associated with pseudomembranous colitis (eg, an aminoglycoside, doxycycline, a macrolide).

2. More severe CDI: Hospitalization is necessary to administer IV fluids, correct electrolyte disturbances, monitor the patient, and prevent complications.

Pharmacotherapy

1. The initial episode or first recurrence of severe forms of CDI, including pseudomembranous colitis:

1) Oral **vancomycin** 125 mg qid for 10 days; this is used in patients with severe CDI, in case of intolerance or ineffectiveness of metronidazole, and in pregnant or breastfeeding women. In patients with **fulminant colitis and toxic megacolon**, consider combined treatment with vancomycin 500 mg qid given orally or via an enteral tube (in patients with bowel obstruction the drug may be administered in enemas 250 mg qid) and IV metronidazole 500 mg tid.

2) Oral **fidaxomicin** 200 mg bid for 10 days. Use may be limited by the relatively high cost of the drug. The rate of clinical cure is similar for vancomycin and fidaxomicin; however, the rate of recurrence may be reduced by 50% with fidaxomicin for non–North American Pulsed Field type 1 (NAP1) strains.◔

3) Oral **metronidazole** 500 mg tid for 10 days for mild to moderate disease (without features of severe disease), or in severe disease only if vancomycin and fidaxomicin are not available or cannot be used. The cost of metronidazole in some jurisdictions may be significantly lower than that of vancomycin and even lower than the cost of fidaxomicin, with the absolute failure rate higher by ~1 per 10 treated patients.◔

2. Fulminant CDI with hypotension, ileus, or megacolon: Oral **vancomycin** 500 mg qid or via a nasogastric tube or 500 mg rectally in 100 mL normal saline qid plus IV **metronidazole** 500 mg every 8 hours.

3. Second episode of CDI or subsequent recurrent CDI: Vancomycin as a prolonged tapered and/or pulsed regimen (eg, 125 mg given orally qid for 10-14 days; 125 mg given orally tid for a week; 125 mg given orally bid for a week; 125 mg given orally once daily for a week and then every 2 or 3 days for 2-8 weeks).

Approximately 50% of patients with multiple recurrent CDI respond to a tapering vancomycin regimen. An alternative to antibiotic therapy for recurrent CDI is **fecal microbiota transplantation (FMT)**, which replenishes the protective colonic microbiota to prevent future episodes of CDI. Patients who have had ≥2 recurrences of CDI and received ≥1 course of a tapering vancomycin regimen may benefit from FMT.

The effects of systemic glucocorticoids in patients with severe pseudomembranous colitis are unknown. Do not administer drugs that reduce peristalsis (loperamide, opioids).

Surgical Treatment

In patients with fulminant CDI, **colectomy**, if performed at an early stage of fulminant colitis, can be life-saving. Laboratory parameters suggestive of fulminant CDI include white blood cell counts >50×10^9/L and serum lactate levels >5.0 mmol/L. The usual practice is subtotal colectomy. However, a retrospective study comparing subtotal colectomy to a colon-sparing procedure of diverting loop ileostomy showed a mortality benefit with loop ileostomy at 19% versus 50% in historical controls and preservation of the colon in >90% of patients treated this way.◔

→ **FOLLOW-UP**

Treatment may be considered effective if abnormal temperature normalizes within 24 to 48 hours and diarrhea resolves within 4 to 5 days. In more severe cases repeated abdominal radiographs should be performed to exclude toxic megacolon. Follow-up testing for *C difficile* toxins is not recommended as there is no laboratory test of cure. Reappearance of signs and symptoms within 8 weeks of onset of a previous CDI episode suggests recurrence of the infection. Patients with suspected recurrence of CDI should be managed according to the clinical presentation.

→ **COMPLICATIONS**

Complications of CDI include fulminant colitis and toxic megacolon (→Chapter 6.1.3.7.2), adynamic ileus, colonic perforation and peritonitis, and edema due to hypoalbuminemia caused by intestinal protein loss.

→ **PREVENTION**

Judicious use of antimicrobial agents.

In hospitals, long-term medical care institutions, and daycare facilities it is necessary to:

1) Follow strict hand hygiene rules (washing hands with soap and water whenever possible).
2) Isolate and implement contact precautions for CDI patients.
3) Wear gown and disposable gloves when caring for CDI patients.
4) Use designated equipment.
5) Use agents effective against *C difficile* spores to disinfect rooms and bathrooms.
6) Properly dispose of used diapers, particularly in the case of CDI patients and carriers of *C difficile*.

1.3.5.6. Gastrointestinal Infections in Immunocompromised Patients

→ **ETIOLOGY AND PATHOGENESIS**

The most frequent sign of gastrointestinal (GI) infection in immunocompromised patients is chronic diarrhea.

Etiologic agents:

1) Viruses: Cytomegalovirus (CMV), herpes simplex virus (HSV), adenoviruses, noroviruses (previously known as Norwalk virus), rotaviruses, and other.
2) Bacteria: *Mycobacterium avium* complex (MAC), *Mycobacterium tuberculosis*, *Clostridium difficile*, *Salmonella* spp, *Shigella* spp, *Campylobacter jejuni*, bacterial overgrowth syndrome.
3) Protozoa: Microsporidia, *Cryptosporidium parvum*, *Cystoisospora belli* (formerly *Isospora belli*), *Giardia intestinalis*, *Entamoeba histolytica*, *Blastocystis hominis*, *Cyclospora* spp, *Toxoplasma gondii*, *Pneumocystis jiroveci* (previously *carinii*), *Leishmania donovani*.
4) Fungi: *Candida albicans*, *Cryptococcus neoformans*, *Histoplasma capsulatum*, *Coccidioides immitis*.

The predominant etiologic agents depend on the type of immunodeficiency (→Chapter 2.5); for instance, the most common pathogens in HIV-infected patients are mycobacteria (predominantly MAC), cryptosporidia, microsporidia, and CMV.

→ CLINICAL FEATURES AND DIAGNOSIS

Frequent diarrhea, usually chronic (→Chapter 1.5).

To confirm etiology, test ≥3 stool samples (bacteriological, virological, and parasitological tests should be performed on each sample). Testing for microsporidiosis and cryptosporidiosis is indicated in significantly immunocompromised patients (CD4$^+$ cell count <0.2×10^9/L). In patients with fever and CD4$^+$ cell counts <0.1×10^9/L, mycobacterial blood culture should be performed. If stool test results do not identify the pathogen and diarrhea does not contain blood, perform upper and lower GI endoscopy. The risk of CMV infection is high in patients with CD4+ cell counts <0.1×10^9/L; in such cases perform colonoscopy and obtain mucosal biopsy specimens for histologic examination and virologic tests.

1. CMV infection: Clinical manifestations range from an asymptomatic CMV carrier status to diffuse ulcerative lesions of the colonic mucosa accompanied by abdominal pain, dysentery, and in some cases also by intestinal perforation.

Diagnosis: Lower GI endoscopy with collection of biopsy specimens for histologic examination; identification of CMV (immunohistochemical studies [characteristic viral inclusion bodies], polymerase chain reaction [PCR]) in specimens.

2. HSV infection: In patients with AIDS, HSV causes persistent chronic proctitis with painful ulcerations (also involving skin in the anal area).

Diagnosis: GI endoscopy with collection of biopsy specimens for histologic examination; detection of HSV antigens (or HSV DNA detection using PCR) in specimens.

3. Infections with intestinal bacteria: In severely immunocompromised patients infections with *Salmonella* spp and frequently also with *C jejuni* may lead to bacteremia and sepsis.

Diagnosis: Based on results of stool cultures.

4. MAC infection: White papules 1 to 3 millimeters in diameter forming in the intestinal mucosa, most frequently in the duodenum (~90% of cases); these are a result of accumulation of macrophages in the lamina propria.

Diagnosis: Diagnosis is difficult to establish and based on detection of mycobacteria in blood and stool specimens (cultures, PCR).

5. Cryptosporidiosis is caused by an intracellular protozoan *C parvum*, which typically infects jejunal enterocytes. The incubation period lasts 7 to 10 days. **Signs and symptoms** include watery diarrhea, abdominal cramping, fever, asthenia, and rarely manifestations from the biliary tract, liver, or pancreas; chronic diarrhea with a significant loss of water and electrolytes develops when the CD4$^+$ cell count falls <0.1×10^9/L.

Diagnosis: Detection of antigens (enzyme-linked immunosorbent assay [ELISA]) and oocysts (modified Ziehl-Neelsen staining) in stool samples or antibodies in serum (ELISA). Histologic examination of intestinal mucosal biopsy specimens is rarely performed.

6. Microsporidiosis is caused by various intracellular protozoa, most commonly *Enterocytozoon bieneusi* and *Encephalitozoon intestinalis*. **Signs and symptoms** include watery diarrhea, low-grade fever, asthenia, nausea, and vomiting.

Diagnosis: Detection of the protozoa by histologic examination of intestinal mucosal biopsy specimens (preferably using electron microscopy); detection of spores in stool.

7. Cystoisosporiasis: Infections in humans are caused by the protozoan *C belli*. The source of infection is water or food contaminated by oocysts. *C belli* multiplies in enterocytes of the small intestine, leading to destruction of the epithelium and intestinal villi. **Clinical features** are similar to cryptosporidiosis.

Diagnosis: Repeated microscopic examinations of stool for the presence of parasites (fecal smear, direct or stained with brilliant green).

8. Candidiasis: Candidiasis is most frequently caused by *C albicans*, *Candida krusei*, *Candida glabrata*, or *Candida tropicalis*. It affects 75% to 90% of patients with AIDS. **Signs and symptoms** include lesions that may develop on the oral mucosa (these may take 4 forms: acute pseudomembranous lesions [thrush], acute atrophic lesions, chronic hypertrophic lesions, chronic atrophic lesions), pharyngeal mucosa, and esophageal mucosa (often asymptomatic; ~50% of patients develop dysphagia and chest pain).

Diagnosis: Esophageal lesions found on endoscopy (characteristic whitish patches that adhere to the surface and may involve the entire esophagus) and oral swab/brush cytology followed by microbiological tests (culture and antifungal susceptibility profile). Isolation of the fungi in the absence of clinical features is not sufficient to diagnose fungal infection and start treatment.

→ **TREATMENT**

1. Symptomatic treatment: As in acute infectious diarrhea.

2. Antimicrobial treatment:

1) *M tuberculosis* (→Chapter 13.18.2): Combined treatment with isoniazid, rifampin (INN rifampicin), pyrazinamide, and ethambutol for 9 to 12 months.

2) **MAC** (→Chapter 13.18.1): Multidrug therapy of symptomatic infection for 9 to 12 months.

3) **CMV**: IV ganciclovir 5 mg/kg every 12 hours (or valganciclovir 900 mg orally bid) as the first-line therapy. An alternative therapy is IV foscarnet 60 mg/kg over 1 hour every 8 hours for 14 to 28 days.

4) **HSV**: Acyclovir (INN aciclovir) 200 mg orally 5 times a day for 5 to 10 days, valacyclovir 1 g orally bid, or famciclovir 500 mg orally tid.

5) *Cryptosporidium* spp: Paromomycin for 14 to 28 days.

6) *Cyclospora* spp: Sulfamethoxazole/trimethoprim or ciprofloxacin for 14 to 28 days.

7) *C belli*: Sulfamethoxazole/trimethoprim, ciprofloxacin, or pyrimethamine for 14 to 28 days.

8) *E intestinalis*: Albendazole. *E bieneusi*: Fumagillin is the drug of choice. Alternative agents include metronidazole and atovaquone. Therapy lasts 14 to 28 days.

9) *Candida* spp: In patients with mild oral candidiasis use nystatin 200,000 to 600,000 IU qid for 7 to 14 days. In patients with moderate or severe candidiasis use oral fluconazole 100 to 200 mg/d for 7 to 14 days (if ineffective, use oral itraconazole, voriconazole, or amphotericin B; IV administration may be considered in patients with recurrent candidiasis). In patients with pharyngeal candidiasis use oral fluconazole 200 to 400 mg/d (in the case of intolerance, administer IV fluconazole; in patients resistant to fluconazole use itraconazole, posaconazole, or voriconazole).

1.3.5.7. Nosocomial Diarrhea

→ **DEFINITION, ETIOLOGY, PATHOGENESIS**

Nosocomial diarrhea refers to diarrhea that develops during a hospital stay or up to 3 days after discharge. Nosocomial diarrhea is typically noninfectious and caused by adverse effects of drugs, enteral feeding with hyperosmotic liquid formulas, or surgery of the gastrointestinal tract. The infectious etiology of nosocomial diarrhea in hospitalized adults is predominantly related to *Clostridium difficile* (responsible for 90% of cases of diarrhea developing within 3 days of hospital admission; →Chapter 6.1.3.5.5).

→ CLINICAL FEATURES AND DIAGNOSIS

Start by excluding or confirming infectious etiology of diarrhea. The infectious etiology should be suspected if the diarrhea occurs in a patient treated with antibiotics (even up to 2 months after the treatment) and is associated with fever, vomiting, and abdominal cramping, or manifests as an epidemic of acute gastroenteritis limited to a particular hospital ward (norovirus infection).

Do not perform routine diagnostics of bacterial infections other than those caused by *C difficile* (results are usually negative), except for hospital epidemics of inflammatory diarrhea or dysentery and patients in whom *C difficile* infection was excluded.

→ TREATMENT AND PREVENTION

Treatment and prevention of *C difficile* infection: →Chapter 6.1.3.5.5.

1.3.5.8. Traveler's Diarrhea

→ DEFINITION, ETIOLOGY, PATHOGENESIS

Traveler's diarrhea refers to signs and symptoms caused by ingestion of food or water contaminated with pathogens. It develops in individuals traveling to regions with poor hygiene and sanitary standards, although in some patients it may be due to travel-related dietary changes or stress.

1. Etiologic agents vary with geographic regions. Approximately 80% of cases are caused by bacteria, predominantly enterotoxigenic *Escherichia coli* and *Campylobacter* spp.

2. Epidemiology (risk of developing the disease depends on the region):

1) **Low risk** (<8% of visiting individuals develop the disease within 1-2 weeks): Japan, Australia, New Zealand, Northern and Western Europe, Canada, the United States.

2) **Moderate risk** (10%-20%): Central and Eastern Europe, Portugal, Greece, the Balkans, Russia, China, Israel, South Africa, Pacific Islands, most of the Caribbean islands, Argentina and Chile, Thailand.

3) **High risk** (20%-56%): Africa, Latin America, South Asia, Middle East.

3. Reservoir, transmission, incubation, and contagious period: →Chapter 6.1.3.5.2.

→ TREATMENT

Treatment is the same as in acute infectious diarrhea. Self-administration of antibiotic therapy is recommended in travelers with moderate or severe diarrhea (≥3 loose stools within 24 hours with other intestinal signs and symptoms) as well as in patients not responding to symptomatic treatment. Since the resistance of *Campylobacter* spp to fluoroquinolones is frequently observed in Asia, the drug of choice in empiric treatment used in this region is **azithromycin** (1 g in a single dose or 500 mg once daily for 3 days). Selected patients—such as those with a limited ability to tolerate dehydration or infection, for instance, immunocompromised hosts, and patients traveling to remote destinations where access to health-care providers is limited—could be prescribed all the necessary drugs prior to departure and could be provided with a written self-treatment strategy in case of infection (→below) as well as guidelines for seeking medical attention when necessary.

→ PREVENTION

1. Hand hygiene and food safety (these are of key importance):

1) Washing hands prior to food preparation and consumption.

2) Avoiding food and water from dubious sources (eg, from street vendors and food stands).

3) Washing and peeling fruit and vegetables, avoiding raw salads.

4) Drinking only bottled water from a known source or carbonated drinks (eg, cola, beer).

5) Consuming only hot (steaming) food (with the exception of jams/preserves, syrups, honey) and drinking hot beverages. Avoiding sauces/dressings stored at room temperatures.

6) Avoiding drinks served with ice.

2. Prophylactic antimicrobial treatment should be considered in patients at high risk for severe bacterial diarrhea and its complications (with achlorhydria, receiving treatment that reduces or neutralizes gastric acid secretion, after gastrectomy, with prosthetic implants, immunodeficiency, irritable bowel syndrome, sickle cell anemia) and those unable to tolerate diarrhea (athletes, individuals on short business trips) who are traveling to high-risk areas:

1) Oral **rifaximin** 200 mg bid or 400 mg once daily with main meals for the entire duration of stay in a high-risk area. The drug is not absorbed from the gastrointestinal tract, is well tolerated, and rarely causes adverse effects. Rifaximin is effective predominantly against enterotoxigenic *E coli* and enteroaggregative *E coli*, but its effectiveness against enteroinvasive bacteria has not been established (if diarrhea occurs in the course of treatment, assume it has been caused by invasive bacteria and administer azithromycin).

2) An oral **fluoroquinolone**, for instance, ciprofloxacin 500 to 750 mg once daily for the entire duration of stay in a high-risk area. The drug is effective against the majority of bacteria responsible for traveler's diarrhea (however, a high percentage of *Campylobacter* strains in Asia are resistant to fluoroquinolones). Patients receiving oral fluoroquinolones are at risk for adverse effects (including diarrhea and pseudomembranous colitis caused by *Clostridium difficile*).

3) Bismuth subsalicylate 2 tablets qid.

1.3.6. Gastrointestinal Obstruction

→ CLINICAL FEATURES AND NATURAL HISTORY

Symptoms of acute gastrointestinal obstruction may include:

1) Abdominal pain.

2) Nausea and vomiting.

3) Retention of gas and stools.

Causes of gastrointestinal obstruction can be broadly characterized as being mechanical or functional in nature. Regardless of the cause, impairment of intestinal transit leads to increase in intestinal secretion and decrease in intestinal reabsorption of fluids. This often results in hypovolemia, which is further exacerbated by diminished oral intake and/or vomiting. Patients with adynamic ileus or mechanical obstruction in whom effective treatment is not started may develop dehydration, hypotension, shock, multiple organ failure, and death.

1.3.6.1. Adynamic Ileus

→ ETIOLOGY AND PATHOGENESIS

Adynamic ileus is defined as cessation of peristalsis. **Causes:**

1) **Peritonitis**, which is most frequently due to:

   a) Acute appendicitis.

   b) Peptic ulcer perforation.

   c) Adnexitis in women.

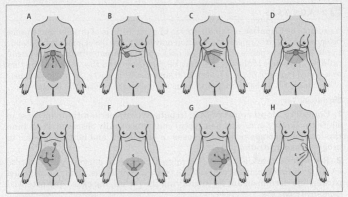

Figure 1-15. The character of pain and abdominal guarding in certain conditions associated with adynamic ileus: **A**, perforation of a peptic ulcer; **B**, biliary colic; **C**, acute cholecystitis; **D**, acute pancreatitis; **E**, appendicitis; **F**, adnexitis; **G**, perforation of a sigmoid diverticulum; **H**, renal colic.

    d) Biliary and pancreatic diseases.

    e) Other types of gastrointestinal (GI) perforation (colonic perforation, abdominal penetrating injury, inflammatory bowel disease).

2) **Renal colic** accompanying kidney stones or urinary tract infection.

3) **Biliopancreatic diseases**.

4) **Metabolic disturbances** (ketoacidosis in patients with diabetes mellitus or ethanol poisoning, uremia, hypokalemia or hyperkalemia, rarely porphyria).

5) **Retroperitoneal or intraperitoneal hematoma** (eg, rupture of an aortic aneurysm or the spleen, vertebral fracture).

6) **Intestinal ischemia,** either acute or chronic. Acute intestinal ischemia can be subcategorized as embolic (eg, atrial fibrillation), thrombotic (due to plaque rupture), venous, or nonocclusive (low-flow). Chronic ischemia refers to progression of atherosclerosis of the abdominal arteries.

7) **Drugs** (opioids, anticholinergics).

8) **Diseases of organs located in the chest**: Myocardial infarction, lower lobar pneumonia.

→ CLINICAL FEATURES

1. Symptoms: The characteristic triad of symptoms of GI obstruction includes abdominal pain, nausea and vomiting, and retention of gas and stools. It is important to qualify the pain as localized or generalized, constant versus intermittent, and dull/crampy versus sharp, as this may help define the underlying cause and determine whether urgent surgical therapy is necessary (→Figure 1-15).

2. Signs:

1) Abdominal distention.

2) Absent peristaltic sounds (silent abdomen).

3) Hyperresonance to percussion.

4) Signs of peritonitis (if this is the cause): Abdominal guarding (increased abdominal muscular tone, which intensifies on slight pressure), pain when attempting to cough, rebound tenderness (pain upon removal of pressure greater than upon application of pressure), and frequently fever.

→ DIAGNOSIS

A prompt confirmation of the diagnosis of peritonitis is of crucial importance because a delay in surgical intervention may lead to the development of systemic inflammatory response syndrome, sepsis, and life-threatening multiple organ failure. The cause of the disease may be suggested by a characteristic history or a typical pattern of pain. Consideration must be given to the various causes of mechanical GI obstruction and ileus in forming a differential diagnosis.

Diagnostic Tests

1. Complete blood count (CBC): In patients with peritonitis an increase in white blood cell counts and neutrophil counts is usually observed. With time, this may be accompanied by increases in hematocrit and hemoglobin due to progressive dehydration.

2. Blood biochemical tests: Electrolytes, pancreatic enzyme levels, glucose levels, liver function tests, coagulation tests, lactate levels, and renal function parameters are important for identifying the underlying cause and potential complications.

3. Imaging studies:

1) **Plain abdominal radiographs** are useful in demonstrating the presence of an ileus. Films taken in the upright position (standing or sitting in acutely ill patients) or when lying on the side (the most sensitive view) may demonstrate free intraperitoneal air, which is evidence of GI perforation (→Figure 1-16). A "transition point," proximal to distension and beyond which there is a paucity of intestinal gas, may help differentiate mechanical obstruction from adynamic ileus. Other radiologic features are less characteristic.

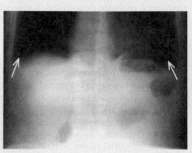

Figure 1-16. Plain abdominal radiograph in the standing position including the diaphragm. Perforation of the gastric ulcer with visible free gas (arrows) under both hemidiaphragms.

2) **Abdominal ultrasonography** is not the test of choice to demonstrate ileus but may reveal a causative process, such as ascites, appendicitis, or nephrolithiasis, as well as abnormalities of the gallbladder and pancreas.

3) **Abdominal and pelvic computed tomography (CT)** provides more detailed information on the causes of adynamic ileus, but may be omitted if previous imaging and signs or symptoms clearly point to the cause (eg, perforation) and treatment will not otherwise be altered.

4. Laparoscopy or laparotomy is sometimes performed in situations of diagnostic uncertainty.

→ TREATMENT

Patients with ileus or obstruction should be almost always referred for surgical consultation. **Medical treatment** is used in patients with metabolic conditions and in some patients with ileus as a result of renal colic (analgesics), acute pancreatitis, or bowel ischemia. Supportive management includes vigilant attention to fluid and electrolyte status, minimization of opioid use, and patient mobilization as appropriate. **Nasogastric decompression**, advised as universal by some surgeons, should be at least considered on a case-by-case basis and may benefit patients who are symptomatic with nausea or vomiting and distention. In other patients with acute intra-abdominal conditions leading to impaired intestinal motility, **laparotomy** or **laparoscopy** with an appropriate surgical procedure is usually performed. Any associated hypovolemia or shock should be aggressively managed while awaiting surgery.

1.3.6.2. Mechanical Intestinal Obstruction

→ ETIOLOGY AND PATHOGENESIS

Mechanical obstructions are typically categorized as involving the small or large bowel and may also be classified as being due to intraluminal, intramural, or extramural causes. **Small bowel obstructions**, which constitute ~75% of mechanical intestinal obstructions, are most commonly caused by intra--abdominal adhesions (from previous surgery, radiation, or other inflammatory processes) or herniae, whereas **large bowel obstructions** comprise the remaining ~25% and are most commonly caused by tumors, volvulus, and strictures.

The most worrisome **complications** of intestinal obstruction include bowel necrosis and perforation. Intestinal strangulation may be caused by incarceration of a hernia or by adhesive bands. (An incarcerated hernia refers to any hernia that is nonreducible, whereas a strangulated hernia implies the development of ischemia and/or necrosis.) This usually affects the small intestine but can also involve the mobile (intraperitoneal) portions of the colon. Necrosis of the bowel may develop due to increased pressure in a bilaterally occluded segment, also known as a "closed loop" obstruction. Examples of this phenomenon include incarcerated herniae or large bowel obstruction in the presence of a competent ileocecal valve. Bowel necrosis may also develop by direct compression of mesenteric vessels at the hernia neck. Necrosis may then lead to perforation, peritonitis (usually with development of adynamic ileus), and sepsis.

Less common forms of intraluminal or intramural obstruction include gallstone ileus (caused by gallstones passing through a cholecystoduodenal fistula) or certain parasitic infections, and in exceptional cases tumors of the small intestine. Impacted feces may also impair intestinal passage and sometimes cause symptoms similar to those of mechanical intestinal obstruction.

→ CLINICAL FEATURES

1. Symptoms: The characteristic triad of symptoms of gastrointestinal obstruction, which may include abdominal pain, nausea and vomiting, and retention of gas and stools. Typically the pain is paroxysmal and crampy. If pain character changes to being constant and either focal or diffuse, it should be suspicious for bowel ischemia or necrosis with accompanying peritonitis.

2. Signs: Attention on general inspection should be paid to signs of toxicity or hypoperfusion. Volume status assessment should be performed. Abdominal examination should be undertaken, with careful inspection of the entire abdomen and inguinofemoral region for signs of either surgical scars or herniae. High-pitched tinkling bowel sounds have been described in small bowel obstruction. Palpation should assess for evidence of herniae and for any evidence of peritoneal irritation. A rapidly deteriorating clinical status or physical examination may indicate intestinal necrosis. It is important to note that by the time the patient manifests evidence of peritonitis, irreversible ischemia or bowel necrosis has usually developed.

→ DIAGNOSIS

It is crucial to promptly establish indications for surgery in patients with strangulation and subsequent intestinal ischemia. Diagnostic clues may be provided by examination of the inguinal areas (hernia), presence of postoperative scars (adhesive bands), and history of alternating constipation and diarrhea, as well as progressive impairment of stool and gas passage (colorectal cancer). Digital rectal examination may reveal an anal or rectal tumor or impacted feces.

Diagnostic Tests

1. Complete blood count (CBC): A progressive increase in hematocrit and red blood cell counts may be observed that is proportional to the degree of dehydration. A rapid increase in white blood cell counts is often observed in patients with intestinal necrosis.

2. Blood biochemical tests: Because intestinal obstruction may lead to fluid and electrolyte disturbances as well as kidney failure and acidosis, it is necessary to measure serum electrolyte levels, kidney function parameters, and blood gas levels. Other tests may include lactic acid levels and coagulation parameters.

3. Imaging studies:

1) **Plain abdominal radiographs** in the upright (eg, standing or, in severely ill patients, sitting), supine, and decubitus positions may reveal fluid levels in the distended intestinal loops (→Figure 1-17). These are caused by a combination of aerophagia and fermentation of stagnant intestinal contents. Bowel loops are typically collapsed distal to the point of obstruction; however, this is not always the case, particularly in early obstruction. A "gasless abdomen" may also be seen in the setting of bowel obstruction in the event that bowel loops are fluid-filled but without significant gaseous distention.

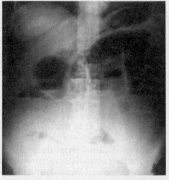

Figure 1-17. Plain abdominal radiograph in the standing position. Obstruction of the small intestine with a significant distention of the small intestine and fluid levels visible in a standing position.

2) **Abdominal computed tomography (CT)** may reveal the probable cause and location of obstruction. It is also the test of choice to demonstrate the presence of complete versus incomplete obstruction and may identify complications such as necrosis or perforation. Oral and IV contrast should be administered if possible. Rectal contrast is sometimes used in the setting of suspected distal large bowel obstruction but need not be administered in all cases of bowel obstruction.

4. Colonoscopy is used for selected causes of large bowel obstruction. In patients with incomplete obstruction it may be possible to introduce the endoscope above the level of obstruction and perform intestinal decompression, which should facilitate preparation for surgery.

→ TREATMENT

Patients should always be referred for surgical consultation because mechanical intestinal obstruction often requires surgical treatment; such patients with mechanical small bowel obstruction should likely be admitted under a surgical service.⊙◯ The need for, and urgency of, intervention should be determined by the surgeon. It may be necessary to prepare the patient for the procedure, particularly by correcting hypovolemia along with associated electrolyte abnormalities. Since surgery may involve exposure to contents of the gastrointestinal tract, IV antibiotics are administered prior to procedure but are not otherwise indicated on the basis of obstruction alone.

1.3.7. Inflammatory Bowel Disease

1.3.7.1. Crohn Disease

→ **DEFINITION, ETIOLOGY, PATHOGENESIS**

Crohn disease (CD) is an inflammatory disease process that may affect any part of the gastrointestinal (GI) tract from the oral cavity to the anus. The disease is characterized by the presence of segments of predominantly granulomatous transmural inflammatory lesions separated by healthy sections of the intestine. Etiology is unknown. The inflammatory process starts in the mucosa and gradually involves all layers of the intestinal wall, leading to its destruction, fibrosis, and the formation of fistulas and strictures.

→ **CLINICAL FEATURES AND NATURAL HISTORY**

1. General symptoms: Fatigue, fever (in ~30% of patients), and weight loss (~60%; secondary to malabsorption or malnutrition).

2. Symptoms dependent on the location, extent, and severity of the GI lesions:

1) **Classic form involving the terminal ileum** (40%-50% of patients): The onset is usually insidious, although in rare cases it may be acute and resemble appendicitis. Presenting symptoms include abdominal pain (~80%; often localized to the right lower quadrant of the abdomen and worsened postprandially), diarrhea, anemia, and fever of unknown origin. Hematochezia and melena are infrequent. In patients with a retrocecal abscess guarded movement of the right hip is seen. Extensive involvement of the small intestine leads to malabsorption syndrome with fatty diarrhea, anemia, hypoproteinemia, vitamin deficiency (particularly cobalamin), and electrolyte disturbances. With time patients develop malnutrition and cachexia, as well as edema in the case of hypoalbuminemia.

2) **Colon** (in 20% of patients lesions are isolated; in 30%-40%, lesions are also present in the small intestine): Symptoms may resemble ulcerative colitis (UC). Diarrhea is the most frequent manifestation (sometimes with visible blood). Abdominal pain is also common, particularly in patients with involvement of the cecum and ileum.

3) **Mouth**: Pain, aphthous ulcers, sores.

4) **Esophagus**: Dysphagia, odynophagia.

5) **Stomach and duodenum**: Abdominal pain, vomiting (symptoms may resemble peptic ulcer disease or pyloric stenosis).

6) **Perirectal area**: Large hemorrhoidal tags, ulcers, fissures, perianal abscesses and fistulas; these occur in 50% to 80% of patients with involvement of the colon and may be the presenting symptoms of CD.

7) **Symptoms of intestinal and extraintestinal complications**: →Complications, below.

3. Natural history: CD has a chronic course typically lasting several decades, usually with alternating periods of flares and remissions. Frequently symptoms are persistent, cause significant disability, and require surgery because of complications (60% of patients after 10 years). Endoscopic recurrence rates after surgery are ~70% at 1 year after resection, and clinical recurrence occurs in 30% to 50% of patients 5 years after resection.

→ **DIAGNOSIS**

Diagnostic Tests

The diagnosis of CD requires correlation and integration of clinical, biochemical, imaging, endoscopic, and histopathologic information.

1. Laboratory tests:

1) Routine studies may reveal anemia, leukocytosis, thrombocytosis, elevated erythrocyte sedimentation rate (ESR), elevated C-reactive protein (CRP) levels, hypoproteinemia with hypoalbuminemia, and electrolyte abnormalities such as hypokalemia. Results of these studies are useful in detecting and determining the severity of disease and degree of malabsorption.

2) Serologic testing, such as anti–*Saccharomyces cerevisiae* antibodies (ASCAs) and antineutrophil cytoplasmic antibodies (ANCAs), may be used as adjunct testing, but generally it is ineffective in routine diagnosis and in differentiating colonic CD from UC.

2. Imaging studies:

1) Depending on which part of the GI tract is being investigated, **barium radiography** (eg, small bowel follow-through [SBFT] and contrast barium enema) can reveal segmental lesions in the small intestine or colon, solitary or multiple strictures, characteristic deep "rose-thorn" or "collar-button" ulcers, or fistulas. SBFT has a sensitivity of ~70% for the diagnosis and detection of complications in CD. Because barium radiography is less sensitive than magnetic resonance or computed tomography (CT) enterography, intestinal ultrasonography, and small bowel capsule endoscopy, it is not the recommended diagnostic method when these alternatives are available.

2) **Ultrasonography, CT, and magnetic resonance imaging (MRI)** can reveal abscesses and fistulas. These studies also visualize the intestinal wall and allow for the assessment of its thickness and diameter of the lumen. Administration of luminal contrast by enteroclysis or enterography improves small bowel visualization. The sensitivity of CT and MRI in the diagnosis of CD is ~80% to 90%. Small intestine contrast ultrasonography (with oral contrast) offers a better detection rate of strictures and associated dilation. Its sensitivity and specificity are comparable to magnetic resonance enterography and CT enterography.

3. Endoscopy: Ileocolonoscopy (colonoscopy with evaluation of the terminal ileum) with ≥2 biopsy specimens from the ileum and from 5 sites around the colon (including the rectum) is suggested to establish the diagnosis of CD. The earliest lesions are small aphthous mucosal ulcers, with subsequent irregular edema and deep ulcers of varying shapes. Typical lesions are transverse and longitudinal linear ulcers with a characteristic "cobblestone" appearance.

1) **Rectoscopy** reveals irregular rectal strictures, islets of mucosal lesions separated by portions of normal mucosa, and ulcers. In ~50% of patients with involvement of the colon, rectal mucosa has a normal appearance but histologic examination of rectal mucosa biopsy specimens may reveal granulomas or a granulomatous reaction in the submucosa.

2) **Ileocolonoscopy** is used to assess the type and extent of inflammatory lesions in the colon and terminal ileum (collecting multiple specimens is recommended).

3) **Capsule endoscopy** is used in patients with suspected inflammatory lesions in the small intestine that are not accessible using classic endoscopy and radiography.

4. Histologic examination: While CD has no pathognomonic histologic features, 60% of patients have noncaseating epithelioid granulomas, giant multinucleated Langerhans-type cells, and lymphocytes in the intestinal wall. However, granulomas are detected only in 10% of patients with CD who have intestinal biopsies.

5. Stool examination:

1) **Microbiology**: In patients with recently diagnosed active CD or a CD exacerbation, microbiological testing of the stool including assessment for *Clostridium* (now *Clostridioides*) *difficile* infection should be performed.

Table 1-7. Differential diagnosis of ulcerative colitis and Crohn disease

Symptoms	Ulcerative colitis	Crohn disease
Bleeding	Common	Rare
Abdominal pain	Not severe	Common and can be severe
Palpable abdominal mass	Very rare	Fairly common
Fistulas	Very rare	Common
Involvement of the rectum	95%	50%
Perianal lesions	5%-18%	50%-80%
Pseudopolyps	13%-15%	Rare
Toxic megacolon	3%-4%	Rare
Intestinal perforation	2%-3%	Rare
Intestinal stricture	Rare	Common

2) **Fecal inflammation markers**: Fecal calprotectin and lactoferrin can be useful in distinguishing inflammatory bowel disease (IBD) from irritable bowel syndrome (IBS) and in predicting relapse. Patients with a calprotectin level <40 μg/g have ≤1% chance of IBD. Fecal lactoferrin has similar utility, as patients with lactoferrin levels ≤10 μg/g have a 2% chance of IBD.◒

Diagnostic Criteria

No strict diagnostic criteria exist for CD. Diagnosis is based on endoscopic, radiologic, and histologic confirmation of segmental inflammatory lesions involving the entire thickness of the intestinal wall, as described in detail above.

There are also no unequivocal criteria for the differentiation between CD and UC; however, several findings may suggest CD over UC, including the presence of granulomatous lesions on biopsy, presence of perianal disease, rectal sparing, and involvement of the small bowel. Nonetheless, in ~10% of patients a diagnosis of indeterminate colitis (IC) or inflammatory bowel disease unclassified (IBDU) is made.

Differential Diagnosis

1. CD of the ileum:

1) **Intestinal tuberculosis**: Difficult to differentiate from CD because of the similar histologic appearance (granulomas) and similar location of lesions in the ileocecal region. Microbiological findings and the presence or absence of caseating necrosis are decisive for the final diagnosis.

2) **Acute ileitis**: A sudden onset with symptoms suggestive of appendicitis. Diagnosis is frequently established during laparotomy. Acute ileitis may be caused by parasites or *Yersinia* spp.

2. CD of the colon:

1) **UC** (→Table 1-7).

2) **Ischemic colitis**: Advanced age, GI hemorrhage as a presenting symptom, rapid course of disease, typical location of lesions near the splenic flexure.

3) **Segmental colitis associated with diverticulosis (SCAD)**: Appearance of localized area of colitis around diverticula with a typical location of disease near the sigmoid colon.

4) **Infectious colitis**: Commonly acute onset, may be associated with symptoms of vomiting and diarrhea.

5) **IBS**: Patients may have some similar manifestations but lack warning (red flag) symptoms (weight loss), have normal laboratory test results (no anemia or elevated CRP levels), and the appearance of the bowel on cross-sectional imaging or colonoscopy is unchanged.

6) **Colorectal cancer**: Cancer may resemble CD when it causes longer intestinal strictures. Most commonly it affects elderly persons without local or general symptoms of inflammation and no lesions typical of CD in the mucosa of the strictures.

→ TREATMENT

General Management

1. Cessation of tobacco smoking is of great importance in the prevention of relapses in active smokers with CD. Previous studies have demonstrated an association of current smoking and CD.◐ Smoking also increases the risk of recurrence after surgery for CD, especially in women and heavy smokers. Smoking cessation likely lowers the risk of symptomatic relapse compared with patients who continue to smoke.◐

2. Avoidance of other factors causing exacerbations, such as infections, nonsteroidal anti-inflammatory drugs (NSAIDs), and stress. High perceived stress levels have been associated with increased risk of IBD flare.◐ Evidence regarding other potential triggers, including NSAIDs, infections, or antibiotic use, is weaker.

3. Correction of metabolic disturbances: Treatment of dehydration; correction of electrolyte disturbances, hypoalbuminemia, and anemia; treatment of cobalamin deficiency in patients with involvement of the ileum or after ileum resection.

Nutritional Management

Nutritional interventions can be used in patients with active disease complicated by malnutrition. Enteral nutrition (EN) with elemental or polymeric formulas is recommended; in patients in whom this is impossible or insufficient (because of GI obstruction, fistulas, or short bowel syndrome), supplementary or total parenteral nutrition should be used.

EN is not regularly used to induce remission in adult patients with CD; however, it can be considered in certain populations (eg, pediatric). A meta-analysis of 10 studies that compared EN with glucocorticoids suggests that glucocorticoid therapy may be more effective than EN for induction of clinical remission in adults with active CD and equally effective for induction of remission in children with active CD.◐◐ Maintenance with EN is typically not performed because of issues with compliance and acceptability.

Specific Pharmacologic Treatment

Treatment of CD is usually directed by gastroenterologists, possibly with interdisciplinary involvement from other allied health-care professionals such as nutritionists. Colorectal and general surgeons are also essential for patients with particular phenotypes of CD, including those with perianal fistulas or structuring disease causing bowel obstructions.

1. Anti-inflammatory drugs:

1) **Glucocorticoids**: Oral **prednisone** or **prednisolone** 40 to 60 mg/d. In patients with lesions involving the ileocecal region, use oral **budesonide** 9 mg/d. In patients with very active disease, use IV **hydrocortisone** 300 mg/d or **methylprednisolone** 60 mg/d. Once an acute flare of CD is under control, taper off the glucocorticoid dose over 2 to 3 months; discontinuation is not always possible.

2) **Aminosalicylates** (5-aminosalicylic acid [5-ASA]): Oral **sulfasalazine** 3 to 4 g/d is sometimes used in mild cases of colonic CD without clear evidence of benefit.◐◐

2. Immunomodulating agents are used in patients with response to gluco-corticoids as maintenance of remission therapy:

1) Oral **azathioprine** 1.5 to 2.5 mg/kg/d, oral **mercaptopurine** 0.75 to 1.5 mg/kg/d. These agents have not been demonstrated to be beneficial for induction but can maintain a glucocorticoid-induced remission.

2) IM **methotrexate**: For induction treatment use 25 mg/wk; for maintenance treatment use 15 mg/wk. Studies examining oral methotrexate have not demonstrated benefit.

3. Biologic agents (standard doses):

1) **Infliximab**: Induction treatment: 3 administrations of 5 mg/kg once a week in a 2-hour IV infusion at weeks 0, 2, and 6; maintenance treatment: repeat the infusion every 8 weeks.

2) **Adalimumab**: Induction treatment: 160 mg subcutaneously followed by 80 mg after 2 weeks; maintenance treatment: 40 mg every 2 weeks.

3) **Vedolizumab**: Induction treatment: 3 administrations of 300 mg once a week in a 30-minute IV infusion at weeks 0, 2, and 6; maintenance treatment: repeat the infusion every 8 weeks.

4) **Ustekinumab**: Induction treatment: 1 weight-based infusion between 260 mg and 520 mg; maintenance treatment: 90 mg subcutaneously every 8 to 12 weeks.

4. Antibiotics: In patients with septic complications and draining perianal fistulas with or without an abscess, you can use metronidazole, ciprofloxacin, or both.

Symptomatic Treatment

1. Analgesics: Acetaminophen (INN paracetamol). In patients with continuous pain who require opioids, use opioids with little effect on motility (eg, tramadol). Cannabinoids may also play a role in the management of patients with CD who have chronic abdominal pain.

2. Antidiarrheal drugs: Diphenoxylate with atropine 2.5 to 5 mg (1-2 tablets) bid or tid or loperamide 2 to 6 mg as needed. In patients with diarrhea caused by impaired absorption of bile acids after resection of the small intestine, use cholestyramine 4 g (1 teaspoon) with main meals.

Treatment Options Depending on CD Location and Severity

Disease severity (based on the 2010 European Crohn's and Colitis Organisation [ECCO] consensus):

1) **Remission**: The patient is asymptomatic, may have responded to medical or surgical therapy, and has no residual active disease. This category does not include patients who require ongoing glucocorticoid treatment.

2) **Mild**: The patient is able to walk, eat, and drink; has lost <10% of body weight; may have mild symptoms but has no GI obstruction, no fever, no dehydration, no palpable mass, and no abdominal tenderness; serum CRP levels may be slightly elevated.

3) **Moderate**: Intermittent vomiting without obstructive findings or >10% body weight loss; ineffective treatment of mild disease or a painful abdominal mass found on physical examination with no clinically overt GI obstruction; usually elevated serum CRP levels.

4) **Severe**: Cachexia (body mass index <18 kg/m^2), GI obstruction, or abscess; symptoms persisting despite intensive treatment; usually elevated serum CRP levels.

Disease Limited to the Ileocecal Region

1. Mild disease: Oral **budesonide** 9 mg/d. The efficacy of mesalamine is low. In patients with mild or no symptoms no pharmacotherapy may be considered.

2. Moderate disease: Oral **budesonide** 9 mg/d or oral **prednisone/prednisolone** 1 mg/kg/d (remission rates after 7 weeks of treatment are >90% but adverse effects are more frequent than with budesonide). Azathioprine/mercaptopurine or methotrexate in combination with glucocorticoids are also appropriate. In patients with glucocorticoid resistance, dependence, or intolerance, biologic drugs may be considered.

3. Severe disease: Use a glucocorticoid, starting from IV **methylprednisolone**. In case of relapse introduce a **biologic drug**, alone or in combination with an immunomodulator; restarting glucocorticoids with an immunomodulator may also be appropriate. In patients with treatment failure, consider surgery.

Colitis

1. Systemic glucocorticoids: Although sulfasalazine is recommended by the American College of Gastroenterology (ACG) guidelines for treating symptoms of colonic CD that is mild to moderately active, it has not been demonstrated to be more effective than placebo for achieving mucosal healing. Sulfasalazine is not recommended by the ECCO guidelines.

2. Recurrent disease of moderate or severe activity: A biologic agent alone or in combination with an immunomodulator. For some patients restarting glucocorticoids with an immunomodulator may also be appropriate.

3. Surgery should be considered before starting treatment with biologic or immunosuppressive agents.

Diffuse Disease of the Small Intestine (>100 cm)

If disease activity is moderate or severe, use oral **prednisone/prednisolone** 1 mg/kg combined with **azathioprine**, **mercaptopurine**, or **methotrexate**. Start **nutritional therapy**. In selected patients consider early **biologic agents** or **surgical treatment**. Aim to avoid surgical treatment in patients with extensive small bowel disease because of the risk of short bowel syndrome.

Disease of the Esophagus, Stomach, and Duodenum

If disease activity is moderate or severe, use oral **prednisone/prednisolone** 1 mg/kg combined with **azathioprine**, **mercaptopurine**, or **methotrexate**. In patients with no response to treatment consider **biologic agents**.

Disease With Fistulas

1. Simple perianal fistulas: If fistulas are asymptomatic, no intervention is needed. If they cause discomfort, seton insertion with or without fistula dissection (fistulotomy) is performed and treatment with metronidazole 750 to 1500 mg/d, ciprofloxacin 1000 mg/d, or both is started.

2. Complex perianal fistulas: First-line treatment includes antibiotics, azathioprine, or mercaptopurine, all combined with surgical treatment. In the case of perianal abscesses, drainage is performed. Second-line treatment includes biologic agents. Biologics are often necessary in patients with complex fistulas because of low response rates to nonbiologic therapies.

3. Enterovaginal fistulas: Low and asymptomatic fistulas may require no surgical treatment, whereas in symptomatic fistulas surgery is usually necessary. Symptomatic **rectovaginal fistulas** that do not respond to medical treatment also warrant surgical treatment. In **fistulas originating in the small intestine or the sigmoid colon** resection of the affected segment of the intestine is required.

4. Enterovesical fistulas require surgical treatment. In high-risk patients (after several surgical interventions or with a significantly shortened intestine) medical treatment should be attempted first.

5. Enterocutaneous fistulas: For fistulas developing after surgery, start with medical treatment (including nutritional management); surgery is performed once a normal nutritional status is restored. For primary fistulas, use surgery (resection of the affected segment of the intestine) or medical treatment.

Remission Maintenance Treatment

1. The use of 5-ASA or glucocorticoids for maintenance treatment is not recommended. In some patients maintenance treatment can be avoided.

2. If remission was achieved with glucocorticoids, maintenance treatment should be considered with azathioprine, mercaptopurine, or methotrexate.

3. In glucocorticoid-dependent patients use azathioprine, mercaptopurine, methotrexate alone or in combination with infliximab, adalimumab, vedolizumab, or ustekinumab.

4. In case of relapse in the course of maintenance treatment with azathioprine or mercaptopurine, first make sure that the patient has been adherent to the prescribed regimen, and then consider switching to methotrexate or a biologic agent.

5. If remission was achieved using infliximab, adalimumab, vedolizumab, or ustekinumab, the same drug should be used for maintenance therapy. Episodic biologic use is likely a less effective strategy compared with regular scheduled use because of sensitization against the biologic.◓

6. Discontinuation of azathioprine may be considered after 2 to 4 years of continuous complete remission. No sufficient data are available to define the duration of maintenance treatment with methotrexate or a biologic drug (our practice is to continue).

7. The need for surgical treatment should be evaluated based on the frequency, extent, and severity of relapses, as well as for adverse effects or failure of maintenance treatments.

8. In patients after resection of the small intestine, use maintenance treatment to prevent relapses; the most effective drugs are anti–tumor necrosis factor agents like infliximab or adalimumab. Azathioprine and mercaptopurine could be considered for initial postoperative recurrence.

9. For maintenance treatment in patients with perianal fistulas, use azathioprine, mercaptopurine, or a biologic drug for ≥1 year.

Surgical Treatment

1. Indications:

1) **Emergency (acute surgery)**: Total GI obstruction due to small intestinal stricture, massive hemorrhage, or intestinal perforation with diffuse peritonitis.

2) **Urgent**: Lack of significant improvement after 7 to 10 days of intensive medical treatment of a severe episode of extensive disease of the colon.

3) **Elective** (most common): Internal and external fistulas, intraabdominal infectious complications, extensive perianal lesions, confirmed or suspected cancer, chronic disability due to persistent troublesome symptoms despite adequate medical treatment, delayed physical development with growth retardation in children.

2. Types of surgical operations:

1) Disease of the small intestine: Resection of as small a portion as possible or surgical dilation of small intestinal strictures (strictureplasty).

2) Disease of the left or right colon: Hemicolectomy.

3) More extensive lesions of the colon: Colectomy with ileoanal anastomosis or proctocolectomy with permanent ileostomy.

→ C O M P L I C A T I O N S

Local Complications

External fistulas (perianal, enterocutaneous) and internal fistulas (communicating between the small intestine and the cecum, another loop of the small intestine, sigmoid, bladder, and vagina), interloop abscesses and significant intestinal strictures with symptoms of partial obstruction; rarely acute intestinal obstruction, massive hemorrhage, perforation with diffuse peritonitis. The risk of colorectal cancer is increased in CD but lower than in UC. Many guidelines recommend endoscopic screening for dysplasia be performed in all patients with Crohn colitis involving more than one-third of the colon after 8 to 10 years from the time of disease onset. Regular surveillance should be considered at 1- to 3-year intervals after the initial screening colonoscopy.

Extraintestinal Complications

As in ulcerative colitis. Additional common complications include cholelithiasis (30% of patients with involvement of the ileum), clubbing of digits (40%-60% of patients with severe CD flares), and nephrolithiasis (10%).

1.3.7.2. Ulcerative Colitis

→ DEFINITION, ETIOLOGY, PATHOGENESIS

Ulcerative colitis (UC) is a diffuse inflammatory condition involving the rectum and extending proximally to a varying degree. UC and Crohn disease are the two major forms of inflammatory bowel diseases (IBD). The etiology of IBD remains uncertain but centers on an overactive intestinal immune response in individuals with a genetic predisposition.

→ CLINICAL FEATURES AND NATURAL HISTORY

1. Signs and symptoms: The most common presenting symptoms are increased stool frequency, rectal bleeding, and urgency. In patients with limited proctitis stool frequency may be normal and even constipation may occur. In such cases rectal bleeding may be the only symptom. Fatigue and weight loss are frequent. Severe flares may be associated with symptoms of dehydration, tachycardia, abdominal tenderness, and fever. Signs and symptoms of specific intestinal and extraintestinal manifestations of IBD are described below.

2. Clinical classification: Inflammatory lesions may be confined to the rectum (proctitis) or extend proximally and contiguously through the colon. In some cases of pancolitis, "backwash" ileitis can also occur. Patients with distal disease can have localized periappendiceal inflammation, referred to as a cecal patch. The following classification of disease extent can have practical implications for the choice of treatment modality (topical vs systemic):

1) **Proctitis**, with inflammation limited to the rectum.

2) **Left-sided colitis**, with inflammation above the rectum but distal to the splenic flexure.

3) **Extensive colitis**, with inflammation proximal to the splenic flexure.

3. Natural history: UC is a chronic condition with periods of active disease ("flares") and periods of remission. Most flares are unexplained, but some are associated with specific triggers, such as stress, changes in diet, nonsteroidal anti-inflammatory drugs (NSAIDs), enteric infections, and antibiotic therapy.

4. Classification of disease activity: A variety of scoring systems have been developed to grade the activity of UC. The most commonly used of these is the Mayo score (→Table 1-8), which combines symptoms with endoscopic findings and physician global assessment (PGA). The score ranges from 0 to 12 points, with higher scores indicating more severe disease. The more recent STRIDE (Selecting Therapeutic Targets in Inflammatory Bowel Disease) consensus advocated eliminating the PGA to leave 2 patient-reported outcomes (stool frequency and bleeding) and endoscopy.

Table 1-8. The Mayo Clinic score for grading the activity of ulcerative colitis

Assessment	Points
Stool frequency	
Patient reporting a normal number of daily stools	0
1-2 more stools than normal	1
3-4 more stools than normal	2
≥5 more stools than normal	3
Rectal bleeding	
None	0
Blood streaks seen with stool less than half of the time	1
Blood with most stools	2
Pure blood passed	3
Endoscopic findings	
Normal or inactive colitis	0
Mild friability, erythema, decreased vascularity	1
Friability, marked erythema, absent vascular pattern, erosions	2
Ulcerations and spontaneous bleeding	3
Physician global assessment	
Normal	0
Mild colitis	1
Moderate colitis	2
Severe colitis	3
Higher scores are correlated with more severe ulcerative colitis.	

Source: N Engl J Med. 1987;317(26):1625-9.

→ DIAGNOSIS

Diagnostic Tests

1. Laboratory tests: No abnormalities are specific for UC. In patients with active disease the following may be observed:

1) Features of inflammation: Elevated serum C-reactive protein (CRP), thrombocytosis, leukocytosis.

2) Anemia, hypoalbuminemia, and electrolyte disturbances (in severe disease).

3) Elevated fecal calprotectin levels.

4) Negative testing for infectious gastroenteritis. Patients with active disease should also be tested specifically for *Clostridium difficile* infection.

2. Imaging studies:

1) **Plain abdominal radiographs** may reveal thumbprinting, signifying mucosal edema. Colonic dilation in patients with active disease (transverse colon >6 cm in diameter in the median plane: →Figure 1-18) is a concerning finding suggestive of toxic megacolon.

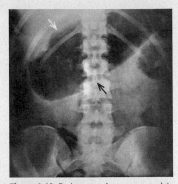

Figure 1-18. Toxic megacolon seen on a plain abdominal radiograph. The transverse colon is 11 cm in diameter in the midline (arrow).

2) **Barium enema** in early disease shows mucosal granularity and shallow mucosal ulceration. Chronic inflammation can lead to inflammatory polyps, loss of haustration, and shortening of the colon (lead-pipe appearance). Barium enema is now performed rarely and should be avoided in severe disease.

3) **Cross-sectional imaging with ultrasonography, computed tomography (CT), or magnetic resonance imaging (MRI)** can show mural thickening with stratification, loss of haustration, and widening of the presacral space. CT is not sensitive for mild mucosal disease. In severe disease CT is useful to exclude perforation and abscess.

3. Endoscopy (→Figure 1-19) can be performed without prior preparation on the first presentation (cathartics such as phosphate enemas may change the endoscopic appearance). Biopsy is important to confirm diagnosis. In active disease the mucosa is erythematous, granular, edematous, and friable; contact bleeding is observed and vascular pattern is absent. In severe forms, ulcers, pseudopolyps, purulent exudate, and blood are seen in the intestinal lumen. In periods of remission the appearance of the mucosa may be normal. Full **colonoscopy** is not needed for diagnosis and may be contraindicated in more active disease. However, colonoscopy is useful to define disease extent, differentiate UC from Crohn disease, and survey for cancer.

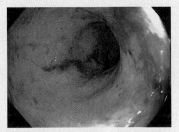

Figure 1-19. Endoscopic findings in moderate ulcerative colitis. Absent vascular pattern and loss of haustration. The mucosa is friable and bleeds on contact with the endoscope.

4. Histologic features depend on the phase of the disease. In active disease increased numbers of granulocytes, lymphocytes, and plasma cells are present in the lamina propria, along with crypt abscesses and reduced numbers of goblet cells. In remission distorted glandular architecture, thinning of muscularis mucosa, and Paneth cell metaplasia are observed. Examination for features of cytomegalovirus (CMV) infection is important in patients with severe disease activity.

Diagnostic Criteria
Diagnosis is based primarily on endoscopic and histologic findings.

Differential Diagnosis
Differential diagnosis includes bacterial (eg, *Salmonella*, *Shigella*, *Campylobacter*, *Yersinia*, gonococci) or parasitic (eg, amebiasis) infection, pseudomembranous colitis, Crohn disease (→Table 1-7), colorectal cancer, ischemic colitis, and radiation proctitis.

→ TREATMENT

1. Classes of medications:

1) Oral **5-aminosalicylic acid (5-ASA) compounds**, administered as pure 5-ASA (**mesalazine**) or its derivatives: **sulfasalazine**, **olsalazine**, and **balsalazide**. Mesalazine can also be administered rectally as suppositories or enemas.

2) Oral **glucocorticoids** include **prednisone**, **prednisolone**, and **budesonide**. IV glucocorticoids include **hydrocortisone** and **methylprednisolone**.

3) **Immunosuppressants** include thiopurines (**azathioprine** and **6-mercaptopurine**) and **cyclosporine** (INN ciclosporin).

4) **Biologic agents** include tumor necrosis factor (TNF)-α antagonists (**adalimumab**, **golimumab**, **infliximab**) and the $\alpha_4\beta_7$ leukocyte integrin antagonist **vedolizumab**.

5) **Janus kinase (JAK) inhibitors**, specifically tofacitinib.

2. Both 5-ASA and glucocorticoids (hydrocortisone, budesonide) can be administered rectally as suppositories or enemas, as monotherapy in patients with distal disease, or as adjuncts to systemic therapies in patients with more extensive disease.

Treatment of Active Disease (Induction of Remission)

Mild to Moderate Disease Activity

1. Outpatient management is typical. In general, there is no restriction of lifestyle and diet. Strategies to maintain and follow bone health should be discussed (prevention and treatment of bone mineral loss: →Chapter 14.13). Vaccinations should be updated, recognizing that live vaccines cannot be administered in patients receiving immunosuppressant or biologic therapy.

2. Selection of drugs:

1) **Proctitis**: 5-ASA suppositories (or enemas) at least 1 g/d as monotherapy or in combination with oral 5-ASA or rectal glucocorticoid.

2) **Left-sided colitis**: 5-ASA enemas◐◕ combined with oral 5-ASA >2 g/d. Oral 5-ASA monotherapy and rectal 5-ASA or glucocorticoid monotherapy can be considered but are less effective.

3) **Extensive colitis**: Oral 5-ASA >2 g/d as monotherapy or preferably in combination with rectal 5-ASA.

4) Consider **oral systemic glucocorticoids** if 5-ASA therapy is optimized and fails. Oral budesonide formulations with colonic delivery can also be used in mild to moderate disease in patients who do not respond to or do not tolerate 5-ASA.

Severe Disease

1. Hospitalization may be required. Perform tests for *C difficile* and CMV as well as plain abdominal radiographs to identify possible complications that require urgent surgical assessment (toxic megacolon or perforation). Prophylaxis against venous thromboembolism (VTE) should be administered (→Chapter 3.19.2).◐○

2. Intensive medical management:

1) Administer **IV hydration**. Blood transfusion may be necessary. Oral or enteral feeding is preferred, but patients unable to tolerate enteric feeds or those who require surgery should be considered for parenteral nutrition.

2) Initiate **IV glucocorticoids** with hydrocortisone 300 mg/d or methylprednisolone 60 mg/d (in the case of glucocorticoid intolerance use infliximab or IV cyclosporine). Evaluate the response to glucocorticoids (stool frequency, CRP, plain abdominal radiography) after 3 days. If effective, continue the glucocorticoid for an additional 4 to 7 days before switching to oral therapy and taper down the dose. Otherwise consider surgery or second-line therapy.

3) Second-line therapy is IV infliximab 5 to 10 mg/kg or IV cyclosporine 2 mg/kg/d. If there is no improvement within 5 to 7 days (or earlier in case of deterioration), consider surgery (colectomy).

4) Do not use antibiotics unless there is evidence of bacterial infection.

3. Manage specific complications (→Complications, below).

Relapses and Refractory Disease

1. For **patients who relapse despite treatment with 5-ASA**, consider 5-ASA dose optimization, concomitant oral/rectal 5-ASA, oral glucocorticoids, or biologic therapy.

2. For **patients with glucocorticoid-refractory disease**, consider biologic therapy ⊘● (alone or in combination with an immunosuppressant) or a JAK inhibitor.

3. For **patients with glucocorticoid-dependent disease**, consider a thiopurine, biologic therapy, or a JAK inhibitor.

4. Always consider surgery.

Maintenance of Remission

Long-term maintenance therapy to prevent relapse should be considered in all patients with UC after successful induction. The choice of agent depends on the extent, frequency, and severity of the disease, effectiveness of previous maintenance therapy, and drug used during previous exacerbations.

1. For **patients responding to oral or rectal 5-ASA or to glucocorticoids**, the maintenance treatment of choice is **oral or rectal 5-ASA**. Once-daily dosing of oral 5-ASA ≥2 g/d is acceptable.⊘● Rectal 5-ASA can be administered daily or titrated to a reduced dose frequency (eg, 3 d/wk). Use rectal treatments in patients with proctitis, oral or rectal treatments in patients with left-sided colitis, and oral treatments in other patients. Apart from maintaining remission, a potential benefit of 5-ASA maintenance therapy is chemoprevention of colorectal cancer. Second-line treatment is a long-term combination of oral and rectal 5-ASA.

2. For **patients who require repeated courses of glucocorticoids**, consider a thiopurine or biologic agent, either alone or in combination with a thiopurine.

3. For **patients in whom remission was induced with an anti-TNF agent**, continue that agent alone or in combination with a thiopurine.

4. For **patients in whom remission was induced with an anti-integrin agent**, continue that agent alone or in combination with a thiopurine.

5. For **patients in whom remission was induced with a JAK inhibitor**, continue that agent as maintenance therapy.

Surgical Treatment

1. Indications for surgical treatment include persistent UC symptoms despite optimal medical treatment. In severe UC not responding to intensive glucocorticoid treatment within 3 to 5 days or within 5 to 7 days of rescue therapy with infliximab or cyclosporine, surgical treatment is urgent. Other indications include cancer or dysplasia, colonic stricture, or (rarely) refractory extraintestinal manifestations.

2. Types of surgery:

1) Total resection of the rectum and colon (proctocolectomy) with formation of a permanent end ileostomy.

2) Restorative proctocolectomy with formation of an ileal pouch and an ileal pouch–anal anastomosis (IPAA). This avoids a permanent stoma but may require up to 3 stages for completion.

→ FOLLOW-UP

---

1. Objective measures of disease activity (complete blood count [CBC], CRP, fecal calprotectin) every 3 to 12 months.

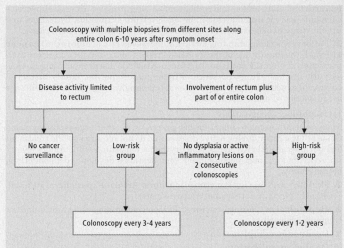

Colonoscopy with multiple biopsies from different sites along entire colon 6-10 years after symptom onset

Disease activity limited to rectum

Involvement of rectum plus part of or entire colon

No cancer surveillance

Low-risk group

No dysplasia or active inflammatory lesions on 2 consecutive colonoscopies

High-risk group

Colonoscopy every 3-4 years

Colonoscopy every 1-2 years

a In patients with >2 of the following risk factors: involvement of the entire colon (pancolitis), active inflammatory lesions, postinflammatory polyps, family history of colorectal cancer.

Figure 1-20. Cancer surveillance in patients with ulcerative colitis. *Based on the 2012 European Crohn's and Colitis Organisation guidelines.*

2. Monitoring for hepatobiliary complications (clinical assessment, liver biochemistry testing) every 12 months.

3. Cancer surveillance (colonoscopy recommended after 6-10 years from the time of diagnosis in various clinical practice guidelines and repeated at intervals depending on previous findings and disease duration: →Figure 1-20). Surveillance colonoscopy is best performed when the patient is in remission. High-definition equipment should be used. In the random biopsy approach, 4-quadrant biopsies are collected from every 10 cm of the intestine along its entire length

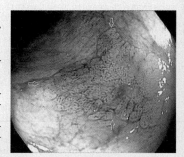

Figure 1-21. A focus of low-grade dysplasia (arrows) revealed by indigo carmine staining.

plus additional samples from suspicious sites (strictures, raised lesions other than postinflammatory polyps). If chromoendoscopy is used (→Figure 1-21), targeted biopsies are taken only from suspicious areas.

→ COMPLICATIONS

Intestinal Complications

1. Toxic megacolon is a potentially fatal complication occurring in ~3% of patients during a severe (often the first) flare. **Clinical manifestations** include abdominal pain and distention, high-grade fever, tachycardia, and abdominal signs of peritoneal inflammation. **Diagnosis** is based on clinical

701

features and plain abdominal radiographs (→Figure 1-18). Intense supportive care (nasogastric decompression, broad-spectrum antibiotics, hydration) and urgent surgical assessment are required due to a high risk of perforation.

2. Patients with long-standing UC are at increased risk of **colorectal cancer**, although the magnitude of the increased risk is controversial and lower than previously thought. **Predisposing factors** include disease duration, disease activity, disease extent, presence of inflammatory polyps, family history of colorectal cancer, and primary sclerosing cholangitis. Dysplasia surveillance is indicated (→Follow-Up, above).

Extraintestinal Complications

Many patients develop inflammatory processes in other organs and systems. Some occur mainly during active disease and do not require specific treatment (eg, peripheral arthritis, iritis, and erythema nodosum), while others (eg, axial arthritis and most hepatobiliary complications) develop independently of colitis activity.

1. Skeletal and articular complications: Arthritis (peripheral or axial; →Chapter 14.20.2), osteopenia, and osteoporosis.

2. Hepatobiliary complications: Primary sclerosing cholangitis and autoimmune hepatitis.

3. Cutaneous complications: Erythema nodosum, pyoderma gangrenosum.

4. Ocular complications: Iritis, episcleritis.

1.3.8. Intestinal Ischemia

→ **DEFINITION AND ETIOLOGY**

Intestinal ischemia refers to reversible and irreversible bowel injury that results from a decrease in blood flow to the small or large intestine. Any process that reduces intestinal blood flow, with or without subsequent reperfusion injury, can cause intestinal ischemia. Causes may be occlusive (arterial embolism, arterial thrombosis, or venous thrombosis) or nonocclusive (eg, due to shock or vasospasm). Intestinal ischemia varies widely in presentation and outcome depending on the time course of disease, degree of blood flow compromise, presence of collateralization, and segment of the bowel affected. Serious consequences such as bowel infarction, perforation, sepsis, and death can occur.

There is variation in terminology in the literature that can cause confusion. **Mesenteric ischemia** refers to small bowel ischemia. **Ischemic colitis** and **colonic ischemia** refer to large bowel ischemia representing variable clinical presentations across the spectrum of severity of the disease. The terms **intestinal ischemia** and **ischemic bowel** can apply to either the small or large bowel.

1.3.8.1. Acute Mesenteric (Small Bowel) Ischemia

→ **ETIOLOGY AND PATHOGENESIS**

Acute mesenteric (small bowel) ischemia results from a sudden occlusion and/or insufficiency of the mesenteric arteries or veins that reduces intestinal perfusion and thus threatens the viability of the small intestine.

Causes include mesenteric artery embolism (45%-50% of cases); nonocclusive mesenteric ischemia (NOMI) (20%-30%) due to low cardiac output secondary to shock, drugs (cocaine, ergotamine, vasopressin analogues, norepinephrine), or after intestinal revascularization interventions; mesenteric arterial thrombosis (15%-25%); or mesenteric venous thrombosis, which by itself may lead to impaired microvascular perfusion (5%).

→ CLINICAL FEATURES AND NATURAL HISTORY

Mesenteric ischemia most commonly occurs in the elderly.

1. Symptoms: Because symptoms are nonspecific, diagnosis requires a high degree of clinical suspicion. The dominant feature is severe abdominal pain that is out of proportion to physical examination and is most frequently located in the periumbilical area. Nausea and vomiting are frequent. Diarrhea, which may be bloody with transmural infarction, may occur.

Initially physical examination may be unremarkable (eg, abdominal distension) or even normal. In the early stages of ischemia bowel sounds may be hyperactive but in later stages they can be reduced to complete cessation. Subsequently fever, diffuse peritonitis, and shock develop if intestinal necrosis or perforation occurs. Only 20% to 25% of patients present with an acute abdomen.

2. Risk factors: Risk factors differ by etiology. Mesenteric arterial embolism commonly occurs in patients with atrial fibrillation, cardiac valvular disease, or recent myocardial infarction. Mesenteric arterial thrombosis frequently occurs in patients with underlying chronic intestinal ischemia from atherosclerosis (→Chapter 6.1.3.8.2). Mesenteric venous thrombosis tends to occur in patients with acquired (eg, secondary to malignancy) or hereditary hypercoagulable states (eg, factor V Leiden mutation, protein C or S deficiency, polycythemia). Trauma, recent abdominal surgery, and inflammatory conditions such as pancreatitis or diverticulitis are also risk factors for mesenteric venous thrombosis. NOMI occurs frequently in critically ill ventilated patients.

→ DIAGNOSIS

Diagnostic Tests

1. Laboratory tests: The most common findings are hemoconcentration and leukocytosis (usually $>20 \times 10^9$/L). In patients developing intestinal necrosis, nonrespiratory (lactic) acidosis, hyperphosphatemia, elevated levels of serum liver and pancreatic enzymes, and elevated creatine kinase levels may be seen as early as in the first few hours.

2. Imaging studies: Abdominal radiographs are nonspecific, and more than 25% radiographs are normal. Radiographic features of intestinal necrosis (including the presence of gas in the intestinal wall) appear late; they are only helpful when findings suggest perforation or a different diagnosis, such as obstruction. **Computed tomography angiography (CTA)** (without oral contrast) has replaced conventional angiography with its high sensitivity and specificity (94% and 95%, respectively). However, **arteriography** is still considered by some to be the definitive diagnostic method if there is uncertainty (with sensitivity of about 90%) or if required for therapeutic purposes. It should not delay surgery, if indicated.

→ TREATMENT

Although specific treatment depends on etiology, the initial management for all patients focuses on resuscitation and prevention of complications.

1. Appropriate treatment of shock (→Chapter 3.16).

2. Conservative management: Medications that may exacerbate mesenteric ischemia, such as vasoconstricting agents, should be avoided. If required, vasopressors with a relatively smaller effect on mesenteric circulation, such as dobutamine, low-dose dopamine, and milrinone, are preferred. Consider nasogastric decompression.

3. Anticoagulation is recommended in occlusive mesenteric ischemia.◐○ It may be the only treatment necessary in mesenteric venous thrombosis.

4. Endovascular treatment (local thrombolysis, percutaneous thrombectomy, balloon angioplasty, stenting) may be considered in selected patients without intestinal necrosis.⊘○ In the case of arterial vasospasm or NOMI found on arteriography, intra-arterial administration of vasodilators may be considered if the patient is not responding to conservative management.

5. Early surgical treatment is indicated if perforation or infarction is suspected. Otherwise surgical treatment is usually reserved for failure of nonoperative management, as endovascular procedures are increasingly performed for revascularization. The goals of surgery include assessment of bowel viability, resection of the nonviable bowel, and revascularization. Revascularization options include embolectomy in patients with embolism and thrombectomy or bypass anastomosis in patients with mesenteric artery thrombosis.

→ PROGNOSIS

In patients with intestinal necrosis mortality rates are up to 90%. However, with early surgical intervention, mortality decreases to ~10% if the patient is operated within 24 hours. Comorbidities, age, and etiology also affect mortality; patients with arterial occlusions have worse survival rates.

1.3.8.2. Chronic Mesenteric (Small Bowel) Ischemia

→ ETIOLOGY AND PATHOGENESIS

Chronic mesenteric ischemia refers to impaired perfusion of the small intestines resulting from chronic occlusion of the mesenteric arteries.

Causes: The majority is due to atherosclerosis of the aorta, superior mesenteric artery, celiac artery, or less commonly inferior mesenteric artery (35%-50% of cases). Less common causes include Dunbar syndrome (compression of the celiac artery by the arcuate ligament [also referred to as median arcuate ligament syndrome]), fibromuscular dysplasia of arteries, aneurysm or dissection of the aorta, or thromboangiitis obliterans (Buerger disease).

→ CLINICAL FEATURES AND NATURAL HISTORY

In patients with atherosclerosis, collateral vessels form over time due to the gradual narrowing of the vessels. Therefore, perfusion to the bowel can be maintained without bowel compromise. Depending on the time course of the disease and whether there is a superimposed acute event, patients can present with mild symptoms or an acute presentation of acute mesenteric ischemia.

1. Symptoms: The characteristic symptoms include:

1) Intestinal angina: Crampy epigastric abdominal pain starting a few minutes after a meal and lasting 1 to 3 hours; the pain is most severe after heavy and fatty meals.
2) Fear of food.
3) Cachexia (weight loss in 80% of patients) due to the fear of pain with eating.
4) Persistent diarrhea.

Less typical symptoms include nausea, vomiting, and early satiety (in 30% of patients; usually in patients with occlusion of the celiac artery). A high index of clinical suspicion is required due to the nonspecific symptoms.

Physical examination is nonspecific. An abdominal bruit may be audible.

2. Risk factors: The disease typically develops in tobacco smokers with clinically manifest atherosclerosis of other vascular beds, especially of the lower extremities, coronary arteries, or renal artery.

3. Natural history: Typically ischemia is transient but acute-on-chronic mesenteric ischemia can occur with thrombus formation. Intestinal necrosis occurs in ~15% of patients.

→ DIAGNOSIS

Diagnostic Tests

1. Laboratory tests: There are no diagnostic laboratory investigations.

2. Imaging studies: Although **dual-modality ultrasonography (with color Doppler)** is a reasonable diagnostic study for high-grade stenotic lesions, **computed tomography angiography (CTA) of the abdomen** is the first-line initial test to identify atherosclerosis and exclude other diseases. **CTA and magnetic resonance angiography (MRA)** have high sensitivity and specificity (>90%). **Arteriography** is used for diagnostic confirmation if noninvasive testing is nondiagnostic or during endovascular procedures.

→ TREATMENT

1. Conservative management: Nutritional assessment and support is important. Smoking cessation and pharmacologic preventive measures to limit atherosclerosis should be considered (eg, antiplatelet therapy).

2. Revascularization: Consider revascularization (percutaneous endovascular or open surgical, endarterectomy, or bypass grafts) in symptomatic patients with documented severe stenosis. Endovascular procedures are being performed more frequently; however, it is unclear whether they are truly superior to open procedures (eg, because of higher recurrence rates).⊙⊙ Revascularization may also be considered in asymptomatic patients undergoing surgical procedures on the aorta or renal arteries for other reasons.

1.3.8.3. Colonic Ischemia

→ DEFINITION, ETIOLOGY, PATHOGENESIS

Colonic ischemia is caused by insufficient perfusion of the intestinal wall that leads to hypoxia, reperfusion injury, and colonic inflammation. Ischemic colitis is the most frequent and less severe form of colonic ischemia. Segments of the intestines that are particularly vulnerable to ischemia include the region of the splenic flexure, descending colon, and rectosigmoid.

In most cases, ischemic colitis results from a low-flow state with no single identifiable cause. It can also result from occlusion of arteries (atherosclerosis, embolism, or thrombosis) and/or rarely of mesenteric veins.

→ CLINICAL FEATURES AND NATURAL HISTORY

Colonic ischemia occurs more frequently in women and older patients.

1. Symptoms: The classic symptoms of ischemic colitis are mild to moderate crampy left lower abdominal pain, urgent need to defecate, and bloody diarrhea within 24 hours of onset. Physical examination is nonspecific.

2. Risk factors include:

1) Medical conditions: Cardiovascular disease (eg, atherosclerosis, peripheral vascular disease, congestive heart failure, atrial fibrillation, hypertension), diabetes mellitus, chronic obstructive pulmonary disease, rheumatoid arthritis.

2) Procedures: Abdominal aortic aneurysm repair, cardiopulmonary bypass, aortoiliac instrumentation.

3) Drugs: Constipation-inducing drugs, immunomodulators (eg, anti–tumor necrosis factor α), drugs of abuse (eg, cocaine).

4) Rare risk factors include long-distance running, sickle cell crisis, and hypercoagulable states.

3. Natural history: Most cases are self-limited. Symptoms usually resolve within a few days and colon healing occurs after a few weeks even when untreated. However, irreversible ischemia can occur in some cases. Necrosis and perforation of the colon wall with diffuse peritonitis and hemodynamic instability may develop rapidly. Long-term complications such as strictures can occur.

4. Mortality: Mortality rates range from 4% to 12%. Increased mortality rates occur in patients with chronic kidney disease or chronic obstructive pulmonary disease, in those requiring surgical management, and in patients with isolated right colon ischemia.

→ D I A G N O S I S

Diagnostic Studies

1. Laboratory tests:

1) **Serology**: There are no specific markers for ischemic colitis. Results are helpful in predicting disease severity. Decreased hemoglobin and albumin levels and the presence of metabolic acidosis predict a more severe disease. In addition, investigations that may suggest advanced tissue damage include increased lactate, lactate dehydrogenase, creatine phosphokinase, and amylase.

2) **Stool tests**: *Clostridium difficile* toxin assay, culture, and ova and parasite tests should be performed to exclude infectious colitis.

2. Imaging: **Abdominal plain films** are usually nonspecific and therefore not very helpful, apart from the cases where they demonstrate signs of advanced ischemia (eg, thumbprinting) or perforation. Nonspecific findings include ileus or colon distension. **Computed tomography (CT)** with IV and oral contrast has replaced barium enema and is the current standard of care. Signs suggestive of ischemic colitis are nonspecific, such as bowel-wall thickening and fat stranding; the results may also be completely normal. **Computed tomography angiography (CTA)** or traditional angiography is only performed when acute mesenteric ischemia is suspected.

3. Colonoscopy: The diagnosis is confirmed with early colonoscopy (or flexible sigmoidoscopy) with biopsies within 48 hours. Contraindications to colonoscopy are peritonitis or signs of irreversible ischemic damage. Endoscopic findings include erythema, edema, hemorrhagic lesions, and/or ulcerations. Pathognomonic features are mucosal infarction and ghost cells. These lesions are frequently segmental with sharp transition between the normal and the affected mucosa. The rectum is relatively unaffected due to its dual blood supply from mesenteric and iliac arteries (as opposed to ulcerative colitis, which involves the rectum).

→ T R E A T M E N T

1. Conservative management: Most cases improve with bowel rest, fluid resuscitation, removal of precipitating factors, and nasogastric tube decompression if ileus is present.

2. Antibiotic therapy: Broad-spectrum empiric antibiotics in moderate to severe disease are recommended.⊘○

3. Anticoagulation: Anticoagulation is only indicated if ischemic colitis is due to mesenteric venous thrombosis or cardiac embolization.

4. Surgical treatment: Resection of the affected segments of the intestines with or without an end stoma is reserved for the most severe cases. Indications for surgery include perforation; clinical, radiologic, or endoscopic features suggestive of gangrene (eg, peritonitis); failure of medical treatment; or rarely massive bleeding in the setting of ischemic colitis. Uncommonly, patients who remain symptomatic or have recurrent episodes for a few weeks after presentation may require surgery. In patients with intestinal strictures resection of the affected segments of the colon is indicated if the patients are symptomatic or there is diagnostic uncertainty (ie, suspicion for cancer).

1.3.9. Irritable Bowel Syndrome (IBS)

→ DEFINITION, ETIOLOGY, PATHOGENESIS

Irritable bowel syndrome (IBS) is the most common chronic disease of the small and large intestine, affecting ~10% of the total population. IBS is a symptom--based condition defined by the presence of abdominal pain associated with defecation or change in bowel habits in the absence of any other condition leading to these symptoms. The etiology is not well understood and is likely multifactorial. Inflammatory, environmental, psychological, and dietary factors as well as intestinal microbiota play an important role in the pathogenesis of IBS. Psychiatric conditions are prevalent, with increased rates of anxiety and depression compared with a healthy control population.○

Classification

According to the Rome IV criteria (→Diagnostic Criteria, below), IBS may be classified into 4 subtypes using the Bristol to determine stool consistency (→Chapter 1.5, Figure 5-1). The scale ranges from 1 to 7, with 1 and 2 corresponding to hard stool; 3 to 5, normal consistency; and 6 to 7, loose and liquid consistency. The IBS subtypes are as follows:

1) **IBS with predominant constipation (IBS-C)**: For >25% of the time stool type 1 or 2 and <25% of the time stool type 6 or 7.

2) **IBS with predominant diarrhea (IBS-D)**: For >25% of the time stool type 6 or 7 and <25% of the time stool type 1 or 2.

3) **IBS with mixed bowel habits (IBS-M)**: For >25% of the time stool type 1 or 2 and >25% of the time stool type 6 or 7.

4) **Unclassified IBS (IBS-U)** meets the diagnostic criteria for IBS but the bowel habits are not accurately described by any of the above subtypes.

IBS subtypes are not separate conditions and the quantity, intensity, and severity of symptoms may vary from patient to patient. Therefore, the IBS subtype should ideally be recategorized as the patient's bowel habits change.

→ CLINICAL FEATURES AND NATURAL HISTORY

The **main symptom is abdominal pain**, which may be constant or recurrent and usually is located in the hypogastric area or in the left lower abdominal quadrant; it may be sharp, spasmodic, and cause significant discomfort but almost never wakes the patient at night. The pain worsens after a meal and is related to bowel movement (either increasing or improving pain). Patients can also have diarrhea or constipation (or both). In most patients symptoms fluctuate over time.

In patients with **diarrhea** the stools are watery or semiliquid (greasy), rarely of increased volume. Bowel movements are more frequent and preceded by a fairly rapid urge to defecate; they occur after meals, in response to stress, and in the morning.

In patients with **constipation**, the frequency of bowel movements is reduced. The stools are hard, lumpy (or in a form of hard nut-like nuggets), and associated with strenuous defecation; a sense of incomplete stool evacuation is common after defecation.

Some patients experience alternating periods of diarrhea and constipation. In both subtypes the stools are typically of small volume. Other symptoms include bloating, presence of mucus in stool, nausea, vomiting, and heartburn.

→ DIAGNOSIS

There are no known biomarkers for IBS diagnosis; therefore, this condition can only be recognized by its symptoms. The diagnosis of IBS requires the presence of specific gastrointestinal (GI) symptoms in the absence of any other GI disease. Physical examination is often normal. Some patients report tenderness in the hypogastrium or flanks.

Diagnostic Criteria

Establishing diagnostic criteria in IBS is important, as it provides a more standardized definition of IBS, which is essential not only for clinical practice but also for research. Since the first reports in 1972, the diagnostic criteria for IBS have evolved over time.

The most current **Rome IV criteria** include recurrent abdominal pain present on average ≥1 day per week in the last 3 months that fulfills ≥2 of the following:

1) Pain related to defecation (which either increases or improves the pain).

2) Pain associated with a change in stool frequency.

3) Pain associated with a change in stool form (appearance).

The criteria are fulfilled if the symptom onset occurred 6 months prior to diagnosis.

Diagnostic Tests

Tests are performed to exclude organic causes of symptoms (→Table 1-9). Commonly advised investigations include routine biochemical blood tests; complete blood count (CBC); thyroid-stimulating hormone (TSH); serologic testing for celiac disease (tissue transglutaminase [tTG] IgA antibodies and total IgA to identify IgA deficiency); and stool tests for bacterial infections, parasitic infections (if diarrhea is predominant), and occult blood. C-reactive protein (CRP) and fecal calprotectin testing are not recommended routinely.

Colonoscopy or flexible sigmoidoscopy is performed in selected cases. Colonoscopy may be indicated in patients aged >50 years even without alarming symptoms or with persistent diarrhea despite empiric treatment (to exclude microscopic colitis) and in younger patients with alarming symptoms. Endoscopy of the upper GI tract is performed in case of dyspepsia or positive serologic testing for celiac disease. A hydrogen breath test with lactose substrate can be performed if lactose intolerance is suspected but currently is not routinely recommended.

Differential Diagnosis

Before making a diagnosis of IBS, other causes of symptoms, particularly of recurrent diarrhea and constipation, should be excluded. IBS is a common condition and may coexist with other GI diseases.

⇥ TREATMENT

Management involves nonpharmacologic and pharmacologic therapies. A stepwise approach is usually preferred. General outline of our management: →Table 1-10.

Nonpharmacologic Treatment

Patient education is of key importance in the management of IBS. There are multiple nonpharmacologic therapies proposed, including lifestyle and dietary interventions, psychological treatment, prebiotics, and probiotics.

1. Diets: Patients with IBS often report worsening of symptoms after the ingestion of certain food components, and >60% of patients relate the occurrence of bloating and abdominal pain with consumption of certain foods, such as wheat and fermentable carbohydrates. Therefore, different elimination diets have been proposed to improve symptoms. It is worth noting that elimination diets are restrictive, expensive, and not easy to follow. The most common restrictive diets recommended in IBS:

1) **Low fermentable oligosaccharides, disaccharides, monosaccharides, and polyols (FODMAP) diet**: Probably effective in relieving IBS symptoms.⊘○ A low FODMAP diet is often recommended for a period of 4 to 8 weeks. This is followed by the second phase, where different foods

Table 1-9. Alarming signs or symptoms not explained by IBS alone that require further investigation	
Alarming symptoms suggestive of organic disease	– Symptom onset >50 years – Progressively worsening symptoms – Unexplained weight loss or loss of appetite – Nocturnal diarrhea – Family history of colon cancer, celiac disease, or IBD – Blood in stool (melena) – Unexplained iron deficiency anemia – Abdominal mass – Ascites – Elevated WBC count – Fever – Recent change in symptoms
Commonly used tests	– CBC – tTG IgA (to exclude celiac disease), duodenal biopsy – CRP and fecal calprotectin (if suspecting IBD; not used routinely) – Colonoscopy (in GI bleeding, unexplained weight loss, family history of colon cancer, and/or abdominal mass, or age >50 years). Consider random biopsies in diarrhea to exclude microscopic colitis – Hydrogen breath test (to exclude SIBO [glucose substrate] or fructose/lactose intolerance [glucose or lactose substrate]; not to be used routinely) – Plain film of abdomen (may be useful to exclude fecal loading) – Motility test (may be useful to identify origin of constipation)

Adapted from JAMA. 2015;313(9):949-58 and United European Gastroenterol J. 2017;5(6):773-788.

CBC, complete blood count; CRP, C-reactive protein; GI, gastrointestinal; IBD, inflammatory bowel disease; IBS, irritable bowel syndrome; SIBO, small intestinal bacterial overgrowth; tTG, tissue transglutaminase; WBC, white blood cell.

containing FODMAP are reintroduced every 6 days to identify symptoms triggered by specific types of food. This phase last 6 to 10 weeks.

2) **Gluten-free diet (GFD)**: There is insufficient evidence to recommend GFD as a first-line therapy in IBS.⊗○

3) **Elimination diet**: There is some suggestion that an elimination diet based on the presence of IgG antibodies to specific food components could improve symptoms in IBS patients. However, the clinical evidence supporting the elimination diet in IBS is of very low quality and the intervention is currently not recommended.

2. Fiber: There is some evidence for the use of different fiber supplements in relieving IBS symptoms, including a modest benefit of psyllium. Current recommendations suggest the use of soluble fiber, specifically psyllium, as first-line therapy, which should be started at a nominal dose and gradually titrated upward over weeks to a total daily intake of 20 to 30 g.◐○

3. Prebiotics, probiotics, and fecal transplantation:

1) Prebiotics refer to food components that remain undigested, such as fructo--oligosaccharides or inulin, and stimulate either the growth or activity of intestinal bacteria. There is no evidence for the positive effect of prebiotics in IBS.

2) Probiotics are live or attenuated microorganisms that may affect the composition or function of the gut microbiota and additionally may have anti--inflammatory and antinociceptive properties. Data have shown consistently

Table 1-10. Algorithm for management of IBS

Initial management	Further pharmacologic treatment (dose)	Mechanism	Indication	Evidence
IBS with predominant constipation (IBS-C)				
– To improve IBS symptoms: Water-soluble fiber (psyllium >12 g daily) – To improve stool consistency, as adjuvant treatment (only as needed): Osmotic laxatives: Poly-ethylene glycol 17 g/d; magnesium hydroxide 15-30 mL/d	Linaclotide (145--290 µg/d) and plecanatide (3-6 mg/d)	Guanylate C agonist	Pain, discomfort, stool consistency, straining	H
	Lubiprostone (8-24 µg bid)	Chloride channel activator	Bloating, pain, straining, frequency, consistency	M
	Antispasmodics: Dicyclomine (20-40 mg qid), pinaverium (50--100 mg tid), trimebutine (200 mg tid)	Anticholinergic or calcium channel blocker	Pain; may worsen constipation	VL
	Antidepressants: Citalopram (20 mg/d), fluoxetine (20 mg/d), paroxetine (20-40 mg/d)	SSRIs	Pain, depression	M
IBS with predominant diarrhea (IBS-D)				
Low FODMAP diet for 4-8 weeks	Loperamide (2-4 mg; max, 12 mg/d; only as needed, not continuously)	Mu-opioid receptor agonist	Diarrhea (no effect on pain) as rescue medication	VL
	Eluxadoline (75--100 mg bid)	Mixed µ-opioid, δ-opioid, and κ-opioid receptor agonist	Diarrhea, pain	M
	Diphenoxylate/atropine[a]: Diphenoxylate 5 mg, then 2.5 mg after each loose bowel movement (max, 20 mg/d)	Mu-opioid receptor agonist and anticholinergic	Diarrhea, pain	M
	Rifaximin (400-550 mg bid for 10-14 days)	Antimicrobial	Diarrhea, pain	M
	Antidepressants (→IBS-C): Amitriptyline (10-20 mg/d), desipramine (25 mg/d), imipramine (25 mg/d)	TCAs	Diarrhea, pain, constipation	H
IBS with mixed bowel habits (IBS-M)				
To improve stool consistency: – Water-soluble fiber (psyllium >12 g daily) – Low FODMAP diet (also improves bloating) – Stop laxatives	→IBS-D and IBS-C	→IBS-D and IBS-C	→IBS-D and IBS-C	→IBS-D and IBS-C

Initial management	Further pharmacologic treatment (dose)	Mechanism	Indication	Evidence
Bloating				
Low FODMAP diet	IBS-C: Linaclotide and lubiprostone	→IBS-C	→IBS-D and IBS-C	→IBS-D and IBS-C
	IBS-D: Rifaximin and eluxadoline	→IBS-D	→IBS-D and IBS-C	→IBS-D and IBS-C

[a] In North America available under trade name Lomotil.

FODMAP, fermentable oligosaccharides, disaccharides, monosaccharides, and polyols; IBS, irritable bowel syndrome; H, high quality; M, moderate quality; SSRI, selective serotonin reuptake inhibitor; TCA, tricyclic antidepressant; VL, very low quality.

that probiotic treatment is effective for IBS, although which individual species and strains are the most beneficial remains unclear. Probiotics help reduce symptom burden, abdominal pain, and duration or intensity of diarrhea☺● and help reduce bloating or distension and improve the frequency and consistency of bowel movements.☺○

3) Fecal transplantation: Although this therapy seems to be promising, there is insufficient evidence of its efficacy in IBS.

4) Psychological treatment: Psychological interventions, such as cognitive behavioral therapy (CBT), hypnosis, and mindfulness-based therapies, have been designed and implemented effectively in IBS. CBT is the most widely studied psychotherapy and is currently suggested by some, when available, as first-line treatment for IBS.☺○ CBT is often provided by mental health practitioners, including counsellors, psychotherapists, psychologists, and psychiatrists.

Pharmacotherapy

When nonpharmacologic treatment has failed, pharmacologic therapies should be initiated, depending on the IBS subtype and predominant symptoms (→Table 1-10).

1. IBS-C:

1) Water-soluble fiber, osmotic laxatives (polyethylene glycol, lactulose), and stimulant laxatives (bisacodyl, senna) are commonly used but generally do not influence the symptoms. They may be used as adjuvants when other symptoms have improved but constipation persists.☺○

2) Agents that target multiple symptoms in IBS-C are linaclotide and plecanatide (guanylate cyclase-C [GCC] agonists) or lubiprostone (a chloride channel activator). Plecanatide binding to GCC receptors is pH-dependent, which is why its activity is mostly confined to the proximal small intestine. Linaclotide binds to GCC receptors in a pH-independent manner and could be active throughout the small intestine and colon. In a recent systematic review, linaclotide, lubiprostone, and plecanatide were superior to placebo for the treatment of IBS-C. Linaclotide was ranked first in efficacy for abdominal pain and achieving complete spontaneous bowel movements and is recommended as first line-therapy in IBS-C.☺●

3) Lubiprostone is a prostaglandin derivative and selective chloride channel activator, which facilitates transport of chloride, sodium, and water into the intestinal lumen. It has been shown to improve IBS-C symptoms, including bloating, bowel frequency, and stool consistency.

4) For patients with IBS-C and predominant pain, antispasmodics (dicyclomine, pinaverium, and trimebutine) have been proposed, as they relax intestinal smooth muscle.⊘◯

5) Antidepressants, including selective serotonin reuptake inhibitors (SSRIs)⊘⊜ and tricyclic antidepressants (TCAs),⊛⊜ are also widely used for IBS treatment, although in doses lower than those used in depression.

6) Prokinetics, such as prucalopride, are an alternative option for the treatment of constipation. Although prucalopride was shown to be effective in idiopathic constipation, the body of evidence for its use in IBS-C is weaker and the agent is not recommended in IBS.⊗◯

2. IBS-D:

1) Diet modification: A low FODMAP diet.

2) Pharmacotherapy:

a) Loperamide, a μ-opioid receptor agonist, decreases diarrhea by slowing intestinal transit and reducing fluid secretion into the intestinal lumen. It is not recommended for continuous use,⊗◯ although it may be useful in specific situations in selected patients.⊘◯

b) Probiotics.⊘◯

c) Eluxadoline is a new therapeutic agent with mixed opioid effects (affecting μ-opioid, κ-opioid, and δ-opioid receptors).⊘⊜

d) Rifaximin is a nonsystemic broad-spectrum antibiotic approved in some countries for IBS-D in adults. The mechanisms of action of rifaximin in IBS are not well understood but may be associated with altering the microbiome and thus reducing gas production. In a recent consensus statement, there were concerns related to the recommendation of rifaximin for the treatment of IBS related to the potential antibiotic resistance and high cost associated with this therapy.

e) Antidepressants, especially TCAs, are widely used to target pain in IBS-D, as they are associated with decreased colonic transit.

f) Diphenoxylate/atropine (in North America available as Lomotil) combines the μ-opioid receptor agonist effect (diphenoxylate) and anticholinergic effect (atropine).

3. IBS-M:

1) A low FODMAP diet, probiotics, and TCAs can be offered to these patients. Treatment will be adjusted according to the predominant symptom of diarrhea or constipation.

2) Ensure the patient is not affected by "pseudo–IBS-M" with overflow diarrhea (feces becoming so hard they cannot be expelled with fecal fluid flowing around the blockage), which requires treatment targeting constipation.

4. Treatment of other symptoms in all patients with IBS:

1) Flatulence: **Simeticone** 80 mg tid; **dimeticone** 100 mg tid.

2) Postprandial pain: **Hyoscine** 10 to 20 mg before meals, **peppermint oil** (recommended for improving IBS symptoms, particularly in patients with pain).⊘◯

1.3.10. Microscopic Colitis

→ **DEFINITION AND CLINICAL FEATURES**

Microscopic colitis is the overarching term for two diseases: **lymphocytic colitis** and **collagenous colitis**; they are diseases of unknown etiology characterized by the presence of distinctive microscopic lesions without macroscopic (endoscopic) or radiologic changes.

Signs and symptoms: Watery diarrhea (high-volume bowel movements, which nevertheless rarely cause dehydration), often not associated with abdominal pain but with abdominal cramps; flatulence; weight loss. The endoscopic appearance of the colon is usually normal, although occasionally it may reveal minor mucosal edema, areas of hyperemia, and petechiae. When performing colonoscopy, it is mandatory to obtain biopsy specimens from the ascending colon and terminal ileum in patients with unexplained watery diarrhea. The results of routine laboratory tests and radiography of the small intestine and colon are normal.

DIAGNOSIS

Diagnosis is based on the results of **histologic examination** of biopsy specimens. An increase in the number of intraepithelial lymphocytes (>20/100 surface epithelial cells) is the cardinal histologic feature of lymphocytic colitis. There is no associated crypt distortion, and the crypt architecture is preserved. The increase in the number of intraepithelial lymphocytes can be maximal on the right side of the colon; therefore, the diagnosis of microscopic colitis can sometimes be missed if the patient only has a flexible sigmoidoscopy as the investigation.

Collagenous colitis has similar histologic features to lymphocytic colitis except that in addition there is thickening of the collagen layer at the base of epithelial cells (defined as thickness >10 µm) accompanied by an increase in the number of lamina propria inflammatory cells.

Differential Diagnosis

Differential diagnosis should include irritable bowel syndrome, celiac disease, Crohn disease, ulcerative colitis, lactose intolerance, abuse of laxatives, amyloidosis, hormone-producing tumors, and disturbances of the bile acid circulation.

MANAGEMENT

The management of microscopic colitis should include a workup for celiac disease (→Chapter 6.1.3.3), because there is an association between the two disorders and both can manifest with diarrhea.

Microscopic colitis is also associated with **nonsteroidal anti-inflammatory drugs (NSAIDs)**, **proton pump inhibitors (PPIs)**, **statins**, and **selective serotonin reuptake inhibitors (SSRIs)**. The benefits of these drugs may outweigh the risks, as microscopic colitis has a benign course, but if the disease is dramatically reducing quality of life and is difficult to treat or there is not a strong indication for these drugs, they should be discontinued. Smoking cessation should also be advised.

Patients with mild diarrhea symptoms should be prescribed **antidiarrheal drugs**, such as loperamide. Other alternatives for mild symptoms include cholestyramine, mesalamine (INN mesalazine), or bismuth salts. Patients with moderate to severe diarrhea should be prescribed budesonide (initially 9 mg/d orally for 6-8 weeks; maintenance treatment with low doses of 3-6 mg/d orally); this therapy is very effective, with a number needed to treat of 2 for collagenous colitis and a number needed to treat of 3 for lymphocytic colitis. In patients not responding to budesonide or other treatment alternatives, **immunosuppressive therapy** such as azathioprine, methotrexate, or anti–tumor necrosis factor agents may be considered with caution. **Surgical treatment** (split ileostomy and subtotal colectomy) is limited only to patients with severe disease not responding to other treatment modalities.

1.3.11. Protein-Losing Enteropathy

DEFINITION, ETIOLOGY, PATHOGENESIS

Protein-losing enteropathy is a clinical syndrome characterized by excessive loss of plasma proteins from the gastrointestinal (GI) tract that leads to hypoproteinemia. Protein loss can occur from abnormalities in the lymphatic system resulting in loss of protein-rich lymph or from mucosal damage (with or without ulceration). The mostly affected proteins are those with long half-lives, such as albumin or immunoglobulins.

Etiology:

1) **Loss of proteins with lymph:**

   a) Primary intestinal lymphangiectasia: Characterized by dilation of lymphatic vessels within the GI tract secondary to congenital obstruction of lymphatics. This leads to a high-pressure system and leakage of protein--rich lymph, causing hypoproteinemia, lymphopenia, and edema. Most patients present before the age of 3 years.

   b) Secondary lymphatic vessel dilation (impaired lymph outflow): Cardiovascular diseases (right ventricular failure, constrictive pericarditis, long-term complications of Fontan procedure [a surgical procedure to correct congenital cardiac abnormalities]), lymphatic dysfunction (eg, cancer, tuberculosis, sarcoidosis, radiotherapy and chemotherapy), cirrhosis, hepatic veno-occlusive disease or hepatic vein thrombosis, chronic pancreatitis with the formation of pseudocysts, Crohn disease, Whipple disease, intestinal lymphatic fistulas, congenital lymphatic malformations, arsenic poisoning, retroperitoneal fibrosis.

2) **Mucosal erosions and ulcerations**: Inflammatory bowel disease, tumors (gastric cancer, lymphomas, Kaposi sarcoma, heavy chain diseases), pseudomembranous colitis, multiple gastric ulcers or gastric erosions, enteropathy induced by nonsteroidal anti-inflammatory drugs or chemotherapy, ulcerative jejunoileitis, graft-versus-host disease.

3) **Increased mucosal permeability**: Celiac disease and tropical sprue, Ménétrier disease, lymphocytic gastritis, *Helicobacter pylori* gastritis, amyloidosis, common variable immunodeficiency–associated gastroenteropathy, infections (small intestinal bacterial overgrowth, complication of acute viral gastroenteritis, parasitic infections, Whipple disease), systemic connective tissue diseases (systemic lupus erythematosus, rheumatoid arthritis, mixed connective tissue disease), hypertrophic hypersecretory gastropathy, allergic gastroenteropathy, eosinophilic gastroenteritis, collagenous colitis.

Proteins lost through the GI tract are usually digested (except for α_1 antitrypsin, thus used as a diagnostic marker [→Diagnostic Tests, below]). In patients with lymphatic stasis, lymphocytes and immunoglobulins are also lost (although this usually does not lead to clinically apparent immunodeficiency) and malabsorption of long-chain triglycerides and fat-soluble vitamins ensues.

→ CLINICAL FEATURES

Clinical manifestations are diverse and largely depend on the underlying condition. The most common signs and symptoms include chronic diarrhea (frequently with steatorrhea), nausea, vomiting, edema (pitting, symmetric, affecting particularly the lower limbs), sometimes lymphedema of various locations, ascites, less frequently pleural or pericardial effusions (fluid may be milky due to the lymph content), malnutrition, cachexia in advanced cases, symptoms of vitamin A and D deficiencies.

→ DIAGNOSIS

Diagnostic Tests

1. Laboratory tests: Hypoalbuminemia; low levels of immunoglobulins (IgG, IgA, IgM), fibrinogen, transferrin, and ceruloplasmin; sometimes lymphopenia, hypocholesterolemia, anemia, and hypocalcemia.

2. Fecal α_1-antitrypsin excretion is increased. α_1 Antitrypsin is produced in the liver and does not undergo secretion, absorption, or digestion; thus, it is only detected intact in stool if there is loss from the GI tract. Alpha$_1$ antitrypsin clearance is measured by collecting 24-hour α_1 antitrypsin levels in stool and serum. A false-negative result may occur in conditions associated with hypersecretion of hydrochloric acid (as α_1 antitrypsin undergoes proteolysis at a pH <3.5); in such cases a proton pump inhibitor should be administered 3 days before the test.⊘○ Intestinal bleeding can increase α_1-antitrypsin clearance.

3. Intestinal scintigraphy and **magnetic resonance imaging (MRI)** may provide additional information and document the loss of radioactively labeled material in some situations (eg, primary protein-losing enteropathy in children with intestinal lymphangiectasia), although the evidence is anecdotal and clinical utility of these tests is not clear.⊘○

Diagnostic Criteria

Increased fecal α_1-antitrypsin excretion in a patient with hypoalbuminemia and edema in whom other causes have been excluded. A fecal clearance >27 mL/24 hours is considered abnormal. In the setting of diarrhea, a fecal clearance >56 mL/24 hours is abnormal.

Differential Diagnosis

Other conditions associated with edema, hypoproteinemia, or chronic diarrhea.

→ TREATMENT

1. Treatment of the underlying condition. In patients with primary lymphangiectasia involving a limited portion of the intestine, resection of the affected segment may be needed.

2. Nutritional management:

1) Restriction of fats containing long-chain triglycerides, as these are mostly absorbed through lymphatic vessels. Alternatively, recommend the use of **formulas containing medium-chain triglycerides (MCTs)** (eg, MCT oils, which are absorbed directly through the portal vein) to reduce the malabsorption of fats as well as to lower the lymphatic pressure and reduce the leakage of lymph to the intestinal lumen in patients with impaired lymphatic drainage.

2) **Protein-rich diet** (2-3 g/kg/d), sometimes supplemented with high-protein formulas.

3) **Vitamin and trace element supplementation** (calcium, iron, magnesium, zinc).

4) **Parenteral nutrition** if necessary.

3. Medications: Specific treatments are limited and pharmacologic therapy is directed either at the underlying conditions or consequences (edema).

1) Patients after Fontan procedure: Certain medications showed potential benefit in very small randomized controlled trials (bosentan)○ or isolated case reports and small case series (sildenafil, budesonide, heparin) with corresponding major uncertainties regarding their usefulness.○

2) Other medications for protein-losing enteropathy tried in isolated cases:

   a) Spironolactone 2.5 mg/kg/d and furosemide 2 mg/kg/d⊘○: A combination of diuretics aimed at decreasing fluid overload. Spironolactone may also reduce proteinuria.

   b) Subcutaneous octreotide 0.1 mg tid⊘○: A somatostatin analogue that aims to reduce splanchnic blood flow and lymph secretion.

1.3.12. Short Bowel Syndrome

→ DEFINITION, ETIOLOGY, PATHOGENESIS

Short bowel syndrome (SBS) develops after surgical resection or bypass of the small intestine, leading to reduced absorption of nutrients and water; in some SBS patients severe malabsorption can lead to intestinal failure such that the patient's well-being cannot be maintained by oral or enteral nutrition alone. The incidence of SBS is ~2 per 1,000,000 per year and the prevalence is ~20 per 1,000,000.

Intestinal failure is unlikely in adults who retain >150 to 200 cm of functional small intestine but patients may tolerate more extensive loss if the colon remains in continuity, as this contributes substantially to the absorption of fluid and nutrients. Anatomically, patients with SBS **at risk of intestinal failure** may be assigned to one of 3 groups:

1) **End jejunostomy (SBS-J) with no residual colon**: The minimum length of residual small intestine required to maintain independence from parenteral nutrition is reported to be ~115 cm.

2) **Jejunocolic anastomosis (SBS-JC) with anastomosis of the remnant jejunum to part of the colon** (most frequently left colon): The minimum length of residual small intestine required to maintain independence from parenteral nutrition is reported to be ~60 cm.

3) **Jejunoileal anastomosis (SBS-JIC) with an intact ileocecal valve and colon**: The minimum length of residual small intestine required to maintain independence from parenteral nutrition is reported to be ~35 cm.

SBS is the most common cause of intestinal failure; the other 4 major pathophysiologic causes, which may be due to a variety of benign or malignant conditions, are intestinal fistula, intestinal dysmotility, mechanical obstruction, and extensive small bowel mucosal disease. Clinically, intestinal failure can be classified by duration:

1) **Acute (type 1) intestinal failure** usually occurs postoperatively and requires short-term IV fluid or nutritional support for days to weeks.

2) **Prolonged acute (type 2) intestinal failure**, in the presence of multiple complications, requires longer-term parenteral support for weeks to months pending resolution of the complications and intestinal adaptation.

3) **Chronic (type 3) intestinal failure** due to incomplete adaptation requires parenteral support for months to years or even permanently.

The most common **causes of intestinal failure**:

1) Extensive intestinal resection due to ischemia, Crohn disease, cancer, trauma, postoperative complications, intestinal torsion or strangulation and necrosis.

2) Extensive small bowel mucosal disease and dysfunction due to, for example, postradiation enteritis or refractory celiac disease.

3) Fistulae, which may be external (causing loss of bowel contents) or internal (bypassing sections of small bowel).

➡ CLINICAL FEATURES

The initial signs and symptoms of SBS—diarrhea, dehydration, cachexia, and electrolyte disturbances—are primarily attributable to the malabsorption of fluid, electrolytes, and macronutrients, and their severity is proportional to the loss of small bowel function. Fluid and electrolyte disturbances are most severe in patients who have end jejunostomy. With time, malabsorption often leads to clinical or subclinical manifestations of vitamin and micronutrient deficiencies, including magnesium, calcium, phosphate, fat-soluble vitamins (A, D, and E, but rarely K), vitamin B_{12}, folic acid, and trace elements (zinc, selenium, chromium, copper).

Long-term complications in patients with type 2 or 3 intestinal failure include:

1) **Psychiatric, neurologic, and visual disturbances** due to vitamin and essential fatty acid deficiencies (particularly vitamins A and E as well as B vitamins, including vitamin B_{12}) exacerbated by bile acid loss after ileal resection. Neurologic disturbances may also occur in patients receiving long-term parenteral nutrition due to the accumulation of manganese (from trace element supplements) in the extrapyramidal system and aluminum (from IV water contaminants).

2) **Arrhythmias, paresthesia, and muscle cramps** due to potassium, magnesium, and calcium deficiency.

3) **Heart failure and myositis** due to selenium and thiamine (vitamin B_1) deficiency.

4) **Gallstones** due to changes in bile composition and gallbladder emptying.

5) **Kidney stones** due to decreased urine volume and, in patients with a retained colon, excessive absorption of oxalate as a result of unabsorbed fatty acids binding to luminal calcium (to the extent that oxalates are absorbed freely from the colon and excreted in urine, where they bind to calcium, producing oxalate nephrolithiasis).

6) **Ascending urinary tract infections**, particularly in women, due to frequent profuse diarrhea and perineal contamination.

7) **Altered mental status, seizures, and ataxia** caused by D-lactic acidosis, predominantly in patients with a retained colon and fermentation of unabsorbed carbohydrates by gram-positive anaerobic bacteria that produce D-lactate.

8) **Diarrhea, bloating, flatulence, anorexia, and malabsorption** due to small bowel bacterial overgrowth caused by loss of the ileocecal valve after surgery.

9) **Esophagitis, peptic ulcer disease, and upper gastrointestinal bleeding** due to gastric hypersecretion caused by loss of neuroendocrine inhibitory feedback.

10) **Anemia** caused by impaired absorption of hematinics, including iron, vitamin B_{12}, folic acid, and copper.

11) **Metabolic bone disease and fractures** caused by multiple factors, including impaired intake and metabolism of calcium, phosphate, magnesium, and vitamin D; abnormal parathyroid hormone secretion; and aluminum accumulation. These factors are exacerbated by protein-energy malnutrition, decreased exercise tolerance, and sarcopenia.

12) **Intestinal failure–related liver disease**, including cholestasis, hepatic steatosis, cirrhosis, and liver failure associated with decreased oral or enteral nutrient intake and parenteral lipid or glucose overload and exacerbated by sepsis and medications.

13) **Blood stream infections, venous thrombosis, catheter breakage, and catheter occlusion**, often due to nonadherence to strict management protocols for venous access management.

→ TREATMENT AND PROGNOSIS

Ideally, SBS should be managed by a multidisciplinary team with nursing, dietetic, and physician members in specialized centers to minimize the risk of catheter-related blood stream infections and ensure coordinated care for patients who often have complex medical problems in addition to the direct effects of small bowel loss. Patients with SBS require close monitoring of their oral intake, with tailored advice regarding the need for hyperphagia and appropriate oral hydration, including rehydration solutions and regular blood tests to ensure appropriate replacement of fluids, electrolytes, macronutrients, micronutrients, and trace elements. Almost all type 3 intestinal failure patients will require long-term parenteral support to provide adequate nutrition, fluid, and electrolytes; even if intestinal adaptation over a period of 6 months to 2 to 4 years permits discontinuation of parenteral support, most patients will require close follow-up. The management of underlying or concomitant conditions, including sepsis, stomas, and fistulae, is complicated by the presence of intestinal failure, while the absorption of oral drugs is often impaired, necessitating careful changes to the dose, formulation, and route of drug administration.

SBS is associated with significant morbidity and impairment of health-related quality of life, partly related to intestinal failure and malabsorption and partly related to the underlying disease as well as the effects of therapy. In general, the 2- and 5-year survival rates for SBS patients, in the absence of malignancy, are ~85% and 70% to 75%, respectively. Efforts to ameliorate the sequelae of intestinal failure have included small bowel transplantation with or without other organs, surgical small bowel lengthening procedures, and most recently the administration of gut trophic hormone analogues. Small bowel transplantation in adults is performed rarely and only at highly specialized centers; unfortunately, the long-term outcomes have been disappointing compared with other organ transplantation procedures. Bowel lengthening procedures have been beneficial in some pediatric patients but there is limited data on their benefit in adults.

Glucagon-like peptide-2 (GLP-2), produced by enteroendocrine L cells in the ileum and colon, plays a key role in maintaining small bowel mucosal mass and function. Recent studies have reported that a long-acting GLP-2 analogue, teduglutide, reduces the need for parenteral support in patients with chronic intestinal failure, allowing up to one-third to discontinue parenteral support completely.◉

2. Liver and Biliary Tract Diseases

2.1. Gallbladder and Bile Duct Diseases

2.1.1. Acute Cholangitis

➔ DEFINITION, ETIOLOGY, PATHOGENESIS

Acute cholangitis is a segmental or diffuse acute inflammation of the intrahepatic or extrahepatic bile ducts caused by impaired or blocked bile outflow (→Figure 2-3). Pathogens most commonly involved include *Escherichia coli*, *Klebsiella* spp, *Enterococcus* spp, *Enterobacter* spp, *Streptococcus* spp, and *Pseudomonas aeruginosa*; anaerobic pathogens are involved in 15% of cases.

Risk factors—causes of cholestasis—include choledocholithiasis, tumors obstructing bile outflow (infiltrates in the bile ducts or the papilla of Vater, external compression), postinflammatory and iatrogenic strictures of the bile ducts, primary sclerosing cholangitis, and compression of the bile ducts by a pancreatic cyst or enlarged lymph nodes.

➔ CLINICAL FEATURES AND NATURAL HISTORY

Typical clinical signs are the **Charcot triad**: severe pain of the biliary colic type located in the right upper abdominal quadrant or in the central epigastrium, fever, and jaundice. When hypotension and impaired mental status are additionally present, the syndrome is termed the Reynolds pentad. Tenderness of the right upper abdominal quadrant with abdominal guarding may also be found on clinical examination. Patients may develop septic shock. Untreated bacterial cholangitis is usually fatal.

➔ DIAGNOSIS

Diagnostic Tests

1. Laboratory tests: Results are similar to those found in patients with choledocholithiasis and additionally include an elevated white blood cell count with a shift to the left in the differential blood count. Severe cholangitis may be accompanied by features of sepsis.

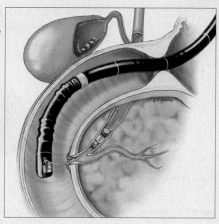

Figure 2-1. Endoscopic retrograde cholangiopancreatography (ERCP) with stone extraction. *Illustration courtesy of Dr Shannon Zhang.*

2. Imaging studies: Ultrasonography may reveal dilated intrahepatic and extrahepatic bile ducts and choledocholithiasis. In patients with acute cholangitis **urgent endoscopic retrograde cholangiopancreatography (ERCP)** (→Figure 2-1) is the optimal diagnostic technique that allows for simultaneous therapeutic intervention.

Diagnostic Criteria

Diagnosis is based on the characteristic clinical features and results of laboratory or imaging studies.

Differential Diagnosis

Other causes of fever and epigastric pain: acute cholecystitis, acute biliary pancreatitis, liver abscess, acute viral hepatitis, diverticulitis, intestinal perforation.

→ TREATMENT

Medical Management

All patients should be assessed for severe sepsis and treated appropriately as needed.

1. Stop oral intake of food and fluids.

2. Administer IV fluids. Usually start with isotonic crystalloids.

3. Analgesics and spasmolytics are used as in biliary colic (→Chapter 6.2.1.3.2).

4. Empiric broad-spectrum antimicrobial treatment: Treatment should include coverage for gram-negative bacteria and anaerobes; our regimens, adjusted for local resistance patterns, may include piperacillin/tazobactam, imipenem, or a combination of a third-generation cephalosporin and metronidazole.

Invasive Treatment

1. The treatment of choice is **ERCP with endoscopic sphincterotomy**. This may apply even to patients with cholangitis without stones shown on imaging studies. When necessary, treatment is combined with stenting of the bile ducts to facilitate normal bile drainage.

2. Percutaneous drainage under ultrasonographic or computed tomographic (CT) guidance is used in patients in whom anatomical abnormalities render endoscopic treatment impossible.

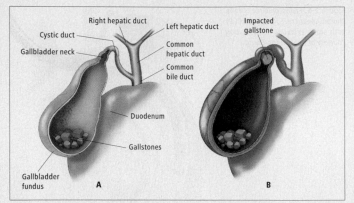

Figure 2-2. Gallstones. **A**, cholelithiasis. **B**, cholecystitis. *Illustration courtesy of Dr Shannon Zhang.*

3. Surgical drainage is used when other forms of biliary drainage are not feasible or have failed; it is performed very rarely.

2.1.2. Acute Cholecystitis

➡ DEFINITION, ETIOLOGY, PATHOGENESIS

Acute cholecystitis is an acute inflammation of the gallbladder and one of the major complications of cholelithiasis (→Figure 2-2). It may be caused by impaired bile outflow from the gallbladder (as a result of occlusion of the cystic duct or edema of the cystic duct mucosa). Approximately 10% of cases of cholecystitis occur in persons without gallstones and usually with serious systemic diseases (acalculous cholecystitis).

➡ CLINICAL FEATURES

Signs and symptoms include persistent biliary colic, fever, rigors, vomiting, poor general condition, severe right upper abdominal quadrant tenderness, positive Murphy sign (→Diagnostic Tests, below), sometimes a palpable tender gallbladder, signs of peritonitis (in some patients), tachycardia, and tachypnea.

➡ DIAGNOSIS

Diagnostic Tests

1. Laboratory tests: Elevated white blood cell (WBC) counts with a shift to the left in the differential blood count; elevated C-reactive protein (CRP) levels; elevated serum aspartate aminotransferase (AST), alanine aminotransferase (ALT), alkaline phosphatase (ALP), and bilirubin (if the case of obstruction of the common bile duct or a concomitant liver disease). Amylase could be elevated in patients with concomitant biliary pancreatitis and cholecystitis.

2. Imaging studies: Ultrasonography may reveal major features of chole-cystitis, including gallstones, edema of the gallbladder wall with an increased gallbladder wall thickness, gas within the gallbladder wall (gangrenous chole-cystitis), and a positive ultrasonographic Murphy sign (tenderness in the right upper abdominal quadrant evoked by pressure from the ultrasound transducer over the visualized gallbladder). Minor features include an enlarged gallbladder, a thickened gallbladder wall, abnormal gallbladder content (eg, sludge), and fluid collections near the gallbladder.◉ **Computed tomography (CT)** is useful in the diagnosis of patients with acute cholecystitis and in the diagnosis of complications.

Diagnostic Criteria

Signs, symptoms, and ultrasonographic features.

→ TREATMENT

1. **Stop oral intake of food and fluids.**

2. **Administer IV fluids**, for example, an isotonic crystalloid.

3. Use **analgesics and spasmolytics** as in biliary colic (→Chapter 6.2.1.3.2).

4. **Empiric broad-spectrum antibiotic treatment** is rarely, if ever, used in Canada in patients who can undergo cholecystectomy in a timely fashion (<8 hours from presentation to the hospital) and without signs of sepsis.⊗◉

5. **Cholecystectomy** is indicated in every patient with acute cholecystitis caused by gallstones within 72 hours of admission to the hospital; in most patients a laparoscopic procedure can be performed.◉◉ If the procedure cannot be performed within 7 days from the onset of symptoms, it should be delayed until ≥6 weeks of the onset. However, it may also need to be delayed from the start in elderly patients with severe cardiovascular and respiratory comorbidities.

→ COMPLICATIONS

Complications that require urgent surgical treatment include empyema, necrosis, or perforation (limited or with diffuse biliary peritonitis) of the gallbladder. Other complications include hygroma of the gallbladder, liver abscess, biliary intestinal fistula (passage of large gallstones to the intestinal lumen may result in gallstone ileus), and Mirizzi syndrome (obstruction of the neck of the gallbladder or the cystic duct by a large gallstone resulting in symptoms of common bile duct compression).

2.1.3. Gallstones

→ DEFINITION AND ETIOLOGY

The presence of gallstones can be classified based on their location as:

1) **Cholelithiasis** (→Figure 2-2), which refers to the presence of gallstones in the gallbladder.

2) **Choledocholithiasis** (→Figure 2-3), which refers to the presence of gallstones in the extrahepatic or intrahepatic bile ducts. Gallstones may originate from the gallbladder (secondary choledocholithiasis) or form in the bile ducts (primary choledocholithiasis; rare in Europe and North America). Ninety-five percent of patients with choledocholithiasis have concomitant cholelithiasis.

Gallstones are classified according to their composition as **cholesterol gallstones** (yellow or yellow-brown), **pigment gallstones** (rare in Europe and North America), or **mixed gallstones**.

Risk factors for cholesterol gallstones include genetic factors, female sex (they are 4 times more common in women than in men), advanced age, estrogen treatment, diabetes mellitus, obesity, hypertriglyceridemia, treatment with fibrates, rapid weight loss (eg, after bariatric surgery), and cystic fibrosis. **Risk factors for pigment gallstones** include hemolytic anemia, Crohn disease, cirrhosis, and long-term total parenteral nutrition.

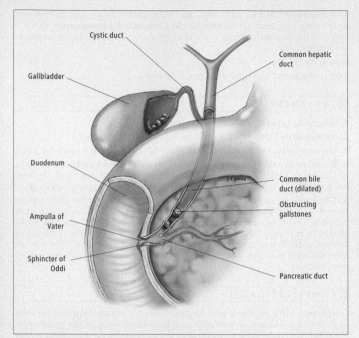

Figure 2-3. Choledocholithiasis. *Illustration courtesy of Dr Shannon Zhang.*

2.1.3.1. Choledocholithiasis

→ **CLINICAL FEATURES AND NATURAL HISTORY**

Choledocholithiasis (→Figure 2-3) is the presence of gallstones in the bile ducts. The gallstones may spontaneously pass to the duodenum, but most of them become blocked in the common bile duct or in the sphincter of Oddi.

Signs and symptoms include right epigastric pain lasting longer than biliary colic, often with concomitant jaundice, nausea, and vomiting. If the common bile duct obstruction persists, pruritus, discolored stools, and dark urine may be present. When symptoms are associated with fever and hypotension, acute cholangitis should be considered. In some cases choledocholithiasis may be asymptomatic.

→ **DIAGNOSIS**

Choledocholithiasis may be suspected mainly in patients with confirmed cholelithiasis who develop jaundice and biliary colic and in patients after cholecystectomy who have recurrent pain or jaundice.

Diagnostic Tests

1. Laboratory tests: Elevated serum alanine aminotransferase (ALT) and aspartate aminotransferase (AST) in the early phase (<72 hours). If obstruction persists longer, patients develop increasing serum levels of alkaline phosphatase (ALP), γ-glutamyl transferase (transpeptidase) (GGT), and bilirubin (most frequently <180 µmol/L [10 mg/dL] with predominance of conjugated bilirubin; this depends on degree of occlusion of the common bile duct).

2. Imaging studies: Ultrasonography is the initial and frequently sufficient diagnostic method. It may reveal gallstones in the bile ducts, but more often it shows only dilatation of the bile ducts due to occlusion. Failure to visualize gallstones in the bile ducts does not exclude choledocholithiasis. **Endoscopic ultrasonography (EUS)** is the most precise diagnostic method that detects stones <5 mm located close to the ampulla of Vater. **Magnetic resonance cholangiopancreatography (MRCP)** has sensitivity and specificity in detecting stones >5 mm in diameter similar to that of EUS. **Computed tomography (CT)** is useful in visualizing calcified gallstones in the common bile duct. It is not the method of choice in the diagnosis of choledocholithiasis but it is useful in differential diagnosis. **Endoscopic retrograde cholangiopancreatography (ERCP)** is not the diagnostic method of choice, as it is invasive and associated with a risk of complications (mainly acute pancreatitis; ~10%). ERCP is indicated if there is a very high probability of choledocholithiasis because it enables therapeutic intervention.

→ TREATMENT

The diagnosis of choledocholithiasis, even in asymptomatic patients, is an indication for invasive treatment, using either endoscopy or surgery.

1. ERCP with sphincterotomy is the treatment of choice with a 90% success rate. Gallstones are retrieved into the duodenal lumen through the incised major duodenal papilla using a balloon or a wire basket. Larger stones must be fragmented prior to evacuation.

2. Extracorporeal shock wave lithotripsy (ESWL) is an auxiliary technique used for fragmentation of gallstones in case of failure of mechanical lithotripsy during ERCP.⊘○

3. Stenting of the common bile duct is used when the above-listed methods are unsuccessful.⊘○

4. Surgical treatment is performed when endoscopic treatment is not feasible or has been unsuccessful. Cholecystectomy is indicated in all patients with cholelithiasis.

→ COMPLICATIONS

Cholestatic cholangitis, acute pancreatitis, rarely biliary intestinal fistula and secondary biliary cirrhosis (in patients with chronic choledocholithiasis).

2.1.3.2. Cholelithiasis

→ CLINICAL FEATURES AND NATURAL HISTORY

Cholelithiasis: →Figure 2-2.

1. Symptoms of cholelithiasis, when present, include paroxysmal acute abdominal pain—so-called **biliary colic**—which is the key symptom of cholelithiasis. It often appears after ingestion of a fatty meal and is caused by elevated pressure in the gallbladder following occlusion of the cystic duct by a gallstone. The pain is located in the right upper abdominal quadrant or in the central epigastrium and can be referred to the right subscapular region. It usually lasts >30 minutes but <5 hours, resolves gradually, and may be accompanied by nausea and vomiting. Other atypical symptoms include heartburn, epigastric discomfort after ingestion of fatty meals, and bloating. Pain persisting >5 hours or fever with rigors may indicate acute cholecystitis, cholangitis, or acute biliary pancreatitis.

surgery. In patients with concomitant cholelithiasis and choledocholithiasis, endoscopic retrograde cholangiopancreatography (ERCP) should be performed with endoscopic sphincterotomy and evacuation of gallstones from the bile ducts before the planned laparoscopic cholecystectomy.⊘●

2. Open cholecystectomy is indicated in patients with contraindications to laparoscopy.

3. Prophylactic cholecystectomy in asymptomatic cholelithiasis is controversial. Suggested indications include sickle cell anemia, immunosuppression, body mass index ≥40 (cholecystectomy during bariatric surgery), and porcelain gallbladder (because of a 25% increase in the risk of cancer).⊘○

Pharmacotherapy

In patients with contraindications to surgery, use oral **ursodiol** (INN ursode-oxycholic acid) 8 to 12 mg/kg/d in 2 to 3 divided doses taken with meals.⊘○ Treatment lasts 6 to 24 months, with the first evaluation of efficacy at 6 months. Continue treatment for 3 months after confirming dissolution of gallstones; discontinue treatment if there is no improvement at 9 months. In ~50% of patients cholelithiasis recurs.

Do not use ursodiol in patients with pigment or calcified gallstones >15 mm in diameter, pregnant women, patients with concomitant liver disease, or patients with severe clinical manifestations of cholelithiasis.

Ursodiol can also be used for prevention of gallstone formation (eg, during the rapid weight loss period following bariatric surgery until the weight stabilizes).

→ COMPLICATIONS

1. Acute cholecystitis (→Chapter 6.2.1.2).

2. Chronic cholecystitis is a morphologic diagnosis based on finding a thick--walled, fibrotic, deformed gallbladder, which is a result of mechanical irritation of the gallbladder by gallstones or recurrent attacks of biliary colic.

Signs and symptoms include pain of varying severity that is located in the right upper abdominal quadrant and central epigastrium and referred to the back and right scapula. Concomitant cholelithiasis may be associated with recurrent biliary colic, episodes of recurrent acute pancreatitis, choledocholithiasis, and cholecystitis.

Diagnosis is based on ultrasonographic findings, which reveal gallstones in the gallbladder and thickened gallbladder walls.

Treatment: In symptomatic patients perform laparoscopic or open cholecystectomy.

2.1.4. Primary Sclerosing Cholangitis

→ DEFINITION AND ETIOLOGY

Primary sclerosing cholangitis (PSC) is a chronic cholestatic liver disease related to chronic inflammation with fibrosis and strictures. It leads to damage and narrowing of intrahepatic and extrahepatic bile ducts.

→ CLINICAL FEATURES AND NATURAL HISTORY

PSC is asymptomatic in 15% to 45% of patients. **Signs and symptoms** include chronic fatigue, pruritus, weight loss, and symptoms of recurrent cholangitis (episodes of jaundice, fever, and right upper abdominal quadrant pain). Clinical examination reveals jaundice of the skin and mucous membranes as well as scratch marks. In advanced stages symptoms of cirrhosis and its complications may be seen. Ulcerative colitis or less commonly Crohn disease coexists in

~70% of patients. Other frequent comorbidities include pancreatitis (10%-25%), diabetes mellitus (5%-15%), and other autoimmune diseases. Within 10 to 15 years of diagnosis, >50% of patients require liver transplantation.

➔ DIAGNOSIS

Diagnostic Tests

1. Laboratory tests:

1) **Blood biochemical tests:** Elevated serum alkaline phosphatase (ALP) levels and/or γ-glutamyl transferase (GGT) levels (usually 3-10×upper limit of normal [ULN]), as well as elevated serum aspartate aminotransferase (AST) and alanine aminotransferase (ALT) levels (usually 2-4×ULN), serum bilirubin levels (although in ~60% of patients bilirubin levels are normal at diagnosis), and hypergammaglobulinemia (elevated IgG and IgM levels in 45%-80% of patients).

2) **Immunologic studies:** Positive antinuclear antibody (ANA) and smooth muscle antibody (SMA) (in 20%-50% of patients) as well as perinuclear antineutrophil cytoplasmic antibody (p-ANCA) (30%-80%).

2. Magnetic resonance cholangiopancreatography (MRCP) is the practical diagnostic gold standard, as it has comparable accuracy to endoscopic retrograde cholangiopancreatography (ERCP), is less invasive, and results in cost savings when used as the initial test strategy for diagnosing PSC.◑◒ It reveals typical strictures with downstream dilatation of the bile ducts; the strictures may be found both in intrahepatic and extrahepatic bile ducts.

3. ERCP is an invasive test. It should be performed only if the diagnosis cannot be confirmed by MRCP or in clinical situations that require immediate therapeutic intervention (sphincterotomy, biliary stenting) and collection of cytologic specimens because of suspected cholangiocarcinoma.◑◒

4. Liver biopsy is indicated if small-duct PSC is suspected (this variant cannot be confirmed by imaging studies), if autoimmune hepatitis overlaps with PSC and diagnosis based on MRCP or ERCP is uncertain, and in patients with clinically suspected cirrhosis (confirmation of advanced fibrosis has significant clinical implications).

Diagnostic Criteria

Typical features of bile ducts consistent with PSC found on ERCP or MRCP. If results of these studies are normal and clinical features suggest PSC, perform histologic examination of liver biopsy specimens (in patients with histologic features typical for PSC, a PSC variant involving only the fine bile ducts is diagnosed).◑◒

Differential Diagnosis

Cholangitis caused by IgG4 antibodies (a manifestation of IgG4-related disease), other chronic liver diseases with cholestasis (eg, primary biliary cholangitis, vanishing bile duct syndrome, eosinophilic cholangitis), secondary sclerosing cholangitis (eg, due to iatrogenic injury of bile ducts or their vasculature), congenital bile duct abnormalities (eg, Alagille syndrome: hypoplasia of intrahepatic bile ducts; Caroli disease: cystic dilatation of intrahepatic bile ducts), infective cholangiopathies (eg, in patients with AIDS or infestation with *Clonorchis sinensis* [the Chinese liver fluke]).

➔ TREATMENT

Pharmacotherapy

1. Oral **ursodiol** (INN ursodeoxycholic acid) 13 to 15 mg/kg/d; ursodiol is not routinely recommended, its effects on clinically important outcomes are unclear, and it may be harmful in higher doses.⊗◒

2. Treatment of pruritus.

3. Prevention and treatment of osteoporosis.

Invasive Treatment

1. Endoscopic treatment: In patients with dominant biliary duct stenosis, endoscopic balloon dilatation and stenting of the biliary ducts may be performed (the success rate is between 60% and 90%).◐◯

2. Liver transplantation: Indications include recurrent episodes of acute cholangitis, no improvement after pharmacologic and endoscopic treatment of advanced biliary duct stenosis, features of end-stage liver failure refractory to medical treatment, and refractory pruritus. In such situations liver transplantation may be the only effective therapeutic option for patients with very advanced primary sclerosing cholangitis and should be explored.◐◯ Five-year survival rates in patients treated with liver transplantation are ~80%. Patients after transplantation may have recurrences of PSC in the transplanted liver.

→ COMPLICATIONS

1. Increased risk of malignancy: Cholangiocarcinoma (in 10%-20% of patients), hepatocellular carcinoma (risk increased in patients with cirrhosis), pancreatic cancer (risk 14 times higher than in the general population), colorectal cancer (PSC additionally increases the risk associated with ulcerative colitis), gallbladder cancer (in 2% of patients).

2. Episodes of acute cholangitis (→Chapter 6.2.1.1).

2.1.5. Sphincter of Oddi Dysfunction

→ DEFINITION, ETIOLOGY, PATHOGENESIS

Sphincter of Oddi dysfunction (SOD) refers to an abnormal function or structure of the sphincter of Oddi that results in abnormalities in the flow of bile and pancreatic juices. Disturbances of motor function of the sphincter of Oddi may affect the biliary portion of the sphincter, pancreatic portion of the sphincter, or both.

SOD is relatively difficult to diagnose and requires exclusion of other biliary/pancreatic disorders. The definitive diagnostic test (manometry) is not widely available.

SOD most frequently develops in patients with a history of cholecystectomy.

→ CLINICAL FEATURES AND NATURAL HISTORY

SOD is classified based on the dominant manifestations as:

1) **Biliary type**, with dominant clinical features of bile duct stenosis (similar to choledocholithiasis).

2) **Pancreatic type**, with dominant clinical features of pancreatitis (acute epigastric pain, usually postprandial) and episodes of acute pancreatitis.

Classification: →Table 2-1.

A typical symptom of dysfunction of the sphincter of Oddi is epigastric or right upper quadrant abdominal pain that lasts from 30 minutes to several hours and is referred to the back or the shoulder. It is triggered by food, narcotic analgesics, or both. Other pain features are discussed under Diagnostic Criteria, below.

The pain may appear shortly or several years after cholecystectomy and may resemble preoperative pain. On physical examination, mild epigastric or right upper quadrant abdominal tenderness is found. Some patients may have episodes of typical acute pancreatitis, which are often recurrent.

Table 2-1. Classification of dysfunction of the sphincter of Oddi	
Type	Criteria
Biliary type	
I	Pain + all additional criteria met:
	1) Elevated (≥2 × ULN) serum AST, ALT, ALP, or bilirubin levels found on ≥2 occasions
	2) Common bile duct dilated >8 mm found on ultrasonography
II	Pain + 1 additional criterion met
III	Only biliary-type pain (as in choledocholithiasis)
Pancreatic type	
I	Pain + all additional criteria met:
	1) Elevated serum amylase or lipase levels found on ≥2 occasions
	2) Pancreatic duct dilated >6 mm in head of the pancreas and >5 mm in tail
II	Pain + 1 additional criterion met
III	Only pancreatic-type pain

ALP, alkaline phosphatase; ALT, alanine aminotransferase; AST, aspartate aminotransferase; ULN, upper limit of normal.

→ DIAGNOSIS

Diagnostic Tests

1. Laboratory tests: Fewer than 50% of patients have elevated blood enzyme levels. Depending on the type of dysfunction, these include liver enzymes (aminotransferases, alkaline phosphatase [ALP]), pancreatic enzymes (amylase, lipase), or both these types; their transient elevation is seen during pain attacks.

2. Imaging studies are used to exclude gallstones and strictures. **Ultrasonography** or **computed tomography (CT)** and **magnetic resonance cholangiopancreatography (MRCP)** may reveal dilatation of bile ducts or of the pancreatic duct, which is used in the classification of SOD (→Table 2-1) and treatment planning.⊘⊖

3. Manometry of the sphincter of Oddi confirms the diagnosis but is rarely available, technically demanding, invasive, and associated with high complication rates (~30% risk of acute pancreatitis). Most commonly, it is performed as a component of **endoscopic retrograde cholangiopancreatography (ERCP)** (ERCP without manometry should not be performed in the diagnostic workup of SOD because of the risk of triggering iatrogenic acute pancreatitis). The criterion of abnormal function of the sphincter of Oddi is a resting pressure >40 mm Hg. Manometry may be justified in type II or type III biliary dysfunction (after an unsuccessful attempt of pharmacologic treatment) and in pancreatic-type dysfunction.⊘⊖ Manometry helps to predict the success of invasive therapy, as patients with a high resting pressure may see improved symptoms with sphincterotomy. If manometry is unavailable or has been unsuccessful, a noninvasive morphine-neostigmine test may be performed.

4. MRCP is performed to exclude gallstones and biliary duct stenosis.

5. Endoscopy: Duodenoscopy with the evaluation of the papilla of Vater is performed to exclude carcinoma of the ampulla of Vater. Biopsy or brush sample collection for microscopy is performed when necessary.

6. Endoscopic ultrasonography (EUS) may be used to detect small gallstones and assess the papilla of Vater to reliably exclude organic lesions.

Diagnostic Criteria

Confirmation of the diagnosis of SOD is possible only on the basis of manometry, but this is rarely performed. In practice, the diagnosis and classification are based on clinical features and results of laboratory tests and imaging studies. According to the **Rome IV diagnostic criteria**, SOD is diagnosed in patients with episodes of epigastric and/or right upper quadrant abdominal pain who fulfill all of the following:

1) The pain increases to reach a constant level and last ≥30 minutes.
2) Symptoms recur at varying intervals (not daily).
3) The pain is severe enough to disturb daily living activities or to make the patient seek urgent medical help.
4) The pain is not significantly (<20%) related to defecation.
5) The pain is not significantly (<20%) reduced by changing the patient's position.
6) The pain is not significantly (<20%) reduced by antacids or gastric acid secretion inhibitors.

Supportive criteria: One or more of the following:

1) The pain is accompanied by nausea and vomiting.
2) The pain is referred to the back or to the right subscapular area.
3) The pain wakes the patient from sleep.

In patients with normal serum amylase and lipase levels, the diagnosis of **biliary-type dysfunction** is made (auxiliary criterion: elevated levels of aminotransferase, ALP, or conjugated bilirubin showing an evident temporal relationship with ≥2 pain episodes). In patients with elevated serum amylase and lipase levels, the diagnosis of **pancreatic-type dysfunction** is made.

Differential Diagnosis

Other causes of abdominal pain. If cholelithiasis and malignancy have been excluded using imaging studies and an attempt of treatment with gastric secretion inhibitors has failed, the likelihood of SOD is significantly increased.

→ TREATMENT

1. Pharmacotherapy: The efficacy of pharmacotherapy is poorly documented. It may be useful mainly in patients with mild SOD and moderate clinical manifestations and in all patients with type III dysfunction. Agents include transdermal or sublingual nitroglycerin, oral nifedipine, and oral trimebutine.⊘⊖

2. Endoscopic treatment: The benefits of endoscopic sphincterotomy are equivocal. To date it has been recommended in patients with type I dysfunction⊘⊖ and in patients with type II or type III dysfunction and elevated sphincter pressures found on manometry.⊘⊖ Between 10% and 20% of sphincterotomies are complicated by acute pancreatitis.

3. Surgical treatment: Transduodenal sphincteroplasty with pancreatic septoplasty, which is rarely performed and used mainly in patients with recurrent stenosis after endoscopic treatment.⊘⊖ Acute pancreatitis is the most common complication of endoscopic sphincterotomy.

2.2. Liver Diseases

2.2.1. Acute Liver Failure

→ DEFINITION, ETIOLOGY, PATHOGENESIS

Acute liver failure (ALF) is a sudden-onset, rapid, and potentially reversible deterioration in liver function in patients without prior liver disease that leads to jaundice, hepatic encephalopathy, and coagulopathy. The condition of patients who develop coagulopathy but do not have any alteration to their level of consciousness is defined as **acute liver injury**.

Causes:

1) Viral hepatitis: Most commonly hepatitis B (HBV), D (HDV), E (HEV) (especially in pregnancy), A (HAV).

2) Less frequently other viral diseases (cytomegalovirus [CMV], hemorrhagic fever, paramyxovirus, Epstein-Barr virus [EBV], herpes simplex virus [HSV], varicella-zoster virus [VZV], dengue virus).

3) Drugs: Acetaminophen (INN paracetamol; the most common cause of drug--induced acute liver failure), halothane, isoniazid, sulfonamides, keto-conazole, and nitrofurantoin; phenytoin and valproate; statins; nonsteroidal anti-inflammatory drugs (NSAIDs); other (including herbal preparations, eg, Chinese herbal remedies).

4) Toxins: α-Amanitin (contained in the *Amanita phalloides* mushroom), tet-rachloromethane, and other substances.

4) Other: Shock; hepatic ischemia; Wilson disease; autoimmune hepatitis; Reye syndrome; sepsis; Budd-Chiari syndrome; portal venous thrombosis; pregnancy associated: acute fatty liver in pregnancy, liver rupture, and HELLP syndrome (**h**emolysis, **e**levated **l**iver enzyme [aminotransferase] levels, **l**ow **p**latelet levels [thrombocytopenia]).

Massive hepatocyte necrosis leads to impaired metabolic function of the liver, including the neutralization of toxins. Pathogenesis of encephalopathy: →Chapter 6.2.2.5.

A prerequisite for establishing the diagnosis of ALF is the absence of previous severe fibrosis or cirrhotic chronic liver disease. Specific exceptions are the acute de novo presentation of autoimmune hepatitis and Budd-Chiari syndrome. In these conditions an underlying chronic disease might not have been recognized or diagnosed previously and there should be no clinical or histologic evidence of cirrhosis. Wilson disease is another exception of a chronic liver disease with splenomegaly that may lead to acute presentation. The precipitating event is often a viral infection or, in adolescents, noncompliance with therapy. Nevertheless, these patients are considered as having ALF because they share the poor prognosis and common clinical picture of ALF and present with significant coagulopathy and encephalopathy.

→ CLINICAL FEATURES AND NATURAL HISTORY

1. Signs and symptoms: Early symptoms are generally nonspecific and may include loss of appetite, diarrhea, fever, and rash. Key clinical manifestations:

1) Encephalopathy: The key symptom, may be of varied severity (→Chapter 6.2.2.5) and dynamics.

2) Jaundice: The presenting symptom in almost all patients. In very rare cases it may develop after the onset of encephalopathy.

3) Symptoms of bleeding disorder (not always present).

4) Hemodynamic instability.

5) Acute kidney injury (hepatorenal syndrome).

6) Ascites (if massive and rapid, suspect Budd-Chiari syndrome).

7) Seizures may occur in some patients (caused by primary brain injury or elevated intracranial pressure).

2. Natural history: The dynamics of ALF may vary. It begins with severe acute liver injury (a 2- to 3-fold increase in serum transaminases, jaundice, and coagulopathy). Depending on the timing of development of hepatic encephalopathy, liver failure may be divided into:

1) **Hyperacute:** Encephalopathy develops within 1 week from the onset of jaundice. It usually occurs with severe coagulopathy and a significant increase

in transaminase activity. Initially there is a small rise in bilirubin. This type is associated with a greater chance of recovery than the subacute form.

2) **Acute**: Encephalopathy develops between day 8 and 28 from the onset of jaundice.

3) **Subacute**: Encephalopathy develops between weeks 5 and 12 from the onset of jaundice. Usually severe jaundice with a slight increase in aminotransferases and mild to moderate coagulopathy are seen. Often there is coexisting enlargement of the spleen, ascites, and reduction in liver volume (this may resemble cirrhosis). Once hepatic encephalopathy develops, these patients have a very low chance of survival without definitive treatment.

A fulminant course is not associated with less favorable outcomes (eg, in acetaminophen poisoning). The majority of patients who do not receive appropriate treatment (including urgent liver transplantation) die due to cerebral edema, coma, and multiorgan failure.

→ DIAGNOSIS

When taking a history always remember to inquire about drugs and herbal preparations that have been used by the patient (including over-the-counter agents), previous surgical procedures, history of autoimmune diseases and heart or lung failure, alcohol consumption, presence of malignancy, blood and blood product transfusions, travel to areas endemic for viral hepatitis, consumption of mushrooms, and family history of liver disease.

Diagnostic Tests

1. Blood tests:

1) Assessment of disease severity: International normalized ratio (INR), bilirubin, sodium, creatinine (included in the Model for End-Stage Liver Disease and Serum Sodium Concentration [MELDNa] score).

2) Assessment of renal function including urine output, creatinine, and urea.

3) Evaluation of etiology:

   a) Acetaminophen level and urine or serum toxicology screen.

   b) Virology: Anti-HAV IgM, hepatitis B surface antigen (HBsAg), IgM antibodies to hepatitis B core antigen (anti-HBc IgM), antibodies to HCV, IgM antibodies to HDV, as well as IgM antibodies to HEV when indicated; IgM antibodies to HSV; IgM antibodies to VZV IgM; polymerase chain reaction (PCR) for VZV, EBV, CMV, parvovirus.

   c) Autoimmune markers: Antinuclear antibodies (ANAs), smooth muscle antibodies (SMAs), soluble liver antigen/liver-pancreas (SLA/LP) antibodies.

4) Other tests: Complete blood count (CBC); serum levels of other electrolytes (potassium, chloride, calcium, magnesium, phosphate), glucose, albumin, lactate, ammonia; levels of other liver function tests (alanine aminotransferase [ALT], aspartate aminotransferase [AST], lactate dehydrogenase [LDH], γ-glutamyl transferase [GGT]); lipase; antineutrophil cytoplasmic antibodies (ANCAs); arterial blood gases; pregnancy test in women of childbearing age.

Interpretation and ordering of the blood tests: Elevated serum aminotransferase levels are very commonly seen (ALT is more specific for viral etiology; very high values [>2000 IU/L] are typical for toxic or ischemic liver injury). Prolonged prothrombin time (PT) (by >4-6 seconds; INR >1.5) is usually present. Hypoglycemia may occur unexpectedly (regular blood glucose measurements are necessary). Elevated blood ammonia levels have some correlation with the presence and severity of hepatic encephalopathy (ammonia should be measured in arterial blood, if possible). Elevated serum lactate level is an early unfavorable prognostic factor in acetaminophen poisoning. Thrombocytopenia is not uncommon. Other abnormalities depending on the etiology, severity, and complications of liver failure (eg, elevated creatinine levels in patients with renal failure).

2. Imaging studies: Computed tomography (CT) of the abdomen allows recognition of previous cirrhosis and facilitates differentiation between ALF and Budd-Chiari syndrome, hepatic steatosis, and disseminated metastases to the liver. CT of the head is also used to exclude other causes of neurologic symptoms.

3. Electroencephalography (EEG): Triphasic waves (encephalopathy grades 1-3); delta waves (grade 4).

4. Liver biopsy may be useful for determining etiology (eg, Wilson disease, autoimmune hepatitis, fatty liver disease in pregnancy, metastases). In patients with contraindications to percutaneous biopsy (coagulopathy), transjugular biopsy may be an option. Liver biopsy carries a small but relevant risk of serious complications and should be used only in case of diagnostic uncertainty.

→ **T R E A T M E N T**

Patients should be admitted to the intensive care unit. Watch for hemodynamic, metabolic, fluid and electrolyte, and septic complications. Early transfer to a tertiary care center is important. Optimally the center should be capable of performing liver transplantation.

General Measures

1. Nutrition therapy: Optimally delivered orally (a nasogastric tube may be needed). Protein ~60 g/d, energy 30 kcal/kg/d; exclude products containing glutamine.

2. N-acetylcysteine: Indicated for use in acetaminophen-induced liver failure, may be also considered for other etiologies of liver failure.

3. Prevention of acute hemorrhagic gastropathy.

4. Antimicrobial and antifungal prophylaxis: In all patients with ALF surveillance cultures should be performed periodically to detect infection as early as possible. There is insufficient evidence to support the routine use of prophylactic antibiotics. However, broad-spectrum antimicrobial agents should be considered in patients with rapidly progressive encephalopathy, hypotension, or systemic inflammatory response syndrome (SIRS) symptoms. The choice of drugs should take into consideration local pathogen resistance profiles.

Symptomatic Treatment

1. Treatment of hepatic encephalopathy: →Chapter 6.2.2.5.

2. Prevention of cerebral edema: Elevate the patient's head and trunk to 30 degrees. In case of seizures, administer **phenytoin** 10 to 15 mg/kg in a slow IV injection (maximum rate, 50 mg/min) followed by a maintenance dose of 100 mg orally or IV every 6 to 8 hours; do not use phenytoin for seizure prevention. Examine the patient frequently for signs of elevated intracranial pressure. Avoid volume overload, fever, and hypoglycemia, and maintain sodium within a range of 140 to 145 mmol/L.

3. Coagulopathy: Despite elevated INR the risk of bleeding is not markedly increased. Do not transfuse fresh frozen plasma prophylactically. Our practice is to administer **vitamin K** 5 to 10 mg (orally, subcutaneously, or IV) and repeat if necessary, although this is frequently not effective. Replacement therapy for thrombocytopenia or prolonged INR is recommended only in the setting of hemorrhage or before invasive procedures. If needed, administer **fresh frozen plasma** 15 mL/kg or alternatively (particularly in case of volume overload) recombinant factor VIIa concentrate. In patients with severe thrombocytopenia (usually <10×10^9/L), patients planned for invasive procedures, and patients with bleeding and platelet counts <50×10^9/L, administer **platelet concentrates**. Target a platelet level ≥60×10^9/L. If blood transfusion is required, aim for a hemoglobin target >70 g/L.

4. Hemodynamic disturbances and renal failure: Maintain appropriate volume status. Usually start with crystalloids (normal saline, then Ringer lactate). Avoid hyperchloremia as it may worsen renal function. Maintain mean arterial pressure (MAP) at 50 to 60 mm Hg (when necessary, administer vasoconstrictors: epinephrine, norepinephrine, less likely dopamine). Consider (rarely) pulmonary artery catheterization for monitoring. Start renal replacement therapy if required (→Chapter 9.2).

5. Metabolic disturbances: Most biochemical parameters (glucose, sodium, phosphate, potassium, magnesium, calcium) require regular monitoring and correction of abnormalities. Hyponatremia is relatively common; correction of sodium levels, including during resuscitation, should be targeted to maintain sodium at 140 to 145 mmol/L, but rapid changes in sodium levels should be avoided (up to 10 mmol/L per 24 hours or 2 mmol/L per hour). Patients with ALF are particularly prone to hypoglycemia, which may require a continuous IV glucose infusion.

6. Infections: Infections are common (most often pneumonia, followed by urinary tract infection, IV catheter infections, spontaneous bacterial peritonitis, and sepsis from other sources).

Treatment of Underlying Conditions

1. Acetaminophen poisoning.

2. Mushroom poisoning (mainly *Amanita phalloides*).

3. Autoimmune hepatitis.

4. Acute fatty liver in pregnancy and HELLP syndrome: Delivery may lead to resolution of liver failure.

5. Ischemic liver injury: Optimize hemodynamic parameters.

Liver Transplantation

Liver transplantation should be considered in patients fulfilling the King's College criteria or those with ALF and a MELDNa score >30.5. The MELDNa score takes into account the need for dialysis and levels of sodium, bilirubin, INR, and creatinine (available at mdcalc.com).

The **King's College criteria** (modified) consider acetaminophen-induced liver injury and other conditions separately:

1) **Patients with acetaminophen-induced liver injury**:
   a) Arterial blood pH <7.3, or arterial lactate >3.0 mmol/L after adequate fluid resuscitation.
   b) All of the following within a 24-hour period: grade 3 or 4 encephalopathy, INR >6.5, serum creatinine >3.4 mg/dL (301 µmol/L).

2) **Patients with liver injury of nonacetaminophen etiology**:
   a) INR >6.5 and encephalopathy present (irrespective of grade); or
   b) ≥3 of the following criteria fulfilled (with encephalopathy, irrespective of its grade): age <10 years or >40 years, duration of jaundice before the onset of encephalopathy >7 days, INR >3.5, serum bilirubin >18 mg/dL (308 µmol/L), unfavorable etiology (such as non-A non-B viral hepatitis, idiosyncratic drug reaction, halothane-induced hepatitis).

Extracorporeal Liver Support

This is most commonly used in patients with hepatic encephalopathy to maintain some metabolic or detoxifying liver functions until liver transplantation or recovery. The techniques include molecular adsorbent recirculating system (MARS) (a combination of albumin dialysis and adsorption), fractionated plasma separation and adsorption (FPSA), and single-pass albumin dialysis (SPAD) combined with continuous venovenous hemodiafiltration (CVVHDF). However, there is no convincing evidence for the effectiveness of these methods and they should only be used in the context of clinical trials.

→ COMPLICATIONS

1. Elevated intracranial pressure and cerebral edema develop in ~30% of patients with grade 3 encephalopathy (→Table 2-4) and in 75% to 80% of patients with grade 4 encephalopathy. Brainstem herniation is the most common cause of death in patients with acute liver failure.

Treatment: Position the patient with the head and trunk elevated to 30 degrees, administer IV **mannitol** 0.5 to 1 g/kg and repeat if necessary, maintain plasma osmolality at 310 to 325 mOsm/kg H_2O (monitor the values using a direct method). Intubate patients with grade 3 or 4 encephalopathy. If mannitol is not effective, consider hyperventilation (in patients with impending brain herniation you may reduce partial pressure of carbon dioxide [$PaCO_2$] down to <25 mm Hg; in all other cases maintain $PaCO_2$ at 30 to 35 mm Hg; the effect is short-term); induction of barbiturate coma is used by some, although evidence for improvement in patient-important outcomes is lacking. Glucocorticoids are not effective. Direct intracranial pressure monitoring is suggested by some but remains controversial. The types of catheters and their use vary. Target pressures are 20 to 25 mm Hg.

2. Gastrointestinal bleeding: The source of bleeding may be gastric stress ulcers or esophageal varices. It may be aggravated by coagulopathy.

3. Disseminated intravascular coagulation.

2.2.2. Alcoholic Liver Disease

→ DEFINITION, ETIOLOGY, PATHOGENESIS

Alcohol-related disorders account for 3.8% of annual global deaths and 48% of all deaths from liver disease in the United States.

Ethanol is absorbed in the stomach (20%) and the small intestine (80%). It is metabolized mainly in the liver via 2 enzymatic steps. Ethanol is first oxidized to acetaldehyde, a highly unstable and toxic intermediate metabolite, by the enzyme called alcohol dehydrogenase. Acetaldehyde is then further metabolized to a nontoxic metabolite called acetic acid by aldehyde dehydrogenase. Acetaldehyde is responsible for many of the systemic toxic effects of ethanol including alcoholic liver disease. In addition, coingestion of alcohol with other drugs (eg, acetaminophen [INN paracetamol], isoniazid) may further enhance its hepatotoxicity.

Liver injury develops in the following stages:

1) **Alcoholic fatty liver**: Alcohol-induced accumulation of macrovesicular steatosis within hepatocytes.

2) **Alcoholic hepatitis**: Macrovesicular steatosis and necroinflammatory changes in the liver.

3) **Alcoholic liver cirrhosis**.

The individual stages of alcoholic liver disease are not clearly distinct and may overlap. Less than 20% of individuals with chronic heavy alcohol use develop end-stage liver disease. Genetic (eg, variations in the *PNPLA3* gene), behavioral, and environmental risk factors are all important in the development of the disease. Women are more susceptible to alcohol-induced liver injury compared with men and tend to have more rapid progression. Obesity and viral hepatitis B and C are also associated with increased risk of accelerated liver injury and cirrhosis in patients with chronic heavy alcohol use.

The "safe" amount of weekly alcohol consumption is not entirely known and may be presented as different thresholds by different resources. The following levels of consumption are thought to carry a low or minimal risk of liver disease: <16 to 21 units per week (<4 units per day on most days) for a healthy male (1 unit = 8 g of alcohol = a half of 341 mL of 5% beer, cider, or cooler = a half of

142 mL of 12% wine = 0.75 oz or 22 mL of distilled alcohol), and <11 to 14 units per week (<3 units per day on most days) for a healthy female. Please note that 1 unit of alcohol is defined differently depending on the country: in the United States, 1 unit is an equivalent of ~14 g of alcohol, which represents a standard small beer, small glass of wine, or 1.5 oz of liquor. The above-listed units (8 g of alcohol) contain about half of that amount. It may be worth pointing out that according to a recent largest epidemiologic study, no amount of alcohol appears safe if other causes of death (eg, accidents) are taken into account.○

→ CLINICAL FEATURES AND NATURAL HISTORY

1. Alcoholic fatty liver disease (alcohol-related steatosis) is present in ~90% of patients with chronic heavy alcohol use. It is often asymptomatic, although sometimes it may cause mild right upper quadrant or epigastric pain, nausea, and anorexia. On physical examination the liver may be enlarged and tender to palpation. The condition often resolves with abstinence, but it may progress to hepatitis and cirrhosis in ~8% to 20% of patients.

2. Alcoholic hepatitis (alcohol-related steatohepatitis) may cause fatigue, nausea, vomiting, loss of appetite, right upper quadrant or epigastric pain, and liver enlargement and tenderness. Up to 80% of patients who present with severe alcohol hepatitis may already have features of cirrhosis. Clinical features of a severe presentation include jaundice, ascites, encephalopathy, and low-grade fever.

3. Alcoholic cirrhosis is not markedly different from cirrhosis of other etiologies. Superimposed alcohol hepatitis may occur and often leads to liver decompensation.

→ DIAGNOSIS

1. Laboratory features: There are no definitive laboratory tests to diagnose alcohol-related liver disease. Alcohol-related fatty liver is diagnosed on the basis of chronic alcohol misuse, elevated serum γ-glutamyl transferase (GGT) levels, and signs of fatty infiltration on ultrasonography. A patient presenting with alcoholic hepatitis may have an elevated serum GGT level, bilirubin >51 µmol/L, elevated aspartate aminotransferase (AST), alanine aminotransferase (ALT) typically <500 IU/L (often <300 IU/L), and an AST/ALT ratio of >1.5 to 2. Additional laboratory abnormalities may include elevated serum alkaline phosphatase (ALP) levels, elevated ferritin, elevated prothrombin time (PT)/international normalized ratio (INR), a variety of electrolyte disturbances (eg, hyponatremia, hypokalemia, hypomagnesemia, hypophosphatemia), respiratory alkalosis, acute kidney injury, macrocytic anemia, thrombocytopenia, and leukocytosis with neutrophilic predominance.

2. Imaging and histopathologic features:

1) **Ultrasonography of the liver** is readily completed to evaluate for signs of cirrhosis and to exclude other etiologies of liver diseases or associated conditions (eg, Budd-Chiari syndrome, portal vein thrombosis). Ultrasonography may reveal nonspecific liver hyperechogenicity secondary to fatty infiltration.

2) **Vibration-controlled transient elastography (VCTE)** is an effective noninvasive test for staging the degree of liver fibrosis. Patients should abstain from alcohol for 1 to 3 weeks prior to completion of this test for improved accuracy, as active alcohol consumption and, in particular, alcohol hepatitis increase liver stiffness measurements and may overestimate the degree of liver fibrosis.

3. Liver biopsy is not routinely recommended if the clinical, laboratory, and imaging data are suggestive of alcohol-related liver disease. Histologic examination of liver biopsy specimens may reveal macrovesicular steatosis, balloon hepatocyte degeneration, Mallory bodies, and in later stages necroinflammatory lesions and cirrhosis.

Diagnostic Criteria

A number of clinical predictive tools have been developed to determine the severity of alcohol-related hepatitis. They include the Model for End-Stage Liver Disease (MELD) score, Maddrey discriminant function (MDF) score, and Glasgow alcoholic hepatitis score (GAHS).

Severe alcoholic hepatitis is defined as MDF ≥32, MELD ≥18, or GAHS ≥8. These scores may be calculated manually or online (eg, at mdcalc.com).

Differential Diagnosis

Differential diagnosis should include (1) other causes of fatty liver (→Chapter 6.2.2.7); (2) hepatitis (as in chronic hepatitis B).

→ TREATMENT

1. Abstinence: Complete abstinence from alcohol may allow for regression of alcohol-related liver changes in patients without cirrhosis and reduces mortality in patients with progression to end-stage liver disease. Psychosocial support and participation in an alcohol abstinence program are highly recommended and may reduce the likelihood of relapse.

2. Nutrition: Management of calorie and protein malnutrition (calorie intake, 35-40 kcal/kg/d; protein intake, 1.2-1.5 g/kg/d) and other dietary deficiencies associated with alcohol misuse is necessary; these most commonly include deficiencies of vitamin A, D, thiamine, folic acid, pyridoxine, and zinc.

3. Pharmacologic therapies can be considered in patients with severe alcoholic hepatitis. Of note, there is considerable discussion regarding each of those therapies and the current North American clinical practice guidelines suggest the use of glucocorticoids⊝○ (preferably prednisolone) and suggest against the use of N-acetylcysteine (NAC)⊗○ and against pentoxifylline.⊗○ All those therapies are used at least by some.

4. Manage complications of cirrhosis and liver failure.

5. Liver transplantation is a definitive therapy for patients eligible in a given jurisdiction with alcoholic cirrhosis or alcoholic hepatitis and account for 15% and 20% of all liver transplantations in the United States and Europe, respectively.

→ PROGNOSIS AND FOLLOW-UP

Severe alcoholic hepatitis is associated with a 1-month mortality rate of 20% to 50%. Long-term outcomes are dependent largely on the presence of cirrhosis and maintenance of abstinence.

The frequency of follow-up visits depends on the stage of liver disease and severity of alcohol misuse. Clinicians should assess biochemical markers of liver function and screen for symptoms of portal hypertension or other complications of cirrhosis. Among patients with cirrhosis, liver ultrasonography should be performed every 6 months as part of screening for hepatocellular carcinoma (→Chapter 6.2.2.5).

2.2.3. Autoimmune Hepatitis

→ DEFINITION, ETIOLOGY, PATHOGENESIS

Autoimmune hepatitis (AIH) is a chronic necroinflammatory hepatitis of unknown etiology that is associated with hypergammaglobulinemia and the presence of circulating autoantibodies. Possible etiologies include environmental, drug, or infectious triggers in genetically predisposed individuals.

→ CLINICAL FEATURES

AIH is rare, with an estimated prevalence of 23/100,000 persons in North America, 19/100,000 persons in Europe, and 13/100,000 persons in Asia. ⊖ The disease may occur at any age but most commonly develops during adolescence and between the ages of 40 and 60 years. Women are affected 4 times more frequently than men. AIH is also associated with other autoimmune conditions, such as autoimmune thyroiditis, type 1 diabetes mellitus, rheumatoid arthritis, ulcerative colitis, and celiac disease.

AIH can present in many ways, ranging from asymptomatic disease to acute liver failure. Two-thirds of patients have either no symptoms or nonspecific symptoms, such as fatigue, anorexia, jaundice, and abdominal pain. Approximately a quarter of patients have features of cirrhosis and its complications at the time of diagnosis. Untreated AIH leads to the development of decompensated cirrhosis in >80% of patients within 5 years.

→ DIAGNOSIS

Diagnostic Tests

1. Laboratory tests:

1) **Biochemical tests:** Elevated serum alanine aminotransferase (ALT) and aspartate aminotransferase (AST) levels (ranging from minor elevations to >50×upper limit of normal [ULN]; the AST/ALT ratio is usually <1), elevated bilirubin, and normal or slightly elevated alkaline phosphatase (ALP) levels.

2) **Immunologic studies:** Elevated serum γ-globulin levels (polyclonal hypergammaglobulinemia, primarily IgG) are found in 85% of patients. Various autoantibodies are also present, most commonly including antinuclear antibody (ANA), smooth muscle antibody (SMA) and rarely antibodies to type 1 liver/kidney microsomal antigen (LKM1) and perinuclear antineutrophil cytoplasmic antibody (p-ANCA). A small proportion of patients have no detectable autoantibodies or have antibodies that are not routinely assessed (eg, antibodies to liver cytosolic antigen type 1 (LC-1) or antibodies to soluble liver antigen/liver-pancreas (SLA/LP).

2. Histology: Histologic examination of liver biopsy specimens is necessary in patients with suspected AIH to confirm the diagnosis and evaluate for cirrhosis. There are no pathognomonic histologic features but typical findings include interface hepatitis (a necrotic process involving hepatocytes at the lobular/portal interface), lymphocytic plasma cell infiltrates of portal areas, emperipolesis (active penetration by one cell into and through a larger cell), and hepatocellular rosette formation.

Diagnostic Criteria

Diagnostic criteria: →Table 2-2.

There are 2 subtypes of autoimmune hepatitis. **Type 1 AIH**, which accounts for 80% of cases, is associated with ANAs or SMAs (or both). **Type 2 AIH** is associated with antibodies to LKM1, LC-1, or both. Type 2 AIH is mainly diagnosed in children.

Among patients with AIH, 10% have an overlap syndrome. This occurs when patients with AIH also have features of either primary sclerosing cholangitis or primary biliary cholangitis.

Differential Diagnosis

Other autoimmune liver diseases (primary biliary cholangitis [formerly known as primary biliary cirrhosis], primary sclerosing cholangitis, and IgG4-associated cholangitis), viral hepatitis (hepatitis virus A, B, and C; Epstein-Barr virus; cytomegalovirus; herpes simplex virus), drug-induced

Table 2-2. Simplified diagnostic criteria for autoimmune hepatitis according to the International Autoimmune Hepatitis Group (2008)

Criteria	Score
Autoantibodies (max, 2 points)	
ANA or SMA titer ≥1:40	1
ANA or SMA titer ≥1:80, anti-LKM1 titer ≥1:40, or positive anti-SLA/LP	2
IgG level	
>ULN (16 g/L)	1
>1.1×ULN (18 g/L)	2
Histology	
Consistent with autoimmune hepatitis	1
Typical for autoimmune hepatitis	2
Viral hepatitis excluded	2
Interpretation: Score 6: Probable autoimmune hepatitis Score 7-8: Definite autoimmune hepatitis	

Based on Hepatology. 2008;48(1):169 76.

ANA, antinuclear antibody; anti-LKM1, antibody to type 1 liver and kidney microsomal antigen; anti-SLA/LP, antibody to soluble liver antigen/liver-pancreas; SMA, smooth muscle antibody; ULN, upper limit of normal.

liver injury, alcoholic liver disease, nonalcoholic fatty liver disease, hereditary hemochromatosis, Wilson disease, α_1-antitrypsin deficiency, celiac disease, systemic lupus erythematosus, cholangiopathy secondary to HIV, and granulomatous hepatitis.

→ **TREATMENT**

General Considerations

1. Immunosuppression is indicated in patients with:

1) AST >10×ULN.

2) AST >5×ULN and γ-globulin level ≥2×ULN.

3) Bridging or multilobular necrosis.

4) Incapacitating symptoms (eg, fatigue, arthralgia).

Immunosuppression is not indicated in patients with cirrhosis without active inflammation (ie, no inflammatory cells on liver biopsy and normal or slightly elevated serum transaminases).

2. Liver transplantation is the treatment of choice in patients with advanced AIH and liver failure.

Pharmacotherapy

Note that there are differences between the usual management of AIH in North America and Europe, mostly reflecting timing of azathioprine introduction and duration of treatment. The information below reflects North American practices. Details regarding European management strategies could be found on the website of the European Association for the Study of the Liver.

The goal of treatment is to achieve biochemical (normalization of serum trans-aminases and IgG) and histologic remission. The cornerstone of AIH therapy includes prednisone/prednisolone monotherapy or prednisone/prednisolone in combination with azathioprine. Combination therapy is preferred unless there are contraindications to azathioprine (eg, severe leukopenia or thrombocytopenia, thiopurine methyltransferase deficiency). In patients who do not respond to or are intolerant of prednisone and azathioprine, treatment with mycophenolate, cyclosporine (INN cyclosporin), or tacrolimus can be considered.⊘○

Combination therapy: Treatment consists of an induction phase followed by a maintenance phase:

1) **Induction**: The induction period lasts 4 weeks and consists of oral pred-nisolone/prednisone 30 mg daily for 1 week followed by 20 mg daily for 1 week and 15 mg daily for 2 weeks. Azathioprine 50 mg daily is administered during the entire 4-week induction period. In Europe, prednisolone is pre-ferred over prednisone and the agents are administered in weight-based doses (prednisolone 0.5-1 mg/kg/d) with azathioprine (1-2 mg/kg/d) usually starting after 2 weeks of glucocorticoid treatment.

   Alternative treatment with oral budesonide (3 mg bid or tid) in combination with azathioprine has been studied and is associated with fewer adverse effects than prednisolone/prednisone but may involve a higher risk of recurrence.⊘⊖

2) **Maintenance**: Maintenance therapy usually consists of prednisone/pred-nisolone 10 mg daily and azathioprine 50 mg daily. Further slow tapering of prednisone/prednisolone by 2.5 mg/week to 5 mg daily may be performed if tolerated by the patient. There is no minimal or maximal duration of treatment. Maintenance therapy should be continued until biochemical remission and histologic normalization are achieved. Typically 18 to 24 months of mainte-nance therapy are required. In Europe, treatment is typically continued for a minimum of 2 to 3 years, including 2 years of complete biochemical remission.

3) **Management of recurrences**: Relapse occurs in 50% to 90% of patients after discontinuation of therapy⊖ and is defined as ALT elevation 3×ULN. Relapse treatment involves the same induction strategy as initial treatment, but maintenance treatment following a relapse should be continued indefinitely.

➡ FOLLOW-UP

Biochemical tests (AST, ALT, IgG) are repeated every 1 to 2 weeks (initially weekly) during remission induction and every 3 to 6 months during maintenance treatment. Elevated autoantibody levels have no prognostic value and are not used for monitoring. Patients not receiving treatment require lifelong annual blood tests, as indicated above, to monitor for disease progression and relapse. Patients receiving long-term glucocorticoid therapy should undergo baseline and annual bone mineral density testing as well as receive osteoporosis prophylaxis.

➡ PROGNOSIS

In patients who receive appropriate treatment, 10-year survival rates are >80% and life expectancy is close to that of the general population. The prognosis is worse in patients with cirrhosis and in those who do not achieve remission after 2 years of treatment.

2.2.4. Budd-Chiari Syndrome (Including Hepatic Vein Thrombosis)

➡ DEFINITION, ETIOLOGY, PATHOGENESIS

Budd-Chiari syndrome (BCS) refers to a partial or complete obstruction of the hepatic venous outflow tract that is not due to heart failure, pericardial disease, or sinusoidal obstruction syndrome.

Based on etiology, BCS is classified into **primary** or **secondary**. Hepatic vein thrombosis and inferior vena cava thrombosis refer to primary BCS. Secondary BCS occurs in the setting of either external compression or infiltration of the hepatic vein or inferior vena cava (or both) by a lesion other than thrombosis or phlebitis (eg, malignancy).

Causes: The underlying etiology can be established in 80% of patients. The most frequent causes of BCS include myeloproliferative neoplasms, neoplastic and nonneoplastic lesions of the liver (hepatocellular carcinoma being the most common neoplastic lesion), and hypercoagulable states including oral contraceptives and inflammatory bowel disease.

→ CLINICAL FEATURES AND NATURAL HISTORY

The presentation of BCS is highly variable. Patients may be initially asymptomatic (15%-20%) for an extended period of time when the disease is limited to one hepatic vein and collateral circulation is well developed. Acute thrombosis of 3 hepatic veins leads to acute liver failure with rapidly developing ascites. However, the course of the disease is often subacute (as collateral hepatic veins develop) or chronic (this may progress to cirrhosis) and includes hepatomegaly, slowly developing ascites, jaundice, features of liver failure, and edema of the lower extremities. Accordingly, clinicians should consider this diagnosis in patients presenting with a clinical picture of acute liver failure, acute hepatitis, or chronic liver disease.

→ DIAGNOSIS

Diagnostic Tests

1. Doppler ultrasonography can often establish the diagnosis of BCS by revealing an abnormal flow pattern and occlusion of hepatic veins. It can also be used to evaluate for chronic BCS by identifying the presence of venous collaterals. Caudate lobe hypertrophy, another sign of chronic BCS identified on ultrasonography, can exacerbate the outflow obstruction through external compression of the intrahepatic component of the inferior vena cava.

2. Computed tomography (CT) is used for diagnosing intrahepatic causes of BCS (eg, tumors or abscesses adjacent to the hepatic veins). CT can visualize abnormalities of hepatic parenchymal perfusion, which may be so severe that they resemble a tumor.

3. Phlebography and magnetic resonance angiography (MRA)—in particular traditional **phlebography** (cavography)—can accurately identify the location and extent of thrombosis or other causes of venous flow obstruction. Phlebography should be considered when noninvasive tests are inconclusive and there is still a strong clinical suspicion for BCS.

Differential Diagnosis

Hepatic veno-occlusive disease, a disease of small intrahepatic veins, has clinical features that closely resemble BCS. It is often observed within 100 days of anticancer chemotherapy or bone marrow transplantation. Heart failure and pericardial disease should also be excluded.

→ TREATMENT

The rates of 3-year survival without treatment are ~10%. The 5-year survival rate with treatment is ~75%.

Key Principles

1. Treatment of the predisposing condition when possible.

2. Initiate **anticoagulation** in all patients who present with BCS, unless there are contraindications. Typically use 5 to 7 days of low-molecular-weight heparin (LMWH) followed by a vitamin K antagonist (VKA). There is less data and experience with direct oral anticoagulants (DOACs), but they may be a reasonable second option.

3. Treatment of complications (ascites, esophageal varices).

Acute Symptomatic Budd-Chiari Syndrome

1. All patients who present with acute liver failure should be referred for a **liver transplantation assessment**.

2. Thrombolysis may be attempted in the first 2 or 3 weeks of the disease if a well-defined clot is present. If there are contraindications to thrombolytics and the patient is symptomatic from the obstruction, angioplasty and stenting may be considered. Other options include transjugular intrahepatic portosystemic shunt (TIPS) and surgical shunts. Failure to improve with the above managements is also an indication for a liver transplantation referral.

Subacute and Chronic Budd-Chiari Syndrome

Treat complications of portal hypertension. Consider referral for liver transplantation, especially in the setting of cirrhosis and hepatocellular carcinoma.

2.2.5. Cirrhosis

→ **DEFINITION, ETIOLOGY, NATURAL HISTORY**

Cirrhosis refers to end-stage liver disease characterized by diffuse fibrosis, which results in distortion of the normal liver architecture and development of structurally abnormal regenerative nodules. Cirrhosis may regress with treatment of the underlying cause but in most cases it is irreversible. Liver transplantation should be considered following the development of complications secondary to liver cirrhosis.

The majority of **complications** associated with cirrhosis are secondary to the development of **portal hypertension**. The pressure gradient between the hepatic vein and the portal vein (hepatic venous pressure gradient [HVPG]) in a healthy liver is ≤5 mm Hg. Portal hypertension refers to an HVPG ≥6 mm Hg. Distortion of hepatic microcirculation via structural (eg, fibrosis) and dynamic changes (increased vasoconstrictors and decreased synthesis of endothelial vasodilators) leads to an increase in HVPG and development of collateral portosystemic circulation in the esophagus, rectum, and abdominal walls. Esophageal varices may develop with an HVPG ≥10 mm Hg. The risk of variceal bleeding and development of ascites increases with an HVPG ≥12 mm Hg.

Portal hypertension may also develop in a variety of situations unrelated to cirrhosis because of disruption of the blood flow due to prehepatic (eg, portal and splenic vein thrombosis), posthepatic (eg, Budd-Chiari syndrome, pericardial disease, heart failure), and many intrahepatic causes (eg, polycystic liver disease, malignancy, granulomatous liver lesions, sinusoidal obstructive syndrome, schistosomiasis). This discussion is beyond the scope of this chapter.

The **etiology** of cirrhosis is identified in up to 90% of patients. The most common causes of cirrhosis in developed countries are nonalcoholic steatohepatitis (NASH), alcoholic liver disease, and viral hepatitis B and C. Other less common causes include hereditary hemochromatosis, autoimmune hepatitis, polycystic liver disease, other infections (syphilis, echinococcosis, brucellosis), metabolic diseases (Wilson disease, α_1-antitrypsin deficiency, cystic fibrosis, porphyria cutanea tarda, galactosemia, hereditary tyrosinemia, glycogenosis [types III and IV], hereditary hemorrhagic telangiectasia [Osler-Weber-Rendu disease], hypervitaminosis A, abetalipoproteinemia); diseases of the bile ducts (extrahepatic biliary tract obstruction, intrahepatic biliary tract obstruction, primary and secondary biliary cholangitis, primary and secondary sclerosing cholangitis); impaired venous flow (hepatic veno-occlusive disease, Budd-Chiari syndrome, right ventricular heart failure); drugs (methotrexate, methyldopa,

Table 2-3. Child-Pugh score

Parameter	Score		
	1	2	3
Encephalopathy	Absent	Grade 1-2	Grade 3-4
Ascites	Absent	Moderate	Tense
Bilirubin (mg/dL [μmol/L]) in PBC	<2 (35) <4 (70)	2-3 (35-50) 4-10 (70-170)	>3 (50) >10 (70)
Albumin (g/dL)	>3.5	2.8-3.5	<2.8
INR	<1.7	1.7-2.3	>2.3
Total score	5-6	7-9	10-15
Child score	A	B	C

Compensated cirrhosis: Class A, no indication for liver transplantation
Decompensated cirrhosis: Class B or C, indications for liver transplantation

Adapted from Br J Surg. 1973;60(8):646-9.

INR, international normalized ratio; PBC, primary biliary cholangitis.

amiodarone, isoniazid); toxins; intestinal bypass anastomosis (treatment of obesity); granulomatous liver disease; and cryptogenic cirrhosis (of unknown cause).

Natural history: Cirrhosis is a progressive disease that over time may lead to biochemical and clinical decompensation. Prognosis depends on etiology, disease severity, and presence of complications and other comorbidities. The most commonly used predictive models for prognostication of patients with cirrhosis are the Child-Pugh score (→Table 2-3) and the Model for End-Stage Liver Disease and Serum Sodium Concentration (MELDNa) score (available at mdcalc.com). The median survival of patients with compensated cirrhosis is ≥12 years. Patients with decompensated cirrhosis have a 1-year mortality of ≥20% depending on severity of decompensation. In one systematic review of patients with decompensated cirrhosis, the median survival of patients with a Child-Pugh score ≥12 or a MELDNa score ≥21 was ≤6 months.

→ **CLINICAL FEATURES**

Clinical features depend on the duration of cirrhosis, amount of preserved functioning liver parenchyma, abnormalities of portal circulation, and treatment. Once the diagnosis is established, it is important to determine whether the patient has compensated or decompensated cirrhosis. Patients with compensated cirrhosis are often asymptomatic or present with nonspecific symptoms. They may have a variety of incidental findings including various laboratory abnormalities (eg, thrombocytopenia, macrocytic anemia, leukopenia), imaging findings (eg, splenomegaly, nodularity of the liver, portosystemic collaterals), or endoscopic features of portal hypertension (eg, portal gastropathy, esophageal and gastric varices). Patients with decompensated cirrhosis may present with one or more of ascites, hepatic encephalopathy, variceal bleeding, hepatic hydrothorax, spontaneous bacterial peritonitis, hepatopulmonary syndrome, and hepatorenal syndrome.

1. General manifestations: Patients with compensated cirrhosis may present with nonspecific symptoms, which include weakness, fatigability, weight loss, and decreased appetite. As the diseases progresses, other general manifestation such as muscle wasting, painful muscular cramps (particularly troublesome at night), and pruritus become more prevalent.

2. Cutaneous manifestations include jaundice, spider angiomas, easy bruising, telangiectasia, palmar and plantar erythema, skin hyperpigmentation, leukonychia, xanthomata, loss of chest and axillary hair in men, hirsutism, and dilated collateral veins on the abdominal walls ("caput medusae"). Petechiae as well as gingival, nasal, and mucosal bleeding may be present. This is because cirrhosis leads to a form of "rebalanced" hemostasis where all stages of the hemostatic process (primary hemostasis, coagulation, and fibrinolysis) may be abnormal and consequently lead to both procoagulant and anticoagulant effects.

3. Gastrointestinal (GI) manifestations include flatulence, nausea, vomiting, smoothing of the tongue, edema of the salivary glands, epigastric tenderness, splenomegaly (~60% of patients), hepatomegaly with palpable nodules on the liver surface, ascites, and hernias of the abdominal wall (most frequently umbilical hernia).

4. Cardiovascular manifestations include decreased mean arterial pressure and cardiac dysfunction called "cirrhotic cardiomyopathy," where patients have increased cardiac output and contractility at rest combined with a blunted response to physiologic, pathologic, or pharmacologic stress.

5. Neurologic manifestations include asterixis (bilateral asynchronous flapping motion of outstretched dorsiflexed hands) and hepatic encephalopathy.

6. Abnormalities of the reproductive system: Men with cirrhosis may develop symptoms of hypogonadism (loss of libido, infertility, testicular atrophy, gynecomastia). Women with cirrhosis also have altered levels of testosterone, lutcinizing hormone, prolactin, and estradiol, which clinically manifest as chronic anovulation or irregular menstrual bleeding.

→ DIAGNOSIS

Common laboratory findings in patients with cirrhosis include thrombocytopenia, macrocytic anemia, and leukopenia. Alanine aminotransferase (ALT) and aspartate aminotransferase (AST) may be normal in end-stage liver disease, as late-stage cirrhosis is representative of a "burnout" state due to the limited volume of remaining viable hepatic tissue. Elevated alkaline phosphatase (ALP) levels (2-3×upper limit of normal [ULN]) are usually seen in patients with cholestatic liver disease. An isolated γ-glutamyl transferase (GGT) elevation may be suggestive of alcoholic cirrhosis. Patients with decompensated cirrhosis may experience pruritus due to progressively worsening conjugated hyperbilirubinemia. Hyponatremia, hypokalemia or hyperkalemia, hypoalbuminemia, and elevated international normalized ratio (INR) may also occur with continued decompensation of liver disease. Although INR increases as synthesis of clotting factors becomes impaired, it poorly reflects the bleeding or clotting tendency in patients with cirrhosis.

In general, factors associated with increased likelihood of cirrhosis include the presence of ascites (odds of cirrhosis increase 7.2-fold if ascites is present; likelihood ratio [LR], 7.2), platelet counts <160×10^9/L (LR, 6.3), and spider angiomas (LR, 4.3).

Diagnostic Tests

1. Noninvasive tests helpful in establishing the presence of cirrhosis:

1) **Blood tests**: Serologic indices rely on a combination of tests, which include usually platelet counts, AST, ALT, and INR. The AST-to-platelet ratio index (APRI) and FIB-4 index can be found online (eg, at mdcalc.com). Other similar scores include the Lok index and Bonacini cirrhosis discriminant index.

2) **Imaging studies**:

   a) **Ultrasonography** may be used to evaluate for hepatocellular carcinoma (HCC) and signs of portal hypertension. It may reveal hypertrophy of the left lobe and caudate lobe, right lobe atrophy, and irregular nodular outline of the liver edge. Features of portal hypertension include dilation of the portal vein >15 mm with monophasic or inverted flow, presence of collateral circulation (particularly in the left gastric, splenic, and umbilical veins), and splenomegaly. An enlarged thick-walled gallbladder and cholelithiasis are frequently observed. HCC usually presents as a hypoechoic focal lesion (for lesions >2 cm in diameter the probability of cancer is ~95%). In one study, high-resolution ultrasonography predicted cirrhosis with a sensitivity and specificity of 91% and 93%, respectively. Computed tomography (CT) is not superior to ultrasonography except for patients with suspected HCC (triphasic helical CT).

b) **Vibration-controlled transient elastography (VCTE)** cutoff scores for cirrhosis vary depending on etiology. A score >11 to 14 kPa has a sensitivity of 87% and a specificity of 91% for diagnosing cirrhosis.

c) **Magnetic resonance elastography** (sensitivity, 94%; specificity, 95%) is one of the most reliable noninvasive tests, but it is more expensive and therefore less readily available.

d) **Ultrasonography-based elastography** (shear wave elastography [SWE] and strain elastography) has similar sensitivity and specificity for diagnosis as VCTE but is less readily available.

2. Invasive tests: Liver biopsy is the gold standard in the diagnosis of cirrhosis. It has a sensitivity of 80% to 100% and can also **aid in establishing etiology.** Liver biopsy is not necessary if noninvasive tests are suggestive of cirrhosis and no change in management is expected.

3. Serologic tests helpful in identifying the etiology of cirrhosis:

1) Viral hepatitis: Hepatitis B surface antigen (HBsAg), hepatitis C antibodies (assess HCV RNA viral load and genotype if the HCV antibody test result is positive).

2) Autoimmune hepatitis: Antinuclear antibodies (ANAs), type 1 liver/kidney microsomal antigen (LKM1), smooth muscle antibodies (SMAs), IgG.

3) Primary biliary cholangitis: Antimitochondrial antibodies (AMAs), IgM.

4) Hemochromatosis: Iron, iron-binding capacity, serum ferritin, transferrin saturation. *HFE* genetic testing is performed if iron studies are indicative of hemochromatosis.

5) Wilson disease: Serum ceruloplasmin, serum copper, 24-hour urinary copper excretion.

6) Deficiency of α_1 antitrypsin: Levels of α_1 antitrypsin.

7) There are no specific serologic markers for the diagnosis of nonalcoholic fatty liver disease and alcoholic liver disease.

→ COMPLICATIONS AND TREATMENT

Liver transplantation is the key treatment option in patients with decompensated cirrhosis. However, complications should be addressed irrespective of transplantation status.

1. Malnutrition: Poor appetite and early satiety are frequently reported and in part due to ascites, delayed gastric emptying, and altered gut motility. Micronutrient and macronutrient deficiencies are common.

Treatment:

1) Cholestatic liver disease reduces digestion of fat and fat-soluble vitamins (A, D, E, K). Supplementation with vitamins is used when indicated.

2) Glycogenolysis and gluconeogenesis are impaired in fasting state and thus protein is used more readily as fuel. This leads to a catabolic state and muscle loss. Nocturnal hypoglycemia may also occur due to impaired hepatic gluconeogenesis. Patients should consume 25 to 35 kcal/kg of their actual

body weight with protein intake optimized at 1.2 to 1.5 g/kg/d and lipids accounting for 20% to 40% of caloric requirements. Late-night snacks with complex carbohydrates are recommended.

2. Ascites: Ascites is the pathologic accumulation of fluid in the peritoneal space. The **pathogenesis** of ascites is complex. The main mechanisms involve underlying portal hypertension, reduced effective arterial blood volume leading to activation of the renin-angiotensin-aldosterone system, and subsequent renal sodium and water retention. The presence of moderately to severely tense ascites is associated with a mortality rate of 50% within 2 years of the onset of ascites.

Treatment and prevention:

1) Where possible, ensure that the underlying cause of cirrhosis is being treated.

2) In patients with mild ascites initiate salt restriction (sodium <2 g/d) as first-line therapy.

3) If ascites persists or worsens, initiate diuretics with, for example, a combination of furosemide 40 mg and spironolactone 100 mg. If the desired effect is not observed after 3 to 5 days (weight reduction 0.3-0.5 kg/d in patients with ascites alone or 0.8-1 kg/d in those with concomitant peripheral edema), double the dose while maintaining the same ratio (maximum doses: spironolactone, 400 mg/d; furosemide, 160 mg/d). After ascites resolves continue the sodium intake restriction and diuretics at levels that prevent repeated fluid accumulation (measure body weight every 1-2 days).

4) The combination of a low-salt diet and diuretics controls ascites in 90% of cases. In patients with refectory ascites, large-volume paracentesis (LVP) may be used. LVP of >5 L can lead to hemodynamic changes and therefore IV albumin (a plasma volume expander) is given at a dose of 8 g/L of ascitic fluid removed.◐○ Other treatment modalities in patients with refractory or recurrent ascites include transjugular intrahepatic portosystemic shunt (TIPS), liver transplantation, and peritoneovenous shunt (the last one is considered in patients who are not candidates for TIPS or transplantation in whom paracentesis cannot be performed safely because of previous surgeries, scar tissue, or obesity).

3. Spontaneous bacterial peritonitis (SBP) develops in 10% to 30% of patients with ascites and in 25% to 65% of patients with ascites and acute GI bleeding. The risk of SBP increases with progression of portal hypertension.

Etiology: SBP is caused by infection of ascitic fluid without an evident intra-abdominal source of infection, most likely due to translocation of bacteria from the GI tract lumen and impaired antimicrobial activity of ascitic fluid.

Typical presentation: Asymptomatic (~10%) or nonspecific symptoms such as fever or hypothermia, abdominal pain, altered mental status/hepatic encephalopathy, and hypotension. It is associated with an 80% in-hospital mortality rate if left untreated.

Diagnosis: Ascitic fluid polymorphonuclear (PMN) cell count >0.25×10^9/L or a positive ascitic fluid culture (collect ≥10 mL of fluid in aerobic and anaerobic culture tubes). Cultures are negative in 20% to 40% of patients despite inflammatory features of ascitic fluid. Differential diagnosis should include secondary peritonitis developing in a patient with ascites.

Risk factors: Previous history of SBP, low total protein concentration in ascitic fluid (<15 g/L), acute upper GI bleeding, and presence of severe liver disease.

Common pathogens: Most common isolates (80% of patients) include gram-negative aerobic bacteria *Escherichia coli* and *Klebsiella* spp. Gram-positive cocci, predominantly *Streptococcus* spp, account for 20% of cases. Less common isolates include *Enterococcus faecalis*, *Enterobacter* spp, *Serratia* spp, *Proteus* spp, and *Pseudomonas* spp.

Treatment: Antibiotic regimens include a third-generation cephalosporin (eg, IV ceftriaxone 2 g, IV cefotaxime 2 g every 8-12 h, or IV ceftazidime 1 g IV every 12-24 h). In patients with serum bilirubin levels >68 µmol/L (4 mg/dL) and serum creatinine levels >88.4 µmol/L (1 mg/dL), administer infusion of albumin solution (1.5 g/kg on day 1 followed by 1 g/kg on day 3). Consider repeat diagnostic paracentesis in 48 to 72 hours. If the PMN count has decreased by >25% or overall it is <0.25×10^9/L, continue therapy for a total of 5 to 7 days; if this does not occur, consider treatment with antibiotics for an extended course, changing antibiotics based on susceptibility, or an alternative diagnosis (secondary bacterial peritonitis).

Screening: Perform diagnostic paracentesis in all patients with cirrhosis presenting with new ascites. All patients with cirrhosis and ascites who present to the hospital for an acute illness should also undergo diagnostic paracentesis irrespective of their symptoms.

Primary prevention: Provide long-term antibiotic prophylaxis to patients with ascites, a low ascitic total protein level (<15 g/L), and evidence of either significant liver or renal dysfunction. Short-term antibiotic prophylaxis (a 7-day course) should be provided to all patients with cirrhosis who present with acute upper GI bleeding to help prevent SBP and bacteremia.

Secondary prevention: This should be provided to patients with a previous history of SBP until resolution of ascites or liver transplantation. Options include oral norfloxacin 400 mg once daily (or another quinolone) or trimethoprim/sulfamethoxazole in double strength once daily or 5 days per week.

4. Portal hypertensive bleeding: The presence of esophageal and gastric varices may result in acute GI bleeding. Portal hypertensive gastropathy may cause occult GI blood losses. Among patients with cirrhosis, 50% have esophageal varices and 33% experience ≥1 episode of variceal hemorrhage. The risk of bleeding within 2 years of endoscopic diagnosis of esophageal varices is ~30%. Variceal bleeding is associated with 30-day mortality rates of 15% to 20%. Additionally, 1 in 3 patients has a recurrent hemorrhage within 6 weeks. Patients who survive the initial 2-week period after initial variceal bleeding have a 1-year survival rate of 52%.

Risk factors for esophageal variceal bleeding include size of varices, endoscopic features of varices (eg, red wale signs, cherry-red spots), severity of liver disease (Child-Pugh class C is at highest risk [→Table 2-3]), and (rarely measured) HVPG (>12 mm Hg; >20 mm Hg is associated with refractory or recurrent bleeding). Risk factors for early rebleeding include age >60 years, renal failure, large varices, and severity of the initial bleeding (hemoglobin <80 g/L).

Primary prevention of esophageal variceal bleeding is imperative. Screening for varices with esophagogastroduodenoscopy (EGD) is done every 1 to 3 years, depending on the severity of liver disease. Nonselective β-blockers (NSBBs), such as propranolol, carvedilol, or nadolol, are recommended as primary prophylaxis against the first variceal bleeding in those with medium to large varices, varices of any size with high-risk features (eg, red wale markings, cherry-red spots), and those with varices of any size and Child-Pugh class B or C cirrhosis. In patients with varices who do not fulfill these criteria, NSBBs may be withheld and repeat screening with EGD is recommended on an annual basis. In those without varices at the initial screening EGD, a repeat procedure is recommended every 2 to 3 years (EGD should be performed annually in those without varices who develop decompensated cirrhosis). There is little evidence to support the use of NSBBs solely as a means to prevent the development of varices. Variceal ligation may be used as primary prevention in those with large high-risk varices or those who do not tolerate NSBBs. There is little evidence to support the combination therapy of NSBBs and variceal ligation for primary prophylaxis.

When NSBBs are indicated, they should be initiated and then titrated to a resting heart rate of 55 to 60 beats/min (systolic blood pressure should remain >90 mm Hg). Repeat endoscopy is not indicated after initiation of NSBBs. NSBBs reduce the risk of first variceal hemorrhage by 50%. Alternatively, in patients not tolerating β-blockers, variceal ligation should be performed every

2 to 8 weeks until all varices have been eradicated. Annual EGD is necessary thereafter for surveillance of esophageal varices.

Secondary prevention following variceal bleeding: An NSBB should be introduced shortly after resolution of variceal hemorrhage. A combination of NSBBs and variceal ligation is more effective than either modality alone for secondary prevention. EGD should be performed at an interval of 2 to 8 weeks until all esophageal varices have been eradicated. TIPS may be a reasonable additional procedure if the above measures are not effective in preventing subsequent bleeding.

Management of bleeding esophageal varices: →Chapter 6.1.3.4.

5. Hepatic encephalopathy (HE): Potentially reversible neurocognitive impairment caused by liver dysfunction, a portosystemic shunt, or both. It is associated with a wide spectrum of clinical manifestations that range from subclinical to a comatose state. Hepatic encephalopathy can be broadly categorized as covert (CHE) or overt hepatic encephalopathy (OHE).

Pathogenesis: HE is most likely caused by the effects of endogenous neurotoxins (ammonia, mercaptans, short- and medium-chain fatty acids, phenols) in conjunction with excessive activation of the GABAergic system.

Natural course: CHE is subclinical and has a prevalence of 20% to 80% in patients with cirrhosis. OHE is diagnosed in 40% of patients with cirrhosis and is one of the most common indications for hospital admission. OHE is associated with a 1-year and 3-year survival probability of 42% and 23%, respectively.

Diagnosis: Because CHE is subclinical, the diagnosis can only be made using specialized neurocognitive testing. The clinical relevance of establishing a diagnosis of CHE is currently not clear and discussion of this subject is beyond the scope of this chapter. A diagnosis of OHE is based on clinical presentation. There are no specific or pathognomonic serologic or radiologic tests available. Although blood ammonia levels are commonly measured, this test is neither sensitive nor specific for the screening or diagnosis of OHE in patients with chronic liver disease. Patients with cirrhosis may have an elevated ammonia level at baseline without evidence of neurocognitive alterations. Conversely, OHE may be present in patients with normal serum ammonia levels (less frequent). Patients presenting with neurocognitive symptoms with known or suspected cirrhosis or other causes of portosystemic shunting should be investigated to exclude other causes of their neurocognitive symptoms and to identify potential precipitants of OHE (eg, infection, bleeding, electrolyte abnormalities, dehydration, HCC, portal vein thrombosis).

Clinical manifestations: Patients often present with varied degrees of impaired consciousness, cognition, behavior, and neuromotor deficits. Of note, severe OHE (in patients with cirrhosis) may result in focal neurologic/upper motor neuron symptoms without associated findings on brain imaging.

The severity of OHE can be quantified by the West Haven criteria (WHC). In clinical practice it is important to communicate the severity of OHE using the WHC grading scale, as it will impact disposition decisions (regarding admission to the hospital [a ward or intensive care unit]) and treatment intensity. WHC and summary of clinical manifestations: →Table 2-4.

HE classification is based on 4 factors: presence of a precipitating factor (precipitant), severity, type, and time course. Most patients have an identifiable precipitant and resolution of HE episode coincides with correction of the suspected underlying precipitant. Common precipitating factors encountered in clinical practice: →Table 2-5. If no precipitant is identified, the patient is said to have spontaneous HE.

Treatment:

1) First-line therapy is oral lactulose 20 g/30 mL to 30 g/45 mL tid to qid titrated to 2 to 3 bowel movements daily. Alternative routes (if oral administration is not possible) include a nasogastric (NG) tube or rectal enemas 300 mL

Table 2-4. West Haven criteria for grading the severity of hepatic encephalopathy

Grade	Neurocognitive manifestations
0/MHE	Increased incidence of motor-vehicle accidents, decreased quality of life, abnormal psychometric or neuropsychological examination
1	Mild cognitive and behavioral impairment that is different from patient's baseline. Manifested by disordered sleep, impaired attention span, mild confusion with intact orientation to time and space. Mild asterixis possible
2	Lethargy, moderate confusion, slurred speech, asterixis, dyspraxia, personality changes, disorientation to time
3	Stupor with intact arousability to stimuli, gross disorientation to time and space, incoherent speech. Clonus, nystagmus, Babinski sign, or rigidity may be seen on physical examination
4	Comatose state that does not respond to any stimuli, including pain

Adapted from Hejazifar N, Bajaj JS. Hepatic Encephalopathy. Reference Module in Biomedical Sciences. Elsevier; 2019. https://doi.org/10.1016/B978-0-12-801238-3.65707-0.

MHE, minimal hepatic encephalopathy.

in 700 mL of water or physiologic saline every 2 to 4 hours titrated to 2 to 3 bowel movements per day.

2) Second-line therapy is oral rifaximin 550 mg bid instituted in case of lactulose intolerance or no clinical improvement with lactulose monotherapy.

3) Other therapies have inconsistent evidence with respect to their efficacy in treating OHE. Consultation with a hepatologist is reasonable to assist in further management of a patient with suspected HE who has no adequate response to the initial and second-line management. A recent randomized clinical trial has suggested that administration of a single 4-L dose of polyethylene glycol (PEG) given by mouth or NG tube over 4 hours may be superior to lactulose for treating an episode of acute HE. NG administration of PEG was not associated with increased risk of aspiration in patients with OHE. Other pharmacologic therapies to be considered may include antibiotics such as metronidazole, branched-chain amino acids (BCAAs), and L-ornithine L-aspartate (LOLA).

Primary prevention: Routine prophylaxis is not indicated but should be considered in high-risk patients (eg, with active GI bleeding).

Secondary prevention:

1) Nonpharmacologic measures: Correct and reduce the risk of recurrence of precipitating factors (titrate doses of diuretic and laxative agents, reconcile all medications [periodically review all drugs to make sure the agents and dosage are correct]), ensure SBP prophylaxis is instituted when indicated, provide appropriate screening and treatment for esophageal varices and HCC.

2) Pharmacologic measures: All patients with a history of OHE should receive maintenance therapy of oral lactulose (20 g/30 mL to 30 g/45 mL given tid to qid and titrated to 2-3 bowel movements daily). If the patient is intolerant of lactulose, rifaximin may be started. If the patient has recurrent OHE while receiving lactulose therapy, oral rifaximin 550 mg bid should be added to lactulose or used as monotherapy in those with lactulose intolerance. The addition of rifaximin to lactulose may decrease mortality in patients with OHE.

6. Hepatorenal syndrome (HRS): Potentially reversible renal failure that occurs in patients with severe acute or chronic liver disease in the absence of shock or intrinsic renal disease. HRS develops in ~7% to 15% of patients admitted for tense ascites.

2. Signs present during biliary colic include right upper quadrant tenderness and pain on palpation in the right upper abdominal quadrant upon deep inspiration.

3. Natural history: Cholelithiasis is asymptomatic in approximately two-thirds of patients. A third of patients have biliary colic, which recurs every few days, weeks, or months.

→ DIAGNOSIS

Diagnostic Tests

1. Imaging studies: Ultrasonography has a diagnostic reliability of >95%. It is used to visualize gallstones ≥3 mm in diameter, evaluate gallbladder enlargement, measure the diameter of intrahepatic and extrahepatic bile ducts, and assess the adjacent organs.◔ Gallstones may be difficult to differentiate from polyps (these are immobile and cause no acoustic echo) and biliary sludge (this contains cholesterol crystals, causes no acoustic echo, and is mobile when the patient's position changes). **Endoscopic ultrasonography (EUS)** and/or **magnetic resonance imaging (MRI)** can be performed in patients with typical symptoms in whom ultrasonography has not detected gallstones. **Plain abdominal radiography** may reveal calcified gallstones (present in <20% of patients with stones) and a porcelain (calcified) gallbladder.

2. Laboratory tests: Results are normal in patients with uncomplicated gallstone disease.

Diagnostic Criteria

Typical gallstones are visualized on ultrasonography.

In patients with symptomatic cholelithiasis who are at low risk for choledocholithiasis, no further imaging studies of the biliary tract are indicated.

In patients with a history of acute pancreatitis, those aged >55 years, and those with elevated alanine aminotransferase (ALT), aspartate aminotransferase (AST), and alkaline phosphatase (ALP) levels, EUS or magnetic resonance cholangiopancreatography (MRCP) is indicated before planned surgery; an alternative is intraoperative cholangiography.

Differential Diagnosis

Other causes of acute epigastric pain: peptic ulcer disease, perforated gastric or duodenal ulcer, acute and chronic pancreatitis, pleurisy, pericarditis, acute appendicitis, acute myocardial infarction, dissecting aortic aneurysm.

Features seen on ultrasonography require differentiation from gallbladder polyps and biliary sludge (→Diagnostic Tests, above).

→ TREATMENT

Treatment of Biliary Colic

1. Analgesics: Acetaminophen (INN paracetamol) and **nonsteroidal anti-inflammatory drugs (NSAIDs)** at typical doses. In patients with severe pain, use opioids: IM or subcutaneous **meperidine** (INN pethidine) 50 to 100 mg or IM **pentazocine** 30 to 60 mg.

2. Spasmolytic agents (hyoscine-N-butylbromide).◔◔

Surgical Treatment

Surgical treatment is indicated in patients with symptomatic cholelithiasis and its complications.

1. Laparoscopic rather than open cholecystectomy is the preferred technique.◔◔ The procedure is contraindicated in patients with multiple prior surgical procedures or with diffuse peritonitis. Approximately ~5% of patients undergoing laparoscopic cholecystectomy require conversion to open

Table 2-5. Nomenclature for hepatic encephalopathy
Spontaneous/precipitated
1) Spontaneous (no obvious precipitating factor)
2) Precipitated:
– Factors causing increase in ammonia (infection, hypokalemia, metabolic alkalosis, GI bleed, excess protein intake)
– Hypovolemic state (diuretic overdose, large volume paracentesis, diarrhea, vomiting)
– Drugs (benzodiazepines, opioids, alcohol), malignancy (primary hepatocellular carcinoma)
– Vascular occlusion (portal and hepatic vein thrombosis), portosystemic shunts
Type
1) Type A: HE associated with acute liver failure
2) Type B: HE associated with portosystemic shunting/bypass in absence of intrinsic hepatocellular disease
3) Type C: HE associated with cirrhosis
Grade
1) West Haven criteria: 0/MHE, 1, 2, 3, 4 (→Table 2-4)
2) ISHEN:
– Cover hepatic encephalopathy: West Haven criteria grades 0/MHE and 1
– Overt hepatic encephalopathy: West Haven criteria grades 2, 3, 4
Time course
1) Episodic: 1 episode in 6 months
2) Recurrent: >1 episode in 6 months
3) Persistent: Persistent altered behavior interspersed with relapses of OHE

Adapted from Hejazifar N, Bajaj JS. Hepatic Encephalopathy. Reference Module in Biomedical Sciences. Elsevier; 2019. https://doi.org/10.1016/B978-0-12-801238-3.65707-0.

GI, gastrointestinal; HCC, hepatocellular carcinoma; ISHEN, International Society for Hepatic Encephalopathy and Nitrogen Metabolism; MHE, minimal hepatic encephalopathy; OHE, overt hepatic encephalopathy.

There are 2 type of HRS. Type 1 HRS develops rapidly (<2 weeks) and is defined by a ≥2-fold increase in serum creatinine (50% reduction in creatinine clearance) to a level ≥221 µmol/L (2.5 mg/dL). It may be associated with oliguria with a urine output <500 mL/d. Type 1 HRS is more likely to occur in patients with acute liver failure, alcoholic hepatitis, or acute decompensation of cirrhosis, most commonly as a consequence of SBP or GI bleeding. Type 2 HRS develops slowly over weeks to months and is most commonly seen in patients with refractory ascites.

Pathogenesis: Portal hypertension leads to increased synthesis of nitric oxide in splanchnic circulation, which leads to vasodilation of systemic and splanchnic circulation. This in turn reduces the effective arterial volume and promotes renal vasoconstriction. Consequently, there is further decline in renal perfusion and glomerular filtration.

Diagnostic criteria:
1) Cirrhosis with ascites.
2) Acute or subacute kidney injury defined as a serum creatinine level >1.5 mg/dL (133 µmol/L) in the absence of shock or hypotension.
3) No improvement of renal function ≥2 days after discontinuation of diuretics and infusion of albumin solution (IV albumin 1 g/kg in divided doses for 48 hours, not exceeding 100 g of albumin per day).

4) No intrinsic renal disease (proteinuria <0.5 g/d, hematuria <50/high-power field, or renal abnormalities observed on ultrasonography) and exclusion of alternative (competing) etiologies of renal impairment.

5) No recent or current use of nephrotoxic drugs.

6) Other findings: Urine sodium concentrations <10 mmol/L.

Treatment:

1) **Nonpharmacologic therapy**:

   a) Discontinue diuretic agents, nephrotoxic drugs, and any agents that may reduce glomerular blood flow, including nonsteroidal anti-inflammatory drugs (NSAIDs), aminoglycosides, angiotensin-converting enzyme inhibitors (ACEIs), and angiotensin receptor blockers (ARBs).

   b) Monitor blood pressure, urine output, and fluid balance.

   c) In patients with ascites perform diagnostic paracentesis to exclude SBP.

   d) In patients with tense ascites consider therapeutic paracentesis while monitoring blood pressure and maintaining volume status using IV albumin infusions.

2) **Pharmacologic and invasive therapies**:

   a) Liver transplantation is the treatment of choice in type 1 and type 2 HRS. Pharmacologic and renal replacement therapy may be used to manage (bridge) patients awaiting liver transplantation and can potentially improve transplantation outcomes. Combined liver and kidney transplantation may be necessary for patients who have required renal replacement therapy for an extended period of time. Liver transplantation is associated with a 3-year survival rate of ~70%.

   b) Terlipressin (a vasopressin analogue decreasing renal and hepatic arterial resistance) 0.5 to 1 mg as an IV bolus every 4 hours or 2 to 12 mg as an IV infusion per day in combination with albumin (1 g/kg IV on day 1, then 40 g/d on subsequent days). If a decrease >25% in serum creatinine levels is not achieved after 3 days of treatment, titrate the dose of terlipressin up to a maximum of 2 mg every 4 hours. Continue treatment until serum creatinine levels decrease to <1.5 mg/dL. Treatment should be discontinued if a complete response is not achieved after 2 weeks of therapy. It is effective in 30% of patients in HRS type 1, although a significant number relapse (15%-50%) with withdrawal of therapy. It is effective in up to 70% of patients with HRS type 2. Terlipressin is currently not available in Canada.

   c) Start and titrate oral midodrine (an α_1 adrenergic agonist/systemic vasoconstrictor) 2.5 to 7.5 mg every 8 hours (maximum dose, 15 mg orally every 8 hours) in combination with subcutaneous octreotide 100 µg (maximum dose, 200 µg subcutaneously every 8 hours, although IV octreotide 25-50 µg/h may be used as well) and IV albumin 50 to 100 g/d. In a retrospective study comparing albumin monotherapy with this treatment modality, combined therapy with midodrine + octreotide + albumin was associated with a higher rate of HRS resolution (40% vs 10%) and lower mortality (43% vs 71%).

7. Hepatopulmonary syndrome (HPS): Characterized by the presence of intrapulmonary arteriovenous right-to-left shunting among patients with cirrhosis or noncirrhotic portal hypertension in the absence of intrinsic lung disease. Patients with HPS have an arterial oxygen tension <80 mm Hg and an alveolar-arterial oxygen gradient >20. Transthoracic contrast echocardiography can be useful in establishing diagnosis.

The **pathogenesis** of HPS is not completely understood. Intrapulmonary vascular dilation occurs possibly secondary to excess synthesis or decreased breakdown of pulmonary vasodilators (eg, nitric oxide) and inhibition of circulating vasoconstrictive substances. The end result is hypoxemia via ventilation-perfusion mismatch, limitation in oxygen diffusion, and in rare instances shunt formation.

Clinical manifestations: Symptoms of HPS include exacerbation of dyspnea and hypoxemia in sitting or standing positions (improving in supine position). Clubbing may develop. HPS should be considered in every patient with the combination of hypoxemia (partial pressure of oxygen [PaO$_2$] <65 mm Hg), underlying cirrhosis, and portal hypertension. It should be differentiated from pulmonary hypertension associated with portal hypertension and from other causes of hypoxemia that are unrelated to cirrhosis and portal hypertension.

Treatment: The only effective treatment of HPS is liver transplantation.

Screening: Screening is required in all patients undergoing liver transplantation.

8. Hypersplenism usually requires no treatment. If it requires frequent transfusions of packed red blood cells or platelet concentrates or if the patient has painful splenomegaly, consider embolization of the splenic artery, TIPS, or splenectomy (rarely performed due to the high risk of complications in patients with cirrhosis).

→ FOLLOW-UP

1. Recommend regular follow-up for monitoring of abstinence from alcohol and early detection of complications of cirrhosis.

2. Perform ultrasonography with or without α-fetoprotein [AFP] every 6 months for HCC screening in patients with Child-Pugh classes A and B. Patients with Child-Pugh class C should undergo HCC screening if they are eligible for liver transplantation.

3. Screen for esophageal varices with upper endoscopy every 1 to 3 years, depending on the severity of liver disease and history of previous varices.

4. Vaccinate against hepatitis A and B, influenza, and pneumococcal infections.

2.2.6. Drug-Induced Liver Injury

→ DEFINITION, ETIOLOGY, PATHOGENESIS

Drug-induced liver injury (DILI) refers to liver injury caused by drugs (prescribed and recreational) and by herbal and dietary supplements. It results in elevated levels of biochemical liver function parameters (alanine aminotransferase [ALT], alkaline phosphatase [ALP], bilirubin). DILI can be divided into **intrinsic drug hepatotoxicity** (dose-dependent, predictable, relatively stable, onset within hours to days; eg, acetaminophen [INN paracetamol]) and **idiosyncratic drug hepatotoxicity** (unpredictable reaction to a drug or its metabolite with onset in days to weeks; rare [1/1000-100,000]; virtually any drug may be involved).

Case definitions for DILI include any of the following:

1) ALT elevation ≥5×upper limit of normal (ULN).
2) ALP elevation ≥2×ULN in the absence of known bone pathology.
3) ALT elevation ≥3×ULN and total bilirubin >2×ULN.

In patients with abnormal liver test results prior to initiation of treatment with a potentially offending agent, replace the ULN with mean baseline values from before the onset of DILI.

→ CLINICAL FEATURES

Major clinical types of DILI:

1) **Transient, asymptomatic elevation of serum aminotransferase levels** (eg, isoniazid, statins, fibrates).
2) **Acute hepatocellular injury** (due to, eg, acetaminophen, cloxacillin, diclofenac, halothane, isoniazid, lovastatin, herbal preparations, cocaine,

amphetamine): Clinical manifestations are similar as in acute viral hepatitis and usually resolve within 1 to 2 months after discontinuation of the offending agent but may lead to hepatic failure requiring liver transplantation. Prognostic factors predictive of acute or subacute liver failure: severe jaundice; water retention (ascites, edema); advanced coagulopathy; encephalopathy, coma, or both with a minor elevation in serum aminotransferase levels.

3) **Acute cholestatic liver injury** (cholestasis may persist for up to 6 months after discontinuation of the offending agent):

a) Intrahepatic cholestasis (eg, oral contraceptives, anabolic steroids, tamoxifen, cytarabine, azathioprine): Pruritus and jaundice, generally with normal aminotransferase levels.

b) Acute cholestatic hepatitis (eg, carbamazepine, sulfamethoxazole/trimethoprim, erythromycin, captopril, ticlopidine): Pruritus, jaundice, right epigastric pain or liver tenderness, elevated aminotransferase levels (but less than ALP levels). If symptoms develop due to hypersensitivity, they may be accompanied by fever, rash, arthralgia, or arthritis.

4) **Mixed (hepatocellular and cholestatic) DILI** (eg, amoxicillin/clavulanic acid, carbamazepine, cyclosporine [INN ciclosporin]) is the most common type of the disease.

5) **Chronic drug-induced liver disease** clinically often resembles autoimmune hepatitis. Other distinctive types of chronic liver disease associated with drug-induced injury:

a) Ductopenic (vanishing bile duct) syndrome (eg, chlorpromazine, carbamazepine, tricyclic antidepressants) has clinical features similar to primary biliary cholangitis with chronic cholestasis and bile duct loss. It is progressive and can lead to cirrhosis.

b) Hepatic veno-occlusive disease (cytotoxic agents, eg, busulfan, including bone marrow transplantation regimens) is characterized by rapidly increasing ascites, painful hepatomegaly, and jaundice. Hepatic encephalopathy, coagulopathy, and renal failure are commonly associated.

c) Acute fatty liver: A clinical syndrome of rapidly developing failure of the liver and other organs associated with extensive microvesicular steatosis (eg, valproate, amiodarone, didanosine, stavudine, zalcitabine). Also known as Reye syndrome in children with salicylate toxicity.

d) Drug-associated fatty liver disease: Nonalcoholic fatty liver disease attributable to exposure to specific agents (eg, methotrexate, 5-fluorouracil, tamoxifen, glucocorticoids).

e) Focal nodular hyperplasia of the liver or hepatic purpura (cytotoxic agents).

f) Drug reaction with eosinophilia and systemic symptoms (DRESS): Drug-induced hypersensitivity involving multiple organs with systemic manifestations (eg, carbamazepine, phenytoin, phenobarbitone).

→ DIAGNOSIS

1. To establish diagnosis, it is necessary to exclude other causes, in particular:

1) Viral hepatitis A, B, C, and E; infections with cytomegalovirus, herpes simplex virus, and Epstein-Barr virus.

2) Bile duct obstruction.

3) Alcoholic liver disease and nonalcoholic fatty liver disease.

4) Heart failure or recent shock.

5) Autoimmune hepatitis.

6) Wilson disease and hemochromatosis.

7) Primary biliary cholangiopathy and primary sclerosing cholangitis.

Biochemical criteria for the diagnosis of DILI and diagnostic tests recommended for differential diagnosis: →Table 2-6.

Table 2-6. Differential diagnosis of drug-induced liver injury according to the 2014 American College of Gastroenterology guidelines

Type	Ratio of ALT[a] to ALP[a] (R)	First-line tests	Second-line tests
Hepato-cellular or mixed	R ≥5 2 <R <5	– Acute viral hepatitis serologic studies, HCV RNA – Autoimmune hepatitis serologic studies – Imaging studies (eg, abdominal US)	On case-by-case basis: – Ceruloplasmin – Serologic studies for less common viruses (HEV, CMV, EBV) – Liver biopsy
Cholestatic	R ≤2	Imaging studies (abdominal US)	On case-by-case basis: – Cholangiography (either endoscopic or MR-based) – Serologic studies for primary biliary cholangiopathy – Liver biopsy

[a] Expressed as a multiple of ULN; R = ALT/ULN$_{ALT}$ to ALP/ULN$_{ALP}$.

Based on Am J Gastroenterol. 2014;109(7):950-66.

ALP, alkaline phosphatase; ALT, alanine aminotransferase; CMV, cytomegalovirus; EBV, Epstein-Barr virus; HCV, hepatitis C virus; HEV, hepatitis E virus; MR, magnetic resonance; ULN, upper limit of normal; US, ultrasonography.

2. To formally establish the causal relationship between a drug and liver injury, the Roussel-Uclaf causality assessment method (RUCAM) (available at the website of the National Institutes of Health) includes weighted scoring of an event according to 7 distinct domains related to:

1) The temporal relationship between exposure to a particular drug and liver injury (both its onset and course).
2) Exclusion of alternative non–drug-related causes.
3) Exposure to other medications that could explain DILI.
4) Risk factors for adverse hepatic reaction.
5) Evidence in the literature regarding DILI caused by the drug in question.
6) Response to repeat exposure to the agent.

The total score, ranging from −9 to +10 points, classifies the event as highly probable (>8), probable (6-8), possible (3-5), unlikely (1-2), or excluded (≤0), according to its likelihood of being the cause of DILI.

→ **TREATMENT**

1. Immediately discontinue the drug suspected to cause liver injury.

2. Management of acetaminophen overdose. Note that the efficacy of N-acetylcysteine (NAC) in reducing the severity of liver injury from drugs other than acetaminophen has not been substantiated. It may be used in DILI-induced acute liver failure.

3. Symptomatic treatment of pruritus caused by cholestasis.

4. Glucocorticoids are beneficial only in the case of immune-mediated DILI and DILI associated with hypersensitivity features, such as eosinophilia, rash, and fever.

5. Management of acute liver failure.

2.2.7. Nonalcoholic Fatty Liver Disease

→ DEFINITION, ETIOLOGY, PATHOGENESIS

Nonalcoholic fatty liver disease (NAFLD) is a spectrum of liver diseases where there is excessive fat accumulation in the liver (hepatic steatosis) in patients without significant alcohol consumption, without long-term use of a steatogenic medication, and without monogenic hereditary disorders. Hepatic steatosis is defined as fat in ≥5% of hepatocytes in a liver specimen or liver fat content >5.6% in proton magnetic resonance spectroscopy (MRS) or phase-contrast magnetic resonance imaging (MRI). NAFLD can be further categorized into:

1) **Nonalcoholic fatty liver (NAFL)**: There is no evidence of hepatocyte damage or fibrosis. The risk of progression to cirrhosis is negligible.

2) **Nonalcoholic steatohepatitis (NASH)**: There is hepatocyte injury such as ballooning and inflammation with or without fibrosis. If untreated, NASH can be associated with a risk of developing cirrhosis, liver failure, and possibly hepatocellular carcinoma (HCC).

NAFLD is associated with metabolic syndrome and with an increased risk of premature atherosclerosis and death from cardiovascular causes. Its pathogenesis includes insulin resistance, abnormal adiponectin regulation, and oxidative stress in patients with overweight or obesity that develop due to a high-calorie diet (particularly in the case of high fructose intake), physical inactivity, and genetic factors.

The **key risk factors** for NAFLD include obesity (particularly visceral obesity), type 2 diabetes mellitus, dyslipidemia, and male sex. Other factors showing a weaker correlation with the development of NAFLD include polycystic ovary syndrome (PCOS), hypothyroidism, hypopituitarism, hypogonadism, and obstructive sleep apnea (OSA). Risk factors for the development of fibrosis and cirrhosis in patients with NAFLD remain unclear but may include NASH histologic subtype (the greatest risk factor), type 2 diabetes mellitus, hyperlipidemia, obesity, hypertension, genetic polymorphism (*PNPLA3*, *TM6SF2*), and age. NASH develops in 15% to 20% of patients with NAFLD. Cirrhosis develops in <5% of patients with NAFLD and in 12% to 35% of patients with NASH.

→ CLINICAL FEATURES AND NATURAL HISTORY

1. Symptoms: The disease is usually asymptomatic, but it may cause fatigue, weakness, malaise, and upper right abdominal discomfort. It is often diagnosed incidentally by ultrasonography performed for another reason or after finding abnormal liver enzyme levels (alanine aminotransferase [ALT], aspartate aminotransferase [AST]) in serum.

2. Signs: Usually obesity, hepatomegaly (up to 75% of patients), splenomegaly (<25%), or other features of portal hypertension (rarely). Liver fibrosis usually progresses slowly over decades (faster in NASH than in NAFL), but in 20% of patients the progression of fibrosis is rapid. In patients with NASH the risk of developing cirrhosis and HCC is increased, but the main cause of death is cardiovascular disease, with liver-related mortality being the second or third cause of death among patients with NAFLD.

→ DIAGNOSIS

Diagnostic Tests

1. Blood biochemical tests: There may be mild to moderate elevations in the serum levels of ALT, AST, and γ-glutamyl transferase (GGT) (~50%). Normal ALT and AST levels do not exclude the diagnosis of NAFLD. Bilirubin is rarely increased. Dyslipidemia and hyperglycemia (or impaired glucose tolerance) may be present. Iron, transferrin saturation, and ferritin are commonly elevated, but if iron studies are suggestive of hemochromatosis, this diagnosis should be excluded with *HFE* genetic testing. Autoantibodies (antinuclear antibody [ANA], smooth muscle antibody [SMA]) may be positive, although their significance is unclear. In patients who develop cirrhosis, there may be hyperbilirubinemia, hypoalbuminemia, prolonged international normalized ratio (INR), thrombocytopenia, and neutropenia.

2. Imaging studies: Ultrasonography (the first-line diagnostic modality) reveals hyperechogenic liver (due to fatty infiltration) and occasional hepatomegaly. In patients with cirrhosis signs of portal hypertension can be observed. Of note, in obese patients ultrasonography can be difficult to perform and cannot detect mild hepatic steatosis or differentiate between simple steatosis and NASH (but it can still assess moderate and severe steatosis). **Computed tomography (CT)** is useful for evaluating the liver and other organs but not recommended for routine use due to ionizing radiation. **MRI** allows for an accurate assessment of mild steatosis (5%-10% of hepatocytes). **Proton MRS** is the only verified method for quantifying fat content in the liver.

3. Noninvasive assessments of liver fibrosis: These may be used to identify patients with less severe fibrosis (F0-F1) in whom liver biopsy may be omitted:

1) Elastography (the accuracy of FibroScan in patients with obesity is limited), magnetic resonance elastography.

2) Scores based on serum biomarkers: NAFLD fibrosis score (available at nafldscore.com), FIB-4 index (available at mdcalc.com), Enhanced Liver Fibrosis (ELF) test (currently available in Europe only), FibroTest.

4. Histologic examination of liver biopsy specimens: This is the diagnostic gold standard for NASH, but it carries a risk of complications. Histologic features are as in alcoholic hepatitis. Biopsy may be indicated in case of diagnostic uncertainty (eg, in patients with high serum iron levels, positive autoantibodies [ANA, SMA, antimitochondrial antibodies, or AMAs], drug abuse) or in patients with another coexisting liver disease.

Diagnostic Criteria

1. Features of hepatic steatosis on imaging studies or histologic examination in a person without a history of significant alcohol consumption (defined in a consensus meeting of the National Institute of Alcohol Abuse and Alcoholism [NIAAA] in 2016 as <21 standard drinks/wk in men and <14 standard drinks/wk in women, each standard drink defined as containing 14 g of pure alcohol).

2. Exclusion of other causes of hepatic steatosis (including hepatitis C, Wilson disease, lipodystrophy, starvation, parenteral nutrition, abetalipoproteinemia, drugs; →Table 2-7).

3. Exclusion of other causes of chronic liver disease (particularly viral hepatitis B or C, autoimmune hepatitis, hemochromatosis, Wilson disease, α_1-antitrypsin deficiency, drug-induced liver injury).

Of note: Differentiation between NAFL and NASH is currently not possible without liver biopsy.

In the diagnostic process, consider alcohol intake; presence and family history of diabetes, hypertension, and cardiovascular diseases; body mass index, lipid levels, thyroid disease, PCOS, and OSA.

Differential Diagnosis

Consider various causes of hepatic steatosis (→Table 2-7). Also →Chapter 6.2.2.10.6.

→ TREATMENT

1. Lifestyle changes: Sustained weight loss, either by diet alone or in combination with exercise. In patients with obesity a reduction in body weight by 3% to 5% may be sufficient to reduce liver steatosis, and a weight loss of 7% to 10% may improve necrotic inflammatory changes and fibrosis.

Table 2-7. Causes of hepatic steatosis
Alcohol
Hepatotoxic substances
– Drugs: Antibiotics (tetracycline, bleomycin, puromycin), cytotoxic agents (methotrexate, asparaginase), vitamins (high-dose vitamin A), other drugs (amiodarone, estrogens, gluco-corticoids, hydralazine, salicylates, sodium valproate, warfarin)
– Chemicals: Chlorinated hydrocarbons, tetrachloromethane, carbon disulfide, phosphate, barium salts
– Mushroom toxins (alfa-amanitin)
Metabolic conditions and nutritional factors
– Overweight, obesity, starvation, protein malnutrition (kwashiorkor)
– Diabetes mellitus
– Cushing syndrome
– Zinc deficiency
– Parenteral nutrition that is long-term or total (or both; choline and carnitine deficiency)
– Hyperlipidemia
Malabsorption syndromes
– Diseases of pancreas
– Intestinal resection
– Intestinal anastomoses (eg, jejunoileal anastomosis)
– Celiac disease
– Inflammatory bowel disease (ulcerative colitis, Crohn disease)
Inherited metabolic disorders
– Abetalipoproteinemia
– Storage diseases involving cholesterol esters (Wolman disease), sphingomyelin (Niemann--Pick disease), gangliosides (Tay-Sachs disease), glucocerebroside (Gaucher disease), copper (Wilson disease), iron (hemochromatosis), glycogen (glycogenoses), galactose, fructose, tyrosine, homocysteine, phytate (Refsum disease)
– Inherited urea cycle abnormalities
Infectious diseases
– Viral hepatitis C
– Fulminant viral hepatitis D
– Effects of endotoxins
Other
– Reye syndrome
– Complications of pregnancy: Acute hepatic steatosis in pregnancy, eclampsia, HELLP syndrome (hemolysis, elevated liver enzyme [aminotransferase] levels, low platelet levels [thrombocytopenia])

1) Diet: There is no specific diet composition. A hypocaloric diet (decrease daily calorie intake by 30% or 750-1000 kcal/d) allowing sustained weight loss is recommended. The Mediterranean diet has been shown to improve steatosis.

2) Exercise: An increase in physical activity (150 min/wk or an increase by >60 min/wk) is associated with a reduction in serum transaminases and body weight in NAFL patients. The effects on NASH and fibrosis are less clear.

2. Treatment of the underlying condition (eg, metabolic syndrome).

3. Bariatric surgery: According to guidelines from the American Association for the Study of Liver Diseases (AASLD), this may be considered in patients who have other indications for bariatric surgery. There is not enough evidence to consider this as an option strictly for NASH. According to guidelines from the European Association for the Study of the Liver (EASL), this is an option for patients not responding to lifestyle changes and pharmacotherapy.

4. Liver protection treatment: This may be considered in patients with NASH documented by liver biopsy. The use of vitamin E (not in cirrhosis or diabetes mellitus) or pioglitazone is suggested by some authorities.

5. Symptomatic treatment of complications of cirrhosis.

6. Liver transplantation may be considered in patients with decompensated cirrhosis or HCC.

→ FOLLOW-UP

As in alcoholic fatty liver disease. Screening is currently not recommended even in populations at increased risk of NAFLD.

2.2.8. Portal Vein Thrombosis

→ DEFINITION, ETIOLOGY, PATHOGENESIS

Thrombosis of the portal vein (PVT) or its intrahepatic branches results in the impairment of blood outflow from the portal venous system and the development of portal hypertension.

Causes: In up to ~50% of cases the cause cannot be determined (idiopathic thrombosis). Possible causes include cirrhosis (the most common known etiology; PVT occurs in <1% of patients with compensated cirrhosis and 8%-25% of those with decompensated cirrhosis), acquired hypercoagulable states (liver or pancreatic cancer, myeloproliferative neoplasms, trauma, inflammatory bowel disease, pancreatitis), inherited prothrombotic states (factor V Leiden; deficiency in protein C, S, or antithrombin protein), and portal vein compression (pancreatic cysts, tumors of the adjacent organs, purulent intra-abdominal lesions).

→ CLINICAL FEATURES

1. Acute PVT: Clinical presentations range from asymptomatic (presenting later as chronic PVT) to severe abdominal pain, abdominal distention secondary to ileus, and bloody diarrhea if complicated by small bowel infarction. A symptomatic patient with acute PVT often presents within days of the initial thrombotic event. PVT must be differentiated from ischemic colitis and other causes of "acute abdomen."

2. Chronic PVT develops over several weeks and may be identified by the development of collateral circulation, splenomegaly, and worsening portal hypertension on imaging. Patients often present due to complications of portal hypertension (eg, ascites and variceal bleeding). However, chronic PVT may also be initially clinically silent (no signs or symptoms) and identified incidentally on imaging studies obtained for other indications.

→ DIAGNOSIS

Diagnostic Tests

1. Doppler ultrasonography visualizes portal vein flow. In patients with acute thrombosis the portal vein may be dilated, but no collateral circulation is seen. In patients with acute or subacute thrombosis, collateral circulation with flow reversal and splenomegaly are observed.

2. Contrast-enhanced computed tomography (CT) or magnetic resonance imaging (MRI) can visualize the portal venous system and identify thrombi and collateral circulation. These techniques have superseded classical angiography, which is now performed only in exceptional cases before surgical treatment or liver transplantation.

Differential Diagnosis

Other causes of "acute abdomen" and portal hypertension (→Chapter 6.2.2.5).

→TREATMENT

1. Management of bleeding esophageal varices: →Chapter 6.1.3.4.

2. Uncomplicated acute PVT: Antithrombotic treatment (low-molecular-weight heparin [LMWH] followed by a vitamin K antagonist [VKA]) for ≥6 months, or for life in patients with risk factors for thrombosis that cannot be eliminated. Direct oral anticoagulants (DOACs) have not been adequately studied in this population but would be a reasonable option for patients in whom VKA treatment is undesirable.

3. Complicated acute PVT: Antithrombotic treatment (LMWH followed by a VKA) alone or with prior thrombolysis. Indications for local catheter-directed thrombolysis may include thrombus extension with worsening symptoms in patients receiving anticoagulant treatment or threatening bowel infarction related to venous stasis. **Intestinal necrosis** is an indication for surgical referral and treatment.

4. PVT in patients with cirrhosis: The evidence for treatment of acute PVT in the setting of cirrhosis is predominantly based on observational and case-series studies (no randomized controlled trials are currently available). The outcomes of these studies suggest that treatment with anticoagulant agents and subsequent recanalization may decrease portal hypertension and associated complications. Guidelines from the American Association for the Study of Liver Diseases (AASLD) state that there is insufficient evidence to recommend for or against routine anticoagulation in patients with compensated cirrhosis or incidental PVT awaiting liver transplantation. The European Association for the Study of the Liver (EASL) does not differentiate the efficacy of anticoagulation based on the presence or absence of cirrhosis.

5. Chronic PVT: Long-term antithrombotic treatment is very rarely needed and used. Treat complications of portal hypertension. Prevention of bleeding esophageal varices: →Chapter 6.2.2.5. In patients with thrombosis limited to the splenic vein (SVT), observation alone may be appropriate. However, splenectomy can be considered in the context of bleeding gastric varices secondary to SVT.

2.2.9. Primary Biliary Cholangitis

→DEFINITION, ETIOLOGY, PATHOGENESIS

Primary biliary cholangitis (PBC) (also referred to as primary biliary cholangiopathy; previously primary biliary cirrhosis) is a chronic autoimmune liver disease of unknown etiology characterized by cholestasis caused by destruction of small intrahepatic bile ducts.

→CLINICAL FEATURES

Most patients are women in their fifth and sixth decades of life. The disease does not occur in children.

1. Symptoms: Chronic fatigue (in ~60% of patients; often the only symptom; not significantly aggravated by increased physical activity and not alleviated by rest), pruritus (in ~50%; may precede other symptoms by many months or years; initially limited to hands and feet). Less common symptoms include oral and conjunctival dryness and constant or intermittent moderate right epigastric pain.

2. Signs: Hepatomegaly (<30% of patients), xanthomata, jaundice (in advanced disease). In late stages of the disease signs of cirrhosis may be present. Signs of other autoimmune diseases may coexist, such as Sjögren syndrome, autoimmune thyroid disease, rheumatoid arthritis, systemic sclerosis, pernicious anemia, celiac disease, and systemic lupus erythematosus.

3. Natural history: The course is unpredictable. In many untreated patients the progression of the disease is minimal for 10 or even 20 years, while in others cirrhosis develops within a few years despite treatment. A mortality risk score for PBC developed at the Mayo Clinic may assist in predicting short-term outcomes (available at mayoclinic.org).

→ DIAGNOSIS

Diagnostic Tests

1. Laboratory tests:

1) **Blood biochemical tests**: Elevated serum alkaline phosphatase (ALP) and γ-glutamyl transferase (transpeptidase) (GGT) levels (the most common abnormality at diagnosis), elevated serum aminotransferase levels, hyperbilirubinemia (in more advanced disease), hypercholesterolemia (in 50%-90% of patients).

2) **Immunologic tests**:

    a) Elevated serum IgM levels.

    b) Positive antimitochondrial autoantibodies (AMAs) (90%-95% of patients).

    c) Antinuclear antibodies (ANAs) (including those specific for PBC: anti--glycoprotein-210 [anti-gp210] and/or anti-Sp100), smooth muscle antibodies (SMAs), or both (in 20%-30% of patients).

2. Ultrasonography should be the first-line imaging study to differentiate intrahepatic from extrahepatic cholestasis. Subsequently **magnetic resonance cholangiopancreatography (MRCP)** or, if MRCP is not available or contraindicated, computed tomography (CT) can be performed to exclude biliary occlusion. Endoscopic ultrasonography (EUS) may be an alternative to MRCP to evaluate distal biliary disease.

3. Histologic examination of liver biopsy specimens can be used for establishing the diagnosis of PBC, histologic staging, and diagnosing cirrhosis or coexisting autoimmune hepatitis, but it is not required for PBC diagnosis. Typical findings include atrophy of the bile ducts (ductopenia) and inflammatory infiltrates in periportal zones.

4. Elastography is useful in assessing the severity of fibrosis.

Diagnostic Criteria

The diagnosis of PBC is made in patients who meet ≥2 out of the 3 following criteria: elevated serum ALP level, positive AMAs (titer ≥1:40) or other antibodies typical for PBC (anti-gp210 or anti-Sp100) if AMAs are negative, and typical histologic features of liver biopsy specimen(s).

Differential Diagnosis

Primary or secondary sclerosing cholangitis, drug-induced cholestasis, overlap syndrome including autoimmune hepatitis, cholestasis in the course of sarcoidosis, idiopathic syndromes presenting with ductopenia and cholestasis.

→ TREATMENT

1. Moderate physical activity and regular weight-bearing exercise may reduce chronic fatigue and decrease the risk of osteoporosis.

2. In patients with dry oral mucosa and conjunctivae, recommend frequent sipping of water and using artificial tears.

3. No pharmacotherapy can achieve radical cure. To slow down the progression of the disease, use **ursodeoxycholic acid (UDCA)** (INN ursodiol) 13 to

15 mg/kg once daily or in 2 divided doses.◉◉ In patients who had an inadequate response (defined by various scoring systems, such as Toronto criteria: ALP >1.67×upper limit of normal [ULN] after 24 months of UDCA therapy), add second-line therapy: obeticholic acid (OCA), if available, in the initial dose of 5 mg once daily and then titrated to 10 mg according to tolerability at 6 months (do not exceed 10 mg bid; this drug may exacerbate pruritus). Patients not tolerating UDCA treatment can be switched to OCA. In patients with decompensated liver cirrhosis (Child-Pugh class B or C), the starting oral dose must not exceed 5 mg once weekly. Bezafibrate therapy may be considered as add-on therapy in patients with an inadequate response to UDCA,◉◉ (although European guidelines predate the main study of that drug and therefore did not formally recommend this therapy at the time of publication).

4. Management of pruritus.

5. Management of chronic fatigue: The only current recommendation from the European Association for the Study of the Liver (EASL) guideline is to seek and treat associated and alternative causes of fatigue (particularly anemia, hypothyroidism, and sleep disturbances) and to develop coping strategies.

6. Liver transplantation is indicated in patients with symptomatic liver failure and features of portal hypertension who do not respond to medical treatment as well as in those with persistent and refractory pruritus, severe chronic fatigue markedly affecting daily activities, hepatocellular carcinoma (HCC) secondary to cirrhosis, or markers of disease severity (eg, persistent elevated bilirubin of 50 µmol/L [3 mg/dL]; or a high Model for End-Stage Liver Disease and Serum Sodium Concentration [MELDNa] score, eg, >15; available at mdcalc.com).

→ COMPLICATIONS

1. Osteoporosis: Prophylaxis and treatment are necessary (→Chapter 14.13). Measurements of bone mineral density every 2 years are indicated.

2. Deficiency of fat-soluble vitamins (A, D, E, and K) due to malabsorption in advanced PBC (chronic hyperbilirubinemia): Administer appropriate vitamin supplements.

3. HCC develops almost exclusively in patients with cirrhosis (~4% of women and ~20% of men). The incidence of HCC in patients with diagnosed PBC is 0.36 per 100 person-years.

→ PROGNOSIS

In asymptomatic patients and in those who were diagnosed early and treated with UDCA, the mean survival time can be close to that of the general population. Ninety-five percent of patients with a good response to UDCA survive 14 years without the need for liver transplantation. In patients with persistent hyperbilirubinemia not treated with liver transplantation, the mean survival time is up to 5 years. In patients with persistent hyperbilirubinemia treated with liver transplantation, the 5-year survival rate is ~85%. In addition to MELDNa, other scores that can be useful in estimating prognosis are the GLOBE score at globalpbc.com and the UK-PBC Risk Score Calculator at uk-pbc.com.

2.2.10. Viral Hepatitis

→ ETIOLOGY

Acute viral hepatitis is characterized by rapidly evolving necrotic and inflammatory hepatic lesions caused by:

1) **Hepatotropic viruses**: Hepatitis A virus (HAV), hepatitis B virus (HBV), hepatitis C virus (HCV), hepatitis D virus (HDV), or hepatitis E virus (HEV).

2) **Viruses causing secondary liver infections** (hepatitis is one of the symptoms of generalized infection associated with specific clinical features): Epstein-Barr virus, cytomegalovirus, herpes simplex virus type 1 and 2, rubella virus, varicella-zoster virus, echovirus, measles virus, yellow fever virus, and adenoviruses. These infections are not discussed further in the subchapters but should be considered in the differential diagnosis of acute hepatitis.

2.2.10.1. Acute Hepatitis A

→ ETIOLOGY AND PATHOGENESIS

1. Etiologic agent: Hepatitis A virus (HAV). Viremia occurs in the incubation period and for up to 30 days of acute disease. Early manifestations are caused by hepatocyte destruction due to the direct cytopathic effect of the virus followed by a cellular response to HAV antigens.

2. Reservoir and transmission: Humans are the nearly exclusive reservoir of HAV (with rare exceptions of chimpanzees and other primates). The virus is extensively shed with feces. Infection is most commonly by the oral route, from physical contact with an infectious individual or sewage contamination in waterborne outbreaks. Sexually transmitted infection that includes direct or indirect oral-anal contact and transmission through contaminated needles are also possible (the latter mainly in injection drug users).

3. Epidemiology: The virus is present worldwide, with endemic areas in the Mediterranean countries, Eastern Europe, Russia, as well as in areas with low hygiene standards.

Risk factors: Traveling to endemic areas, close contact with infected individuals (eg, household contacts), close contact (household or professional) with children attending nursery or preschool, consumption of seafood (notably crustaceans and raw oysters), anal sex (especially men who have sex with men [MSM]), waste or sewage management, as well as maintenance of equipment used for such purposes. Epidemics caused by the consumption of contaminated food and water may also occur.

4. Incubation and contagious period: Incubation period is usually from 15 to 50 days (on average ~28 days). The virus is shed with feces for 1 to 2 weeks before and ~1 week after the onset of signs and symptoms (the contagious period). Patients are no longer contagious 7 days after jaundice occurs.

→ CLINICAL FEATURES AND NATURAL HISTORY

The disease is often asymptomatic or subclinical (particularly in children). In symptomatic patients it may be **icteric**, **anicteric** (most frequently in children), or **cholestatic**.

Signs and symptoms: Infected patients commonly present with jaundice, fatigue, nausea, vomiting, abdominal pain, and muscle and joint pain. Skin pruritus is prominent in cholestatic disease. In the prodromal period minor liver enlargement may be observed. In icteric disease dark urine and light-colored stools are seen. Fulminant hepatitis with acute liver failure is very rare but may be observed in patients with preexisting liver disease (→Chapter 6.2.2.1). The disease is more severe in patients >50 years and in malnourished individuals.

Acute symptoms resolve within several days and elevated aminotransferase levels persist for 3 to 4 weeks on average. Recurrences are observed within 3 months of the first episode. In patients with jaundice the disease lasts on average 6 weeks and symptoms rarely persist >3 months (cholestatic hepatitis). HAV does not cause chronic hepatitis. Patients with uncomplicated hepatitis A may be expected to return to normal daily activities and work within 6 months.

→ DIAGNOSIS

Diagnostic Tests

1. Serologic tests: The basis for diagnosis is the finding of positive serum anti-HAV IgM antibodies (detected using enzyme-linked immunosorbent assay [ELISA]). The antibodies confirm a recent infection. They may persist for up to 4 to 6 months and are gradually replaced by anti-HAV IgG antibodies, which persist for life.

2. Other laboratory tests: Elevated plasma alanine aminotransferase (ALT) and aspartate aminotransferase (AST) levels (with a greater increase in ALT), hyperbilirubinemia (most commonly mixed, with elevated unconjugated and conjugated bilirubin levels); in patients with cholestatic disease also elevated alkaline phosphatase (ALP) and γ-glutamyl transferase (GGT).

3. Liver biopsy is performed only in exceptional circumstances in case of diagnostic uncertainties.

Differential Diagnosis

Acute hepatitis caused by other pathogens (viruses [hepatitis virus B, D, and C; viruses causing secondary liver infections] or bacteria [leptospirosis, listeriosis, brucellosis, tularemia, bartonellosis, and tuberculosis]), exacerbation of chronic hepatitis, toxic liver injury (drug-induced, alcohol-induced, *Amanita phalloides* poisoning), cholelithiasis causing obstruction of the common bile duct, cirrhosis, autoimmune hepatitis, nonalcoholic fatty liver disease, Wilson disease, acute liver ischemia, acute fatty liver in pregnancy, and liver metastases.

→ TREATMENT

No antiviral treatment is available. Hospital admission may be required in patients with severe or complicated disease. The goal of treatment is to maintain appropriate nutrition and volume status. The specifics of treatment reflect our pattern of practice and judgment and represent a number of suggestions.

1. Rest: Physical activity restricted to that which is easily tolerated in patients with acute disease and during the first month of convalescence.

2. Nutrition and fluid management: Adjust diet to energy requirements. A normal diet may be resumed within 6 months. In case of severe vomiting and signs of dehydration, administration of fluids and enteral nutrition (via a gastric or intestinal tube) or parenteral nutrition may be necessary. Alcohol abstinence is strongly recommended for 6 months and should be significantly restricted for up to 1 year.

3. Management of pruritus.

4. Avoidance of drugs metabolized by the liver or causing cholestasis in patients with acute disease and convalescents.

→ FOLLOW-UP

Monitor for the development of acute liver failure by following liver synthetic functions, including international normalized ratio (INR) as required (once a week with adjustments as needed). Clinical follow-up should include assessment of potential encephalopathy. After resolution of acute disease, monitor levels of aminotransferases and when relevant also of serum bilirubin until resolution.

→ COMPLICATIONS

1. Fulminant hepatitis or acute liver failure is very rare (~0.2% of patients) and more common in those aged >50 years or with chronic liver disease.

2. In rare cases patients may develop kidney injury caused by immune complexes or autoimmune hepatitis.

→ PREVENTION

Specific Prophylaxis

Vaccination is the key method of primary prevention.

General Preventive Measures

1. Strict hand hygiene. Avoid sharing food during the contagious period and limit food-handling activities. Symptomatic patients who are food handlers, child-care staffs, and health-care workers should be excluded from high-risk settings for 2 weeks after symptoms begin. Contacts of infected individuals should be educated and should self-monitor for symptoms. Breastfeeding may be continued throughout the disease.

2. Disease reporting is subject to local regulations.

2.2.10.2. Acute Hepatitis B

→ ETIOLOGY AND PATHOGENESIS

1. Etiologic agents: Hepatitis B virus (HBV). The surface of HBV contains glycoprotein S (HBs antigen [HBsAg]), while the DNA core contains HBc antigen (HBcAg) (undetectable in serum, in contrast to HBV core antigen, which is found in serum or plasma). The infected hepatocyte releases noninfectious HBsAg particles and complete infectious virions. Blood, body fluids, and secretions also contain HBe antigen (HBeAg), sharing a part of the common protein structure with HBcAg (some mutant strains do not produce HBeAg). HBeAg and HBV DNA are markers of intense viral replication and high infectivity of the patient.

Symptoms of hepatocyte damage result from a strong immune response (cytotoxic and cytokine-mediated), whereas the development of chronic hepatitis is caused by a poor immune response to viral antigens. Some of the extrahepatic symptoms and complications of hepatitis B (eg, polyarteritis nodosa, glomerulonephritis, as well as serum sickness–like symptoms observed in the prodromal period) are caused by the formation of immune complexes (particularly those formed by HBsAg and anti-HBs antibodies).

2. Reservoir and transmission: The only HBV reservoir is individuals with active disease or carriers. Routes of transmission include parenteral (contact with infected blood and blood-contaminated instruments), sexual, and perinatal transmission.

3. Epidemiology: The virus is present worldwide, with endemic (high-risk) areas in Eastern Europe, southeast Asia, China, Russia, the former Soviet republics in Asia, Africa, Latin America, South America, and the Pacific islands. **Risk factors**, depending on the local conditions, are found in ~70% of patients and include close contact with a person with HBV infection (household contacts, sexual contacts, invasive diagnostic or therapeutic procedures, treatment with blood products, hemodialysis, multiple sexual partners, IV drug use, occupational exposure to blood and body fluids (health-care professionals), employment in long-term care facilities, and being a prison inmate. The risk of vertical mother--to-child transmission without interventions (→Chapter 6.2.2.10.6) is ~90% for HBeAg-positive mothers and ~10% for HBeAg-negative HBsAg-positive mothers.

4. Incubation and contagious period: The incubation period is from 28 to 160 days (average, 70-80 days). Patients with positive serum HBeAg tend to be more contagious because of the presence of high levels of HBV DNA in the blood.

→ CLINICAL FEATURES AND NATURAL HISTORY

Clinical manifestations of acute hepatitis B are similar to those of acute hepatitis A, but the development of signs and symptoms is generally slower while the course of the disease is more severe. In 5% to 15% of patients clinical manifestations of the prodromal period may resemble serum sickness, including persistent muscle and joint pain, which resolve with the onset of jaundice. An asymptomatic course is also possible.

Hyperbilirubinemia usually lasts ~4 weeks and elevated alanine aminotransferase (ALT) levels persist for up to 8 to 16 weeks. In patients with cholestatic disease symptoms persist for up to 24 weeks. In some patients, particularly the elderly, several flares of subacute hepatitis may be observed in the first 3 months of the disease.

→ DIAGNOSIS

Viral hepatitis is suspected in patients with jaundice or elevated plasma aminotransferase levels (or both).

Diagnostic Tests

1. Identification of HBV DNA is the first detectable indicator of infection, occurring on average around week 12 after infection.

2. Serologic tests: Depending on the time from infection and phase of the disease, HBV antigens (HBsAg, HBeAg) and specific antibodies (anti-HBc IgM and IgG, anti-HBe, anti-HBs) can be detected in serum in variable combinations, with anti-HBc IgM positivity being an important marker of acute hepatitis B in the "window period" (the period between disappearance of HBsAg and appearance of anti-HBs antibodies). Assuming there is no progression to chronic hepatitis B, serum HBeAg remains positive for up to ~10 weeks and HBsAg for up to 3 months. As their levels gradually decrease, anti-HBe IgG and anti-HBc IgG appear. Anti-HBs are observed during convalescence. Over time, the antibodies gradually disappear, beginning from anti-HBe and followed by anti-HBs. Anti-HBc IgG persist for life.

3. Laboratory tests: Serum ALT levels become elevated within several days or weeks after the appearance of HBV antigens in serum. Elevation of bilirubin may follow. Mixed hyperbilirubinemia may be present.

4. Liver biopsy is generally not required for the diagnosis of acute hepatitis B but may be needed if it progresses to chronic hepatitis B or in case of diagnostic uncertainty.

Differential Diagnosis

As in acute hepatitis A.

→ TREATMENT

Supportive therapy as in acute hepatitis A. Glucocorticoids are generally contraindicated due to the increased risk of developing chronic hepatitis. Adult patients in most instances do not require hepatitis B therapy, given the high rates of spontaneous HBV clearance. However, in patients with fulminant hepatitis B treatment should be focused on the management of acute liver failure; use of nucleoside analogues (NAs), such as entecavir or tenofovir, may be of benefit.

→ FOLLOW-UP

As in hepatitis A. Perform follow-up serologic tests at 6 months to exclude chronic hepatitis even in patients with normal ALT levels.

→ COMPLICATIONS

1. Fulminant hepatitis is the most serious complication (~1% of patients, more frequently in young women and in 30%-40% of patients with hepatitis D virus

[HDV] coinfection; the risk is also higher in patients with preexisting hepatitis C virus [HCV] infection).

2. Extrahepatic complications (caused by immune complexes) include systemic vasculitides (eg, polyarteritis nodosa), polymyalgia rheumatica, erythema nodosum, glomerulonephritis and nephritic syndrome (more common in children), mixed cryoglobulinemia, myocarditis, and Guillain-Barré syndrome.

→ PROGNOSIS

Acute hepatitis B may progress to chronic hepatitis B in 90% of neonates and infants, ~30% of children aged 1 to 5 years, and in 2% to 5% (according to some authors <10%) of older children and adults. **Risk factors** include perinatal or early childhood infection, high exposure to the virus, anicteric acute hepatitis, mild acute hepatitis, low ALT levels during acute disease, male sex, advanced age, immunosuppression, and use of glucocorticoids. Mortality is <1% and is mainly due to fulminant liver failure. The course is more severe in patients with HCV or HDV coinfection.

→ PREVENTION

Specific Prophylaxis

1. Vaccination is the key method of primary prophylaxis.

2. Passive immunoprophylaxis with hepatitis B immunoglobulin (HBIG) is used mostly to prevent vertical transmission to the newborn.

General Preventive Measures

1. Strict adherence to the principles of infection prevention, both in health--care and other facilities (hair salons, tattoo parlors). This involves the use of disposable equipment and appropriate handling of materials contaminated with blood or other body fluids, use of condoms, as well as testing of blood donors and limiting indications for transfusion.

2. No isolation precautions are required in HBV-infected patients. Educate patients and carriers about reducing the risk of transmitting the infection to other persons by preventing contact with the patient's personal belongings that may be contaminated with infected blood (eg, toothbrushes, razors, as well as needles and syringes in the case of IV drug users). Sexual abstinence is recommended until the elimination of HBV infection or until the partner completes the vaccination cycle.

3. Disease reporting is subject to local regulations.

2.2.10.3. Acute Hepatitis C

→ ETIOLOGY AND PATHOGENESIS

1. Etiologic agent: Hepatitis C virus (HCV). Hepatocyte damage is mainly caused by a strong cell-mediated immune response (and probably also by nonspecific responses).

2. Reservoir and transmission: The only HCV reservoir is patients with hepatitis C. The routes of transmission include contact with blood, blood products (nonsterile medical instruments or nonmedical equipment, such as razor blades, tubes for inhaling cocaine, needles and syringes in injection drug users, toothbrushes), and sexual contacts. Perinatal infection is possible.

3. Epidemiology. In 2013, the estimated prevalence of chronic hepatitis C infection in Canada was ~250,000. **Risk factors** are present in <50% patients and most commonly associated with injection drug use. The risk of HCV transmission to a sexual partner is ~1.5% per year of nontraumatic sexual activity or 1% to 11% for partners in long-term relationships. The risk of neonatal infection from a seropositive mother is ~2%; 4% to 7% in the case of mothers with positive serum HCV RNA on the day of delivery; and 15% in mothers with HIV coinfection.

4. Incubation and contagious period: The incubation period is 15 to 160 days (average, 50 days). Patients are contagious starting ≥1 week before the onset of symptoms and remain contagious as long as HCV RNA is positive. HCV particles are contagious on environmental surfaces for up to 6 weeks.

→ CLINICAL FEATURES AND NATURAL HISTORY

Most patients with HCV infection are asymptomatic. In others the clinical features resemble mild hepatitis A or B. In the prodromal period serum sickness–like symptoms associated with immune complexes may be observed; these improve with the onset of jaundice. Physical examination may reveal moderate hepatomegaly.

HCV clearance in acute hepatitis C is observed in 15% to 50% of patients, particularly those with symptomatic disease. Patients with uncomplicated acute hepatitis C return to normal daily activities and work within 6 months. The remaining patients develop chronic hepatitis C, out of which 5% to 20% may progress to liver cirrhosis within 20 to 25 years.

→ DIAGNOSIS

Diagnostic Tests

1. Virologic tests: HCV RNA can be detected in serum as early as 1 to 3 weeks from infection (because it is detectable intermittently, HCV infection cannot be excluded on the basis of a single test result and repeat testing is necessary).

2. Serologic tests: Anti-HCV antibodies are detected 4 to 10 weeks from infection (average, 7 weeks). At the onset of symptoms, anti-HCV are detectable in 50% to 70% of patients, and at 3 months, in >90%. The results may be negative in patients who are immunocompromised or treated with hemodialysis.

3. Other laboratory tests: Abnormalities are as in acute hepatitis A but less severe.

4. Liver biopsy is not routinely indicated.

Diagnostic Criteria

Criteria:

1) Documented exposure to HCV (based on risk factors; →Etiology and Pathogenesis, above) within the prior 4 months.

2) Documented anti-HCV seroconversion (2 results of serologic tests with the first result negative and the second positive).

3) A positive HCV RNA test result.

4) Serum alanine aminotransferase (ALT) levels ≥10×upper limit of normal (ULN) with documented results within normal values from the prior 12 months.

Because the above criteria are rarely met simultaneously in a given patient, it is sometimes difficult to distinguish acute from chronic hepatitis C. Histologic examination of specimens obtained during liver biopsy that is performed after resolution of acute hepatitis may be helpful in such situations if it is needed for prognosis or treatment. Gradual resolution of features of inflammation and absence of fibrosis indicate resolving acute hepatitis, whereas presence of fibrosis is generally a proof of chronic hepatitis.

Differential Diagnosis

As in hepatitis A.

→ TREATMENT

1. General measures and symptomatic treatment as in hepatitis A.

2. Antiviral treatment was previously recommended after 24 weeks of diagnosis and the regimen was similar to chronic hepatitis C. However, the 2017 guidelines from the European Association for the Study of the Liver (EASL) recommend treatment at the time of diagnosis with a direct-acting antiviral (DAA) regimen that is similar to that used in chronic hepatitis C but with a shortened duration of 8 weeks (→Chapter 6.2.2.10.7).

→ FOLLOW-UP

As in hepatitis A. Perform follow-up virologic studies (HCV RNA levels) at 6 months to exclude chronic hepatitis even if ALT levels are normal. Patients should be tested for hepatitis B virus, HIV, and other sexually transmitted infections, if appropriate. Provide education and counseling regarding prevention of further transmission, especially avoiding blood donation and avoiding sharing needles in IV drug users. Encourage vaccination against hepatitis A and B if the patient is not immune.

→ COMPLICATIONS

1. Fulminant hepatitis (<1% of patients).

2. Complications caused by immune complexes: Glomerulonephritis, mixed cryoglobulinemia (more frequent in patients with chronic hepatitis C).

3. Progression to chronic hepatitis C.

→ PROGNOSIS

Mortality is low and mainly due to the rare fulminant hepatitis (primarily in patients with HCV and hepatitis virus A or B coinfection). **Risk factors** for the development of chronic hepatitis C include infection caused by transfusion of blood or blood products (in developed countries this has been extremely rare since 1989), asymptomatic acute HCV infection, multiphasic course of ALT activity, male sex, infection at an age >40, and immunosuppression.

→ PREVENTION

1. No specific vaccines or immunoglobulins are available.

2. The key prevention method is adherence to the general rules of prevention of blood-borne infections. Instruct the patient how to reduce the risk of infecting others by preventing contact with the patient's personal belongings that may be contaminated with blood (eg, toothbrushes, razors, needles, syringes and other paraphernalia in the case of persons who inject drugs). Patients should adhere to safe-sex practices. HCV-positive women may continue breastfeeding. Contact notification is recommended with permission of the infected patient.

3. Disease reporting is subject to local regulations.

2.2.10.4. Acute Hepatitis D

→ ETIOLOGY AND PATHOGENESIS

1. Etiologic factor: Hepatitis D (delta) virus (HDV), a defective RNA virus (viroid) with a capsule consisting of hepatitis B surface antigen (HBsAg) that is capable of replication only in the presence of hepatitis B virus (HBV). It probably has cytopathic effects on hepatocytes. Acute hepatitis D may be a result of coinfection (simultaneous infection with HBV and HDV) or HDV superinfection in an HBV carrier. The virus is present worldwide, affecting about 5% of all HBV patients. The reservoir, route of transmission, and risk factors are as in hepatitis B.

2. Incubation: 21 to 140 days (average, 35 days).

3. Clinical features and natural history: The course of HBV/HDV coinfection is similar to that of hepatitis B. HDV superinfection in a patient with chronic HBV infection leads to exacerbation of the disease, resulting in progression to fulminant hepatitis and acute liver failure (particularly in asymptomatic HBV carriers). Chronic HDV infection develops in 70% to 90% of patients with superinfection.

DIAGNOSIS

The protein encoded by the HDV genome (hepatitis delta antigen [HDAg]) is present in the blood only in the first few days of disease and can be detected using specialized techniques. The diagnosis of HBV/HDV coinfection is made in patients with high serum anti-HBc and anti-HDV IgM levels (detected using enzyme-linked immunosorbent assay [ELISA]). Anti-HDV IgM persist for ~6 weeks (in exceptional cases for 12 weeks) and are then replaced by anti-HDV IgG. Levels of HBsAg are low or undetectable (due to suppression by HDV; often this also affects anti-HBc IgM). In the case of HDV superinfection in an HBV-infected patient, anti-HDV IgM are detected, which are subsequently replaced by anti-HDV IgG; for some time both antibody classes can be detected in serum. Anti-HBc IgM are not detected. In patients with chronic HDV infection associated with active hepatitis, anti-HDV IgM persist in the blood. In HDV infection convalescents, anti-HDV IgG continue to be detectable.

Differential diagnosis is as in hepatitis A.

MANAGEMENT

There are no guidelines for the treatment of acute HDV infection. In patients with chronic HDV infection, the recommended treatment is pegylated interferon α-2a administered for 48 weeks. In those with HBV DNA, nucleoside analogue (NA) therapy may be of benefit. The prognosis is worse in individuals with HBV-HDV coinfection compared with HBV infection alone in terms of rapid progression to cirrhosis and development of hepatocellular carcinoma.

PREVENTION

As in hepatitis B.

2.2.10.5. Acute Hepatitis E

DEFINITION, ETIOLOGY, PATHOGENESIS

1. Etiologic agent: Hepatitis E virus (HEV), a Hepeviridae family virus in the *Orthohepevirus A* species. Eight genotypes are known in this group. Genotypes 1 and 2 cause human infections only and are transmitted in contaminated water sources by the fecal-oral route. Outbreaks tend to occur in areas with poor hygiene. Genotypes 3 and 4 are zoonotic, most commonly found in pigs (true primary host) and wild boars. Humans become infected when they consume infected meat. Genotypes 5 and 6 are found in wild boars and genotypes 7 and 8, in camels. Pathogenesis is not fully known. The primary site of viral replication is probably the gastrointestinal tract.

2. Incubation period: From 15 to 60 days.

3. Clinical features, natural history, and prognosis: In the majority of patients (up to 80%) HEV infection is asymptomatic. Manifestations of symptomatic HEV infection are as in other types of acute viral hepatitis. Jaundice is more common in patients with HEV genotype 1 or 2 infection. Cholestatic disease may occur. Overt acute hepatitis caused by HEV genotype 1 or 2 infection in endemic regions is most common in young adults (15-35 years), 2 to 5 times more frequent in men, and associated with estimated mortality rates of 0.2% to 4% (up to ~10% in children <2 years and 10%-25% in pregnant women due to obstetric complications and fulminant liver failure). In middle-aged and elderly men, acute infections with HEV genotype 3 or 4 are usually symptomatic, mild, and only rarely fatal. The antibodies that develop after HEV clearance are nonprotective and reinfections can occur. Chronic infections (only in the case of HEV genotype 3) may occur, particularly in immunosuppressed patients.

→ DIAGNOSIS

Laboratory test results are the same as in other types of acute viral hepatitis. Diagnosis is usually based on the detection of serum anti-HEV antibodies (IgM antibodies appear in the prodromal period and are then replaced by IgG antibodies). The most reliable finding for hepatitis E is a positive serum HEV RNA test result, especially in immunocompromised patients (fecal tests are also performed but access is limited). Chronic infection is diagnosed in patients with serum HEV RNA persisting >3 months.

Differential diagnosis is as in hepatitis A.

→ MANAGEMENT

Treatment, monitoring, and effects on daily activities are as in hepatitis A. Probably the most common diagnostic omission is classification of liver disease caused by HEV infection as drug-induced.

Most cases of acute HEV infection are self-limiting and do not require antiviral therapy. In patients with severe acute HEV or acute-on-chronic liver failure, the use of ribavirin may be considered for 3 months. In addition, patients with primary liver disease infected with HEV genotype 3 and those receiving immunosuppressive drugs in doses that cannot be reduced or in whom dose reduction is ineffective may consider ribavirin 600 to 800 mg/d for ≥3 months as monotherapy or in combination with peginterferon α.

→ COMPLICATIONS

Arthritis, aplastic anemia, mesangioproliferative or membranous glomerulonephritis, pancreatitis, peripheral neuropathies, polyradiculopathies, Guillain--Barré syndrome, ataxia, and Bell palsy. These manifestations may be the dominant clinical features and may not be attributed to HEV infection.

→ PREVENTION

1. In endemic regions improvement of hygiene standards, including water supply, is necessary. In developed countries preventive measures include appropriate disposal of sewage from animal farms, thermal processing of pork at 71°C for ≥20 minutes, and avoiding consumption of raw shellfish by immunocompromised persons. Hepatitis E vaccine against genotype 4 HEV is approved in China but does not provide immunity.

2. Disease reporting is subject to local regulations.

2.2.10.6. Chronic Hepatitis B

→ **DEFINITION, ETIOLOGY, PATHOGENESIS**

Chronic hepatitis B is a chronic (>6 months) liver disease that is characterized by necroinflammatory lesions caused by persistent hepatitis B virus (HBV) infection (→Chapter 6.2.2.10.2). HBV DNA can integrate into the host's genome of hepatocytes and other cells and may also be present in the form of HBV covalently closed circular DNA (cccDNA) that is capable of HBV replication. Chronic HBV infection causes hepatocellular carcinoma (HCC).

→ **CLINICAL FEATURES AND NATURAL HISTORY**

1. Signs and symptoms: Early disease is usually asymptomatic, and most patients have no symptoms for a long time. If symptoms occur early, they may include fatigue (most common) and depressed mood (relatively frequent). Developing manifestations may include:

1) Potentially mild hepatomegaly and in more severe cases moderate jaundice (constant or intermittent).
2) Presentations in some patients are due to:
   a) Cirrhosis and portal hypertension (causing splenomegaly and other symptoms).
   b) Extrahepatic complications caused by immune complexes: Polyarteritis nodosa, leukocytoclastic vasculitis, glomerulonephritis, and polymyalgia rheumatica.

2. Natural history can be separated into distinct phases during which hepatitis B surface antigen (HBsAg) is positive and anti-HBs antibody is negative until phase 5 (this employs the new nomenclature for describing chronic states as used in the 2017 European Association for the Study of the Liver [EASL] guidelines):

1) **Phase 1** (previously labeled "immune tolerant"): Chronic HBV infection, positive HBeAg. HBV DNA is present in high concentrations, alanine aminotransferase (ALT) is normal, and there is minimal fibrosis and inflammation.
2) **Phase 2** (previously "immune active"): Chronic HBV infection, positive HBeAg. HBV DNA levels are declining, ALT is elevated, and inflammation, necrosis, and fibrosis of varying severity occur. The clinical evolution may include seroconversion with clearance of HBeAg and production of anti-HBe antibodies (although in some patients HBeAg reversion may occur). If seroconversion does not occur, inflammation, necrosis, and fibrosis continue to progress.
3) **Phase 3** (previously "inactive HBV carrier"): Chronic HBV infection, negative HBeAg. Anti-HBe antibodies are present, HBV DNA levels are low, and ALT decreases. Improved immune control signifies a better prognosis in patients without cirrhosis.
4) **Phase 4** (previously "HBeAg-negative chronic hepatitis B"): Chronic HBV infection, negative HBeAg. The levels of HBV DNA and ALT fluctuate and liver damage progresses. This is usually related to the development of a mutation allowing the virus to escape anti-HBe control.
5) **Phase 5**: Negative HBsAg. This phase is also referred to as "occult hepatitis." It occurs if HBsAg is cleared (occurring spontaneously in <1% of phase 4 patients per year) and anti-HBs antibody may appear. Phase 5 signifies functional cure (persistent HBV cccDNA remains in the liver).

Treatment is indicated in phases 2 and 4 (as opposed to all infection phases).

→ **DIAGNOSIS**

Diagnostic Tests

1. Laboratory and serologic tests include hepatitis B surface antigen (HBsAg, positive in phases 1-4), hepatitis B surface antibody (HBsAb) (may be positive in phase 5), hepatitis B e antigen (HBeAg, positive in phases 1-2), anti-HBe antibody, and serum aminotransferase levels. In patients with more advanced disease, intermittent or constant mixed hyperbilirubinemia may be observed.

2. Virologic tests: Measurements of serum HBV DNA levels (polymerase chain reaction [PCR]) and quantitative assessment of HBsAg (in Canada available for research purposes only) allow for the evaluation of viral replication (viral load).

3. Fibrosis assessment: Liver biopsy with histologic examination of specimens may be indicated in patients meeting the criteria of chronic hepatitis. This includes evaluation of liver injury (characterized by periportal mononuclear cell infiltrates, hepatocyte necrosis, and fibrosis) and allows for the exclusion of other causes of the disease. Noninvasive testing, such as FibroScan and FibroTest, may be used instead if only fibrosis assessment is required.

Differential Diagnosis

Differential diagnosis for elevated liver enzymes includes:

1) Acute hepatitis, chronic hepatitis C, coinfection with hepatitis D virus.
2) Autoimmune hepatitis, primary biliary cholangitis, primary sclerosing cholangitis.
3) Drug-induced liver injury, alcoholic liver disease, nonalcoholic fatty liver disease.
4) Wilson disease, hemochromatosis, α_1-antitrypsin deficiency.

→ TREATMENT

General Measures

Abstinence or minimal consumption of alcohol (alcohol increases liver injury and accelerates progression to cirrhosis). Hepatitis A vaccination in patients susceptible to hepatitis A virus infection. There are no contraindications to work or regular daily activities including sports, unless the presence of blood-borne infection precludes specific activities (eg, some medical exposure-prone procedures).

Antiviral Treatment

1. The **objective of antiviral treatment** is **sustained suppression of HBV replication**, with the ultimate ideal goal of **HBsAg clearance** to prevent the development of cirrhosis and HCC. Specific treatment objectives depend on the phase and severity of the disease:

1) In chronic hepatitis without cirrhosis, the objective is regression of fibrosis and reduction of inflammation and necrosis.
2) In compensated cirrhosis, delaying the progression to decompensated cirrhosis and possible reduction of fibrosis to a noncirrhotic stage after prolonged antiviral therapy.
3) In patients with decompensated cirrhosis and contraindications to liver transplantation, the objective is to prolong survival and revert to compensated cirrhosis.

2. Intermediate treatment objectives:

1) Normalization of levels of biochemical markers of hepatitis.
2) In HBeAg-positive patients, seroconversion to anti-HBe.

3. Qualification for treatment of both HBeAg-positive and HBeAg-negative patients requires documented positive HBsAg for ≥6 months, detectable HBV DNA, and fulfilment of ≥2 out of the 3 following criteria, according to guidelines from the EASL and the Canadian Association for the Study of the Liver (CASL):

1) HBV DNA >2000 IU/mL (~10,000 copies/mL).
2) Serum ALT levels > upper limit of normal (ULN).
3) Histologic features of chronic hepatitis and fibrosis in a liver biopsy specimen or significant fibrosis detected with noninvasive fibrosis testing.

Another group of patients who should be evaluated for treatment are those who are planned for cancer chemotherapy or immunosuppressive treatment and who are HBsAg-positive only or anti-HBc–positive only regardless of HBV DNA presence.

Pregnant HBsAg-positive mothers should be evaluated before the third trimester. If HBV DNA is >200,000 IU/mL, antiviral therapy should be started, ideally by 28 weeks' gestation. In addition, hepatitis B immunoglobulin (passive immunization) and neonatal hepatitis B vaccination (active immunization) should be given to the newborn within 12 hours of life. Physicians should also ensure the remainder of neonatal vaccinations are completed at 1 and 6 months of life to minimize the risk of vertical transmission from mother to child.

4. Drugs:

1) This field is evolving. Current treatments usually focus on **viral suppression**. Oral **nucleoside or nucleotide analogues (NAs)** are typically used indefinitely (→below) and include adefovir (ADF) (now rarely used), entecavir (ETV), lamivudine (LAM), telbivudine (used predominantly in Asia), tenofovir (TDF), and tenofovir alafenamide (TAF). These drugs are generally well tolerated; nephrotoxicity may rarely occur with ADF and TDF. ETV, TDF, and TAF are used preferentially if resources permit. The use of LAM is limited by the emergence of resistant strains (up to over 50% within 5 years).

2) Subcutaneous **pegylated interferon (PEG-IFN) α** (this does not induce HBV resistance) for 48 weeks: Now used very rarely and reserved for patients who value the important advantage of receiving therapy of finite duration.

    Contraindications: Autoimmune diseases (including untreated hyperthyroidism), major depression (resistant to treatment), severe heart failure, decompensated cirrhosis, prior organ transplantation, thrombocytopenia ($<100\times10^9$/L), and pregnancy. Not recommended in patients with extrahepatic manifestations of hepatitis B.

    Adverse effects: Most commonly influenza-like symptoms, fatigue, loss of appetite, weight loss, and transient severe alopecia. Less common symptoms include myelosuppression (neutropenia, thrombocytopenia), anxiety, nervousness, and depression (including suicidal ideations).

5. Other treatment considerations: Ideally treatment with TDF, ETV, or TAF should be used, although access to therapy may dictate initial options. In Canada, certain provinces have mandated the use of LAM as first-line therapy despite the known high rate for genetic barrier of resistance. ETV should not be used in patients who had an inadequate response to LAM because of the considerably increased risk of developing resistance to ETV.

The duration of therapy in the majority of patients is indefinite, given the low incidence of achieving HBsAg clearance with currently available treatments. However, in HBeAg-positive patients who developed HBeAg loss and anti-HBe antibody positivity, after a minimum of 12 months of ongoing therapy a trial of discontinuation may be considered as long as careful serial monitoring is arranged and therapy is resumed in the setting of relapse or HBeAg reversion.

Current guidelines recommend that HBV carriers receiving or planned for cancer chemotherapy or immunosuppressive treatment should be given NA therapy continued for ≥12 months after completion of cancer treatment. The risk of HBV reactivation depends on the chemotherapy or immunosuppression regimen and treatment duration should be tailored accordingly.

→ FOLLOW-UP

1. Monitoring for HCC is usually done every 6 months (→Complications, below).

2. In patients not currently meeting the criteria for therapy, monitoring of liver function tests and liver enzymes (ALT) should be performed every 3 to

6 months and HBV DNA every 6 months. Ideally, evaluation of liver fibrosis should be updated every 1 to 3 years, depending on the HBeAg status and HBV DNA.

3. Monitoring of antiviral treatment:

1) **Patients treated with PEG-IFN**: After 1 week of treatment and then every 4 weeks monitor white blood cell, neutrophil, and platelet counts; if any of these falls below normal, reduce the dose of PEG-IFN or skip a dose. Severe leukopenia, neutropenia, or thrombocytopenia (<2% of patients) requires discontinuation of treatment. Measure ALT levels every 4 weeks as well as thyroid-stimulating hormone (TSH) and HBV DNA levels every 12 weeks. Assess the efficacy of treatment at 24 weeks and after the end of therapy.

2) **Patients treated with NAs**: Liver enzymes and liver function testing should be performed every 3 to 6 months and HBV DNA every 6 to 12 months. Renal function should also be checked every 6 to 12 months, and patients with worsening renal function (higher risk associated with ADF and TDF) should change agents to those with fewer renal adverse effects (TAF, ETV) or have dose adjustments based on their glomerular filtration rate if other treatment is not available.

→ **COMPLICATIONS**

1. Cirrhosis develops within 5 years in 8% to 20% of patients with chronic hepatitis B. Risk factors include intensive HBV replication; HCV, HDV, or HIV coinfection; middle-aged or elderly patients; male sex; frequent exacerbations; low ALT levels; and alcohol use.

2. HCC: The risk is highest among HBsAg-positive patients with cirrhosis (with the cumulative 5-year incidence up to 20%). In patients without cirrhosis, those of Asian or African descent traditionally are at higher risk compared with white populations. Other known factors include age, male sex, immunosuppression, close family members with HCC, high serum HBV DNA and high ALT, prolonged time to HBeAg seroconversion, concurrent viral infections, excessive alcohol use or smoking, and nonalcoholic steatohepatitis.

3. Diseases caused by immune complexes are rare and most frequently include glomerulonephritis, polyarteritis nodosa, or mixed cryoglobulinemia.

Screening

In patients with cirrhosis screening begins when the diagnosis of chronic hepatitis B is made. In Asian male patients, those with a family history of HCC, and those with HIV coinfection, screening should be started at the age of 40 years. In Asian female patients, the threshold for starting screening is 50 years. In patients of African descent, screening was previously recommended to start at the age of 20 years, but recently this has become a controversial recommendation.

Screening modality: Abdominal ultrasonography every 6 months remains the standard. α-Fetoprotein (AFP) is not advised as a stand-alone screening tool due to the lack of accuracy.

→ **PROGNOSIS**

Serious complications (cirrhosis, liver failure, or HCC) develop in 15% to 40% of patients with chronic HBV infection. The 5-year mortality rate is 14% to 20% in patients with compensated cirrhosis and may be >80% in patients with decompensated cirrhosis.

→ **PREVENTION**

As in acute hepatitis B.

2.2.10.7. Chronic Hepatitis C

→ **DEFINITION, ETIOLOGY, PATHOGENESIS**

Chronic hepatitis C is a chronic (>6 months) disease characterized by hepatic necroinflammatory changes caused by persistent hepatitis C virus (HCV) infection (→Chapter 6.2.2.10.3). The chronic infection results in inflammation, necrosis, and regeneration of hepatocytes that develop over time and may lead to the development of cirrhosis and, potentially, hepatocellular carcinoma (HCC).

→ **CLINICAL FEATURES AND NATURAL HISTORY**

Clinical manifestations are similar to chronic hepatitis B. The majority of patients remain asymptomatic. Of those who are symptomatic, nearly 70% may report ≥1 of the following extrahepatic symptoms: fatigue, myalgia, arthralgia, paresthesia, pruritus, dry mucosae, secondary Raynaud phenomenon, or depressed mood.

In contrast to acute HCV infection, spontaneous HCV clearance rates in patients with chronic infection are extremely rare (~0.03% per year). The progression of the disease is slow and depends on the dynamics of liver fibrosis and cirrhosis. However, it is twice as rapid in patients with elevated alanine aminotransferase (ALT) levels (~40% of infected patients).

→ **DIAGNOSIS**

Diagnostic algorithm: →Figure 2-4.

Diagnostic Tests

1. Laboratory tests include complete blood count (CBC), liver enzymes (aspartate aminotransferase [AST], ALT, alkaline phosphatase [ALP]), other tests of liver function (bilirubin, international normalized ratio [INR], albumin), and creatinine levels. ALT levels are normal in ~30% of patients, and in some they are only periodically elevated (increases may follow a sinusoidal pattern). Thrombocytopenia, elevated bilirubin, or elevated INR suggests advanced fibrosis or cirrhosis.

2. Serologic and virologic tests include antibodies to HCV, HCV RNA, HCV genotype (this helps determine treatment type). Additional investigations should include testing for possible coinfections: hepatitis B surface antigen (HBsAg), anti-HBs antibody, anti-HBc antibody, HIV.

False-negative results of HCV antibodies may be seen over the first 4 to 10 weeks of infection or in immunocompromised patients, including those treated with hemodialysis (in this group consider measurements of HCV RNA as part of the initial diagnostic workup). In the acute phase there may be also periods of undetectable HCV RNA. If testing for HCV antibodies is positive and HCV RNA is negative, retest for HCV RNA (or HCV core antigen, if available) 12 and 24 weeks later to confirm the negative result.

To determine treatment, it is helpful to establish the viral genotype by a molecular method (polymerase chain reaction [PCR]) and, in the case of genotype 1, establish the subgenotype (GT1a or GT1b).

3. Noninvasive assessment of the extent of fibrosis:

1) Transient elastography (specialized ultrasonography measuring the degree of fibrosis).

2) Biochemical markers (AST to platelet ratio index [APRI], FIB-4 index; both available at mdcalc.com).

In all patients it is important to identify cirrhosis because of increased risk of HCC and decreased treatment response. The finding is also used to guide surveillance.

4. Liver biopsy with histologic examination of specimens: This may be indicated in case of suspected liver comorbidity, discrepancy between the

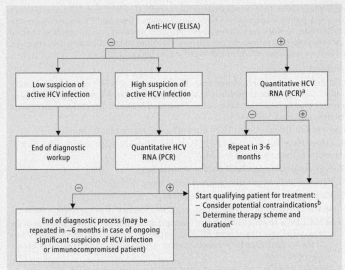

⊕ Positive result. ⊖ Negative result.

a In general patients identified with positive HCV RNA (with acute or chronic infection) should be treated, but the ultimate decision may differ across jurisdictions. For example, as of August 2019, the Ontario government guidelines mandate 2 HCV RNA positive tests 6 months apart (confirmation of chronic HCV infection) in order for the patient to be eligible for drug reimbursement.

b Treatment of currently pregnant patient is not recommended. Some patients may have limited life expectancy for reasons unrelated to HCV infection. Patient compliance or financing of treatment may affect its deferral (compliance has to be judged adequate and financial coverage has to be established, as government drug plans do not cover all patients and under private plans the patient may be charged copayment).

c Consider HCV genotype, potential drug-drug interactions, stage of liver fibrosis, renal function, and previous treatment history.

ELISA, enzyme-linked immunosorbent assay; HCV, hepatitis C virus; PCR, polymerase chain reaction.

Figure 2-4. Diagnostic algorithm in patients with hepatitis C virus infection.

results of noninvasive tests and the patient's clinical status, or discrepancy between test results.

5. Clinical scores designed to measure the severity of liver disease, for example, the Model for End-Stage Liver Disease and Serum Sodium Concentration (MELDNa) score (available at mdcalc.com).

Diagnostic Criteria

Positive HCV RNA in blood for >6 months from infection (the World Health Organization [WHO] definition). Biopsy is not required.

Differential Diagnosis

As in chronic hepatitis B.

→ **TREATMENT**

General Measures

Abstinence from alcohol (as alcohol increases liver injury and accelerates progression to cirrhosis) and smoking cessation is recommended. Hepatitis A or B vaccination in patients susceptible to infection with hepatitis A or B virus. In obese patients introduce a body-weight reduction plan. There are no contraindications to work (except for heavy physical work) or regular daily activities including sports, unless the presence of blood-borne infection precludes specific activities (eg, some medical exposure-prone procedures).

Antiviral Treatment

Guidelines from North American, European, and WHO expert panels may reflect local judgment and availability regarding treatment. Input from local experts may be helpful in some cases. Presented below are general considerations based on such guidelines.

Any patient infected with HCV should be considered for treatment.

1. Objective: Eradication of HCV, as this significantly reduces the risk of developing liver cirrhosis and HCC.

2. Key priority populations for treatment:

1) Patients with a new diagnosis or recurrence of hepatitis C.

2) Patients awaiting liver transplantation:

   a) MELDNa score <18-20: Start treatment before liver transplantation.

   b) MELDNa score ≥18-20: Liver transplantation is performed without prior antiviral treatment and HCV infection is treated after the operation. If the waiting time for transplantation is >6 months, start treatment before the operation.

3) Patients after liver transplantation with reactivation of HCV infection.

4) Patients treated for chronic renal disease (including hemodialysis), especially those awaiting renal transplantation.

5) Patients with HBV or HIV coinfection (or both).

6) Patients at risk of rapid liver dysfunction progression due to a coexisting liver disease or with extrahepatic manifestations of chronic hepatitis (→Complications, below),

7) Individuals at risk of transmitting HCV:

   a) People who inject drugs.

   b) Men who have sex with men (MSM) with high-risk sexual practices.

   c) Women of childbearing age who wish to get pregnant (currently antiviral treatment of patients who are pregnant is not recommended).

   d) Incarcerated individuals.

3. Treatment regimens depending on HCV genotype (based on the 2018 Canadian Association for the Study of the Liver [CASL] guidelines): A combination of direct-acting antiviral (DAA) agents is the current standard of therapy. It relies on combining nucleoside reverse transcriptase inhibitors (NRTIs), nonnucleoside reverse transcriptase inhibitors (NNRTIs), protease inhibitors, entry and integrase inhibitors (a combination of 2-4 agents among nonstructural protein 3 [NS3], 5A [NS5A], and 5B [NS5B] inhibitors), and/or adding ribavirin. DAA monotherapy is unacceptable due to the risk of selection of resistant strains. In the past, treatment used to include interferon, but it has been mostly replaced by DAA therapy. The choice of regimen and duration of treatment are determined by:

1) HCV genotype.

2) Stage of liver fibrosis and presence of cirrhosis.

3) Previous treatment and its outcomes (no response, partial response, or relapse without a sustained virologic response).

4) Coexisting diseases (eg, renal failure) and the possibility of discontinuation of other drugs that have interactions with the planned treatment.

5) Local conditions (eg, the possibility of funding).

Available common regimens (see 2018 CASL guidelines for details [available from the website of the *Canadian Medical Association Journal*]):

1) **Genotype-specific regimens**:

   a) Elbasvir/grazoprevir (genotypes 1 and 4).

   b) Sofosbuvir/ledipasvir (genotypes 1, 4, 5, 6; genotype 3 requires ribavirin in conjunction).

   c) Paritaprevir/ritonavir/ombitasvir/dasabuvir (genotypes 1 and 4; now rarely used).

   d) Sofosbuvir/daclatasvir (genotypes 1, 2, and 3; daclatasvir is not available in Canada).

2) **Pangenotypic regimens**:

   a) Glecaprevir/pibrentasvir.

   b) Sofosbuvir/velpatasvir.

If previously treated with DAA agents, patients with or without cirrhosis can try sofosbuvir/velpatasvir/voxilaprevir. In European guidelines this combination is also recommended in treatment-naive and treatment-experienced patients with compensated cirrhosis.

Important contraindications:

1) Agents inducing cytochrome P450 and P-glycoprotein (carbamazepine, phenytoin) are contraindicated because of the risk of significantly decreased DAA concentrations and the resulting high risk of virologic failure.

2) Do not use NS3/4A protease inhibitors (grazoprevir, glecaprevir, paritaprevir, voxilaprevir, simeprevir) in patients with Child-Pugh B or C decompensated cirrhosis (→Table 2-3) or in those with previous episodes of decompensation, as higher concentrations of these agents result in increased risk of toxicity.

3) In patients with an estimated glomerular filtration rate (eGFR) <30 mL/min/1.73 m^2, sofosbuvir should be used only if no alternative treatment is available.

4. Criteria of response to treatment:

1) Negative serum HCV RNA levels (<15 IU/mL) at 12 weeks or 24 weeks after the end of treatment.

2) Alternatively, negative serum HCV core antigen <3.0 fmol/L, if available, at 24 weeks after the end of treatment.

5. Potential drug interactions: Interaction checker from the University of Liverpool available at www.hep-druginteractions.org.

→ FOLLOW-UP

DAA and ribavirin toxicity should be monitored. Liver enzymes and creatinine levels should be measured every 4 weeks and as clinically indicated. In patients with severe adverse reactions treatment should be discontinued (dose reduction is not used); this includes a >10-fold increase in ALT at any time; or a <10-fold increase in ALT with symptoms or significantly elevated bilirubin, ALP, or INR. If there is a <10-fold increase in ALT and the patient is asymptomatic, repeat testing should be performed every 2 weeks and therapy should be discontinued if the levels remain elevated. For regimens with ribavirin, it is also important to monitor hemoglobin, initially after 1 week and then every 4 weeks. In cases of severe hemolytic anemia (<2% of patients), treatment should be discontinued.

Annual HCV RNA testing is recommended in patients with ongoing exposure risks. Assessment of fibrosis should also be completed every 1 to 2 years. Patients with cirrhosis should be monitored for HCC every 6 months. If cirrhosis is identified, esophagogastroduodenoscopy should be completed to screen for esophageal varices.

→ COMPLICATIONS

1. Cirrhosis: Without effective treatment, cirrhosis can develop in ~20% of patients with chronic HCV infection over a period of 20 to 50 years. **Risk factors** for accelerated progression to cirrhosis include alcohol, male sex, infection age >40 years, overweight or obesity, tobacco smoking, elevated serum iron levels, fatty liver disease, infection with HCV genotype 3, diabetes mellitus, HBV/HIV coinfection, and blood transfusion–related infection. Liver transplantation may be indicated in patients with liver failure caused by cirrhosis.

2. Extrahepatic, autoimmune, and immune complex–related diseases:

1) Renal: Membranoproliferative or membranous glomerulonephritis (from asymptomatic hematuria and proteinuria to nephrotic syndrome and chronic kidney disease).

2) Dermatologic: Purpura (inflammation of small vessels of the skin), lichen planus, porphyria, psoriasis (especially in patients treated with interferon).

3) Hematologic: Immune thrombocytopenia, mixed cryoglobulinemia, lymphoma.

4) Neurologic: Peripheral neuropathy (usually sensory), cerebral vasculitis.

5) Rheumatologic: Arthritis (symmetric inflammation of numerous small joints similar to rheumatoid arthritis or inflammation of ≥1 large joint), Sjögren syndrome, antiphospholipid syndrome, systemic lupus erythematosus.

6) Cardiovascular: Vasculitis, arterial hypertension.

3. HCC: HCC may develop within 20 years in ~3% to 5% of patients with chronic hepatitis C. The risk is significantly increased (1%-2% per year) in patients with cirrhosis (HCC without liver fibrosis is rare) and decreased with successful antiviral treatment. Additional risk factors include age >60 years, increased ALP, and thrombocytopenia.

→ PROGNOSIS

Sustained virologic response with DAA combination regimens is achieved in >90% of participants of clinical studies; in some subgroups the response rate may approach 100% of patients.

In patients with compensated cirrhosis the 5-year and 10-year risks of esophageal variceal bleeding are ~2.5% and 5%, respectively. The risk of decompensation of cirrhosis (ascites) in these patients is 7% and 20%, respectively, and the 10-year risk of encephalopathy is ~2.5%. Within 10 years, progression to end-stage liver failure occurs in 30% of patients with compensated cirrhosis. Mortality rates are 20% after 10 years in patients with compensated cirrhosis and 50% after 5 years in patients with symptomatic liver failure. In each case the prognosis is markedly improved after successful virus eradication, although cirrhosis and portal hypertension usually persist, particularly if other causes are still present (eg, alcohol use, nonalcoholic steatohepatitis).

→ PREVENTION

As in acute hepatitis C. Treatment of acute hepatitis C reduces the risk of developing chronic hepatitis C.

→ SCREENING

Screening is recommended in the following situations:

1) **Risk factor–based screening**:

   a) History (present or past) of injection drug use.

   b) Received blood transfusion, blood products, or organ transplantation before 1992 in Canada.

c) History (present or past) of incarceration.

d) People who were born or lived in areas endemic for hepatitis C (prevalence >3%): Central/East/South Asia; Australasia and Oceania; Eastern Europe; sub-Saharan Africa; North Africa; Middle East.

e) Offspring of an HCV-infected mother.

f) History of sexual contact with HCV-positive individuals.

g) HIV positivity.

h) Chronic hemodialysis.

i) Elevated ALT.

2) **Population-based screening**: In Canada, individuals born between 1945 and 1975.

2.2.11. Wilson Disease

→ DEFINITION, ETIOLOGY, PATHOGENESIS

Wilson disease is characterized by an excessive cytotoxic accumulation of copper in tissues caused by an autosomal recessive defect of a hepatocyte membrane–bound copper transporting protein. This is related to a mutation of the *ATP7B* gene located on chromosome 13 of which there are >500 known genetic variants. The resulting impaired biliary excretion of copper and its accumulation in the liver, brain, kidney, and cornea lead to damage to these organs. One in every 30,000 Canadians is estimated to be living with Wilson disease.

→ CLINICAL FEATURES AND NATURAL HISTORY

The onset of symptoms usually occurs between 5 and 40 years of age, rarely (~3% of patients) later in life. Clinical manifestations are varied and may involve many systems and organs, as outlined below. When untreated, the disease is progressive and may lead to cirrhosis. Patients may also present with acute liver failure, which is associated with high mortality rates and may require urgent liver transplantation. Early diagnosis and treatment is the key to preventing copper accumulation and its complications.

1. Hepatic features are seen in ~40% to 50% of patients. Depending on progression of the disease, patients present with various features secondary to steatosis, hepatitis, cirrhosis, or acute liver failure. These include fatigue, abdominal pain, hepatomegaly, splenomegaly, jaundice, portal hypertension, hepatic encephalopathy, and upper gastrointestinal bleeding.

2. Neuropsychiatric features are present in ~40% to 50% of patients and include dystonia, dysarthria, parkinsonism (tremor, bradykinesia, rigidity, dysarthria), salivation, seizures, personality changes, cognitive impairment, mood disorders, and psychosis. Clinicians should be careful not to mistake hepatic encephalopathy for the above findings.

3. Other organ abnormalities: Kayser-Fleischer rings (copper deposits in the Descemet membrane of the cornea, visible on slit lamp examination as a gold-brown corneal rim), sunflower cataract, Coombs test–negative hemolytic anemia (~15% of patients), Fanconi syndrome, cardiomyopathy, arrhythmia, osteomalacia, osteoporosis, arthritis, pancreatitis, delayed puberty, infertility, amenorrhea, repeated miscarriages, hypothyroidism, or hypoparathyroidism.

→ DIAGNOSIS

Diagnostic Tests

1. Blood tests: Elevated serum aminotransferase levels (essentially all patients), occasionally low alkaline phosphatase levels, low serum ceruloplasmin levels, and decreased total serum copper levels (used more for monitoring than diagnosis).

2. Urine tests: In ~80% of patients 24-hour urine copper excretion is >100 µg (1.6 µmol).

3. Imaging studies: Depending on stage of the disease, ultrasonography may reveal hepatomegaly or features of portal hypertension (splenomegaly). In patients with neurologic symptoms, magnetic resonance imaging (MRI) and computed tomography (CT) can reveal lesions in the basal ganglia.

4. Histologic examination of liver biopsy specimens: Nonspecific abnormalities, elevated copper levels (≥250 µg/g of dry tissue in >90% of patients).

5. Genetic tests: Direct sequencing of the *ATP7B* gene and haplotype analysis are diagnostic options in challenging cases and in siblings of patients with Wilson disease.

Diagnostic Criteria

The diagnosis of Wilson disease is made most often on the basis of a combination of clinical and laboratory findings. The presence of Kayser-Fleischer rings (although their absence does not exclude Wilson disease) and serum ceruloplasmin levels <200 mg/L or 24-hour urinary cooper excretion >100 µg/24 h in a patient with symptoms of liver disease and associated neurologic or psychiatric manifestations represent a classic presentation of Wilson disease. In reality, many cases are not that straightforward and the Leipzig scoring system (→Table 2-8) is used to aid diagnosis.

Differential Diagnosis

Other causes of liver dysfunction, such as alcoholic liver disease, fatty liver disease, hepatitis B or C, α_1-antitrypsin deficiency, autoimmune hepatitis, hemochromatosis, and medication hepatotoxicity. Neuropsychiatric conditions to consider include parkinsonism, essential tremor, Huntington disease, idiopathic dystonias, and adverse effects of antipsychotic medications.

→ TREATMENT

1. Recommend **abstinence from alcohol and avoidance of foods that are high in copper**, such as nuts, chocolate, soy, mushrooms, liver, and seafood.

2. Use **pharmacotherapy** indefinitely in all patients, even in pregnancy:

1) For asymptomatic patients start with a copper chelator (this increases urinary copper excretion). Initially use oral penicillamine 250 to 500 mg/d with the dose titrated up by 250 mg every 4 to 7 days to a total of 1 to 1.5 g/d in 4 divided doses. During therapy the patient should receive pyridoxine supplementation (25-50 mg/d). When treated with penicillamine, 30% of patients develop adverse effects (dysgeusia, nausea, myelosuppression) and may be switched to another chelator: trientine 1 to 1.5 g/d. Reduce the dose of chelators by 25% to 50% during pregnancy.

   The cost of trientine in some jurisdictions may exceed $1000 per day and access to the drug is thus limited.

2) For maintenance treatment we recommend oral zinc 75 to 250 mg/d in 2 or 3 divided doses (zinc acts to inhibit gastrointestinal copper absorption). This can be in addition to the copper chelator or as monotherapy in asymptomatic patients and patients in whom chelators are poorly tolerated or contraindicated.

3. Liver transplantation is indicated in patients with acute liver failure due to Wilson disease (formerly known as "fulminant Wilson disease") and a prognostic index of ≥11 (→Table 2-9) or in patients with refractory decompensated cirrhosis.

→ FOLLOW-UP

Regular follow-up is necessary after starting copper chelation, initially every week over the first month, 1 to 3 months per the first year of therapy, then 1 to 2 times per year. Follow-up should include history and physical examination,

Table 2-8. Scoring system developed at the 8th International Meeting on Wilson disease (Leipzig 2001)

Clinical findings	Serum/blood tests	Urine copper	*ATP7B* mutation	Liver biopsy	Score
			Homozygous		4 points
− KF rings − Severe neurologic symptoms[a]	Ceruloplasmin <0.1 g/L	− >2×ULN − Normal but >5×ULN after peni-cillamine		Copper >5×ULN (>4 μmol/g)	2 points each
Mild neuro-logic symp-toms	− Ceruloplasmin 0.1-0.2 g/L − Hemolytic anemia	− 1-2×ULN	Heterozygous	− Copper 0.8--4 μmol/g − Rhodanine--positive granules[b]	1 point each
				Normal copper (<0.8 μmol/g)	−1 point

Interpretation:

Score ≥4: Wilson disease probable

Score 3: Inconclusive

Score ≤2: Wilson disease unlikely

[a] Or typical abnormalities on brain MRI.

[b] If no quantitative liver copper available.

Based on Liver Int. 2003;23(3):139-42.

KF, Kayser-Fleischer; MRI, magnetic resonance imaging; ULN, upper limit of normal.

Table 2-9. Prognostic index of acute liver failure in patients with Wilson disease

Score	1	2	3	4
Serum bilirubin (μmol/L)	100-150	151-200	201-300	>300
AST (IU/L)	100-150	151-300	301-400	>400
INR	1.3-1.6	1.7-1.9	2.0-2.4	>2.4
WBC (1 × 10⁹/L)	6.8-8.3	8.4-10.3	10.4-15.3	>15.3
Serum albumin (g/L)	34-44	25-33	21-24	<21

A total score ≥11 indicates a high risk of death if the patient is not treated with liver transplan-tation. Data from children populations.

Adapted from Liver Transpl. 2005;11(4):441-8.

AST, aspartate aminotransferase; INR, international normalized ratio; WBC, white blood cell.

complete blood count (CBC) with differential count (→Diagnostic Tests, above), liver and kidney function parameters, serum copper level, urinalysis, and 24-hour urinary copper excretion (should be 200-500 µg/24 h in a controlled state; at the beginning of therapy initially may be much higher). Nephrotoxicity and myelosuppression are rare but important adverse effects of penicillamine that are often detected on routine blood tests. The thresholds for concern about myelosuppression and decision to stop the drug should follow the manufacturer's guidelines and may depend on baseline values and time trend of changes, but such thresholds are usually suggested as below 3×10^9 and 3.5×10^9 white blood cells/L, ~2×10^9 neutrophils/L, and 100×10^9 to 120×10^9 platelets/L.

→ **PROGNOSIS**

Acute liver failure is life-threatening (scoring of severity: →Table 2-9). The prognosis for patients receiving treatment with other clinical presentations and complications of Wilson disease is generally good, including those with advanced live disease. The risk of hepatocellular carcinoma is controversial.

3. Pancreatic Diseases

3.1. Acute Pancreatitis

→ **DEFINITION, ETIOLOGY, PATHOGENESIS**

Acute pancreatitis is an acute inflammatory condition associated with premature activation of pancreatic zymogens (primarily trypsin), a varying degree of damage to the adjacent tissues, and, in some cases, also to distant organs.

Causes: The most frequent causes include diseases of the gallbladder and alcohol use (these are responsible for ~80% of cases), idiopathic etiology (~10% of cases), iatrogenic factors (endoscopic retrograde cholangiopancreatography [ERCP], abdominal surgical procedures), hypertriglyceridemia (in particular chylomicronemia syndrome) >1000 mg/dL (11.3 mmol/L), hyperparathyroidism, drugs (including asparaginase, pentamidine, azathioprine, glucocorticoids, cytarabine), congenital malformations (pancreas divisum), abdominal trauma, postoperative complications; and very rarely, viral infection (coxsackievirus, mumps virus, cytomegalovirus, HIV), parasites (ascaris), genetic factors (eg, mutations of the *SPINK1* gene, which encodes a trypsin inhibitor; cystic fibrosis), autoimmune diseases (systemic lupus erythematosus, Sjögren syndrome).

Acute pancreatitis is classified into 2 types:

1) **Interstitial pancreatitis**, which affects 80% to 90% of patients and is not associated with necrosis of the pancreas or the adjacent tissues.
2) **Necrotizing pancreatitis**.

→ **CLINICAL FEATURES AND NATURAL HISTORY**

1. Signs and symptoms: Abdominal pain (usually the presenting sign; the pain has a sudden onset, is very severe, and is located in the epigastrium or left upper abdominal quadrant; sometimes may be referred to the spine), nausea and vomiting that bring no relief of discomfort, fever (a frequent manifestation; the time of onset is important for the determination of the cause and clinical importance of fever: onset in the first week suggests fever caused by systemic inflammatory response syndrome [SIRS], which resolves once the intensity of the inflammatory reaction has decreased; onset of fever in the second or third week is usually associated with infection of the necrotic tissues), epigastric pain, weak or absent peristalsis (paralytic ileus), increased abdominal wall muscle tone, palpable tender epigastric mass (observed in some patients with severe acute pancreatitis; this is caused by expanding necrosis and peripancreatic inflammatory infiltrates), altered mental status (a sign of developing shock, hypoxemia, and endotoxemia; disturbances of consciousness and restlessness can progress to pancreatic encephalopathy), tachycardia (common), hypotension (usually results from hypovolemia), sometimes shock (10% of cases), jaundice (in 20%-30% of patients, particularly with acute pancreatitis caused by biliary disease), rarely cutaneous manifestations (patients with severe acute pancreatitis and shock may develop facial erythema, cyanosis of the face and extremities, bruising around the umbilicus [Cullen sign] or in the lumbar area [Turner sign]), pleural effusion (in ~40% of patients; this is most frequently left-sided).

2. Two overlapping phases of acute pancreatitis have been described: an **early phase** (characterized by systemic responses to the local pancreatic injury) and a **late phase** (with infection of necrotic tissues and septic complications). The early phase usually lasts 1 week, but sometimes may persist for 2 weeks. The onset of the second phase of acute pancreatitis, which lasts from a few weeks to a few months, confirms the diagnosis of a moderate to severe disease.

→ DIAGNOSIS

Diagnostic Tests

1. Laboratory tests:

1) **Abnormalities typical for acute pancreatitis**: Elevated levels of pancreatic enzymes (usually >3×upper limit of normal):

   a) **Serum lipase** (this has the highest sensitivity and specificity in diagnosing acute pancreatitis).

   b) **Serum and urine amylase**: After 48 to 72 hours, serum amylase levels often return to normal despite the ongoing disease; however, total urine amylase and serum pancreatic isoenzyme levels continue to be elevated.

2) **Abnormalities related to the severity of acute pancreatitis or to its complications**: Elevated white blood cell counts with a left shift in the differential count, elevated C-reactive protein (CRP) levels (this correlates with the severity of acute pancreatitis, particularly within the first 48 to 72 hours), elevated serum procalcitonin levels (this correlates with the severity of acute pancreatitis as well as with the risk of organ failure and infected pancreatic necrosis), elevated blood urea/blood urea nitrogen (BUN) levels (this may indicate inadequate fluid resuscitation in the initial stages of the disease or deterioration of renal function; it is an independent risk factor of death), biochemical markers of liver injury (hyperbilirubinemia, elevated levels of alanine aminotransferase, aspartate aminotransferase, alkaline phosphatase; these suggest a biliary etiology of acute pancreatitis), elevated lactate dehydrogenase levels, hypoalbuminemia, relative erythrocytosis (due to dehydration [vomiting] and effusions [third space]) or anemia (due to bleeding), hypoxemia, hyperglycemia, hypertriglyceridemia, and hypocalcemia.

2. Imaging studies: Abdominal ultrasonography is the first-line study, but it often fails to visualize the pancreas (due to intestinal gas or obesity). In patients with acute pancreatitis ultrasonography may reveal pancreatic edema, an indistinct pancreatic outline, reduced and heterogeneous echogenicity of the pancreatic parenchyma; it may also visualize cholelithiasis and complications of acute pancreatitis (eg, fluid collections). Ultrasonography with IV contrast enhancement is used to visualize the pancreatic parenchyma. **Contrast-enhanced computed tomography (CT)** of the abdomen, the gold standard in diagnosing acute pancreatitis, is used to assess the extent of pancreatic necrosis as well as necrosis of the peripancreatic fat and connective tissues. This study should not be routinely performed in patients in whom the diagnosis of acute pancreatitis is straightforward and the disease is mild and uncomplicated. CT should be performed in patients who do not improve within 48 to 72 hours (eg, those who have persistent pain, fever, and nausea, and in whom oral nutrition is not possible) to diagnose possible local complications, such as pancreatic necrosis. Abdominal CT performed between days 5 and 7 of the onset of the disease is optimal for the assessment of the extent of necrosis. CT should be performed immediately in every patient with suspected acute pancreatitis who is critically ill or requires surgery. Follow-up studies are performed in case of clinical deterioration, progressive organ failure, or signs and symptoms of sepsis. **Chest radiographs** may demonstrate bibasilar atelectasis, pleural effusion (particularly left-sided), or acute respiratory distress syndrome. **Plain abdominal radiographs** may reveal fluid levels or intestinal loop distension (symptoms of paralytic ileus: →Chapter 6.1.3.6.1). **ERCP with therapeutic sphincterotomy** should be performed as an emergency procedure in selected patients with coexisting cholangitis or persistent cholestasis◉◉ (→below). **Magnetic resonance cholangiopancreatography** (MRCP) is performed in the acute phase of the disease in patients with equivocal diagnosis; however, it is mainly used as part of the diagnostics of cholelithiasis and assessment of the pancreatic duct in patients with fluid collections or cysts and fistulae in advanced stages of the disease.

3. Endoscopic ultrasonography is useful in the identification of etiologic factors in patients with a history of acute pancreatitis or idiopathic recurrent acute pancreatitis as well in the identification of fluid collections in patients with advanced disease.

Diagnostic Criteria

Diagnosis is confirmed in patients in whom 2 out of the following 3 criteria are fulfilled:

1) Typical clinical manifestations (epigastric pain of sudden onset, often referred to the back).
2) Levels of pancreatic enzymes elevated >3×the upper limit of normal.
3) Results of imaging studies (abdominal ultrasonography, dynamic CT, or magnetic resonance imaging [MRI]) typical for acute pancreatitis.

Assessment of the Severity and Prognosis in Acute Pancreatitis

1. The Atlanta Classification (2012):

1) **Mild acute pancreatitis**: No organ failure, no local complications (except for an acute peripancreatic fluid collection), and no systemic complications.
2) **Moderate acute pancreatitis**: Transient (<48 hours) organ failure, local complications (necrosis, acute necrotizing collection, walled-off pancreatic necrosis), and/or exacerbation of comorbidities.
3) **Severe acute pancreatitis**: Persistent (>48 hours) organ failure and usually ≥1 local complication. **Definitions of multiple organ dysfunction (a modified Marshall score)**: →Table 3-1. Patients who develop organ failure within the first 24 hours of hospitalization in whom the failure cannot be classified as transient or persistent should be initially managed as patients with severe acute pancreatitis; reevaluate the severity of acute pancreatitis after 24 hours, 48 hours, and 7 days from admission.

2. Clinical features observed on admission that indicate the risk of development of severe acute pancreatitis:

1) Age >55 years.
2) Obesity (body mass index >30 kg/m^2).
3) Altered consciousness status.
4) Comorbidities.
5) SIRS (→Chapter 8.14).
6) Abnormal laboratory test results:
   a) BUN >20 mg/dL (blood urea level, 42.86 mg/dL [7.14 mmol/L]) or rising.
   b) Hematocrit >44% or rising.
   c) Increased serum creatinine levels.

Table 3-1. Modified Marshall scoring system

Organ system	Score				
	0	1	2	3	4
Respiratory (PaO_2/FiO_2)	>400	301-400	201-300	101-200	≤101
Renal (serum creatinine, μmol/L)[a]	≤134	134-169	170-310	311-439	>439
Cardiovascular (systolic blood pressure, mm Hg)[b]	>90	<90 Fluid responsive	<90 Not fluid responsive	<90, pH <7.3	<90, pH <7.2

A score of ≥2 in any system defines the presence of organ failure.

[a] The score for patients with preexisting chronic renal failure depends on the extent of further deterioration of baseline renal function. No formal correction exists for a baseline serum creatinine ≥134 μmol/L or ≥1.4 mg/dL.

[b] Off inotropic support.

Source: Gut. 2013;62(1):102-11.

7) Abnormal results of imaging studies:
   a) Pleural effusion.
   b) Pulmonary infiltrates.
   c) Multiple or extensive extrapancreatic fluid collections.

Other criteria: Computed tomography severity index (CTSI), Acute Physiology and Chronic Health Evaluation (APACHE) II score. The severity of the elevation of serum and urine levels of pancreatic enzymes is of no prognostic value.

Differential Diagnosis

Differential diagnosis should include gastrointestinal perforation (gastric or duodenal ulcer, intestinal perforation), acute appendicitis, acute intestinal ischemia, dissecting aortic aneurysm, ectopic pregnancy, and myocardial infarction (particularly posterior wall infarction).

→ TREATMENT

Treatment of the acute phase of the disease includes fluid resuscitation, pain management, and nutrition therapy. Other interventions depend on the severity of the disease and its complications.

Medical Treatment

1. Initial management:

1) In the first 12 to 24 hours of hospitalization in all patients without concomitant cardiovascular disease or kidney disease start intensive IV fluid resuscitation using an isotonic electrolyte solution (eg, Ringer lactate) at a rate of 250 to 500 mL/h; adjust the infusion rate to the patient's volume status, response to fluid, cardiovascular function, and renal function (these should be assessed on the basis of the heart rate, arterial blood pressure, urine output [≥0.5 mL/h], and central venous pressure [in some patients]). In patients with severe hypovolemia (hypotension, tachycardia) a more rapid fluid administration (bolus) may be necessary.

2) Immediately treat electrolyte disturbances, in particular hypokalemia.

3) Use blood transfusion as per guidelines in critically ill patients.

4) In patients with hyperglycemia >13.9 mmol/L (250 mg/dL), administer insulin.

2. Pain management: There is no difference in the complication risk between opioids and other analgesic options. Opioids (IV morphine or hydromorphone) may be an appropriate choice in the treatment of pain in acute pancreatitis.◐◑

3. Nutrition therapy: In mild acute pancreatitis oral feedings can be started immediately if there is no nausea and vomiting. Initiation of feeding with a low-fat solid diet appears as safe as a clear liquid diet.◐◑ In patients with severe acute pancreatitis start enteral nutrition within the first 24 to 48 hours (if possible) and add parenteral nutrition if enteral nutrition is not tolerated.

1) **Enteral nutrition** is administered using a nasogastric or nasojejunal tube. The preferred enteral formula might be a semielemental nutrition, which is low in fat and higher in predigested protein than regular feeding formulas. It should be started at a low rate (10-20 mL/h) and slowly increased until the desired caloric intake is reached.◐◯ Complications are rare and minor (dislocation or obstruction of the tube, diarrhea, nausea, and flatulence caused by too rapid administration of the nutrition formulas).

2) **Total parenteral nutrition (TPN)** should be avoided in patients with mild and severe acute pancreatitis and used only if enteral nutrition is not possible. Monitor and treat metabolic disturbances (hypoglycemia and hyperglycemia, hypocalcemia, hypokalemia and hyperkalemia, hypophosphatemia, hypomagnesemia, and acid-base disturbances). Discontinue TPN promptly once enteral nutrition becomes feasible.

4. Antibiotic therapy: Do not use routine antibiotic prophylaxis in patients with severe acute pancreatitis or in patients with sterile pancreatic necrosis to prevent its infection.●◑ Antibiotics are indicated in the treatment of infected pancreatic necrosis (→Complications, below) and extrapancreatic infections: cholangitis, catheter-related infections, bacteremia, urinary tract infections, pneumonia. Infected pancreatic necrosis should be suspected in the setting of positive blood cultures or evidence of gas within a pancreatic fluid collection on CT imaging. Antifungal therapy should not be routinely used in patients treated with antibiotics.

Invasive Treatment

1. ERCP with sphincterotomy is indicated within 24 hours of admission in patients with coexisting acute cholangitis. It is not necessary in the majority of patients with biliary acute pancreatitis without laboratory or clinical features of persistent biliary obstruction. In patients without cholangitis and/or jaundice but with a well-grounded suspicion of biliary duct stones, MRCP should be performed rather than a diagnostic ERCP.◐◑

2. Cholecystectomy: In patients with mild biliary acute pancreatitis, cholecystectomy should be performed before discharge unless it is contraindicated for other reasons. In patients with severe biliary acute pancreatitis, cholecystectomy is performed after the resolution of active inflammation and resorption or stabilization of fluid collections.◐◯

3. Debridement of pancreatic necrosis: Infection of the necrosis is an indication for invasive procedures to evacuate the infected tissues. In stable patients with infected necrosis, surgical, endoscopic, or radiologic drainage procedures preferably should be delayed for >4 weeks to allow the development of a fibrous wall around the necrosis. Minimally invasive methods of necrosectomy are usually preferred to open necrosectomy.◐◑

⇥ FOLLOW-UP

In patients with severe acute pancreatitis intensive care is required:

1) Monitor arterial blood pressures, pulse, and fluid balance hourly.
2) Monitor arterial blood gas and serum electrolyte levels frequently (a reasonable rate is every 4-12 hours).
3) Perform physical examination at least every 12 hours.

4) Monitor pancreatic enzyme levels, the complete blood count, prothrombin time (PT), activated partial thromboplastin time (aPTT), biochemical kidney function tests, CRP, total protein and albumin levels, and, if necessary, also a 24-hour glucose profile on a daily basis.

5) Assess organ failure using the Marshall score on a daily basis over the first 7 days.

6) Periodically perform ultrasonography or CT.

7) Fine-needle aspiration (FNA) should only be used in selected situations where there is no clinical response to antibiotics, such as when a fungal infection is suspected.◐○

→ COMPLICATIONS

1. Acute peripancreatic fluid collection (APFC) develops early, usually in the first 24 to 48 hours of interstitial pancreatitis, and has no distinct wall visible on ultrasonography or CT. The contents are liquid. APFC results from rupture of the pancreatic ducts or from accumulation of inflammatory exudate. APFC is usually reabsorbed within 4 weeks, but in rare cases it may transform into a pseudocyst.

2. Pseudocysts develop from APFCs that have not been reabsorbed within 4 weeks. The wall of a pseudocyst is usually a capsule made of fibrous connective tissue lined with granulation tissue. Pseudocysts may also involve parts of the adjacent organs, such as the stomach, intestines, or pancreas. Similarly to APFC, the contents of pseudocysts are liquid.

3. Acute necrotic collection (ANC) develops in the early phase of necrotizing acute pancreatitis and may undergo complete reabsorption (if necrosis affects <30% of the pancreas) or gradual liquefaction with subsequent formation of a capsule. The contents of ANCs consist of varying amounts of solid debris (necrotic tissue), which differentiate ANC from APFC and pseudocysts. ANC may become infected. MRI, endoscopic ultrasonography (EUS), and abdominal ultrasonography are useful in differential diagnosis.

4. Walled-off necrosis (WON) is a late ANC that contains a variable amount of liquid and solid debris encapsulated in a thick wall, which reduces the probability of spontaneous reabsorption. WON usually develops ≥4 weeks from the onset of necrotizing acute pancreatitis. It may be asymptomatic or manifest with abdominal pain, duodenal obstruction, and/or biliary obstruction.

5. Infected necrosis of the pancreas and adjacent tissues usually develops during week 3 of the disease; mortality rates are as high as 50%. It should be suspected in patients with pancreatic or extrapancreatic necrosis who deteriorate or who do not improve within 7 to 10 days of hospital treatment. **Diagnosis** is based on positive blood cultures or evidence of gas in the necrotic tissue on a CT scan or alternatively with percutaneous FNA. An acceptable approach in patients with suspected pancreatic necrosis (after day 10-15) is IV **empiric antimicrobial therapy** with a carbapenem (**doripenem**, **ertapenem**, **imipenem/cilastatin** 1 g every 8 hours, or **meropenem** 500 mg every 8 hours) or a quinolone (**ciprofloxacin** 200 mg every 12 hours, **moxifloxacin** or **pefloxacin**) in combination with **metronidazole** 500 mg every 8 hours. Invasive procedures are usually necessary (→Invasive Treatment, above); in selected, relatively stable patients, the invasive procedures may be delayed or spared, as long as strict monitoring can be ensured.

6. Fistulae: A late complication of necrotizing acute pancreatitis, which results from the loss of continuity of the pancreatic ducts. Most frequently, fistulae communicate with the duodenum or transverse colon. **Diagnosis**: MRCP (noninvasive) or ERCP (this offers a possibility of therapeutic stenting to improve healing). In patients with enteric fistulae, perform oral-contrast–enhanced CT. **Treatment**: Most fistulae close spontaneously without the need of surgical intervention.

7. **Vascular complications**:

1) Prehepatic portal hypertension caused by compression or occlusion of the splenic vein or the superior mesenteric vein.

2) Bleeding or pseudoaneurysm due to direct erosion of the pancreatic or peripancreatic arteries or veins (or both). Rupture of a pseudoaneurysm leads to a massive hemorrhage to the pseudocyst, peritoneal cavity, or into the gastrointestinal tract. In patients with pseudoaneurysms communicating with the pancreatic duct, gastrointestinal bleeding may occur via the ampulla of Vater.

3) Thrombosis of the splenic vein, splenic artery, or portal vein (→Chapter 6.2.2.8).

Diagnosis: CT, MRI, Doppler ultrasonography, selective splanchnic angiography (this allows for stopping the bleeding and occlusion of the pseudoaneurysm). Depending on the location, surgery may be required.

8. Organ complications: Early complications result from SIRS (→Chapter 8.14): shock, acute respiratory distress syndrome, acute kidney injury, disseminated intravascular coagulation, sepsis, and abdominal compartment syndrome.

3.2. Chronic Pancreatitis

➡ DEFINITION, ETIOLOGY, PATHOGENESIS

Chronic pancreatitis is a chronic inflammatory disorder resulting in progressive irreversible changes of the pancreatic parenchyma (atrophy, fibrosis) and a gradual development of exocrine and endocrine pancreatic insufficiency. The pathogenesis has not been fully explained; most probably, the disease is a consequence of recurrent acute pancreatitis with subsequent fibrosis.

Causes (according to the **TIGAR-O** classification system):

1) **T**oxic-metabolic: Alcohol (in up to 85% of cases), tobacco smoking, hypercalcemia (hyperparathyroidism), hyperlipidemia (a rare and controversial cause), chronic kidney disease.

2) **I**diopathic.

3) **G**enetic: Gene mutations: *PRSS1* (cationic trypsinogen), *CFTR* (cystic fibrosis), *SPINK1* (serine protease inhibitors), or α_1-antitrypsin deficiency.

4) **A**utoimmune.

5) **R**ecurrent and severe acute pancreatitis: Prior severe necrotizing acute pancreatitis, recurrent acute pancreatitis, vascular diseases, or radiation-induced ischemia.

6) **O**bstructive: Pancreas divisum, functional disorders of the sphincter of Oddi (controversial), obstruction of the pancreatic duct (eg, tumor), injury to the pancreatic duct, periampullary duodenal cysts.

➡ CLINICAL FEATURES AND NATURAL HISTORY

Chronic pancreatitis is an indolent condition. The dominant clinical features include abdominal pain (although in rare cases, particularly those of autoimmune etiology, the disease may be painless) and in more advanced disease also symptoms of exocrine and endocrine pancreatic insufficiency.

1. Pain: Located in the epigastrium, may be referred to the back, occurs after meals or often following alcohol use. It may last from several hours to several days (usually <10 days) and recur with varying frequency or be constant with exacerbations. The pain may improve or disappear with the development of exocrine insufficiency.

2. Signs and symptoms of exocrine pancreatic insufficiency: Flatulence, sensation of epigastric distention, sometimes vomiting, chronic diarrhea (usually steatorrhea due to an impaired secretion of pancreatic lipase). Since meals exacerbate the symptoms, patients often limit their food intake, which together with the coexisting impaired digestion (and secondary malabsorption) and loss of appetite (frequent in alcoholism) results in body weight loss, malnutrition, or even cachexia.

3. Symptoms of endocrine pancreatic insufficiency: Impaired glucose tolerance or diabetes mellitus in advanced stages of chronic pancreatitis. Patients with diabetes are prone to hypoglycemia associated with insulin therapy and glucagon deficiency. In rare cases, ketoacidosis develops.

4. Signs: Epigastric tenderness (primarily during exacerbations); some patients develop a palpable abdominal mass (eg, a pseudocyst) or jaundice (usually mild, recurrent, caused by pancreatic head edema or stricture of the terminal portion of the common bile duct, which may be due to compression by the enlarged or fibrotic pancreatic head, or by pseudocysts).

→ DIAGNOSIS

Diagnostic Tests

1. Laboratory tests: Serum amylase and lipase levels may be slightly elevated but are usually normal. In patients without a clear etiology in whom autoimmune pancreatitis is suspected clinically, tests for IgG4 levels or IgG4-positive plasma cells should be ordered as screening tests.

2. Imaging studies:

1) **Diagnostic findings** (morphologic features that unequivocally confirm the diagnosis of chronic pancreatitis): Varying (in calcific chronic pancreatitis) or uniform (in obstructive chronic pancreatitis) dilation of the pancreatic duct to >4 mm in diameter (ultrasonography); dilation of secondary pancreatic ducts (most frequently observed on endoscopic retrograde cholangiopancreatography [ERCP], magnetic resonance cholangiopancreatography [MRCP]); pancreatic calcifications (sometimes visualized on plain abdominal radiographs); stones in pancreatic ducts.

2) **Nondiagnostic findings** (these are frequently observed in chronic pancreatitis but may occur in other diseases of the pancreas): Diffuse pancreatic edema (as in acute pancreatitis), pancreatic parenchymal fibrosis; pseudocysts; focal necrosis of the pancreas; pancreatic abscesses; portal vein thrombosis; pancreatic atrophy.

Ultrasonography and **computed tomography (CT)** are the first-line studies used in the assessment of the pancreatic parenchyma (size, presence of calcifications), the pancreatic duct (diameter, outline), and detection of pseudocysts. **Endoscopic ultrasonography**, **MRCP** (optimally with prior intravenous administration of secretin), and **ERCP** are more sensitive and specific than other imaging studies; due to a higher risk of complications, endoscopic ultrasonography (EUS) and ERCP are only performed in the case of diagnostic uncertainty or for therapeutic measures.

3. Functional tests: These are indicated when the diagnosis of chronic pancreatitis cannot be established on the basis of imaging studies:

1) The **secretin-cholecystokinin test** is the most sensitive test but extremely costly and labor-intensive and therefore rarely done as part of routine clinical practice. The lower limit of exocrine pancreatic sufficiency is defined as 20 mmol HCO_3^- per hour, trypsin 60 IU/h, lipase 130,000 IU/h, amylase 24,000 IU/h.

2) **Fecal elastase 1 levels**: 100 to 200 μg/g of feces with mild and moderate exocrine insufficiency and <100 μg/g with severe insufficiency.

Diagnostic Criteria

Diagnostic criteria in advanced chronic pancreatitis: a typical history (usually involving alcohol abuse, abdominal pain), typical abnormalities observed on imaging studies of the pancreas (eg, calcifications and stones [→Diagnostic Tests, above]), or symptoms of exocrine or endocrine pancreatic insufficiency (chronic steatorrhea, diabetes mellitus). Confirmation of diagnosis in the early stages of the disease may be difficult, as imaging studies usually reveal no abnormalities (except for EUS); in such cases the secretin-cholecystokinin test may prove useful. Sometimes diagnosis is made only after a longer follow-up.

Differential Diagnosis

Differential diagnosis should include other causes of abdominal pain and of other symptoms.

→ TREATMENT

General Considerations

1. Treatment of the underlying condition: This is possible only in patients with autoimmune chronic pancreatitis, where oral glucocorticoid therapy results in improvement of symptoms, resolution of abnormalities observed on imaging studies, and improvement of laboratory test results. One should have a high index of suspicion of pancreatic cancer and cholangiocarcinoma before starting treatment of chronic pancreatitis.

2. Symptomatic treatment: Pain control, pancreatic enzyme replacement,⊘⊖ management of impaired glucose tolerance or diabetes mellitus, prevention of malnutrition, treatment of complications.

3. Treatment of exacerbations: Treatment as in acute pancreatitis is frequently necessary.

Long-Term Treatment

1. General measures:

1) **Avoidance of alcohol**.

2) **Cessation of tobacco smoking**.

3) A **high-calorie** (2500-3000 kcal/d) **and high-protein diet**. The fat intake should be adjusted to the individual tolerance of a patient receiving adequate enzyme replacement. In the case of severe fatty diarrhea persisting despite enzyme replacement, recommend a reduced fat intake (up to 60-70 g/d) and consumption of 5 or 6 smaller meals per day. If this management does not yield expected results, try medium-chain triglyceride (MCT) preparations and supplement essential unsaturated fatty acids. Patients receiving enzyme replacement therapy should avoid high-fiber foods, as fiber may inhibit the activity of exogenous pancreatic enzymes.⊘⊖

2. Pain management: Introduce the following treatment methods in a stepwise manner: general recommendations (→above); pancreatic enzyme replacement; analgesics; invasive methods (→below). In case of changes in the nature of pain or development of constant pain, exclude other causes of abdominal pain.

1) **Pancreatic enzyme preparations** (→below): These might reduce pancreatic stimulation and consequently alleviate the pain.⊘⊖

2) **Nonnarcotic analgesics (acetaminophen** [INN paracetamol], **nonsteroidal anti-inflammatory drugs [NSAIDs])** and **spasmolytics**; in patients not responding to treatment, use **opioid analgesics** (these must be administered with special care particularly in alcohol abusers due to the risk of developing dependence); coanalgesics may prove useful (→Chapter 1.20). The use of antioxidants might slightly reduce pain; however, the clinical relevance is uncertain.⊘⊖

3) **Endoscopic treatment** may include sphincterotomy of the major duodenal papilla (and sometimes also the minor papilla), stenting of the pancreatic duct, dilation of the pancreatic duct strictures, stone extraction, drainage of pseudocysts, and treatment of the common bile duct strictures.

4) **Surgical treatment** is indicated in patients with chronic persistent pain that is refractory to medical and endoscopic treatment. A celiac plexus block under CT or EUS guidance or thoracoscopic bilateral dissection of sympathetic nerve fibers yields satisfactory effects in some patients, but the pain is often recurrent. For patients with obstructive chronic pancreatitis with a dilated pancreatic duct, surgical drainage procedures are preferred to endoscopic or conservative management.⊘●

3. Treatment of exocrine pancreatic insufficiency:

1) **Pancreatic enzyme replacement therapy** is indicated in patients with a progressive body weight loss or fatty diarrhea. Therapy improves digestion and absorption of nutrients, reduces pain, and improves diabetes control. The body weight is the optimal clinical parameter used to assess the efficacy of the treatment. **Lipase** plays a key role; administer ≥25,000 to 50,000 IU during or immediately after meals and 25,000 IU during snacks between the main meals. It is recommended to use preparations that release their contents in the duodenum. The efficacy of pancreatic enzyme replacement can be enhanced by coadministration of gastric acid inhibitors: proton pump inhibitors (PPIs) or H_2 blockers (agents and dosage: →Chapter 6.1.2.4), which reduce the inactivation of enzymes in the acidic environment (sometimes also in the duodenum).⊘●

2) **Supplementation of fat-soluble vitamins** (particularly vitamins A and D) in patients with steatorrhea.

4. Treatment of endocrine pancreatic insufficiency:

1) Nutritional treatment of diabetes mellitus, generally without caloric restrictions.

2) If the diet alone is ineffective, start oral antidiabetic drugs. Use insulin with caution, as patients have low requirements for exogenous insulin and are prone to hypoglycemia; usually, the 2-injection regimen is followed, although in some patients with an inadequate diabetes control a more intensive insulin therapy may be required.

→ COMPLICATIONS

Complications of chronic pancreatitis develop at various stages of the disease and in most cases require endoscopic or surgical treatment.

1. Pancreatic pseudocysts (→Chapter 6.3.3) develop in 20% to 40% of patients.

2. Stenosis or obstruction of the common bile duct occurs in 5% to 10% of patients; it causes postprandial abdominal pain and cholestatic liver injury (elevated liver enzyme levels with conjugated hyperbilirubinemia). Patients with **duodenal stenosis** experience early satiety.

3. Pancreatic ascites is caused by pancreatic duct rupture resulting in the formation of a peritoneal (or pleural) fistula, or rupture of a pseudocyst draining into the peritoneal (or pleural) cavity. High amylase levels (>1000 IU/L) in the ascites fluid are typically observed.

4. Splenic vein thrombosis develops in 2% to 4% of patients; it causes secondary isolated portal hypertension and gastric varices, with possible upper gastrointestinal bleeding.

5. Pseudoaneurysms of peripancreatic vessels (eg, the splenic, gastroduodenal, or pancreaticoduodenal arteries) are rare.

6. Pancreatic cancer develops in 4% of patients with chronic pancreatitis and in up to 44% of patients with hereditary chronic pancreatitis <70 years (patients with hereditary chronic pancreatitis should be under oncologic surveillance).

3.3. Pancreatic Cysts and Pseudocysts

→ DEFINITION, ETIOLOGY, PATHOGENESIS

Pancreatic cysts are fluid collections located within or outside the pancreas that usually contain pancreatic secretions. They may be classified as true cysts or postinflammatory cysts (pseudocysts).

1. True cysts have an epithelial lining. They may be further divided into:

1) **Retention cysts**, which result from dilation of the pancreatic duct due to obstruction (this is frequent in chronic pancreatitis).

2) **Neoplastic cysts** (these account for >50% of all pancreatic cysts): Mucinous cystic neoplasms (MCN) (may be malignant), serous cystadenoma (SCA) (almost always nonmalignant), intraductal papillary mucinous neoplasms (IPMN) (some are considered to be precancerous lesions).

3) **Parasitic cysts**, which develop as a result of echinococcosis, ascariasis, or schistosomiasis.

4) **Dermoid** (congenital) **cysts and teratomas**.

2. Postinflammatory cysts or pseudocysts are a complication of acute pancreatitis.

This chapter will mainly focus on the diagnosis and management of pseudocysts.

→ CLINICAL FEATURES AND NATURAL HISTORY

Pseudocysts

Patients with pseudocysts have a history of acute or chronic pancreatitis (or risk factors for these) or trauma.

Signs and symptoms: Abdominal discomfort, tenderness, or acute pain. In some patients nausea, vomiting, loss of appetite, progressive weight loss, fever. Patients may have palpable epigastric or abdominal mass. Presenting signs and symptoms may already result from complications (→Complications, below). Small cysts may be asymptomatic. Within 6 to 12 weeks of the onset of acute pancreatitis, up to 80% of postinflammatory fluid collections are spontaneously reabsorbed. However, the likelihood of reabsorption is lower in the case of multiple collections; large collections (≥4 cm); collections located in the pancreatic tail; thick-walled collections; collections communicating with the pancreatic duct; collections enlarging in the course of follow-up; collections with concomitant stenosis of the proximal pancreatic duct; collections caused by biliary or postsurgical acute pancreatitis or chronic pancreatitis due to alcohol abuse.

→ DIAGNOSIS

Diagnostic Tests

1. Laboratory tests: Elevated serum and urine α-amylase levels, elevated serum lipase levels; periodically elevated white blood cell (WBC) counts and serum C-reactive protein (CRP) levels; elevated serum alkaline phosphatase (ALP) levels and hyperbilirubinemia in patients with compression of extra-hepatic bile ducts.

2. Imaging studies: In patients with pseudocysts results of **ultrasonography** and **endoscopic ultrasonography** (EUS) reveal an encapsulated fluid collection, usually with hyperechoic structures observed in the lumen. The presence of solid structures within the cyst lumen is not typical for a pseudocyst and should be further investigated to exclude malignancy. **Computed tomography (CT)** visualizes a smooth-walled, round, hypodense lesion with homogeneous low density typical of the fluid contents. **Magnetic resonance cholangiopancreatography (MRCP)** is the best method of documenting the

Table 3-2. Differential diagnosis of pancreatic cysts		Pseudocyst	SCA	MCN	IPMN
History of acute pancreatitis		+++	–	–/+	+
Imaging studies	Number of chambers	1	>6	<6	–
	Calcifications	++ (calcific chronic pancreatitis)	+ (central)	+ (peripheral)	+/– (obstructive chronic pancreatitis)
	Ampulla of Vater	Normal	Normal	Normal	Gaping
	Pancreatic duct	Often features of chronic pancreatitis	Normal	Normal	Partially dilated
	Communication with the pancreatic duct	>60%	0.6%	10%	100%
Fluid sample examination	Amylase and lipase activity	↑↑↑	Low	Low	↑
	CEA	↓	<0.5 ng/mL	>192 ng/mL	↓ (dilution)
	Viscosity	↓	↓	↑ (>1.63)	↑ (>1.63)

CEA, carcinoembryonic antigen; IPMN, intraductal papillary mucinous neoplasms; MCN, mucinous cystic neoplasms; SCA, serous cystadenoma.

communication of a cyst with the pancreatic duct. **Endoscopic retrograde cholangiopancreatography (ERCP)** should be performed in patients in whom endoscopic treatment is planned (eg, stenting of the pancreatic duct). **Selective splanchnic angiography** is performed in the case of suspected pseudoaneurysm, as it allows for embolization.

3. Examination of the cyst contents via EUS and fine-needle aspiration (FNA): If the diagnosis of pseudocysts is not confirmed by imaging studies or if an infection is suspected, the fluid cyst can be aspirated. The fluid of pseudocysts may be clear, watery, yellow, or brown; high α-amylase and lipase levels, markedly higher than the serum levels, are frequently seen. Microbiological examination of the contents should be performed if infection is being considered. Patients with neoplastic cysts could have markedly elevated carcinoembryonic antigen and positive mucin staining. In these patients cytology may help identify dysplastic or malignant cells.

Diagnostic Criteria

Differential diagnosis should be focused on differentiating the nonneoplastic and neoplastic cysts: →Table 3-2.

⇒ TREATMENT

Management algorithm: →Figure 3-1.

1. Endoscopic drainage is indicated in the case of severe symptoms of compression caused by the cyst. Methods of drainage are as follows:

1) **Endoscopic internal drainage** has similar efficacy to surgical drainage; however, it is less invasive and therefore it is the preferred first approach.⊘○

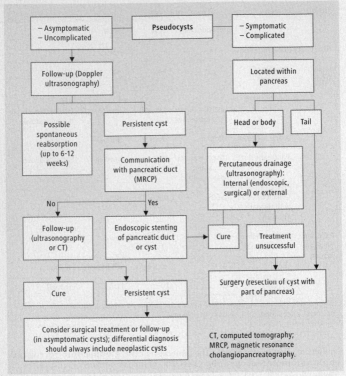

Figure 3-1. Treatment algorithm for pancreatic pseudocysts.

In patients with disrupted continuity of the pancreatic duct, endoscopic stenting might be performed with some success; otherwise, the stent may be introduced directly into the cyst via a gastric or duodenal approach. Before or during the drainage of persistent cysts communicating with the pancreatic duct, consider administration of octreotide 100 to 250 mg subcutaneously every 8 to 12 hours to reduce pancreatic secretion.

2) **Image-guided external drainage** could be performed if the endoscopic or surgical internal drainage is not feasible and the patient remains symptomatic due to compression caused by the pseudocyst.

2. Surgical treatment should be considered in patients with symptomatic persistent pseudocysts (>12 weeks) who are not eligible for endoscopic treatment. Methods of surgical treatment:

1) **Complete resection of the cyst** (this is often possible in cysts located in the pancreatic tail, in which case the cyst is resected with the pancreatic tail and the spleen is preserved if technically feasible).

2) **Surgical internal drainage** (ie, anastomosis of the cyst with the gastrointestinal tract: pancreatocystogastrostomy, pancreatocystoduodenostomy, or pancreatocystojejunostomy; complete cure rates are 70%-80%).

3) **Surgical external drainage** (the least favorable method, which often results in pancreatic cutaneous fistulae).

3. The persistence of large (≥4 cm) pseudocysts 12 weeks after the onset of acute pancreatitis is not an indication for therapeutic intervention if they remain asymptomatic; there is also no need for follow-up imaging.⊘○

→ FOLLOW-UP

In patients who are symptomatic, periodical measurements of biochemical parameters (serum and urine α-amylase levels, serum lipase, ALP, and bilirubin levels), WBC counts, and abdominal ultrasonography are warranted to evaluate the resolution of the pseudocyst. Differential diagnosis should always include neoplastic cysts.

→ COMPLICATIONS

1. Cyst rupture resulting in its drainage to the peritoneal cavity, which may lead to signs of peritonitis and ascites. Management is complex and may require a combination of percutaneous drainage and operative intervention.

2. Extrahepatic cholestasis or duodenal obstruction due to external duodenal compression by the cyst; in patients with cholestasis, perform MRCP and in some cases also ERCP with biliary stenting (when endoscopic treatment is indicated).

3. Bleeding from varices of the gastric fundus or esophagus, which form as a result of splenic or portal vein thrombosis or compression by the cyst. Doppler ultrasonography may be diagnostic.

4. Bleeding into the cyst lumen from the adjacent vessels, which manifests on ultrasonography as hyperechogenic contents of the cyst.

5. A **pseudoaneurysm** results from damage to peripancreatic arteries (splenic, gastroduodenal, pancreatoduodenal, and hepatic arteries) with persistent communication between the artery and the cyst lumen. Doppler ultrasonography may demonstrate blood flow within the cyst. The rupture of a pseudoaneurysm may cause bleeding to the peritoneal cavity or the retroperitoneal space, depending on the location. A rare complication of pseudoaneurysms is gastrointestinal bleeding via the pancreatic duct. Angioembolization is the preferred initial approach for bleeding pseudoaneurysms.

1. Anemia: General Considerations

→ **SUMMARY**

Anemia is defined as a decrease in hemoglobin levels (Hb), hematocrit values (Ht), and red blood cell (RBC) counts.

Classification based on the severity of anemia:

1) **Mild anemia**: Hb 10 to 120 g/L in women and to 135 g/L in men.
2) **Moderate anemia**: Hb 80 to 99 g/L.
3) **Severe anemia**: Hb 65 to 79 g/L.
4) **Life-threatening anemia**: Hb <65 g/L.

Causes: Loss of RBCs due to hemorrhage (acute or chronic), hemolysis, sequestration, or impaired erythropoiesis.

Systemic manifestations are independent of the cause and type of anemia. They include weakness, fatigue, concentration and attention deficits, headache, dizziness/vertigo, tachycardia and dyspnea (in severe anemia), and pallor of the skin and mucous membranes (or jaundice in hemolytic anemia). In severe cases manifestations of systemic hypoxia lead to cardiovascular collapse, acidosis, and death.

RBC parameters (→Table 1-1) may be used for the initial differentiation between the causes of anemia.

Table 1-1. Classification of anemias based on the reticulocyte count, mean corpuscular volume, and red cell distribution width

MCV	RDW	RC ≥100×10^9/L	RC <100×10^9/L
Microcytic MCV↓	N	β Thalassemia	Anemia of chronic disease (some cases)
	↑	β Thalassemia	– Iron deficiency anemia – Inherited sideroblastic anemia (some cases)
Normocytic MCV (N)	N		– Anemia of chronic disease (most cases) – Anemia in chronic kidney disease – Aplastic anemia
	↑	– Anemia due to acute blood loss – Most of hemolytic anemias	– Early stage of iron deficiency anemia – Cobalamin or folate deficiency – Mixed-type anemia (eg, combined iron and cobalamin deficiency) – Myelodysplastic syndrome
Macrocytic MCV↑	N	Chronic liver disease	– Chemotherapy – Alcohol dependency – Aplastic anemia
	↑	– Some autoimmune hemolytic anemias (due to reticulocytosis) – Chronic liver disease	– Cobalamin or folate deficiency – Myelodysplastic syndrome

↑, increased; ↓, decreased; MCV, mean corpuscular volume; N, normal; RC, reticulocyte count; RDW, red cell distribution width.

2. Aplastic Anemias

2.1. Aplastic Anemia

→ DEFINITION, ETIOLOGY, PATHOGENESIS

Aplastic anemia (AA) is type of bone marrow failure that leads to pancyto-penia, life-threatening infections in the setting of neutropenia, bleeding due to thrombocytopenia, and severe anemia leading to transfusion dependence.

The primary cause of AA is either an inherited anomaly or acquired injury of hematopoietic stem cells or the bone marrow microenvironment, which leads to the inhibition of cellular proliferation and differentiation.

Classification of AA:

1) **Congenital or inherited causes** are responsible for ≥25% of cases among children and up to 10% of cases among adults. Examples: Fanconi anemia, dyskeratosis congenita, Shwachman-Diamond syndrome, Diamond-Blackfan anemia, familial aplastic anemia. Patients may exhibit dysmor-phic features, hyperpigmentation, skeletal abnormalities, or other physical stigmata. Pancytopenia and the associated symptoms may be the presenting features.

2) **Acquired AA** (up to 80% of cases):

    a) Infectious causes: Hepatitis virus A, B, C; Epstein-Barr virus (EBV); HIV; parvovirus B19 (eg, in the setting of sickle cell disease); mycobac-teria.

    b) Exposure to ionizing radiation.

    c) Transfusion-associated graft-versus-host disease (GVHD): Donor T cells cause GVHD in patients with hematologic malignancies who receive purine analogues such as bendamustine or fludarabine; after autologous or allogeneic hematopoietic stem cell transplantation (HSCT).

    d) Chemicals such as benzene, organic solvents, trinitrotoluene, pesticides, and herbicides.

    e) Autoimmune or connective tissue diseases.

    f) Anorexia nervosa, severe nutritional deficiencies (vitamin B_{12}, folate).

    g) Paroxysmal nocturnal hemoglobinuria (PNH).

    h) Drugs: Nonsteroidal anti-inflammatory drugs (NSAIDs), busulfan, cyclo-phosphamide, anthracyclines, methotrexate, antibiotics such as chloram-phenicol and sulfonamides, gold compounds, chloroquine, chlorpropamide, phenytoin, allopurinol, and thiazides.

    i) Idiopathic factors.

    j) Pregnancy (rare).

→ CLINICAL FEATURES

Symptoms of AA may develop rapidly (within several days) or slowly (several weeks or months). Clinical manifestations of AA result from anemia, neutro-penia, and thrombocytopenia.

→ DIAGNOSIS

Diagnostic Tests

1. Complete blood count (CBC) and peripheral smear: Normocytic (sometimes macrocytic) and normochromic anemia, very low reticulocyte counts, leukopenia with neutropenia (usually $<1.5 \times 10^9$/L), thrombocytopenia ($<50 \times 10^9$/L).

2. Exclude other causes: Measurements of vitamin B_{12}, folate, copper (ceruloplasmin), and zinc to exclude nutritional deficiency; liver function tests to exclude hepatitis; hemolytic screen; viral serology (→above); chromosomal studies to exclude Fanconi anemia. Exclude autoimmune diseases; test for antinuclear antibodies and double-stranded DNA (dsDNA). Imaging studies are used to assess for infections or lymphoma; chest radiography and abdominal ultrasonography may be helpful.

3. Bone marrow examination: Cell markers and flow cytometry to detect a PNH clone, large granulocytic lymphocytes, or MDS. Aspirate usually reveals decreased numbers of hematopoietic cells (<30%), a proportion of fat cells to hematopoietic cells >3, and no malignant cells. Trephine biopsy specimens reveal few cellular fields in a generally hypocellular marrow.

Diagnostic Criteria

Peripheral blood cytopenia (affecting ≥2 of 3 lineages) and hypocellular bone marrow without infiltrative or fibrotic process after other causes have been excluded (→below). At least 2 out 3 cytopenias: hemoglobin (Hb) <100 g/L, platelet count <50×10^9/L, and/or absolute neutrophil count (ANC) <1.5×10^9/L.

Severity of AA as per the modified Camitta criteria:

1) Severe AA: Marrow cellularity <30% with ≥2 of the following: ANC <0.5×10^9/L; platelet count <20×10^9/L, reticulocyte count <20×10^9/L.

2) Very severe AA: ANC <0.2×10^9/L.

Differential Diagnosis

Acute leukemia (particularly acute lymphoblastic leukemia), hairy cell leukemia, MDS, PNH, hypersplenism, bone marrow infiltrates (cancer), lymphomas.

→ TREATMENT

1. General measures:

1) Promptly refer the patient to a hematology center.

2) Transfusion support: Leukoreduced packed red blood cells (PRBCs) and platelets used only when this is considered essential. HSCT may be compromised by prior transfusion therapy. Seek consultation with a transfusion medicine specialist regarding transfusion of phenotype-matched blood to reduce the risk of alloimmunization.

3) Iron chelation therapy is used when indicated due to iron load with transfusions. Patients who undergo successful HSCT may receive regular phlebotomies.

4) Initiate prophylactic antifungal treatment in patients with prolonged neutropenia (<0.2×10^9/L for >1 week). Antiviral treatment should be offered to patients receiving immunosuppressive therapy. Defer initiation of granulocyte colony-stimulating factor (G-CSF) therapy until the patient is seen by a hematologist and bone marrow examination is completed to exclude acute leukemia. Broad-spectrum antibiotics with antipseudomonal coverage should be started in case of febrile neutropenia.

2. Allogeneic HSCT is the treatment of choice for otherwise eligible patients up to 50 years of age with severe AA for whom a human leukocyte antigen (HLA)-matched sibling donor is available. Allogeneic HSCT is curative in 60% to 90% of patients. In case of no response to 6-month immunosuppressive treatment, allogeneic HSCT should be considered. Related donors are generally preferred to unrelated donors.

3. Immunosuppressive treatment is indicated in patients who are not considered for allogeneic HSCT. It results in improvement in 60% to 80% of cases. Use antithymocyte globulin (ATG) combined with cyclosporine (INN ciclosporin). In patients treated with ATG, all transfused PRBCs and platelets must be irradiated to avoid transfusion-associated GVHD.

4. Androgens (eg, oxymetholone 2.5 mg/kg/d) may be effective in patients with Fanconi anemia or acquired AA with refractoriness or contraindications to immunosuppressive treatment; however, the drugs should be discontinued if no improvement is achieved within 4 to 6 months. In patients with good response to treatment, the dose is tapered down slowly to discontinuation.

5. Alemtuzumab: In patients with recurrent AA the drug has efficacy similar to ATG combined with cyclosporine.

→ PROGNOSIS

In patients with severe AA who are not treated with allogeneic HSCT, 2-year mortality rates are 80%. The most frequent causes of death are severe bacterial or fungal infections. AA may transform to MDS, acute leukemia, or PNH.

2.2. Pure Red Cell Aplasia

→ DEFINITION AND ETIOLOGY

Pure red cell aplasia (PRCA) refers to aplasia of the erythroid lineage leading to severe normocytic (in some cases macrocytic) and normochromic anemia. It may be inherited (Diamond-Blackfan syndrome) or acquired. In the latter case, it develops due to viral infections (parvovirus B19, Epstein-Barr virus, hepatotropic viruses), immunologic disorders (thymoma, myasthenia gravis, systemic lupus erythematosus, rheumatoid arthritis), chronic lymphocytic leukemia and other hematologic disorders including large granular lymphocytosis, treatment with an erythropoiesis-stimulating agent (ESA), or drugs (phenytoin, carbamazepine, valproate, azathioprine, chloramphenicol, sulfonamides, isoniazid). Many cases are idiopathic. PRCA may precede myelodysplastic syndrome.

→ CLINICAL FEATURES

The diagnosis of PRCA is usually made in patients >40 years. Clinical features include severe anemia with low reticulocyte count, normal serum erythropoietin levels, and low bone marrow erythroblast counts (<0.5%). Clinical subtypes include acute transient PRCA (caused by viral infections or drugs) and chronic PRCA (idiopathic, thymoma, systemic lupus erythematosus, rheumatoid arthritis).

→ TREATMENT

Successful treatment of the underlying condition (eg, withdrawal of the ESA) frequently leads to the resolution of PRCA. In other cases, immunosuppressive treatment is used (most frequently with glucocorticoids; in steroid-resistant patients, cyclosporine [INN ciclosporin], antilymphocyte globulin, cyclophosphamide, high-dose intravenous immunoglobulin, rituximab, and alemtuzumab are used). Patients requiring frequent packed red blood cell transfusions may develop iron overload.

3. Hemolytic Anemias

3.1. Hemolytic Anemia: General Considerations

→ DEFINITION, ETIOLOGY, PATHOGENESIS

Hemolytic anemia (HA) refers to a heterogeneous group of diseases characterized by an abnormal, premature destruction of red blood cells (RBCs). Hemolysis may be either intravascular or extravascular (in the spleen and/ or the liver).

1. Hereditary HAs are caused by primary intracorpuscular defects:

1) **Membrane defects**: For example, hereditary spherocytosis and hereditary elliptocytosis.

2) **Enzymopathies**: Glucose-6-phosphate dehydrogenase (G6PD) deficiency, pyruvate kinase (PK) deficiency.

3) **Hemoglobinopathies**: Some forms, for example, sickle cell disease, methemoglobinemia, HbC.

4) **Thalassemia syndromes**: Quantitative abnormalities of globin chain synthesis (most frequently affecting β-globin).

2. In **acquired HAs**, RBCs are constitutively normal, and hemolysis is caused by extracorpuscular factors (except for paroxysmal nocturnal hemoglobinuria [PNH], which is acquired and intracorpuscular):

1) **Immune HA** (with antibodies against red cell antigens; in some cases, only complement may be detected on the RBC surface):

   a) **Warm antibody autoimmune HA (AIHA)** (idiopathic or associated with other conditions [including systemic lupus erythematosus, chronic lymphocytic leukemia, non-Hodgkin lymphoma, immunodeficiency syndromes], drug-induced [methyldopa, cephalosporins, purine analogues], after solid organ transplantation or allogeneic hematopoietic stem cell transplantation [in the case of blood group mismatch of the donor and the host], after packed red blood cell [PRBC] transfusions). A variant of AIHA is seen in patients with common variable immunodeficiency.

   b) **Cold agglutinin disease** (idiopathic or associated with infection [mycoplasma, Epstein-Barr virus] or lymphomas).

   c) **Posttransfusion hemolytic reactions**.

   d) **Neonatal alloimmune hemolysis**.

2) **Nonimmune HA**:

   a) **RBC destruction** (mechanical due to the effect of fibrin deposition, artificial valves or native valvular disease, stents, "march hemoglobinuria," thrombotic thrombocytopenic purpura [TTP], hemolytic-uremic syndrome [HUS], disseminated intravascular coagulation [DIC]).

   b) **Infections** (malaria, babesiosis, toxoplasmosis, leishmaniasis, *Clostridium perfringens*).

   c) **Chemical or physical factors** (methemoglobinemia, drugs [mitomycin C; cyclosporine, or INN ciclosporin; tacrolimus; ticlopidine; sulfonamides; sulfasalazine; dapsone; platinum analogues], drugs of abuse [cocaine], metals [lead, copper], venoms [*Loxosceles* spiders, bee, wasp, cobra, viper], severe burns).

   d) **PNH**.

   e) **Hypersplenism**.

→ CLINICAL FEATURES AND NATURAL HISTORY

Patients with low-grade hemolysis, particularly chronic hemolysis, usually reveal no symptoms of HA. General symptoms of anemia are usually observed in patients with a hemoglobin (Hb) level <80 g/L or rapidly progressive anemia. Jaundice is observed in the periods of increased RBC destruction but is frequently absent in patients with chronic hemolysis. An enlarged spleen (in some patients accompanied by an enlarged liver) is observed only in some types of HA and usually suggests a systemic underlying condition (lymphoproliferative or autoimmune disorders).

Characteristic clinical features of selected types of HA:

1) **Hereditary spherocytosis (HS)** is the most frequent hereditary HA in white patients; it typically involves an enlarged spleen, hemolytic and/or aplastic crises, and cholelithiasis due to increased heme catabolism (affects ~50% of adult patients).

2) **G6PD deficiency**: Men are more frequently affected than women. Acute attacks of hemolysis (acute jaundice, dark urine, abdominal pain) are triggered by certain drugs (see www.g6pd.org and www.g6pddeficiency.org) and foods (fava beans). No spleen enlargement is observed.

3) **PK deficiency**: Typically presents in early childhood, or in adulthood in heterozygous individuals.

4) **Methemoglobinemia** may be hereditary (HbM) or acquired (much more frequent); the latter is caused by agents that oxidize heme iron (sodium nitroprusside, phenacetin, sulfonamides, lidocaine, benzocaine, dapsone, rasburicase, nitrates, nitroglycerin, nitric oxide, nitrites, aniline, chlorites). Cyanosis is observed at methemoglobin levels >15 g/L.

5) **Thalassemia syndromes**: Spleen enlargement is typically observed. Severe HA develops in homozygotes or double heterozygotes and presents in the first year of life.

6) **Sickle cell disease**: Recurrent severe pain of hands and feet, jaundice, spleen enlargement, cholelithiasis, ankle ulcers, and a tendency to thromboembolism causing ischemia and functional impairment of various organs, including cerebral ischemia.

7) **Cold agglutinin disease** (incidence, ~1/1,000,000 per year): Symptoms of lymphoma, infectious mononucleosis, or pneumonia are typically present. Acrocyanosis (purple discoloration of distal body parts on exposure to cold) and livedo reticularis may occur.

8) **PNH** (incidence, ~1/1,000,000 per year): Hemolytic anemia, thrombosis in an atypical location (~50%), pancytopenia in patients with overlapping bone marrow failure (aplastic anemia or myelodysplastic syndrome).

→ DIAGNOSIS

Diagnostic Tests

1. Complete blood count (CBC): Anemia is typically normocytic and normochromic, although in some patients it may be macrocytic due to reticulocytosis. Reticulocyte counts are usually increased (typically 5%-20%). In patients with thalassemia, microcytic and hypochromic anemia is observed. Spherocytes and elliptocytes may be observed in HS and AIHA, sickled RBCs are present in sickle cell disease, acanthocytes in PK deficiency, target cells in thalassemia syndromes, and RBC fragments in DIC, HUS, and TTP. Erythroblasts may be present in severe anemia associated with increased erythropoiesis. Elevated mean corpuscular hemoglobin concentration (MCHC) is observed in HS.

2. Biochemical tests: Elevated lactate dehydrogenase (LDH) levels, decreased (or undetectable) haptoglobin levels, elevated serum unconjugated bilirubin levels (usually <4 mg/dL).

3. Urinalysis: Elevated urobilinogen levels, hemoglobinuria (positive dipstick test).

4. Other studies specific for individual types of HA:

1) **HS**: Positive acidified glycerol lysis test (AGLT) and/or positive eosin-5-maleimide (EMA) binding test on immunohistochemical analysis.

2) **G6PD deficiency**: Heinz bodies in RBC cytoplasm, decreased G6PD activity in RBCs (the measurements should not be performed in periods of acute hemolysis).

3) **PK deficiency**: Decreased PK activity in RBCs.

4) **Methemoglobinemia**: Elevated methemoglobin levels.

5) **β-Thalassemia syndromes**: Absence of hemoglobin A (HbA) and elevated hemoglobin F (HbF) levels in Hb electrophoresis in homozygotes. Heterozygotes may produce small amounts of HbA and in 50% of cases have increased HbF; all have increased hemoglobin A_2 (HbA$_2$) fractions.

6) **Sickle cell disease**: Howell-Jolly bodies in RBCs, absence of HbA, increased sickle hemoglobin (HbS) and HbF levels in Hb electrophoresis, presence of sickle cells.

7) **Warm antibody AIHA**: Positive direct antiglobulin test (with anti-IgG or anti-C3d antibodies).

8) **Cold agglutinin disease**: Positive direct antiglobulin test (with anti-C3d antibodies), RBC agglutination observed by light microscopy, increased mean corpuscular volume (MCV) (apparent macrocytosis caused by RBC aggregates), monoclonal protein testing.

9) **PNH**: Deficiency of glycosylphosphatidylinositol-associated proteins (GPI-AP) in granulocytes and RBCs observed on flow cytometry.

5. Bone marrow examination: Increased erythropoiesis, frequently with megaloblastic features.

6. Imaging studies: Spleen enlargement and/or cholelithiasis are observed on ultrasonography in some types of hemolytic anemia.

Diagnostic Criteria

Anemia of varying severity, typically normocytic and normochromic (exceptions: above), with increased serum LDH and unconjugated bilirubin levels, decreased haptoglobin levels, and increased reticulocyte counts.

Differential Diagnosis

Anemia of chronic disease.

→ TREATMENT

General Measures

1. Secondary HA: Treat the underlying condition. Discontinue the drugs that may cause hemolysis.

2. Severe symptomatic anemia: Transfusion of PRBCs.

3. Chronic HA: Lifelong administration of folic acid 1 mg/d. Iron therapy only in patients with a documented absolute iron deficiency (→Chapter 7.5.2) (however, it is contraindicated in the majority of cases).

Specific Treatment of Individual Types of Hemolytic Anemia

1. Warm antibody AIHA: Administer glucocorticoids (oral prednisone 1 mg/kg/d) for several weeks, then taper the dose down to the lowest level that maintains remission and negative antiglobulin test results. Hb levels usually increase after 1 to 3 weeks of treatment. In patients with a more severe hemolysis, initiate high-dose intravenous methylprednisolone. In steroid-resistant, steroid-intolerant, or steroid-dependent (>15 mg/d after a few months of therapy) individuals, consider splenectomy; in the case of contraindications to or ineffectiveness of splenectomy, consider IV rituximab 375 mg/m^2 once a week for 4 consecutive weeks or a trial of another immunosuppressive agent (oral azathioprine 100-150 mg/d, oral cyclophosphamide 100 mg/d or 500-700 mg/d IV every 3-4 weeks, cyclosporine [INN ciclosporin] in doses adjusted to serum drug levels, oral mycophenolate mofetil 0.5-1 g bid). In steroid-resistant patients, particularly in the case of hemolytic crisis, plasmapheresis with intravenous immunoglobulin (IVIG) administration (1 g/kg for 2 days or 1 dose of 2 g/kg) may be used. Syk inhibitors may be effective in refractory cases.

2. Cold agglutinin disease: Treat the underlying condition. In the majority of patients avoidance of exposure to cold and wearing appropriately warm clothing is sufficient to prevent hemolysis. Warm PRBCs and IV fluids; avoid blood products with a high amount of complement (platelets, fresh-frozen plasma). In patients with severe disease consider a trial of immunosuppressive treatment with oral cyclophosphamide 100 mg/d, chlorambucil, IV rituximab 375 mg/m^2 once a week for 4 consecutive weeks (this is most effective as monotherapy or in combination with fludarabine). If urgent suppression of antibody titers is necessary, perform plasmapheresis. IVIG may also reduce hemolysis in acute crises. Acute cold agglutinin disease due to mycoplasma infection usually responds promptly to glucocorticoids and/or IVIG and rarely produces long-lasting disease.

3. Methemoglobinemia: Discontinue the drugs that may have caused methemoglobinemia. In severe cases (>20% of total Hb) administer methylene blue 1 to 2 mg/kg (1% solution in 0.9% saline) in an IV infusion over 5 minutes and consider hyperbaric oxygen therapy. In patients with life-threatening methemoglobinemia (>50% of total Hb), perform exchange transfusion. In patients with chronic methemoglobinemia, administer oral ascorbic acid 0.3 to 1 g/d in divided doses and oral riboflavin 20 mg/d; in exacerbations use oral methylene blue 100 to 300 mg/d.

4. Thalassemia syndromes (→Chapter 7.3.3): In all patients with thalassemia major and some patients with thalassemia intermedia, chronic PRBC transfusions are usually necessary to eliminate symptomatic anemia. Monitor iron parameters and treat iron overload. Supplement with folic acid. Consider splenectomy in the case of >50% increase in PRBC transfusion requirements over a 1-year period. In selected cases, consider allogeneic hematopoietic stem cell transplantation (HSCT).

5. Sickle cell disease (→Chapter 7.3.2): In the majority of patients, treatment is symptomatic (analgesics, antithrombotic treatment, physiotherapy). PRBC transfusions are used in the case of aplastic crisis and in situations posing a risk of exacerbation (to achieve HbS levels ≤30% as a result of dilution). Monitor iron parameters and start appropriate treatment in case of absolute deficiency (→Chapter 7.5.2) or treat iron overload. Administer folic acid. Treatment with hydroxyurea (INN hydroxycarbamide) 15 to 20 mg/kg/d is recommended with dose increments until reduction in the white blood cell count is achieved. Chronic transfusion therapy may be indicated for prevention of cerebrovascular diseases. In selected cases consider allogeneic HSCT. Red cell exchange transfusion may be indicated in patients with acute severe complications of sickle cell disease.

6. PNH: In the classic form of the disease (GPI-AP absent in >50% of granulocytes; overt intravascular hemolysis) treatment is necessary in patients with clinically significant symptoms and complications. Eculizumab is the drug of choice. Allogeneic HSCT is the only "curative" treatment that can eradicate the PNH clone. In case of thromboembolic complications, use standard antithrombotic treatment, with secondary prophylaxis with a vitamin K antagonist and primary prophylaxis with heparin. In patients with moderate or severe anemia, consider danazol 200 to 600 mg/d in 3 divided doses. Supportive treatment includes PRBC transfusions, supplementation of iron and folic acid, and growth factors (erythropoietin and granulocyte colony-stimulating factor

[G-CSF] in the case of bone marrow failure). In atypical forms of the disease treatment depends on the coexisting type of bone marrow failure (aplastic anemia, myelodysplastic syndrome).

3.2. Sickle Cell Disease

→ DEFINITION, ETIOLOGY, PATHOGENESIS

Sickle hemoglobin (HbS) was the first hemoglobin (Hb) variant to be discovered. The β-globin gene mutation that gives rise to HbS is a single nucleotide substitution in the sixth codon of the β-globin gene that converts glutamic acid, which is relatively hydrophilic, to valine, which is hydrophobic. This single amino acid substitution results in an Hb molecule that polymerizes when deoxygenated, resulting in formation of sickle cells. Sickling of red blood cells (RBCs) causes shortened RBC life-span due to destruction (hemolysis) and blockage of blood flow (vaso-occlusion), resulting in diverse acute and chronic disease manifestations.

The inheritance of a single sickle cell gene (heterozygous HbS) is known as "sickle cell trait" and occurs in >20% of the population of equatorial Africa, 20% of the eastern provinces of Saudi Arabia and central India, and 5% of people living in various regions of the Mediterranean, Middle East, and North Africa. Owing to the autosomal recessive pattern of inheritance of the HbS gene, sickle cell trait is typically a silent carrier state.

The term sickle cell disease (SCD) encompasses all genotypes resulting in a combination of hemolysis and vaso-occlusive complications, which are hallmarks of the condition. Genotypes include homozygous HbS (HbSS) or compound heterozygous states, including HbS and another β-globin gene mutation (eg, sickle cell-HbC [HbSC], sickle cell–$β^0$-thalassemia, sickle cell–$β^+$-thalassemia, and less commonly, sickle cell-O_{Arab} [HbSO$_{Arab}$] or sickle cell-D$_{Punjab}$ [HbSD$_{Punjab}$]).

→ CLINICAL FEATURES

Clinical features of SCD are the result of 2 main pathophysiologic processes: hemolysis and vaso-occlusion.

The average RBC life-span in SCD is shortened from the typical 120 days to anywhere from 10 to 25 days, resulting in chronic hemolytic anemia, with Hb concentrations in patients with HbSS genotype typically ranging from 60 to 90 g/L.

Sickled RBCs also result in microvascular obstruction, leading to local tissue hypoxia, ischemia, and even infarction. Disease manifestations in SCD are highly varied and can be divided broadly into acute and chronic complications.

1. Acute complications:

1) **Pain crisis** (also referred to as vaso-occlusive crisis): The most common complication of SCD. It is caused by local obstruction of the bone marrow microcirculation by sickled RBCs and other reactive cells, leading to local tissue hypoxia and infarction. It may occur in the long bones, sternum, ribs, and spine. Pain crisis may be precipitated by physiologic stress, including hypoxia, fever, dehydration, cold temperatures, or pregnancy. Many episodes occur with no clear trigger.

2) **Acute chest syndrome**: Defined by (1) respiratory symptoms (cough, dyspnea, chest pain, tachypnea, hypoxia) and/or fever with (2) a new infiltrate on chest radiography. It is a leading cause of hospitalization in patients with SCD and a major risk factor for early mortality. Causes include infection (viral, bacterial, mixed), pulmonary vaso-occlusion, and fat embolism. Pulmonary embolism is an important alternative cause that should be considered as part of differential diagnosis.

3) **Stroke and cerebrovascular diseases**: SCD places individuals at risk of stroke (hemorrhagic and ischemic), transient ischemic attacks, cerebral vasculopathy, and moyamoya syndrome. Moyamoya (Japanese for "hazy puff of smoke") refers to a unique pattern on cerebral angiography characterized by large-vessel occlusion affecting the circle of Willis and corresponding formation of collateral vessels. Moyamoya syndrome is a rare complication of SCD that results from progressive damage to the intimal layers of large cerebral vessels and significantly predisposes to ischemic stroke.

4) **Priapism**: A prolonged painful erection of the penis due to sickle cell vaso-occlusion. It occurs in 30% to 45% of male patients with SCD. Minor episodes can last from minutes to hours and are often self-limited, while major episodes can last up to several days and compromise tissue viability.

5) **Hypercoagulability**: SCD is recognized as a prothrombotic state due to endothelial dysfunction, chronic inflammation leading to white blood cell (WBC) activation, increased platelet activity, and oxidative damage from free Hb. Thrombosis in SCD ranges from microvascular and small-vessel arterial thrombosis to venous thromboembolism.

6) **Aplastic crisis**: A transient arrest of RBC production in patients with SCD can cause a sudden decrease in their reticulocyte count and Hb level. It is most commonly provoked by parvovirus B19 infection, which directly infects RBC precursors in the bone marrow.

7) **Hepatic and splenic sequestration**: Trapping of blood cells in the spleen, liver, or both. There is typically increase in size of the liver or spleen, depending on the organ involved, and accompanying severe decrease in Hb concentration and platelet counts; reticulocyte counts are often increased. This represents an acute and potentially life-threatening complication of SCD.

8) **Infection**: Worldwide, infection is the most common cause of mortality among patients with SCD. Patient predisposition towards infection in SCD is multifactorial. Patients develop functional asplenia early in life due to splenic infarction, typically by the age of 5 years, and thus become predisposed to infection by encapsulated microorganisms. Abnormal clearance of viral and bacterial pathogens is caused by dysfunctional complement activity in patients with SCD.

9) **Acute cholecystitis and other biliary tract diseases**: Chronic hemolysis and associated increased bilirubin turnover can result in the formation of pigment gallstones and biliary sludge, which can predispose to acute and chronic cholecystitis.

2. Chronic complications:

1) **Leg ulcers**: These can be chronic and disabling, tending to form over the medial and lateral malleoli of the ankles, and less commonly over the anterior tibial areas and dorsal aspects of the feet.

2) **Avascular necrosis (AVN)**: Bone pain is common in SCD. If it is present chronically in the hips or shoulders, AVN should be considered. Magnetic resonance imaging (MRI) is the most sensitive diagnostic imaging modality.

3) **Chronic pain**: Most commonly arises from chronic tissue injury (eg, AVN of bone, skin ulcers). Additionally, following recurrent pain crises, SCD patients are at risk of developing central hypersensitivity to pain. Patients who have been treated with high doses of opioids or received prolonged opioid therapy can develop a combination of opioid dependence and opioid-induced hyperalgesia. A detailed assessment by a care team with expertise in SCD and chronic pain is essential to individualized optimization of chronic pain management.

4) **Osteoporosis**: Reduced bone mineral density is common in children and adults with SCD. Associated factors include low vitamin D levels, low body weight, low Hb concentration, male sex, elevated ferritin, and low zinc concentration.

5) **Retinopathy**: Proliferative retinal vascular disease is the most common ocular manifestation of SCD. Patients may be asymptomatic or describe floaters or visual field loss. Eye examinations should be performed as part of routine screening in patients with SCD.

6) **Pulmonary complications**: Patients with SCD are at increased risk of developing multiple pulmonary complications, such as pulmonary hypertension, asthma, restrictive lung defects, and sleep-disordered breathing. While the pathophysiology of specific SCD-associated lung diseases remains poorly understood, recurrent episodes of acute lung inflammation, as seen in acute chest syndrome, and chronic subclinical inflammation from sickle cell–related vasculopathy can predispose to airway inflammation and intraparenchymal scarring.

7) **Renal complications**: RBC sickling and vaso-occlusion primarily affect the kidneys at the level of the medulla and glomeruli. Over time, this results in renal tubular damage, hematuria, and inability to form concentrated urine (hyposthenuria). When sickle vasculopathy affects the glomeruli, this is known as sickle glomerulopathy, which manifests as proteinuria and sometimes even nephrotic syndrome.

→ DIAGNOSIS

Diagnostic Tests

1. Complete blood count (CBC): Varying degrees of anemia along with elevated reticulocyte counts. Review of the peripheral blood smear reveals sickled RBCs and Howell-Jolly bodies.

2. Hemolytic markers: Elevated indirect bilirubin and lactate dehydrogenase, reduced haptoglobin levels.

3. Hb separation techniques: Automated methods using high-performance liquid chromatography (HPLC) or capillary electrophoresis (CE) separate and quantify the various fractions of Hb that are present. Normal hemoglobins in adults are hemoglobin A (HbA) and hemoglobin A_2 (HbA$_2$), with a possible small quantity of hemoglobin F, also known as fetal hemoglobin (HbF). In most SCD genotypes HbA is absent and HbS is present, with or without other variant Hbs that comprise compound heterozygous SCD (eg, HbC in HbSC genotype).

4. Molecular studies and DNA analysis: These can be further pursued to confirm positive characterization of the Hb variant(s).

→ TREATMENT

Strategies to treat SCD are generally divided into 4 categories: curative treatment, disease-modifying therapy, preventive measures, and management of acute complications.

1. Curative treatment:

1) Hematopoietic stem cell transplantation (HSCT) is the only curative treatment currently available for patients with SCD. The decision to proceed to HSCT is challenging due to the significant potential risks of HSCT, including acute and chronic graft-versus-host disease (GVHD), infertility, and transplant-related death. HSCT has been more extensively studied in children than with adult patients with SCD and has better outcomes in children, particularly with human leukocyte antigen (HLA)-matched related donors. HSCT in older SCD patients is primarily considered with progressive vaso-occlusive complications or organ dysfunction despite optimal use of disease-modifying therapies.⊘◯

2) Gene therapy is a curative therapy under active study.

2. Disease-modifying therapy:

1) **Hydroxyurea** has been shown to reduce the incidence of painful vaso-
-occlusive crises, hospitalization, and need for RBC transfusion in adults
and children with SCD. Mechanisms of action of hydroxyurea in SCD are
multifactorial and include promoting the production of HbF, reducing WBC
count, and improving RBC hydration. Hydroxyurea is recommended for
adults with SCD and ≥3 painful episodes in a year.🗹● Hydroxyurea can also
reduce the incidence of acute chest syndrome and improve mortality in SCD
patients.🗹○ CBC with WBC differential count should be measured at least
every 4 weeks during periods of dose adjustments to monitor for peripheral
blood cytopenias. If the absolute neutrophil count decreases $<2\times10^9$/L and/
or platelet count decreases $<80\times10^9$/L, hydroxyurea should be withheld
until the counts recover and subsequently reinstituted at a dose 5 mg/kg/d
lower than the previous dose. Once a stable dose is established, monitoring
can be performed every 2 to 3 months.

2) **RBC transfusions** can be used either prophylactically, to reduce the incidence of SCD-related complications (eg, preoperatively), or for the treatment
of acute complications, such as aplastic crisis and acute chest syndrome.
The target Hb concentration with simple transfusion depends on the indication. RBC exchange transfusion involves removal of the patient's RBCs
and replacement with donor RBCs, targeting an HbS level <30%. The
advantage of RBC exchange over simple RBC transfusion is the avoidance
of hyperviscosity and volume overload.

a) Prophylactic RBC transfusion: Simple RBC transfusion targeting an Hb
concentration of 100 g/L is recommended for patients requiring surgery
under general or regional anesthesia, with consideration of exchange
transfusion in high-risk patients (eg, previous history of stroke, recurrent
acute chest syndrome).🗹○

b) Chronic RBC transfusion: This is recommended for children with silent
cerebral infarction or 2 transcranial Doppler (TCD) ultrasonography
velocity measurements ≥200 cm/s within a 1- to 2-week period.🗹● Despite
the absence of high-quality evidence, chronic transfusion therapy may
be indicated for patients with recurrent acute chest syndrome, priapism,
and refractory painful vaso-occlusive episodes.

c) Blood transfusion as acute treatment: Simple RBC transfusion may be
indicated for patients with symptomatic anemia due to decreased oxygen
delivery. The target Hb should not exceed 100 g/L to avoid the risks of
hyperviscosity. Exchange transfusion is usually reserved for SCD patients
with multiorgan failure, respiratory compromise, or severe acute chest
syndrome.🗹○

3. Preventive measures:

1) Penicillin prophylaxis is advised for all children with SCD up to the age of
5 years for the prevention of pneumococcal infections.🗹●

2) Age-appropriate vaccinations, including those against encapsulated organisms (*Streptococcus pneumoniae*, *Haemophilus influenzae*, and *Neisseria
meningitidis*), seasonal influenza virus, and hepatitis B virus.

3) Screening TCD ultrasonography should be performed in children to identify
those at high risk of stroke who would benefit from chronic RBC transfusions.

4. Management of SCD-related acute complications:

1) **Acute painful crisis**: Patients should have a clear management plan and
regular follow-up regarding the effectiveness of their home analgesic therapy with guidance on alarming signs of serious SCD complications. Home
medications usually include short-acting opioids, long-acting opioids, and
nonopioid adjuncts such as nonsteroidal anti-inflammatory drugs (NSAIDs)
and acetaminophen (INN paracetamol). If pain is intense or unresponsive
to oral analgesics, hospital admission with the administration of IV opioids

is warranted. IV morphine or hydromorphone are commonly used to treat painful crises in the emergency department. It is important to review the previous effective dose used for prior pain episodes. Constant assessment of pain should be performed, as many patients will not have relief following their initial dose of analgesic. Adequate IV hydration is recommended but consider further monitoring for patients with acute chest syndrome as volume overload may worsen hypoxemia.

2) **Acute chest syndrome**: Empiric broad-spectrum IV antibiotics, supplemental oxygen, and fluids to target euvolemia are the cornerstones of treatment. Simple transfusion is recommended for mild acute chest syndrome, targeting an Hb concentration of 95 to 100 g/L, while exchange transfusion is recommended for moderate to severe acute chest syndrome, targeting an Hb concentration of 95 to 100 g/L and HbS concentration <30%.

3) **Stroke**: Suspicion for an acute neurologic event in patients with SCD requires urgent neuroimaging with computed tomography (CT) to identify intracranial hemorrhage followed by MRI to identify ischemia if the CT result is normal. Ischemic and hemorrhagic strokes are acutely managed by RBC exchange transfusion, targeting an HbS percentage <30%.

▶ PROGNOSIS

SCD is associated with a decreased life expectancy, previously estimated at 48 years of age in women and 42 years of age in men with HbSS genotype in North America. However, novel therapeutic strategies are changing clinical expectations and outcomes in SCD, and newer studies are needed to better understand life expectancy in SCD in the current therapeutic landscape.

3.3. Thalassemia

▶ DEFINITION, ETIOLOGY, PATHOGENESIS

Thalassemia is a chronic inherited anemia, most commonly caused by reduced (+) or absent (0) synthesis of α-globin and/or β-globin chains, the key protein components of the adult hemoglobin (Hb) tetramer, HbA ($\alpha_2\beta_2$) ($\rightarrow$Table 3-1).

The thalassemias comprise the most common monogenetic disorder worldwide, resulting from inheritance of mutant or deleted copies of globin genes (2 α-globin genes on each chromosome 16 [4 genes], one β-globin gene on each chromosome 11 [2 genes]). Thalassemia prevalence is highest in populations from Southeast Asia, the Middle East, North and Central Africa, and Mediterranean regions.

The imbalanced production of globin chains leads to excess of the unaffected globin chain (eg, excess α-globin chains in β thalassemia), which is unstable, resulting in ineffective intramedullary erythropoiesis (decreased Hb production) and extramedullary hemolysis (reduced red blood cell [RBC] survival).

▶ CLINICAL FEATURES

The clinical spectrum of thalassemia is broad, ranging from clinically silent (no symptoms or signs) to severe, lifelong, potentially fatal anemia ($\rightarrow$Table 3-1). Disease manifestations may include:

1) Anemia.

2) Ineffective erythropoiesis stimulating extramedullary hematopoiesis and leading to proliferation of marrow cavities (eg, frontal bossing), hepatosplenomegaly, and increased risk of osteoporosis.

3) Chronic hemolysis (jaundice, gallstones, splenomegaly, leg ulcers, aplastic crisis).

Table 3-1. Examples of genotype and phenotype correlation in thalassemia

	Phenotype	Genotype	Clinical manifestations
β Thalassemia	Trait/minor	$β/β^+$	Mild microcytic anemia
	Intermedia (non–transfusion-dependent thalassemia)	$β^+/β^0$ $β^+/β^+$	Moderate to severe microcytic anemia
	Major (transfusion-dependent thalassemia)	$β^0/β^0$	Severe anemia; transfusion-dependent
α Thalassemia	Carrier	-α/αα	Asymptomatic; MCV normal or mild microcytosis
	Trait/minor	--/αα -α/-α	Mild anemia with microcytosis
	Hemoglobin H disease	--/-α	Mild to moderate microcytic anemia
	Bart hydrops fetalis	--/--	May be fatal in utero or neonatal period

$β^0$, no β-globin chain production; $β^+$, reduced β-globin chain production; α, functional α chain; -, loss of α chain; MCV, mean corpuscular volume.

4) Increased intestinal iron absorption with or without chronic blood transfusions can result in iron overload (cirrhosis, cardiomyopathy, endocrinopathies including hypopituitarism, diabetes mellitus, testicular or ovarian failure).

5) Affected offspring.

➔ DIAGNOSIS

In patients with suspected thalassemia perform complete blood count (CBC), peripheral blood film, and Hb electrophoresis. The diagnosis of thalassemia is confirmed with globin gene testing (molecular studies).

Diagnostic Tests

1. CBC: Low Hb level, low mean corpuscular volume (MCV).

2. Peripheral blood film: Microcytosis, hypochromia, target cells, basophilic stippling, nucleated RBCs.

3. Hb electrophoresis: Increased levels of hemoglobin A_2 (HbA_2) >3.5% (β thalassemia), hemoglobin H (HbH) preparation (presence of HbH inclusion bodies suggests α thalassemia); this test does not detect α-thalassemia silent carrier or trait (ie, a defect in 1 or 2 out of 4 genes; molecular testing is needed) but does detect thalassemic-variant hemoglobins (eg, HbE, Hb Constant Spring, Hb Lepore).

4. Molecular genetic testing for thalassemia.

5. Other studies: Ferritin, zinc protoporphyrin IX (normal in thalassemia, elevated in iron-deficient erythropoiesis) to distinguish thalassemia from iron deficiency anemia or anemia of chronic disease.

Differential Diagnosis

Iron deficiency, anemia of chronic disease, enzymopathies (pyruvate kinase deficiency).

➡ TREATMENT

Management should be tailored to the patient's disease phenotype and clinical manifestations. Patients with thalassemia trait usually have a mild anemia that does not require hematology consultation or treatment.

1. General measures:

1) Referral to a hematology center for individuals with moderate or severe anemia.

2) Genetic counseling and prenatal family planning.

2. RBC transfusions: Patients with thalassemia major require chronic transfusions. A pretransfusion Hb level target of 90 to 105 g/L is used with the aim of preventing extramedullary hematopoiesis. Patients with non–transfusion--dependent thalassemia may require transfusion support during acute illness or physiologic stress (eg, pregnancy).

3. Iron overload: Ferritin levels should be measured on a regular basis. Liver and myocardial iron content should be assessed. This can be done through biopsy or, preferably, by specialized noninvasive techniques such as R2 or T2* magnetic resonance imaging (MRI). Patients with non–transfusion--dependent thalassemia can also develop iron overload through increased intestinal iron absorption. Chelators used in the treatment of iron overload include deferoxamine, deferiprone, and deferasirox. Therapy should be tailored to individual patient characteristics, including the area of iron deposition, preferred route of chelator administration, and coexisting medical concerns. Chelator therapy is considered at the time of starting chronic transfusions or detecting marked elevations of ferritin or iron stores in organs that exceed predefined levels.

4. Splenectomy: Possible indications include a significant increase in transfusion requirements, symptomatic splenomegaly, and hypersplenism causing cytopenias. Splenectomy should only be considered in carefully selected patients given the risks that include infection, hypercoagulability, and pulmonary hypertension.

5. Allogeneic hematopoietic stem cell transplantation: This can be considered in selected patients as a curative therapy.

➡ FOLLOW-UP

Consider the following investigations for patients with thalassemia major and intermedia:

1. Annual blood tests: CBC, reticulocyte count, creatinine, urine albumin--to-creatinine ratio, ferritin, calcium, vitamin D, thyroid-stimulating hormone (TSH), follicle-stimulating hormone (FSH), luteinizing hormone (LH), estradiol (women), testosterone (men), fasting glucose, liver enzymes, HIV testing, and hepatitis B and C serologic testing.

2. Imaging studies:

1) Hepatic and cardiac MRI: Performed as needed for the assessment of iron overload.

2) Bone mineral density: Performed at baseline, then every 1 to 5 years as needed.

3) Echocardiography: Performed at baseline, then every 1 to 3 years as needed.

3. Regular **audiometry and ophthalmology evaluations** in patients treated with iron chelators.

4. Hemostasis Disorders

4.1. Acquired Coagulation Disorders

4.1.1. Acquired Hemophilia A

→ **DEFINITION, ETIOLOGY, PATHOGENESIS**

Acquired hemophilia A (AHA) is an autoimmune disease caused by antibodies to factor VIII (factor VIII inhibitors). AHA is very rare and affects both men and women. Etiology is unknown in 50% of patients. AHA may develop in mothers within 6 months of delivery as well as in patients with autoimmune diseases, malignancy, allergic diseases, or drug-induced reactions.

→ **CLINICAL FEATURES AND NATURAL HISTORY**

AHA manifests as acute severe coagulopathy with cutaneous, mucous membrane (gastrointestinal, urinary, genital), dental site, and surgical site bleeding. Less common features include retroperitoneal hematoma, intracranial bleeding, and bleeding into skeletal muscles. Very rarely, patients may have spontaneous bleeding into the joints (a manifestation typical for hemophilia A).

In ~30% of patients (and more frequently for postpartum cases) AHA resolves spontaneously within one year. Relapses occur in ~20% of patients in whom remission has been achieved with prior immunosuppressive treatment.

→ **DIAGNOSIS**

Diagnostic Tests

1. Screening tests: Activated partial thromboplastin time (aPTT) is usually prolonged. Prothrombin time (PT), thrombin time (TT), platelet counts, and serum fibrinogen levels are normal (unless consumption or dilutional coagulopathy has developed or the inhibitor antibody affects multiple coagulation factors).

2. Studies confirming the diagnosis: Absence of aPTT normalization in a 1:1 mixture of the patient's plasma and normal plasma (the aPTT mixing test, which requires prolonged incubation to detect acquired inhibitors), decreased factor VIII activity (usually 2-10 IU/dL), a positive factor VIII inhibitor test result. Confirmation of the antibody should be performed in a laboratory with specific expertise, given the variability in the activity of the antibodies that cause this disorder.

Diagnostic Criteria

AHA is diagnosed on the basis of typical clinical manifestations as well as results of the screening tests and studies confirming the diagnosis (→Figure 4-1).

Differential Diagnosis

A combination of screening test results consistent with AHA may also be seen in hemophilia A, inherited deficiency of factor XI or factor XII, or in patients with lupus anticoagulant (in which case thrombosis may be present). Various acquired coagulopathies can present with similar signs and symptoms (eg, well-compensated chronic disseminated intravascular coagulation).

→ **TREATMENT**

Management of a patient with AHA: →Figure 4-2.

Treatment Goals

1. Short-term treatment goals include treatment of bleeding.
2. The long-term treatment goal is eradication of factor VIII inhibitors.

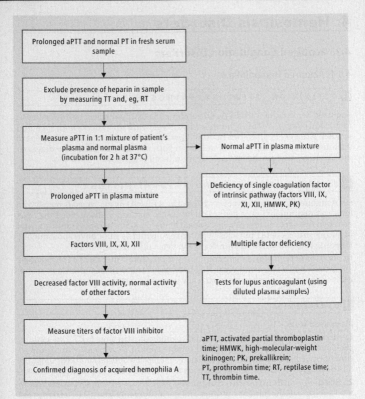

Figure 4-1. Diagnostic algorithm of acquired hemophilia.

General Measures

1. Promptly diagnose and treat underlying conditions, if any.

2. Avoid invasive procedures, IM injections, administration of acetylsalicylic acid (ASA) or nonsteroidal anti-inflammatory drugs (NSAIDs). Be conservative in performing fasciotomy for compartmental syndromes provoked by muscular hematomas.

Pharmacotherapy

1. Treatment of bleeding (all patients should be treated at an expert center or in consultation with experts in this area):

1) The first-line treatment is recombinant activated factor VII concentrate (rFVIIa) ≥90 µg/kg IV every 2 to 24 hours, activated prothrombin complex concentrate (aPCC) 50 to 100 IU/kg IV every 8 to 12 hours (up to a maximum dose of 200 IU/kg per day), or recombinant porcine factor VIII 50 to 200 IU/kg per day.

2) Desmopressin may be effective in cases of AHA with low titers of factor VIII inhibitors and minor bleeding.

3) Emicizumab has recently become available in many jurisdictions for the treatment of hemophilia A with inhibitors. This agent should be highly

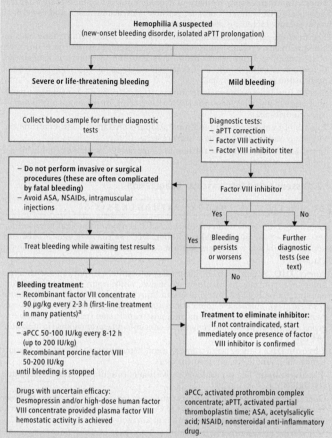

Figure 4-2. Management of a patient with acquired hemophilia A.

effective in patients with acquired inhibitors, although published evidence is currently confined to individual case reports. If its use is considered, dosing should be formulated in consultation with an expert in the management of hemophilia A.

4) In case of failure of the above treatments, consider:

a) Plasmapheresis or extracorporeal immunoadsorption followed by the administration of factor VIII (this type of treatment has low efficacy).

b) Sequential treatment with both first-line agents, for instance, an alternate administration of rFVIIa in a dose ≥90 µg/kg and aPCC in a dose of 50 to 100 IU/kg every 6 hours.

2. Immunosuppressive treatment should be started immediately after the diagnosis of AHA is made. Consider possible contraindications and the risk of adverse events, including severe infections:

1) The first-line treatment is oral prednisone 1 to 2 mg/kg/d; it may be combined with oral cyclophosphamide 1.5 to 2 mg/kg/d. The maximum duration of treatment is 4 to 6 weeks before a second-line treatment is introduced. Remission is achieved in ~70% of patients, for whom very slow tapering of prednisone is recommended.

2) Second-line treatments include rituximab, azathioprine, vincristine, mycophenolate mofetil, cyclosporine (INN ciclosporin), intravenous immunoglobulin, cladribine.

3) In patients not responding to immunosuppressive treatment, continue the follow-up and treat bleeding when present.

4) In patients with relapse use the immunosuppressive treatment that achieved the first remission.

4.1.2. Disseminated Intravascular Coagulation

→ DEFINITION, ETIOLOGY, PATHOGENESIS

Disseminated intravascular coagulation (DIC) is a syndrome that may develop in the course of various clinical conditions. DIC is a result of generalized activation of coagulation with a concomitant activation or inhibition of fibrinolysis.

1. Causes:

1) **Acute DIC**: Sepsis, severe infection (particularly in patients with hyposplenism), trauma (particularly extensive, multiorgan trauma or trauma causing fat embolism), internal organ injury (eg, acute pancreatitis, acute liver failure), obstetric complications (premature placental abruption, amniotic fluid embolism, preeclampsia), posttransfusion reactions, transplant rejection, snake bites, and sometimes cancer (acute promyelocytic leukemia [APL]).

2) **Chronic DIC**: Cancer (solid tumors), giant hemangiomas (Kasabach-Merritt syndrome), and large aortic aneurysms.

2. Pathogenesis: The generalized activation of coagulation may develop due to the following:

1) General effects of proinflammatory cytokines, for instance, in sepsis or major trauma, which lead to impairment of the anticoagulant effects of protein C, activation of platelets, and inhibition of fibrinolysis.

2) Circulating procoagulants, for instance, in the case of obstetric complications or cancer (in patients with APL or prostate cancer, activation of coagulation may be offset by a very severe activation of fibrinolysis).

3. Consequences:

1) Multiple thrombi in the microcirculation and (less frequently) in major vessels, which cause ischemic multiorgan injury.

2) Consumption of platelets, fibrinogen, and other coagulation factors, which leads to their deficiency and bleeding.

→ CLINICAL FEATURES AND NATURAL HISTORY

Acute DIC has a rapid clinical course associated with severe bleeding (from surgical wounds, nasal and oral mucosa, genitourinary tract, and sites of vascular access), ischemic organ injury (renal failure, liver failure, respiratory insufficiency), and in some cases with shock and stroke (either hemorrhagic or ischemic).

Chronic DIC is associated with a spectrum of bleeding complications and may be clinically innocuous.

→ DIAGNOSIS

Diagnosis is based on serial measurements of parameters of hemostasis in a patient with a condition that may cause DIC. There is no single diagnostic laboratory test. Diagnosis of the cause of DIC (underlying condition) is essential.

1. Acute DIC: Unexplained thrombocytopenia (generally 50×10^9/L-100×10^9/L); prolonged prothrombin time (PT)/international normalized ratio (INR), activated partial thromboplastin time (aPTT), and thrombin time; low serum levels of fibrinogen (in patients with sepsis this feature may be absent or develop late, because fibrinogen is an acute-phase protein and its levels may be transiently elevated) and other coagulation factors; elevated D-dimer levels.

2. Chronic DIC: Usually suspected due to a mild to moderate platelet count reduction. Other laboratory measures are similar to acute DIC, although findings may be less marked.

Differential Diagnosis

Immune thrombocytopenia (including heparin-induced thrombocytopenia), thrombotic thrombocytopenic purpura, and hemolytic-uremic syndrome (these are differentiated by severe thrombocytopenia with normal coagulation profiles), primary or secondary hyperfibrinogenolysis, catastrophic antiphospholipid syndrome. Purpura fulminans mimics DIC but has very different treatment requirements.

→ TREATMENT

1. Treatment of the underlying condition (eg, sepsis).

2. Transfusions of blood products when indicated:

1) **In patients with significant blood loss**, transfuse packed red blood cells.

2) **In patients with active bleeding (or those requiring an invasive procedure) and a prolonged aPTT or PT/INR (>1.5 × normal)**, administer fresh-frozen plasma.

3) **In patients with a plasma fibrinogen level <1 g/L and bleeding**, administer cryoprecipitate or fibrinogen concentrate; administration can be titrated against the fibrinogen level.

4) **In patients with platelet counts $<50 \times 10^9$/L and severe bleeding**, administer platelet concentrate. Prophylactic transfusion is not indicated except in cases of very severe thrombocytopenia ($<10 \times 10^9$/L), as the transfused platelets will be rapidly consumed and repeated exposure to donor platelets will cause refractoriness to subsequent transfusion. Poor response to platelets should be expected.

3. Drugs that may be considered:

1) The role of **heparin** (or low-molecular-weight heparin [LMWH]) in the treatment of DIC is controversial. Heparin is indicated in chronic, compensated DIC with predominant thrombosis. It may be effective in pregnant patients with fetal death syndrome and hypofibrinogenemia before induction of delivery or in patients with severe hemorrhage from a giant hemangioma or aortic aneurysm before planned resection. Consider using therapeutic doses of heparin in patients with DIC with predominant arterial or venous thrombosis or with severe fulminant purpura with symptomatic occlusion of cutaneous vessels. Unfractionated heparin (UFH) is administered IV (without an initial bolus) at a dose of 500 IU/hour (or 10 IU/kg/h). Subcutaneous injections of prophylactic doses of UFH or LMWH reduce the severity of bleeding in patients with chronic DIC and are indicated in the prevention of venous thromboembolism in severely ill patients with acute DIC without active bleeding.

2) **Tranexamic acid** (a fibrinolysis inhibitor) 10 to 15 mg/kg IV is indicated only in very rare cases of DIC with severe fibrinolysis (in patients with APL,

prostate cancer, and in some patients with Kasabach-Merritt syndrome). Absolute contraindications include hematuria, renal failure, features of ischemic organ injury, and chronic DIC.

A variety of experimental treatments are used in patients with DIC, such as antithrombin concentrates; however, evidence to support their use is limited. These treatment options should be confined to expert centers in patients with measured deficiency of these factors.

4.2. Inherited Coagulation Disorders Associated with Bleeding

→SUMMARY

Inherited coagulation disorders are most frequently caused by a deficiency or dysfunction of one of the plasma coagulation factors (hemophilia A [factor VIII] or B [factor IX]). Inherited deficiencies of factor XII, prekallikrein, and high-molecular-weight kininogen cause prolongation of the activated partial thromboplastin time but are asymptomatic and require no treatment. Rare deficiencies of fibrinogen, prothrombin, and factors V, VII, X, XI, or XIII cause bleeding of varied severity. Treatment is based on replacement of the deficient coagulation factors.

4.2.1. Hemophilia A and Hemophilia B

→DEFINITION, ETIOLOGY, CLASSIFICATION

Hemophilia A and **hemophilia B** are inherited coagulation disorders. Mutations of the genes of factor VIII or factor IX, located on chromosome X, may result—mostly in men, as in X-linked disorders—in a decrease or absence of synthesis of these factors or in the synthesis of defective factors. Hemophilia A is caused by reduced activity of factor VIII, whereas hemophilia B is caused by reduced activity of factor IX.

A **classification of hemophilia** based on factor VIII or factor IX activity levels:
1) <1% of normal (<0.01 IU/mL): Severe hemophilia.
2) 1% to 5% of normal (0.01-0.05 IU/mL): Moderate hemophilia.
3) >5% to 40% of normal (>0.05-0.4 IU/mL): Mild hemophilia.

→CLINICAL FEATURES AND NATURAL HISTORY

Features of bleeding disorder usually appear at the age of 1 to 2 years. In patients with severe hemophilia the dominant features are spontaneous joint hemorrhages; these most frequently affect the knees, elbows, and ankles, and lead to joint destruction, deformation (termed hemophilic arthropathy), and secondary muscle atrophy. Other manifestations include bleeding into muscles (often in the iliopsoas), hematuria, gastrointestinal bleeding, intracranial bleeding (frequently fatal), and bleeding to the posterior pharyngeal wall or lower wall of the oral cavity. A typical feature is delayed and persistent bleeding after surgery or tooth extraction. Spontaneous bleeding is rare in patients with moderate hemophilia and virtually absent in patients with mild hemophilia.

→DIAGNOSIS

Diagnostic Tests

1. Screening tests: Activated partial thromboplastin time (aPTT) is prolonged in most patients with hemophilia A or B; however, it may be normal in patients with mild hemophilia and factor VIII or IX activity >30%.

2. Studies confirming the diagnosis: Reduced plasma activity of factor VIII or IX, genetic studies.

Diagnostic Criteria

A documented decrease in the plasma activity of factor VIII or factor IX.

Differential Diagnosis

1. Von Willebrand disease.

2. Acquired hemophilia (→Chapter 7.4.1.1).

3. Other causes of a prolonged aPTT in a patient with a normal pro-thrombin time (PT), such as lupus anticoagulant (→Chapter 14.4).

→ TREATMENT

General Measures

1. Patients with hemophilia should always carry identification indicating their diagnosis, emergency management, and contact details of their physician. Patients can engage in physical activity but should take particular care to avoid injuries and may require pharmacologic prophylaxis (situational prophylaxis). Patients with moderate to severe hemophilia should be followed in a hemophilia treatment center, and their management should be overseen by that center.

2. Do not use antiplatelet agents; in particular, do not use acetylsalicylic acid (ASA). In the treatment of pain (eg, pain caused by hemarthrosis) use acetaminophen (INN paracetamol), selective cyclooxygenase-2 (COX-2) inhibitors, and opioids. Patients with medical conditions requiring antiplatelet treatment are better referred to specialized centers.

3. Avoid intramuscular injections.

4. Prophylactic treatment (→Pharmacotherapy, below) prevents complications of the disease and is recommended in most patients with severe hemophilia where available.

5. Treatment of most cases of bleeding as well as prophylactic treatment may be self-administered at home by a trained patient. In the case of joint bleeding, RICE (**r**est, **i**ce, **c**ompression, **e**levation) may help contain the pain. The effect on duration of symptoms and arthropathy is unknown.

6. Surgical procedures and treatment of life-threatening hemorrhages should always be conducted in centers that are capable of daily laboratory monitoring of treatment results (measurements of factor VIII or IX activity, titers of factor VIII or IX inhibitors).

Pharmacotherapy

1. Plasma-derived or recombinant factor VIII or factor IX concentrates administered as IV injections:

1) **Long-term prophylactic treatment**: The goal of the treatment is to maintain the deficient factor plasma level above 1% to 2%. In patients with **hemophilia A**, use factor VIII concentrates 25 to 40 IU/kg 3 times a week or every other day. In patients with **hemophilia B**, use factor IX concentrates 25 to 50 IU/kg 2 to 3 times a week. Measurements of plasma factor levels at the end of the treatment interval (trough levels) are recommended to tailor the dose to the individual needs. The frequency of prophylactic administration can be adapted to the schedule of physical activity, particularly in children and adolescents.

2) **Prophylactic treatment before planned surgical procedures** (including tooth extraction; →Table 4-1): Such procedures should only be managed in expert centers with immediate access to monitoring of coagulation factor levels. In case of emergency surgery, administer factor VIII or IX to raise the level >80% (0.8 IU/mL) trough for the entire duration of the procedure and at least 3 postoperative days.

3) **Treatment of bleeding**: In patients with **hemophilia A**, administer a factor VIII concentrate every 8, 12, or 24 hours. In patients with **hemophilia B**,

Table 4-1. Dosage of factor VIII and factor IX in the treatment of moderate to severe hemophilia

Indication	Hemophilia A, dose of factor VIII concentrate (IU/kg)	Hemophilia B, dose of factor IX concentrate (IU/kg)	Treatment duration (days)[a]
Bleeding to joints and/or muscles, epistaxis, gingival bleeding	20-30	40-60	1-2 days; in case of unsatisfactory effects increase dose and prolong treatment
Tooth extraction[b]	25	40	Once before procedure
Bleeding: to lower wall of oral cavity and to neck; gastrointestinal; to iliopsoas; intracranial; retroperitoneal hematomas; surgical procedures	40-50	60-80	For 1-7 days after onset of bleeding, then reduce dose

[a] Depending on the clinical situation, administer a factor VIII concentrate every 8, 12, or 24 hours (hemophilia A) and factor IX concentrate every 12, 18, or 24 hours (hemophilia B).

[b] For 7 days from the extraction, administer tranexamic acid 10-15 mg/kg every 8 hours.

administer a factor IX concentrate when needed, for instance, every 12, 18, or 24 hours. Dosage: →Table 4-1. Start treatment as soon as possible (optimally within 2 hours); in patients with life-threatening bleeding (head, neck, chest, or gastrointestinal hemorrhage), treatment should be started before completing diagnostics and does not require a factor VIII level prior to its initiation.

IV administration of 1 IU of lyophilized factor VIII concentrate/kg increases plasma factor VIII activity by ~2% of normal (0.02 IU/mL). IV administration of 1 IU of lyophilized factor IX concentrate/kg increases plasma factor IX activity by ~1% of normal (0.01 IU/mL). In patients with a poor clinical response to treatment, suspect factor VIII or factor IX inhibitors.

A variety of long half-life factor VIII and IX variants are available. These products allow extended dosing intervals, increasing convenience of therapy for patients. Their availability varies from jurisdiction to jurisdiction and they should be prescribed only on advice from a hemophilia treatment center. Individual patient pharmacokinetic analysis may assist in dosing of both normal half-life and long half-life factor concentrates. Note that routine laboratory testing may be inaccurate in patients treated with these products.

2. Desmopressin is the drug of choice in patients with mild hemophilia A (dosage: →Chapter 7.4.2.2). Desmopressin causes a 2- to 5-fold increase in plasma factor VIII activity by releasing it from tissue stores. This pool can be exhausted after 3 to 7 days of continuous desmopressin treatment; in such situations, consider the administration of a human-derived factor VIII concentrate. In patients treated with desmopressin (especially children, pregnant women, and the elderly) the drug can induce water retention, hyponatremia, and occasionally seizures. Desmopressin has no effect on plasma factor IX and is not used in hemophilia B.

3. Tranexamic acid is used for clot stabilization in patients with oral bleeding, epistaxis, and urogenital bleeding. Dosage: →Chapter 7.4.2.2.

4. Novel treatments: A variety of novel treatments are being explored for the treatment of hemophilia, including implantable microcapsules of genetically modified human-derived cells that secrete a modified factor VIII, use of emicizumab (→below) in patients who do not have inhibitors, small interfering RNA (siRNA) therapies that downregulate anticoagulant proteins in blood (including tissue factor pathway inhibitor and antithrombin), and gene therapy, which has shown promise in both hemophilia A and B.

→ COMPLICATIONS

1. Development of inhibitors of factor VIII or factor IX: IgG antibodies against factor VIII (factor VIII inhibitors) develop in about 30% of patients with severe hemophilia A and in 5% to 10% of patients with moderate or mild hemophilia A (in some patients spontaneous clearance of the inhibitor occurs). Antibodies to factor IX develop in <5% of patients with severe hemophilia B and may cause allergic reactions after the administration of factor IX. In prevention and treatment of bleeding in patients with inhibitor titers <5 Bethesda units/mL (BU/mL), administer high doses of factor VIII/IX concentrates while monitoring plasma factor VIII/IX activity. In patients with inhibitor titers >5 BU/mL, use an activated prothrombin complex concentrate (aPCC) 50 to 100 IU/kg every 6 to 12 hours or recombinant factor VIIa 90 to 120 µg/kg every 2 to 3 hours. If specific treatment is not available, a standard prothrombin complex concentrate (PCC) can be used to treat emergency bleeding. Treatment strategies to eliminate inhibitors should only be used in centers with focused skills in this area; referral to such centers should be strongly considered in all patients with inhibitors. In many jurisdictions the availability of emicizumab has greatly simplified care of patients with factor VIII inhibitors; administered once monthly, a subcutaneous injection of this bispecific antibody nullifies the impact of the inhibitor and causes cessation of bleeding. It should only be used in consultation with an expert who is familiar with its use.

2. Chronic synovitis, hemophilic arthropathy: Adult patients with severe hemophilia are at risk of arthropathy leading to disability if they have not received effective prophylaxis.

3. Viral infections related to treatment with blood products: Since the late 1980s and the introduction of virally inactivated plasma-derived factor concentrates, the risk of transmission of hepatitis C and B viruses as well as HIV with plasma-derived clotting factor concentrates has been minimal.

4.2.2. Von Willebrand Disease

→ DEFINITION, ETIOLOGY, PATHOGENESIS

Von Willebrand disease (vWD) is the most frequent inherited bleeding disorder. It is caused by a deficiency or dysfunction of von Willebrand factor (vWF), which affects both primary and secondary hemostasis (vWF is a cofactor in the adhesion of platelets to the exposed subendothelium and protects factor VIII from inactivation).

Classification:

1) **Type 1 vWD** (65%-75% of patients): Partial quantitative vWF deficiency with preserved function (plasma levels of antigen and activity are similar). The level of factor VIII is normal or decreased.

2) **Type 2 vWD** (20%-25% of patients): vWF dysfunction (depending on type of dysfunction, this is classified as subtype 2A, 2B, 2M, or 2N), which causes a reduction in vWF activity that is disproportionate to the decrease in its concentrations. The level of factor VIII is normal (2A, 2B, 2M) or decreased (2N).

3) **Type 3 (severe) vWD**: Undetectable activity of vWF with the factor VIII level usually <10% of normal.

→ CLINICAL FEATURES

Mucocutaneous bleeding (recurrent epistaxis and gingival bleeding, easy bruising, heavy and prolonged menstrual bleeding); hemorrhages after tooth extraction and surgical procedures; gastrointestinal bleeding (all types); bleeding into joints (hemarthrosis) and muscles almost exclusively in patients with type 3 vWD (this may cause arthropathy). Types 1 and 2 are mostly due to autosomal dominant gene defects, with many family members affected and a variable clinical phenotype.

➔ DIAGNOSIS

Diagnostic Tests

1. Screening tests: Prothrombin time (PT)/international normalized ratio (INR) and thrombin time (TT) are normal. Activated partial thromboplastin time (aPTT) may be prolonged and it corrects at mixing studies. Bleeding time and platelet function analyzer (PFA)-100 closure time are always prolonged in patients with type 3 vWD and may be prolonged or normal in patients with type 1 or type 2 vWD. The platelet count is normal, except for type 2B vWD, which may rarely cause intermittent thrombocytopenia during stress conditions or after desmopressin administration.

2. Studies confirming the diagnosis: Decreased concentration and activity of vWF (an activity-to-antigen ratio ≥0.7 suggests type 1 vWD while <0.7 indicates type 2 vWD), decreased or normal activity of factor VIII.

3. Specialized studies: Specialized testing, including genetic analyses and analysis of the multimeric composition, are available and should be interpreted by experts, as the laboratory findings in vWD are pleomorphic.

Diagnostic Criteria

Diagnosis is made on the basis of the laboratory tests (→above). The types and subtypes of vWD are confirmed by specialized studies. Laboratory confirmation of mild vWD is fraught with controversy; many patients with a mild bleeding disorder phenotype are misdiagnosed with vWD based on inappropriate laboratory testing.

Differential Diagnosis

Hemophilia A (particularly the mild variant), acquired von Willebrand syndrome (most frequently occurring in the course of autoimmune diseases, valvular heart disease, lymphoid neoplasms, polycythemia vera, or essential thrombocytosis), platelet-type (pseudo-) vWD (inherited abnormalities of the glycoprotein Ib platelet receptor causing its increased affinity to vWF, leading to thrombocytopenia and bleeding), platelet function disorders.

➔ TREATMENT

General Measures

1. Do not use antiplatelet agents; in particular, do not use acetylsalicylic acid (exceptions as in hemophilia A and hemophilia B).

2. Avoid intramuscular injections.

3. Major surgical procedures and treatment of severe bleeding should be performed, if possible, in a hospital capable of 24-hour measurements of vWF and factor VIII activity.

Pharmacotherapy in Case of Bleeding or Surgery

1. Desmopressin: A 30 minute IV infusion of 0.3 mg/kg every 12 to 24 hours. Desmopressin is the drug of choice in patients with type 1 vWD. It is also effective in some patients with type 2 vWD; however, in patients with type 2B disease it may rarely cause thrombocytopenia, and in most patients with type 3 vWD it is ineffective. Desmopressin causes a 2- to 5-fold increase in plasma vWF and factor VIII activity by releasing them from tissue stores. This pool can be exhausted after 3 to 7 days of continuous desmopressin treatment; in such situations, consider the administration of a factor VIII concentrate containing vWF (intermediate-purity plasma-derived factor VIII). In patients treated with

Table 4-2. Typical doses of factor VIII concentrate containing von Willebrand factor (vWF) in the prevention and treatment of bleeding in patients with severe vWF and factor VIII deficiency (<10%)

Type of bleeding	Dose (IU/kg)[a]	Frequency of administration	Suggested plasma activity of factor VIII or vWF (% of normal)
Major surgery[b]	50	Before procedure, then every 12-24 h until wound is completely healed	>50% for 5-7 days, then dose may be reduced
Minor surgery	40	Before procedure, then every 24-48 h until wound is completely healed	>30% for 1-5 days
Tooth extraction[c]	30	Once before procedure	>50% for 12 h
Minor bleeding	25	Repeat every 24 h if necessary	>30% until bleeding stops
Delivery	40	Every 24 h	>50% on day of delivery and for subsequent 3-4 days

[a] In children increase each dose by 20% because of the higher relative plasma volume.

[b] In patients with severe bleeding (eg, central nervous system hemorrhage) use the same doses as for major surgery. To reduce the risk of thrombosis, maintain plasma factor VIII activity <250% of normal.

[c] For 3 to 7 days after the extraction, additionally administer tranexamic acid 10 to 15 mg/kg orally every 8 hours.

desmopressin (especially children, pregnant women, and the elderly) the drug can induce water retention, hyponatremia, and occasionally seizures.

2. Plasma-derived concentrates containing vWF are used in patients in whom desmopressin is ineffective or contraindicated. IV administration of 1 IU of vWF/kg increases plasma vWF activity by ~2% of normal. Dosage: →Table 4-2. In selected patients with recurrent bleeding, consider regular prophylaxis. A phase 3 study on recombinant vWF is ongoing.

3. Oral or IV **tranexamic acid** is used in patients with mucosal bleeding at a dose 10 to 15 mg/kg every 8 hours.

4. Combined (estrogen-progestogen) oral contraceptives or levonorgestrel-releasing intrauterine systems may prevent heavy menstrual bleeding.

4.3. Platelet Disorders

→ **DEFINITION, ETIOLOGY, PATHOGENESIS**

Disorders of platelets may be caused by abnormal platelet counts (thrombocytopenia, rarely thrombocythemia) or abnormal platelet function.

1. Thrombocytopenia is usually defined as a **platelet count <150 × 10⁹/L**. It may be classified as:

1) Thrombocytopenia caused by **decreased platelet production**:

   a) **Inherited**: Rare, sometimes familial, it may present in childhood. Examples include Bernard-Soulier syndrome, Fanconi anemia, Alport syndrome. In some cases platelets are reduced in number and are morphologically abnormal.

   b) **Acquired**: More frequent, it may be caused by drugs (myelosuppressive agents, thiazide diuretics, interferons, and many others), alcohol and other toxins, viral infections, cobalamin and/or folate deficiency, bone marrow disorders (leukemia, lymphoid neoplasm, myelodysplastic syndrome, cancer metastasis, Gaucher disease, tuberculosis, myelofibrosis), aplastic anemia, radiation, selective megakaryocytic aplasia, or cyclic thrombocytopenia (regular decreases in platelet counts every 21-39 days, most frequently in young women).

2) Thrombocytopenia caused by **excess destruction of platelets and decreased platelet production**; this is termed immune thrombocytopenia (ITP).

3) Thrombocytopenia caused by **excess destruction of platelets**:

a) **Immune**: Caused by transfusion, drugs (eg, heparin [nonimmune thrombocytopenia caused by heparin is usually asymptomatic, while immune heparin-induced thrombocytopenia—HIT— is associated with thrombosis, not bleeding], abciximab, quinidine, sulfonamides, nonsteroidal anti--inflammatory drugs, antibiotics, gold compounds), infections, autoimmune diseases (eg, systemic lupus erythematosus, antiphospholipid syndrome), non-Hodgkin lymphomas, or treatment with antilymphocyte immunoglobulin or antithymocyte immunoglobulin, among many other causes.

b) **Nonimmune**: Thrombotic thrombocytopenic purpura (TTP), hemolytic--uremic syndrome (HUS), sepsis, disseminated intravascular coagulation (DIC), Kasabach-Merritt syndrome, cyanotic congenital heart disease, and others.

4) Thrombocytopenia caused by **sequestration of platelets**: Hypersplenism; rarely at other sites, such as large hemangiomas.

5) Thrombocytopenia caused by **dilution** developing after massive transfusion or fluid resuscitation.

6) Pregnancy (platelet counts are usually $>70 \times 10^9/L$; the condition requires no treatment and resolves spontaneously after delivery).

Pseudothrombocytopenia is a laboratory artifact caused by in vitro platelet agglutination in the blood collected in a tube containing ethylenediaminetetraacetic acid (EDTA); it can cause significant underestimation of platelet counts; however, most automated analyzers will recognize platelet clumping and not report a falsely reduced level. Platelet counts in the blood collected in tubes containing heparin or citrate are usually unaffected by this artifact.

2. Thrombocytosis is defined as a **platelet count $>400 \times 10^9/L$**:

1) **Primary thrombocytosis** (essential thrombocythemia) is a myeloproliferative neoplasm (→Chapter 7.8.15).

2) **Secondary (reactive) thrombocytosis** may be caused by surgery, solid tumors, iron deficiency anemia, hemolytic anemia, chronic inflammatory or infectious diseases, acute blood loss, splenectomy, chronic alcohol abuse, or multiple blood donations. It is usually asymptomatic, causes no bleeding or thrombosis, and resolves after successful treatment of the underlying condition.

3. Qualitative disorders of platelet function cause prolonged bleeding times and impaired platelet aggregation as assessed using aggregometry in patients with normal or slightly decreased platelet counts:

1) **Inherited**: Rare abnormalities of platelet surface receptors, membrane, cytoskeleton, or degranulation.

2) **Acquired**: Most commonly drug-induced (acetylsalicylic acid, ticlopidine, clopidogrel, prasugrel, ticagrelor, glycoprotein IIb/IIIa antagonists, fibrinolytic agents, or other drugs) or caused by uremia, myeloproliferative neoplasms, acute leukemia, or monoclonal gammopathy.

Note: In patients with severe bleeding you may use desmopressin 0.3 µg/kg or platelet concentrate (usually in patients not responding to desmopressin).

The effects will vary. Repeated doses of desmopressin are limited by tachyphylaxis and hyponatremia. Neither of these agents has been validated in clinical trials as effective.

→ CLINICAL FEATURES

Cutaneous and mucosal bleeding: petechiae on the skin of extremities, trunk (rarely the face), and oral mucosa; gingival bleeding; epistaxis; menorrhagia and urinary and/or genital bleeding. Life-threatening gastrointestinal or intracranial hemorrhages may occur, and excessive bleeding after tissue injury may be observed. In patients with thrombocytopenia bleeding usually occurs with platelet counts $<20 \times 10^9$/L.

4.3.1. Immune Thrombocytopenia

→ DEFINITION AND ETIOLOGY

Immune thrombocytopenia (ITP), formerly termed idiopathic thrombocytopenic purpura, is an acquired immune disease characterized by isolated thrombocytopenia (here defined as platelet counts <100,000 μL) with no known causes. Etiology is unknown.

→ CLINICAL FEATURES AND NATURAL HISTORY

ITP is classified on the basis of its duration as newly diagnosed ITP, persistent ITP (3-12 months), or chronic ITP (≥12 months). In adults the disease is usually chronic and asymptomatic, and it is associated with remissions and relapses. In ~10% of adult patients ITP resolves spontaneously. Typical manifestations include epistaxis, gingival bleeding, and heavy and prolonged menstrual bleeding; in some patients the only features are cutaneous petechiae and bruising. Petechiae are usually located on the mucous membranes and the skin of distal portions of extremities. Tissue injury causes excessive bleeding, but gastrointestinal and central nervous system hemorrhages are rare.

→ DIAGNOSIS

Diagnostic Tests

1. Complete blood count (CBC): Isolated thrombocytopenia, increased mean platelet volume (MPV), increased numbers of young platelets.

2. Bone marrow aspiration or biopsy might be considered in patients aged >60 years to exclude myelodysplastic syndrome, as well as in patients with treatment resistance who are planned for splenectomy or patients with relapse after splenectomy. Bone marrow examination is not generally useful in patients with suspected ITP.

3. Other studies: Tests for HIV, hepatitis C virus, *Helicobacter pylori*, parvovirus B19, Epstein-Barr virus, and cytomegalovirus infections; antinuclear antibodies (to exclude systemic lupus erythematosus); pregnancy test. Immunologic testing (detection of antiplatelet antibodies) is of no value in the diagnosis of ITP.

Diagnostic Criteria

Isolated thrombocytopenia with an otherwise normal CBC in a patient in whom other causes have been excluded.

Differential Diagnosis

Other causes of thrombocytopenia: →Chapter 7.4.3.

→ TREATMENT

Treatment is not necessary in patients who are not bleeding.
"Prophylactic treatment" might be considered in patients with extreme thrombocytopenia (eg, $<20 \times 10^9$/L-30×10^9/L) or prior to a procedure.

First-Line Treatment

1. Glucocorticoids: Cycles of dexamethasone 40 mg/d for 4 days every 14 or 28 days (1-4 cycles) or alternatively oral prednisone 1 to 1.5 (usually 1) mg/kg/d for 2 to 4 weeks, until platelet counts increase to $>50 \times 10^9$/L, then taper the dose. In most patients glucocorticoids must be discontinued because of adverse effects. Use long-term prednisone therapy in patients in whom low-dose prednisone (≤ 10 mg/d) maintains a platelet count that provides effective hemostasis and attempts to discontinue the treatment cause bleeding. In patients treated with glucocorticoids for >3 months, prevention of osteoporosis is necessary (→Chapter 14.13). In patients not responding to prednisone, the drug should be discontinued within 4 weeks.

2. Patients with *H pylori* infection should be considered for *H pylori* **eradication therapy**, as this may lead to an improvement in the platelet counts (→Chapter 6.1.2.4).

3. Intravenous immunoglobulin (IVIG) might be considered as a first-line therapy in patients with life-threatening hemorrhage, those with inability to take glucocorticosteroids, those requiring immediate surgery, or in pregnant patients with imminent delivery.

Second-Line Treatment

1. Splenectomy: Indications for splenectomy are considered on a case-by-case basis in patients with ITP and primary resistance to glucocorticoids or those who need long-term glucocorticoid therapy to maintain adequate platelet counts. Before splenectomy a trial of second-line pharmacotherapy may be used (→below). In the majority of cases splenectomy is performed after ≥ 6 months of diagnosing the disease, as spontaneous remissions have been observed even after 6 months of diagnosis. In the case of symptomatic severe thrombocytopenia ($<10 \times 10^9$/L) in a patient treated with appropriate doses of glucocorticoids for >2 weeks, earlier splenectomy (before 6 months) may be justified. The most common complications of splenectomy include infections and venous thrombosis. Splenectomy leads to remission in up to 65% of patients. In the remaining patients continued glucocorticoid therapy at the lowest possible dose is necessary, and if this is ineffective, other second-line agents are used. To optimize the preoperative platelet count (usual goal $>50 \times 10^9$/L), IVIG or anti-D immunoglobulin may be administered; use of a thrombopoietin-receptor agonist may also be considered in the perioperative period. At least 2 weeks before splenectomy (and if this is not feasible, as soon as possible after splenectomy) the patient should receive vaccines against *Streptococcus pneumoniae*, *Neisseria meningitidis*, and *Haemophilus influenzae*; the vaccinations should be repeated every 5 years.

2. Second-line agents:

1) **IVIG**: 1 g/kg/d for 1 to 2 days. In some patients glucocorticoids may enhance the response to IVIG; their combined use may reduce infusion-associated reactions and prevent aseptic meningitis.

2) **Rituximab** is widely used as a second-line agent in patients with ITP. Although associated with a good initial response in many patients, long--term results of rituximab use have been disappointing, with recrudescent thrombocytopenia in the majority of patients.

3) **Anti-D immunoglobulin**.

4) **Thrombopoietin-receptor agonists**: Romiplostim, eltrombopag.

5) **Other drugs** used in the case of resistance to glucocorticoids or contraindications to glucocorticoids and splenectomy: Immunosuppressive agents

(cyclophosphamide, azathioprine, cyclosporine [INN ciclosporin], vincristine, vinblastine, mycophenolate mofetil, rituximab), danazol, and dapsone.

Acute Treatment

In patients being prepared for surgery or after a massive hemorrhage, use intravenous methylprednisolone 1 g/d for 3 days or IVIG 1 g/kg/d for 2 days; in patients with severe hemorrhagic complications, both agents may be used in combination. In the case of life-threatening complications, administer platelet concentrate, optimally in combination with IVIG treatment.

Treatment of Pregnant Patients

Oral glucocorticoids are generally used as first-line agents in patients requiring therapy. IVIG might be considered in selected patients. Vaginal delivery is recommended (platelet counts should be $\geq 30 \times 10^9$/L), and cesarean section should only be performed for obstetric indications. Epidural analgesia is usually not administered to patients with platelet counts $<80 \times 10^9$/L.

4.3.2. Thrombocytopenia Caused by Decreased Platelet Production

→ DIAGNOSIS

Thrombocytopenia found in complete blood count in a patient with a certain clinical condition (causes: →Chapter 7.4.3). Bone marrow aspiration and biopsy reveal reduced megakaryocyte counts or their abnormal morphology. Other diagnostic studies depend on the suspected underlying condition.

→ TREATMENT

Repeated platelet transfusion is likely to be associated with refractoriness; thus, transfusion should be used sparingly.

1. Treatment of inherited disease: Platelet concentrate transfusions.

2. Treatment of acquired disease: Eliminate the causative factor or factors, treat the underlying condition, and administer platelet concentrate when necessary.

4.3.3. Thrombocytopenia Caused by Excess Destruction of Platelets

Typical features of thrombocytopenia caused by excess destruction of platelets include increased mean platelet volume and bone marrow megakaryocyte counts as well as a reduced platelet life-span, which lead to low peripheral platelet counts despite a marked increase in bone marrow platelet production.

4.3.3.1. Hemolytic-Uremic Syndrome

→ DEFINITION, ETIOLOGY, PATHOGENESIS

Hemolytic-uremic syndrome (HUS) is a very rare severe nonimmune hemolytic anemia caused by thrombotic microangiopathy with thrombocytopenia. The dominant clinical feature is kidney dysfunction. In >90% of cases HUS is caused by verotoxin-producing bacteria: enterohemorrhagic *Escherichia coli* (EHEC) strains (serotype O157:H7 or O104:H4) or *Shigella* spp (more frequent in children). Other causes responsible for the development of atypical HUS include hereditary abnormalities in complement proteins, viral infections, and certain drugs. Epidemics of HUS are well described and associated with food or water contamination with pathognomonic bacteria.

In patients with atypical HUS, uncontrolled activation of the alternative complement pathway takes place (the majority of patients have inherited mutations of genes coding elements of the pathway).

→ CLINICAL FEATURES AND NATURAL HISTORY

HUS may be preceded by bloody diarrhea, urinary tract infection, or skin infection. Dominant clinical features include hemolytic anemia, thrombocytopenia, and renal failure, which are frequently associated with hypertension and fever. Neurologic symptoms are rare. The course of atypical HUS is markedly more severe than that of the typical syndrome.

→ DIAGNOSIS

Diagnostic Tests

1. Complete blood count (CBC): Normocytic anemia, erythroblasts and schistocytes present in peripheral blood smears, reticulocyte count increase, thrombocytopenia.

2. Blood biochemical tests: Elevated serum unconjugated bilirubin and lactate dehydrogenase levels, features of impaired renal function.

3. Urinalysis: Proteinuria, microscopic hematuria.

4. Coagulation parameters: Elevated serum levels of fibrin degradation products, sometimes also elevated D-dimer levels. Otherwise coagulation parameters are normal.

5. Serologic studies: Normal or slightly decreased ADAMTS-13 (von Willebrand factor–cleaving protease) levels, negative testing for autoimmune hemolytic anemia.

6. Documentation of Shiga toxin–producing infections: Classically *E coli* serotype H7:O157 (rarely identified but pathognomonic if found).

Diagnostic Criteria

Diagnosis is based on clinical features.

Differential Diagnosis

Disseminated intravascular coagulation, Evans syndrome, catastrophic antiphospholipid syndrome, bacterial sepsis, thrombotic thrombocytopenic purpura (TTP), atypical HUS due to complement component mutations (→Table 4-3).

→ TREATMENT

In most patients supportive care, early renal replacement therapy, and packed red blood cell transfusions are necessary. Plasmapheresis is administered in many patients in whom differentiating TTP and HUS is difficult. Atypical HUS with documented complement mutations may respond to complement-directed therapies. In epidemic cases public health intervention is required to identify and mitigate the source of the contamination.

→ PROGNOSIS

Mortality rates are up 25%. Chronic kidney disease develops in ~25% of surviving patients.

4.3.3.2. Thrombotic Thrombocytopenic Purpura

→ DEFINITION, ETIOLOGY, PATHOGENESIS

Thrombotic thrombocytopenic purpura (TTP) is a thrombotic microangiopathy with thrombocytopenia caused by the formation of intravascular platelet aggregates, which develop due to endothelial injury and the presence of ultra large von Willebrand factor (vWF) molecules in plasma (in healthy persons these are degraded by a plasma metalloproteinase: ADAMTS-13 [vWF-cleaving

Table 4-3. Clinical and laboratory features which may assist in differentiating among DIC, TTP, HUS, and CAPS

Clinical features	DIC	TTP	HUS	CAPS
CNS manifestations	+/−	++	+/−	++
Renal impairment	+/−	+/−	+++	++
Liver impairment	+/−	+/−	+/−	+
Hypertension	−	−/+	+/−	−
Fever	+/−	+/−	−/+	−/+
Hemolysis	+	+++	++	+
Thrombocytopenia	+++	+++	++	++
Coagulopathy	+++	−	−	+/−

Adapted from Br J Haematol. 2003;120(4):556-73.

CAPS, catastrophic antiphospholipid syndrome; CNS, central nervous system; DIC, disseminated intravascular coagulation; HUS, hemolytic-uremic syndrome; TTP, thrombotic thrombocytopenic purpura.

protease]). Hemolytic anemia and schistocytes result from red blood cell damage related to platelet aggregates in microcirculation.

Chronic TTP is associated with an inherited ADAMTS-13 deficiency, while acute TTP can be caused by autoantibodies to ADAMTS-13. In some patients, particularly those with a history of organ transplantation, the etiology is unknown (ADAMTS-13 levels are normal). TTP may also develop in patients with bacterial infections; HIV infection; in the course of treatment with various drugs, including calcineurin inhibitors, quinine, interferon α, ticlopidine, clopidogrel, simvastatin, trimethoprim, gemcitabine, and bleomycin; in pregnancy; or in patients with cancer. Platelet aggregates present in microcirculation cause hemolytic anemia with schistocytes in peripheral blood smears and features of ischemia of various organs and systems, most frequently the central nervous system. Thrombi form in capillaries and arterioles in all organs, with particularly extensive involvement of the vessels of the brain, heart, kidneys, pancreas, and adrenal glands.

CLINICAL FEATURES AND NATURAL HISTORY

TTP is more prevalent in women, usually between the ages of 30 to 40 years. The onset is acute and may be preceded by a mild upper respiratory tract infection. Manifestations include signs and symptoms of thrombocytopenia, hemolysis (anemia and jaundice), neurologic symptoms (these may include behavioral abnormalities, headache, visual disturbances, paresthesias, aphasia, coma), fever, abdominal pain, myalgia (frequent), and enlargement of the liver and spleen.

DIAGNOSIS

Diagnostic Tests

1. Complete blood count (CBC): Normocytic anemia, erythroblasts and schistocytes present in peripheral blood smears, thrombocytopenia, increased reticulocyte counts.

2. Blood biochemical tests: Elevated serum unconjugated bilirubin and lactate dehydrogenase (LDH) levels. Features of impaired renal function in some patients.

3. Urinalysis: Proteinuria, microscopic hematuria, casts.

4. Other studies: Markedly decreased concentrations and decreased activity of ADAMTS-13 (<10%) as well as positive antibodies to ADAMTS-13 may be seen. Coombs test results are negative.

Diagnostic Criteria

Diagnosis is usually based on clinical features. Confirmation of microangiopathic hemolytic anemia and thrombocytopenia without an identifiable cause is sufficient for establishing the diagnosis. Documenting reduced ADAMTS-13 levels and positive antibodies to ADAMTS-13 may be performed if available.

Differential Diagnosis

Disseminated intravascular coagulation, Evans syndrome, catastrophic antiphospholipid syndrome, bacterial sepsis, hemolytic-uremic syndrome, and other microangiopathies.

→ TREATMENT

1. Plasmapheresis (plasma exchange) of 1 to 1.5 total plasma volume per day (the most effective treatment). Continue plasmapheresis until the resolution of neurologic symptoms and normalization of platelet counts and LDH levels. If plasma exchange is not immediately available, a plasma infusion (25-30 mL/kg of frozen plasma per day) can be used as a temporizing measure. Because plasma infusion is poorly tolerated, due to fluid overload, plasma exchange is preferred.

2. Rituximab 375 mg/m^2 once weekly for 4 to 8 weeks, particularly in patients not responding to plasmapheresis or glucocorticoids, or with relapse. Rituximab is being used with increasing frequency in newly presenting patients, as it may facilitate recovery and reduce the rate of relapse.

3. Immunosuppressive drugs: These are used in patients who deteriorate despite other treatments. Glucocorticoids are frequently used; however, there is little evidence of efficacy. From day 4 of treatment agents may include IV vincristine 1.4 mg/kg every 3 days, cyclophosphamide, azathioprine, or other agents, including bortezomib.

4. Splenectomy may lead to improvement in some patients. Optimally it should be performed in remission after the first relapse.

5. Packed red blood cell transfusions are used to control anemia.

6. Platelet concentrates are administered only in patients with life--threatening hemorrhages.

7. Caplacizumab is an inhibitor of the interaction between vWF and glycoprotein Ib. It has been approved for use in some countries and has been shown to hasten resolution of acute TTP when used in combination with other therapies.

8. Chronic TTP: Administer FFP 20 mL/kg every 3 to 4 weeks.

→ PROGNOSIS

Mortality rates are 90% in untreated patients and 10% to 20% in patients treated with plasma exchange. TTP relapses in 30% of patients, and in half of these cases relapse occurs within 2 months of the first episode. Rituximab therapy may reduce the rate of relapse.

4.4. Thrombophilia (Hypercoagulable States)

→ DEFINITION, ETIOLOGY, PATHOGENESIS

Thrombophilia is a genetic or acquired tendency to the development of venous (VTE) or arterial thromboembolism.

Classification:

1) **Inherited thrombophilia**: Factor V Leiden (majority of cases of resistance to activated protein C), the G20210A variant of the prothrombin gene, protein C deficiency (reduced concentration or activity), protein S deficiency (reduced concentration or activity), antithrombin (AT) deficiency (reduced concentration or activity), and a large number of rare abnormalities of various procoagulant (eg, dysfibrinogenemia) and anticoagulant proteins (eg, plasminogen deficiency). The most prevalent of thrombophilia—factor V Leiden—variably increases the risk of VTE and occurs in 5% of the European population, 20% of unselected patients with VTE, and 40% of patients with recurrent VTE or a strong family history of VTE.

2) **Acquired thrombophilia**: Procoagulant states are associated with antiphospholipid syndrome; increased activity of factor VIII (>150%), factor IX, or factor XI; acquired plasminogen deficiency; cancer; trauma; pregnancy; paroxysmal nocturnal hemoglobinuria; heparin-induced thrombocytopenia; *JAK2* 617VF mutation; immobilization; and a wide variety of other states.

In a third of cases, a thromboembolic event in a patient with thrombophilia develops in the presence of a concomitant acquired risk factor (→Chapter 3.19.1) (eg, trauma, immobilization, pregnancy, oral contraceptive use, malignancy). Thrombophilia is usually associated with an increase in the production of thrombin or with its impaired inactivation.

→ CLINICAL FEATURES

The majority of types of thrombophilia are associated with an increased risk of VTE. The risk of thrombosis is highest in patients with AT deficiency. Hereditary thrombophilia is also associated with an increased risk of cerebral sinus vein thrombosis, abdominal venous thrombosis (most frequently affecting the portal vein and hepatic veins), and upper extremity VTE. The risk of recurrent thrombosis varies with thrombophilias and is only slightly higher in patients heterozygous for factor V Leiden and the G20210A mutation than in the general population.

A rare complication of protein C or protein S deficiency is skin necrosis.

An increased risk of arterial thromboembolism, and particularly of ischemic stroke, is observed in patients with antiphospholipid syndrome; a small increase in risk may also be attributable to other thrombophilias.

→ DIAGNOSIS

1. Indications for diagnostic workup of thrombophilia: There are few indications for routine thrombophilia screening. It might be considered in patients with a strong history of VTE in first-degree relatives, in patients with VTE in atypical locations (eg, abdominal veins), and in selected patients planning pregnancy or combined contraceptive use. Testing may be indicated in selected patients who are considering discontinuation of anticoagulation where the presence of the thrombophilia (particularly the lupus anticoagulant) may influence the discontinuation discussion. Experts also advise a focused work-up in patients aged <50 years with arterial thrombosis despite no risk factors, such as young patients with myocardial infarction. Testing in these patients should include antiphospholipid antibody testing, homocysteine, and lipoprotein(a), as well as testing for more conventional risk factors for premature arterial thrombosis including lipids.

2. Investigations recommended in patients suspected of thrombophilia include resistance to activated protein C (mostly indicating the presence of factor V Leiden), the 20210A variant of the prothrombin gene, protein C activity, free protein S concentration, AT activity, the lupus anticoagulant, and IgG anticardiolipin antibodies. Additional testing might be considered, but only under the advice of a specialist in this area.

3. Investigations should be performed 3 to 6 months after a thrombo-embolic event, because it will both allow adequate counseling of patients, and because the thrombosis and its treatment may alter the results of functional assays. None of the functional assays should be performed in patients receiving any form of anticoagulation; if required, patients should temporarily interrupt anticoagulants to ensure they are tested after the anticoagulant effect has lapsed. In patients on warfarin, a switch to low-molecular-weight heparin is advised for 10 to 14 days; in patients on direct oral anticoagulants (DOACs), a delay of at least 24 hours since the last dose is recommended.

→ TREATMENT

1. Treatment modalities and outcomes of acute VTE in patients with thrombophilia are the same as in other patients with venous thrombosis. In patients with severe deficiency of natural anticoagulants, additional options (substitution) should be considered. The presence of a thrombophilia may influence the duration of treatment.

2. In patients with protein C or protein S deficiency avoid high loading doses of vitamin K antagonists (VKAs) and simultaneously administer heparin/low-molecular-weight heparin (LMWH) until the international normalized ratio (INR) has been in the range of 2 to 3 for 48 hours to reduce the risk of skin necrosis. DOACs may be preferred in such patients, as the agents do not reduce the levels of proteins C and S.

3. In patients who would otherwise be discontinuing anticoagulants, lifelong secondary antithrombotic prevention with a VKA or DOAC could be considered after the first episode of VTE in patients with AT deficiency, homozygotes for factor V Leiden, or patients with the 20210A variant of the prothrombin gene, as well as patients with coexisting heterozygosity for these conditions, or in patients with antiphospholipid syndrome with an unprovoked VTE event. After the first episode of unprovoked thrombosis in patients with types of thrombophilia other than those mentioned above, anticoagulant treatment should be continued for ≥3 months. Consideration for extended--duration therapy in such patients (particularly men) is reasonable if the risk of bleeding is low to moderate.

→ PREVENTION

Thrombophilia in a patient with no episodes of thrombosis requires no prophylactic treatment outside periods of a particularly high risk (eg, major surgery). It may be considered in patients—and particularly in pregnant women—with AT deficiency and a positive family history of thrombosis. All pregnant patients with the diagnosis of thrombophilia should be monitored for VTE on a regular basis; if there are additional thrombosis risk factors, preventative therapy may be administered (antithrombotic prevention in pregnant women with different types of thrombophilia: →Chapter 3.19.2).

4.5. Vascular Purpuras

Bleeding disorders caused by abnormalities of the vessel wall develop due to vascular malformation or damage. They are associated with cutaneous or mucosal flat or palpable purpura.

Of note, the commonly used but nonspecific word "purpura" is usually used to describe subcutaneous bleeding, which may be related to blood vessel wall abnormalities (described here) or platelet abnormalities.

1. Inherited vascular purpuras:

1) **Hereditary hemorrhagic telangiectasia** (Osler-Weber-Rendu disease).

2) **Purpura associated with congenital connective tissue diseases**: Ehlers-Danlos syndrome, Marfan syndrome, osteogenesis imperfecta.

2. Acquired vascular purpuras:

1) **IgA vasculitis** (Henoch-Schönlein purpura) and other forms of vasculitis (eg, serum sickness).

2) **Purpura caused by elevated venous pressure**: Small, point-like petechiae on the face and upper trunk, which may be caused by cough, vomiting, interpersonal violence, or lifting heavy objects, may develop in women after delivery, or may appear on the lower extremities due to venous stasis.

3) **Senile purpura.**

4) **Purpura caused by Cushing syndrome.**

5) **Ascorbic acid deficiency ("scurvy").**

6) **Purpura in dysproteinemia (cryoglobulinemia, Waldenström macroglobulinemia) and amyloidosis**.

7) So-called **simple purpura** (mild purpura occurring in young women, which exacerbates during menstruation and is probably related to female sex hormones).

8) **Purpura related to trauma or sunburn**.

9) **Purpura associated with infection**: This is usually due to meningococcal, streptococcal, *Salmonella* spp, or other rare bacterial infections such as *Capnocytophaga canimorsus, Pasteurella multocida,* varicella-zoster virus, influenza virus, measles virus, or malaria. It may also develop in patients with gram-negative sepsis, for instance, Waterhouse-Friderichsen syndrome, pneumococcal sepsis, endocarditis, purpura fulminans (a rapid severe purpura in the course of infections, which initially manifests as fever, rigors, massive symmetric purpura on the lower extremities and trunk, and progresses to bullous and necrotic lesions that may lead to gangrene or even autoamputation of fingers). The risk of such infections is increased significantly by splenectomy, functional hyposplenism, or the use of selected medications, such as eculizumab.

10) **Purpura related to thromboembolism**: Hemorrhagic and necrotic lesions in patients with disseminated intravascular coagulation, heparin induced thrombocytopenia, cutaneous necrosis caused by vitamin K antagonists, antiphospholipid syndrome, embolism caused by atherosclerotic plaques, and severe hereditary deficiency of protein C.

11) **Drug-induced purpura**: Purpura located mainly on the skin of the trunk and extremities. It appears after several days to over 2 weeks of administration of certain drugs (eg, allopurinol, cytarabine, atropine, barbiturates, quinidine, phenytoin, isoniazid, methotrexate, morphine, naproxen, nitrofurantoin, penicillins, piroxicam, sulfonamides, iodine) and disappears within several days of their discontinuation.

12) **Psychogenic purpura**: Typical manifestations are painful edematous petechiae and erythema on the upper extremities and thighs, which are preceded by pruritus, burning sensation, or pain. The condition is usually mild and follows a pattern of remissions and relapses. No effective treatment is available; psychotherapy may sometimes lead to improvement.

5. Iron Deficiency and Other Hypoproliferative Anemias

5.1. Anemia of Chronic Disease

→ **DEFINITION, ETIOLOGY, PATHOGENESIS**

Anemia of chronic disease (ACD) (also termed anemia of inflammation) is caused by decreased red blood cell (RBC) production due to an activated cellular immune response and by increased production of proinflammatory cytokines and hepcidin. It is the second most common anemia after iron deficiency anemia. Its incidence increases with age and it is frequently found in patients with acute or chronic inflammatory conditions.

Causes: Acute or chronic infections, malignancy, autoimmune diseases (most frequently rheumatoid arthritis, systemic lupus erythematosus, and vasculitis syndromes), occult inflammatory conditions, selected drug therapies (eg, interferon treatment)

→ **CLINICAL FEATURES AND NATURAL HISTORY**

ACD usually manifests within a few months of the development of the underlying condition. Its severity increases with the severity of the causative disorder. Clinical manifestations include signs and symptoms of the underlying condition as well as general symptoms of anemia.

→ **DIAGNOSIS**

Diagnostic Tests

1. Complete blood count (CBC) (→Table 5-1, →Table 5-2), normal or low reticulocyte counts, normal red cell distribution width.

2. Parameters of iron metabolism: →Table 5-1, →Table 5-2.

3. Other tests: Abnormalities caused by the underlying condition, frequently increased levels of the markers of inflammation. Endogenous erythropoietin levels do not correspond to the severity of anemia. Serum transferrin receptor (sTfR) is a protein that can be assayed in the blood. It generally should be normal in patients with ACD and increased in patients with iron deficiency anemia.

Diagnostic Criteria

Normocytic and normochromic anemia after other causes of anemia (particularly coexisting iron deficiency) have been excluded.

Differential Diagnosis

Iron deficiency anemia (→Table 5-1), other types of anemia (→Table 1-1).

→ **TREATMENT**

1. Treatment of the underlying condition

2. Severe anemia: Transfusion of packed red blood cells (PRBCs).

3. Patients with anemia in the course of anticancer chemotherapy and selected other patients with low serum erythropoietin levels: Consider the use of an erythropoiesis-stimulating agent (ESA): subcutaneous **human recombinant erythropoietin α** 40,000 IU once weekly, subcutaneous **human recombinant erythropoietin β** 30,000 IU once weekly, or subcutaneous **darbepoetin** 500 µg every 3 weeks. Doses are titrated to increase hemoglobin

Table 5-1. Differential diagnosis of hypochromic anemia

Parameter	Iron deficiency anemia	Anemia of chronic disease	Thalassemia α or β	Sideroblastic anemia
Anemia severity	Any	Rarely Hb <90 g/L	Mild (in trait)	Any
MCV	↓ or ↓↓	N or ↓	↓↓	N, ↓, or ↑
Serum ferritin	↓ (may be normal or increased with inflammation/liver disease)	N or ↑	N	↑
TIBC	↑	↓	N	N
Iron				
Serum	↓	↓	N	↑
Bone marrow	↓ or absent	present	present	present

↓, decreased; ↑, increased; Hb, hemoglobin; MCV, mean corpuscular volume; N, normal; TIBC, total iron binding capacity.

Table 5-2. Differential diagnosis of anemia of chronic disease and iron deficiency anemia

Parameter	Anemia	
	Anemia of chronic disease	Iron deficiency anemia
Severity	Hb usually ≥90 g/L	Variable
Symptoms	Variable	Variable
Coincident illness	Always (anemia may be the presenting manifestation)	Variable
RBCs	Usually normochromic and normocytic, but in patients with severe and long-lasting anemia it may be hypochromic and microcytic	Hypochromic and microcytic
Other cell lines	Usually normal but may reveal leukocytosis and high platelet counts (due to underlying condition)	Sometimes high platelet counts
Serum iron	↓	↓↓
TIBC	↓	↑
Serum ferritin	N or ↑	↓ (may be N or ↑ in the setting of coincident inflammation)
Serum soluble transferrin receptor	N	↑
Bone marrow iron	N or ↑	↓ or absent

↑, increased; ↓, decreased; Hb, hemoglobin; N, normal; RBC, red blood cell; TIBC, total iron binding capacity to the lowest level sufficient to avoid PRBC transfusion. Contraindications and adverse effects: →Chapter 9.2.

4. Absolute or relative iron deficiency may be observed in some patients with ACD and should be treated with IV iron. Controversy exists regarding what ferritin and transferrin saturation level should be provided. However, a low serum ferritin level is an absolute indication for iron therapy (→Chapter 7.5.2).

5.2. Iron Deficiency Anemia

→ DEFINITION, ETIOLOGY, PATHOGENESIS

Iron deficiency anemia (IDA) is caused by an impaired heme synthesis due to systemic iron deficiency. It is characterized by the presence of microcytic red blood cells (RBCs) with a decreased hemoglobin (Hb) concentration (microcytic and hypochromic anemia) and abnormal parameters of iron metabolism (low ferritin levels, unless the patient has another reason for having an elevated ferritin level, such as systemic inflammation or liver disease).

Causes of iron deficiency:

1) **Blood loss** (the most frequent cause): Bleeding from the gastrointestinal (GI) (including bleeding caused by aspirin and other nonsteroidal anti-inflammatory drugs), urogenital (hematuria), or respiratory tract (chronic hemoptysis), trauma (including surgical procedures), multiple blood donations. Blood loss leading to iron deficiency is almost always clinically inapparent.

2) **Increased iron demand with inadequate supply**: Adolescence, pregnancy, breastfeeding, increased erythropoiesis in the course of treatment of cobalamin deficiency.

3) **GI malabsorption of iron**: After gastrectomy or various forms of bariatric surgery, *Helicobacter pylori* infection, autoimmune gastritis (~20 years before B_{12} deficiency manifestation), celiac disease, after intestinal resection, in low-protein diets, or due to high dietary contents of substances that decrease iron absorption (phosphates, oxalates, phytates, tannin).

4) **Low dietary iron contents**: Vegetarians.

5) **Iron-refractory iron deficiency anemia (IRIDA)**: A rare autosomal-recessive disorder.

6) **Chronic gastric acid suppression**: A growing body of evidence suggests that long-term use of gastric acid suppressive therapy is associated with subsequent iron deficiency.

→ CLINICAL FEATURES

1. Systemic manifestations of anemia (→Chapter 7.1).

2. Signs and symptoms of chronic iron deficiency (these may be absent in a substantial proportion of patients): Perverted appetite (pica; clay, starch, ice, dirt), pain/tingling and smoothing of the tongue, dry skin, painful cheilosis, abnormalities of nails (pale, fragile nails with longitudinal stripes and furrows) and hair (fine, fragile hair with split ends).

3. Manifestations of the underlying condition (eg, colorectal cancer).

→ DIAGNOSIS

Diagnostic Tests

1. Complete blood count (CBC): →Table 5-1; →Table 5-2; decreased Hb levels (the decrease is more pronounced than the fall in red blood cell [RBC] counts), variable microcytosis, reticulocyte counts decreasing with the increasing severity of anemia. Differential blood count can reveal RBCs of varied sizes (anisocytosis) and shapes (poikilocytosis) in the case of partial treatment; leukopenia may be present (in ~10% of patients, usually those with severe iron deficiency). Reactive thrombocytosis is commonly seen and normalizes with treatment.

2. Parameters of iron metabolism: →Table 5-1; →Table 5-2. A decreased ferritin level is the best indicator of iron deficiency unless there is coincident inflammation.

3. Other tests used to diagnose the cause of IDA:

1) Upper and lower GI tract endoscopy: In every man and postmenopausal woman; in premenopausal woman in case of GI tract symptoms or signs, positive family colorectal cancer history, or iron refractoriness; additionally, where indicated by accepted age-specific and sex-specific colon cancer screening strategies.

2) GI tract imaging if endoscopy is contraindicated.

3) Screening for celiac disease (anti–tissue transglutaminase [tTG] antibody or IgA endomysial antibody) with endoscopic confirmation where appropriate.

4) Urine analysis to detect hematuria.

In case of unexplained and refractory IDA, consider *H pylori* testing; measurements of serum gastrin, antiparietal, or intrinsic factor antibodies; and capsule endoscopy.

Diagnostic Criteria

→Definition, Etiology, Pathogenesis, above.

Differential Diagnosis

Other types of anemia, particularly microcytic, and anemia of chronic disease (→Table 5-1; →Table 5-2).

→ TREATMENT

This includes treatment of the underlying cause of iron deficiency as well as iron replacement therapy aimed at restoring normal ferritin levels. All patients with unexplained iron deficiency should be assumed to have GI malignancy until this is excluded with endoscopy. In case of severe symptomatic anemia, transfuse packed red blood cells (PRBCs).

1. Patients with no known malabsorption: Administer **oral iron preparations** in doses equivalent to 150 to 200 mg of elemental iron per day or every other day (lower doses [even 30 mg] may be effective as well) in the form of tablets, chewing gum, or syrup; alternatively, use fixed combinations of iron and ascorbic acid 100 to 200 mg/d (ascorbic acid increases GI iron absorption). Preparations vary in their requirement for being taken on an empty stomach. If possible, avoid long-term gastric acid suppression therapy. The effectiveness of the therapy is evidenced by an increase in reticulocyte counts after 5 to 10 days of starting treatment and a slow increase in Hb concentration after 1 to 2 weeks of therapy. The treatment should be continued for 3 months after the normalization of Hb and ferritin levels.

2. Patients with intolerance of or refractoriness to oral iron supplements, persistent significant iron loss (eg, due to GI bleeding), treated with an erythropoiesis-stimulating agent in the setting of chemotherapy, with malabsorption, inflammatory bowel disease, chronic inflammatory disease, or chronic kidney disease: Use **parenteral iron**, usually IV or in exceptional cases IM while strictly observing the administration instructions recommended by the manufacturer. A variety of dosing regimens are currently available; for convenience, administration of larger doses at lower frequency over smaller doses is generally desirable, where appropriate medications are available. A total dose of 1 to 1.2 g is generally given and response monitored using the ferritin and hemoglobin levels.

Due to the risk of severe hypersensitivity reaction (HSR), iron infusions should be given only at appropriately staffed sites equipped with resuscitation facilities. In case of HSR, stop the infusion. You may resume the iron infusion at 50% of the initial infusion rate after ≥15 minutes in case of mild HSR with spontaneous resolution.

→ SPECIAL CONSIDERATIONS

Pregnant and breastfeeding women should receive prophylactic iron supplements in the dose of 30 mg/d, and in case of iron deficiency, 100 to 200 mg/d. Parenteral iron should be used with caution due to the risk of HSR.

5.3. Sideroblastic Anemia

→ DEFINITION, ETIOLOGY

Sideroblastic anemia refers to a heterogeneous group of disorders of heme synthesis characterized by the presence of hypochromic red blood cells and accumulation of iron in the cytoplasm of erythroblasts (sideroblasts). It may be inherited or acquired. Acquired sideroblastic anemia may be further divided into clonal (classified as myelodysplastic syndrome) or metabolic (reversible), caused by copper or pyridoxine deficiency, zinc or lead poisoning, drugs (isoniazid, cycloserine, chloramphenicol), or alcohol dependency.

→ CLINICAL FEATURES

Clinical features are nonspecific and include general symptoms of anemia (in patients with severe disease) as well as manifestations of the underlying condition. Complete blood count (CBC) and biochemical tests: →Table 5-1. Bone marrow examination reveals increased iron deposition and ring sideroblasts (the diagnostic criterion is >10% of ring sideroblasts).

→ TREATMENT

Treatment of the underlying condition in acquired reversible cases. In inherited anemia attempt a course of treatment with pyridoxine 50 to 200 mg/d; if this is ineffective, use symptomatic treatment (packed red blood cell transfusions, treatment of iron overload).

6. Iron Overload

6.1. Hereditary Hemochromatosis

→ DEFINITION, ETIOLOGY, PATHOGENESIS

Hereditary hemochromatosis (HH) is a genetically determined disease in which excessive absorption of iron in the small intestine leads to iron overload, that is, accumulation of iron in the parenchymal organs (especially in the liver, heart, pancreas, other endocrine glands, and joints) resulting in tissue and organ damage. HH can be caused by mutations in the *HFE* gene (*HFE*-related hereditary hemochromatosis) (*HFE*-HH) or other genes encoding hemojuvelin, hepcidin, transferrin receptor 2, or ferroportin (non–*HFE*-related hemochromatosis)

HFE-HH is an autosomal recessive condition. In ≥80% of patients it is caused by the C282Y mutation in the gene encoding hemochromatosis protein (HFE), a membrane protein. This protein is one of the factors stimulating hepatic synthesis of hepcidin, an acute phase protein that inhibits gastrointestinal iron absorption and release of iron from macrophages. Clinical penetration of this mutation is low (~28% in men and ~1% in women, which is attributed to the protective effects of blood loss during menstruation and iron demands of pregnancy). In the remaining cases, *HFE*-HH is caused by other mutations in the *HFE* gene (eg, H63D or S65C).

The following **4 pathophysiologic mechanisms** are implicated in primary hemochromatosis:

1) Increased upper intestinal absorption of dietary iron.

2) Decreased expression of hepcidin for iron regulation.

3) Altered HFE protein function.

4) Tissue injury and fibrogenesis related to iron overload, particularly liver damage.

→ CLINICAL FEATURES AND NATURAL HISTORY

HH is classified into the following stages:

1) Stage 1: Genetic disorder with no increase in iron stores but with genetic susceptibility.

2) Stage 2: Genetic disorder with phenotypic evidence of iron overload but no end-organ damage.

3) Stage 3: Genetic disorder with iron overload and end-organ damage.

The prevalence of clinically overt *HFE*-HH is higher in men than in women. The onset of symptoms is usually >40 years of age in men and >50 years in women. Early manifestations include fatigue, loss of libido, and arthralgia (most commonly affecting the hands and wrists). Later signs and symptoms result from chronic hepatitis or cirrhosis, cardiomyopathy, pancreatic damage (diabetes mellitus in ~70% of patients), accumulation of iron and melanin in the skin (increased pigmentation), and hormonal abnormalities (hypopituitarism, mainly gonadotropic, and rarely hypothyroidism). However, increasingly patients are being identified in the asymptomatic stage if ferritin testing is included in routine blood screening tests. Untreated hemochromatosis is progressive. Approximately a third of patients with cirrhosis develop hepatocellular carcinoma (HCC).

Juvenile hemochromatosis, caused by mutations in genes encoding hepcidin or hemojuvelin, has a more severe and rapid course. The onset of symptoms (hypogonadism and heart failure) occurs between the ages of 15 and 20 years.

→ DIAGNOSIS

Diagnostic Tests

1. Blood tests: Elevated ferritin levels and significantly elevated transferrin saturation (>45%). In hepatic iron overload elevated serum alanine aminotransferase (ALT) and aspartate aminotransferase (AST) levels may be seen.

2. Imaging studies: Features of cirrhosis and its complications. In advanced disease computed tomography (CT) and magnetic resonance imaging (MRI) reveal increased hepatic iron content. Elastography may be used to assess the severity of liver fibrosis.

3. Histologic examination of liver biopsy specimens is not necessary if ferritin is <1000 µg/L. If ferritin is >1000 µg/L, biopsy may be required for determining the stage of the disease and grading fibrosis (for prognosis evaluation). It may be used to assess hepatocyte iron content, fibrosis, and cirrhosis. The decision to biopsy should involve the patient, a hematologist, and a hepatologist. If biopsy is performed, hepatic iron concentration and histopathologic iron staining may help determine the degree and cellular distribution of iron loading.

4. Genetic studies confirm the diagnosis of HH by demonstrating specific mutations using a polymerase chain reaction (PCR) assay. The studies are indicated in (1) patients with simultaneously elevated serum ferritin levels (>200 µg/L in women, >300 µg/L in men), elevated transferrin saturation (>45%), and unexplained chronic liver disease; (2) first-degree relatives of patients with HH.

Diagnostic Criteria

Diagnostic criteria for *HFE*-HH:

1) Iron overload confirmed by elevation of serum ferritin and transferrin saturation (>45%).

2) Documented homozygosity for the C282Y mutation of the *HFE* gene in a patient with high transferrin saturation and high serum ferritin level (this is the diagnostic gold standard in *HFE*-HH) or compound heterozygosity for the C282Y/H63D mutations. Other polymorphisms of the *HFE* gene (including homozygosity for the H63D mutation) should be interpreted with caution as they are less likely to have clinical significance. Alternative causes for high ferritin levels should be investigated.

3) Liver biopsy is not required for diagnosis and usually not performed unless the diagnosis is in doubt.

Differential Diagnosis

1. High ferritin with normal transferrin saturation:

1) Other causes of liver disease including alcoholic liver disease, viral hepatitis, nonalcoholic steatohepatitis, and Wilson disease.

2) Nonhepatic inflammatory conditions: Chronic infections (eg, osteomyelitis, tuberculosis), connective tissue disease (eg, systemic lupus erythematosus, rheumatoid arthritis), malignancy.

2. Secondary iron overload states.

➡ TREATMENT

---

1. Phlebotomy is the treatment of choice to remove excess iron from the body. Early identification and initiation of phlebotomy preemptively before the development of cirrhosis or diabetes mellitus significantly reduces hemochromatosis--related morbidity and mortality. Symptomatic patients and those with existing end-organ damage should be treated to prevent progressive organ damage. Asymptomatic individuals with homozygous disease and biochemical or biopsy--proven evidence of iron overload should be treated. Phlebotomy reduces tissue iron stores and improves survival in the precirrhotic and prediabetic settings, quality of life, cardiac function, diabetes control, physical symptoms (abdominal pain, skin pigmentation, arthropathy, testicular atrophy), and biochemical and structural liver abnormalities (elevated transaminases, hepatic fibrosis, portal hypertension).

Phlebotomy is routinely performed in quantities up to 500 mL (equivalent to ~250 mg of iron) every 1 to 2 weeks until the ferritin level is reduced to 50 to 100 ng/mL (µg/L) and transferrin saturation is <50%. Phlebotomies should be done weekly, as tolerated, targeting the above serum ferritin levels and stopped at levels lower than these. It remains the treatment of choice when compared with red blood cell (RBC) removal (erythrocytapheresis).⊘○ Hematocrit and hemoglobin (Hb) levels should be allowed to decrease by a maximum of 20% from their prior level between phlebotomies. Complete blood count (CBC) and ferritin should be checked before each phlebotomy (at Hb <100 g/L the frequency of phlebotomies should be reduced; Hb before phlebotomy should be within the normal reference range or at minimum 110-120 g/L). The initial course of phlebotomy treatment should be continued until the target ferritin level is reached, with most patients requiring maintenance phlebotomy every 2 to 4 months, guided by serial serum Hb, hematocrit, and ferritin levels. In many jurisdictions patients with HH are encouraged to donate blood to the public blood supply, provided they meet other donor criteria.

2. In patients treated with phlebotomy, reduction of meat consumption is not necessary. Alcohol intake should be limited (<20 g/d; in patients with cirrhosis total abstinence is needed) and avoidance of iron and vitamin C supplements is advised, including avoidance of cooking with iron pots and skillets. Data suggesting beneficial effects of controlling iron intake are very limited.○

3. All patients should receive hepatitis A and B vaccinations. All patients with cirrhosis should receive pneumococcal and influenza vaccinations.

→ FOLLOW-UP

In the course of treatment, serum Hb and hematocrit should be assessed prior to each phlebotomy and ferritin levels (target, 50-100 µg/L) should be assessed prior to each phlebotomy or monthly. Transferrin saturation should be measured after every 10 to 12 phlebotomies (approximately every 3 months). During maintenance therapy ferritin should be assessed before every second phlebotomy.

Screening with iron studies and *HFE* mutation analysis should be done for all first-degree relatives of patients with HH. Genotypic and phenotypic testing should be performed simultaneously. For children identified through a proband (first identified patient), testing of the other parent is indicated to evaluate homozygosity or heterozygosity; further testing is warranted in homozygosity and not warranted in heterozygosity (unless there is compound heterozygosity).

Ongoing screening for cirrhosis and development of HCC should be arranged for patients regardless of whether phlebotomy is used.

→ PROGNOSIS

Approximately one-third of untreated patients survive 5 years from diagnosis. Effective treatment (before the onset of cirrhosis and other irreversible complications) is associated with survival similar to that of the general population.

6.2. Secondary Iron Overload

→ DEFINITION, ETIOLOGY, PATHOGENESIS

Secondary iron overload encompasses the following etiologies:

1) **Iron-loading anemias**, including thalassemias, sickle cell disease, sideroblastic anemias, chronic hemolytic anemia, pyruvate kinase deficiency, dehydrated hereditary stomatocytosis.

2) **Iron overload secondary to excessive intake** (iatrogenic or transfusional): Chronic or frequent red blood cell (RBC) transfusions, inappropriate iron therapy (oral or IV).

3) Miscellaneous causes: Porphyria cutanea tarda, aceruloplasminemia, congenital atransferrinemia.

→ CLINICAL FEATURES AND NATURAL HISTORY

Clinical features are similar to primary hemochromatosis.

Natural history is specific to the etiology of secondary iron overload and will not be explored in detail in this chapter.

→ DIAGNOSIS

As in primary hemochromatosis, serum ferritin is a useful screening test for iron overload. Magnetic resonance imaging (MRI) or liver biopsy (or both) are used to quantify hepatic iron concentration and guide therapy.

1. Blood tests: A general cutoff of ferritin >1000 µg/L can be applied for most cases of secondary iron overload, although it is increasingly recognized that in non–transfusion-dependent thalassemias (NTDTs) (eg, β thalassemia intermedia and hemoglobin H disease) and other inherited hemolytic anemias iron overload can be present at ferritin levels ≥300 µg/L. Transferrin saturation is useful in confirming the presence of iron overload.

2. MRI: MRI R2 or R2* scans of the liver with validated image analysis provide noninvasive quantification of hepatic iron overload and are considered the standard of care in the assessment of iron overload in transfusion-dependent thalassemia, NTDT, and sickle cell disease. Selected patients may also require specialized MRI iron assessment of other organs (eg, the heart, pancreas, or pituitary).

3. Liver biopsy for hepatic iron concentration and histopathologic iron staining can be used to directly assess hepatic iron concentration while also examining the liver tissue for findings of fibrosis. If noninvasive MRI assessment is available, liver biopsy is less likely to be used because of the procedural risks and potential for inaccurate estimation of the total hepatic iron content when hepatic iron distribution is patchy.

→ TREATMENT

Treatment should be focused on the underlying condition whenever possible.

Phlebotomy is useful for certain types of secondary iron overload. It is clearly indicated in porphyria cutanea tarda (reduction in skin manifestations), and small volume phlebotomy ("miniphlebotomy") can often be safely and successfully used in patients with NTDTs with normal or near-normal baseline hemoglobin.

In patients who are ineligible for phlebotomy, including all who are transfusion-dependent, pharmacologic iron chelation strategies are used. Deferoxamine is a parenteral therapy that can be administered via a continuous subcutaneous or IV infusion 8 to 24 hours per day at a total daily dose of 20 to 60 mg/kg/d. Options of oral iron chelation include deferasirox 10 to 40 mg/kg/d or deferiprone 75 to 100 mg/kg/d (total daily dose divided into tid dosing). Selection of iron chelation regimens depends on coexisting comorbidities, medication availability, and patient preference for administration route and frequency, as well as organs affected by iron overload and severity of iron loading. In our experience, iron chelation is typically managed by specialized medical teams.

→ FOLLOW-UP

Patients with iron overload require ferritin monitoring at regular intervals (eg, every 1-4 months). Selected patients, as outlined (→Diagnosis, above), also benefit from MRI monitoring of hepatic iron concentrations. Specialized liver MRI will often be completed annually to monitor therapeutic effects.

→ PROGNOSIS

Previously, when the availability of iron chelation agents was limited, complications of organ iron overload were one of the main causes of early mortality in patients with transfusion-dependent thalassemia. With the advent and growing availability of a variety of iron chelation drugs, it is expected that patients with these conditions will now have dramatically improved life expectancy.

7. Megaloblastic Anemias

7.1. Cobalamin Deficiency

➔DEFINITION, ETIOLOGY, PATHOGENESIS

Cobalamin (vitamin B_{12}) deficiency leads to an impaired production of erythroblasts, premature destruction of erythroblasts in bone marrow (ineffective erythropoiesis), as well as to a reduced red blood cell (RBC) life-span, consequently causing megaloblastic anemia. The minimum daily intake of cobalamin is ≤ 5 µg (mean, 2.4 µg). Its main sources are meat and milk products. The body stores of cobalamin cover a 4-year requirement. Cobalamin deficiency manifests in tissues characterized by rapid cell turnover (eg, the gastrointestinal [GI] mucosa) as well as in changes affecting the nervous system (demyelination and peripheral neuropathy).

Causes:

1) **Inadequate cobalamin dietary intake**: Vegetarian or vegan diet, alcohol dependency.

2) **Cobalamin malabsorption**: Pernicious anemia (autoimmune gastritis); congenital intrinsic factor deficiency or intrinsic factor abnormalities; gastrectomy, bariatric surgery, *Helicobacter pylori* infection, or ileal resection; Crohn disease; bacterial overgrowth syndrome; chronic pancreatitis; Zollinger-Ellison syndrome; congenital selective cobalamin malabsorption; drugs (metformin, inhibitors of gastric acid secretion, nitric oxide used in anesthesia); fish tapeworm and other GI infestations.

3) **Transcobalamin II deficiency**.

➔CLINICAL FEATURES AND NATURAL HISTORY

1. General symptoms: General symptoms of anemia are observed in advanced disease (→Chapter 7.1).

2. GI manifestations are observed in ~50% of patients and involve loss of taste; an enlarged, smoothened, and dark-red tongue; tingling of the tongue; nausea, constipation or diarrhea.

3. Nervous system manifestations: Paresthesias affecting the upper and lower extremities (usually the presenting symptom is a tingling sensation in the fingertips), numbness, gait abnormalities, miction abnormalities (these may progress to urinary tract obstruction), autonomic symptoms (orthostatic hypotension, urinary incontinence, sexual dysfunction). The first symptom of so-called "subacute combined degeneration" (demyelination of the dorsal and lateral columns of the spinal cord) is usually loss of position sense in the second toe combined with loss of vibration sense. Patients with severe chronic cobalamin deficiency have abnormal tendon and extrapyramidal reflexes (hyperreflexia or hyporeflexia), decreased muscle tone, visual abnormalities (optic atrophy), or hearing impairment. Psychiatric symptoms include cognitive dysfunction, depression, mania, mood instability, and delusions; in elderly patients, dementia may be the leading feature. Severe untreated cobalamin deficiency leads to irreversible neurologic deficits. The severity of anemia is not always correlated with the degree of neurologic dysfunction.

4. Cutaneous manifestations: Mild jaundice (lemon-yellow or wax-yellow skin), premature graying of hair, in some patients acquired vitiligo, less commonly petechiae.

→ DIAGNOSIS

Diagnostic Tests

1. Complete blood count (CBC): Macrocytosis (this precedes the development of anemia), normochromic RBCs (mean corpuscular hemoglobin, 27-31 pg/L), oval macrocytes. Other features include a low reticulocyte count, leukopenia with neutropenia, increased numbers of hypersegmented neutrophils (1% neutrophils with ≥6 nuclear lobes or 5% neutrophils with ≥5 nuclear lobes; this is the earliest feature of cobalamin deficiency), moderate thrombocytopenia, and occasionally the presence of large platelets.

2. Biochemical and immunologic studies: Low serum cobalamin levels (note that the proportion of false-positive and false-negative results is high). Supplementary findings include increased serum or plasma homocysteine and/or methylmalonic acid (MMA) levels (>400 nmol/L), features of moderate hemolysis (increased serum lactate dehydrogenase levels, decreased haptoglobin levels, minor elevations of unconjugated bilirubin levels), and increased serum iron levels. In patients with pernicious anemia autoantibodies against parietal cells and intrinsic factor are present.

3. Bone marrow biopsy reveals hypercellular bone marrow with megaloblastic changes, features of dyserythropoiesis and intramedullary hemolysis, multiple giant metamyelocytes and bands, hypersegmented granulocytes, and large multinucleated megakaryocytes.

4. Gastroscopy: Features of atrophic gastritis.

5. Response to treatment: Prompt normalization of hematologic parameters after administration of vitamin B_{12} supports the diagnosis of cobalamin deficiency. Care should be exercised to ensure that coexisting B_{12} and folate deficiency are not present, as treatment of only folate deficiency can exacerbate underlying B_{12} deficiency.

The Schilling test is of historical interest as a test for B_{12} absorption; it may still be available in some jurisdictions but is no longer available in most countries. It tests for the ability to absorb radiolabeled vitamin B_{12}.

Diagnostic Criteria

Diagnosis is based on the clinical features, low serum cobalamin levels, and/or elevated MMA levels.

Differential Diagnosis

Folate deficiency, other types of anemia associated with dyserythropoiesis (sideroblastic anemia, myelodysplastic syndromes), other conditions associated with RBC macrocytosis (alcohol dependency, cirrhosis, purine inhibitors [methotrexate, mercaptopurine, cyclophosphamide, zidovudine, trimethoprim], hydroxyurea, hypothyroidism).

→ TREATMENT

1. Parenteral or oral **cyanocobalamin**:

1) IM or deep subcutaneous cyanocobalamin 1 mg daily for 7 to 14 days followed by administration once a week until the resolution of anemia (4-8 weeks). Maintenance treatment (especially in patients with neurologic manifestations) includes lifelong IM administration of 1 mg of cyanocobalamin once per month. In cases of severe deficiency the first dose of parenteral cobalamin can be associated with severe symptomatic hypokalemia reported to be associated with cardiac dysrhythmia and death.

2) The efficacy of high-dose oral cyanocobalamin (1-2 mg/d) is the same as in parenteral treatment. A replacement oral dose as low as 1 mg/mo may be enough once stability is achieved.

2. Symptomatic anemia: Transfusion of **packed red blood cells**.

→ **P R O G N O S I S**

Treatment leads to the resolution of anemia and hematologic abnormalities. An increase in reticulocyte counts and decrease in mean corpuscular volume are observed after 4 to 5 days of treatment. Hemoglobin levels, hematocrit values, and RBC counts start to increase as early as after 7 days of treatment and return to normal after ~2 months of treatment. Peripheral neuropathy may partially improve (usually within 6 months), but demyelination of the spinal cord is irreversible. Pernicious anemia is associated with a 2- to 3-fold increase in the risk of gastric adenocarcinoma.

→ **P R E V E N T I O N**

Prophylactic administration of cyanocobalamin may be necessary in patients after gastric surgery. Vegetarians, and particularly vegans, should take supplements.

7.2. Folate Deficiency

→ **D E F I N I T I O N , E T I O L O G Y , P A T H O G E N E S I S**

Folate deficiency leads to abnormalities of DNA synthesis, resulting in megaloblastic anemia. Minimum daily dietary folate requirements in adults are 0.1 to 0.15 mg (0.6 mg in pregnant women and 0.5 mg in breastfeeding women). The main sources of folate are green vegetables, citrus fruits, nuts, yeast, and animal products (liver). The body stores of folate cover up to a 4-month requirement. After being absorbed in the gastrointestinal (GI) tract, folate is converted to tetrahydrofolate; the conversion occurs only in the presence of cobalamin (vitamin B_{12}). In many nations dietary folate supplementation has completely eliminated this disorder.

Causes of folate deficiency:

1) **Inadequate dietary intake**: Low consumption of fresh foods or foods boiled for a short time (boiling for >15 minutes causes the degradation of folate), in particular of green vegetables, and total parenteral nutrition without folate supplementation.

2) **Inadequate absorption**: Crohn disease.

3) **Chronic liver disease** (mainly cirrhosis).

4) **Drugs**: Phenytoin, sulfasalazine, folate antagonists (methotrexate, trimethoprim).

5) **Alcohol dependency**.

6) **Zinc deficiency**.

7) **Increased folate demand**: Pregnancy, breastfeeding, inflammatory conditions, malignancy.

8) **Increased folate loss**: Renal replacement therapy, chronic hemolytic anemia.

→ **C L I N I C A L F E A T U R E S**

Clinical features are the same as in cobalamin deficiency (→Chapter 7.7.1); nervous system manifestations and jaundice are not observed in folate deficiency. Focal cutaneous and mucosal hyperpigmentation (the former particularly on the dorsal areas of fingers) also may be observed. Folate deficiency may cause infertility.

→ DIAGNOSIS

Diagnostic Tests

1. Complete blood count (CBC): As in cobalamin deficiency.

2. Biochemical studies: Decreased plasma (or red blood cell [RBC]) folate levels, features of moderate hemolysis (elevated serum lactate dehydrogenase levels, decreased haptoglobin levels, minor increases in unconjugated bilirubin levels), increased serum iron levels.

3. Bone marrow biopsy: As in cobalamin deficiency.

Diagnostic Criteria

Reduced folate levels. RBC folate may be more reliable than serum folate.

Differential Diagnosis

Cobalamin deficiency, other types of anemia associated with dyserythropoiesis (sideroblastic anemia, myelodysplastic syndromes), other conditions associated with RBC macrocytosis (alcohol dependency, cirrhosis, purine inhibitors [methotrexate, mercaptopurine, cyclophosphamide, zidovudine, trimethoprim, hydroxyurea], hypothyroidism).

→ TREATMENT

1. Treatment of the underlying condition.

2. A diet rich in high-folate food (→Definition, Etiology, Pathogenesis, above).

3. Oral **folic acid** 0.8 to 1.2 mg/d (up to 5 mg/d in patients with malabsorption) for 1 to 4 months, until the normalization of hematologic parameters or as long as the cause of folate deficiency persists. The effectiveness of treatment is evidenced by a rapid increase in reticulocyte counts on days 4 to 7 of treatment. In the early stages of treatment, hypokalemia may occur. Starting folate treatment alone in a patient with coexisting cobalamin deficiency may cause an acute onset of neurologic manifestations (or their worsening, if already present).

4. A common practice is to give folate in patients with an expected increased need, for example, those with hemolytic anemia or those with a recovering marrow after a bleeding event; the evidence for this is weak.

8. Neoplastic and Other Proliferative Disorders

8.1. Acute Lymphoblastic Leukemia

→ DEFINITION, ETIOLOGY, PATHOGENESIS

Acute lymphoblastic leukemia (ALL)/lymphoblastic lymphoma (LBL) are malignancies originating from B-lymphocyte or T-lymphocyte precursor cells (lymphoblasts). The lymphoblasts are present mainly in bone marrow and peripheral blood (B-cell ALL, T-cell ALL) or less frequently in lymph nodes and extranodal sites (B-cell LBL, T-cell LBL). In children <15 years ALL/LBL constitute ~25% of all malignancies and ~75% of all leukemias. In adults they usually develop before 30 years of age and account for ~20% of acute leukemias.

The 2016 World Health Organization (WHO) classification is based on cell origin and biology. In B-cell and T-cell subtypes genetically and molecularly distinct clinical entities are defined, while other types are jointly classified as "ALL/LBL, not otherwise specified." Burkitt-type ALL is a leukemic manifestation of Burkitt lymphoma, which is currently classified as a mature B-cell malignancy.

The immunophenotypic classification is of key importance for clinical practice. It includes:

1) **B-cell ALL**: Pro-B (pre-pre-B) ALL, common ALL (CD10+, the most frequent type), pre-B ALL.

2) **T-cell ALL**: Pro-T and pre-T ALL (CD1a−, cyCD3+), cortical ALL (CD1a+, relatively good prognosis), medullary T-cell ALL (CD1a−, sCD3+).

➡ CLINICAL FEATURES AND NATURAL HISTORY

1. Signs and symptoms are similar to acute myeloid leukemia but lymphadenopathy, splenomegaly, or both are observed in as many as 50% of patients, and manifestations of the involvement of erythropoietic and megakaryopoietic lineages are less severe. Twenty five percent of patients develop bone and joint pain. ALL can present as an oncologic emergency, such as febrile neutropenia, tumor lysis syndrome, or leukostasis. Central nervous system (CNS) involvement is relatively more common than in AML and ranges from 3% in B-cell ALL to 8% in T-cell ALL. In patients with T-cell ALL mediastinal lymph node enlargement as well as high white blood cell (WBC) counts are frequent.

2. Natural history: In patients with early disease the abnormalities may be limited to the complete blood count (CBC). Patients with advanced disease present with bleeding, infection, or with signs of CNS, mediastinal, and other organ involvement, which untreated lead to death within a few weeks.

➡ DIAGNOSIS

Diagnostic Tests

1. CBC: Leukopenia may be observed in patients with certain subtypes of ALL (particularly in early disease); leukocytosis (very high and rapidly increasing in patients with T-cell ALL subtypes). In ~25% of patients with pro-B ALL, WBC counts are $>100 \times 10^9$/L. Anemia, neutropenia, and thrombocytopenia are usually seen. Lymphoblasts may be seen in peripheral blood. Eosinophilia may be also present (in T-cell ALL).

2. Biochemical tests to assess renal function or evidence of tumor lysis (uric acid, phosphate, potassium) in addition to coagulation tests.

3. Bone marrow examination: Bone marrow aspiration with microscopic examination and immunophenotyping.

4. Immunophenotyping using flow cytometry (peripheral blood or bone marrow) is the basis for confirming the diagnosis and the immunophenotypic classification, which facilitates the assessment of prognosis as well as identification of the abnormalities that are used in monitoring minimal residual disease (MRD) during treatment.

5. Cytogenetic and molecular studies: In the majority of patients with ALL, lymphoblasts have an abnormal karyotype, including abnormalities in the chromosome numbers and structure. Translocation t(9;22), also termed the Philadelphia (Ph) chromosome, is found in 20% to 30% of all ALL cases, more frequently in patients with common ALL and in elderly patients (up to 50%), and is associated with the highest risk. Quantitative molecular studies (real-time quantitative polymerase chain reaction) are also used for MRD monitoring (eg, identification of the *BCR-ABL1* fusion gene in patients with Ph+ ALL). A number of other genetic abnormalities, beyond the scope of this text, are recognized and tested for in specialized settings to determine prognosis and optimal treatment.

6. Imaging studies: In ~50% of patients with T-cell ALL subtypes, upper mediastinal mass caused by involvement of the thymus and mediastinal lymph nodes is seen. Imaging is useful in assessing the size of the lymph nodes and spleen. A biopsy from extramedullary disease can be obtained for diagnostic purposes.

7. Lumbar puncture: In the case of CNS involvement lumbar puncture may reveal increased cerebrospinal fluid (CSF) cell counts with blasts detected by cytologic examination.

Diagnostic Criteria

Bone marrow microscopy and immunophenotyping are essential for diagnosis. The presence of lymphoblasts must be documented and ≥2 B-cell or T-cell markers must be found to confirm the diagnosis. In ~20% of patients, features of LBL are predominant, with infiltrates affecting mainly lymph nodes and <20% to 25% blasts in bone marrow; in such cases examination of a lymph node may be necessary.

Differential Diagnosis

Poorly differentiated AML; infectious mononucleosis; other viral infections, particularly causing lymphocytosis, thrombocytopenia, or hemolytic anemia; other conditions causing pancytopenia; non-Hodgkin lymphomas.

→ TREATMENT

Choice of therapy based on patient-related and disease-related factors helps in management decisions. Older patients with comorbidities do not receive the same chemotherapy medications as younger patients with good performance status. In patients with Philadelphia chromosome the use of tyrosine kinase inhibitors (TKIs) is indicated.

1. Initial treatment is aimed at decreasing leukemic cell burden to reduce the risk of tumor lysis syndrome; this may involve the use of prednisone or dexamethasone. Prophylaxis of tumor lysis syndrome should be provided to all patients initiating therapy (→Chapter 9.1.1). This includes IV fluids and allopurinol, a xanthine oxidase enzyme inhibitor that is considered to be one of the most effective drugs used to decrease urate levels. In patients with high disease burden and increased urate levels, rasburicase, a recombinant urate oxidase enzyme that catalyzes uric acid and helps its elimination, may be used.

2. Remission induction is aimed at removing tumor burden; this includes 3-drug to 4-drug combination chemotherapy regimens (eg, vincristine, an anthracycline, glucocorticoids [prednisone or dexamethasone], and pegylated asparaginase; usually for 4 weeks). Assessment for response to therapy at the end of induction determines if further combination chemotherapy is required for refractory or measurable disease.

3. Remission consolidation is aimed at removing MRD; this includes sequential cycles of high-dose or intermediate-dose antineoplastic agents. These usually include vinca alkaloids, glucocorticoids, thiopurines, and asparaginase.

4. Postconsolidation treatment:

1) In standard-risk patients and in patients who are not eligible for hematopoietic stem cell transplantation (HSCT), **maintenance treatment is continued for 2 years**, provided the MRD-negative status is maintained.

2) In high-risk patients (>80% of adult patients; →Prognosis, below), **allogeneic HSCT** from a human leukocyte antigen (HLA)-compatible sibling or an unrelated donor should be considered.

5. Treatment of Ph+ ALL: Chemotherapy combined with TKIs (imatinib, dasatinib) with the goal of allogeneic HSCT in patients who qualify for this therapy. Because genetic mutations such as T135I may infer resistance to TKI therapy, ponatinib would be the TKI of choice.

6. Prevention and treatment of CNS involvement: All patients receive intrathecal chemotherapy during induction for prophylaxis. Those with CNS disease receive therapeutic intrathecal chemotherapy doses as well as—depending on the risk profile, age, and comorbidities—CNS radiation.

7. Management of patients with no response to the first-line treatment or with relapses: New agents, drugs with no cross-resistance with the first-line agents, other drug combinations, HSCT (all decided in specialized settings only).

8. Supportive treatment as in acute myeloid leukemia.

9. Complications:

1) Early complications: Cytopenias and infection, toxicities of CNS-directed therapy, osteonecrosis, deep vein thrombosis, and pancreatitis.

2) Late complications: Obesity and metabolic syndrome, peripheral neuropathy, cardiotoxicity, neurocognitive deficits, and secondary malignant neoplasms.

→ PROGNOSIS

Risk groups:

1) **Standard-risk group**:

   a) Age <35 years.

   b) WBC $<30 \times 10^9$/L in B-cell ALL or $<100 \times 10^9$/L in T-cell ALL.

   c) Immunophenotype: Common/pre-B ALL or cortical (CD1a$^+$) T-cell ALL.

   d) Complete remission (CR) achieved within <4 weeks.

2) **High-risk group**: All patients not included in points 1 and 3.

3) **Very high-risk group**: Karyotype t(9;22) [Ph+, *BCR-ABL1*+].

The importance of risk groups may change in the course of treatment. Apart from the above cytogenetic abnormalities, the most important adverse prognostic factor that is the basis for the classification of patients into standard-risk and high-risk groups is the MRD status monitored using cytogenetic or molecular studies at subsequent stages of treatment. CR is achieved in >90% of adult patients with ALL. Overall 5-year survival rates in adults: 54% in patients <30 years of age; 35% in patients 30 to 44 years of age; 24% in patients 45 to 60 years of age; and 13% in patients >60 years of age.

Patients with the Ph chromosome historically had a poor prognosis but the use of TKI (imatinib) has improved the rates of event-free survival in this group.

8.2. Acute Myeloid Leukemia

→ DEFINITION, ETIOLOGY, PATHOGENESIS

Acute myeloid leukemia (AML) is a heterogeneous hematologic malignancy that is characterized by the presence of a clone of transformed myeloid cells originating at early stages of myelopoiesis. The cells predominate in bone marrow and peripheral blood and infiltrate various organs, affecting their function.

Risk factors include exposure to ionizing radiation, benzene, and cytotoxic agents (alkylating drugs, topoisomerase inhibitors).

Classification had been based on morphology until some recurrent cytogenetic abnormalities were identified, which helped with better understanding of disease biology and choice of therapy. AML can be classified into de novo AML or secondary AML with antecedent blood cancer. There is also a subset that is therapy-related where prior radiation therapy or chemotherapy cause the emergence of a malignant clone.

AML with myelodysplasia-related changes (AML-MRC) is known to be of poor prognosis due to the higher incidence of cytogenetic abnormalities associated with poor risk, commonly in older patients with comorbidities, transfusion dependence, risk of catastrophic bleeding, and/or iron overload.

→ CLINICAL FEATURES AND NATURAL HISTORY

1. General symptoms: Constitutional symptoms including fevers, weight loss, and drenching sweats in addition to fatigue and bone and joint pain.

2. Manifestations of anemia; thrombocytopenia with associated mucocutaneous bleeding, petechial rash, urogenital and/or gastrointestinal bleeding. Other features involve those of immunodeficiency with recurrent infection symptoms, including bacterial sepsis and fungal infections.

3. Manifestations of leukostasis associated with white blood cell (WBC) counts >100×10⁹/L: Altered mental status, headache, visual disturbances, angina, features of hypoxemia caused by impaired pulmonary perfusion, and priapism.

4. Manifestations of leukemic infiltrates in various tissues and organs, more commonly seen in patients with monocytic leukemia: Leukemia cutis, gingival infiltrates, pulmonary infiltrates, splenomegaly and/or hepatomegaly, and/or lymphadenopathy. Central nervous system (CNS) leukemia is common in patients with higher WBC counts who present with various symptoms including headaches, visual changes, and nausea or vomiting.

→ DIAGNOSIS

Diagnostic Tests

1. Complete blood count (CBC): Any degree of pancytopenia with leukopenia, anemia and thrombocytopenia. Leukocytosis is also possible with accompanying left shift and pathognomonic circulating blasts.

2. Bone marrow aspiration and biopsy: Assessment by morphology, cytochemistry, immunophenotyping, cytogenetic analysis, and molecular studies to detect mutations using the myeloid next-generation sequencing panel. Such mutations could carry a prognostic significance or would indicate targeted therapy (→Treatment, below). Bone marrow biopsy gives an idea on cellularity, stromal abnormalities, or antecedent myeloid malignancy. The presence of Auer rods on bone marrow examination is pathognomonic of AML.

3. Other laboratory studies: Coagulation parameters, serum lactate dehydrogenase, uric acid, electrolytes, calcium, magnesium, and phosphate levels. Tumor lysis is common in patients with high WBC counts at presentation, hyperuricemia, hyperkalemia, hypocalcemia, and hyperphosphatemia. Acute kidney injury can be seen due to tumor lysis or leukostasis. Patients with high WBC counts may develop artifactual hyperkalemia, hypoxemia, and hypoglycemia due to the effects of leukemic cells after the samples are drawn.

Diagnostic Criteria

The diagnosis of AML is established in patients with ≥20% blasts (including myeloblasts and their equivalents: monoblasts, promonocytes, and megakaryoblasts). In certain situations the diagnosis of AML can be made regardless of the percentage of blasts: in patients with core-binding factor AML with inv(16) or t(8;21) or those with acute promyelocytic leukemia with t(15;17) as well as patients with granulocytic sarcoma.

Classification of risk groups (according to the European LeukemiaNet) is based on the results of cytogenetic and molecular studies. The adverse-risk group also includes secondary AML in patients after radiotherapy and/or chemotherapy, AML preceded by myelodysplastic syndrome (MDS), and AML with primary treatment resistance.

Differential Diagnosis

Infectious mononucleosis, acute lymphoblastic leukemia, large B-cell lymphoma, high-risk MDS, myeloproliferative neoplasms with high blast counts, leukemoid reaction, and recovering marrow (particularly in patients with recently treated vitamin B_{12} deficiency).

→ TREATMENT

Therapeutic choice is tailored to patient-related and disease-related factors. Scoring systems such as the AML composite model for risk assessment and hematopoietic cell transplantation–specific comorbidity index (available at www.hctci.org) are helpful to evaluate the patient's eligibility for therapy. These decisions should be used in specialized settings.

Individualized therapy is offered based on the patient's Eastern Cooperative Oncology Group (ECOG) performance status (available at ecog-acrin.org), comorbidities, disease biology, molecular mutations, and cytogenetics. Such tools assist the clinician in decision-making with regard to therapeutic choices and eligibility for allogeneic hematopoietic stem cell transplantation (HSCT) after remission induction.

1. Remission induction depends on the patient's fitness for intensive chemotherapy. All patients receive induction treatment using the 3 + 7 regimen (a combination of daunorubicin and cytarabine). More intensive induction treatment using fludarabine, cytarabine, granulocyte colony-stimulating factor (G-CSF), and idarubicin—the FLAG-IDA regimen—may be offered to patients with secondary AML or therapy-related AML. In elderly patients or those with poor performance status hypomethylating agents (azacitidine or decitabine) can be used with palliative intent; this line of therapy provides good quality of life and transfusion independence. A specialized hematologist should be making decisions regarding therapy and patients should be cared for in an expert center familiar with the current best practices in treatment.

Outcomes of induction treatment: Complete remission (CR), CR with minimal residual disease (CR-MRD), CR with hematologic recovery (CR-H), CR with incomplete hematologic recovery (CR-i), partial remission (PR), or treatment failure in the case of nonresponse or progressive disease.

Criteria for CR: Bone marrow blasts <5%; absence of circulating blasts and blasts with Auer rods; absence of extramedullary disease; absolute neutrophil count (ANC) $\geq 1 \times 10^9$/L; platelet count $\geq 100 \times 10^9$/L.

2. Remission consolidation: Postremission treatment is aimed at eradicating residual disease, including minimal residual disease (MRD) (presence of leukemic cells at a level producing no clinical manifestations and detectable only using sensitive methods [flow cytometry, molecular studies]). Regimens include high-dose cytarabine administered in 3 cycles.

3. Allogeneic hematopoietic stem cell transplantation (HSCT) for patients in the adverse-risk or intermediate-risk group who have good performance status and have both access to a bone marrow transplant center and donor available. This results in 5-year disease-free survival (DFS) rates of 40% to 60%. There is up to 20% transplant-related mortality at 1 year. In patients who are elderly or have poor performance status, allogeneic HSCT with a nonmyeloablative conditioning protocol can be used.

4. Supportive treatment:

1) Tumor lysis prophylaxis should be provided to all patients initiating therapy. This includes IV fluids and allopurinol, a xanthine oxidase enzyme inhibitor that is considered to be one of the most effective drugs used to decrease urate levels. In patients with high disease burden and increased urate levels, use rasburicase, a recombinant urate oxidase enzyme that catalyzes uric acid and helps its elimination (→Chapter 9.1.1).

2) Hyperleukocytosis (>100×10^9/L): Hydroxyurea (INN hydroxycarbamide) 50 to 60 mg/kg/d until WBC counts decrease to <10×10^9/L.

3) Transfusion support: Packed red blood cells (PRBCs) to maintain hemoglobin (Hb) >70 g/L, platelet concentrates to maintain platelet >10×10^9/L or in patients with bleeding or coagulopathy.

4) Prevention of infections: Antifungal prophylaxis using posaconazole during the induction phase, antiviral prophylaxis using acyclovir until WBC count recovery. Preemptive antibacterial prophylaxis is not indicated.

5) Treatment of infections: →Chapter 8.7.

6) Symptom management: Antiemetic drugs and bowel routine.

7) Multidisciplinary team approach: Involve clinical dietitians for appropriate nutritional management, either enteral or parenteral, social workers for psychological counseling and coping mechanisms, and physiotherapy and occupational therapy for mobilization and prevention of deconditioning.

→ COMPLICATIONS

Severe or life-threatening complications may include neutropenic septicemia, end-organ damage or multiorgan failure, prolonged pancytopenia, and refractory thrombocytopenia with subsequent transfusion dependence. Iron overload, coagulopathy, and risk of intensive care unit (ICU) transfer for mechanical ventilation may all occur.

→ FOLLOW-UP

Clinical follow-up including examination and a CBC with differential count should be performed monthly for up to 6 months, then every 3 months for 1 year, then every 6 months for 2 years, and subsequently once a year.

→ PROGNOSIS

Cure rates are highest in patients aged <60 years with favorable cytogenetic features and no unfavorable molecular features who achieve rapid CR during induction therapy. Combination chemotherapy alone may achieve cure in some favorable-risk patients with AML (60% cure rate). In selected low-risk adult patients highly intensive chemotherapy regimens may produce 5-year survival rates of 40%, while HSCT is associated with >60% cure rates in eligible patients who survive to transplantation and who do not die as a result of transplantation. In other individuals, who constitute the majority of the patient population, cure rates are 10% to 15%.

8.3. Chronic Lymphocytic Leukemia

→ DEFINITION, ETIOLOGY, PATHOGENESIS

Chronic lymphocytic leukemia (CLL) is a neoplasm originating from morphologically mature B cells present in peripheral blood, bone marrow, lymphatic tissue, and other organs. Etiology is unknown. CLL is the most common type of leukemia.

→ CLINICAL FEATURES AND NATURAL HISTORY

The large majority of patients are asymptomatic at diagnosis, as most patients are diagnosed after observing asymptomatic lymphocytosis on complete blood count (CBC).

1. Symptoms: Constitutional symptoms (present in 5%-10% of patients; the first 3 are so-called B symptoms): At least 10% weight loss over the previous

Table 8-1. Rai classification of chronic lymphocytic leukemia

	Stage				
	0	I	II	III	IV
Lymphocytosis	+	+	+	+	+
Lymphadenopathy	–	+	+/–	+/–	+/–
Splenomegaly or hepatomegaly	–	–	+	+/–	+/–
Anemia (hemoglobin <110 g/L)	–	–	–	+	+/–
Thrombocytopenia (<100 × 10^9/L)	–	–	–	–	+
Percentage of patients[a]	30	25	25	10	10
Median survival (years)	12.5	8.4	6	1.5	

[a] At the moment of diagnosis.

Based on Blood. 1975;46(2):219-34 and Ann Oncol. 2005;16 Suppl 1:i50-1.

Table 8-2. Binet classification of chronic lymphocytic leukemia

Stage	Percentage of patients[a]	Clinical and hematological features	Median survival (years)
A	60	<3 areas of lymphoid enlargement[a]	>10
B	30	≥3 areas of lymphoid enlargement[a]	5
C	10	Anemia (hemoglobin <100 g/L) or thrombocytopenia (<100 × 10^9/L)	2

[a] Out of 5 areas: cervical lymph nodes (unilateral or bilateral), axillary lymph nodes, inguinal lymph nodes, spleen, liver.

Based on Cancer. 1977;40(2):855-64 and Ann Oncol. 2005;16 Suppl 1:i50-1.

6 months, fever (>38°C) persisting ≥2 weeks (with no infection), drenching night sweating for >2 weeks (with no infection), marked fatigue (≥2 in Eastern Cooperative Oncology Group [ECOG] performance status [available at ecog--acrin.org]), a subjective feeling of abdominal distention and abdominal pain (manifestations of splenomegaly).

2. Signs: Lymphadenopathy; enlargement of the spleen, rarely of the liver or other lymphatic organs (Waldeyer ring, tonsils); very rarely involvement of extralymphatic organs (most frequently skin).

3. Complications: Infections, autoimmune cytopenia (in particular autoimmune hemolytic anemia or immune thrombocytopenic purpura), acquired immunodeficiency states.

4. Natural history: The course of CLL may be predicted on the basis of the Rai staging system (→Table 8-1) or the Binet staging system (→Table 8-2). Other prognostic features include the lymphocyte doubling time; biochemical (including lactate dehydrogenase), cytogenetic, and molecular markers; *IGHV* mutation status; CD38 and ZAP-70 expression. In <10% of patients, CLL undergoes transformation to a more aggressive lymphoma (Richter syndrome). CLL and small lymphocytic lymphoma fall on a spectrum and may be indistinguishable in some patients.●

→ DIAGNOSIS

Diagnostic Tests

1. CBC: Lymphocytosis ($>5 \times 10^9$/L) with predominant small, morphologically mature lymphocytes as well as anemia and thrombocytopenia (in patients with advanced disease this is due to the suppression of normal hematopoiesis by a leukemic clone; at every stage of the disease cytopenias may also be autoimmune). Peripheral blood smear may show characteristic "smudge cells."

2. Immunophenotyping (peripheral blood or bone marrow) is used to establish diagnosis and for prognosis evaluation. It reveals clonality (kappa or lambda light chain restriction) and characteristic coexpression of B-cell antigens (CD19, CD22, CD23) and a T-cell antigen (CD5).

3. Cytogenetic (fluorescent in situ hybridization in peripheral blood) **and molecular studies**: No single cytogenetic abnormality is typical for CLL. The most frequent abnormalities of prognostic value are del(13q), trisomy 12, del(11q), del(17p), and *TP53* mutations; del(17p) and *TP53* mutations are associated with poor prognosis.

4. Other laboratory studies: Positive direct antiglobulin test results (Coombs test; in 35% of patients), hypogammaglobulinemia.

Diagnostic Criteria

1. Peripheral blood lymphocytosis $\geq 5 \times 10^9$/L with a predominant population of morphologically mature small lymphocytes.

2. Clonal nature of the circulating B cells documented by a characteristic immunophenotype observed by flow cytometry.

Differential Diagnosis

Monoclonal B-cell lymphocytosis (this is associated with the presence of a clone of lymphocytes with the phenotype characteristic for CLL, cell counts $<5 \times 10^9$/L, and no clinical symptoms or signs; the annual risk of progression to CLL is 1%-2%), prolymphocytic leukemia, hairy cell leukemia, large granular cell leukemia, mantle cell lymphoma, follicular lymphoma, Waldenström macroglobulinemia.

→ TREATMENT

1. Indications to start treatment:

1) Significant constitutional symptoms.

2) Significant anemia or thrombocytopenia caused by bone marrow involvement.

3) Massive, progressive, or symptomatic lymphadenopathy, or massive, progressive, or symptomatic spleen enlargement.

4) Very high lymphocyte counts (usually $>500 \times 10^9$/L) causing symptoms of leukostasis, or rapidly progressive lymphocytosis (>50% increase over 2 months, or lymphocyte doubling time <6 months in patients with initial lymphocyte counts $>30 \times 10^9$/L).

5) Autoimmune cytopenias refractory to initial treatment with glucocorticoids. In patients who do not require treatment, follow-up visits are recommended every 3 to 12 months (physical examination, CBC).

2. First-line treatment: CLL is a disease of active research interest with rapid advances being made in therapy. Treatment should be provided in expert clinical centers. There may be significant differences in available therapy between centers, jurisdictions, and countries.

1) Purine analogues (fludarabine, pentostatin) in monotherapy or as part of combination regimens. In young patients and in the elderly with no comorbidities, the recommended first-line regimen is FCR (fludarabine, cyclophosphamide, rituximab) repeated every 28 days.

2) Chlorambucil in monotherapy or in combination with an anti-CD20 antibody (rituximab, obinutuzumab, ofatumumab) is recommended in elderly patients or patients with comorbidities.

3) Bendamustine in monotherapy or in combination with rituximab is recommended in elderly patients with no serious comorbidities who nevertheless cannot be treated according to the FCR regimen.

4) Alemtuzumab in monotherapy or as part of combination regimens is recommended in patients with del(17p) or *TP53* mutation.

5) Ibrutinib is recommended in patients with del(17p) or *TP53* mutation.

3. Management of patients with relapse or failure of the first-line treatment:

1) If relapse or progression occurred 12 to 24 months from the end of monotherapy or 24 to 36 months from the end of immunochemotherapy, repeat the first-line treatment.

2) If relapse or progression occurred sooner, treat the patient with an alternative agent, such as venetoclax or idelalisib.

3) In selected cases allogeneic hematopoietic stem cell transplant (HSCT) may be considered.

4. Patients with purine analogue resistance, del(17p), or Richter transformation: Reduced-intensity allogeneic HSCT for transplant-eligible patients. In patients with Richter transformation, multiagent chemotherapy is required (eg, rituximab plus cyclophosphamide, doxorubicin, vincristine, and prednisone [R-CHOP] as in diffuse large B-cell lymphoma), and autologous HSCT may be preferred.

5. Prevention of infections: Influenza and pneumococcal vaccination. Oral acyclovir (INN aciclovir) 400 to 800 mg bid and sulfamethoxazole/trimethoprim 800 mg/160 mg daily 3 times a week in patients treated with purine analogues and alemtuzumab. In patients with hypogammaglobulinemia (<500 mg/dL) and recurrent respiratory tract infections requiring intravenous antimicrobial therapy and/or hospitalization, consider intravenous immunoglobulin (IVIG) or subcutaneous immunoglobulin (SCIG).

6. Treatment of autoimmune cytopenia: Glucocorticoids. Second-line treatments include splenectomy, IVIG, immunosuppressive agents, and monoclonal antibodies. If there is no response to glucocorticoids, definitive treatment of the underlying CLL is required.

→ PROGNOSIS IN PATIENTS REQUIRING TREATMENT

Treatment with purine analogues combined with cyclophosphamide and rituximab results in the highest remission rates and longest progression-free survival rates. The most frequent causes of death are infections, and many older patients die "with" the disease rather than "from" it. In younger patients (who are not expected to die of other disease), 10-year survival is >80%. The risk of developing another malignancy (solid tumors or hematologic diseases) is 2-fold to 7-fold higher than in the general population.

8.4. Chronic Myeloid Leukemia

→ DEFINITION, ETIOLOGY, PATHOGENESIS

Chronic myeloid leukemia (CML) is a myeloproliferative neoplasm involving clonal proliferation of a malignant multipotential hematopoietic stem cell. As a result of reciprocal translocation of the long arms of chromosomes 9 and 22, the Philadelphia (Ph) chromosome is formed, and the subsequent fusion of the *BCR* and *ABL1* genes leads to the development of a new mutant *BCR-ABL1* gene. This gene encodes the BCR-ABL1 fusion protein, which due to its constitutive tyrosine kinase activity causes an increased clonal proliferation of hematopoietic stem cells, inhibition of apoptosis, and impaired adhesion of leukemic cells to the bone marrow matrix.

→ CLINICAL FEATURES AND NATURAL HISTORY

Clinical manifestations include weight loss, constitutional symptoms, and manifestations of splenomegaly (left upper quadrant pain, early satiety) and hepatomegaly. Rarely patients present with leukostasis (leukocytes >200×10^9/L--300×10^9/L) that alters microcirculation, manifesting as altered mental status, visual disturbances, headache, symptoms of hypoxemia, and priapism. In ~40% of patients CML is an incidental finding in a complete blood count (CBC) performed for other reasons.

The chronic phase of CML always progresses (sometimes rapidly) to blast crisis. The progression usually follows through an intermediate accelerated phase or less often it may be direct. In patients with blast crisis, peripheral blood or bone marrow blast counts increase to >20%, consistent with acute leukemia (in ~50% of patients CML transforms into myeloid leukemia; in ~30%, into lymphoblastic leukemia; in ~10%, into megakaryoblastic leukemia; and in the remaining cases blast crisis has features of myelofibrosis). The accelerated phase and blast crisis in CML are characterized by multiple cytogenetic abnormalities, resistance to treatment, and a poor prognosis.

→ DIAGNOSIS

Diagnostic Tests

1. CBC: White blood cell (WBC) counts are elevated in all patients with CML, with mature and immature granulocytes at all stages of development, thrombocytosis (in a third of patients), and basophilia. Differential blood count reveals a left shift that may extend to blasts and includes promyelocytes, myelocytes, metamyelocytes, less frequently erythroblasts. Hemoglobin levels at diagnosis are typically normal.

2. Bone marrow examination: Required to confirm the chronic phase. Bone marrow aspiration and trephine biopsy reveal increased bone marrow cellularity with an elevated proportion of cells of neutrophilic (similar to that observed in peripheral blood) and megakaryopoietic lineages.

3. Cytogenetic and molecular studies of bone marrow (Ph chromosome) are performed both to establish diagnosis and exclude additional cytogenetic abnormalities.

4. Molecular studies of peripheral blood: These studies are used to confirm the diagnosis of CML (qualitative) and monitor response to therapy (quantitative).

Diagnostic Criteria

The diagnosis is based, at all stages, on the documented presence of the Ph chromosome using cytogenetic studies or the *BCR-ABL1* gene using molecular studies.

1. The **World Health Organization (WHO) diagnostic criteria of accelerated phase** (≥1 feature must be present):

1) 10% to 19% blasts in peripheral blood or bone marrow.
2) ≥20% of basophils in peripheral blood.
3) Sustained thrombocytopenia <100×10^9/L (unrelated to treatment).
4) Clonal cytogenetic evolution (emergent chromosomal aberrations) during treatment.
5) Progressive splenomegaly or leukocytosis not responding to treatment.

2. The **WHO diagnostic criteria of blast crisis** (≥1 feature must be present):

1) ≥20% blasts in peripheral blood or bone marrow.
2) Extramedullary blastic infiltrates (in organs other than spleen).
3) Large aggregates or clusters of blasts in bone marrow.

Differential Diagnosis

1. Conditions associated with elevated neutrophil counts:

1) Other myeloproliferative and myelodysplastic-myeloproliferative neoplasms.
2) Leukemoid reaction: Infection (WBC count ≤100×10^9/L), particularly in patients with bacterial pneumonia, meningitis, diphtheria, tuberculosis, or fungal infections.
3) Other neoplasms that produce granulocyte growth factors: Small cell lung cancer, ovarian cancer, melanoma, Hodgkin lymphoma.
4) Other conditions (WBC count, 30×10^9/L-40×10^9/L): Tissue necrosis, myocardial infarction, myositis, acute hemorrhage, glucocorticoid therapy.
5) Exogenous administration of granulocyte colony-stimulating factor or granulocyte and macrophage colony-stimulating factor.

2. Conditions associated with thrombocytosis:

1) Other myeloproliferative neoplasms (eg, essential thrombocythemia).
2) Reactive thrombocytosis: Infection, malignancy, chronic inflammatory disorders, tissue damage.
3) Iron deficiency.
4) Medications: Glucocorticoids, epinephrine, vincristine, tretinoin, methimazole.

→ TREATMENT

1. Long-term treatment with tyrosine kinase inhibitors (TKIs):

1) **Imatinib** 400 mg orally once daily.
2) **Dasatinib** 100 mg orally once daily; this is effective in all patients with resistance to imatinib caused by *BCR-ABL1* gene mutations except for T315I/A, F317L, and V299L mutations.
3) **Nilotinib** 300 mg orally bid; this is effective in all patients with resistance to imatinib caused by *BCR-ABL1* gene mutations except for T315I, Y253H/F, E255V/K, and F359V mutations.
4) **Bosutinib** 400 mg orally once daily.
5) **Ponatinib** 45 mg orally once daily; this is effective in patients with the T315I mutation.

The first-line agents include imatinib, nilotinib, bosutinib, and dasatinib. In the case of imatinib resistance or intolerance, dasatinib, nilotinib (800 mg/d), or bosutinib may be used. No significant data in favor of any of these agents are available, except for the *BCR-ABL1* mutations causing resistance to any one of them. The choice of the agent should be based on the availability, cost, toxicity profile, as well as the patient's comorbidities and possible interactions with other administered drugs.

Criteria for response to treatment:

1) Complete hematologic response (CHR): WBC $<10 \times 10^9$/L, no immature granulocytes on peripheral blood film, basophils <5%, platelet count $<450 \times 10^9$/L, nonpalpable spleen. No CHR or presence of >95% Ph+ cells on cytogenetic examination following 3 months of TKI therapy is considered treatment failure.

2) Major hematologic response (MCyR) (≤35% of Ph+ cells on cytogenetic examination) and/or achieving ≤10% of *BCR-ABL1* transcript on the International Scale (IS) in real-time quantitative polymerase chain reaction after 3 months of treatment is considered optimal.

3) Complete cytogenetic response (CCyR) (no Ph+ cells on cytogenetic examination) and/or <1% of *BCR-ABL1* transcript on the IS after 6 months of treatment is optimal, 1% to 10% requires closer follow-up, and >10% warrants a change in therapy.

4) Major molecular response (MMR) (<0.1% of *BCR-ABL1* transcript on the IS) 12 months from treatment initiation or anytime afterwards is optimal. Maintaining this level of response ensures progression-free survival.

2. Allogeneic hematopoietic stem cell transplantation (HSCT) should be considered in patients in the chronic phase with the T315I mutation of *BCR-ABL1* (after a trial of ponatinib therapy) or after the failure of ≥2 TKIs.

3. Interferon α is used in pregnant women (monotherapy) and in patients with TKI treatment failure who are not eligible for allogeneic HSCT (in combination with cytarabine or another agent).

4. Hydroxyurea (INN hydroxycarbamide) is used as a short-term treatment to reduce WBC counts prior to confirming the diagnosis. It has no disease--modifying effect and no influence on survival.

5. Treatment of accelerated phase and blast crisis requires higher doses of TKIs. In patients with disease progression in the course of treatment, switch to another TKI (→above). For patients in accelerated phase/blast crisis, allogeneic HSCT should be considered, optimally after achieving a chronic phase. The only exception is TKI-naive patients with accelerated phase diagnosed de novo in whom the optimal response to TKI treatment has been achieved.

6. Treatment-free remission (TFR) is ongoing molecular remission in the absence of TKI therapy. Patients can only be considered for a trial of TFR if high-quality monitoring can be assured. Following ≥3 years of TKI therapy patients may attempt TFR if they have achieved a deep molecular response (*BCR-ABL1* transcript ≤0.01% on the IS or deeper) and maintained it for ≥2 years. Patients attempting TFR must undergo molecular monitoring for relapse (>0.1% of *BCR-ABL1* transcript on the IS) every 4 weeks for ≥6 months.

→ PROGNOSIS

The response to TKI treatment is the most important prognostic factor. In patients treated with imatinib, 7-year rates of progression-free survival and survival free of accelerated phase/blast transformation are 81% and 93%, respectively. In patients undergoing allogeneic HSCT (from a related donor), the 3-year survival rate is reported as up to 76%.◓

8.5. Chronic Myelomonocytic Leukemia

→ DEFINITION, ETIOLOGY, PATHOGENESIS

Chronic myelomonocytic leukemia (CMML) is a rare (0.3 cases/100,000 people/year) clonal hematologic disorder characterized by persistent monocytosis in peripheral blood, the absence of the Ph chromosome and *BCR-ABL1* gene, and

≤20% blasts in bone marrow. CMML combines myeloid cell proliferation with myeloid cell dysplasia and ineffective hematopoiesis.

→ CLINICAL FEATURES AND NATURAL HISTORY

General symptoms are weakness, fatigue, weight loss, fever, and night sweats.

Signs and symptoms of cytopenias include features of anemia (easy fatigability, tachycardia, pale skin), neutropenia (increased susceptibility to infections), and thrombocytopenia (bleeding).

Signs and symptoms caused by extramedullary leukemic infiltrates: Hepatosplenomegaly, lymphadenopathy, cutaneous lesions; pleural, pericardial, and peritoneal effusions in patients with high monocyte counts.

Natural history depends on the stage of the disease (CMML-1 or CMML-2). The risk of transformation to acute myelogenous leukemia (AML) is 15% to 30%. The median survival is between 20 and 40 months.

→ DIAGNOSIS

Diagnostic Tests

1. Complete blood count (CBC): Monocytosis $>1 \times 10^9$/L, white blood cell (WBC) counts normal or slightly decreased (neutropenia) in ~50% of patients, otherwise slightly increased; mild basophilia and eosinophilia; moderate thrombocytopenia is frequent, and in some patients atypical giant platelets may be observed; normocytic (rarely macrocytic) anemia.

2. Bone marrow examination: In 75% of patients bone marrow aspiration reveals increased bone marrow cellularity, usually with dominant neutrophil or erythroid lineage and evident monocytic proliferation; >50% of patients have dysplastic changes, and in >80% of patients megakaryocytes with abnormal nuclear segmentation are observed. In ~30% of cases trephine biopsy also reveals bone marrow fibrosis.

3. Cytogenetic and molecular studies, immunophenotyping: Nonspecific clonal cytogenetic abnormalities are observed in 20% to 40% of patients. About 20% of patients with CMML have the *JAK2* mutation.

4. Imaging studies: Abdominal ultrasonography may reveal hepatosplenomegaly, lymphadenopathy, and ascites. **Chest radiographs** may show pleural effusions. **Echocardiography** may reveal pericardial effusion.

Diagnostic Criteria

1. The **World Health Organization (WHO) diagnostic criteria:**

1) Persistent peripheral blood monocytosis $\geq 1 \times 10^9$/L with monocytes accounting for ≥10% of WBC count.

2) Not meeting WHO criteria for chronic myeloid leukemia, primary myelofibrosis, polycythemia vera, or essential thrombocythemia. The presence of features of myeloproliferative neoplasm (MPN) in bone marrow (eg, increased numbers of enlarged, mature megakaryocytes with hyperlobulated nuclei) and/or mutations in *JAK2*, *CALR*, or *MPL* tend to support MPN with monocytosis rather than CMML.

3) In cases with eosinophilia, no evidence of *PDGFRA*, *PDGFRB*, or *FGFR1* rearrangement or *PCM1-JAK2*.

4) Less than 20% blasts (myeloblasts, monoblasts, and promonocytes) in bone marrow and peripheral blood.

5) Dysplasia in >1 myeloid lineages.

6) If dysplasia is absent or minimal, the diagnosis of CMML may still be made if the other requirements are met and an acquired clonal cytogenetic or molecular genetic abnormality is present in myeloid cells or when the

monocytosis has persisted for ≥3 months and all other causes of monocytosis have been excluded.

2. CMML subgroups:

1) CMML-0 (<2% blasts in peripheral blood and <5% in bone marrow).

2) CMML-1 (2%-4% in peripheral blood and/or 5% to 9% in bone marrow).

3) CMML-2 (5%-19% blasts in peripheral blood and/or 10%-19% in bone marrow and/or Auer rods present).

Differential Diagnosis

1. Infection: Bacterial infections (tuberculosis, syphilis, endocarditis), viral infections (cytomegalovirus, varicella/zoster, herpes simplex), fungal infections (acute and chronic).

2. Diseases of the gastrointestinal system: Inflammatory bowel disease (Crohn disease, ulcerative colitis), alcoholic liver disease, celiac disease.

3. Systemic connective tissue diseases, for instance, rheumatoid arthritis, systemic lupus erythematosus, systemic vasculitis syndromes, polymyositis.

4. Granulomatous diseases, such as sarcoidosis.

5. Hematopoietic disorders: Acute monocytic and myelomonocytic leukemias, chronic myelogenous leukemia, myeloid neoplasms with the *PDGFRB* gene rearrangement, myeloproliferative neoplasms, and myelodysplastic syndrome.

6. Other: Glucocorticoid therapy, splenectomy, tetrachloroethane poisoning, convalescence phase of acute infections, bone marrow regeneration after radiotherapy or chemotherapy, use of granulocyte colony-stimulating factor (G-CSF) or granulocyte and macrophage colony-stimulating factor (GM-CSF).

→ TREATMENT

1. Supportive treatment as in myelodysplastic syndromes (eg, use of erythropoietin analogues, prophylactic antibiotics, and iron chelation).

2. Allogeneic hematopoietic stem cell transplantation (HSCT) is the only curative treatment; it may be considered in younger patients. The results of HSCT are similar to those achieved in patients with myelodysplastic syndrome with a median overall survival of 3 years.

3. Cytoreductive treatment: Usually with hydroxyurea (INN hydroxycarbamide) to control myeloproliferation.

4. Hypomethylating agents: Azacitidine is used in patients with CMML and ≥10% blasts in bone marrow.

→ PROGNOSIS

Chemotherapy rarely achieves complete remission. Prognosis can be calculated using multiple risk stratification scores, including a CMML-specific prognostic scoring system that incorporates molecular information (the CPSS-Mol; simplified form available at QxMD). This distinguishes low, intermediate-1, intermediate-2 and high risk groups with median overall survivals ranging from 17 to 68 months. Allogeneic HSCT is considered for patients from intermediate-2 and high risk groups.

8.6. Essential Thrombocythemia

→ DEFINITION, ETIOLOGY, PATHOGENESIS

Essential thrombocythemia (ET) is a myeloproliferative neoplasm characterized by markedly elevated platelet counts and an increased megakaryocyte proliferation in bone marrow.

→ CLINICAL FEATURES AND NATURAL HISTORY

1. Signs and symptoms depend on the stage of the disease as well as the number and severity of functional abnormalities in the platelets; they include features of both small-vessel and large-vessel occlusion: paresthesias, transient visual impairment, seizures, hemiparesis, symptoms of ischemic heart disease, erythromelalgia, headache, and vertigo or dizziness. Rare symptoms include mucosal and gastrointestinal bleeding caused by abnormalities of platelet function and/or acquired von Willebrand disease. Splenomegaly is seen in <50% of patients. Many patients have asymptomatic disease discovered on routine complete blood cell analysis that demonstrates thrombocytosis with or without elevations or other cell lines.

2. Natural history: The disease may remain asymptomatic for many years before the development of thrombotic (most frequently), hemorrhagic complications, or both. In ~8% of patients transformation to myelofibrosis occurs. Transformation to acute leukemia or myelodysplastic syndrome (MDS) is less frequent (~1%).

→ DIAGNOSIS

Diagnostic Tests

1. Complete blood count (CBC): Persistent elevation of platelet counts ($\geq 450 \times 10^9$/L), abnormal platelet shape and size, and various abnormalities of platelet function (most frequently impaired aggregation) can be seen.

2. Bone marrow examination: Bone marrow aspiration and/or trephine biopsy reveal increased marrow cellularity with proliferation of the megakaryocytic lineage and an increased proportion of large, mature megakaryocytes. No proliferation or immature cells of granulocytic or erythropoietic lineages are observed. Bone marrow aspiration and biopsy are important to confirm the diagnosis of ET and to distinguish it from other myeloproliferative neoplasm, particularly prefibrotic myelofibrosis.

3. Molecular studies: Most patients are found to harbor the *JAK2* V617F mutation or other clonal genetic markers (*MPL* or *CALR* mutations).

Diagnostic Criteria

To establish the diagnosis of ET, all the following criteria must be fulfilled:

1) Persistently elevated platelet counts $\geq 450 \times 10^9$/L.

2) Bone marrow biopsy showing proliferation mainly of the megakaryocyte lineage with increased numbers of enlarged, mature megakaryocytes with hyperlobulated nuclei. No significant left shift of neutrophil granulopoiesis or erythropoiesis and very rarely minor (grade 1) increase in reticulin fibers is seen.

3) Exclusion of polycythemia vera (PV), primary myelofibrosis, chronic myelogenous leukemia (CML), MDS, and other myeloid neoplasms.

4) Presence of the *JAK2* V617F mutation or other clonal genetic markers; if these are absent, exclude reactive thrombocytosis.

Differential Diagnosis

1. Thrombocytosis associated with other myeloproliferative neoplasms: PV, CML, primary myelofibrosis, MDS 5q-, refractory anemia with ring sideroblasts and thrombocytosis (RARS-T).

2. Reactive thrombocytosis: Solid tumors (mainly lung or pancreatic cancers), iron deficiency anemia, chronic inflammatory or infectious conditions, acute hemorrhage, splenectomy, chronic alcohol abuse, frequent blood donations, as well as hemolytic or drug induced anemias.

3. Familial thrombocytosis (mutations of the thrombopoietin gene).

4. Apparent thrombocytosis: Cryoglobulinemia, fragmented erythrocytes, or malignant cells in peripheral blood.

→ TREATMENT

The **choice of treatment** depends on the presence of risk factors for thrombotic complications: age >60 years, mutational status, and prior thrombosis (arterial or venous). Patients who are <60 years, have no thrombosis history, and do not harbor the *JAK2* mutation (very low risk) are treated with observation alone unless cardiovascular risk factors or vasomotor symptoms are present, in which case acetylsalicylic acid (ASA) may be used. All other patients should receive ASA unless they are receiving therapeutic anticoagulation or have acquired von Willebrand disease. In patients >60 years or with a history of thrombosis add cytoreductive treatment. This may also be considered in patients with platelet counts >1500×10^9/L, progressive myeloproliferation (eg, progressive enlargement of the spleen), uncontrolled systemic symptoms, or evidence of microcirculatory impairment due to platelet clumping that is clinically resistant to ASA.

1. Cytoreductive treatment: Hydroxyurea (INN hydroxycarbamide) is the first-line drug. Second-line treatments are used in:

1) Patients in whom no significant reduction of platelet counts has been achieved using adequate hydroxyurea doses.

2) Patients with intolerance of hydroxyurea.

Second-line agents:

1) Anagrelide.

2) Interferon α.

3) Busulfan (consider these in patients with short life expectancy).

2. Antiplatelet agents: ASA 50 mg to 100 mg once daily (bid administration may be considered in patients not responding to the once-daily treatment) in all patients with microcirculation abnormalities (eg, erythromelalgia), except for patients with acquired von Willebrand disease. The second-line agents are clopidogrel 75 mg once daily or ticlopidine 250 mg bid. Patients requiring therapeutic anticoagulation (eg, atrial fibrillation, venous thrombosis) do not require ASA unless there are compelling indications (eg, recent coronary artery stenting).

3. Appropriate preventative measures should be used in patients with either additional risk factors for thrombosis or a history of thrombosis: →Chapter 3.15; →Chapter 3.19.

→ FOLLOW-UP

Examination of platelet counts as required to monitor cytoreductive therapy (to ensure that underdosing or overdosing does not occur). The frequency at which monitoring is required in asymptomatic patients is unknown but should be increased as the platelet count rises >1000×10^9/L.

→ PROGNOSIS

Prognosis is established on the basis of International Prognostic Score for ET:

1) Age >60 years: Score 2.

2) White blood cell count >11×10^9/L: Score 1.

3) A previous thrombotic event: Score 1.

The mean survival in patients without the above risk factors is similar to that of general population; in patients with scores 1 or 2, the mean survival is 25 years; and in patients with score 3, it is 14 years.

8.7. Hemophagocytic Lymphohistiocytosis

→ DEFINITION, ETIOLOGY, PATHOGENESIS

Hemophagocytic lymphohistiocytosis (HLH) is a disturbance of immune regulation caused by proinflammatory cytokines in a person with a concomitant dysfunction of immune cells (natural killer [NK] cells and cytotoxic T cells). The dysfunction may be congenital (familial or primary HLH, observed mainly in children; mild types of the disease may be diagnosed in adults) or acquired (secondary HLH in the setting of severe infection [most commonly Epstein-Barr virus], autoimmune disease, or malignancy [particularly lymphoma]; 6%-18% of cases are idiopathic). Hypersecretion of proinflammatory cytokines causes a pathologic inflammatory reaction that leads to generalized organ damage.

A variety of hematologic malignancies may present as HLH, including highly aggressive T cell lymphomas.

A subtype of HLH is **macrophage activation syndrome** (MAS) (→Chapter 14.21), which is differentiated from HLH on the basis of high serum C-reactive protein levels. MAS develops rarely in the course of Still disease, systemic lupus erythematosus, and in patients after bone marrow transplantation.

→ CLINICAL FEATURES AND NATURAL HISTORY

Individual differences in clinical manifestations exist, which may include persistent fever, enlargement of the liver and the spleen, and bleeding disorder; erythematous, papular, or bullous rash, which may be hemorrhagic; effusions in body cavities; and altered mental status. Untreated disease is 100% fatal.

→ DIAGNOSIS

Diagnostic Tests

1. Laboratory tests:

1) Complete blood count (CBC): Pancytopenia (usually including lymphopenia).

2) Biochemical tests (→Diagnostic Criteria, below).

3) Disseminated intravascular coagulation may be present.

2. Histologic/cytologic studies of bone marrow specimens, the spleen, lymph nodes, and sometimes of other organs or cerebrospinal fluid (CSF) (in patients with central nervous system [CNS] involvement) reveal prominent hemophagocytes. These are macrophages containing phagocytosed red blood cells (RBCs), and sometimes also other cells, for instance, white blood cells or platelets, or their fragments.

3. Other studies are performed for differential diagnosis (→Differential Diagnosis, below).

Diagnostic Criteria

Molecular diagnosis (identification of the causative mutation) or fulfilling ≥ 5 out of the 8 following criteria (according to the HLH-2004 trial):

1) Fever $\geq 38.5°C$.

2) Splenomegaly.

3) Peripheral cytopenia affecting ≥ 2 out of 3 lineages (hemoglobin <90 g/L, platelet count $<100 \times 10^9$/L, neutrophil count $<1 \times 10^9$/L).

4) Elevated triglyceride levels (fasting triglycerides ≥ 3 mmol/L [265 mg/dL]) and/or decreased fibrinogen levels (<1.5 g/L).

5) Elevated ferritin levels (≥ 500 µg/L).

6) Prominent hemophagocytes found in bone marrow, CSF, or lymph nodes.

7) Reduced or absent NK-cell activity (measured by cytotoxicity assays, such as chromium release or flow cytometry, for expression of perforin, granzyme B, or CD107a).

8) sCD25 (α chain of the interleukin-2 receptor) levels $\geq$2400 U/mL.

In patients with ferritin levels >2000 µg/L, fulfillment of only 4 criteria may be sufficient for diagnosis.

Another scoring system, HScore, available online at saintantoine.aphp.fr, can be used to estimate an individual's risk of having acquired HLH.

Differential Diagnosis

The most important condition to be differentiated from HLH is sepsis (although these two may also coexist). Other conditions that cause fever, pancytopenia, liver abnormalities, or neurologic findings (eg, hematologic malignancies) should be considered. Conditions with possible elevated ferritin levels include iron overload (repeated RBC transfusions), infections, cancers, rheumatologic/inflammatory disorders (particularly Still disease), liver diseases, and renal failure; however, the negative predictive value of a normal ferritin level for HLH diagnosis remains extremely high.

To differentiate between various causes of abnormalities that serve as diagnostic criteria of HLH, perform the following studies:

1) Laboratory tests: Reticulocyte count, erythrocyte sedimentation rate (ESR), biochemical tests (lactate dehydrogenase, aminotransferase, bilirubin, creatinine, urea/blood urea nitrogen [BUN], C-reactive protein), coagulation parameters, serum protein electrophoresis, serum immunoglobulin levels, antiglobulin (Coombs) tests.

2) Virologic studies, including diagnostics for Epstein-Barr virus infection (immunohistochemistry for latent membrane protein 1 in biopsy).

3) Neurologic examination. In patients with CNS symptoms, perform also CSF examination including a smear.

4) Ultrasonography and/or computed tomography (CT) of the spleen and the liver, and CT or magnetic resonance imaging (MRI) of the head if indicated.

5) Cytologic and histologic examination of bone marrow and/or other pathologic tissues, such as enlarged lymph nodes or liver biopsy in cases of abnormal liver function tests.

→TREATMENT

1. Treatment of HLH: Use the HLH-2004 regimen (etoposide, dexamethasone, cyclosporine [INN ciclosporin]) for 8 weeks, also in patients with relapse. In patients with CNS involvement, administer intrathecal methotrexate. In treatment-resistant patients, consider use of lymphoma chemotherapy regimens or alemtuzumab, as well as anti–interleukin-6 monoclonal antibodies (if available). In patients with HLH caused by lymphoma or other cancers, replace the HLH-2004 regimen with a standard regimen used in the causative malignancy. In inherited, refractory, or recurrent disease, allogeneic hematopoietic stem cell transplantation should be considered. Treatment of MAS: →Chapter 14.21.

Emapalumab-lzsg can be considered, where available, for the treatment of pediatric and adult patients with HLH with refractory, recurrent, or progressive disease or those who do not tolerate conventional HLH therapy.

2. Symptomatic treatment: Many patients are critically ill and require aggressive therapies to maintain life. Treatments for secondary conditions (such as suspected sepsis) should be administered.

→PROGNOSIS

Despite treatment, this disorder has very high mortality rates in adults (up to 50%-75%). These rates are largely dependent on the underlying pathology.

Table 8-3. Lugano (2014) staging system for primarily nodal lymphomas	
Clinical stage (CS)	Definition
I	One node or a group of adjacent nodes, or single extranodal lesions without nodal involvement
II[a]	≥2 nodal groups on the same side of the diaphragm, or CS I/II by nodal extent with limited contiguous extranodal involvement
III	Nodes on both sides of the diaphragm, or nodes above the diaphragm with spleen involvement
IV	Additional noncontiguous extralymphatic involvement

The tonsils, Waldeyer ring, and spleen are considered nodal tissue.

Additionally in Hodgkin lymphoma: **A**, no general symptoms; **B**, general symptoms: unexplained fever (>38°C), drenching night sweats, or weight loss >10% of body weight in the prior 6 months.

[a] CS II bulky: CS II as above and bulky disease (a single nodal mass of ≥10 cm or >1/3 of the transthoracic diameter at any level of thoracic vertebrae as determined by computed tomography).

Based on J Clin Oncol. 2014;32(27):3059-68.

8.8. Hodgkin Lymphoma

→ DEFINITION, ETIOLOGY, PATHOGENESIS

Hodgkin lymphoma (HL) is a form of lymphoma in which a small number of malignant B cells (called Reed-Sternberg cells and Hodgkin cells) reside in an abundant heterogeneous background of nonneoplastic inflammatory cells. The etiology of HL is unknown. Most patients are young adults. Unique clinicopathologic features and treatment requirements differentiate it from other lymphomas (called non-Hodgkin lymphomas [NHLs]).

→ CLINICAL FEATURES AND NATURAL HISTORY

1. General symptoms: Nonspecific symptoms (B symptoms: →Table 8-3; in ~30% of patients). Sometimes patients have pruritus or pain in the lymph nodes after consumption of alcohol.

2. Lymphadenopathy: Lymph nodes are painless. The most commonly involved nodes are supradiaphragmatic nodes: cervical and mediastinal (60%-80% of patients); as well as axillary nodes (20%-40% of patients). Subdiaphragmatic inguinal and retroperitoneal nodes are affected less frequently.

3. Symptoms related to lymphadenopathy:

1) **Mediastinal mass**: Dyspnea, cough. Extremely severe lymphadenopathy may cause superior vena cava syndrome.

2) **Retroperitoneal lymph nodes**: Abdominal discomfort, urine retention, flatulence, constipation, gastrointestinal obstruction in advanced disease.

4. Extranodal lesions: Hepatomegaly, splenomegaly; extralymphatic lesions in bones kidneys, uterus, ovaries, urinary bladder, skin, central nervous system, and testes. Unlike in NHL, involvement of the Waldeyer ring (pharyngeal lymphoid ring), gastrointestinal tract, liver, and bone marrow is uncommon.

5. Natural history: Early HL spreads locally to adjacent regions. In advanced disease, hematogenous spread to remote lymphatic regions and internal organs occurs. In untreated patients 5-year survival rates are ~5%.

6. Staging: The Ann Arbor HL classification with Lugano (2014) modification (→Table 8-3).

7. Histologic classification of HL (World Health Organization, 2016):

1) **Classical HL** includes nodular sclerosis HL (NSHL) (70%-80% of HL cases), mixed-cellularity HL (MCHL), lymphocyte-depleted HL (LDHL), and lymphocyte-rich HL (LRHL). Most patients present with early disease, which is associated with upper cervical lymphadenopathy, usually without constitutional symptoms.

2) **Nodular lymphocyte-predominant HL (NLPHL)** is observed in ~5% of patients with HL; it affects peripheral lymph nodes (usually in one lymphatic region only). The course is usually very slow, with no clinical progression over many years. Patients with relapse have a good response to treatment.

➡ DIAGNOSIS

Diagnostic Tests

1. Complete blood count (CBC): Nonspecific abnormalities may include elevated neutrophil and/or eosinophil counts, lymphocytopenia, thrombocytopenia, normocytic anemia with low serum iron levels (the usual pathogenesis is that of anemia of chronic disease), or less frequently autoimmune hemolytic anemia.

2. Bone marrow biopsy: Cells typical for HL are found in ~6% of patients.

3. Histologic and immunohistochemical examination of an involved lymph node (examination of a complete node is recommended) or other involved tissues.

4. Other laboratory tests: Abnormalities may include elevated serum lactate dehydrogenase or alkaline phosphatase, increased erythrocyte sedimentation rate (ESR), elevated γ globulin and β_2-microglobulin levels, and low serum albumin levels.

5. Imaging studies: Contrast-enhanced computed tomography (CT) (of the neck, chest, abdomen, and lesser pelvis), chest radiographs. Positron emission tomography (PET)-CT can be useful in initial staging.

6. Other studies: Pretreatment electrocardiography (ECG), echocardiography, and pulmonary function tests, HIV and hepatitis testing, pregnancy test in younger women.

Diagnostic Criteria

Diagnosis is based on histologic and immunohistochemical examination of an involved lymph node or other involved tissue specimens.

Adverse prognostic factors in clinical stages I and II: Large mediastinal mass (>1/3 of the maximum horizontal chest diameter), ESR >50 mm/h (>30 mm/h if B symptoms are present), age ≥50 years, ≥3 nodal areas, extranodal disease.

Adverse prognostic factors in clinical stages III and IV: Serum albumin level <4 g/dL, hemoglobin <105 g/L, male sex, age ≥45 years, clinical stage IV, white blood cell count $\geq 15 \times 10^9$/L, lymphocytopenia $<0.6 \times 10^9$/L or <8%.

Differential Diagnosis

Other causes of lymphadenopathy. Classical HL (especially NSHL) should be differentiated from primary mediastinal large B-cell lymphoma.

➡ TREATMENT

Treatment of Classical Hodgkin Lymphoma

1. First-line treatment: Chemotherapy (ABVD [doxorubicin, bleomycin, vinblastine, dacarbazine] or BEACOPPesc [bleomycin, etoposide, doxorubicin, cyclophosphamide, vincristine, procarbazine, prednisone]), usually in combination with radiotherapy of residual lesions or of the primarily involved field.

2. Progression or relapse: In most cases salvage chemotherapy regimens are used and followed by high-dose chemotherapy and autologous hematopoietic stem cell transplantation (HSCT) with or without radiotherapy. In patients not eligible for HSCT or those with late relapses (after 12 months), combination treatment (chemotherapy with radiotherapy) should be considered. In patients not eligible for intensive chemotherapy, consider palliative chemotherapy and/or radiotherapy, and after ≥2 lines of chemotherapy, consider brentuximab vedotin. Options in case of relapse after autologous HSCT include allogeneic HSCT, clinical trials, brentuximab vedotin, checkpoint (PD-1) inhibitors (nivolumab, pembrolizumab), and palliative treatment.

Treatment of NLPHL

1. Stage IA or IIA disease (excluding cases with >2 involved sites or extensive infradiaphragmatic disease): Surgical resection of the involved lymph nodes followed by radiotherapy.

2. More advanced disease: Chemotherapy (ABVD, CHOP [cyclophosphamide, doxorubicin, vincristine, prednisone], CVP [cyclophosphamide, vincristine, prednisone]) ± rituximab ± radiotherapy.

3. Relapse: Radiotherapy (local relapse), combination chemotherapy (symptomatic advanced-stage relapse), watch-and-wait approach (asymptomatic advanced-stage relapse).

→ PROGNOSIS

Using current treatment strategies, 80% to 90% of patients with HL are cured. In relapsed or refractory patients undergoing autologous HSCT, cure is possible in ~50% of cases.

8.9. Hypereosinophilia (Including Chronic Eosinophilic Leukemia)

→ DEFINITION, ETIOLOGY, PATHOGENESIS

Hypereosinophilia (HE) is defined as particularly high peripheral eosinophil counts (≥1.5 × 10^9/L) and/or eosinophilic infiltration of one or more target tissues or organs. In the case of target organ damage, **hypereosinophilic syndrome (HES)** is diagnosed. HE/HES may be nonneoplastic (reactive, congenital, or idiopathic) or neoplastic (clonal; very rare).

Chronic eosinophilic leukemia (CEL) is a myeloproliferative neoplasm and subtype of HES in which uncontrolled clonal proliferation of eosinophil precursors causes hypereosinophilia of peripheral blood with eosinophilic infiltration of bone marrow and other tissues. In the 2016 World Health Organization classification of chronic myeloproliferative neoplasms, cases with *PDGFRA*, *PDGFRB*, and *FGFR1* mutations were excluded from this clinical entity, which is now called chronic eosinophilic leukemia not otherwise specified (CEL-NOS).

Primary HE/HES: Conditions with eosinophils present as part of a malignant clone (myeloproliferative neoplasms, acute myeloid leukemia [AML]).

Secondary (reactive) HE/HES: Parasitic infections, allergic reactions including skin and food allergies, allergic and nonallergic asthma, drug-induced (allergic or toxic) reactions. Less commonly pulmonary eosinophilia, graft-versus-host disease, Hodgkin lymphoma, peripheral T-cell lymphomas, Langerhans cell histiocytosis, indolent systemic mastocytosis, solid tumors, allergic bronchopulmonary aspergillosis, chronic inflammatory diseases (eg, inflammatory bowel disease), systemic connective tissue diseases (allergic angiitis and granulomatosis [Churg-Strauss syndrome], other systemic vasculitis syndromes, deep eosinophilic fasciitis with eosinophilia), lymphocytic variant HES (caused by clonal T-cell cytokine production).

→ **CLINICAL FEATURES AND NATURAL HISTORY**

1. Symptoms:

1) **General symptoms** are caused by a massive release of cytokines from eosinophils and include fatigue, fever, sweating, anorexia, and weight loss.

2) **Cardiovascular symptoms** (observed in ~20% of patients) are caused by myocardial and endocardial necrosis and fibrosis, as well as by subendocardial thrombosis. They include valvular regurgitation (most commonly mitral and tricuspid), features of restrictive cardiomyopathy, arrhythmias, conduction disturbances, thromboembolic events, and heart failure.

3) **Respiratory symptoms** (~50% of patients) are caused by eosinophilic infiltrates, pulmonary fibrosis, heart failure, or pulmonary embolism and include chronic nonproductive cough and dyspnea.

4) **Cutaneous symptoms** (~60% of patients) include angioedema, erythema, urticaria, subcutaneous papules and nodules, and pruritus. This is very common in lymphocyte-type HES.

5) **Gastrointestinal symptoms** (~30% of patients) are associated with mucosal ulcerations, bleeding, perforation, cholecystitis, and eosinophilic gastritis/gastroenteritis; they include diarrhea and abdominal pain.

6) **Neurologic symptoms** (~55% of patients) include behavioral abnormalities, memory impairment, ataxia, and features of peripheral polyneuropathy.

7) **Other symptoms** include hepatomegaly and/or splenomegaly, myalgia and arthralgia (caused by release of proinflammatory cytokines from eosinophils), and visual disturbances (caused by retinal thrombosis).

2. Natural history: The disease is chronic. In some cases, the course may be mild, but most frequently it is progressive and may rapidly lead to death due to organ involvement (usually heart failure) or transformation to acute leukemia.

→ **DIAGNOSIS**

Diagnostic Tests

1. Complete blood count (CBC): Eosinophilia (arbitrarily classified absolute eosinophil counts: mild, 0.5×10^9/L to 1.5×10^9/L; moderate, 1.5×10^9/L to 5×10^9/L; severe, $>5 \times 10^9$/L; the average peak eosinophil count in HES is ~6.6×10^9/L), anemia (~50% of patients), thrombocytopenia (~30%) or thrombocytosis (~15%), monocytosis, and moderate leukocytosis (in particular in patients with CEL).

2. Bone marrow examination: Aspiration reveals increased proportions of eosinophils, which in some patients are accompanied by dysplasia of megakaryocytes and granulocytes. Trephine biopsy reveals hypercellular marrow, expansion of megakaryopoietic and neutrophil granulocytic lineages, as well as increased amounts of reticulin fibers. Immunophenotyping and immunohistochemical (positive tryptase) studies are also performed. These may include abnormal T-cell receptor rearrangements.

3. Cytogenetic and molecular studies are performed to document clonal expansion (→Diagnostic Criteria, below). These are best performed on bone marrow samples rather than in peripheral blood. In some patients the *FIP1L1-PDGFRA* fusion gene is found (by polymerase chain reaction [PCR] and by fluorescent in situ hybridization [FISH]). Other cytogenetic parameters could be examined in specialized settings.

4. Other laboratory tests: Abnormal population of lymphocytes in peripheral blood (eg, CD3$^+$CD4$^-$CD8$^-$ or CD3$^-$CD4$^+$CD8$^+$) may suggest lymphocyte-variant HES. IgE levels are elevated in patients with idiopathic hypereosinophilia (including the majority of patients with lymphocytic variant) and usually normal in patients with CEL-NOS. The activity of granulocyte alkaline phosphatase is increased (>100 IU) in patients with CEL-NOS.

5. Histology: Inflammatory eosinophilic infiltrates are found in biopsy samples of the affected organs.

Diagnostic Criteria

1. CEL-NOS:

1) Eosinophilia $\geq 1.5 \times 10^9$/L.

2) Absence of the Ph chromosome, *BCRABL1* fusion gene, and exclusion of other myeloproliferative (polycythemia vera, essential thrombocytosis, primary myelofibrosis) or myelodysplastic-myeloproliferative (chronic myelomonocytic leukemia, atypical chronic myelogenous leukemia) neoplasms.

3) Absence of t(5;12)(q31-35;p13) or other *PDGFRB* gene rearrangements.

4) Absence of the *FIP1L1-PDGFRA* fusion gene or other *PDGFRA* gene rearrangements.

5) Absence of *FGFR1* gene rearrangements.

6) Less than 20% blasts in peripheral blood and bone marrow, absence of inv(16)(p13q22), t(16;16)(p13;q22), or other features that warrant the diagnosis of AML.

7) Presence of a clonal or cytogenetic abnormality, >2% blasts in peripheral blood, or >5% blasts in bone marrow.

2. Neoplasms with a *PDGFRA* gene rearrangement:

1) A myeloid (most frequently CEL, less often AML) or less commonly lymphoid (T-lymphoblastic lymphoma) neoplasm with significant eosinophilia.

2) Presence of the *FIP1L1-PDGFRA* fusion gene.

Differential Diagnosis

Disorders of the organs affected in HES (→Clinical Features, above).

→ TREATMENT

1. In patients with eosinophil counts $<5 \times 10^9$/L and no organ involvement, cytoreduction is not necessary.

2. HE with the *FIP1L1-PDGFRA* gene: Imatinib. Patients with cardiac involvement should receive concomitant glucocorticoids when therapy with imatinib is initiated to prevent acute cardiac injury.

3. HES without a *PDGFRA* rearrangement: Glucocorticoids, for instance, prednisone 1 mg/kg until eosinophil counts decrease $<1.5 \times 10^9$/L and symptom control is achieved; then slowly taper the dose. Patients at risk for infection with *Strongyloides* as a cause of HES should receive ivermectin (200 µg/kg/d for 2 days) concomitantly with glucocorticoids to avoid dissemination of infection. Monoclonal antibodies against interleukin 5 (IL-5) (mepolizumab and benralizumab) are safe and effective in reducing blood and tissue eosinophils, improving clinical outcomes, and helping to reduce the dose of maintenance glucocorticoids.⊘●

4. In patients not responding to treatment and patients with CEL-NOS: Cytotoxic agents (hydroxyurea [INN hydroxycarbamide]; if ineffective, interferon α, then vincristine or etoposide). In patients with no response to these agents consider less established treatments (mepolizumab, alemtuzumab)⊘○ or consider allogeneic hematopoietic stem cell transplantation. In patients with high eosinophil counts use glucocorticoids, as above. Rarely leukapheresis may be considered.

→ FOLLOW-UP

CBC (target eosinophil counts $<1.5 \times 10^9$/L); other studies relevant to organ involvement (including echocardiography) every 6 to 12 months. In patients with the *FIP1L1/PDGFRA* gene, perform molecular studies every 3 months if indicated to monitor response to therapy or to determine if remission is durable in patients obtaining a complete molecular response.

→ **PROGNOSIS**

The majority of patients with idiopathic HES have a good response to gluco-corticoids in monotherapy and in combination with hydroxyurea, and patients who are refractory to these treatments respond to other modalities listed above (5-year survival rates are up to 90%). Patients with the *FIP1L1/PDGFRA* gene have a very good response to imatinib. In the case of CEL-NOS, the prognosis is poor; in half of these patients, transformation to AML occurs and the mean survival is 22 months.

8.10. Mastocytosis

→ **DEFINITION, ETIOLOGY, PATHOGENESIS**

Mastocytosis is a group of disorders characterized by the proliferation and accumulation of mast cells in one or more organs. **Types of mastocytosis** include:

1) **Cutaneous mastocytosis (CM)**, which may have the form of a maculo-papular rash (urticaria pigmentosa), diffuse CM, or mastocytoma of skin.

2) **Systemic mastocytosis (SM)**, which may be indolent SM, smoldering SM, SM with an associated hematologic neoplasm, aggressive SM, or mast cell leukemia.

3) Mast cell sarcoma.

→ **CLINICAL FEATURES AND NATURAL HISTORY**

1. Cutaneous manifestations: Yellow-brown or red-brown macules and pruritic papules, Darier sign (urticaria appearing within minutes after stimulation of the skin affected by the lesions).

2. Symptoms caused by mast cell mediator release: Hypotension, tachycardia, syncope, headache, and shock (due to vasodilation); dyspnea (due to bronchoconstriction); flushing; bone pain, osteopenia and osteoporosis; fatigue, weight loss, cachexia; dyspepsia, diarrhea, and symptoms of peptic ulcer disease; depression, mood changes, lack of concentration, increased somnolence; bleeding.

Triggering factors: Drugs (eg, acetylsalicylic acid [ASA], morphine, nonsteroidal anti-inflammatory drugs [NSAIDs]), physical factors (heat, cold, pressure), physical activity, alcohol, insect venom, iodinated contrast agents, stress, invasive procedures.

3. Symptoms caused by tissue and organ infiltration: Hepatosplenomegaly, lymphadenopathy, diarrhea, and weight loss (due to malabsorption); features of anemia; bleeding; pathologic fractures; other organ-specific signs and symptoms.

→ **DIAGNOSIS**

1. CM: Histologic examination of skin biopsy specimens.

2. SM: Bone marrow examination, biopsy of the skin or other affected organs, molecular studies (*KIT* D816V mutation), high serum tryptase levels.

3. Mast cell leukemia: Over 20% mast cells in bone marrow, >10% mast cells in peripheral blood, or organ infiltrates, frequently without cutaneous lesions.

Differential Diagnosis

Differential diagnosis should include nonclonal mast cell activation syndromes, idiopathic anaphylaxis, chronic spontaneous urticaria, hereditary or acquired angioedema, carcinoid syndrome, pheochromocytoma, and vasoactive intestinal peptide-secreting tumors.

→ TREATMENT

1. General measures:

1) Due to the risk of anaphylactic shock, the patient should be advised of the factors that may trigger mast cell degranulation, learn the ways to avoid them, and carry at least 2 epinephrine autoinjectors.

2) Agents that may trigger mast cell degranulation (eg, opioids, ASA and NSAIDs, radiocontrast dye, some muscle relaxants) should be used with caution.

3) β-Blockers can make anaphylaxis more severe and more difficult to manage and should be avoided where possible.

4) Before invasive medical or surgical procedures, administration of a prophylactic H_1 antagonist, H_2 antagonist, and glucocorticoid is suggested. A leukotriene antagonist can also be used.

5) If the patient has a coexisting insect venom allergy, they should be treated with venom immunotherapy.

2. CM, indolent and smoldering SM: Symptomatic treatment only, including H_1 antihistamines, H_2 antihistamines, leukotriene modifiers, omalizumab, proton pump inhibitors in the case of dyspepsia or peptic ulcer disease, topical glucocorticoids, psoralens with ultraviolet light in the A range (PUVA) photochemotherapy, mast cell stabilizers (cromolyn), calcium and vitamin D, and bisphosphonates. Interferon α-2b is used in the case of severe bone disease or progressive hepatosplenomegaly.

3. SM with an associated hematologic neoplasm: Treatment of the associated hematologic disorder.

4. Aggressive SM: The first-line agents are midostaurin, cladribine and interferon α-2b. Imatinib mesylate may be considered in patients who are negative for *KIT* D816V mutation. Allogeneic hematopoietic stem cell transplantation (HSCT) is used in selected patients.

5. Mast cell leukemia: Midostaurin, multidrug chemotherapy (as in acute myeloid leukemia) or cladribine, which may be combined with interferon α (chemotherapy is of limited efficacy); allogeneic HSCT.

→ PROGNOSIS

In adults, spontaneous remissions are rare. Patients with CM, indolent SM, or smoldering SM in general respond well to symptomatic treatment and have normal life expectancy. The prognosis in patients with aggressive SM is variable, with a median survival of a few years. In patients with mast cell leukemia, the prognosis is poor.

8.11. Multiple Myeloma

→ DEFINITION, ETIOLOGY, PATHOGENESIS

Multiple myeloma (MM) or plasma cell myeloma (PCM) is a hematologic malignancy that involves the proliferation and accumulation of monoclonal plasma cells, which produce monoclonal immunoglobulin or its fragments (M protein). Neoplastic cells most probably originate from memory B cells. Etiology is unknown.

→ CLINICAL FEATURES AND NATURAL HISTORY

Clinical manifestations are caused by the proliferation of neoplastic plasma cells, which secrete monoclonal (abnormal) proteins as well as cytokines. Manifestations include:

1) **Bone pain** (the most common symptom, present at some stage in a majority of patients) in the lumbar spine, pelvis, ribs, or less commonly in the skull and long bones. This is caused by osteolytic lesions and pathologic fractures (eg, vertebral compression fractures).

2) **Features of hypercalcemia and its complications**: Symptoms may occur in up to 20% of patients.

3) **Features of renal failure**: These are present at the time of diagnosis of MM in ~30% of patients.

4) **Symptoms of anemia** (seen in a majority of patients).

5) **Neurologic signs and symptoms**: These may include limb paresis or paralysis (due to spinal cord or nerve compression caused by vertebral body fracture or extramedullary plasma cell tumor [plasmacytoma]) and rarely features of peripheral neuropathy. The manifestations are seen in ~10% of patients.

6) **Recurrent respiratory and urinary tract infections**.

7) **Features of hyperviscosity syndrome** (in <10% of patients): Somnolence, headache, hearing impairment, altered mental status, heart failure, and bleeding (usually epistaxis or gingival bleeding).

8) Rarely extramedullary plasmacytoma and enlargement of the liver, peripheral lymph nodes, and spleen.

In ~10% to 15% of patients the disease is indolent and requires no treatment (so-called smoldering MM). However, in the majority of patients the disease is progressive or relapses after subsequent lines of treatment.

→ DIAGNOSIS

Diagnostic Tests

1. Complete blood count (CBC) in the majority of patients reveals normocytic (less commonly macrocytic) normochromic anemia, with the formation of red blood cells in the form of rouleaux in 50% of patients. Less commonly, leukopenia or thrombocytopenia are observed.

2. Bone marrow examination: More than 10% of clonal plasma cells.

3. Cytogenetic studies may be performed for risk stratification.

4. Other laboratory tests: Hypergammaglobulinemia; decreased levels of normal immunoglobulins; monoclonal protein identified in blood and urine electrophoresis and immunofixation; presence of abnormal light chains in blood and/or urine (monoclonal urinary light chains are referred to as Bence Jones proteinuria); hypercalcemia; increased serum uric acid, creatinine, β_2-microglobulin, C-reactive protein, and lactate dehydrogenase levels; rarely cryoglobulinemia. Hyperproteinemia and the erythrocyte sedimentation rate (this may be markedly elevated) are nonspecific tests.

5. Skeletal imaging studies (radiography, computed tomography [CT] and/or magnetic resonance imaging [MRI], or positron emission tomography [PET]-CT) reveal focal osteolytic lesions, most commonly in the flat and long bones, as well as osteoporosis and pathologic fractures. Radiographs should include the skull, brachial and femoral bones, pelvis, spine, and all painful locations.

Diagnostic Criteria

1. According to the 2014 International Myeloma Working Group criteria, **MM is diagnosed in patients with clonal bone marrow plasma cells ≥10% or biopsy-proven bony or extramedullary plasmacytoma** and at least one of the following myeloma-defining events:

1) Evidence of end-organ damage that can be attributed to the underlying plasma cell proliferative disorder, specifically:

   a) Hypercalcemia: Serum calcium >0.25 mmol/L above the upper limit of normal or >2.75 mmol/L.

b) Renal insufficiency: Creatinine clearance <40 mL/minute or serum creatinine >177 μmol/L.

c) Anemia: Hemoglobin level >20 g/L below the lower limit of normal or <100 g/L.

d) Bone lesions: One or more osteolytic lesions on skeletal radiography, CT, or PET-CT.

2) Any one or more of the following biomarkers of malignancy:

a) Clonal bone marrow plasma cells ≥60%.

b) An involved to uninvolved serum free light chain (FLC) ratio ≥100 if the involved FLC concentration is ≥100 mg/L.

c) More than 1 focal lesion ≥5 mm in diameter on MRI studies.

2. Smoldering MM:

1) Serum monoclonal protein (IgG or IgA) ≥30 g/L or urinary monoclonal protein ≥500 mg/24 hours and/or clonal bone marrow plasma cells 10% to 60%.

2) Absence of myeloma-defining events or amyloidosis.

3. Solitary plasmacytoma: A solitary tumor of the bone or (in 1%-2% of patients) other organs, with normal results of bone marrow aspiration and trephine biopsy, normal skeletal radiographs and MRI (or CT) of the spine and pelvis (except for the primary lesion), negative CRAB (hypercalcemia, renal failure, anemia, bone lesions) criteria, and absence or low levels of serum and urine monoclonal immunoglobulin.

4. Plasma cell leukemia: A peripheral blood malignant plasma cell count >2×10^9/L or >20% of the circulating white blood cells. This is an aggressive disease with a poor prognosis and short survival.

5. POEMS syndrome (peripheral neuropathy, organomegaly, endocrinopathy, monoclonal gammopathy, skin changes) is a very rare manifestation of MM.

Differential Diagnosis

1. Other types of monoclonal gammopathy (diseases characterized by the proliferation of a single clone of plasma cells producing the M protein):

1) Monoclonal gammopathy of undetermined significance: The presence of a monoclonal protein alone is an observation that requires no treatment but may transform to MM at a rate of ~1% per year. It can be associated with other conditions (malignancy, connective tissue diseases [rheumatoid arthritis, systemic lupus erythematosus, polymyositis], nervous system diseases [multiple sclerosis, myasthenia, Gaucher disease], bacterial [eg, bacterial endocarditis] or viral [cytomegalovirus, hepatitis C and B viruses] infections) as well as develop in patients after solid organ or hematopoietic stem cell transplantation.

2) Other plasma cell dyscrasias: Amyloidosis, immunoglobulin light chain deposition disease, heavy chain deposition diseases, lymphoplasmacytic lymphoma/Waldenström macroglobulinemia.

2. Reactive polyclonal plasmacytosis in patients with infection (eg, rubella, infectious mononucleosis), chronic inflammation, and liver disease (usually <10% plasma cells in bone marrow, absence of M protein, polyclonal plasma cells).

3. Bone metastases of cancer (eg, renal cancer, breast cancer, non–small cell lung cancer, prostate cancer).

→ TREATMENT

Antineoplastic Treatment

1. Patients with asymptomatic (smoldering) myeloma require follow-up only.

2. Patients aged <70 years and patients ≥70 years with no comorbidities are candidates for high-dose chemotherapy (myeloablative dose of melphalan) followed by autologous peripheral blood stem cell transplantation (PBSCT) after achieving a response to induction chemotherapy (usually 4 cycles of multiagent therapy such as VTd [bortezomib, thalidomide, dexamethasone], CyBorD [cyclophosphamide, bortezomib, dexamethasone], or VRd [bortezomib, lenalidomide, dexamethasone]).

3. Patients not qualified for autologous PBSCT: Chemotherapy, usually using VMP (bortezomib, melphalan, prednisone), Rd (lenalidomide, dexamethasone), or MPT (melphalan, prednisone, thalidomide).

4. Patients with treatment resistance or relapse: Immunomodulators (thalidomide, lenalidomide, pomalidomide), proteasome inhibitors (bortezomib, carfilzomib), bendamustine, monoclonal antibodies (daratumumab). ◐
In selected patients a second autologous transplant or allogeneic PBSCT may be performed.

5. Solitary plasmacytoma: Surgery or radiation and close monitoring for progression to systemic myeloma.

Supportive Treatment

1. Treatment of kidney failure:

1) Appropriate hydration (fluid intake >3 L/d).

2) Prompt initiation of antimyeloma therapy.

3) Avoidance of nephrotoxic drugs (eg, nonsteroidal anti-inflammatory drugs, aminoglycosides) and contrast media.

4) Treatment of hyperuricemia with allopurinol (→Chapter 14.8).

5) Plasmapheresis is an expensive and invasive treatment that has been shown to not modify outcomes, ◑◯ except rarely in patients with hyperviscosity.

2. Prevention of bony complications and treatment of osteolysis is based on bisphosphonates administered for 2 years or longer in patients with lytic lesions (to be resumed in case of disease progression or relapse). The agents include:

1) Pamidronate disodium (INN pamidronic acid) 60 to 90 mg as a 3- to 4-hour IV infusion in 500 mL 0.9% saline every 4 weeks with consideration given to lower doses for patients with renal insufficiency.

2) Zoledronate (INN zoledronic acid) 2 to 8 mg as a 5- to 15-minute IV infusion in 500 mL of 0.9% saline every 4 weeks.

In patients with vertebral compression fractures, consider vertebroplasty or kyphoplasty. Calcium and vitamin D supplementation is used in the case of deficiencies.

3. Treatment of hypercalcemia and hypercalcemic crisis.

4. Treatment of hyperproteinemia and coagulopathy: Plasmapheresis with substitution of albumin or clotting factors.

5. Treatment of symptomatic anemia: Erythropoiesis-stimulating agents or transfusions if required (→Chapter 7.5.1; →Chapter 13.7.7).

6. Analgesic treatment: Acetaminophen (INN paracetamol), opioids (avoid nonsteroidal anti-inflammatory drugs), radiotherapy, surgery (vertebroplasty).

7. Prevention of infections: Influenza and pneumococcal vaccinations; acyclovir (INN aciclovir) in patients treated with bortezomib. Consider intravenous immunoglobulin or subcutaneous immunoglobulin in patients with severe recurrent infections.

8. Antithrombotic prophylaxis: Acetylsalicylic acid (ASA) 75 to 100 mg/d or low-molecular-weight heparin (LMWH) (→Chapter 3.19, Table 3.19-10) in patients treated with thalidomide or lenalidomide in combination with dexamethasone.

⇥ PROGNOSIS

Outcomes in MM vary depending on staging and risk stratification. Overall 5-year survival rates are >45%.

8.12. Myelodysplastic Syndromes

▶ DEFINITION, ETIOLOGY, PATHOGENESIS

Myelodysplastic syndromes (MDS) are clonal hematologic disorders characterized by peripheral blood cytopenia, dysplasia of ≥1 hematopoietic lineage, ineffective hematopoiesis, and risk of transformation to acute myeloid leukemia. It could be preceded by acquisition of somatic mutations that drive clonal expansion in the absence of abnormal counts or dysplasia, referred to as clonal hematopoiesis of indeterminate potential (CHIP), which are precursor states for hematologic neoplasms but are usually benign and do not progress. This can be analogous to monoclonal gammopathy of undetermined significance (MGUS) and monoclonal B-cell lymphocytosis.

Risk factors include exposure to chemicals (eg, benzene, toluene) and heavy metals; tobacco smoke; ionizing radiation; chemotherapy/cytotoxic agents; and radiation therapy. The median age of onset is between 60 and 75 years of age with an incidence of ~2/100,000 population per year.

▶ CLINICAL FEATURES AND NATURAL HISTORY

Patients may present with signs and symptoms due to low counts, symptomatic anemia, recurrent infections in neutropenia, or bruises and ecchymosis in cases with thrombocytopenia. It could be detected on routine blood tests in asymptomatic individuals.

▶ DIAGNOSIS

Diagnostic Tests

1. Complete blood count (CBC): Pancytopenia is common. Macrocytic anemia with increased red cell distribution width (RDW); leukopenia with neutropenia; and severe thrombocytopenia. Circulating blasts may be seen. Blood smears may show dysmorphic or bilobed neutrophils, polychromasia, poikilocytosis, anisocytosis, and severe thrombocytopenia. Inappropriately low reticulocyte counts are common due to poor bone marrow reserve.

2. Bone marrow examination reveals features of hypercellular marrow for age. In 10% of cases MDS may be hypoplastic with decreased cellularity. Unilineage or multilineage dysplasia, dyserythropoiesis with appearance of ring sideroblasts (iron laden mitochondria visible as perinuclear granules with Prussian iron stain), dysplastic granulocytes, and increased monocytes can be seen. Classification based on appearance of myeloblasts or Auer rods is known as MDS with excessive blasts type 1 (MDS-EB-1) (5%-9%) or type 2 (MDS-EB-2) (10%-19%).

3. Cytogenetic testing: Normal cytogenetic findings or common abnormalities such as loss of the Y chromosome do not exclude the diagnosis of MDS. Fluorescence in situ hybridization (FISH) may be used for selected specific mutations, such as del(5q), which is seen in elderly female patients. Other abnormal karyotypes including del(7) or del(17p) are diagnostic for MDS in the absence of cytopenias or dysplasia.

4. Molecular studies: *NPM1* or wild-type, *FLT3*-ITD/TKD; *BCR-ABL1* to exclude chronic myelogenous leukemia; *JAK2* V617F to exclude myeloproliferative neoplasm (MPN). The next generation sequencing panel is now used to detect epigenetic driver mutations or splicing mutations that are associated with poor risk and progression to acute myeloid leukemia (AML) or *TP53* mutation, which is known for resistance to conventional chemotherapy.

5. Other laboratory studies: Any of elevated serum iron, fetal hemoglobin (HbF), and endogenous erythropoietin levels may be seen (lower erythropoietin levels are predictors of better response to erythropoietin-stimulating agents [ESAs]).

Diagnostic Criteria

In patients with cytopenia and no documented features of MDS or with dysplasia not accompanied by cytopenia, the diagnosis of **idiopathic cytopenia of undetermined significance (ICUS)** or **idiopathic dysplasia of uncertain significance (IDUS)** is made. These conditions may progress to MDS.

Differential Diagnosis

Megaloblastic anemia, aplastic anemias, nutritional causes of leukopenia with neutropenia, primary immune thrombocytopenia, acute leukemia, primary myelofibrosis, or metastatic disease involving bone marrow.

→ **TREATMENT**

Treatment, conducted in specialized centers, depends on performance status and age of the patient as well as on the risk category according to the International Prognostic Scoring System (IPSS) (this takes into consideration the proportion of blasts in bone marrow, karyotype, and number of lineages affected by cytopenia) or newer prognostic systems (World Health Organization [WHO]-adapted Prognostic Scoring System [WPSS]: www.mds-register.de/ipss; or revised IPSS [IPSS-R]: www.mds-foundation.org/ipss-r-calculator).

1. ESAs are used in patients with low-risk to intermediate-risk IPSS score.

2. Combined immunosuppressive treatment (antithymocyte immunoglobulin, cyclosporine [INN ciclosporin] in patients with hypoplastic MDS).

3. Lenalidomide is used in patients with del(5q).

4. Hypomethylating agents (azacitidine, decitabine, and more recently guadecitabine) are effective in disease control, prevent progression to AML, and result in transfusion independence and improved quality of life.

5. Intensive induction chemotherapy (using the same agents as in AML) and/or allogeneic hematopoietic stem cell transplantation (HSCT) (the only curative treatment) are reserved for younger symptomatic patients with excellent physiologic reserve and low comorbidity index scores.

6. Supportive treatment is the mainstay of therapy:

1) Packed red blood cell (PRBC) transfusions (using leukocyte-depleted preparations).

2) ESAs in patients with low to intermediate-1 risk with hemoglobin <100 g/L, endogenous erythropoietin <500 mIU/mL, and/or requiring transfusion of <2 units of PRBCs per month.

3) Management of febrile neutropenia (→Chapter 8.7). The use of granulocyte colony-stimulating factor (G-CSF) is controversial, as it may lead to progression to AML.

4) Platelet transfusions are used to improve thrombocytopenia.

5) Iron-chelating agents (deferoxamine or deferasirox) can be considered in selected younger patients with low-risk disease and predicted long-term survival.

→ **PROGNOSIS**

Intermediate-2 or high-risk disease based on IPSS or IPSS-R scores are associated with risk of progression to AML and early mortality within 5 to 12 months. Poor risk or complex cytogenetic abnormalities, in addition to mutations in *TP53*, *EZH2*, *ETV6*, *RUNX1*, and *ASXL1*, are associated with poor overall survival.

In patients undergoing allogeneic HSCT, 3-year to 5-year disease-free survival rates are 30% to 50%. Overall prognosis without intensive treatment is determined by the risk score at presentation and frequency and type of complications.

8.13. Non-Hodgkin Lymphoma

→ **DEFINITION, ETIOLOGY, PATHOGENESIS**

Non-Hodgkin lymphomas (NHLs) are a group of neoplasms characterized by the clonal proliferation of lymphoid cells at various stages of B-cell or less commonly T-cell or natural killer (NK)-cell differentiation. NHLs are the sixth most prevalent type of cancer in adults. Factors showing a documented causal relationship with the development of NHL include environmental factors (exposure to benzene, ionizing radiation), viral infections (human T-lymphotropic virus type I, Epstein-Barr virus [EBV], HIV, human herpesvirus 8, hepatitis C virus), bacterial infections (*Helicobacter pylori*), autoimmune diseases, immunodeficiencies (including immunosuppressive treatment after transplantation), and prior chemotherapy (particularly when combined with radiotherapy).

The **World Health Organization (WHO) histologic classification** includes >30 NHL subtypes:

1) **B-lymphoblastic and T-lymphoblastic leukemia/lymphoma** (B/T-ALL/LBL) (→Chapter 7.8.1).

2) **Mature B-cell neoplasms (80%-90%)**: Chronic lymphocytic leukemia/small lymphocytic lymphoma (CLL/SLL), hairy cell leukemia (HCL), marginal zone lymphoma (MZL), follicular lymphoma (FL), lymphoplasmacytic lymphoma/Waldenström macroglobulinemia (LPL/WM), mantle cell lymphoma (MCL), diffuse large B-cell lymphoma (DLBCL) and its variants, Burkitt lymphoma (BL), and other types.

3) **Mature T-cell and NK-cell neoplasms**: Peripheral T-cell lymphoma not otherwise specified (PTCL-NOS), large granular lymphocytic leukemia (LGL), mycosis fungoides (MF), and other types.

→ **CLINICAL FEATURES AND NATURAL HISTORY**

1. General symptoms: →Table 8-3.

2. Lymphadenopathy: Lymph nodes are usually painless and the overlying skin is unchanged. Typically, they are >1 cm in diameter and have a tendency to form conglomerates. Lymph nodes usually enlarge slowly, and temporary decreases in their size may be observed. Massive lymphadenopathy may cause superior vena cava syndrome as well as pleural effusions, ascites, and edema of the lower extremities. Rapid enlargement should suggest high-grade characteristics, as seen, for example, with BL.

3. Manifestations of extranodal tumors: Abdominal pain caused by enlargement of the spleen or liver; jaundice caused by liver infiltration; gastrointestinal bleeding, obstruction, and malabsorption that may be caused by gastrointestinal NHL; and other symptoms caused by infiltrates in various organs (eg, skin, central nervous system [CNS]).

4. Staging: →Table 8-3.

5. Natural history: The prognosis and clinical management in NHL are based on the following classification:

1) **Indolent NHLs** (about half of cases): The majority of small B-cell NHLs, including FL, CLL/SLL, LPL/WM, MZL, and a few T-cell NHLs (MF, LGL); these develop mainly in the elderly and present with generalized lymphadenopathy, bone marrow and peripheral blood involvement, and (frequently) splenic and hepatic involvement. General symptoms are rare. Indolent NHL may transform into aggressive NHL, and it is usually characterized by slow progression of signs and symptoms, with survival for most types measured in years. The most common indolent NHL is FL (10%-20% of NHLs).

2) **Aggressive NHLs** (about half of cases): DLBCL (most common, 30%-35% of NHLs) and MCL, as well as the majority of T-cell lymphomas. Untreated patients survive from a few to several months.

3) **Highly aggressive NHLs**: ALL/LBL and BL. Untreated patients survive from several weeks to a few months.

→ DIAGNOSIS

Diagnostic Tests

1. Histologic and immunohistochemical examination of an involved lymph node or organ specimens (excisional biopsy or multiple core biopsies).

2. Studies performed to identify nodal and extranodal lesions (required for staging):

1) Contrast-enhanced computed tomography (CT) of the chest, abdomen, and pelvis (in fluorodeoxyglucose [FDG]-avid NHL and as the only imaging test in primarily extranodal NHL, CLL/SLL, LPL/WM, MZL).

2) Positron emission tomography (PET)-CT should be considered in the case of FDG-avid NHL.

3) Bone marrow aspiration and biopsy.

4) Depending on the subtype and signs/symptoms, it may be necessary to perform endoscopy, cerebrospinal fluid examination, or other studies.

3. Laboratory studies:

1) Complete blood count (CBC).

2) Other: Renal and liver function tests and lactate dehydrogenase levels, β_2--microglobulin; serum protein electrophoresis and immunoglobulins concentration, direct antiglobulin (Coombs) tests; HIV, hepatitis B or C virus, EBV.

4. Electrocardiography (ECG) and echocardiography are indicated in every patient in whom treatment with anthracyclines is planned and in the elderly.

5. Cytogenetic studies and molecular studies are performed for those lymphomas that have identifiable abnormalities.

Diagnostic Criteria

Diagnosis is made on the basis of histologic and immunohistochemical examination of an entire lymph node or a specimen of an involved organ.

Differential Diagnosis

Other causes of general symptoms, lymphadenopathy, or splenomegaly.

→ TREATMENT

The choice of treatment modalities depends on the histologic type and stage of NHL as well as the presence of certain prognostic factors at the onset of the disease (→Table 8-4), performance status, and comorbidities.

Treatment of Indolent NHL

Currently available treatment modalities cannot achieve a radical cure in this group of patients. Exceptions are localized lymphomas (clinical stage I or II), which sometimes may regress spontaneously or may be successfully treated by eradicating the etiologic factor using antimicrobial agents (eg, *H pylori* in patients with gastric mucosa-associated lymphoid tissue lymphoma) and/or surgical resection of the primary lesion (eg, spleen in patients with splenic MZL) combined with adjuvant radiotherapy and/or chemotherapy. Localized follicular lymphoma can sometimes be cured with radiation alone. Blood and marrow transplant can be used with curative intent in a subset of patients.

Indications for systemic treatment (chemotherapy or immunochemotherapy): Significant constitutional symptoms, progressive bulky disease, significant

Table 8-4. International prognostic index for non-Hodgkin lymphomas	
International prognostic index (IPI) for aggressive NHL	
Risk factors	**Cutoff value**
Age	≤60 years vs >60 years
ECOG performance status (see ecog-acrin.org)	<2 vs ≥2
Clinical stage (→Table 8-3)	I/II vs III/IV
Number of extranodal sites involved	≤1 vs >1
Serum LDH level	≤ULN vs >ULN
Risk groups	**Number of risk factors**
Low risk	≤1
Low-intermediate risk	2
High-intermediate risk	3
High risk	≥4
Follicular lymphoma-specific international prognostic index (FLIPI) for indolent NHL	
Risk factors	**Cutoff value**
Age	≤60 years vs >60 years
Number of extranodal sites involved	≤4 vs >4
Clinical stage (→Table 8-3)	I/II vs III/IV
Hemoglobin level	<120 g/L vs ≥120 g/L
Serum LDH level	≤ULN vs >ULN
Risk groups	**Number of risk factors**
Low risk	≤1
Intermediate risk	2-3
High risk	4-5

ECOG, Eastern Cooperative Oncology Group; LDH, lactate dehydrogenase; NHL, non-Hodgkin lymphoma; ULN, upper limit of normal.

cytopenia, threatened end-organ function (CNS, gastrointestinal system). In patients who do not require immediate treatment, it should be delayed until symptomatic progression of the disease is observed. Cutaneous NHL may require skin-directed therapy.

Treatment of Aggressive Lymphomas

Lymphoma treatment is an area of active interest with novel agents entering clinical practice. Clinicians are encouraged to enter patients into clinical trials and to refer patients to expert centers where recent advances in therapy are more likely to be available.

1. First-line treatment: Start multiagent chemotherapy as soon as possible in combination with rituximab (in B-cell NHL) and involved field radiotherapy (if necessary).

2. In patients with refractoriness or relapse, use alternative chemotherapy regimens with or without radiotherapy of the remaining active neoplastic tissue followed by autologous hematopoietic stem cell transplantation (HSCT) in transplant-eligible patients. Chimeric antigen receptor (CAR) T cells have shown promise for patients with relapsed refractory disease.

Treatment of Highly Aggressive Lymphomas

1. BL: Urgent initiation of intensive multiagent chemotherapy with CNS prophylaxis. Before this treatment, start prevention of tumor lysis syndrome (→Chapter 9.1.1).

2. ALL/LBL: →Chapter 7.8.1.

→ PROGNOSIS

Indolent lymphomas: Remissions are frequent (>75%) but short-lasting (although up to several years), and cure is very rare. High-grade transformations should be treated as aggressive lymphomas and may result in complete remission of high-grade lesions.

Aggressive lymphomas: Complete remissions are achieved in >75% of treated patients, and long-term survival rates are ~50%. In general, "cure" rates are highest with the most aggressive forms of B-cell lymphomas and lower in the elderly and in patients with comorbid conditions that restrict the use of aggressive chemotherapy regimens.

8.14. Polycythemia Vera

→ DEFINITION, ETIOLOGY, PATHOGENESIS

Polycythemia vera (PV) is a myeloproliferative neoplasm characterized by marked increase in red blood cell (RBC) counts, frequently accompanied by increased production of white blood cells (WBCs) and platelets. The disease is caused by a malignant proliferation of a mutant clone derived from a multipotential hematopoietic stem cell of the bone marrow. The incidence is 2 to 3/100,000 population per year.

→ CLINICAL FEATURES AND NATURAL HISTORY

Signs and symptoms depend on the number of blood cells, degree of increase in the circulating blood volume, and presence of thrombotic and hemorrhagic complications. In many patients PV is an incidental diagnosis made as a result of a routine complete blood count (CBC).

1. Symptoms include manifestations of hyperviscosity (headache, vertigo, tinnitus, visual disturbances), erythromelalgia, aquagenic pruritus (pruritus worsening after a hot bath; present in ~40% of patients), arterial or venous thrombosis (stroke, myocardial infarction, superficial or deep vein thrombosis, pulmonary embolism; the overall risk is ~20% over a 10-year period), hypertension, or gout. Nonspecific symptoms also occur including weakness, weight loss, abdominal distention, or pain due to splenomegaly. Bleeding may occur, due to acquired von Willebrand disease (particularly when the platelet count is >1500 × 10^9/L), acquired platelet function defect, or by coincident drug use, such as antiplatelet agents.

2. Signs: Splenomegaly; plethora of the face, hands, feet, and ears; lip cyanosis; hepatomegaly; hyperemia and erythema of oral mucosa and conjunctivae; characteristic venous stasis seen in fundoscopy.

3. Natural history: The disease may remain asymptomatic for many years. Symptoms are associated with increasing RBC counts and circulating blood volumes, thrombocytosis, and extramedullary hematopoiesis leading to hepatosplenomegaly. Progression to myelofibrosis is manifested by severe anemia, thrombocytopenia, and emerging extramedullary hematopoiesis in the liver and spleen. In ~10% of patients transformation to either acute myelogenous leukemia or more frequently to myelodysplastic syndrome occurs. The most common cause of death in patients with PV is thrombosis.

→ DIAGNOSIS

Diagnostic Tests

1. CBC: Increased RBC, hemoglobin (Hb), and hematocrit (Ht) levels; thrombocytosis (>400 × 10^9/L in ~60% of patients), frequently abnormal size, shape, and function of platelets; leukocytosis (>10 × 10^9/L in ~40% of patients) consisting mainly of neutrophils.

2. Bone marrow aspiration: Hypercellular marrow with hyperplastic erythropoietic, granulopoietic, and megakaryopoietic lineages; megakaryocytes are frequently of abnormal shape and variable size. The results of biopsy additionally reveal minor features of fibrosis that are more pronounced in a more advanced disease.

3. Molecular studies: Mutations of *JAK2* gene including V617F (96% of cases) or mutations in exon 12 (3%). The absence of *JAK2* or related mutations almost excludes the diagnosis of a primary polycythemia.

4. Other studies may be performed to establish the etiology of secondary erythrocytosis (→Differential Diagnosis, below).

Diagnostic Criteria

The diagnosis of PV requires meeting either all 3 major criteria or the first 2 major criteria and the minor criterion:

1) **Major criteria**:
   a) Hb >165 g/L (or Ht >49%) in men or Hb >160 g/L (or Ht >48%) in women; or increased red cell mass.
   b) Bone marrow biopsy showing hypercellularity for age with trilineage growth (panmyelosis) including prominent erythroid, granulocytic, and megakaryocytic proliferation with pleomorphic mature megakaryocytes (differences in size).
   c) Presence of *JAK2* V617F or *JAK2* exon 12 mutation.
2) **Minor criterion**: Subnormal serum erythropoietin level.

Differential Diagnosis

Differential diagnosis of erythrocytosis: →Table 8-5.

1. Familial erythrocytosis (rare): Hypersensitivity of erythropoietic progenitors to normal serum levels of erythropoietin.

2. Secondary erythrocytosis due to the following:

1) Hypoxia and erythropoietin hypersecretion caused by pulmonary or cardiovascular diseases (particularly heart defects with right-to-left shunts), obstructive sleep apnea, high altitude, tobacco smoking (owing to the presence of carboxyhemoglobin), high-affinity hemoglobins (causing relative hypoxia due to the inability to normally release oxygen in the periphery).
2) Erythropoietin hypersecretion not related to tissue hypoxia: Polycystic kidneys; Cushing syndrome; primary hyperaldosteronism; use of anabolic steroids; long-term glucocorticoid therapy; use of exogenous erythropoiesis-stimulating agents; erythropoietin-secreting tumors such as hepatocellular carcinoma, renal cancer, hemangioblastoma, uterine myoma, and pheochromocytoma.
3) Unknown etiology: After kidney transplantation.

3. Relative erythrocytosis: Hemoconcentration due to fluid loss (vomiting, diarrhea, increased diuresis including diuretic treatment), decreased fluid intake, obesity, excessive alcohol consumption, or protein loss (enteropathy, extensive burns).

Table 8-5. Differential diagnosis of polycythemia vera, secondary erythrocytosis, and relative erythrocytosis

Feature	Polycythemia vera	Secondary erythrocytosis	Relative erythrocytosis
RBC mass	↑	↑	N
WBC count	N or ↑	N	N
Platelet count	N or ↑	N	N
Bone marrow	Trilineage hyperplasia	Erythropoietic lineage hyperplasia	N
Splenomegaly	+++	−	−
Pruritus	+/-	−	−
SaO$_2$	N	N or ↓	N
Serum vitamin B$_{12}$ levels	N or ↑	N	N
Granulocyte alkaline phosphatase	↑	N	N
Serum erythropoietin levels	↓ or N	↑	N
Endogenous growth of erythroid colonies	+	−	−

↑, increased; ↓, decreased; N, normal; RBC, red blood cell; SaO$_2$, direct measurement of hemoglobin oxygen saturation in arterial blood; WBC, white blood cell.

→ TREATMENT

The choice of treatment depends on the presence of risk factors for thrombotic complications (age >60 years and prior thrombosis). Phlebotomy is the primary therapy used in patients with marked erythrocytosis with the goal of Ht <45%.◐◐ We recommend antiplatelet therapy (acetylsalicylic acid [ASA]) for all patients, unless oral anticoagulants are indicated. All patients should have cardiovascular risk factors addressed and modified.

1. Phlebotomy: Usually 200 to 500 mL every 2 to 3 days until Ht <45% is achieved (in elderly patients with cardiovascular diseases, phlebotomies should be less frequent and of lower volumes, ie, 100-150 mL). A 500 mL phlebotomy eliminates 200 mg of iron. After iron stores become depleted (based on serum ferritin), iron replacement therapy should be avoided and the frequency of phlebotomy can be reduced.

2. Cytotoxic therapy is indicated in the following patients:

1) At high risk of thrombotic complications (age >60 years or history of thrombosis).
2) Intolerant of or dependent on frequent phlebotomies.
3) With progressive symptomatic splenomegaly.
4) With severe symptoms of PV.
5) With persistent platelet counts >1500×10^9/L.

First-line agents: Hydroxyurea (INN hydroxycarbamide) (starting dose, 15-20 mg/kg/d; maintenance dose, 500-1500 mg/d) or interferon α. In the event of intolerance of or resistance to one of these agents, the patient may be switched to the other.

Hydroxyurea resistance/intolerance: Patients meeting the European Leukemia Network criteria for hydroxyurea resistance or intolerance may be considered for treatment with the JAK inhibitor ruxolitinib.

3. Antiplatelet therapy is recommended in all patients with no contraindications; ⊘⊖ use ASA 50 to 100 mg/d. Antiplatelet therapy should be used with caution in patients with a bleeding diathesis, including the form of acquired von Willebrand disease that can be seen in patients with marked thrombocytosis. In the case of contraindications to ASA, such as allergy, consider oral ticlopidine 250 mg bid or clopidogrel 75 mg once daily.

4. Treatment of hyperuricemia: Daily consumption of ~2 L of fluids; allopurinol (→Chapter 14.8) or other uric acid reduction strategies.

5. Symptomatic treatment:

1) Pruritus: Avoidance of aggravating factors; use cyproheptadine or cimetidine. If these are unsuccessful, administer paroxetine, interferon α 3 million IU/d subcutaneously 3 times per week, or photochemotherapy using psoralen and ultraviolet A light (PUVA).

2) Erythromelalgia can be treated with ASA used bid.

6. Modification of cardiovascular risk factors: Prevention or treatment of hypertension, diabetes, obesity, and hypercholesterolemia; smoking cessation.

7. Treatment of hemorrhagic complications: A short course of tranexamic acid, usually 10 to 15 mg/kg orally or IV every 8 hours, discontinuation of antiplatelet therapy. In acquired von Willebrand disease, desmopressin 0.3 µg/kg and vWF concentrates may be used (→Chapter 7.4.2).

→ MONITORING

After achieving normal Hb levels, schedule follow-up visits as necessary for ongoing phlebotomy (if required), to monitor for recurrent cytosis, and to address complications such as progressive splenomegaly or progression.

→ PROGNOSIS

In patients with PV aged >65 years life expectancy is similar to that of the age-matched general population, while in younger patients life expectancy is shorter, mainly due to the development of secondary myelofibrosis, transformation to acute leukemia, or thrombosis (the 10-year risk being, respectively, ~10%, 3%, and >20%).

8.15. Primary Myelofibrosis

→ DEFINITION, ETIOLOGY, PATHOGENESIS

Primary myelofibrosis (PMF) is a myeloproliferative neoplasm characterized by anemia, presence of immature forms of granulocytic lineage in peripheral blood, bone marrow fibrosis, splenomegaly, and extramedullary hematopoiesis. Etiology is unknown. Estimated incidence is 1.5/100,000 population per year.

→ CLINICAL FEATURES AND NATURAL HISTORY

1. General symptoms: Fatigue (in 50%-70% of patients), anorexia (<20%), weight loss, low-grade fever, dyspnea, tachycardia, night sweats, pruritus, muscle and joint pain, cachexia.

2. Symptoms of bone marrow fibrosis and extramedullary hematopoiesis: Splenomegaly (observed at presentation in >90% of patients; severe in two-thirds of patients), pain due to splenic infarcts; hepatomegaly (in 40%-70% of patients), portal hypertension; thrombocytopenia, features of anemia; symptoms of mass effect due to extramedullary hematopoiesis.

3. Natural history: Asymptomatic PMF is followed by progression with worsening symptoms of anemia, thrombocytopenia, hepatosplenomegaly, and extramedullary hematopoiesis. Median survival is ~5 years. Transformation to acute myelogenous leukemia occurs in 20% of patients.

→ DIAGNOSIS

Diagnostic Tests

1. Complete blood count (CBC): Normocytic anemia; a variable white blood cell (WBC) count including marked leukocytosis; thrombocytosis may be seen in early disease but advanced patients demonstrate thrombocytopenia; morphologic and functional abnormalities of the platelets. Differential blood counts reveal anisocytosis, poikilocytosis, teardrop-shaped red blood cells (RBCs), erythroblasts, and immature granulocyte forms (leukoerythroblastosis).

2. Bone marrow examination: In early PMF marrow is hypercellular with atypical megakaryocytes. In later stages of the disease marrow fibrosis and osteosclerosis make aspiration infeasible and trephine biopsy must be performed. The results reveal fibrosis (increased marrow reticulin and collagen fibers) with reduced or absent hematopoiesis.

3. Molecular studies reveal *JAK2* V617F mutation (in ~50% of patients), *CALR*, or *MPL* gene mutations.

Diagnostic Criteria

A diagnosis of overt PMF requires meeting all 3 major criteria and ≥1 minor criterion:

1) **Major criteria**:
   a) Presence of megakaryocytic proliferation and atypia accompanied by either reticulin and/or collagen fibrosis grade 2 or 3.
   b) Not meeting World Health Organization criteria for essential thrombocythemia (ET), polycythemia vera (PV), *BCR-ABL1* chronic myelogenous leukemia (CML), myelodysplastic syndromes, or other myeloid neoplasms.
   c) Presence of *JAK2*, *CALR*, or *MPL* mutation or, in the absence of these mutations, presence of another clonal marker, or absence of reactive myelofibrosis.

2) **Minor criteria**: Presence of ≥1 of the following, confirmed on 2 consecutive determinations:
   a) Anemia not attributed to a comorbid condition.
   b) Leukocytosis $>11 \times 10^9$/L.
   c) Palpable splenomegaly.
   d) Lactate dehydrogenase (LDH) increased to above the upper limit of normal.
   e) Leukoerythroblastosis.

Differential Diagnosis

1. Myelofibrosis caused by malignant conditions: PV, ET, CML, acute megakaryoblastic leukemia, acute panmyelosis with myelofibrosis, MDS, chronic myelomonocytic leukemia (CMML), hairy cell leukemia, multiple myeloma (MM), Hodgkin lymphoma, and some metastatic solid tumors (breast cancer, prostate cancer, non–small cell lung cancer). In early disease it may be difficult or impossible to differentiate myelofibrosis from PV, CML, or especially ET when the only presenting observation is thrombocytosis.

2. Myelofibrosis caused by nonneoplastic conditions: Paget disease, secondary hyperparathyroidism in patients with vitamin D deficiency, renal osteodystrophy, systemic lupus erythematosus; less frequently, other systemic connective tissue diseases, tuberculosis, syphilis, chronic benzene poisoning; thrombopoietin-receptor agonists; radiation exposure.

→ TREATMENT

The only curative treatment for PMF is allogeneic hematopoietic stem cell transplantation (HSCT). The choice of treatment depends on the patient's predicted survival based on the Dynamic International Prognostic Scoring

System (DIPSS) Plus score. The score is used both at the time of diagnosis and in the course of treatment and includes 8 risk factors:

1) Age >65 years.

2) Constitutional symptoms.

3) Hemoglobin (Hb) <100 g/L.

4) WBC count $>25 \times 10^9$/L.

5) Peripheral blood blasts $\geq$1%.

6) Packed red blood cell transfusion dependence.

7) Thrombocytopenia $<100 \times 10^9$/L.

8) Unfavorable karyotype.

Asymptomatic patients classified as low-risk or intermediate-1-risk group (0 or 1 risk factor present) are observed. In patients with symptoms and/or splenomegaly consider conventional symptomatic treatment or JAK inhibition. Patients classified as intermediate-2-risk or high-risk group ($\geq$2 risk factors) may be considered for allogeneic HSCT or treatment with JAK inhibitors if they are symptomatic or have splenomegaly; if this is not feasible, patients receive conventional treatment.

Types of treatment:

1) **Allogeneic HSCT**: The only potentially curative treatment, which could be considered in suitable patients who have predicted survival <5 years (high--risk or intermediate-2-risk group), are transfusion-dependent, or have an unfavorable karyotype. The 5-year survival rates in highly selected patients treated with myeloablative allogeneic HSCT regimens are 45% to 50%.

2) **Cytoreductive treatment** (using doses lower than in other myeloproliferative neoplasms) is indicated in patients with high WBC counts, symptomatic thrombocytopenia, severe splenomegaly, and severe general symptoms. The agents used include hydroxyurea (INN hydroxycarbamide) and interferon α. Rarely melphalan, busulfan, or cladribine may be used.

3) **Treatment of anemia (Hb <100 g/L)**: Transfusion, erythropoiesis--stimulating agents (ESAs), androgens (danazol, testosterone enanthate, fluoxymesterone), glucocorticoids (prednisone), thalidomide, lenalidomide (in patients with 5q- deletion).

4) **Splenectomy** is indicated in patients with severe or painful splenomegaly refractory to cytoreductive treatment, radiation, or both; selected patients with transfusion-dependent anemia; and patients with severe symptomatic portal hypertension. Perioperative mortality is 5% to 10%.

5) **Splenic irradiation**: Indications are the same as in splenectomy.

6) **Irradiation of symptomatic foci of extramedullary hematopoiesis**.

7) **JAK inhibitors (eg, ruxolitinib)** may be of benefit in patients with symptomatic splenomegaly and severe general symptoms.

→ **FOLLOW-UP**

CBC and clinical evaluation should be performed based on the stage of the disease and manifest complications. In early disease, follow-up can be infrequent. Patients may require acute assessments at the time of splenic infarcts to differentiate surgical causes of abdominal pain from complications of the disease.

→ **PROGNOSIS**

PMF has the least favorable prognosis of myeloproliferative neoplasms. Mean survival varies from 15.4 years in the low-risk group to 1.3 years in the high--risk group. Most patients die of infection, hemorrhage, or transformation to leukemia.

9. Porphyria, Acute Intermittent

→ **DEFINITION, ETIOLOGY, PATHOGENESIS**

Acute intermittent porphyria (AIP) is a hereditary autosomal dominant disorder of heme synthesis. Potential disease-causing mutations occur in ~1 in 1700 Europeans. It is a result of deficiency of hepatic porphobilinogen (PBG) deaminase, which leads to the accumulation of porphyrin precursors PBG and δ-aminolevulinic acid (ALA) in situations associated with increased heme synthesis. This is a probable cause of intermittent peripheral neuropathy and sympathetic overactivity. An acute attack of porphyria is often triggered by factors that increase the synthesis of porphyrins, such as hepatocyte cytochrome P450 inducers (most commonly alcohol, steroid sex hormones [eg, progesterone], barbiturates, sulfonamides, carbamazepine, valproic acid, griseofulvin, and ergot derivatives), fasting (including weight-loss diets with a significantly reduced calorie and carbohydrate intake), tobacco and marijuana smoking, infection, stress, and surgery.

→ **CLINICAL FEATURES**

Over 90% of persons with PBG deaminase deficiency never develop any features of the disease. The onset of symptoms is usually between the ages of 20 and 40 years. The disease manifests as attacks, ranging from one in a lifetime to several per year, which are most common in young women. The most frequent symptom is paroxysmal severe abdominal pain with concomitant nausea, vomiting, and constipation (or less commonly diarrhea). The syndrome often resembles the "acute abdomen," but on physical examination the abdomen is soft and signs of peritonitis are absent. Pain can also occur in the back or chest. Patients are often tachycardic and hypertensive and may be febrile. During the attack various neurologic abnormalities develop. These may include paresis or paralysis (usually proximal and symmetric), hyperesthesia, paresthesia, neuropathic pain, and psychiatric symptoms (altered affect, insomnia, confusion, anxiety, hallucinations, paranoia), which either precede or occur simultaneously with the attack. Paresis of respiratory muscles can occur and is life-threatening. During an attack dark urine or darkening of urine when exposed to light may be observed.

→ **DIAGNOSIS**

Diagnostic Tests

1. Laboratory tests:

1) **Blood tests**: Hyponatremia, hypomagnesemia, nonspecific and mild white blood cell (WBC) count elevation.

2) **Urine tests**: Increased urinary PBG and ALA excretion is always seen during an attack. Levels may be measured in a random urine sample; 24-hour collection is not necessary. Levels remain high for months to years after an attack.

2. Plain abdominal radiographs may reveal features of adynamic ileus during an attack.

Diagnostic Criteria

1. During an attack: Increased urinary excretion of ALA and PBG, adjusted to urine creatinine (a normal result excludes porphyria as the cause of symptoms). Preserve a urine sample and send plasma and stool samples for quantitative determination of PBG, ALA, and porphyrins (to help differentiate the various types of porphyrias).

2. Confirmatory tests that may also be used for screening:

1) Enzyme tests: Decreased activity (~50%) of PBG deaminase in red blood cells (RBCs) or lymphocytes (sometimes also measured in dermal fibroblasts).

2) Genetic testing: The specific type of acute porphyria can be established through sequencing of 4 target genes (ie, *ALAD*, *HMBS*, *CPOX*, and *PPOX*).

→ **TREATMENT**

General Measures

1. Recommend avoidance of known factors causing porphyria attacks, including drugs. Detailed lists of safe and unsafe drugs can be found on European websites (porphyria.eu, www.drugs-porphyria.org) and North American websites (drug database at porphyriafoundation.com, porphyriadrugs.com) discussing porphyria. Patients should avoid tobacco smoking, marijuana smoking, and heavy alcohol intake.

2. Provide dietary counseling to ensure a well-balanced diet with appropriate carbohydrate intake (~60%-70% of total caloric intake).

3. Encourage the patient to always carry information about their diagnosis (eg, on a wrist bracelet).

Management of Porphyria Attacks

1. Admit the patient to the hospital and closely monitor their heart rate, blood pressure, neurologic status, fluid balance, and serum electrolyte and creatinine levels (at least daily).

2. Discontinue all drugs and eliminate all other factors that may cause porphyria attacks (→Definition, Etiology, Pathogenesis, above).

3. If diagnosis is uncertain or IV hemin (→below) is not available, start IV infusion of **10% glucose (dextrose)** at a rate of up to 15 g/h (usually 100-125 mL/h and usually <300 g of glucose per day); this may control only a mild porphyria attack (mild pain, no paresis or hyponatremia). Be aware that hypotonic fluids can potentiate dangerous hyponatremia.

4. If available and feasible, as soon as possible start IV **hemin** at a dose of 3 to 4 mg/kg daily (maximum, 250 mg/d) for 3 to 6 days. Clinical improvement is usually seen after 2 to 4 administrations. Of note, the evidence supporting the use of this drug comes from a small case series.○

5. Start **symptomatic treatment** using drugs that can be safely administered in porphyria:

1) Treat dehydration and electrolyte disturbances (→Chapter 4).

2) Manage pain using acetaminophen (INN paracetamol) and opioid analgesics.

3) Manage nausea or vomiting using ondansetron and phenothiazines (eg, chlorpromazine).

4) Manage symptomatic tachycardia and hypertension using β-blockers.

5) Treat infection using penicillins, cephalosporins, and aminoglycosides.

6) Other safe drugs include atropine, gabapentin, glucocorticoids, insulin, and acetylsalicylic acid. Some low-dose short-acting benzodiazepines (eg, low-dose lorazepam) are probably safe, yet it is likely safer to avoid the use of this class of drugs altogether. Clinicians are encouraged to check all medications against published lists of safe and unsafe drugs.

→ **PROGNOSIS**

The rate of attack resolution depends on the severity of nerve injury. If treatment is started promptly, the symptoms usually improve within several days. Features of severe motor neuropathy persist for months or even years. Susceptibility to triggering factors and the frequency of attacks decrease with age. Individuals with AIP are more likely to develop cirrhosis, hepatocellular carcinoma, and chronic renal insufficiency. Monitoring of liver enzymes and renal function, abdominal ultrasonography, and blood pressure measurement should be done regularly (eg, annually).

1. Acquired Immunodeficiency Syndrome (AIDS)

→ **ETIOLOGY AND PATHOGENESIS**

1. Etiologic agent: Human immunodeficiency virus (HIV), a retrovirus that infects CD4-positive cells (T-helper cells, macrophages, monocytes, dendritic cells).

2. Reservoir and transmission: The reservoir of HIV is humans (however, the virus originated in nonhuman primates and was later transmitted to humans). The source of infection is another HIV-infected individual. Principal virus transmission routes include sexual contacts, blood, and mother-to-child transmission, that is, transmission to infants during pregnancy, birth, and breastfeeding.

3. Epidemiology: HIV is present worldwide, with the majority of the epidemic principally affecting sub-Saharan Africa. A significant proportion of infected individuals remain undiagnosed until clinically apparent immunodeficiency develops.

4. Risk factors: Sexual intercourse (estimated median risk of HIV transmission per exposure ranges from 1.1% for receptive anal to 0.082% for insertive vaginal intercourse; receptive oral sex, 0.02%); IV drug use (0.67% per needle-sharing event); needlestick injury (0.3% risk); transmission to a newborn from the HIV-positive mother (risk of ~30% without prophylaxis; this may be reduced to <1% if prophylactic treatment is provided to mother and child).

5. Incubation and contagious period: Primary HIV infection, 1 to 8 weeks; development of acquired immunodeficiency syndrome (AIDS) in individuals not receiving antiretroviral therapy (ART), 1.5 to 15 years (on average 8-10 years) from the time of infection. An HIV-infected individual becomes contagious within a few days of contracting the virus.

→ **CLINICAL FEATURES AND NATURAL HISTORY**

HIV infection progresses through various stages, which are characterized by distinctive clinical features and immunologic parameters and may be classified as one of 5 HIV infection stages (0, 1, 2, 3, or unknown) based on the CD4+ T-cell count or diagnosis of an opportunistic infection (→Table 1-1 and →Table 1-2). Irrespective of infection stages, clinical presentations may include the following:

1. Primary HIV infection [clinical stage 0]): Infection within prior 6 months with a documented sequence of negative/indeterminate results prior to the confirmed HIV positive test. Clinically, a primary HIV infection may manifest as acute retroviral syndrome (ARS) with clinical features of a mononucleosis-like illness. The symptoms may be minor and resolve spontaneously within 2 weeks; the most common ARS symptoms include fever, generalized lymphadenopathy, pharyngitis, rash, and myalgia/arthralgia. HIV infection is commonly associated with the history of other sexually transmitted infections, especially syphilis. Primary HIV infection may be suspected in the following cases:

1) The patient has a history of high-risk sexual exposure or has been exposed to infected blood in the previous few weeks (currently blood products are rarely a source of infection, as they are screened for HIV).

2) An adult patient has a recent episode of "mononucleosis."

3) The patient has signs and symptoms or history of other sexually transmitted diseases (syphilis, gonorrhea).

2. Chronic HIV infection may manifest as the following conditions:

1) **Asymptomatic HIV infection** occurs after the primary infection and results from establishing a relative balance between HIV replication and

Table 1-1. Stages of HIV infection based on the CD4+ T-cell counts in adults and children ≥6 years[a]

Immunologic categories (CD4+ T-cell count)	Clinical categories	
	CD4+ T-cell count	CD4+ T-cell%[b]
Stage 0	Sequence of discordant test results indicative of early HIV infection in which a negative or indeterminate result was obtained within 180 days of a positive result, regardless of CD4 T-lymphocyte test results and opportunistic illness diagnoses	
Stage 1	$\geq 0.5 \times 10^9$/L	≥26
Stage 2	0.2×10^9/L-0.499×10^9/L	14-25
Stage 3	$<0.2 \times 10^9$/L	<14

[a] If the criteria for stage 0 are not met and information on the criteria for other stages is missing, the stage is classified as unknown.

[b] CD4+ T-cell percentage is taken into consideration only if the CD4+ T-cell count is missing.

If the criteria for stage 0 are not met and an opportunistic illness defining stage-3 disease has been diagnosed (→Table 1-2), the patient is classified as stage 3 regardless of CD4+ T-cell test results.

Based on: Centers for Disease Control and Prevention (CDC). 1993 Revised classification system for HIV infection and expanded surveillance case definition for AIDS among adolescents and adults. MMWR Recomm Rep. 1992 Dec 18;41(RR-17):1-19.

HIV, human immunodeficiency virus.

the antiviral immune response. Patients not receiving ART may remain asymptomatic for 1.5 to 15 years.

2) **Persistent generalized lymphadenopathy (PGL)** is observed in the asymptomatic stage and includes enlarged lymph nodes (>1 cm in diameter) in ≥2 regions (except for inguinal nodes) persisting >3 months (key diagnostic criterion).

3) **Chronic fatigue; headache; splenomegaly** (~30%); **increased incidence of nonopportunistic skin, respiratory, and gastrointestinal infections.**

4) **Symptomatic infection with clinical features not fulfilling the criteria for the AIDS-defining condition**; these include infections resulting from decreased CD4+ T-cell counts (→Table 1-2): herpes zoster (shingles) involving >1 dermatome or recurrent bacillary angiomatosis (red papillary skin lesions caused by *Bartonella henselae* infection with features resembling Kaposi sarcoma); oral hairy leukoplakia (lesions similar to oral candidiasis, located mainly on the lateral aspects of the tongue); oropharyngeal (thrush) candidiasis or vulvovaginal candidiasis (persistent, recurrent, or resistant to treatment); cervical dysplasia and cervical carcinoma in situ (human papillomavirus [HPV] infection); fever lasting >1 month; persistent diarrhea lasting >1 month; clinical manifestations of thrombocytopenia; listeriosis; peripheral neuropathy; pelvic inflammatory disease.

3. Clinical features of AIDS: Conditions and opportunistic infections indicative of the stage 3 disease as listed in the AIDS surveillance case definition (opportunistic infections and neoplasms: →Table 1-2). AIDS diagnosis usually requires prompt ART, as the patient may die of opportunistic infections or neoplasms.

Table 1-2. AIDS-indicator diseases

Stage-3 defining opportunistic infections	– Bacterial infections, multiple or recurrent[a] – Candidiasis of bronchi, trachea, or lungs – Candidiasis of esophagus – Cervical cancer, invasive[b] – Coccidioidomycosis, disseminated or extrapulmonary – Cryptococcosis, extrapulmonary – Cryptosporidiosis, chronic intestinal (>1 month's duration) – Cytomegalovirus disease (other than liver, spleen, or nodes), onset at age >1 month – Cytomegalovirus retinitis (with loss of vision) – Encephalopathy attributed to HIV – Herpes simplex: chronic ulcers (>1 month's duration) or bronchitis, pneumonitis, or esophagitis (onset at age >1 month) – Histoplasmosis, disseminated or extrapulmonary – Isosporiasis, chronic intestinal (>1 month's duration) – Kaposi sarcoma – Lymphoma, Burkitt (or equivalent term) – Lymphoma, immunoblastic (or equivalent term) – Lymphoma, primary, of brain – *Mycobacterium avium* complex or *Mycobacterium kansasii*, disseminated or extrapulmonary – *Mycobacterium tuberculosis* of any site, pulmonary,[b] disseminated, or extrapulmonary – Mycobacterium, other species or unidentified species, disseminated or extrapulmonary – *Pneumocystis jirovecii* (previously known as *Pneumocystis carinii*) pneumonia – Pneumonia, recurrent[b] – Progressive multifocal leukoencephalopathy – Salmonella septicemia, recurrent – Toxoplasmosis of brain, onset at age >1 month – Wasting syndrome attributed to HIV
Neoplastic diseases	– Kaposi sarcoma – Lymphoma (Burkitt, primary lymphoma of brain, immunoblastic) – Invasive cervical carcinoma
Clinical syndromes	– HIV-related encephalopathy – HIV-related wasting

[a] Only among children aged <6 years.
[b] Only among adults, adolescents, and children aged ≥6 years.

Adapted from: Centers for Disease Control and Prevention (CDC). Revised surveillance case definition for HIV infection--United States, 2014. MMWR Recomm Rep. 2014 Apr 11;63(RR-03):1-10.

AIDS, acquired immunodeficiency syndrome; HIV, human immunodeficiency virus.

→ DIAGNOSIS

The patient must give his/her informed consent prior to HIV testing. The patient has the right to anonymous testing.

HIV testing should be considered part of differential diagnosis in patients with a condition of unknown etiology that has an atypical course, is resistant

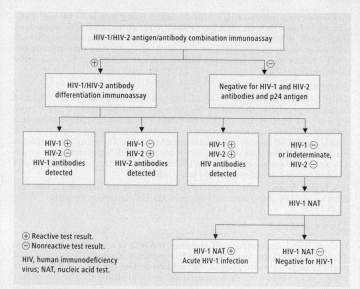

Figure 1-1. Recommended laboratory HIV testing algorithm for serum or plasma specimens. *Based on: Centers for Disease Control and Prevention. Laboratory Testing for the Diagnosis of HIV Infection: Updated Recommendations. Published June 27, 2014. Accessed November 23, 2015.*

to treatment, or recurs, and is potentially related to a known clinical presentation. HIV testing is particularly recommended in the case of a confirmed AIDS-indicator disease (→Table 1-2), syphilis, molluscum contagiosum, genital herpes simplex, anogenital warts, lymphogranuloma venereum, hepatitis B or C, pneumonia not responding to antimicrobial treatment, aseptic meningitis, Guillain-Barré syndrome, transverse myelitis, encephalopathy of unknown etiology, progressive dementia in patients <60 years, vaginal dysplasia, recurrent vulvovaginal candidiasis, HPV infection and other sexually transmitted diseases, pregnancy (including partners of the pregnant women), lung cancer, seminoma, head and neck cancer, Hodgkin lymphoma, Castleman disease, thrombocytopenia, neutropenia or lymphopenia of unclear etiology, loss of body weight for unknown reasons, esophageal or oral candidiasis, persistent diarrhea of unclear etiology, colitis of unclear etiology, cachexia of unclear etiology, herpes simplex virus retinitis, varicella-zoster virus infection, *Toxoplasma gondii* infection, retinopathy of unclear etiology, glomerular and tubular nephropathies of unclear etiology, seborrheic dermatitis, psoriasis without a positive family history, herpes zoster (recurrent, involving large areas of the skin).

Diagnostic Tests

1. Serology (the basis of screening) (→Figure 1-1): Serum anti-HIV antibodies (enzyme-linked immunosorbent assay [ELISA] or enzyme immunoassay [EIA]). Anti-HIV antibodies appear within 2 to 9 weeks of infection (after 8 days at the earliest) and are usually detectable within 12 weeks. A positive result must be confirmed by a Western blot assay (performed exclusively by reference centers). In the case of inconclusive results, fourth-generation tests detecting p24 antigen and anti-HIV antibodies may be used (these allow for the detection of HIV already at the stage of primary HIV infection).

2. Decreased CD4+ T-cell counts; a CD4+/CD8+ T-cell ratio <1.

3. Virology (detection of HIV RNA in serum using molecular biology methods, including DNA and RNA detection, viral culture, or HIV sequence): Diagnostics of seronegative/indeterminate individuals suspected of primary HIV infection, newborns of HIV-positive mothers. Quantitative assays (number of HIV RNA copies/mL) are used to determine viral load and to monitor the effectiveness of ART.

Diagnostic Criteria

Confirmed HIV infection (→Figure 1-1) and fulfillment of the clinical and immunologic criteria that determine the stage of the disease (→Table 1-1 and →Table 1-2). Pretest and posttest counseling is necessary. In patients with primary HIV infection, the screening and confirmatory serologic tests detecting anti-HIV antibodies may be negative or inconclusive. Therefore, the diagnosis may be established solely on the basis of serum HIV RNA detection, or serum p24 antigen if the assays detecting the virus are not available (negative p24 antigen test results do not exclude acute infection).

It is highly recommended to test sexual partners of the individuals who test positive for HIV, are diagnosed with primary HIV infection, or both.

→ **TREATMENT**

1. Combined antiretroviral therapy (cART) is a combination of three drugs acting synergistically to inhibit HIV replication, which allows for at least partial functional restoration of the immune system (increase in CD4+ T-cell counts, sometimes even up to normal values) and elimination of active HIV replication (serum/plasma HIV RNA levels below the limit of detection using the molecular assay), but it does not eradicate the virus nor achieve a total virologic clearance. cART significantly reduces the risk of HIV transmission and improves survival and quality of life. It is used as a long-term treatment option to suppress HIV replication for as long as possible.

2. Indications for cART: The judgement on when to start cART has changed in the light of the START trial. Evidence is accumulating that starting ART on the same day of HIV diagnosis is feasible and acceptable to HIV-positive persons. cART is recommended in all adults with chronic HIV infection irrespective of CD4+ cell counts.◐● An exception to this rule is cryptococcal meningitis, where a delay of ≥2 weeks and possibly up to 10 weeks is suggested, especially in individuals with a low white cell count in cerebrospinal fluid (CSF) or with elevated intracranial pressure (ICP). Another exception is tuberculosis, where starting cART is suggested in pregnant women as early as feasible and in individuals with CD4+ cell count $<0.05\times10^9$/L within 2 weeks, but in those with CD4+ counts $\geq0.05\times10^9$/L it could be delayed for up to 8 weeks. Patients with tuberculous meningitis are at higher risk of adverse event and deaths with early initiation of treatment.

3. Classes of drugs used in cART:

1) Nucleoside/nucleotide reverse transcriptase inhibitors (NRTIs): Abacavir, emtricitabine, lamivudine, tenofovir, zidovudine.

2) Nonnucleoside reverse transcriptase inhibitors (NNRTIs): Efavirenz, etravirine, nevirapine, rilpivirine.

3) Protease inhibitors (PIs): Darunavir, fosamprenavir, indinavir, lopinavir, nelfinavir, saquinavir, tipranavir, atazanavir.

4) Integrase inhibitors (integrase strand transfer inhibitors [INSTIs]): Raltegravir, elvitegravir/cobicistat, dolutegravir, bictegravir.

5) Entry inhibitors: Enfuvirtide.

6) CCR5 inhibitors: Maraviroc.

Recommended combinations of drugs in ART-naive patients: 2 NRTIs + NNRTI; 2 NRTIs + PI (+ low-dose ritonavir); 2 NRTIs + INSTI (most current preferred regimens are INSTI-based).

→ PROGNOSIS

The implementation of cART in HIV-infected individuals results in the restoration of immune function (lymphocyte CD4$^+$ counts, proportions, and function), suppression of HIV replication, decrease in the risk of AIDS-related and non–AIDS-related conditions, as well as improvement in survival rates (life expectancy of an HIV-positive patient receiving cART in whom stable lymphocyte CD4$^+$ counts $>0.5\times10^9$/L have been restored is similar to individuals who are HIV-negative).◔

→ PREVENTION

1. Avoiding exposure to HIV. No vaccine is available.

2. Postexposure prophylaxis: →Chapter 8.10.

3. Preexposure prophylaxis (PrEP): Daily oral PrEP with fixed-dose combination of tenofovir disoproxil fumarate 300 mg and emtricitabine 200 mg has been shown to be safe and effective in reducing the risk of acquisition of HIV in adults. PrEP is recommended as a prevention option in:

1) Men who have sex with men (MSM) who are sexually active and at substantial risk of acquiring HIV infection.

2) Adult heterosexually active men and women who are at substantial risk of acquiring HIV infection

3) Adult persons who inject drugs (injection drug users) at substantial risk of acquiring HIV infection.

PrEP provides a significant decrease in the transmission rate in persons with high risk of sexual transmission (male to male), in whom we recommend its use,◉◔ and in injection drug users, in whom we suggest its use.◔◔ On-demand preexposure prophylaxis is being investigated.

2. Antimicrobial Agents

2.1. Anthelmintic Agents

Pregnancy risk categories: →Table 2-1.

1. Benzimidazoles: Albendazole, mebendazole, triclabendazole:

1) **Spectrum of activity**:

   a) Albendazole: Albendazole has a broad range of activity against intestinal roundworms (*Ascaris lumbricoides*, *Enterobius vermicularis*, *Trichuris trichiura*, *Ancylostoma duodenale*, *Necator americanus*, *Strongyloides stercoralis*), extraintestinal roundworms (cutaneous larva migrans, *Trichinella* spp, *Loa loa*), tapeworms (*Echinococcus* spp, *Taenia solium* cysticerci), and flatworms (*Clonorchis sinensis*). It is also used as alternative therapy for *Giardia lamblia* infection.

   b) Mebendazole: Mebendazole shows similar activity to albendazole but is used predominantly in the treatment of intestinal nematodes, paragonimiasis, and cutaneous larva migrans.

   c) Triclabendazole: The drug of choice for the treatment of liver fluke infections due to *Fasciola hepatica*.

2) **Adverse effects**: Hypersensitivity reaction. Hematologic effects, such as bone marrow suppression (anemia, leukopenia, pancytopenia). Hepatic effects, such as reversible transaminase elevations. Gastrointestinal effects, such as abdominal pain, nausea, and vomiting. Alopecia (albendazole).

3) **Pregnancy risk**: C.

2. Diethylcarbamazine:

1) **Spectrum of activity**: Diethylcarbamazine has activity against lymphatic filariasis, loiasis, and visceral larva migrans.

2) **Adverse reactions**: Inflammatory reactions secondary to death of adult worms (fever, urticaria, asthma, gastrointestinal upset). Other adverse effects include headache, dizziness, and transient exacerbation of lymphangitis.

3) **Pregnancy risk**: Safety not established.

3. Ivermectin:

1) **Spectrum of activity**: Ivermectin is considered first-line therapy for the treatment of *Strongyloides stercoralis* and *Onchocerca volvulus*. It has activity against intestinal nematodes (*A lumbricoides*, *E vermicularis*, *Trichuris trichiura*) but albendazole is usually used as the first-line therapy. Ivermectin is also used in the treatment of cutaneous larva migrans and ectoparasitic infections, such as head lice and scabies. Ivermectin has poor efficacy against hookworms (*A duodenale*, *N americanus*).

2) **Adverse reactions**: Hypersensitivity reaction. Inflammatory reactions related to death of adult worms (Mazzotti reaction). Loiasis must be excluded and treated before initiating treatment for onchocerciasis as serious and/or fatal encephalopathy has been reported with ivermectin use in coinfected patients.

3) **Pregnancy risk**: C.

4. Niclosamide:

1) **Spectrum of activity**: Niclosamide is an alternative treatment option for tapeworms, as it has activity against *Taenia* spp, *Hymenolepis* spp, and *Diphyllobothrium* spp. It is also active against flukes (flatworms), including *C sinensis*, *F hepatica*, *Fasciolopsis buski*, and *Paragonimus* spp.

2) **Adverse reactions**: Anorexia and/or nausea and vomiting.

3) **Pregnancy risk**: B.

5. Praziquantel:

1) **Spectrum of activity**: Praziquantel is considered first-line therapy for infections secondary to flukes (*Schistosoma* spp, *Clonorchis*, *Paragonimus*, and *F buski*) and intestinal tapeworms (*Taenia* spp [including cysticerci], *Hymenolepis* spp, and *Diphyllobothrium* spp). It is not active against *F hepatica*.

2) **Adverse reactions**: Well tolerated. Mild adverse effects include drowsiness, nausea/vomiting, rash, and fever. Contraindicated in ocular cysticercosis.

3) **Pregnancy risk**: B.

6. Pyrantel:

1) **Spectrum of activity**: Pyrantel is active against intestinal roundworms (*A lumbricoides*, *E vermicularis*) and hookworms (*A duodenale*, *N americanus*). Pyrantel is often considered as alternative therapy for the infections listed above and is the drug of choice for pregnant women, as it has minimal systemic absorption.

2) **Adverse reactions**: Mild adverse effects, including gastrointestinal upset, nausea/vomiting, rash, and fever.

3) **Pregnancy risk**: C.

2.2. Antibacterial Agents

Pregnancy risk categories: →Table 2-1.

→ PENICILLINS

Penicillin allergy: →Special Considerations, below.

1. Penicillins: Penicillin G (INN benzylpenicillin) (IV), penicillin V (INN phenoxymethylpenicillin) (oral). Penicillin G has two formulations:

Table 2-1. US Food and Drug Administration pregnancy risk categories

Category	Interpretation
A	Controlled human studies show no risk
B	No evidence of risk in studies. Either animal studies have not demonstrated a fetal risk and no controlled human studies exist or animal studies have shown an adverse effect that was not confirmed in controlled human studies
C	Risk cannot be excluded. Either animal studies have revealed adverse effects on the fetus and there are no controlled human studies or studies in women and animals are not available. Only administer the drug if the potential benefits outweigh the potential risk to the fetus
D	Evidence of human fetal risk. Only administer the drug if the potential benefits outweigh the known risk to the fetus
X	Contraindicated in pregnancy

penicillin G sodium and penicillin G potassium. The potassium-based preparations are preferred in patients with heart failure, and the sodium preparations are favored in patients who experience infusion-related phlebitis.

1) **Mechanism of action**: Penicillin G binds to penicillin-binding proteins on the cell wall and interferes with bacterial cell wall synthesis resulting in bacterial death.

2) **Spectrum of activity**: Active against β-hemolytic streptococci (group A, B, C, D, F, and G), *Listeria monocytogenes*, *Neisseria meningitides*, and *Treponema pallidum*. Activity against other important bacterial species (*Enterococcus faecalis*, *Streptococcus pneumoniae*, viridans-group streptococci, anaerobic bacteria) may vary. Penicillins are inactive against most *Staphylococcus* species, including *Staphylococcus aureus* and coagulase-negative staphylococci, due to β-lactamase (penicillinase) production. In addition, penicillin G and V are inactive against the majority of aerobic gram-negative bacilli as well as *Bacteroides* species.

3) **Adverse reactions**: Anaphylactoid/hypersensitivity reaction. Central nervous system (CNS) effects (increased risk of myoclonus and seizures especially in patients with high drug levels and renal insufficiency). Prolonged use associated with hematologic abnormalities, including hemolytic anemia, neutropenia, thrombocytopenia, interstitial nephritis, hepatitis, and serum sickness.

4) **Pregnancy risk**: B.

2. Semisynthetic antistaphylococcal penicillins: Cloxacillin (oral, IV):

1) **Mechanism of action**: Semisynthetic antistaphylococcal penicillins bind to penicillin-binding proteins on the cell wall and interfere with bacterial cell wall synthesis resulting in bacterial death.

2) **Spectrum of activity**: The drug of choice for penicillinase-producing staphylococci (ie, methicillin-susceptible *S aureus* [MSSA]). Also active against β-hemolytic streptococci and *S pneumoniae*. Inactive against methicillin-resistant *S aureus* (MRSA), *Enterococcus* spp, *L monocytogenes*, aerobic gram-negative bacilli, penicillin-resistant pneumococci, and all anaerobes.

3) **Adverse reactions**: Anaphylactoid/hypersensitivity reaction, CNS effects (increased risk of myoclonus and seizures may occur especially in patients with high drug levels and renal insufficiency), hematologic effects (neutropenia, thrombocytopenia), hepatitis, interstitial nephritis.

4) **Pregnancy risk**: B.

3. Aminopenicillins: Ampicillin (IV), amoxicillin (oral):

1) **Mechanism of action**: Aminopenicillins bind to penicillin-binding proteins on the cell wall and interfere with bacterial cell wall synthesis resulting in cell wall death.

2) **Spectrum of activity**: Compared to penicillins, aminopenicillins have a similar spectrum of activity but with additional aerobic gram-negative coverage including strains of *Haemophilus* that do not produce β-lactamase and some Enterobacteriaceae. Ampicillin is the drug of choice in the treatment of *L monocytogenes* and *E faecalis* infections. It is also active against β-hemolytic streptococci, *S pneumoniae*, *Borrelia burgdorferi*, and most gram-positive anaerobes with the exception of *Clostridium difficile*. The prevalence of resistant strains among *Escherichia coli*, *Proteus mirabilis*, *Salmonella* spp, and *Shigella* spp is variable. Resistance to commonly isolated gram-negative bacilli include all *Klebsiella* spp, the Enterobacteriaceae producing extended-spectrum β-lactamases (ESBLs) and AmpC chromosomal-induced cephalosporinases (SPICE organisms: *Serratia*, *Proteus* [indole-positive], *Citrobacter*, *Enterobacter*), as well as nonfermenting gram-negative bacilli (*Pseudomonas* spp, *Acinetobacter* spp, and *Stenotrophomonas* spp).

3) **Adverse reactions**: Hypersensitivity/anaphylactoid reactions. Rash noted in 65% to 100% of patients with Epstein-Barr Virus (EBV) infection. Hematologic effects (neutropenia, thrombocytopenia).

4) **Pregnancy risk**: B.

4. Carboxypenicillins: Ticarcillin (IV):

1) **Mechanism of action**: Carboxypenicillins bind to penicillin-binding proteins on the cell wall and interfere with bacterial cell wall synthesis resulting in cell wall death. They are able to penetrate the outer cell membrane of selected gram-negative bacteria.

2) **Spectrum of activity**: A penicillin derivative with extended activity against aerobic gram-negative bacilli compared to aminopenicillins. The most important feature of carboxypenicillins is their activity against *Pseudomonas aeruginosa*. Compared with ampicillin, ticarcillin has increased activity against indole-positive *Proteus* spp (*Proteus vulgaris* and *Proteus rettgeri*) and *Morganella morganii*. Otherwise ampicillin is the preferred drug of choice for other Enterobacteriaceae in addition to aerobic gram-positive bacteria, as it is a more active drug. Gram-positive and gram-negative anaerobic coverage is variable.

3) **Adverse reactions**: Hypersensitivity/anaphylactoid reactions. CNS effects similar to penicillin, including seizures when high drug doses are used. Hematologic effects, including bleeding related to platelet dysfunction and neutropenia. Hepatitis.

4) **Pregnancy risk**: B.

5. Ureidopenicillins: Piperacillin (IV):

1) **Mechanism of action**: Ureidopenicillins bind to penicillin-binding proteins on the cell wall and interfere with bacterial cell wall synthesis resulting in cell wall death. They are able to penetrate the outer cell membrane of selected gram-negative bacteria.

2) **Spectrum of activity**: Piperacillin is available alone or more commonly combined with tazobactam (see piperacillin/tazobactam, below). It is a penicillin derivative with extended activity against aerobic gram-negative bacilli, similar to ticarcillin, with activity against *P aeruginosa*. Piperacillin has variable activity to the Enterobacteriaceae family owing to the production of β-lactamases. Gram-positive bacterial coverage is similar to that of ampicillin; however, ampicillin remains the drug of choice secondary to increased activity. Gram-positive and gram-negative anaerobic coverage is variable.

3) **Adverse reactions**: Hypersensitivity/anaphylactoid reactions. CNS effects similar to penicillin, including seizures when high drug doses are used.

Hematologic effects, including bleeding related to platelet dysfunction and neutropenia. Hepatitis.

4) **Pregnancy risk**: B.

→ C E P H A L O S P O R I N S

Enterococcus spp and *L monocytogenes* have natural resistance to all cephalosporins.

Mechanism of action: All cephalosporins bind to penicillin-binding proteins on the cell wall and interfere with bacterial cell wall synthesis resulting in cell wall death.

1. First-generation cephalosporins: Cefazolin (IV) and cephalexin (oral):

1) **Spectrum of activity**: Highly active against MSSA and coagulase-negative staphylococci. Other gram-positive coverage includes β-hemolytic streptococci, *S pneumoniae*, and viridans-group streptococci. Aerobic gram-negative coverage is limited due to the production of β-lactamase–producing bacteria; however, these antibiotics can be susceptible to *E coli*, *Klebsiella* spp, and *P mirabilis*. Resistance is seen to ESBL- and AmpC-producing bacteria, aerobic gram-negative nonfermenters (*Pseudomonas* spp, *Acinetobacter* spp, and *Stenotrophomonas* spp), and most anaerobic bacteria.

2) **Adverse reactions**: Hypersensitivity reactions. Hematologic effects, such as neutropenia and thrombocytopenia. Transient elevations in transaminases or serum alkaline phosphatase have been noted.

3) **Pregnancy risk**: B.

2. Second-generation cephalosporins: This generation of cephalosporins can be divided into two groups: one with activity against *H influenzae* and the other, cephamycins, with activity against *Bacteroides*. The antistaphylococcal activity of second-generation cephalosporins is inferior to that of first-generation cephalosporins.

1) **Cefaclor (oral), cefprozil (oral):**

   a) **Spectrum of activity**: Compared to first-generation cephalosporins, cefaclor and cefprozil have better activity against most streptococci, such as *S pneumoniae* and β-hemolytic streptococci. Aerobic gram-negative coverage is similar to first-generation cephalosporins with the addition of *H influenzae* and *M catarrhalis*. Cefprozil appears to be more active against gram-negative bacteria compared to cefaclor. Resistance is seen to ESBL- and AmpC-producing bacteria, aerobic gram-negative nonfermenters (*Pseudomonas* spp, *Acinetobacter* spp, and *Stenotrophomonas* spp), and most anaerobic bacteria.

   b) **Adverse reactions**: Hypersensitivity reactions including serum sickness, particularly in young children receiving cefaclor. Cefaclor and cefprozil have the same side chain as ampicillin, thus cross-allergenicity may occur.

   c) **Pregnancy risk**: B.

2) **Cefuroxime (IV and oral [cefuroxime axetil]):**

   a) **Spectrum of activity**: This agent is active against most streptococci, such as penicillin-sensitive *S pneumoniae* strains and β-hemolytic streptococci. Cefuroxime has good coverage against *H influenzae* and *M catarrhalis* (including strains producing β-lactamases). Unique among second-generation cephalosporins is cefuroxime's activity against *B burgdorferi*, the causative agent in Lyme disease. Activity against the Enterobacteriaceae is variable and includes *E coli*, *Klebsiella* spp, and *P mirabilis*. Resistance is similar to that of cefaclor and cefprozil.

   b) **Adverse effects**: Hypersensitivity reactions.

   c) **Pregnancy risk**: B.

3) **Cephamycin group**: Cefoxitin (IV):

   a) **Spectrum of activity:** The activity of cefoxitin against gram-positive bacteria is similar to that of other second-generation cephalosporins. Aerobic gram-negative coverage is enhanced with activity against the Enterobacteriaceae including ESBL- but not AmpC-producing strains. Unlike the first-generation cephalosporins, cephamycins are active against many gram-positive and gram-negative anaerobes, including some strains of *Bacteroides*. Unique to cephamycins is the activity against rapidly growing mycobacteria (*Mycobacterium abscessus, Mycobacterium chelonae,* and *Mycobacterium fortuitum*).

   b) **Adverse reactions**: Hypersensitivity reactions.

   c) **Pregnancy risk**: B.

3. Third-generation cephalosporins: In general, compared to first--generation cephalosporins, third-generation cephalosporins have a broader range of activity against gram-negative bacteria and decreased activity against staphylococci.

1) **Cefotaxime (IV) and ceftriaxone (IV)**:

   a) **Spectrum of activity**: These antibiotics are highly active against the Enterobacteriaceae (*E coli, P mirabilis,* indole-positive *Proteus, Klebsiella* spp, *Providencia* spp, *Enterobacter* spp, *Serratia* spp, and *Citrobacter* spp); however, they are susceptible to inactivation by ESBLs and AmpC chromosomal-induced cephalosporinases. Enhanced activity is seen against *Salmonella, Shigella,* and *Yersinia* species, as well as against *Vibrio* spp, *H influenzae, N meningitides,* and *Neisseria gonorrhoeae*. Excellent gram-positive coverage is seen against *S pneumoniae,* β-hemolytic streptococci, and viridans-group streptococci. In addition, both antibiotics have activity against MSSA, but cefazolin and semisynthetic antistaphylococcal penicillins remain the drugs of choice for treatment of bacteremia. Ceftriaxone remains the drug of choice for Lyme disease with CNS involvement. For neurosyphilis, ceftriaxone can be considered as an alternative therapy for those with mild nonanaphylactic allergy to penicillin. These antibiotics are inactive against gram-negative nonfermenters (*Pseudomonas* spp, *Acinetobacter* spp, and *Stenotrophomonas* spp) and to most anaerobic bacteria.

   b) **Adverse reactions**: Hypersensitivity reactions. Pseudocholelithiasis secondary to sludge in the gallbladder and hyperbilirubinemia seen with ceftriaxone only. Hematologic effects (anemia, thrombocytopenia, neutropenia).

   c) **Pregnancy risk**: B.

2) **Cefixime (oral)**:

   a) **Spectrum of activity**: The spectrum of activity of cefixime is not quite as wide as that of the third-generation cephalosporins listed above. While it retains reasonable activity against β-hemolytic streptococci and viridans--group streptococci, variable activity exists for *S pneumoniae* and resistance is seen towards the staphylococcal bacteria. Among the Enterobacteriaceae, *E coli, Klebsiella* spp, *Proteus* spp, *Salmonella* spp, *Shigella* spp, and *Yersinia* spp remain susceptible. Coverage of *Neisseria* species includes *N gonorrhea* only, although increasing resistance has been noted. Cefixime is inactive against gram-negative nonfermenters and most anaerobes.

   b) **Adverse reactions**: Hypersensitivity reactions.

   c) **Pregnancy risk**: B.

3) **Ceftazidime (IV)**:

   a) **Spectrum of activity**: Similar activity to that of ceftriaxone and cefotaxime for the gram-negative bacteria Enterobacteriaceae. Ceftazidime is also particularly active against the gram-negative nonfermenters, including *Pseudomonas, Acinetobacter, Burkholderia,* and *Stenotrophomonas* species. Markedly lower activity against gram-positive cocci compared to ceftriaxone and cefotaxime is noted. Resistance is seen towards ESBL- and AmpC-producing gram-negative bacteria and anaerobes.

b) **Adverse reactions**: Hypersensitivity reactions. Side chains of ceftazidime and aztreonam are identical, resulting in cross-allergenicity. CNS effects, such as seizures, have been associated with high ceftazidime levels in patients with renal insufficiency.

c) **Pregnancy risk**: B.

4. Fourth-generation cephalosporins: Cefepime (IV):

1) **Spectrum of activity**: Cefepime has similar activity to ceftriaxone and cefotaxime with respect to *S pneumoniae* and MSSA. In addition, while similar activity also exists against the Enterobacteriaceae and *H influenzae*, activity of this agent against *Pseudomonas* spp and gram-negative bacilli producing AmpC β-lactamases is high, although there is regional variability with respect to *Pseudomonas* susceptibility. Cefepime is inadequate in the case of ESBL--producing strains, as variable susceptibility has been noted. Cefepime has poor to no activity against other gram-negative nonfermenters, *Burkholderia*, *Acinetobacter*, and *Stenotrophomonas* species, as well as anaerobes.

2) **Adverse reactions**: Hypersensitivity reactions. CNS effects with risk of encephalopathy, myoclonus, seizures, and nonconvulsive status epilepticus.

3) **Pregnancy risk**: B.

5. Fifth-generation cephalosporins:

1) **Ceftaroline (IV):**

   a) **Mechanism of action**: Avid binding to penicillin-binding protein 2a, which results in activity against MRSA.

   b) **Spectrum of activity**: Active against most gram-positive bacteria with notable activity against MRSA and coagulase-negative staphylococci. In vitro activity is seen against vancomycin-intermediate *S aureus* (VISA), hetero-VISA, and vancomycin-resistant *S aureus* (VRSA). Activity against aerobic gram-negative bacilli is similar to that of ceftriaxone and cefotaxime. In addition, ceftaroline has activity against Streptococcus pneumoniae that is intermediate or resistant to penicillin or ceftriaxone. Ceftaroline is inactivated by ESBL and AmpC and is inactive against *Pseudomonas* spp, *Acinetobacter* spp, enterococci, and most anaerobes.

   c) **Adverse reactions**: Hypersensitivity reactions. Positive direct Coombs test without clinical hemolysis.

   d) **Pregnancy risk**: B.

2) **Ceftobiprole (IV):**

   a) **Mechanism of action**: Avid binding to penicillin-binding protein 2a, which results in activity against MRSA. It can also bind penicillin-binding protein 2×in penicillin-resistant S pneumonia.

   b) **Spectrum of activity**: An advanced generation cephalosporin with activity against some aerobic gram-positive and gram-negative bacteria including MRSA and enterococci. Its in-vitro activity is similar to ceftaroline. Ceftobiprole is inactivated by ESBL and AmpC.

   c) **Adverse reactions**: Hypersensitivity reactions/anaphylaxis. Positive direct Coombs test without clinical hemolysis. Hyponatremia.

   d) **Pregnancy risk**: B.

→ MONOBACTAMS

Aztreonam (IV):

1) **Mechanism of action**: Aztreonam binds to penicillin-binding proteins on the cell wall and interferes with bacterial cell wall synthesis resulting in cell wall death.

2) **Spectrum of activity**: Only gram-negative bacteria are susceptible to aztreonam. Most notable activity is against *Pseudomonas* spp; however, antipseudomonal β-lactams are more active. This antibiotic is also active against a wide range of the Enterobacteriaceae (*E coli*, *Proteus* spp, *Klebsiella* spp, *Providencia* spp, *Enterobacter* spp, *Serratia* spp, *Citrobacter* spp, *Salmonella* spp, and *Shigella* spp), although they are susceptible to inactivation by ESBLs and AmpC chromosomal-induced cephalosporinases.

3) **Adverse reactions**: Hypersensitivity reactions. Clinical cross-allergenicity with other β-lactams has not been demonstrated except for ceftazidime, where in vitro cross-allergenicity exists due to their identical side chains.

4) **Pregnancy risk**: B.

➤ CARBAPENEMS

Ertapenem, meropenem, imipenem, doripenem (IV):

1) **Mechanism of action**: Carbapenems bind to penicillin-binding proteins on the cell wall and interfere with bacterial cell wall synthesis resulting in cell wall death.

2) **Spectrum of activity**: These agents have the broadest spectrum of activity of all antibiotics and cover multiple gram-positive, gram-negative (β-lactamase–producing *H influenzae* and the Enterobacteriaceae) and anaerobic bacteria (including *Bacteroides*). Carbapenems are the drug of choice for ESBL- or AmpC-producing gram-negative bacteria. Notable differences between carbapenems include ertapenem resistance in *Pseudomonas* and *Acinetobacter* species, meropenem susceptibility in *Burkholderia* species, and imipenem susceptibility in *Nocardia* species. Carbapenems are generally inactive against *S maltophilia*, *Enterococcus faecium*, and MRSA. Imipenem has the highest activity against *E faecalis*.

3) **Adverse reactions**: Hypersensitivity/anaphylactoid reactions. CNS toxicity including seizures, with imipenem associated with the highest risk. Doripenem should not be used for treatment of pneumonia given its higher mortality rates compared to other carbapenems, such as imipenem.

4) **Pregnancy risk**: B.

➤ BETA-LACTAMASE INHIBITOR COMBINATIONS

Amoxicillin/clavulanic acid and piperacillin/tazobactam are more commonly used in routine practice than ticarcillin/clavulanic acid and ampicillin/sulbactam.

1. Amoxicillin +clavulanic acid (oral):

1) **Mechanism of action**: Amoxicillin binds to penicillin-binding proteins on the cell wall and interferes with bacterial cell wall synthesis resulting in cell wall death. Clavulanic acid acts as a β-lactamase inhibitor.

2) **Spectrum of activity**: The combination of amoxicillin and clavulanic acid retains the antimicrobial activity of amoxicillin with the addition of selected β-lactamase–producing bacteria that are susceptible to the inhibition of clavulanic acid as well as broader anaerobic coverage. Gram-positive coverage includes MSSA, β-hemolytic streptococci, *S pneumoniae*, *E faecalis*, and viridans-group streptococci. Gram-negative β-lactamase–producing strains of *H influenzae* and *Moraxella catarrhalis* are susceptible to amoxicillin/clavulanic acid. Amoxicillin/clavulanic acid is the drug of choice for animal and human bites as it has excellent activity against *Pasteurella* spp, *Capnocytophaga* spp, and other oral pathogens. This antibiotic retains high activity against the vast majority of clinically important gram-positive and gram-negative anaerobic bacteria with the exception of *C difficile*. Similar to amoxicillin, resistance is common against the Enterobacteriaceae producing

ESBL and AmpC β-lactamase–producing strains as well as nonfermenting gram-negative bacilli.

3) **Adverse reactions**: Hypersensitivity/anaphylactoid reactions. Incidence of diarrhea higher than with amoxicillin alone and primarily attributed to the clavulanic acid component. Rash in patients with EBV-mediated infectious mononucleosis. Hepatotoxicity linked to clavulanic acid, usually resulting in a cholestatic reaction.

4) **Pregnancy risk**: B.

2. Piperacillin + tazobactam (IV):

1) **Mechanism of action**: Piperacillin binds to penicillin-binding proteins on the cell wall and interferes with bacterial cell wall synthesis resulting in cell wall death. Tazobactam acts as a β-lactamase inhibitor.

2) **Spectrum of activity**: The activity of this combination is similar to ampicillin/clavulanic acid with additional coverage against nonfermenting gram--negative bacilli (*Pseudomonas* spp and *Acinetobacter* spp). *Stenotrophomonas maltophilia* is resistant.

3) **Adverse reactions**: Hypersensitivity/anaphylactoid reactions. Use with caution in patients with a history of seizure disorder, as high drug levels may increase the risk of seizures. Serious skin reactions, such as toxic epidermal necrolysis, Stevens-Johnson syndrome, and drug reaction with eosinophilia and systemic symptoms (DRESS) have been reported. Hematologic effects, including bleeding related to platelet dysfunction and neutropenia.

4) **Pregnancy risk**: B.

3. Ticarcillin + clavulanic acid (IV):

1) **Mechanism of action**: Ticarcillin binds to penicillin-binding proteins on the cell wall and interferes with bacterial cell wall synthesis resulting in cell wall death. Clavulanic acid acts as a β-lactamase inhibitor.

2) **Spectrum of activity**: Similar to that of piperacillin/tazobactam with the addition of *S maltophilia* coverage.

3) **Adverse reactions**: Hypersensitivity/anaphylactoid reactions. CNS effects similar to penicillin, including seizures when high drug doses are used. Hematologic effects, including bleeding related to platelet dysfunction and neutropenia. Hepatitis.

4) **Pregnancy risk**: B.

4. Ampicillin + sulbactam:

1) **Mechanism of action**: Ampicillin binds to penicillin-binding proteins on the cell wall and interferes with bacterial cell wall synthesis resulting in cell wall death. Sulbactam acts as a β-lactamase inhibitor.

2) **Spectrum of activity**: The addition of the β-lactamase inhibitor sulbactam expands the spectrum of ampicillin to include MSSA, β-lactamase producing *H influenzae* and *M catarrhalis*, some Enterobacteriaceae including *Klebsiella* species, and added anaerobic coverage including *Bacteroides* species. Importantly, ampicillin/sulbactam has activity against many strains of *Acinetobacter baumannii.*

3) **Adverse reactions**: Hypersensitivity/anaphylactoid reactions. Hepatic effects, such as hepatitis and cholestatic jaundice, have been noted. Rash in patients with EBV-mediated infectious mononucleosis.

d) **Pregnancy risk**: B.

5. Ceftolozane + tazobactam (IV):

1) **Mechanism of action**: Ceftolozane binds to penicillin-binding proteins on the cell wall and interferes with bacterial cell wall synthesis resulting in cell wall death. Tazobactam acts as a β-lactamase inhibitor.

2) **Spectrum of activity**: A novel cephalosporin whose main activity is against aerobic gram-negative bacteria, including ESBL-producing strains

and AmpC producers. A unique spectrum exists for multidrug-resistant *P aeruginosa*. Although activity does exist for streptococcal species, this antibiotic is generally inactive to staphylococcal and enterococcal species. Anaerobic coverage includes *Bacteroides* species.

3) **Adverse reactions**: Hypersensitivity reactions.

4) **Pregnancy risk**: B.

6. Ceftazidime + avibactam (IV):

1) **Mechanism of action**: Ceftazidime binds to penicillin-binding proteins on the cell wall and interferes with bacterial cell wall synthesis resulting in cell wall death. Avibactam acts as a β-lactamase inhibitor and protects ceftazidime from degradation.

2) **Spectrum of activity**: A novel cephalosporin whose main activity is against aerobic gram-negative bacteria, including *Pseudomonas* spp, ESBL--producing strains and AmpC producers, and some carbapenemase-producing Enterobacteriaceae (CPE) such as *Klebsiella pneumoniae* carbapenemases and OXA-type carbapenemases. Ceftazidime-avibactam does not have activity against Acinetobacter species or CPE that produce metallo-β-lactamases. It is less active against anaerobes compared with other β-lactam/β-lactamase combinations.

3) **Adverse reactions**: Hypersensitivity reactions. Neurotoxicity (asterixis, coma, encephalopathy, myoclonus, seizures).

4) **Pregnancy risk**: B.

7. Meropenem-vaborbactam (IV):

1) **Mechanism of action**: Meropenem binds to penicillin-binding proteins on the cell wall and interferes with bacterial cell wall synthesis resulting in cell wall death. Vaborbactam acts as a β-lactamase inhibitor and protects meropenem from degradation.

2) **Spectrum of activity**: The main role of this antibiotic is its use against K pneumoniae carbapenemase-producing Enterobacteriaceae. It is not active against class B or D carbapenemases (ie, metallo-β-lactamases and OXA--type enzymes).

3) **Adverse reactions**: Hypersensitivity reactions. Neurotoxicity (seizures, myoclonus).

4) **Pregnancy risk**: No data available.

→ MACROLIDES AND AZALIDES

Discussed agents include **macrolides erythromycin** and **clarithromycin (oral)**; **azalides azithromycin (oral and IV)**; the **ketolide telithromycin (oral)**; and **spiramycin**.

1) **Mechanism of action**: These agents bind to the 50S subunit of bacterial ribosomes leading to inhibition of protein synthesis.

2) **Spectrum of activity**: **Clarithromycin** and **azithromycin** have broader activity compared to erythromycin. The macrolides are used quite extensively for respiratory tract infections. These agents have good activity against *S pneumoniae*, *Haemophilus* spp, *M catarrhalis*, and atypical pneumonia pathogens, including *Legionella pneumophila*, *Chlamydophila pneumoniae*, and *Mycoplasma pneumoniae*. **Erythromycin** is inactive against *H influenzae*. Additional activity includes aerobic gram-positive coverage including MSSA and β-hemolytic *Streptococcus* (group A, B, C, G), although increasing resistance has been noted and susceptibility testing is required before using macrolides for these infections. **Azithromycin** is the macrolide of choice for treatment of sexually transmitted infections, including *Chlamydia trachomatis*, *Mycoplasma genitalium*, and *T pallidum*. Resistance has been noted for *N gonorrhea*. The gram-negative spectrum includes activity against *E coli*,

Salmonella spp, *Yersinia enterocolitica*, *Shigella* spp, *Campylobacter jejuni*, *Vibrio cholerae*, and *Helicobacter pylori*. Unique to both azithromycin and clarithromycin is the activity against nontuberculous mycobacteria, including being first-line therapy for *Mycobacterium avium* complex. **Telithromycin** has a unique spectrum of activity in that it was designed to target macrolide--resistant respiratory pathogens including multidrug-resistant *S pneumoniae*. **Spiramycin** is predominantly used for treatment of suspected or confirmed *Toxoplasma gondii* infection acquired during pregnancy.

3) **Adverse reactions**: Hypersensitivity reactions. Hepatotoxicity and gastrointestinal adverse effects, such as nausea and diarrhea. Cardiac effects, including QT prolongation with risk of torsades de pointes. **Azithromycin** may increase the risk of cardiovascular death in patients with predisposing factors. Transient reversible hearing loss has been associated with azithromycin use. In the case of **telithromycin**, hepatic effects including severe liver injury and acute failure, and cautious use is advised in patients with underlying liver disease. Telithromycin is contraindicated in patients with myasthenia gravis.

4) **Pregnancy risk**: Azithromycin and erythromycin, category B. Clarithromycin and telithromycin, category C.

LINCOSAMIDES

Clindamycin (oral and IV):

1) **Mechanism of action**: Clindamycin binds to the 50S subunit of bacterial ribosomes leading to inhibition of protein synthesis.

2) **Spectrum of activity**: This agent is active against aerobic gram-positive cocci (MSSA, β-hemolytic *Streptococcus*, viridans-group streptococci, *S pneumoniae*), gram-positive and gram-negative anaerobic bacteria (including *Bacteroides* species), and certain protozoa (*Plasmodium falciparum*, *T gondii*, *Pneumocystis jiroveci*). However, increasing rates of resistance have been noted for gram-positive cocci and *Bacteroides* species. Clindamycin is intrinsically inactive against *Enterococcus* and all aerobic gram-negative bacteria.

3) **Adverse reactions**: The most common adverse reactions include diarrhea, including the risk of *C difficile* infection, and hypersensitivity reactions (fever, rash, erythema multiforme, DRESS).

4) **Pregnancy risk**: B.

STREPTOGRAMINS

Quinupristin/dalfopristin (IV):

1) **Mechanism of action**: Quinupristin/dalfopristin binds to the 50S subunit of bacterial ribosomes leading to inhibition of protein synthesis.

2) **Spectrum of activity**: This agent is active against multidrug-resistant strains of gram-positive cocci, including *S aureus* (MRSA, VISA, VRSA), penicillin-resistant *S pneumoniae*, and vancomycin-resistant *E faecium* (VRE). Quinupristin/dalfopristin is inactive against *E faecalis* (due to natural resistance) and all aerobic gram-negative bacilli.

3) **Adverse reactions**: Hypersensitivity reactions. Arthralgias and myalgias. Hyperbilirubinemia. Phlebitis has been noted when the antibiotic is infused through a peripheral line.

4) **Pregnancy risk**: B.

OXAZOLIDINONES

1. Linezolid (oral and IV):

1) **Mechanism of action**: Linezolid binds to the 50S subunit of bacterial ribosomes leading to inhibition of protein synthesis.

2) **Spectrum of activity**: This agent is active against multidrug-resistant strains of gram-positive cocci, including *S aureus* (MRSA, VISA, VRSA), penicillin-resistant *S pneumoniae*, vancomycin-resistant *E faecium* and *E faecalis* (VRE). It is also active against β-hemolytic streptococci and viridans-group streptococci. The unique coverage includes *Nocardia* and a variety of mycobacterial species.

3) **Adverse reactions**: Hypersensitivity reactions. Hematologic effects, such as myelosuppression, dependent on duration of therapy (>2 weeks). Lactic acidosis, peripheral and optic neuropathy with an extended therapy course >4 weeks. Because linezolid is a monoamine oxidase inhibitor, serotonin syndrome may occur with concomitant proserotonergic drug use.

4) **Pregnancy risk**: C.

2. Tedizolid (oral and IV):

1) **Mechanism of action**: Tedizolid binds to the 50S subunit of bacterial ribosomes leading to inhibition of protein synthesis.

2) **Spectrum of activity**: Tedizolid is similar to linezolid with respect to the spectrum of activity. Data on its efficacy for MRSA bacteremia is limited.

3) **Adverse reactions**: Hypersensitivity reactions. Hematologic effects, such as myelosuppression; however, it may be less myelotoxic compared with linezolid. Because tedizolid is a monoamine oxidase inhibitor, serotonin syndrome may occur with concomitant proserotonergic drug use.

4) **Pregnancy risk**: C.

▶ GLYCOPEPTIDES

Vancomycin (IV, oral only indicated for *C difficile*), teicoplanin (IV):

1) **Mechanism of action**: These agents bind to target peptidoglycan (D-alanyl--D-alanine) terminus and inhibit cell wall synthesis.

2) **Spectrum of activity**: Activity is most notable against gram-positive aerobes and anaerobes, and particularly against MSSA and MRSA, enterococci, streptococci, *Corynebacterium* spp, and *Clostridium* spp. Vancomycin's activity is unique in that it has activity against *C difficile* and is recommended as first-line therapy for severe infections. Natural resistance to glycopeptides is found in *Lactobacillus* spp, *Leuconostoc* spp, *Pediococcus* spp, and in *Erysipelothrix rhusiopathiae*. Neither antibiotic has activity against aerobic or anaerobic gram-negative bacteria.

3) **Adverse reactions**: Hypersensitivity reactions, not to be confused with infusion-related reaction red man syndrome (hypotension, flushing, urticaria) due to rapid (<1 hour) IV administration. Rash (erythema multiforme, Stevens-Johnson syndrome, toxic epidermal necrolysis). Nephrotoxicity (acute tubular necrosis and interstitial nephritis) and ototoxicity consisting of tinnitus and vertigo. Hematologic effects, such as neutropenia and thrombocytopenia, noted after prolonged therapy or associated with high drug doses and levels in the blood.

4) **Pregnancy risk**: B (oral), C (IV).

▶ LIPOGLYCOPEPTIDES

Telavancin, oritavancin, dalbavancin (IV) are all new antibiotics.

1) **Mechanism of action**: Inhibition of bacterial cell wall synthesis.

2) **Spectrum of activity**: Currently these antibiotics are only indicated for complicated skin and skin tissue infections caused by susceptible strains of gram-positive bacteria including *S aureus* (MRSA and MSSA), β-hemolytic *Streptococcus* (A and B), and the *Streptococcus anginosus* group. Telavancin and oritavancin are approved for infections with *E faecalis*

(vancomycin-susceptible isolates only). These agents have no activity against aerobic and anaerobic gram-negative bacteria.

3) **Adverse reactions**: **Telavancin** is associated with infusion-related reactions similar to vancomycin, QT prolongation, and nephrotoxicity. **Oritavancin** is associated with infusion-related reactions and increased risk of osteomyelitis. **Dalbavancin** is associated with hypersensitivity reactions, infusion-related reactions, and elevation in liver enzymes.

4) **Pregnancy risk**: C for all 3 drugs.

→ LIPOPEPTIDES

Daptomycin (IV):

1) **Mechanism of action**: Daptomycin produces irreversible alterations in the cell membrane leading to loss of ions such as potassium and eventually leading to cell death.

2) **Spectrum of activity**: Activity is most notable against gram-positive aerobes and particularly against resistant staphylococci (MRSA, VISA, VRSA), *E faecalis* and *E faecium* including VRE, and streptococci. Daptomycin is not to be used for primary pneumonia, as it is inactivated by pulmonary surfactant. It shows no activity against aerobic and anaerobic gram-negative bacteria.

3) **Adverse reactions**: Hypersensitivity reactions. Risk of myopathy and increased creatinine kinase. Peripheral neuropathy. Eosinophilic pneumonia after 2 to 4 weeks of therapy.

4) **Pregnancy risk**: B.

→ FLUOROQUINOLONES

Agents discussed include **second-generation fluoroquinolones ciprofloxacin (oral, IV), norfloxacin (oral), and ofloxacin (oral); third-generation fluoroquinolone levofloxacin (oral, IV)**; and **fourth-generation fluoroquinolone moxifloxacin (oral, IV)**.

1) **Mechanism of action**: Inhibition of DNA gyrase and topoisomerase IV leading to direct inhibition of DNA synthesis.

2) **Spectrum of activity**: The greatest activity of these agents is against aerobic gram-negative bacilli from the Enterobacteriaceae family, including ESBL and AmpC producers, *H influenzae*, *M catarrhalis*, and nonfermenters including *Pseudomonas, Acinetobacter, Burkholderia*, and *Stenotrophomonas* species. Among fluoroquinolones, ciprofloxacin has the most potent activity against gram-negative bacteria, especially against *P aeruginosa*. The third- and fourth-generation agents have better activity against gram-positive bacteria and respiratory pathogens compared to that of second-generation fluoroquinolones; this includes coverage against *S aureus* (MSSA) and *S pneumoniae*, as well as *C pneumoniae*, *M pneumoniae*, and *L pneumophila*. *Enterococcus* species can be susceptible to fluoroquinolones; however, these agents must only be used for urinary infections and not for systemic infections. Unique to moxifloxacin is its enhanced activity against anaerobic bacteria such as *Bacteroides* species, although higher rates of resistance have been noted. Fluoroquinolones also have activity against tuberculous and nontuberculous mycobacteria and are often used in combination therapy.

3) **Adverse reactions**: Hypersensitivity reactions. Exercise caution when using in children aged <16 years due to joint cartilage injury. Gastrointestinal effects, such as diarrhea and *C difficile* infection. CNS toxicity ranging from headaches and lightheadedness to seizures. These agents have neuromuscular--blocking activity and may exacerbate muscle weakness in individuals with

myasthenia gravis. Increased risk of tendinopathy and retinal detachment. Cardiac effects, such as QT prolongation. Dysglycemia in patients with diabetes mellitus with moxifloxacin conferring the highest risk.

4) **Pregnancy risk**: C.

→ **TETRACYCLINES**

Agents discussed include **the first-generation drug tetracycline (oral)**; **second-generation tetracyclines doxycycline (oral, IV) and minocycline (oral, IV)**; and **third-generation tetracycline tigecycline (IV)**.

1) **Mechanism of action**: These agents bind to the 30S ribosomal subunit of bacteria and inhibit protein synthesis. **Doxycycline** is one of the most active tetracyclines and as such is more often used than tetracycline.

2) **Spectrum of activity**: As for **first- and second-generation tetracyclines**, these agents have a broad spectrum of activity, including aerobic gram-positive and gram-negative bacteria. They are also active against MRSA. Major uses of these antibiotics, especially doxycycline, are for infections due to atypical bacteria (*Chlamydia* spp, *Ureaplasma* spp, *Chlamydophila* spp, *M pneumoniae*, *L pneumophila*), spirochetes (*Leptospira* spp, *Borrelia* spp, *Treponema* spp), and *Rickettsia* and *Plasmodium* species.

Third-generation tetracyclines have a narrow spectrum of use, as tigecycline is currently Health Canada–approved only for treatment of complicated skin and soft tissue infections and intra-abdominal infections. Tigecycline is often used for treatment of multidrug-resistant bacteria as it shows activity against VRE, MRSA, and ESBL-, AmpC-, and carbapenemase-producing bacteria. Resistance to tigecycline is frequently observed in *A baumannii*, *Burkholderia cepacia*, *M morganii*, *Providencia* spp, *Proteus* spp, and *S maltophilia*. *Pseudomonas* species have inherent resistance to tigecycline.

3) **Adverse effects**: Contraindicated in children aged <8 years due to deposition in developing teeth and bones. Hypersensitivity reactions. Erosive esophagitis, especially if taken orally at bedtime. Photosensitivity. Risk of intracranial hypertension (eg, pseudotumor cerebri). Increased blood urea nitrogen due to the catabolic effect; therefore, use with caution in patients with renal impairment. Hepatotoxicity more common with tetracycline than with doxycycline.

4) **Pregnancy risk**: D.

→ **AMINOGLYCOSIDES**

Amikacin, gentamicin, tobramycin, streptomycin, spectinomycin (IV, IM, inhaled):

1) **Mechanism of action**: These agents bind to the 30S ribosomal subunit of bacteria and inhibit protein synthesis.

2) **Spectrum of activity**: The spectrum of antimicrobial activity of aminoglycosides includes mainly aerobic gram-negative bacteria including ESBL-, AmpC-, and carbapenemase-producing bacteria and *P aeruginosa*. In severe invasive infections caused by gram-negative bacilli, aminoglycosides are often used in combination with another active antibiotic from a different class, such as β-lactams. Similarly, among gram-positive bacteria such as staphylococci, streptococci, and enterococci, the use of aminoglycosides must always be part of combination therapy with β-lactams or glycopeptides.◐○ **Streptomycin** and **amikacin** demonstrate favorable activity against mycobacteria. **Spectinomycin** is used predominately for second-line treatment against *N gonorrhoeae* in patients with cephalosporin allergy. Aminoglycosides are not active against *Burkholderia* spp, *S maltophilia*, and anaerobic bacteria.

Among all aminoglycosides, resistance to **amikacin** is least frequently seen. **Tobramycin** is most active against *P aeruginosa*. **Gentamicin** is most established among aminoglycosides in combination treatment of infections caused by gram-positive bacteria.

3) **Adverse reactions**: Primary toxicities include nephrotoxicity and ototoxicity (cochlear and vestibular toxicity). Neuromuscular blockade can occur and as such aminoglycosides are contraindicated in patients with myasthenia gravis.

4) **Pregnancy risk**: D.

➔ RIFAMYCINS

1. Rifampin (INN rifampicin), rifapentine, and rifabutin (oral):

1) **Mechanism of action**: Inhibition of bacterial DNA-dependent RNA polymerase.

2) **Spectrum of activity**:

   a) Rifampin: The most common rifamycin used. The primary use of rifampin is in the prophylaxis or treatment of tuberculous and nontuberculous mycobacteria. It is also the drug of choice for *H influenzae* type b and *Neisseria meningitidis* prophylaxis. As treatment, rifampin is given as combination therapy. The ability for rifampin to penetrate biofilms and its activity against staphylococci make it a preferable drug for use in combination therapy for deep-seated staphylococcal infections (endocarditis and prosthetic joints). Monotherapy with rifampin outside of latent tuberculosis and *H influenzae* type b prophylaxis is not recommended due to the rapid emergence of resistance.

   b) Rifabutin: Relative to rifampin, the main advantage of rifabutin is its reduced potential for drug interactions. It is therefore used as a substitute for rifampin in treatment of selected mycobacterial infections in patients receiving medications that exhibit significant interactions with rifampin.

   c) Rifapentine: Currently approved for latent tuberculosis treatment only. An advantage of rifapentine is its long half-life, which means it can be given once a week.

3) **Adverse reactions**: Hypersensitivity reaction. Orange or red discoloration of body fluids. Influenza-like syndrome seen with use of high drug doses and especially with the use of rifapentine and isoniazid. Hematologic effects, such thrombocytopenia, leukopenia, or anemia, with rifabutin having the higher risk. Hepatotoxicity with increased risk in patients with underlying liver disease or with use of concomitant hepatotoxic medications. Significant drug-drug interactions due to CYP3A4 induction.

   Rifabutin-specific reactions: Uveitis (rare).

   Rifapentine-specific reactions: Hyperuricemia.

4) **Pregnancy risk**: C.

2. Rifaximin (oral):

1) **Spectrum of activity**: A nonabsorbable antibiotic that is indicated in the treatment of traveler's diarrhea (*E coli*) and hepatic encephalopathy. It may also be used (off-label) in the treatment of *C difficile* diarrhea in patients not responding to first-line and second-line antimicrobial drugs.

2) **Adverse reactions**: Hypersensitivity reaction.

3) **Pregnancy risk**: C.

➔ OTHER ANTIBACTERIAL AGENTS

1. Sulfamethoxazole/trimethoprim (oral, IV):

1) **Mechanism of action**: The combination of sulfamethoxazole/trimethoprim inhibits enzyme systems involved in the bacterial synthesis of folic acid.

2) **Spectrum of activity**: This agent is effective against a wide variety of aerobic gram-positive and gram-negative bacteria. Out of gram-positive bacteria, sulfamethoxazole/trimethoprim is most active against MSSA and MRSA. Its activity against β-hemolytic streptococci is quite variable. Gram--positive bacilli coverage includes *L monocytogenes* and *Nocardia* species. Gram-negative coverage is notable for the Enterobacteriaceae family (*E coli*, *Proteus* spp, *Klebsiella* spp, *Salmonella* spp, *Shigella* spp, *Y enterocolitica*) including both ESBL and AmpC producers, and *Burkholderia species*. Sulfamethoxazole/trimethoprim is the drug of choice for *S maltophilia* and *P jiroveci*. Resistance is seen against *P aeruginosa* and most anaerobes.

3) **Adverse reactions**: Hypersensitivity reaction/anaphylaxis. Rash, including increased risk for Stevens-Johnson syndrome, erythema multiforme, and toxic epidermal necrolysis. Hematologic effects (agranulocytosis, anemia, thrombocytopenia). Renal effects (increased creatinine due to inhibition of tubular secretion, hyperkalemia, interstitial nephritis). Hepatic toxicity.

4) **Pregnancy risk**: D.

2. Nitrofurantoin (oral):

1) **Mechanism of action**: Nitrofurantoin shows multiple actions, including inhibition of ribosomal translation, bacterial DNA damage, and interference with the Krebs cycle.

2) **Spectrum of activity**: Nitrofurantoin is used exclusively in the treatment of lower urinary tract infections. The spectrum of activity includes gram--positive bacteria (predominantly *Staphylococcus saprophyticus* and entero-cocci, including VRE) and gram-negative bacilli from the Enterobacteriaceae family (including ESBL and AmpC producers). Nitrofurantoin is not active against *P aeruginosa* or anaerobes.

3) **Adverse reactions**: Hypersensitivity reaction, including DRESS syndrome. Contraindicated in patients with renal dysfunction and creatinine clearance <60 mL/min. Due to the risk of hemolytic anemia, use with caution in patients with glucose-6-phosphate dehydrogenase deficiency. Hepatic and pulmonary toxicity with interstitial pneumonitis after prolonged therapy. Neurologic effects, such as peripheral neuropathy and optic neuritis.

4) **Pregnancy risk**: B. Due to the risk of hemolytic anemia, nitrofurantoin is contraindicated at term (38-42 weeks' gestation) and in neonates <1 month of age.

3. Fosfomycin (oral, IV):

1) **Mechanism of action**: Inhibition of cell wall synthesis.

2) **Spectrum of activity**: The oral formulation of fosfomycin is currently available in Canada. It is approved for treatment of uncomplicated lower tract urinary infections secondary to *E coli* and *E faecalis*. Its coverage includes resistant organisms, such as VRE (*E faecalis* only), and ESBL- and carbapenemase-producing gram-negative bacilli.

3) **Adverse reactions**: Hypersensitivity reactions.

4) **Pregnancy risk**: B.

4. Imidazole derivatives: Metronidazole, tinidazole (oral, IV):

1) **Mechanism of action**: These agents are cytotoxic to anaerobic bacteria.

2) **Spectrum of activity**: Metronidazole is more commonly used than ti-nidazole. The primary spectrum of activity includes gram-positive and gram-negative anaerobic bacteria, although they are more active against gram-negative bacteria such as *Bacteroides* spp and *Fusobacterium* spp. Among gram-positive anaerobic bacilli, the majority of *Actinomyces* spp, *Propionibacterium* spp, and *Lactobacillus* spp are resistant. Metronidazole is the drug of choice for treatment of nonsevere *C difficile* diarrhea. These agents are also active against many protozoa (*Trichomonas vaginalis*, *Giardia lamblia*, *Entamoeba histolytica*).

3) **Adverse reactions**: Hypersensitivity reactions. A disulfiram-like reaction when metronidazole is administered systemically to patients drinking ethanol. CNS effects, such as peripheral neuropathy, aseptic meningitis, and optic neuropathy, have been reported with prolonged drug use.

4) **Pregnancy risk**: B.

5. Fidaxomicin (oral):

1) **Mechanism of action**: Fidaxomicin inhibits RNA polymerase, resulting in inhibition of protein synthesis and cell death.

2) **Spectrum of activity**: Currently indicated for treatment of *C difficile* infections in adults.

3) **Adverse reaction**: Hypersensitivity reaction. Due to cross-reactivity with macrolides, it should be used with caution in patients with a history of macrolide allergy.

4) **Pregnancy risk**: B.

6. Mupirocin (topical):

1) **Mechanism of action**: Mupirocin binds to bacterial RNA synthetase resulting in inhibition of protein synthesis.

2) **Spectrum of activity**: A topical antibiotic used to eradicate nasal carriage of *S aureus* including MRSA strains and treat uncomplicated skin infections (eg, impetigo).

3) **Adverse reactions**: Hypersensitivity reaction.

4) **Pregnancy risk**: B.

7. Colistin (polymyxin E) (IV, inhaled):

1) **Mechanism of action**: Colistin acts as a detergent and damages the bacterial cell membrane.

2) **Spectrum of activity**: Colistin has a narrow spectrum of activity and is primarily used for infections with multidrug-resistant bacteria, such as *P aeruginosa*, *Acinetobacter* spp, *S maltophilia*, and carbapenemase-producing *E coli* and *Klebsiella* spp. Some aerobic gram-negative bacilli are intrinsically resistant (*Serratia* spp, *Proteus* spp, *Providencia* spp, and *Morganella* spp). Other resistant organisms include all gram-positive bacteria and most anaerobes.

3) **Adverse reactions**: The most important adverse effect of colistin is nephrotoxicity resulting in acute tubular necrosis. CNS toxicity with dizziness, paresthesia, slurred speech, and vertigo may occur. Use of inhaled colistin may result in bronchoconstriction.

4) **Pregnancy risk**: C.

→ SPECIAL CONSIDERATIONS

Penicillin Allergy

Penicillin allergy is the most common patient-reported drug allergy, with 5% to 10% of patients identifying themselves as allergic. In large studies it has been found that ~90% of these patients will have negative penicillin allergy skin tests and will tolerate penicillin.

For self-identified penicillin-allergic patients, it is suggested they be referred to an allergist for assessment and diagnosis, ideally when they are not acutely ill. Penicillin skin testing is useful in the prediction of Gell and Coombs type 1 hypersensitivity (IgE-mediated allergy). Typical symptoms of these reactions include hives, angioedema, shortness of breath, and drop in blood pressure. Approximately 1% to 3% of skin test-negative patients will react on subsequent challenge to penicillin and these reactions are typically mild.● There is no utility of skin testing in predicting type 4 (cell-mediated) drug reactions. Red flags for these types of reactions include joint pain, fever, and desquamating or bullous rash. Penicillin should be avoided in the future if the patient has a history of these symptoms.

Penicillins and cephalosporins share a common β-lactam ring, which often leads to avoidance of cephalosporins in penicillin-allergic patients. Data suggest that R-group chains are more important in predicting cross-reactivity of these drugs that the β-lactam ring itself.

Clear estimates of cross reactivity are limited by lack of high-quality controlled studies and by the fact that cephalosporins manufactured before 1980 are known to have been contaminated with penicillin. In a group of studies including only patients with confirmed penicillin allergy, on skin testing the reaction rate to cephalosporins was ~3.4%; this falls to 2% if studies published before 1980 are excluded. It must be remembered that cephalosporin allergy can occur independently of penicillin allergy.

Use of cephalosporin in patients with confirmed or reported allergy to penicillin may depend on the available choices and severity of reaction and should consider the above probability.

2.3. Antifungal Agents

Pregnancy risk categories: →Table 2-1.

→ A Z O L E S

Mechanism of action: Azoles act on the cell membrane of fungi. They inhibit cytochrome P450-dependent 14-α-demethylase, which is the enzyme responsible for converting lanosterol to ergosterol.

1. Fluconazole (oral, IV):

1) **Spectrum of activity**: The most important activity is against yeast, including most *Candida* spp (with the exception of decreased activity against *Candida glabrata* and full resistance in *Candida krusei*), *Cryptococcus* spp, and endemic fungi (*Histoplasma, Blastomyces, Coccidioides*, and *Paracoccidioides* spp). It is not active against molds (eg, *Aspergillus* spp). Fluconazole can also be used for the treatment of cutaneous leishmaniasis.

2) **Adverse reactions**: All azoles are associated with hepatic toxicity; the effects may range from mild elevations in transaminases to severe hepatic reactions. QT prolongation, especially in patients with underlying risk factors. Alopecia noted in patients receiving long-term therapy (>3 months).

3) **Pregnancy risk**: C.

2. Itraconazole (oral, IV):

1) **Spectrum of activity**: Activity is similar to that of fluconazole with respect to *Candida* species; however, it offers a broader spectrum of activity against endemic fungi where it is the preferred drug over fluconazole for first-line treatment. In addition, itraconazole has added activity against *Sporothrix schenckii* and certain molds, such as *Aspergillus* species.

2) **Adverse reactions**: Hepatotoxicity risk similar to that of fluconazole. Contraindicated in patients with underlying ventricular dysfunction, as itraconazole has been associated with hypertension, hypokalemia, and peripheral edema leading to congestive heart failure. Central nervous system (CNS) effects, such as delirium and peripheral neuropathy, have been noted.

3) **Pregnancy risk**: C.

3. Voriconazole (oral, IV):

1) **Spectrum of activity**: The spectrum of antifungal activity is broadest among all azoles and includes fluconazole-resistant *C krusei*. Voriconazole is most often used as first-line therapy for mold infections including *Aspergillus* spp, *Scedosporium* spp, and most *Fusarium* spp. Voriconazole is also active against amphotericin-resistant strains of *Aspergillus terreus*. Voriconazole

has no activity against Mucorales species. It has very good vitreous, retinal, and CNS concentrations. One of the major limitations of voriconazole is the significant intraindividual and interindividual pharmacokinetic variability that can lead to clinical failures. Therapeutic drug monitoring (if available) should be carried out to ensure adequate blood levels are achieved.

2) **Adverse reactions**: Hepatotoxicity and QT prolongation similar to fluconazole. Ocular effects, such as visual changes, blurred vision, bright spots, and photophobia, have been noted but tend to subside after the first week of treatment. Dermatologic reactions including rash, photosensitivity, and other exfoliative reactions (Stevens-Johnson syndrome). Long-term use has been associated with painful periostitis and rare cases of malignancy (melanoma, squamous cell carcinoma) have been reported in patients with underlying risk factors. Intravenous formulation contains cyclodextrin, which has a relative contraindication of creatinine clearance <50 mL/min.

3) **Pregnancy risk**: D.

4. Posaconazole (oral [delayed release, suspension; tablet], IV):

1) **Spectrum of activity**: Posaconazole has a spectrum of antifungal activity comparable to that of voriconazole. Additionally, it shows in vitro activity against Mucorales species. For most mold infections, posaconazole is usually reserved for treatment of refractory infections. It is, however, first-line treatment for invasive fungal infection prophylaxis in patients with acute myeloid leukemia or myelodysplastic syndrome undergoing chemotherapy and those with grade 2 and higher graft-versus-host disease receiving immunosuppressive medications.

2) **Adverse reactions**: Risk of hepatotoxicity low compared to other azoles. Use with caution in patients at high risk of QT prolongation. The intravenous formulation contains cyclodextrin, which has a relative contraindication of creatinine clearance <50 mL/min.

3) **Pregnancy risk**: C.

5. Isavuconazole (IV, oral):

1) **Spectrum of activity**: The spectrum is similar to voriconazole with added activity against Mucorales species. A unique benefit of isavuconazole is that the intravenous formulation is free of cyclodextrin and as such can be used in patients with creatinine clearance <50 mL/min.

2) **Adverse reactions**: Hypersensitivity reactions including anaphylaxis and severe skin reactions (Stevens-Johnson syndrome). Hepatotoxicity.

3) **Pregnancy risk**: C.

6. Ketoconazole (oral, topical):

1) **Spectrum of activity**: The antifungal spectrum of ketoconazole is limited to dermatophytes causing skin and nail infections. Ketoconazole is also active against *Candida* spp, but compared with fluconazole it has lower clinical efficacy and more adverse effects.

2) **Adverse reactions**: With ketoconazole applied topically, severe irritation and pruritus may occur. Systemic adverse effects include severe hepatotoxicity and adrenal suppression.

3) **Pregnancy risk**: C.

→ POLYENES

Amphotericin B (standard and lipid formulations: amphotericin B lipid complex, amphotericin B colloidal dispersion, liposomal amphotericin B; IV, inhaled):

1) **Mechanism of action**: Amphotericin B acts on the fungal cell membrane. It binds to ergosterol and causes leakage of intracellular contents, leading to cell death. The lipid composition of all 3 of the lipid formulations is different and contributes to their different pharmacokinetic parameters.

2) **Spectrum of activity**: This agent has a broad spectrum of activity that includes the yeast *Candida* spp, *Cryptococcus neoformans*, endemic fungi (*Histoplasma*, *Blastomyces*, *Coccidioides*, *Paracoccidioides* spp), and *S schenckii*. Mold activity includes *Aspergillus* and Mucorales species. Amphotericin is not active against *Candida lusitaniae*, *Candida guilliermondii*, and *Aspergillus terreus*. *Aspergillus ustus* complex has variable susceptibility. Amphotericin can be used for the treatment of both cutaneous and visceral leishmaniasis.

The use of aerosolized or nebulized amphotericin is limited to patients with cystic fibrosis and prophylaxis in certain high-risk populations, such as lung transplant recipients.

3) **Adverse reactions**: Infusion-related complications (nausea, vomiting, fever, chills) are common with the administration of amphotericin B deoxycholate and liposomal formulations. Fewer infusion-related adverse effects are observed with lipid formulations of amphotericin. The most important adverse effect is nephrotoxicity. Use with caution in patients with underlying renal insufficiency or in patients receiving concomitant renal-toxic medications. Amphotericin B deoxycholate is more nephrotoxic than the lipid-based formulations. Electrolyte abnormalities, including hypokalemia, hypomagnesemia, and hypocalcemia, have been noted and warrant frequent electrolyte monitoring throughout the duration of therapy.

4) **Pregnancy risk**: B (all formulations).

➔ ECHINOCANDINS

Discussed agents include **caspofungin (IV)**, **anidulafungin (IV)**, and **micafungin (IV)**.

1. Mechanism of action: These agents act on fungal cell wall and inhibit synthesis of $(1,3)$-β-D-glucan, which results in loss of cell integrity and cell lysis.

2. Spectrum of activity: Echinocandins have limited yeast and mold activity compared with azoles and polyenes. They are predominantly used for the treatment of *Candida* infections and have the added advantage over azoles in that they are active against *C krusei* and *C glabrata*, although increasing resistance has been noted in *C glabrata*. Echinocandins, however, have higher minimum inhibitory concentrations with *Candida parapsilosis* and *C guilliermondii. Most Candida auris isolates are susceptible to echinocandins.* All of the echinocandins have in vitro activity against *Aspergillus* species and are reserved for use as an alternative therapy. They are not active against dimorphic fungi (*Histoplasma*, *Blastomyces*, *Coccidioides*, *Paracoccidioides* spp) or *C neoformans*. While in vitro activity against Mucorales species has been noted, this has not been supported by clinical data. These agents do not cross the blood-brain barrier or concentrate in the urine and therefore should not be used for treatment of CNS or urinary infections, respectively. All echinocandins can be used in end-stage renal disease and Child-Pugh B liver cirrhosis with no dose adjustments. Only anidulafungin has been studied in Child-Pugh C liver cirrhosis.

3. Adverse reactions: Echinocandins are well tolerated and all 3 have a similar adverse effect profile. Hepatotoxicity with increases in transaminases and alkaline phosphatase with rare clinically significant hepatitis and hepatic failure may develop. Infusion-related symptoms (rash, pruritus, fever).

4. Pregnancy risk: C.

➔ NUCLEOSIDE ANALOGUES

1. Flucytosine:

1) **Spectrum of activity**: This drug is primarily used in combination therapy with amphotericin in the treatment of *C neoformans* and *Candida* meningitis. Flucytosine has no activity against *Aspergillus* species or Mucorales species.

2) **Adverse reactions**: Hematologic effects (leukopenia, thrombocytopenia). Hepatotoxicity (elevation in transaminases). Use with extreme caution in patients with renal dysfunction; dosage adjustment required.

3) **Pregnancy risk**: C.

2. Terbinafine (oral, topical):

1) **Spectrum of activity**: Topical and oral preparations are indicated for use in the treatment of onychomycosis. The use of oral terbinafine has been also emerging for combination therapy in the treatment of multidrug-resistant molds, such as *Scedosporium prolificans* and *A ustus* complex.

2) **Adverse effects**: Hypersensitivity reactions. Gastrointestinal effects, such as taste disturbance. Hematologic effects (lymphopenia and neutropenia). Hepatic effects (acute failure, cholestatic injury).

3) **Pregnancy risk**: B.

2.4. Antiprotozoal Agents

Pregnancy risk categories: →Table 2-1.

1. Antibiotics: Metronidazole, tinidazole, sulfamethoxazole/trimethoprim, clindamycin, spiramycin (→Chapter 8.2.2).

2. Atovaquone:

1) **Spectrum of activity**: Used as an alternative therapy for prophylaxis or treatment of *Pneumocystis jiroveci* (formerly *carinii*) pneumonia in patients who do not tolerate sulfamethoxazole/trimethoprim. It also shows activity against toxoplasmosis and is used in combination therapy with azithromycin for the treatment of babesiosis.

2) **Adverse reactions**: Hypersensitivity reaction. Gastrointestinal effects, such as vomiting and diarrhea. Use with caution in patients with severe liver impairment as rare cases of cholestatic hepatitis and liver failure have been reported. Methemoglobinemia.

3) **Pregnancy risk**: C.

3. Benznidazole (oral):

1) **Spectrum of activity**: Primary therapy for American trypanosomiasis (Chagas disease).

2) **Adverse reactions**: Angioedema. Cutaneous effects (rash, photosensitivity, exfoliative dermatitis, Stevens-Johnson syndrome). Peripheral neuropathy (dose-dependent). Hematologic effects, such as bone marrow suppression. A disulfiram-like reaction can occur with concomitant alcohol use (nausea, vomiting, flushing, headache).

3) **Pregnancy risk**: Not classified. Avoid in pregnancy.

4. Furazolidone:

1) **Spectrum of activity**: A nitrofuran derivative. It is used as alternative therapy for the treatment of resistant *Giardia lamblia* infection and also considered as alternative therapy for *Vibrio cholera* infection.

2) **Adverse reactions**: Hypersensitivity reaction. Gastrointestinal effects, such as vomiting and diarrhea. A disulfiram-like reaction can be seen when taken with alcohol.

3) **Pregnancy risk**: Safety in the childbearing age has not been established.

5. Iodoquinol:

1) **Spectrum of activity**: Iodoquinol is used predominantly for the treatment of noninvasive *Entamoeba histolytica* infection, *Dientamoeba fragilis* infection, and considered an alternative treatment for *Balantidium coli* infection.

2) **Adverse reactions**: Hypersensitivity reaction. Because iodoquinol contains iodine, caution should be used in patients with thyroid disease. Prolonged use may result in optic neuritis and peripheral neuropathy.

3) **Pregnancy risk**: Safety in the childbearing age has not been established.

6. Miltefosine (oral):

1) **Spectrum of activity**: Miltefosine is indicated for the treatment of visceral and cutaneous leishmaniasis.

2) **Adverse reactions**: Gastrointestinal adverse effects (nausea, vomiting, and diarrhea). Central nervous system effects include headache and vertigo.

3) **Pregnancy risk**: D.

7. Nitazoxanide:

1) **Spectrum of activity**: Nitazoxanide is used for the treatment of *Cryptosporidium* infection. It also has activity against *E histolytica* and *G lamblia*.

2) **Adverse reactions**: Hypersensitivity reaction. Gastrointestinal effects, such as abdominal pain, vomiting, and diarrhea.

3) **Pregnancy risk**: B.

8. Nifurtimox (oral):

1) **Spectrum of activity**: Primary therapy for American trypanosomiasis (Chagas disease).

2) **Adverse reactions**: Gastrointestinal adverse effects are common and include abdominal pain, nausea, vomiting, and diarrhea. Central nervous system effects are also common and include insomnia, irritability, depression, tremors, and peripheral neuropathy. Cutaneous effects (erythema, pruritus). Avoid alcohol use during treatment as it may increase the risk of adverse effects.

3) **Pregnancy risk**: Not classified. Avoid use in pregnancy.

9. Paromomycin (oral, topical):

1) **Spectrum of activity**: Paromomycin is an aminoglycoside antibiotic showing no gastrointestinal absorption. It is used in the treatment of noninvasive *E histolytica* and to eliminate luminal cysts after treatment of invasive disease. It also has activity against *D fragilis*, *Cryptosporidium parvum*, and *G lamblia*. As topical therapy, it has been used for the treatment of cutaneous leishmaniasis.

2) **Adverse reactions**: Hypersensitivity reaction. Gastrointestinal effects, such as abdominal pain, vomiting, and diarrhea.

3) **Pregnancy risk**: B.

10. Pentamidine (IV, inhaled):

1) **Spectrum of activity**: Inhaled and parenteral pentamidine is used for prophylaxis and treatment of *P jiroveci* pneumonia. It is also active against *Leishmania* spp, *Trypanosoma brucei gambiense* (West African sleeping sickness), and free-living amoebas (*Acanthamoeba* and *Balamuthia*).

2) **Adverse reactions**: Hypersensitivity reaction. Because pentamidine may cause QT prolongation, avoid it in patients with underlying risk factors for prolonged QT; other cardiac effects include hypotension and arrhythmias. Reversible nephrotoxicity and electrolyte abnormalities, including hyponatremia, hyperkalemia, hypomagnesemia, and hypocalcemia. Hematologic effects (neutropenia, thrombocytopenia). Pentamidine can be toxic to pancreatic islet β cells, causing hypoglycemia and pancreatitis.

3) **Pregnancy risk**: C.

11. Pentavalent antimonials: Sodium stibogluconate (IV, IM) and meglumine antimoniate (IV, IM):

1) **Spectrum of activity**: These agents are indicated for the treatment of visceral and cutaneous leishmaniasis.

2) **Adverse reactions**: Gastrointestinal effects, such as nausea and vomiting, hepatitis, and pancreatitis. Arthralgias and myalgias. Cardiotoxicity including QT prolongation. Bone marrow suppression.

3) **Pregnancy risk**: Not classified.

12. Pyrimethamine:

1) **Spectrum of activity**: Pyrimethamine in combination therapy is used for the treatment of toxoplasmosis (pyrimethamine/sulfadiazine) and prophylaxis of *Pneumocystis* pneumonia (pyrimethamine/dapsone). It also has activity against *Cystoisospora belli*.

2) **Adverse reactions**: Hypersensitivity reaction. Hematologic effects, such as hemolytic anemia (especially in patients with glucose-6-phosphate dehydrogenase deficiency), megaloblastic anemia (in those with folate deficiency), neutropenia, and thrombocytopenia. In patients receiving high doses of pyrimethamine, administer concomitant folinic acid.

3) **Pregnancy risk**: C.

13. Antifungal agents: Fluconazole and amphotericin B (→Chapter 8.2.3).

2.5. Antiviral Agents

Pregnancy risk categories: →Table 2-1.

→ NUCLEOSIDE AND NUCLEOTIDE ANALOGUES

1. Acyclovir (INN aciclovir) (oral, IV) and valacyclovir (INN valaciclovir) (oral):

1) **Spectrum of activity**: Valacyclovir is an ester prodrug of acyclovir with improved bioavailability compared to acyclovir. These agents are mainly used in the treatment of herpes simplex virus (HSV) and varicella-zoster virus (VZV) infections. Their activity against Epstein-Barr virus (EBV) and human herpesvirus 6 (HHV-6) is lower. Cytomegalovirus (CMV) is resistant at clinically achievable levels.

2) **Adverse reactions**: With intravenous administration, central nervous system (CNS) effects, such as headache, lethargy, confusion, and tremors, seen more commonly in patients with renal insufficiency. Renal toxicity due to crystalline nephropathy and interstitial nephritis. Adequate prehydration may prevent nephrotoxicity. Oral formulations are generally well tolerated. Neurotoxicity and nephrotoxicity are less common.

3) **Pregnancy risk**: B.

2. Famciclovir (oral):

1) **Spectrum of activity**: An ester prodrug of penciclovir with improved bioavailability. Activity mainly includes HSV and VZV infections. Activity against EBV is lower. CMV is resistant at clinically achievable levels.

2) **Adverse reactions**: Oral formulations are generally well tolerated. Toxicity is similar to that of oral acyclovir with neurotoxicity and nephrotoxicity.

3) **Pregnancy risk**: B.

3. Ganciclovir (IV, ophthalmic) and valganciclovir (IV, oral):

1) **Spectrum of activity**: Valganciclovir is the prodrug of ganciclovir. These agents are mainly used in the treatment of CMV infections. In vitro activity also exists against other herpesviruses, including HSV, EBV, VZV, and HHV-6, although acyclovir, famciclovir, or valacyclovir are usually preferred over ganciclovir for the treatment of HSV and VZV infections. Ganciclovir is the drug of choice for the treatment of simian herpes B virus.

2) **Adverse reactions**: Hematologic effects (neutropenia, anemia, and thrombocytopenia) with onset commonly observed in the second week of treatment; the effects tend to be reversible. CNS effects (headache, insomnia, confusion, paresthesia).

3) **Pregnancy risk**: C.

4. Cidofovir (IV):

1) **Spectrum of activity**: Cidofovir demonstrates activity against a number of DNA viruses, including CMV, EBV, HHV-6, HHV-8, polyomaviruses

(BK virus), and adenoviruses. Clinically, cidofovir is used in the treatment of CMV infections refractory or resistant to ganciclovir and foscarnet.

2) **Adverse reactions**: The most important toxicity is dose-dependent nephrotoxicity. Cidofovir may cause Fanconi-type syndrome with proteinuria, glucosuria, and metabolic acidosis. It should not be used in patients with creatinine clearance <55 mL/min. Hematologic effects, with the most common adverse effect being neutropenia. Ocular toxicity (iritis, uveitis, reduced intraocular pressure).

3) **Pregnancy risk**: C.

5. Foscarnet (IV):

1) **Spectrum of activity**: A pyrophosphate analogue. Foscarnet is principally used in the treatment of ganciclovir-resistant CMV infections. It also shows activity against HSV (acyclovir-resistant strains), VZV, EBV, and HHV-8.

2) **Adverse reactions**: The most important adverse effects include nephrotoxicity, electrolyte abnormalities (hypocalcemia, hypomagnesemia, and hypokalemia), and infusion-related nausea. Genital ulcerations have been linked to foscarnet therapy and are thought to be caused by high urinary foscarnet concentrations.

3) **Pregnancy risk**: C.

6. Ribavirin (oral, IV, inhaled):

1) **Spectrum of activity**: The main use of ribavirin is in the treatment of hepatitis C virus (HCV) infection; for HCV, ribavirin is always used in combination therapy. Clinically, it has also been used for treatment of respiratory syncytial virus (RSV) bronchiolitis and pneumonia (especially in the immunocompromised population) and several hemorrhagic fever syndromes (Lassa, Crimean-Congo).

2) **Adverse reactions**: In the case of intravenous and oral formulations, the most important adverse effect is dose-dependent hemolytic anemia, which may be exacerbated by cardiac disease and lead to myocardial infarctions. Avoid use in patients with significant/unstable cardiac disease. In the case of inhaled formulations, conjunctival irritation, rash, and bronchospasm may develop.

3) **Pregnancy risk**: X.

→ NUCLEOSIDE AND NUCLEOTIDE REVERSE-
-TRANSCRIPTASE INHIBITORS

Agents used exclusively in the treatment of HIV infection are not included.

1. Adefovir:

1) **Spectrum of activity**: Used in the treatment of hepatitis B virus (HBV) infections. The main advantage is in the treatment of lamivudine-resistant strains.

2) **Adverse effects**: Nephrotoxicity. Lactic acidosis and hepatomegaly. Adefovir may cause the development of HIV drug resistance in patients with unrecognized or untreated HIV infection.

3) **Pregnancy risk**: C.

2. Entecavir:

1) **Spectrum of activity**: Used in the treatment of HBV infections. Cross-resistance can be seen in patients with lamivudine-resistant strains.

2) **Adverse reactions**: Lactic acidosis and hepatomegaly. Entecavir may cause the development of HIV drug resistance in patients with unrecognized or untreated HIV infection.

3) **Pregnancy risk**: C.

3. Lamivudine:

1) **Spectrum of activity**: Used in the treatment of both HIV and HBV infections. The major limitation for the use of lamivudine in HBV infections is the high rates of resistance that will develop while on therapy.

2) **Adverse reactions**: Lactic acidosis and hepatomegaly. Lamivudine may cause the development of HIV drug resistance in patients with unrecognized or untreated HIV infection.

3) **Pregnancy risk**: C.

4. Telbivudine:

1) **Spectrum of activity**: Used in the treatment of HBV infection, although its role in primary therapy is limited.

2) **Adverse reactions**: Lactic acidosis and hepatomegaly. Myopathy and peripheral neuropathy.

3) **Pregnancy risk**: B.

5. Tenofovir disoproxil fumarate:

1) **Spectrum of activity**: Used in the treatment of both HIV and HBV infections. Considered first-line therapy for treatment-naive patients including those with drug-resistant viruses.

2) **Adverse reactions**: Decreased bone density. Nephrotoxicity (classically Fanconi syndrome). Lactic acidosis and hepatomegaly.

3) **Pregnancy risk**: B.

6. Tenofovir alafenamide: A prodrug of tenofovir, converted intracellularly to tenofovir.

1) **Spectrum of activity**: Used in treatment of both HIV and HBV infections. Considered first-line therapy for treatment-naive patients including those with drug-resistant viruses.

2) **Adverse reactions**: The advantages over tenofovir disoproxil fumarate are less nephrotoxicity and less effect on bone mineral density.

3) **Pregnancy risk**: B.

→ ANTIVIRALS AGAINST INFLUENZA VIRUS

1. Neuraminidase inhibitors: Oseltamivir (oral), zanamivir (dry powder inhaler, IV), peramivir (IV):

1) **Spectrum of activity**: These agents are used in the treatment of or prophylaxis against influenza A and B.

2) **Adverse reactions**: Rare hypersensitivity reactions, including anaphylaxis and severe cutaneous reactions (Stevens-Johnson syndrome, erythema multiforme). Rare CNS effects, such as confusion, delirium, or hallucinations, have been reported. Inhaled zanamivir has been associated with bronchospasm. Use with caution in patients with obstructive lung disease, such as asthma or chronic obstructive pulmonary disease.

3) **Pregnancy risk**: C.

2. Adamantanes: Amantadine (oral) and rimantadine (oral):

1) **Spectrum of activity**: These agents are only active against influenza A infections; however, widespread emergence of adamantane-resistant influenza A strains has limited their use. Adamantanes are no longer recommended for the treatment of influenza A infections.

2) **Adverse reactions**: CNS effects, such as anxiety, difficulty concentrating, and lightheadedness, have been noted during the first week of treatment. More serious adverse effects, such as seizures and delirium, are associated with high drug levels resulting from renal insufficiency, especially in those with preexisting seizure or psychiatric disorders.

3) **Pregnancy risk**: C.

ANTIVIRALS AGAINST HCV

There are 5 main categories of currently available HCV medications (a shift toward interferon-sparing regimens):

1. HCV NS3/4A protease inhibitors: Boceprevir, telaprevir, simeprevir, paritaprevir, grazoprevir, voxilaprevir, glecaprevir, asunaprevir.

2. NS5B RNA-dependent RNA polymerase inhibitors: Sofosbuvir, dasabuvir.

3. NS5A HCV protein inhibitors: Daclatasvir, ledipasvir, ombitasvir, elbasvir, velpatasvir, pibrentasvir.

4. Pegylated interferon α 2a and α 2b.

5. Ribavirin (→Nucleoside and Nucleotide Analogues, above).

For more information, please see the chapter on chronic hepatitis C. You may also visit www.hcvguidelines.org.

OTHER ANTIVIRALS

Letermovir is a viral terminase inhibitor.

1) **Spectrum of activity**: Used in primary prophylaxis for CMV infection in patients treated with hematopoietic stem cell transplantation.

2) **Adverse reactions**: Nausea, vomiting, cough, peripheral edema, headache, cough, fatigue, abdominal pain, atrial arrythmias.

3) **Pregnancy risk**: B.

3. Bacterial Neurotoxin-Mediated Diseases

3.1. Botulism

DEFINITION, ETIOLOGY, PATHOGENESIS

Botulism is a group of systemic signs and symptoms associated with flaccid muscle paralysis caused by botulinum toxin, a bacterial neurotoxin.

1. Etiologic agent: A *Clostridium* spp bacillus (most frequently *Clostridium botulinum*) that is an obligate anaerobe producing spores and releasing botulinum toxin, a neurotropic exotoxin and one of the most toxic known substances; more rarely, botulism has also been associated with *Clostridium baratii* and *Clostridium butryricum*. After being absorbed into the bloodstream, botulinum toxin blocks the release of acetylcholine from motor nerve endings, causing flaccid muscle paralysis and autonomic dysfunction. Botulinum toxin affects only the peripheral nerves, does not enter the central nervous system (CNS), and does not penetrate intact skin.

To date, 7 serotypes of botulinum toxin have been identified (A-G). The majority of cases of botulism in humans are caused by serotype A or B, less frequently by serotype E. Serotype F is very rare. However, serotype E is the leading cause of food-borne botulism in North America and is primarily associated with food practices in northern aboriginal communities.

Dissolved botulinum toxin is colorless, odorless, and tasteless. It is inactivated by exposure to a temperature of 100°C for 10 minutes. Spores are destroyed at temperatures of 116°C to 121°C (pressure cooking).

2. Reservoir and transmission: Spores are ubiquitous and survive in soil for years. The most frequent source of infection is food contaminated with spores, which contains replicating bacteria that produce high amounts of botulinum toxin. The most common route of transmission is via the gastrointestinal (GI) tract (food-borne botulism). Preserved foods (most commonly homemade) become an anaerobic environment of low acidity and low content of salt, nitrites, and sugar that may promote growth of *Clostridium* spp (eg, canned meat or vegetables, foil-wrapped vegetables and potatoes, garlic in oil, onions, meat, fish, sauces/dressings). Exceptionally rare forms of botulism are wound botulism, infant botulism, and inhalation botulism (the latter may be caused by the aerosolized toxin released into the air during a bioterrorist attack).

3. Incubation and contagious period: The rate of development and severity of the clinical manifestations depend on the rate of absorption and amount of ingested botulinum toxin. After contaminated food is consumed, the onset of symptoms occurs within 2 hours to 8 days (usually 12-72 hours). The shorter the incubation period, the more severe the course of disease. The patient is not contagious.

→CLINICAL FEATURES

Clinical features are similar in all types of botulism. The principal manifestation is **flaccid muscle paralysis**, which has an acute onset and symmetric progression. It always starts and is most pronounced in the muscles with bulbar innervation (affecting cranial nerve motor nuclei, usually multiple), with subsequent descending progression. Characteristic features of bulbar palsy (the 4 D's) are diplopia, dysarthria, dysphonia, and dysphagia (including impaired gag reflex on physical examination). Infants with botulism often present with generalized hypotonia. The clinical manifestations may vary from relatively mild to severe, including respiratory failure and coma-like state (with preserved consciousness). No sensory disturbances, fever, or altered mental status are observed. Other signs and symptoms:

1) Very frequent (≥90% of patients): Xerostomia (dry mouth).

2) Frequent (>60%-89%): Fatigue, constipation, weakness of the arms and lower extremities, blurred vision, nausea, ptosis, oculomotor nerve palsy, facial nerve palsy.

3) Moderately frequent and rare (≤60%): Dyspnea, vomiting, sore throat, vertigo/ dizziness, abdominal cramps, paresthesias, tongue weakness, mydriasis or rigid pupils, hyporeflexia or areflexia, diarrhea, nystagmus, ataxia.

→DIAGNOSIS

Diagnosis is based on the patient's medical history and clinical features. Neurologic examination may be necessary to exclude other CNS disorders (→Table 3-1). In every case of suspected botulism, attempt to confirm or exclude the diagnosis on the basis of laboratory tests; consultation with a reference laboratory is usually required. Public health authorities generally require immediate notification of all cases of botulism (a 24-hour service is usually available).

Diagnostic Tests

Detection of botulinum toxin in blood samples or culture of toxigenic strains from other samples is the primary method of laboratory confirmation of botulism. Testing should be performed in every case. Samples may include serum (collected before antitoxin administration), feces, gastric contents, enema fluid, and potentially the food product of interest. For infant botulism, the key sample is feces; if not available (infants with botulism are often constipated), enema samples or rectal swabs may be acceptable.

Differential Diagnosis

Differential diagnosis: →Table 3-1.

Table 3-1. Differential diagnosis of botulism

Condition	Distinguishing features
Guillain-Barré syndrome[a]	History of recent infection; paresthesias; frequently ascending paralysis; early deep areflexia; in advanced disease elevated CSF protein levels; abnormal EMG results
Myasthenia gravis	Recurrent paresis; abnormal EMG results; sustained response to cholinesterase inhibitors
Stroke	Frequently asymmetric paresis; CNS abnormalities observed on neuroimaging studies
Poisoning with substances having neurodepressant effects[b]	History of exposure to toxic agents; high levels of drugs or toxins in body fluids
Lambert-Eaton syndrome	Increased muscle strength with prolonged contraction; confirmed small cell lung cancer; EMG results similar to botulism
CNS infections[c]	Altered mental status; CNS abnormalities on neuroimaging studies and EEG; abnormal CSF
CNS tumor	Frequently asymmetric paresis; CNS abnormalities on neuroimaging studies
Inflammatory myopathies	Increased creatine kinase levels
Complications of diabetes mellitus	Sensory neuropathy; paresis involving only few cranial nerves
Hypothyroidism	Abnormal test results

[a] Including variants of Guillain-Barré syndrome, particularly Miller-Fisher syndrome.

[b] For instance, acute ethyl alcohol intoxication, poisoning with organic phosphates, carbon monoxide, nerve gas, magnesium.

[c] Particularly involving the brainstem.

CNS, central nervous system; CSF, cerebrospinal fluid; EEG, electroencephalography; EMG, electromyography.

The diagnosis of botulism is highly improbable in patients without paralysis affecting multiple cranial nerves. Electromyography (EMG) is useful in differential diagnosis.

→ TREATMENT

Specific Treatment

1. Botulinum antitoxin is indicated in all cases with the exception of infant botulism. It should be administered as soon as possible in patients with a justified suspicion of botulism or with confirmed wound botulism and immediately after making the clinical diagnosis in patients with neurologic symptoms. There are various antitoxin preparations and the administered product generally depends on the available supplies, except for infant botulism. Do not delay treatment to perform microbiological tests! Prior to administration, perform a **hypersensitivity skin test** to botulinum antitoxin (equine protein), following the manufacturer's label. If the test result is positive or equivocal, administer antitoxin according to a desensitization protocol, following the manufacturer's instructions. When performing the skin test and administering antitoxin, have all necessary equipment and drugs ready in case of anaphylaxis (hypersensitivity may occur in as many as 9% of patients but is rarely severe).

918

Botulinum antitoxin minimizes nerve damage and disease severity; however, it does not reverse paralysis that has already developed. Treatment may be discontinued if the intensity of paralysis has peaked and symptoms begin to resolve. Do not administer botulinum antitoxin in patients who are allergic to equine proteins or have received equine proteins in the past, unless botulism is severe and life-threatening; if administration of botulinum antitoxin is necessary in such individuals, use a desensitization protocol or administer parenteral glucocorticoids prior to antitoxin.

2. Human Botulism Immune Globulin Intravenous (BIG-IV) is recommended for most cases of infant botulism. Delay in BIG-IV administration is associated with worse outcomes (prolonged mechanical ventilation). The benefits of this product—primarily significant reductions in duration of mechanical ventilation, intensive care unit stay, and overall hospital stay—are most pronounced in infants who receive treatment within 7 days of the onset of symptoms. There is currently only a single product available (BabyBIG®), which is active against *C botulinum* type A or B and usually can be acquired in consultation with public health authorities.

3. Elimination of botulinum toxin from the GI tract (gastric lavage, deep enemas): →Prevention, below.

4. Antibiotic therapy is indicated only in cases of wound botulism (IV penicillin G [INN benzylpenicillin] 3 million U every 4 hours or IV metronidazole 500 mg every 8 hours for several days). Do not use aminoglycosides and clindamycin, as these may increase the neuromuscular blockade.

General Measures and Symptomatic Treatment

1. Start **mechanical ventilation** in case of severe respiratory failure. In some patients it may need to be continued for several months.

2. Place the patient in a **supine position** with the bed rest elevated to 20 to 25 degrees while supporting the cervical spine, as this improves ventilation and reduces the risk of aspiration. Avoid placing the patient in a supine or semirecumbent position without head elevation, which may impair mobility of the diaphragm and airway clearance.

3. Provide **appropriate patient care** (including prophylaxis of pressure ulcers) and **rehabilitation** in case of severe paralysis.

4. Maintain **adequate volume status and nutritional support**. If necessary, use a nasogastric tube, percutaneous endoscopic gastrostomy (PEG), or parenteral nutrition.

→ FOLLOW-UP

Monitor the patient's respiratory function (blood gas analysis, pulse oximetry), positioning (prophylaxis of aspiration), and ability to swallow and eat.

→ COMPLICATIONS

Complications include respiratory failure, death (rare, mostly due to complications related to mechanical ventilation; however, mortality in patients >60 years is ~30%), aspiration, and persistent paresis.

→ PROGNOSIS

Recovery is complete in the majority of patients (in adults within several weeks to several months). Abnormalities in neuromuscular conduction may resolve as late as after 3 to 6 months, while fatigue and dyspnea may persist for years. In untreated patients with severe botulism, the disease leads to death due to airway obstruction (paresis of the pharyngeal and upper airway muscles) and low tidal volumes (paresis of the diaphragm and accessory muscles of respiration).

→ **PREVENTION**

General Preventive Measures

1. Avoidance of suspicious food. If food and water cannot be obtained from trusted sources, they should be boiled before consumption at 85°C to 100°C for 10 minutes. Every food product that may contain soil (particularly homemade preserved food) is potentially contaminated. Products that are spoiled or expired should be discarded. Canned food should be inspected prior to opening: if the lid is bulging (this suggests an accumulation of gas produced by *C botulinum*), the cans should be boiled for a long time and discarded or destroyed. Gas bubbles that appear after opening a jar suggest contamination of the preserved food.

2. Prompt notification of authorities of a justified suspicion or confirmed cases of botulism facilitates a timely epidemiologic investigation.

Specific Prevention

Prophylactic postexposure administration of botulinum antitoxin is not recommended.

3.2. Tetanus

→ **DEFINITION, ETIOLOGY, PATHOGENESIS**

Tetanus is an acute disease of the nervous system caused by a bacterial neurotoxin, which typically manifests as an increased tone and severe spasms of skeletal muscles. This disease is now very rare in developed countries (<1 case per 1 million people per year), primarily thanks to the use of tetanus vaccine.

1. Etiologic agent: *Clostridium tetani*, a gram-positive, rod-shaped, obligate anaerobe producing spores and releasing a neurotoxin (an exotoxin referred to as tetanospasmin). Tetanus toxin enters the subsynaptic zone of central inhibitory neurons (spinal cord, brainstem) and irreversibly blocks the secretion of neurotransmitters (glycine, γ-aminobutyric acid [GABA]). This abolishes their inhibitory effects on the skeletal muscles and results in the increased muscle tone. *C tetani* spores are resistant to environmental factors, disinfectants, and high temperatures; they may survive in soil for many years.

2. Reservoir and transmission: Gastrointestinal tracts of various animals are reservoirs for *C tetani* (the bacteria are excreted with feces into the environment). Infection usually develops as a result of contamination of a wound (the site of entry) with soil fertilized with manure or other material containing spores of *C tetani* (eg, while tending to horses or cattle). The anaerobic conditions in the wound lead to local growth of the bacteria (no systemic dissemination) and production of tetanospasmin.

3. Risk factors: Sustaining wounds while working with soil (particularly soil fertilized with manure), plants, horses, or other livestock, as well as while using tools contaminated with soil; IV substance abuse; incompletely vaccinated or unvaccinated individuals (adults are recommended to receive booster immunization every 10 years). Wounds at exceptionally high risk for tetanus include crush wounds, deep penetrating wounds, gunshot wounds, and wounds with a retained foreign body; wounds highly contaminated with soil, excrements, saliva, or by-products of meat production; wounds infected with aerobic bacteria (which use up oxygen in the wound) that are not cleaned/debrided within 24 hours; and wounds in patients with shock (ischemia), burns, or frostbites. Wounds at low risk for tetanus are superficial wounds with good perfusion and without necrosis that have been sustained indoors.

4. Incubation and contagious period: This may last from 2 to 21 days (usually ~7 days, in rare cases up to several months), depending on type of wound and degree of contamination. Tetanus cannot be spread from person to person.

→ CLINICAL FEATURES

1. Prodromal phase (preceding symptomatic tetanus): Anxiety, malaise, increased muscle tone, sweating, headache, insomnia, pain and paresthesia in the areas adjacent to the wound.

2. Generalized tetanus (the most frequent form):

1) Increased muscle tone and muscle spasms (most severe during the first 2 weeks) without altered mental status. Initially dysphagia and difficulty chewing, followed by trismus (lockjaw, or increased tone of the masseter muscle) and risus sardonicus (increased tone of the orbicularis oris muscle—"sardonic smile"). Increased tone of the abdominal muscles and opisthotonus (trunk arching backward with upper extremities flexed and lower extremities hyperextended). Severe paroxysmal spasms involving various muscle groups of the trunk and extremities, which are triggered by external stimuli (noise, light, touch) and cause severe pain. Some patients develop respiratory obstruction or respiratory arrest (diaphragm spasm).

2) Autonomic instability (predominantly sympathetic) that appears within a few days, peaks during week 2, and is the most frequent cause of death. It manifests as hypertension and tachycardia alternating with hypotension and bradycardia, arrhythmias, cardiac arrest, mydriasis, hyperthermia, laryngospasm, and urinary retention.

3. Localized tetanus: Stiffness of the muscles adjacent to the entry wound. It may resolve spontaneously (as a result of partial immunity to the toxin) or, most frequently, is a prodromal symptom of generalized tetanus. Cephalic tetanus is a rare form of the disease that develops following a head injury and affects the muscles innervated by cranial nerves (most frequently nerve VII). Patients often have facial muscle weakness (due to lower motor neuron damage).

4. Neonatal tetanus: A severe generalized form that develops in newborns of tetanus-susceptible mothers (having no protection by maternal antibody transfer), usually between 4 to 14 days of life. Typically it occurs as a result of umbilical stump infection. Neonatal tetanus is observed predominantly in developing countries.

→ DIAGNOSIS

In medical practice the diagnosis of tetanus is based exclusively on the patient's medical history and clinical presentation. Microbiological and serologic tests are not useful. Tetanus is generally considered reportable to public health units.

Classification of disease severity:

1) **Mild tetanus**: Trismus and risus sardonicus; relatively mild, isolated muscle spasms.

2) **Moderate tetanus**: Trismus and risus sardonicus, dysphagia, stiffness, periodic muscle spasms.

3) **Severe tetanus**: Generalized muscle spasms, respiratory failure, tachycardia, blood pressure fluctuations.

Differential Diagnosis

1. Strychnine poisoning: The only condition with an almost identical clinical presentation as that of tetanus (due to the inhibition of glycine-dependent signaling pathways). Medical history and toxicology test results are conclusive for diagnosis.

2. Meningitis or encephalitis: Nuchal rigidity, usually accompanied by fever and altered mental status.

3. Tetany: This is usually due to abnormalities in electrolytes such as calcium (the most common cause of tetany), phosphate, or magnesium. It can be quickly be identified through measurement of electrolytes and parathyroid hormone (PTH) levels.

4. Dystonic reactions caused by antipsychotic agents (eg, haloperidol) or phenothiazines (eg, promethazine), which may be associated with nuchal stiffness and torticollis (this is rare in patients with tetanus).

5. Inflammation or an abscess of oropharyngeal cavity (eg, a peritonsillar abscess) **or the temporomandibular joint**: This may be associated with trismus; other features typical for tetanus are absent.

6. Stiff person syndrome: An immune-mediated movement disorder that is associated with muscle stiffness with superimposed muscle spasms. It can be considered as part of the differential diagnosis for tetanus, although it generally has a less acute presentation and does not present with trismus.

→ TREATMENT

Patients with moderate or severe tetanus should be treated in an intensive care unit (ICU).

1. Diagnosis and patient stabilization (the first hour):

1) Maintain the airway and ventilation.

2) Place the patient in a dark and quiet room (preferably in an ICU).

3) Perform biochemical and toxicologic testing (calcium level, strychnine, antipsychotic agents, phenothiazines).

4) Take the patient's medical history. Establish the site of entry and immunization history.

5) Administer IV benzodiazepines, for instance, **diazepam** 10 to 40 mg every 1 to 8 hours or midazolam as needed, to sedate the patient, decrease muscle stiffness, and prevent spasms. The dosage should be subsequently tapered down to prevent withdrawal symptoms.

2. Early antitoxin administration and symptomatic treatment (the first 24 hours):

1) IM **human tetanus immunoglobulin (HTIG)** 3000 to 6000 U in a single dose (no test dose is administered; dosage according to the manufacturer's label); it has been suggested (in one small observational study) that a dose of 500 U may be as effective. When HTIG is not available, another potential option is intravenous immunoglobulin (IVIG) at a dose of 200 to 400 mg/kg.

2) IV **metronidazole** 500 mg every 6 hours or 1000 mg every 12 hours for 7 to 10 days eradicates tetanus bacilli from the wound. Penicillin is a second-line option.

3) **Surgical wound debridement and cleaning**.

4) In case of persistent airway obstruction, **intubate the patient and start mechanical ventilation**.

5) **Enteral feeding via a nasogastric tube**.

6) In patients with muscle spasms that are severe or interfere with mechanical ventilation, supportive care and pharmacotherapy (eg, muscle relaxants or paralytic agents) could be used to help control tetanic spasms.

7) Schedule and start tetanus vaccination once the patient is stable, if possible along with the administration of HTIG. In unvaccinated patients administer a complete vaccination series.

3. Intermediate treatment phase (symptomatic treatment; weeks 2-3):

1) In patients with sympathetic hyperactivity, you may administer IV **magnesium sulfate** 40 mg/kg over 30 minutes followed by a continuous infusion and IV **labetalol** 0.25 to 1 mg/min or IV morphine 0.5 to 1 mg/kg/h in a continuous infusion. You may also consider an epidural block (case reports only).

2) In case of hypotension, administer IV crystalloids.

3) In patients with bradycardia, start cardiac pacing (→Chapter 3.2).

4) Prophylaxis of venous thromboembolism (→Chapter 3.19.2).

5) Prophylaxis of pressure ulcers.

4. Convalescence (subsequent 2-6 weeks):

1) Once muscle spasms have resolved, start rehabilitation (physiotherapy and psychotherapy).

2) All patients should undergo active immunization with a full series of tetanus toxoid–containing vaccine during convalescence. Having acute tetanus does not confer immunity against subsequent episodes because of the extremely small quantities of toxin in disease pathogenesis.

→ COMPLICATIONS

Bone fractures, aspiration pneumonia, pulmonary embolism, dehydration, respiratory failure, cardiac arrest, bacterial superinfections (including pneumonia and sepsis), rhabdomyolysis and myoglobinuria resulting in kidney failure, severe tetanus-related psychiatric sequelae (requiring psychotherapy).

→ PROGNOSIS

In patients with mild and localized tetanus, the prognosis is good. Severe generalized tetanus and neonatal tetanus are associated with a poor prognosis.

Historically, mortality rates ranged from ~6% (mild and moderate tetanus) to 60% (severe tetanus) and may be as high as 90% in neonatal tetanus. Currently, the most frequent direct causes of death include autonomic instability and bacterial superinfections (pneumonia, sepsis).

Additional factors worsening the prognosis are incubation period <9 days, time from the onset of symptoms to the first generalized muscle spasm <48 hours, multiple bone fractures, and substance abuse.

The signs and symptoms persist for 4 to 6 weeks, whereas the increased muscle tone and periodic mild muscle spasms may occur for months.

→ PREVENTION

Specific Prevention

1. Vaccination is the key prevention method.

2. Postexposure prophylaxis: Vaccination, passive immunization (HTIG), or both.

General Preventive Measures

Cleaning wounds with soap and water, surgical debridement (removal of necrotic tissues, foreign bodies, purulent exudates).

4. Candidiasis

→ ETIOLOGY AND PATHOGENESIS

1. Etiologic agent: *Candida albicans* is the most frequently isolated species of *Candida*; however, non–*C albicans* species are increasing in frequency and include *C glabrata*, *C parapsilosis*, *C tropicalis*, *C krusei*, *C guilliermondii*, *C lusitaniae*, and *C dubliniensis*. *C auris* is an emerging fungal pathogen that has now been found worldwide with most strains resistant to azoles and echinocandins and some resistant to all classes of antifungals.

2. Reservoir and transmission: *C albicans* is widely present in the environment and can be found in soil, in hospitals, on animals, on objects, and in food. *Candida* spp are saprophytes that reside in the human body and are present on the skin, in the gastrointestinal tract, and in the female genital tract. The majority of *Candida* infections are endogenous from translocation through gut mucosa or breaches of the skin, but transmission can occur between humans and also from the environment. *C auris* can persist in the environment and the clonal nature of spread within clades supports hospital acquisition.

3. Risk factors for infection: Risk factors for systemic candidiasis: Antibacterial treatment, chemotherapy, mechanical ventilation, immunosuppressive treatment (including glucocorticoids), malignancy (particularly hematologic), neutropenia or neutrophil function disorders, abdominal surgery, thoracic surgery, central vascular lines, parenteral nutrition, extensive burns, prematurity or low birth weight in neonates, HIV infection with low CD4$^+$ cell counts, IV drug use, cirrhosis.

4. Incubation and contagious period: The duration of incubation and contagious periods varies and depends on a number of parameters, including the immunologic status of the patient, risk factors, and environment.

→ CLINICAL FEATURES AND NATURAL HISTORY

Patients may develop candidemia (presence of *Candida* spp in blood) without internal organ involvement, candidemia with internal organ involvement, or systemic candidiasis without candidemia.

1. Candidemia: Presence of *Candida* spp in blood cultures.

2. Cardiovascular candidiasis: Endocarditis (→Chapter 3.10) and myocarditis, pericarditis, vascular bed infection (usually associated with catheters or prosthetic grafts).

3. Respiratory candidiasis.

4. Urinary tract candidiasis.

5. Candidiasis of joints, bones, and bone marrow.

6. Central nervous system candidiasis.

7. Candidiasis of other organs: The peritoneum, liver, spleen, pancreas, gallbladder, thyroid, and eye may be involved.

8. Systemic candidiasis: Various organs may be affected (with formation of microabscesses), most frequently the kidney, brain, heart, or eye, and less frequently the lungs, gastrointestinal tract, skin, and endocrine glands.

→ DIAGNOSIS

Diagnostic Tests

1. Identification of the etiologic agent:

1) Blood cultures: In patients with systemic candidiasis blood cultures can be negative in ~50% due to the absence of viable organism, insufficient concentration in blood, or intermittent release. If *Candida* spp are isolated from blood, repeat blood cultures should be performed every day or every other day until clearance is documented, as this will impact the duration of treatment.

2) Serologic studies: Tests for detection of *Candida* spp antigen and antibodies are not widely available and their results should be interpreted with caution, as they do not allow for definite differentiation between systemic infection and contamination. β-D-glucan is found in the cell wall of *Candida* spp in addition to *Aspergillus* and *Pneumocystis jiroveci*. Some consider testing for this antigen helpful in making the decision to start empiric antifungal therapy (high sensitivity but low specificity for invasive candidiasis).

3) Histologic examination with fungal stains (Gomori methenamine silver [GMS] or periodic periodic acid–Schiff [PAS] stain): This is the most reliable method for identifying systemic candidiasis in internal organs.

4) Molecular studies: Polymerase chain reaction [PCR] and sequencing are additional methods to detect *Candida* species.

5) Identification of *Candida* species: Identification from culture is usually performed by automatic methods (eg, Vitek 2, MicroScan) or manual strips (analytical profile index [API] strips) based on enzymatic and assimilation reactions. Matrix-assisted laser desorption/ionization time of flight (MALDI--TOF) is an accurate identification method with rapid results in <30 minutes. Misidentification of *C auris* as *C haemulonii* or *C famata* or no identification can occur with many identification methods. Recent updates in the database libraries for MALDI-TOF have improved the accuracy of identification of *C auris*.

6) Antifungal susceptibility testing: Species-specific clinical breakpoints are available for multiple antifungal agents. In patients with candidemia or severe systemic candidiasis consider performing antifungal susceptibility for azole antifungals. *C krusei* is intrinsically resistant to fluconazole and should always be reported as resistant. Susceptibility testing for echinocandins should be considered in patients with a history of treatment with these drugs as well as and in the case of *C glabrata* or *C parapsilosis* infection and for other species where local antibiogram data suggest increasing resistance. Antifungal susceptibility testing to all 3 classes of antifungals should be performed with *C auris*.

2. Other tests:

1) Imaging studies and endoscopy: These are performed depending on the location of infection.

2) Ophthalmoscopy: Candidiasis causes typical lesions seen on fundoscopy. In the case of ophthalmitis of unknown etiology, it is recommended to perform diagnostic vitreous aspiration. In all patients with confirmed candidemia dilated ophthalmologic examination should be performed in the first week of treatment.

3) Echocardiography: Limited studies support considering echocardiography to evaluate for endocarditis.

→ TREATMENT

Treatment should take into account risk factors, clinical manifestations, coexisting neutropenia, and the strain of *Candida* causing the infection. If candidiasis is suspected in a patient with risk factors, start empiric treatment and continue until the diagnosis is confirmed or excluded. If the isolated species is other than *C albicans*, patient has a history of fluconazole treatment, or infection is severe, the recommended agents include an echinocandin or amphotericin B. Amphotericin B (AmB) includes 1 conventional preparation (AmB deoxycholate) and 3 lipid formulations of AmB (LFAmB): AmB lipid complex, liposomal AmB, and AmB colloidal dispersion. LFAmB is less nephrotoxic than conventional AmB.

Candidemia in Patients Without Neutropenia

1. Preferred treatment: Echinocandins: Caspofungin every 24 hours, first dose 70 mg, subsequent doses 50 mg; micafungin 100 mg every 24 hours; or anidulafungin, first dose 200 mg, subsequent doses 100 mg every 12 hours.◐◐

2. Alternative treatment:

1) Fluconazole 800 mg (12 mg/kg of body weight) followed by a maintenance dose of 400 mg (6 mg/kg) per day. Fluconazole should be considered in patients without severe infection with a *Candida* strain of confirmed susceptibility to fluconazole.

2) LFAmB 3 to 5 mg/kg/d. This regimen should be used in case of intolerance or unavailability of echinocandins or resistance to other classes of antifungal agents.

3. Treatment duration: Treatment should be continued for 14 days from obtaining negative blood culture results provided the infection has not spread to other organs. In clinically stable patients infected by a *Candida* strain susceptible to fluconazole, after 5 to 7 days of treatment with echinocandins or LFAmB switch to fluconazole. In the case of infection with *C glabrata*, if testing indicates dose-dependent susceptibility to fluconazole, maintenance therapy with fluconazole 800 mg (12 mg/kg) per day is recommended. For maintenance treatment in patients with candidemia caused by *C krusei*, use voriconazole in standard doses if susceptible.

4. Removal of intravascular catheters should be performed unless this may cause severe consequences for the patient.🗹○

Candidemia in Patients With Neutropenia

1. Preferred treatment: Echinocandins: Caspofungin every 24 hours, first dose 70 mg, subsequent doses 50 mg; micafungin 100 mg every 24 hours; or anidulafungin, first dose 200 mg, subsequent doses 100 mg every 12 hours.

2. Alternative treatment:

1) LFAmB 3 to 5 mg/kg/d.

2) Fluconazole (in patients who not previously treated with this agent) 800 mg (12 mg/kg) followed by 400 mg (6 mg/kg) per day or voriconazole 400 mg (6 mg/kg) every 12 hours for one day followed by 200 mg (3 mg/kg) every 12 hours. In the case of *C krusei* infection the preferred agents are echinocandins, LFAmB, or voriconazole.

3. Pharmacotherapy duration: 14 days from obtaining a negative blood culture result and clinical improvement provided the infection has not spread to other organs.

4. Supportive treatment: Granulocyte colony-stimulating factor (G-CSF) in patients with chronic candidemia.

5. Removal of intravascular catheters: Should be considered on an individual basis (in patients with neutropenia sources other than intravascular catheters are more frequent).

6. Patients with candidemia and endophthalmitis: Echinocandins should not be used as these drugs do not penetrate into the affected tissue. Management should involve an ophthalmologist as the patient may require intravitreal injection of deoxycholate AmB or voriconazole.

Suspected Candidiasis in Patients Without Neutropenia: Empiric Treatment

Empiric treatment in such cases should be considered in critically ill patients with risk factors for systemic candidiasis and with fever of unknown origin.

1. Preferred treatment: Echinocandins: Caspofungin every 24 hours, first dose 70 mg, subsequent doses 50 mg; micafungin 100 mg every 24 hours; or anidulafungin, first dose 200 mg, subsequent doses 100 mg every 12 hours.

2. Alternative treatment:

1) Fluconazole 800 mg (12 mg/kg) followed by 400 mg (6 mg/kg) per day. This should be used in patients who have not been previously treated with imidazole antifungals; do not use fluconazole in patients colonized with strains resistant to imidazole antifungals.

2) LFAmB 3 to 5 mg/kg/d.

3. Pharmacotherapy duration: 2 weeks. In patients without confirmed fungal infection and no clinical improvement in 4 to 5 days, consider discontinuation of treatment.

Suspected Candidiasis in Patients With Neutropenia: Empiric Treatment

Treatment should be started in patients with persistent fever after 4 days of antimicrobial treatment.

1. Preferred treatment: LFAmB 3 to 5 mg/kg/d, caspofungin at a loading dose of 70 mg followed by 50 mg/d, or voriconazole 400 mg (6 mg/kg) every 12 hours followed by 200 mg (3 mg/kg) every 12 hours.

2. Alternative treatment: Fluconazole 800 mg (12 mg/kg) followed by 400 mg (6 mg/kg) per day or itraconazole 200 mg (3 mg/kg) every 12 hours.

Chronic Systemic Candidiasis, Hepatosplenic Candidiasis

1. Preferred treatment: Start with LFAmB3 to 5 mg/kg/d or echinocandins (caspofungin every 24 hours, first dose 70 mg followed by 50 mg; micafungin 100 mg every 24 hours; or anidulafungin, first dose 200 mg followed by 100 mg every 12 hours) administered for a few weeks. Then continue treatment with oral fluconazole 400 mg (6 mg/kg) in patients with no resistance to fluconazole.

2. Pharmacotherapy duration: The duration is not determined. Usually treatment lasts a few months until regression of lesions; it should be continued for the whole duration of immunosuppression, including chemotherapy and hematopoietic stem cell transplantation (HSCT).

3. Supportive treatment: In patients with persistent fever consider nonsteroidal anti-inflammatory drugs (NSAIDs) or glucocorticoids for 1 to 2 weeks.

Fungal Endocarditis

1. Preferred treatment: LFAmB 3 to 5 mg/kg/d (with or without flucytosine 25 mg/kg every 6 hours) or echinocandins (caspofungin 150 mg/d, micafungin 150 mg/d, or anidulafungin 200 mg/d). Treatment may be continued with fluconazole 400 to 800 mg (6-12 mg/kg) per day provided that susceptibility to fluconazole has been confirmed. In clinically stable patients in whom candidemia has been resolved as well as in those infected with a fluconazole-resistant strain, it is recommended to use oral voriconazole 200 to 300 mg (3-4 mg/kg) every 12 hours or oral posaconazole 300 mg every 24 hours provided that susceptibility to these agents has been confirmed.

2. Surgical treatment: Assessment by a cardiac surgeon required (for valve replacement).

3. Duration of treatment: At least 6 weeks following surgery or longer in the case of a perivalvular abscess or other complications. In patients with contraindications to valve replacement and infection with fluconazole-susceptible *Candida* strains, start long-term treatment with fluconazole 400 to 800 mg/d. In patients with prosthetic valve infection, treatment is the same as in those with native valve infection; continue treatment with fluconazole 400 to 800 mg/d to prevent recurrences.

Fungal Myocarditis or Pericarditis

1. Pharmacologic treatment: LFAmB 3 to 5 mg/kg/d, fluconazole 400 to 800 mg/d (6-12 mg/kg/d), or an echinocandin.

2. Surgical treatment: Pericardiectomy may be considered.

3. Pharmacotherapy duration: Usually a few months.

Fungal Thrombophlebitis

1. Pharmacologic treatment: LFAmB 3 to 5 mg/kg/d, fluconazole 400 to 800 mg/d (6-12 mg/kg/d), or an echinocandin (caspofungin 150 mg/d, micafungin 150 mg/d, or anidulafungin 200 mg/d). In the case of infections with strains susceptible to imidazole antifungals, once response to primary treatment is achieved consider continuing treatment with fluconazole 400 to 800 mg/d (6-12 mg/kg).

2. Surgical treatment: Surgical treatment is recommended whenever possible.

3. Pharmacotherapy duration: Treatment should be continued for 14 days from obtaining negative blood culture results.

Fungal Infections of a Cardiac Pacemaker, ICD, or VAD

1. Preferred treatment: LFAmB 3 to 5 mg/kg/d (with or without flucytosine 25 mg/kg every 6 hours) or echinocandins (caspofungin 150 mg/d, micafungin

150 mg/d, or anidulafungin 200 mg/d). Treatment may be continued with fluconazole 400 to 800 mg (6-12 mg/kg) per day provided that susceptibility to fluconazole has been confirmed. In clinically stable patients in whom candidemia has resolved as well as in those infected with a fluconazole-resistant strain, it is recommended to use oral voriconazole 200 to 300 mg (3-4 mg/kg) every 12 hours or oral posaconazole 300 mg every 24 hours provided that susceptibility to these agents has been confirmed.

2. Pharmacotherapy duration: 4 weeks following removal of the device in patients with pocket infection, ≥6 weeks in patients after electrode replacement. In patients with a ventricular assist device (VAD), use long-term treatment with fluconazole for the whole duration of VAD treatment.

3. Surgical treatment: Removal of the pacemaker or implantable cardioverter--defibrillator (ICD). Reinsertion is based on the presence/absence of concomitant valvular endocarditis and clearance of fungemia.

Asymptomatic Candiduria
→Chapter 8.16.2.

Symptomatic Fungal Cystitis
Removal of the urinary catheter is a starting point.

1. Preferred treatment: In the case of infections with *Candida* strains susceptible to fluconazole, use fluconazole 200 mg (3 mg/kg) per day for 14 days. In the case of infections with *C glabrata* strains resistant to fluconazole, use AmB deoxycholate 0.3 to 0.6 mg/kg for 1 to 7 days or flucytosine 25 mg/kg every 6 hours for 7 to 10 days. In the case of infections with *C krusei*, use AmB deoxycholate 0.3 to 0.6 mg/kg for 1 to 7 days.

2. Alternative treatment: Intravesical administration of AmB deoxycholate (50 mg/L of sterile water per day) is used only in the case of infection with strains with primary resistance to fluconazole (eg, *C glabrata*, *C krusei*). Treatment duration is 5 days.

Fungal Pyelonephritis
1. Preferred treatment: In the case of infections with strains susceptible to fluconazole, use fluconazole 200 to 400 mg (3-6 mg/kg) per day for 14 days. In the case of infections with *C glabrata* strains resistant to fluconazole, use AmB deoxycholate 0.3 to 0.6 mg/kg for 1 to 7 days as monotherapy, AmB deoxycholate in combination with flucytosine 25 mg/kg every 6 hours, or flucytosine as monotherapy for 14 days. In the case of infections with *C krusei*, use AmB deoxycholate 0.3 to 0.6 mg/kg for 1 to 7 days.

2. Surgical treatment: Removal of urinary tract obstruction. In patients with nephroureteral stents or nephrostomy catheters, consider their replacement.

Urinary Tract Candidiasis With Fungus Balls
1. Pharmacologic treatment: As in pyelonephritis. Additionally perform irrigation with a nephrostomy catheter using AmB deoxycholate 25 to 50 mg dissolved in 200 to 500 mL of sterile water.

2. Surgical treatment: Mechanical removal of the fungus balls.

Fungal Osteomyelitis
1. Preferred treatment:
1) Fluconazole 400 mg (6 mg/kg) per day for 6 to 12 months.
2) Echinocandins (caspofungin 50-70 mg/d, micafungin 100 mg every 24 hours, or anidulafungin 100 mg/d) for ≥2 weeks followed by fluconazole 400 mg (6 mg/kg) per day for 6 to 12 months.

2. Alternative treatment: LFAmB 3 to 5 mg/kg/d for ≥2 weeks followed by fluconazole for up to 6 to 12 months.

3. Surgical treatment: Debridement and/or removal of the lesion are frequently necessary.

Fungal Arthritis

→Chapter 14.9.

Central Nervous System Candidiasis

→Chapter 8.5.3.

C auris **Infection**

1. Pharmacologic treatment: Anidulafungin, first dose 200 mg IV followed by 100 mg IV every 24 hours; caspofungin, first dose 70 mg/d IV followed by 50 mg/d IV; or micafungin 100 mg/d IV. In case of lack of response or fungemia persisting >5 days, use LFAmB 5 mg/kg/d.

2. Pharmacotherapy duration and surgical treatment: As recommended for the specific type of infection. Specialist consultation is required.

→ PROGNOSIS

In patients with systemic candidiasis the prognosis is poor. Patients with hepatosplenic candidiasis are at a very high risk of death.

→ PREVENTION

Prophylactic use of antifungal agents to prevent invasive candidiasis is controversial. It may be considered in:

1) Recipients of allogeneic HSCT (fluconazole, posaconazole, micafungin).
2) Patients treated in intensive care units, particularly those after surgery (fluconazole).
3) Patients with chemotherapy-induced neutropenia until granulocyte counts increase.
4) Patients with HIV infection, recurrent candidiasis, and low CD4$^+$ counts.

Candida auris has been associated with clonal spread and nosocomial transmission causing hospital outbreaks. Due to the persistence of *C auris* in the environment, consider surveillance for carriage of *C auris* in high-risk patients. Contact precautions are recommended to limit nosocomial transmission.

5. Central Nervous System Infections

5.1. Encephalitis

→ DEFINITION, ETIOLOGY, PATHOGENESIS

Encephalitis is an inflammatory process involving the nervous tissue in the brain and frequently also the meninges (meningoencephalitis) and the subarachnoid space. It is caused by the presence of microorganisms in the brain parenchyma (among others, this may be due to the progression of meningitis).

1. Etiologic agents: Encephalitis is usually caused by viruses, including herpes simplex virus (HSV) and varicella-zoster virus (VZV); flaviviruses such as West Nile (WNV), St Louis, and Powassan viruses; and rarely by measles, mumps, or rubella viruses, cytomegalovirus (CMV), enteroviruses (type 71), rabies virus, HIV, Epstein-Barr virus (EBV), influenza viruses, human herpesvirus 6 (HHV-6), or fungi (*Candida* spp, *Cryptococcus neoformans*, *Aspergillus* spp).

2. Reservoir and transmission: These vary with etiologic agents. The reservoir is predominantly humans; the only exception is rabies virus, in which case the reservoir is wild animals (foxes, squirrels, bats), dogs, and less frequently cats. In flaviviruses, such as WNV, birds may be the reservoirs and infections are spread via mosquito or tick vectors. Depending on the pathogen, transmission occurs through airborne droplets, direct contact with sick individuals or human secretions, or vectors; in rabies, transmission is through a bite of an infected animal or direct contact of injured skin or mucosa with animal saliva.

3. Epidemiology: The incidence of viral encephalitis in some countries is between 1 to 2 cases per 100,000 persons per year. In the case of certain viruses (VZV, enteroviruses, tick-borne encephalitis virus [TBEV] [in endemic areas outside North America]) occurrence is seasonal. **Risk factors**: Enclosed areas, public beaches and swimming pools, hypogammaglobulinemia, impaired cell-mediated immunity, contact with stray or wild animals (rabies), living in regions endemic for TBEV, contact with sick individuals. Risk factors for fungal central nervous system (CNS) infections: →Chapter 8.5.3.

→ CLINICAL FEATURES AND NATURAL HISTORY

In many patients neurologic features are preceded by prodromal manifestations (influenza-like symptoms: diarrhea, fever, lymphadenopathy), manifestations of an underlying condition (eg, measles, mumps, varicella), or both. A particularly severe and highly dynamic course of the disease is associated with herpes simplex encephalomyelitis (herpetic skin and mucosal lesions are usually absent). The dominant clinical features include **altered mental status**, **fever** of various grades, and **focal neurologic deficits**: alterations of mental status that may be qualitative (psychotic and personality disorders) and quantitative (various degrees of impairment, which may progress to coma); headache, nausea and vomiting, bradycardia (clinical features of cerebral edema and increased intracranial pressure [→Chapter 10.7]); focal and generalized seizures; spastic paresis or paralysis and other features of involvement of the pyramidal neurons (motor neuron disease); paresis or paralysis of the cranial nerves (most frequently III, VI, IV, and VII); flaccid paralysis (indicating brainstem injury); cerebellar signs (predominantly in the course of cerebellitis associated with varicella); memory impairment, including severe amnestic disorders; motor or mixed aphasia; autonomic hyperactivity—excessive sweating, alternating bradycardia and tachycardia, hypothermia or hyperthermia, and hypersalivation (sialorrhea; eg, in the course of rabies).

→ DIAGNOSIS

Diagnostic Tests

1. Magnetic resonance imaging (MRI) (preferred) or **computed tomography (CT) of the head** is mandatory in every patient suspected of encephalitis. Abnormalities may be observed even in early stages of the disease (particularly on MRI); their location and features may be suggestive of etiology or exclude other causes. Patients with acute encephalitis may have features of cerebral edema.

2. Analysis of cerebrospinal fluid (CSF): Elevated opening pressure with a slight predominance of mononuclear cells, increased protein levels, or both. In patients with meningoencephalitis, CSF abnormalities depend on etiology. Increased intracranial pressure (eg, in cerebral edema) is a contraindication to lumbar puncture; if features of cerebral edema or focal deficits are present, the patient's eligibility for lumbar puncture should be determined on the basis of MRI or CT.

3. Microbiological studies: As in meningitis. The basis for establishing the etiology of viral CNS infections is detection of viral genetic material in CSF by polymerase chain reaction (PCR) or reverse transcription polymerase chain reaction (RT-PCR); if clinical features suggest herpes simplex encephalitis and PCR results are negative, consider repeat PCR testing after 3 to 7 days.

4. Serologic studies (not useful in immunocompromised patients): Specific IgM levels in CSF (HSV, VZV, EBV, WNV, TBEV where endemic), alternatively specific IgG levels in CSF and serum (CSF levels 20-fold higher than serum levels confirm a CNS infection). Results are usually negative during the first 1 or 2 weeks of encephalitis.

5. Electroencephalography (EEG) is always indicated. The EEG patterns are relatively specific in herpes simplex encephalitis, showing a temporal slowing pattern, and are often detectable earlier than neuroimaging abnormalities.

Differential Diagnosis

Meningitis, intracranial mass (abscess, subdural empyema, intracranial hematoma, primary or metastatic brain tumor, cysticercosis or echinococcosis of the brain), stroke or subarachnoid hemorrhage, cerebral vasculitis (isolated or in the course of systemic diseases), metabolic disturbances (hypoglycemia or hyperglycemia, hyponatremia, hypocalcemia), poisoning (medications, illicit drugs), hepatic or uremic encephalopathy, epilepsy, status epilepticus, psychosis, postinfectious encephalitis (an autoimmune process associated with a viral disease [eg, measles or rubella] or extremely rarely caused by certain vaccines [eg, against rabies or measles], leading to multifocal demyelination, usually mild or moderately severe [low mortality]; CSF negative for viruses; necessary differentiation from multiple sclerosis; MRI essential for diagnosis).

→ TREATMENT

Infection Treatment

1. IV **acyclovir** (INN aciclovir) 10 mg/kg every 8 hours should be initiated promptly on an empiric basis in all patients with encephalitis (particularly if severe), without waiting for virologic confirmation of the diagnosis (in herpes simplex encephalitis the effectiveness of treatment is correlated with its prompt initiation). Continue the treatment for 3 weeks in those with virologically confirmed HSV.

2. In the case of justified suspicion or a confirmed specific etiology, consider the following:

1) **CMV**: IV **ganciclovir** (5 mg/kg by infusion every 12 hours for 3 weeks) in combination with IV **foscarnet** (60 mg/kg every 8 hours or 90 mg/kg every 12 hours).

2) **VZV**: IV **acyclovir** 10 to 15 mg/kg by infusion every 8 hours for 10 to 14 days; alternatively you may use ganciclovir.

3) **HHV-6** in patients with impaired cell-mediated immunity: Our pattern of practice involves **ganciclovir** or foscarnet. Cidofovir may also be considered.

4) **Fungal infections**: →Chapter 8.5.3.

Supportive Treatment

As in meningitis. Supportive treatment is crucial in encephalitis. Empiric glucocorticoids are not used.

→ FOLLOW-UP

The effectiveness of treatment is confirmed by the resolution of signs and symptoms and improvement in the patient's general clinical condition. It is not necessary to perform a routine follow-up CSF examination. In case of a lack of improvement or development of complications, repeat CSF analysis and neuroimaging studies (preferably MRI). Postinflammatory CSF abnormalities may persist for considerable time after the resolution of the acute phase of the disease.

→ COMPLICATIONS

In acute encephalitis: status epilepticus, brain herniation (as a result of raised intracranial pressure), syndrome of inappropriate antidiuretic hormone secretion (SIADH).

Late complications include permanent paresis or paralysis, epilepsy, psychotic disorders, memory impairment, dementia, and aphasia.

→ PROGNOSIS

Prognosis is poor. Mortality rates are particularly high in herpes simplex encephalitis (in patients receiving no specific antiviral treatment, mortality rates are 70%-80%; in patients in whom treatment is initiated early, prior to loss of consciousness, the mortality rate is 30%). Encephalitis or cerebellitis in the course of varicella. Fungal CNS infections: →Chapter 8.5.3.

→ PREVENTION

1. Vaccination against measles, mumps, rubella, VZV, influenza, poliomyelitis, rabies in high-risk individuals (long-term travelers, veterinary workers, those interacting with wild animals).

2. Passive immunoprophylaxis: In special cases administer varicella-zoster immunoglobulin (VZIG), rabies immunoglobulin (RIG), or antimeasles virus immunoglobulin.

3. Avoidance of any contact with wild animals and stray dogs and cats (prophylaxis of rabies).

4. In endemic areas outside North America **nonspecific protection against ticks**: →Chapter 8.15.1 (prophylaxis of TBEV).

5.2. Focal Infections of the Central Nervous System

5.2.1. Brain Abscess

→ DEFINITION, ETIOLOGY, PATHOGENESIS

A brain abscess is a focal infection of the brain parenchyma. It spreads directly by continuity or via a hematogenous route (even from remote primary foci, such as the endocardium). An early inflammatory infiltrate disintegrates after ~2 weeks, forming a reservoir of purulent material enclosed in a thin, well-vascularized capsule that is surrounded by a zone of cerebral edema.

Etiology varies with the location of the primary site of infection as well as other **risk factors**:

1) Sinusitis: Aerobic or anaerobic streptococci, *Haemophilus* spp, *Bacteroides* spp, *Fusobacterium* spp, *Streptococcus anginosus*.

2) Otitis media or mastoiditis: Streptococci, aerobic gram-negative intestinal bacilli (particularly *Proteus* spp), *Bacteroides* spp, *Pseudomonas aeruginosa*.

3) Endocarditis: Viridans-group streptococci.

4) Trauma: *Staphylococcus aureus*.

5) Impaired cell-mediated immunity: Fungi *Candida* spp, *Aspergillus* spp, rarely *Cryptococcus neoformans*; in patients with AIDS predominantly *Toxoplasma gondii*, fungi (*Cryptococcus neoformans*).

6) Tuberculous brain abscess (tuberculoma) filled with caseous mass.

7) Other: Dental infections, surgery-related infections, bronchiectasis, pulmonary abscess, sepsis.

Headache is the presenting symptom; it is often dull, generalized, and in 50% of patients accompanied by fever. Signs and symptoms of elevated intracranial pressure and cerebral edema develop gradually. Focal neurologic deficits are present in 50% of patients and include paresis, paralysis, aphasia, and seizures. Twenty-five percent of patients have papilledema.

Mortality rates are up to 25%. Permanent neurologic deficits (paresis, paralysis, seizures) develop in 30% to 50% of patients.

1. Laboratory tests: Nonspecific findings in routine cerebrospinal fluid (CSF) analysis (elevated opening pressure; other parameters may be normal). Blood and CSF cultures are usually negative. Culture of needle-aspirated abscess material has the highest diagnostic yield (cultures should always include both aerobic and anaerobic bacteria and fungi). Due to the risk of brain herniation, consultation with a neurosurgeon and careful consideration of brain biopsy versus lumbar puncture after performing computed tomography (CT) and/or magnetic resonance imaging (MRI) of the head is needed.

2. CT and MRI: Characteristic features include a hypodense enhancing inflammatory infiltrate with a well-enhancing capsule and a peripherally located hypodense zone of cerebral edema. The adjacent brain structures are displaced and compressed (mass effect).

1. Surgical treatment is the method of choice. It includes needle aspiration or surgical resection (particularly in the case of abscesses located in the posterior cranial fossa and those of fungal and tuberculous etiology).

Contraindications: Multiple brain abscesses, a difficult surgical approach, small abscesses <2 cm in diameter.

2. Antimicrobial therapy: An IV third-generation cephalosporin + IV metronidazole for 8 weeks in combination with surgery or alone in patients in whom surgery is not feasible. Fungal CNS infections: →Chapter 8.5.3.

3. Supportive treatment: →Chapter 8.5.3.

4. Monitoring: In our practice, assuming clinical improvement, we repeat the radiologic assessment after 4 to 6 weeks. A deterioration or even lack of response may dictate the need to repeat the assessment earlier.

Perforation of the abscess into the brain ventricles is the most serious complication. It manifests as a sudden deterioration of the patient's general condition and is associated with mortality rates of 80% to 100%.

5.2.2. Neurocysticercosis

Neurocysticercosis is a parasitic infection leading to cyst formation in the central nervous system (CNS). It most commonly presents as seizures and is likely the main global cause of seizures. Neurocysticercosis is probably the most common CNS infection in the world.

Etiology: *Taenia solium*, a tapeworm (cestode), is the causative agent. While the infection is classically acquired through the ingestion of contaminated pork, this leads only to shedding of proglottid segments (eggs) in the stool of the infected individuals. Ingestion of contaminated human stool, either by autoinoculation or fecal-oral contamination of food or water, results in oncosphere hatching and eventual cyst formation in end-organ tissue. This can occur in the CNS, eyes, subcutaneous tissues, and muscle.

▶ CLINICAL FEATURES AND NATURAL HISTORY

The typical presentation is generalized tonic-clonic seizures, which are a consequence of the cyst itself or the patient's immunologic response to the cyst. As cysts degenerate, the subsequent edema and calcification can also be a nidus. In patients with a high cyst burden, encephalitis may be the initial presentation. Involvement of the ventricles may lead to obstructive hydrocephalus. Involvement of the retinas may result in visual loss.

▶ DIAGNOSIS

1. Laboratory tests: Taking a detailed history of potential exposure is paramount to diagnosis. Serologic studies that detect cysticercosis can be helpful, with sensitivity decreasing with 1 to 2 cysts and increasing with >2 cysts. Treatment is typically initiated based on a relevant history and radiologic findings. In treatment-refractory patients, brain biopsy for pathology may be considered to confirm the diagnosis.

2. Computed tomography (CT) and magnetic resonance imaging (MRI): Characteristic features include a single or multiple ring-enhancing lesions, occasionally with a live scolex inside. Cerebral edema is typically associated with neurocysticercosis. When cysts degenerate, the ring-enhancing lesions may look atypical and eventually form a calcification, which signifies a noninfectious process. Obstructive hydrocephalus may occur with infection of the ventricles.

▶ TREATMENT

1. Antiseizure therapy: The mainstay of therapy includes antiseizure drugs, as the lesions may become a focus for recurrent seizures. Specific medications should follow local practice for epilepsy.

2. Glucocorticoids/anthelmintic therapy: Anthelmintic therapy may be considered when cysts are viable (ie, they have a visible scolex or are not calcified). Glucocorticoids should be initiated in all patients with cerebral edema, and this should be done before anthelmintic drugs. Our practice is to use dexamethasone 0.1 mg/kg/d started 24 hours before anthelmintic therapy and tapered off after completion of therapy.

Anthelmintic therapy should be offered to patients with single or multiple viable lesions, but it is contraindicated in the setting of intraventricular disease, encephalopathy, or severe subarachnoid disease, until surgical and glucocorticoid therapy is initiated. Typical treatment is oral albendazole 400 mg bid used for 10 to 14 days. In patients with ≥3 lesions, praziquantel 50 mg/kg/d tid in divided doses for 10 to 14 days should be considered. Also →Chapter 8.2.1.

3. Surgery: Surgery is reserved for patients with intraventricular disease. In patients with a high burden or signs of hydrocephalus prior to or during treatment, a ventriculoperitoneal shunt may be considered.

4. Monitoring: Imaging studies should be repeated in 4 to 6 weeks or earlier if there is clinical deterioration. Ocular lesions should be followed by fundoscopy.

→ **COMPLICATIONS**

Worsening cerebral edema, encephalopathy, or hydrocephalus may result from degeneration of the cysts secondary to anthelmintic therapy. In such cases patients should be managed aggressively for intracranial pressure and glucocorticoids should be reinitiated. Seizures may occur at any point during the infection or resolution. The patient should be monitored for response to antiepileptic therapy.

5.2.3. Subdural Empyema

→ **DEFINITION, ETIOLOGY, PATHOGENESIS**

Subdural empyema is an accumulation of purulent material between the dura and arachnoid membranes of the brain.

1. Etiologic factors: Aerobic (35%) or anaerobic (10%) streptococci, *Staphylococcus aureus* (10%), *Staphylococcus epidermidis* (2%), aerobic gram-negative bacilli (10%).

2. Risk factors: Sinusitis (>50% of cases), otitis media (30%), head injury (30%), cranial osteitis, surgery.

→ **CLINICAL FEATURES AND NATURAL HISTORY**

Subdural empyema has a nonspecific clinical course. Initially the only symptoms caused by the formation of empyema are headache and fever. Subsequently the patient develops nausea, vomiting, and signs of meningitis (nuchal rigidity). The progressive accumulation of purulent material in the subdural space leads to worsening features of cranial edema and focal neurologic deficits. Delayed treatment leads to permanent neurologic deficits (most commonly spastic paresis or paralysis, seizures, aphasia) or death, with a mortality rate of 40%.

→ **DIAGNOSIS**

1. Laboratory tests: Nonspecific findings in cerebrospinal fluid (CSF) analysis (usually moderate pleocytosis with a predominance of granulocytes; ~40% of patients have lymphocyte predominance). CSF culture may be negative.

2. Computed tomography (CT) or magnetic resonance imaging (MRI): The most important diagnostic test. Diagnosis is confirmed by the presence of characteristic lesions in the subdural space, accumulation of liquid matter, and meningeal enhancement, as well as features of compression of the brain (mass effect).

→ **TREATMENT**

1. Empiric antimicrobial therapy: Administer 3 antimicrobial drugs IV in maximum doses: penicillin G (INN benzylpenicillin), a third-generation cephalosporin (eg, cefotaxime, ceftriaxone), and metronidazole (7.5 mg/kg every 6 hours). If you suspect methicillin-resistant *S aureus* (MRSA) etiology, replace penicillin with vancomycin. Continue antibiotic treatment for 2 to 4 weeks in patients after drainage of the empyema and for 6 to 8 weeks in patients in whom drainage was not performed.

2. Surgical treatment: Surgical drainage is the treatment of choice (especially with thicker empyemas >9 mm)

3. Supportive treatment: →Chapter 8.5.3.

4. Monitoring: In the course of treatment perform a follow-up CT or MRI of the head every 7 to 14 days.

5.3. Meningitis

Meningitis is an inflammatory disease involving the arachnoid mater, pia mater, and subarachnoid space. It is caused by penetration of pathogens to the cerebrospinal fluid (CSF). Untreated infection spreads to the cerebral parenchyma (meningoencephalitis).

The most common source of infection is hematogenous spread from other locations. Bacterial and fungal infections may also spread by continuity from a fractured skull or injured meninges or as a complication of acute otitis media or sinusitis. Although meningitis is typically community acquired, nosocomial meningitis may occur through neurosurgical manipulation.

1. Etiology:

1) **Viral (aseptic) meningitis**: The most commonly involved pathogens are enteroviruses, herpes simplex virus (HSV), and varicella-zoster virus (VZV). Less common pathogens include Epstein-Barr virus, cytomegalovirus, human herpesvirus 6, adenoviruses (in individuals with impaired cell-mediated immunity), and HIV. A number of other flaviviruses, such as West Nile virus, may cause seasonal transmission of aseptic meningitis. Tick-borne encephalitis virus (TBEV), also a flavivirus, is endemic in some areas, mostly outside North America.

2) **Bacterial meningitis**: The most common pathogens in adults are *Neisseria meningitidis, Streptococcus pneumoniae, Haemophilus influenzae* type b (Hib) (rare in adults, becoming less common in children thanks to vaccination), *Listeria monocytogenes* (particularly in adults with impaired innate immune systems), and occasionally *Staphylococcus aureus*. In newborns, the predominant pathogens are *Escherichia coli, Streptococcus agalactiae, L monocytogenes,* and other gram-negative intestinal bacilli; in infants and children aged <5 years, *N meningitidis, H influenzae,* and *S pneumoniae*; and in children >5 years, *N meningitidis* and *S pneumoniae*.

In patients with meningitis associated with neurosurgery, the common pathogens include organisms such as *S aureus,* coagulase-negative staphylococci, *Candida* spp, and gram-negative bacilli, particularly *Pseudomonas aeruginosa*.

3) **Bacterial aseptic meningitis**: Acid-fast mycobacteria, particularly *Mycobacterium tuberculosis* (tuberculous meningitis); spirochetes *Borrelia* spp (neuroborreliosis [→Chapter 8.15.1]) or *Leptospira* spp (leptospirosis), *L monocytogenes* (more commonly causing purulent meningitis), *Treponema pallidum* (neurosyphilis), *Francisella tularensis* (tularemia), and coccobacilli *Brucella* spp (brucellosis).

4) **Fungal meningitis (aseptic or purulent)**: Predominantly *Cryptococcus neoformans* (among patients with impaired cell-mediated defenses and HIV), *Cryptococcus gattii,* rarely dimorphic fungi such as *Histoplasma* and *Blastomyces,* and occasionally *Aspergillus* spp among severely immunocompromised individuals.

2. Reservoir and transmission vary with etiologic factors. The reservoir is predominantly humans (sick individuals or carriers) and rarely wild or domestic animals (eg, *L monocytogenes, Borrelia* spp), including birds (*Cryptococcus* spp), or the environment (molds). Depending on the pathogen, transmission occurs through respiratory droplets, direct contact, vectors such as mosquitoes and ticks, fecal-oral route, and rarely via other routes (eg, *L monocytogenes* is transmitted by consumption of infected dairy products, undercooked meat, salads, or seafood).

3. Epidemiology: Viral meningitis: 3 to 5 cases per 100,000 persons per year; bacterial purulent meningitis: ~3 cases per 100,000 persons per year. Tuberculous meningitis is rare. Other types are very rare. **Risk factors**: →Table 5-1.

Table 5-1. Risk factors for meningitis

Risk factor	Prevalent pathogens
Crowded residences (school or college dormitories, military barracks)	*Neisseria meningitidis*, viruses (enteroviruses, measles, mumps)
Public beaches and swimming pools	Enteroviruses
Age >60 years	*Streptococcus pneumoniae* and *Listeria monocytogenes*
Sinusitis, acute or chronic purulent otitis media, mastoiditis	*S pneumoniae*, Hib
Alcohol abuse	*S pneumoniae*, *L monocytogenes*, *Mycobacterium tuberculosis*
Impaired cell-mediated immune response (HIV and AIDS, immunosuppressive therapy—particularly after transplantation—or glucocorticoid treatment, cancer treatment), diabetes, hemodialysis, liver cirrhosis, cachexia in end-stage cancer or other diseases	*L monocytogenes*, *M tuberculosis*, fungi
Fractures of the skull base or ethmoidal cells involving the anterior cranial fossa and tears of the dura mater resulting in CSF leakage	*S pneumoniae*, Hib, group A β-hemolytic streptococci
Penetrating head injuries	*Staphylococcus aureus*, *Staphylococcus epidermidis*, aerobic gram-negative bacilli including *Pseudomonas aeruginosa*
Neurosurgical procedures	*Klebsiella pneumoniae*, other Enterobacteriaceae, *P aeruginosa*, *Acinetobacter baumannii*, *S aureus*, *S epidermidis* (hospital-acquired meningitis)
CSF shunts	*S epidermidis*, *S aureus*, *P aeruginosa*, other aerobic gram-negative bacilli, *Propionibacterium acnes*, fungi
Complement deficiencies	*N meningitidis* (frequently familial or recurrent meningitis), *Moraxella* spp, *Acinetobacter* spp
Neutropenia <1 × 10^9/L	*P aeruginosa*, other gram-negative bacilli
Impaired humoral immune response	*S pneumoniae*, Hib, less commonly *N meningitidis*
Asplenia	*S pneumoniae*, Hib, *N meningitidis*
Cranial or vertebral osteomyelitis	*S aureus*, gram-negative bacilli
Sarcoidosis	*M tuberculosis*
Burns, severe illness, invasive ICU procedures (intubation, tracheostomy, vascular access procedures, parenteral nutrition), prosthetic heart valves or other prostheses, treatment with broad-spectrum antibiotics	Fungi

CSF, cerebrospinal fluid; Hib, *Haemophilus influenzae* type b; ICU, intensive care unit.

4. Incubation and contagious period: In meningococcal infection, the incubation period is from 2 to 10 days; in Hib infection, it is 2 to 4 days; and in viral infections, it differs depending on the species from a few days up to 3 weeks. Incubation periods for other pathogens are not well established and may vary from 2 to 14 days. Infectivity and contagious periods are specific for individual pathogens; infectivity is highest in viral meningitis, such as enteroviral meningitis, and lower or low in bacterial meningitis (eg, transmission of meningococcal infection requires prolonged close contact with an infected individual) and fungal meningitis.

→ CLINICAL FEATURES AND NATURAL HISTORY

1. Clinical features:
1) Signs of meningeal irritation are the key signs of meningitis; they may be absent in elderly patients. Manifestations include neck stiffness, photophobia, and phonophobia.
2) Signs and symptoms of increased intracranial pressure: Headache (severe, throbbing or dull, not responding to analgesics and nonsteroidal anti-inflammatory drugs [NSAIDs]), nausea and vomiting, bradycardia, respiratory failure.
3) Fever >39°C.
4) Other signs and symptoms of encephalitis: Agitation, altered mental status (this may progress to coma), focal or generalized seizures, spastic paresis or other manifestations of pyramidal tract involvement, paresis or paralysis of the cranial nerves (particularly in tuberculous meningitis, which most commonly affects nerves VI, III, IV, and VII), clinical features of brainstem or cerebellar involvement (particularly in advanced *L monocytogenes* meningitis).
5) Other signs and symptoms: Labial or facial herpes; petechiae and purpura, predominantly on extremities (these suggest meningococcal meningitis); symptoms of systemic inflammatory response syndrome, disseminated intravascular coagulation, shock, and multiple organ dysfunction syndrome.

2. Natural history: Although the dynamics of the disease and intensity of signs and symptoms vary with etiology, the causative factor cannot be established on the basis of clinical features alone. Results of routine CSF analysis confirm meningitis and help narrow down the diagnosis to a particular group of pathogens. **Bacterial purulent meningitis** is associated with a sudden onset and rapid progression; patients are usually severely ill and within <24 hours the disease becomes life-threatening. **Viral meningitis** usually has a milder course. In **bacterial aseptic meningitis** (eg, tuberculous) and **fungal meningitis**, the onset is nonspecific and the course is usually subacute or chronic. In untreated or inadequately treated patients, the inflammation spreads to the brain, leading to altered mental status and focal neurologic deficits (encephalitis).

→ DIAGNOSIS

Management Algorithm

If you suspect meningitis, stabilize the patient, collect blood specimens for cultures, and determine if there are any contraindications to lumbar puncture. If it is not contraindicated, promptly perform lumbar puncture, collect CSF for a routine analysis (eg, glucose, protein, and cell count) and for microbiological studies, including culture, sensitivity, and viral polymerase chain reaction (PCR)/culture if available, and start empiric treatment. If there is a significant delay to lumbar puncture owing to contraindications and the clinical suspicion is sufficient, our pattern is to do blood cultures and initiate antimicrobial therapy immediately afterwards, followed by lumbar puncture as soon as feasible. Adjust treatment after receiving the results of microbiological studies (including cultures) of CSF, blood, or both and of drug susceptibility analysis.

Diagnostic Tests

1. Routine CSF analysis: CSF opening pressure is usually elevated (>200 mm H_2O), particularly in patients with bacterial or cryptococcal meningitis. Alteration in the CSF cell count is a distinguishing feature, with a predominantly neutrophilic pleocytosis characteristic for bacterial meningitis and lymphocytic predominance typical for viral, tuberculous, and cryptococcal meningitis. Protein levels may be elevated in all conditions; a significant protein elevation in CSF may be suggestive of tuberculous meningitis. Low glucose levels are often seen with bacterial meningitis and should be correlated with serum glucose levels. In patients with significant immunosuppression, such as in advanced HIV disease, there may be fairly minimal changes to the CSF cell count and chemistry results because of the lack of inflammatory response.

2. Microbiology:

1) **CSF**: Microscopic examination of a gram-stained centrifuged sediment serves as the preliminary identification of bacteria and fungi; India ink staining is used in the preliminary identification of *Cryptococcus* spp, and acid-fast staining is used for the identification of *M tuberculosis*. The **latex agglutination test**, where available, can help with detecting antigens of Hib, *S pneumoniae*, *N meningitidis*, and *C neoformans*; results can be obtained within 15 minutes. This test is particularly useful in patients who have already been treated with antibiotics or in those with negative results of the Gram stain or cultures. **Bacterial and fungal cultures** allow for a definitive diagnosis of the causative factor of meningitis and determination of drug sensitivity of the isolated pathogen. In bacterial infections, the results are usually obtained within 48 hours (except for tuberculosis). In fungal infections, repeated cultures may be necessary until fungal growth is obtained. **PCR** (bacteria, viruses, fungi) is used to establish etiology when cultures are negative (eg, in patients treated with antibiotics prior to lumbar puncture); this is the key diagnostic method in viral meningitis. **Serologic studies**: Detection of specific IgM (in some cases also IgG) using the enzyme-linked immunosorbent assay (ELISA) is helpful in diagnosing certain cases of viral meningitis and neuroborreliosis.

2) **Blood cultures** (bacteria, fungi) should be performed prior to antibiotic treatment in all patients with suspected meningitis (sensitivity is 60%-90%).

3) **Throat and rectal swabs**: Viral culture is recommended if enteroviral etiology is suspected.

3. Computed tomography (CT) or magnetic resonance imaging (MRI) of the head are not essential for the diagnosis of isolated meningitis (although the results may suggest tuberculous meningitis). The studies are helpful in excluding cerebral edema or a brain tumor prior to lumbar puncture and in detecting early and late complications of meningitis in patients with persisting neurologic signs and symptoms (eg, focal deficits, altered mental status), with positive follow-up CSF cultures, or with recurrent meningitis. Imaging should be performed both with and without contrast enhancement. MRI is able to diagnose sagittal sinus thrombosis, a rare complication of purulent meningitis.

4. In case of suspected tuberculous etiology, search for the primary source, such as in the lungs, and perform microbiological studies from that site. This may yield a higher positivity rate than staining and culture of CSF. The tuberculin skin test is not useful in this setting.

Differential Diagnosis

Differential diagnosis includes:

1) Subarachnoid hemorrhage.

2) Focal central nervous system (CNS) infections (abscess or empyema) and brain tumor.

3) Meningeal irritation in the course of an infection located outside the CNS or of noninfectious etiology (signs and symptoms of increased intracranial pressure may be present but CSF is always normal).

4) Carcinomatous meningitis resulting from metastases or lymphoproliferative infiltrates in the meninges (CSF features are usually similar to bacterial aseptic meningitis; detection of tumor cells in CSF cytology and identification of the primary tumor are essential for diagnosis).

5) Drugs: NSAIDs (particularly in patients with rheumatoid arthritis and other systemic connective tissue diseases), sulfamethoxazole/trimethoprim, carbamazepine, cytarabine, IV immunoglobulin. Clinical features are similar to aseptic meningitis.

6) Systemic connective tissue diseases (including systemic vasculitis). Clinical features are similar to aseptic meningitis.

→ TREATMENT

Patients with acute meningitis should be treated in a monitored setting with intensity of care depending on the acuity and severity of presentation. Management may require admission to an intensive care unit (ICU) or a center with expertise in the diagnosis and treatment of CNS infections.

Treatment of Bacterial Meningitis

Start antibacterial treatment immediately after obtaining specimens for microbiological studies. Results of microscopic evaluation of CSF and of the latex agglutination test may be helpful in the immediate initiation of targeted antimicrobial treatment. If necessary, modify empiric treatment after obtaining culture results. If clinical features and CSF analysis results indicate tuberculous meningitis, start empiric treatment of tuberculosis before confirming the diagnosis with microbiological tests.

Treatment of Viral Meningitis

Treatment of viral meningitis is typically not indicated unless there are signs and symptoms of concomitant encephalitis. In such patients acyclovir (INN aciclovir) at a dose of 30 mg/kg/d administered in 3 divided doses should be considered while pending definitive cause identification.

1. Empiric antimicrobial therapy:

1) **Adults aged <50 years**: IV ceftriaxone 2 g every 12 hours + vancomycin 15 mg/kg every 8 hours for 10 to 14 days; this is the basic panel covering the most common pathogens. Alternatively use IV meropenem 2 g every 8 hours if the patient has a known significant allergy to ceftriaxone.

2) **Adults aged ≥50 years or with other risk factors for *L monocytogenes* infection** (→Table 5-1): As in adults aged <50 years + IV ampicillin 2 g every 4 hours. If the patients has a significant allergy to ampicillin, use IV sulfamethoxazole/trimethoprim at a dose of 20 mg/kg/d of the trimethoprim component divided every 6 to 12 hours.

3) **Patients with basal skull fracture**: Treat as adult patients <50 years.

4) **Patients after penetrating head trauma, after neurosurgical procedures, or with CSF shunts**: IV vancomycin 15 mg/kg every 8 hours for 10 to 14 days; IV ceftazidime or IV meropenem, both at a dose of 2 g every 8 hours, may be added to vancomycin. Serum levels of vancomycin should be monitored during treatment and the trough level should be maintained at 15 to 20 µg/mL.

2. Targeted antimicrobial therapy:

1) ***S pneumoniae***: For penicillin-sensitive strains (minimum inhibitory concentration [MIC] ≤0.064 mg/L), use IV penicillin G (INN benzylpenicillin) at a dose of 4 million U every 4 hours for 10 to 14 days. For strains with decreased sensitivity to penicillin (MIC >0.064 mg/L), use ceftriaxone

(→above) or meropenem (→above). For cephalosporin-resistant strains (MIC ≥2 μg/mL), use vancomycin 15 mg/kg every 8 hours + oral rifampin (INN rifampicin) 600 mg every 24 hours.

2) *N meningitidis*: For penicillin-sensitive strains (MIC <0.1 mg/mL), use penicillin G or ampicillin, as in treatment against *S pneumoniae*; alternatively use ceftriaxone. For strains with decreased sensitivity to penicillin, use ceftriaxone, or alternatively meropenem as second-line therapy (→above).

3) *L monocytogenes*: Use IV ampicillin 2 g every 4 hours in combination with IV amikacin 5 mg/kg every 8 hours (or another aminoglycoside) for ≥21 days. Alternatively use IV penicillin G, meropenem, or sulfamethoxazole/trimethoprim for 21 days.

4) *S aureus*: For methicillin-sensitive strains, use IV cloxacillin 2 g every 4 hours for 14 days; alternatively use vancomycin or ceftriaxone (→above). For methicillin-resistant strains, use vancomycin (→above); alternatively use IV linezolid 600 mg every 12 hours or IV ceftaroline 600 mg every 12 hours for 10 to 14 days.

5) *S epidermidis*: Vancomycin + rifampin (→above); alternatively IV or oral linezolid 600 mg every 12 hours for 10 to 14 days.

6) *Enterococcus* spp: For ampicillin-sensitive strains, use IV ampicillin + gentamicin 5 mg/kg/d in divided doses every 8 hours. For ampicillin-resistant strains, use vancomycin + gentamicin. For ampicillin-resistant and vancomycin-resistant strains, use linezolid.

7) **Gram-negative bacilli, antibiotic-resistant strains** (hospital-acquired purulent meningitis): Use IV meropenem 2 g every 8 hours (if there is no response, consider intrathecal amikacin 20-25 mg/d). For carbapenem-resistant strains, use colistin 100,000 U via the intrathecal and/or intraventricular route every 24 hours for 14 to 21 days, IV aztreonam 2 g every 6 to 8 hours for 21 days (intrathecal and intraventricular routes of administration are off-label).

8) **Gram-negative bacilli, antibiotic-sensitive strains** (community-acquired purulent meningitis): Use IV ceftazidime 2 g every 8 hours combined with IV amikacin 5 mg/kg in a slow infusion every 8 hours for 14 days, or IV cefepime 2 g every 8 hours; alternatively use IV meropenem 2 g every 8 hours or IV ceftriaxone 2 g every 12 hours.

Treatment of Fungal Meningitis

Administer IV antifungal drugs for the first 6 weeks of treatment followed by oral fluconazole or voriconazole until the resolution of all CNS signs and symptoms (including neuroimaging features). Removal or replacement of a CSF shunt, if present, is recommended. In patients with severe disease not responding to treatment, consider intrathecal drug administration (except for aspergillosis). Because itraconazole, caspofungin, and anidulafungin penetrate poorly to the CSF and brain parenchyma, these agents should not be used in fungal CNS infections, and particularly not as monotherapy.

1. Candidiasis: Administer IV amphotericin B 0.8 to 1 mg/kg/d in 500 mL of 5% glucose (dextrose) as an infusion over 4 to 5 hours (or as a liposomal formulation 5 mg/kg/d) as monotherapy or in combination with IV flucytosine 25 mg/kg every 6 hours for the first few weeks, followed by oral fluconazole 800 mg/d for 6 days, then 400 mg/d. Alternatively use IV fluconazole 800 mg/d or IV voriconazole 6 mg/kg every 12 hours on the first day followed by 4 mg/kg every 12 hours for a minimum of 2 to 3 weeks, depending on organism clearance and normalization of CSF parameters.

2. Cryptococcosis: Administer amphotericin B (a liposomal formulation may also be used) and flucytosine (→above) for a minimum of 2 weeks, based on organism clearance and clinical response. Consolidation therapy with fluconazole 400 mg/d is continued for 10 weeks and subsequently followed by long-term oral fluconazole 200 mg/d for 6 to 12 months (under supervision of an infectious disease specialist). Therapy may be discontinued in HIV patients on antiretroviral therapy when CD4 counts are >200. Antiretroviral therapy should not be initiated for 6 to 8 weeks as the risk of mortality is higher in this population.

3. Aspergillosis: Use voriconazole 6 mg/kg IV every 12 hours on day 1, followed by 4 mg/kg IV every 12 hours, and subsequently 200 mg orally every 12 hours. Alternatively administer IV amphotericin B up to 1 mg/kg/d (in a liposomal formulation 5-7 mg/kg/d) as an infusion (→above) or combine both agents. Therapy should be continued for a minimum of 6 weeks with reassessment of clinical and radiologic improvement.

Supportive Treatment

1. General recommendations:

1) **IV fluid therapy**, depending on the patient's hemodynamic parameters, and restoration of water and electrolyte balance. Routine limitation of fluid intake below daily requirements is not recommended, except for patients with syndrome of inappropriate antidiuretic hormone secretion (SIADH).

2) **Enteral or parenteral nutrition**.

3) **Physical therapy**: As soon as cerebral edema has decreased and signs and symptoms of increased intracranial pressure are reduced, start passive physical therapy and move on to active therapy.

2. Treatment reducing cerebral edema and inflammation: In every patient with purulent meningitis use IV **dexamethasone** 8 to 10 mg every 6 hours (up to 1 mg/kg/d in patients with cerebral edema). Administer the first dose 15 to 20 minutes prior to or at the moment of initiating antimicrobial treatment and continue for 2 to 4 days if pneumococcal meningitis is confirmed.◉◉ The benefit of this intervention in other forms of purulent bacterial meningitis is less clear.

3. Treatment and prevention of complications: Increased intracranial pressure or cerebral edema: →Chapter 10.7. In patients with hypogammaglobulinemia, consider IV immunoglobulin. Antithrombotic prophylaxis: →Chapter 3.19.2. Prevention of acute hemorrhagic gastropathy (stress ulcers): →Chapter 6.1.2.4; and combine this with initiation of enteral nutrition as soon as possible. Also →Chapter 13.16.1; →Chapter 8.14; →Chapter 7.4.1.2.

→ **FOLLOW-UP**

1. Bacterial meningitis: Routine follow-up examinations of CSF are not necessary if signs and symptoms resolve and the patient's general condition is improving. The **effectiveness of treatment of causative pathogens** is indicated by clinical improvement, a decrease in CSF inflammatory marker levels, and an increase in CSF mononuclear cell counts and glucose levels. Follow-up CSF culture should be negative.

2. Fungal meningitis: Monitor the patient's condition, resolution of signs and symptoms (including neuroimaging features), CSF markers of inflammation, and clearance of fungi from CSF and blood. Repeat lumbar puncture for culture is suggested at 2 weeks before switching to consolidation therapy, and earlier if the patient deteriorates or for relief of elevated intracranial pressure. We do not recommend serial antigen testing for monitoring the response to treatment.

3. Tuberculous meningitis: Monitor the resolution of signs and symptoms, CSF markers of inflammation, and structural abnormalities in the brain detected by CT or MRI. The first indicators of effective therapy may be observed as late as after 2 to 4 weeks of treatment.

➔ COMPLICATIONS

Purulent and bacterial aseptic meningitis (tuberculosis, listeriosis) as well as fungal meningitis are characterized by a higher risk and severity of complications than viral meningitis. Complications may include status epilepticus (in acute disease) and epilepsy, hydrocephalus, cerebral edema, SIADH, spastic paresis or paralysis (in tuberculous meningitis often affecting the cranial nerves), cognitive impairment and speech impairment, mental retardation, and hearing impairment or loss (particularly in pneumococcal meningitis). Rare complications include brain abscess (particularly in infections with gram-negative bacilli, eg, *Enterobacter* spp and *Citrobacter* spp), inflammatory aneurysm, transverse myelitis, and sphincter dysfunction (particularly in tuberculous meningitis with spinal cord involvement).

➔ PROGNOSIS

1. Viral meningitis: Prognosis is good. Usually the disease has a mild course and resolves completely without permanent sequelae. The mortality rate is <1%.

2. Bacterial purulent meningitis: Prognosis is worse in the case of advanced age, immunodeficiency, higher pathogen virulence (pneumococci, gram-negative bacilli, antibiotic-resistant strains), delayed initiation of effective treatment (including treatment of cerebral edema), shock, altered mental status, and seizures in acute disease. Permanent neurologic deficits occur in 9% of patients, or more often in higher-risk populations. Mortality rates depend on etiologic factors and are on average ~20%.

3. Tuberculous meningitis: The mortality rate is ~30%. Permanent neurologic deficits develop in 40% of patients. Delayed diagnosis and initiation of effective treatment increases the risk of death and permanent neurologic sequelae.

4. Fungal meningitis: The disease has a poor prognosis and is associated with high mortality rates.

➔ PREVENTION

Specific Prevention

1. Vaccination against pneumococcal, meningococcal, and Hib infections, as well as against tuberculosis (only in children), mumps, VZV, and poliomyelitis. The preferred pneumococcal vaccine is the 13-valent conjugate vaccine in children and high-risk individuals and the polysaccharide 23-valent vaccine in those aged >65 years and high-risk individuals who have received conjugate vaccines. Meningococcal vaccination includes serogroup C meningococcal conjugate vaccine, quadrivalent meningococcal vaccine (targeting serogroups A, C, W-135, and Y), and serogroup B meningococcal vaccine in high-risk individuals and children.

High-risk individuals include, among others, those with chronic heart, lung, kidney, or liver disease; diabetes mellitus; a history of solid organ or stem cell transplantation; immunodeficiency or immunosuppression (including HIV and treatment with steroids); malignancies.

2. Postexposure chemoprophylaxis is indicated in selected persons after close contact with a patient diagnosed with purulent meningococcal or Hib meningitis. All individuals who have had contact with such persons and who develop signs and symptoms suggestive of meningitis or sepsis should seek immediate medical attention.

1) *N meningitidis*. One dose of oral ciprofloxacin 500 to 750 mg or oral rifampin 600 mg every 12 hours for 2 days, or a single dose of IM ceftriaxone 250 mg (this is the agent of choice in pregnant women). **Indications**: Individuals who were in close contact with a patient with invasive meningococcal disease

(sepsis, purulent meningitis) within 7 days before the onset of signs and symptoms, such as household contacts, persons sleeping in the same room as the infected person (dormitories, shelters), persons who remained in close direct contact with the patient (kissing), persons sharing cooking facilities with the patient (college campuses, dormitories, shelters, hostels, hotels), military, and other personnel living in barracks. Patients with invasive meningococcal disease who were treated with penicillin G (not a third-generation cephalosporin) are at higher risk for recurrent bacterial colonization of the upper respiratory tract and becoming a carrier; chemoprophylaxis is recommended prior to discharge from the hospital.

2) **Hib**: Oral rifampin 20 mg/kg (maximum 600 mg) once daily for 4 days (contraindicated in pregnancy), or a single dose of IM ceftriaxone 250 mg (this is the agent of choice in pregnant women). **Indications**: Individuals who were in close contact with a patient within 30 days before the onset of signs and symptoms, such as personnel of a daycare facility that supervised an infected child if the facility supervises any other children aged ≤4 years who were not vaccinated or incompletely vaccinated against Hib infection as well as all household contacts of the patient if there is a child ≤4 years who was not vaccinated or incompletely vaccinated against Hib infection or an immunocompromised individual (regardless of age and vaccination status) living in the same household. Patients with Hib meningitis are at higher risk for recurrent bacterial colonization of the upper respiratory tract and becoming a carrier; chemoprophylaxis is recommended prior to discharge from the hospital.

3. Chemoprophylaxis of *L monocytogenes* infections: The risk of listeriosis in recipients of solid organ or bone marrow transplants is possibly reduced by long-term administration of sulfamethoxazole/trimethoprim used in these patients for *Pneumocystis carinii* pneumonia prophylaxis.

General Preventive Measures

1. Personal protection measures: Use a face mask and gloves while in contact with a patient with meningococcal infection. Maintain good hand hygiene after contact with the patient or their secretions. Precautions should be maintained until 24 hours after the resolution of clinical symptoms in the patient.

2. Nonspecific protection against ticks in endemic areas (not part of Canadian practice): →Chapter 8.15.2.

3. Reportable diseases: In many jurisdictions, including Canada, meningitis cases have to be reported to the public local health authorities.

5.4. Myelitis

→ DEFINITION, ETIOLOGY, PATHOGENESIS

Myelitis is an inflammatory process involving the nervous tissue of the spinal cord. It is caused by the presence of microorganisms in the tissue. The most common causative factor is a viral infection, including infections caused by enteroviruses (coxsackieviruses A and B, echovirus, poliovirus, enteroviruses type 70 and 71), herpesviruses (herpes simplex virus [HSV], varicella-zoster virus [VZV], cytomegalovirus [CMV], Epstein-Barr virus [EBV]), and HIV. Myelitis may develop in the course of neuroborreliosis, leptospirosis, neurosyphilis, and central nervous system (CNS) tuberculosis.

→ CLINICAL FEATURES AND NATURAL HISTORY

The presenting symptom may be weakness, back pain, or both.

1. Involvement of anterior horn cells: Currently, etiologic factors are predominantly enteroviruses. The involvement manifests as acute progressive asymmetric flaccid paralysis, which usually affects all extremities, is associated with muscle weakness, persists for several days, and is accompanied by fever and myalgia. No sensory deficits are present. Bulbar involvement may lead to dysphagia and respiratory failure.

2. Transverse myelitis: Ascending flaccid paralysis, sensory deficits, and sphincter dysfunction.

3. Myelitis in the course of meningitis, encephalitis, or meningoencephalitis: A combination of signs and symptoms typical for the respective clinical syndrome. In some patients features of a particular viral disease may also be present (although their absence does not exclude viral myelitis).

Many patients develop permanent neurologic deficits, including sensory deficits and paresis and paralysis of various extent and patterns. Any delay in the initiation of treatment increases the risk of permanent neurologic sequelae.

➡ DIAGNOSIS

Magnetic resonance imaging (MRI) should be performed as soon as possible in every patient with suspected myelitis (this also allows to exclude noninflammatory abnormalities leading to spinal cord compression). For **microbiological and serologic studies**, see encephalitis and meningitis. **Routine cerebrospinal fluid (CSF) analysis** reveals features of inflammation; viral etiology is characterized by a predominance of mononuclear cells and significantly elevated protein levels (patients with poliomyelitis initially have pleocytosis with normal protein levels; after ~2 weeks cell numbers return to normal while protein levels increase). Tuberculosis is associated with very high protein levels.

➡ TREATMENT AND PREVENTION

See encephalitis and meningitis. Treatment of inflammation and edema (dexamethasone) is of vital importance. In case of spinal cord compression by an epidural abscess, perform emergency surgery (decompression).

6. Epiglottitis

➡ DEFINITION, ETIOLOGY, PATHOGENESIS

1. Definition: The epiglottis is part of the structures comprising the superior portion of the larynx, which are collectively referred to as the supraglottis (→Figure 6-1). Epiglottitis describes inflammation of the mucosa of the epiglottis (→Figure 6-2). It is frequently associated with inflammation of other parts of the supraglottis, in which case the condition is referred to as supraglottitis.

2. Etiology: Epiglottitis may be either infectious or noninfectious. Infectious epiglottitis has historically been related to *Haemophilus influenzae* type b (Hib) infection. However, since the introduction of Hib vaccination, Hib infection is rare in vaccinated populations. Data on relevant pathogens in the vaccine era are incomplete; non–type b *Haemophilus influenzae* and *Streptococcus* species appear to be the most prevalent pathogens, although a wide variety of bacteria have been implicated. *Staphylococcus aureus* can rarely be a causative organism.

Noninfectious epiglottitis can be caused by a number of factors, among which trauma is the most common. Thermal trauma of the epiglottis is especially common in patients using makeshift filters to smoke crack cocaine but may occur with any type of inhalation burn. Blunt trauma to the neck may cause swelling of the supraglottic structures. Iatrogenic trauma, typically from a traumatic intubation, also causes injury to supraglottic structures. Finally,

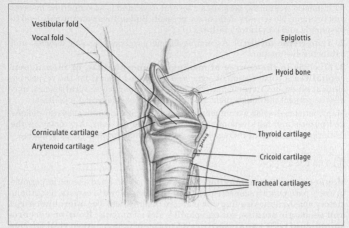

Figure 6-1. Larynx anatomy. *Illustration courtesy of Dr Shannon Zhang.*

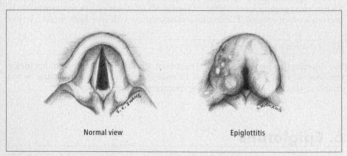

Normal view   Epiglottitis

Figure 6-2. Epiglottitis. *Illustration courtesy of Dr Shannon Zhang.*

external beam radiation treatments for cancers of the upper aerodigestive tract often cause long-standing inflammation of the supraglottis.

Angioedema is another potential noninfectious cause of epiglottitis. Angioedema of the epiglottitis may be caused by a hypersensitivity reaction, various protein deficiencies (sometimes lumped together under the term hereditary angioedema), or medications, such as angiotensin-converting enzyme inhibitors.

3. Pathogenesis: Swelling of the upper airway causes airway obstruction in two ways. First, it reduces the airway lumen. Second, it is often associated with thickened secretions and impaired clearance of secretions. Epiglottitis may lead to deep neck space infections or abscesses. These infections can spread through the neck to cause septic thrombophlebitis of the internal jugular vein and inferiorly to cause mediastinitis.

→ CLINICAL FEATURES

The clinical presentation of epiglottitis depends on etiology. Infectious epiglottitis may present with a viral prodrome, fever, odynophagia, muffled voice, and drooling.

The key clinical feature of epiglottitis is respiratory distress, and its degree can vary significantly. Determining the severity of distress is the most important part of the clinical assessment.

Patients in severe distress are unable to lie flat, often sitting up and leaning forward ("tripoding"). They have markedly increased work of breathing with recruitment of accessory muscles of respiration and nasal flaring. Stridor is usually inspiratory and varies with the degree of obstruction and respiratory effort. Patients have difficulty managing their secretions and may be drooling.

Critically, patients may have normal oxygen saturations, and only as they tire will their oxygen saturations begin to decrease. This reduction in oxygen saturation presages imminent respiratory arrest. Consequently, using oxygen saturations as a marker of severity in epiglottitis may lead to disaster.

Patients with less severe obstruction and respiratory distress have little or no increased work of breathing. They are able to speak in complete sentences and easily tolerate lying on their back. They should have no difficulty handling their secretions.

→ DIAGNOSIS

The diagnosis of epiglottitis is primarily made on the basis of the initial history and physical examination. Assessing the patient's level of respiratory distress and stabilizing the airway take precedence over performing any diagnostic tests. Furthermore, before the patient is transferred from the safety of an emergency room setting to the radiology department, it is critical that their condition is stable for the transfer. Radiology departments are often poorly equipped to handle respiratory arrests.

Diagnostic Tests

1. Fiberoptic nasolaryngoscopy: Fiberoptic endoscopy of the upper airway is usually performed by the otolaryngology consultant service. It allows excellent visualization of the supraglottic structures and is key to diagnosing epiglottitis. It can be performed in the emergency room in awake patients in almost all situations. Special consideration is likely necessary in the very rare pediatric patient presenting with epiglottitis, in whom the theoretical risk of inducing laryngospasm requires that any endoscopic assessment of the airway should be performed in the operating room.

2. Lateral neck radiography: A lateral neck radiograph may show thickening of the epiglottis (the "thumb" sign). However, this finding is not pathognomonic of epiglottitis. The gold-standard investigation remains fiberoptic visualization. Suspicious clinical findings require further investigation with fiberoptic endoscopy regardless of the results of lateral neck radiography. Lingual tonsillitis may give the false impression of a positive thumb sign by obliterating the vallecular space.

3. Complete blood count, electrolytes.

4. Chest radiographs: Chest radiographs are performed to exclude concomitant intrathoracic problems.

5. Computed tomography (CT) scan of the neck and upper mediastinum: A contrast-enhanced CT scan of the neck can be useful to exclude the possibility of a deep neck abscess, especially in patients whose infection fails to respond to standard intravenous antibiotics or who have significant restriction of neck movement. It should only be ordered in patients stable enough to be transferred to the radiology department.

Differential Diagnosis

1. Croup: A consideration only in children. Epiglottitis is extremely rare in children, especially in infants and toddlers, the demographic most affected by croup. Croup typically presents with a viral prodrome, has a gradual onset, and is associated with barking cough. Conversely, when it does occur in children, epiglottitis has a rapid onset and causes significant airway distress.

2. Airway foreign body: A consideration mostly in children. Any history of aspiration should be taken seriously. Usually the diagnosis requires laryngoscopy or bronchoscopy in the operating room.

3. Lingual/palatine tonsillitis: Patients with tonsillitis may present with a muffled voice and noisy, snoring-like breathing. Infection of the palatine tonsils is visible on intraoral examination.

4. Laryngeal cancer: Laryngeal cancer may present as an obstructing lesion. It should be considered part of diagnosis in individuals with a smoking history. Occasionally, these patients may be misdiagnosed as having an exacerbation of obstructive pulmonary disease. Diagnosis requires fiberoptic endoscopy.

5. Subglottic stenosis: This usually presents with a gradual onset of worsening stridor and shortness of breath. It is often but not always associated with a history of prolonged intubation.

6. Paradoxical vocal fold movement: An idiopathic disorder. It requires fiberoptic endoscopy for diagnosis. Speech language therapy is the most common form of treatment.

7. Laryngomalacia: The most common cause of stridor in infants. This is almost always non–life-threatening. Diagnosis requires fiberoptic endoscopy.

➔ TREATMENT

Airway Management

Management of epiglottitis revolves around management of the airway. Patients with severe respiratory distress require immediate transfer to the operating room for an awake intubation or awake tracheostomy. Both anesthesia and otolaryngology services should be consulted. A team approach should be used to decide whether intubation or tracheostomy will be chosen as the primary management strategy. The team should also have at least one back-up plan in case the first strategy fails.

If specialty services do not exist and the patient is in extremis and unsafe to transfer to another institution, local airway expertise should be sought urgently and the airway should be controlled in whatever manner is deemed the safest and most expeditious.

While management of a severely distressed patient can be very difficult, the need for aggressive intervention is usually obvious. Sometimes equally challenging is deciding how to manage patients in less extreme distress; often they can be monitored in a step-down unit or intensive care unit and managed conservatively. The decision to use conservative management is based on both the history of how fast any airway distress is progressing and on the current status of the patient.

Pharmacotherapy

1. Antibiotics: Third-generation cephalosporins are the usual choice for treatment of infectious epiglottitis. Both cefotaxime and ceftriaxone are commonly used, as they have a broad spectrum of action. Knowledge of local flora is helpful in guiding antibiotic management. Some authors advocate the addition of vancomycin to the standard antibiotic regime as empiric treatment for methicillin-resistant *Staphylococcus aureus*.

2. Glucocorticoids: Only very limited evidence is available.◯ The use of glucocorticoids is controversial, yet it is common in the initial period, especially if a conservative approach is being taken towards the airway. The goal of glucocorticoid use is to reduce airway swelling but it is not without risk, as it may worsen glucose control in patients with diabetes mellitus and reduce immune competency. The decision to use glucocorticoids should be taken carefully.

Dexamethasone is commonly chosen because of its high glucocorticoid potency. The dose varies greatly and depends on the patient's premorbid conditions; an average first dose of 4 to 8 mg and a daily dose of 8 to 16 mg may be reasonable. Typically, the use of glucocorticoids is reassessed daily based on the patient's symptoms and findings on fiberoptic examination.

3. Racemic epinephrine: The use of inhaled racemic epinephrine may allow temporary stabilization of airway distress to facilitate transfer to the operating room for definitive airway management. Racemic epinephrine is usually given as a nebulized solution (commonly a 2.25% solution with the usual dose of 0.5 mL).

4. Heliox: Heliox is a mixture of helium and oxygen, which allows for less turbulent inhalations in patients with epiglottitis. Like racemic epinephrine, heliox should only be used to temporarily stabilize a patient prior to definitive airway control.

Supportive Treatment

1. Intubated patients require care in an intensive care unit. Tracheotomized patients require care in a step-down unit or specialized head and neck surgery unit.

2. Patients who are not intubated require close observation in a specialized unit with a tracheostomy tray at the bedside.

3. Intravenous rehydration and venous thromboembolism prophylaxis are used as necessary.

COMPLICATIONS

Epiglottitis may lead to **abscess formation** within the structures of the larynx or in the adjacent deep neck spaces. Retropharyngeal abscess can cause descending mediastinitis.

PROGNOSIS

Prognosis is excellent. Early recognition and prompt treatment of airway distress in the vaccine era has led to a mortality rate <1%.

7. Febrile Neutropenia

DEFINITION, ETIOLOGY, PATHOGENESIS

Neutropenia is the most common hematologic complication of cancer treatment. It may result from the myelotoxic effects of chemotherapy or radiation therapy or from bone marrow infiltration by malignant cells. In patients with febrile neutropenia the causative pathogen can be identified only in 20% to 30% of cases. Prior to the introduction of empiric therapy for febrile neutropenia, the most frequently identified etiologic agents were *Pseudomonas* spp and Enterobacteriaceae (eg, *Escherichia coli*, *Klebsiella* spp) followed by gram-positive cocci (most commonly *Staphylococcus aureus*). In the era of empiric therapy, there has been a shift in the microbiology of pathogens to predominantly gram-positive organisms (coagulase-negative staphylococci being the most common) followed by Enterobacteriaceae and then by nonfermenting gram-negative bacilli, such as *Pseudomonas aeruginosa*.

Febrile neutropenia is defined as:

1) Oral temperature ≥38.3°C in a single measurement or ≥38°C sustained over ≥1 hour; and

2) Absolute neutrophil count (ANC) <0.5×10⁹/L or an expected decrease in ANC <0.5×10⁹/L within 48 hours.

Table 7-1. The MASCC risk-index score for identification of neutropenic patients at low risk of infection and complications

Characteristic	Score
Burden of illness (select only one):	
– No or mild symptoms	5
– Moderate symptoms	3
– Severe illness or terminal condition	0
No hypotension	5
No COPD	4
Solid tumor or hematologic malignancy with no previous fungal infection	4
No dehydration requiring parenteral fluids	3
Outpatient at the onset of fever	3
Age <60 years (not applicable to age ≤16 years)	2
Interpretation: Score ≥21: Low risk	

Source: J Clin Oncol. 2000;18(16):3038-51.

COPD, chronic obstructive pulmonary disease; MASCC, Multinational Association of Supportive Care in Cancer.

→ MANAGEMENT

1. Assess the risk of complications and death using the Multinational Association of Supportive Care in Cancer (MASCC) score (→Table 7-1) or a simplified classification:

1) High risk: Expected long-term (>7 days) and profound neutropenia (ANC ≤0.1 × 10^9/L) and/or clinically significant complications.

2) Low risk: All other patients.

2. Collect ≥2 separate specimens for blood cultures, every time from each lumen of a central vascular catheter, peripheral vein, and from other sites, depending on the suspected etiology (→Chapter 16.11.2).

3. Immediately start empiric febrile neutropenia therapy (→Figure 7-1) using an escalation strategy. This strategy, avoiding initial combination therapies and carbapenems, could be used in patients with no previous infections or colonization with resistant bacteria and in centers where infections due to resistant pathogens are rarely seen.

4. With the escalation strategy being the standard of care, in some cases a **de-escalation strategy** may be employed. Examples include initial therapy involving carbapenems as the first-line regimens (in seriously ill patients, eg, with septic shock; known previous colonization with ESBL-producing Enterobacteriaceae or gram-negative bacteria resistant to narrow-spectrum β-lactam antibiotics or centers with high prevalence of such strains) or combinations with aminoglycosides (septic shock, resistant *Pseudomonas* or *Acinetobacter* strains likely due to colonization or local epidemiology, or use of carbapenems within the previous month). Subsequent management is directed to treat the identified infection (even if it is culture-negative) and to narrow the coverage (→Figure 7-2).

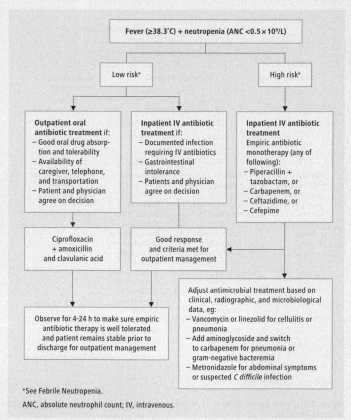

Figure 7-1. Initial management of patients with fever and neutropenia. *Source: Clin Infect Dis. 2011;52(4):e56-93.*

Indications for adding **vancomycin** or another antibiotic active against gram-positive bacteria to the initial empiric therapy:

1) Hemodynamic instability or other signs of severe sepsis.

2) Radiographically confirmed pneumonia.

3) Cultures positive for gram-positive bacteria (prior to the definitive identification of the causative pathogen and obtaining drug susceptibility test results).

4) Clinical suspicion of a severe vascular catheter-associated infection (eg, chills during an infusion via the catheter or signs of infection in the area adjacent to the catheter).

5) Skin or soft tissue infection.

6) Documented colonization by methicillin-resistant *S aureus* (MRSA) or penicillin-resistant pneumococci.

7) Severe mucositis in patients who received prophylactic fluoroquinolones and their current empiric therapy includes ceftazidime.

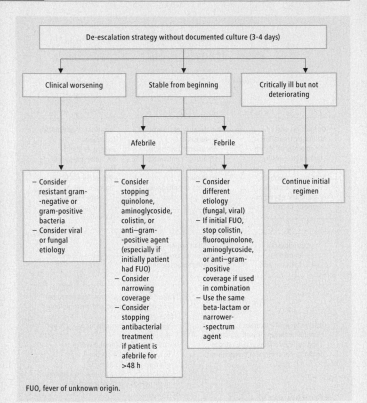

FUO, fever of unknown origin.

Figure 7-2. De-escalation strategy in febrile neutropenia. *Adapted from Haematologica. 2013;98(12):1826-35.*

Modification of the empiric febrile neutropenia therapy in the case of suspected or confirmed infection with a resistant strain (according to 2011 Infectious Diseases Society of America and 2013 European Conference on Infections in Leukemia guidelines):

1) MRSA: Vancomycin, linezolid, or daptomycin.

2) Vancomycin-intermediate *S aureus* (VISA): Linezolid, tigecycline, dapto-mycin, quinupristin/dalfopristin.

3) Vancomycin-resistant enterococci (VRE): Linezolid, tigecycline, daptomycin, quinupristin/dalfopristin (*Enterococcus faecium*).

4) Extended-spectrum β-lactamase (ESBL)–producing strains: Carbapenem.

5) Carbapenem-resistant Enterobacteriaceae strains: Colistin, tigecycline, or an aminoglycoside.

6) Carbapenemase-producing *Klebsiella pneumoniae*: Colistin or tigecycline.

7) β-Lactamase–resistant *P aeruginosa*: Colistin or aminoglycosides.

8) β-Lactamase–resistant *Acinetobacter* spp: Colistin or tigecycline.

9) *Stenotrophomonas maltophilia*: Sulfamethoxazole/trimethoprim, fluoro-quinolones (ciprofloxacin, moxifloxacin), ticarcillin/clavulanate.

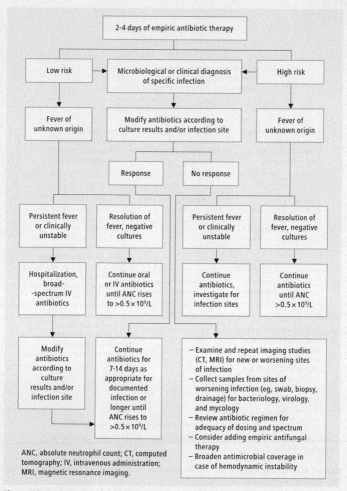

Figure 7-3. Reassessment of patients with febrile neutropenia after 2 to 4 days of empiric antibiotic therapy. *Source: Clin Infect Dis. 2011;52(4):e56-93.*

Patients in whom the etiologic agent responsible for the infection has been identified should receive a targeted therapy. However, it is recommended that empiric febrile neutropenia coverage be maintained until the resolution of fever and neutrophil recovery (ANC >0.5×10⁹/L).

Between days 2 through 4 of empiric antibiotic therapy reevaluate the patient: →Figure 7-3. Patients with persistent neutropenia who have completed a course of antibiotics should stay in the hospital for an observation lasting ≥24 to 48 hours. Management of high-risk patients with fever persisting for >4 days of empiric antibiotic therapy should include either the addition of empiric antifungal therapy or preemptive therapy (therapy as directed by testing indicating

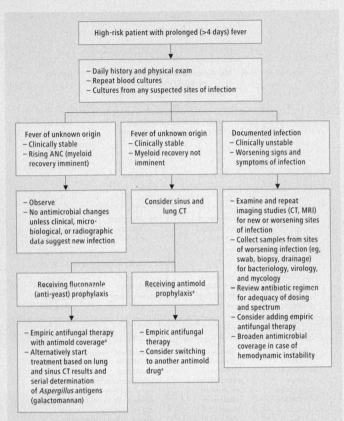

Figure 7-4. Management of high-risk patients with fever after 4 days of antibiotic therapy. *Source: Clin Infect Dis. 2011;52(4):e56-93.*

the possibility of fungal infection [bronchoalveolar lavage, galactomannan, high-resolution computed tomography]) in selected patients: →Figure 7-4.⊘◌

5. Prophylaxis in afebrile neutropenic patients:

1) Follow universal precautions, particularly hand hygiene and cough etiquette (masks covering the face and nose), for all patients. Institute reverse isolation with laminar flow or high-efficiency particulate air (HEPA) filtration only for hematopoietic stem cell transplantation patients and those receiving standard therapy for acute leukemia or aplastic anemia.

2) Recommend a fluoroquinolone (ciprofloxacin or levofloxacin) or sulfamethoxazole/trimethoprim only in high-risk patients, defined as hematologic patients on standard chemotherapy, hematopoietic stem cell transplantation patients, and patients with solid tumors (breast, lung, ovary, germ cell tumors).⊘●

3) Recommend antifungal and antiviral agents only in patients undergoing allogeneic hematopoietic stem cell transplantation or induction or reinduction chemotherapy for acute myeloid leukemia.✅⊘●

4) Recommend sulfamethoxazole/trimethoprim in patients with risk factors for *Pneumocystis jiroveci* infection, for instance, in the course of glucocorticoid therapy lasting ≥1 month or therapy with purine analogues and allogeneic transplant recipients after engraftment.

5) Consider granulocyte colony-stimulating factor or granulocyte and macrophage colony-stimulating factor in patients with prolonged bacteremia and confirmed infections.

6) Avoid prolonged contacts with environment contaminated with fungal spores (eg, large-scale construction/renovation works).

8. Intravascular Catheter-Related Infections

→ DEFINITION, ETIOLOGY, PATHOGENESIS

Intravascular catheter-related infections may present as: (1) catheter-related bloodstream infections; or (2) infections localized to the catheter exit site (or subcutaneous tissue along tunneled central venous catheters [central lines]). Localized exit-site infections may eventually result in bloodstream infections.

Etiologic agent: Skin flora that migrates along the catheter or enter the bloodstream through the port during drug infusion or injection. Most frequently, the etiologic pathogens are coagulase-negative staphylococci, *Staphylococcus aureus*, *Enterococcus* spp, *Candida* spp, and gram-negative bacilli.

→ CLINICAL FEATURES AND NATURAL HISTORY

1. Catheter-related bloodstream infection (CRBSI): Manifestations may range from fever alone to features of sepsis. CRBSI should be suspected in every patient with a vascular catheter and unexplained fever. A simultaneous exit-site infection is found in <30% of patients.

2. Exit-site infection: Erythema, pain, edema, warmth of the skin, sometimes with purulent drainage.

→ DIAGNOSIS

Cultures:

1) **CRBSI**: Simultaneously obtain ≥2 blood samples for culture: draw one from a peripheral venipuncture site and the other via the catheter. If the catheter has multiple ports, consider drawing cultures from each port. A CRBSI is diagnosed if the same microorganism is cultured from both the peripheral blood and the catheter with a time-to-positivity ≥2 hours earlier in the sample drawn via the catheter.

   In cases where blood cultures are inconclusive, catheter-associated infection is still suspected, and catheter removal is an option, consider catheter-tip culture. After removal, cut off the tip of the catheter and send it to the microbiology laboratory for semiquantitative or quantitative culture. Isolation of the same pathogen from blood and the catheter tip confirms a catheter-related infection.

2) **Exit-site infection**: If purulent drainage is present at the catheter exit site, consider sending a swab of the drainage for additional cultures. Interpret the results in the context of blood and catheter-tip cultures.

→ **TREATMENT**

1. Antimicrobial treatment: Collect blood cultures, as possible and feasible, before starting antimicrobial therapy. De-escalate treatment based on cultures and susceptibility testing as results become available (→Table 8-1).

For empiric therapy, administer the following:

1) Vancomycin. Alternatively, an antibiotic active against methicillin-susceptible *Staphylococcus* spp (intravenous cloxacillin or cefazolin) could be considered if the facility has a low prevalence of methicillin-resistant *S aureus* (MRSA), if the patient is not MRSA-colonized, if the patient has no recent history of intensive care unit stay or long-term hospitalization, and if the patient is not severely sick from the infection.

2) Add empiric gram-negative (including antipseudomonal) coverage in severe infections, in immunocompromised patients (particularly those with neutropenia), and in patients with femoral catheters. If a patient is known to be colonized with a multidrug resistant gram-negative species, consider including empiric coverage for that pathogen.

3) Add empiric antifungal coverage for patients with sepsis who are immunocompromised, who are receiving total parenteral nutrition, who have femoral catheters, or who have been on prolonged broad-spectrum antibiotics. Use an echinocandin (such as caspofungin or anidulafungin); alternatively, consider fluconazole if the patient has had no exposure to azoles in the previous 3 months and in settings where the risk of *Candida krusei* or *Candida glabrata* infection is very low.

2. Catheter removal is ideally performed in all cases of CRBSI, but especially in the following situations:

1) When the source of infection is a **short-term central venous catheter or arterial catheter**. In exceptional cases, salvaging the catheter may be considered if the pathogen is coagulase-negative staphylococci (other than *Staphylococcus lugdunensis*). In the case of exit-site infection, remove the catheter.

2) When the source of infection is a **long-term line, tunneled line, or a totally implantable device** and the infection is complicated by an abscess, septic thrombophlebitis, or metastatic infection (eg, endocarditis, septic arthritis, septic emboli); persistent bacteremia is present after 72 hours of appropriate antibiotic treatment; or when the patient's condition is critical. Additionally, routine catheter removal is recommended in cases where infection is caused by *S aureus*, *Pseudomonas aeruginosa*, and *Candida*◐◖ or other fungi. In cases of attempted catheter salvage, consider antibiotic lock therapy in conjunction with systemic antibiotics.

3. Duration of treatment:

1) If the catheter has been removed:

   a) Coagulase-negative staphylococci (other than *S lugdunensis*): 5 to 7 days.

   b) Enterococci or gram-negative bacilli: 7 to 14 days.

   c) *S aureus*: 14 days (consider 4-6 weeks in patients with diabetes mellitus, immunodeficiency, intravascular devices, endocarditis, thrombophlebitis, or if fever and bacteremia fail to resolve within 72 hours of appropriate antibiotic treatment). If available, consider infectious disease consultation in cases of *S aureus* bloodstream infection.

   d) *Candida*: ≥14 days. Exclude endophthalmitis with an ophthalmologic examination. Consider infectious disease consultation when possible.

2) If the catheter has been salvaged, in the absence of complications: Coagulase-negative staphylococci for 10 to 14 days (in combination with antibiotic lock therapy).

Table 8-1. Organism-based treatment of catheter-related bloodstream infections[a]

Pathogen	Antibiotic and routine dosage	Alternative antibiotics
Staphylococcus aureus and methicillin-susceptible coagulase-negative staphylococci	Cloxacillin 2 g IV every 4 h Cefazolin 2 g IV every 8 h	Vancomycin
MRSA and methicillin-resistant coagulase-negative staphylococci	Vancomycin 15-20 mg/kg every 12 h[b]	Daptomycin (use for MRSA if vancomycin MIC ≥2 µg/mL)
Ampicillin-sensitive *Enterococcus* spp	Ampicillin 2 g IV every 6 h	Vancomycin
Ampicillin-resistant *Enterococcus* spp	Vancomycin (as above)	Daptomycin
VRE	Linezolid 600 mg IV every 12 h	Daptomycin
Pseudomonas aeruginosa	Ceftazidime 2 g IV every 8 h or piperacillin/tazobactam 4.5 g IV every 6-8 h, or Ciprofloxacin 400 mg IV every 8 h	Aminoglycosides Imipenem Meropenem Cefepime
"SPICE" organisms (*Serratia* spp, *Providencia* spp, *Proteus vulgaris*, *Citrobacter* spp [non-*koseri*], *Enterobacter* spp), ESBL-producing organisms	Ertapenem 1 g IV daily	Meropenem Imipenem
Other gram-negative organisms (eg, *Escherichia coli*, *Klebsiella* spp)	Based on susceptibilities, eg, ceftriaxone 2 g IV every 24 hours	
Candida spp	Anidulafungin 200 mg IV on day 1 then 100 mg IV daily Caspofungin 70 mg IV on day 1 then 50 mg IV daily	Fluconazole[c] Amphotericin

[a] Recommendations should be further guided by susceptibility testing as available. Doses indicated assume normal renal function and body mass.

[b] Serum trough levels suggested with first trough prethird or prefourth dose: levels should be 15-20 µg/mL for *S aureus* infection and 10-20 µg/mL for other pathogens.

[c] Fluconazole is suboptimal therapy in *Candida krusei* and *Candida glabrata*; use an echinocandin instead. For *Candida parapsilosis*, use fluconazole instead of an echinocandin.

ESBL, extended-spectrum β-lactamase; IV, intravenous; MIC, minimum inhibitory concentration; MRSA, methicillin-resistant *Staphylococcus aureus*; VRE, vancomycin-resistant enterococci.

→ PREVENTION

1. Maintain good hand hygiene prior to establishing new vascular access and while changing dressings.

2. Disinfect the skin with alcoholic chlorhexidine (>0.5%) in preparation for peripheral catheter insertion and during dressing changes.⊘⊖ In patients with contraindications to chlorhexidine, use iodine, iodophor, or 70% alcohol.

3. During insertion or exchange of central venous catheters, maintain aseptic technique and use maximal sterile barrier precautions, including a cap, mask, sterile gown, sterile gloves, and sterile full-body drape. If possible, use ultrasound guidance for central line insertion.

4. Avoid using the femoral vein for central venous catheters if possible.⊗⊖

5. While inserting a peripheral catheter, clean disposable gloves can be used instead of sterile gloves as long as the insertion site is not touched after skin disinfection.

6. Protect all catheter insertion sites with a sterile dressing. For adults with short-term, nontunneled central venous catheters, use chlorhexidine-impregnated dressings.◉● Replace dressings when wet, damaged, detached, or soiled.

7. For central venous catheters, routinely replace gauze dressings every 48 hours and transparent/semipermeable dressings every 7 days.

8. Before accessing catheter ports for injection or infusion, disinfect them with 70% alcohol.

9. Consider the routine use of ethanol or antibiotic lock to prevent catheter--related infections, especially in patients on hemodialysis with tunneled central venous catheters or in patients with a history of multiple catheter-related infections.◉○

10. Do not routinely replace central venous catheters or long-term lines. There is no need to routinely replace peripheral catheters to reduce infection risk.

11. Remove all catheters promptly when no longer needed.

9. Mediastinitis

→ DEFINITION, ETIOLOGY, PATHOGENESIS

Mediastinitis involves an infection in the mediastinum. The infection occurs through inoculation of organisms into the mediastinal space, typically through contiguous spread from nearby tissue spaces, and the subsequent inflammatory response.

Etiology:

1) Acute esophageal perforation: This may be a consequence of spontaneous rupture or due to complications from esophageal or gastric surgery. Organisms typically involved include oral aerobes and anaerobes and *Candida* spp.

2) Inoculation from the neck: Typically due to an odontogenic infection. Organisms include oral flora (as above).

3) Cardiac surgery: This is a consequence of inoculation of organisms due to contamination of the surgical bed or infection of the wound. Organisms include skin flora, such as staphylococci, streptococci, and gram-negative aerobes in patients requiring prolonged hospitalization.

4) Other organisms through extension from the lung: Inhalational anthrax leads to hemorrhagic mediastinitis after inoculation of pulmonary lymph nodes. Actinomyces and fungal agents causing mucormycosis may invade through pulmonary tissue planes into the mediastinal space.

5) Chronic fibrosing mediastinitis: A long-term inflammatory response to pulmonary histoplasmosis leading to complications from extrinsic compression of local structures.

Symptoms:

1) **Acute mediastinitis** presents as severe retrosternal chest pain that intensifies with breathing or coughing; tenderness around the sternum and sternocostal joints; symptoms of pneumomediastinum and subcutaneous emphysema; and symptoms of inflammation (systemic inflammatory response syndrome) or sepsis. In post–cardiac surgery mediastinitis there is instability or inflammatory changes of the sternal wound. Hemorrhagic mediastinitis after anthrax exposure leads to acute respiratory failure and acute respiratory distress syndrome (ARDS).

2) **Chronic mediastinitis** may present with signs of extrinsic compression of the mediastinal structures from advanced (overwhelming) fibrosis. This may lead to airway obstruction, superior vena cava syndrome, esophageal compression, or constrictive pericarditis.

→ **DIAGNOSIS**

Diagnosis is made by diagnostic imaging of the mediastinum. Chest radiography may show air in the mediastinum, subcutaneous emphysema, or other complications from esophageal perforation. Computed tomography (CT) is typically used for confirmation. The presence of air, fluid, or distinct collections in the mediastinum is suggestive of acute mediastinitis. In chronic mediastinitis CT scans may show evidence of fibrosis of the mediastinum with compression of nearby anatomic structures.

→ **TREATMENT**

In **patients with acute esophageal rupture or after cardiac surgery**, debridement of the mediastinal space along with repair of any perforated viscus is needed. Given that there are often different organisms involved, broad--spectrum antimicrobial therapy directed against gram-positive, gram-negative, and anerobic organisms, and occasionally against yeast, is required. A regimen such as vancomycin and piperacillin/tazobactam could be considered while waiting for cultures. Antimicrobial therapy should be subsequently tailored to the results of bacterial cultures.

Anthrax requires a combination treatment including ciprofloxacin, meropenem, linezolid, and monoclonal antibody therapy.

In **chronic fibrosing mediastinitis** the disease is mainly due to fibrosis as a consequence of inflammation derived from histoplasmosis. However, at this stage of mediastinitis, treatment has not been shown to alter its course and management is directed at reducing compression of the anatomic structures.

10. Occupational Exposures to Blood--Borne Viral Infections

The key blood-borne pathogens are hepatitis B virus (HBV), hepatitis C virus (HCV), and human immunodeficiency virus (HIV).

→ **INFECTION RISK ASSESSMENT**

The risk of infection following exposure depends on the type of exposure, type of potentially infectious biological material, susceptibility to infection of the exposed individual, etiologic agent, and status of the source patient (infected vs not infected, level of infectiousness).

1. Types of exposure (incidents that pose a risk of virus transmission):

1) Skin injury with infected sharp objects (needle, scalpel).

2) Contact of mucosa (conjunctiva, oral mucosa) or nonintact skin (skin with lacerations, abrasions, inflammatory lesions, wounds) with a potentially infectious material: the source patient's blood, tissues, or body fluids (risk of infection is minimal if the skin is intact).

3) Each direct contact with a concentrated viral stock of HBV, HCV, or HIV in research facilities.

4) Very rarely, a human bite (both the bitten and the biting individual can be the source of infection).

2. Infectious material is a biological material containing the minimal amount of infectious particles required for transmitting infection that has been described as potentially infectious. The highest risk of transmitting HBV, HCV, and HIV is through blood. Other infectious materials include cerebrospinal fluid (CSF), synovial fluid, pleural fluid, peritoneal fluid, pericardial fluid, amniotic fluid, unfixed tissue, virus culture, saliva (only in HBV infection following percutaneous exposure [bite]), vaginal secretions, and semen. In clinical practice, noninfectious material (ie, material that does not contain a particular microorganism or risk of transmission has not been described) is defined as feces, urine, vomit, sputum, nasal discharge, tears, and sweat, unless blood-stained.

3. Etiologic factors:

1) **HBV**: In individuals susceptible to HBV infection, the risk of infection due to needlestick or another sharp object injury depends on the serologic status of the source patient (source of exposure) ($\rightarrow$Table 10-1):

   a) In the case of HBsAg(+) and HBeAg(+), the risk of clinically overt hepatitis B is from 22% to 31%, and the risk of asymptomatic hepatitis B is from 37% to 62%.

   b) In the case of HBsAg(+) and HBeAg(−), the risk of clinically overt hepatitis B is from 1% to 6%, and the risk of asymptomatic hepatitis B is from 23% to 37%.

2) **HCV**: The risk of infection following occupational exposure to blood is relatively low—on average 1.8% after needlestick injury and even lower after mucosal exposure. No infection through nonintact or intact skin has ever been reported. The risk of transmitting the disease via body fluids other than blood is very low.

3) **HIV**: Apart from blood, HIV may be present in saliva, tears, urine, and other body fluids; however, infections in medical personnel following occupational exposure to these biological materials have not been documented. Similarly, there were no reports of infections transmitted through vomit or through aerosols that may be generated during certain procedures (dental, surgical, autopsy).

   The risk of HIV infection:

   a) By needlestick or injury with other sharps (eg, scalpel) is ~0.3%.

   b) As a result of mucosal or intact skin contact with blood is ~0.1%.

   c) If the source patient is adequately treated (suppressed HIV viral load on antiretroviral treatment), the risk is ≥79-fold lower than after exposure to the blood of an untreated patient.

   High-risk factors include high viral load in the source patient (detectable prior to seroconversion and in late-stage HIV infection), deep injury, blood visible on the object that caused injury, and injury with a large-diameter hollow-bore needle.

→ **POSTEXPOSURE PROPHYLAXIS**

Every health-care worker, including a trainee, who is in contact with patients or potentially infectious body fluids (particularly blood) and has a negative history of HBV infection should receive a hepatitis B vaccination series (3 doses;) together with evaluation of the immune response to vaccination.

Protocols for nonspecific protection against potential occupational infections in health-care facilities should be strictly implemented. They include, among others, proper storage and disposal of equipment, avoiding unnecessary contact with blood and blood-contaminated objects (eg, designated sharps containers,

10. Occupational Exposures to Blood-Borne Viral Infections

Table 10-1. Recommended HBV postexposure prophylaxis

Vaccination status of exposed individual and immunity induced by hepatitis B vaccine	Decision on further management based on HBsAg status of source patient[a]		
	HBsAg(+)	HBsAg(−)	Exposure source unknown[h] or HBsAg measurement not feasible
History of HBV[b] or ongoing infection (HBsAg[+] in exposed person)	No need for additional specific prophylaxis	No need for additional specific prophylaxis	No need for additional specific prophylaxis
Unvaccinated	1 dose of HBIG[c] + start hepatitis B vaccine series[d]	Start hepatitis B vaccine series[d]	Start hepatitis B vaccine series[d] Consider HBIG if source considered at high risk (eg, drug use history, men who have sex with men)
Vaccinated with response to vaccination evaluated 1-2 months after scheduled vaccination			
Sufficient serologic response[e]	No need for additional specific prophylaxis	No need for additional specific prophylaxis	No need for additional specific prophylaxis
Insufficient serologic response[f]	1 dose of HBIG[c] + start hepatitis B vaccine series[d]	No need for additional specific prophylaxis[g]	Administer booster dose of vaccine Consider HBIG if high risk
Multiple vaccinations with confirmed lack of response to vaccination	2 doses of HBIG at 1-month interval	No need for additional specific prophylaxis	No need for additional specific prophylaxis If clinical and epidemiologic data indicate high risk of HBV infection, follow guidelines for exposure to HBsAg(+) blood
Vaccinated without evaluation of response to vaccination 1-2 months after scheduled vaccination; in such cases measure anti-HBs as part of qualification for prophylaxis			
Anti-HBs ≥10 mIU/mL	No need for additional specific prophylaxis	No need for additional specific prophylaxis	No need for additional specific prophylaxis
Anti-HBs <10 mIU/mL	Booster dose + 1 dose of HBIG	No need for additional specific prophylaxis	Administer booster dose of vaccine; consider HBIG if high risk

Recommendations presented in this table are graded as strong recommendations based on low quality of evidence.◉○

[a] Measure HBsAg in patients whose blood or body fluids were the source of infection.

[b] Individuals who have recovered from an earlier HBV infection acquire sustained immunity and require no postexposure prophylaxis.

[c] IM or IV, depending on the preparation (dosage as per manufacturer's prescribing information), as soon as possible after exposure, preferably within 12 hours. HBIG should be administered simultaneously with the first dose of hepatitis B vaccine (IM preparations should be injected in separate sites).

[d] As soon as possible (preferably within 12-24 hours). Safe in pregnant and breastfeeding women. Vaccination schedule: month 0, 1, then month 6; or month 0, 1, and 2, then month 12.

[e] Serum anti-HBs levels ≥10 mIU/mL in individuals tested within 1-2 months of completion of a primary (scheduled, pre-exposure) vaccination series.

[f] Serum anti-HBs levels <10 mIU/mL in individuals tested within 1-2 months of completion of a primary (scheduled, pre-exposure) vaccination series, without a repeated vaccination dose.

[g] A repeated scheduled vaccination should be administered 1-2 months following the last dose. Serologic response should be evaluated.

Anti-HBs, serum antibodies against HBsAg; HBIG, hepatitis B immunoglobulin; HBsAg, HBs antigen; HBV, hepatitis B virus; IM, intramuscular; IV, intravenous.

disposal of needles without recapping them, following relevant procedures), using personal protective equipment (gloves, masks, safety eyewear), maintaining good hand hygiene, and disinfecting objects and surfaces contaminated with body fluids.

General Postexposure Recommendations

1. We recommend that **the site of the needlestick injury** is cleaned by washing it with soap and large amounts of water without attempting to stop the bleeding or squeezing the wound. Do not use disinfectants. Mucosa exposed to potentially infectious material should be flushed with 0.9% saline or water. The incident should be reported to the designated responsible individual and appropriate assessment and management should be provided by a clinician with expertise in postexposure procedures.

2. The risk of infection should be assessed on the basis of (1) type of exposure (injury with a needle or other contaminated object, contamination of mucosa or injured skin, bite resulting in bleeding); (2) type of potentially infectious material (blood, blood-stained body fluid, other potentially infectious fluids or tissues, highly concentrated viral stock).

3. We recommend, where feasible, to **check the source patient for infection** (if exposure was associated with a significant infection risk) on the basis of (1) clinical and epidemiologic data; (2) serum HBsAg, HCV antibody, and HIV antibody levels. Do not test the sharps (eg, needle, scalpel) that caused the injury for HBV, HCV, or HIV.

4. It is good practice to **examine the exposed worker**: Assess the worker's HBV immunity status (vaccination status, anti-HBs levels 1 or 2 months after completing a full vaccination series) and take history of current illnesses, medications, pregnancy, and breastfeeding.

5. We recommend to **start appropriate prophylaxis** if the risk of infection is significant. The exposed individual should be provided with appropriate recommendations and monitoring appointments and follow-up tests should be scheduled.

Specific Management

1. HBV: We recommend, where feasible, to measure HBsAg in the source patient and perform serologic tests in the exposed individual to evaluate the susceptibility to infection (HBsAg, anti-HBc; in the case of previously immunized persons, anti-HBs levels if they were not measured after the primary vaccination). Prophylaxis involves use of HBV vaccine, HBV vaccine and hepatitis B immunoglobulin (HBIG), or HBIG alone. The choice of prophylaxis depends on the vaccination history of the exposed individual and the availability of the exposure source and their serologic status (→Table 10-1). Prophylaxis should be instituted as soon as possible, optimally within 24 hours and not later than after 7 days of exposure. If active-passive prophylaxis is indicated, it is recommended to administer HBV vaccine and HBIG on the same day. The exposed worker at risk of HBV infection should be monitored by measuring anti-HBc 6 months after the exposure.

2. HCV: There is no specific postexposure HCV prophylaxis; no vaccine or specific anti-HCV immunoglobulin is available. Human polyclonal immunoglobulins and antiviral drugs are not recommended for postexposure HCV prophylaxis.

Management:

1) It is good practice to assess serum HCV antibody levels in the exposed individual on the day of exposure (to exclude previously undiagnosed hepatitis C); if there is a risk of infection, it is recommended to repeat the tests after 3 and 6 months, or earlier if the patient develops symptoms suggestive of acute hepatitis C. A positive result of the HCV antibody test should be confirmed by qualitative polymerase chain reaction detecting serum HCV RNA. One can also measure HCV RNA levels within 4 to 6 weeks of exposure instead of performing serologic tests.

Table 10-2. Types of occupational HIV exposure in which postexposure prophylaxis is recommended	
Type of exposure	Serologic status of source patient
Percutaneous exposure (needlestick, cut)	HIV(+) or status unknown but HIV infection risk factors present (eg, multiple sexual partners, history of IV drug use, highly endemic country)
Contact with mucosa or nonintact skin: a small amount of infectious material (a few drops)	HIV(+)
Contact with mucosa or nonintact skin: a large amount of infectious material or prolonged time of contact (>15 min)	HIV(+) or status unknown but HIV infection risk factors present
HIV, human immunodeficiency virus; IV, intravenous.	

2) If the exposed individual develops acute hepatitis C, you may consider antiviral treatment in consultation with appropriate specialist (→Chapter 6.2.2.10.3).

3. HIV:

1) We recommend consultation with an expert in HIV treatment for complicated cases: An HIV-exposed individual should consult a specialist with expertise in HIV treatment within a few hours of exposure, particularly in complicated cases (eg, underlying health issues or pregnancy in the exposed individual, resistant strain of virus in the source patient).

2) An HIV antibody blood test should be offered to the exposed individual to establish the baseline serologic status. In addition to HIV antibody testing in the source patient, consideration may be given to plasma HIV RNA testing of the source patient in certain settings, such as possible acute seroconversion or an inconclusive HIV antibody result.

3) Where there is a risk of HIV transmission (depending on the type of exposure and underlying probability of HIV in the source patient) (→Table 10-2), it is recommended to start a postexposure prophylaxis antiviral regimen as soon as possible (optimally within 1-2 hours, but not later than 48 hours after the exposure, or 72 hours in exceptional cases). Our current practice is to use a 3-drug antiretroviral regimen: a 2 nucleoside/nucleotide analogue reverse transcriptase inhibitor combination (eg, tenofovir + emtricitabine) + an integrase inhibitor as a preferred choice⊘○; alternative regimens may also be considered in special circumstances by specialists or if certain drugs are not available. Medications included in an HIV postexposure prophylaxis regimen should be selected to optimize adverse-effect and toxicity profiles and a convenient dosing schedule to encourage completion of the regimen.

4) If the exposed individual may be pregnant, it is recommended to obtain a pregnancy test. It is currently recommended that dolutegravir be avoided in pregnant women early in their pregnancy or in women who may become pregnant (eg, sexually active without effective birth control). It is good practice to perform a complete blood count (CBC) and tests of kidney function at baseline and repeat them at 2 and 4 weeks if any abnormalities were detected.

5) It is recommended to perform serologic tests for HIV on the day of exposure and then after 6 weeks, 3 months, and 6 months using a fourth-generation HIV Ag/Ab assay. Follow-up testing for HIV RNA is not generally recommended but may be considered in cases of clinical features suggestive of acute retroviral syndrome.

6) A follow-up visit should be scheduled within the first 72 hours of starting drug prophylaxis to provide for modification of the treatment according to incoming results (eg, anti-HIV test results in the source patient).

7) The exposed individual should be considered infectious until HIV infection has been excluded. To minimize the potential risk of transmission, we recommend that the exposed individual should refrain from sexual contacts (or use condoms); refrain from blood, sperm, and organ donation; and refrain from becoming pregnant, or stop breastfeeding, if applicable.

8) Postexposure prophylaxis should be discontinued if HIV infection has been excluded in the source patient.

9) Treatment should be continued for 4 weeks if the source patient is positive or the HIV status of the source patient is unknown.

11. Pharyngitis (Tonsillitis)

→ **DEFINITION, ETIOLOGY, PATHOGENESIS**

Acute pharyngitis refers to inflammation of the mucosa of the pharynx, which frequently includes the tonsils (tonsillitis) and is caused by infection or irritation.

1. Etiology: Etiology depends on the patient's age. In adults, pharyngitis is most commonly caused by viruses—respiratory (eg, rhinovirus, enteroviruses, influenza, parainfluenza, respiratory syncytial virus, human metapneumovirus, adenovirus, coronaviruses), herpesviruses (Epstein-Barr virus [EBV], infectious mononucleosis, cytomegalovirus [CMV], herpes simplex virus [HSV]), and other (eg, HIV). Less often, this syndrome is caused by bacteria. *Streptococcus pyogenes* (group A streptococcus [GAS]) is responsible for the majority of cases of bacterial pharyngitis; group C or G streptococci are also commonly isolated. Rarer bacterial causes include *Mycoplasma pneumoniae*, *Arcanobacterium haemolyticum*, *Fusobacterium necrophorum*, *Neisseria gonorrhoeae*, and *Corynebacterium diphtheriae*.

2. Reservoir and transmission: The majority of pathogens listed above infect the human respiratory tract and are spread by droplets or close contact. Many people with these active viral or bacterial infections may not be overtly symptomatic but can still transmit infection. Note that the detection of GAS in the throat does not imply active infection; many individuals can be colonized with GAS for prolonged periods.

3. Epidemiology: Given that most pharyngitis is caused by respiratory viruses, this infection is most commonly observed in the fall, winter, and early spring. Risk factors are very dependent on etiology. Contact with young children predisposes to infection with respiratory viruses and herpesviruses. Sexual contact is an obvious risk factor for HIV and *N gonorrhoeae* infection (the latter occurs via oral-genital contact). *Arcanobacterium haemolyticum* is more commonly found in adolescents and young adults. *Corynebacterium diphtheriae* is extremely rare and usually occurs in unvaccinated individuals who travel to areas where diphtheria is still endemic.

4. Incubation and contagious period:

1) **Respiratory viral infection**: The incubation period varies between 1 and 6 days, depending on the pathogen. The patients are often contagious from 1 or 2 days before the onset of symptoms and can often shed virus for up to several weeks.

2) **Herpesvirus infections**: EBV has an incubation period from 30 to 50 days. The incubation period for CMV is not well defined.

3) **GAS**: The incubation period for pharyngitis is 2 to 5 days. The patients are contagious up to 24 hours after the start of an effective antimicrobial treatment or for ~7 days after the resolution of symptoms in the case of no antimicrobial treatment. The risk of transmission to household contacts is ~25%.

→ CLINICAL FEATURES

Individuals with infectious pharyngitis often develop fever, malaise, and sore throat. Unfortunately, it is difficult to reliably differentiate bacterial pharyngitis from viral pharyngitis. History of close contact with an individual with a defined cause of pharyngitis is often helpful. In general:

1. Viral pharyngitis is more likely to be associated with myalgia and respiratory symptoms, such as rhinorrhea and cough. Adenoviral infection commonly also causes conjunctivitis. Enteroviral infection, most common during the summer, can cause ulcerations on the posterior pharynx ("herpangina"). Many viruses can cause generalized rash. Infectious mononucleosis (most frequently EBV or CMV infection) can cause exudative pharyngitis, generalized lymphadenopathy, and splenomegaly. HSV infection often causes erosions and ulcers in the anterior part of the oral cavity.

2. GAS pharyngitis is much less likely to have associated rhinorrhea, cough, or rash. It is much more likely to have pharyngeal and tonsillar inflammation (mucosal erythema and edema), palatal petechiae, well-demarcated pharyngeal/tonsillar exudates (→Figure 11-1), and associated cervical lymphadenopathy. Fever is more often high grade. Abdominal pain, nausea, and vomiting can occur in children.

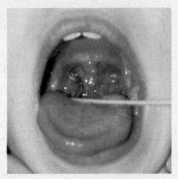

Figure 11-1. Streptococcal pharyngitis.

3. Natural history: The vast majority of pharyngitis cases, bacterial or otherwise, resolve spontaneously within 3 to 7 days. Untreated GAS pharyngitis is associated with an increased risk of rheumatic fever (primarily in children) and a slightly higher risk of suppurative complications (eg, peritonsillar abscess).

→ DIAGNOSIS

Diagnostic Tests

1. Rapid GAS antigen-detection tests: Material: throat swab (→below). The tests have moderate sensitivity and high specificity. A positive result confirms GAS infection, whereas a negative result excludes infection in immunocompetent adult patients; in children, or in patients in whom the likelihood of GAS infection is high, a negative rapid test result requires confirmation using culture or a nucleic acid amplification test (NAAT).

2. Throat swab culture is performed in patients with suspected GAS infection (based on symptoms such as sore throat, fever, red and swollen tonsils when a rapid test is not feasible) or to detect another bacterial etiology; in latter case, notification of the microbiology laboratory is necessary to ensure the appropriate transport media and processing of specimens. Swab specimens should be collected from both tonsils and the posterior wall of the pharynx, avoiding the tongue and cheeks. Culture is the only method that permits GAS susceptibility testing.

3. Nucleic acid amplification methods (eg, polymerase chain reaction [PCR]) are becoming more affordable and available. These methods are both sensitive and specific, so culture is only required if antibiotic susceptibility data are needed; furthermore, they are much more rapid than culture (though not quite as fast as commercially available rapid tests).

Diagnostic Criteria

Clinical scoring systems are often used to determine who requires microbiologic testing to confirm or exclude the diagnosis of GAS pharyngitis. Note that in some scenarios the likelihood of GAS infection is high enough to make scoring or diagnostic testing irrelevant (eg, a child with fever and sore throat with a sibling with confirmed GAS pharyngitis).

1. Centor score: For this score, validated in adults, one point is given for each of the following (total score, 0-4): fever by history, absence of cough, tender anterior cervical adenopathy, and tonsillar exudates.

2. MacIsaac score adjusts the Centor score for age-related probability of GAS infection; one point is added to the Centor score for patients aged 3 to 14 years and one point is subtracted for those aged >45 years. For scores 0 and 1, only symptomatic treatment is suggested, whereas for scores 4 or 5, treatment with antibiotics is recommended. For scores 2 or 3, the preferred option in reliable patients is to perform a rapid antigen test; if negative, it is followed by throat culture. If follow-up cannot be ensured, you may consider treatment with antibiotics for score 2 or higher.

Differential Diagnosis

Simple bacterial and/or viral pharyngitis should be differentiated from the following:

1) **Infectious mononucleosis** caused by EBV infection (clinical features very similar to streptococcal pharyngitis). In addition to exudative pharyngitis, it is often accompanied by disseminated lymphadenopathy and splenomegaly. A similar clinical picture may be caused by CMV and *Toxoplasma gondii*.

2) **Rhinitis** with postnasal drip causing sore throat (extremely common).

3) **Epiglottitis or tracheitis**: These conditions are potentially life-threatening due to airway obstruction that is not easily managed with endotracheal intubation. Patients are often toxic-appearing with high fevers and audible stridor. Epiglottitis is predominantly caused by *Haemophilus influenzae* b and is seen primarily in countries without universal immunization against this pathogen, where these infections are endemic.

4) **Infectious esophagitis**, predominantly caused by *Candida* and HSV.

5) **Gastroesophageal reflux disease, thyroiditis, throat cancer**: Chronic sore throat (sometimes with inflammation) is the dominant symptom.

→ TREATMENT

Antimicrobial Treatment

Do not use antimicrobial agents in viral pharyngitis. Therapeutic options are available for streptococcal pharyngitis, primarily to prevent the development of rheumatic fever⊘○; treatment will also diminish the likelihood of the development of suppurative sequelae. **Options** (with adult doses):

1) Oral **penicillin V** (INN phenoxymethylpenicillin) 500 mg (1 million U) bid to tid or oral amoxicillin 1000 mg once daily or 500 mg bid for 10 days. Alternatively, a single dose of 1.2 million U of IM benzathine penicillin G (INN benzathine benzylpenicillin) can be used. These agents should always be used unless contraindicated because of allergy, as GAS is universally susceptible to penicillins.

2) For patients with type I hypersensitivity to penicillin (eg, anaphylaxis, generalized urticaria): Use **macrolides** (oral clarithromycin 250 mg bid for 10 days or oral azithromycin 500 mg on day 1, then 250 mg every 24 hours for 4 days) or oral **clindamycin** 300 mg tid for 10 days. In many countries, macrolide resistance is much more frequent (10%-20%) than clindamycin resistance (<5%) but macrolides have a more favorable adverse-effect profile.

3) For patients with non–type I hypersensitivity (eg, rash): You can use **cephalosporins**, such as oral cephalexin 500 mg bid or oral cefadroxil 1000 mg once daily for 10 days.

Trimethoprim/sulfamethoxazole and tetracyclines are generally believed to be ineffective.

Supportive Treatment

1. Bed rest as needed, ample fluids (particularly in patients with fever).

2. Acetaminophen (INN paracetamol) or nonsteroidal anti-inflammatory drugs (eg, ibuprofen) to control pain and fever.

3. A single dose of oral glucocorticoids (dexamethasone or prednisone) was found to be associated with a modest decrease in the time to complete pain resolution, but glucocorticoids did not help with all patient-reported outcomes (such as time missed from school/work).⊝○

→ **FOLLOW-UP**

There is almost never an indication to do routine throat swab testing for GAS after treatment or in the absence of sore throat, as GAS throat colonization is common, and resistance among GAS to penicillins has not been documented. For those with recurrent pharyngitis that is associated with positive microbiologic testing for GAS, eradication can be attempted; for this, cephalosporins or clindamycin for 10 to 21 days may be more effective than penicillin.

→ **COMPLICATIONS**

Streptococcal pharyngitis can result in the following:

1) **Suppurative complications (early)**: Retropharyngeal abscess, suppurative cervical lymphadenitis, suppurative otitis media and/or mastoiditis, suppurative sinusitis.
2) **Late immunological complications (very rare in adults)**: Rheumatic fever, acute glomerulonephritis.
3) **Other complications (very rare)**: Bacteremia, pneumonia, toxic shock.

→ **PROGNOSIS**

Prognosis is good. Even when untreated, streptococcal pharyngitis resolves spontaneously. Complications in adults are rare.

12. Rheumatic Fever

→ **DEFINITION, ETIOLOGY, PATHOGENESIS**

Acute rheumatic fever (ARF) is an autoimmune disease caused by an excessive immune response to group A β-hemolytic streptococcus (GABHS) infection, which occurs in ~3% of patients with untreated streptococcal pharyngitis and tonsillitis. The immune response is directed against epitopes similar to proteins found in the myocardium, heart valves, synovia, skin, hypothalamus, and caudate nucleus. The disease is rare in developed countries, but the incidence is higher in low- and middle-income countries, in particular in Africa, and in some indigenous populations, such as those in Australia and New Zealand. It is usually diagnosed in children aged between 5 and 15 years.

→ CLINICAL FEATURES AND NATURAL HISTORY

1. Signs and symptoms of streptococcal pharyngitis (→Chapter 8.11).

2. Signs and symptoms of rheumatic fever usually develop 2 to 3 weeks after pharyngitis:

1) Polyarthritis affecting large joints (35%-66% of patients) is always asymmetric and accompanied by characteristic swelling, severe pain, tenderness, and erythema. Untreated arthritis persists for 2 to 3 weeks and does not lead to permanent joint damage.

2) Carditis (50%-70% of patients) may involve the endocardium, myocardium, and pericardium, but valvulitis is the most common feature. Although murmurs of aortic or mitral regurgitation may be heard, diagnosis by echocardiography in the absence of auscultatory findings is increasingly being recognized.

3) Sydenham chorea (10%-30% of patients) manifests as involuntary movements of the trunk or extremities. It is associated with muscle weakness and emotional lability.

4) Erythema marginatum (<6% of patients) is a pink rash that develops on the trunk and proximal parts of extremities.

5) Painless subcutaneous nodules (0%-10% of patients) on the extensor surfaces of elbows and knees are usually seen in patients with heart involvement.

3. Natural history: In patients without cardiac involvement, the disease has a mild course. The majority of relapses occur within 2 years of the first episode. Each recurrence of rheumatic fever increases the risk of mitral or aortic valve disease.

→ DIAGNOSIS

Diagnostic Tests

1. Laboratory tests:

1) A positive throat swab or rapid antigen test for acute GABHS infection (→Chapter 8.11).

2) Elevations in the erythrocyte sedimentation rate (ESR) and serum C-reactive protein (CRP) levels, which persist for up to several months.

3) Increasing antistreptolysin O (ASO) or other streptococcal antibodies (anti-deoxyribonuclease B [anti-DNase B]).

2. Echocardiography to detect evidence of valvular dysfunction, most commonly mitral or aortic regurgitation (valvular stenosis is usually a late sequelae).

Diagnostic Criteria

1. Jones criteria:

1) **Major manifestations**: Carditis, polyarthritis, chorea, erythema marginatum, subcutaneous nodules.

2) **Minor manifestations**: Polyarthralgia, fever, elevated ESR or serum CRP levels, a prolonged PR interval.

2. The first episode of rheumatic fever is diagnosed in patients with a documented prior GABHS infection (most frequently diagnosed on the basis of elevated ASO titers) and ≥2 positive major Jones criteria or 1 major + 2 minor Jones criteria.

→ TREATMENT

1. Patients with suspected ARF are typically admitted to hospital for evaluation

2. Start anti-inflammatory agents for arthritis. Acetylsalicylic acid (ASA) has been typically used. A glucocorticoid can be added in patients who cannot tolerate nonsteroidal anti-inflammatory drugs.

3. Treat for acute streptococcal pharyngitis with antibiotics to eradicate bacteria from the oropharynx. The risk of heart involvement is almost completely eliminated if the antibiotics are started within 10 days from the onset of the symptoms of pharyngitis.

→ **PREVENTION**

1. Primary prevention: Effective treatment of streptococcal pharyngitis.

2. Secondary prevention: In patients with confirmed rheumatic fever, prevention of relapses should be the goal using continuous antimicrobial prophylaxis for up to 5 years or until the age of 21 for rheumatic fever without carditis, for up to 10 years or until 21 years of age for rheumatic fever with carditis but no residual heart disease, and for up to 10 years or until 40 years when there is carditis and residual heart disease. Intramuscular **benzathine penicillin G** (INN benzathine benzylpenicillin) is the antibiotic of choice. Secondary choices include oral penicillin V (INN phenoxymethylpenicillin); in patients with serious allergies to penicillin, a macrolide can be used (azithromycin or erythromycin). The dosing changes by age and region and usually requires consultation with an infectious disease specialist.

13. Rhinosinusitis

→ **DEFINITION, ETIOLOGY, PATHOGENESIS**

Rhinosinusitis refers to inflammation of the mucosa, nasal cavities, and sinuses (formerly called sinusitis). It is classified as:

1) **Acute rhinosinusitis** (<4 weeks' duration, complete resolution of symptoms) or **recurrent acute rhinosinusitis** (≥4 episodes per year).

2) **Chronic rhinosinusitis (CRS)** (>12 weeks' duration; as defined by Canadian guidelines, >8 weeks' duration) with nasal polyps (CRSwNP) or without nasal polyps (CRSsNP).

3) **Subacute rhinosinusitis** (4-12 weeks' duration).

The etiology of acute rhinosinusitis is usually infectious (viral: common cold, usually lasting <5 days; nonviral: worsening of symptoms after 5 days of illness or symptoms lasting ≥10 days). The complex interaction between inflammatory cells, obstruction of the sinus ostia, impairment of mucociliary clearance, and involvement of the adjacent bones all play a role in the development of rhinosinusitis. Causes of obstruction of the sinus ostia include allergic and nonallergic rhinitis, infections, anatomic defects of the nasal cavity (eg, nasal septal deviation), and other factors. Etiologic factors causing acute rhinosinusitis include rhinoviruses (up to 50%), other viruses, *Streptococcus pneumoniae*, *Haemophilus influenzae*, *Moraxella catarrhalis*, and (rarely) other bacteria or fungi.

→ **CLINICAL FEATURES AND NATURAL HISTORY**

1. Symptoms: Nasal purulent discharge, postnasal discharge, nasal obstruction (congestion), hyposmia or anosmia, headache, halitosis (unpleasant breath odor), dental pain, cough (caused by postnasal drip), or facial pressure localized to the affected sinus.

2. Physical findings: Fever (may be low grade), mucosal reddening and edema, nasal discharge, postnasal drip, tenderness of the areas of affected sinuses.

3. Natural history: Acute viral rhinosinusitis usually resolves spontaneously (improvement as early as after 48 hours). Superimposed bacterial infection should be suspected in case of worsening of symptoms at 5 days or no improvement after 7 to 10 days. The course of chronic rhinosinusitis may include periods of remission and recurrence.

→ DIAGNOSIS

Diagnostic Criteria

Diagnosis according to the 2011 Canadian clinical practice guidelines:

1) **Acute bacterial rhinosinusitis (ABRS)**: Diagnosis requires:
   a) ≥2 symptoms of PODS (facial **p**ain/pressure/fullness; nasal **o**bstruction; nasal purulence/discolored postnasal **d**ischarge; hyposmia/anosmia [**s**mell]), one of which must be O or D; and
   b) Symptom duration >7 days without improvement.
2) **CRS**: Diagnosis requires:
   a) ≥2 symptoms of CPODS (facial **c**ongestion/fullness; facial **p**ain/pressure; nasal **o**bstruction/blockage; purulent anterior/posterior nasal **d**rainage; hyposmia/anosmia [**s**mell]); and
   b) ≥1 objective finding on endoscopy or computed tomography (CT).

   CRS may be overdiagnosed (incorrectly diagnosed when not present) due to the overlap of symptoms with other disease entities.

Following the above criteria, there is a need for an objective finding to confirm diagnosis. Of note, a large proportion of patients diagnosed in the past as having rhinosinusitis do not fulfill these criteria when evaluated by a nonotolaryngologist.⊖

Diagnostic Tests

1. Laboratory tests: Elevated erythrocyte sedimentation rate (ESR) and white blood cell counts in bacterial rhinosinusitis. Elevated serum IgE in allergic CRS.

2. Imaging studies: Indicated in CRS and in the case of suspected complications. **CT of the sinuses** (possibly radiography) reveals sinus opacifications, fluid levels, mucosal thickening or polyps, anatomic defects predisposing to rhinosinusitis, and complications of the disease. This test is not recommended in the case of uncomplicated ABRS, as patients with a viral upper respiratory tract infection will likely have sinus opacification. **Magnetic resonance imaging (MRI)** is used in the diagnostic workup of fungal rhinosinusitis or malignancy.

3. Microbiology: Routine nasal culture is not recommended for the diagnosis of ABRS. When required because of an unexpected clinical course (resistance to treatment), sinus aspirates can be obtained, usually by endoscopically guided culture or, rarely, by maxillary tap.

4. Other studies used in the diagnostics of causes and complications of rhinosinusitis include anterior rhinoscopy, endoscopy of the nasal cavity and sinuses, as well as diagnostic tests for allergies, immune deficiencies, and cystic fibrosis.

Differential Diagnosis

This includes differential diagnosis of rhinitis, headache, and chronic cough.

→ TREATMENT

1. ABRS: Management algorithm: →Figure 13-1.
1) Nasal lavage using isotonic or hypertonic saline.
2) Nonsteroidal anti-inflammatory drugs in case of pain.
3) Nasal decongestants (→Chapter 2.1): There is limited evidence supporting the use of nasal decongestants. They should be used only for a short course (<5 days) to avoid rhinitis medicamentosa.

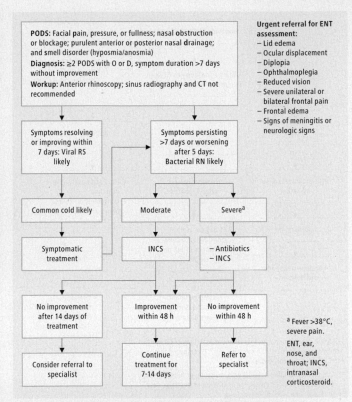

PODS: Facial **p**ain, pressure, or fullness; nasal **o**bstruction or blockage; purulent anterior or posterior nasal **d**rainage; and **s**mell disorder (hyposmia/anosmia)

Diagnosis: ≥2 PODS with O or D, symptom duration >7 days without improvement

Workup: Anterior rhinoscopy; sinus radiography and CT not recommended

Urgent referral for ENT assessment:
– Lid edema
– Ocular displacement
– Diplopia
– Ophthalmoplegia
– Reduced vision
– Severe unilateral or bilateral frontal pain
– Frontal edema
– Signs of meningitis or neurologic signs

Symptoms resolving or improving within 7 days: Viral RS likely

Symptoms persisting >7 days or worsening after 5 days: Bacterial RN likely

Common cold likely

Moderate

Severe[a]

Symptomatic treatment

INCS

– Antibiotics
– INCS

No improvement after 14 days of treatment

Improvement within 48 h

No improvement within 48 h

Consider referral to specialist

Continue treatment for 7-14 days

Refer to specialist

[a] Fever >38°C, severe pain.

ENT, ear, nose, and throat; INCS, intranasal corticosteroid.

Figure 13-1. Management algorithm of adults with acute rhinosinusitis. *Adapted from Rhinology. 2012 Mar;50(1):1-12.*

4) Antibiotics should not be used in patients with acute uncomplicated rhinosinusitis. Indications: →Figure 13-1. The literature suggests antibiotic treatment of ABRS may shorten the time to symptom resolution, although most studies show similar disease progression with ultimately similar rates of resolution in patients receiving antibiotics or placebo. However, there are no high-quality data on individuals with severe sinusitis or immunocompromised status. First-line therapy is amoxicillin 1.5 to 2 g every 12 hours. Second-line therapy includes amoxicillin/clavulanic acid (amoxicillin 1.5-2 g every 12 hours) and cephalosporins (eg, cefuroxime 0.5 g every 12 hours); in case of allergic reactions to β-lactam antibiotics, administer macrolides (eg, clarithromycin 0.5 g every 12 hours or azithromycin 0.25-0.5 g every 24 hours for 3 days or a single dose of 2 g).

5) Intranasal corticosteroids (INCSs): Indications: →Figure 13-1. There is significant evidence to suggest that INCSs improve symptoms and the time to symptom resolution. They are recommended as monotherapy for mild to moderate ABRS and are useful for preventing future episodes in patients with recurrent ABRS.

6) Antihistamines: Useful only in patients with allergies.

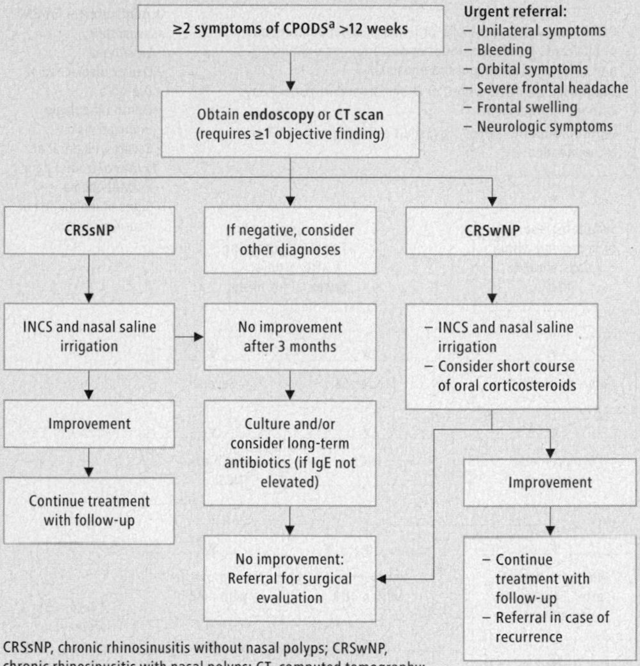
≥2 symptoms of CPODS[a] >12 weeks
Urgent referral:
– Unilateral symptoms
– Bleeding
– Orbital symptoms
– Severe frontal headache
– Frontal swelling
– Neurologic symptoms
Obtain endoscopy or CT scan (requires ≥1 objective finding)
CRSsNP
If negative, consider other diagnoses
CRSwNP
INCS and nasal saline irrigation
No improvement after 3 months
– INCS and nasal saline irrigation
– Consider short course of oral corticosteroids
Improvement
Culture and/or consider long-term antibiotics (if IgE not elevated)
Improvement
Continue treatment with follow-up
No improvement: Referral for surgical evaluation
– Continue treatment with follow-up
– Referral in case of recurrence

CRSsNP, chronic rhinosinusitis without nasal polyps; CRSwNP, chronic rhinosinusitis with nasal polyps; CT, computed tomography; INCS, intranasal corticosteroid.

[a] Congestion or fullness; facial pain, pressure, or fullness; nasal obstruction or blockage; purulent anterior or posterior nasal drainage; and smell disorder.

Figure 13-2. Management algorithm of adults with chronic rhinosinusitis. *Adapted from Can Fam Physician. 2013;59(12):1275-81 and Rhinology. 2012;50(1):1-12.*

2. CRS: Management algorithm: →Figure 13-2.

1) INCSs are the mainstay of CRS treatment with significant evidence for benefit in CRSwNP (decrease in polyp size and prevention of regrowth); studies involving patients with CRSsNP are more limited. The 2012 European Position Paper on Rhinosinusitis and Nasal Polyps concluded INCSs are effective and not associated with major adverse effects. Agents and dosage: →Chapter 2.1.

2) Oral corticosteroids: A short course is effective in reducing polyp size in patients with refractory CRS. There is limited evidence for corticosteroid use in patients with CRSsNP, although such therapy may be beneficial in those with severe symptoms.

3) Antibiotics may be beneficial in the setting of bacterial CRSsNP, but there is very limited evidence for short-course antibiotics compared with placebo. Long-term low-dose macrolide therapy has some evidence of benefit in patients with normal serum IgE and CRSsNP. The benefits are currently thought to be due to the anti-inflammatory rather than anti-infective properties of macrolides.

4) Topical or oral antihistamines: Used only in patients with allergies.

5) The benefits of nasal lavage are not entirely clear○ with suggestions of little benefit of low-volume (5 mL) nebulized saline spray compared with INCSs and some benefit of daily large-volume (150 mL) saline irrigations with a hypertonic solution compared with placebo.

Ear, nose, and throat (ENT) specialist consultation is indicated when diagnostic doubts are present or treatment is not effective. In selected patients polypectomy or endoscopic sinus surgery (ESS) is used.

→ COMPLICATIONS

The complications of bacterial rhinosinusitis include orbital cellulitis, orbital abscess, osteomyelitis of the sinus walls, cavernous sinus thrombosis, meningitis, and brain abscess.

14. Sepsis and Septic Shock

→ DEFINITION, ETIOLOGY, PATHOGENESIS

The most widely used definition for the sepsis spectrum was based on the 2001 International Sepsis Definitions Conference criteria. In 2016, the Third International Consensus Definitions for Sepsis and Septic Shock (Sepsis-3) were published.

2001 International Sepsis Definitions Conference Criteria

Systemic inflammatory response syndrome (SIRS) refers to an acute onset of ≥2 of the following symptoms:

1) Temperature >38.3°C or <36°C.

2) Heart rate >90 beats/min (this may be absent in patients treated with β-blockers).

3) Respiratory rate >20 breaths/min or partial pressure of carbon dioxide in arterial blood ($PaCO_2$) <32 mm Hg.

4) White blood cell (WBC) count >12×10^9/L or <4×10^9/L, or >10% of immature neutrophils in the differential WBC count.

Infection is an inflammatory response to microorganisms in tissues, body fluids, or cavities that are sterile under normal conditions.

Microbiologically documented infection refers to isolation of a pathogen from the normally sterile body fluid or tissue (or, alternatively, detection of its antigens or genetic material).

Clinically suspected infection refers to the presence of clinical features strongly suggestive of infection, for instance, leukocytes found in the normally sterile body fluid (other than blood), visceral perforation, radiographic features of pneumonia accompanied by purulent respiratory secretions, or an infected wound.

Sepsis is defined as a systemic inflammatory response caused by infection.

Severe sepsis is sepsis causing failure or severe malfunction of ≥1 organs or systems (other causes must be excluded; diagnostic criteria are relative) including:

1) **Cardiovascular system**: Hypotension (systolic blood pressure [SBP] <90 mm Hg, mean arterial pressure [MAP] <70 mm Hg, or an SBP drop >40 mm Hg).

2) **Respiratory system**: PaO_2/FiO_2 <300 mm Hg (<200 mm Hg in patients with primary diseases of the respiratory tract).

3) **Kidneys**: Urine output <0.5 mL/kg/h over >2 hours with adequate fluid intake/resuscitation or a serum creatinine level increase by >0.5 mg/dL (44.2 µmol/L).

4) **Metabolism**: Elevated serum lactate levels.

5) **Hemostasis**: Platelet count <100×10^9/L or international normalized ratio (INR) >1.5.

6) **Liver**: Serum bilirubin levels >34.2 µmol/L (2 mg/dL).

7) **Central nervous system (CNS)**: Features of encephalopathy (anxiety, confusion, agitation, delirium, coma).

Septic shock is severe sepsis with persistent hypotension refractory to fluid resuscitation, requiring administration of vasopressors.

Multiple organ dysfunction syndrome (MODS) refers to severe functional organ disturbances in an acutely ill patient, which are indicative of the failure to maintain homeostasis without therapeutic intervention.

Bacteremia is the presence of live bacteria in the bloodstream. **Viremia** is the presence of a replication-competent virus in the bloodstream. **Fungemia** is the presence of live fungi in the bloodstream (candidemia: presence of live *Candida* spp in the bloodstream).

Sepsis-3 Definition and Diagnostic Criteria

Quick sequential organ failure assessment (qSOFA) includes prognostic criteria that predict poor outcomes. It should not be used to screen patients for sepsis (as it may lead to substantial underdiagnosis) but it may prompt clinicians to monitor and assess the patient for the possibility of sepsis. A positive qSOFA score implies >2 of the following 3 criteria are met: altered mental status, SBP <100 mm Hg, and respiratory rate ≥22/min.

Sepsis is now defined as a life-threatening organ dysfunction caused by a dys-regulated host response to infection. **Clinical diagnostic criteria for sepsis**: a suspected or documented infection and ≥2 points increase from the baseline on the sequential (sepsis-related) organ failure assessment (SOFA) score.

The SOFA score (available at mdcalc.com) assesses dysfunction of different organs by measuring degree of hypoxia and hypotension, platelet count, bil-irubin level, urine output and creatinine level, and neurologic function (the Glasgow Coma Scale [GCS]). One point is granted after meeting each of the following thresholds:

1) MAP <70 mm Hg (1 point) and then additional points for use of low (2 points), medium (3 points), or high dose of vasopressors (4 points).

2) Ratio of arterial partial pressure of oxygen to fraction of inspired oxygen (PaO_2/FiO_2) <400 mm Hg (1 point), then an additional point for each of <300 mm Hg, 200 mm Hg, and 100 mm Hg.

3) GCS score of 13 to 14 (1 point), then an additional point for each score in the range of 10 to 12, 6 to 9, and <6 points.

4) Platelet count <150×10^9/L (1 point), then an additional point for each of <100×10^9/L, <50×10^9/L, and <20×10^9/L.

5) Bilirubin >20 µmol/L (1.2 mg/dL) (1 point), then an additional point for each of >32 µmol/L (1.9 mg/dL), >101 µmol/L (5.9 mg/dL), and >204 µmol/L (12 mg/dL).

6) Creatinine level >110 µmol/L (1.2 mg/dL) (1 point), then additional points for each of 171 µmol/L (2.0 mg/dL), 300 µmol/L (3.5 mg/dL), and >440 µmol/L (5.0 mg/dL). Urine output <200 mL/d carries 4 points and <500 mL/d, 3 points.

Septic shock is now defined as a subset of sepsis in which underlying circulato-ry and cellular metabolism abnormalities are profound enough to substantially increase mortality. **Clinical diagnostic criteria for septic shock** include the presence of sepsis, vasopressor therapy needed to elevate MAP ≥65 mm Hg, and lactate level >2 mmol/L (18 mg/dL) despite adequate fluid resuscitation.

Comparison of 2001 and 2016 definitions and concepts: →Table 14-1.

Table 14-1. Definitions and criteria for the diagnosis of sepsis and septic shock

Consensus criteria	Previous (1991, 2001)	Current (2016)
Sepsis	Systemic inflammatory response caused by infection. Criteria for SIRS are considered to be met if ≥2 of the following occur: 1) Body temperature >38°C or <36°C 2) Heart rate >90/min[a] 3) Respiratory rate >20/min or $PaCO_2$ <32 mm Hg 4) Leukocyte count >12 × 10⁹/L or <4 × 10⁹/L or >10% immature neutrophil	Life-threatening organ dysfunction caused by a dysregulated host response to infection, which causes organ damage (corresponds to the previous concept of severe sepsis)
Severe sepsis	Sepsis causing failure or severe malfunction of ≥1 organ or system (corresponds to the current concept of sepsis)	Sepsis, as above
Organ dysfunction	– Cardiovascular system: Hypotension (SBP <90 mm Hg, MAP <70 mm Hg, or SBP drop >40 mm Hg) – Respiratory system: PaO_2/FiO_2 <300 mm Hg (<200 mm Hg in patients with primary diseases of the respiratory tract) – Kidneys: Urine output <0.5 mL/kg/h over >2 h with adequate fluid intake/resuscitation or serum creatinine level increase by >0.5 mg/dL (44.2 μmol/L) – Metabolism: Elevated serum lactate levels – Hemostasis: Platelet count <100 × 10⁹/L or INR >1.5 – Liver: Serum bilirubin levels >34.2 μmol/L (2 mg/dL) – CNS: Features of encephalopathy (anxiety, confusion, agitation, delirium, coma)	Patient with suspected or documented infection and ≥2 points increase from baseline on SOFA (see text)[b]
Septic shock	Severe sepsis with acute circulatory failure characterized by persistent hypotension (SBP <90 mm Hg, mean <65 mm Hg or decrease in SBP by >40 mm Hg) despite adequate fluid resuscitation (thus requiring use of vasoconstrictive drugs)	Subset of sepsis with underlying circulatory and cellular metabolism abnormalities profound enough to substantially increase mortality. Clinical criteria include presence of sepsis and vasopressor therapy needed to elevate MAP ≥65 mm Hg and lactate level >2 mmol/L (18 mg/dL) despite adequate fluid resuscitation
Scale proposed for early isolation of patients at risk of death	Not specified; SIRS, organ dysfunction, and extended criteria for diagnosis of sepsis were used	qSOFA: ≥2 of: 1) Disturbance of consciousness 2) SBP ≤100 mm Hg 3) Respiratory rate ≥22/min

[a] This may not occur in patients receiving β-blockers.

[b] In patients without acute organ dysfunction the SOFA score is usually 0.

Based on Intensive Care Med. 2003;29(4):530-8 and JAMA. 2016 23;315(8):801-10.

CNS, central nervous system; FiO_2, fraction of inspired oxygen; INR, international normalized ratio; MAP, mean arterial pressure; $PaCO_2$, partial pressure of carbon dioxide in arterial blood; PaO_2, arterial partial pressure of oxygen; qSOFA, quick sequential organ failure assessment; SBP, systolic blood pressure; SIRS, syndrome of systemic inflammatory response; SOFA, sequential organ failure assessment.

Etiology

The etiology of sepsis does not always determine its clinical course. Pathogens may be undetectable in the bloodstream or other tissues. In the majority of patients there is no history of immunodeficiency (although it is an important risk factor for sepsis).

Infection and inflammation that eventually lead to the development of sepsis initially affect various sites, such as the abdominal organs (eg, peritonitis, acute pancreatitis), urinary system (eg, pyelonephritis), respiratory system (eg, pneumonia, empyema), CNS (eg, meningitis, encephalitis), musculoskeletal system (eg, septic arthritis, osteomyelitis), and skin and subcutaneous tissue (eg, injury-related and surgical wounds, pressure ulcers). Location of the primary infection site is frequently occult (eg, periodontal sites, sinuses, tonsils, endocardium, gallbladder and biliary tract, reproductive system including gestational sac infections).

Iatrogenic risk factors include intravascular catheters, urinary catheters, implantable prostheses and devices, endotracheal tube, parenteral nutrition, surgical wounds, and drug-induced immunodeficiency.

Pathophysiology

Sepsis is a pathologic response to infection involving several factors such as pathogen antigens, endotoxins, as well as proinflammatory and anti-inflammatory mediators produced by the host (cytokines, chemokines, eicosanoids, and other mediators causing SIRS) and substances causing cell damage (eg, free radicals).

Septic shock (hypotension and tissue hypoperfusion) is a consequence of inflammatory mediators, which cause relative hypovolemia (inadequate intravascular volume resulting from vasodilation and reduced systemic vascular resistance), absolute hypovolemia (increased vascular permeability), or, less commonly, myocardial dysfunction (in septic shock the stroke volume is usually increased as long as the intravascular volume is maintained). Hypotension and hypoperfusion lead to decreased tissue oxygen delivery and hypoxia. Ultimately, this results in increased cellular anaerobic metabolism and lactic acidosis. Other manifestations of septic shock may include acute respiratory distress syndrome; acute kidney injury (acute kidney injury, initially in the form of prerenal acute kidney injury); altered mental status resulting from CNS hypoperfusion and the effects of inflammatory mediators; gastrointestinal system disturbances, including ileus or gut ischemia, that predispose to intestinal mucosal disruption, which causes bleeding (acute hemorrhagic gastropathy and stress ulcers, ischemic colitis) or bacterial translocation from the intestinal lumen to the bloodstream; acute hepatic insufficiency or failure; relative adrenal insufficiency; and disturbances of hemostasis (disseminated intravascular coagulation; usually beginning with thrombocytopenia).

→ CLINICAL FEATURES AND NATURAL HISTORY

Clinical manifestations of SIRS and severe sepsis: →Definition, Etiology, Pathogenesis, above and →Table 14-2. Additional signs and symptoms depend on the involvement of particular organs and systems. If the spread of infection and/or the host response to infection is not attenuated at an early stage, functional impairment of other organs and systems will follow (→Definition, Etiology, Pathogenesis, above). If adequate treatment is not started, the symptoms of septic shock can progress to MODS and death.

→ DIAGNOSIS

Diagnostic Tests

1. Laboratory tests: Assessment of organ dysfunction including arterial and venous blood gases, serum lactate level (when possible, it should be measured even within the first hour of the onset of symptoms of [severe] sepsis), coagulation tests, kidney and liver function tests, and inflammatory markers (complete blood

Table 14-2. Clinical consequences and diagnostic features of sepsis

Infection (documented or suspected) and some of the following:

General variables:
- Fever >38.3°C or hypothermia <36°C
- Tachycardia >90/min
- Tachypnea >30/min (or mechanical ventilation)
- Sudden deterioration of mental status
- Significant edema or positive fluid balance (>20 mL/kg/d)
- Hyperglycemia (>7.7 mmol/L [140 mg/dL]) in the absence of diabetes

Inflammatory variables:
- Leukocytosis (WBC count >12 × 10⁹/L) or leukopenia (WBC count <4 × 10⁹/L)
- More than 10% of immature neutrophil forms in WBC differential counts
- Plasma CRP >2 SD above mean value
- Plasma procalcitonin >2 SD above mean value

Hemodynamic and tissue perfusion variables:
- Arterial hypotension (SBP <90 mm Hg, MAP <70 mm Hg, or SBP drop >40 mm Hg)
- Serum lactate levels >ULN
- Decreased capillary refill

Emerging or worsening organ dysfunction variables:
- Hypoxemia (PaO_2/FiO_2 <300 mm Hg; <200 mm Hg in patients with primary diseases of the respiratory tract)
- Acute oliguria (urine output <0.5 mL/kg/h over >2 hours with adequate volume status)
- Increase in creatinine levels by ≥44.2 μmol/L (≥0.5 mg/dL) over 48 hours
- Coagulation abnormalities (platelet count <100 × 10⁹/L, INR >1.5, aPTT >60 seconds)
- Total serum bilirubin levels >70 μmol/L (4 mg/dL)
- Ileus (absent bowel sounds)

Adapted from Crit Care Med. 2013;41(2):580-637.

aPTT, activated partial thromboplastin time; CRP, C-reactive protein; INR, international normalized ratio; MAP, mean arterial pressure; SBP, systolic blood pressure; SD, standard deviation; ULN, upper limit of normal; WBC, white blood cell.

count [CBC], C-reactive protein [CRP], or procalcitonin [PCT]). Negative PCT or similar markers may support the decision to shorten the course of empiric antimicrobial therapy in patients suspected of sepsis.⊘◯

2. Microbiology:

1) Blood: ≥2 samples including ≥1 from a noncatheterized vessel (separate venipuncture) and 1 from each vascular catheter (especially if inserted prior to the development of sepsis).

2) Other samples: Depending on the suspected etiology, the samples should be obtained from the respiratory tract, urine, other body fluids (cerebrospinal fluid, pleural effusion), or wound discharge.

3. Imaging studies (as suggested by symptoms, signs, and laboratory tests): Radiography (particularly chest radiographs), ultrasonography, and computed tomography (CT) (particularly of the abdomen).

→ TREATMENT

Antimicrobial and other supportive treatment should be started urgently and simultaneously. Prognosis is determined primarily by the prompt administration of antibiotics and IV fluids.

It was recently proposed that during the first hour after clinical recognition of sepsis several aspects of diagnosis and management are performed: obtaining blood cultures, measuring lactate level, delivery of antibiotics, beginning of fluid resuscitation, and application of vasopressors if needed to maintain SBP >65 mm Hg. The ability to achieve all this in clinical practice is questioned by many clinicians.

Treatment of Infection

1. Antimicrobial treatment: Start empiric antimicrobial therapy as soon as possible, that is, **within 1 hour of presentation (each hour of delay may increase mortality by 8%, especially in septic shock)**.◐● It is important to collect appropriate samples for microbiological testing before the treatment (but only if it does not delay treatment by more than a short period of time, eg, up to 30-45 minutes; →Diagnosis, Etiology, Pathogenesis, above). In sepsis administer at least one IV broad-spectrum antibiotic; consider the coverage of the most likely etiologic organisms (bacteria, fungi) and the penetration of the antibiotic to the sites of infection, as well as local pathogen resistance patterns. Treatment may be modified after 48 to 72 hours, depending on available microbiology results and the clinical course. Targeted treatment should be implemented as soon as possible. Monotherapy is preferred; combination therapy may be used, for instance, in the case of suspected or confirmed *Pseudomonas* or *Acinetobacter* infection. In septic shock with bacteremia caused by *Streptococcus pneumoniae*, combine a β-lactam with a macrolide. The duration of treatment is usually 7 to 10 days (it may be longer in the case of delayed clinical response to treatment, if local infection sites cannot be adequately drained or eradicated, if patients are immunodeficient, or if the infections are due to particularly virulent pathogens). Antimicrobial treatment in patients with neutropenia: →Chapter 8.7.

2. Source control should include infected tissues or organs (eg, gallbladder, necrotic segment of bowel), infected catheters, implantable prostheses and devices. Drainage of any abscesses, empyema, and other infected collections in closed spaces is also of key importance, as long as the likely benefits and risks of procedures are considered. The preferred treatment should generally be kept as noninvasive as maintaining efficacy allows (eg, percutaneous drain rather than open abdominal washout). In the case of infected pancreatic necrosis, a stepwise approach rather than a complete removal of infected tissue is suggested.◐●

Supportive Treatment

1. Initial treatment of shock should be started as soon as possible (prior to the intensive care unit admission). A prompt recognition and initiation of treatment by clinicians experienced in resuscitation with frequent reassessment are likely at least as important as following any specific algorithm or obtaining specific values. For clinicians who are less experienced or who prefer to use an algorithm for resuscitation, the reasonable early goal-directed therapy (EGDT) hemodynamic targets are:

1) Central venous pressure (CVP) 8 to 12 mm Hg (11-16 cm H_2O) or 12 to 15 mm Hg (16-20 cm H_2O) in patients treated with positive airway pressure mechanical ventilation or with elevated abdominal pressures (intra--abdominal hypertension or abdominal compartment syndrome). Bedside ultrasonography may also be used to identify patients with hypovolemia.◐○

2) MAP ≥65 mm is standard of treatment.◐● Possible exceptions may occur in patients with hypertension in whom higher MAP (up to 80 mm Hg) may be acceptable.◐○

3) Spontaneous urine output ≥0.5 mL/kg/h.

4) Central venous oxygen saturation (superior vena cava) ($ScvO_2$) ≥70% or mixed venous oxygen saturation ≥65% (measurement of lactate levels has a similar clinical significance and could be used instead).◐● Recently

managing patients according to capillary refill assessed every half hour was again shown to be equivalent.🗹🟢

To achieve these goals, use **fluid resuscitation** (→below). In patients in whom despite achieving the target CVP and MAP (including the patients treated with vasopressors; →below) the target $ScvO_2$ or lactate clearance has not been obtained within 6 hours, it is suggested to use, depending on the circumstances (heart rate, left ventricular function, previous hemodynamic response to fluid, hemoglobin [Hb] level) one or more of the following: continued fluid resuscitation, transfusion of packed red blood cells (PRBCs) to achieve a hematocrit ≥30%, dobutamine (maximum dose, 20 µg/kg/min).⊘🔾

Clinicians trained in resuscitation and sepsis management can use bedside dynamic volume status and perfusion assessment (eg, echocardiography, ultrasonography, cardiac index, capillary refill time, urine output, and others), and laboratory values such as serum lactate level when available, avoiding measurement of $ScvO_2$, transfusing PRBCs only for Hb <70 g/L, and with lower use of dobutamine.🗹🟢 The key is frequent assessment of the patient.

2. Treatment of cardiovascular dysfunction:

1) **Maintain adequate intravascular volume**. In patients with tissue hypoperfusion and suspected hypovolemia, **start with a rapid infusion of crystalloids** (reasonable amount may be ≥30 mL/kg; alternatively clinicians use 500-1000 mL boluses with frequent reassessment) while watching for volume overload (part of this volume may be substituted by equivalent volumes of albumin); repeat depending on the effects on arterial pressure, urine output, and possible adverse effects (symptoms of volume overload). Some patients may require rapid administration of higher fluid volumes. Administration of colloids other than albumin, and particularly of hydroxyethyl starch (HES), may result in kidney injury and increased mortality, and thus it is recommended not to use HES in patients with sepsis and/or septic shock.🛇🔾 Until further data are available, we also suggest avoiding a rapid use of larger volumes (eg, >2 L) of unbalanced crystalloids with a high concentration of chloride (typically 0.9% NaCl).🛇🔾

2) **Vasopressors**: If hypotension persists in spite of adequate fluid resuscitation, we recommend **norepinephrine** (rather than dopamine) as a first-line vasopressor.🗹🟢 **Vasopressin** (dosage: →Chapter 3.16) could be used when reduction of the dose of norepinephrine is attempted⊘🟢 or as an early addition to norepinephrine (rather than major increase in the dose of norepinephrine) as it may reduce the risk of death, atrial fibrillation, and need for renal replacement therapy at the expense of increased risk of digital ischemia.⊘🟢 **Epinephrine** can be used as an alternative to **norepinephrine** if the patient is unresponsive to vasopressors or if additional vasopressors are required to support hemodynamics.

Administer the vasopressor agent as soon as practical through a central venous catheter under invasive intra-arterial pressure monitoring (arterial catheterization is necessary). The use of dopamine should be limited to patients with bradycardia, reduced stroke volumes, and those at low risk of arrhythmias.

3) **Inotropic therapy**: **Dobutamine** (dosage: →Chapter 3.16) may be tried on the basis of physiologic rationale in patients with low stroke volumes in spite of adequate fluid resuscitation, although the benefit of such action is unclear. Coexisting or developing hypotension may require the addition of a vasopressor.

3. Treatment of respiratory failure (→Chapter 13.16.1). Usually mechanical ventilation is necessary. Also →Chapter 13.14.

4. Treatment of renal failure: Hemodynamic stabilization (normalization of arterial pressure) is essential. Use renal replacement therapy (RRT) when necessary; the effects of early versus late institution of RRT in critically ill patients are not clear as is not clear the choice between intermittent and continuous RRT, although the latter may result in less hemodynamic instability.☺

5. Treatment of acidosis: The main goal of acidosis treatment should be directed at removing the underlying cause. The use of IV NaHCO$_3$ to raise pH in patients with significant acidosis has been controversial, but the recent evidence suggests that its use is likely beneficial, particularly among patients with metabolic acidosis and renal dysfunction.☺●

6. Glucocorticoids: In patients with persistent hypotension despite adequate fluid resuscitation and vasopressor therapy, low-dose IV hydrocortisone (200 mg/d) may be used☺◯ (at least until the symptoms of shock resolve).

7. Glucose control: In the case of severe sepsis associated hyperglycemia (>10 mmol/L [180 mg/dL]), it is recommended to control glucose with target levels <10 mmol/L (180 mg/dL) rather than <6.1 mmol/L (110 mg/dL).☺● If IV insulin infusion is used, in the initial phase of insulin therapy check glucose levels every 1 to 2 hours, and after stabilization of blood glucose, every 4 to 6 hours. Avoid hypoglycemia. In patients with hypoperfusion the glucose levels in capillary blood should be interpreted with caution; venous or arterial blood measurements are more reliable.

8. Other supportive treatment:

1) **Transfusions of blood products:**

   a) Transfuse PRBCs in patients with a Hb <70 g/L (rather than with a Hb <100 g/L) to achieve a target Hb of 70 g/L to 90 g/L.☺● Exceptions may include transfusion of PRBCs in patients with a Hb >70 g/L and tissue hypoperfusion (acute septic shock may represent such a situation), active bleeding, or significant coronary artery disease.

   b) Platelet transfusion: It is suggested to transfuse platelets in patients with platelet counts <10 × 10^9/L; it may be also beneficial in patients with platelet counts 10 × 10^9/L to 20 × 10^9/L and increased risk of bleeding (including severe sepsis and septic shock). A reasonable target platelet count for larger invasive procedures may be ≥50 × 10^9/L.☺◯

   c) Fresh-frozen plasma (FFP) and cryoprecipitate are used mainly in the case of active bleeding or preparation for invasive procedures.☺◯

2) **Nutrition** should preferably be via the enteral route. The volumes should not exceed the level tolerated by the patient (covering the full caloric requirement initially is not mandatory). The patient-important consequences of using prokinetics are not clear.☺

3) **Stress ulcer prophylaxis** is administered in patients with risk factors of bleeding.☺● Proton pump inhibitors may be preferred over H$_2$-receptor antagonists.☺◯

4) **Deep vein thrombosis prophylaxis** (→Chapter 3.19.1) should be used unless the risk of bleeding is judged prohibitive.☺● We suggest low-molecular--weight heparin rather than unfractionated heparin.☺◯

5) **Management of patients treated with mechanical ventilation:** Administer sedatives in the lowest possible doses to achieve the target (lowest well-tolerated) level of sedation. Avoid long-term administration of neuromuscular blocking agents; however, in patients with acute respiratory distress syndrome and PaO$_2$/FiO$_2$ <150 mm Hg, consider using neuromuscular blocking agents for 48 hours of mechanical ventilation.☺◯ Maintain the head of the bed elevated at 30 to 45° and, until future evidence helps to clarify current controversies, consider the use of oropharyngeal decontamination with chlorhexidine gluconate or selective decontamination of the digestive tract to prevent ventilator-associated pneumonia.

6) Treatment of **disseminated intravascular coagulation** (→Chapter 7.4.1.2). Treatment of the underlying causes of sepsis is crucial.

15. Tick-Borne Diseases

15.1. Lyme Borreliosis

Lyme borreliosis is a multiorgan bacterial inflammatory disease involving the skin, joints, nervous system, and heart.

1. Etiologic agent: Gram-negative spirochetes *Borrelia* spp transmitted by ticks. In Canada and the US, the most common species is *Borrelia burgdorferi*; in Europe, it is most commonly *Borrelia afzelii*, *Borrelia garinii*, and rarely *B burgdorferi*. After being injected into the skin, the spirochetes migrate locally and form an early skin lesion (erythema migrans). Over the course of several days to weeks, the spirochetes may spread to several organs with blood or lymph.

2. Reservoir and transmission: Wild animals, especially rodents and white--tailed deer. Infection occurs through the bite of an infected *Ixodes* (hard, black legged) tick. The incidence of tick-borne diseases varies geographically and follows seasonable patterns that depend on the activity of ticks, which feed on human and animal blood and are active from spring until late fall.

3. Epidemiology: Epidemiology changes quickly as ticks migrate with the animal hosts. Readers are recommended to review their local epidemiology on a regular basis.

1) Canada: Southern British Columbia; Manitoba; Quebec; New Brunswick; southern, eastern, and northwestern Ontario; and part of Nova Scotia.
2) United States: Predominantly in the Northeast with smaller foci in the upper Midwest and Pacific Northwest.
3) Europe: Central Europe, Scandinavia, and endemic regions in Russia.

4. Risk factors: Residence, tourism, or work in tick-infested endemic areas. Ticks must feed on the host for >24 hours in order to transmit Lyme disease. Stimulation of ticks attached to the skin (eg, by squeezing, applying gasoline or oil, burning) may increase transmission rate.

5. Incubation and contagious period: The incubation period refers to the early infection (stage 1; →below) and lasts from 3 to 30 days (in some cases up to 3 months) from the time of tick attachment. The patient is not infectious for contacts.

Stages of the disease (these may overlap or occur simultaneously; usually not all signs and symptoms are present):

1. Early localized infection (stage 1):

1) **Erythema migrans** usually appears within ~7 (3-30) days after the tick bite. It is initially a red--colored spot or macula, which rapidly increases in diameter (>5 cm) and develops a bright-red outer border with partial central clearing (though it may be uniformly red) with clearly demarcated margins (→Figure 15-1). The lesion is flat, painless, and does not cause itching. It rarely ulcerates. Multiple

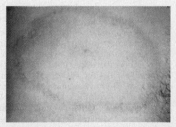

Figure 15-1. Typical features of erythema migrans, a sign of the early phase of Lyme borreliosis.

erythema migrans rashes are indicative of disseminated infection. Early infection may include flu-like symptoms.

2) **Borrelial lymphocytoma** is a rare manifestation of Lyme borreliosis; it is a painless, bluish-red nodule, which most frequently develops on the pinna, nipple, or scrotum.

Erythema migrans and early systemic clinical features resolve spontaneously within 4 to 12 weeks regardless of antimicrobial treatment.

In some untreated patients relatively mild clinical symptoms persist for several years, while others develop signs and symptoms of late infection (these symptoms, such as arthritis, may be the first and only manifestation of the disease, even years after the tick bite).

2. Early disseminated infection (stage 2) may develop over several weeks to a few months after exposure:

1) **Carditis** (~5% of patients): Sudden-onset atrioventricular block or arrhythmia and other conduction disturbances. The block resolves with antibiotic treatment.

2) **Inflammatory neurologic involvement (neuroborreliosis)**: Simultaneous or gradual involvement of different levels of the central and peripheral nervous systems, which may manifest as lymphocytic meningitis (usually mild; headache may be the only manifestation) and cranial neuritis (paralysis or paresis; most commonly facial nerve palsy, which may be bilateral).

3. Late localized infection (stage 3) may develop weeks to months after exposure:

1) **Arthritis**: Most frequently involves one large joint (knee (90%), ankle, elbow), although sometimes several joints may be affected. Typically no severe systemic inflammatory reaction is present in spite of a major joint effusion. Recurrent flares lasting several days to weeks may occur; their frequency and severity diminishes over time. Early flares may respond to a repeat course of antibiotics. Late flares may be antibiotic resistant (inflammatory rather than infectious) and may require anti-inflammatory therapy. Patients with HLA-DRB1 are more prone to develop a chronic inflammatory arthritis even after successful treatment for Lyme disease.

2) **Chronic neuroborreliosis** (very rare): Radiculitis and peripheral neuritis, peripheral polyneuropathy, chronic encephalomyelitis.

3) **Acrodermatitis chronica atrophicans**: Reddish-violaceous skin lesions on distal limbs, usually asymmetric and appearing several years after the tick bite. Initially this manifests as inflammatory edema; later skin atrophy becomes the predominant sign (skin becomes thin, hairless, and has violaceous discoloration). The lesions are frequently accompanied by pain of adjacent joints and by paresthesias.

4. Lyme disease in pregnancy: There are rare case reports of perinatal transmission of Lyme disease but no studies or expert consensus. Pregnant women diagnosed with Lyme disease should be treated appropriately for their stage at presentation. Tetracyclines should be avoided.

5. Concepts of chronic Lyme disease versus post-Lyme syndrome: The term chronic Lyme disease is sometimes used to describe nonspecific symptoms persisting for >3 months in a patient with negative Lyme antibodies. Current literature does not support active infection in the setting of a negative antibody results for patients with symptoms lasting >12 weeks and another etiology for their symptoms should be investigated. Post-Lyme syndrome refers to persistent symptoms lasting >6 to 12 months after appropriate antibiotic therapy in patients positive for Lyme antibody. Signs and symptoms of active inflammation should be excluded. Most patients do not require repeated or prolonged antibiotic therapy in the absence of documented inflammation, such as arthritis or uveitis.

→ DIAGNOSIS

Erythema migrans rash with the appropriate epidemiologic risk factors is diagnostic of early (stage 1) Lyme disease. Patients with an erythema migrans rash in the right setting should be treated empirically, as antibodies are only positive 50% of the time.

A negative history of tick bite in a patient with erythema migrans does not preclude the diagnosis of Lyme disease. At most 80% of patients remember a prior tick bite.

Antibody testing for chronic symptoms in low-risk areas is not recommended due to the low positive predictive value.

Diagnostic Tests

Laboratory diagnosis is necessary to diagnose stage 2 or 3 Lyme disease.

Diagnosis involves a two-step process:

1) **Enzyme-linked immunosorbent assay (ELISA)**: Measurement of specific serum IgM levels. The ELISA is sensitive but not specific for Lyme disease. A negative ELISA result excludes Lyme disease unless the exposure was acute, for example, within the last 3 to 30 days. An inconclusive or positive ELISA must be confirmed with a Western blot.

2) **Western blot**: The Western blot confirms that a positive ELISA is actually due to Lyme disease. The Western blot measures both IgM and IgG:

   a) IgM: Specific IgM antibodies are detectable in blood within 3 to 4 weeks from the moment of infection (they peak after 6-8 weeks) and gradually disappear over the next 4 to 6 months. Rarely, IgM may persist for years. A positive Western blot IgM result with a negative Western blot IgG result may represent early disease. An isolated positive IgM after >8 weeks of symptom onset is considered a false positive and other causes for the patient's symptoms should be investigated; these patients do not require antibiotic therapy for Lyme disease.

   b) IgG: Specific IgG antibody is detected within 6 to 8 weeks of the tick bite and remains positive for many years even in patients successfully treated with antibiotics. It should be interpreted within the context of clinical symptoms.

   c) Central nervous system disease: In patients with neuroborreliosis, specific IgM or IgG may be detected in cerebrospinal fluid (CSF). Lymphocytic pleocytosis may be found both in early and late neuroborreliosis; however, in early cranial neuritis and late neuroborreliosis with peripheral nervous system involvement, CSF is usually normal.

The diagnosis of late Lyme borreliosis is made in patients who have a positive Lyme ELISA result with a confirmatory IgG Western blot and who have signs and symptoms of the disease persisting for ≥12 months.

→ TREATMENT

Antimicrobial Treatment

1. Antibiotic treatment: The choice of the antibiotic and duration of treatment vary with disease manifestations (→Table 15-1). Antibiotics are warranted for patients presenting with an erythema migrans rash and a risk of exposure to Lyme disease or those with a longer duration of symptoms who have a positive antibody for Lyme disease. No antibiotics are necessary for asymptomatic patients with an incidental positive IgG antibody.

2. Relapse versus reinfection versus persistent inflammation: Relapses are rare but may be more frequent in patients with arthritis who are HLA-B27–positive. Reinfection, which requires a new round of treatment, is possible and must be distinguished clinically from relapse, which requires extension of the

Table 15-1. Antibiotic treatment in various stages of Lyme borreliosis[a]

Clinical features	Drug, route of administration (choose one)	Dosage	Treatment duration (days)
Tick bite where rate of tick infections is <10% and/or tick was on for <24 h	Monitoring[b]		
– Erythema migrans – Borrelial lymphocytoma – Cranial neuritis[c] (palsy)	Doxycycline,[b] PO	100 mg bid or 200 mg once daily	14-21
	Amoxicillin, PO	500 mg tid (children 50 mg/kg/d)	14-21
	Cefuroxime axetil, PO	500 mg bid (children 30 mg/kg/d)	14-21
Arthritis (first episode)	Doxycycline, PO	100 mg bid or 200 mg once daily	14-28
	Amoxicillin, PO	500-1000 mg tid (children 50 mg/kg/d)	14-28
	Cefuroxime axetil, PO	500 mg bid (children 30 mg/kg/d)	14-28
– Neuroborreliosis – Arthritis (relapse) – Carditis	Ceftriaxone, IV	2000 mg once daily (children 50-75 mg/kg/d)	14-28
	Cefotaxime, IV	2000 mg tid (children 150--200 mg/kg/d in 3-4 divided doses)	14-28
Acrodermatitis chronica atrophicans	Doxycycline, PO	100 mg bid or 200 mg once daily	14-28
	Amoxicillin, PO	500-1000 mg tid	14-28
	Ceftriaxone, IV	2000 mg once daily	14-28
	Cefotaxime, IV	2000 mg tid	14-28

[a] Based on guidelines from the Infectious Diseases Society of America and the Polish Society of Epidemiology and Infectious Diseases (2008).

[b] Tetracyclines are contraindicated in pregnancy and for children aged <8 years. Macrolides are considered third-line therapy and should be reserved for patients with contraindications to both β-lactams and doxycycline.

[c] Evaluate for signs and symptoms of meningitis.

bid, 2 times a day; IV, intravenous; PO, oral; tid, 3 times a day.

recently completed treatment. Many patients can have persistent inflammatory symptoms in the absence of active infection and require only symptomatic support. Symptoms after appropriate treatment for the late stages of Lyme disease, particularly neuroborreliosis or arthritis, may persist for months to years.

Symptomatic Treatment

Symptomatic treatment is used when necessary and may include, for instance, nonsteroidal anti-inflammatory drugs and arthrocentesis with evacuation of joint effusion. Some patients with persistent postinfectious arthritis require disease-modifying agents.

→ PROGNOSIS

Early appropriate antibiotic treatment is curative in >90% of patients. In the remaining group, late neurologic, articular, and cutaneous sequelae may develop.

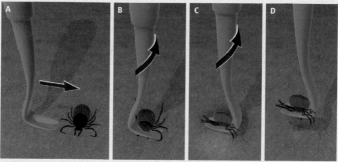

Figure 15-2. Tick removal using a plastic hook: **A, B**, slide the hook between the skin and the tick, keeping it as close to the skin as possible, **C**, until the tick is caught between the prongs. **D**, gently lift the hook while rotating it 2 to 3 times around its longer axis.

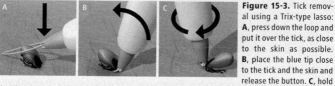

Figure 15-3. Tick removal using a Trix-type lasso: **A**, press down the loop and put it over the tick, as close to the skin as possible. **B**, place the blue tip close to the tick and the skin and release the button. **C**, hold the blue tip close to the skin, tilt the tool perpendicularly to the skin surface, and rotate it between the fingers in any direction, at the same time removing the tick. To minimize the risk of tearing the tick, do not pull it upwards (along the longer axis of the tool).

→ PREVENTION

Nonspecific Protection Against Ticks (Mainstay of Prevention)

1. Covering the skin while hiking or working in meadows and forests, for instance, by wearing long-sleeved shirts, long pants tucked into socks, a baseball cap or a wide brim sun-hat, light-colored clothes (ticks are easier to spot), and high-top shoes.

2. Repellents: Tick repellents, preferably containing diethyltoluamide (DEET) (they should be sprayed over clothes and exposed skin, except for the face) or permethrin (kills ticks on contact, should be sprayed onto clothes only).

3. Thorough full-body check upon each return from forests or meadows (particularly including inguinal and axillary areas, skin behind the ears, and skin folds). Ticks must be attached for ≥24 hours in order to transmit Lyme disease to humans. Prompt removal of ticks that have been feeding for <24 hours does not result in Lyme transmission.

4. Prompt mechanical tick removal using a small hook (→Figure 15-2), a lasso (→Figure 15-3), or thin-tipped tweezers (→Figure 15-4). If tick mouthparts remain in the skin (this does not increase the risk of infection), apply disinfectant

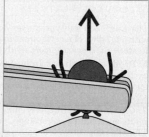

Figure 15-4. Tick removal using tweezers.

to the affected area. Do not twist, scratch, squeeze, or burn the tick, and do not apply greasy liquids, alcohol, or gasoline, as this is actually associated with a higher risk of infection due to increasing the amount of tick's vomit and saliva injected to the bloodstream. Disinfect the wound. After removing the tick, instruct the patient how to recognize the signs and symptoms of the disease, and advise to monitor the bite site for the next 30 days for signs of erythema migrans.

5. Protection of domestic animals (dogs, cats), which may bring ticks into the home: Tick repellents for animals, skin inspection, mechanical tick removal.

6. Postexposure prophylaxis: A single oral dose of 200 mg doxycycline is warranted **only** in the case of multiple tick bites in an adult who is not a permanent resident of an area endemic to Lyme borreliosis. To date, this approach has not been validated in children.

7. Vaccine is not available.

15.2. Tick-Borne Encephalitis

→ DEFINITION, ETIOLOGY, PATHOGENESIS

Tick-borne encephalitis (TBE) is a viral central nervous system (CNS) infection that usually follows a biphasic course.

1. Etiology: Tick-borne encephalitis virus (TBEV), a neurotropic virus that is a member of the Flaviviridae family. TBEV is divided into European, Siberian, and Far Eastern (also known as Russian spring-summer) subtypes.

2. Reservoir and transmission: Small rodents and Ixodes ticks (transmitting the infection to next generations). The virus is usually transmitted via a bite of an infected tick, and rarely via oral route by consumption of unpasteurized milk from infected animals (this may cause small-scale epidemics). The incidence of tick-borne diseases varies geographically and follows seasonable patterns that depend on the activity of ticks, which feed on human and animal blood and are active from spring until late fall.

3. Epidemiology: The disease is found in endemic areas across large regions of Europe (central and eastern) and Asia (southern Russia, northern Kazakhstan, China, Mongolia, and Japan). Epidemiology is changing with climate changes, with TBE being reported, for example, in Scandinavia. Readers are encouraged to seek information regarding local epidemiology.

4. Risk factors: Longer stays or work in forests in endemic areas, consumption of unpasteurized milk from animals kept in endemic areas.

5. Incubation and contagious period: Incubation period is usually from 7 to 14 days (occasionally up to 4 weeks). The patient is not infectious for contacts.

→ CLINICAL FEATURES

The European subtype causes acute disease and follows a biphasic course with 5 to 7 days of no symptoms in between the 2 phases. The Siberian and Far Eastern subtypes are more likely to be monophasic.

1. Prodromal phase: Influenza-like symptoms, nausea, vomiting, and diarrhea persist for up to 7 days and in the majority of patients are followed by spontaneous recovery. In some patients features of CNS involvement appear after a few days of remission.

2. CNS infection phase: Meningitis (the most common manifestation; usually mild), encephalitis, cerebellitis, or myelitis. Most patients recover completely. The Siberian subtype is associated with a higher risk of chronic neurologic symptoms.

→ DIAGNOSIS

Features of viral infection found on cerebrospinal fluid examination (CSF) and presence of specific serum IgM (enzyme-linked immunosorbent assay [ELISA]). To confirm diagnosis in uncertain cases, measure specific IgM levels in CSF.

→ TREATMENT

Antiviral treatment is not available. General recommendations and symptomatic treatment are the same as in other viral CNS infections.

→ PROGNOSIS

In the majority of patients the recovery is complete. In patients with encephalitis and myelitis, sensory disturbances, paresis, and impairment of memory and concentration may persist for several months. Paresis is usually accompanied by muscle atrophy. The mortality rate is ~1% in the European type and it is higher in the Siberian and especially Far Eastern types (5%-10%; the disease is fatal predominantly in patients with paralysis of limbs and respiratory compromise).

→ PREVENTION

1. Nonspecific protection against ticks: →Chapter 8.15.1.
2. Vaccination.

16. Urinary Tract Infections (UTIs)

→ DEFINITION, ETIOLOGY, PATHOGENESIS

The term **urinary tract infection** (UTI) is defined as the presence of microorganisms in the urinary tract above the bladder sphincter in symptomatic patients.

Significant bacteriuria is defined as bacteriuria with proposed thresholds ranging from $\geq 10^3$ to 10^5 bacterial colony forming units (CFU)/mL in a clean-catch voided urine or $\geq 10^2$ CFU/mL in a single catheterized specimen.

Asymptomatic bacteriuria (ABU) (historically "asymptomatic UTI") is defined as $\geq 10^5$ bacterial CFU/mL in a culture of urine in patients without signs or symptoms of UTI. The presence of white blood cells (WBCs) or nitrites has no implications for the differentiation between ABU and symptomatic UTI.

Uncomplicated UTI may be diagnosed in a nonpregnant female patient without genitourinary abnormalities and without impairment of the local and systemic immune responses (ie, without UTI risk factors; →below). It is caused by microorganisms typical for UTI.

Complicated UTI: The rationale for separating complicated UTI from uncomplicated UTI is that these cases are more likely not to respond to first-line treatment or are more prone to relapse. Complicated UTI refers to the following:
1) UTI in a female patient with anatomical abnormalities, functional abnormalities, or both that affect urine flow (including pregnancy), or with impaired systemic or local immune response.
2) All UTIs in male patients (according to most guidelines).
3) UTI caused by uncommon or multiresistant microorganisms.

Recurrent UTI may be caused by **relapse or reinfection**.

Relapse of UTI is a recurrent UTI that develops after prior antimicrobial treatment and is caused by the microorganism(s) responsible for the previous UTI episode, which persist in the urinary tract. In clinical practice, a recurrent UTI is regarded as a relapse if the onset of signs and symptoms occurs within ≤2 weeks of completing the treatment of the previous UTI and the same etiologic agent is isolated in both instances.

Reinfection is a recurrent UTI caused by a microorganism that originates from outside of the urinary tract and is an entirely new etiologic agent. In clinical practice, a recurrent UTI is regarded as a reinfection if the onset of signs and symptoms occurs after >2 weeks of completing the treatment of a previous UTI, even if the etiologic agent remains the same.

Physiologically, the urinary tract remains sterile, with the exception of the distal part of the urethra, which is colonized by saprophytic coagulase-negative staphylococci (eg, *Staphylococcus epidermidis*), vaginal coccobacilli (*Gardnerella* [formerly *Haemophilus*] *vaginalis*), nonhemolytic streptococci, corynebacteria, and lactobacilli. Pathogenic colonization of the urinary tract is predominantly ascending. The first stage of an ascending UTI involves colonization of the urethral opening by uropathogenic bacteria; women are more susceptible to this process due to the constant presence of uropathogenic microorganisms in the vaginal vestibule, as well as due to the closer proximity of the urethral opening to the anus and the short urethra. Sexual intercourse can facilitate ascending colonization in female patients. Subsequently, the microorganisms enter the bladder. In immunocompetent individuals, microbial colonization typically does not extend beyond the bladder. The risk of kidney involvement increases as the bacteria continue to persist in the bladder or in the presence of risk factors (→below). Hematogenous and lymphatic spread of infection is responsible for only ~2% of all cases of UTI, but these have the most severe course and usually affect patients who are seriously ill, immunodeficient, or both.

Risk factors for developing a complicated course of UTI: Urinary retention, nephrolithiasis, vesicoureteral reflux, catheterization, diabetes mellitus (particularly poorly controlled), advanced age, pregnancy, postpartum period, hospitalization for unrelated reasons.

Etiologic agents:

1) Bacteria:

   a) **Uncomplicated and recurrent cystitis**: *Escherichia coli* (70%-95% of patients), *Staphylococcus saprophyticus* (5%-10% of patients, predominantly sexually active women), *Proteus mirabilis*, *Klebsiella* spp, *Enterococcus* spp, and other pathogens (≤5% of patients).

   b) **Uncomplicated acute pyelonephritis**: As above, but the proportion of *E coli* infections is higher and no *S saprophyticus* infections are observed.

   c) **Complicated UTI**: *E coli* (≤50% of patients); compared to uncomplicated UTI, more cases are due to infection with *Enterococcus* spp (≤20%), *Klebsiella* spp (10%-15%), *Pseudomonas* spp (~10%), *P mirabilis*, and mixed bacterial flora.

   d) **ABU**: In women most frequently *E coli*; in patients with a long-term indwelling urinary catheter, usually mixed bacterial flora, in particular *Pseudomonas* spp, *Candida* spp, and urease-positive bacteria (eg, *Proteus* spp).

2) Microorganisms undetectable using standard methods typically result in urethritis and include *Chlamydia trachomatis*, *Neisseria gonorrhoeae*, and viruses (predominantly herpes simplex virus).

3) Fungi: Most frequently *Candida albicans* and other *Candida* spp, *Cryptococcus neoformans*, and *Aspergillus* spp; these cause ~5% of complicated UTI. Fungal UTI most frequently affects patients receiving immunosuppressive treatment, as well as patients with diabetes mellitus, those treated with antibiotics, with indwelling urinary catheters, and after instrumental procedures in the urinary tract. However, in most instances yeasts are colonizers not causing symptomatic UTI (→Chapter 8.16.2).

→ **CLINICAL FEATURES AND NATURAL HISTORY**

On the basis of natural history and necessary diagnostic and therapeutic procedures, the following types of UTI are distinguished:

1) Acute cystitis in women.
2) Recurrent cystitis in women.
3) Uncomplicated acute pyelonephritis in women.
4) Complicated UTI.
5) ABU.

→ **DIAGNOSIS**

Diagnostic Tests

1. Urinalysis: Leukocyturia, WBC casts (suggestive of pyelonephritis), microscopic hematuria (frequent in female patients with cystitis). Note that neither leukocyturia nor detection of nitrites produced from nitrates by Enterobacteriaceae are sufficiently sensitive or specific to diagnose UTIs. The findings need to be correlated with the patient's symptoms.

2. Urine culture:

1) The most common cause of uncomplicated cystitis in female outpatients are *Escherichia coli* or *Staphylococcus saprophyticus*; thus, treatment can be started without performing urine cultures.

2) Perform **urine cultures** in all other patients with UTI, as well as in women with signs and symptoms of cystitis not responding to a standard empiric treatment, hospitalized patients, patients with suspected complicated UTI, and patients in whom the current episode of UTI occurred within <1 month of the previous episode.

3) The results of a standard urine culture are negative in patients with nonbacterial cystitis or urethritis.

3. Other diagnostic tests not to be routinely used:

1) **Blood tests**: Elevated WBC counts, erythrocyte sedimentation rate (ESR), and C-reactive protein (CRP) or procalcitonin levels.

2) **Blood cultures** may be positive in patients with severe UTI.

3) **Imaging studies** are indicated in complicated UTI as well as in uncomplicated acute pyelonephritis in women if the signs and symptoms of infection persist or worsen in spite of standard treatment. **Abdominal ultrasonography** can detect abnormalities of the urinary tract (eg, nephrolithiasis, urinary retention, cysts, malformations) and complications of UTI (renal or perinephric abscess). **Urography** is indicated predominantly in patients with suspected abnormalities of the pyelocalyceal system or the ureters. **Contrast-enhanced CT**, needed infrequently, has the highest sensitivity for detecting perinephric abscesses; it may also visualize focal bacterial nephritis.

Diagnostic Criteria

UTI is diagnosed on the basis of clinical features. Always attempt to confirm the diagnosis with urine cultures (except for uncomplicated cystitis in women, which may be diagnosed solely on the basis of the clinical features). Significant bacteriuria is only indicative of UTI if the patient is symptomatic (versus ABU).

Differential Diagnosis

Differential diagnosis should include other conditions causing voiding problems, dysuria, pelvic pain (diseases of the reproductive tract in women, diseases of the prostate in men), renal colic, and inflammation of other abdominal organs.

→ TREATMENT

The goal of treatment of a clinically overt UTI is eradication of pathogens from the urinary tract using antimicrobial agents. Initially the choice of drugs is empiric, and subsequent adjustments are based on the results of urine cultures (if indicated). Always attempt to eliminate modifiable risk factors for UTI (if any).

General Measures

1. Administration of oral or intravenous fluids to maintain appropriate volume status.

2. Treatment of fever, pain, or both, for instance, with acetaminophen (INN paracetamol) or nonsteroidal anti-inflammatory agents.

Antimicrobial Treatment

Antimicrobial treatment depends on the type of UTI (see treatment descriptions in relevant chapters).

→ PROGNOSIS

1. Uncomplicated UTI: The prognosis is good.

2. Chronic or recurrent UTI in patients with persistent anatomic urinary tract abnormalities (eg, nephrolithiasis, vesicoureteral reflux) may result in chronic kidney disease.

3. Complications of UTI: Some complications, such as urosepsis (particularly in elderly patients), are associated with high mortality rates.

→ PREVENTION

Recurrent UTI typically manifests as uncomplicated cystitis, much less frequently as uncomplicated acute pyelonephritis. Methods of preventing uncomplicated UTI are listed below. Recurrences of complicated UTI are a distinct clinical issue and have usually been associated with urinary tract abnormalities, impaired immunity, or drug-resistant pathogens.

Nonpharmacologic Prevention

An increase in fluid intake by 1.5 L per day may prevent recurrent UTIs.⊘⊖

Other measures that are supported by limited evidence and may also be considered for female patients with recurrent UTIs:

1) Voiding immediately after feeling the urge or at regular intervals every 2 to 3 hours as well as shortly before bedtime and immediately after sexual intercourse.
2) Avoiding the use of feminine hygiene deodorants, diaphragms, and vaginal spermicides.
3) Avoiding bubble baths and bath cosmetics.
4) Daily intake of cranberry juice or supplements.

Pharmacologic Prevention

Pharmacologic prevention may be considered if nonpharmacologic measures are not successful:

1. Vaginal suppositories containing lactobacilli.⊘⊖

2. Vaginal estrogen cream (in postmenopausal women).

3. Antimicrobial prophylaxis (options):

1) **Self-treatment of female patients at the onset of signs and symptoms** as in uncomplicated cystitis. Advise the patient to seek medical attention if the signs and symptoms do not resolve within 48 hours or are atypical.

2) **Postcoital prophylaxis**: A single antimicrobial dose after sexual intercourse. Agents and dosage as in long-term prophylaxis. This strategy may
be recommended for patients with a well-established temporal relationship
of UTI episodes with sexual activity.

3) **Long-term prophylaxis**: Oral sulfamethoxazole/trimethoprim 240 mg,
trimethoprim 100 mg, norfloxacin 200 mg or ciprofloxacin 125 to 250 mg,
cephalexin 125 to 250 mg, daily at bedtime or 3 times/wk, initially for
6 months. Nitrofurantoin 50 to 100 mg (there is a risk of chronic lung disease with prolonged use). If UTI continues to recur, consider extension of
prophylaxis to ≥2 years.

4. Prophylaxis of catheter-associated UTI:

1) Antibiotic prophylaxis in patients using clean intermittent self-catheterization
may be beneficial in terms of reducing UTI recurrence rates over 12 months;
however, emergence of antimicrobial resistance may preclude longer-term
management using this approach. Antibiotics that can be considered include
once-daily nitrofurantoin 50 mg, trimethoprim 100 mg, or 250 mg cephalexin
[INN cefalexin].

16.1. Asymptomatic Bacteriuria

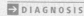

Asymptomatic bacteriuria (ABU) is diagnosed when significant bacteriuria
is detected in properly collected urine samples and is not accompanied by
clinical signs or symptoms of urinary tract infection. Except for certain cases,
ABU must not be treated with antibiotics, as the potential harm outweighs
the potential benefits.

TREATMENT

ABU requires no treatment, except for:

1) Pregnant patients (→Chapter 8.16.11).

2) Patients scheduled for urologic procedures when bleeding is anticipated,
including transurethral resection of the prostate. In such individuals start
antibacterial prophylaxis on the evening prior to the procedure using an
antibiotic selected on the basis of culture results (preferably a fluoroquinolone)
and continue only in case of delayed catheter removal.

16.2. Candiduria

Diagnosis of candiduria is based on the presence of *Candida* spp in 2 consecutive
urine cultures. Risk factors include diabetes mellitus, indwelling catheters,
and antibiotics. The presence of *Candida* spp in urine usually indicates colonization rather than infection. However, these two clinical situations cannot be
distinguished from each other solely on the basis of quantitative urine cultures
and the presence or absence of leukocyturia, as the latter can be present in the
absence of an active infection.

In the majority of patients, asymptomatic candiduria requires no treatment,
with the exception of those who undergo invasive surgical procedures involving
the urinary tract, and may be considered for severely immunocompromised
patients such as neutropenic patients. In patients at risk for disseminated
candidiasis in whom continued catheterization is indicated, replacement of the
catheter or intermittent catheterization instead of the indwelling catheter can
be considered. Asymptomatic candiduria usually resolves following removal of
the catheter or discontinuation of antibiotic therapy.

In rare cases, candiduria may be a sign of kidney infection, which almost always results from hematogenous spread secondary to candidemia and manifests as multiple microabscesses that can be visualized on computed tomography (CT) scans.

→ **TREATMENT**

Treatment of symptomatic candiduria: Oral fluconazole 200 mg/d for 7 to 14 days or IV amphotericin B 0.3 to 0.7 mg/kg for 3 to 7 days.

16.3. Catheter-Associated Urinary Tract Infection

→ **DEFINITION, ETIOLOGY, PATHOGENESIS**

A single catheterization of the bladder is associated with a 1% to 3% risk of developing bacteriuria. The risk increases by 3% to 10% with every additional day the catheter remains in the bladder; after 30 days of continuous catheterization, the incidence of bacteriuria is almost 100%. Intestinal bacilli are the pathogens most commonly isolated from urine samples, but colonizations by *Pseudomonas* spp, *Enterococcus* spp, *Staphylococcus* spp, and fungi are also frequent. Since symptomatic urinary tract infection (UTI) is rare in patients with an indwelling urinary catheter and bacteriuria, it is not recommended to diagnose and treat asymptomatic bacteriuria in catheterized patients, as the resolution of bacteriuria is transient and followed by rapid selection of drug-resistant microorganisms. Usually, bacteriuria resolves spontaneously once the catheter has been removed; only <1% of patients develop symptomatic UTI. The most common signs and symptoms of UTI include fever, deterioration of the patient's general condition, leukocytosis, bacteriuria >10^5 colony-forming units (CFU)/mL (frequently more than one pathogen is identified).

→ **TREATMENT**

On the basis of urine culture results, use an antibiotic with as narrow an antibacterial spectrum as possible for 7 to 10 days in patients without bacteremia and for 10 to 14 days in patients with bacteremia.

→ **PREVENTION**

Antibiotic prophylaxis in patients using clean intermittent self-catheterization may be beneficial in terms of reducing UTI recurrence rates over 12 months; however, emergence of antimicrobial resistance may preclude longer-term management using this approach. Antibiotics that can be considered include once-daily nitrofurantoin 50 mg, trimethoprim 100 mg, or 250 mg cephalexin [INN cefalexin].⊘●

16.4. Complications of Urinary Tract Infections

1. Renal parenchymal abscess: Solitary or multiple abscesses are most frequently a complication of pyelonephritis in patients with coexisting vesicoureteral reflux or urinary obstruction. A computed tomography (CT) scan is the imaging study of choice. Early antibiotic treatment may achieve complete recovery, but larger or not resolving abscesses may require surgical intervention—most frequently drainage, rarely partial or complete nephrectomy.

2. Multiple renal cortical abscesses develop as a result of hematogenous spread from a distant infection site (most frequently skin, bone, or endocardial infection) that is undetectable in approximately one-third of patients at the time of the diagnosis of renal involvement. In 90% of patients, *Staphylococcus aureus* is identified as the etiologic agent. Microabscesses form in the renal cortex and then coalesce into larger abscesses, which may occasionally spontaneously drain into the renal collection system. Blood and urine cultures are usually negative. A CT scan is the imaging study of choice.

Treatment: Antibiotics and surgical procedures as in renal parenchymal abscess.

3. Perinephric abscess refers to an accumulation of purulent exudate between the renal capsule and the renal fascia. It may be caused by pyonephrosis (→below; particularly in the course of nephrolithiasis) or by pyelonephritis complicated by renal parenchymal abscess or renal cortical abscesses; hematogenous spread is rare. Patients with diabetes mellitus account for approximately a quarter of all cases. The clinical manifestations include fever, rigors, flank pain, sometimes also a palpable mass in the lower back. Blood cultures are positive in 10% to 40% of patients. A CT scan is the imaging study of choice (ultrasonography results are false negative in ~30% of cases).

Treatment: Surgical or percutaneous drainage in combination with targeted antibiotic therapy based on the culture results (urine, blood, and abscess contents).

4. Pyonephrosis (pus collected in renal pelvis) usually develops as a result of an ascending infection in patients with hydronephrosis, frequently as a complication of nephrolithiasis.

Treatment: Urologic intervention.

5. Emphysematous pyelonephritis is a severe multifocal bacterial infection that leads to necrosis and production of gas in the renal parenchyma or perinephric tissues. Approximately 95% of cases involve patients with diabetes mellitus and coexisting impaired urine flow; women are more frequently affected than men. Emphysematous pyelonephritis manifests clinically as particularly severe pyelonephritis with features of septic shock. Sometimes physical examination reveals crackles over the affected area. Emphysematous pyelitis is a milder form of the disease, with the production of gas limited to the pyelocalyceal system. Imaging studies reveal the presence of gas.

Treatment: Surgical drainage and antibiotic therapy, and nephrectomy when necessary. Despite therapeutic interventions, the mortality rates are high and range between 11% to 42%.

6. Renal papillary necrosis: Ascending infection may lead to necrosis of the renal papillae and their sloughing into the pyelocalyceal system. The sloughed papillae may cause renal colic. Papillary necrosis affects predominantly patients with coexisting diabetes mellitus. The clinical manifestations are similar to severe acute pyelonephritis.

Treatment: Antibiotics are usually effective; invasive procedures are necessary in the case of urinary obstruction by necrotic tissues.

7. Chronic pyelonephritis: Chronic tubulointerstitial nephritis caused by chronic or recurrent kidney infections. This almost exclusively affects patients with significant anatomic abnormalities of the urinary tract, such as urinary obstruction, staghorn kidney stones, or vesicoureteral reflux (the most frequent cause of chronic pyelonephritis in children). A characteristic feature is focal scarring of the renal parenchyma causing a rough surface of the kidney on imaging studies. The disease may be limited to one kidney. With time, patients develop progressive fibrosis, tubular atrophy, glomerular sclerosis, and glomerular atrophy. The dominant clinical features are the signs and symptoms of recurrent urinary tract infection (UTI) (→Chapter 8.16), and in the case of severe renal impairment, features of chronic renal failure. Urinalysis usually reveals leukocyturia, occasionally with white blood cell casts. Negative culture results do not exclude the diagnosis of chronic pyelonephritis. Proteinuria (usually <2 g/d) is indicative of progressive renal impairment. Ultrasonography usually reveals small kidneys, sometimes with a rough surface, as well as features of the underlying condition (kidney stones, urinary obstruction). Urography shows deformations of some or all renal calices (widening, blunting). Renal scintigraphy has the highest sensitivity for detecting parenchymal scarring. Voiding cystography may be helpful in detecting vesicoureteral reflux.

Treatment includes management of the underlying condition and slowing the progression of chronic kidney disease.

8. Xanthogranulomatous pyelonephritis is a severe chronic renal parenchymal infection, which leads to kidney damage and perirenal fibrosis. It is almost always caused by chronic urinary obstruction, and three-quarters of patients have concomitant staghorn stones and chronic or recurrent UTI symptoms. The clinical presentation is typical for chronic inflammation, with recurrent fever, lower back pain, and weight loss. Exacerbations manifest as severe UTI and may lead to the development of cutaneous or intestinal fistulas if left untreated. Usually the diagnosis is made following nephrectomy, which is often performed due to misdiagnosed renal cancer. A CT scan is the imaging study of choice. Ultrasonography findings revealing large kidneys with staghorn stones may suggest xanthogranulomatous pyelonephritis.

Treatment: Nephrectomy.

9. Acute prostatitis is almost always caused by pathogens ascending from the urethra. It may be accompanied by urethritis or UTI. The most frequent etiologic agents are Enterobacteriaceae and other pathogens causing urethritis. Clinical features include rapidly increasing fever, pelvic or perineal pain, dysuria, and cloudy urine. Prostatic edema may cause urinary retention. When examined by palpation (this should be done gently due to the risk of causing bacteremia), the prostate is swollen, soft, warm, and very tender. Urine cultures should be performed in every patient. Blood cultures should be obtained in all hospitalized patients (these are positive in 20% of patients).

Treatment: Same as in complicated UTI. Once culture results are available, modify the treatment if necessary. Acute prostatitis is usually treated for 2 (maximum 4) weeks; in patients with chronic prostatitis, treatment is extended to 4 (maximum 6) weeks. Lack of improvement after one week of treatment may suggest prostatic abscess.

10. Acute epididymitis is the most frequent cause of the so-called acute scrotum in adult male patients. Infection is the result of reflux of infected urine from the prostatic segment of the urethra through the spermatic cord into the epididymis. In young men, the most common etiologic agents are *Chlamydia trachomatis* and *Neisseria gonorrhoeae* (sexually transmitted diseases), while in older patients the incidence of infections with Enterobacteriaceae increases. One-sided scrotal pain is a characteristic symptom of acute epididymitis; it may be accompanied by fever and rigors, dysuria, or signs and symptoms of acute prostatitis. Physical examination reveals inflamed, swollen, and very tender epididymis. Orchitis may occur later in the course of the disease and lead to the development of hydrocele.

Treatment: Empiric therapy should be started before receiving microbiology results (culture, nucleic acid amplification test) and should be adjusted once the results become available. Empiric treatment of patients <35 years must cover *Neisseria gonorrhoeae* and *Chlamydia trachomatis*: a single dose of IM ceftriaxone 250 mg and doxycycline 100 mg bid for 10 days. Because Enterobacteriaceae are much more common in patients >35 years, empiric treatment consists of starting IV ceftriaxone 2 g once daily. A single-dose treatment is sufficient for the treatment of epididymitis due to *N gonorrhea* or *C trachomatis* (→Chapter 8.16.9), while the duration of treatment of epididymitis caused by Enterobacteriaceae is 10 to 14 days.

11. Urosepsis: →Chapter 8.14.

16.5. Complicated Urinary Tract Infection

→ CLINICAL FEATURES AND DIAGNOSIS

The most frequently observed factors contributing to the diagnosis of complicated urinary tract infection (UTI) include male sex, diabetes mellitus, pregnancy, nephrolithiasis, and urinary obstruction.

Clinical features range from mild cystitis to urosepsis. In each case of a diagnosed or suspected complicated UTI, perform urinalysis, urine cultures, and blood biochemical tests to assess kidney function. Order blood cultures in all febrile hospitalized patients. Consider ultrasonography and abdominal radiographs in patients in whom it is necessary to exclude nephrolithiasis and urinary obstruction. Indications for additional imaging studies: suspected renal and perinephric complications of UTI (→Chapter 8.16.4), other coexisting pelvic or abdominal abnormalities, previously diagnosed urinary tract abnormalities that have contributed to the complicated UTI.

→ TREATMENT

1. Depending on the intensity of symptoms and the presence of comorbidities, the patient may either be treated as an outpatient or be admitted to the hospital. Potential **indications for hospital admission**: urinary tract abnormalities, immunocompromised patients, renal failure, serious comorbidities, other factors as in uncomplicated acute pyelonephritis.

2. Urologic intervention is the mainstay of treatment in the setting of an underlying obstruction. The key objective is to correct potential abnormalities in the urinary tract; in such cases antimicrobial treatment is only an adjunctive therapy.

3. Empiric treatment of complicated UTI as in uncomplicated acute pyelonephritis. If the empiric treatment is ineffective and microbiology results are unavailable, start a broad-spectrum antimicrobial agent active against *Pseudomonas* spp (eg, piperacillin + tazobactam, ceftazidime, or a carbapenem). Selection of oral antibiotics and duration of treatment as in uncomplicated acute pyelonephritis.

4. Outpatient treatment as in uncomplicated pyelonephritis.

5. Treatment in young men with no additional risk factors for complicated UTI: The usual duration is 7 days for a case of cystitis and up to a maximum of 14 days in the case of acute pyelonephritis.

6. Follow-up urine cultures are performed within 1 to 2 weeks of treatment discontinuation.

16.6. Cystitis

16.6.1. Nonbacterial Cystitis

→ DEFINITION, ETIOLOGY, PATHOGENESIS

Nonbacterial cystitis refers to a range of signs and symptoms typical for infectious cystitis, which affect women of childbearing age. Routine microbiological studies do not reveal the presence of any uropathogens. Some cases of nonbacterial cystitis are caused by viruses (herpes simplex virus type 1 or type 2, BK polyomavirus, cytomegalovirus, and adenovirus), chlamydia (*Chlamydia trachomatis*), fungal infection (→Chapter 8.16.2), or mycobacteria. Cystitis may also be a complication of prior pelvic irradiation or cancer chemotherapy or a manifestation of autoimmune diseases. In the remaining cases, the etiology remains unknown, and such patients are usually diagnosed with interstitial cystitis on the basis of cystoscopy and urodynamic tests. Spontaneous resolution of signs and symptoms over time is frequently observed.

→ TREATMENT

1. Infectious etiology: Appropriate antimicrobial treatment based on microbiological testing, including polymerase chain reaction (PCR) for viruses and chlamydial infection.

2. Noninfectious etiology: Treat the underlying disease (eg, autoimmune disease), consider symptomatic treatment, or both. Symptomatic treatment: oral oxybutynin 5 mg bid or tid, oral hydroxyzine 10 to 50 mg/d, oral amitriptyline 25 mg bid or tid, and behavioral therapy. A recent trial among women with moderate to severe refractory interstitial cystitis/bladder pain syndrome suggested a benefit of certolizumab pegol, an anti–tumor necrosis factor (TNF)-α agent used in the treatment of rheumatoid diseases; such treatment may be tried in selected patients in a specialized setting.◓

16.6.2. Recurrent Cystitis in Women

→ CLINICAL FEATURES AND DIAGNOSIS

Recurrent cystitis affects 10% to 20% of women without any risk factors for complicated urinary tract infection (UTI). Etiologic agents are the same as in uncomplicated sporadic cystitis. Reinfections are markedly more frequent than relapses. In some patients an evident relationship between sexual intercourses and subsequent episodes of UTI may be observed. Additional diagnostic tests (including imaging studies) are generally not recommended, unless risk factors for complicated UTI are suspected or rare uropathogens (eg, *Proteus* spp) are detected.

→ TREATMENT

1. The same drugs may be used as in uncomplicated cystitis.

2. In some cases a recurrent UTI is actually a relapse. This occurs most frequently in patients in whom the previous episode of cystitis was accompanied by asymptomatic pyelonephritis that has not been successfully treated with a short course of antimicrobial therapy. In patients with a relapse of UTI, perform urine cultures and start empiric treatment with a different class of antibiotics until culture results are available.

16.6.3. Uncomplicated Cystitis

→ CLINICAL FEATURES AND DIAGNOSIS

Typical clinical features of uncomplicated cystitis include dysuria, frequency, and suprapubic pain, sometimes also urgency/incontinence and hematuria (in ~40% of patients), as well as suprapubic tenderness. Additionally, leukocyturia and bacteriuria >10^5 colony-forming units (CFU)/mL (in some patients 10^2-10^4 CFU/mL) are seen. Untreated uncomplicated cystitis may last from a few to over 10 days. Urine cultures are usually performed and imaging studies can be considered if the symptoms persist despite treatment or recur within 1 to 4 weeks.

→ TREATMENT

1. First-line agents:

1) Oral nitrofurantoin 100 mg bid for 3 to 5 days (preferred agent due to low resistance rates and similar efficacy as sulfamethoxazole/trimethoprim).◓◓

2) Other options include sulfamethoxazole/trimethoprim 960 mg bid for 3 days or trimethoprim 100 mg bid for 3 days, fosfomycin 3 g in a single dose (in particular if an extended-spectrum β-lactamase [ESBL]–producing strain is suspected).

3) In areas where >20% of *Escherichia coli* strains are resistant to sulfamethoxazole/trimethoprim and resistance rates to fluoroquinolones are <20%, consider a 3-day course of ciprofloxacin 250 to 500 mg bid, norfloxacin 400 mg bid, or ofloxacin 200 mg bid.

2. Second-line agents: Oral amoxicillin + clavulanic acid 625 mg bid for 3 to 7 days, cephalexin (INN cefalexin) 500 mg qid for 3 to 7 days, amoxicillin 500 mg tid for 7 to 10 days.

3. Ibuprofen is inferior to antibiotic treatment, but two-thirds of women with uncomplicated cystitis recover without antibiotics. Therefore, ibuprofen can be considered if patients would prefer to avoid exposure to antibiotics.

4. Follow-up: In female patients with no symptoms persisting after treatment, no follow-up urine testing is indicated.

16.7. Genitourinary Tuberculosis

Genitourinary tuberculosis results from hematogenous spread and may manifest within 5 to 15 years of the primary infection.

→ CLINICAL FEATURES

In the majority of patients, the disease presents with signs and symptoms of cystitis. Systemic manifestations are rare.

→ DIAGNOSIS

Urinalysis reveals leukocyturia with negative culture results (sterile pyuria); proteinuria and occasionally hematuria develop later in the course of the disease. Imaging studies may reveal a deformed pyelocalyceal system, ureteral stenosis or obstruction, increased bladder wall thickness, and decreased bladder capacity. Confirming the diagnosis usually requires multiple cultures for *Mycobacterium tuberculosis*; less frequently, the diagnosis is based on histologic examination and cultures of tissue samples collected during endoscopic examination of the urinary tract.

→ TREATMENT

Administration of antituberculous drugs for 6 months (as in pulmonary tuberculosis) with dosage adjusted to the patient's kidney function.

16.8. Uncomplicated Acute Pyelonephritis

→ CLINICAL FEATURES AND DIAGNOSIS

Uncomplicated acute pyelonephritis results from an ascending infection that originates in the lower urinary tract. Infection and inflammation involve the pyelocalyceal system and the adjacent renal parenchyma. The clinical features may vary, ranging from symptoms of cystitis (subclinical acute pyelonephritis) to urosepsis. In typical cases, signs and symptoms occurring within the first 24 hours include flank pain of varying intensity, malaise, fever, and rigors; dysuria, nausea, and vomiting may also be present. Physical examination reveals flank pain on percussion (Murphy kidney punch; usually unilateral) and in some patients also lower abdominal tenderness caused by the ongoing cystitis that preceded pyelonephritis.

In each case, samples for urinalysis and urine cultures should be obtained prior to starting treatment; in individuals admitted to the hospital, blood cultures should also be performed. Leukocyturia is almost always present and urine cultures are positive in 90% of patients (typically revealing bacteriuria ≥10^5 colony-forming units [CFU]/mL). Imaging studies should be considered if or when diagnosis is not conclusive, fever persists for >48 hours while on appropriate antibiotic treatment, the patient's clinical condition deteriorates during treatment, or the patient has a recurrent episode of acute pyelonephritis.

→ TREATMENT

Treatment should always be based on urine culture results and continued for 7 to a maximum of 14 days. Empiric treatment should be continued until urine culture results become available.

Because resistance rates of community-acquired *Escherichia coli* strains to fluoroquinolone are >10% in many areas in Canada, it can no longer be recommended as the first-line choice for empiric treatment.

1. Compliant patients in good clinical condition with mild symptoms may be treated on an outpatient basis:

1) IV ceftriaxone 1 to 2 g followed by (if susceptible):

   a) First-line agents: **Sulfamethoxazole/trimethoprim** 960 mg bid for 7 to 14 days or oral **fluoroquinolones** for 7 days (eg, ciprofloxacin 500 mg bid or levofloxacin 250 mg once daily).

   b) Alternative oral agents (if the first-line drugs cannot be used) for 10 to 14 days: **Cephalexin** (INN cefalexin) 500 mg qid, **cefpodoxime** 200 mg bid, **amoxicillin + clavulanic acid** 1 g bid.

2) A single daily dose of an aminoglycoside can be used (eg, IV gentamicin 5-7 mg/kg) for empiric treatment in patients with contraindications to ceftriaxone. If resistance rates in community-acquired *Escherichia coli* strains are <10%, antibiotics listed above under a) and b) can be considered for empiric treatment before culture results are available.

2. Patients requiring hospitalization: Hospitalization is indicated in the case of persistent nausea and vomiting, lack of improvement or worsening of symptoms in the course of outpatient treatment, inconclusive diagnosis, or pregnancy. Drugs are typically administered IV, starting with empiric treatment using one of the following antimicrobial agents:

1) IV **ceftriaxone** 1 to 2 g once daily.

2) **Aminoglycosides**: IV gentamicin 5 to 7 mg/kg once daily or 1 mg/kg every 8 hours **as monotherapy or in combination with IV ampicillin** 1 g every 6 hours.

3) **In the case of a pathogen susceptible to fluoroquinolones**: IV ciprofloxacin 500 mg bid or 200 to 400 mg every 12 hours if the patient is not a candidate for oral treatment.

Treatment should be modified according to the results of urine and blood cultures. If fever has resolved and clinical improvement is observed (usually within 72 hours), therapy with an oral antimicrobial agent selected on the basis of microbiology results should be started (the drug may be different from the IV agent).🗸◓

16.9. Urethritis

Urethritis is usually a sexually transmitted disease (STD). **Gonococcal urethritis** is caused by *Neisseria gonorrhoeae*, while the more common **nongonococcal urethritis** is predominantly due to infection with *Chlamydia trachomatis* but also secondary to infections by *Ureaplasma urealyticum*, *Mycoplasma genitalium*, *Trichomonas vaginalis*, or less frequently other microorganisms.

Signs and symptoms usually develop within a few days for gonococcal urethritis, and between 1 and 3 to a maximum of 5 weeks for nongonococcal urethritis. Symptoms include pain in the distal urethra at voiding (intensity is highest in the morning); occasional itching around the external opening of the urethra between mictions; frequency and urgency in patients with concomitant cystitis or prostatitis; purulent, occasionally blood-stained urethral discharge, which is sometimes observed only after massaging the urethra; and vaginal discharge in women. Systemic signs and symptoms of infection are absent. Note that the majority of chlamydial infection are asymptomatic, in particular in female patients, potentially leading to pelvic inflammatory disease and its sequelae.

Microscopic examination of a Gram-stained urethral smear or first-void urine combined with nucleic acid amplification test (NAAT) (tests for gonorrhea and chlamydia) are the diagnostic tests of choice. In the microscopic examination, the presence of neutrophils confirms the diagnosis of urethritis, while intracellular gram-negative diplococci within neutrophils are the evidence of gonococcal etiology.

Due to the limited availability of diagnostic tests for microorganisms typically causing urethritis, empiric treatment for gonococcal and nongonococcal urethritis is usually started as soon as possible and involves a single dose of IM ceftriaxone 250 mg (alternatively, a single dose of oral cefixime 400 mg) plus either doxycycline 100 mg bid for 7 days or a single dose of oral azithromycin 1 g. All sexual partners at risk of potential infection should also undergo testing and treatment.

16.10. Urinary Tract Infections in Patients With Spinal Cord Injury

Patients with spinal cord injury require either multiple repeated bladder catheterizations or long-term catheterization. The majority eventually develop asymptomatic bacteriuria, which may resolve spontaneously and recur and requires no diagnostics or treatment. Symptomatic urinary tract infection (UTI) is very frequent (~2.5 UTI episodes a year per patient). In these patients, uropathogens typically form a thick biofilm on the bladder walls that prevents their eradication; thus, ≥90% of patients continue to have bacteriuria 30 days after discontinuation of treatment. The most frequently isolated pathogens are *Proteus* spp, *Pseudomonas* spp, *Klebsiella* spp, *Serratia* spp, and *Providencia* spp. In ~70% of patients, more than one pathogen is identified.

Antibacterial treatment is started in patients with clinical signs and symptoms of UTI. Management is as in patients with complicated UTI and catheter--associated UTI.

16.11. Urinary Tract Infections in Pregnant Women

1. Asymptomatic bacteriuria increases the risk of acute cystitis, acute pyelonephritis, premature birth, and a low birth weight. Urine cultures should be performed at least once in the early stages of pregnancy (during the first obstetric visit or between weeks 12 and 16 of pregnancy) and treatment should be started if significant bacteriuria is detected.

Treatment according to the results of urine culture (as in cystitis) should last from 3 to 7 days. After discontinuation of treatment, follow-up urine cultures should be performed periodically to detect possible relapses (these affect a third of patients).

2. Cystitis: Diagnosis may be delayed due to the frequent occurrence of features typical for cystitis (frequency, urgency, lower abdominal discomfort) during normal pregnancy. The recommended oral treatment includes amoxicillin 500 mg tid; amoxicillin + clavulanic acid 625 mg bid; cephalexin (INN cefalexin) 250 to 500 mg qid; fosfomycin 3 g in a single dose; sulfamethoxazole/trimethoprim 960 mg bid (do not use in the first trimester or shortly before delivery).

Duration of treatment: 3 to 7 days. Urine cultures must be performed in every patient and the treatment regimen must be adjusted on the basis of the culture results.

3. Acute pyelonephritis affects from 1% to 2% of all pregnant women. It most frequently occurs during the second or third trimester due to impairment of the urinary flow. Typical clinical manifestations include high-grade fever, flank pain, frequently dysuria and vomiting (this may cause dehydration).

Treatment should be started in hospital as in acute pyelonephritis in nonpregnant patients. Note that fluoroquinolones are contraindicated in pregnant women due to their teratogenic effects.

17. Viral Diseases

17.1. Common Cold (Nonspecific Infections of the Upper Respiratory Tract)

→ DEFINITION, ETIOLOGY, PATHOGENESIS

The term common cold (viral rhinopharyngitis; viral rhinosinusitis) refers to signs and symptoms associated with a mucosal inflammation of the nasal cavities, pharynx, and sinuses usually caused by an acute viral infection.

1. Etiologic agents: Over 20 types and 250 subtypes of viruses, most commonly rhinoviruses (30%-50%), coronaviruses (10%-15%), influenza and parainfluenza viruses, respiratory syncytial virus, adenoviruses, and enteroviruses (eg, coxsackievirus). Occasionally, bacteria such as *Mycoplasma pneumonia*, *Chlamydophila pneumonia*, and *Bordetella pertussis* can cause symptoms of the common cold. The respiratory viruses penetrate the upper respiratory epithelium and begin to replicate. This induces a local inflammatory response, which leads to vasodilation (edema, exudate), an increase in mucus secretion, and sometimes also to a damage to epithelial cells.

2. Reservoir and transmission: The reservoir for the etiologic agents of the common cold are sick individuals; it is transmitted mainly by contact with droplets of infected respiratory secretions but may also involve a direct contact with a sick person or an enteral route, depending on the type of the virus.

3. Incubation and contagious period: The incubation period varies between viruses but is generally from 1 to 4 days. Virus shedding is highest during the first 3 days of the illness but may continue for up to 2 weeks after the onset of the disease.

→ CLINICAL FEATURES

The common cold usually has a mild onset. The signs and symptoms may include some or all of the following:

1) **Sore throat**.

2) **Rhinitis**: Initially clear nasal discharge and postnasal drip, followed by nasal congestion, olfactory impairment, and sneezing. Nasal discharge may subsequently become thicker, greenish, or even purulent, although this does not generally indicate a bacterial etiology.

3) **Cough**: Initially dry, later may become productive from postnasal drip.

4) **Chills and fever (usually low grade)**, although body temperature is frequently normal. Fever is more common in children and is an infrequent symptom in adults with the common cold. Fever >38°C may be indicative of influenza.

5) **Malaise, headache, lethargy, and myalgia** may occur. Myalgia is more typical of influenza infection than of the common cold.

6) **Pharyngitis**: Erythema and inflammatory papules on the posterior pharyngeal wall, sometimes papules or vesicles on the soft palate, discharge on the posterior pharyngeal wall.

7) **Conjunctivitis** (adenoviruses) and **rash** (adenoviruses, enteroviruses) may be present.

Patients with the common cold recover spontaneously. The signs and symptoms peak within 2 to 3 days and usually resolve after 7 to 10 days. In a portion of patients, some symptoms may persist for 2 to 3 weeks or longer.

The significant overlap in symptoms associated with the common cold and influenza may make it difficult to distinguish between the two infections. The common cold is generally a milder illness. Runny or stuffed nose and sneezing are more frequently associated with the common cold, whereas a sudden onset of fever, myalgia, intense exhaustion, and cough are more likely associated with influenza.

→ DIAGNOSIS

Diagnosis is based on the medical history and physical examination. As the course of the disease is usually mild, diagnostic tests are not necessary.

Differential Diagnosis

1. Acute pharyngitis of other etiology, predominantly streptococcal (→Chapter 8.11).

2. Bacterial sinusitis; distinguishing between viral and bacterial etiologies on the basis of the clinical presentation and even some investigations may be difficult (imaging studies reveal sinus abnormalities in almost 90% of patients).

3. Influenza, laryngitis, bronchitis, and pneumonia.

4. The prodromal phase of various systemic infectious diseases (eg, measles, varicella, mumps, pertussis).

5. Allergic rhinitis: Persistent signs and symptoms of rhinitis.

→ TREATMENT

Antiviral Treatment

No specific antiviral treatment is available.

Symptomatic Treatment

In symptomatic patients:

1) **Echinacea preparations** may be considered⊘⊖; they may reduce the duration of symptoms. The wide variation in available echinacea preparations makes it difficult to recommend a particular form or dose. **Vitamin C** after the onset of symptoms is not effective in treatment.⊗⊖ The use of **zinc lozenges** may be considered within 24 hours of symptom onset, as these have been shown to reduce the duration of the cold;⊘⊖ their use may be associated with a bad taste or nausea.

2) When necessary, **nasal decongestants or saline nasal irrigation** (isotonic or hypertonic [2.5%-3% sea salt solutions]) may be used.⊘◯ **Analgesics and antipyretics** (acetaminophen [INN paracetamol], nonsteroidal anti-inflammatory drugs) may also be used to relieve discomfort.⊘◯ **Cough suppressants**: →Chapter 1.3.

3) **Increased fluid intake** in febrile patients and limitation of physical activity to a tolerated level.⊘◯

COMPLICATIONS

Complications of the common cold include bacterial sinusitis and bacterial otitis media (particularly in children). Prophylactic antimicrobial treatment in patients with the common cold does not reduce the risk of these complications.

PREVENTION

Maintaining good hand hygiene after contact with a sick individual as well as patient isolation are the essential prevention methods.⊘⊖ Other nonspecific measures reducing the risk of infection may include echinacea preparations⊘◯ and moderate but regular exercise.

17.2. Herpes Simplex Virus Infections

ETIOLOGY, PATHOGENESIS

1. Etiologic agents: Herpes simplex virus (HSV), a DNA virus, exists as either type 1 (HSV-1) or type 2 (HSV-2). The virus enters the body through a mucosal surface or through breaks in the skin and replicates, causing viremia; first-episode primary infection typically has the most severe course. Subsequently, the virus enters neuronal cells and is transported via axons to sensory ganglia (in the case of HSV-1, more frequently to the trigeminal ganglion; in the case of HSV-2, more commonly to the sacral nerve root ganglia [S2 to S5]), where it remains latent. Reactivation of the virus with subsequent viral shedding is extremely common; HSV-1 more commonly reactivates at the orolabial mucosa, whereas HSV-2 frequently reactivates at the genital mucosa.

2. Reservoir and transmission: Humans are the only reservoir for HSV. Both individuals with active lesions and those with no detectable illness can shed the virus and can transmit infection through direct contact. Vertical transmission from the mother is possible either in utero (congenital infection of the fetus) or, more commonly, via infectious vaginal secretions intrapartum (perinatal infection of the newborn).

3. Epidemiology: HSV infections are prevalent worldwide. HSV-1 infections often occur during childhood, whereas HSV-2 infections are more often sexually transmitted; the incidence of both is higher in populations with a lower socioeconomic status. Perinatal or congenital transmission is rare. A history of HSV-1 infection does not confer immunity against HSV-2.

4. Incubation and contagious period: This depends on the form of disease (→Clinical Features, below). The incubation period for primary gingivostomatitis is generally 3 to 6 days.

CLINICAL FEATURES

Symptoms develop as a result of a primary or recurrent infection (reactivation of the latent virus). In both cases, a characteristic **vesicular rash** appears, which is preceded by initial localized prodromal signs and symptoms (pain, burning, itching, tingling sensations). Subsequently, inflammatory papules appear and continue to evolve into vesicles (which may then turn into pustules), eventually leading to erosions or ulcerations. Primary infections are characterized by a highly dynamic development of coalescing cutaneous eruptions. Recurrent infections typically involve more pronounced prodromal symptoms, while skin lesions are less numerous and clustered on smaller areas. Regional lymphadenopathy is common.

Clinical Spectrum

Note that the differentiation of HSV-1 and HSV-2 infections based on the clinical presentation is extremely difficult, though HSV-1 more commonly recurs at orolabial sites, whereas HSV-2 commonly recurs at genital sites.

1. Oral-facial infections:

1) **Primary infection** (may be asymptomatic):

a) **Acute gingivostomatitis** (orolabial infection): Predominantly affects children and young adults. The infection has a sudden onset and is associated with fever, malaise, anorexia, edema, gingival pain, and erythema, in addition to vesicles and/or erosions of the oral and lingual mucosa as well as of the lips and skin around the mouth. Regional lymphadenopathy is also common. Acute symptoms persist for 5 to 7 days, with the lesions healing after ~2 weeks. Viral shedding in the saliva is observed for 3 weeks, occasionally longer.

b) **Acute pharyngitis/tonsillitis**: More frequent in adults. Symptoms initially include fever, malaise, headache, sore throat, myalgia, and are later followed by the appearance of vesicles on the tonsils and posterior pharyngeal wall. As the vesicles rupture, grey erosions and ulcerations are formed. Lesions on the lips are present in <10% of patients. In ~30% of patients, a primary HSV-2 infection is accompanied by meningeal signs, and in 5% of patients, it causes meningitis with a mild course.

2) **Recurrent infection** (usually HSV-1): **Herpes labialis** is the most common presentation of recurrent oral infection. Symptoms of recurrent infection are typically much less severe than those associated with the first episode and persist for a shorter duration. Many individuals shed the virus in the absence of demonstrable orolabial lesions.

2. Genital herpes simplex:

1) **Primary infection**: Typically has a severe course. General symptoms are present in ~70% of women and ~40% of men and include fever, headache, and myalgia. Cutaneous lesions start as vesicles and evolve rapidly into ulcers, which can coalesce; they are very painful. In men, the cutaneous lesions appear on the penis, less frequently on the scrotum and inner thighs. In women, the cutaneous lesions appear on the labia, perineum, vagina, cervix, and thighs. Tender inguinal lymphadenopathy is common, and dysuria occurs. Anal intercourse may lead to proctitis. In women, the cutaneous lesions are more extensive and persist for ~20 days (~16 days in men). Viral shedding continues for 10 to 12 days.

2) **Recurrent infection** (usually HSV-2): Mild or associated with minor symptoms. Local prodromal symptoms may persist from 2 hours up to 2 days. General symptoms are usually absent. In women, vesicular lesions on the labia (major and minor) and perineum (may be very painful) are observed. In men, the lesions occur predominantly on the penis. Viral shedding continues for ~5 days.

3. Ocular herpes simplex: Lesions may involve the conjunctiva, cornea, or both (ulcerations develop predominantly as a result of autoinoculation). Inadequate treatment or frequent recurrences may lead to corneal scarring (or even blindness). Patients can develop vesicular lesions in other skin areas in dermatome V1, including the tip of the nose and the eyelids.

4. Central nervous system (CNS) infections:

1) **Meningitis** commonly develops within 2 weeks of primary genital infection, especially the one caused by HSV-2. Presenting symptoms include headache,

vomiting, photophobia, and nuchal rigidity. The natural history of this syndrome is self-limiting.

2) **Meningoencephalitis**, which can be associated with either a primary infection or recurrence, is much rarer than aseptic meningitis and associated with significantly higher morbidity and mortality. Dramatic changes in the level of consciousness, seizures, and focal neurologic signs are frequent.

5. Other cutaneous infections: Lesions located outside the face and genital region are rare. Primary infection may be caused by rubbing in of the infected material:

1) **Herpetic whitlow** often develops in individuals with preexisting HSV infection who expose their fingertips to infected secretions. It has a sudden onset. Signs and symptoms include edema, erythema, pain, and vesicles/pustules involving 1 or several fingertips.

2) **Herpes gladiatorum**: Associated with contact sports. Lesions typically involve chest, ears, face, and hands.

3) **Eczema herpeticum**: A distinct manifestation developing in patients with atopic dermatitis. It is associated with a generalized vesicular rash that rapidly adopts a crusted "punched-out" appearance, has a severe course, and may be life-threatening.

6. Perinatal infection is common in women with primary genital infection at the time of labor, though much less so in women with recurrent disease. Caesarian delivery is protective and indicated for any woman with active lesions at the time of labor. There are 3 main neonatal HSV infection syndromes:

1) **Skin-eye-mouth** manifests as grouped vesicular lesions anywhere on the skin surface; conjunctivitis and oral ulcerations can also occur.

2) **Disseminated disease** often presents as severe sepsis, with hemodynamic compromise, respiratory insufficiency, hepatitis, and coagulopathy. Mortality is high.

3) **CNS infection**, which can present with protean manifestations, often with fever and irritability; many patients also have cutaneous lesions. Neurodevelopmental sequelae are common.

→ DIAGNOSIS

Diagnosis is usually based on the clinical presentation. The finding of grouped small vesicles (in early stages) or ulcers (later on) is often very suggestive of HSV infection.

Diagnostic Tests

Diagnostic tests are recommended to confirm the involvement of HSV. Identification of the type of HSV in patients with genital herpes is used to predict the risk of recurrence.

1. HSV isolation in cell cultures (specimens: vesicular fluid, cervical swab): Culture of HSV from mucosal samples is relatively rapid; sensitive and specific results are usually obtained within days. Older lesions may not yield the virus.

2. Detection of HSV DNA by polymerase chain reaction (PCR) (specimens: vesicular fluid, cervical swab, vaginal discharge, and cerebrospinal fluid [CSF]) is the most sensitive and therefore primary test for detecting HSV in CSF samples. It is increasingly being used for detection in other samples as well (eg, blood, mucosal swabs).

3. Serology is less useful on a routine basis for the diagnosis of HSV-associated infectious syndromes, as culture or PCR results are usually available sooner. Specific anti-HSV antibodies appear in the blood within a few weeks of infection; note that HSV-1 seropositivity in the general population is relatively high (and increases with age) due to the high prevalence of orolabial HSV infection, which is why detection of HSV antibodies does not necessarily imply active

HSV infection/shedding. Detection of anti-HSV-2 antibodies usually indicates genital herpes (sensitivity, 80%-98%; specificity ≥96%).

Differential Diagnosis

1. Oral-facial herpes: Candidiasis, aphthous stomatitis, enteroviral oropharyngeal infections (including herpangina), erythema multiforme major, Stevens-Johnson syndrome, Behçet syndrome.

2. Genital herpes: Syphilis, chancroid, granuloma inguinale, herpes zoster.

→ TREATMENT

Antiviral Treatment

Systemic antiviral treatment (**acyclovir** [INN aciclovir], **valacyclovir** [INN valaciclovir]) reduces the symptoms associated with primary and recurrent infections; however, the drugs do not eradicate the latent virus, do not make patients less contagious, and do not reduce the frequency or severity of the future recurrences after the treatment is discontinued. Valacyclovir is a pro-drug for acyclovir and is generally preferred over oral acyclovir due to more favorable pharmacokinetics.

1. Genital herpes: Topical drugs are not effective.

1) In patients with a **primary infection**, use oral acyclovir 400 mg every 8 hours or 200 mg every 4 to 5 hours (5 times a day) for 7 to 10 days, or oral valacyclovir 1000 mg every 12 hours for 7 to 10 days. Treatment may be extended in patients in whom the lesions have not resolved completely after 10 days.

2) In patients with **recurrent infections** (periodic treatment of recurrences), it is preferable to start treatment during the prodromal stage, not later than at the onset of cutaneous eruptions; oral acyclovir 400 mg every 8 hours or 800 mg every 12 hours for 5 days, or oral acyclovir 800 mg every 8 hours for 3 days, oral valacyclovir 500 mg every 12 hours for 3 days, or 1000 mg every 24 hours for 5 days.

2. Meningoencephalitis: IV acyclovir 10 mg/kg every 8 hours for 14 to 21 days; therapy is often continued until CSF HSV PCR is negative.

3. Oral-labial herpes or gingivostomatitis/pharyngitis:

1) In patients with a **primary infection**, if the infection is highly dynamic, severe, or the patient is immunocompromised (irrespective of the etiology of immunosuppression), use oral acyclovir 200 to 400 mg every 4 to 5 hours (5 times a day) for 3 to 5 days, or oral valacyclovir 2000 mg every 12 hours for 1 day (2 doses) or 1000 mg every 12 hours for 7 to 10 days.

2) In patients with **recurrent infections** (periodic treatment of severe recurrences), it is preferable to start treatment during the prodromal phase, no later than at the onset of cutaneous eruptions. You may use oral acyclovir 200 mg every 4 to 5 hours (5 times a day) for 3 to 5 days, or oral valacyclovir 2000 mg every 12 hours for 1 day (2 doses). In patients with mild oral-labial herpes, topical acyclovir in the form of a cream (applied 5 times a day) can also be effective.

4. In **pregnant women**, acyclovir can be used (it is considered safe for the fetus). Treatment of primary infection or recurrences: above. In pregnant women with a history of recurrent genital herpes, it is recommended to start prophylactic administration of acyclovir in the third trimester of pregnancy, as antivirals have been shown to reduce HSV shedding and the recurrence of genital lesions at delivery (and therefore caesarian section rates), though no trials have been powered to show a significant decrease in neonatal infection rates (no events among >1000 women).◉◔ Cesarean section is preferred in women with active genital lesions or in women with a history of genital herpes and prodromal symptoms (burning, pain).

5. In patients with **ocular herpes simplex**, immediate referral to an ophthalmologist is indicated for monitoring and treatment with topical antivirals.

Symptomatic Treatment

Analgesics and antipyretics may be used when necessary.

→ COMPLICATIONS

Complications of HSV infections include secondary bacterial or fungal infections of the cutaneous lesions. Disseminated infection can occur (which may involve the esophagus, adrenal glands, lungs, joints, and CNS), especially in immunocompromised individuals. Erythema multiforme has commonly been reported in association with HSV infection.

→ PROGNOSIS

HSV infection is a lifelong recurring disease. Deaths are rare and affect predominantly newborns, severely immunocompromised individuals, and patients with meningoencephalitis.

→ PREVENTION

Vaccine is not available.

1. Primary prevention: Avoiding high-risk sexual contacts. Using a latex condom during intercourse will decrease the risk of infection, but does not eliminate it, since lesions may often be located outside the covered area. Infected individuals should inform their partners about the infection prior to initiating sexual contacts (risk of infection is also present in the asymptomatic phase of the disease). Patients with active genital lesions or in the prodromal stage of the disease should not have sexual contacts with healthy individuals; however, avoidance of contact at this time will not eliminate transmission, as asymptomatic shedding is not uncommon. Pregnant women with a history of genital herpes should inform their doctors. Healthy women whose partners have a history of genital herpes should refrain from sexual contacts during the third trimester of pregnancy.

2. Secondary prevention (long-term antiviral therapy): In patients with frequent and distressing recurrences, use oral acyclovir 400 mg every 12 hours or oral valacyclovir 500 mg or 1000 mg every 24 hours (acyclovir has been confirmed to be safe and effective when administered daily for 6 years; valacyclovir, for 1 year). The treatment reduces the frequency of recurrences and improves the quality of life. Prophylactic antiviral therapy will also decrease the risk of transmission of genital HSV.

17.3. Herpes Zoster

→ DEFINITION, ETIOLOGY, PATHOGENESIS

Herpes zoster (shingles) is a viral infection caused by the local reactivation of a latent varicella-zoster virus (VZV) after a prior primary infection. Herpes zoster is associated with characteristic cutaneous signs and symptoms.

1. Etiologic agent: VZV (→Chapter 8.17.11); the virus remains latent in the cells of dorsal root ganglia and cranial nerve ganglia following the primary VZV infection, and may reactivate under certain conditions (eg, in immunocompromised patients, with advanced age).

2. Reservoir and transmission: →Chapter 8.17.11.

3. Risk factors: Age >50 years, malignancy, immunosuppressive treatment, HIV infection, and other factors leading to a significant impairment of cell-mediated immune response.

4. Incubation and contagious period: →Chapter 8.17.11; patients with herpes zoster are significantly less contagious than patients with varicella. Susceptible individuals who have a history of exposure to vesicular zoster lesions on uncovered areas of the skin are at risk for developing varicella.

→ CLINICAL FEATURES

1. Prodromal phase (observed in 70%-80% of cases): Pain within a single dermatome, which may be constant or intermittent, frequent or sporadic, burning, piercing, pulsating, sometimes triggered mostly by touch. The clinical presentation may be dominated by pruritus, a tingling sensation, or other paresthesias. The pain occurs throughout the day and night. It usually precedes skin eruptions by 3 to 4 days and may persist for a week or longer after the lesions have resolved. Other symptoms may include low-grade or high-grade fever, malaise, and headache.

2. Rash: Polymorphic eruptions most commonly limited to 1 or 2 adjacent dermatomes (localized zoster), commonly appearing on the trunk along a thoracic dermatome (→below); usually, the rash does not cross the body's midline. The rash evolves from erythematous macular lesions (transient and easy to overlook) to clustered papules. Over 1 to 2 days the papules turn into vesicles filled with a clear or turbid fluid, and then into pustules. After 4 to 5 days the vesicles rupture, leaving painful erosions and ulcerations, which crust in 7 to 10 days. Successive crops of lesions continue to appear over ~7 days. The crusts fall off within 3 to 4 weeks, frequently leaving scars and areas of hypo- and hyperpigmentation. Mucosal lesions (erosions and minor ulcerations) may also be observed. In the course of typical zoster, clustered lesions appear within the area innervated by 1 sensory nerve branch (a dermatome), unilaterally, most frequently on the trunk (dermatomes Th3 to L3) or on the head within the areas innervated by cranial nerves: V (in particular the first branch: V_1), VII, and VIII. Involvement of the extremities is less frequent. The rash is accompanied by pain and pruritus (similar to the prodromal phase) as well as general symptoms (observed in <20% of patients): fever, headache, malaise, and fatigue.

3. Other manifestations: Paresis (in 5%-15% of patients), most frequently affecting the extremities as a result of motor nerve involvement. Paresis may manifest as Bell palsy (due to the involvement of the cranial nerve VII [peripheral facial nerve paresis]) or Ramsay Hunt syndrome (involvement of the geniculate ganglion and cranial nerve VII, which results in unilateral peripheral facial nerve paresis and auricular herpes zoster; it may be accompanied by disturbances of taste and of secretion of tears and saliva).

4. Distinct clinical presentations of herpes zoster:

1) **Herpes zoster ophthalmicus**: Eruptions are located along the trigeminal nerve (particularly V1), involving the skin of the forehead and eyelids as well as conjunctiva and cornea. The course may be severe and may lead to the development of corneal ulcerations. Untreated herpes zoster ophthalmicus may result in vision impairment (or even blindness) and ocular motor nerve paralysis.

2) **Herpes zoster oticus**: Lesions form along the peripheral nerves of the geniculate ganglion, involving the skin of the auricle and retroauricular area, external auditory canal, and tympanic membrane. The eruptions are accompanied by severe otalgia, tinnitus, impaired hearing, and vertigo (due to the involvement of cranial nerve VIII); this may also be accompanied by peripheral paralysis of cranial nerve VII (Ramsay Hunt syndrome).

3) **Disseminated herpes zoster** develops most commonly in patients who are immunocompromised (eg, as a result of hematologic or solid organ malignancy, or due to immunosuppressive medications). The rash involves 3 or more dermatomes and may even involve the entire body; it is similar to the

course of varicella but painful. Patients may develop pneumonia, hepatitis, and encephalitis.

4) **Recurrent herpes zoster** (in ≤5% of patients) may indicate a malignancy or impaired cell-mediated immune response.

→ DIAGNOSIS

In typical cases, herpes zoster is diagnosed in patients with a history of varicella and a typical clinical presentation.

Diagnostic Tests
→Chapter 8.17.11.

Diagnostic tests are recommended in immunocompromised patients as well as in atypical or equivocal cases.

Differential Diagnosis

1. Prodromal pain (particularly if persistent): Other possible causes of pain affecting the same area.

2. Skin lesions: Herpes simplex (herpes simplex virus [HSV] infection), contact dermatitis, toxic dermatitis, and skin lesions resulting from multiple insect bites.

3. Disseminated herpes zoster: Varicella, disseminated HSV infection, allergic rash, papular urticaria, acne vulgaris.

4. Herpes zoster ophthalmicus: HSV infection, erysipelas.

→ TREATMENT

Antiviral Treatment

1. In immunocompetent patients ≥50 years of age, patients with moderate or severe pain, or patients with skin eruptions that are of at least moderate severity or extend beyond the trunk, use oral **acyclovir** (INN aciclovir) 800 mg 5 times a day for 7 to 10 days, or oral **valacyclovir** (INN valaciclovir) 1000 mg every 8 hours for 7 days. Start treatment as soon as possible after the onset of rash (optimally within 24 hours).✓●●

2. In immunocompromised patients, organ transplant recipients, patients with malignancy, or with disseminated herpes zoster, use IV **acyclovir** 10 mg/kg (500 mg/m^2 body surface area) every 8 hours (guidance for IV administration of acyclovir: →Chapter 8.17.11). In patients whose condition improves (no new lesions, resolution of symptoms including pain), oral acyclovir may be continued until the improvement of immune function.

Symptomatic Treatment

1. Treatment of pain:

1) In patients with **mild or moderate pain**, use acetaminophen (INN paracetamol) or nonsteroidal anti-inflammatory drugs; adding a weak opioid (eg, tramadol) may be also considered.

2) In patients with **severe pain**, consider a strong opioid (eg, fentanyl or transdermal buprenorphine). If this is not effective, consider adding one of the following: oral gabapentin (start from 300 mg at bedtime and titrate up to tid administration, up to a maximum of 3600 mg/d) or oral pregabalin (start from 75 mg at bedtime and titrate up to bid administration, up to a maximum of 600 mg/d); oral amitriptyline (start from 10 mg at bedtime and titrate up to a maximum of 150 mg/d); a glucocorticoid (only in combination with antiviral treatment; eg, oral prednisone 30 mg bid on days 1 to 7 followed by 15 mg bid on days 8 to 14 and then by 7.5 mg bid on days 15 to 21).

2. Topical agents (antiviral agents, antibiotics, and analgesics) in a form of powders or pastes are not recommended.

→ COMPLICATIONS

Complications are more frequent in patients with impaired cell-mediated immune response.

1. Local complications:

1) **Postherpetic neuralgia** (occurs in 20%-50% of patients, more frequently in the elderly): Pain persisting for >30 days from the onset of the infection or recurring after approximately 4 weeks; it may persist for months or even years. Postherpetic neuralgia is a common complication of herpes zoster ophthalmicus; this can be a disabling complication because of the severity of pain. Treatment of pain: →Symptomatic Treatment, above.

2) **Postherpetic pruritus** may persist for several months after the skin lesions have resolved; it is sometimes accompanied by neuralgia. Postherpetic pruritus is a neuropathic phenomenon.

3) **Scarring, hyper- or hypopigmentation of the skin**.

4) Complications of herpes zoster ophthalmicus include **conjunctivitis, keratitis, uveitis, optic neuritis**.

5) **Bacterial superinfection of lesions** due to *Staphylococcus aureus* or group A streptococcus.

2. Neurologic complications:

1) **Aseptic meningitis**: Characterized by a mild course; resolves spontaneously within 1 to 2 weeks. Asymptomatic cerebrospinal fluid abnormalities typical for aseptic meningitis are observed in as many as one-third of immunocompetent patients with herpes zoster.

2) **Acute encephalitis** (rare): Usually develops a few days after the onset of rash (less frequently, a few weeks before or after). Risk factors: immunocompromised patients, involvement of dermatomes innervated by cranial nerves, and disseminated herpes zoster. The risk of death is up to 25%, depending on the immune status.

3) **Chronic encephalitis**: Affects almost exclusively patients with impaired cell-mediated immune response, particularly with AIDS. Chronic encephalitis develops a few months after recovering from herpes zoster (in 30%-40% of patients, no prior skin manifestations are seen). The prognosis is poor, as the disease is progressive and fatal.

4) **Stroke**: A rare complication of herpes zoster ophthalmicus, which results from segmental inflammation, stenosis, or thrombosis of the proximal branch of the middle or anterior cerebral artery; it may also affect immunocompetent individuals, typically occurring ~7 weeks (sometimes up to 6 months) after herpes zoster. The mortality rates are 20% to 25%; permanent neurologic sequelae are seen.

5) **Myelitis**: A rare complication that develops predominantly in patients with impaired cell-mediated immune response (particularly with AIDS). Myelitis is usually a complication of herpes zoster affecting the thoracic dermatomes, but it may also occur in patients without prior skin manifestations. Signs and symptoms: motor paresis (in the case of involvement of the pyramidal tracts) of the segment affected by skin lesions and/or hypoesthesia of the dermatomes below the affected one (involvement of the sensory tracts). The symptoms appear ~12 days after the onset of rash. Severe forms of myelitis: hemisection of the spinal cord (Brown-Séquard syndrome) or complete transverse spinal cord injury. The prognosis is variable.

6) **Retinitis**: Acute retinal necrosis in immunocompetent patients; in patients with AIDS: retinitis, progressive outer retinal necrosis, or rapidly progressive herpetic retinal necrosis. Retinitis usually develops simultaneously or a few weeks or months after the onset of rash. The disease may progress to involve both eyes. Ophthalmoscopic examination reveals granular yellowish ischemic patches that are expanding and coalescent; retinal detachment may

1009

eventually develop. The rapid progression of the disease leads to confluent necrosis and blindness (in 75%-85% of patients).

7) **Facial nerve palsy**.

3. Disseminated herpes zoster, viremia, cutaneous dissemination: These are usually observed in patients with severe impairment of cell-mediated immune response; high risk of death in patients with visceral dissemination.

→ PROGNOSIS

Prognosis is good in immunocompetent patients, although postherpetic neuralgia may persist for months. Immunocompromised patients and patients with complications of herpes zoster are at risk for permanent sequelae and death, depending on the course of the disease (→Complications, above).

→ PREVENTION

Specific Prevention

Vaccination:

1) Varicella vaccine is the key prevention method.

2) Herpes zoster vaccine is indicated in persons >50 years of age.◐●

General Preventive Measures

1. Isolation of patients (particularly from high-risk individuals): Immunocompromised patients as well as immunocompetent patients with disseminated herpes zoster should be isolated for the entire duration of the disease. Immunocompetent patients with localized herpes zoster should be isolated until all lesions have dried and crusted.

2. Covering the affected areas of the skin (eg, with clothing) reduces the risk of VZV infection in persons who have direct contact with a sick individual.

17.4. Infectious Mononucleosis

→ DEFINITION, ETIOLOGY, PATHOGENESIS

Infectious mononucleosis is a syndrome characterized by fever, pharyngitis/tonsillitis, lymphadenopathy, and peripheral atypical lymphocytosis.

1. Etiologic agents: Ninety percent of cases of typical mononucleosis are caused by the Epstein-Barr virus (EBV) (Herpesviridae family). The virus first infects oropharyngeal epithelial cells and B cells. Some of these B cells are transformed into immortal plasma cells and are triggered to produce polyclonal γ globulins, which are detected as nonspecific heterophile antibodies. The activated B cells, which are visualized as atypical lymphocytes, stimulate proliferation of T cells, leading to the enlargement of the lymph nodes, tonsils, spleen, and liver. After the primary infection, EBV remains latent in B cells and oral epithelial cells; EBV reactivation may lead to uncontrolled monoclonal lymphoproliferation. Shedding of active EBV virus takes place intermittently thereafter from the asymptomatic host.

There are other pathogens that cause infectious mononucleosis indistinguishable from EBV, the most common of which is cytomegalovirus (CMV) (Herpesviridae family), which has been estimated to account for 7% of cases of infectious mononucleosis. Like EBV, CMV infects B lymphocytes, establishing a reservoir of latent virus that persists for life. Other pathogens that are rarer causes of infectious mononucleosis-like symptoms include human herpesvirus 6 (HHV-6), human herpesvirus 7 (HHV-7), HIV, and the protozoan pathogen *Toxoplasma gondii*.

2. Reservoir, transmission, incubation period: Humans are the only reservoir for EBV. EBV is common worldwide; over 95% of adults are seropositive for this virus. In industrialized countries, half of children are infected by the age of 5 years; in lower-income settings, people acquire infection more rapidly. EBV is spread via direct contact, and transmission is usually mediated through saliva, which contains large amounts of the virus. Transmission is also possible by blood transfusion as well as bone marrow and solid organ transplantation.

3. Incubation period: The incubation period is 30 to 50 days.

→ CLINICAL FEATURES

EBV infection can often be asymptomatic, especially in young children.

1. Infectious mononucleosis, as noted above, refers to a clinical syndrome featuring fever, pharyngitis, lymphadenopathy, and peripheral atypical lymphocytosis. This is often preceded by a prodromal phase of fever, headache, and malaise indistinguishable from that associated with other viral pathogens. This classic syndrome is less often seen in very young children and elderly adults.

2. Pharyngitis associated with EBV can be accompanied by severe sore throat and fever up to 40°C (this usually resolves within 1 to 2 weeks, in exceptional cases may persist for 4 to 5 weeks). Classically, the tonsils are enlarged and covered with a characteristic exudate reminiscent of streptococcal pharyngitis (→Chapter 8.11); the pharyngeal mucosa is erythematous, and frequently palatal petechiae and halitosis are detected. Signs may also include skin edema around the eyelids, at the nasal root, and above the eyebrows (more frequent in children). EBV infection can present with pharyngitis alone in the absence of other features of infectious mononucleosis.

3. Lymphadenopathy and splenomegaly: Lymph nodes may be significantly enlarged, even >3 cm in diameter, and are elastic, movable, tender, do not form aggregates, and are often surrounded by edema. Lymphadenopathy is the longest-persisting symptom (may be observed for up to 6 months following the acute infection). Children usually develop generalized lymphadenopathy; in adolescents and adults, lymphadenopathy is more often limited to posterior and anterior cervical and submandibular lymph nodes, and generalized lymphadenopathy with the involvement of axillary and inguinal lymph nodes is less frequent. Note that cervical lymphadenopathy, if massive, can cause airway obstruction. Splenomegaly occurs during the second and third week of the infection in 50% of patients and resolves after 7 to 10 days.

4. Hepatitis occurs in 20% to 90% of patients. It is usually without jaundice but may be accompanied by hepatomegaly (in 10%-15% of cases). Hepatitis persists for up to 4 weeks.

5. Rash develops in 3% to 15% of patients and can vary in appearance; morbilliform, macular, petechial, scarlatiniform, urticarial, or erythema multiforme rashes occur. A more severe and generalized rash can result after the administration of antibiotics, especially aminopenicillins (ampicillin or amoxicillin). Though this is generally assumed to occur in >90% of individuals with infectious mononucleosis treated with aminopenicillins, recent data suggest that it is much less common.

6. Other nonspecific symptoms associated with infectious mononucleosis: Headache (typically retro-orbital), abdominal pain, nausea and vomiting. During the period of convalescence, asthenia, malaise, fatigue, exhaustion, and impaired concentration occur. Fatigue resolves more slowly than other symptoms associated with infectious mononucleosis; one study documented persistent fatigue in 13% of patients at 6 months.

7. EBV-associated lymphoproliferative disorder affects immunocompromised individuals, particularly patients with AIDS and transplant recipients; the clinical spectrum can be quite variable, ranging from the development of masses (enlargement of the lymph nodes and other lymphatic organs) to the development of lymphomas.

8. EBV-associated hematologic disorders: EBV-associated hemophagocytic lymphohistiocytosis and chronic active EBV infection are rare types of EBV infection associated with proliferation of T cells or natural killer (NK) cells. The pathogeneses of these conditions are different, but both can be associated with persistent fever, lymphadenopathy, splenomegaly, hepatitis, and pancytopenia; chronic active EBV infection (CAEBV) also presents with interstitial pneumonia, uveitis, and the dermatosis hydroa vacciniforme.

9. Other infectious syndromes: EBV can also be a rare cause of meningoencephalitis (especially in pediatric populations), transverse myelitis, cranial nerve palsies, Guillain-Barré syndrome, glomerulonephritis, myocarditis, pancreatitis, and mesenteric adenitis.

→ DIAGNOSIS

Diagnostic Tests

1. Complete blood count: In 98% of cases of infectious mononucleosis, moderate leukocytosis (up to 20×10^9/L) with a significant proportion of lymphocytes (>50% of all white blood cells or $>4.5 \times 10^9$ lymphocytes/L) is observed. "Atypical lymphocytosis" is defined as having ≥10% of lymphocytes on blood smear with atypical features (loosely arranged chromatin, eccentric nucleus).

2. Serology:

1) **Specific anti-EBV antibodies** are most helpful in determining whether an infection with EBV has occurred. As EBV is a ubiquitous pathogen, serologies are often positive; the timing of positivity and negativity for the antigens listed below enable the determination of whether infection was acquired within days, weeks, or months.

   a) IgM antibodies against viral capsid antigen (anti-VCA IgM) appear first and are detectable in 95% of patients with a primary infection. The titers increase rapidly within a few days of the acute phase onset and decrease to zero after 2 to 3 months. Anti-VCA IgG appear within a few days of EBV infection and persist for life. Anti-VCA antibodies are highly sensitive and specific for EBV infection.

   b) Antibodies against the early antigen (EA) develop later than anti-VCA IgG (within 2 weeks, peaking at 3-4 weeks) after the development of clinical symptoms and persist for 3 to 6 months; however, up to 30% of individuals may not have detectable anti-EA.

   c) Antibodies against Epstein-Barr nuclear antigen (EBNA) appear in the later phases of the disease, within weeks (3-6) of acute infection. These persist for life.

2) **Nonspecific heterophile antibodies** (mainly IgM; Paul-Bunnell--Davidsohn reaction, rapid agglutination tests, monospot test) may be helpful in the diagnostic workup if specific serologic tests are not available; this testing is often readily available and easily done. The antibodies appear at the end of the second week of the disease (in 80%-90% of adult patients) and persist for ≥3 to 6 months. A positive result is usually conclusive (specificity, ~90%), though false negatives are common in early infection. The sensitivity of heterophile antibodies is dramatically reduced in children under the age of 5 years, so much so that the test should generally not be used in this population.

3. Detection of EBV DNA (polymerase chain reaction [PCR]; specimens: serum, blood [lymphocytes], tissues): Useful in immunocompromised patients (who lack specific antibodies) or in tracking EBV infection in patients with cancer, after transplantation, with lymphoproliferative disorders, and with chronic active EBV infection. There is little benefit to the routine use of EBV PCR in immunocompetent patients, as the diagnosis of EBV infection is readily made by the use of serologic testing.

Differential Diagnosis

As noted above, infectious mononucleosis-like illness not attributable to EBV can be due to CMV, HHV-6, HHV-7, HIV, and toxoplasmosis. Pharyngitis can be caused by respiratory viruses (eg, influenza, parainfluenza, rhinovirus, enterovirus), though these do not typically cause exudative pharyngitis, which is commonly due to group A streptococcus and extremely rarely due to diphtheria. Hepatitis associated with EBV is similar to that resulting from other viruses (eg, CMV, adenovirus, enterovirus) and toxic ingestions. Lymphadenopathy and splenomegaly can also be seen with infections such as enteric (typhoid) fever, brucellosis, bartonellosis, as well as in a number of other infections, rheumatologic diseases, and immunologic disorders.

→TREATMENT

Antiviral Treatment

Ganciclovir is active against EBV but has no role in the treatment of any EBV-associated infections in immunocompetent individuals. It is sometimes used for active EBV infections in severely immunosuppressed patients; however, the evidence base for this practice is scant, and this should only be undertaken in consultation with an expert in infectious diseases.

Other Treatment Modalities

1. General recommendations: The mainstay of treatment is supportive. Acetaminophen (INN paracetamol) or nonsteroidal anti-inflammatory drugs can be used for pain. The vast majority of patients do not require hospitalization or intravenous therapy to maintain adequate fluid status.

2. Glucocorticoid therapy should not be routinely prescribed to patients with infectious mononucleosis, given the results of a meta-analysis that did not find any significant benefit >12 hours after their administration.⊗◯ A more recent meta-analysis, including many more patients with pharyngitis in higher-quality trials, showed a significant increase in the rate of resolution of throat pain at 24 hours after treatment with glucocorticoids, but individuals with infectious mononucleosis were specifically excluded.

Treatment with glucocorticoids should generally be reserved for those with severe lymphadenopathy and impeding airway obstruction in an effort to avoid the necessity of operative intervention, though no randomized trials have evaluated this practice.◯◯ Isolated case reports have documented the use of glucocorticoids for severe persistent neutropenia, thrombocytopenia, or hemophagocytic lymphohistiocytosis following EBV infection.

3. Minimization of immunosuppression, administration of rituximab, and use of EBV-specific cytotoxic lymphocytes are advocated for the treatment of posttransplant EBV-associated lymphoproliferative disorders; treatment of this condition should only be done in consultation with specialists in hematology-oncology.

→COMPLICATIONS

Complications of infectious mononucleosis are rare, but potentially severe, and include the following:

1) Splenic rupture, mainly subcapsular (0.5% of patients), may occur during the second or third week of the disease, is preceded by severe abdominal pain, and may require surgery. It is suggested that athletes refrain from contact sports for 4 weeks and sports where chest/abdominal trauma is possible for 3 weeks,◯◯ simply due to the fact that splenic rupture is less likely >21 days after the onset of symptoms.

2) Malignancy: A very rare late complication; EBV infection is associated with Hodgkin lymphoma, Burkitt lymphoma, T-cell or NK-cell leukemia, nasal-type

extranodal NK/T-cell lymphoma, lymphoproliferative disorders associated with immune deficiency, and nasopharyngeal cancer.

→ PROGNOSIS

The prognosis of infectious mononucleosis is good in the vast majority of patients. The disease resolves spontaneously, although some symptoms may persist for several months. In patients who develop very rare hematologic and neurologic complications, the prognosis is unfavorable. Deaths related to infectious mononucleosis are rare and usually result from splenic rupture, secondary bacterial infections, or myocarditis.

→ PREVENTION

Individuals with a recent history of confirmed EBV infection or disease reminiscent of infectious mononucleosis should not donate blood or organs for transplantation. No vaccine is available.

17.5. Influenza

→ DEFINITION, ETIOLOGY, PATHOGENESIS

Influenza is an acute respiratory illness caused by influenza viruses. **Seasonal influenza** outbreaks occur annually and are caused by seasonal human influenza virus strains. **Pandemic influenza** occurs every several years to decades and is caused by novel reassortant strains of influenza A to which humans have not been previously exposed, for instance, the Spanish influenza pandemic in the 1920s. Pandemic influenza by definition implies global spread, and the incidence of infection is typically several-fold higher than during seasonal influenza epidemics. An influenza pandemic is declared by the World Health Organization (WHO) on the basis of widespread geographic distribution of infections with the new virus strain, regardless of the severity of the disease.

1. Etiologic agent: Epidemic outbreaks in humans are caused by influenza virus type A or B. Influenza A virus is divided into subtypes defined on the basis of antigenic specificity of 2 surface proteins: hemagglutinin (HA) and neuraminidase (NA). Seasonal influenza epidemics are most frequently caused by the H1N1 and H3N2 subtypes of influenza A virus, with a lower frequency of circulation of influenza B virus. Influenza A virus is characterized by a high antigenic variation that is associated with a relative lack of protective immunity in subsequent seasons and therefore warrants an annual update of immunization against influenza H1N1 and H3N2 strains. Influenza B viruses are separated into 2 distinct genetic lineages (Yamagata and Victoria). Because they undergo antigenic drift less rapidly than influenza A viruses, they are not categorized into subtypes. Influenza B viruses from both lineages may cocirculate, but frequently one lineage predominates. In the Northern hemisphere, the influenza season typically extends from fall to early spring (October to April). Sporadic human infections with avian influenza viruses (potentially pandemic subtypes) associated with high morbidity and mortality rates have been reported predominantly in Asia and Egypt (H5N1), and most recently in China (H7N9, H10N8). However, so far there has been no evidence of ongoing sustained person-to-person spread of these avian influenza virus subtypes. In June 2009, the WHO declared a pandemic caused by a new influenza H1N1 2009 subtype, which dominated the 2009/2010 influenza season, almost entirely displacing the prior seasonal subtypes. Influenza virus replicates in the epithelium of the upper and lower respiratory tract and rarely causes viremia; the systemic signs and symptoms of the infection are caused by cytokines released due to inflammatory response.

2. Reservoirs and transmission: The reservoirs of influenza viruses are humans and certain animals (eg, pigs, domesticated and wild birds). Transmission is by droplets of human secretions (although transmission by direct contact with virus-contaminated surfaces is also possible). In **avian influenza** the reservoirs are infected birds; transmission to humans may be via a direct close contact with a sick person or through a close contact with infected birds.

3. Incubation period: 1 to 7 days (2 days on average). In adults, the virus shedding lasts from 1 day prior to the onset of symptoms to 3 to 5 days after the onset of symptoms (in some cases up to 10 days). Young children may shed the virus from a few days before the onset of symptoms to ≥10 days after the onset of symptoms. Severely immunocompromised patients may shed the virus for several weeks or months.

4. Risk factors for infection:

1) Prolonged close contact (within 1.5-2 meters) with a sick individual without a protective barrier (face mask) or direct face-to-face contact without protective measures.
2) Direct contact with a sick or infected individual, or with objects contaminated by influenza virus.
3) Inadequate hand hygiene.
4) Touching mouth, nose, or eyes with contaminated hands.
5) Staying in crowded spaces during the influenza season.

→ CLINICAL FEATURES

The disease onset in healthy hosts is typically rapid and includes the following:

1) **Systemic signs and symptoms**: Fever, chills, myalgia, headache (most commonly frontal and retro-orbital), fatigue, and malaise.
2) **Respiratory symptoms**: Sore throat, rhinitis (usually mild), and dry cough.
3) **Less common symptoms**: Nausea, vomiting, and/or mild diarrhea (particularly in children). Usually the patients recover spontaneously within 3 to 7 days; cough and malaise may persist for ≥2 weeks. Up to 50% of cases are asymptomatic.

In the elderly, the presentation is frequently more subtle and may include fever, malaise, cough, or sore throat alone.

→ DIAGNOSIS

Diagnostic Tests

1. Virology: Detection of the genetic material of the virus (reverse transcription polymerase chain reaction [RT-PCR]), immunofluorescence assays (direct [DFA] or indirect [IFA] fluorescence antibody staining), isolation of the virus using cell cultures and rapid influenza antigen detection tests (rapid influenza diagnostic test [RIDT]) on nasal and pharyngeal specimens (aspirate, wash, swab; the nose and throat samples should be pooled). Typically, virology testing is done early in the season when there is uncertainty about influenza, but usually it is not necessary during the peak influenza season. However, it should be considered in patients with risk factors for complications or severe course of influenza (→below), or in cases of severe (complicated) and progressive influenza-like illness (ILI) or any other indication for hospitalization (→below). Results of the testing may be useful in determining whether the infecting strain is resistant to treatment. The test with the highest diagnostic accuracy is RT-PCR. Respiratory samples should be collected as early as possible after the onset of symptoms (ideally within 48-72 hours) to maximize influenza testing sensitivity. Any errors related to the type of samples, time and method of sampling, and storage and transport conditions may cause false-negative results. If the clinical suspicion is high, consider repeating the test if negative. In the case of lower respiratory tract infections, testing tracheal and bronchial aspirates has superior diagnostic value. RIDTs are highly specific, with pooled specificity of 98%, but moderately sensitive, with pooled sensitivity of 62%👁; therefore, negative results do not exclude infection. As with any other test, the number of false-negative results increases with increasing disease prevalence in the community while the negative predictive value decreases. Testing time varies among virologic testing methods: conventional cell culture takes between 3 and 10 days, rapid cell culture (eg, shell vials) from 1 to 3 days, immunofluorescence (DFA, IFA) from 1 to 4 hours, RT-PCR between 1 and 6 hours, and RIDT <30 minutes.

2. Serologic testing is of little practical importance.

Diagnostic Criteria

1. Diagnosis of infection (laboratory-confirmed influenza). The diagnosis of influenza is based on positive results of virology tests.

2. In the influenza season, the diagnosis of influenza should be considered in every patient with fever and respiratory signs and symptoms (sore throat, cough, or both). Although clinical presentation alone only allows for a diagnosis of ILI (infection with several microorganisms may produce similar signs and symptoms), during the peak influenza season ILI is predictive of influenza and therefore testing in healthy or nonseverely ill patients is not generally needed.

3. Classification of disease severity:

1) **Severe or complicated influenza (warrants hospital admission)** is associated with typical manifestations plus ≥1 of the following:

   a) Clinical (tachypnea and other manifestations of dyspnea, hypoxia) and/or radiologic features (pneumonia) of lower respiratory tract infection, central nervous system (CNS) manifestations (seizures, encephalitis, encephalopathy), severe dehydration.

   b) Secondary complications: Renal failure, multiple organ dysfunction, sepsis and septic shock, myocarditis, rhabdomyolysis.

   c) Exacerbation of primary chronic diseases including asthma, chronic obstructive pulmonary disease, coronary artery disease, chronic heart failure, chronic liver or kidney disease, diabetes.

   d) Other serious conditions not listed above that require hospitalization.

   e) Any signs and symptoms of disease progression (→below).

2) **A progressive (worsening) course of the disease**: Emerging signs and symptoms of severe or complicated influenza in patients who have been previously seen by a physician for uncomplicated influenza. The patient's clinical status may deteriorate very rapidly (eg, within 24 hours); signs and symptoms of progressive influenza warrant reevaluation of the prior treatment and, in most cases, are an indication for hospital admission (below, items a-c). The **signs and symptoms of progressive disease**:

   a) Signs and symptoms of lower respiratory tract involvement or heart failure: Dyspnea, cyanosis, hemoptysis, chest pain, hypotension, decreased hemoglobin oxygen saturation measured by pulse oximetry (SpO_2).

   b) Symptoms suggestive of CNS involvement: Altered mental status, loss of consciousness, somnolence, seizures (significantly decreased muscle strength, paralysis or paresis).

   c) Features of severe dehydration: Dizziness and orthostatic hypotension, somnolence and altered mental status, low urine output.

   d) Laboratory and/or clinical features of persistent viral infection or secondary invasive bacterial infection (eg, high-grade fever and other acute signs and symptoms persisting >3 days).

4. Risk factors for a severe course and complications of influenza (including hospitalization and death):

1) Age >65 years or <5 years (particularly <12 months).

2) Pregnancy (particularly the second and third trimesters).

3) Extreme obesity (body mass index ≥ 40 kg/m^2).

4) Certain chronic conditions (irrespective of age): Respiratory (eg, chronic obstructive pulmonary disease, asthma), cardiovascular (eg, coronary artery disease, congestive heart failure), renal, liver, metabolic (including diabetes), hematologic (including hemoglobinopathies), immunodeficiency (primary, HIV infection, immunosuppressive therapy), other conditions affecting respiratory function or the ability to clear respiratory secretions (eg, cognitive impairment, spinal injury, seizures, and neuromuscular disorders).

Differential Diagnosis

Common cold and other viral respiratory tract infections, bacterial respiratory tract infections.

 TREATMENT

Management algorithms: →Figure 17-1 and →Figure 17-2.

Symptomatic Treatment

1. Bed rest as required, adequate hydration, patient isolation (particularly to prevent contact with individuals at high risk for complications of influenza).

2. Antipyretics and analgesics: Acetaminophen (INN paracetamol), nonsteroidal anti-inflammatory drugs (NSAIDs) (eg, ibuprofen); do not use acetylsalicylic acid in children and adolescents <18 years of age due to the risk of Reye syndrome.

3. Cough suppressants, nasal decongestants, and **isotonic or hypertonic saline nasal spray solution** may be used as required.

4. Popular **over-the-counter medications**, such as vitamin C and rutoside, are not effective. There is no firm evidence of the beneficial effects of homeopathic remedies.

Antiviral Treatment

With different options available and lack of direct comparisons, our default choice is **oseltamivir** (longer period of availability and most data).

1. Antiviral agents for the treatment of influenza:

1) Neuraminidase inhibitors (active against influenza A and B viruses): **Oseltamivir** (oral), **zanamivir** (dry powder inhaler), peramivir (IV).

2) M2 inhibitors (only active against influenza A viruses): **Amantadine** and **rimantadine**.

3) Endonuclease inhibitor: **Baloxavir**.

Because the spectrum of resistance to antiviral agents changes every year, recommendations for empiric treatment are updated prior to each influenza season (or during the season, when necessary). The currently circulating influenza A (H3N2) and H1N1 2009 viruses are resistant to M2 inhibitors; therefore, these medications are not recommended for use against influenza A virus infections. However, almost all current influenza A and B virus strains are, with rare exceptions, susceptible to the neuraminidase inhibitors. Sporadic oseltamivir-resistant H1N1 2009 virus infections have been identified, but the public health impact has been limited to date. Oseltamivir and peramivir should not be used if an oseltamivir-resistant influenza strain is suspected. All oseltamivir-resistant H1N1 2009 strains are susceptible to zanamivir. Early initiation of antiviral treatment (optimally within 48-72 hours of onset) in uncomplicated cases can reduce the symptom duration of influenza by <24 hours. However, data for the reduction of complications of influenza are quite limited, with more evidence derived from observational studies than from randomized trials.

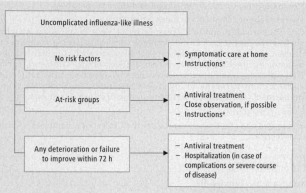

Figure 17-1. Initial clinical management of patients with uncomplicated influenza-like illness or influenza. See text for comments. *Based on the World Health Organization and Centers for Disease Control and Prevention guidelines.*

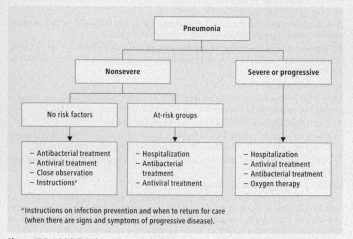

Figure 17-2. Initial clinical management of influenza-associated pneumonia. See text for comments. *Based on the World Health Organization and Centers for Disease Control and Prevention guidelines.*

Adverse events:

1) **Oseltamivir**: Nausea and vomiting (might be less severe if oseltamivir is taken with food), transient neuropsychiatric events (self-injury or delirium; the majority of reports were among Japanese adolescents and adults). It may impair the immune response to influenza vaccines. In patients with creatinine clearance of 10 to 30 mL per minute, a reduction of the treatment dosage to 75 mg once daily and in the chemoprophylaxis dosage to 75 mg every other day is recommended.

2) **Zanamivir**: Bronchospasm (zanamivir is licensed only for use in persons without an underlying respiratory or cardiac disease). It does not impair the immune response to inactivated influenza vaccines. No dose adjustment of inhaled zanamivir is recommended for a 5-day course of treatment in patients with either mild-to-moderate or severe impairment in renal function.

3) **Peramivir**: Diarrhea. Serious skin reactions and transient neuropsychiatric events have been reported.

4) **Baloxavir**: The most common adverse event is diarrhea, but no adverse event was more common in baloxavir compared with placebo or oseltamivir in a phase 3 clinical trial.

2. Indications for treatment with oseltamivir:

1) In patients with suspected or confirmed influenza of a severe or progressive course, or complications of influenza (→Diagnostic Criteria, above), we recommend starting oseltamivir as soon as possible (this includes also pregnant women).◐○ If oseltamivir is not available or is contraindicated, or in the case of documented resistance of the isolated virus to oseltamivir, treat the patient with zanamivir.

2) In the case of a strong clinical suspicion of influenza or laboratory-confirmed influenza in a patient at high risk for a severe course or complications of influenza (→Diagnostic Criteria, above), we suggest starting oseltamivir as soon as possible after the onset of disease, regardless of the severity of clinical manifestations.◐○

In the majority of patients with mild to moderate influenza who are not at high risk of complications, as well as in patients who present in the convalescence phase, antiviral treatment is generally not necessary. For situations where it is important to reduce symptom duration (still within 24 hours), we suggest oseltamivir.◐○ Clinical judgment should be an important component of outpatient-treatment decisions. Long-term treatment with oseltamivir may lead to the development of drug resistance, particularly in immunocompromised patients.

3. Dosage and treatment regimens:

1) **Oseltamivir** (oral) in patients >40 kg or >12 years of age: 75 mg bid, usually for 5 days. If the treatment is not effective, continue oseltamivir for a longer time. There are probably no virologic or clinical advantages of a double dose of oseltamivir compared with a standard course in patients with severe influenza admitted to hospital.

2) **Zanamivir** (dry powder inhaler): The recommended dosage is 2 inhalations (2 × 5 mg) bid for 5 days. Do not use zanamivir in nebulization because it contains lactose, which may affect the functioning of the nebulizer.

3) **Peramivir**: A single IV dose of 600 mg.

4) **Baloxavir**: A single dose: 40 mg for patients <80 kg, 80 mg for patients ≥80 kg.

Hospital Management

Hospitalization is indicated in patients with severe or progressive influenza (→Diagnostic Criteria, above).

1. Initial patient assessment:

1) SpO_2 should be monitored in every patient and maintained >90% in patients with pneumonia. In some patients (pregnant women, children), the recommended SpO_2 is 92% to 95%.

2) In patients with dyspnea, perform a chest radiograph.

3) Perform (or repeat) RT-PCR assay for the influenza virus. A negative result in a patient with a strong clinical suspicion of influenza requires repeating the test every 48 to 72 hours.

4) Frequently reevaluate the patient, as the clinical deterioration may progress rapidly over hours.

2. Immediately after admission, **start empiric treatment with oseltamivir** (or an alternative first-line antiviral agent if seasonal recommendations have changed). In patients hospitalized because of complications of influenza, oseltamivir is usually continued for >5 days or ≥10 days (or until the resolution of signs and symptoms and/or virology test results confirm that the virus no longer replicates). If severe symptoms of influenza persist despite oseltamivir treatment in a patient with documented influenza, consider IV zanamivir or peramivir.

3. In patients with influenza-associated pneumonia (particularly if severe), combine oseltamivir with empiric antibiotic therapy according to the current recommendations for treatment of community-acquired pneumonia. Bacterial pneumonia in patients with influenza is most frequently caused by *Staphylococcus aureus* and pneumococci, but standard microbiologic diagnostics should be carried out in each patient. Prophylactic antibiotic use is not recommended. If clinical features do not suggest bacterial infection in a patient with laboratory-confirmed influenza, consider discontinuation of antibiotic treatment.

4. Mechanical ventilation is used when necessary (eg, in acute respiratory distress syndrome).

5. Glucocorticoids: High doses should be avoided in viral pneumonia due to the risk of serious adverse effects, including opportunistic infections and prolonged viral replication. Administration of low-dose glucocorticoids may be considered in the case of septic shock requiring vasopressor therapy (→Chapter 8.14).

→ COMPLICATIONS

Complications of influenza:

1) **Pneumonia:**
   a) **Primary influenza-associated pneumonia**: Persistent signs and symptoms of influenza. This is the most prevalent severe viral pneumonia during influenza seasons, which may progress to acute respiratory distress syndrome.
   b) **Secondary bacterial pneumonia** caused by *Streptococcus pneumoniae*, *Staphylococcus aureus*, or *Haemophilus influenzae* develops during recovery or convalescence (recurrence of fever, increasing dyspnea, cough, fatigue).
2) **Streptococcal pharyngitis.**
3) **Exacerbation of concomitant chronic diseases.**
4) **Rare complications**: Meningoencephalitis, encephalopathy, transverse myelitis, Guillain-Barré syndrome, myositis (in extreme cases with myoglobinuria and renal failure), myocarditis, pericarditis, sepsis, and multiple organ dysfunction.
5) An extremely rare complication (affecting mainly children): Reye syndrome, usually associated with the use of acetylsalicylic acid.

→ SPECIAL CONSIDERATIONS

Pregnancy and Breastfeeding

Pregnant women are at higher risk for complications from influenza, including an unfavorable pregnancy outcome (miscarriage, premature birth, and fetal distress). Carefully monitor pregnant women with suspected or confirmed influenza and consider antiviral treatment prior to obtaining virology results regardless of intensity of symptoms. Administer acetaminophen (INN paracetamol) for pain and fever (acetylsalicylic acid and NSAIDs are contraindicated in pregnancy). There are no adequate data on using doses of oseltamivir higher than 75 mg every 12 hours. Oseltamivir and zanamivir are safe during breastfeeding (the principles of infection control have to be followed).

→ PREVENTION

1. Vaccination is the basis of influenza prevention (there is no high quality evidence on its effects on patient-important outcomes, especially in high-risk groups).◉

2. Hand hygiene: During the influenza season, hands should be washed frequently (10 times a day for 20 seconds) with soap and water—or, preferably, an alcohol-based antiseptic—and dried with disposable paper towels, particularly in the case of close contact with sick individuals (eg, household, workplace, hospital, and outpatient contacts). Hand washing should be performed after every contact with a sick person, after using the toilet, before eating or touching the mouth or nose, upon returning home, after clearing the nose or covering the mouth while sneezing or coughing.

3. Wearing a **protective face mask** (eg, surgical, dental) when in close contact (within 1.5-2 meters) with a sick person. The patient should also wear a face mask to minimize the risk of infecting others. Face masks should be discarded after each contact with a sick individual and replaced with new ones. Wearing prophylactic face masks by healthy persons when outdoors is not recommended. During medical procedures generating aerosols of respiratory secretions (eg, bronchoscopy, suctioning of respiratory secretions), face masks with an N95 respirator (or equivalent) as well as protective eyewear, gowns, and gloves should be used.

4. Other recommendations for hygiene during the influenza season include covering the mouth with a tissue while sneezing or coughing, disposing of the tissue in a waste basket, and washing hands thoroughly (if tissues are not available, it is recommended to sneeze or cough into an elbow or upper sleeve, not into the hands); avoiding face-to-face contact with other people; avoiding public gatherings; avoiding touching the mouth, nose, and eyes with unwashed hands; and frequent and thorough ventilation of rooms.

5. Patient isolation for 7 days from the onset of symptoms, and in the case of persistent symptoms, until 24 hours after the resolution of fever and acute respiratory symptoms. Longer isolation is needed in immunocompromised patients.

6. Chemoprophylaxis (oral oseltamivir [75 mg once daily] or zanamivir [10 mg once daily] for a total of no more than 10 days after the most recent known exposure) may be used in high-risk persons within 48 hours after a close contact (eg, within household) with a suspected or confirmed case, but it is not recommended as a routine procedure. Antiviral treatment of infected high-risk individuals is preferred (→Diagnostic Criteria, above), and this should be started as soon as possible after the onset of symptoms of influenza. Unvaccinated health care workers who sustain occupational exposures and were not using an adequate personal protective equipment at the time of exposure are also potential candidates for chemoprophylaxis. Clinical judgment is an important factor in making postexposure chemoprophylaxis decisions, which should take into account the exposed person's risk for influenza complications (→Diagnostic Criteria), the type and duration of contact (→Diagnostic Criteria), and recommendations from local or public health authorities. Chemoprophylaxis is not a substitute for influenza vaccination when influenza vaccine is available and not contraindicated.

17.6. Measles

→ DEFINITION, ETIOLOGY, PATHOGENESIS

Measles is an acute systemic viral disease virtually always characterized by a generalized rash.

1. Etiologic agent and pathogenesis: Rubeola (measles) virus is an enveloped single-stranded RNA virus that is a member of the Paramyxoviridae family. It infects the upper respiratory and conjunctival epithelial cells. The virus replicates in the local lymph nodes as well as lymphatic tissue and causes secondary viremia, which leads to other organ involvement (eg, skin).

2. Reservoir and transmission: Humans and other primates are the only reservoir for measles virus. Transmission is via direct contact and airborne droplet nuclei, occurring because of the production of aerosolized particles from respiratory secretions of infected hosts.

3. Incubation and contagious period: The time from exposure to the onset of first prodromal symptoms is 8 to 12 days; the rash generally appears 7 to 18 days after exposure (14 days on average). The disease is highly contagious—susceptible individuals are at a very high risk of developing measles after being exposed to measles virus. The patient is contagious from the onset of the prodromal phase for up to 5 days after the appearance of rash.

→ CLINICAL FEATURES

Infection is almost always symptomatic. The signs and symptoms appear in the following order:

1) **Prodromal signs and symptoms** (lasting a few days): Fever up to 40°C (1-7 days); dry cough (this may persist for 1-2 weeks), pronounced rhinitis. Bilateral, nonpurulent conjunctivitis (causing photophobia) may be significant (particularly in adults) and accompanied by eyelid edema; it resolves with the resolution of fever.

2) **Koplik spots** (→Figure 17-3): Multiple gray-white papules on the buccal mucosa adjacent to the premolars, which appear 1 to 2 days before the onset of rash and persist for 1 to 2 days after its resolution. Although Koplik spots are a pathognomonic sign, their absence does not exclude measles.

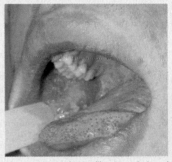

Figure 17-3. Measles. Koplik spots on the buccal mucosal membrane.

3) **Rash**: Erythematous maculopapular eruptions (dark red to purple in color), 0.1 to 1 cm in diameter, appear over 2 to 4 days. The rash typically starts on the head (forehead, at the hairline, behind the ears; excluding the scalp) and gradually progresses to include the trunk and extremities (→Figure 17-4). Individual lesions usually become confluent. Within 3 to 7 days, the rash begins to fade away and gradually disappears in the order in which it appeared, leaving brownish discolorations and fine desquamation.

4) **Other less common signs and symptoms**: Anorexia, diarrhea, generalized lymphadenopathy.

→ DIAGNOSIS

Measles can be suspected on the basis of clinical manifestations, but generally the diagnosis should be confirmed by diagnostic testing. However, measles may also be diagnosed conclusively on the basis of the typical clinical manifestations in a patient who had contact with an individual in whom the infection was confirmed by laboratory test results.

Diagnostic Tests

Diagnostic tests are recommended in each case of suspected measles. Obtain specimens for virology and molecular studies.

1. Serology (enzyme-linked immunosorbent assay [ELISA]): The diagnosis is confirmed by serum measles virus-specific IgM antibodies in a person who

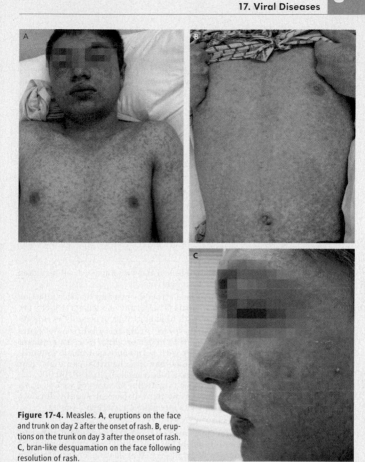

Figure 17-4. Measles. **A**, eruptions on the face and trunk on day 2 after the onset of rash. **B**, eruptions on the trunk on day 3 after the onset of rash. **C**, bran-like desquamation on the face following resolution of rash.

has not been vaccinated within the previous 2 to 3 months. The antibodies are detectable within 2 to 3 days of the onset of the rash and disappear over 4 to 5 weeks. Blood samples should be collected after >7 days from the onset of the rash (which is when the highest titers of specific IgM are observed). If the blood samples have been obtained too early and the result is negative, the test should be repeated. If IgM measurement is not feasible, the diagnosis of measles can be confirmed on the basis of a 4-fold increase in the specific IgG antibodies titer observed over a 4-week period (acute phase vs convalescence).

2. Detection via molecular techniques or culture: Clinical specimens (blood, urine, throat swab, nasopharyngeal swab/aspirate) should be collected, preferably within 1 to 4 days of the onset of the rash. Detection is now most easily done using molecular techniques (eg, polymerase chain reaction) on respiratory samples or urine at a reference laboratory, but isolation of measles virus from urine or peripheral blood mononuclear cells can still be undertaken. Sampling multiple sites increases sensitivity (eg, respiratory and urine).

Differential Diagnosis

Differential diagnosis should include other diseases associated with rash:

1) **Infections**: Scarlet fever (group A streptococcus), rubella, enteroviruses, adenoviruses, parvovirus B19, Epstein-Barr virus (particularly in patients with ampicillin/amoxicillin-triggered eruptions), *Mycoplasma*, leptospirosis.

2) **Noninfectious diseases**: Allergic and drug-induced cutaneous reactions, Kawasaki disease.

→ TREATMENT

Antiviral Treatment

No specific antiviral treatment is available.

Symptomatic Treatment

Treatment is symptomatic only and includes antipyretics, adequate hydration, and nutrition. Vitamin A treatment in doses up to 200,000 U daily for 2 days reduces mortality in deficient patients.◔ Bacterial complications (eg, pneumonia) require antimicrobial treatment.

→ COMPLICATIONS

Infants and adults (particularly malnourished and with impaired cell-mediated immunity) are at a higher risk for complications:

1) **Sinopulmonary infections** can result from the primary measles infection or bacterial superinfection. Otitis media (7% 9%) and pneumonia (1%-6%) are common; the latter is associated with high mortality, especially in infants.

2) **Neurologic complications** can be severe. Acute encephalitis only occurs in 0.1% of patients but is associated with high mortality (15%); a significant proportion of patients (25%) are left with permanent neurologic sequelae. Seizures (0.5%) and blindness (retrobulbar optic neuritis) can also occur. Subacute sclerosing panencephalitis, a rare complication (1-4/100,000; the prevalence increases to 1/8000 cases in patients <2 years of age), is a progressive, neurodegenerative, uniformly fatal disease; it usually develops several years after the measles virus infection (on average 7 years).

3) **Myocarditis, hepatitis** (rare).

4) **Secondary bacterial infections and exacerbation of latent tuberculosis** (measles virus induces transient but significant immunosuppression): These are often severe and may be fatal; persistent (lasting longer than a few days) or recurrent fever indicates possible complications.

→ PROGNOSIS

Measles usually has a mild or moderately severe course. Patients recovering from measles develop a lifelong immunity. Measles may have a particularly severe course and involve a high risk of complications in malnourished infants and young children (particularly vitamin A-deficient) and other immunodeficient patients. Deaths are rare and predominantly caused by complications (particularly in infants, malnourished individuals, and patients with impaired cell-mediated immunity).

→ PREVENTION

Specific Prevention

1. Vaccination is the key prevention method. Vaccination should be offered to nonimmune immunocompetent individuals after contact with a sick individual within 72 hours of exposure.

2. Passive immunoprophylaxis: Either IM or IV immunoglobulin (particularly for those >30kg) can be offered to susceptible contacts for whom vaccination is contraindicated (eg, immunocompromised individuals, pregnant women). It should be given within 6 days of exposure.

General Preventive Measures

1. Immunocompetent susceptible contacts should be in **airborne and contact isolation** from day 5 after the first exposure to day 21 after the last exposure to an infectious patient with measles. Immunocompetent individuals with measles should be isolated until 5 days after the onset of rash, and immunocompromised individuals with measles should be isolated for the duration of the illness.

2. Mandatory reporting and epidemiologic investigation: Each suspected case of measles should be reported to local public health authorities; as noted above, its transmissibility can quickly lead to outbreak situations.

17.7. Molluscum Contagiosum

→ DEFINITION, ETIOLOGY, PATHOGENESIS

Molluscum contagiosum is a chronic inflammatory viral skin disease that causes characteristic papular epidermal lesions.

1. Etiologic agent: Molluscum contagiosum virus (MCV), which replicates exclusively in squamous epithelial cells, does not spread into the deeper layers of skin, and does not cause viremia.

2. Reservoir and transmission: Humans are the only reservoir for MCV. Infection spreads through direct contact with the infected skin (including sexual contacts) or via contaminated clothing, towels, and other objects. Autoinoculation is frequent; this causes the lesions to spread to unaffected areas and leads to the persistent course of the disease.

3. Incubation and contagious period: The incubation period is 2 to 12 weeks (up to 6 months). The patient is contagious for the entire duration of cutaneous lesions.

→ CLINICAL FEATURES AND NATURAL HISTORY

The primary cutaneous lesions are firm, smooth, flesh-colored or lighter papules, measuring from 1 to 5 mm in diameter (in immunocompromised individuals >5 mm [so-called giant molluscum contagiosum]). Older lesions may be characteristically umbilicated with a dimple at the center, which is particularly visible when the lesion is illuminated from the side by a strong light source. The papule may be surrounded by a discolored or erythematous rim. In immunocompetent individuals, the number of lesions ranges from 1 to 30. In adolescents and adults, they are most frequently found on the inner thigh, external genital area, pubic area, and lower abdomen; in young children, on the face, eyelids, trunk, and extremities; in immunocompromised patients, the lesions are disseminated and numerous (up to several hundred). The lesions are otherwise asymptomatic, only rarely producing discomfort upon healing (in the case of intense inflammation or eczema).

In immunocompetent individuals, the infection resolves spontaneously over 6 to 18 months, occasionally persisting for up to 4 years. Receding lesions may be accompanied by a local inflammatory reaction (mild erythema, irritation), which indicates an active cell-mediated immune response (the clinical manifestation of recovery). Healed lesions may leave the dimples, which subsequently disappear or evolve into point-like scars.

Autoinoculation, secondary bacterial infection (in particular if the lesions are being scratched), and scarring may complicate the course of the disease.

→ **DIAGNOSIS**

Diagnosis is based on the clinical presentation. In equivocal cases, a microscopic examination of smears of the contents of the lesions or skin biopsy material stained with Wright or Giemsa stain may reveal cytoplasmic inclusions ("molluscum bodies").

Differential Diagnosis

1. Spitz nevus, epitheliomas (eg, basal cell carcinoma), juvenile xanthogranuloma, common warts, condylomata acuminata, milia, keratosis pilaris, lichen nitidus, and sebaceous or sudoriferous cysts.

2. Disseminated lesions in patients with impaired cell-mediated immune response should be differentiated from disseminated cryptococcosis or histoplasmosis.

3. In patients with inflammatory molluscum contagiosum, exclude bacterial skin infections (eg, folliculitis, furuncle).

→ **TREATMENT**

Most lesions in low-risk patients are self-limiting and do not require treatment. If judged needed (eg, for esthetic reasons, or in the case of multiple, persistent, or refractory lesions, repeated development of new lesions, or autoinoculation) a number of treatments may be tried. However, most evidence is of low quality and cannot be recommended with confidence.⊘◯ According to authors of one Cochrane review, "no randomised trials for several commonly used treatments, such as expressing lesions with an orange stick or topical hydrogen peroxide" could be found. And "since most lesions resolve within months, unless better evidence for the superiority of active treatments emerges, molluscum contagiosum can be left to heal naturally."

Antiviral Treatment

1. Pharmacologic treatment (please note above the comment regarding questionable, if any, efficacy):

1) Topical imiquimod (cream) 3 times per week for 4 to 16 weeks: Apply to the affected areas overnight (6-10 hours), wash off in the morning.

2) Topical podophyllotoxin cream or solution may also be considered, particularly in men; use with caution in women of childbearing age.

3) Highly active antiretroviral therapy (HAART) is associated with the resolution of lesions in HIV-positive patients (data is limited).

2. Invasive treatment (according to authors of the Cochrane review, the evidence for effectiveness of physical destruction of molluscum is very limited and, until this changes, awaiting spontaneous resolution of molluscum lesions remains a strong option):

1) Laser therapy: Effective, associated with a low risk of scarring or discoloration.

2) Liquid nitrogen spray cryotherapy in the case of a limited number of lesions; possible complications include blisters and scars. In some patients the procedure may need to be repeated every 2 to 4 weeks.

3) Curettage or needle extraction under local anesthesia may be used in patients with a limited number of lesions.

→ **FOLLOW-UP**

In the case of reasonable suspicion, examine adolescents and adults for the presence of other sexually transmitted diseases. If a treated lesion becomes tender or reveals erythema, edema, crusting, or purulent exudate (suggesting a secondary bacterial infection), administer topical antimicrobial treatment (less frequently, oral antimicrobial treatment is necessary). Disseminated lesions (in particular giant molluscum contagiosum) and lesions appearing on the face, neck, and scalp in adult patients are an indication for HIV testing.

→ PROGNOSIS

In immunocompetent individuals the lesions resolve spontaneously. In severely immunocompromised patients the disease is protracted and produces giant, generalized, confluent, and disfiguring lesions, which are difficult to treat unless a normal immune function is restored.

→ PREVENTION

Sharing of clothing and towels as well as maintaining sexual contacts with infected individuals should be avoided. Examination of household contacts is recommended (the infection is frequently transmitted among household contacts). Lesions should not be rubbed or scratched (risk of autoinoculation).

17.8. Mumps

→ ETIOLOGY AND PATHOGENESIS

1. Etiologic agent: Mumps virus, an enveloped RNA virus in the Paramyxoviridae family. It enters the respiratory system (initially replicating in the respiratory epithelium), causes viremia, and infects multiple organs and tissues (including the salivary glands and central nervous system).

2. Reservoir and transmission: Humans are the only reservoir for mumps virus. The virus is transmitted from a person with mumps or asymptomatic infection via droplets as well as by direct or indirect contact with contagious biological material (blood, saliva, cerebrospinal fluid, urine) or contaminated objects.

3. Incubation and contagious period: The incubation period is from 12 to 25 days (typically 16-18 days). Patients may have viral shedding in the saliva up to 7 days before the onset of parotitis and up to 9 days afterwards (virus shedding in urine is observed for up to 2 weeks).

→ CLINICAL FEATURES

In up to a third of patients, mumps is either asymptomatic or subclinical with only mild respiratory tract symptoms. Symptomatic mumps virus infections have a sudden onset and acute course. All of the following signs and symptoms may occur simultaneously, separately, or in various combinations.

1. Prodromal phase (influenza-like symptoms): Rarely observed in children, but more frequent in adults; it occurs 1 to 7 days prior to parotitis.

2. Parotitis is the most common presentation (60%-70%); the submandibular salivary glands are affected less frequently (10%). Although it may often present with unilateral swelling, ultimately most cases progress to bilateral involvement (~70%). The clinical manifestations of parotitis include the following:
1) Pain and swelling of the salivary glands, which is most pronounced on day 2 or 3; typically the gland is soft (pitting edema), though occasionally it may be firm. The skin above the gland is taut, but of otherwise normal appearance. The swelling gradually extends to the surrounding tissues (temporal area, zygomatic arch, mastoid process, neck) causing an outward displacement of the earlobe. The symptoms begin to subside within 3 to 4 days and resolve within ~7 days.

2) Characteristic appearance of the buccal mucosa: Erythema and edema around the orifice of the parotid duct.

3) Earache on the side of involvement.

4) Decreased production of saliva ("dry mouth" sensation), parotid pain exacerbated by consumption of acidic foods (or any other products that stimulate the production of saliva).

5) Difficulties in chewing, swallowing (dysphagia), and opening the mouth.

6) Fever (38°C-39°C) appears simultaneously with glandular swelling and persists for 3 to 4 days; it recurs when a new salivary gland becomes involved or complications develop. Young children may remain afebrile.

7) Other signs and symptoms: Malaise and fatigue, headache, appetite loss, vomiting.

3. Mumps meningitis: Cerebrospinal fluid pleocytosis is observed in over half of patients with mumps parotitis, most of whom do not have symptoms of meningitis or encephalitis. The majority of cases are either associated with minor symptoms or asymptomatic. Clinical features of meningitis occur in 5% to 10% of patients, more frequently in adults and males, usually between day 4 and day 8 of infection (less commonly before the onset of parotitis or during convalescence). Signs and symptoms are usually mild and resolve within 1 week; however, more severe sequelae can occur (eg, deafness, paresis, hydrocephalus) and mortalities have been reported at a rate of ~1%. Up to half of meningitis cases occur in the absence of parotitis.

➲ DIAGNOSIS

Typical cases can be diagnosed on the basis of supportive medical history, exposure history, and physical examination, but given the current rarity of the infection and that other infectious agents can cause similar presentations, laboratory confirmation is generally sought. Given that even the administration of 2 doses of the vaccine is not 100% effective, in regions of high vaccination coverage many cases occur in fully vaccinated individuals and therefore vaccination history cannot be used to exclude the diagnosis.

Diagnostic Tests

1. Biochemistry: Increased serum and urinary amylase levels support the involvement of salivary glands.

2. Complete blood count: The white blood count is often low with a relative lymphocytosis.

3. Serum serology: This is only reliable in nonvaccinated individuals. Positive IgM response in the acute phase of the disease and/or a ≥4-fold increase in specific IgG levels between acute and convalescent sera are generally diagnostic. In vaccinated patients who develop mumps, IgG levels may be elevated in the acute period and IgM may not appear, and therefore serologic diagnosis is often not possible.

4. Detection of mumps virus: Mumps virus is detected either through culture or detection of viral RNA using reverse transcription polymerase chain reaction (RT-PCR). Suitable specimens include buccal (around the duct of Stensen) or pharyngeal swabs, blood, urine, and cerebrospinal fluid. The sooner the sample is collected after the symptom onset, the higher the yield.

Differential Diagnosis

1. Other infectious causes of parotitis: Viral (parainfluenza virus, influenza virus, cytomegalovirus, enteroviruses, lymphocytic choriomeningitis virus, HIV, Epstein-Barr virus); bacterial, including abscess (most frequently *Staphylococcus*, less commonly *Mycobacterium*, *Actinomyces*; purulent drainage may be present around the orifice of the parotid duct, appearing spontaneously or after applying pressure to the involved gland); cat-scratch disease (anterior auricular lymphadenopathy, Parinaud syndrome); toxoplasmosis.

2. Noninfectious causes of parotid gland enlargement: Sialolithiasis, ductal obstruction (in patients with recurrent obstruction, perform ultrasonography, sialography, or both); cyst, angioma, or salivary gland tumor (perform ultrasonography, histologic examination, or both); Sjögren syndrome, Waldenström macroglobulinemia, sarcoidosis; drug-induced allergic reactions (iodides, guanethidine, phenylbutazone, thiouracil); trauma; cystic fibrosis; amyloidosis.

3. Diseases affecting the adjacent tissues and organs: Lymphadenopathy, bone tumors (eg, mandibular tumor), arthritis of the temporomandibular joint, hypertrophy of the sternocleidomastoid muscle.

4. In patients with meningitis and no signs of parotitis: Other types of aseptic meningitis (of a viral or tuberculous etiology).

→ TREATMENT

Antiviral Treatment

No specific antiviral treatment is available.

Symptomatic Treatment

Antipyretics and analgesics when necessary (acetaminophen [INN paracetamol], nonsteroidal anti-inflammatory drugs). Adequate hydration, mouth rinsing, avoidance of sour-tasting foods.

→ COMPLICATIONS AND LESS COMMON PRESENTATIONS

Adults are at higher risk of complications of mumps than children. Complications may develop during the acute disease phase, convalescence, or even later; rarely, they may precede parotitis or are the only manifestation of the disease. Note: Recurrence of fever and vomiting in the course of mumps suggests the development of complications.

1. Epididymo-orchitis: Unilateral or bilateral, it affects 30% to 40% of pubertal boys and young men with mumps and usually occurs at the end of the first week of the disease (frequently accompanied by meningitis). Epididymo-orchitis may affect spermatogenesis and cause infertility (this is a rare complication, usually resulting from bilateral infection).

Signs and symptoms: Sudden onset, fever, severe testicular pain with referred perineal pain, testicular edema, erythema and warming; lower abdominal pain, headache, chills, nausea, and vomiting. The symptoms usually persist for 4 days. Orchitis can occur prior to or in the absence of parotitis. Mumps virus RNA can be detected in seminal fluid weeks after infection. Differential diagnosis: bacterial epididymo-orchitis (chlamydia, syphilis, gonorrhea, tuberculosis), testicular torsion, injury.

Treatment: Symptomatic treatment includes analgesics (in some cases even opioids may be necessary), suspensory garment (or tight underwear), bed rest, which may alleviate the pain, and ice packs. Glucocorticoids are not effective and may worsen the course of parotitis and increase the risk of secondary bacterial infection.

2. Oophoritis: Unilateral or bilateral, it affects 5% to 7% of postpubertal girls and women. Signs and symptoms are less severe than in the case of epididymo-orchitis and are more like those of acute appendicitis (lower abdominal pain or tenderness). Oophoritis is not believed to cause infertility.

3. Pancreatitis: Affects <10% of patients, usually occurs in the later phases of the disease (up to a few weeks after parotitis). Approximately one-third of patients with pancreatitis have no concomitant parotitis.

Signs and symptoms: Acute upper abdominal pain (may be accompanied by referred left abdominal and back pain), nausea and vomiting, fever and chills, diarrhea; increased serum lipase levels (in parotitis, blood and urine amylase levels are also increased). Usually, pancreatitis resolves spontaneously within 7 days.

Symptomatic treatment: →Chapter 6.3.1. Opioid analgesics may be necessary in some cases.

4. Other (rare) complications:

1) **Neurologic**: Guillain-Barré syndrome, transverse myelitis, polyneuropathies, labyrinthitis, facial nerve palsy, hearing loss.

2) **Ophthalmologic**: Conjunctivitis, dacryoadenitis, scleritis, keratitis, uveitis/iritis, optic neuritis.

3) **Hematologic**: Thrombocytopenia, paroxysmal nocturnal hemoglobinuria.

4) **Other**: Thyroiditis, arthritis (0.4% risk, usually affects large joints), myocarditis, thymitis, hepatitis with acute cholecystitis, mastitis, nephritis; infection during the first trimester of pregnancy increases the risk of miscarriage.

➡ PROGNOSIS

In the majority of cases, the prognosis is favorable and depends on the type of complications (→Complications and Less Common Presentations, above). Mumps usually confers lifelong immunity; a second mumps infection is extremely rare. Recurrent parotitis most frequently develops in patients with ductal obstruction (perform sialography) or immunodeficiency (cytomegalovirus or human immunodeficiency virus infection, Sjögren syndrome). Infection during pregnancy does not increase the risk of malformations.

➡ PREVENTION

1. Vaccination is the key prevention method. Two doses of mumps-containing vaccine administered after 1 year of age are recommended given the reduced effectiveness of 1 dose (estimated at ~80%). There is also evidence of some waning immunity with age.

2. Exposed individuals: Mumps vaccine given after exposure has not been shown to reduce the risk of developing disease.

3. Suggest **limitation of social contacts** to decrease the propagation of infection for 5 days following the onset of parotitis.

4. Hospitalized patients: Droplet precautions are recommended until 9 days after parotid swelling.

17.9. Parvovirus B19–Related Diseases

Parvovirus B19 causes erythema infectiosum ("fifth disease" or "slapped--cheek disease") in children as well as the papular-purpuric "gloves-and-socks" syndrome (PPGSS). Infection may also cause polyarthritis, hydrops fetalis in pregnancy, aplastic anemia in persons with underlying hematological disorders, and chronic anemia in immunocompromised persons.

➡ ETIOLOGY, PATHOGENESIS

1. Etiologic agent: Human parvovirus B19 (Parvoviridae family) is a DNA virus that causes viremia and replicates exclusively in erythroid progenitor cells.

2. Reservoir and transmission: Humans are the only reservoir for parvovirus B19; the source of infection is an infected individual. Parvovirus B19 is transmitted predominantly via respiratory droplets but may also spread via blood products (very rarely) and transplacental infection from mother to fetus.

3. Incubation and contagious period: The disease is highly contagious, with attack rates of up to 60%. The incubation period is 4 to 14 days. In erythema infectiosum, viral loads peak within 6 to 10 days of infection, when the risk of transmission is highest, and decrease with the onset of rash. Viral shedding lasts ~1 week and patients are unlikely to be infectious after the appearance of rash. However, patients with PPGSS are contagious for the entire duration of rash, and patients with aplastic crisis are contagious before the onset of symptoms and for at least 1 week after symptoms have appeared.

→ CLINICAL FEATURES

The course of parvovirus B19 infection is frequently asymptomatic or associated with mild influenza-like symptoms. Symptomatic disease most commonly manifests as erythema infectiosum.

1. **Erythema infectiosum**:

1) **Initial prodromal symptoms are associated with viremia** and include upper respiratory tract infection (rhinitis, pharyngitis, cough), fever, malaise, headache, myalgia, and nausea. The symptoms resolve with the appearance of specific IgM antibodies.

2) **Rash** (immune complex–mediated) develops within 7 to 10 days of the onset of the disease (upon the appearance of specific IgG antibodies); this is the most characteristic sign of infection (observed in most children but in <50% of adults). Initially, a bright red, slightly elevated and well-demarcated erythema appears on the cheeks, sparing the nasal bridge and area around the mouth. Over the next 1 to 4 days, erythematous macules and papules appear on the arms, trunk, buttocks, and lower extremities, subsequently evolving into erythematous coalescent blotches with a lacy, net-like appearance, particularly distinct on the extensor surfaces and trunk. The palms and soles remain free of rash. The rash may remit and relapse over a period of 1 to 3 weeks or longer, but usually lasts ~10 days. In adults, it may be pruritic. The rash may worsen with increased physical activity or increased body temperature.

3) **Arthritis** (immune complex–mediated) develops predominantly in adults, more frequently in women (children are affected in ~10% of cases). Arthritis may coincide with the onset of rash or appear as the only manifestation of the disease. The clinical presentation is dominated by pain (affecting 77% of patients >20 years); swelling is less frequent (observed in 57% of patients >20 years) and usually affects the small joints of the hand, wrist, knee, and ankle. The disease is self-limiting (usually resolves within 3 weeks, but may persist for several months) and does not cause joint damage.

2. **PPGSS**:

1) A **mild prodromal phase**: Fever, loss of appetite, arthralgia.

2) The **onset of rash** during the prodromal phase with viremia; painful edema and erythema involves both hands and feet and is associated with petechial and purpuric eruptions. The lesions may also involve the dorsal surfaces of hands and feet, with sharp demarcation at the wrists and ankles, and are frequently accompanied by a burning sensation and pruritus. The rash usually disappears within 1 to 3 weeks.

3) Development of **oral mucosal lesions**: Erosions, vesicles, lip edema, petechiae on the hard palate and the pharyngeal and lingual mucosa. The lesions of the oral mucosa may appear concomitantly with skin lesions and resolve spontaneously after 7 to 14 days.

3. **Chronic anemia** results from an inadequate or absent antibody response that allows the virus to persist, leading to red cell aplasia. Chronic anemia occurs in immunocompromised patients (with primary immunodeficiency syndromes, malignancy, HIV infection, transplant recipients, and other causes of immunosuppression) as a consequence of a chronic parvovirus B19 infection of erythroid progenitor cells.

4. Aplastic crisis: This may occur in patients with hemolysis or decreased red blood cell production (sickle cell disease, thalassemia, hereditary spherocytosis), in whom viral replication results in a further decrease of red blood cell production and rapid hemolysis with an abrupt fall in hemoglobin concentrations. Aplastic crisis is associated with the clinical features of severe anemia.

5. Hydrops fetalis: Parvovirus infection in pregnant women may result in fetal anemia and hydrops fetalis, or may lead to miscarriage, particularly when infection occurs before 20 weeks' gestation.

6. Rarely, parvovirus manifests as hepatitis, myocarditis, vasculitis, or encephalitis. Hepatitis affects ~4% of patients with parvovirus B19 infection and resolves spontaneously.

→ DIAGNOSIS

Diagnosis is based on the clinical features. Diagnostic tests are usually not needed. When necessary, the diagnosis is confirmed by the following:

1) In **immunocompetent patients**: A **positive serology result**; detection of parvovirus B19 IgM antibodies in serum indicates an infection within the previous 7 to 120 days; detection of a 4-fold increase of IgG also indicates acute infection. Specific IgG antibody appears within 2 weeks of infection and persists for many years (indicating a past infection). The presence of low-avidity antibodies suggests a recent infection.

2) In **immunocompromised patients or patients with aplastic crisis**: **Detection of parvovirus B19 DNA** in the blood by molecular testing (polymerase chain reaction [PCR]). Serologic tests may be negative. PCR may remain positive for 9 months after infection, and therefore is unhelpful in diagnosing acute infection.

Bone marrow examination reveals features of hypoplasia and the presence of characteristic giant pronormoblasts.

Differential Diagnosis

1. Erythema infectiosum: Rash of other viral (echovirus 12, rubella, measles, enterovirus, or adenovirus infections) or bacterial (scarlet fever) etiology, erythema multiforme, arthritis and vasculitis in connective tissue diseases, and drug-induced reactions (including serum sickness).

2. PPGSS: Thrombocytopenia; IgA-associated vasculitis (Henoch-Schönlein purpura); hand-foot-and-mouth disease (HFMD) (coxsackievirus or enterovirus infection); infectious mononucleosis; cytomegalovirus infection; human herpesvirus 6 (HHV-6) infection; hepatitis B.

3. Chronic anemia and aplastic crisis (→Chapter 7.2.1).

→ TREATMENT

Antiviral Treatment

No antiviral treatment is available. In immunocompromised patients with chronic infection, intravenous immunoglobulin (IVIG) is suggested.☺○ No standard dosage has been established; the recommended doses are 1 to 1.5 g/kg for 3 days or 400 mg/kg for 5 to 10 days.

Symptomatic Treatment

When needed, use antipyretics (acetaminophen [INN paracetamol], ibuprofen) or other nonsteroidal anti-inflammatory drugs (to reduce arthralgia). It is recommended that antiretroviral therapy and IVIG is administered to patients with HIV infection, and that patients with aplastic crisis and chronic anemia are administered packed red blood cells and IVIG.

→ **FOLLOW-UP**

Follow-up visits are recommended in immunocompromised patients and patients with chronic hemolysis to monitor for severe anemia.

It is recommended that pregnant women exposed to parvovirus B19 should be tested for specific serum IgG. If parvovirus IgG is present and IgM is negative, the woman is immune. While a negative IgG indicates susceptibility to infection, the absolute risk of fetal infection is low. A diagnosis of an acute parvovirus B19 infection during pregnancy (positive IgM) would be an indication for ultrasonography repeated every 1 or 2 weeks for 10 to 12 weeks to detect the development of fetal anemia and hydrops.

→ **COMPLICATIONS**

Complications of parvovirus B19 infection include transient anemia and reticulocytopenia (rare in otherwise healthy individuals, usually asymptomatic); erythema multiforme; severe anemia with hydrops fetalis (the most frequent cause for nonimmune generalized fetal edema), miscarriage, or fetal death. The rate of transplacental transmission of parvovirus B19 is ~30%; the risk of pregnancy loss due to infection is 8% to 10%, highest before 20 weeks' gestation. The overall incidence of hydrops fetalis following maternal infection is 2.9%, but it is higher if infection occurs earlier in pregnancy. Rare complications include myocarditis, vasculitis, glomerulonephritis, encephalitis, and primary immune thrombocytopenic purpura.

→ **PROGNOSIS**

In low-risk patients the course of infection is mild and infection resolves spontaneously without sequelae. Rash may continue to recur over several months; arthritis can persist for several months, occasionally even years. Immunocompetent individuals acquire long-term immunity upon recovery. Immunocompromised patients are at risk of chronic infection.

→ **PREVENTION**

In health-care settings droplet precautions are recommended for symptomatic individuals, in particular patients with aplastic crisis or immunocompromised persons who remain contagious for a longer time. Pregnant women should avoid contact with patients with prolonged viral replication. Vaccine is not available.

17.10. Rubella

→ **DEFINITION, ETIOLOGY, PATHOGENESIS**

Rubella (German measles) is an acute systemic viral disease, typically accompanied by a generalized rash. Congenital rubella syndrome (CRS) is a constellation of congenital malformations in infants caused by maternal infection with rubella virus during the first 4 months of pregnancy. Congenital infection is possible after the first 4 months of pregnancy, but clinical manifestations are rare in this situation.

1. Etiologic agent: Rubella virus, which is a single-stranded RNA virus in the Togaviridae family. The virus infects the upper respiratory tract, spreads to the local lymph nodes, and replicates there, causing viremia. Rubella virus can infect the majority of cells and tissues (eg, lymphocytes, monocytes, conjunctiva, synovium, cervix, placenta).

2. Reservoir and transmission: Humans are the only reservoir for rubella virus. It is transmitted by respiratory droplets, direct contact with infectious material (particularly respiratory secretions, but also urine, blood, feces), and via the placenta (congenital infection).

3. Incubation and contagious period: The incubation period is from 14 to 23 days (usually 16-18 days). Rubella is most contagious from a few days before the appearance of rash until 7 days after the appearance of rash; however, viral shedding can occur up to 7 days before and 14 days after the appearance of rash. Congenitally infected infants can shed virus for a year or longer. Fetal infection occurs during primary viremia in the mother; the risk of infection is from 85% to 100% when the rash appears during the first 12 weeks of pregnancy; 54% when it appears in weeks 13 to 16; and 25% when it appears in weeks 17 to 22. Fetal involvement in the course of recurrent infection is possible, however the risk is very low.

→ CLINICAL FEATURES

Rubella is frequently asymptomatic (in ~50% of patients) or manifests with minor symptoms. In other patients, the signs and symptoms appear in the following order (although some may be absent):

1. Prodromal signs and symptoms (persisting for a few days): Malaise, headache and myalgia, pharyngitis, rhinitis, dry cough, conjunctivitis (without photophobia), low-grade fever, loss of appetite.

2. Painful lymphadenopathy affecting the occipital, posterior auricular, posterior, or anterior cervical lymph nodes. It develops 1 day prior to the onset of rash and may be the only symptom of the disease. Lymphadenopathy persists for several weeks.

3. Rash: A variable generalized macular or maculopapular rash. Initially, it appears on the face (typically behind the ears) and trunk, then spreads to the extremities over 1 or 2 days. The rash on the face may look like that in measles (the lesions are confluent), but it also involves the skin between the nasolabial folds. The lesions on the trunk are similar to scarlet fever. The rash may be accompanied by pruritus. Lesions disappear after 2 to 3 days and do not leave discolorations; fine desquamation is possible.

4. Other (less common): Splenomegaly, pharyngitis, petechiae on the soft palate, transient hepatitis.

5. CRS: Clinical manifestations depend on the time of infection (the week of pregnancy), with more severe manifestations associated with infections early in gestation. Miscarriage is a frequent result of infection in the first few weeks. The following is a list of potential manifestations of CRS:

1) Intrauterine growth retardation.
2) Central nervous system: Meningoencephalitis, microcephaly, large anterior fontanelle, sensorineural hearing loss, developmental delays.
3) Ophthalmologic: Cataracts, infantile glaucoma, pigmentary retinopathy, microphthalmos.
4) Dermatologic: Dermal erythropoiesis ("blueberry muffin" syndrome).
5) Cardiac: Patent ductus arteriosus, peripheral pulmonary artery stenosis.
6) Respiratory: Interstitial pneumonitis.
7) Gastrointestinal: Hepatosplenomegaly, jaundice, hepatitis, diarrhea.
8) Other: Radiolucent bone lesions (in the long bones), adenopathy, hemolytic anemia, thrombocytopenia.

→ DIAGNOSIS

Diagnosis of rubella made solely on the basis of the clinical presentation is highly unreliable. Therefore, laboratory diagnosis should be made particularly in suspected cases in pregnant women and newborn infants. In vaccinated patients (even with only 1 vaccine dose), rubella is unlikely.

1. Serology (enzyme-linked immunosorbent assay, indirect immunofluorescence) is the key method of confirming the diagnosis of an acquired infection that is used in epidemiologic investigations:

1) Rubella-specific serum IgM antibodies (false-positive and false-negative results are possible) appear on day 2 after the onset of the rash, persist for ~1 month, and reappear in the case of reinfection.

2) A more than 4-fold increase in rubella-specific serum IgG antibodies over a period of 2 to 4 weeks or seroconversion between acute and convalescent serum titers are both diagnostic of postnatal infection. Stable IgG titers indicate a history of infection and a resulting immunity.

2. Isolation of the virus (culture) or viral RNA (reverse transcription polymerase chain reaction [RT-PCR]) from various specimens: throat or nasopharynx, urine, blood, or cerebrospinal fluid; this is particularly useful in diagnosing CRS.

Other diseases associated with a generalized rash:

1) **Infections**: Measles, scarlet fever (group A streptococcus), enteroviruses, adenoviruses, parvovirus B19, Epstein-Barr virus, *Mycoplasma*.

2) **Noninfectious diseases**: Drug-induced and allergic reactions.

Congenital infections that can have similar presentations as CRS: Cytomegalovirus, toxoplasmosis, herpes simplex virus, HIV, syphilis, lymphocytic choriomeningitis virus, Chagas disease (*Trypanosoma cruzi*).

→ TREATMENT

Specific antiviral treatment is not available.

Treatment is symptomatic only:

1) Arthritis: Nonsteroidal anti-inflammatory drugs.

2) Clinically significant thrombocytopenia: Prednisone (1 mg/kg) or platelet concentrates.

3) Encephalitis.

→ COMPLICATIONS

1. Arthritis: More common in adolescents and adults, particularly in girls and young women (prevalence, 1%-25%). Arthritis may develop at the end of the rash phase and up to several weeks after its resolution; it predominantly involves small joints of the hand and wrist, less commonly other joints (eg, the knee). The symptoms persist for 5 to 10 days (rarely extending to several weeks) and resolve spontaneously without sequelae.

2. Thrombocytopenia (incidence <1/3000): Persists for several days (rarely up to 6 months), resolves spontaneously.

3. Encephalitis (incidence, 1/5000): Develops within 7 days of the onset of rash and usually resolves within a week without sequelae. Prognosis is good. Mortality rates are low.

4. Other (rare): Myocarditis, optic neuritis, Guillain-Barré syndrome, bone marrow aplasia.

→ **PROGNOSIS**

The prognosis in patients with acquired rubella is good; the vast majority acquires lifelong immunity. CRS is associated with worse outcomes (mortality rates are >15%; complications include psychomotor developmental delay, malformations, and other permanent sequelae).

→ **PREVENTION**

Specific Prevention

1. Vaccination is the key prevention method.

2. Passive immunoprophylaxis (immunoglobulin) is controversial and may be used in exceptional situations. In particular, immunoglobulin may be considered as postexposure prophylaxis for susceptible women who have had exposure early in pregnancy, although the efficacy of this intervention is not clear⊘⊝.

General Preventive Measures

1. Isolation of hospitalized patients (particularly from women of childbearing age): Acquired rubella: droplet isolation for up to 7 days after the appearance of the rash; congenital rubella: contact isolation of children until at least 12 months of age, or until after 3 months of age if no virus was isolated from the nasopharynx and urine on 2 subsequent occasions. Children hospitalized due to a congenital cataract should be considered as potentially infectious until the age of 3.

2. Serologic screening of young unvaccinated women (for whom vaccination records are not available): Prompt vaccination of patients with negative specific IgG unless they are known to be pregnant.

3. Prenatal screening of women: If routine prenatal screening identifies a woman as nonimmune, she should be provided with vaccination immediately after birth (prior to discharge).

17.11. Varicella

→ **DEFINITION, ETIOLOGY, PATHOGENESIS**

Varicella (chickenpox) is an acute systemic viral infection associated with a characteristic vesicular rash.

1. Etiologic agent: Varicella-zoster virus (VZV), which enters the upper respiratory tract and/or conjunctiva and spreads to the reticuloendothelial system where it replicates, thus leading to viremia. VZV infects the epidermal and mucosal cells (as well as many other organs and tissues) and remains latent in dorsal root ganglia. After many years, a latent VZV may reactivate, resulting in herpes zoster (shingles).

2. Reservoir and transmission: Humans are the only reservoir for VZV. The source of infection is a patient with varicella or herpes zoster. Patients with varicella transmit the virus very effectively via droplets and direct contact; secondary attack rates approach 90%, and in temperate countries prior to universal immunization infection was ubiquitous in childhood. Those with zoster are only contagious via direct contact with skin lesions. Varicella can also infect the fetus through transplacental transmission.

3. Risk factors for a severe course of varicella and complications: Pregnancy (susceptible women only), in particular the second and third trimesters; immunosuppressive treatment including prolonged high-dose glucocorticoid therapy (prednisone >20 mg/d, or 2 mg/kg/d for ≥14 days); leukemia, lymphoma, or chemotherapy treatment; primary immune deficiency; newborns of mothers who developed varicella between 5 days prior to delivery and up to

48 hours after delivery; all hospitalized premature infants born before 28 weeks' gestation; and hospitalized premature infants born after 28 weeks' gestation to a susceptible woman. Other risk factors for moderate-to-severe disease include age ≥13 years, chronic pulmonary or skin disorders, chronic salicylate therapy, and prolonged aerosolized or low-dose glucocorticoid therapy.

4. Incubation and contagious period: The incubation period is 10 to 21 days (usually 14-16 days); it is prolonged to 28 days in immunocompromised patients who receive postexposure prophylaxis with varicella hyperimmunoglobulin and shorter (2-16 days) in newborns exposed in the perinatal period. Individuals are infectious from 24 to 48 hours prior to the onset of rash until all vesicles have dried and crusted over (usually after ~7 days).

→ CLINICAL FEATURES

Varicella is rarely asymptomatic, though it is not uncommon for seropositive adults (and their immediate family members) to have no recollection of childhood illness.

1. Prodromal phase: One to 2 days prior to the onset of rash nonspecific symptoms appear, including fever, malaise, headache, myalgia, pharyngitis, rhinitis, and loss of appetite. Occasionally, abdominal pain and diarrhea can be observed.

2. Rash:

1) A generalized, very pruritic vesicular rash, which begins as erythematous macules that evolve into papules 5 to 10 mm in diameter, with subsequent formation of vesicles filled with fluid that is initially clear and later becomes turbid. After 2 to 3 days, the lesions evolve into pustules, which dry and crust over the next 3 to 4 days. The crusts eventually fall off, leaving discolorations that disappear in patients with uncomplicated disease. Hemorrhagic lesions may develop in immunocompromised subjects. Because successive crops of skin eruptions appear over the initial

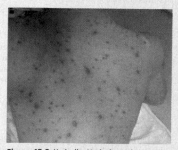

Figure 17-5. Varicella. Vesicular rash at various stages of evolution ("starry sky" appearance).

3 to 4 days, the fully developed rash is polymorphic, that is, consists of "crops" of lesions at various stages of evolution ("starry sky" appearance: →Figure 17-5). Eruptions appear on the head (including the scalp) and trunk, later on the arms, and eventually involve the lower extremities (rarely the hands and feet). A vesicular rash that begins peripherally and does not exhibit "crops" in different stages of development is unlikely to be varicella. The number of lesions varies, ranging from less than 10 to several hundred. In 10% to 20% of patients, the lesions are found on the oral, pharyngeal, and genital mucosa, as well as the conjunctiva and cornea (fine ulcerations). Rash in immunized individuals ("breakthrough varicella") almost always involves many fewer lesions, which usually appear atypical (ie, are not vesicular) and cause much less pruritus.

2) Fever (usually within 4 days from the onset of the rash) and lymphadenopathy are common with primary varicella and very unusual with breakthrough disease.

3. Perinatal/neonatal varicella results from infection of the fetus around the time of delivery. Infants born to mothers in whom the onset of rash occurred within 5 days before delivery or 48 hours after delivery do not receive protective maternal antibody and develop transplacental viremia; consequently, they frequently develop severe disseminated disease (including pneumonitis, hepatitis, and meningoencephalitis) and outcomes are very poor.

4. Congenital varicella results from transplacental infection of the fetus early in gestation. Infection in the first and second trimesters leads to fetal death or congenital varicella syndrome (in 1%-2% of newborns born to mothers who acquired varicella within the first 20 weeks of pregnancy): limb hypoplasia, violaceous cicatricial skin scarring, central nervous system defects (microcephaly, developmental delay, seizures), cataract, retinitis, and uveitis. As symptoms and signs are the result of the disruption of normal embryogenesis from a long-ago infection, these neonates are not usually acutely unwell, though the overall neurodevelopmental prognosis is not good. Infants born to mothers who acquired varicella after the 20th week of pregnancy do not develop congenital varicella syndrome but may develop herpes zoster early in life.

→ DIAGNOSIS

Diagnosis is usually based on the clinical presentation of a polymorphic vesicular rash and a history of contact with a sick person, though this is substantially more difficult in the era of universal immunization.

Diagnostic Tests

Diagnostic tests are recommended in equivocal cases and in those with the possibility of severe disease (risk factors: →Definition, Etiology, Pathogenesis, above) who might benefit from antiviral therapy.

1. Detection of VZV using viral culture or polymerase chain reaction (PCR). Culture usually takes up to a week and is less sensitive; consequently, PCR is generally preferred. New vesicles should be de-roofed and swabbed to obtain specimens for testing. Genotyping can also be used to distinguish vaccine from wild-type strains.

2. Detection of VZV antigens in epithelial cells using a direct immuno-fluorescence assay (specimen: scrapings from the base of the vesicles); this is less sensitive and specific than PCR.

3. Serology is not useful as a rapid diagnostic test. Detection of specific serum IgG is usually helpful in confirming prior infection and acquired immunity. Many commercially available (whole-cell lysate) enzyme-linked immunosorbent assays do not have good sensitivity for the detection of vaccine-induced immunity, so such testing of immune responses is not routinely recommended.

Differential Diagnosis

Other infections that can lead to generalized vesicular rashes include enteroviruses and disseminated herpes simplex ("eczema herpeticum"), especially in individuals with preexisting atopic dermatitis. Smallpox and monkeypox present in a similar fashion to varicella but are extremely rare and are associated with specific features on history. Bullous impetigo (often caused by staphylococcal infections) typically features bullae, not small vesicular lesions. Noninfectious causes of vesicular lesions include drug rashes, atopic dermatitis, and papular urticaria.

→ TREATMENT

In immunocompetent patients ≤12 years of age and in patients with mild varicella, no specific therapy is indicated.⊗◖ Antiviral treatment for previously healthy children aged <18 years demonstrated that acyclovir (INN aciclovir) started early in infection reduces the duration of fever by ~1 day and reduces the overall number of lesions, but leads to no other improvements in outcomes (including the duration of pruritus). Daily baths or showers followed by careful drying of the skin with a towel are recommended in all cases. Antihistamines can reduce pruritus. Acetylsalicylic acid (ASA) should be avoided; ASA therapy during varicella has been associated with the development of Reye syndrome.

Antiviral Treatment

Antiviral treatment is indicated for patients at high risk of complications or those with severe varicella or complications. Valacyclovir, a prodrug of acyclovir, has 3 to 5 times higher bioavailability than acyclovir and is therefore generally preferred to acyclovir.

1) In those with risk factors for **moderate to severe disease** (including age ≥13 years, chronic pulmonary or skin disorders, chronic salicylate therapy, and low-dose systemic or aerosolized glucocorticoid therapy) and pregnant women, use oral valacyclovir 1000 mg tid for 5 days or acyclovir 800 mg qid for 5 to 7 days, starting ideally within 24 hours of the onset of rash.

2) In patients at **high risk for severe disease** (including malignancy, immunosuppressive medications, primary immunodeficiency, or neonates with perinatal transmission) or those with severe or complicated VZV infection (including pneumonia or central nervous system infection), administer IV acyclovir 10 mg/kg every 8 hours for 7 to 10 days.

Due to the risk of crystal precipitation in the kidneys, maintaining an appropriate hydration (urine volume) is mandatory in the course of the treatment. Thus, crystalloid infusion prior to IV drug administration is recommended (eg, isotonic fluid with a volume at least equal to the volume of drug infusion); serum creatinine and urine output should be monitored regularly. In patients with renal failure, the dosage should be adjusted.

→ COMPLICATIONS

1. Bacterial superinfections of the skin lesions are common complications of varicella. The risk of bacterial superinfection is increased by the use of nonsteroidal anti-inflammatory drugs, topical preparations (eg, powder), and poor hygiene. Bacterial superinfections may be the following:

1) **Localized** (*Streptococcus pyogenes*, *Staphylococcus aureus*): Abscess, phlegmon, erysipelas, wound-associated scarlet fever.

2) **Precursor to invasive infection** (*S pyogenes*): Necrotizing fasciitis, bacteremia, toxic shock syndrome.

2. Pneumonia:

1) **Varicella pneumonia** (interstitial pneumonitis) is the most common complication in adults (incidence, 1/400 cases), particularly in pregnant women in the second and third trimesters and in immunocompromised patients. Tachypnea, cough, and shortness of breath usually develop on days 3 to 5 of VZV infection, and outcomes are frequently poor.

2) **Secondary bacterial pneumonia** (most frequently caused by *S aureus*, sometimes by *Streptococcus pneumoniae*, *Haemophilus influenzae*) may complicate the course of varicella pneumonia or develop independently (even during convalescence). Secondary bacterial pneumonia is difficult to distinguish from varicella pneumonia; thus, it should be always taken into consideration when establishing the diagnosis.

3. Neurologic complications:

1) **Cerebellitis** (cerebellar ataxia) is most common in children <15 years (incidence, 1/4000 cases), usually develops in the first 3 weeks of VZV infection, and has a benign course, resolving within 3 to 4 weeks.

2) **Encephalitis** occurs predominantly in adults (incidence, 1-2/1000 cases) and has a severe course, usually lasting ≥2 weeks; mortality rates are 5% to 20%, and up to 15% of survivors can have permanent neurologic sequelae.

3) **Reye syndrome** (encephalopathy with hepatic dysfunction) is most commonly seen with ASA use, especially in children; it is now very rare. Reye syndrome is associated with rapid progression to coma and a poor prognosis.

4) **Meningitis, transverse myelitis, Guillain-Barré syndrome, cranial nerve paresis, retinitis** (may occur even a few weeks after the onset of varicella).

4. Other (rare): Myocarditis, arthritis, nephritis, symptomatic hepatitis, thrombocytopenia, urethritis and/or cystitis (dysuria).

→ PROGNOSIS

In immunocompetent patients, varicella usually has a mild course; the infection confers life-long immunity. In high-risk groups, the course of varicella is protracted, more severe, and associated with an increased risk of complications. Deaths related to varicella complications are rare (1/50,000 cases; in adults, 1/3000); however, mortality rates are up to 15% in immunocompromised patients and ~40% in pregnant women who develop pneumonia.

→ PREVENTION

Specific Prevention

1. Vaccination is the key prevention method. Two doses of varicella-containing vaccine are recommended after 1 year of age given the higher risk of breakthrough infection seen in one-dose regimens.

2. Active postexposure immunization should be provided as soon as possible (up to 120 hours after exposure) for nonimmune individuals >1 year of age, provided there are no contraindications.

3. Passive postexposure immunoprophylaxis (varicella-zoster immunoglobulin [VZIG]) should be administered as soon as possible, but up to 10 days after close contact with an individual with active varicella for patients at high risk for severe varicella; ◐○ patients at high risk for severe varicella:

1) Newborns of mothers who developed varicella from 5 days before to 2 days after delivery.

2) Susceptible pregnant women.

3) Individuals with malignancies or undergoing chemotherapy or immune suppression without a history of VZV infection or completed immunization.

4) Patients after hematopoietic stem cell transplant, including immune individuals who are highly immunosuppressed (due to high-dose steroid therapy or T-cell depletion).

5) Hospitalized premature newborns born <28 weeks' gestation or born >28 weeks' gestation to susceptible women.

4. Prophylactic pharmacotherapy: In the patients at high risk for severe varicella (above), if VZIG is not available or >10 days have elapsed since exposure, oral valacyclovir 1000 mg tid for 5 days or acyclovir 800 mg qid for 7 days starting on day 7 after exposure can be considered. ◐● The rationale for this is to optimize the efficacy of treatment by ensuring that there is no delay in the institution of antiviral therapy.

General Preventive Measures

1. Isolation of the following groups of patients (particularly from high-risk individuals):

1) **Patients with varicella**: For at least 5 days after the onset of rash and until all lesions have crusted over. In the case of a maculopapular rash in vaccinated individuals, isolation should continue until no more new lesions appear and/or lesions start to resolve (fade, but not necessarily disappear).

Cases of breakthrough varicella with <50 lesions are approximately 33% as infectious as typical varicella.

2) **Susceptible individuals who had contact with a patient with varicella**: Between days 7 and 21 following the exposure, or up to day 28 if VZIG or intravenous immunoglobulin (IVIG) was administered. If possible, the exposed patients should be discharged, while the exposed susceptible health-care personnel should be temporarily reassigned to areas other than patient care.

2. Serologic screening of unvaccinated health-care personnel and high-risk individuals without a history of varicella infection or for whom vaccination records are not available: Prompt vaccination of patients with negative varicella titers (IgG, above a certain level, indicating past infection), unless specifically contraindicated.

1. Acute Kidney Injury

→ **DEFINITION, ETIOLOGY, PATHOGENESIS**

Acute kidney injury (AKI) is a clinical syndrome arbitrarily defined by either an abrupt increase in serum creatinine concentration by ≥26.5 µmol/L (0.3 mg/dL) within 48 hours, a ≥1.5-fold increase in serum creatinine over the prior 7 days, or urine output <0.5 mL/kg/h for 6 hours (→Table 1-1). This definition, as per the latest Kidney Disease: Improving Global Outcomes (KDIGO) 2012 consensus guidelines, takes into account the RIFLE (risk, injury, failure; loss, end-stage renal disease) criteria created by the Acute Dialysis Quality Initiative (ADQI) and the Acute Kidney Injury Network (AKIN) definition. It also highlights the increased mortality resulting from even small increases in creatinine.

The yearly incidence of AKI is about 200 per 1,000,000 patients, occurring in 5% of hospitalized patients and 30% of patients in intensive care units. The occurrence of AKI is linked to increased mortality. Age, sex, and medical co-morbidities are risk factors for the development of AKI, with older men being at the highest risk.

The diagnostic approach is broadly divided into 3 groups: prerenal, intrinsic (renal), and postrenal (→Figure 1-1).

1. Prerenal AKI is characterized by a decrease in glomerular filtration rate (GFR) in response to impaired renal perfusion with intact renal parenchyma. However, intact tubular function with high urine osmolality and low urine sodium concentrations should not necessarily be interpreted as prerenal AKI, as many intrinsic etiologies, such as glomerulonephritis or AKI due to sepsis, may initially have intact tubular function. **Etiology**:

1) Decreased effective circulatory volume (hypovolemia):

    a) Hemorrhage: Traumatic, surgical, postpartum, gastrointestinal GI).

    b) GI fluid loss: Vomiting, diarrhea, surgical drainage.

    c) Kidney loss: Diuretic therapy, osmotic diuresis in diabetes, and adrenal insufficiency.

    d) Vasodilatory loss of the extravascular compartments: Sepsis syndromes, acute pancreatitis, peritonitis, severe trauma, burns, and severe hypo-albuminemia.

Table 1-1. Staging of acute kidney injury according to the 2012 KDIGO guidelines

Stage	Serum creatinine	Urine output
1	Increase 1.5-1.9 × baseline or Increase by ≥26.5 µmol/L (≥0.3 mg/dL)	<0.5 mL/kg/h for 6-12 hours
2	2-2.9 × baseline	<0.5 mL/kg/h for ≥12 hours
3	3 × baseline or Serum creatinine ≥353.6 µmol/L (≥4.0 mg/d) or Initiation of RRT	<0.3 mL/kg/h for ≥24 hours or Anuria for ≥12 hours

Based on: Kidney Disease: Improving Global Outcomes (KDIGO) Acute Kidney Injury Work Group. KDIGO Clinical Practice Guideline for Acute Kidney Injury. Kidney Inter., Suppl. 2012; 2: 1-138.

KDIGO, Kidney Disease: Improving Global Outcomes; RRT, renal replacement therapy.

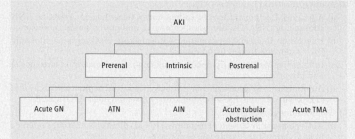

AIN, acute interstitial nephritis; AKI, acute kidney injury; ATN, acute tubular necrosis; GN, glomerulonephritis; TMA, thrombotic microangiopathy.

Figure 1-1. Basic classification of causes of acute kidney injury.

2) Reduced cardiac output: Diseases of the myocardium, valves, and pericardium; arrhythmias; massive pulmonary embolism; positive-pressure mechanical ventilation.

3) Vascular abnormalities:

   a) Vasodilation: Sepsis, hypotension caused by antihypertensive medications (including drugs that reduce afterload), and general anesthesia.

   b) Vasoconstriction: Hypercalcemia, norepinephrine, epinephrine, tacrolimus, cyclosporine (INN cyclosporin), and amphotericin B.

4) Impaired renal autoregulation and hypoperfusion: Cyclooxygenase inhibitors (nonsteroidal anti-inflammatory drugs [NSAIDs]), angiotensin-converting enzyme inhibitors (ACEIs), angiotensin receptor blockers (ARBs), and direct renin inhibitors.

5) Hyperviscosity syndrome: Multiple myeloma, Waldenström macroglobulinemia, and polycythemia.

6) Renal vessel occlusion:

   a) Renal artery occlusion: Atherosclerosis, thromboembolism, dissecting aneurysm, and systemic vasculitis.

   b) Renal vein occlusion: Thromboembolism and external compression.

2. Intrinsic AKI is characterized by a decrease in GFR with loss of renal parenchymal integrity due to both inflammatory and noninflammatory factors. **Etiology**:

1) Small vessel disease: Thrombotic microangiopathy (TMA) (hemolytic-uremic syndrome [HUS], thrombotic thrombocytopenic purpura [TTP]), cholesterol crystal embolization, disseminated intravascular coagulation (DIC), preeclampsia or eclampsia, malignant hypertension, systemic lupus erythematosus (SLE), and progressive systemic sclerosis (scleroderma renal crisis).

2) Acute tubular necrosis (ATN):

   a) Ischemia: Prolonged prerenal AKI.

   b) Exogenous toxins: Radiographic contrast agents, cyclosporine, antibiotics (eg, aminoglycosides), chemotherapy (cisplatin), ethylene glycol, methanol, and NSAIDs.

   c) Endogenous toxins: Myoglobin, hemoglobin, monoclonal proteins (eg, in multiple myeloma).

   d) Crystals: Uric acid, oxalic acid (a metabolite of ethylene glycol), acyclovir (INN aciclovir) (particularly IV), methotrexate, sulfonamides, and indinavir.

3) Acute interstitial nephritis (AIN):

    a) Allergic: β-Lactam antibiotics, sulfonamides, trimethoprim, rifampin (INN rifampicin), NSAIDs, diuretics, captopril, and proton pump inhibitors.

    b) Infectious: Bacterial (legionella, leptospirosis), viral (cytomegalovirus, BK virus), and fungal (candidiasis).

    c) Infiltrative: Malignant (lymphoma, leukemia), granulomatous (sarcoidosis), and idiopathic.

    d) Autoimmune: Sjögren syndrome, tubulointerstitial nephritis with uveitis (TINU) syndrome, IgG4-related kidney disease (IgG4-RKD), SLE.

4) Glomerulonephritis (GN):

    a) Anti–glomerular basement membrane (GBM) disease (sometimes referred to as Goodpasture syndrome or disease).

    b) Antineutrophil cytoplasmic antibody (ANCA)-associated GN (granulomatosis with polyangiitis [formerly Wegener granulomatosis]), Churg-Strauss syndrome, microscopic polyangiitis).

    c) Immune complex–mediated GN (SLE, postinfectious, cryoglobulinemia, and primary membranoproliferative GN).

5) Acute graft rejection following renal transplantation.

6) Other rare causes: Acute renal cortical necrosis, Chinese herb nephropathy, acute phosphate nephropathy, warfarin-related nephropathy, loss of the solitary functioning kidney.

3. Postrenal AKI or obstructive nephropathy develops in the case of obstructed urinary flow from either structural or functional impediment in the urinary tract. **Etiology**:

1) Obstruction of either both ureters or a single ureter in a solitary functioning kidney:

    a) Occlusion: Calculi, blood clots, sloughed renal papillae.

    b) External compression: A tumor or retroperitoneal fibrosis.

    c) Damage: Inadvertent ligation or incision during surgical procedures.

2) Diseases of the bladder: Neurogenic bladder, bladder neck obstruction by a tumor (bladder cancer), calculi, blood clots.

3) Diseases of the prostate: Benign prostatic hypertrophy or cancer.

4) Urethral disease: Obstruction by a foreign body or calculi and trauma.

→ **CLINICAL FEATURES AND NATURAL HISTORY**

The clinical presentation of AKI varies depending on the cause, severity, and associated diseases related to renal injury. Most patients with mild to moderate AKI are asymptomatic and identified by laboratory testing. Patients with severe AKI may have symptoms of uremia including fatigue, loss of appetite, weight loss, pruritus, nausea, vomiting, muscle cramps, and changes in mental status.

Oliguria or anuria occurs in ~50% of patients and is frequently seen with prerenal AKI, acute renal cortical necrosis, thromboembolism, and thrombotic microangiopathy. Normal or even increased urine output can be seen in intrinsic etiologies of AKI.

There are **4 phases** that can be distinguished in the natural history of AKI:

1) **Initiation phase**: This phase presents with normal urine output as it commences from the initial impact of the insult (cause) until the point of actual kidney damage. The duration of this phase is usually several hours and varies depending on the causative factor.

2) **Oliguria (urine output 100-400 mL/d) or anuria (urine output <100 mL/d)**: This phase occurs when urine output is typically between 50 and 400 mL/d. It develops in ~50% of patients and lasts an average of 10 to 14 days but can vary from 1 day to 8 weeks.

3) **Polyuria**: This phase begins with rapidly increasing urine output over several days after a period of oliguria or anuria. It occurs due to tubular dysfunction and is manifested by sodium wasting and polyuria. Serum creatinine and urea levels may not decrease for several days. The duration of polyuria is proportional to the duration of oliguria/anuria and may last up to several weeks. This phase of AKI is associated with considerable risk of dehydration and severe loss of electrolytes, particularly potassium and calcium.

4) **Recovery phase**: During this phase urine output gradually returns to normal and serum creatinine and urea begin to normalize. It may take up to several months for complete recovery or for a new baseline function to be established.

AKI is associated with increased risks of adverse outcomes such as progression to chronic kidney disease (CKD), end-stage renal disease (ESRD), and mortality. Therefore, early diagnosis, treatment, and proper follow-up are essential.

→ **D I A G N O S I S**

Diagnostic Tests

1. Blood laboratory tests:

1) Serum creatinine and urea/blood urea nitrogen (BUN): Increased levels of serum creatinine and urea are important in assessing renal injury. However, a comparison of the currently increased serum creatinine and urea levels with previous levels aids in determining the duration and severity of kidney injury. In intrinsic AKI the daily serum creatinine increments are 44 to 88 µmol/L (0.5-1 mg/dL). In conditions associated with tissue catabolism, such as sepsis or crush syndrome, daily serum creatinine increments are significantly higher (as high as >176 µmol/L [2 mg/dL]) and are usually accompanied by severe acidosis and significant hyperkalemia. Estimation of GFR using the Cockcroft-Gault or Modification of Diet in Renal Disease (MDRD) formulas (→Chapter 9.2) is not useful in describing or monitoring AKI.

2) Potassium: Hyperkalemia usually occurs in patients with reduced urine volumes and can be life-threatening if levels are >6.5 mmol/L. It is necessary to assess potassium concentrations in the context of the associated acid-base balance, because acidosis causes shifts of K^+ from the intracellular compartment to the extracellular compartment. Also →Chapter 4.2.4.1.

3) Hypocalcemia and hyperphosphatemia may be significant in patients with crush syndrome, whereas hypercalcemia is usually seen in patients with a malignancy (eg, myeloma). Also →Chapter 4.2.1.1.

4) Uric acid: Hyperuricemia may be a sign of gout or tumor lysis syndrome.

5) Creatine kinase (CK) and myoglobin levels: Increased CK and myoglobin levels are seen in patients with crush syndrome or rhabdomyolysis (eg, caused by statins, trauma, hyperthermia, electrical shock, and severe viral and bacterial infections).

6) Arterial blood gases: Metabolic acidosis may be associated with AKI. If severe metabolic acidosis is observed, then the plasma anion gap (PAG) and osmolar gap (OG) should be calculated to determine if AKI resulted from the ingestion of toxic substances.

7) Anemia: Often a common feature of CKD. In AKI it may develop due to hemolysis or blood loss. Schistocytes are often seen on peripheral smear in the case of HUS or TTP.

8) Thrombocytopenia: Associated with HUS, TTP, and DIC.

2. Urine evaluation (→Table 1-2, →Table 1-3): This is a particularly important noninvasive test in the initial evaluation of AKI. The following parameters should be assessed: urine output, urinalysis, urine sediment, urine

Table 1-2. Urinalysis in the evaluation of acute kidney injury

Component	Interpretation
Specific gravity	Estimates urine osmolality – Values <1.010: Hydrated state – Values <1.005: Diabetes insipidus or water intoxication – Values >1.035: Dehydration, high glucose levels, IV contrast
pH	Normal range: 4.5-8.0 – High urine pH: Distal RTA, infections with urea-splitting organisms, vegetarians – Low urine pH: Metabolic acidosis, dehydration, high-protein diet
RBCs	Positive result may indicate hematuria, hemoglobinuria, or myoglobinuria
WBCs	Suggest inflammation: UTI, GN, or AIN
Ketones	Not normally found in urine. Dipstick tests for presence of acetoacetic acid but not acetone or β-hydroxybutyric acid. Positive results are associated with uncontrolled diabetes, pregnancy with diabetes, carbohydrate-free diets, and starvation
Glucose	Nearly all glucose filtered by glomeruli is reabsorbed in proximal tubules and undetectable in healthy patients. Positive results are associated with hyperglycemia, pregnancy, and Fanconi syndrome
Bilirubin	Unconjugated bilirubin is not present in urine. Conjugated bilirubin appears in liver disease or obstruction of bile ducts

AIN, acute interstitial nephritis; GN, glomerulonephritis; RBC, red blood cell; RTA, renal tubular acidosis; UTI, urinary tract infection; WBC, white blood cell.

Table 1-3. Urine microscopy features in the evaluation of acute kidney injury

Features	Comments

Cells	1) >3 RBCs/HPF: Quantity and morphology assessment required; dysmorphic RBCs are associated with GN
	2) WBCs: Associated with infection or inflammation:
	  a) PMNs associated with infection
	  b) Eosinophilia associated with AIN, cholesterol emboli, or schistosomiasis
	3) Epithelial cells:
	  a) Squamous cells are usually contaminants
	  b) Transitional cells usually due to bladder irrigation or catherization, rarely due to malignancy
	  c) Renal tubular cells seen in ATN

Casts	1) Hyaline cast: Nonspecific, seen in strenuous exercise and dehydration 2) Granular cast (muddy-brown cast): Seen in ATN 3) Waxy cast: Seen in CKD 4) Fatty cast: Seen in nephrotic syndrome, mercury and ethylene glycol poisoning 5) RBC cast: Seen in GN 6) WBC cast: Seen in AIN, pyelonephritis, and GN
Crystals	1) Acidic urine: Uric acid or calcium oxalate 2) Alkaline urine: Triple phosphate or calcium phosphate

AIN, acute interstitial nephritis; ATN, acute tubular necrosis; GN, glomerulonephritis; HPF, high-power field; RBC, red blood cell; PMN, polymorphonuclear neutrophil; WBC, white blood cell.

electrolytes, and urine osmolality. This will aid in differential diagnosis and guide further workup.

3. Electrocardiography (ECG): This should be performed particularly if there are significant electrolyte disturbances, as cardiac activity may be affected.

4. Imaging studies: Routine studies include ultrasonography and radiography. Renal ultrasonography can be used to exclude obstruction and evaluate kidney size and parenchyma. However, false-negative results of obstruction can occur in patients with severe volume depletion or with retroperitoneal fibrosis. Chest radiographs are helpful in evaluating pulmonary congestion and infiltrates.

5. Kidney biopsy: Biopsy should be obtained in situations when prerenal and postrenal causes of AKI have been excluded and the cause of intrinsic renal injury is unclear. Specifically, biopsy should be performed in patients in whom the probable or possible diagnosis will alter treatment, such as patients with oliguria who have rapidly worsening AKI with hematuria and high suspicion for GN, systemic vasculitis, acute interstitial nephritis, or who need immuno-suppressive medications.

Diagnostic Criteria

AKI is diagnosed if either of the following criteria is met:

1) A rapid increase in serum creatinine concentrations, that is, by ≥ 26.5 μmol/L (0.3 mg/dL) within 48 hours or a ≥ 1.5-fold increase in serum creatinine within the prior 7 days.
2) Urine volume <0.5 mL/kg/h for 6 hours.

Identification of causes of AKI is based on a thorough medical history, physical examination, and results of laboratory tests.

Differential Diagnosis

It is important to differentiate prerenal and postrenal AKI from intrinsic AKI, as rapid improvement of renal perfusion or release of obstruction leads to improved renal function. Markers may be useful for distinguishing prerenal and intrinsic causes and for differential diagnosis (→Table 1-4). In patients with AKI superimposed on a preexisting CKD, the causes and differential diagnosis can vary (→Table 1-5). Postrenal AKI is confirmed by ultrasonographic evidence of urinary flow obstruction in the renal pelvis, ureters, or bladder.

→ TREATMENT

General Measures

1. All efforts should be made to eliminate the causes of AKI and to avoid factors that could worsen renal function, particularly nephrotoxic drugs.

2. Monitoring of fluid balance, including urine output, fluid intake, and daily body weight.

3. Frequent monitoring (at least daily) of serum creatinine, urea, potassium, sodium, and bicarbonate. Complete blood count (CBC), blood gases, calcium, phosphate, and uric acid should be checked when deemed necessary. If severe metabolic acidosis is observed, the PAG and OG should be calculated.

4. Adjust drug dosage to the severity of renal failure (note that GFR assessment in patients with AKI may not be reliable).

5. Provide appropriate nutrition: We recommend that protein intake should not be restricted to prevent or delay starting renal replacement therapy (RRT) in AKI as malnutrition has been associated with an increased likelihood of death, complications, and use of health-care resources.⊗○ Dietary protein or amino acids should be 0.8 to 1 g/kg/d in AKI patients without significant hypercatabolism not requiring RRT or 1 to 1.5 g/kg/d (maximum, 1.7 g/kg/d) in those with hypercatabolism or undergoing RRT. Carbohydrates, which are

Table 1-4. Selected differential features of prerenal azotemia and intrinsic AKI

	Prerenal AKI	Intrinsic AKI
Daily urine output (mL)	<400	Variable
Urine osmolality (mOsm/kg H_2O)	>500	<350
Urine specific gravity (g/mL)	>1.023	≤1.012
Ratio of urea (mmol/L) to serum creatinine (µmol/L)	>1:10	<1:10
Ratio of urinary to serum creatinine concentration	>40	<20
Urinary [Na^+] concentration (mmol/L)[a]	<20	>40
Fractional excretion of sodium[b]	<1%	>2%
Urine sediment	No abnormal findings or hyaline casts only	Epithelial cells, pigmented muddy-brown granular casts or tubular epithelial cell casts

[a] Urinary sodium concentration (this should be measured before administering furosemide).

[b] Fractional excretion of sodium: FE_{Na} = [(urinary Na concentration in mmol/L × serum creatinine concentration in mg/dL) / (serum Na concentration in mmol/L × urinary creatinine concentration in mg/dL)] × 100%.

AKI, acute kidney injury.

Table 1-5. Selected differential features of AKI and CKD

	AKI	CKD
History suggestive of CKD	No	Yes
Kidney size	Normal	Small
Dynamics of serum creatinine increases	High	Low
CBC	Normal	Anemia
Calcium-phosphate metabolism	Mild or moderate disturbances (depending on AKI etiology)	High phosphate level, increased alkaline phosphatase level, radiographic signs of renal osteodystrophy and/or soft tissue calcifications
Fundoscopy	Usually normal	Frequently lesions typical of diabetes mellitus or chronic hypertension

AKI, acute kidney injury; CBC, complete blood count; CKD, chronic kidney disease.

the principal source of energy, should be up to 5 g of glucose per kg a day. Fat should be between 0.8 to 1.2 g/kg/d. The maximum energy intake should be 35 kcal/kg/d. Standard commercially available diets are appropriate for the majority of patients with AKI who do not have significant hypercatabolism.⊘○

Treatment of Underlying Conditions

In some patients further kidney injury can be prevented by appropriate treatment of underlying conditions.

1. Prerenal AKI: Treatment is aimed at addressing the underlying causes: shock and heart failure. In patients without hemorrhagic shock, volume restoration with crystalloids or albumin (rather than synthetic colloids) is recommended for initial management to restore effective circulatory volume.◐◑ Normal renal perfusion can prevent the transition of prerenal azotemia to intrinsic AKI and may lead to normalization of renal function within 1 to 3 days. Albumin can be considered to aid in reaching resuscitation goals, avoid excessive fluid administration in patients requiring large-volume resuscitation, or in specific patient subgroups (eg, a patient with cirrhosis and spontaneous peritonitis, patients with burns). Withdrawal of nephrotoxic agents such as diuretics, NSAIDs, ACEIs, and ARBs is important to avoid further damage.

2. Intrinsic AKI: Treatment is aimed at addressing the underlying cause of kidney disease. Supportive care is necessary to eliminate any life-threatening complications, such as hypotension or severe metabolic complications.

3. Postrenal AKI: Treatment is aimed at rapid resolution of the urinary tract obstruction. In the postobstructive phase, specific attention should be paid to urine output, volume status, and electrolytes. Usually patients with polyuria should receive in the beginning 0.45% saline at a replacement rate of approximately two-thirds of the urinary losses. The replacement fluid rate can be decreased over several days and the concentration of administered saline can be adjusted depending on the results of serum biochemical testing.

Renal Replacement Therapy

The most commonly used types of RRT are intermittent or daily hemodialysis (HD), continuous renal replacement (CRRT), sustained low-efficiency dialysis (SLED), and peritoneal dialysis (PD). The decision on when to start RRT remains controversial and is based on clinical and biochemical features. It may depend on the time course of disease progression and involves individual clinical judgement.◑

1. Clinical indications: Volume overload (pulmonary edema) refractory to diuretic agents, uremic encephalopathy (altered mental status or seizures), pericarditis, uremic coagulopathy, and drug overdose.

2. Biochemical indications (approximations, ie, there is no decisive difference between a pH of 7.21 and 7.19): Refractory hyperkalemia (serum potassium >6.5 mmol/L), refractory metabolic acidosis (pH <7.2; bicarbonate level [HCO_3^-] <8 mmol/L), refractory hypercalcemia (>4.5 mmol/L), uremia 20 to 40 mmol/L (based on observational trials), refractory hypermagnesemia (3-5 mmol/L), severe dysnatremia (eg, <116 or >160 mmol/L; levels are reasonable examples only), or severe hyperuricemia in tumor lysis syndrome.◐◑

3. Modality: Numerous studies and meta-analyses failed to show benefits of CRRT as compared with standard intermittent RRT.◑ More studies are ongoing. Currently CRRT can be considered in patients with hemodynamic instability, acute brain injury, and increased intracranial pressure or generalized brain edema.

Treatment of Complications

1. Volume overload: Restrict salt and water intake and administer a loop diuretic, eg, IV furosemide 40 mg. If this is ineffective, use additional doses up to a maximum of 500 mg/d of furosemide. Note that high doses of loop diuretics may cause hearing loss. Addition of a thiazide diuretic can be considered, such as oral metolazone 5 to 10 mg bid, to augment diuresis. The practice pattern on when to start RRT to remove excess water is variable.

2. Hyperkalemia: →Chapter 4.2.4.1.

3. Metabolic acidosis: Sodium bicarbonate ($NaHCO_3$) is recommended in patients with severe acidosis to maintain a serum [HCO_3^-] >8 mmol/L or arterial pH >7.2.◐◑ Possible adverse effects are hypocalcemia and hypokalemia.

4. Hyperphosphatemia: →Chapter 4.2.3.1.

5. Anemia: Transfusion of packed red blood cells should be guided by the patient's symptoms and clinical situation. Erythropoietic agents are not indicated in the treatment of AKI.

6. Coagulopathy leading to bleeding:

1) Desmopressin 0.3 µg/kg in an IV or subcutaneous infusion over 15 to 30 minutes or 3 µg/kg intranasally; the dose may be repeated after 6 hours. The effect of desmopressin on improving platelet function is short lasting, with bleeding times returning to baseline within 24 hours. Adverse effects include tachyphylaxis after one dose, headache, facial flushing, and rare thrombotic events.

2) Cryoprecipitate is a source of factor VIII, factor XIII, multimeric form of von Willebrand factor, fibrinogen, and fibronectin. Use 10 units IV over 30 minutes every 12 to 24 hours. Adverse effects include risk of transfusion--related infection, fever, and allergic reaction. Rare but severe reactions include anaphylaxis, pulmonary edema, and intravascular hemolysis.

3) Esterified estrogens 0.6 mg/kg IV over 30 to 40 minutes once daily for 5 days. The duration of action is up to 2 weeks. Esterified estrogens can be administered in men and if given for short periods have been associated with hot flashes only.

→ PROGNOSIS

The overall mortality in patients with AKI is high, and AKI is considered an independent risk factor for mortality. Mortality rates are population-dependent, ranging between 10% and 80%. Patients with uncomplicated AKI have mortality rates of ~10%. Patients presenting with AKI and multiorgan failure have mortality rates >50%. In patients requiring RRT mortality rises to >80%. Death is usually a result of the severity of the underlying disease causing AKI rather than the renal injury itself. It has been shown that from 20% to 50% of patients with AKI progress to CKD and 3% to 15% develop ESRD, even those who initially recover sufficient kidney function to discontinue dialysis.

→ PREVENTION

1. Patients at increased risk of AKI should be identified and appropriate preventative measures should be undertaken as early as possible to treat the underlying diseases.

2. Institute early and intensive treatment of conditions causing reduction of effective circulating blood volume with appropriate IV fluids and close monitoring of volume and patient response.

3. Monitor urine output and periodically evaluate renal function in patients at increased risk of AKI.

4. Avoid nephrotoxic drugs, particularly in patients with impaired renal function.

5. Identify patients at increased risk for contrast nephropathy (→Special Considerations, below).

6. Patients at risk of AKI caused by myoglobinuria should be identified and hydration with 0.9% sodium chloride or sodium bicarbonate should be initiated.

→ SPECIAL CONSIDERATIONS

1. Contrast-induced nephropathy (CIN) is defined as an impairment of renal function and measured as either a 25% increase in serum creatinine levels from baseline or an increase of 44 µmol/L (0.5 mg/dL) in the absolute serum creatinine value that develops within 1 to 3 days of administration of radiographic contrast agents. Its treatment, prevention, and definition itself remain controversial.

The exact **pathophysiology** of CIN is unclear and appears to be multifactorial. Several theories suggest intrarenal vasoconstriction leading to medullary hypoxia, which is mediated by decreased production of nitric oxide and prostaglandin and increased levels of endothelin and adenosine. In addition, there is increased viscosity within the medullary vascular bed, which may further contribute to medullary hypoxia and renal injury. The second mechanism of injury is the generation of reactive oxygen species, leading to cytotoxic effects on the renal parenchyma. Lastly, the contrast media itself may be cytotoxic, leading to direct damage.

Patient **risk factors** for the development of CIN include CKD, diabetes mellitus, intravascular volume depletion, decreased cardiac output, and concomitant use of nephrotoxic drugs. Other factors include high doses of radiocontrast, multiple procedures within 72 hours, intra-arterial administration, and high--osmolar contrast media.

Diagnosis is based on an early increase of serum creatinine levels of administration of a contrast agent (within 1-3 days) and exclusion of other potential causes, such as prerenal azotemia, AIN, cholesterol crystal embolization, and renal artery thromboembolism. Cholesterol crystal embolization can be distinguished from CIN by abnormal renal function occurring at ~4 weeks after contrast exposure. Patients may have fever, headaches, intestinal ischemia, myalgia, livedo reticularis, and "blue toe syndrome."

Prevention is the mainstay of therapy for CIN and the following strategies should be considered:

1) **Nonpharmacologic prevention strategies**:

   a) Identification of high-risk individuals and screening for both acute kidney disease and CKD is highly recommended.

   b) Administer the lowest possible doses of contrast agents. Dosing per kilogram of body weight is recommended to reduce the amount of contrast media, particularly in patients with a low body mass index.✅◒

   c) Use of either iso-osmolar or low-osmolar iodinated contrast media is recommended over high-osmolar iodinated contrast media.✅◒

   d) Avoidance of concomitant use of nephrotoxic drugs.

2) **Pharmacologic prevention strategies**: Note that this is a subject of ongoing debate, with meta-analyses generally showing low quality of evidence◒ and more recent randomized controlled trials not showing benefit of bicarbonates or N-acetylcysteine.◒ Among patients at high risk of developing CIN consideration is given to the use of:

   a) Volume resuscitation with the use of IV hydration with either 0.9% saline or $NaHCO_3$ (154 mmol/L in 5% glucose [dextrose]) 1 to 1.5 mL/kg/h for 3 to 6 hours before and 6 to 12 hours after the administration of a contrast agent.

   b) N-acetylcysteine 1200 mg orally or IV bid for 48 hours, beginning 1 day prior to the procedure.

   c) Prophylactic intermittent HD or hemofiltration for contrast media removal is not recommended for the prevention of AKI as it may increase its risk.❌◒

2. Acute phosphate nephropathy is a form of AKI that is caused by rapidly developing nephrocalcinosis following oral administration of phosphate--containing agents (usually sodium phosphate) used for bowel preparation before colonoscopy. Renal failure is usually seen within a few days of phosphate administration. Some patients may have a subacute presentation and develop AKI over weeks to months after ingestion of these preparations. Acute phosphate nephropathy is frequently preceded by symptoms of acute hyperphosphatemia and hypocalcemia, including tetany, altered mental status, and hypotension.

Table 1-6. Causes and contributing factors in abdominal compartment syndrome

Primary	– Massive intrabdominal, retroperitoneal, or pelvic bleeding
	– Liver transplantation
	– Mechanical intestinal obstruction
	– Postoperative closure of abdomen under tension
Secondary	– Large-volume fluid replacement
	– Pancreatitis
	– Severe intra-abdominal infection
	– Ascites
	– Ileus
	– Major burns
	– Continuous ambulatory peritoneal dialysis

Renal deposition of calcium phosphate precipitants along with tubulointerstitial inflammation is seen on biopsy and is irreversible.

Risk factors associated with the development of acute phosphate nephropathy include advanced age, preexisting CKD, dehydration, use of renin--angiotensin-aldosterone (RAA) system blockade, NSAIDs, diuretics, and high-dose phosphates.

Prevention: The most important prevention strategy is identification of high-risk patients and avoidance of phosphate agents in this group. Patients at increased risk are elderly, with hypertension, and have low estimated GFR (<60 mL/min/1.73 m^2). Rigorous attention should be paid to adequate hydration and avoidance of RAA system blockade, diuretics, and NSAIDs on the day before and day of the procedure.

Treatment: There is no specific treatment for acute phosphate nephropathy. Patients should be treated with supportive care.

3. Warfarin-related nephropathy (WRN): This is a poorly understood and fairly underreported cause of AKI associated with glomerular hemorrhage and renal tubular obstruction by red blood cell casts. Clinically it is characterized by a sudden and unexplained irreversible deterioration of renal function without hematuria in patients treated with warfarin and having significant prolongation of prothrombin time (international normalized ratio [INR] >3.0) in the preceding week.

WRN may develop in up to 20% of patients with excessive anticoagulation, most frequently within 1 year after initiation of therapy. The majority of reported cases involve patients with preexisting CKD. Additional risk factors include advanced age, diabetes mellitus, hypertension, and cardiovascular disease. At this time, little is known about the exact pathophysiology or therapeutic approach. Minimizing exposure to warfarin and avoiding excessive INR is recommended, especially in patients with CKD, to reduce the risk of this condition.

4. Abdominal compartment syndrome (ACS) refers to organ dysfunction caused by increased intra-abdominal pressure leading to impairment of blood supply to various organs, including kidneys. This condition is likely underdiagnosed among critically ill patients.

The causes of ACS can be categorized as primary (sometimes requiring surgery), secondary (medical), and recurrent (→Table 1-6). Primary conditions are disorders that may require surgical intervention. Secondary conditions are usually managed medically. Recurrent conditions are disorders in which ACS redevelops after either medical or surgical treatment. ACS should be suspected in patients who develop oliguria in the course of intestinal obstruction and respiratory failure. Diagnosis is confirmed by sustained intra-abdominal pressure >20 mm Hg (with or without abdominal perfusion pressure <60 mm Hg) associated with new organ dysfunction or failure. Once the diagnosis of intra--abdominal hypertension (IAH) has been established, the goal is to decrease the intra-abdominal pressure to <15 mm Hg.

5. Hepatorenal syndrome: →Chapter 6.2.2.5.

6. Acute renal cortical necrosis (ARCN) is a very rare cause of AKI. It is caused by diminished renal arterial perfusion that leads to cortical ischemia. It is prevalent in pregnant women, usually in advanced pregnancy, as a result of accidental hemorrhage or placental abruption. Rare causes include complications of intrauterine fetal death, sepsis, preeclampsia, or amniotic fluid embolism. The precipitating event is probably intravascular coagulation or severe renal ischemia.

ARCN presents with sudden decrease of urine volume or anuria, which is frequently accompanied by hematuria, lumbar pain, and hypotension. The presence of the **triad of symptoms**, including anuria, hematuria, and lumbar pain, differentiates ARCN from other forms of AKI in pregnancy.

Diagnosis is suspected on the basis of the triad of symptoms. Imaging studies can confirm the diagnosis of ARCN is some patients. CT angiography is preferred despite the risk of contrast nephropathy. Alternatively isotopic penta-acetic acid scanning can be used. In the acute phase imaging studies show patchy or diffuse densities in the renal cortex, which appear as hypoechogenic areas on ultrasonography and hypodensity on CT scans. After 1 to 2 months calcifications in the renal cortex may be seen on plain abdominal radiographs. Renal biopsy is rarely needed and performed only if the diagnosis is unclear.

Prognosis is poor, with mortality rates at 1 year >20% and partial renal recovery rates ≤40%.

Treatment is aimed at addressing the underlying condition. Patients should be treated with supportive management.

1.1. Tumor Lysis Syndrome

→ **DEFINITION, ETIOLOGY, PATHOGENESIS**

Tumor lysis syndrome (TLS) is an oncologic emergency with life-threatening metabolic disturbances resulting from a rapid lysis of tumor cells. It may develop following exposure to chemotherapy (tumor chemosensitivity) or occur spontaneously in some malignancies that have high tumor burden or a rapid proliferation rate. The most common malignancies associated with TLS include acute lymphoblastic leukemia (ALL) and high-grade non-Hodgkin lymphoma (NHL), specifically Burkitt lymphoma. Though uncommon, TLS can also occur in multiple myeloma and solid tumors, particularly with the advent of novel systemic therapies. The rapid lysis of tumor cells leads to release of large amounts of potassium, purines (further broken down to uric acid), and phosphate.

Several clinical factors, in addition to tumor properties, can increase the risk of TLS. These include preexisting kidney injury or chronic kidney disease, baseline hyperphosphatemia, volume depletion, and concurrent use of nephrotoxic agents.

→ **CLINICAL FEATURES AND DIAGNOSIS**

Clinical manifestations of TLS are associated with consequences of metabolic disturbances. Tumor cell phosphate storage capacity is several-fold higher than that of nonmalignant cells. As TLS occurs, a large amount of released phosphate binds the circulating calcium, leading to precipitation in the myocardium and renal tubules. Calcium phosphate product, along with uric acid crystal deposition, leads to severe renal vasoconstriction and tubular damage, causing acute kidney injury (AKI). Calcium phosphate crystal deposition and hyperkalemia (secondary to tumor cell release) collectively can lead to significant cardiac arrhythmias and sudden death. Lastly, circulating serum calcium binding to the released phosphate reduces serum calcium concentration and can progress to symptomatic hypocalcemia.

Diagnostic Criteria

The diagnosis of TLS includes both laboratory and clinical criteria. **Laboratory TLS** can be diagnosed according to the Cairo-Bishop definition in a patient with high tumor burden who within 3 days prior or 7 days after initiation of treatment develops ≥2 of:

1) Hyperphosphatemia (≥1.45 mmol/L in adults, ≥2.1 mmol/L in children, or 25% increase from the baseline value).
2) Hyperkalemia (≥6.0 mmol/L or 25% increase from baseline).
3) Hyperuricemia (≥476 mmol/L or 25% increase from baseline).
4) Hypocalcemia (≤1.75 mmol/L or 25% reduction from baseline).

Clinical TLS can be diagnosed when criteria for laboratory TLS are met in the presence of AKI, cardiac arrhythmias/sudden cardiac death, or seizures.

Several **risk stratification scores** allow patients to be placed in low-, intermediate-, and high-risk categories; details of risk stratification are beyond the scope of this chapter. However, the highest risk is marked by Burkitt lymphoma (stage III-IV); acute myeloid leukemia with a white blood cell (WBC) count >100 × 10^9/L; ALL with a WBC >100 × 10^9/L and lactate dehydrogenase (LDH) >2 × upper limit of normal; chronic lymphocytic leukemia with high lymph node burden undergoing treatment and elevated LDH; heavy tumor burden or bulky lymphadenopathy in diffuse large B-cell lymphoma; adult T-cell leukemia; transformed lymphoma; or mantle cell lymphoma.

→ PREVENTION

1. Hydration: IV hydration and volume repletion are the cornerstone of TLS prevention. This allows for renal perfusion and excretion of calcium phosphate and uric acid, preventing precipitation and kidney injury. IV fluids with a target of 2 to 3 L/m^2 daily to achieve a target urine output of ≥80 to 100 mL/m^2/h are recommended; however, this should be done carefully to avoid volume overload, which could further predispose to cardiac arrhythmia. Loop diuretics can be attempted to increase urine output if adequate volume repletion has been achieved.

2. Uric acid reduction: Oral allopurinol at 100 mg/m^2 tid (maximum, 800 mg/d) is used in patients at intermediate risk for TLS. If oral allopurinol is unavailable, IV allopurinol can be attempted (maximum, 600 mg/d; the cost may be a factor). In patients at high risk, rasburicase (0.15-0.2 mg/kg once daily or a fixed one-time 3-mg dose) can be used, if available. Rasburicase is contraindicated in patients with glucose-6-phosphate dehydrogenase (G6PD) deficiency, as it can precipitate hemolysis. Testing for G6PD is recommended for those at risk (ie, males of African, Mediterranean, or South-Asian ancestry). The duration of therapy can vary from 1 to 7 days (the cost of this treatment may be prohibitive). On the basis of available evidence, febuxostat is currently not recommended for TLS prevention.

→ TREATMENT

In patients with suspected or confirmed TLS, the following therapies can be used (if available):

1) **Uric acid lowering with rasburicase**, if not already done for prevention (and using the same dose), **along with IV hydration** (and diuretics if necessary to promote diuresis; →Prevention, above). Allopurinol prevents new uric acid formation by inhibiting xanthine oxidase, whereas rasburicase results in rapid metabolism of existing uric acid (within hours). Allopurinol may be used if rasburicase is not available or cannot be used (G6PD deficiency);

however, owing to its mechanism of action, it will not affect preexisting uric acid levels. Furthermore, it may lead to accumulation of nonsoluble xanthine, increasing the risk of renal injury.

2) **Electrolyte disturbance management**: Restrict phosphate and potassium in all patients. Those with hyperkalemia should have cardiac monitoring and serial 4- to 8-hour measurements of levels of uric acid creatinine and electrolytes (including potassium, calcium, and phosphate). Hyperkalemia should be managed with routine hyperkalemia management strategies, including shifting (insulin with glucose [dextrose] and β-agonists), bowel excretion (via sodium polystyrene sulfonate), and renal excretion (with diuretics if adequately volume replete). Phosphate binders (calcium carbonate) can be used for the management of hyperphosphatemia and IV calcium replacement for hypocalcemia. Also →Chapter 4.2.

3) A calcium-phosphate (Ca×P) product ≥70 mg^2/dL^2 (5.6 mmol^2/L^2), refractory hyperkalemia, refractory fluid overload, and refractory severe symptomatic hypocalcemia can be considered indications for **renal replacement therapy** (→Chapter 9.2).

2. Chronic Kidney Disease (CKD)

→ DEFINITION, ETIOLOGY, PATHOGENESIS

Chronic kidney disease (CKD) is defined according to the 2012 Kidney Disease: Improving Global Outcomes (KDIGO) guideline as abnormalities of the kidney structure or function present for >3 months with implications for health. CKD diagnostic criteria: →Table 2-1.

The severity of CKD is classified based on glomerular filtration rate (GFR) (G categories, expressed in mL/min/1.73 m^2; →Table 2-2) and albuminuria (A categories; →Table 2-3). Estimated GFR (eGFR) is based on serum creatinine levels. Albuminuria is measured as the urine albumin-to-creatinine ratio (UACR) or on the basis of 24-hour urinary albumin excretion. In patients with nephrotic range proteinuria or suspected glomerular disease, 24-hour urinary protein excretion is commonly used and informs decisions about biopsy and treatment. KDIGO recommends the UACR as the initial test in a patient with a newly discovered low GFR. A complete CKD diagnosis includes the name of the kidney disease (ie, the cause of CKD, if known) and the appropriate G and A categories.

The term "**chronic renal failure**" was formerly used to refer to the current CKD categories G3 to G5. Category G5 CKD is termed **kidney failure**. **Uremia** is a clinical syndrome of fatigue, nausea, anorexia, and itching that occurs in category G5 and sometimes category G4 CKD; it does not refer to the concentration of serum urea (the term for elevated serum urea is azotemia). Canadian guidelines recommend distinguishing patients treated with dialysis by using the suffix "-D" and those with functioning transplants with a "-T." The term **end-stage renal disease (ESRD)** does not correspond exactly to any category within the KDIGO classification and usually means patients treated with dialysis or transplantation, known together as renal replacement therapy (RRT). CKD G5ND refers to patients with G5 CKD who are not receiving RRT. It does not distinguish between patients in whom RRT has not yet been thought indicated, those in whom it has been offered and declined, and those for whom it is not available.

Recommended GFR estimating equations: Equations with the best measurement properties are the **Chronic Kidney Disease Epidemiology Collaboration (CKD-EPI) equation** and the **Modification of Diet in Renal**

Table 2-1. Diagnostic criteria for CKD according to the 2012 KDIGO guideline

Criterion	Comment
1. Duration >3 months	Necessary for diagnosis of CKD
2a. GFR <60 mL/min/1.73 m^2 (CKD categories G3a-G5)	eGFR (mL/min/1.73 m^2) calculated with equations[a] using S_{Cr}: **1) CKD-EPI creatinine equation:** eGFR = 141 × min(S_{Cr}/κ, 1)^α × max(S_{Cr}/κ, 1)$^{-1.209}$ × 0.993^{age} × 1.018 [if female] × 1.159 [if black] Where: S_{Cr} = serum creatinine in mg/dL κ = 0.7 for females and 0.9 for males α = −0.329 for females and −0.411 for males min = the minimum of S_{Cr}/κ or 1 max = the maximum of S_{Cr}/κ or 1 **2) Abbreviated MDRD equation:** eGFR = 186 × [S_{Cr}]$^{-1.154}$ × [age]$^{-0.203}$ × [0.742 if female] × [1.21 if black] Where: S_{Cr} = serum creatinine level
2b. Albuminuria or proteinuria (albuminuria categories: →Table 2-3)	− Urine albumin excretion ≥30 mg/d, or − Albumin-to-creatinine ratio ≥30 mg/mmol
2c. Urine sediment abnormalities	− Isolated microscopic hematuria with dysmorphic RBCs − RBC casts, WBC casts, fatty casts, granular casts, or renal tubular epithelial cells
2d. Renal tubular disorders	Renal tubular acidosis, nephrogenic diabetes insipidus, renal potassium and magnesium wasting, Fanconi syndrome, cystinuria, nonalbumin proteinuria
2e. Structural abnormalities detected by imaging	Polycystic kidneys,[b] dysplastic kidneys, hydronephrosis due to obstruction, cortical scarring due to infarcts, pyelonephritis or vesicoureteral reflux, renal masses or infiltrative diseases, renal artery stenosis, small hyperechoic kidneys (commonly revealed by ultrasonography in severe CKD due to many parenchymal diseases)
2f. Pathologic abnormalities detected by histology or inferred	− Glomerular diseases (glomerulonephritis, diabetes mellitus, autoimmune diseases, amyloidosis, systemic infections, drugs, neoplasia) − Vascular diseases (atherosclerosis, hypertension, ischemia, vasculitis, thrombotic microangiopathy, cholesterol embolism) − Tubulointerstitial diseases (urinary tract infections, stones, obstruction, sarcoidosis, drug toxicity, environmental toxins) − Cystic and congenital diseases (Alport syndrome, Fabry disease)
2g. History of kidney transplantation	In most patients biopsies of transplanted kidneys reveal abnormalities even with GFR >60 mL/min/1.73m^2 and no albuminuria

To meet the CKD criteria, a duration >3 months and any of 2a to 2g are required.

[a] Online calculator for both equations at www.kidney.org.
[b] Simple renal cysts are not a criterion for diagnosing CKD.

Based on: Kidney Disease: Improving Global Outcomes (KDIGO) Acute Kidney Injury Work Group. KDIGO Clinical Practice Guideline for Acute Kidney Injury. Kidney Inter., Suppl. 2012; 2: 1-138.

CKD, chronic kidney disease; CKD-EPI, Chronic Kidney Disease Epidemiology Collaboration; eGFR, estimated glomerular filtration rate; GFR, glomerular filtration rate; KDIGO, Kidney Disease: Improving Global Outcomes; MDRD, Modification of Diet in Renal Disease; P_{Cr}, plasma creatinine level; RBC, red blood cell; S_{Cr}, serum creatinine level; WBC, white blood cell.

Table 2-2. GFR categories in CKD according to the 2012 KDIGO guideline

GFR category	GFR (mL/min/1.73 m^2)	Terms
G1	≥90	Normal or high GFR
G2	60-89	Mildly decreased GFR
G3a	45-59	Mildly to moderately decreased GFR
G3b	30-44	Moderately to severely decreased GFR
G4	15-29	Severely decreased GFR
G5	<15	Kidney failure

Based on: Kidney Disease: Improving Global Outcomes (KDIGO) Acute Kidney Injury Work Group. KDIGO Clinical Practice Guideline for Acute Kidney Injury. Kidney Inter., Suppl. 2012; 2: 1-138.

CKD, chronic kidney disease; GFR, glomerular filtration rate; KDIGO, Kidney Disease: Improving Global Outcomes.

Table 2-3. Albuminuria categories in CKD according to the 2012 KDIGO guideline

Category	Albumin excretion rate (mg/24 h)	Albumin/creatinine ratio (mg/mmol)
A1	<30	<3
A2	30-300	3-30
A3	>300	>30

Based on: Kidney Disease: Improving Global Outcomes (KDIGO) Acute Kidney Injury Work Group. KDIGO Clinical Practice Guideline for Acute Kidney Injury. Kidney Inter., Suppl. 2012; 2: 1-138.

CKD, chronic kidney disease; KDIGO, Kidney Disease: Improving Global Outcomes.

Disease (MDRD) Study equation (both available online at the National Kidney Foundation). Although useful in clinical practice, it is worth knowing that these equations are accurate to within approximately 30% of the calculated value 85% of the time (ie, in 15% of patients the true GFR is >30% different from the eGFR value). The Cockcroft-Gault formula is computationally easier but less accurate and biased. It has been extensively used in original pharmacokinetic studies of medications. There is currently no clinically useful method that is more accurate than these equations. Measured creatinine clearance based on a 24-hour urine collection is intrusive, often done incorrectly, and even in research settings performs worse than eGFR. Isotope measurements are generally not useful in clinical practice, with the exception of establishing GFR when the absolute value, rather than the trend, is critically important (eg, in potential transplant donors).

For drug dosing, **absolute clearance, expressed in mL/min**, is needed, rather than clearance corrected for the body surface area (BSA), in mL/min/1.73 m^2. Creatinine clearance (CrCl) is useful in dose adjustment of drugs excreted by the kidneys. It can be estimated using the **Cockcroft-Gault formula**:

$$\text{CrCl in mL/min} = \frac{(140 - \text{age}) \times \text{mass (kg)} \; [\times 0.85 \text{ if female}]}{72 \times \text{serum creatinine (mg/dL)}}$$

In SI units:

$$\text{CrCl in mL/min} = \frac{(140 - \text{age}) \times \text{mass (kg)} \; [\times 1.23 \text{ if male or } \times 1.04 \text{ if female}]}{\text{serum creatinine (µmol/L)}}$$

Alternatively, eGFR in mL/min can be calculated from the MDRD or CKD--Epi formula, which provide a value in mL/min/1.73 m^2, and the patient's BSA calculated from height in centimeters (H) and weight in kilograms (W) using the **DuBois and DuBois formula**:

$$\text{BSA in m}^2 = (W^{0.425} \times H^{0.725}) \times 0.007184$$

eGFR is then calculated as:

$$\text{eGFR in mL/min} = \frac{\text{MDRD or CKD-Epi (mL/min/1.73 m}^2) \times \text{BSA (m}^2)}{1.73}$$

Given the accessibility of eGFR estimates in routine clinical practice and the inherent inaccuracies of all assessment methods, simply using eGFR in place of CrCl in adults with relatively normal body habitus is likely a sensible approach.

Etiology: Common causes of CKD are diabetic nephropathy, hypertensive nephropathy, glomerulonephritis, tubulointerstitial diseases of the kidney, and polycystic kidney disease. Rare causes include myeloma, ischemic nephropathy, obstructive nephropathy, systemic connective tissue diseases, vasculitis, sarcoidosis, amyloidosis, and some congenital diseases.

The majority of chronic renal diseases may cause a gradual loss of nephrons, resulting in an overload of the remaining viable nephrons, in particular due to hyperfiltration. Initial glomerular hypertrophy is followed by glomerular sclerosis associated with interstitial fibrosis, resulting in the impairment of renal function. As CKD progresses, uremic toxins accumulate in blood (these include the low- and medium-molecular-weight products of protein metabolism). Hundreds of putative uremic toxins have been proposed, but none of them are measurable in clinical practice. Urea and creatinine are useful markers of filtration, but neither is responsible for uremic syndrome. Renal erythropoietin production is reduced, which together with other factors (iron deficiency, occult or overt blood loss, bone marrow depression, erythropoietin resistance caused by uremic toxins, and reduced red blood cell [RBC] life-span) leads to the development of anemia. Reduced 1-α-hydroxylation of vitamin D in the kidneys and failure to excrete phosphate are thought to be 2 of the root causes of secondary hyperparathyroidism and derangements in calcium and phosphate homeostasis that lead to metabolic bone disease and vascular, valvular, and ectopic (tissue) calcification (calciphylaxis). The kidneys lose their ability to maintain normal water balance, electrolyte levels, and pH. As a result of the impaired renal excretion of sodium and water, excessive renal release of vasoconstrictors (angiotensin II, endothelin-1), low levels of vasodilators (such as nitric oxide, prostaglandins), sympathetic activation, hormonal and metabolic disturbances, and stiffness of the walls of large arteries, hypertension develops in >90% of patients with significantly impaired renal function.

Modifiable factors associated with an accelerated progression of CKD: Proteinuria, hypertension, hyperglycemia, hyperlipidemia, tobacco smoking, metabolic acidosis, obesity.

Factors causing deterioration of renal function (acute kidney injury [AKI]) in people with CKD: Exacerbation of the underlying condition; dehydration; hypotension, especially in the context of angiotensin-converting enzyme inhibitors (ACEIs), angiotensin receptor blockers (ARBs), or neprilysin inhibitors; iodinated contrast media; nephrotoxic drugs, especially nonsteroidal anti-inflammatory drugs (NSAIDs), trimethoprim (causing crystal nephropathy, particularly when the dose is not adjusted for GFR), aminoglycosides, and amphotericin; urinary obstruction; pyelonephritis and its complications; malignant hypertension; exacerbation of congestive heart failure; rhabdomyolysis; renal artery thromboembolism; renal vein thrombosis.

→ CLINICAL FEATURES AND NATURAL HISTORY

Clinical manifestations depend on the severity of CKD and underlying conditions. In G2 and G3 CKD, it is unusual to have symptoms directly referable to the low GFR, although it likely contributes in a multifactorial way to fatigue and weakness in some patients. The lower GFR present in G4 and G5 CKD is associated with the development of clinical manifestations and complications involving various organs and systems:

1) **General symptoms**: Weakness, fatigue, hypothermia, loss of appetite, increased susceptibility to infection.

2) **Cutaneous manifestations**: Pale, dry, hyperpigmented skin; prolonged bleeding times and easy bruising (uremic coagulopathy); pruritus and secondary excoriations; uremic frost (cutaneous urea deposits—extremely rare in countries with patient access to dialysis and transplantation).

3) **Cardiovascular abnormalities**: Hypertension, left ventricular (LV) hypertrophy, LV dilatation, systolic dysfunction, congestive heart failure, arrhythmias, accelerated atherosclerosis, vascular calcifications, uremic pericarditis, sudden death.

4) **Respiratory abnormalities**: Pulmonary edema, Kussmaul respiration (→Chapter 1.21) from metabolic acidosis, uremic pleurisy.

5) **Gastrointestinal abnormalities**: Gastric or duodenal ulcers, angiodysplasia, gastrointestinal bleeding. In patients with advanced CKD, uremic fetor (urine-like odor of the breath), nausea and vomiting, ileus.

6) **Neuromuscular abnormalities** (in patients with advanced CKD): Concentration and memory impairment, headache, somnolence or insomnia, behavioral disturbances (eg, apathy or irritability), seizures and coma (signs of severe encephalopathy or cerebral edema), restless legs syndrome (discomfort of the feet relieved by frequent leg movement), areflexia, muscle weakness, low-frequency tremor, fasciculations or twitching of muscles, sarcopenia, recurrent hiccups, distal polyneuropathy, mononeuropathies (median, fibular), flaccid quadriparesis in patients with the most severe neuropathy.

7) **Reproductive system abnormalities**: Menstrual disturbances (oligomenorrhea, secondary amenorrhea), female infertility, sexual dysfunction (loss of libido, erectile dysfunction), decreased sperm numbers and motility. If a patient with G4 or G5 CKD becomes pregnant, there is a risk of hypertension, preeclampsia, eclampsia, and loss of kidney function for the mother, and prematurity, low birth weight, and fetal demise for the fetus. (Patients who have undergone transplantation and have good kidney function are at increased risk for these outcomes compared with patients without CKD, but they also achieve much better outcomes than those with G4 or G5 GFR and those on dialysis.)

8) **CKD–mineral and bone disorder (CKD MBD)**: Abnormalities of calcium (hypocalcemia or hypercalcemia) and phosphate (hyperphosphatemia) metabolism, vitamin D deficiency, and parathyroid hormone (PTH) hypersecretion (secondary or tertiary hyperparathyroidism), which together cause disturbances of bone metabolism and calcifications of blood vessels or soft tissues (calciphylaxis). CKD MBD is a progressive disorder affecting the bone structure and resulting from either excessively rapid (due to hyperparathyroidism, sometimes called osteitis fibrosa cystica) or excessively low (adynamic bone disease) bone turnover.

Other causes of bone disease in patients with severe CKD include β_2-microglobulin (usually in patients with a long history of ESRD) or aluminum (in patients dialyzed without adequate removal of aluminum from the water used in treatment or in patients treated for long periods with aluminum-based phosphate binders [now rare]) in the bones. The disorder manifests as bone and joint pain and pathologic fractures.

9) **Fluid, electrolyte, and acid-base disturbances**: Laboratory tests (→Diagnostic Tests, below).

Clinical Manifestations of CKD According to GFR Category

1. G1 (GFR ≥90 mL/min/1.73 m^2): Symptoms of the underlying condition (diabetes mellitus, hypertension, glomerulonephritis, or other). Blood pressure may be elevated. To be classified as having CKD, these patients need to have other evidence of kidney abnormalities, most commonly albuminuria. Diagnosis of the cause and minimizing the risk factors for disease progression are the cornerstones of care.

2. G2 (GFR 60-89 mL/min/1.73 m^2; mildly decreased): Often normal serum urea and creatinine levels. The ability of the renal tubules to concentrate urine is impaired, thus increasing the patient's susceptibility to dehydration. Phosphate retention occurs, but it is very unusual to see hyperphosphatemia or hyperparathyroidism.

3. G3 (GFR 30-59 mL/min/1.73 m^2): Hypertension occurs in >50% of patients. Most patients are asymptomatic, although isosthenuria (inability to concentrate or dilute urine), polyuria, nocturia, and polydipsia may occur. Some patients have anemia but hemoglobin (Hb) level <100 g/L on the basis of the kidney disease alone is unusual; in those with IIb <100 g/L, an alternative etiology should be sought. Phosphate retention occurs but it is very unusual to see hyperphosphatemia. Hyperparathyroidism may be seen, but the PTH level is rarely more than 3 times the upper limit of normal (ULN).

4. G4 (GFR 15-29 mL/min/1.73 m^2; severely decreased): Particularly at the lower end of this category uremic symptoms may develop or worsen. These include dysgeusia (dysfunction of the sense of taste), loss of appetite, and rarely nausea and vomiting. Fatigue and itching may also occur. Hypertension occurs in >80% of patients; many of them have LV hypertrophy, and some have symptoms of heart failure. Although many patients have anemia, the majority, especially with higher GFR within this category, will still maintain an Hb level >90 g/L without erythropoietin. Metabolic acidosis may occur and is usually asymptomatic. Hyperphosphatemia occurs, particularly at the lower GFR threshold of this category. Hyperparathyroidism of any degree may occur, and it is usually worst in those who have had a low GFR for a long time. At the lower end of this eGFR range, hypocalcemia may be seen. Hypercalcemia is often present, sometimes secondary to tertiary (autonomous) hyperparathyroidism but more commonly as a result of therapy (calcium-containing phosphate binders, nutritional vitamin D, activated vitamin D [eg, alfacalcidol]).

5. G5 (GFR <15 mL/min/1.73 m^2; kidney failure): Any of the signs and symptoms of uremia may be present. At the lower end of this category patients may develop uremic pericarditis or uremic encephalopathy, including seizures. Patients may have severe, symptomatic anemia (Hb <90 g/L), acidosis, hyperphosphatemia, hypocalcemia or hypercalcemia, and hyperparathyroidism. Some patients, especially those with diabetes and those on peritoneal dialysis, have low PTH levels, associated with adynamic bone disease. Ectopic calcification (vascular, valvular, and soft tissue) may develop. Where resources are available, nephrologists, guided by the patient's symptoms, decide with the patient on the optimal timing for the initiation of dialysis. There is no benefit to starting dialysis early, based on a particular level of GFR. When available, most people start dialysis before their GFR is 5 mL/min/1.73 m^2; a minority choose either maximal medical therapy without dialysis or a fully palliative approach.

→ **DIAGNOSIS**

Screening for CKD is recommended only in people with diabetes. However, case-
-finding (identifying patients among those who clinically are at increased risk
of developing a given disease) based on the patient's history of cardiovascular
disease or systemic disease, symptoms suggestive of uremia, or a systemic disease that may have a renal component is a key identification method of people
with a low GFR or albuminuria. In developed countries screening in people
with hypertension is suggested, with the recognition that this is not based
on strong evidence (eg, lowest grade of recommendation in the Hypertension
Canada guidelines).⊘⊖ Case-finding also appropriately occurs in the context
of hospitalization, major intercurrent illnesses, and whenever contemplating
the use of drugs that require dose adjustment for GFR or which are nephrotoxic. As the next step, KDIGO recommends evaluation of albuminuria using
UACR. Urinalysis may also be helpful in diagnosis, particularly in patients
with a newly identified low GFR in whom there is a clinical suspicion of an
acute or a subacute course. The timing of the second creatinine measurement
to establish chronicity in someone with a newly identified low GFR is based
on the clinical scenario and the physician's assessment of the likelihood of the
acute or subacute component (in which case testing may be repeated in days to
weeks). The best marker of renal function is the eGFR rather than the serum
creatinine level, which also depends on age and muscle mass. In patients with
a family history of polycystic kidney disease and in those with clinical suspicion
of obstruction, ultrasonography examination may be useful. The cause of CKD
may be suggested by signs and symptoms, comorbidities, prior and current
abnormal test results, and family history of kidney disease.

Diagnostic Tests

1. Urinalysis: Albuminuria, proteinuria, microscopic or gross hematuria,
casts, leukocyturia, low specific gravity of urine.

2. Blood tests: Anemia (typically normocytic and normochromic); increased
serum levels of creatinine, urea, uric acid, potassium, phosphate, PTH, triglycerides, cholesterol; hypocalcemia; metabolic acidosis.

3. Imaging studies: Ultrasonography usually reveals a reduced kidney
size (frequently <10 cm in the long axis); exceptions (normal-sized kidneys
despite CKD) are patients with amyloid nephropathy, diabetic nephropathy, or
HIV nephropathy. Patients with polycystic kidney disease who have a low GFR
usually have overall enlarged kidneys and multiple cysts on each side; they may
also have liver cysts and cysts of other abdominal organs. Because of the risk
of contrast nephropathy, the risks and benefits of contrast-enhanced imaging
studies (eg, computed tomography [CT]) must be considered if an abnormality,
such as a renal mass, is identified that would usually be evaluated in this way.

4. Specialized laboratory tests: These are selected based on the clinical
presentation and results of standard laboratory tests of blood and urine and
are not ordered together as part of the initial screen. Depending on the clinical context, they include serum protein electrophoresis and immunofixation,
serum free light chains, serum immunoglobulins, C3, C4, antinuclear antibodies (ANAs), antibodies to double-stranded DNA (dsDNA), antiphospholipid
antibodies (APLAs), cryoglobulins, hepatitis B and C serologies, HIV serology,
anti–phospholipase A_2 receptor antibody, and cytoplasmic (c-ANCA) and perinuclear (p-ANCA) antineutrophil cytoplasmic antibodies.

5. Kidney biopsy: This is usually done only after consultation with a nephrologist. Check the patient's coagulation status (international normalized ratio
[INR], partial thromboplastin time [PTT]), Hb level, and platelets. Consider
giving IV desmopressin as bleeding prophylaxis. Several cores of kidney tissue
are taken and studied with light microscopy, electron microscopy, and immunofluorescence. Histology is useful in the diagnosis of glomerular diseases causing
nephritic or nephrotic syndrome, tubulointerstitial disease, vasculitis, and

infiltrative diseases such as amyloidosis, light chain deposition disease, and diabetes. Risks associated with kidney biopsy are gross hematuria (developing in ~20% of patients), perinephric hematoma, bleeding requiring transfusion (~5%), and bleeding requiring embolization or nephrectomy (6/10,000 patients); very rarely the bleeding is fatal. The risk of not obtaining useful kidney tissue is ~5%.

6. Angiography: The definitive test for renal artery stenosis, which presents in some patients as CKD often accompanied by hypokalemia and difficult-to--control hypertension, is a formal renal angiogram. The need for this test has fallen with recent trials showing that intervening for diagnosed renal artery stenosis with angioplasty, with or without stenting, is associated with no clear benefit and in some studies with harm. Given the lack of a distinct treatment plan and the risks of angiography (contrast nephrotoxicity and cholesterol embolization syndrome), it is not necessary to pursue this diagnosis definitively in most patients in whom it is suspected.🟢🔵 Highly selected patients with hypertension that is truly resistant to medical therapy may still benefit from stenting, but evidence for this intervention is lacking.

Diagnostic Criteria

CKD is diagnosed in patients with abnormalities of kidney structure and function, a GFR <60 mL/min/1.73 m^2, or both if present for >3 months (→Definition, above). Diagnostic criteria: →Table 2-1.

→ **TREATMENT**

Management of patients with CKD involves treatment of the underlying condition, prevention of CKD progression, prevention and treatment of CKD complications, preparing the patient for RRT, and administration of RRT.

General Principles

1. Treatment of the underlying disease, if evidence-based treatment is available (eg, for patients with glomerulonephritis or interstitial nephritis).

2. Treatment of comorbidities.

3. Prevention of cardiovascular diseases (a high risk in patients with CKD), including the use of statins🟢🔵 and smoking cessation.

4. Avoidance of nephrotoxic drugs: Avoid aminoglycosides and amphotericin where possible. Sulfamethoxazole/trimethoprim should be dosed according to GFR and avoided if there is a concomitant risk of AKI. Avoid NSAIDs, with the exception of short courses in patients with G1 to G3 CKD, recognizing that some patients will be prepared to accept the risks (hypertension, volume overload, chronic heart failure, CKD progression, AKI) because of symptom benefit if alternatives cannot be identified.

5. Avoidance of iodinated contrast: Give careful thought to the risks and benefits of investigations that require contrast. Administer IV saline prophylactically before procedures where possible.

6. Avoidance of gadolinium: In patients with G4 or G5 CKD, gadolinium is associated with a severe and progressive skin disease, nephrogenic systemic fibrosis, which can lead to contractures, ulcerations, sepsis, and death; the risk increases the lower the GFR and is highest in dialysis patients. If the use of gadolinium is recommended, explain the risks and benefits, along with alternative strategies, to the patient, use a macrocyclic chelate preparation (such as gadoteridol, gadobutrol, or gadoterate) in the lowest possible dose, and consider performing hemodialysis treatment immediately after the study for hemodialysis patients. Consider also performing hemodialysis in patients receiving peritoneal dialysis and patients with a GFR <20 mL/min/1.73 m^2, particularly if they have an existing vascular access.

7. Immunization: These recommendations are based on generalization from observational studies of the efficacy of vaccination in the general population combined with evidence of high respiratory and infectious morbidity in patients with CKD:

1) Yearly influenza vaccination in all patients with CKD.
2) Polyvalent pneumococcal vaccine in all patients with G4 or G5 CKD, diabetes, nephrotic syndrome, and those who are immunosuppressed.
3) Hepatitis B vaccination in all patients with an eGFR <20 mL/min/1.73 m^2 or higher in the case of a progressive GFR decrease, because of the risk of hepatitis B acquisition during dialysis.

8. Nutritional management: The key goal is to ensure sufficient calorie and protein intake to avoid malnutrition, which in adults with CKD and a normal body weight is 35 kcal/kg (30-35 kcal/kg in patients aged >60 years). Dietary protein restriction has not been definitely shown to be safe or effective and we usually do not advise it.⊗◯ While patients with a high protein intake (>1.5 g/kg/d) should probably be advised to moderate it, protein restriction for patients with a normal protein intake should be limited to highly motivated, well-nourished patients with access to a wide variety of foods and expert dietary supervision, after discussion of the uncertain effectiveness of the intervention.

For patients with a high sodium intake, reduction towards about 3.3 g of sodium per day (8 g of salt) is recommended. Routine further reductions in dietary sodium to <2 g/d, although widely recommended, are not supported by randomized evidence; however, they may be clinically indicated in patients with refractory hypertension, edema, or chronic heart failure. We do not recommend the commercially available low-sodium salt substitutes for patients with G4 or G5 CKD or patients with a history of hyperkalemia, as sodium is often replaced by potassium in these products, which may increase the risk of life-threatening hyperkalemia.

It is not necessary to restrict potassium intake unless there is documented hyperkalemia. Low GFR, drugs (ACEIs, ARBs, direct renin inhibitors, potassium-sparing diuretics, and potassium supplements), high-potassium diets, and diabetic hyporeninemic hypoaldosteronism may all contribute to hyperkalemia.

In patients with serum inorganic phosphate or PTH levels above the ULN, possible approaches that are common in clinical practice are restriction of daily phosphate intake (to 800-1000 mg), which cannot be achieved without a degree of protein restriction, and the use of phosphate binders. Evidence of changes in clinically important outcomes from these interventions is lacking. Supplementation with nutritional vitamin D, in keeping with general population recommendations, is likely appropriate for people with G1 to G3 CKD. In G4 and G5 disease, reductions of 1-α-hydroxylation by the kidneys may lead to deficiency of alfacalcidol. However, no clinical trials have elucidated the role of nutritional vitamin D or alfacalcidol in preventing clinically important outcomes. In patients with G4 or G5 CKD, the use of either nutritional vitamin D or alfacalcidol is a common accepted practice, but direct evidence of benefit is lacking.

Protein-calorie malnutrition that develops in some patients due to the spontaneous decrease in protein intake in patients with a low GFR, excessive dietary protein and caloric restriction, anorexia, and nausea and vomiting usually resolves after the institution of RRT and nutritional management, although sometimes comorbidities are responsible, in which case specific investigations and management are required. Protein-calorie malnutrition, accompanied by increased inflammation and accelerated atherosclerosis (malnutrition-inflammation-atherosclerosis [MIA] syndrome), occurs most frequently in patients with G5 CKD, usually undergoing RRT, and is associated with high cardiovascular mortality rates.

9. Sick day rules: A sick day is defined as a day of intercurrent illness sufficiently severe that one would not work or attend school, if applicable. On such days there is a risk of AKI, particularly because of dehydration if nausea, vomiting, or diarrhea are among the symptoms. Based on evidence that some drugs contribute to AKI in the context of volume contraction (ACEIs, ARBs, direct renin inhibitors, diuretics, NSAIDs) and other drugs are cleared by the kidney and may accumulate if there is AKI (sulfonylureas and metformin), patients should be advised, including written instructions to take home, to stop taking these drugs while they are unwell, and to resume them afterwards; the acronym SADMANS (**s**ulfonylureas, **A**CEIs, **d**iuretics/direct renin inhibitors, **m**etformin, **A**RBs, **N**SAIDs, **s**odium-glucose cotransporter 2 [SGLT-2] inhibitors) may be used as a mnemonic for health-care professionals. This strategy is impractical for some elderly patients and for patients whose medications are prepackaged for them on a weekly basis by a pharmacist or family member. Patients and their families should also be educated about the importance of having a low threshold for coming to a hospital for IV fluids if they are becoming dehydrated. Direct evidence that these strategies are effective in preventing AKI or other clinically important adverse outcomes is lacking.

10. Preparation for RRT, advance decision-making, and end-of-life issues: Most people with CKD will not require RRT in their lifetime. However, the possibility of a future need for RRT should be considered. Concrete plans are usually not necessary until the GFR is <20 mL/min/1.73 m^2, although in addition to the current GFR this should depend on the patient's age, competing risk of death, rate of progression of CKD, and prognostic markers for progression, such as the underlying condition and proteinuria. The kidney failure risk equation is a validated tool that predicts the need for RRT from age, sex, serum creatinine level, and UACR; it is empirically derived and takes into account the competing risk of death. (Online calculator available at QxMD.) Avoidance of transfusion whenever possible prevents sensitization that can make kidney transplantation more complicated and worsen the outcomes. Selected patients at high risk for RRT should be advised to save the veins in the nondominant arm for possible future access creation (ie, avoid venipuncture and intravenous cannulas on that side).

Start more concrete preparations when the patient's GFR is 15 to 20 mL/min/1.73 m^2. We suggest that such patients are best managed in a multidisciplinary clinic where care from a number of health-care workers (including doctors, nurses, pharmacists, social workers, diabetes educators, and dietitians) can be integrated.

Education about the different available methods of performing dialysis and about transplantation may need to be repeated and delivered in a variety of ways sensitive to the patient's learning needs, remembering that cognitive impairment is prevalent in patients with G4 or G5 CKD. In every patient with no prior RRT, consider kidney transplantation from a living donor as the first-line treatment bearing in mind that risks of renal transplantation likely outweigh benefits in many patients aged >75 years at the time of transplantation. Preparation for hemodialysis includes establishing an adequate vascular dialysis access (preferably an upper extremity arteriovenous fistula [AVF]); these often require more than one operation to create and some months to mature. It is usual to start the process at a GFR 15 to 20 mL/min/1.73 m^2 anticipating possible problems, unless the patient appears to have nonprogressive CKD. Patients whose anatomy is deemed unsuitable for a fistula may be able to have a graft inserted (a less durable form of access, more prone to stenosis and thrombosis than a fistula), but this is usually done weeks to months before the need for hemodialysis, rather than even earlier as is the case with fistula creation. In patients whose plan is peritoneal dialysis, a peritoneal dialysis catheter is inserted, usually closer to the time when its use is anticipated (evidence of progression or early uremic symptoms). Peritoneal dialysis catheters affect body image, limit activities such as bathing and swimming, and are associated with a risk of infection whether in use or not.

Discussion should include realistic goals of care based on an individualized prognosis. For patients contemplating RRT, the alternatives of maximal conservative therapy and a fully palliative philosophy should be discussed. Patients should also be aware that they may choose to stop dialysis at any time, ideally after careful consideration and team discussion, and what the likely consequences of that would be at different stages in their disease. Advance care planning including other aspects of care should be integrated into these discussions and may result in the patient identifying (formally or informally) a substitute decision-maker in the event of future inability to participate in decision-making, and the patient composing an advance care directive.

Pharmacotherapy

1. Use of ACEIs or ARBs: ACEIs and ARBs reduce the progression of kidney disease (loss of GFR), especially in patients with proteinuria >1 g/d.◉◉ In patients with established vascular disease or diabetes and nephropathy or retinopathy, there is also a cardiovascular benefit (based on the large randomized HOPE [Heart Outcomes Prevention Evaluation] study of ramipril 10 mg daily). The usual full doses should be used, with the caveat that some drugs require adjustment for low GFR. Check potassium and creatinine levels after starting, perhaps at 2 weeks. Stop if creatinine is persistently elevated by >20% from baseline or if unmanageable hyperkalemia occurs (our opinion and current practice). Do not use ACEIs and ARBs in combination because of the increased risk of AKI and hyperkalemia without any cardiovascular or renal benefit.◉◉ Sacubitril/ARB combinations may be used in patients with a specific evidence-based indication (eg, ejection fraction <40%; →Chapter 3.8.2) but they are not known to be superior to ACEIs or ARBs alone to reduce progression in patients whose indication is CKD.◉ Agents and dosage: →Chapter 3.9, Table 9-5. Monitoring: →Chapter 3.9.3.

2. Treatment of hypertension: The strongest randomized evidence is for a blood pressure target of 140/90 mm Hg for all patients, regardless of the presence or absence of diabetes or proteinuria. Because there is a lack of clarity and consistency in the evidence for lower targets for specific subgroups (eg, proteinuric disease, patients with diabetes), we do not recommend this approach. A target of systolic blood pressure <120 mm Hg may be discussed with patients: compared with a target of <140 mm Hg, this leads to fewer major cardiovascular events and fewer deaths. The absolute difference in the number of events was small and there was an increase in hypotension, syncope, electrolyte abnormalities, and acute kidney injury or failure, but not of injurious falls in patients treated to the lower target.◉

3. Management of lipids: In patients with G1 to G3 CKD, assess the lipid profile in the context of the overall cardiovascular risk. In patients with G4 or G5 CKD (not on dialysis), consider using a statin plus ezetimibe regardless of lipid levels in keeping with randomized evidence of the cardiovascular (but not renal) benefit of this intervention in this population;◉◉ evidence for this treatment in patients on dialysis is less compelling.◉◉ An alternative, based on generalization from other evidence about the efficacy of lowering cholesterol and of statins, is a statin alone in a higher dose.

In patients with G4 or G5 CKD, including patients treated with RRT and kidney transplant recipients, the following daily doses of statins are used: fluvastatin 80 mg, atorvastatin 20 mg, rosuvastatin 10 mg, pravastatin 40 mg, simvastatin 40 mg, and a combination of simvastatin 20 mg and ezetimibe 10 mg.

No direct randomized evidence supports the use of fibrates in people with CKD. However, generalizing from their use in the general population, fibrates may be administered in patients at cardiovascular risk who do not tolerate statins. They may be considered for patients with hypertriglyceridemia refractory to lifestyle changes, especially in those with extreme hypertriglyceridemia who are at risk for pancreatitis. Dose reductions are needed for fenofibrate (50% for G1 CKD; 75% for G2 to G4 CKD; complete avoidance for G5 CKD and patients on dialysis) but not for gemfibrozil. Fenofibrate and, to a lesser extent, gemfibrozil cause small increases in serum creatinine that are reversible on discontinuation; they are not nephrotoxic.

Do not use statins and fibrates in combination because of a very high risk of rhabdomyolysis in these patients.

4. Management of diabetes mellitus: →Chapter 5.2. Specific CKD-related issues:

1) In patients who are able to maintain their target glycated hemoglobin (HbA$_{1c}$) <7.0, this strategy reduces major cardiovascular events and new albuminuria, does not reduce cardiac death or death from all causes, and leads to an increase in major hypoglycemic events. Our pattern of practice is to aim for higher, individualized targets in the range 7.0 to 8.5 in patients with recurrent severe hypoglycemia, unawareness of hypoglycemia, limited life expectancy, dementia, frailty, or functional dependence. In patients with type 2 diabetes mellitus and G1 to 3 CKD, use metformin initially. This may reduce cardiovascular events in patients who are overweight and is associated with less weight gain than some other agents. The dose should be adjusted according to GFR and the drug should be stopped once GFR is persistently <25 to 30 mL/min/1.73 m^2 (metformin is associated with life-threatening lactic acidosis in patients with a low GFR).

2) In patients with type 2 diabetes mellitus, consider addition of an SGLT-2 inhibitor. In patients with G1 to 3 CKD and in those with high cardiovascular risk, SGLT-2 inhibitors reduce major cardiovascular events and progression of kidney disease. SGLT-2 inhibitors cause loss of glucose in urine; they should not be used in patients who are underweight or catabolic. Because there may be an increased risk of limb amputation, they should not be used in patients with foot ulceration. Patients should receive diabetic foot care, as would be routine in many settings, and stop SGLT-2 inhibitors if foot ulceration develops. Glycosuria leads to an increased risk of fungal genital infections (thrush) and urinary tract infections. There is a risk of ketoacidosis with normal glucose levels. SGLT-2 inhibitors have hypoglycemic and diuretic effects. When starting treatment, consider reducing other hypoglycemic agents and diuretic doses. Check the patient clinically 2 weeks after starting for postural hypotension and to adjust hypoglycemic medications, diuretics, and other antihypertensive drugs. Serum potassium is not affected by starting SGLT-2 inhibition. Canagliflozin specifically can be started at 100 mg daily in patients with G1 to 3 CKD and continued through G4 and G5ND CKD.⊘●

In patients with G1 to 3 CKD, glucagon-like peptide-1 (GLP-1) receptor agonists also reduce major cardiovascular events and albuminuria.● Rates of serious adverse events are similar to placebo. Gastrointestinal upset can occur and may require the drug to be stopped. GLP-1 receptor agonists are not available as oral agents and the daily subcutaneous injection may be a barrier for some patients. However, compared with insulin, they are associated with weight loss rather than weight gain and have been shown to affect patient-important outcomes, which insulin has not.

Insulin, dipeptidyl peptidase-4 (DPP-4) inhibitors, sulfonylureas, meglitinides, and α-glucosidase inhibitors all reduce glucose and HbA$_{1c}$ but have not been shown to reduce the rates of cardiovascular or kidney outcomes. In choosing a sulfonylurea, avoid first-generation and second-generation agents such as chlorpropamide and tolbutamide because of their long half-life. Among third-generation agents, glyburide has unique pharmacodynamic properties that result in a very long effective half-life in patients with and without CKD. In unselected patients it is associated with higher rates of hypoglycemia than other sulfonylureas. Unless resources and cost are a key issue, it should not be used.⊗● Glipizide and gliclazide are safer choices in patients with or without CKD.

Thiazolidinediones have likewise not been shown to decrease any patient--important outcomes and are associated with swelling and possibly chronic heart failure.

5. Management of salt and water balance: Use diuretics as second-line antihypertensive agents and to control clinically apparent volume overload, peripheral edema (when judged to be caused by volume overload), and congestive heart failure. Use a thiazide diuretic in patients with G1 to G3 CKD and a loop diuretic in those with G4 or G5 CKD. Chlorthalidone is approximately twice as potent as hydrochlorothiazide, but the risk of hypokalemia is likewise increased. Of loop diuretics, ethacrynic acid is particularly ototoxic and should not be used except in patients with true allergy to furosemide. Use a bid dose if edema or chronic heart failure is the underlying problem, giving the second dose in the late afternoon to minimize the effect of nocturia on sleep. Combine a loop diuretic with a thiazide diuretic in patients with refractory volume overload resistant to high-dose loop diuretics alone. Consider whether a high sodium intake (sodium >3.3 g/d) is contributing to refractory hypertension and restrict towards this level or lower the intake, if needed. Fluid restriction is usually not necessary except in patients on dialysis and those who have previously been accustomed to a high fluid intake. Do not restrict salt in people with salt-wasting nephropathies, and do not restrict fluid in patients with diabetes insipidus.

6. Metabolic acidosis: In G4 and G5 CKD, oral sodium bicarbonate 0.5 to 1 g/10 kg/d in 3 to 5 divided doses may be used to maintain serum HCO_3^- levels 23 to 28 mmol/L. Sodium bicarbonate (baking soda—not baking powder) sold for cooking may be used as an alternative (500 mg sodium bicarbonate = 1/8 teaspoon). Maintaining the serum HCO_3^- level in this range reduces catabolism (linked to malnutrition) and may reduce the rate of progression of renal disease.☺◯ Potential harms include alkalosis and edema. In patients with renal tubular acidosis (RTA), sodium or potassium citrate is sometimes used, because it is metabolized to bicarbonate and its duration of action is longer. It may not be possible to normalize the serum HCO_3^- level in patients with RTA.

7. Treatment of calcium and phosphate metabolism disturbances and hyperparathyroidism: Disturbances of calcium and phosphate metabolism are rare in patients with G1 to G3 CKD. Calcium, phosphate, and PTH should be monitored at intervals in patients with G4 or G5 CKD, more frequently in patients with lower GFR, on dialysis, with previous abnormalities, or who are taking drugs that affect calcium levels. Therapeutic decisions should be based on the joint interpretation of serum concentrations of calcium, inorganic phosphate, and PTH.

Objectives:

1) Reduce serum inorganic phosphate levels towards the normal range in patients with category G5D CKD (category G5 patients treated with dialysis).

2) Maintain serum calcium levels in the normal range in all CKD patients.

Treatment: No evidence-based interventions that demonstrate reductions in clinically important outcomes have been identified. These recommendations are based on trials of phosphate binders and of drugs—usually alfacalcidol or other vitamin D metabolites or analogues in patients with elevated serum PTH levels—and on translational and basic science investigations of the pathways involved. Dietary phosphate restriction may be attempted but is difficult in the context of other dietary restrictions and the need to avoid malnutrition. Its use in patients with G3 or G4 CKD is controversial, because extrapolations of presumed therapeutic benefits lead to very high numbers needed to treat (NNT) to prevent an outcome; in patients with G5 CKD, especially G5D disease, dietary phosphate restriction is a routine, although not evidence-based, practice. In patients with persistent hyperphosphatemia, phosphate binders are commonly used, also without evidence of benefit in clinically important outcomes (→Chapter 4.2.3.1).

Optimal levels of PTH are not known but are generally postulated to be 2 to 9 times the ULN in G5D CKD. Optimal levels are likely closer to the usual normal range in patients with G3 and G4 CKD. Because of the risk of adynamic bone disease and vascular calcification, avoid suppressing PTH levels below this range. However, some patients will have low PTH levels without active pharmacologic suppression. To reduce PTH levels, mostly in G5D CKD, use vitamin D analogues (alfacalcidol, calcitriol, paricalcitol), or, if available, calcimimetics such as cinacalcet. The choice of initial treatment depends on calcium and inorganic phosphate levels; in patients with hypercalcemia or uncontrolled hyperphosphatemia, calcimimetics are the first choice, if available. Reduce the dose or discontinue vitamin D or vitamin D analogues in patients who develop hypercalcemia or hyperphosphatemia. Reduce the dose or discontinue calcimimetics in patients who develop hypocalcemia. Generalizing from evidence from the general population, in patients with G1 to G3 CKD routine vitamin D supplementation may be used (eg, cholecalciferol 400-2000 U/d). This may also be used in G4 to G5D CKD, although direct evidence for the safety and efficacy of this intervention in these patients, in whom multiple and severe disturbances of calcium-phosphate homeostasis are known to occur, is lacking.

Some patients with G4 or G5 CKD develop severe hyperparathyroidism that is resistant to pharmacologic treatment and is associated with high levels of PTH, hypercalcemia, hyperphosphatemia, and clinical complications (refractory anemia, pruritus, tissue calcifications). In such cases consider parathyroidectomy (→Chapter 5.5.1.3).

In patients with concurrent osteoporosis, do not use bisphosphonates or denosumab in those with G4 or G5D CKD, as neither safety nor efficacy has been shown in this group. Denosumab is associated with hypocalcemia.

8. Treatment of anemia: Target Hb levels are 90 to 110 g/L, based on randomized trials showing quality-of-life benefit and avoidance of transfusion.◐◐ Trials of Hb normalization compared with this target show equivocal and inconsistent evidence of further quality-of-life benefit, doubling of the risk of stroke, and tripling of the costs of **erythropoiesis-stimulating agents (ESAs)**. Start with treatment of iron deficiency and optimization of iron stores, with the objective of maintaining transferrin saturation levels >30% and serum ferritin levels >500 ng/mL (500 μg/L). Iron deficiency is not a consequence of kidney disease; when it is diagnosed, consideration must be given, as usual, to the identification of the underlying cause. Iron supplements may be used in patients with normal iron stores to optimize the response to endogenous or exogenous erythropoietin. Oral iron supplementation (usually 100-200 mg of elemental iron per day, often given as a single bedtime dose to avoid interactions, especially with phosphate binders, if used) may be insufficient due to impaired intestinal absorption; this treatment is also frequently associated with dyspepsia, cramps, and diarrhea or constipation. Consider giving iron on alternate days or thrice weekly to maximize absorption.◐◐ In patients with no response to oral treatment or persistent adverse effects, administer IV iron. Markers of iron deficiency and formulations: →Chapter 7.5.2. All patients treated with ESAs who have serum ferritin levels ≤500 μg/L and transferrin saturation ≤30% should receive iron supplements. In patients on dialysis, high-dose IV iron, 400 mg of iron sucrose per month, temporarily suspended if ferritin was >700 μg/L or transferrin saturation was >40% on monthly bloodwork measured 3 weeks later, was safe compared with lower doses titrated more frequently and led to a 24% reduction in the ESA dose for the same achieved Hb.◐

ESAs:

1) Recombinant human **erythropoietin α** (epoetin α) and **erythropoietin β** (epoetin β): The usual starting dose is 50 U/kg IV (epoetin β may be administered subcutaneously) 3 times a week.

2) **Darbepoetin α**: Start from 0.45 μg/kg IV or subcutaneously once a week.

3) **Methoxy polyethylene glycol-epoetin β**: Start from 0.6 μg/kg IV or subcutaneously every 2 weeks. After an Hb level >100 g/L is achieved, continue to administer the agent once a month.

The subcutaneous route is usually used in patients with CKD who are not on hemodialysis, including those on peritoneal dialysis. ESAs are used in patients with an Hb <100 g/L after causes of anemia other than CKD have been excluded and following an initial trial of iron supplementation, or in combination with iron supplementation. The dose is adjusted to maintain an Hb increase of 10 to 20 g/L per month, and after the target Hb is achieved, to maintain its levels within that target range. Nurse-led algorithms are at least as good as usual care.

Adverse effects of ESAs include hypertension (20%-30% of patients), hyperco-agulability with fistula thrombosis (5%-10%), seizures (~3% of patients, most frequently in the course of hypertensive encephalopathy), and pure RBC aplasia (PRCA) caused by antibodies to erythropoietin (a rare complication of subcuta-neous epoetin administration). Do not start ESAs in patients with uncontrolled hypertension because of the potential for hypertension to worsen with increased red cell mass. Normalization of Hb levels, compared with more moderate tar-gets such as those described above, is associated with a doubling of the risk of stroke. In patients with cancer, ESAs are associated with worse cancer-related outcomes. Use ESAs in patients with cancer only after a clear discussion of the risks (including an increased risk of cancer-related death) and benefits (reduced need for transfusions and risk of transfusion-related complications).

Contraindications: Uncontrolled hypertension; PRCA; history of stroke (a relative contraindication); an active, potentially treatable malignancy; drug hypersensitivity.

9. Treatment of hyperkalemia: Low GFR, drugs (ACEIs, ARBs, direct renin inhibitors, potassium-sparing diuretics, and potassium supplements), high-potassium diets, and diabetic hyporeninemic hypoaldosteronism (type IV RTA) may all contribute to hyperkalemia. Treatment is primarily dietary restriction, though direct evidence of benefit is lacking. Thiazide or loop di-uretics may be useful if there is an additional indication for their use, such as hypertension or volume overload. Discontinuation of potassium-sparing diuretics and, if needed, discontinuation of ACEIs or ARBs may be necessary. Daily or 3-times-weekly doses of a potassium-binding resin such as sodium polystyrene sulfonate (which exchanges potassium for sodium and sometimes causes volume overload; eg, 5-15 g/d) or calcium resonium (which exchanges potassium for calcium and sometimes causes hypercalcemia) are used by some nephrologists as an alternative to the discontinuation of ACEIs and ARBs, especially in patients whose ability to benefit in terms of vascular and renal protection is high (ie, established vascular disease, diabetes with complications, proteinuria >1 g). However, evidence that resins lower serum potassium is limited to small short-term studies, and evidence of effectiveness in lowering potassium in this long-term role is completely lacking. Newer binders such as patiromer and zirconium cyclosilicate (ZS-9) reduce potassium levels in the medium term. ZS-9 exchanges potassium for sodium and may cause edema in some patients. The safety of these binders has yet to be shown in phase 3 and postmarketing studies, and no impact on patient-important outcomes has yet been demonstrated. In the clinical trials that demonstrated efficacy of ACEIs and ARBs, patients with hyperkalemia discontinued the ACEI or ARB.

Renal Replacement Therapy

1. Types of RRT:

1) **Hemodialysis** is a 3- to 4-hour procedure performed 3 times a week, either by the patient or a caregiver at home or in a dialysis center. Some patients choose to perform shorter treatments (around 2 hours) more frequently (5 or 6 days a week), or nighttime treatment (around 8 hours) 3 to 6 days a week. More frequent dialysis is associated with reductions in surrogate outcomes as well as improved quality of life and metabolic parameters; evidence of a difference in cardiovascular or mortality outcomes is lacking. Recovery time from a dialysis session, which may be 4 to 8 hours in patients on the conventional 3-times-weekly dialysis, is generally much shorter in those who dialyze more frequently, whether for short hours or overnight. Increasing the amount of dialysis based on clearance measurements within a conventional 3-times-weekly hemodialysis schedule does not improve outcomes.✗● When providing outpatient or inpatient care to a patient treated with hemodial-ysis in another center, contact the center and obtain clinical information along with their usual dialysis and medication prescriptions. The vessels of the extremity with the AVF can only be punctured for hemodialysis or

for life-saving indications. Do not measure blood pressure on the extremity with the AVF or graft.

Because of the lead time required to obtain a functioning AVF, and because some individuals have unsuitable vascular anatomy, some patients will have instead a synthetic graft inserted between an artery and a vein and used for venipuncture sites for hemodialysis. Others—more than 50% of prevalent dialysis patients in some countries—dialyze through double-lumen dialysis catheters, usually tunneled subcutaneously to reduce the risk of bacteremia. Nonetheless, the risk of bacteremia in a patient on dialysis through a catheter is 10 times that of a patient with a fistula. Because of the risk of bacteremia, because of the precious status of this access as prerequisite for life-sustaining therapy, and because of the risk of air embolism (the lumen size greatly exceeds that of a standard central venous access), these catheters are usually accessed only by dialysis health-care workers with appropriate training. Each lumen of the catheter is closed by both clamp and Luer-lock caps.

If you need to use a patient's dialysis catheter in a life-threatening emergency, start with the clamp closed. Remove the Luer-lock cap and make a connection with a 10-mL Luer-locked syringe, open the clamp, withdraw 10 mL of blood, reclamp, remove the syringe, and discard its contents. This will remove the catheter-locking solution that is instilled in the catheter after each hemodialysis treatment (usually heparin, citrate, or tissue plasminogen activator [tPA]—to minimize the risk of catheter thrombosis). Repeat with a clean syringe if blood is needed for laboratory testing. Reclamp and attach the IV line to be used, again using a Luer-locked connection. Unclamp and run the IV fluid quickly at first to flush the line and prevent thrombosis; the catheter is designed to support flow rates >500 mL/min, so a very rapid infusion is possible when indicated. Minimize the number of new connections and the number of people who access the line. Not following these recommendations may lead to inadvertent instillation of an anticoagulant into a critically ill patient, blood tests that are uninterpretable owing to dilution and the presence of high concentrations of anticoagulants, and the risk of potentially fatal air embolism.

2) **Peritoneal dialysis**: Continuous ambulatory peritoneal dialysis (CAPD) involves instilling approximately 2 L of sterile fluid into the peritoneal cavity using an indwelling tunneled peritoneal dialysis catheter that exits from the abdominal wall. The fluid is usually exchanged 4 times a day. Because of the frequency of the procedure, it is done by the patient or by a trained caregiver. Automated peritoneal dialysis (APD) is performed overnight by a machine that cycles fluid in and out of the peritoneal cavity, most frequently over 8 to 10 hours. Usually a last fill is needed to provide adequate clearance of uremic toxins. This last fill may be held in the peritoneal cavity until the next dialysis, drained in the middle of the day, or changed in the middle of the day, using an exchange similar to that used in CAPD. Because this technique requires 2 or 3 patient contacts during the day, rather than 4, it is the preferred technique for assisted peritoneal dialysis, in which a health-care worker visits the patient's home and performs dialysis. Assisted peritoneal dialysis allows the benefits of home dialysis to be extended to those who are unable to perform their own dialysis and lack a caregiver who is able to perform it for them. As in 3-times-weekly hemodialysis, in peritoneal dialysis increasing the dose of dialysis based on measurements of clearance does not improve outcomes and we recommend against it.🟢🔵 When providing outpatient or inpatient care to a patient treated in another center with peritoneal dialysis, contact the center and obtain clinical information along with their usual dialysis and medication prescriptions.

Peritoneal dialysis–related peritonitis is a complication usually presenting as draining a cloudy dialysate accompanied by clinical manifestations including abdominal pain, nausea, vomiting, and change in bowel habit; signs of peritoneal irritation are generally much less severe than in surgical causes of peritonitis. Typically empiric broad-spectrum antibiotics (eg, cefazolin and tobramycin) are given intraperitoneally to provide high local concentrations and are then adjusted based on culture and sensitivity results.

3) **Kidney transplantation**: This method of RRT is associated with the least intrusiveness, highest quality of life, longest survival, and it is cost-effective. All patients with functioning transplants are treated under the supervision of a transplantation center. The usual maintenance immunosuppression is 2 or 3 agents: often a calcineurin inhibitor (cyclosporine [INN ciclosporin] or tacrolimus) or rapamycin, an antimetabolite (azathioprine or mycophenolate), and prednisone. Some patients are on prednisone-free immunosuppression. When patients with a kidney transplant are hospitalized or present for emergency care, pay close attention to their immunosuppression to ensure that they do not miss doses. If patients are unable to take medications orally, it is a priority to switch them to parenteral drugs. In patients on, or recently on, prednisone, give stress-dose glucocorticoids if shock is present or suspected. Infection is one of the common presentations of patients with kidney transplants, sometimes relatively straightforward, such as a urinary tract infection, wound infection, or community-acquired pneumonia. However, immunosuppression leads to the possibility of opportunistic infection, and patients may present or become gravely ill. Some antibiotics, most notably macrolides, interact with calcineurin inhibitors. When a patient with a kidney transplant is hospitalized or seen as an outpatient, contact the transplant center for clinical information to ensure that immunosuppressive agents are correct, and, unless the treating team is familiar with the management of renal transplant patients, to seek advice about ongoing management.

2. Indications: RRT should be started before the symptoms of uremia and target organ damage are severe (usually in patients with a GFR 5-15 mL/min/1.73 m^2). Indications for starting RRT are signs and symptoms of uremia (uremic pericarditis, uremic bleeding, uremic encephalopathy or neuropathy [a distal, symmetric, mixed sensorimotor polyneuropathy, more often involving lower extremities]), chronic nausea and vomiting, uncontrolled volume overload or hypertension, or progressive protein-calorie malnutrition. Starting dialysis based on the value of GFR, compared with waiting for symptoms or other early clinical indications for dialysis, is associated with increased resource use and increased time on dialysis but no improvement in clinically important outcomes.⊗● In the majority of patients these problems appear at a GFR of 5 to 10 mL/min/1.73 m^2.

3. Alternatives to RRT: In patients with advanced comorbidity and frailty, initiation of dialysis will generally be associated with further decline rather than reversal. When nursing home residents start dialysis, 60% die in the first year. Some patients whose prognosis on dialysis for survival would be relatively good may choose not to be dialyzed. Frank and realistic education of patients, their families, and substitute decision-makers, where applicable, is critical to making the best decisions around whether to start dialysis or to pursue nondialytic options. Alternatives to RRT are maximal conservative therapy, which might include continued bloodwork and ESAs along with symptom management, and full palliation, in which symptom management alone is the priority.

4. Contraindications: Severe cognitive impairment or other irreversible psychiatric disorders that make it impossible to achieve compliance with the requirements of RRT.

→ **FOLLOW-UP**

An approximate suggested frequency of follow-up serum creatinine measurements:

1) Categories G1 and G2 and stable category G3 patients (a GFR decrease <2 mL/min/1.73 m^2 per year): Once a year.

2) Category G3 patients with progression (a GFR decrease >2 mL/min/1.73 m^2 per year) and stable category G4 patients: Every 6 months.

3) Category G4 and G5 patients: Every 1 to 3 months.

In patients with an eGFR <30 mL/min/1.73 m^2, measure the Hb and serum calcium, inorganic phosphate, bicarbonate, and PTH levels. If the results are normal, they may not need to be repeated unless kidney function changes or there is a clinical change that suggests an abnormality. An abnormal result indicates complications, and the frequency of subsequent determinations depends on treatment. It is unusual for the Hb level to be <100 g/L, for serum phosphate to be elevated, for bicarbonate to be decreased, or for calcium to be decreased until GFR is <30 mL/min/1.73 m^2; any of these findings may warrant further investigations of an alternative etiology. PTH elevation may be seen as early as in G3 CKD. Patients with an eGFR <30 mL/min/1.73 m^2 with proteinuria >1 g/d (or albuminuria >60 mg/mmol [UACR], or a protein--to-creatinine ratio >100 mg/mmol) should be referred to a nephrologist. Other reasons for referral include uncertainty about the diagnosis, suspected polycystic kidney disease or hereditary nephritis, inability to meet blood pressure goals, severe electrolyte abnormalities, recurrent nephrolithiasis, an unexplained or unexpected low GFR (especially in the nonelderly patients), and a rapid change in GFR.

→ **P R O G N O S I S**

The projected 2- and 5-year risk of renal progression to RRT in patients with CKD stage 3 to 5 can be estimated using the 4-variable kidney failure risk equation (available at QxMD), which has been validated in >700,000 people across >30 countries. For example, a 65-year-old North American with an eGFR of 35 mL/min/1.73 m^2 and a UACR of 5 mg/mmol has an estimated 2-year risk of 1.93% and 5-year risk of 5.91%.

In patients with CKD not on dialysis, the majority will die without requiring RRT, the main causes of death being cardiovascular complications and infections. In dialysis patients typical 3-year survival rates are ~65%; this is better in younger adults and in those without diabetes. Transplantation involves a selected subset of those with ESRD whose prognosis is better than average, and it likely directly improves their prognosis: typical 3-year patient survival is ~95% and graft survival is ~90% in recipients of a first transplant.

In a study of US nursing home residents who started dialysis, dialysis was associated with a further significant functional decline, and 60% of patients died in the first year. In a UK cohort of patients who chose either maximal conservative therapy or dialysis, median survival was 14 months in the maximal conservative therapy group compared with 42 months in the dialysis group, but the maximal conservative therapy group experienced fewer days of hospitalization per year of survival and were 4 times more likely to die at home or in a palliative care setting rather than in a hospital.

3. Glomerular Diseases

→ **D E F I N I T I O N   A N D   C L A S S I F I C A T I O N**

Glomerular diseases, or glomerulopathies, belong to a heterogeneous group of kidney diseases that affect mainly the glomeruli, causing structural and functional abnormalities. They have a varied presentation and course, ranging from asymptomatic and benign to rapidly life-threatening. The diseases can be limited to the glomeruli or be part of a systemic disease affecting multiple organ systems. The term **glomerulonephritis** is often used to reflect the involvement of inflammation in many of the diseases that affect the glomerulus.

Classification, etiologies, and clinical features of glomerulopathies: →Table 3-1.

Table 3-1. Classification, etiologies, and clinical features of glomerulopathies

Glomerulopathy	Etiology/secondary causes	Clinical features
Postinfectious GN	– Primarily streptococcal and staphylococcal infections – Less commonly gram-negative bacteria, viral, fungal, or protozoal	Nephritic syndrome ~1-3 weeks after streptococcal infection, 4 weeks after staphylococcal infection
IgA nephropathy	– Seen with Henoch-Schönlein purpura – Associated with cirrhosis, celiac disease, inflammatory bowel disease, HIV, and seronegative arthritis	Microscopic hematuria, "synpharyngitic" gross hematuria, hypertension, proteinuria
Membranoproliferative GN		
Immune complex–mediated	Hepatitis C with cryoglobulinemia, hepatitis B, HIV, endocarditis, shunt nephritis, malaria, schistosomiasis, autoimmune disorders (SLE, Sjögren syndrome), malignancies (dysproteinemias, rarely lymphomas, carcinomas)	Varied presentation: microscopic and nonnephrotic proteinuria, nephrotic syndrome, occasionally rapidly progressive renal failure, commonly hypertension
Complement-mediated	C3 nephritic factor, factor H deficiency (inherited or autoimmune)	
Minimal change disease	– Most commonly primary/idiopathic – Secondary causes include NSAIDs, interferon, lithium, gold, lymphoproliferative disorders (Hodgkin lymphoma)	Nephrotic syndrome
Membranous nephropathy	– Most commonly primary/idiopathic – Secondary causes include autoimmune conditions (primarily SLE), infections (hepatitis B and C), medications (NSAIDs, gold, penicillamine), malignancies	Nephrotic syndrome
FSGS	– Primary/idiopathic – Secondary causes include HIV, parvovirus B19, CMV, EBV, pamidronate, heroin, lithium, obesity, reflux, sickle cell disease	Hypertension, proteinuria, and microscopic hematuria; nephrotic syndrome and abrupt development more common in primary/idiopathic FSGS

CMV, cytomegalovirus; EBV, Epstein-Barr virus; FSGS, focal segmental glomerulosclerosis; GN, glomerulonephritis; NSAID, nonsteroidal anti-inflammatory drug; SLE, systemic lupus erythematosus.

The classification and diagnosis of glomerular diseases are primarily based on histologic patterns seen on renal biopsy, although specific histologic patterns can have multiple causes, requiring interpretation based on other presenting factors and laboratory investigations. Diagnosis is therefore further classified by etiology. **Primary diseases** are idiopathic in nature and lack a known associated secondary cause. Ongoing research is increasingly isolating specific markers and antibodies associated with some of the primary glomerular diseases. Multiple **secondary causes** exist, depending on the underlying histologic lesion. Distinguishing between primary and secondary causes of a glomerular disease is important, as the pathophysiology and subsequent management of the disease can differ substantially. Primary diseases are

Table 3-2. Worldwide incidence of various primary glomerular diseases

Glomerular disease	Incidence (per 100,000 people)
IgA nephropathy	0.2-2.9
Membranous nephropathy	0.3-1.4
Focal segmental glomerulosclerosis	0.2-1.1
Minimal change disease (in adults)	0.2-0.8
Membranoproliferative disease	0.1-0.9

mostly immune-mediated and often require immunosuppression, whereas secondary diseases require treating the underlying inciting cause. Lastly, glomerular diseases can be **congenital**, and in such cases they are almost always evident prior to adulthood.

While diagnosis is dependent on the histologic pattern and renal biopsy may be necessary in case of diagnostic uncertainty, not all patients require or benefit from biopsy. The decision to biopsy a patient requires careful consideration of the risks and benefits and a clear understanding of how the information provided would change management. For example, a biopsy is often required in patients with adult-onset nephrotic syndrome or rapidly progressive glomerulonephritis to assist with the diagnosis and management, whereas in individuals with microscopic hematuria and normal renal function it is not necessary because of the usually benign nature of presentation. Similarly, individuals with a classic presentation for diabetic nephropathy without concern for other pathologies usually do not require a biopsy despite potentially severe proteinuria.

Glomerular diseases are relatively uncommon, and there is significant geographic variation in the incidence of the various diseases. Worldwide incidence: →Table 3-2.

→ CLINICAL FEATURES

Glomerular diseases can be asymptomatic and only identifiable on blood or urine tests. However, many can be associated with systemic signs and symptoms, which may assist in providing evidence for an underlying diagnosis. Additionally, in the setting of secondary glomerular diseases, past medical history and medications may strongly suggest a diagnosis. In the majority of patients with a glomerular disease, one of the following clinical forms is often present, although significant overlap can exist and individual diseases can have different clinical presentations:

1) **Nephrotic syndrome**.
2) **Nephritic syndrome**: Characterized by hypertension, oliguria, and edema (which is usually mild to moderate). Proteinuria is <3.5 g/d and urine microscopy shows active or nephritic urine sediment (dysmorphic erythrocytes, red blood cell casts, or both). Glomerular filtration rate (GFR) is often reduced at presentation.
3) **Asymptomatic microscopic hematuria with or without proteinuria**: Persistent or recurrent microscopic hematuria, or gross hematuria during exacerbations, with varying degrees of proteinuria that do not exceed the nephrotic range. Often no other clinical manifestations of glomerular disease are present. With time, chronic kidney disease (CKD) may develop.
4) **Chronic glomerulonephritis**: Progressive CKD caused by occult glomerulonephritis lasting several years. The progression of CKD is a result

of long-term damage affecting a significant number of glomeruli and of progressive secondary fibrosis of the interstitium with tubular atrophy. The disease is often undiagnosed, as patients can be asymptomatic and do not present until CKD is advanced or discovered incidentally. Clinical features are typical of chronic kidney disease and depend on its stage. Urinalysis reveals proteinuria and microscopic hematuria.

5) **Rapidly progressive glomerulonephritis**: Nephritic syndrome accompanied by rapidly progressive renal failure.

3.1. Nephrotic Syndrome

→ **DEFINITION, ETIOLOGY, PATHOGENESIS**

Nephrotic syndrome is a clinical condition characterized by proteinuria >3.5 g/d, hypoalbuminemia, and edema. In contrast to nephritic syndrome, patients can often have normal glomerular filtration rate (GFR) at presentation. Normal daily urinary protein excretion is <150 mg (on average 50 mg). Damage to the podocytes, which are the epithelial cells responsible for forming the glomerular filtration barrier, leads to urinary loss of plasma proteins.

In children minimal change disease (MCD) is the most common cause of nephrotic syndrome, such that it is treated empirically without a renal biopsy. In adults, the etiology of nephrotic syndrome is more varied and requires a biopsy for diagnosis. Focal segmental glomerulosclerosis (FSGS) is the most common cause of nephrotic syndrome in African Americans. Primary FSGS routinely presents with nephrotic syndrome, whereas in secondary FSGS the degree of proteinuria is typically less severe. Membranous nephropathy is the most common cause of nephrotic syndrome in white populations and is usually primary or idiopathic. Other causes of nephrotic syndrome in adults include MCD, membranoproliferative glomerulonephritis (MPGN), IgA nephropathy, amyloid, and diabetes mellitus.

→ **CLINICAL FEATURES**

Edema often occurs when protein loss is >5 g/d and serum albumin concentration is ≤25 g/L, although variability occurs. Two proposed mechanisms exist for the development of volume overload and edema. One mechanism—overfill theory—involves a collecting tubule defect leading to a significant impairment of sodium and volume excretion. The second mechanism—underfill theory—suggests that the reduction of oncotic pressure from significant hypoalbuminemia leads to the loss of fluid from the intravascular into the extravascular compartment, leading to the activation of the renin-angiotensin-aldosterone system and subsequent sodium and volume retention.

Clinically, foaming of urine (due to the high protein content) may be observed. Pitting edema is usually symmetric and its location depends on the body position (facial edema is frequently observed in the morning, edema of the feet and lower legs in the evening), although edema is often severe enough that lower limb edema is persistent. Orthostatic hypotension may occur in elderly patients with severe hypoalbuminemia.

Hyperlipidemia and hypertriglyceridemia develop mainly as a result of the decreased rate of catabolism of lipoproteins, increased synthesis of very low–density lipoprotein in response to hypoalbuminemia, and urinary losses of high-density lipoprotein cholesterol. Hyperlipidemia can often be severe and contributes to an increased risk of coronary artery disease if prolonged. Xanthelasma can be seen in severe hypercholesterolemia.

Nephrotic syndrome leads to a significant increase in the risk of both venous and arterial thrombosis. The mechanism is not completely understood but likely involves urinary loss of antithrombin III and plasminogen as well as increased hepatic synthesis of procoagulant factors. Increased platelet activation has also been described. Thrombosis occurs in 10% to 50% of patients (more commonly in primary membranous nephropathy). Renal venous thrombosis may be asymptomatic, but it can also present with acute kidney injury, flank pain, or hematuria. Additionally, patients with nephrotic syndrome are at risk of infection. Urinary loss of IgG is the main cause for increased susceptibility to infection. This particularly decreases the ability to respond to encapsulated organisms such as pneumococcus, and both conjugate and polysaccharide pneumococcal vaccinations are recommended.

→ DIAGNOSIS

1. Urinalysis/microscopy: Severe proteinuria and microscopic hematuria may be seen. Lipiduria is manifested by oval fat bodies or "Maltese crosses" on microscopy.

2. Twenty-four–hour urine collection: While urinalysis and the urine albumin-to-creatinine ratio (ACR) will demonstrate significant proteinuria, a 24-hour urine collection should be done to quantify the degree of proteinuria.

3. Blood tests: Hypoalbuminemia and hyperlipidemia are hallmarks of nephrotic syndrome. Other abnormalities may include increased creatinine and urea, hypocalcemia (primarily a reduction in the concentration of protein-nonionized calcium), vitamin D deficiency, and hypogammaglobulinemia. Additional investigations to assess for the cause of nephrotic syndrome should include antinuclear antibodies (ANAs), antibodies to phospholipase A_2 receptors, serum and urine electrophoresis, quantitative immunoglobulins, fasting glucose, chronic hepatitis serologies, complement levels, and HIV testing.

4. Imaging studies: Renal ultrasonography is rarely diagnostic but should be done prior to renal biopsy.

5. Renal biopsy: In the majority of cases, renal biopsy is required in adults to determine the cause of nephrotic syndrome, unless it is obvious (eg, patients with diabetes with retinopathy and/or neuropathy and a history of progressive proteinuria).

→ TREATMENT

Treatment includes diagnosis and management of the underlying condition as well as addressing complications of nephrotic syndrome. Edema can be significant and should be treated with **sodium restriction** (<2 g/d), although **loop diuretics** are usually required. Loop diuretics are protein-bound, which leads to decreased delivery to the kidney in hypoalbuminemia and increased binding of the medication in the tubules because of albuminuria, resulting in the requirement of larger than usual doses to achieve diuresis. Combination with a thiazide diuretic or addition of IV albumin may assist with diuresis.

Reduction of proteinuria results in decreased progression of chronic kidney disease regardless of the underlying etiology. As a result, angiotensin-converting enzyme inhibitors (ACEIs)/angiotensin receptor blockers (ARBs) are recommended in nephrotic syndrome and can reduce proteinuria by ~50%.◐●

Statins, or 3-hydroxy-3-methylglutaryl coenzyme A (HMG-CoA) reductase inhibitors, are routinely used to treat the hyperlipidemia associated with nephrotic syndrome. In the absence of specific recommendations for targets in nephrotic syndrome, general cardiovascular guidelines are used.

Thromboembolic events should be treated as per usual therapy. The role of **prophylactic anticoagulation** is controversial; it is not routinely done, although it can be considered in patients with primary nephrotic syndrome and severe hypoalbuminemia (<20 g/L).

3.2. Rapidly Progressive Glomerulonephritis

→ DEFINITION, ETIOLOGY, PATHOGENESIS

Rapidly progressive glomerulonephritis (RPGN) is a clinical syndrome of rapid deterioration of renal function within weeks, with histologic features of extra-capillary proliferation; this forms cellular crescents in Bowman space and can be referred to as crescentic glomerulonephritis. RPGN can be kidney-limited or associated with systemic diseases.

The causes of RPGN are often categorized into 3 classes of underlying conditions:

1) **Anti–glomerular basement membrane (anti-GBM) disease**: Presence of autoantibodies against type IV collagen. Historically, the term "Goodpasture syndrome" referred to lung (pulmonary hemorrhage) and kidney involvement.

2) **Immune complex deposition**: Immune complexes deposited in the glomer-ulus can be seen either on immunofluorescence or electron microscopy. Serum complement levels may be low. Immune complex deposition is associated with infectious or autoimmune conditions. Common causes include systemic lupus erythematosus (SLE), IgA nephropathy, postinfectious glomerulonephritis, and endocarditis. Signs and symptoms are reflective of the underlying disease.

3) **Pauci-immune RPGN**: Histologically characterized by the absence of immune deposits in the vessel wall or glomerulus. The majority of patients have circulating antineutrophil cytoplasmic antibodies (ANCAs). Causes of pauci-immune glomerulonephritis include granulomatosis with polyangiitis (GPA), microscopic polyangiitis (MPA), and less commonly Churg-Strauss syndrome. Pulmonary hemorrhage can also occur. Other areas of vasculitis involvement include the eyes, skin, and nervous system.

Patients occasionally have both antibodies to the GBM and ANCAs and are then considered "double-antibody positive."

→ CLINICAL FEATURES

RPGN often manifests as nephritic syndrome with hypertension, mild edema, dysmorphic red blood cells/red cell casts on microscopy, non–nephrotic range proteinuria, and decreased glomerular filtration rate (GFR). In some patients the onset of symptoms is insidious, and presenting manifestations are weakness, fatigue, fever, and arthralgias. When RPGN is secondary to an underlying condition, symptoms of that disease can be observed. Nephrotic syndrome can occur but is uncommon.

In untreated patients, end-stage renal disease (→Chapter 9.2) can develop rapidly.

→ DIAGNOSIS

1. Urinalysis/microscopy: Active urine sediment, proteinuria usually below the nephrotic range.

2. Blood tests: Increased creatinine/urea and other abnormalities consis-tent with acute kidney injury. Tests for diagnosis include anti-GBM antibody, cytoplasmic antineutrophil cytoplasmic antibody (c-ANCA), perinuclear anti-neutrophil cytoplasmic antibody (p-ANCA), antinuclear antibody (ANA), anti–double-stranded DNA (anti-dsDNA) antibody, complements, antistreptolysin O (ASO) titer, and cryoglobulins.

3. Diagnostic imaging: Renal ultrasonography. Consider echocardiography and chest radiography.

4. Renal biopsy: Biopsy is usually required for diagnosis and shows crescent formation in the glomeruli.

→ **TREATMENT**

Treatment of RPGN varies depending on the underlying cause but should be started quickly, as permanent renal damage develops rapidly. Involvement of nearly all glomeruli, fibrotic crescents, diffuse interstitial fibrosis, and diffuse renal tubular atrophy are biopsy signs of irreversible damage, and in such cases aggressive immunosuppressive therapy has only marginal benefits and is outweighed by the risk. Dialysis is the only treatment option for such patients unless nonrenal indications for treatment exist (pulmonary hemorrhage).

1. Anti-GBM disease⊘⊖:

1) Glucocorticoids: IV methylprednisolone 0.5 to 1 g/d for 3 days followed by oral prednisone 1 mg/kg/d titrated to 10 mg/d after 4 months and discontinued after 6 months.

2) Oral cyclophosphamide 2 mg/kg/d for 3 months (in IV pulses if the patient is unable to take oral formulations). Dose adjustment is required for reduced renal function.

3) Daily plasmapheresis with an exchange of 4 L of plasma per procedure for 14 days or until anti-GBM antibodies are undetectable.

Prolonged immunosuppression (>3 months) is not usually necessary. Individuals who present requiring dialysis very rarely derive benefit from treatment and are not usually treated with immunosuppression in the absence of pulmonary hemorrhage.

2. Immune complex disease: Treatment and the evidence supporting treatment varies depending on the underlying cause of the immune complexes. SLE is treated with glucocorticoids and either cyclophosphamide or mycophenolate mofetil. Glucocorticoids can be also considered for postinfectious glomerulonephritis and endocarditis.

3. Pauci-immune RPGN (with or without positive ANCA titer results):

1) IV methylprednisolone 0.5 to 1 g/d for 3 days followed by oral prednisone 1 mg/kg for 1 month and then tapered over 3 to 4 months. Evidence varies on the appropriate duration of glucocorticoid maintenance therapy.

2) Cyclophosphamide IV 15 mg/kg initially every 2 weeks or daily orally 1.5 to 2 mg/kg. IV cyclophosphamide may have fewer adverse effects than the oral formulation but it may be associated with higher rates of relapse. The appropriate duration of cyclophosphamide is unclear but suggested as 3 to 6 months.⊘⊖

3) Rituximab has been shown to be noninferior to cyclophosphamide and can be considered in patients with contraindications to cyclophosphamide.⊘⊖

4) Plasmapheresis is currently recommended in guidelines for those with advanced renal disease (creatinine >500 µmol/L) and suggested for those with pulmonary hemorrhage, although recent research questions the long-term efficacy.⊘⊖ A large ongoing randomized controlled trial (PEXIVAS [Plasma Exchange and Glucocorticoids for Treatment of Anti-Neutrophil Cytoplasm Antibody–Associated Vasculitis]) is further investigating the utility of plasmapheresis.

5) The appropriate duration of maintenance therapy is unknown, with suggestions ranging from 12 to 24 months. Azathioprine and rituximab both have evidence supporting their use as maintenance agents.⊘⊖

Unlike in anti-GBM disease, patients with pauci-immune RPGN requiring dialysis at presentation can recover renal function and should be treated even in the absence of extrarenal manifestations unless renal biopsy demonstrates a near complete loss of glomeruli and interstitial scarring. If patients remain dialysis-dependent and have no extrarenal manifestations, maintenance therapy is not necessary.

Relapses

1. Anti-GBM disease relapses rarely but should be treated in the same way as at first presentation.

2. Relapses of pauci-immune glomerulonephritis are more common. If severe (life- or organ-threatening), they require a repeat of the initial therapy, although rituximab can be considered over cyclophosphamide, depending on the previous cumulative dose of cyclophosphamide.

→ PROGNOSIS

The prognosis of RPGN is dependent on the underlying pathology and severity of the initial presentation. Anti-GBM disease is usually quickly fatal if untreated. Patient survival is greatly improved with treatment and is as high as 90%. Renal survival, unfortunately, is much poorer. Mortality in untreated pauci--immune vasculitis is 90% without therapy, although treatment is effective and has reduced mortality to between 10% and 20%. Permanent renal replacement is required in 20% to 40% of patients.

3.3. Selected Congenital Glomerulopathies

3.3.1. Alport Syndrome

→ DEFINITION, ETIOLOGY

Alport syndrome (AS) is a hereditary nephropathy caused by abnormal synthesis of type IV collagen α chains, which leads to damage of the glomerular basement membrane. AS is mostly commonly X-linked (in ~80% of patients). A fully symptomatic disease occurs in men, while women are carriers or have a milder form of the disease. Other types of AS have autosomal inheritance, occur in both sexes, and have a course similar to X-linked AS.

→ CLINICAL FEATURES

Microscopic hematuria and proteinuria are observed. End-stage renal disease (→Chapter 9.2) occurs in almost all men and usually develops by their early- to mid-30s. Most patients have high-frequency sensorineural hearing loss. Various ocular lesions, such as anterior lenticonus, can occur.

→ TREATMENT

There is no specific therapy for AS.

3.3.2. Fabry Disease

→ DEFINITION

Fabry disease is a hereditary X-linked disease caused by α-galactosidase A deficiency, which leads to tissue accumulation of glycosphingolipids and multiple organ dysfunction.

→ CLINICAL FEATURES

Renal disease manifests as proteinuria and eventually worsening renal function. Nephrotic range proteinuria and nephrotic syndrome occur in <20% of patients but when present, they lead to increased risk of developing end-stage renal disease (→Chapter 9.2). Common presenting findings include angiokeratomas and severe neuropathic pain. Cardiac involvement occurs in up to

80% of patients and can manifest as myocardial infarction, left ventricular hypertrophy, and conduction problems. Other frequent abnormalities include hypohidrosis, nonspecific abdominal complaints, ocular abnormalities, and hearing impairment.

→ DIAGNOSIS

Diagnosis is based on reduced or absent α-galactosidase A activity. Renal biopsy findings include pronounced vacuoles in the glomerular epithelial cells containing glycosphingolipids.

→ TREATMENT

Treatment is enzyme replacement with recombinant α-galactosidase A infusions.

3.3.3. Thin Basement Membrane Disease

→ DEFINITION, ETIOLOGY

Thin basement membrane disease (TBMD) (also called benign familial hematuria) is a congenital glomerulopathy characterized by thinning (<250 nm) of the glomerular basement membrane. Patients with familial TBMD have autosomal dominant inheritance, although they may not have a known family history, given the asymptomatic nature of the condition.

→ CLINICAL FEATURES

Patients develop microscopic hematuria, which is frequently detectable as early as in childhood. Typically proteinuria and hypertension are absent and patients do not develop renal failure. Hematuria is not aggravated by comorbidities and extrarenal symptoms do not occur.

→ DIAGNOSIS

Diagnosis is based on electron microscopy examination demonstrating thin basement membranes without other pathologies.

→ TREATMENT

Specific treatment is neither available nor necessary.

3.4. Specific Pathologies

3.4.1. Focal Segmental Glomerulosclerosis

→ DEFINITION, ETIOLOGY, PATHOGENESIS

Focal segmental glomerulosclerosis (FSGS) is a histologic pattern characterized by initial damage of the podocytes with progressive glomerulosclerosis and accompanying expansion of mesangial matrix. Sclerotic lesions are focal (some but not all glomeruli are involved) and segmental (only part of the glomerulus is involved), and multiple different histologic subtypes exist.

FSGS can be primary/idiopathic or secondary to a diverse group of causes. The cause of primary FSGS is unknown, although it is thought likely to be due to a circulating factor. Causes of secondary FSGS include hyperfiltration (reflux nephropathy, malignant hypertension, reduction of renal mass, obesity, and sickle cell anemia), drugs (heroin, pamidronate, lithium, calcineurin inhibitors, sirolimus), and viral infections (HIV, parvovirus B19, and less commonly cytomegalovirus or Epstein-Barr virus).

→ CLINICAL FEATURES

FSGS is more prevalent in African Americans and in males. Edema and proteinuria are the most common clinical manifestations. Nephrotic syndrome is often found and occurs in up to 80% of patients. Substantial edema and nephrotic range proteinuria are more common in primary FSGS. Microscopic hematuria, hypertension, and decreased glomerular filtration rate (GFR) are also frequently present.

Spontaneous remissions have been reported and are associated with preserved renal function, lower degrees of proteinuria at presentation, and the histologic "tip lesion."

→ DIAGNOSIS

Diagnosis is based on histologic examination of kidney biopsy specimens. At least 20 glomeruli are required to exclude FSGS, given the focal nature of lesions.

→ TREATMENT

All patients without contraindications should be treated with **sodium restriction** and **renin-angiotensin system blockade** to reduce proteinuria and control hypertension.

In addition to the renin-angiotensin system blockade, **glucocorticoids** are used to treat patients with primary FSGS There is some controversy over when to initiate immunosuppressive therapy but most elect only to treat those with nephrotic syndrome. Dosing and duration are based on observational data. Current recommendations are to use immunosuppression only in patients with nephrotic syndrome. Suggested doses are prednisone 1 mg/kg/d or 2 mg/kg every other day for 4 to 16 weeks until remission is achieved (daily proteinuria <300 mg/d) and then titrated over 6 months after remission. Remission is usually achieved slowly and will often take 3 to 4 months of glucocorticoid therapy. In patients who fail to respond or require alternative therapies to glucocorticoids, calcineurin inhibitors may be considered.

Secondary causes of FSGS are treated by addressing the underlying cause. There is no role for immunosuppression in secondary FSGS.

→ PROGNOSIS

Without treatment most patients have progressive renal failure. Proteinuria is a strong predictor of progression: More than 50% of patients with proteinuria >3.5 g/d who do not respond to therapy progress to end-stage renal disease by 10 years, whereas patients with non–nephrotic range proteinuria have renal survival of 95%. Remission, even partial, is associated with significantly better renal outcomes. Other predictors of poor outcomes include African American populations, increased creatinine at presentation, and collapsing variant on histology.

3.4.2. IgA Nephropathy

→ DEFINITION, ETIOLOGY, PATHOGENESIS

IgA nephropathy is the most common primary glomerulopathy. In addition to diffuse proliferation of mesangial cells and expansion of mesangial matrix, it is characterized by deposition of IgA in the glomeruli on immunofluorescence.

It represents 10% to 45% of primary glomerular diseases and is more common in Asian and white populations.

Secondary causes of IgA nephropathy are most frequently associated with IgA-related vasculitis (also referred to as Henoch-Schönlein purpura), cirrhosis and other severe liver diseases, celiac disease and other autoimmune conditions, or HIV infection. Their treatment and prognosis are related to the underlying condition.

→ CLINICAL FEATURES

IgA nephropathy is characterized by hematuria that can be microscopic, recurrent macroscopic, or both. Macroscopic hematuria most frequently accompanies viral or bacterial upper respiratory tract infections or gastrointestinal infections. This so-called synpharyngitic hematuria differentiates IgA nephropathy from the longer 10-to-21-day delay of postinfectious glomerulonephritis. Macroscopic hematuria may last from several hours to several days and may be accompanied by flank pain. Non–nephrotic range proteinuria is often present, although nephrotic range proteinuria and nephrotic syndrome occur in 5% to 10% of patients. The degree of proteinuria is the strongest prognostic indicator. Hypertension is present in up to 40% of patients. IgA levels are increased in approximately 50% of patients, but this is neither sensitive nor specific.

→ DIAGNOSIS

Biopsy is required for a definitive confirmation.

Diagnosis is based on pathologic findings including predominant mesangial IgA deposition on immunofluorescence.

→ TREATMENT

Hypertension is associated with progression of renal disease and should be controlled (→Chapter 3.9.3). **Renin-angiotensin system blockers** are the first-line therapy given the usual presence of proteinuria. In patients with proteinuria >1 g/d, renin-angiotensin system blockers should be titrated to reduce proteinuria to <1 g/d, as blood pressure permits, and additional titration to <500 mg/d can be considered.

Evidence for **glucocorticoids** for patients who continue to have proteinuria >1 g/d despite appropriate renin-angiotensin system blockade is uncertain.⊗○ Older studies demonstrated benefit but were criticized for multiple reasons, including lack of universal renin-angiotensin system blockade. More recently, the STOP IgAN (Supportive Versus Immunosuppressive Therapy of Progressive IgA Nephropathy) trial has not shown improvement in estimated glomerular filtration rate (eGFR) with glucocorticoid use (although the trial excluded patients with proteinuria >3.5 g/d). The Therapeutic Evaluation of Steroids in IgA Nephropathy Global (TESTING) did show an improvement in worsening eGFR but was stopped early due to increased adverse events (serious infections) in the treatment arm. Additional studies are ongoing.

Patients presenting with rapidly progressive glomerulonephritis/crescents on biopsy can be considered for cyclophosphamide and glucocorticoids.

→ PROGNOSIS

Between 15% and 40% of patients will develop end-stage renal disease at 25 years after diagnosis. The degree of proteinuria is the most significant indicator of poor prognosis, with hypertension and decreased GFR at presentation also associated with worse outcomes.

Table 3-3. Classification, biopsy findings, and prevalence of lupus nephritis

Lupus nephritis class	Biopsy findings	Prevalence
I (minimal mesangial)	– Normal light microscopy – Mesangial immune deposits on immunofluorescence	0%-1%
II (mesangial proliferative)	Mesangial hypercellularity or expansion	9.8%-18.1%
III (focal proliferative)	– Endocapillary or extracapillary glomerulonephritis involving <50% of glomeruli – Subendothelial immune deposits – Active or chronic	8.7%-10%
IV (diffuse proliferative)	– Endocapillary or extracapillary glomerulonephritis involving ≥50% of glomeruli – Subendothelial deposits – Active or chronic – Segmental or global	36.9%-37.1%
V (membranous)	– Subepithelial deposits – May occur with classes III or IV	11.7%-40.2%
VI (global glomerulosclerosis)	≥90% of globally sclerosed glomeruli	2.7%-4.3%

Source: Kidney Int. 2004;65(2):521-30.

3.4.3. Lupus Nephritis

→ **DEFINITION, ETIOLOGY, PATHOGENESIS**

Lupus nephritis (LN) is a common complication of systemic lupus erythematosus (SLE), with approximately 50% to 60% of patients with SLE developing renal involvement during the course of the disease, although some studies suggest that the rate of renal involvement without clinical manifestations may be much higher. Approximately one-third of patients have renal involvement at the time of SLE diagnosis. Patients with LN have an overall worse prognosis than patients without renal involvement. The risk to patients is greater than just that caused by renal disease, suggesting that LN is an indicator of overall disease severity. LN is most common and more severe in African Americans and least common and severe in whites. Male SLE patients are more likely to acquire LN, although most patients are female, given the large gender difference in the overall SLE prevalence.

LN is primarily an immune complex disease of the glomerulus. Anti–double-stranded DNA (anti-dsDNA) immune complexes are found deposited in various parts of the glomerulus, resulting in an inflammatory response and disease. Immune complexes can deposit in the mesangial, endothelial, and epithelial spaces, with varying presentations depending on location. Other renal diseases can occur in SLE, including thrombotic microangiopathy and tubulointerstitial nephritis.

Classification: LN is divided into 6 different classes based on the International Society of Nephrology and the Renal Pathology Society classification system (→Table 3-3), which correspond to differing levels of severity and treatment requirements:

1) **Class I (minimal mesangial LN)**: Normal light microscopy and mesangial immune deposits on immunofluorescence or electron microscopy. This is not

usually seen on biopsy since these patients often have few clinical abnormalities necessitating biopsy.

2) **Class II (mesangial proliferative LN)**: The earliest stage to show light microscopy changes, which consist of mesangial hypercellularity or expansion. These patients often have proteinuria and hematuria but usually normal renal function.

3) **Class III (focal LN)**: Endocapillary or extracapillary glomerulonephritis in <50% of the glomeruli. This is typically associated with subendothelial immune deposits. Patients usually have proteinuria, hematuria, and decreased glomerular filtration rate (GFR). Class III can be subdivided into active or chronic lesions.

4) **Class IV (diffuse LN)**: The most common and most severe form of LN. It is manifested by endocapillary or extracapillary glomerulonephritis in >50% of the glomeruli. Patients will usually have proteinuria, hematuria, and decreased GFR. Class IV can also be subdivided into active or chronic lesions.

5) **Class V (membranous LN)**: Thickening of the glomerular basement membrane (GBM) and subepithelial immune deposits. Patients typically present with nephrotic syndrome. Class V can overlap with classes III and IV.

6) **Class VI (advanced sclerosing LN)**: Glomerulosclerosis in >90% of the glomeruli without evidence of active inflammation. It represents permanent damage from previous class III, IV, or V disease and is unlikely to respond to therapy.

Patients can switch between classes of disease, so changes in clinical situations may necessitate a repeat biopsy to determine if a class switch has occurred and subsequent alteration of management is required.

→ CLINICAL FEATURES

Renal disease in LN is often asymptomatic, although the patient may exhibit other signs and symptoms of SLE (such as rash, arthritis, fatigue, fever, or weight loss). Proteinuria is almost universal in LN. Microscopic hematuria and red cell casts are very common, while gross hematuria is relatively rare and can represent both renal and nonrenal disease (eg, lupus cystitis). Patients are often hypertensive, with hypertension worsening with the severity of the disease. Nephrotic syndrome can occur with associated significant edema; it is suggestive of membranous LN. Patients often have decreased renal function, hypocomplementemia (both C3 and C4), increased erythrocyte sedimentation rate (ESR), and elevated titers of anti-dsDNA antibodies.

→ DIAGNOSIS

A diagnosis of LN is strongly suggested based on the presence of microscopic hematuria/red cell casts and proteinuria in a patient with SLE and is confirmed on biopsy.

→ TREATMENT

General Considerations

In all patients with nephropathy blood pressure should probably be managed according to the current general guidelines (→Chapter 3.9.3).

In patients with proteinuria, administer an angiotensin-converting enzyme inhibitor (ACEI) or angiotensin-receptor blocker (ARB). Patients with nephrotic syndrome: →Chapter 9.3.1.

Immunomodulatory treatment: In all patients with lupus nephritis, including those in remission, antimalarial therapy is recommended. Otherwise, specific treatment is based on the underlying class of LN seen on biopsy.

Specific Treatment

Treatment is based on the underlying class of LN seen on biopsy. Class I is not associated with long-term renal impairment and is not specifically treated (patients in this class are also typically not biopsied). Class II also does not usually require immunosuppression, although it can be considered in individuals with nephrotic range proteinuria. SLE in classes I and II should be treated according to the patient's extrarenal manifestations.

Classes III and IV are associated with very poor outcomes if left untreated. These patients are provided with initial **immunosuppression** followed by maintenance immunosuppression. Initial immunosuppression consists of glucocorticoids and either cyclophosphamide or mycophenolate mofetil (MMF), based on a number of different studies.◐● Glucocorticoids should consist of prednisone 1 mg/kg/d tapered over 6 to 12 months with pulse solumedrol often being used initially in the setting of severe disease. Additional immunosuppression includes one of the following regimens:

1) IV cyclophosphamide 0.5 to 1 g/m^2 monthly for 6 months.
2) IV cyclophosphamide 500 mg every 2 weeks for 3 months.
3) Oral cyclophosphamide 1 to 1.5 mg/kg/d for 2 to 4 months.
4) Oral MMF up to 3 g/d for 6 months.

MMF may be more useful than cyclophosphamide in African Americans and Latin Americans, and cyclophosphamide may be more useful in severe disease. The patient's preferences may also play a role in treatment decisions, as many SLE patients are young and cyclophosphamide has potential for gonadal toxicity.

Maintenance therapy should consist of either MMF 1 to 2 g/d or azathioprine 1.5 to 2.5 mg/kg/d combined with low-dose prednisone. Some evidence suggests that MMF may be better than azathioprine at preventing the progression of chronic kidney disease or flares of disease. Maintenance therapy is suggested for at least 1 year after remission is achieved, although its appropriate duration is unknown.

There is significantly less evidence for treatment of class V compared with class III or IV. Patients with non–nephrotic range proteinuria can be treated with antiproteinuric (eg, angiotensin-converting enzyme inhibitor [ACEI]/angiotensin receptor blocker [ARB]) and antihypertensive medications. In those with nephrotic range proteinuria, glucocorticoids in addition to another immunosuppressive medication (cyclophosphamide, calcineurin inhibitor, or MMF) can be used. In contrast to idiopathic membranous nephropathy, membranous LN rarely resolves spontaneously.

Patients with a combination of class V and class III or IV have significantly worse outcomes than those assigned to class V alone and should be treated similarly to those in class III or IV. Class VI represents advanced chronic damage that does not benefit from immunosuppression; such patients should be treated according to extrarenal manifestations and with therapies aimed at reducing the progression of chronic kidney disease/delaying end-stage renal disease.

→ PROGNOSIS

Survival has improved substantially with the introduction of immunosuppressive therapy for LN. Whereas previously <50% of patients with class IV LN survived >5 years, the 10-year survival rate for patients with LN is now approximately 88% (compared with 92% for SLE patients without LN). Estimates on the rate of end-stage renal disease vary between 3% and 36% for patients with LN.

Achieving a complete renal response to therapy is an important marker of prognosis. Definitions of complete response vary between studies but it usually consists of stabilization of creatinine to previous disease activity levels and substantial reduction of proteinuria. The Lupus Nephritis Collaborative Study

Group demonstrated renal survival of 94% at 10 years in those with a complete renal response to therapy compared with only 31% in those that did not.

3.4.4. Membranoproliferative Glomerulonephritis

→ **DEFINITION, ETIOLOGY, PATHOGENESIS**

Membranoproliferative glomerulonephritis (MPGN) is characterized by diffuse proliferation of the mesangium and thickening of the capillary walls. It is a rare disease, accounting for <10% of glomerular diseases.

MPGN is classified on the basis of the underlying pathology into either immune complex–mediated MPGN or complement-mediated MPGN. In both cases complement ultimately causes damage to the glomerulus. However, in immune complex–mediated MPGN the initiating event is immune complex deposition, which activates complement, whereas with complement-mediated MPGN there is underlying inappropriate and continuous complement activation due to dysregulation of the complement system.

The majority of immune complex–mediated MPGN is caused by infections, with most of those being caused by hepatitis C with cryoglobulinemia. Less common causes of immune complex–mediated MPGN include monoclonal gammopathies and autoimmune conditions (most commonly lupus). Complement-mediated MPGN is less common than immune complex–mediated MPGN and is usually due to either an acquired (genetic) defect or autoimmune removal (antibodies) of complement or complement regulatory proteins. An older classification system separated MGPN into classes I, II, and III based on the appearance on electron microscopy and this classification can still be found in the literature.

→ **CLINICAL FEATURES**

MPGN that is acquired or autoimmune occurs mainly between the ages of 5 and 30 years. Presentation varies and can include asymptomatic hematuria and proteinuria, nephrotic syndrome, and rarely rapidly progressive glomerulonephritis. Hypertension is common and present in most patients. Levels of C3 are low and C4 may be low.

MPGN that is secondary to another condition is associated with signs and symptoms of the underlying condition. When MPGN is associated with hepatitis C–induced cryoglobulinemia, it is often accompanied by weakness, arthralgias, and purpura, which preferentially affects the lower extremities.

→ **TREATMENT**

There is no universally accepted treatment regimen for MPGN, as the evidence is of generally low quality. For idiopathic immune complex–mediated MPGN, patients with proteinuria >3.5 g/d and/or a progressive decline of glomerular filtration rate (GFR), **immunosuppressive treatment** may be attempted, with the appropriate choice of medication being unclear.

Treatment for immune complex–mediated MPGN secondary to an underlying condition should be targeted towards the underlying condition. Evidence for complement-mediated MPGN is less clear given the rarity of the disease. Immunosuppression and complement inhibitors may be attempted in those with significant proteinuria or declining renal function.

→ **PROGNOSIS**

Idiopathic MPGN is usually progressive. Approximately 50% of patients reach end-stage renal disease by 10 years. In secondary MPGN effective treatment of the underlying condition usually leads to at least partial remission.

3.4.5. Membranous Nephropathy

➡️ **DEFINITION, ETIOLOGY, PATHOGENESIS**

Membranous nephropathy (MN) is a histologic diagnosis characterized by thickening of the glomerular basement membrane (GBM) on light microscopy without cellular proliferation. It is an immune-mediated disease with immune complex deposition near or on the foot processes of the podocytes. Deposition and subsequent complement activation lead to GBM damage and podocyte effacement, resulting in substantial proteinuria.

The majority (approximately two-thirds) of cases are idiopathic. The inciting event for antibody deposition in primary MN is unknown. Circulating antibodies against phospholipase A_2 receptors on the podocyte are observed in 70% to 80% of patients with primary MN but not in those with secondary causes. Causes of secondary MN include malignancy (primarily solid tumors, including lung and gastrointestinal tumors), connective tissue diseases (especially systemic lupus erythematosus), hepatitis B and C infections, drugs (penicillamine, gold salts, nonsteroidal anti-inflammatory drugs, captopril), and sarcoidosis.

➡️ **CLINICAL FEATURES**

MN may develop in patients of all ages but is most frequently seen in middle--aged individuals and is rare in children. It is more common in males and in whites. The majority of patients present with nephrotic syndrome, with the remainder having non–nephrotic range proteinuria. Microscopic hematuria occurs in approximately 30% of patients. Hypertension and decreased glomerular filtration rate (GFR) at presentation are uncommon but can develop over the course of the disease. Reported rates of thromboembolic events vary considerably and range between 5% and 50%. Approximately one-third of patients have spontaneous remissions, which are more likely in individuals with lower degrees of proteinuria.

➡️ **DIAGNOSIS**

Diagnosis is based on histology. The classic finding is thickening of the GBM with "spikes" of the GBM projecting around immune complex deposits on light microscopy with the silver stain. Assays are available for antibodies to phospholipase A_2 receptors, which can assist in differentiating primary MN from secondary MN.

➡️ **TREATMENT**

Treatment of primary MN is based upon the risk of progression of renal disease. Patients with proteinuria <4 g/d and normal renal function over 6 months of observation progress rarely. Individuals with normal or near-normal renal function and proteinuria between 4 and 8 g per day despite conservative management are at increased risk (approximately 55% are at risk of progressing to chronic kidney disease), and those with persistent proteinuria >8 g/d or worsening renal function are at high risk of progression.

Conservative management for all patients should include **renin-angiotensin system blockade** to control hypertension and proteinuria. Patients should also be treated for complications of nephrotic syndrome. Treating the underlying cause of secondary MN usually results in remission.

Immunosuppressive therapy for primary MN is recommended in patients who have any of the following:

1) Persistent proteinuria >4 g/d despite maximal conservative management for 6 months.

2) Severe symptoms or complications of nephrotic syndrome.

3) Rising serum creatinine levels (>30%) within 6 to 12 months of diagnosis.

When initiating immunosuppression, glucocorticoids alone are ineffective at treating MN. The Ponticelli regimen is the recommended initial therapy, which consists of alternating months of IV methylprednisolone followed by oral prednisone for 1 month and then an alkylating agent (oral cyclophosphamide or chlorambucil) for 1 month◐◑; cyclophosphamide is preferred due to fewer adverse effects. This cycle is repeated for 6 months. Calcineurin inhibitors (eg, tacrolimus) with low-dose prednisone or tacrolimus without prednisone can be considered as alternatives.

→ **PROGNOSIS**

In the majority of patients successful treatment of the underlying condition leads to the resolution of secondary MN. In drug-induced MN discontinuation of the causative agent almost always leads to resolution of MN, although remission can be delayed (up to years with gold and penicillamine). The prognosis in idiopathic MN depends largely on the degree of proteinuria, with end-stage renal disease occurring after 15 years in ~40% of patients.

3.4.6. Minimal Change Disease

→ **DEFINITION, ETIOLOGY, PATHOGENESIS**

Minimal change disease (MCD) is a frequent cause of nephrotic syndrome. It is so named because of the normal-appearing histologic results on light microscopy. Electron microscopy demonstrates significant foot process effacement.

The cause of primary MCD is unknown. Secondary MCD is rare, with known associations including drugs (nonsteroidal anti-inflammatory agents, interferon, and lithium) and lymphoproliferative disorders, specifically Hodgkin lymphoma.

→ **CLINICAL FEATURES AND NATURAL HISTORY**

Typically MCD causes nephrotic syndrome, which develops over days to weeks. Primary MCD is by far the most common cause of nephrotic syndrome in patients <16 years of age (70%-90%), such that nephrotic syndrome in children is usually treated empirically as MCD without biopsy. In adults it may occur at any age and accounts for 10% to 25% of cases of nephrotic syndrome. Hypertension can occur in adults. Renal function is usually normal. Proteinuria is frequently severe, averaging ~10 g/d. Microscopic hematuria is observed in 20% to 30% of patients.

The natural history of primary MCD may vary. It can present with acute kidney injury but usually does not progress to chronic kidney disease. Patients often have periods of remission alternating with relapses of nephrotic syndrome. Relapses are more common in children but still occur in >50% of adults.

→ **DIAGNOSIS**

In adults diagnosis is based on normal histologic results on light microscopy with foot process effacement on electron microscopy.

→ **TREATMENT**

The goal of treatment is to achieve remission promptly and thus avoid the complications of severe nephrotic syndrome.

Evidence is sparse for the treatment of MCD in adults and is largely based on pediatric approaches. **Glucocorticoids** are recommended ◐◑ with suggested initial doses of either daily or alternating-day prednisone 1 mg/kg once daily or 2 mg/kg every other day for at least 4 weeks and then tapered slowly over 6 months.⊙○ The initial dose of prednisone can be continued for up to 16 weeks if remission is not achieved.

For patients with infrequent relapses, a repeat course of glucocorticoids can be used. Unfortunately, up to 30% of adults have frequent relapses or are steroid-dependent. For these patients oral **cyclophosphamide** for 8 weeks is suggested. If patients are unresponsive to or unable to take cyclophosphamide, other potential treatments include calcineurin inhibitors (cyclosporine [INN ciclosporin] and tacrolimus) or mycophenolate mofetil.

In patients who fail to respond to therapy, a repeat biopsy can be considered to reassess the underlying diagnosis, as focal segmental glomerulosclerosis (FSGS) lesions can be missed on biopsy given their focal nature; there is also some suggestion that MCD may evolve into FSGS.

Secondary causes of MCD, while uncommon, are usually responsive to treatment of the underlying cause.

3.4.7. Monoclonal Immunoglobulin Deposition Disease

Glomerulopathy in monoclonal immunoglobulin deposition disease (MIDD) develops as a result of granular deposition of subunits of monoclonal immunoglobulins, which can be light chain, heavy chain, or both, with the subsequent development of nodular glomerulosclerosis. These deposits differ from amyloid deposits (→Chapter 9.3.4.9) by negative metachromatic staining on immunofluorescence and random rather than organized arrangement.

The disease is caused by monoclonal gammopathies and occurs in approximately 5% of patients with multiple myeloma.

Renal involvement presents as renal insufficiency and proteinuria of varying degrees. It may improve with effective therapy.

3.4.8. Postinfectious Glomerulonephritis

→ **DEFINITION, ETIOLOGY, PATHOGENESIS**

Postinfectious glomerulonephritis (PIGN) is a rapidly developing glomerular disease with circulating immune complexes associated with an ongoing or a recent infection. Classically, it is related to streptococcal infections, although it develops also with staphylococcal infections, especially in elderly patients. PIGN is less commonly linked to other bacterial and viral pathogens.

→ **CLINICAL FEATURES**

PIGN previously affected mostly children, and it is still more common in this group in developing countries. However, the incidence has decreased in the developed world, likely reflecting the quicker and more widespread use of antibiotics, such that PIGN is now significantly more common in adults and preferentially affects the elderly as well as patients with diabetes mellitus or alcoholism.

The disease develops acutely, usually 1 to 2 weeks after streptococcal pharyngitis or 2 to 3 weeks after streptococcal skin infections. PIGN due to staphylococcal infections is slightly more delayed, occurring approximately after 4 weeks.

The usual presentation is nephritic syndrome, with most patients having edema (85% of individuals), hypertension (60%-80%), and abnormal urinalysis/microscopy results (microscopic hematuria and red blood cell casts). Proteinuria is usually not in the nephrotic range. Systemic symptoms include malaise, loss of appetite, nausea, and vomiting. While acute kidney injury (AKI) usually exists, it does not commonly progress to the need for renal replacement. PIGN can present as both nephrotic syndrome and rapidly progressive glomerulonephritis (RPGN), although both are rare. Patients can also be asymptomatic; such cases are estimated to be 4 to 5 times more common than symptomatic ones.

→ DIAGNOSIS

1. Urinalysis/microscopy: Non–nephrotic range proteinuria and active urine sediment.

2. Blood tests: Increased antistreptolysin O (ASO) titers are observed in 90% of patients after streptococcal throat infections and in up to 80% of patients after streptococcal skin infections. Hypergammaglobulinemia along with low serum hemolytic complement activity, low C3 levels, and normal C4 levels are often present.

3. Kidney biopsy: Biopsy is not usually done and only considered in patients who do not recover renal function or have an abnormal presentation.

→ TREATMENT

Treatment of active infection with antibiotics is necessary if infection is present, but given the delay between infection and renal disease, the infection has often already resolved or been treated. Treatment of nephritic syndrome includes sodium and fluid restriction and loop diuretics as necessary. Hypertension should be controlled. Renin-angiotensin system blockers should be used with caution in the setting of AKI. Glucocorticoids can be considered in the setting of PIGN presenting as RPGN, although observational data suggest that they do not change outcomes and potentially increase risk, especially if there is an ongoing infection.⊗○

→ PROGNOSIS

The vast majority of children have complete recovery of their renal function, whereas up to 70% of adults will develop chronic kidney disease, with patients with diabetes being at greater risk of this complication. Recurrences of PIGN are rare.

3.4.9. Renal Amyloidosis

Renal amyloidosis is a glomerulopathy resulting from glomerular deposition of insoluble fibrillar proteins in the mesangium of the glomerulus.

Definition, classification, epidemiology, clinical presentation, diagnosis, and treatment of amyloidosis: →Chapter 14.3.

Diagnosis is confirmed by the presence of amyloid protein on immunofluorescence and electron microscopy. Many different types of amyloid protein exist, but the two most common subtypes are AL and AA amyloid:

1) **AL amyloidosis** is the most common renal amyloidosis. It results in organized deposits of light chains in the glomerulus. Renal involvement occurs in approximately 50% of patients and manifests as decreased renal function and proteinuria. Nephrotic syndrome can occur. Hypertension is usually absent and the kidneys are often enlarged. Renal treatment response is related to the degree of improvement in light chain production from the underlying condition. Proteinuria and renal function improve with successful therapy.

2) **AA amyloidosis** is a secondary amyloidosis. It develops as a response to chronic inflammatory conditions such as rheumatoid arthritis. In contrast to AL amyloidosis, renal involvement is almost universal and presents with varying levels of proteinuria. Treatment of the underlying condition may lead to reduction of proteinuria, stabilization of renal function, and in some cases even to a reduction in the amount of amyloid deposited in the kidneys.

4. Nephrolithiasis

→ **DEFINITION, ETIOLOGY, PATHOGENESIS**

Nephrolithiasis refers to the presence of insoluble stones in the urinary tract, which form in a complex cascade of events when the concentration of stone--forming salts in urine exceeds the threshold of solubility and precipitation occurs. These precipitates form crystals or nuclei that may become retained in the kidney or flow into the urinary tract and become a nidus for stone aggregation and growth.

The main factors contributing to the formation of kidney stones depend on the underlying etiology, with the common factors being:

1) High urine concentrations of lithogenic substances, such as oxalate, calcium, phosphate, uric acid, and cystine.

2) Impaired urinary flow.

3) Urinary tract infection (UTI).

Most frequently kidney stones are formed of calcium oxalate, less commonly of calcium phosphate, urate, struvite (magnesium ammonium phosphate), or cystine. Etiology and pathogenesis of main types of nephrolithiasis: →Table 4-1.

The stones may form at various levels of the urinary tract, most frequently in the renal calyces and renal pelvis. They may subsequently move downstream to the ureters and the bladder, where they may either continue to grow or be passed with urine. Some stones reach considerable sizes, but stones of any size can lead to obstructive uropathy resulting in kidney injury.

→ **CLINICAL FEATURES AND NATURAL HISTORY**

Nephrolithiasis typically manifests as **renal colic**, that is, flank pain referred to the pubic region, genitalia, and inner thighs; in patients with urethral obstruction, the pain is referred to the suprapubic region. The pain starts when the stone passes through the narrow lumen of the ureter. It may be accompanied by nausea and vomiting, urinary urgency, urinary frequency, rigors, fever, hypotension (sepsis), and even syncope (in patients with severe pain). Hematuria is also occasionally observed. In patients presenting with rigors, fever, or hypotension, care must be taken to exclude urosepsis secondary to obstructive uropathy, which is associated with significant mortality if unrecognized and will require urgent urologic consultation and management. Physical examination reveals flank pain and increased muscle tone on the side of the colic. The pain is relieved when urine flow is restored (as a result of passage of the stone to the bladder and/or spontaneous passage of the stone with urine).

The underlying cause of stone formation determines the risk for disease recurrence. A highly recurrent disease is observed in 10% of patients with nephrolithiasis. Approximately half of all stone-forming patients will have a subsequent recurrence of renal colic within the next 10 years.

→ **DIAGNOSIS**

Diagnosis of Acute Nephrolithiasis

Diagnosis is based on the clinical signs and symptoms from detailed medical history and physical examination as well as results of imaging studies. In some patients kidney stones are diagnosed incidentally, when imaging studies are performed for unrelated reasons.

In patients evaluated for acute flank pain, initial diagnostic imaging studies should include ultrasonography or noncontrast computed tomography

Table 4-1. Etiology and pathogenesis of common types of nephrolithiasis

Calcium oxalate and apatite stones

Hypercalciuria with hypercalcemia	– Primary hyperparathyroidism: hypercalciuria caused mainly by increased bone resorption – Granulomatous diseases (eg, tuberculosis, sarcoidosis, certain types of lymphoma): hypercalciuria caused by excessive synthesis of $1,25(OH)_2D_3$ – Malignancy: bone metastases or increased bone resorption caused by secreted cytokines, synthesis of PTH and PTHrP by some types of cancer

Hypercalciuria without hypercalcemia	– Type 1 distal RTA: nonrespiratory acidosis causing decrease in citrate excretion and reducing reabsorption of calcium (increasing calcium excretion)
	– Idiopathic hypercalciuria:
	  a) With increased calcium absorption: GI calcium absorption ~50% higher than in general population
	  b) With increased calcium resorption: increased bone resorption without clinically relevant bone disease; increased bone turnover
	  c) Renal

Hypocitraturia	– Type 1 distal RTA: nonrespiratory acidosis causing decrease in citrate excretion and reducing reabsorption of calcium (increasing calcium excretion) – Nephrolithiasis associated with chronic diarrhea: chronic diarrhea with loss of bases causing acidosis; may also cause hypokalemia – Intracellular acidosis caused by chronic hypokalemia: chronic hypokalemia leading to intracellular acidosis, which directly causes hypocitraturia
Hyperoxaluria	– Enzyme defects causing increased synthesis of oxalate – Acquired: excessive dietary oxalate intake, long-term administration of vitamin C, low-calcium diet (lack of binding of oxalate by calcium in GI tract), chronic diseases of small intestine; bariatric bypass surgery

Cystine stones

Cystinuria	Genetic defects of reabsorption of amino acids: cystine, ornithine, arginine, lysine; stones formed from the least soluble cystine

Struvite (magnesium ammonium phosphate) stones

Alkaline urine	UTIs caused by urease-producing bacteria; degradation of urea causing increase in urine pH, which leads to precipitation of struvite stones

Uric acid stones

Hyperuricosuria	– Gout, Lesch-Nyhan syndrome: abnormalities of purine metabolism – Myeloproliferative neoplasms and other malignancies: increased degradation of nucleic acids – Excess dietary purine intake – Treatment with uricosuric agents – Idiopathic

GI, gastrointestinal; PTH, parathyroid hormone; PTHrP, parathyroid hormone-related peptide; RTA, renal tubular acidosis; UTI, urinary tract infection.

(CT). Ultrasonography is the first-line imaging study of choice for pediatric patients and patients who are or may be pregnant. A noncontrast CT scan offers better sensitivity and specificity compared with ultrasonography but has risks associated with radiation exposure. In patients with a body mass index (BMI) <30, a low-dose CT scan should be offered, which substantially decreases radiation exposure while maintaining high specificity and sensitivity.

A contrast-enhanced CT may be used to assess for suspected anatomic renal collecting system abnormalities as part of operative planning.

Other diagnostic tests evaluated during an episode of acute nephrolithiasis include urinalysis and bloodwork (a complete blood count [CBC] and evaluation of serum electrolytes and creatinine). On urinalysis, three-quarters of patients show microscopic or gross hematuria, and ~3% have leukocyturia and bacteriuria due to a coexisting UTI. In bloodwork no specific abnormalities are typical for nephrolithiasis. An elevated creatinine level may be observed in patients with acute renal injury secondary to obstructive uropathy particularly in patients with a solitary kidney.

Differential Diagnosis

Differential diagnosis should include cholelithiasis, acute abdomen, acute pyelonephritis, and other causes of urinary tract obstruction (eg, thrombi or necrotic fragments of renal parenchyma in patients with acute renal papillary necrosis or tuberculosis).

Diagnosis of Causes of Nephrolithiasis

All first-time stone-forming patients should undergo a limited metabolic evaluation to exclude potential systemic disorders as an underlying cause of stone formation. Patients with clearly identifiable risk factors for recurrent stone formation should undergo a more thorough metabolic evaluation.

Risk factors for recurrent stone formation include stones in children (<18 years of age); bilateral or multiple stones; recurrent stones (having ≥2 kidney stone episodes in the past); noncalcium stones (eg, uric acid, cystine); pure calcium phosphate stones; any complicated stone episodes that resulted in severe acute kidney injury (AKI); sepsis; hospitalization or complicated hospital admission; any stones requiring percutaneous nephrolithotomy treatment (usually staghorn stones—stones involving the entire renal pelvis and extending calyces); stones in the setting of a solitary kidney (anatomic or functioning); patients with chronic kidney disease; and history of kidney stones and a systemic disease that increases the risk of kidney stones, such as gout, osteoporosis, bowel disorders with associated malabsorptive states, hyperparathyroidism, renal tubular acidosis, and type 2 diabetes mellitus.

Diagnostic Tests

1. Limited metabolic evaluation: A basic evaluation including urinalysis, culture, and bloodwork should be done for all patients with acute renal colic. Stone analysis should be completed for any collected stones to determine their composition. Following the first episode of renal colic, a limited metabolic stone workup should be performed in all patients in the absence of risk factors for recurrent stone disease. This basic workup is done when the patient is free of the acute symptoms of colic, usually 2 to 3 months after the episode or urologic intervention due to renal colic (the patient should follow his/her usual diet) and in persons incidentally diagnosed with asymptomatic kidney stones:

1) **Urinalysis**: Presence of specific crystals such as uric acid, cystine, calcium oxalate, or calcium phosphate in urine may indicate the type of renal stones.

2) **Urine culture**: Confirms or excludes a concomitant infection.

3) **Serum levels** of creatinine, sodium, potassium, bicarbonate, calcium, phosphorus, and uric acid.

2. In-depth metabolic evaluation: In addition to the limited metabolic evaluation, patients with risk factors for recurrent stone disease as well as occupational risk factors, where public safety is at risk (pilots, air traffic controllers, police officers, firemen, military personnel), should undergo an in-depth metabolic evaluation including the following:

1) **Two 24-hour urine collections**: Urine collections should be evaluated for volume, creatinine, calcium, sodium, potassium, oxalate, citrate, uric

acid, magnesium (and cystine in case of suspected cystine stones or if stone analysis has identified cystine).

2) **Spot urine collection**: pH, specific gravity, urinalysis.

3) **Serum levels** of creatinine, sodium, potassium, chloride, calcium, albumin, uric acid, bicarbonate, parathyroid hormone (PTH) (if serum calcium level is elevated), and vitamin D (if serum calcium is low or if serum PTH is elevated).

Stone analysis of any captured kidney stones should be performed whenever possible to determine stone composition. Further evaluation may be needed depending on the underlying etiology of the formed stones (→Table 4-1). Repeat imaging studies may be required in patients at high risk of stone recurrence to assess stone burden.

→ TREATMENT

The principles of treatment for acute renal colic are recognition of any emergent sequelae of the stones requiring urgent management, pain control, and identification and treatment of the underlying causes.

Indications for an urgent urologic consultation and treatment include:

1) Signs or symptoms of sepsis with obstruction.

2) Oliguria or anuria.

3) Obstructing stones in a solitary kidney.

4) Failure to control pain using pharmacotherapy.

Specific treatment of various types of nephrolithiasis: →Table 4-2.

Medical Treatment of Acute Renal Colic

The management of pain should not be delayed. It should follow a stepwise fashion with nonsteroidal anti-inflammatory drugs (NSAIDs) being the first option whenever possible.

1. Acute treatment of pain:

1) Oral or rectal **NSAIDs**, for example, ketoprofen 50 to 100 mg, ibuprofen 600 to 800 mg, diclofenac 50 to 100 mg, naproxen 500 to 750 mg.

2) Oral **acetaminophen** (INN paracetamol) 325 to 650 mg every 4 hours.

3) α-**Blockers**, for example, oral tamsulosin 0.4 mg once daily (this allows for an increased rate of stone passage and decreases overall analgesic use).✓⦾

2. Acute treatment of severe pain:

1) **Oral acetaminophen** and **NSAIDs** should be first-line options whenever possible.

2) IV or IM NSAIDs, for example, ketoprofen 100 mg, diclofenac 75 mg, or ketorolac 30 mg, are as effective as opioids in relieving severe renal colic and additionally reduce edema and inflammation surrounding a blocked stone. Relieving pain may facilitate the passage of the stone downstream to the bladder. Care must be taken in patients with AKI when prescribing NSAIDs, as these agents may exacerbate AKI.

3) **Opioids**:

   a) IV or IM **tramadol** 100 mg.

   b) IV **morphine sulfate** 2 to 5 mg every 4 hours, with extra doses for breakthrough pain used as necessary.

   c) IV **hydromorphone** 0.5 to 2 mg every 4 hours, with extra doses for breakthrough pain used as necessary.

Conservative Treatment

Depending on stone location and size as well as the patient's tolerance, conservative management of nephrolithiasis may be an option. Natural history of kidney stones depending on size and likelihood of spontaneous passage: →Table 4-3.

Active Treatment

1. Extracorporeal shock wave lithotripsy (ESWL): In situ fragmentation of stones in the kidney or other part of the urinary tract using external (electrohydraulic, electromagnetic, or piezoelectric) shock waves. The procedure is performed under sedation with analgesia, usually in an outpatient setting. Contraindications: pregnancy, bleeding disorders (anticoagulants and antiplatelet drugs should be temporarily discontinued), poorly controlled hypertension. Special caution is needed in patients with a cardiac pacemaker or abdominal aortic aneurysm.

2. Ureteroscopic lithotripsy (URSL): Manipulation and removal of stones using a ureteroscope (an endoscope introduced through the urethra and the bladder into the ureter).

3. Percutaneous nephrolithotomy (PCNL): Removal of stones from the kidney or upper urinary tract using an endoscope (nephroscope) introduced directly into the renal pelvis. PCNL is reserved for patients with large stone burden (particularly patients with staghorn stones) or those in whom it is not possible to perform ESWL or URSL.

4. Surgical removal of the stone (in exceptional cases total nephrectomy may be needed; rarely done).

→ **PROGNOSIS**

In patients with incidentally diagnosed urinary stones, the 5-year risk of developing symptomatic nephrolithiasis is ~50%. The risk of a second episode of renal colic in patients who have not received prophylactic treatment is ~15% within a year, up to 40% within 5 years, and 50% within 10 years. Early diagnosis of the underlying conditions along with the introduction of targeted treatment improves prognosis, in particular in patients with recurrent nephrolithiasis or with nephrolithiasis developing at a young age. In rare cases nephrolithiasis may lead to end-stage renal failure (2%-4% of patients require renal replacement therapy; 40% of these have struvite nephrolithiasis associated with the formation of staghorn stones).

→ **PREVENTION**

General Measures

1. Increased **fluid intake** (maintain daily urine output ≥2.5 L).⊘⊖

2. Moderation of **animal protein intake** and avoidance of **purine-rich foods** such as fish, red meats, and shellfish (particularly in patients with recurrent calcium oxalate and uric acid stones).

3. Salt intake restricted if possible to 1500 mg (65 mmol) daily and not exceeding 2300 mg (100 mmol) due to the calciuretic effects of sodium.⊘⊖

4. The goal of **dietary calcium intake** should be 1000 to 1200 mg/d.⊘⊖

5. For patients receiving **vitamin C supplementation**, the daily dose should not be >1000 mg because of the associated risk of hyperoxaluria and stone formation, although robust studies are lacking.

6. Vitamin D supplementation may be considered in calcium oxalate stone–forming patients with vitamin D deficiency with urinary monitoring over the subsequent 24 hours for hypercalciuria, although robust studies are lacking.

7. A **high-fiber diet** may protect against kidney stone formation.

8. Specific measures will depend on the underlying etiology of the stone.

Details on treatment and prevention strategies: →Table 4-2.

Table 4-2. Treatment of underlying causes of various types of nephrolithiasis

Idiopathic hypercalciuria

Treatment of hypercalciuria	– Diet: Normal calcium intake 1-1.2 g/d (note: dietary calcium restriction causes increased intestinal absorption of oxalate and subsequent hyperoxaluria and is also a risk factor for osteoporosis), sodium restriction to 1500 mg/d (65 mmol/d), protein restriction to 0.8-1 g/kg of body mass/d; low-sugar meals and drinks – Thiazide diuretics to inhibit urinary calcium excretion, eg, hydrochlorothiazide 12.5-50 mg/d, chlorthalidone 25 mg/d, indapamide 2.5 mg/d (always combined with potassium supplementation either through a high-potassium diet or as potassium supplements, preferably potassium citrate)

Hypocitraturia

Raising urine pH	Potassium citrate; maintain urine pH in the range 6.4-6.8 (raising urine pH causes increased urinary citrate excretion)
Citrate supplementation	Potassium citrate increases urinary citrate excretion and reduces calciuria

Hyperoxaluria due to increased oxalate intake

Reducing dietary oxalate intake	Low-fat, low-oxalate diet[a] (dietary fats increase oxalate absorption)
Binding oxalate in GI tract	– Normal dietary calcium intake; in case of inadequate dietary calcium intake use calcium supplements (calcium 1-1.5 g/d in divided doses with meals); magnesium supplementation: recommended Mg^{+2} intake is 21-25 mmol/d in the form of magnesium citrate (with meals; do not use magnesium oxide) – Cholestyramine (binds oxalate in GI tract)

Primary hyperoxaluria

Pyridoxine 250-1000 mg/d	Increases glyoxylate conversion to glycine (this lowers the amount of glyoxylate available for conversion to oxalate)
Correction of enzyme defect	Liver transplantation combined with kidney transplantation

Cystine stones

Increasing cystine solubility	– Intake of fluids to maintain urine output >3 L/d; high amounts of fluids should also be consumed at bedtime and nighttime (after every voiding at nighttime patient should drink 300-500 mL of fluids and take an additional dose of urine-alkalizing agents) – Raising urine pH using potassium citrate; during treatment frequent urine pH monitoring required (self-monitoring using dipstick tests); recommended pH is >7.5 – Tiopronin 0.8-1 g/d, penicillamine 1-2 g/d (these agents form soluble cysteine-drug complexes)
Reduction of methionine (source of cystine) intake	Dietary protein restriction to 0.8 mg/kg/d

Struvite stones (associated with infection)

Treatment to achieve sterile urine	Antimicrobial treatment based on results of susceptibility testing
Total removal of stones	ESWL, percutaneous nephrolithotomy

Ensuring adequate urine flow	Correction of anatomic or functional abnormalities of the urinary tract (urinary retention is the main risk factor for recurrent UTIs)
Urease inhibition	Acetohydroxamic acid 12 mg/kg/d; only after all surgical treatment options have been exhausted
Uric acid stones	
Reduction of purine intake	Low-purine diet
Raising urine pH	Potassium citrate; recommended pH is >6.5
Reduction of uric acid excretion	In patients with hyperuricosuria: allopurinol 100-300 mg/d
[a] Avoid spinach, rhubarb, soy products, nuts, almonds, chocolate, strong coffee or tea, beetroots, and excess meat.	
ESWL, extracorporeal shock wave lithotripsy; GI, gastrointestinal; UTI, urinary tract infection.	

Table 4-3. Natural history of spontaneous stone passage rates

Stone size (mm)	Number of days to pass stone (mean)	Likelihood of eventual need for intervention
≤2	8	3%
3	12	14%
4-6	22	50%
>6	–	99%

5. Obstructive Nephropathy

→ **DEFINITION, ETIOLOGY, PATHOGENESIS**

Obstructive nephropathy refers to a group of anatomic and functional abnormalities of the urinary tract that cause impaired urine flow due to a partial or total blockade of the urinary tract.

Etiology:

1) **Mechanical**: Benign prostate hyperplasia or prostate cancer, bladder neck stenosis, other pelvic tumors (uterine, ovarian, colorectal cancers; retroperitoneal tumors), uterine prolapse, retroperitoneal fibrosis, stenosis of the ureteropelvic junction (acquired or congenital subpelvic ureteral stenosis) or ureterovesical junction (acquired or congenital ureteral stenosis), posterior urethral valve, ureterocele, nephrolithiasis.

2) **Functional (neurologic)**: Spinal cord injury, neurogenic bladder (bladder neck spasm), congenital spinal malformations.

A special form of obstructive nephropathy is **reflux nephropathy**, a complication of vesicoureteral reflux.

Functional abnormalities include impaired transport of hydrogen and potassium ions, impaired ability to concentrate urine, contraction of blood vessels, reduced renal blood flow, and reduced glomerular filtration rate. Chronic obstruction leads to distention of the collecting system, tubulointerstitial fibrosis, and loss of the renal parenchyma. A typical sign is enlargement of the renal pyelocalyceal system, referred to as hydronephrosis. In patients with a coexisting urinary tract infection, the presence of bacteria and their endotoxins in the renal parenchyma aggravates the existing damage.

→ CLINICAL FEATURES AND NATURAL HISTORY

Clinical manifestations are not characteristic and can be highly varied, depending on the site of obstruction and rate and degree of hydronephrosis progression. Slowly progressive hydronephrosis may be painless, although pain may be associated with an underlying condition or infection. A rapidly developing urinary tract obstruction may cause renal colic. Urine output may be normal, increased, or decreased. Conditions with bilateral obstruction or obstruction in a solitary kidney can result in anuria. In patients with partial obstruction, polyuria may alternate with oliguria. Once the obstruction has been eliminated, patients often develop polyuria, which can be due to osmotic diuresis and a decreased response to vasopressin. This "postobstructive" diuresis needs close monitoring until it resolves because of the possibility of profound serum electrolyte abnormalities that may result (mostly potassium and sodium abnormalities). In patients with hydronephrosis, an epigastric mass (unilateral or bilateral) may be palpable. Hydronephrosis may sometimes also cause local flank pain on percussion. In patients with distension of the bladder, a suprapubic mass may be palpable.

→ DIAGNOSIS

Diagnostic Tests

1. Urinalysis: Abnormalities depend on the cause of urinary tract obstruction. Decreased urine specific gravity, microscopic or gross hematuria, and leukocyturia are often observed. Mild proteinuria (<1.5 g/d) may occur.

2. Blood tests: Increased serum urea and creatinine levels (in renal failure); acidosis and hypokalemia (in distal renal tubular acidosis).

3. Imaging studies: Ultrasonography reveals the presence of hydronephrosis and sometimes also location of the obstruction. The absence of hydronephrosis does not always exclude urinary tract obstruction or even a complete blockade. This is particularly true in patients who are dehydrated or have poor kidney function (ie, small kidney or advanced chronic kidney disease) on the affected side. In such individuals a computed tomography (CT) scan without contrast may be considered if the clinical suspicion for obstruction remains high (ie, flank pain, history of nephrolithiasis, history of retroperitoneal lymphoma or radiation). Other studies (urography, voiding cystourethrography, ascending pyelography) are useful in locating the obstruction and determining its nature. Radionuclide renography (with or without furosemide) is sometimes helpful in differentiating functional dilation of the pyelocalyceal system from hydronephrosis caused by an anatomic obstruction.

→ TREATMENT

Treatment depends on the location of obstruction and the cause and degree of renal impairment. A total obstruction of the urinary tract causing acute kidney injury requires urgent intervention. Urologic consultation is advised to bypass the obstruction for treatment. This may involve placement of a Foley or suprapubic catheter for lower urinary tract obstructions and possible stenting or nephrostomy tube placement for upper urinary tract obstructions. Serum chemistry abnormalities as a consequence of acute kidney injury due to obstruction should be monitored closely and treated appropriately (→Chapter 9.1).

6. Renal Cysts

6.1. Acquired Cystic Kidney Disease

→ DEFINITION, ETIOLOGY, PATHOGENESIS

Acquired cystic kidney disease refers to the presence of ≥4 cysts involving both kidneys with atrophy and a reduction of overall kidney size after development of advanced chronic kidney disease (CKD). Acquired cystic kidney disease may develop regardless of CKD etiology and should not be confused with polycystic kidney disease. Acquired cystic kidney disease is common in patients undergoing renal replacement therapy, with incidence rising with dialysis vintage (length of time on dialysis). While etiology is unknown, proximal tubular cell proliferation is thought to be important. In the majority of cases cysts remain asymptomatic, but they may cause episodes of hematuria, chronic flank pain, or renal colic. Acquired cystic kidney disease is associated with risk of renal cell carcinoma, which may occur in 4% of patients. In 25% to 50% of renal cell carcinoma cases it is multifocal and bilateral.

→ DIAGNOSIS

Diagnosis is based on ultrasonography followed by computed tomography (CT) or magnetic resonance imaging (MRI) for questionable lesions. Screening would occur during evaluation for transplantation. Screening is not recommended in patients with limited life expectancy but can be considered in patients who have long life expectancies 3 to 5 years following the initiation of renal replacement therapy.

→ TREATMENT

No specific treatment is required. Episodes of hematuria are treated symptomatically. Interventional radiologic or surgical treatment may be necessary in case of retroperitoneal bleeding from a cyst, persistent or severe hematuria, cyst infection not responding to medical treatment, and suspected or confirmed renal cell carcinoma.

6.2. Autosomal Dominant Polycystic Kidney Disease

→ DEFINITION, ETIOLOGY, PATHOGENESIS

Autosomal dominant polycystic kidney disease (ADPKD) is the most frequent genetic kidney disease (~1/1000) leading to innumerable bilateral kidney cysts, increased total kidney volume, and progressive chronic kidney disease. ADPKD accounts for ~7% of cases of end-stage renal failure requiring renal replacement therapy. Hypertension, flank pain, polyuria, kidney stones (~20% of patients), hematuria, cyst infections, liver cysts (up to 90% of patients but usually asymptomatic), diverticulosis, hernias, and vascular abnormalities including intracranial aneurysms (~8% of patients) are more common in patients with ADPKD. Despite autosomal dominant inheritance, family history may be missing in 10% to 25% of cases. In clinically ascertained samples, 60% of patients with ADPKD have a *PKD1* mutation, 26% have a *PKD2* mutation, and 15% have no mutation detected. Less than 1% of families have mutations in *GANAB* or *DNAJB11*. Families with mutations in *PKD1* tend to be the most severely affected, and protein-truncating mutations are more severe than nontruncating mutations. The exact mechanism by which these mutations lead to loss of intracellular inhibitory signaling and subsequent proliferation of renal tubular epithelial cells remains unclear.

→ DIAGNOSIS

For those with a family history of ADPKD, ultrasound-based diagnostic criteria for ADPKD have been formulated●:

1) Patients 15 to 39 years of age: ≥3 unilateral or bilateral kidney cysts.
2) Patients 40 to 59 years of age: ≥2 cysts in each kidney.
3) Patients ≥60 years: ≥4 cysts in each kidney.

Genetic testing is not routinely required but can be considered if there is diagnostic uncertainty: atypical presentation, no family history, requirement for early diagnosis (age <25); or for preimplantation genetic diagnosis.

→ TREATMENT

First-line therapy includes maintenance of a healthy body habitus, smoking cessation, blood pressure control, and supportive management of hematuria, cyst infections, and pain. Episodes of hematuria are treated with conservative expectant observation. Renin-angiotensin-aldosterone (RAA) system inhibitors are recommended but dual RAA system blockade provides no additive benefit.⊗● A blood pressure target of <110/75 mm Hg may benefit those with estimated glomerular filtration rate (eGFR) >60 mL/min/1.73 m². ⊘● Maintenance of a high water intake (>3 L/d) to suppress antidiuretic hormone may be of benefit for slowing disease progression and is unlikely to be harmful. ⊘○ Specialist consultation for the evaluation of rate of ADPKD progression and potential for initiation of tolvaptan (a vasopressin V_2 receptor antagonist) is recommended.⊗● Patients with ADPKD and end-stage renal failure are good candidates for kidney transplantation.

6.3. Autosomal Dominant Tubulointerstitial Kidney Disease

→ DEFINITION, ETIOLOGY, PATHOGENESIS

Autosomal dominant tubulointerstitial kidney disease (ADTKD), formerly medullary cystic kidney disease (MCKD) or familial juvenile hyperuricemic nephropathy, is a rare adolescent-onset or adult-onset condition leading to progressive chronic kidney disease and end-stage kidney disease caused by mutations in either *UMOD, MUC1*, or *REN*. Tubulointerstitial fibrosis and bland urine (absence of hematuria or proteinuria) are hallmarks of ADTKD, but small medullary cysts may also be present.

ADTKD-*UMOD* is the most common form of ADTKD, caused by mutations in uromodulin (Tamm-Horsfall mucoprotein), the most abundant protein in normal urine and hyaline casts. Patients often develop gout as early as adolescence. ADTKD-*MUC1* is caused by mutations in mucin 1 and has a similar presentation as ADTKD-*UMOD*, but gout is often later in onset. ADTKD-*REN* is the rarest form of ADTKD, caused by mutations in the renin signal sequence leading to hyperkalemia, hypotension, anemia, and increased propensity to acute kidney injury.

→ TREATMENT

There is no specific treatment for ADTKD. Hyperuricemia may be treated with allopurinol in ADTKD-*UMOD* or ADTKD-*MUC1*, and symptomatic hypotension may be treated with a high-salt diet or fludrocortisone in ADTKD-*REN1*. End-stage kidney disease requiring renal replacement therapy typically develops between the ages of 20 and 70 years.

6.4. Medullary Sponge Kidney

→ DEFINITION, ETIOLOGY, DIAGNOSIS

Medullary sponge kidney (MSK) is usually identified following imaging evaluation of flank pain, kidney stones, hematuria, or urinary tract infections. On IV pyelography or computed tomography (CT) imaging MSK is associated with nephrocalcinosis, small 1 to 7 mm medullary cysts, and enlargement of the pyramids without overall renal enlargement. Factors increasing the risk for calcium stone formation, such as hypercalciuria, hyperuricosuria, hypocitraturia, and hyperoxaluria, are present. The cause of MSK remains unknown. About half of patients with MSK have a positive family history but no definitive genetic cause has been found.

MSK follows a benign course and does not progress to chronic kidney disease. The main complications include kidney stones and urinary tract infections. There is an association with reduced bone mineral density. In asymptomatic patients no specific monitoring is required. In those with a history of a kidney stone, a full diagnostic workup is indicated, with stone prophylaxis based on the results.

6.5. Simple Renal Cyst

→ DEFINITION, ETIOLOGY, PATHOGENESIS

Simple renal cysts are found in >10% of adults aged >50 years, more commonly in men, with increasing prevalence with age. Simple renal cysts may increase in size with age and are usually asymptomatic; however, large cysts (>5 cm) may cause abdominal distention, flank or lower back pain, or nonspecific gastrointestinal symptoms. Possible complications of simple renal cysts include hematuria and infection. Polycystic kidney disease should be considered in those with renal enlargement, multiple cysts, bilateral involvement and positive family history.

→ DIAGNOSIS

Simple renal cysts are often incidental findings on imaging. On ultrasonography, a simple cyst must have smooth round walls, no solid component or internal vascularity, and clearly defined back wall. Cysts with these characteristics or small cysts with <1 mm thin septations do not require further imaging.🟢🔴 Cysts that do not meet these criteria should be investigated with computed tomography (CT) scanning and classified with the Bosniak renal cyst classification system.

→ TREATMENT

Patients with asymptomatic simple renal cysts require no further monitoring or imaging. Bosniak 2F cysts should be compared with previous images if available. Contrast-enhanced magnetic resonance imaging (MRI) may be performed in equivocal cases, and if truly 2F, the cyst should be followed with yearly ultrasonography. Changes in the cyst should be reinvestigated with CT.🟢🔴 Bosniak 3 and 4 cysts should be referred to a urologist, who may elect to biopsy a category 3 cyst or follow it closely. In rare cases where large simple cysts are symptomatic, treatment with cyst drainage and foam sclerotherapy or surgical resection of the cyst are possible.

7. Tubulointerstitial Nephritis

→ **DEFINITION, ETIOLOGY**

Interstitial nephritis is characterized by inflammation of the renal interstitium. It may be secondary to glomerular or renal vascular damage and usually coexists with renal tubular damage, which is why it is often termed **tubulointerstitial nephritis (TIN)**.

Acute interstitial nephritis (AIN) is associated with acute kidney injury (AKI), which develops over a period of days to several weeks and is often reversible. Most often AIN is an immunologically induced hypersensitivity reaction to an antigen (most commonly a drug or an infectious agent).

Chronic interstitial nephritis (CIN) develops over months or years and is associated with progressive fibrosis of the tubulointerstitium, leading to chronic kidney disease. Tubulointerstitial injury can be caused by exogenous or endogenous toxins, infections, immune-mediated mechanisms, obstruction, or ischemia.

7.1. Acute Interstitial Nephritis

→ **ETIOLOGY AND PATHOGENESIS**

Classification of acute interstitial nephritis (AIN) based on etiology:

1) **Drug-induced AIN** (the most common cause of AIN):
   a) Nonsteroidal anti-inflammatory drugs (NSAIDs): Most frequently fenoprofen, phenylbutazone, ibuprofen, indomethacin, naproxen, piroxicam, cyclooxygenase-2 (COX-2) inhibitors.
   b) Antibiotics: Ampicillin, methicillin, penicillin, rifampicin, sulfonamides, vancomycin, ciprofloxacin, erythromycin, tetracycline.
   c) Other drugs: Proton pump inhibitors, cimetidine, allopurinol, interferon, antiviral drugs, 5-aminosalicylic acid.

2) **Infection-induced AIN**:
   a) Primary renal infections: Acute bacterial pyelonephritis (→Chapter 8.16.8), renal tuberculosis, fungal nephritis.
   b) Systemic infections: Bacterial (*Legionella* spp, *Brucella* spp, *Salmonella* spp, *Streptococcus* spp), viral (Epstein-Barr virus, cytomegalovirus, hantavirus, adenoviruses), fungi (histoplasmosis, coccidioidomycosis), or other etiology (mycoplasma, protozoa).

3) **AIN associated with systemic diseases**:
   a) Immune-mediated: Systemic lupus erythematosus, Sjögren syndrome, tubulointerstitial nephritis with uveitis (TINU), tubulointerstitial nephritis with hypocomplementemia.
   b) Hematologic/neoplastic: Light-chain deposition disease associated with or without plasma cell dyscrasias, lymphoproliferative disorders, IgG4-related disease.

AIN accounts for 5% to 18% of kidney biopsies performed in the setting of acute kidney injury (AKI). In developed countries drug-induced AIN is the leading cause of biopsy-proven AIN (>70%), whereas in developing countries infectious AIN can account for 40% to 50% of all AIN cases. In patients with a genetic predisposition or hypersensitivity antigens trigger immune reactions in the renal interstitium. The reactions primarily involve cellular processes associated with the presence of T cells in the interstitium and secretion of proinflammatory cytokines, and, less frequently, humoral processes, associated with the activation of the complement system by antibodies.

CLINICAL FEATURES

AIN is associated with AKI, which develops over a period of days to several weeks. There is no pathognomonic sign or symptom of AIN. The following occur at varying frequencies: dull flank pain, oliguria, maculopapular rash, hematuria, fever (often in case of a relapse), joint pain, edema, and hypertension. The triad of fever, rash, and eosinophilia occurs in 10% of drug-induced AIN. On average, the symptoms appear within 3 weeks of starting the offending drug (ranging from day 1 to >2 months). In AIN associated with generalized infection the dominant symptoms are those of the underlying disease and AKI. Idiopathic AIN manifests clinically as AKI of unknown etiology.

DIAGNOSIS

Most frequently the (probable) diagnosis is made on the basis of clinical manifestations (sudden onset of symptoms of kidney injury in a patient with generalized infection or treated with drugs that may cause AIN, in particular when extrarenal allergic symptoms occur simultaneously) after other causes of AKI have been excluded.

Diagnostic Tests

1. Urinalysis: Proteinuria, often mild (<1 g/d) or moderate (~2 g/d); nephrotic range proteinuria (≥3.5 g/d) suggests NSAID-induced AIN; microscopic hematuria and leukocyturia in most patients. Eosinophiluria (>1%) has historically been considered a useful diagnostic test for drug-induced AIN, but it lacks sensitivity and specificity and cannot be relied upon.⊗○

2. Blood tests: In patients with drug-induced AIN peripheral eosinophilia may occur.

3. Imaging studies: Ultrasonography reveals enlarged or normal kidneys with increased cortical echogenicity.

4. Renal biopsy: Renal biopsy confirms diagnosis. It is performed in case of significant uncertainty as to the cause of kidney disease, particularly when the existing AKI could have been caused by a condition that may be effectively treated (eg, rapidly progressive glomerulonephritis).

TREATMENT

1. Elimination of known or suspected causes: Aggressive treatment of systemic infections, discontinuation of drugs that might have caused AIN.

2. Management of AKI: →Chapter 9.1.

3. Glucocorticoids may be considered in patients with biopsy-proven drug-induced AIN after withdrawal of the offending drug.⊙○ When started early (within 2 weeks of withdrawal of the drug), glucocorticoids may limit the extent of renal fibrosis and may increase the probability of complete renal recovery. Consider a course of oral **prednisone** 1 mg/kg/d tapered off over 4 to 6 weeks. The role of other immunosuppression therapy (mycophenolate mofetil, cyclosporine [INN ciclosporin], cyclophosphamide) cannot be informed by the current state of evidence. Indications for immunosuppressive therapy in other forms of AIN are less evident; therapy should be preceded by kidney biopsy.

PROGNOSIS

In patients in whom AIN was diagnosed early and its cause has been successfully eliminated, the rate of complete resolution is ~50%. Other patients have varying degrees of chronic kidney disease and some may require chronic renal replacement therapy.

7.2. Chronic Interstitial Nephritis

→ DEFINITION, ETIOLOGY, PATHOGENESIS

Chronic interstitial nephritis (CIN) is a common description referring to a number of various nephropathies characterized by chronic inflammation that originates in the renal interstitium. It is associated with a progressive loss of glomerular filtration rate (GFR) over time and commonly also with tubular dysfunction.

Classification of CIN based on etiology:

1) Drug-induced: Analgesics (phenacetin and acetaminophen [INN paracetamol], either alone or in combination with acetylsalicylic acid [ASA] and caffeine, nonsteroidal anti-inflammatory drugs [NSAIDs]), lithium, calcineurin inhibitors (cyclosporine [INN ciclosporin], tacrolimus), 5-aminosalicylic acid.

2) Toxic: Lead, cadmium, mercury.

3) Chronic pyelonephritis.

4) Renal tuberculosis.

5) Metabolic diseases: Gout, hypercalcemia, hypokalemia.

6) Immune-mediated: Sjögren syndrome, systemic lupus erythematosus, anti–glomerular basement membrane disease, antineutrophil cytoplasmic antibody (ANCA)-associated vasculitis, chronic rejection of kidney transplant.

7) Hematologic/malignant: Sickle cell disease, light-chain diseases, lymphoproliferative disorders, multiple myeloma.

8) Vascular diseases: Ischemic nephropathy due to atherosclerosis of the renal arteries.

9) Structural abnormalities of the urinary tract: Obstructive nephropathy, reflux nephropathy.

10) Hereditary: Polycystic kidney disease, Autosomal dominant tubulointerstitial kidney disease, cystinosis, Dent disease, primary hyperoxaluria.

11) Other: Balkan endemic nephropathy, aristolochic acid nephropathy, radiation nephropathy.

→ CLINICAL FEATURES AND NATURAL HISTORY

CIN can remain asymptomatic for a long time, and the early clinical signs suggestive of kidney damage are often neglected by patients and physicians. Clinical features of chronic kidney disease develop gradually, along with a progressive impairment of GFR. A particular complication of some forms of CIN is papillary necrosis, which may be asymptomatic or manifest as renal colic. Common etiologies and features of CIN: →Table 7-1.

→ DIAGNOSIS

Diagnosis is usually established on the basis of clinical manifestations and noninvasive diagnostic tests.

Diagnostic Tests

1. Urinalysis: Specific gravity <1.02 (frequently close to 1.01), proteinuria (<1-2 g/d), leukocyturia of varying severity, sometimes white blood cell casts, less commonly microscopic hematuria.

2. Blood tests: Normocytic anemia, often disproportionately severe for the actual degree of GFR reduction; increased serum creatinine levels and other abnormalities typical for patients with a low GFR; various electrolyte disturbances (hypokalemia or hyperkalemia, hypocalcemia, hypomagnesemia, hyponatremia) and a non–anion gap metabolic acidosis due to renal tubular acidosis, which results from renal tubular dysfunction.

Table 7-1. Etiology/types and features of chronic tubulointerstitial nephritis

Type or etiology	Causes/risk factors	Features
Analgesic nephropathy	Excessive analgesic use >3 years in various combinations, including NSAIDs; more frequent in women	Hypertension, nocturia, sterile leukocyturia, hemolytic anemia; characteristic papillary calcifications on CT; small kidneys with irregular outlines, features of papillary necrosis; increased incidence of urinary system cancers
Lithium-associated nephropathy	Treatment with lithium for ~15 years	Proteinuria >1 g/d, hypertension, possibly NDI
Lead nephropathy	Long-term exposure to lead (lead smelters, paint or battery manufacturing/recycling plants, oil refineries)	Serum lead may not be elevated but urinary lead excretion (>0.6 mg/d after IV infusion of sodium versenate) is evidence of increased lead burden; high serum uric acid, gout (~50%)
Uric acid (gouty) nephropathy	Long-standing inconsistently treated hyperuricemia	Hypertension, proteinuria <1 g/d, decreased urinary concentrating ability, frequently uric acid nephrolithiasis
Hypercalcemic nephropathy	Chronic hypercalcemia	NDI (~20%), renal sodium loss, distal RTA; possible nephrocalcinosis and urolithiasis; acute hypercalcemia may be cause of AKI
Hypokalemic nephropathy	Chronic hypokalemia	Extrarenal symptoms of hypokalemia; NDI, renal cysts
Hyperoxaluric nephropathy	Congenital metabolic defect (primary hyperoxaluria); complication of extensive small bowel resection or gastric/bariatric bypass surgery or in patients with IBD	Nephrocalcinosis, nephrolithiasis
Sjögren syndrome		Symptoms of underlying condition (CIN develops within 2-4 y of disease onset); NDI (~10%), distal RTA (~5%), renal potassium loss
Radiation nephritis	Several years after exposure to cumulative radiation dose >23 Gy (2300 rad)	Hypertension, proteinuria, slow reduction in GFR
Aristolochic acid nephropathy (Chinese herbal nephropathy)	Chinese herbal preparations (made of *Aristolochia* plant, traditional Chinese names: Mu Tong, Fang Ji) that contain aristolochic acid (nephrotoxic alkaloid; used for weight loss or skin diseases)	Moderate proteinuria, glucosuria, no abnormalities of urinary sediment; severe anemia; diagnosis confirmed by detection of metabolites of aristolochic acid in DNA of renal cells; rapid GFR impairment, which may be partially inhibited by glucocorticoids; RRT necessary in >80% of patients within 2 years; urinary system cancers develop in 40%-50%
Balkan endemic nephropathy	Endemic along tributaries of the Danube River (Bulgaria, Romania, Bosnia and Herzegovina, Croatia, Serbia); long-term exposure to aristolochic acid contained in cereal products plus genetic predisposition	Progressive anemia and GFR reduction, rarely hypertension; ESRD develops within 15-20 years; ~100-fold increase in incidence of urinary system cancers

Type or etiology	Causes/risk factors	Features
Hereditary interstitial kidney diseases	Include autosomal recessive disorders (nephronophthisis) diagnosed in children and autosomal dominant disorders (ADTKD) typically diagnosed in adulthood	– Nephronophthisis (form of ciliopathy); ESRD in teenagers to patients in their 20s, salt wasting, urinary concentrating defect, occasional medullary cysts on US, extrarenal involvement (CNS, liver) – ADTKD: Slowly progressive kidney failure, bland urinalysis, unremarkable renal US; strong family history of ESRD in patients in their 30s-60s. More common mutations include *UMOD* gene encoding uromodulin (may present with history of gout), *MUC1* gene encoding mucin 1, and *REN* gene encoding renin (may present with mild hypotension and hyperkalemia)
Papillary necrosis	Ischemic or toxic kidney damage (analgesics, NSAIDs); risk factors: diabetes, urinary obstruction, UTI, analgesics, NSAIDs	Polyuria, nocturia, renal colic; urinalysis: proteinuria, leukocyturia, microscopic hematuria; diagnosis: urography, antegrade pyelography

ADTKD, autosomal dominant tubulointerstitial kidney disease; AKI, acute kidney injury; CIN, chronic interstitial nephritis; CNS, central nervous system; CT, computed tomography; ESRD, end-stage renal disease; GFR, glomerular filtration rate; IBD, inflammatory bowel disease; NDI, nephrogenic diabetes insipidus; NSAID, nonsteroidal anti-inflammatory drug; RRT, renal replacement therapy; RTA, renal tubular acidosis; US, ultrasonography; UTI, urinary tract infection.

3. Imaging studies: Ultrasonography typically reveals a decreased kidney size and increased echogenicity, sometimes with irregular outlines and scarring.

4. Kidney biopsy is not performed routinely and is reserved for cases of diagnostic uncertainty.

→ **TREATMENT**

1. Elimination of the cause: In early disease this may lead to a significant improvement or even to normalization of renal function (in patients with no interstitial fibrosis and glomerular atrophy).

2. Treatment of CKD: →Chapter 9.2.

→ **PROGNOSIS**

Prognosis depends on the degree of renal dysfunction (GFR reduction) at the time of diagnosis as well as on treatment options for the underlying condition.

8. Tubulopathies

→ **DEFINITION, ETIOLOGY, CLINICAL FEATURES**

Tubulopathy is an umbrella term that encompasses various disease processes affecting the renal tubules. Some of these include renal tubular acidosis (RTA) (with type 1, type 2, and type 4), tubular channel defects leading to salt-losing nephropathies, and nephrogenic diabetes insipidus. A majority of these diseases are acquired as a result of another disease process damaging the kidneys, and very rarely the etiology is genetic or inherited.

Tubulopathies can present in a variety of ways. Some patients are completely asymptomatic, whereas others may present with respiratory failure related to severe hypokalemic periodic paralysis.

Clinicians often consider RTA when a non–anion gap metabolic acidosis (NAGMA) is discovered in a patient with other electrolyte derangements and normal renal function or when the acidosis is found to be out of proportion to the degree of renal function. NAGMA can be caused by etiologies that are renal, extrarenal, or both.

RTA is characterized by tubular inability to maintain acid-base balance despite relatively well-preserved renal function. This can be due to either net bicarbonate loss or inability to excrete acid.

→ DIAGNOSIS

RTA is usually suspected following the establishment of a hyperchloremic NAGMA. Diagnosis requires measurement of urinary pH and urinary anion gap (UAG) to estimate urinary ammonium excretion. A low urinary ammonium excretion, indicated by a positive UAG, helps distinguish RTA from other causes of NAGMA that would also present with hypokalemia, such as diarrhea.

8.1. Bartter and Gitelman Syndromes

→ ETIOLOGY AND CLINICAL FEATURES

Bartter and Gitelman syndromes result from loss-of-function mutations in 2 membrane transport proteins in the thick ascending limb of the loop of Henle and the distal convoluted tubule, respectively. Bartter syndrome is caused by mutations in the sodium-potassium-chloride cotransporter (NKCC) channel in the ascending loop of Henle, whereas Gitelman syndrome is a result of the sodium-chloride cotransporter (NCC) mutations in the distal convoluted tubule.

There are 5 subtypes of Bartter syndrome. Type 1 Bartter syndrome, described above, is caused by the loss-of-function mutation in the NKCC channel, which is sensitive to loop diuretics. The other subtypes develop due to mutations in various other proteins in the same loop of Henle cells involved in sodium and potassium trafficking, which maintains tubular and cellular electrical charge.

Bartter syndrome may present in various ways. Some patients are asymptomatic and are diagnosed with milder forms of the disease on the basis of hypokalemia, metabolic alkalosis, and mild hypotension. Subtypes of Bartter syndrome can also be associated with excessive thirst, polydipsia, and polyuria. More severe forms lead to neonatal death.

Both Bartter syndrome and Gitelman syndrome are quite rare and inherited in an autosomal recessive fashion.

→ DIAGNOSIS

Diagnosis in Bartter syndrome and Gitelman syndrome is one of exclusion. Patients usually present with unexplained hypokalemia and metabolic alkalosis with a low-to-normal blood pressure. Other causes of such manifestations, including surreptitious vomiting and diuretic use, must be excluded.

A tentative diagnosis is usually made on the basis of detailed history, physical examination, and assessment of other serum and urinary studies (→Table 8-1). Although not needed for diagnosis, serum renin and aldosterone levels are elevated.

Table 8-1. Differences between Bartter and Gitelman syndromes

	Bartter syndrome	Gitelman syndrome
Age of onset	Neonatal to childhood	Late childhood to adulthood
Serum magnesium	Low to normal	Low
Urinary calcium	High	Low
Urinary concentration ability	Reduced	Normal

→ **TREATMENT**

The goal of therapy in Bartter and Gitelman syndromes involves management of hypokalemia, which can be done both by oral potassium supplementation and by the use of potassium-sparing diuretics, particularly spironolactone. Because of the rise in prostaglandin levels related to the loop of Henle dysfunction in Bartter syndrome, nonsteroidal anti-inflammatory drugs can also be used and have been shown to be effective in reducing polyuria and hypokalemia.

8.2. Cystinosis

→ **DEFINITION, ETIOLOGY, CLINICAL FEATURES**

Cystinosis is caused by mutations in the *CTNS* gene (found on chromosome 17), which encodes a lysosomal cystine/proton symporter termed cystinosin. In the absence of a functional cystinosin protein, cystine accumulates and crystallizes in the lysosomal lumen. Like in other tissues, cystine accumulates in the renal tubules and the interstitium, leading to tubular dysfunction and end-stage renal disease (ESRD).

Cystinosis has 3 forms:

1) The **infantile form**, also called nephropathic, is the most severe and presents at the age of 3 to 6 months, manifesting as Fanconi syndrome (→Chapter 9.8.7); such children develop ESRD by the age of 10 years.

2) The **late-onset form**, also known as juvenile, occurs usually around the age of 10 years, and the presentation as Fanconi syndrome is less common. Nephrotic range proteinuria can be a presenting feature. Patients develop ESRD around the age of 15 years.

3) The **adult-onset form**, which is usually a benign form of the disease, may have only ocular manifestations of photophobia or ocular discomfort.

→ **DIAGNOSIS**

Diagnosis is made by measuring intraleukocyte cystine content, slit-lamp examination of the eye, and/or testing for the *CTNS* gene sequence.

→ **TREATMENT**

Recommended therapy following confirmation of the diagnosis is cysteamine, a chaperone protein that allows for effective excretion of cystine from the cells, preventing tissue deposition and damage. This has been shown to preserve renal function and prevent other end-organ manifestations of the disease.

Patients who undergo transplantation for ESRD resulting from cystinosis, as long as they remain on cysteamine thereafter, have a very indolent course of cystinuria with no recurrence.

8.3. Cystinuria

→ DEFINITION, ETIOLOGY, PATHOGENESIS

Cystinuria is an autosomal recessive hereditary disorder of cystine and other dibasic amino acid (ornithine, arginine, lysine) transport system in the renal tubules and gastrointestinal tract. Excretion of excessive amounts of poorly soluble cystine in urine is the cause of cystine urolithiasis, which may develop as early as in infancy but usually occurs in patients >20 years of age.

Cystine is a homodimer of the amino acid cysteine (linked through a disulfide bond), which is freely filtered across the glomerulus and then subsequently absorbed in the proximal convoluted tubule via the cystine transporter. The absorption apparatus requires a carrier protein that assists with the expression of the protein transport channel. Mutations in the carrier protein and others in the channel are responsible for the disease phenotype. The precipitation of cystine leads to heavy stone burden, infections, and eventually to chronic kidney disease.

The same apparatus is responsible for transport of other dibasic amino acids, but their excretion does not result in stone formation because of higher urinary solubility.

→ DIAGNOSIS

Cystinuria should be suspected in patients who present with stones early in life and in those with a family history. Diagnosis can be made on the basis of results of urine microscopy revealing pathognomonic hexagonal cystine crystals, stone analysis, and a 24-hour urine collection for cystine. Under physiologic conditions, urinary excretion of cystine is <0.13 mmol/d (30 mg/d), whereas the majority of patients with cystinuria excrete >1.7 mmol/d (400 mg/d). Genetic testing is not recommended.

→ TREATMENT

The goal of therapy is decreasing urinary concentration and increasing urinary solubility and excretion of cystine.

1. Reduction in urinary concentrations can be achieved by limiting salt and animal protein intake, which results in lower excretion of cysteine. The mechanisms explaining why reduced salt or sodium intake results in reduced cystine elimination are not understood.

2. Urinary solubility can be improved by increasing fluid intake and urinary alkalinization. Urine pH can be increased by potassium citrate supplementation; sodium citrate and acetazolamide are generally avoided due to their adverse effect profile. The dose of potassium citrate is weight dependent. Usually a dose of 3 to 4 mEq/kg is effective. Treatment can be started with 20 mEq orally tid and the dose subsequently increased to target a urine pH >7.0 (maximizing cystine solubility).

3. In patients refractory to the above therapy, thiol-containing drugs can be used, including D-penicillamine or tiopronin. Thiol breaks down the cystine disulfide bond, allowing for free cysteine formation and excretion. Adverse effects from both drugs can be minimized by starting with low doses (200 mg orally tid) and titrating up (usually a maximum of 400 mg orally tid). Captopril is an alternative agent that has been shown to induce similar changes as thiol compounds, forming captopril-cysteine bonds that have a significantly higher solubility than cystine alone. However, this is achieved only with high doses and may lead to significant antihypertensive effects. Evidence for clinical efficacy of captopril is very limited.○

Progressive disease and lack of response to therapy can lead to heavier stone burden and may require urological intervention.

Table 8-2. Etiologies of distal (type 1) renal tubular acidosis

Autoimmune diseases	Sjögren syndrome,[a] systemic lupus erythematosus, rheumatoid arthritis, primary biliary cirrhosis
Drugs/toxins	Lithium,[a] antibiotics (amphotericin B[a]), chemotherapeutics (ifosfamide)
Tubulointerstitial disorders	Status post renal transplantation, obstructive uropathy
Other	Nephrocalcinosis (hypercalciuria, vitamin D toxicity, hyperparathyroidism), sickle cell disease

[a] The more common causes.

8.4. Distal (Type 1) Renal Tubular Acidosis

→ **DEFINITION AND ETIOLOGY**

Distal renal tubular acidosis (dRTA), also known as type 1 renal tubular acidosis, results from reduction of H^+ secretion in the distal nephron, which prevents urinary acidification and thereby minimizes urinary bicarbonate losses (fractional excretion of bicarbonate [$FE_{HCO_3^-}$] <3%-5%). A constant feature of dRTA is the inability to acidify urine to pH <5.5 in the presence of nonrespiratory acidosis. Impaired H^+ secretion results in urinary sodium loss, secondary activation of the renin-angiotensin aldosterone system, and increased urinary potassium loss. Hypercalciuria and hypocitraturia (causative factors for nephrocalcinosis and urolithiasis) frequently occur.

dRTA can be caused by a number of illnesses (→Table 8-2). Rare autosomal dominant and autosomal recessive channelopathies will not be discussed, as they are beyond the scope of this chapter.

→ **DIAGNOSIS**

In patients with dRTA urinary pH is persistently high, independently of acidifying challenge testing. To make a diagnosis of dRTA in a patient with hyperchloremic metabolic acidosis, urinary pH should be ≥5.5 regardless of serum bicarbonate levels with a positive urinary anion gap (UAG).

→ **TREATMENT**

If renal tubular acidosis (RTA) persists following treatment of the underlying cause, it can be managed with supplemental doses of alkali therapy.

Treatment of patients with dRTA requires relatively lower doses of supplemental bicarbonate therapy (1-2 mEq/kg/d) compared with proximal RTA. Children have higher requirements than adults because of their overall net acid production being higher on a daily basis. Sodium bicarbonate or sodium citrate is usually adequate to raise serum bicarbonate concentration back to the normal range. Potassium--based citrate, alone or with sodium citrate, can be used if hypokalemia persists.

8.5. Hyperkalemic (Type 4) Renal Tubular Acidosis

→ **DEFINITION, ETIOLOGY**

Type 4 renal tubular acidosis (RTA) is also referred to as hyperkalemic RTA. The hallmark of this disease is hypoaldosteronism manifested by hyperkalemia

Table 8-3. Etiologies of type 4 renal tubular acidosis

Aldosterone deficiency	
Low renin levels	– Systemic disorders: diabetic nephropathy,[a] HIV, CIN – Drugs: NSAIDs,[a] calcineurin inhibitors
Normal-to-high renin levels	– Systemic disorders: primary adrenal insufficiency, severe critical illness – Drugs: ACEIs, ARBs, UFH, direct renin inhibitors, ketoconazole

Aldosterone resistance
– Systemic disorders: sickle cell disease, SLE, obstructive uropathy – Drugs: potassium-sparing diuretics[a] (aldosterone antagonists, ENaC inhibitors such as amiloride and triamterene), antibiotics (trimethoprim, pentamidine, calcineurin inhibitors)

[a] The most common causes.

ACEI, angiotensin-converting enzyme inhibitor; ARB, angiotensin receptor blocker; CIN, chronic interstitial nephritis; ENaC, epithelial sodium channel; HIV, human immunodeficiency virus; SLE, systemic lupus erythematosus; UFH, unfractionated heparin.

and a very mild hyperchloremic metabolic acidosis, usually resulting from aldosterone deficiency or tubular resistance to aldosterone.

The etiologies of type 4 RTA can be divided into aldosterone underproduction and aldosterone resistance. Selected etiologies of type 4 RTA: →Table 8-3.

DIAGNOSIS

Hyperkalemia and a mild hyperchloremic metabolic acidosis are the major manifestations of type 4 RTA. The diagnosis of type 4 RTA should be considered in any patient with these findings present persistently in the absence of other etiologies of hyperkalemia, such as chronic kidney disease or the use of potassium supplements.

Careful examination of the medical history and medication list should be carried out to ensure the patient is not taking any medications or does not have an undiagnosed disorder known to cause type 4 RTA.

Diagnostic Tests

Various etiologies can be differentiated by measurement of plasma renin activity (PRA) and serum aldosterone and cortisol concentrations. These tests should be performed following the administration of a loop diuretic or after assuming the upright position for 3 hours, which are known to increase renin and aldosterone release in healthy individuals.

Careful assessment of these values should be performed to elucidate the underlying etiology. Renin and aldosterone concentrations depending on etiology: →Table 8-3.

A general approach to RTA based on results of urinary studies: →Table 8-4.

TREATMENT

Unlike in other RTAs, no bicarbonate replacement therapy is required, as acidosis is only mild.

Management of type 4 RTA depends on underlying disease, which should be treated if possible. Hyporeninemic hypoaldosteronism can be treated with fludrocortisone in doses significantly higher than those used for adrenal insufficiency. However, most of these patients have hypertension and edema,

Table 8-4. Approaches to renal tubular acidosis

Feature	pRTA (type 2 RTA)	dRTA (type 1 RTA)	Type 4 RTA
Degree of acidosis	Moderate	Severe	Mild
Minimal urine pH (during acidosis)	<5.5	>5.5	<5.5
Fractional HCO_3^- excretion (FE_{HCO3}) with normal serum HCO_3^- (after $NaHCO_3$ load)	>15%	<3%-5%	<3%-15%
Nephrocalcinosis	Rarely	Often	Never

dRTA, distal renal tubular acidosis; pRTA, proximal renal tubular acidosis; RTA, renal tubular acidosis.

Table 8-5. Etiologies of nephrogenic diabetes insipidus

Inherited/ hereditary	Vasopressin V_2-receptor gene mutations (X-linked),[a] *AQP2* gene mutations (autosomal dominant/autosomal recessive)
Acquired	– Systemic disorders: hypercalcemia,[a] amyloidosis, Sjögren syndrome, polycystic kidney disease, sickle cell disease – Drugs: lithium,[a] cidofovir, foscarnet, amphotericin B – Other: hypokalemia, pregnancy

[a] The most common causes.

which can be exacerbated with mineralocorticoid replacement. In such cases a low-potassium diet combined with a loop diuretic or thiazide-type diuretic can be used to control hyperkalemia. Patients with primary adrenal insufficiency should receive glucocorticoid and mineralocorticoid replacement.

8.6. Nephrogenic Diabetes Insipidus

→ **DEFINITION AND ETIOLOGY**

Nephrogenic diabetes insipidus (NDI) refers to the inability to appropriately concentrate urine that results from resistance to circulating antidiuretic hormone (ADH). This can be due to a defect at the site of action of ADH, interference with the countercurrent mechanism, or decreased sodium chloride reabsorption at the level of the thick ascending limb of the loop of Henle.

The etiology of NDI can be divided into **hereditary** and **acquired** causes. Hereditary causes are more common in children, whereas acquired causes are more common in adults. Selected etiologies of NDI: →Table 8-5.

→ **DIAGNOSIS**

A broad approach to **polyuria** should be undertaken when considering the diagnosis of NDI in any patient. This should involve collecting a careful history looking at various etiologies of central and nephrogenic diabetes insipidus.

NDI is suspected if there is a failure of response to water restriction and desmopressin in raising urine osmolarity or reducing plasma sodium concentration. However, patients strongly suspected of having NDI (children with very dilute urine, patients on chronic lithium therapy) should not undergo water restriction and can rather have direct administration of desmopressin followed by a response assessment. A suboptimal response to desmopressin, represented by minor or no elevation in urine osmolality, is the hallmark of complete NDI. A small (<45%) elevation in urine osmolality in response to desmopressin occurs in partial NDI.

→ TREATMENT

Secondary etiology should be corrected when identified and offending medications should be stopped, if feasible. All patients should receive advice to stay on a low-salt diet and perform double voiding to prevent bladder distension. Special recommendations for children with NDI are beyond the scope of this chapter.

If the patient is unable to control polyuria with a low-salt diet, a nonsteroidal anti-inflammatory drug or thiazide diuretic can be tried. The effect of thiazide diuretics is likely due to the increase in proximal sodium and water reabsorption, which is induced by hypovolemia. This diminishes water delivery to the ADH--sensitive sites in the collecting tubules, reducing urine output. Amiloride can be also attempted if inadequate response is achieved with initial therapies; this can be particularly helpful in patients with NDI in whom lithium cannot be discontinued. However, we advise careful and frequent monitoring of lithium levels, as this approach may result in their increase.

In patients in whom the therapy discussed above is unsuccessful, we suggest a trial of desmopressin.

8.7. Proximal (Type 2) Renal Tubular Acidosis

→ DEFINITION AND ETIOLOGY

Proximal renal tubular acidosis (pRTA), also known as type 2 renal tubular acidosis, can occur as an isolated defect in bicarbonate reabsorption or in association with other defects in proximal tubular function, leading to impaired reabsorption of other solutes, such as phosphate, glucose, uric acid, and amino acids. These patients usually have an isolated non–anion gap acidosis.

If acidosis develops in association with loss of other solutes, the patient may have hypophosphatemia, hypouricemia, renal glucosuria (with normal serum glucose concentrations), and/or aminoaciduria; this is termed **Fanconi syndrome**.

Isolated hereditary pRTA is rare and can be autosomal dominant or autosomal recessive. Rare sporadic cases have been reported. Acetazolamide and topiramate are two commonly reported drugs also known to cause isolated pRTA.

More commonly pRTA is found in conjunction with Fanconi syndrome, which may be caused by several genetic and acquired systemic diseases. Etiologies of pRTA and Fanconi syndrome: →Table 8-6.

→ DIAGNOSIS

Patients with pRTA develop an increase in their urinary pH following an alkali load. Their urine pH may rise from 5.5 at baseline to 7.5 when serum bicarbonate levels are normalized following the administration of sodium bicarbonate.

→ TREATMENT

If renal tubular acidosis (RTA) persists following treatment of the underlying cause, it can be managed with supplemental doses of alkali therapy.

Treatment of patients with pRTA requires treatment of acidemia and rarely of hypokalemia and hypophosphatemia. Compared with patients with distal RTA, the requirement for alkali therapy is usually significantly higher (up to 10-15 mEq/kg/d) to exceed the urinary bicarbonate losses (although doses of

Table 8-6. Etiologies of proximal (type 2) renal tubular acidosis and Fanconi syndrome	
Familial	Cystinosis,[a] Wilson disease, hereditary fructose intolerance, tyrosinemia, galactosemia, Lowe disease, Dent disease
Dysproteinemias	Multiple myeloma (LCDD),[a] amyloidosis
Drugs	NRTIs (tenofovir,[a] adefovir, didanosine, lamivudine), chemotherapeutics (ifosfamide)
Heavy metals	Lead,[a] mercury, copper (Wilson disease)
Tubulointerstitial diseases	Status post renal transplantation, Balkan/Chinese herb nephropathy (aristolochic acid toxicity), medullary cystic kidney disease
Other	Vitamin D deficiency
Familial causes are more prevalent among the pediatric population but can remain undiagnosed until later in life.	
[a] The more common etiologies.	
LCDD, light chain deposition disease; NRTI, nucleoside reverse transcriptase inhibitor.	

about 2 mEq/kg/d may be sufficient, with 100 mEq translating into 8.4 g of oral sodium bicarbonate). This can be done with sodium bicarbonate, sodium citrate, or potassium citrate. It is not uncommon to use a combination of potassium-based and sodium-based alkali to ensure potassium replacement and compensate for the urinary potassium losses. These losses are related to increased water and salt delivery to the distal tubule and negatively charged urinary bicarbonate ions stimulating secretion of potassium into urine. Thiazide diuretics may be occasionally used, as inducing mild volume depletion leads to increased proximal sodium and bicarbonate reabsorption.

1. Ataxia

→ CAUSES AND PATHOGENESIS

Ataxia is an impairment of motor coordination that makes it difficult to perform smooth and precise movements. It is due to disorders causing damage to the cerebellum or cerebellar systems (**cerebellar ataxia**) or damage to the afferent proprioceptive pathways at the level of peripheral nerves or dorsal columns of the spinal cord (**sensory ataxia**).

Causes of cerebellar ataxia:

1) Toxic (alcohol and drugs [eg, phenytoin, barbiturates, lithium]).

2) Vascular (ischemic or hemorrhagic stroke).

3) Infectious or postinfectious (viral cerebellitis, HIV infection, Creutzfeldt-
-Jakob disease).

4) Inflammatory (multiple sclerosis, ataxia associated with anti–glutamic acid decarboxylase [GAD] antibody, glucocorticoid-responsive encephalopathy associated with autoimmune thyroiditis).

5) Neoplastic (metastatic tumors, primary tumors, paraneoplastic syndromes).

6) Metabolic (vitamin E deficiency, vitamin B_1 deficiency [Wernicke encepha-lopathy], celiac disease, hypothyroidism, hypoparathyroidism).

7) Neurodegenerative (multiple system atrophy, cerebellar type; Wilson disease; spinocerebellar ataxias; Friedreich ataxia [mixed cerebellar and sensory ataxia]).

8) Structural (Arnold-Chiari malformation).

Causes of sensory ataxia:

1) Toxic (drug-induced neuropathy [vincristine, isoniazid], neuropathy related to heavy metal poisoning).

2) Infectious (tabes dorsalis [neurosyphilis-related degeneration of posterior columns of the spinal cord]).

3) Inflammatory (Guillain-Barré syndrome, chronic inflammatory demyelinating polyneuropathy, Sjögren syndrome–related neuronopathy [damage to dorsal root ganglia], spinal cord lesions in multiple sclerosis).

4) Neoplastic (paraneoplastic neuronopathies, neuropathy secondary to mono-clonal gammopathy).

5) Metabolic (diabetic neuropathy, subacute combined degeneration [vitamin B_{12} deficiency]).

6) Neurodegenerative (Friedreich ataxia).

→ DIAGNOSIS

1. History and physical examination:

1) **Cerebellar ataxia**:

   a) Appendicular ataxia (dysmetria [abnormal finger-to-nose and heel-to-shin tests, overshooting or undershooting with finger chase]).

   b) Dysdiadochokinesia (irregular amplitude and rhythm with rapid alter-nating movements [eg, pronating and supinating the forearm]).

   c) Tremor (often intention tremor, with increased amplitude of tremor as the limb nears the target]).

   d) Axial ataxia (wide-based gait, truncal titubation).

   e) Dysarthria (slurred speech, scanning speech).

   f) Abnormal eye movements (ocular dysmetria [overshooting or undershoot-ing with saccades], nystagmus).

Table 1-1. Differentiation between cerebellar and sensory ataxia

Manifestations	Cerebellar ataxia	Sensory ataxia
Nystagmus	Present	Absent
Dysarthria	Present	Absent
Proprioception	Normal	Abnormal
Deep tendon reflexes	Normal or pendular	Decreased or absent
Truncal ataxia	Present	Absent
Can be compensated by visual control	No	Yes

2) **Sensory ataxia**: Loss of proprioception, symptoms of peripheral nerve or spinal cord damage, positive Romberg test (stand behind the patient ready to catch them in case of fall and ask the patient to stand erect with the feet together, arms stretched forward, and eyes closed; the test is positive if the patient begins to fall).

Differentiation between cerebellar and sensory ataxia: →Table 1-1.

2. Diagnostic studies: Investigations depend on the presumed neurologic localization and pathophysiology and may include brain imaging studies (computed tomography [CT], magnetic resonance imaging [MRI]) in cerebellar ataxia, MRI of the spinal cord in sensory ataxia (in the case of suspected dysfunction of the dorsal columns of the spinal cord), and electrophysiologic studies (in case of suspected peripheral neuropathy). Other studies depend on the suspected cause.

2. Headache

→ **CAUSES AND PATHOGENESIS**

Headache is a symptom that may be caused by various diseases. It may develop through a wide range of pathogenetic mechanisms that depend on the underlying condition. The International Headache Society (IHS) classifies headache using a hierarchical organization and specific diagnostic criteria based on symptoms, signs, and associated medical conditions. Classification is an important step in accurately identifying the probable headache etiology, natural history, and treatment.

The IHS divides headache into 2 groups: primary (not caused by an underlying disease process) or secondary (caused by an underlying disease process). The pathogenesis of primary headache, such as migraine, is not completely understood, although proposed mechanisms include various neuronal, vascular, receptor, and electrophysiologic changes. The pathogenesis of secondary headache usually involves irritation, ischemia, or stretching of pain-sensitive structures around the brain (meninges, vessels) or pain-sensitive structures around the head (muscle, bone, peripheral nerve, joint, and sinus).

1. Primary headache: The most common primary headache types are migraine (with or without aura), tension-type headache, and cluster headache (trigeminal autonomic cephalalgias).

1) **Migraine**: Features: →Table 2-1. The headache cannot be better explained by another diagnosis. A particularly disabling form of migraine is chronic migraine, which is diagnosed in patients with a headache present ≥15 days

Table 2-1. Features of migraine headaches

Frequency/duration	≥5 attacks with headache attacks lasting 4-72 hours (when untreated or treated unsuccessfully)
Characteristics (≥2 of 4)	Unilateral location, pulsating quality, moderate or severe pain intensity, aggravated by or leading to avoidance of physical activity
Associated symptoms (≥1 of 2)	≥1 of nausea/vomiting, photophobia, and phonophobia

Table 2-2. Features of tension headaches

Frequency	≥10 episodes of headache occurring on average on 1-14 days per month (12-180 days per year)
Duration	Lasting from 30 minutes to 7 days
Characteristics (≥2 out of 4)	– Bilateral location – Pressing or tightening (nonpulsating) quality – Mild or moderate intensity – Not aggravated by routine physical activity (eg, walking or climbing stairs)
Further features	– No nausea or vomiting – Photophobia or phonophobia may be present (but not both)

in a month for ≥3 subsequent months, provided that on ≥8 days of each month the headache fulfills the criteria for migraine and the patient has a history of ≥5 migraine attacks (with or without aura).

2) **Tension-type headache**: Features: →Table 2-2. The headache cannot be better explained by another diagnosis.

3) **Trigeminal autonomic cephalalgias**: These headaches include cluster headache (episodic or chronic), paroxysmal hemicrania (episodic or chronic), and short-lasting unilateral neuralgiform headache attacks with conjunctival injection and tearing (SUNCT). The classification of trigeminal autonomic cephalalgias is mainly based on the frequency and duration of individual attacks. In patients with paroxysmal hemicrania, headache episodes occur more frequently (≥20 times a day) but generally last a shorter time (2-30 minutes). The attacks in SUNCT are even more frequent (up to 100 times a day) and most often last <1 minute.

a) Characteristics of **cluster headache**: →Table 2-3. The headache cannot be better explained by another diagnosis.

b) **Paroxysmal hemicrania** refers to attacks of severe strictly unilateral pain, which is orbital, supraorbital, temporal, or any combination of these sites, lasts 2 to 30 minutes, and occurs several or many times a day.

4) Other (rare) types of primary headache: Primary stabbing headache, primary cough headache, primary exertional headache, primary headache associated with sexual activity, hypnic headache, primary thunderclap headache, new-onset daily persistent headache, nummular headache, and hemicrania continua.

2. Secondary headache: Causes of secondary headache are multiple and include (as listed by the IHS) head or neck trauma (immediate or delayed); cranial or cervical vascular disorders (aneurysm, arterial dissection, cerebral vein and sinus thrombosis [CVST]); nonvascular intracranial disorders (tumor, after seizures); substance abuse or withdrawal (medication overuse headache);

Table 2-3. Features of cluster headache	
Frequency	≥5 attacks, may occur from every other day to up to 8 per day
Duration	Lasting from 15 to 180 minutes (if untreated)
Characteristics	– Severe or very severe unilateral pain in the orbital, supraorbital, and/or temporal area And ≥1 of: – Conjunctival injection and/or lacrimation – Nasal congestion and/or rhinorrhea – Eyelid edema – Forehead and facial sweating and/or flushing – Miosis and/or ptosis – Restlessness or agitation

infections (meningitis, encephalitis); disorders of cerebrospinal fluid (CSF) flow (intracranial hypertension or hypotension); disorders of the neck, eyes, ears, nose, sinuses, teeth, mouth, or other facial or cranial structures (cervical radiculopathy or myofascial pain, sinusitis); psychiatric disorders (depression, anxiety, posttraumatic stress disorder).

3. Additional considerations:

1) **Medication overuse headache** is a common cause of chronic headache that occurs on ≥15 days per month in a patient with a preexisting headache disorder and with regular overuse for >3 months of ≥1 drug that can be taken for acute or symptomatic treatment of headache. The headache cannot be explained by another diagnosis. Discontinuation of the involved drug (offending agent) can often improve the headache and also increases responsiveness to treatments for other headache etiologies.

2) **Severe sudden-onset headache**: Sudden-onset headache is a common presentation in the emergency room or primary care setting. Only a small percentage is a result of a life-threatening illness; more than half of the life-threatening diseases are due to vascular causes (subarachnoid hemorrhage, intracranial hemorrhage, CVST, arteriovenous malformation, giant cell arteritis, arterial dissection); the other causes include tumors and meningitis.

Patients with a severe sudden-onset headache require urgent evaluation, as the headache may be a symptom of subarachnoid hemorrhage or another life-threatening condition.

→ DIAGNOSIS

1. History and physical examination: Start from excluding secondary headache that may be life-threatening. Pay special attention to **alarming symptoms (red flags)**, which may suggest a serious etiology of the headache and require urgent diagnostics (→Table 2-4). "SNOOP4" is a useful bedside mnemonic for secondary causes: **s**ystemic symptoms/signs/disease, **n**eurologic symptoms/signs, **o**nset sudden, **o**nset after the age of 50 years, **p**attern change. After excluding the most common and most serious causes of secondary headache, reevaluate the patient, paying particular attention to atypical features of the headache or comorbidities.

2. Diagnostic studies: Available tests include neuroimaging (computed tomography [CT], magnetic resonance imaging [MRI], in some cases angiography [CTA, MRA]), lumbar puncture, and blood tests, each depending on the suspected secondary headache (its presence and potential causes).

Table 2-4. Alarming features (red flags) in a patient with headache

Feature	Most frequent causes	Recommended diagnostic studies
Sudden-onset headache (± signs of meningeal irritation)	Subarachnoid hemorrhage, bleeding from tumor or arteriovenous malformation, brain tumor (particularly in posterior fossa)	Neuroimaging,[a] CSF analysis[b]
Headache of constantly increasing severity	Brain tumor, subdural hematoma, medication overuse	Neuroimaging[a]
Headache with accompanying systemic symptoms (fever, nuchal rigidity, rash)	Meningitis, encephalitis, Lyme neuroborreliosis, systemic infection, connective tissue disease (including systemic vasculitis)	Neuroimaging,[a] CSF analysis,[b] blood tests as needed
Focal neurologic signs or symptoms, or symptoms other than typical visual or sensory aura	Brain tumor, arteriovenous malformation, connective tissue disease (including systemic vasculitis)	Neuroimaging,[a] diagnostic workup for connective tissue diseases with vascular involvement
Papilledema	Brain tumor, idiopathic intracranial hypertension, encephalitis, meningitis	Neuroimaging,[a] CSF analysis[b]
Headache on coughing, exercise, or Valsalva maneuver	Subarachnoid hemorrhage, brain tumor (particularly in posterior fossa)	Neuroimaging[a]; consider CSF analysis[b]
Headache during pregnancy or in postpartum period	Cerebral vein or sinus thrombosis, carotid artery dissection, pituitary apoplexy	Neuroimaging[a]
New-onset headache in patient with cancer	Cancer metastasis	Neuroimaging,[a] CSF analysis[b]

[a] Computed tomography or magnetic resonance imaging.

[b] After a mass lesion causing raised intracranial pressure has been excluded by neuroimaging.

CSF, cerebrospinal fluid.

Neuroimaging is indicated in the following situations:

1) Severe sudden-onset headache that is new or associated with red flag symptoms.

2) Nonacute headache with abnormal neurologic signs.

Neuroimaging is suggested in:

1) Nonacute headache with red flag symptoms.

2) Patients with possible migraine that do not meet all the criteria for migraine or have some atypical symptoms.

Neuroimaging is generally not necessary if the patient's history of headaches is consistent with typical and common headache disorders (migraine, tension-type headache) and no abnormal findings have been identified on physical (including neurologic) examination.

→ TREATMENT

Treatment of Migraine

The approach to treating migraine is dependent on the severity and frequency of attacks and, most importantly, on the impact on the quality of life of the patient. Acute treatment is used at the start of migraine attacks; prophylactic treatment is used when the frequency, severity, or impact on the patient is such that prevention of attacks is warranted; and rescue therapy is used when acute treatment has not aborted the migraine attack and symptomatic treatment for pain and nausea or vomiting is required.

1. Acute attacks of migraine: Mild to moderate acute attacks of migraine may respond to oral analgesics and nonsteroidal anti-inflammatory drugs (NSAIDs): acetylsalicylic acid (ASA) 1000 mg, acetaminophen (INN paracetamol) 1000 mg, ibuprofen 200 to 600 mg, diclofenac 50 to 100 mg, or a combination of these drugs taken as soon as possible with the onset of headache.

In patients with moderate to severe acute attacks of migraine or in those not responsive to analgesics or NSAIDs, triptan therapy is more effective. Various triptan drugs are available with different speed of onset, duration, and tolerability. Subcutaneous sumatriptan 6 mg has the most rapid mode of onset and highest probability of decreasing pain. Patient preference, individual response, and adverse effects guide the choice of a particular triptan drug and whether another should be tested. Triptans are contraindicated in patients with coronary artery, cerebrovascular, and peripheral vascular disease.

As migraine attacks are very often accompanied by nausea or vomiting, administer an **antiemetic** as soon as possible: metoclopramide 10 to 20 mg orally or 10 mg IM or IV or domperidone 10 mg orally.

Emergency room treatment of migraine, including status migrainosus (a migraine attack with a prolonged headache phase that lasts >72 hours; the headache may temporarily resolve but not for >4 hours), is often necessary when oral treatment has failed at home. Treatment in this situation can include IV rehydration in the context of nausea and vomiting, IV metoclopramide 10 to 40 mg, subcutaneous sumatriptan 6 mg, IV lysine acetylsalicylate 1000 mg, and IV dexamethasone 4 to 8 mg.

2. Prophylactic treatment of migraine: Migraine-preventive treatment should last ≥3 months, optimally ~6 months.

1) **First-line agents**: Metoprolol 50 to 200 mg/d, propranolol 40 to 240 mg/d, bisoprolol 5 to 10 mg/d, flunarizine 5 to 10 mg/d, valproic acid 500 to 1500 mg/d, topiramate 25 to 100 mg/d, amitriptyline 50 to 75 mg/d may all be effective.◐◐

2) **Second-line agents** (drugs that are less effective or cause more adverse effects than first-line agents): Opipramol 50 to 150 mg/d, ASA 300 mg/d, magnesium 600 mg/d, magnesium + vitamin B_2 400 mg/d + coenzyme Q10 150 mg/d, lisinopril 10 mg/d, candesartan 16 mg/d, or telmisartan 80 mg/d.◐◐○

Nonpharmacologic treatments that may be considered, either used alone or in combination with other options, include biofeedback, relaxation therapy, and cognitive behavioral therapy.

3. Chronic migraine: Options include topiramate 100 to 200 mg/d, valproic acid 500 to 1500 mg/d, botulinum toxin type A 155 to 195 IU (a total dose per 1 series) administered to muscles around the head according to an appropriate regimen.

Treatment of Cluster Headache

Treatment of individual attacks is difficult because they are relatively short-lived and resolve spontaneously, which means that almost no traditional analgesics become effective before the spontaneous cessation of pain.

1. Acute attacks of cluster headache:

1) **First-line agents**: Sumatriptan 6 mg subcutaneously, zolmitriptan 5 to 10 mg as nasal spray, oxygen 6 to 12 L/min.

2) **Second-line agents**: Sumatriptan 20 mg as nasal spray, zolmitriptan 5 to 10 mg orally.

2. Prophylactic treatment of cluster headache:

1) **First-line agents**: Suboccipital steroid injection, civamide 0.025% nasally daily.

2) **Second-line agents** (limited data): Lithium 900 mg/d, verapamil 360 mg/d, warfarin with a target international normalized ratio (INR) of 1.5 to 1.9, melatonin 10 mg/d.

Treatment of Paroxysmal Hemicrania

The drug of choice is indomethacin 150 to 225 mg/d. A very good response to indomethacin additionally supports the diagnosis of paroxysmal hemicrania.

Treatment of Medication Overuse Headache

Agents used for abortive treatment of headache are strictly contraindicated because their overuse may be the underlying cause of the headache. Explain to the patient what has caused the pain and why they need to discontinue the overused drugs. An abrupt discontinuation is recommended in the case of overuse of simple analgesics, ergotamine, or triptans, while tapering the dose down to discontinuation is recommended in the case of overuse of opioids, benzodiazepines, and barbiturates. In some patients discontinuation of analgesic agents may be facilitated by using a preventive medication, such as topiramate 100 mg/d (maximum, 200 mg/d), a short course of glucocorticoids (prednisone or prednisolone ≥60 mg/d), or amitriptyline (maximum, 50 mg/d).

3. Impaired Consciousness

→ **DEFINITION AND ETIOLOGY**

The level of consciousness depends on the activity of the reticular activating system (RAS) of the brain stem and cerebral cortex. Loss of consciousness may be caused by any pathologic state that interferes with the function of the RAS (eg, brainstem stroke), both cerebral cortices (eg, encephalitis), or both the RAS and cortices (eg, cardiac syncope). Between normal consciousness and complete loss of consciousness, states of partially preserved consciousness with limited ability to respond to external stimuli can be identified (→Table 3-1). Also →Chapter 10.4.

Table 3-1. Disturbances of consciousness

Descriptive term	Symptoms
Confusion	Patients seem fully awake but their thoughts and actions are incoherent and chaotic; likely disoriented to time or place; exclude aphasia, which may mimic confusion
Delirium	Sudden onset and fluctuating symptoms that feature inattention or easy distractibility and disorganized thinking, or fluctuations in consciousness from a hypervigilant state to lethargic
Lethargy (excessive drowsiness)	Patients wake in response to verbal stimuli, provide verbal responses, and make voluntary movements
Stupor	Patients wake after a strong pain stimulus, show no or minimal response to verbal commands
Coma	No response even to strong pain stimuli; reflexive movements can occur

Table 3-2. Glasgow Coma Scale		
Type of reaction	**Response**	**Score**
Eye opening	Spontaneous	4
	To verbal command	3
	To pain stimuli	2
	No response	1
Verbal response	Normal, patient is fully oriented	5
	Responds but is disoriented	4
	Uses inappropriate words	3
	Inarticulate sounds	2
	No response	1
Motor response	To verbal command	6
	Can locate pain stimuli	5
	Undirected and nonpurposeful movements of the limbs	4
	Abnormal flexion posturing of arms, legs in extension (decorticate)	3
	Abnormal extension posturing of arms, legs in extension (decerebrate)	2
	No response	1
Adapted from Lancet. 1974;2(7872):81-4.		

→ **DIAGNOSIS AND TREATMENT**

Determination of the level of consciousness may be very difficult, for instance, in patients with aphasia, depression, or those treated with muscle relaxants. In such situations the neurologic assessment may be limited and interpretation of signs may not be accurate. Responses to the following stimuli are of diagnostic and prognostic importance in the assessment of a patient with a decreased level of consciousness: eye opening, verbal response, and motor response to pain stimuli. The Glasgow Coma Scale is most often used (→Table 3-2). In the assessment take into account the best response. Repeat the examination periodically and monitor the dynamics of changes in the level of consciousness. A more detailed neurologic examination assessing brainstem functions (eg, pupillary function, extraocular movements, gag response) and cortical brain functions (eg, visual fields, language function) may identify the brain localization and possible etiology of the decreased level of consciousness.

Management: →Chapter 10.4.

4. Loss of Consciousness

Loss of consciousness may be caused by syncope (the patient usually recovers within a minute) or may signal the onset of coma. Altered mental status: →Chapter 10.3.

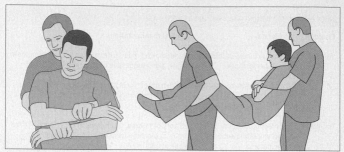

Figure 4-1. Safe transfer of an unconscious nontrauma patient by 2 persons.

➤ BASIC MANAGEMENT

1. Evaluate the patient using the ABCD scheme. Basic life support: →Chapter 3.3. Assess the patient's response to verbal and tactile stimuli. If a pulse is absent, begin cardiopulmonary resuscitation (CPR). If available, ask a bystander to call for help (or if in hospital, consider activating the emergency response team). Advanced life support: →Chapter 3.3.

2. Clear the airway (→Chapter 3.3; in trauma patients, particularly after head or neck injury, do not tilt the head backwards or in other directions), administer 100% oxygen via a face mask, check the capillary blood glucose level, and establish a peripheral intravenous line.

3. Monitor the vital signs. If blood pressure is low, administer 1 L crystalloid solution (eg, 0.9% NaCl) or, if not available, elevate the lower limbs to 45°.

4. If the loss of consciousness is a result of trauma or a head or neck injury is suspected, stabilize the cervical spine (apply a rigid cervical collar if available) and carry out a rapid trauma survey.

5. Protect the patient from environmental extremes. If the loss of consciousness may have been caused by external factors (eg, hyperthermia, hypothermia, or gas poisoning [most frequently carbon monoxide]), and it is safe for you to do so, remove the patient from the environment (transferring a nontrauma patient: →Figure 4-1). If the patient is already in hospital, ensure he or she is moved to an area capable of providing appropriate support.

6. If the loss of consciousness (in a nontrauma patient) is prolonged but the patient is hemodynamically stable (heart rate, blood pressure, and respiratory rate are within normal limits), you may place the patient in the recovery position (→Figure 3.3-4).

7. If the patient does not regain consciousness, continue the management you have already initiated. Call for advanced help as required, depending on the patient's requirements as well as your level of expertise and comfort (eg, unstable arrhythmia, refractory hypotension, a persistent Glasgow Coma Scale score <8 [→Table 3-2]), and investigate for causes of coma (→Table 4-1).

8. If the patient recovers rapidly, investigate for causes of the transient loss of consciousness.

4.1. Coma

➤ DEFINITION AND CAUSES

Coma is a prolonged loss of consciousness with reduced response to external stimuli. **Causes:** →Table 4-1.

Table 4-1. Typical manifestations of coma based on etiology

Etiology	Causes	Typical manifestations
Vascular	Subarachnoid or intracranial hemorrhage	Sudden onset, headache, vomiting, focal neurologic signs, signs suggestive of meningitis
	Extensive stroke affecting bilateral cerebral hemispheres or brainstem	Sudden onset, focal neurologic signs, progressive clinical deterioration
Trauma	Direct brain injury or accumulating subdural hematoma	History of trauma, lacerations or other signs of head trauma, bleeding from ears or CSF leakage from nose or ears
Increased intracranial pressure	Brain tumor or abscess, subdural hematoma	History of escalating headache, progressive impairment of mental status, papilledema, focal neurologic signs
Inflammatory	Meningitis	History of headache and fever, subacute course, signs suggestive of meningitis
	Encephalitis	As above plus signs of disseminated encephalopathy, seizures, involuntary movements
Metabolic	Hypoglycemia	Hyperhidrosis, dilated pupils, seizures, hyporeflexia, Babinski sign, sometimes focal neurologic signs
	Hyperglycemia	Hyperventilation, Kussmaul breathing
	Uremia	Progressive apathy, progressive obtundation, tremor, seizures
	Liver disease	Coma preceded by memory impairment, confusion, and somnolence with subsequent development of pyramidal, extrapyramidal, and cerebellar signs and low frequency tremor
	Hypercalcemia	Signs of hypercalcemia
	Hyponatremia	Cerebral edema caused by changes in CSF and cell tonicity, can also be provoked by overly rapid correction in patient with chronic derangement
	Hypernatremia	Signs of hypernatremia
	Myxedema	History of hypothyroidism, gradual deterioration over weeks, common hypercapnia
Epilepsy	Epilepsy	Sudden abnormalities in behavior or mental status, seizures, sometimes extremity paresis
Hypoxia	Cardiac and respiratory arrest	Sudden onset, decortication or decerebration, myoclonus, epileptic seizures
Hypercapnia	Carbon dioxide retention in patients with respiratory insufficiency	Gradual deterioration of mental status, prior headache, shallow respiration, conjunctival injection
Extreme body temperatures	Hypothermia	Signs of hypothermia
	Hyperthermia	Signs of hyperthermia

Etiology	Causes	Typical manifestations
Toxins	Toxic alcohols, ethanol	Signs of alcohol intoxication
	Anticholinergics, sedative hypnotics, antipsychotics, opioids, carbon monoxide poisoning	Signs of poisoning and intoxication
Psychiatric	Catatonia, pseudocoma	History of psychiatric diagnosis and deterioration, normal cold caloric testing

CSF, cerebrospinal fluid.

→ **MANAGEMENT**

1. Assess the patient (→Chapter 10.4).

2. Assess consciousness (depth of coma): Check responsiveness (to voice, touch, and pain) using the Glasgow Coma Scale (GCS) (→Table 3-2). Reevaluate the GCS score often to monitor for any fluctuation in the patient's mental status.

3. Perform a complete head-to-toe assessment:

1) **Vital signs**: Tachycardia, bradycardia, hyperthermia, hypothermia, hyperventilation, hypoventilation, hypertension, hypotension.

2) **Eyes**: Pupil size and reactivity, nystagmus, gaze deviation, scleral icterus; fundoscopy for papilledema.

3) **Head and neck**: Meningismus, tongue biting (especially the lateral aspects of the tongue), Battle sign.

4) **Neurologic examination**: Ability to follow commands, tone, deep tendon reflexes, Babinski reflex, asterixis, posturing (decerebrate/extensor or decorticate/flexor), convulsions, myoclonus.

5) **Cardiovascular examination**: Murmurs, arrhythmias, volume status.

6) **Respiratory examination**: Pattern of breathing (Cheyne-Stokes, Kussmaul), decreased breath sounds, wheezes, crackles.

7) **Abdominal examination**: Distension, ascites, peritoneal signs, distended bladder.

8) **Dermatologic examination**: Cellulitis, sacral or heel ulceration, signs of IV drug use.

4. Initiate universal and specific antidotes (as applicable):

1) Thiamine 100 mg IM or IV (administer before glucose [dextrose]).

2) Glucose (1 ampoule of 50% dextrose in water).

3) Naloxone 0.4 mg IV (if opioid overdose is suspected).

4) Supplemental oxygen (100% fraction of inspired oxygen [FiO_2] if carbon monoxide poisoning is suspected).

5. Order diagnostic tests:

1) **Electrocardiography (ECG)**.

2) **Laboratory tests**:

   a) **Complete blood count**: An elevated white blood cell count may indicate a central nervous system infection.

   b) **Serum biochemistry tests**: Serum levels of glucose (low or elevated in hyperosmolar hyperglycemic nonketotic coma and diabetic ketoacidosis), sodium, potassium, ammonia (usually elevated in hepatic coma), urea/blood urea nitrogen (BUN) and creatinine (elevated in uremia), lactate (elevated in hypoxia and shock), calcium (elevated in hypercalcemic crisis), phosphate, magnesium.

   c) **Arterial blood gas analysis** may reveal hypercapnia, hypoxemia, and acidosis.

d) **Serum and urine osmolality** (elevated in toxic alcohol ingestions).

e) **Toxicology screen** if ingestion suspected.

f) Levels of **acetylsalicylic acid (ASA) and paracetamol** (INN acetaminophen) (in all patients with suspected overdose, as ingestion is common).

g) **Thyroid-stimulating hormone (TSH) levels** (high in myxedema coma).

h) **Urinalysis**: Elevated ketone bodies (and sometimes glucose) in ketoacidosis.

i) **Lumbar puncture and cerebrospinal fluid examination** if meningitis or encephalitis are suspected.

3) **Imaging studies**: **Computed tomography (CT)** of the head with no contrast enhancement allows visualization of intracranial bleeding and cerebral edema. **Chest radiographs** are used to assess for atelectasis due to aspiration (perform a therapeutic bronchoscopy if necessary).

6. Perform a differential diagnosis of coma (→Table 4-1), determine the cause, and treat the underlying condition, if possible.

4.2. Syncope and Other Causes of Transient Loss of Consciousness

→ DEFINITION AND CAUSES

Syncope is a transient loss of consciousness caused by global cerebral hypoperfusion. It is characterized as a loss of postural tone with a rapid onset, short duration, and spontaneous recovery without neurologic deficits. Syncope can be classified into several broad categories (→Table 4-2). In **presyncope** (a syncopal prodrome) the patient has a sensation of imminent loss of consciousness but true syncope does not occur.

Other causes of symptoms that can mimic syncope include sudden-onset conditions not associated with loss of consciousness, such as a fall or psychogenic pseudosyncope (appearance of a transient loss of consciousness in the absence of true loss of consciousness), or conditions associated with a partial or complete loss of consciousness not primarily related to cerebral hypoperfusion (metabolic disturbances [eg, hypoglycemia], hypoxia, hyperventilation with hypocapnia, seizure, drug or alcohol intoxication).

→ GENERAL APPROACH TO SYNCOPE

1. Management of patients with loss of consciousness: →Chapter 10.4.

2. Exclude other causes of transient loss of consciousness.

3. Identify clinical features suggestive of cardiac etiology.

4. Stratify patients into low risk and high risk (requiring prompt diagnostic testing).

5. Provide a provisional diagnosis and management plan.

6. Identify when driving privileges should be held (follow local laws and regulations).

Initial Evaluation of a Patient With Syncope

1. Detailed and comprehensive history:

1) **Context at the onset of symptoms**: After standing; with dehydration (decreased oral intake, bleeding, diarrhea, vomiting); with drug administration (suggestive of an orthostatic cause); related to strong emotions like fear, pain, or sight of blood (vasovagal); related to specific situations such as micturition, defecation, coughing, sneezing, or exercise (situational); on exertion; with head turning (carotid artery occlusion); or when supine.

2) **Prodromal symptoms**: Weakness, presyncope, visual blurring, diaphoresis, nausea, terminal warmth (vasovagal), palpitation, or lack of prodromal symptoms (cardiac).

Table 4-2. Syncope: causes and management suggestions

Causes	Triggers	Diagnosis	Management
VVS			
– Inappropriate reflex response leading to vasodilation or bradycardia – Most common type of syncope in all ages (46% of all events) – Usually benign and not requiring specific treatment. Ensure adequate salt intake and hydration	– Sudden, unexpected, or unpleasant stimulus (sight, sound, smell, pain) – Following long periods of standing in crowded hot places – After meals; concomitant nausea or vomiting	– Typical history – Calgary Syncope Symptom Score (→Table 4-4) – Tilt table testing can be considered in case of diagnostic uncertainty	– Avoidance of triggers – Advise on episodic management (sitting down, isometric exercises) – Orthostatic training (unproven benefit) – In selected patients with episodes of prolonged asystole dual-chamber pacemaker is indicated
Carotid sinus syndrome			
– Hypersensitivity of afferent or efferent limbs of carotid sinus leading to bradycardia and/or vasodilation – ...rely in adults ...<50 years	– Syncope after head turning (eg, changing traffic lanes)	– Carotid sinus massage – Asystole >3 s or fall in SBP >50 mm Hg	– Dual-chamber pacemaker – Pharmacotherapy only in exceptional cases with specialist consultation (unproven benefit)
...ic hypotension			
...n auto-...athetic ...stem ...d to ...osed ...tion, ...nsion	– Primary causes: Parkinson disease, MSA, pure autonomic failure – Secondary causes (more common): volume depletion: alcohol, drugs (diuretics, β and α blockade, vasodilators)	– Sustained drop in BP (≥20 mm Hg drop in SBP, or SBP <90 mm Hg) within 3 min of standing – Consistent medical history	– Discontinue offending drugs – Avoid circumstances that may trigger syncope – Increase intravascular volume with fluids or drugs: fludrocortisone 0.1-0.4 mg/d PO or midodrine 5-40 mg/d PO
Cardiac sy...			
Can be structu... or arrhythmog... leading to decre... cardiac output an... drop in cerebral pe... fusion	– Significant organic heart disease; syncope during physical exercise or in supine position; syncope preceded by palpitations; family history of SCD – ...atients at high ...sk for VTE	– ECG or telemetry changes of conduction delay, QT prolongation, IHD, hypertrophy – Echocardiography	– Referral to cardiologist for management of underlying cardiac disease – Interrogate pacemaker if in situ

Cerebrovascular syncope			
Causes	**Triggers**	**Diagnosis**	**Management**
– Decreased cerebrovascular blood flow, can occur with: 1) Subclavian steal syndrome 2) TIA affecting vertebral and posterior arteries 3) Migraine variant	– Subclavian steal syndrome: stenosis of subclavian artery proximal to vertebral artery causing reversal of flow during strenuous upper limb exercise – Ischemic risk factors (hypertension, dyslipidemia, prior CVA, smoker, DM) – Migraine triggers	– Subclavian and/or carotid artery bruit, BP differential – Ultrasonography of carotids – Vertebral and subclavian angiography – MRA/MRI	– Referral to specialists for management of underlying disease depending on etiology (eg, neurologist for migraines, TIA; vascular surgeon for subclavian steal)

BP, blood pressure; CVA, cerebrovascular accident; DM, diabetes mellitus; ECG, electrocardiography; IHD, ischemic heart disease; MRA, magnetic resonance angiography; MRI, magnetic resonance imaging; MSA, multiple system atrophy; PO, oral; SBP, systolic blood pressure; SCD, sudden cardiac death; TIA, transient ischemic attack; VTE, venous thromboembolism; VVS, vasovagal syncope.

3) **Symptoms following the event**: Rapid return of consciousness (cardiac) versus confusion, focal weakness, or delayed return to baseline (seizure).

4) **Collateral history of the event**: Appearance during the event, including the overall duration, presence of seizure symptoms, signs of pseudosyncope (slumping to the floor, lack of trauma, closed eyes, lack of diaphoresis).

5) **Associated conditions**: Primary autonomic failure (Parkinson disease, dementia with Lewy bodies, pure autonomic failure, multiple system atrophy) or secondary autonomic failure (diabetes mellitus, amyloidosis, spinal cord injuries, autoimmune autonomic neuropathy, paraneoplastic autonomic neuropathy, kidney failure); bradyarrhythmias such as sinus node dysfunction, heart block; tachyarrhythmias such as atrial fibrillation, long QT syndrome, Brugada syndrome, and other supraventricular tachyarrhythmias; structural heart disease like history of myocardial infarction and cardiomyopathy, valvular heart diseases like aortic stenosis; pulmonary embolism.

2. Physical examination:

1) **Vital signs** including orthostatic blood pressure and heart rate.

2) **Neurologic examination**: Screening examination for focal deficits. Examination of the lateral aspects of the tongue for signs of tongue biting indicating a seizure.

3) **Cardiovascular examination**: Jugular veins, enlarged/displaced apical beat, murmurs, bruits, signs of congestive heart failure.

4) **Carotid sinus massage**: Indicated in all patients aged >40 years with syncope of unknown origin compatible with a reflex mechanism. Carotid sinus hypersensitivity is defined as a ventricular pause lasting >3 seconds, a decrease in systolic blood pressure >50 mm Hg, or both. Done, unilateral

5) **Other**: Signs of pulmonary embolism such as parasternal heave, unilateral leg swelling, tenderness, and erythema.

3. Investigations:

1) **12-lead electrocardiography (ECG)** is performed in all patients to look for signs of conduction disturbances, ischemia, preexcitation syndromes (long QT, delta wave, or Brugada syndrome [right bundle branch block with ST-segment elevation in leads V_1-V_3]).

Table 4-3. Risk assessment following syncope

Major risk factors	
Abnormal ECG	Any bradyarrhythmia, tachyarrhythmia, or conduction disorder, ischemia, or history of myocardial infarction
History of cardiac disease	Ischemic, arrhythmic, obstructive, valvular
Hypotension	Systolic blood pressure <90 mm Hg
Minor risk factors	
Cerebrovascular disease	
Family history of sudden cardiac death	At age <50 years
Specific situations	Syncope while supine, during exercise, or no prodromal symptoms
ECG, electrocardiography.	

Table 4-4. Calgary Syncope Symptom Score

Individual items of the Calgary Syncope Symptom Score	Points if "YES"
Is there a history of ≥1 of the following: bifascicular block, asystole, supraventricular tachycardia, diabetes mellitus?	−5
At times, have bystanders noted you to be blue during your faint?	−4
Did your syncope start when you were 35 years of age or older?	−3
Do you remember anything about being unconscious?	−2
Do you have lightheaded spells or faint with prolonged sitting or standing?	1
Do you sweat or feel warm before a faint?	2
Do you have lightheaded spells or faint with pain or medical settings?	3
The diagnosis of vasovagal syncope is made if the score is ≥−2.	
Source: Eur Heart J. 2006;27(3):344-50.	

2) **Echocardiography** is performed in patients with signs of possible structural heart disease including aortic stenosis, hypertrophic cardiomyopathy, pulmonary embolism, pulmonary hypertension, and ischemia.

3) Other investigations are used to identify etiology of the syncopal event as dictated by the history, physical examination, and ECG. These include tilt table testing (orthostatic hypotension), extended ECG monitoring and electrophysiologic study (arrhythmia-related cardiac syncope), and in-hospital video recording (seizure).

→ **RISK OF SERIOUS OUTCOMES**

Patients with syncope who present to medical attention may have a significant risk of adverse outcomes during follow-up; however, the gravity of this risk varies widely depending on etiology (→Table 4-3). The Calgary score may be useful in the identification of patients with vasovagal syncope (→Table 4-4).⊙○ The Canadian

Table 4-5. Risk stratification scores after syncope

Canadian Syncope Risk Score	San Francisco Syncope Rule	OESIL risk score
Risk factors		
– Predisposition to vasovagal symptoms (−1) – Heart disease history (+1) – SBP <90 or >180 mm Hg (+2) – Elevated troponin (+2) – Abnormal QRS axis (+1) – QRS duration >130 ms (+1) – Corrected QT interval >480 ms (+2) – Vasovagal syncope (−2) – Cardiac syncope (+2)	– SBP <90 mm Hg – Shortness of breath – ECG: Nonsinus rhythm or new changes – Hematocrit <30%	– Age >65 years – History of CVD – Syncope without prodrome – Abnormal ECG findings
Assessed endpoint		
30-day morbidity and mortality after presentation to ED:	7-day morbidity and mortality after presentation to ED:	1-year mortality:
– Score −3 to 0: 0.4%-1.9% – Score 1-3: 3.1%-8.1% – Score 4-5: 12.9%-19.7% – Score 6-11: 28.9%-83.6%	– No factors present: 0.3% – ≥1 factor present: 15.2%	– 0-1 factor (low risk): 0.6% – 2-4 factors (high risk): 31%
Score accuracy		
– Score ≥−2: Sensitivity 99%, specificity 26% – Score ≥−1: Sensitivity 98%, specificity 46%	– Sensitivity 98% – Specificity 56% – LR+: 2.9 – LR−: 0.03	– Sensitivity 97% – Specificity 73% – LR+: 3.6 – LR−: −0.11

Adapted from CMAJ. 2016;188(12):E289-98, Ann Emerg Med. 2004;43(2):224-32, and Eur Heart J. 2003;24(9):811-9.

CVD, cardiovascular disease; ECG, electrocardiography; ED, emergency department; LR+, positive likelihood ratio; LR−, negative likelihood ratio; OESIL, Osservatorio Epidemiologico sulla Sincope nel Lazio; SBP, systolic blood pressure.

Syncope Risk Score can be used to identify patients at high risk for serious adverse events after an emergency department visit for syncope. Other risk scores include the Osservatorio Epidemiologico sulla Sincope nel Lazio (OESIL) score and the San Francisco Syncope Rule (→Table 4-5).⊙○ The Canadian Cardiology Society provides a list of major and minor risk factors predictive of short-term morbidity (→Table 4-3). They recommend that higher-risk patients (>1 major risk factor) should be considered for further cardiac assessment (eg, echocardiography and cardiologist consultation within 2 weeks).⊙○ The subsequent management depends on the suspected cause of the syncope (→Table 4-2).

→ DIAGNOSTIC UNCERTAINTY AND RECURRENCE

Recurrences of syncope are frequent. In patients with diagnostic uncertainty, further investigations can be considered. Tilt table testing, which provides a strong orthostatic stress to provoke vasovagal syncope, can be used in instances of undiagnosed recurrent syncope felt not to be of cardiac or cerebrovascular origin.

Standard 24- to 48-hour Holter monitoring can also be considered; however, unless the episodes are happening daily to weekly, there is little chance that a syncopal event will be recorded. A 1-month event recorder or an implant-able loop recorder (ILR) could be used in selected patients soon after the initial encounter if there is diagnostic uncertainty with ongoing symptom reoccurrence.◐◑

5. Muscular Weakness (Paresis and Paralysis)

→ DEFINITION AND PATHOGENESIS

Muscular weakness is one of the most common neurologic presentations.

Paresis is a reduction in muscle strength with a limited range of voluntary movement. **Paralysis** (-plegia) is a complete inability to perform any movement.

Dysfunction may be of the upper motor neurons (cerebral motor cortex, subcorti-cal structures, brainstem, and corticospinal tracts) or lower motor neurons (motor nuclei of the cranial nerves or motor neurons of the ventral horn of the spinal cord; or peripheral nerve, muscle, or neuromuscular junction). Clinically, any dysfunction above the motor neurons in the brainstem or spinal cord is termed upper motor neuron weakness or spastic weakness and any dysfunction at the motor neurons or below, including the nerve, muscle, or neuromuscular junc-tion, is termed lower motor neuron weakness or flaccid weakness (→Table 5-1).

1. Spastic weakness: Upper motor neuron dysfunction. Commonly caused by stroke (ischemic or hemorrhagic), mass lesions (tumor, abscess), demyelination, or trauma. Acute upper motor neuron dysfunction (eg, stroke, traumatic spinal cord injury) may initially present as flaccid paresis.

2. Flaccid weakness: Lower motor neuron dysfunction. Caused by neuropathy (Guillain-Barré syndrome, heavy metal poisoning, adverse effects of drugs [vincristine, isoniazid], neuropathy in patients with autoimmune diseases or diabetes, acute intermittent porphyria, nerve compression), neuromuscular junction disorders (myasthenia gravis, botulism, effects of muscle relaxants, organophosphate poisoning), or muscle disorders (inflammatory myopathy, periodic paralysis [in patients with hypokalemia or hyperkalemia]).

3. Concomitant spastic and flaccid weakness: Caused by amyotrophic lateral sclerosis, transverse myelitis, and other diseases of the spinal cord (spastic weakness below the level of injury caused by disruption of the cor-ticospinal tract; flaccid weakness at the level of injury due to destruction of the motor cells of the ventral horns). Vitamin B_{12} deficiency can present with spastic weakness due to dysfunction of the corticospinal tracts of the spinal cord and flaccid weakness due to dysfunction of the peripheral nerves (areflexic weakness with bilateral Babinski signs).

→ DIAGNOSIS

1. History and physical examination: The nervous system is distributed throughout the body and therefore weakness on its own cannot accurately define the location of the dysfunction (eg, weakness in a leg could be due to a peripheral nerve injury or stroke affecting the cortical neurons controlling the leg). However, the pattern of weakness can help localize the abnormality:

1) In patients with muscular weakness in the arms and legs, assess the pattern of weakness and if there are upper or lower motor neuron signs:

   a) **Quadriparesis** (all 4 limbs affected) suggests cervical cord injury (upper motor neuron signs) or Guillain-Barré syndrome (lower motor neuron signs).

Table 5-1. Manifestations of upper and lower motor neuron dysfunction

Manifestation	Upper motor neuron	Lower motor neuron
Weakness	Often hemiparetic pattern	Often proximal in muscular weakness and distal in peripheral nerve weakness
Tendon reflexes	Hyperreflexia	Reduced or absent
Clonus (eg, foot clonus)	Present	Absent
Pathologic signs	Present (Babinski sign)[a]	Absent
Muscle atrophy	Absent; secondary atrophy possible due to lack of use of weak muscles	Develops relatively rapidly
Muscle tone	Increased (spastic)	Normal or reduced (flaccid)
Abdominal skin reflexes	Absent	Present
Pathologic movements (eg, chorea)	Present	Absent
Fasciculations	Absent	Occasionally present

[a] Babinski sign: dorsiflexion (extension) of the big toe on scratching the sole of the foot (with a blunt object moved along the outer aspect of the foot from the heel towards the front and the big toe).

b) **Hemiparesis** (affecting the upper and lower limbs on the same side of the body) suggests injury at the contralateral brainstem level or higher in the neuraxis.

c) **Paraparesis** (paresis of the lower limbs only) suggests thoracic or lumbar spinal cord injury.

d) **Monoparesis** (only one limb affected) suggests injury to peripheral nerves or peripheral nerve plexus unless there are upper motor neuron signs.

2) In patients with weakness of the muscles of the head and neck, evaluate distribution and severity:

a) **Eye movement abnormalities**: Injury to cranial nerves III, IV, VI.

b) **Weakness of the muscles of mastication**: Trigeminal nerve injury.

c) **Weakness of the facial muscles**: Weakness of the entire half of the face with inability to close the eye suggests a peripheral facial nerve injury such as Bell palsy. Weakness of the lower part of the face and a relatively preserved ability to close the eye suggests contralateral upper motor neuron dysfunction above the level of the facial nerve nucleus in the brainstem, such as stroke.

d) **Dysphagia, dysphonia**: Vagus nerve injury (vocal cord) or glossopharyngeal nerve injury (palate).

e) **Weakness of the sternocleidomastoid and trapezius muscles**: Accessory nerve injury.

f) **Weakness of the muscles of the tongue**: Injury to the hypoglossal nerve.

3) Pathognomonic signs can accurately identify the neurologic localization. Aphasia, agnosia, neglect, hemianopsia, and changes in cognition or behavior can only occur as a result of cortical hemispheric dysfunction. A cranial nerve abnormality as above with a contralateral limb paresis can only occur as a result of a brainstem dysfunction. A sensory level across the trunk can only occur as a result of a spinal cord dysfunction (→Chapter 10.6).

4) Establish the circumstances in which the weakness has occurred (acute, subacute, or gradual onset); stroke is sudden, mass lesions and demyelination are subacute, neuropathy can have gradual onset. Establish the associated clinical features, such as history of trauma, fever, previous stroke or transient ischemic attack, and other medical conditions, to identify the possible pathophysiology of the neurologic disturbances.

2. Diagnostic studies: Diagnostic tests depend on the presumed neurologic localization and pathophysiology. Blood tests are performed in the case of toxic exposure or metabolic disturbances; imaging studies (computed tomography [CT], magnetic resonance imaging [MRI]), in the case of brain or spinal cord injury; electrophysiologic studies (EPSs) (nerve conduction, electromyography), in the case of nerve or muscle dysfunction; and lumbar puncture, in the case of infection.

6. Sensory Disturbances

→**CAUSES AND PATHOGENESIS**

Sensory disturbances may present as either or both of sensory decrease (negative symptoms; eg, impairment or loss of one or more types of sensory perception) and positive symptoms (eg, abnormal sensory perception in the form of paresthesia [pins and needles] or hypersensitivity to sensory stimuli [hyperesthesia and/or pain]).

Causes: Conditions that damage peripheral receptors located in various tissues and organs, sensory fibers in peripheral nerves, ascending tracts in the spinal cord or brainstem, the thalamus, or cortical centers in the parietal lobe.

Sensory disturbances can occur separately but can also be associated with motor weakness or other neurologic signs that help identify the location of the disturbance (eg, lower motor neuron signs, such as hypotonia and loss of reflexes, suggest a peripheral nerve dysfunction; →Chapter 10.5). The presence of pain suggests irritation of a peripheral nerve, plexus, nerve root, or dorsal horn ganglion as the location of the sensory disturbance.

Patterns and causes of specific types of sensory symptoms based on the location of nervous system lesions: →Table 6-1. Brief and transient paresthesias are not suggestive of nervous system damage.

→**DIAGNOSIS**

1. History and physical examination: Determine the type and severity of sensory symptoms, location and distribution of sensory abnormalities, and circumstances in which they have occurred. The **sense of touch** is examined by touching the patient's body with your finger or cotton swab. The **sense of pain** is examined with a sharp pin. The **sense of temperature** is examined with a cold and hot object. The **sense of vibration** is examined with a 128 Hz tuning fork. The **sense of position** is examined by moving a joint. When examining for sensory abnormalities, compare the symmetric parts of the body, precisely determine the boundaries of sensory abnormalities, compare them with the areas of innervation by specific peripheral nerves and with dermatomes (→Figure 6-1), compare them with the patterns of sensory loss based on the location of the lesion (→Table 6-1), and identify associated motor or pathognomonic signs (→Chapter 10.5).

2. Diagnostic studies: Imaging studies (computed tomography [CT], magnetic resonance imaging [MRI]) of the brain or spinal cord (or both) as well as electrophysiologic tests (sensory conduction, somatosensory evoked potentials), depending on the suspected location of the lesion.

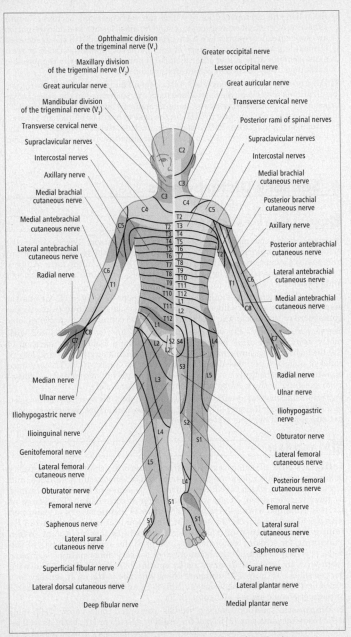

Figure 6-1. Segmental innervation of the skin and cutaneous fields of peripheral nerves.

Table 6-1. Manifestations and causes of sensory abnormalities based on the location of the lesion

Lesion location	Pattern of sensory disturbances	Possible causes
Peripheral nerve	Pain and paresthesia in area innervated by affected nerve followed by sensory loss involving all sensory functions	Mononeuropathy (compression, injury)
Nerve root	Pain worsened by activities increasing intraspinal pressure (eg, cough, defecation), paresthesia within areas innervated by respective nerve roots followed by sensory loss involving all sensory functions	Radiculopathy (disc herniation, acute inflammatory demyelinating polyradiculopathy, severe degenerative lesions of spine, tumor)
Spinal cord lesion	– Sensory loss below lesion level – Hemicord syndrome: Ipsilateral loss of vibration and position sense with contralateral loss of pain and temperature sense	Trauma, tumor, demyelination, infection, ischemia or hemorrhage, of spinal cord
Anterior spinal artery syndrome	Sensory loss below lesion level, dissociated sensory loss: loss of pain and temperature with preserved vibration and position sense (with paralysis)	Anterior spinal artery thrombosis
Posterior columns of spinal cord	Loss of vibration and position sense with preserved pain and temperature (with loss of reflexes)	Subacute combined degeneration of spinal cord (in vitamin B_{12} deficiency), tabes dorsalis (neurosyphilis)
Trigeminal nerve or nucleus	Sensory loss in face in distribution of the trigeminal nerve or branches	Inflammation, demyelination, tumor
Thalamus or posterior limb of internal capsule	Sensory loss of pain and temperature on contralateral side of face, arm, and leg, including trunk; chronic thalamic pain syndrome may occur later	Ischemic or hemorrhagic stroke, tumor, demyelination
Parietal cortex	Inability to assess stimulus intensity and location, impaired graphesthesia (ability to recognize letters or numbers traced on skin), loss of 2-point discrimination (ability to recognize 2 simultaneously applied stimuli as separate), extinction (inability to recognize 1 of 2 simultaneously applied tactile stimuli on symmetric body regions), astereognosis (inability to recognize objects held in hand without visual inspection)	Ischemic or hemorrhagic stroke, tumor

7. Stroke

→ DEFINITION, ETIOLOGY, PATHOGENESIS

Stroke is defined as an abrupt onset of focal brain, spinal cord, or retinal injury due to abnormalities of cerebral blood flow with clinical symptoms or signs lasting >24 hours and/or radiologic abnormalities of infarction or hemorrhage present on imaging studies. Subarachnoid hemorrhage (SAH) is also considered in the category of stroke although cerebral dysfunction is usually generalized.

Focal neurologic signs and symptoms that resolve spontaneously within 24 hours and without radiologic abnormalities are referred to as a **transient ischemic attack (TIA)**.

On the basis of **pathomechanism and etiology**, stroke can be classified as:

1) **Ischemic stroke** (accounting for ~80% of stroke cases), which is usually due to an occlusion (often a transient occlusion with embolic strokes) of an artery and the resulting reduction of focal cerebral perfusion. Ischemic stroke may be caused by:

   a) Atherosclerotic plaques (in situ plaque rupture with occlusion or artery--to-artery embolism) in the major arteries supplying the brain (aortic arch, carotid and vertebral arteries) or in large- and medium-size intracranial arteries.

   b) Degenerative lesions/microatherothrombosis (in situ occlusion) in small penetrating arteries of the brain (lacunar stroke [LACI]).

   c) Cardiac embolism from atrial fibrillation (most frequently), ischemic heart disease (left ventricular aneurysm or cardiomyopathy), mitral or aortic valvular heart disease (rheumatic valvular disease, endocarditis, or artificial bioprosthetic or mechanical valves).

   d) Less common causes, such as patent foramen ovale (PFO) (paradoxical embolism), arterial dissection, or coagulopathies.

   Despite recent diagnostic advances, ~17% of ischemic strokes are found to be cryptogenic (embolic stroke of undetermined source) after diagnostic evaluation.

2) **Hemorrhagic stroke** (accounting for ~15%-20% of stroke cases), which may be caused by:

   a) **Intracerebral hemorrhage**: Most commonly occurs due to bleeding from a ruptured penetrating intracranial vessel in the context of hypertension (weakened vessel due to degenerative changes and microaneurysmal formation), bleeding from rupture of a lobar vessel in the elderly (weakened vessel due to amyloid deposition), or rupture from an arteriovenous malformation.

   b) **SAH** (~5% of stroke cases): Most frequently occurs as a result of rupture of a saccular aneurysm at the base of the brain in the subarachnoid space and presents clinically with generalized brain dysfunction (headache, decreased level of consciousness [LOC]).

   Hemorrhagic transformation of ischemic infarction occurs in 7% of patients after thrombolysis, but it can occur spontaneously in patients with cardioembolic stroke and large infarction. Hemorrhagic infarct is often asymptomatic because it is due to bleeding into the already damaged tissue, but if severe, it can manifest clinically as deterioration in neurologic function and is managed as spontaneous intracerebral hemorrhage.

3) **Cerebral venous thrombosis** (<1% of stroke cases), which occurs as a result of thrombosis of the intracranial venous sinuses, deep venous system, and cortical veins, causing cerebral ischemia, infarction, and hemorrhage. The clinical presentation can be variable and includes headache, seizures, focal signs, and decreased LOC.

Risk factors: Hypertension, diabetes mellitus, dyslipidemia, tobacco smoking, physical inactivity, cardiac diseases, alcohol abuse, oral contraceptives, hormonal replacement therapy, pregnancy, migraine.

→ CLINICAL FEATURES AND NATURAL HISTORY

1. Symptoms of ischemic stroke depend on the **location of the lesion**. The Oxford classification identifies ischemic stroke subtypes based on location and vascular territory:

1) **Total anterior circulation infarct (TACI)** involves the area supplied by the anterior and middle cerebral arteries and causes total anterior circulation syndrome (TACS): significant hemiparesis or sensory disturbances

affecting one side of the body in ≥ 2 out of 3 areas (face, upper extremities, lower extremities), aphasia, and homonymous hemianopsia.

2) **Partial anterior circulation infarct (PACI)** involves part of the anterior cerebral circulation and causes partial anterior circulation syndrome (PACS): motor or sensory symptoms in 1 or 2 out of the 3 areas mentioned above, or isolated aphasia.

3) **LACI** develops in the areas supplied by the penetrating arteries, most frequently in the basal ganglia, internal capsule, thalamus, or brainstem, and causes lacunar stroke syndrome (LACS), which is usually limited to paresis or sensory disturbances in 2 out of 3 areas (face, upper extremities, lower extremities). Isolated weakness involving all of the face, arm, and leg (pure motor stroke) is a relatively specific LACS.

4) **Posterior circulation infarct (POCI)** affects the vertebrobasilar system and manifests with cerebellar, brainstem, or occipital lobe signs and symptoms (posterior circulation syndrome [POCS]), including ataxia and nystagmus, cranial nerve palsies with contralateral motor or sensory deficits (or both), or isolated homonymous hemianopia.

Symptoms of hemorrhagic stroke depend on the **type and location of bleeding**:

1) **Intracerebral hemorrhage** results in a variety of focal deficits depending on the location of bleeding. It is typically associated with a prominent headache due to intracranial hypertension, but the headache does not usually have a thunderclap quality. It is not possible to differentiate it on clinical grounds from cerebral infarction and imaging is required.

2) **SAH** should always be carefully excluded in each patient with a sudden and intense (thunderclap) headache (often described as "the worst ever in my life"). Usually, there are few focal neurologic signs, but more commonly, a change in the LOC is seen.

Cerebral venous thrombosis causes a wide range of clinical manifestations and the area of injury does not correspond to the area of arterial blood supply. Cerebral venous thrombosis may lead to focal neurologic symptoms or partial seizures, symptoms of increased intracranial pressure, and altered mental status; and with involvement of the cavernous sinus, to abnormal eye movement (palsies of cranial nerves III and VI) with accompanying exophthalmos, retrobulbar pain, and eyelid edema.

2. Natural history: In the first hours or days following a stroke, the patient's neurologic status may change. Up to 20% of patients with cerebral infarction will have worsening of their impairments in the first 24 to 48 hours (stroke in progression). In 5% to 10% of patients with ischemic stroke, a second stroke occurs early (new neurologic symptoms develop; it may be associated either with a new or the same blood supply area as the first stroke). In up to 10% of large cerebral infarctions (TACIs), hemorrhagic transformation may occur, usually in the first 48 hours, with possible neurologic worsening. In addition, large cerebral infarctions (TACIs) may show clinical worsening or decreased LOC due to cerebral edema between days 3 and 5. In the absence of these complications, most patients start to improve after the initial few days and the majority of motor recovery occurs over the first 2 to 3 months. The risk of stroke is ~10% in the first 30 days after a TIA, with half of the events occurring in the first few days. Rapid identification of stroke etiology and implementation of risk-reduction strategies in patients with an acute TIA are imperative.◉●

→ DIAGNOSIS

Diagnostic Workup

1. Take a history. Carefully establish the exact time of the onset of symptoms, as this is crucial for determining indications for thrombolytic treatment or endovascular clot retrieval. Almost all stroke patients present with sudden and focal neurologic signs and symptoms.

Table 7-1. Example of application of the NIHSS as used in Hamilton Health Sciences.
For a full scale, visit www.nihstrokescale.org

1a. LOC	0	Alert
	1	Drowsy
	2	Stuporous
	3	Comatose
1b. LOC questions	0	Answers both questions correctly
	1	Answers 1 question correctly
	2	Answers neither question correctly
1c. LOC commands	0	Performs both tasks correctly
	1	Performs 1 task correctly
	2	Performs neither task correctly
2. Best gaze	0	Normal
	1	Partial gaze palsy
	2	Forced deviation
3. Visual fields	0	No visual loss (or in coma)
	1	Partial hemianopia
	2	Complete hemianopia
	3	Bilateral hemianopia
4. Facial palsy	0	Normal
	1	Minor
	2	Partial
	3	Complete
5. Best motor: right arm	0	No drift
	1	Drift
	2	Some effort against gravity
	3	No effort against gravity
	4	No movement
6. Best motor: left arm	0	No drift
	1	Drift
	2	Some effort against gravity
	3	No effort against gravity
	4	No movement
7. Best motor: right leg	0	No drift
	1	Drift
	2	Some effort against gravity
	3	No effort against gravity
	4	No movement

8. Best motor: left leg	0	No drift
	1	Drift
	2	Some effort against gravity
	3	No effort against gravity
	4	No movement
9. Limb ataxia	0	Absent (or in coma)
	1	Present in 1 limb
	2	Present in ≥2 limbs
10. Sensory	0	Normal
	1	Partial loss
	2	Dense loss (or in coma)
11. Best language	0	No dysphasia
	1	Mild
	2	Severe dysphasia
	3	Mute
12. Dysarthria	0	Normal articulation
	1	Mild to moderate dysarthria
	2	Unintelligible or worse
13. Neglect	0	No neglect (or in coma)
	1	Partial neglect
	2	Complete neglect

NIHSS total score

NIHSS scoring for aphasic and comatose patients:
1b) **LOC questions:** Aphasic and stuporous patients unable to state age or month = 2 points.
 2. **Best gaze:** Conjugate gaze deviation overcome by voluntary or reflex movement = 1 point. Isolated eye nerve palsy = 1 point.
 3. **Visual fields:** Visual field clear cut asymmetry = 1 point. Total blindness = 2 points.
 4. **Facial palsy:** Facial asymmetry can be assessed in response to noxious stimuli.
5-8. **Motor testing:** Motor testing can be pantomimed for aphasic patients.
 9. **Limb ataxia:** If cannot be demonstrated = 0 points.
10. **Sensory:** Asymmetry = 1 point. Bilateral sensory loss = 2 points. Patient in coma and with no response to pain = 2 points.
11. **Best language:** Patient in coma = 3 points.
12. **Dysarthria:** Scored only if audible speech is heard.
13. **Neglect:** Present if obviously more than blindness or sensory loss.

NIHSS, National Institute of Health Stroke Scale; LOC, level of consciousness.

2. Assess the vital signs (airway, breathing, circulation [ABC]): Respiration rate, blood pressure, heart rate (including electrocardiography [ECG]), and oxygen saturation (SaO_2) (pulse oximetry).

3. Perform an efficient general examination: Look for evidence of trauma or other signs that may require immediate medical intervention. In patients with SAH symptoms and signs of meningeal irritation (stiff neck) can be present.

4. Perform a focused neurologic examination: A standardized stroke scale, such as the National Institutes of Health Stroke Scale (NIHSS) (→Table 7.1), is a tool that can quantify the degree of impairment, identify stroke location, quantify change in neurologic impairments, and predict the outcome. The NIHSS is useful in determining prognosis after stroke and has become a common and reliable communication tool among clinicians.◗

5. Assess blood glucose levels. Patients with hypoglycemia can present with a focal stroke-like picture.

6. Collect blood samples for a complete blood count (CBC), international normalized ratio (INR), activated partial thromboplastin time (aPTT), serum electrolytes, renal function tests, and serum biomarkers of myocardial infarction. Measure thrombin time (TT) if the patient is suspected to be treated with a direct thrombin inhibitor or ecarin clotting time (ECT) if a direct factor Xa inhibitor is suspected. In selected patients there may be specific indications to order liver function tests, toxicology screen, blood alcohol level, and pregnancy test.

7. Perform nonenhanced computed tomography (NECT) or magnetic resonance imaging (MRI) of the brain as soon as possible; these studies accurately differentiate ischemic stroke from hemorrhagic stroke, which cannot be reliably done on clinical grounds, and are crucial for both acute and chronic management. While MRI offers better resolution, NECT takes a shorter time to complete, can be performed in patients with metal implants, is less susceptible to motion artifacts, and in most cases provides enough information to make emergency treatment decisions. To decide about potential clot retrieval, computed tomography angiography (CTA) or magnetic resonance angiography (MRA) is subsequently necessary to identify the presence of a large vessel occlusion in patients who are potential candidates for endovascular clot retrieval for large vessel occlusion (carotid artery, middle cerebral artery, anterior cerebral artery).

The sensitivity of computed tomography (CT) scanning in the first few hours after SAH is almost 100%. If the results of head CT scanning are normal or inconclusive and SAH is suspected based on clinical presentation, perform a diagnostic lumbar puncture. Do not perform lumbar puncture until you have excluded an intracranial space-occupying lesion with brain CT or MRI.

8. Further studies should be guided by the need to identify the pathomechanism of stroke: carotid ultrasonography and/or CTA/MRA for large vessel atherosclerosis and stenosis; echocardiography (transthoracic and/or transesophageal) for a cardioembolic source; prolonged cardiac monitoring for suspected atrial fibrillation. Other studies are guided by the clinical indication: chest radiography for suspected aspiration pneumonia or electroencephalography (EEG) for suspected epileptic disorders mimicking stroke.

Differential Diagnosis

Differential diagnosis includes a broad spectrum of diseases that may occasionally present with and produce focal neurologic symptoms or signs. Even in expert hands >10% of patients diagnosed with ischemic stroke at the initial evaluation are found to have another disorder (most commonly seizure, migraine, or psychosomatic conversion disorder).

CT or MRI brain scanning reliably differentiates ischemia or infarction from hemorrhage. Most mass lesions, such as tumor, subdural hematoma, or abscess, are evident on brain imaging. Toxic and metabolic disorders simulating stroke become evident from their atypical presentation, examination, laboratory analyses, and progression of the disorder.

▶ TREATMENT

Stroke is a medical emergency, a life-threatening condition that often results in severe and permanent neurologic impairment and disability. Therefore, it requires urgent diagnosis and immediate treatment. A patient with suspected stroke should be urgently transported to a hospital that is experienced in

Table 7-2. Treatment of hypertension in patients with recent ischemic stroke who are eligible for fibrinolytic treatment (examples; other medications are possible)

Before fibrinolytic treatment	
– Do not administer rtPA if BP cannot be maintained ≤185/110 mm Hg	
Patient eligible for rtPA administration except for SBP >185 mm Hg and/or DBP >110 mm Hg	– IV labetalol 10-20 mg over 1-2 min, may be repeated once
	or
	– IV nicardipine 5 mg/h, titrate up by 2.5 mg/h every 5-15 min (maximum rate, 15 mg/h). When target BP is achieved, adjust to maintain appropriate BP range
	or
	– IV clevidipine 1-2 mg titrated by doubling the dose every 2-5 min until target is reached (maximum, 21 mg/h)
	or
	– Other agents (eg, hydralazine, enalaprilat) may be considered

During or after fibrinolytic treatment	
– Maintain BP ≤180/105 mm Hg (use IV labetalol 10 mg followed by infusion 2-8 mg/h, nicardipine (maximum, 15 mg/h), or clevidipine (maximum, 21 mg/h)	
– Monitor BP every 15 min for 2 h following the start of rtPA administration, then every 30 min for 6 h, and then every hour for 16 h	
BP cannot be controlled with labetalol or nicardipine or DBP >140 mm Hg	– Admission to ICU
	– IV sodium nitroprusside 0.5 µg/kg/min

BP, blood pressure; DBP, diastolic blood pressure; ICU, intensive care unit; rtPA, recombinant tissue plasminogen activator; SBP, systolic blood pressure.

providing stroke care, and preferably directly to a hospital with a dedicated stroke unit.◐◑

General Medical Treatment

1. Control the vital parameters: Immediately assess and stabilize airway, breathing, and circulation (ABC). Patients with stroke may require mechanical ventilation and treatment of cardiac dysfunction in an intensive care unit (ICU) setting.

2. Control blood pressure: In the early phase of stroke blood pressure is frequently elevated and then spontaneously decreases after a few days. An excessive lowering of blood pressure may lead to a reduction in cerebral blood flow, resulting in expansion of the ischemic lesion and deterioration of the patient's neurologic status. Avoid rapid lowering of blood pressure.

1) **Usual indications for the use of antihypertensive drugs**:
   a) Patients with ischemic stroke **eligible for thrombolysis**: Systolic blood pressure (SBP) >185 mm Hg or diastolic blood pressure (DBP) >110 mm Hg (→Table 7-2).
   b) Patients with ischemic stroke **not eligible for thrombolysis**: SBP >220 mm Hg or DBP >120 mm Hg (→Table 7-3). The available evidence has failed to show benefit of lowering SBP below certain thresholds (ie, 180 or 160 mm Hg).◑
   c) Patients with intracerebral hemorrhage: SBP lowering to 140 mm Hg is suggested as it is safe and probably beneficial (→Table 7-4). It is probably safe to rapidly lower the SBP to 140 or less; however, the efficacy is unproven.
   d) Patients with SAH: SBP >160 mm Hg.

Table 7-3. Treatment of hypertension in patients with recent ischemic stroke not receiving fibrinolytic treatment (examples; other medications possible)

Blood pressure	Management[a]
SBP <220 mm Hg and DBP <120 mm Hg	Do not use antihypertensive agents. Hold 50% of previously used β-blockers, hold other antihypertensive medications. Consider antihypertensive treatment in patients with severe heart failure, aortic dissection, or symptoms of hypertensive encephalopathy (choice of agents: →Table 7-2)
SBP >220 mm Hg or DBP of 120--140 mm Hg	Benefit of lowering is uncertain but suggested. Lowering BP by 15% within the first 24 h and use of medications (→Table 7-2) is reasonable (IV labetalol, nicardipine, clevidipine, hydralazine, enalaprilat [0.625-1.25 mg every 6 h])
DBP >140 mm Hg	– ICU admission – IV sodium nitroprusside 0.5 µg/kg/min

[a] Target BP reduction is 10%-15%. Continuous BP monitoring is necessary. Onset, duration of action, and adverse effects of the drugs: →Chapter 3.9, Table 9-3.

BP, blood pressure; DBP, diastolic blood pressure; ICU, intensive care unit; SBP, systolic blood pressure.

Table 7-4. Treatment of hypertension in patients with recent intracerebral hemorrhage (examples; other medications could be used [also →Table 7-2; →Table 7-3])

Blood pressure	Management
Systolic BP at presentation >140-150 mm Hg. ICP normal. Maintain BP ≤140/80 mm Hg	IV nicardipine 5 mg/h, titrate up by 2.5 mg/h every 5-15 min (maximum rate, 15 mg/h). IV labetalol, enalapril, or nitroprusside could be used
If ICP is elevated, maintain cerebral perfusion pressure	ICU admission with ICP monitoring

BP, blood pressure; ICP, intracranial pressure; ICU, intensive care unit.

e) Patients with elevated blood pressure associated with acute coronary syndrome, aortic dissection, heart failure, renal injury, or markedly reduced coagulability in the course of anticoagulant treatment: Blood pressure targets are based on the condition and urgency of the situation.

2) **Choice of agents**: Blood pressure is best controlled with IV drugs; examples: →Table 7-2, →Table 7-3, →Table 7-4. Stroke is rarely accompanied by **hypotension**, which is usually associated with ischemic heart disease or may be a result of dehydration, bleeding (usually from the gastrointestinal tract), or pharmacotherapy. Correct the underlying cause of hypotension, administer fluids, and, if necessary, manage the patient in an ICU setting with vasopressors.

3. Correct any existing fluid and electrolyte disturbances (→Chapter 4).

4. Monitor blood glucose levels: Both hyperglycemia and hypoglycemia have adverse effects on the brain in the setting of acute stroke. In patients with **hyperglycemia** restrict dietary carbohydrates. In patients with glucose levels ≥10 mmol/L consider insulin treatment but with caution, to avoid hypoglycemia. In patients with **hypoglycemia** (<3.3 mmol/L) administer 25 mL of 50% glucose (dextrose) in a slow IV injection (low tonicity of a 5% glucose solution may cause brain edema).

5. Reduce body temperature if it is >37.5°C. Fever is frequent in the first 48 hours after stroke and is associated with a less favorable prognosis. The source of fever, in particular infection, should be identified. Use acetaminophen (INN paracetamol) (up to 4000 mg/d) and surface cooling.

6. Monitor urine output: Urinary incontinence is common after acute stroke, and as many as 20% of patients with stroke have urinary retention. Bladder scanning, in-out catheterization, or both should be ordered. Temporary catheterization may be indicated to monitor urine output and in the case of urinary retention; however, prolonged catheterization should be avoided if possible, as it is associated with increased risk of infections.

7. Insert a **nasogastric tube** to provide oral medications otherwise not available IV in patients with dysphagia. Dysphagia is common after stroke; however, early feeding does not change the probability of a good outcome and may be deferred as long as hydration is maintained.

8. Start **prophylaxis of venous thromboembolism** for immobile patients with low-molecular-weight heparin (LMWH) (eg, enoxaparin 40 mg/d) rather than unfractionated heparin (UFH). Consider pneumatic compression if anticoagulation is contraindicated.◐● (→Chapter 3.19.2).

9. Good nursing care and positioning can reduce the risk of aspiration pneumonia, other infections, and pressure ulcers.

10. Management of **increased intracranial pressure or seizures**: →Complications, below.

Specific Therapy for Ischemic Stroke

1. Acetylsalicylic acid (ASA): Administer ASA immediately in patients who are not treated with fibrinolysis or 24 hours following fibrinolytic treatment; intracranial hemorrhage must be excluded by brain CT. Start with 160 to 325 mg/d, then reduce the dose to 81 mg/d.◐● In patients after a minor ischemic stroke or TIA, add clopidogrel 300 to 600 mg as a loading dose followed by 75 mg/d for ~30 days.◐● Due to increased risk of bleeding, it is preferred to postpone ASA in patients receiving fibrinolytic treatment (for 24 hours) or undergoing clot retrieval (unless a stent is placed during the procedure), but with that consideration both interventions can be used in a person who has already received ASA.

2. Fibrinolytic treatment: Recombinant tissue plasminogen activator (rtPA) 0.9 mg/kg (10% of the dose in IV injection over 1-2 minutes followed by the remaining 90% of the dose as IV infusion over 1 hour; maximum total dose, 90 mg).◐●

1) rtPA may be used within 4.5 hours from the onset of an ischemic stroke that has caused clinically significant and measurable neurologic deficits. Note that the benefits of fibrinolytic therapy decrease as more time elapses from the onset of stroke to the administration of rtPA.

2) Recognizing the increased risk of bleeding, rtPA may be used in patients who are currently treated with ASA or have taken it recently, or in patients in whom subsequent clot retrieval is considered.

3) **Exclusion criteria**: →Table 7-5.

4) **Complications**: The risk of symptomatic intracranial hemorrhage is increased in patients who receive rtPA (7% vs 1%), as is early death; however, death or dependency at 3 to 6 months is still decreased in patients treated with rtPA. The risk of bleeding increases with the time from the onset of symptoms and with severity of stroke.●

3. For **patients with occlusions of the proximal intracranial vessels** (carotid artery, middle cerebral artery, anterior cerebral artery) as seen on CTA and within 6 hours of the onset of ischemic stroke, including those who underwent fibrinolytic therapy, intra-arterial clot extraction with stent retrievers significantly improves the probability of good recovery; consideration

Table 7-5. Thrombolytic therapy for ischemic stroke. An example of exclusion criteria as used in Hamilton Health Sciences

Exclusion criteria for thrombolytic therapy with tPA for acute stroke order set
Goal: Door-to-needle time: 60 minutes

Absolute exclusion criteria: All answers must be "NO"

Onset of symptoms or the "last seen normal" is >4.5 hours	Yes	No
CT evidence of cerebral hemorrhage	Yes	No
Clinical presentation consistent with subarachnoid hemorrhage even if CT scan normal	Yes	No
Blood pressure >185/110 mm Hg and not treatable	Yes	No
Blood glucose level <2.7 mmol/L (48.6 mg/dL)	Yes	No
Significant head trauma, brain surgery, or spinal surgery within 3 months	Yes	No
History of intracranial hemorrhage (in previous 6 months)	Yes	No
Recent minor stroke (1 month) or moderate to severe stroke (3 months)	Yes	No
Active internal, gastrointestinal, or urinary bleeding within 21 days	Yes	No
Arterial puncture at a noncompressible site in previous 7 days	Yes	No
Platelet count <100 × 10^9/L	Yes	No
IV heparin received within 48 hours, resulting in abnormally elevated aPTT >40 seconds	Yes	No
Low-molecular-weight heparin at full anticoagulant levels	Yes	No
Warfarin use with INR >1.7	Yes	No
Direct oral anticoagulants (rivaroxaban, dabigatran, apixaban) taken within previous 24 hours	Yes	No

Relative contraindications: Consider eligibility on an individual basis based on benefits and risks

Rapidly improving neurologic signs or NIHSS <4	Yes	No
History of arteriovenous malformation or aneurysm	Yes	No
Profound stroke with obtundation, fixed eye deviation, and complete hemiplegia, or NIHSS >24	Yes	No
Acute cerebral infarct with ASPECT score ≤5	Yes	No
Recent large myocardial infarction or pericarditis within 3 months	Yes	No
Blood glucose level >22.2 mmol/L (399.6 mg/dL)	Yes	No
Recent major surgery or trauma (cardiac, thoracic, abdominal, orthopedic) within 14 days	Yes	No
History of bleeding diathesis or liver failure	Yes	No
Seizure at onset of stroke with residual postictal neurologic deficits	Yes	No
Pregnancy	Yes	No
Age <18 years	Yes	No

Summary eligibility assessment: All answers must be checked		
1. The patient meets inclusion criteria: acute ischemic stroke symptom and symptom onset <4.5 hours.	Yes	No
2. The patient does not have any of the absolute exclusion criteria.	Yes	No
3. The patient may have one or more of the relative contraindications, but potential benefits of alteplase exceed potential risks.	Yes	No
Alteplase (rtPA) to be given (YES or NO):	Yes	No

aPTT, activated partial thromboplastin time; ASPECT, Alberta Stroke Program Early CT Score; CT, computed tomography; INR, international normalized ratio; NIHSS, National Institutes of Health Stroke Scale; PO, oral; tPA, tissue plasminogen activator.

should be given to treatment or transfer to an interventional stroke center if feasible.🟢🟤 Patients with occlusion of the proximal intracranial vessels as seen on CTA and within 6 to 24 hours of the onset of ischemic stroke may be candidates for intra-arterial clot extraction if imaging with CT perfusion identifies a significant mismatch between infarcted and potentially salvageable brain tissue.🟢🟤

4. Heparin:

1) **Ischemic stroke**: Administration of UFH or LMWH at therapeutic doses (the majority of immobilized patients require the use of heparin at prophylactic doses) is indicated only in exceptional cases: possibly in patients with stroke caused by cardioembolism who are at high risk of a second embolism as well as in patients with arterial dissection. However, even in these circumstances there is no generally accepted evidence that the benefit from treatment outweighs the risk of increased bleeding.

2) **Cerebral venous thrombosis**: Start with heparin (UFH or LMWH) at therapeutic doses (→Chapter 3.19, Table 19-2), then continue treatment with a vitamin K antagonist (VKA) (warfarin) for 3 to 6 months (INR, 2.0-3.0). Repeat venous imaging should be used to guide discontinuation of anticoagulation.🟢🟤

3) **Contraindications**: Extensive ischemic infarction (eg, involving >50% of the area supplied by the middle cerebral artery), uncontrolled hypertension, hemorrhagic transformation of ischemic infarction, and stroke complicating infective bacterial endocarditis.

Specific Therapy for Intracerebral Hemorrhage and SAH

SAH requires surgical clipping of the ruptured vessel and/or endovascular embolization using coils inserted into the aneurysm. Neurosurgical consultation should be obtained in all patients with SAH.

Surgical evacuation of an intracerebral hemorrhage is generally not recommended, except for selected patients with cerebellar hematoma to prevent fatal brain stem compression and in patients with a large spontaneous superficial intracerebral hemorrhage with impending herniation. Neurosurgical consultation is recommended for most patients with intracerebral hemorrhage.

Rehabilitation

Rehabilitation plays a crucial role in the resolution of neurologic deficits caused by stroke. The goals of rehabilitation are to prevent complications, minimize loss of function (impairment), and maximize activity and participation (disability and handicap). Patients should be admitted to and managed in a rehabilitation stroke unit by a multidisciplinary stroke team that includes the core disciplines of physiotherapy, occupational therapy, and speech language therapy.

→ **COMPLICATIONS**

Progressive stroke, brain edema, hemorrhagic transformation, and recurrent infarction are the neurologic causes of clinical deterioration.

1. Increased intracranial pressure and brain edema, which develops as early as 24 to 48 hours of stroke, after vascular reperfusion, usually peaks after 3 to 5 days. Increasing edema is a frequent cause of worsening neurologic deficits (affecting about 10% of patients); it may lead to cerebral herniation and death.

Treatment:

1) Elevate the head of the bed at 20° to 30°.

2) Provide a comfortable environment and prevent secondary complications (eg, adequate pain management, appropriate body positioning, shoulder protection in hemiplegic patients).

3) Prevent hypoxemia and maintain a normal body temperature.

4) Short-term hyperventilation (unproven efficacy for improving outcomes) may be used (provided cerebral perfusion is good). Lowering partial pressure of carbon dioxide ($PaCO_2$) by 5 to 10 mm Hg may decrease intracranial pressure by 25% to 30%.

5) Pharmacologic treatment (unproven efficacy) might be considered only in the case of massive cerebral edema: IV mannitol 0.25 to 0.5 g/kg over 20 minutes (this may be repeated every 6 hours) or hypertonic saline. Glucocorticoids have not been shown to be effective.

6) In younger patients (<60 years) with massive hemispheric cerebral infarction (>2/3 of the middle cerebral artery territory), early decompressive craniectomy decreases mortality from ~80% to 30% but with potentially severe residual disability; the decision should be guided by patient values and preferences.⊘● In older individuals (>60 years) decompressive craniectomy increases survival but only at the expense of severe disability.●

7) Cerebellar infarction or hemorrhage is particularly dangerous and prone to life-ending herniation. Close monitoring and early neurosurgical consultation should be obtained. Patients may require early craniectomy or ventricular drainage.

2. Epileptic seizures, which are usually partial or secondarily generalized partial seizures (rarely status epilepticus), may occur early or later after stroke in 5% to 15% of patients; recurrence is not uncommon. Treatment of seizures may require immediate control with IV lorazepam 2 to 4 mg (maximum, 8 mg), followed by phenytoin 15 to 20 mg/kg by IV infusion (maximum rate, 50 mg/min). Long-term treatment is preferred with either lamotrigine, levetiracetam, carbamazepine, or gabapentin; drug choice is dependent on other patient factors.

3. Venous thromboembolism and pulmonary embolism: Prevention and treatment: →Chapter 3.19.1; →Chapter 3.19.3; →Chapter 3.19.2.

4. Infections:

1) **Urinary tract infections** occur in up to 15% of patients within the first 2 weeks of stroke and may be prevented by maintaining adequate fluid volume and avoiding unnecessary catheterization.

2) **Respiratory infections** most often occur in the context of dysphagia and more severe strokes in up to 7% of patients and are associated with increased mortality and poor functional outcomes. Assessment and monitoring for dysphagia, early mobilization, and early treatment of infection can improve outcomes.

5. Urinary and fecal incontinence: Urinary incontinence is present in up to 50% of patients early after stroke and persists in up to a third of patients 1 year later. Avoid aggravating factors (eg, diuretics), treat urinary tract infections with appropriate antibiotics, and monitor for urinary retention. Constipation may occur in up to 50% of patients within the first month of stroke. Proper hydration, monitoring, and mobilization may prevent complications.

6. Pressure ulcers: Due to immobility and incontinence, patients with stroke are at high risk of skin breakdown. Monitoring, skin protection, and positioning are the key preventive measures.

7. Spasticity is a velocity-dependent increase in tone that occurs after stroke. It can cause pain and decrease in function and interfere with recovery. Positioning, stretching, a range of motion exercises, and other physiotherapeutic interventions are the mainstay of treatment. Antispasmodic medication (avoiding benzodiazepines) and botulinum toxin injections are part of a comprehensive spasticity-management program.

8. Shoulder pain syndrome: A painful shoulder has many causes, including trauma, bursitis/tendonitis/capsulitis, rotator cuff tears, spasticity, and complex regional pain syndrome 1 or 2. Appropriate shoulder protection is necessary as a prophylactic measure; start physiotherapy and use analgesics if needed (glucocorticoid injections are not recommended unless there is a specific indication). Advise the patient and the caregiver how to get up from the bed without straining the affected shoulder and how to support the affected limb, especially if the limb is flaccid. Treatment of spasticity and restoration of a normal range of motion require specialized procedures (avoid exercises using weights suspended over the head).

9. Falls: Falls may occur in 15% to 65% of stroke patients. Strategies for the prevention of falls are necessary.

10. Malnutrition: Patients unable to eat on their own or with dysphagia are at risk for dehydration and malnutrition. Maintain adequate hydration and nutrition; introduce nasogastric or percutaneous endoscopic gastrostomy (PEG) feedings if necessary and desired. Note that early nasogastric feeding is not associated with better outcomes.

11. Depression (affects ~30% of patients at different periods following stroke): Treatment with selective serotonin reuptake inhibitors (SSRIs) should be considered. The use of SSRIs improves depression but does not improve functional outcomes.🗹🔵

12. Delirium is common after stroke and affects up to a quarter of patients. An underlying cause aside from stroke should be sought and treated if found.

→ PREVENTION

Secondary Stroke Prevention

1. Management of risk factors:

1) Hypertension: Start treatment with an angiotensin-converting enzyme inhibitor (ACEI) in stable patients after a few days (on average 7) targeting an SBP <140 mm Hg and a DBP <90 mm Hg🗹🔵; for patients with LACI a treatment target of an SBP <130 mm Hg is indicated.🗹🔵 Initiate treatment with an ACEI (perindopril or ramipril) and/or diuretic (eg, indapamide).

2) Glucose intolerance and diabetes mellitus: These are best assessed by measuring glycated hemoglobin (HbA_{1c}). Follow treatment guidelines for nonstroke and mixed patient populations.

3) Hypercholesterolemia: High-dose statin treatment (eg, atorvastatin 80 mg/d) should be initiated in all patients with an ischemic stroke or TIA presumed to be of atherosclerotic origin.🗹🔵 The efficacy of treating to target is unproven.

4) Cessation of smoking: Continued smoking is associated with stroke recurrence. Behavioral therapy and pharmacotherapy are effective in treating tobacco dependence.

5) Screening for obesity, weight loss measures: Although screening is recommended, weight loss is of uncertain benefit.

6) Regular physical activity: Those patients who can and have no other contraindications should participate in moderate to vigorous intensity exercise 3 to 4 times per week for 40 minutes.

7) Obstructive sleep apnea (OSA): There is a high prevalence of OSA in patients with TIA and stroke. Although treatment with continuous positive airway pressure (CPAP) reduces sleepiness and other symptoms of OSA, it does not prevent cardiovascular events in patients with moderate to severe OSA.◒

8) Alcohol: Light to moderate amounts of alcohol may have protective effects (2 drinks per day for men, 1 drink per day for women). Heavier use is associated with an increased risk of ischemic and hemorrhagic stroke.

2. Antithrombotic treatment: Treatment is dependent on the presumed cause of stroke.

1) Noncardioembolic sources of TIA or stroke (extracranial atherosclerotic arterial disease, intracranial atherosclerotic arterial disease, lacunar disease): Use antiplatelet treatment, not anticoagulation.◓◖ Options include ASA 81 to 325 mg/d, clopidogrel 75 mg/d, or ASA 25 mg + extended-release dipyridamole bid. The combination therapy (ASA + dipyridamole) and clopidogrel have similar efficacy. A combination of ASA 81 mg/d and clopidogrel 75 mg/d may be used for the first 30 days after TIA or stroke or 90 days in patients with intracranial disease; long-term treatment without other indications is associated with increased risk of bleeding and should not be used. Triple antiplatelet therapy (ASA + clopidogrel + dipyridamole) is associated with increased risk of major bleeding without benefit over clopidogrel alone or the combination of ASA and dipyridamole.✖◖

2) Cardioembolic sources of TIA or stroke (atrial fibrillation, cardiomyopathy, left ventricular thrombus, valvular heart disease [native, bioprosthetic, mechanical]): In patients with atrial fibrillation long-term anticoagulation is indicated to prevent recurrent stroke.◓◖ Use a VKA or non-VKA oral anticoagulants (direct oral anticoagulants [DOACs]; apixaban, dabigatran, rivaroxaban). The target INR for a VKA is 2.5 (range, 2.0-3.0). DOACs are chosen based on the patient's preference, tolerability, drug interactions, renal dysfunction, and time in range for VKA treatment. ASA 81 mg/d is indicated if anticoagulation is not possible; ASA 81 mg/d with clopidogrel 75 mg/d may also be considered if anticoagulation is not possible.◓◖ Single antiplatelet therapy may be added to anticoagulation in patients with atrial fibrillation and acute coronary syndrome or a coronary stent; dual antiplatelet therapy plus anticoagulation is associated with increased risk of bleeding without a decrease in the rate of thromboembolic events.✖◖ Anticoagulation with a VKA is indicated for a left ventricular thrombus; the target INR is 2.5 (range, 2.0-3.0).

3) Long-term anticoagulation with a VKA is recommended for the prevention of stroke in patients with mechanical heart valves; the intensity of anticoagulation varies by the valve position (aortic: INR, 2.0-3.0; mitral: INR, 2.5-3.5). The addition of ASA 81 to 100 mg/d in patients at a lower risk of bleeding decreases the risk of embolism. DOACs should not be used in patients with mechanical valves as these agents increase the risk of embolism and bleeding.✖◖ The risk of embolism and recurrent embolism is lower with bioprosthetic valves, and long-term anticoagulation over antiplatelet treatment may not be indicated.

4) Patients with dilated or restrictive cardiomyopathy (left ventricular ejection fraction ≤35%) with sinus rhythm and without a thrombus have a relatively low risk of recurrent embolism. Antiplatelet treatment rather than a VKA or DOAC may be reasonable.◓◖

5) Other, less common sources of stroke are arterial dissection, aortic arch disease, PFO, and cerebral vein and sinus thrombosis. One recent randomized trial compared antiplatelet treatment with anticoagulation treatment in cervical (carotid or vertebral) arterial dissection and found no difference between these treatments; however, the study was associated with major imprecision that precluded a clear recommendation.◒ Aortic arch disease has been associated with increased risk of stroke, and in such cases antiplatelet

therapy with statin therapy is suggested over anticoagulation.⊘○ A PFO can be a source of embolism with or without paradoxical embolism but is often an "innocent bystander" (found in 23% of the general population); antiplatelet and anticoagulant therapy seem equally effective in preventing recurrence of stroke. PFO closure is associated with a small increased risk of periprocedural new-onset atrial fibrillation but with a long-term reduction in recurrent stroke in carefully selected patients <60 years of age with confirmed stroke, TIA, or systemic embolism and high probability of PFO-associated event.⊘● Cerebral vein and sinus thrombosis is treated acutely with therapeutic doses of LMWH despite the possibility of hemorrhagic conversion of venous infarctions.⊘○ Long-term anticoagulation of this condition (3 months vs longer) is based on indirect evidence from other venous thrombosis territories and depends on the individual patient's circumstances (presence of precipitating factors or thrombophilias).

In the absence of carotid artery stenosis warranting revascularization or a major-risk cardioembolic source requiring anticoagulation (such as atrial fibrillation or a left ventricular thrombus), the 3 most important mainstays of secondary ischemic stroke risk reduction are blood pressure control, antiplatelet therapy, and high-dose statins.

3. Invasive treatment of carotid artery stenosis: →Chapter 3.18.2.

1. Dyspnea in Palliative and End-of-Life Care

Also →Chapter 1.8.

→ SYMPTOMATIC TREATMENT

1. Nonpharmacologic treatment involves establishing good trust-based communication with the patient (dyspnea is accompanied by anxiety and determined by the patient's previous experiences), providing an optimal environment (appropriate room ventilation and humidity), education (teaching how to breathe and expectorate effectively), airway suctioning (in patients with ineffective evacuation of respiratory secretions), appropriate body positioning (eg, a sitting position in pulmonary edema; a lateral recumbent position to reduce agonal respirations), appropriate fluid intake (to dilute respiratory secretions), prevention of constipation (elevation of the diaphragm and increased abdominal pressure at defecation may precipitate dyspnea), psychological techniques (eg, relaxation), and occupational therapy (this may prevent the patient from dwelling on the threat of dyspnea).

2. Pharmacotherapy in palliative care (patients with advanced cancer or in the terminal, irreversible stage of chronic respiratory, cardiovascular, or neurologic disease):

1) **Oxygen therapy**: Used to relieve dyspnea in patients with hypoxemia. In patients without hypoxemia, the beneficial effects of oxygen are similar to administering air. Inducing air movement using a fan may provide comfort to the patient.

2) **Opioids**: Oral or parenteral agents may be used (→Table 1-1).

3) **Bronchodilators**: Inhaled β-agonists or anticholinergic agents improve dyspnea in most patients with chronic obstructive pulmonary disease (COPD) or obstructive airway disease.

4) **Glucocorticoids**: Used, among others, in lymphangitis carcinomatosis, superior vena cava syndrome, bronchospasm (in asthma or COPD), and radiation-induced pneumonitis.

5) **Benzodiazepines**: Used predominantly to stop the vicious circle of anxiety leading to dyspnea (eg, in a respiratory panic attack). Usually benzodiazepines are administered in combination with opioids. Principles of using benzodiazepines: →Table 1-2.

Overuse of opioids and benzodiazepines can lead to somnolence and respiratory depression and therefore these drugs should be administered with caution. When administered in other than end-of-life care, their antagonists (naloxone and flumazenil, respectively) must be available for immediate use.

→ SPECIAL CONSIDERATIONS

Special Clinical Considerations in Palliative Care

1. Respiratory panic attacks are attacks of dyspnea accompanied by fear of suffocating. If possible, encourage the patient to control hyperventilation by taking slow deep breaths. Try to eliminate any factors that exacerbate the dyspnea. Administer a short- or intermediate-acting benzodiazepine (midazolam or lorazepam: →Table 1-2) to stop the attack.

Long-term management after a respiratory panic attack: Establish good trust-based communication with the patient and together try to identify the psychosocial factors behind the respiratory panic attacks. Evaluate the patient for any underlying causes of dyspnea and start appropriate treatment (targeted

Table 1-. Suggested dosage of morphine for symptomatic treatment of dyspnea in palliative and end-of-life care

Clinical setting	Dosage[a]
Opioid-naive patient with moderate to severe dyspnea at rest	PO morphine: 1) Test dose of immediate-release morphine 2.5-5 mg (or hydromorphone 0.5-1 mg). Patient must be monitored for 60 min after the first dose. If ≥2 doses are required for dyspnea within 24 h, regular morphine is usually started and dose titrated depending on effect, duration, and adverse effects. 2) Immediately start regular morphine (2.5-5 mg every 4 h) or hydromorphone (0.5-1 mg every 4 h) using immediate-release formulation and consider rescue doses[b] (eg, morphine 1-1.5 mg or hydromorphone 0.25-0.5 mg every 1-2 h). Patient must be monitored for 60 min after the first dose. If necessary, titrate the dose further. Use caution to avoid excessive sedation.
Patient receiving PO morphine every 4 h for dyspnea after establishing dose requirements	Switching to controlled-release formulation + rescue doses[b] may be considered.
Patient treated with PO or SC morphine for pain who develops further dyspnea	Additional dose of immediate-release morphine depending on the severity of dyspnea (eg, in mild to moderate dyspnea add 25%-50% of regular analgesic dose every 4 h): 1) If response is good, use only if dyspnea worsens (and continue regular analgesic doses). 2) After assessing the initial dose, the current analgesic dose of morphine used every 4 h may be increased (eg, by 25%) and further titrated.
Patient treated with PO morphine for dyspnea who needs to be switched to parenteral route (eg, dysphagia, vomiting)	Converting PO opioid to SC opioid: →Chapter 1.20 Usually SC morphine = 1/3 to 1/2 of PO morphine Usually SC hydromorphone = 1/3 to 1/2 of PO hydromorphone
Patient with increasing dyspnea at rest and anxiety (most often end-of-life; usually oral intake no longer possible)	1. Morphine or hydromorphone used regularly and in case of dyspnea: Switch from PO to SC (reduce daily dose 3 times, sometimes 2 times) and titrate the dose. If anxiety and dyspnea persist, consider adding benzodiazepine; eg, if patient receives morphine, add midazolam, starting from low doses (eg, 1-2.5 mg SC if needed).[c] 2. Opioid-naive patients: Use initial dose of SC morphine (eg, 1.25-2.5 mg) or hydromorphone (0.5-1 mg); use SC every 4 h and make sure rescue doses are available. Consider adding benzodiazepine (→above).[c] Continue morphine titration.

Clinical setting	Dosage[a]
Acute dyspnea (eg, dying patient)	No universal dosage regimens exist. Individual approach and close monitoring are necessary. Morphine/hydromorphone is the mainstay of treatment. Adding midazolam is often necessary (most frequently in continuous infusion with parenteral rescue doses).[c] Rapid titration with low doses of morphine is also possible (in-hospital and under close monitoring): 1) Administer morphine/hydromorphone in low doses[d] (0.5-1 mg) IV every 10-15 min or SC every 20-30 min until dyspnea begins to resolve or adverse effects (somnolence) appear. There may be delayed increase in drug concentration in CNS (slow penetration of blood-brain barrier). 2) Usually benzodiazepine is recommended, eg, parenteral midazolam (eg, 0.5 mg IV or 1-2 mg SC)[e]; repeated dosing may be needed. **Comments:** 1) If parenteral morphine/hydromorphone and midazolam are used (especially IV), make sure their antagonists are available if clinical situation warrants reversal. 2) In patients with compromised peripheral perfusion (eg, dehydration, shock, hypothermia), absorption of drugs used in SC boluses during rapid titration and their effects on dyspnea may be delayed. If peripheral perfusion improves (rehydration, reversal of subcutaneous vasoconstriction, warming up), the drug may undergo rapid absorption from subcutaneous tissue.

[a] No universal dosage regimen exists. Dosage is individual and requires close monitoring. Doses are at discretion of the physician caring for the patient.

[b] Rescue doses of immediate-release morphine (PO or SC) must also be titrated. When the daily morphine requirement is stabilized, rescue doses are usually 10% of the total daily use. There are no recommendations on dosing frequency. Based on morphine pharmacokinetics and physician expertise in the management of breakthrough pain, the recommended dosing interval of subsequent doses is ≥60 to 90 minutes for PO morphine and 60 minutes for SC morphine.

[c] Consult the manufacturer's prescribing information to establish whether a particular formulation of midazolam may be mixed in one syringe with morphine or if it should be administered separately.

[d] One of many available regimens; the choice is made on an individual basis and requires close monitoring. Elderly patients, patients with cachexia, with COPD, and those treated with benzodiazepines are more susceptible to opioids. Dosage should be adjusted on a case-by-case basis.

[e] Because response to the drug varies from patient to patient, it must be administered very slowly and with caution. This is only one of many available regimens. Elderly patients, patients with cachexia, with COPD, and those treated with opioids are more susceptible to benzodiazepines.

CNS, central nervous system; COPD, chronic obstructive pulmonary disease; PO, oral; SC, subcutaneous.

Table 1-2. Principles of using benzodiazepines in dyspnea accompanied by anxiety in patients receiving palliative care

Clinical setting	Dosage[a]
Outpatient with dyspnea attacks accompanied by anxiety	Oral lorazepam starting from 0.5 mg[b]
Patient at end of life treated with oral morphine for constant dyspnea with anxiety	Oral lorazepam (starting from single dose 0.5 mg)[b] administered on regular basis and/or in case of dyspnea and anxiety (eg, 0.5-1 mg, if necessary up to 3 times/d); further titration may be required

[a] No strict dosage regimens exist. Dosage is determined on an individual basis and needs close monitoring. Consider dose reduction in elderly patients, patients with cachexia, frail patients, and in patients with severe pulmonary comorbidities (eg, COPD).

[b] In patients with coexistent COPD some authors recommend titration of the rescue dose starting from 0.25 mg.

COPD, chronic obstructive pulmonary disease

at both the underlying condition and symptoms). Depending on prognosis, antidepressant therapy may be used, usually in the form of a selective serotonin reuptake inhibitor, for 2 to 3 weeks and, while waiting for the full effect of the antidepressant to develop, an intermediate- or long-acting benzodiazepine (eg, lorazepam or clonazepam) may be added. Relaxation techniques may also be beneficial to the patient.

2. Agonal respirations are mostly a consequence of accumulation of saliva in the laryngopharynx in patients who are dying. When approaching a patient with agonal respirations, exclude pulmonary edema and other causes of pseudo-agonal breathing (below). Anticholinergic agents such as scopolamine or glycopyrrolate may be used. Scopolamine can be administered subcutaneously (0.4-0.6 mg every 4-8 hours as needed) or transdermally (1-mg patch applied every 72 hours for mild symptoms). Glycopyrrolate can be administered subcutaneously (0.2-0.4 mg every 4-8 hours as needed).

Agonal breathing can be distressing to family members or caregivers. It is important to explain that these are not likely to cause discomfort to an unconscious patient. Airway suctioning may be beneficial. Pseudo-agonal breathing is caused by the inability to expectorate excess airway secretions (eg, due to infection, pulmonary edema, airway hemorrhage) and is not necessarily an indicator of impending death. As pseudo-agonal breathing is less dependent on the secretion of saliva, anticholinergic drugs are less effective. Also →Chapter 11.2.

2. Last Days and Hours

→ TERMINAL PHASE OF LIFE

The final stages of life may last from several hours to several days (unless death is sudden, eg, from cardiac arrhythmia, hemorrhage, or pulmonary embolism). It is important to recognize that dying is an active process. As the underlying disease progresses and organs shut down, new symptoms arise and changes in therapy are needed. When the cause of death is progression of a complex terminal illness, such as heart failure, patients may need more frequent reassessments than someone in whom the goals are curative.

As an individual nears death, some common signs and symptoms may be present:

1) **Alterations of mental status** leading to fatigue, drowsiness, and decreased levels of consciousness. Delirium and even agitation may occur.

2) **Decreased perfusion** leading to cool extremities, mottled skin tone, and decreased urine output.

3) **Changes in respiratory control** leading to fluctuation in the patient's breathing pattern. Apnea is common and can be present paroxysmally in the last days of life.

4) **Muscle weakness and incoordination** leading to inability to swallow. Oral secretions begin to pool in the posterior pharynx and vibrate with respirations. In the past, end-of-life respiratory secretions were referred to as the "death rattle." It is not painful to the patient but can be distressing to those around.

5) **Loss of the ability to control body temperature**, which can result in fever in the last hours of life. This fever responds to antipyretics and is associated with absence of an acute infectious source.

PRINCIPLES OF END-OF-LIFE CARE

The primary goal of the last stages of end-of-life care is to provide comfort for the patient and family or caregivers during this impactful time. The definition of comfort and its exact needs will differ for every patient and family. For most, comfort includes freedom from symptoms such as dyspnea and pain. For some, comfort includes psychosocial and/or spiritual support. For others, comfort includes attention to legal and financial documents. Health-care professionals should explore the needs of each patient and family to insure they are addressing their expectations. This is best done in the setting of a multidisciplinary team.

In general, quality end-of-life care includes:

1) Adequate management of symptoms such as pain, fear, and discomfort.

2) Prevention of unnecessary prolongation of the dying process.

3) Clear, coherent, sensitive, and compassionate communication to facilitate meaningful decision-making in the least stressful and burdensome manner.

4) Focus on patient-centered care such that the patient and/or family/substitute decision-makers are actively involved in decision-making and planning.

5) Opportunity to focus on personal relationships while reducing burdens on others.

6) Access to care, support, and resources to provide an optimal quality-of-life experience as defined by the patient.

INTERVENTIONS AND CARE MANAGEMENT

1. Pain, suffering, and symptom management: The end of life can be associated with a considerable burden of physical symptoms. Every effort must be made by the patient's physicians and care team to relieve these symptoms.

Despite conservative goals of care, it may sometimes be prudent to perform simple investigations (eg, blood tests, radiographs) to best guide symptom management. Discussion with patients and their caregivers can determine if this is appropriate. Overall, however, treatment should be individualized based on the needs, goals of care, location of care, and life expectancy. In the last hours and days it is usually most appropriate to simply conduct a trial of medications for symptom management based on clinical scenario.

1) **Pain control** should continue as initiated prior to transition into the terminal phase. The route of administration of medications should be changed from oral to subcutaneous (preferably) or IV (less preferred) when swallowing is not possible. Assessment of pain control should focus on the presence or

absence of grimacing, calling out, or moaning as the patient becomes unable to communicate.

2) **Dyspnea** should be managed with opioids (similar dosing to that used for pain management). Opioids reduce the sensation of work of breathing. In small doses that are titrated as needed to comfort, opioids have not been shown to cause respiratory depression or hasten death. Dyspnea that is resistant to opioids should be treated with a combination of opioids and benzodiazepines (eg, midazolam 0.5-2 mg subcutaneously or IV every 4 hours).

3) **Delirium** at the end of life should be treated for comfort of the patient and family. Antipsychotics are the first-line therapy for terminal delirium (haloperidol 0.5-2 mg orally or subcutaneously every 4-8 hours; quetiapine 12.5-50 mg orally every 12 hours). Patients with delirium resistant to antipsychotic agents or at high risk of causing harm should be treated with benzodiazepines for their sedating properties (eg, midazolam 0.5-2 mg subcutaneously).

4) **Fever** can be treated with acetaminophen (INN paracetamol) orally or rectally.

5) **Oral secretions** can be managed with gentle oral suctioning, frequent turning (to allow the fluids to redistribute), or anticholinergic medications (eg, scopolamine [hyoscine hydrobromide] 0.3-0.6 mg or glycopyrrolate 0.2-0.4 mg [max, 1.2 mg/d] subcutaneously every 4 hours as needed). Anticholinergic medications can worsen or cause agitation/delirium and should be used with caution.

Relief of symptoms may also include minimally invasive procedures such as insertion of a nasogastric tube for the management of nausea and noninvasive ventilation for dyspnea. These more invasive options should be considered only if symptoms are refractory to all less invasive pharmacologic and nonpharmacologic therapies.

Early consideration of consultation and collaboration with specialists who can address difficult instances of pain, anxiety, dyspnea, confusion, or gastrointestinal complaints must be a priority for health-care providers. A small number of patients may encounter refractory distressing symptoms necessitating assessment and consideration of palliative sedation.

2. Nonphysical symptoms: Nonphysical symptoms are a common source of suffering at the end of life. These may include (but are not limited to) grief, financial concerns, spiritual struggles, anxiety, existential suffering, and depression. Nonphysical symptoms must be assessed and treated with the same intensity as one would in the case of physical symptoms. Early consultation and collaboration with expert clinicians in other disciplines (eg, palliative care, spiritual care, social work, psychology, psychiatry, bioethics) must be a priority for health-care providers.

3. Personal care: Care of the actively dying patient should include routine personal care, with hand and face washing and bathing. For highly symptomatic patients even bathing can be uncomfortable due to pain, dyspnea, or agitation. Scheduling bathing around medication administration, availability of additional bedside staff, and family visits may help to improve comfort.

4. Prevention of bedsores: Actively dying patients are at high risk of bedsores, especially those with the additional burdens of edema, cachexia, incontinence, and obesity. Close monitoring of skin integrity is imperative. Early consideration should be given to frequent repositioning and use of friction-reducing mattresses. Patients at end of life who develop bedsores should be treated in the same fashion as patients not at the end of life. a wound care specialist should be consulted when appropriate.

5. Mouth care: Patients at the end of life require aggressive mouth care to prevent dry mouth and chapped lips and to reduce the risk of aspiration pneumonia. Limited evidence in patients with cancer and stroke suggests that maintaining a moist mouth reduces the sensation of thirst.

6. Bowel and bladder care: Constipation at the end of life is common. Even when not consuming food, the body produces cellular waste that is excreted through the gastrointestinal tract. At the end of life the patient should have a small to moderate bowel movement every 1 to 3 days. Oral laxatives should be used when the patient is able to swallow. For those unable to swallow, a suppository should be available every 2 to 3 days to ensure constipation does not develop.

If the patient is able to void and tolerates personal care, a Foley catheter is not needed. However, catheters provide protection from skin breakdown, improved pain control in patients who have pain on turning, and relief of discomfort for patients with urinary retention and should be considered in these situations.

7. Monitoring of vital signs: At the end of life it is usually not necessary nor appropriate to monitor all vital signs. However, in some situations provision of comfort might require monitoring of certain vital signs. Elevated temperature can easily be treated with antipyretics. Dyspnea can be treated with opiates and benzodiazepines. Patients who have a tendency toward symptomatic rapid heart rhythms may need to have their heart rate checked regularly to prevent chest pain or dyspnea. It is appropriate to consider what would be done for abnormal readings prior to making the decision to discontinue vital signs monitoring. Selective ordering of vital signs in every case is advised.

8. Artificial hydration and nutrition: The eventual but normal inability to take in food or water at the end of life can be challenging for patients and families. Artificial hydration and nutrition at the end of life do not prolong life and do not provide improved quality of life. In the very last hours and days of life artificial hydration and nutrition can cause discomfort to the patient. As the body becomes less able to process foods and fluids, enteral nutrition can cause bloating, vomiting, and aspiration. Artificial hydration leads to peripheral and pulmonary edema as cardiac output decreases. Careful ongoing conversations to discuss this normal process with patients and families are vital to their ability to grow in their understanding and acceptance of this situation. Some families, despite this information, preparation, and support, may wish to continue preexisting feeding or hydrating despite the lack of evidence for improved life expectancy or increased energy. In such cases it is important to identify situations in which the intervention will need to be stopped to prevent further harm (eg, aspiration of feeds leading to respiratory failure).

9. Grief: Grief is a natural response to real or threatened loss. The nature of loss can have a profound impact on the grief process and experience of bereavement. Allowing families and friends ongoing support and opportunity to express their impressions of the patient's comfort and to work with the health-care team to address concerns and fears can help them grieve in a healthy fashion.

10. Organ and tissue donation: The discussion of organ and tissue donation with dying patients and their families is becoming a standard part of care. This must be done in a sensitive manner that both respects the patient and family in a difficult time while also ensuring that they are not denied the opportunity to donate. For many patients and their families organ donation can provide a positive orientation to a sad time. In Ontario, Canada, it is mandatory to report all actual or impending deaths in the hospital to the Trillium Gift of Life Network (TGLN), which assesses whether the patient would be eligible for donation. This avoids offering donation as an option in ineligible patients and also allows trained experts from the TGLN to approach the patient or family if they are eligible to discuss it. Notification in advance of death helps facilitate this process, but the TGLN does not approach families prior to death without the consent of the clinicians involved. Consent for donation is obtained in 68% of situations when the discussion is led by TGLN facilitators compared with 15% when done by the hospital staff.○ Having a TGLN facilitator handle this aspect of end-of-life care also allows the hospital staff to remain free of perceived conflicts of interest and focus on the direct care of the patient. Most physicians think of organ donation in the setting of brain death. However, many organ donation programs are beginning to develop protocols for organ donation in the setting of circulatory/cardiac death, such as when life sustaining therapies are withdrawn in the setting of critical nonneurologic illness. Additionally, tissues such as skin, bone, heart valves, and corneas have a longer viability window after death and can readily be harvested on the basis of more traditional criteria, making this a relevant consideration for all dying patients.

11. Diagnosis of death: →Chapter 11.2.1.

2.1. Diagnosis of Death

→ DIAGNOSIS OF DEATH

Death is defined as the irreversible loss of bodily functions that support a living organism. In the majority of cases (when respiratory and circulatory functions are not artificially supported), the traditional criteria of death apply.

Brain death is defined as the irreversible loss of brain stem functions needed to support a living organism. Brain death is important in the setting of organ donation and when artificial ventilation is used.

The traditional criterion for the diagnosis of death involves identification of:

1) **Cessation of circulatory function**: Absence of pulse on large arteries (carotid arteries) and no heart sounds on auscultation for ≥2 minutes. Difficulties in palpating the pulse may be caused by advanced atherosclerosis or presence of stents in the carotid arteries. If the examination of pulse or auscultation of heart sounds is too short, it is possible to overlook preserved cardiac function in patients with profound bradycardia.

2) **Cessation of spontaneous respiratory function**: Auscultate and observe the chest for 1 minute. An insufficiently long observation of breathing in patients with irregular and slow respirations in the course of acid-base disturbances, drug poisoning, encephalitis, brain tumors, and brain edema can miss extreme bradypnea. Contractions of the neck and chest muscles can imitate breathing even for several minutes after cessation of circulatory function; thus, observation must be combined with auscultation.

3) **Dilated pupils unresponsive to light**: Assess both eyes, as the lack of pupillary response to light may be a result of iris trauma, diseases of the retina and optic nerve, treatment with mydriatics, and presence of ocular prosthesis.

→ SPECIAL CONSIDERATIONS

Diagnosis of Brain Death

This requires more rigorous testing than determination of death. It is usually done in the setting of anticipated organ donation. In Canada, criteria for determination of clinical brain death in the adult patient include:

1) Cause of death that is capable of causing brain death.
2) Absence of reversible causes of coma:
   a) Untreated shock.
   b) Hypothermia (<34°C).
   c) Untreated metabolic disturbances.
   d) Peripheral nerve or muscle dysfunction due to disease or neuromuscular blocking agents.
   e) Central nervous system depressants.
3) Absence of brain stem reflexes:
   a) Pupillary response to light.
   b) Corneal reflex.
   c) Gag reflex.

d) Cough reflex (use bronchial suctioning to try to elicit the reflex).

e) Oculovestibular reflex (cold calorics): With the head of the bed at 30°, 50 mL ice cold water is syringed into the patient's ear canal. Any movement of the eyes excludes neurologic death. Repeat in both ears.

4) Absence of response to stimuli in all extremities and above clavicles.

5) Absence of respiratory effort: Apnea testing: In the setting of normal arterial blood gas values the patient is preoxygenated with 100% oxygen. The ventilator is disconnected but oxygen is delivered to the patient (through an endotracheal tube or tracheostomy). The patient is monitored continuously for respirations. Arterial blood gas measurement is repeated at 10 to 15 minutes, and the patient is reconnected to the ventilator. Apnea is confirmed if partial pressure of carbon dioxide in arterial blood ($PaCO_2$) is >60 mm Hg, has risen >20 mm Hg above baseline, and pH is ≤7.28. Testing is aborted if the patient becomes hemodynamically unstable.

6) Two physicians who are fully licensed for independent practice must confirm that the above criteria are met. These physicians must not have a relationship with the potential organ recipients. They may perform the examination simultaneously or separately, although the apnea test is usually only done once with both physicians present.

7) Ancillary testing to confirm the lack of cerebral blood flow is necessary only when any of the above physical examination steps cannot be completed or interpreted. Radionucleotide imaging, 4-vessel cerebral angiography, computed tomography (CT), and magnetic resonance angiography (MRA) are acceptable modalities of ancillary testing.

Diagnosis of Death in a Patient With Pacemaker

A pacemaker may continue to provide electrical stimulation for a short time after death. This ongoing electrical activity will be detected on electrocardiography (ECG) but will not create a systemic pulse or systemic circulation.

Diagnosis of Death in a Hypothermic Individual

Death can be diagnosed in a cadaver at subzero temperatures in the presence of postmortem lividity, rigor mortis, and body decomposition. If you approach a hypothermic person without circulatory function and cannot confirm the above criteria, start and continue resuscitation (→Chapter 3.3) while warming the patient. Death can be diagnosed when resuscitation is ineffective in spite of normalizing the body temperature. In some situations, achieving normothermia is impossible and death will have to be declared despite ongoing low core body temperatures.

When diagnosing death on the basis of postmortem lividity, it is important to remember that cyanotic discoloration of the skin, which develops in advanced congestive heart failure, may be mistaken for postmortem lividity (cyanotic areas blanch under pressure, postmortem lividity does not).

3. Palliative Sedation. Canadian Perspective

 DEFINITIONS

Administration of medications to reduce consciousness or induce sleep in patients suffering from refractory symptoms that are difficult to control is becoming more common in the palliative care setting, particularly in the end-of-life care. **Palliative sedation** refers to the intentional administration of medications that reduce the patient's level of consciousness in situations where death is imminent (hours to days) in order to relieve their intolerable and intractable suffering. It involves the use of appropriate, carefully selected and dosed medications and is aimed at relieving suffering—not shortening or ending the patient's life. This sedation may be intermittent (the patient desires the ability to rouse) or continuous. By contrast, **medical assistance in dying (MAiD)** (as it is referred to in Canada) refers to the prescription and administration of medications with the explicit intent of ending a patient's life in order to relieve their suffering. Palliative sedation can be performed in the hospital and community settings with sufficient family and nursing support.

From the Canadian professional and ethical standpoints, medical practitioners have the obligation to offer or use palliative sedation **in justified situations**, when the patient's suffering is intolerable and symptoms are refractory to other palliative treatment options. This responsibility is often neglected either for fear of being accused of shortening the patient's life (ie, palliative sedation is confused with MAiD) or due to the lack of skills in administering sedation. Nevertheless, palliative sedation may have 2 kinds of effects: beneficial, of relieving refractory symptoms, and adverse, as deep sedation makes it impossible for patients to communicate, maintain interpersonal contacts, eat, or drink.

When used in the last days and hours of life, palliative sedation has not been shown to shorten life. However, if implemented early in the disease process, it has the potential to contribute to an unintended shortening of a patient's life if no artificial nutrition or hydration is offered. Timing of palliative sedation should be discussed explicitly as part of the informed consent process (→below).

→ INDICATIONS

Indications for sedation in palliative care:

1) Relief of distressing and intolerable symptoms that are **refractory** to all other forms of treatment. Such symptoms may include dyspnea, anxiety or panic attacks, agitated delirium, pain, persistent nausea and hiccups, myoclonus, or seizures. This sedation is typically continuous but may still be intermittent if the patient desires the ability to rouse up.

2) Respite from brief painful procedures such as insertion of a central venous catheter or some nursing interventions (eg, painful dressing changes) or while awaiting another treatment option (eg, epidural for pain control). This sedation is typically intermittent and timed around the required procedure.

→ PROCEDURE

1. The decision to administer sedation should be preceded by a thorough clinical assessment, which includes the patient's general clinical status, possible alternative therapies, reversibility of symptoms, and life expectancy.

2. In competent and conscious patients informed consent must be obtained. This requires holding a frank discussion with the patient to explain the aims and methods used in sedation. It is important to make the patient aware that sedation impairs consciousness, induces deep sleep (making communication with family or caregivers impossible), prohibits any involvement in making decisions or in further preparations for the end of life. Any decisions around other aspects of care, such as artificial hydration or nutrition, must be made prior to initiating sedation. Goals of care have to be focused on comfort. Do-not-resuscitate (DNR) and allow-natural-death (AND) orders have to be documented. The patient should be aware of imminent death and have the opportunity to say goodbye to family or caregivers before continuous palliative sedation is instituted. If the patient's condition makes obtaining informed consent impossible, the consent should be sought from a substitute decision-maker (SDM), such as the family or an appointed power of attorney, who needs to be fully aware of the consequences of sedation. If the patient requires urgent suppression of consciousness (in case of a massive hemorrhage or choking/respiratory distress), sedation may be used for the immediate relief of suffering without the consent of the patient, family, or caregivers.

3. It is recommended that all patients being considered for palliative sedation have a consultation with a palliative care physician to ensure that all possible treatment strategies have been tried prior to the initiation of sedation. The administration of palliative sedation should be guided by a physician experienced in this procedure. This is typically a palliative care physician, anesthesiologist, or critical care physician.

4. Pain management should be continued (usually with opioids [→Chapter 1.20]) throughout sedation.

5. Sedatives are administered in a continuous IV or continuous subcutaneous infusion or via intermittent or repeated injections (every 4 hours and as needed) to maintain sedation.

6. The degree of sedation should be proportional to the degree of refractory symptom being managed. sedation should be re-assessed regularly, usually several times a day. Particular focus should be paid to the depth of sedation (the patient being roused by painful stimuli) and effectiveness (presence of distressing symptoms). The goal of sedation with any medication is to ensure comfort. There is usually no need for routine administration of oxygen, monitoring oxygen saturation (SaO_2), or routine vital sign checks.

Commonly Used Sedative Agents

The dosages below are examples only. Individual patients may respond to smaller or may require higher doses.

1. Midazolam: A short-acting benzodiazepine with sedative, anxiolytic, hypnotic, and skeletal muscle relaxing properties. For continuous sedation start with an IV or subcutaneous injection of 0.25 to 1 mg followed by a continuous infusion at the rate of 0.25 to 1 mg/h (or higher if needed). Higher initial doses (2.5-5 mg) may be required in severely distressed patients (eg, with agitated delirium). For intermittent sedation start with 0.5 to 2 mg subcutaneously every 2 to 4 hours. Patients who have been receiving benzodiazepines prior to initiation of sedation should start at doses at least equivalent to their baseline dose. The onset of action is within 1 to 3 minutes (IV) or 10 to 15 minutes (subcutaneous administration). The duration of action is 15 to 30 minutes after discontinuation of infusion. Depending on dose and infusion rate, midazolam may lead to central respiratory depression, particularly when used in combination with opioids. The duration of action may be markedly prolonged with repeated intermittent injections.

2. Methotrimeprazine: A sedating neuroleptic useful for agitated delirium. The initial dose is 6.25 to 12.5 mg in subcutaneous injections every 4 to 8 hours and then titrated as needed; the dose may need to be titrated up to 25 to 50 mg. The agent suppresses nausea and vomiting and may have weak analgesic properties, but it also lowers the seizure threshold and has potential extrapyramidal adverse effects.

3. Phenobarbital: A sedating anticonvulsant useful for all types of seizures and as a third-line sedating agent. Doses range between 30 and 120 mg subcutaneously every 8 to 12 hours and then titrated as needed.

4. Propofol: An anesthetic agent recommended in patients not responding to other therapies. Propofol should be used in a monitored setting (in many hospitals it can be used exclusively in critical care areas). Initial doses of 5 to 20 mg are administered every 90 seconds to 2 minutes and followed by a continuous IV infusion at the rate of 10 to 70 mg/h. The onset of action is within several seconds and duration of action is 2 to 3 minutes. Propofol also suppresses vomiting and hiccups.

5. Haloperidol: Haloperidol may be used in addition to midazolam for delirium or for other symptoms such as nausea or emesis. The initial doses are 0.5 to

2 mg in subcutaneous intermittent injections every 4 to 6 hours. Haloperidol is **not recommended** as a single agent for palliative sedation as it is not a sedating neuroleptic and with high doses potentially increases the risk of extrapyramidal adverse effects.

Opioids should not be used for sedation. While it is important to initiate and continue them along with sedatives to ensure comfort and analgesia, opioids are not appropriate as the single agent for inducing palliative sedation because sedating doses cause many adverse effects.

1. Agitated Patient

→ DEFINITIONS AND ETIOLOGY

Physicians may encounter agitated patients in emergency rooms, on inpatient units, and in nursing home settings. Agitation may be expressed in many ways. Patients may be uncooperative, angry, threatening, or they may express their agitation through behavior with restlessness, pacing, self-injurious behavior, and violence. Agitation may be a reflection of an underlying medical disorder, psychiatric disorder, substance use disorder, or a maladaptive response to a challenging environment. In a hospital setting, agitated and violent behavior may occur in patients with delirium, dementia, personality disorders, substance intoxication and withdrawal, and in those with serious mental illnesses, such as schizophrenia and bipolar disorder. Appropriate assessment and treatment are needed to ensure agitation is resolved in a manner that ensures the safety of the patient and health-care workers and promotes the patient's engagement in treatment. For patients with agitation due to primary psychiatric or substance use disorders, the clinical encounter may be their first presentation to medical professionals for conditions that will likely require ongoing treatment. How the physician manages the encounter and the resultant experience of the patient may have a lasting impact on the patient's willingness to engage with health-care professionals in the future.

Clinical Considerations

There are a number of factors that increase the risk that individuals in the general population will be violent. These include being male, having a lifetime history of violence or criminal behavior, being of late teen or young adult age, alcohol and drug intoxication or withdrawal, delirium, and mental illness. In individuals with mental illness, the risk of violence is greatly increased by concurrent substance abuse, personality disorders, and recent medication nonadherence. In patients with psychotic disorders, the presence of persecutory delusions, command hallucinations, and low intellectual functioning also contribute to the risk of violence.

→ TREATMENT

General Principles

When assessing an agitated patient, it is critical to be aware of the goals that need to be achieved in the interaction:

1) Safety—of yourself, the agitated patient, other patients, and hospital staff.
2) Careful assessment of the patient to ensure that any urgent medical problems contributing to the agitation are identified in order to minimize morbidity and mortality.
3) Determination of medical or surgical referrals that are required for further investigation and management of the patient.
4) Reducing the patient's distress.

In most cases agitation can be de-escalated with verbal interventions and support. When these are not effective, pharmacologic intervention may be required. A number of steps should be taken when initiating contact with an agitated patient. Make sure that:

1) The patient has been searched for any objects that could be dangerous, including weapons.
2) You have someone accompany you if you feel uncomfortable or intimidated.
3) The door to the examination room is kept open.
4) You are positioned so that you maintain a safe distance from the patient and can safely leave the room.

5) You have a clear plan for how to get urgent help if needed.

6) You convey a sense of calm, reassurance, and being in control when you approach the patient.

Restraint and seclusion may be required for highly agitated patients (→Chapter 12.9). Restraints are more commonly available in medical settings, with seclusion being an additional option in psychiatric settings. For violent patients, the use of restraints eliminates the risks to staff of entering a seclusion room with a patient who remains violent. Major international efforts have been focused on reducing and eliminating the use of restraint and seclusion in psychiatric settings, as these techniques are traumatic for patients and are associated with physical risk to staff and medical risks to patients. The latter include complications that may be severe and potentially life-threatening, including fractures, rhabdomyolysis, strangulation, asphyxia, deep vein thrombosis, and pulmonary embolism.

The management of an agitated patient, irrespective of etiology, begins with a focused assessment that will include vital signs, appropriate history, physical and mental state examination, and laboratory testing (→Chapter 12.11). In some cases a more complete medical assessment may need to be delayed until acute agitation is resolved. Once a rapid focused assessment is obtained, an individualized intervention can be made based on the patient's medical and psychiatric history, physical and mental status examination, and results of any laboratory investigations.

Pharmacologic Management

The specific goals of pharmacologic intervention need to be identified. These include calming the patient, ensuring safety, addressing the underlying cause of agitation, and facilitating completion of the medical evaluation needed to inform the patient's clinical management. Giving patients some control over the route of administration of medications prescribed for agitation often helps to calm them. Offering patients sedating medication in the form of pills, rapidly dissolving tablets, or liquid formulations should be considered as the first choice for all but the most agitated patients, as these are experienced as less threatening than injectable medications.

The choice of specific medications for the agitated patient is determined by the etiology of agitation. The causes of agitation can be classified into 3 broad categories: primary medical disorders (most commonly delirium), substance intoxication or withdrawal, and those due to primary psychiatric disorders. Two broad categories of tranquilizing agents generally used in the acute management of agitation are **benzodiazepines** and **antipsychotic medications**. Benzodiazepines potentiate the effects of endogenous γ-aminobutyric acid (GABA), the most abundant inhibitory neurotransmitter. The agents include lorazepam, diazepam, and clonazepam. Benzodiazepines are available for oral use (in pill form, rapidly dissolving sublingual tablets, and liquid formulations) and for IM and IV injections. Antipsychotic medications act by blocking dopamine D_2 receptors in the brain. Both first-generation antipsychotics (FGAs) and second-generation antipsychotics (SGAs) are used for managing agitation and are available in a range of oral and injectable formulations. Depending on the etiology of agitation and degree of tranquilization required, benzodiazepines and antipsychotics may be used individually or in combination.

1. Agitation due to a primary medical disorder: Delirium is a medical emergency for which it is critical that the underlying etiology be identified and treated. Achieving these goals may well require that the patient's agitation be resolved. If it is clear that the delirium is not due to alcohol or benzodiazepine withdrawal, benzodiazepines should be avoided as they may worsen delirium and, when given parenterally, may lead to respiratory depression and hypotension. Benzodiazepines should also be avoided in elderly patients considered to be at high risk of developing delirium. Antipsychotic medications are preferred for the management of agitated patients with delirium, and both FGAs and SGAs have been used for this indication. SGAs are generally associated with a lower risk of acute extrapyramidal symptoms (EPSs) (ie, acute dystonia, parkinsonism, and akathisia) than FGAs. Risperidone (1-2 mg) or olanzapine (5-10 mg) are SGAs that can be given in rapidly dissolving tablets or pill form. Haloperidol (1-2 mg) is the most commonly used FGA for acute agitation. It has minimal anticholinergic activity and low potential for causing hypotension. Haloperidol can increase QTc intervals, as can all other antipsychotics to varying degrees; cases of torsade de pointes have been reported with its use. When IM injections are required, olanzapine (5-10 mg) and haloperidol (2-5 mg) are the SGA and FGA, respectively, that have been most studied. The increased likelihood of anticholinergic effects with olanzapine should be weighed against the higher risk of acute EPSs with haloperidol. These risks will vary with dose and age of the patient (youths and the elderly being at higher risk for EPSs).

Patients with acute agitation of medical etiology who are psychotic in the absence of delirium should also be managed with antipsychotic medication. If the agitated medical patient is neither delirious nor psychotic, benzodiazepines are recommended. Lorazepam (1-2 mg orally, sublingually, IM, or IV), diazepam (5-10 mg orally), or clonazepam (0.5-1 mg orally) are commonly used.

2. Agitation due to substance intoxication or withdrawal: The emergency management of the agitated intoxicated patient will vary depending on the cause of intoxication. Agitation due to acute alcohol intoxication should be treated with antipsychotics, as benzodiazepines can contribute to the risk of respiratory depression. Haloperidol has been used extensively for this indication. It is critical that alcohol withdrawal be distinguished from alcohol intoxication, as benzodiazepines—not antipsychotics—are indicated in the management of agitated patients who are in alcohol withdrawal.

Patients agitated as a result of being intoxicated with stimulants (eg, cocaine, amphetamine, methamphetamine) should be treated with benzodiazepines. Stimulants can also induce acute psychotic symptoms, in which case antipsychotics may be required.

3. Agitation due to a primary psychiatric disorder: In the emergency setting, agitation due to an underlying psychiatric disorder occurs most commonly in patients who are experiencing psychosis (hallucinations, paranoid ideation, delusions) due to schizophrenia or a manic episode of bipolar disorder. As discussed above, both FGAs and SGAs can be used for managing acute agitation in a psychotic patient. Antipsychotic medications can bring about measurable improvement in overall symptoms within 2 hours and in psychotic symptoms within 24 hours.◉ SGAs are associated with a lower risk of EPSs than haloperidol and are generally considered to be first-line agents. Risperidone has been shown to be safe and effective in the management of acute agitation and is available in pill, rapidly dissolving tablet, and liquid forms. Liquid risperidone (2 mg) used in combination with oral lorazepam (2 mg) has been shown to be as effective as the combination of IM haloperidol (5 mg) and IM lorazepam (2 mg).◉ Risperidone is not available for acute IM injections; the long-acting injectable forms of risperidone and its primary metabolite, paliperidone, are not used in the management of acute agitation. Oral olanzapine has been shown to be as effective as oral risperidone in acutely agitated patients and is available in both pill and rapidly dissolving tablet forms. In Canada, olanzapine is the only SGA available for acute IM injections for those patients who will not accept oral medications. IM olanzapine given in a dose of 5 to 10 mg has been shown to be as effective as IM haloperidol 7.5 mg in the management of acute agitation. Olanzapine is associated with a lower risk of acute dystonic reactions than haloperidol but with a slightly higher frequency of hypotension.◉ Parenteral benzodiazepines should not be administered within an hour before or after IM olanzapine due to the risk of hypotension and cardiorespiratory depression that have been associated with reported fatalities.

The FGA most commonly used and most extensively studied for the management of agitation is haloperidol. It is available for oral, IM, and IV administration. The combination of IM haloperidol (5 mg) and IM lorazepam (2 mg) given concomitantly reduces agitation more quickly than either drug administered alone.👄 When acute dystonic reactions (eg, oculogyric crisis, torticollis, opisthotonus) do occur, IM benztropine 2 mg should be given immediately. Subsequent doses of haloperidol can be accompanied by oral or IM doses of benztropine in order to prevent further dystonic reactions. Acute akathisia (objective or subjective motor restlessness) is extremely distressing and can be managed with IM or oral benzodiazepines. Haloperidol, like other antipsychotics, is associated with prolongation of the QTc interval and, in rare cases, torsade de pointes. The risk is thought to be greatest with the use of higher doses and IV administration.

2. Anxiety and Related Disorders in Medical Settings

➡ DEFINITION

The fifth edition of the American Psychiatric Association's *Diagnostic and Statistical Manual of Mental Disorders* (*DSM-5*) defines anxiety disorders as "disorders sharing features of excessive fear and anxiety and related behavioral disturbances. Fear is the emotional response to real or perceived imminent threat, whereas anxiety is the emotional response in anticipation of future threat. Fear is more often associated with surges of autonomic arousal necessary for fight or flight, thoughts of immediate danger and escape behaviors, and anxiety more often associated with muscle tension and vigilance in preparation for future danger and cautious or avoidant behaviors."

DSM-5 introduced a number of changes in the classification of anxiety disorders. The major change was to move the obsessive-compulsive and related disorders and the trauma-related and stressor-related disorders into separate chapters.

In May 2019, the World Health Organization (WHO) ratified the 11th revision of the *International Classification of Diseases and Related Health Problems* (*ICD-11*). In *ICD-11*, the anxiety category includes disorders in which anxiety or fear are the primary clinical feature. Separation anxiety disorder and selective mutism have been moved from the childhood disorders section to the anxiety category. As with *DSM-5*, a new category has been introduced: obsessive-compulsive and related disorders (OCRD), which in *ICD-11* includes obsessive-compulsive disorder (OCD), body dysmorphic disorder, olfactory reference disorder, hypochondriasis (illness anxiety disorder), and hoarding disorder. These conditions have symptoms of repetitive unwanted thoughts and related repetitive behaviors as the primary clinical feature.

For the sake of continuity, this brief chapter will include OCD and posttraumatic stress disorder (PTSD).

Anxiety and fear are experienced by everyone in daily life and are essential in protecting us from realistic dangers. In anxiety disorders the emotions of anxiety and fear are triggered without there being any realistic threat of harm or the threat is perceived to be out of proportion. The diagnosis of an anxiety disorder is made when the symptoms arise and there is impairment in usual behavior. Commonly, the impairment leads to frequent escapes from uncomfortable situations or avoidance of places or tasks that used to be part of the person's repertoire.

Symptoms of anxiety occur commonly in multiple psychiatric conditions. The term "anxiety disorder" refers to those conditions in which the experience of anxiety forms the central symptom. Anxiety disorders are common, with prevalence rates between 2% and 9%, although social anxiety ranges from 13% to 16%. Anxiety disorders can cause significant disability and frequently have a chronic course.

→ ETIOLOGY

A relatively consistent finding in neuroimaging studies of anxiety is hyperactivity of the amygdala and impairment of frontal emotion regulation circuits. In OCD there is evidence of altered activity in the orbitofrontal-limbic-basal ganglia-thalamic circuitry. Several neurotransmitters have been implicated in anxiety, especially serotonin and γ-aminobutyric acid (GABA).

Genetic predisposition, inborn temperamental traits, early childhood development, attachment quality, and family and social environment also contribute to etiology.

Psychological theories initially were based on classical learning theories. Avoidance of anxiety-provoking situations is a major perpetuating factor. Dysfunctional thought patterns leading to misinterpretations and misattributions are evident in all anxiety disorders.

→ CLINICAL FEATURES AND DIAGNOSIS

Diagnostic Features

1. Generalized anxiety disorder (GAD):
1) Key symptoms: Excessive worry focused on plausible possibilities that are highly magnified, leading to distress and preoccupation.
2) Associated physical symptoms: Feeling on edge, restlessness, fatigue, churning, impaired concentration, muscle tension, irritability, and insomnia.

2. Panic disorder (PD):
1) Key symptoms: Rapid surges of intense anxiety that peak within minutes. Intense anxiety in the form of a panic attack is the main feature of PD and may occur in many mental disorders.
2) Associated physical symptoms: Rapid heart rate, palpitations, sweating, subjective shortness of breath, chest pain, trembling, nausea, light-headedness, feeling hot or cold, numbness, tingling.
3) Psychological symptoms: Fear that one is going to die or lose one's mind; feelings of unreality and detachment (depersonalization).

3. Agoraphobia: Key symptoms are marked anxiety about specific situations: open, crowded, or enclosed spaces, such as shopping malls, standing in line or on buses. The patient avoids these situations or endures them with intense anxiety. Frequently associated with panic attacks.

4. Social anxiety disorder (SAD): Key symptoms are intense anxiety in social situations, feeling of being judged by others, embarrassment, and inadequacy. Occurs when meeting new people, being at social gatherings, making a presentation, or eating in public. In learners frequently leads to avoidance of going to school, which impedes progression in education.

5. Specific phobia: Key symptoms are intense anxiety about a specific object or situation, for instance, fear of injections, flying, or specific animals. Panic attacks may occur with severe fear. The patient avoids the situation or object. In the medical setting, fear of blood taking and injections has the most clinical relevance.

6. OCD:
1) Key symptoms: Intrusive unwanted thoughts, images or urges of violence, suicide, harm to others; disturbing sexual or blasphemous thoughts. The thoughts are recognized by the patient to arise in himself or herself but they are uncontrollable and may be very alarming.
2) Compulsive behaviors: Behaviors such as repetitive checking, counting, handwashing, touching, rereading, or ordering occur and are aimed at reducing the anxiety triggered by the thoughts or urges. The ritualistic behaviors may occupy many hours each day and lead to very severe impairment in many spheres.

7. PTSD: Key symptoms are intense physiological and emotional hyperarousal: intrusive vivid memories, flashbacks or bodily sensations of the traumatic event.

Symptoms are triggered by reminders or cues of the event leading to marked avoidance. Frequently accompanied by mood dysregulation, anger, depression, and suicidal ideation.

Differential Diagnosis

Anxiety disorders are frequently comorbid with other mental disorders, most commonly depression and alcohol and substance use disorders. Additionally, anxiety disorders commonly co-occur in a patient, including OCD and trauma--related disorders and other disorders within the anxiety disorder category.

It is important to exclude endocrine and cardiac disorders. Investigations including a complete blood count (CBC), liver function tests, γ-glutamyl transferase (GGT) (alcohol), thyroid indices (thyroid-stimulating hormone [TSH]), and electrocardiography (ECG) may be considered.

→ SCREENING

Initial screening for anxiety disorders of patients who appear to be very stressed or jittery can be performed by asking questions about the person's experience in the previous 2 weeks. There are many brief questionnaires that focus on the specific disorders. As a general brief screen, it is important to ask the following questions: Have you been bothered by the following problems: (1) Feeling nervous, anxious, frightened, worried, or on edge? (2) Feeling panic or being frightened? (3) Avoiding situations that make you anxious?

If there is a positive response, then follow up with questions about the nature of the anxiety, when and where it occurs, and about its impact on functioning.

→ TREATMENT

After assessment and necessary investigations (→Chapter 12.11), the first step in the treatment of anxiety disorders is to provide the patient with information about the diagnosis, available evidence-based treatments, and ways to access further information suited to the patient's needs and wishes.

Stepped-Care Approach

Stepped care involves increasing levels of intervention based on nonresponse. The first-step interventions are offered to all patients with diagnosed or suspected cases of the specific anxiety disorder and consist of self-management strategies and access to self-help and educational resources.

1. Step 1: **Self-management**:

1) Reduce or eliminate stimulants, including caffeine-containing drinks such as tea, coffee, and cola drinks.

2) Reduce alcohol to a minimal amount. Alcohol should not be used by patients in attempts to control their anxiety.

3) Reduce or eliminate tobacco use and cannabis intake.

4) Sleep hygiene as well as regular sleeping and waking times reduce anxiety. Educate the patient on the effects of regular aerobic exercise.

5) Introduce relaxation training and mindfulness meditation.

6) Provide the patient with information about the management of anxiety disorders. There are many reliable books, manuals, and websites for each of the anxiety and related disorders (eg, www.anxietyBC.ca, www.adaa.org). This information can be used by the patient alone or worked through in brief guided sessions together with a therapist.

7) Internet-delivered cognitive behavior therapy (iCBT) is evidence-based and available via the internet. It may be guided, with a health-care professional, or unguided, in which case the patient follows the program unassisted.

8) Low-intensity psychoeducational groups, which may be provided by community organizations and peer support services.

Table 2-1. First-line medication for specific anxiety and related disorders

Disorder	First-line medications
Panic disorder	Paroxetine, sertraline, escitalopram
Social anxiety disorder	Paroxetine, sertraline, escitalopram, pregabalin
Generalized anxiety disorder	Paroxetine, sertraline, pregabalin
Obsessive-compulsive disorder	Fluoxetine, fluvoxamine, sertraline
Posttraumatic stress disorder	Prazosin, paroxetine, sertraline

2. Step 2: **Psychotherapy** (for those not responsive to step 1): Psychotherapy is an effective treatment modality and should be considered in all patients with sufficient disorder severity,◐○ with **cognitive behavioral therapy (CBT)** likely being the most effective.○ CBT is usually delivered in a structured format and can be used in an individual or group setting. A course of therapy varies between 12 to 20 sessions delivered ideally once or twice a week. Booster sessions once a month after the initial course help to maintain and reinforce the gains made. CBT requires that the patient take a very active part in the treatment. McMaster University supports an online resource that provides details about the nature and use of CBT at Psychotherapy Training e-Resources.

The specific anxiety and related disorders are treated using variations of CBT methods. OCDs and trauma related disorders require specialized therapy focused on the core symptoms of the disorders, such as repeated washing, flashbacks, or nightmares that do not occur commonly in other anxiety disorders.

3. Step 3: A **combination of psychotherapy and medication** (for those with more severe levels of symptoms, comorbidity, and marked impairment of functioning):

1) First-line medications: The medications recommended for anxiety disorders are classified in the **antidepressant** category but have been found to be effective in anxiety disorders. Antidepressants should be initiated at low doses to lessen adverse effects but may need to be titrated up to doses that are in the higher approved ranges. Specific selective serotonin reuptake inhibitors (SSRIs) are first-line agents (→Table 2-1). The effectiveness of the serotonin--norepinephrine reuptake inhibitors (SNRIs) venlafaxine and duloxetine is less well established. The tricyclic antidepressant clomipramine is one of the most effective medications for OCD but is mostly used as a second-line option because of the greater tolerability of SSRIs. **Medications with dopaminergic and noradrenergic effects can exacerbate anxiety**; this includes bupropion, venlafaxine, methylphenidate, and other stimulants.

2) Second-line medications:

   a) **Benzodiazepines** can be very effective for acute management of PD and GAD. Drawbacks include tolerance, cognitive adverse effects, and mood changes. Benzodiazepines can reduce the effectiveness of CBT due to their impact on memory consolidation. Additionally, they should be used sparingly, if at all, in the management of PTSD.

   b) **GABA derivatives** (pregabalin or gabapentin) may be prescribed if the first-line medications do not provide sufficient symptom relief and return of function. Although evidence on this is preliminary, gabapentin can be used as an alternative to benzodiazepines to reduce anxiety symptoms and enhance slow-wave sleep.

   c) **Buspirone** is a mild anxiolytic but has the advantage of not causing dependence. Interestingly, it is one of the only medications that alleviates bruxism (involuntary grinding of teeth), which can be an adverse effect of SSRIs.

d) **Propranolol** can be effective for performance anxiety, which is a subtype of social anxiety. Contrary to the widespread view, propranolol does relieve psychic anxiety in addition to the physiologic symptoms, such as tremor and tachycardia. **Asthma is an absolute contraindication**.

e) **Medical cannabis**: As yet, there is limited evidence about the benefits and risks of using cannabidiol (CBD) in anxiety disorders. In jurisdictions where it is legal, patients have been using CBD oil with mixed results.

Management

After obtaining the patient's consent and having educated the patient about the expected effects and adverse effects of the medications, a drug suggested for the anxiety disorder can be chosen (→Table 2-1). It is also necessary to make sure that there are no contraindications for use with any other medications that the patient is taking. It is advisable to use a drug interaction program as a general principle when patients are taking multiple medications.

Currently it is recommended that the first choice of medication in the primary care setting should be an SSRI (→Table 2-1). Patients with anxiety disorders can be very sensitive to adverse effects and it is important to begin treatment with a low dose followed by a gradual increase to a therapeutic dose range. Escitalopram can be initiated at 5 mg daily for 1 week and then increased in 5-mg daily doses to 20 mg daily. Similarly, sertraline is started at 25 mg daily increasing in 25-mg doses up to 200 mg daily. There is usually a delay in the response and it may be 4 to 6 weeks before patients report that they are feeling less anxious. If the response is insufficient after 2 trials of an SSRI, the family practitioner may wish to seek the opinion of a psychiatrist about the next steps. When there is a good response to the medication, it is necessary to continue its use for at least 6 months and frequently for longer.

In addition to the above, **prazosin** is now well established as a first-line agent for treatment of PTSD. Prazosin reduces nightmares, hyperarousal, and sleep disturbances. It improves total sleep time and sleep quality.◯

The use of antipsychotics is controversial but quetiapine or olanzapine have been used in low doses, with caution and attention paid to the risk of serious adverse effects, such as metabolic syndrome, diabetes mellitus, and tardive dyskinesia. These medications should be reserved for treatment-resistant patients under psychiatric care.as quetiapine or olanzapine, can be used in low doses and with caution and attention due to the risk of serious adverse effects, such as metabolic syndrome, diabetes mellitus, and tardive dyskinesia. These medications should be reserved for treatment-resistant patients under psychiatric care.

3. Delirium

➲ DEFINITION, ETIOLOGY, PATHOGENESIS

Delirium is an acute clinical syndrome characterized by fluctuating confusion, inattention, disorganized thinking, and altered levels of consciousness. Affecting up to 50% of hospitalized seniors and up to 90% of intensive care unit (ICU) patients, it is a common and important cause of patient morbidity and mortality, including those in emergency department, general medical, ICU, surgical, oncology, and palliative care settings. In fact, it is the most common complication of hospitalization for older adults.

Although preventable in 30% to 40% of cases,◔ delirium can lead to significant short-term and long-term consequences, including accelerated cognitive and functional decline, increased hospital length of stay, institutionalization, and death. The impact of delirium on health-care systems is profound, with hundreds of billions of annual health-care costs attributed directly to delirium. Prevention is critical as delirium can take weeks to months for resolution. A moderate-quality systematic review of hospitalized patients showed that persistent delirium was still present in 44.7% at discharge and in 21% at 6 months postdischarge.◔

Etiology

Although a single factor can precipitate delirium, the etiology is usually multifactorial. Evidence of a medical cause can usually be elucidated through focused history, physical examination, and diagnostic investigations. Common predisposing and precipitating factors for delirium: →Table 3-1. Delirium development is dependent on complex interactions between the patient's baseline vulnerability for delirium (based on predisposing risk factors) and their exposure to precipitating factors or noxious insults (→Figure 3-1, →Figure 3-2). Precipitants alone do not usually cause delirium. Delirium occurs when the stress associated with the precipitant/insult exceeds the brain's reserve to compensate and maintain normal functioning. As a result, a small insult might be enough to precipitate delirium in a frail older adult with multiple morbidities, while a combination of large insults may be necessary in a younger healthier individual.

The mnemonic "DELIRIUM Plus" is a useful way of considering the various etiologies in the differential diagnosis of delirium that may be contributing to its onset (→Table 3-2).

Clinically, the implications of a multifactorial etiology are 2-fold: (1) identifying and addressing the specific underlying cause or causes in each case is important; and (2) multicomponent strategies for preventing delirium are more likely to be effective.

High-risk drug use is an important predisposing risk factor and precipitant for delirium. There is a large list of drugs and their metabolites that precipitate delirium, but the most common ones are those with known psychotropic or anticholinergic effects (→Table 3-3). Studies have shown that use of 2 or more psychotropics and starting 3 or more drugs lead to a 4.5-fold and 3.9-fold increased relative risk of delirium, respectively.

Pathophysiology

The pathophysiology of delirium is poorly understood. There are several proposed hypotheses, but accumulating evidence suggests that there are likely multiple interacting factors disrupting normal neuronal brain function. Delirium appears to be the final common pathway and expression of multiple different pathologies that disrupt multiple brain regions and neurotransmitter systems. These include, but are not limited to, altered neurotransmission due to cholinergic deficiency and/or dopamine excess, stress-induced inflammation and cytokine release, cerebral hypoxia, disturbances in tryptophan metabolism, chronic physiological stress (eg, hypercortisolism) and genetic factors (eg, apolipoprotein E genotype variance leading to disturbance of normal physiological processes). Different mechanisms may be more prominent depending on the circumstance (eg, postoperative, ICU, general medical illness).

→ CLINICAL FEATURES

The cardinal features of delirium are an acute onset and fluctuating course of disorganized thinking or disturbances in consciousness with poor attention. Other supporting features include disorientation, memory impairment, perceptual disturbances (hallucinations, illusions, misperceptions), delusions, psychomotor agitation or retardation, and sleep-wake cycle disturbances. Physical signs such as asterixis (flapping of outstretched, dorsiflexed hand), multifocal myoclonus (nonrhythmic, asynchronous muscle jerking), carphologia

Table 3-1. Common predisposing and precipitating factors for delirium

Predisposing factors	Precipitating factors
– Advanced age – Neurodegenerative or cerebrovascular disease (eg, dementia, stroke) – History of delirium – History of alcohol abuse – Severe illness – Multimorbidity – Frailty and functional decline – Malnutrition – Vision and/or hearing impairment – Polypharmacy – Use of psychoactive medications – Uncontrolled pain	– Any medical illness – Infection – Acute organ dysfunction (eg, cardiac, respiratory, renal, or hepatic failure) – Metabolic disturbance (eg, electrolyte abnormalities, endocrine disorders, hypoglycemia and hyperglycemia) – Alcohol and/or drug intoxication or withdrawal – Use of higher-risk medications associated with delirium (eg, psychoactive drugs, anticholinergics, opioids) – Dehydration and/or malnutrition – Iatrogenic events (eg, surgery) – Uncontrolled pain – Use of physical restraints – Use of indwelling bladder catheters – Immobilization

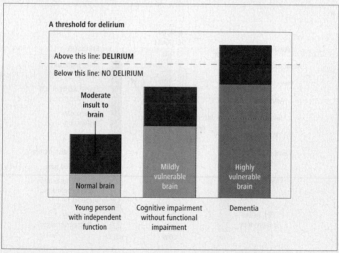

Figure 3-1. Framework for delirium risk.

(involuntary picking or grasping of real or imaginary objects), and postural action tremor can often be observed in metabolic and toxic delirium.

Similar to dementia, responsive behaviors are common. These behaviors are actions, words, and gestures that are expressed by patients in response to unmet needs or stimuli (perceived or real) in their personal, social, or physical environment. Due to effects of delirium on memory, judgement, orientation, mood, and behavior, they often manifest as agitation, aggression, wandering, anxiety, calling out, or sexual behavior.

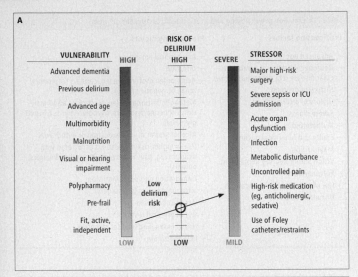

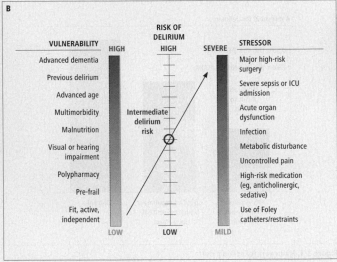

Figure 3-2. Four scenarios illustrating interactions between vulnerability, stressor, and delirium risk. A line connecting the perceived vulnerability and stress levels determines the point of intersection on the delirium risk scale. **Scenario A**, an older adult that is fit, active, and independent with activities of daily living (low vulnerability) is prescribed a daily benzodiazepine for primary insomnia (mild stressor). The risk for developing delirium with short-term or long-term use of this high-risk drug is anticipated to be low. **Scenario B**, an older adult that is fit, active, and independent with activities of daily living (low vulnerability) is scheduled for coronary artery bypass grafting (severe stressor). The risk for developing postoperative delirium is anticipated to be intermediate.

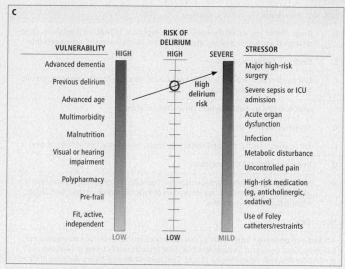

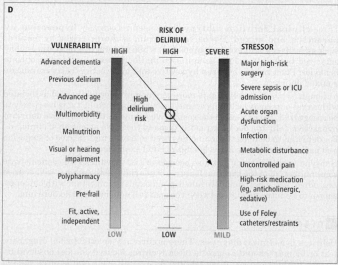

Scenario C, a frail 95-year-old adult with multimorbidity (high vulnerability) is scheduled for coronary artery bypass grafting (severe stressor). The risk for developing postoperative delirium is anticipated to be very high. **Scenario D**, an older adult with advanced dementia who is dependent for all activities of daily living (high vulnerability) is prescribed a daily benzodiazepine for primary insomnia (mild stressor). The risk for developing postoperative delirium is anticipated to be very high. *Inspired by JAMA. 1996;275(11):852-7.*

Table 3-2. Differential diagnosis of delirium

D	Drugs: Excess (eg, anticholinergics, sedative-hypnotics, opioids, corticosteroids, dopaminergics) and withdrawal (eg, alcohol, nicotine, benzodiazepines, antidepressants)
E	Electrical: Seizure, postictal
L	Low oxygen: Myocardial infarction, heart failure, stroke, pulmonary embolus, chronic obstructive pulmonary disease
I	Infection: Urinary tract infection, pneumonia, cellulitis
R	Retention: Urine or stool
I	Intracranial: Trauma, subdural hematoma, tumor, malignancy, hemorrhage, stroke
U	Underhydration and undernutrition
M	Metabolic: Hyponatremia or hypernatremia, hypocalcemia or hypercalcemia, hypoglycemia or hyperglycemia, hypothyroidism or hyperthyroidism, uremia, liver failure, vitamin B_{12} deficiency, anemia
Plus	Pain

Adapted with permission from the Saint Louis University Geriatrics Evaluation Mnemonics and Screening Tools, Division of Geriatric Medicine, Saint Louis University School of Medicine, and the Geriatric Research, Education and Clinical, Saint Louis VA Medical Center. Available at slu.edu.

Three **clinical delirium subtypes** have been recognized: **hypoactive, hyperactive**, and **mixed**. Hypoactive delirium is characterized by features such as lethargy and excess somnolence, while hyperactive delirium is characterized by features such as agitation, hallucinations, and inappropriate behavior. Fluctuations between hypoactive and hyperactive features indicate a mixed delirium.

Although hypoactive delirium is more common in older adults and associated with worse outcomes including an increased risk of mortality, it is less likely to be recognized. In contrast to the responsive behaviors of hyperactive delirium, hypoactive delirium does not readily demand the extra attention of clinicians. For delirium to be detected, clinicians need to have a high degree of suspicion and patients need to be actively engaged and examined.

"Subsyndromal delirium" has also been described in patients who demonstrate some but not all of the cardinal features of delirium. Although not well defined or studied, subsyndromal delirium is prognostically important with outcomes shown to be intermediate between those in full delirium and no delirium.

➔ DIAGNOSIS

Delirium is a clinical diagnosis. There is currently no established diagnostic test or biomarker and diagnosis often requires focused clinical observation, history taking, and cognitive testing. As a result, delirium is often missed and goes undetected in >50% of patients. Timely detection is critical because delirium is a potential medical emergency. Delayed or missed diagnosis has been associated with a 7-fold increased risk for mortality.

The reference standard for the diagnosis of delirium has typically been defined by the American Psychiatric Association's *Diagnostic and Statistical Manual of Mental Disorders*. According to the 5th edition (*DSM-5*), delirium is diagnosed by 5 key features:

1) A disturbance in attention (reduced ability to direct, focus, sustain, and shift attention) and awareness.

Table 3-3. Common drugs associated with delirium

Drugs	Examples
Analgesics	Opioids (especially meperidine)
Anticholinergics	– Tricyclic antidepressants (eg, amitriptyline, doxepin) – Antihistamines (eg, diphenhydramine, dimenhydrinate, hydroxyzine) – Antimuscarinics (eg, scopolamine) – Incontinence agents (eg, oxybutynin)
Anticonvulsants	– Carbamazepine – Phenytoin – Valproic acid
Sedative/hypnotics	– Benzodiazepines (eg, triazolam, lorazepam, flurazepam, temazepam) – Barbiturates
Muscle relaxants	– Cyclobenzaprine – Baclofen
Antipsychotics	– Typical antipsychotics (eg, chlorpromazine) – Atypical antipsychotics (eg, olanzapine)
Substance toxicity	– Ethanol
Glucocorticoids	– Prednisone (in high doses)
Antiparkinson agents	– Pramipexole – Ropinirole – Amantadine – Levodopa
Cardiac agents	Digoxin
Respiratory agents	Theophylline
Gastrointestinal agents	– Metoclopramide – Loperamide
Herbal preparations	– Jimson weed – St. John's wort – Valerian – Kava kava

This table should be used in context of each specific patient and one's professional clinical judgment. In many clinical situations the drugs specified may be clinically appropriate and indicated.

2) The disturbance develops over a short period of time (usually hours to days), represents a change from baseline, and tends to fluctuate during the course of the day.

3) An additional disturbance in cognition (memory deficit, disorientation, language, visuospatial ability, or perception).

4) The disturbances are not better explained by another preexisting, evolving, or established neurocognitive disorder and do not occur in the context of a severely reduced level of arousal, such as coma.

5) There is evidence from history, physical examination, or laboratory findings that the disturbance is caused by a medical condition, substance intoxication or withdrawal, or adverse effects of medications.

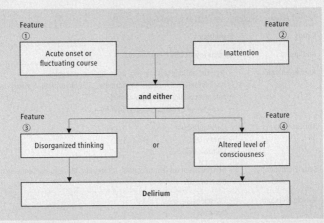

Figure 3-3. Confusion assessment method (CAM) delirium screening algorithm. Score based on cognitive testing. *Adapted from Ann Intern Med. 1990; 113: 941-948 and Inouye SK. Confusion Assessment Method: Training Manual and Coding Guide. Available at www.hospitalelderlifeprogram.org.*

A formal diagnosis using this reference standard typically involves an in-depth patient interview and cognitive testing by an experienced clinician.

Several bedside screening and diagnostic instruments have been developed to improve identification and better guide which patients should receive formal consultation and intervention. Recent systematic reviews suggest the Confusion Assessment Method (CAM) has the best evidence to support its use. Taking 5 minutes to administer and available at www.hospitalelderlifeprogram.org, the CAM has a sensitivity of 94% to 100%, specificity of 90% to 95%, positive likelihood ratio of 9.6, and negative likelihood ratio of 0.16 for diagnosing delirium. It identifies 4 delirium features: acute onset or fluctuating course, inattention, disorganized thinking, and altered level of consciousness. The diagnosis of delirium requires the presence of features 1 and 2 with either feature 3 or 4 (→Figure 3-3).

The CAM has become the most widely used instrument for clinical and research purposes and it performs well in emergency department, postoperative, and mixed inpatient settings. It has also been adapted for use in nonverbal or intubated patients in the form of the CAM-ICU. However, specific training is recommended to ensure optimum performance. The CAM must be applied after cognitive testing.

A common clinical challenge is **differentiating delirium from dementia**, given some overlapping symptoms and strong associations with each other. Delirium is associated with an increased risk of developing dementia, and dementia is associated with an increased risk of developing delirium. Dementia with Lewy bodies is particularly difficult to distinguish, given that it has features of both delirium and dementia. The key feature that helps to distinguish delirium from dementia is the time course of its presentation and progression. Delirium typically has an acute and rapid onset, whereas dementia almost always progresses more gradually. Evidence-based tools for detecting delirium superimposed on dementia are very limited, although some existing tools show promise, including the CAM, CAM-ICU, and the 4 A's test.

The 4 A's test, available at www.the4at.com, consists of 4 items that take 2 to 3 minutes to administer: 2 brief cognitive tests and assessments of level of consciousness and acute changes in mental status. A single validation study has shown a sensitivity and specificity of 90% and 84% in older hospital inpatients and 94% and 91% in patients with dementia, respectively.⊖ Although it requires further study, the reported advantages of the 4 A's test are ease and speed of use without requiring specific operator training.

→ MANAGEMENT

The mainstay of delirium management is reversal of the underlying cause and prevention of its complications. Pharmacologic treatment should only be considered in circumstances where the patient is at risk of harming themselves or others.

Treatment of the Underlying Cause

Reviewing the patient's medical history, physical examination, medications, and laboratory investigations usually points to one or more causes of delirium. Common causes: →Table 3-4.

Nonpharmacologic Management

After reversing the underlying cause of delirium, nonpharmacologic strategies should be instituted to prevent worsening (→below), relieve symptoms, and reduce complications. Nonpharmacologic measures are also used to prevent injuries to the patient and others. The following strategies should be used:

1) Familiar faces and environment can often alleviate agitation in a delirious patient. We recommend informing family members and other caregivers when a patient is agitated and offer them a chance to comfort the patient, either in person, by phone, or other means (eg, video chat through Skype or FaceTime). We also recommend putting familiar pictures and belongings (eg, pillows, blankets, photographs) in the patient's room.

2) Validation is a technique used to explore and comfort patients with confusion. For example, older patients with delirium will sometimes ask for their parents, who are often deceased. Instead of confronting them with the truth, it is often helpful to explore their disorientation and validate their fears. Validation is often used in dementia but it can be applied to delirium as well. More details available at vfvalidation.org.

3) De-escalation and redirection are important techniques when encountering an agitated patient. Attending a local training course is recommended. Programs such as Gentle Persuasive Approach (www.ageinc.ca/GPA/basics.html) is an example from the Advanced Gerontological Education based in Hamilton, Canada.

4) A sitter is a trained staff (either health-care professional or volunteer) or family member who provides constant observation for patients in delirium. Sitters should be actively engaged in the patient's care and not just passively observing. Sitters provides care (eg, hydration, toileting, reorientation) and can alert health-care staff about imminent dangers (eg, falls, agitation, wandering) at the bedside in a timely manner. Although there are associated costs, sitters can prevent complications of delirium and reduce physical restraint use. We recommend a sitter providing constant observation to patients in delirium, particularly those with hyperactive subtype.

5) Physical restraints should be avoided unless all possible measures have failed and imminent harm is likely. Restraints are associated with worsening of delirium, falls, serious injuries, increased length of stay, and death.⊗⊖ We recommend expert consultation (eg, geriatric medicine or psychiatry specialists) when physical restraint use is unavoidable in a delirious patient.

Pharmacologic Management

Assuming that the underlying cause of delirium is treated appropriately, there are circumstances when pharmacologic treatment of delirium is warranted. Antipsychotic medications may be appropriate if an agitated patient is causing imminent harm to self or others. Antipsychotic medications may also be

Table 3-4. Common causes of delirium

Etiology	Investigations to consider	Treatment suggestions
Infections All settings: UTI, pneumonia, abdominal, cellulitis, skin ulcers, meningitis ICU: Venous catheter--associated infection, sepsis Surgical: Wound and surgical site infections	Culture and image appropriately. Asymptomatic bacteriuria is common in older people and positive urine culture alone does not indicate UTI. Look for other causes of delirium	Appropriate use of empiric antibiotics with adjustment based on culture and sensitivity
Medication changes (new additions or withdrawal)	Medication reconciliation, pill count	Either taper/stop offending medications or treat medication withdrawal accordingly
Alcohol withdrawal	Alcohol level, anion gap, osmolar gap	Treat with benzodiazepines, thiamine, and use CIWA to guide management
Pain	Pain scale, eg, PAINAD in those with cognitive impairment	Appropriate pain management with acetaminophen and low-dose opioid medications (eg, hydromorphone). Consider peripheral nerve block or adjunct pain management strategies as appropriate
Metabolic abnormality (eg, hypercalcemia, hyponatremia, hypernatremia)	Blood test including sodium and calcium	Determine cause and correct as indicated
Urinary retention	Bedside bladder US to determine PVR. Given the prevalence of urinary retention in the elderly, we typically check PVR in all cases of delirium.	Urinary catheter for obstruction relief, UTI testing/treatment, urologic consultation if needed
Constipation Surgical: Ileus	Abdominal radiographs if indicated	Treatment of constipation
Hypoxia ICU: Ventilatory failure, ventilator-associated pneumonia	Chest radiographs, arterial blood gas, ventilation settings	Treat underlying cause (eg, COPD, heart failure, pulmonary embolism, pneumonia, aspiration)
Serotonin syndrome	Medication review	Stop offending medications and treat with benzodiazepines
Hepatic encephalopathy	Ammonia level in appropriate situations	Lactulose or polyethylene glycol, treatment underlying cause
Uremic encephalopathy	Creatinine and urea	Consider dialysis

Etiology	Investigations to consider	Treatment suggestions
Subdural hematoma, intracranial hemorrhage, stroke	Neurologic deficits should prompt urgent CT or MRI of the head. Cardiac and vascular surgeries have particularly high risk for postoperative stroke	Initiate ischemic or hemorrhagic stroke management. Neurosurgical consultation for CNS bleeding
Postoperative complications	Thorough history and physical exam looking for anastomotic leak, DVT, fluid overload, hematoma	Treat causes
Excess sedation (in ICU)	Validated tools (eg, Richmond Agitation-Sedation scale) should be used to assess depth of sedation	Avoid excess sedation
Nonconvulsive status epilepticus	In patients with persistent decreased level of consciousness not explained by structural cause EEG should be performed to exclude nonconvulsive status epilepticus	Treatment of seizure with neurologic consultation
Trauma	Sometimes an unwitnessed fall leads to fracture or concussion that is manifested by delirium. Thorough physical examination is critical. Imaging of injured areas can be considered	Treat as per injury

CIWA, Clinical Institute Withdrawal Assessment; CNS, central nervous system; COPD, chronic obstructive pulmonary disease; CT, computed tomography; DVT, deep venous thrombosis; EEG, electroencephalography; ICU, intensive care unit; MRI, magnetic resonance imaging; PVR, postvoid residual volume; US, ultrasonography; UTI, urinary tract infection.

appropriate if the patient is experiencing distressing hallucinations or delusions. Before considering the use of antipsychotics, we recommend the following:

1) Since delirium is a sign of underlying illness, it is not wise to conceal the symptoms of delirium by use of sedatives or antipsychotics without investigating the cause. Every attempt should be made to find and treat the underlying cause or causes.

2) From our experience, untreated or undertreated pain is a frequent contributor to delirium, particularly in postoperative or ICU patients. Patients with cognitive impairment or delirium may not reliably express pain, so a nonverbal pain assessment tool such as the PAINAD can be used to assess pain in these patients.

3) Be aware of the risk of antipsychotic use in patients with Parkinson disease. Dopamine antagonism will worsen stiffness and discomfort in this group. If an antipsychotic must be used, quetiapine at low doses is possibly the safest choice. Otherwise, low-dose trazodone or benzodiazepine may be considered. Although benzodiazepines may precipitate delirium, its use can be considered for sedation when antipsychotics are contraindicated in an agitated or violent patient.

4) Antipsychotics are a form of chemical sedation, and consent should be obtained before use when possible. Substitute decision-makers (SDMs) should be informed about the risks of untreated agitation as well as the risks of antipsychotic use. Ideally, electrocardiography (ECG) should be performed before starting antipsychotics to assess for QT prolongation. In general, giving low doses more frequently with monitoring is better than giving a single higher dose.

Antipsychotics and sedative-hypnotics that can be considered when indicated: →Table 3-5.

Table 3-5. Antipsychotics and sedative-hypnotics used in delirium

Psychotropics	Dose	Comments
Haloperidol	– Initial dose: 0.25 mg in frail older patients (0.5-1 mg in robust or younger patients) – May be given PO, SC, IM, or IV – May be given every 4 hours, not exceeding 2 mg in a 24-h period in older patients	– FDA "black-box warning" for risk of arrhythmia and death when dose is >10 mg in a 24-h period in patients of all ages – Parenteral route available – May cause QT prolongation
Risperidone	– Initial dose: 0.25 mg in frail older adults (0.5 mg in robust or younger patients) – May be given bid, not exceeding 2 mg in a 24-h period in older patients	– PO only – May cause QT prolongation
Quetiapine	– Initial dose: 6.25-12.5 mg in frail older patients (25 mg for robust or younger patients) – May be given bid	– PO only – Increased risk of sedation – May cause QT prolongation – Least likely to cause extrapyramidal adverse effects. Can be considered in patients with Parkinson disease
Lorazepam or other benzodiazepine	– For lorazepam, initial dose 0.5 mg – May be given PO, SC, IM, or IV	– Use for alcohol withdrawal – Consider in patients with Parkinson disease

bid, 2 times a day; FDA, US Food and Drug Administration; IM, intramuscular; IV, intravenous; PO, oral; SC, subcutaneous.

➔ PREVENTION

Delirium prevention is considered a standard of care in high-risk settings, such as medical/surgical wards, orthopedic wards, and the ICU.

Nonpharmacologic Delirium Prevention

Multicomponent intervention: There is consistent evidence that a multicomponent nonpharmacologic intervention reduces the risk of delirium in both medical and surgical inpatient settings. In several randomized controlled trials proactive geriatric medicine consultation or multidisciplinary geriatric surgical units can effectively reduce delirium incidence by addressing a wide range of predisposing and precipitating factors.

An alternative cost-effective solution is a multicomponent intervention delivered by volunteers. There are 6 key delirium prevention interventions derived from the Delirium Prevention Trial, which resulted in the Hospital Elder Life Program (www.hospitalelderlifeprogram.org):

1) Ensure frequent reorientation of the patient.

2) Maintain adequate hydration.

3) Clean and put on eyeglasses for those with visual impairment.

4) Put on hearing aids or use personal amplifier for those with hearing impairment.

5) Ensure early and daily ambulation.

6) Provide nonpharmacologic sleep promotion, such as a warm drink (noncaffeinated), back rub, and a dark and quiet sleep environment.

Other interventions as part of a multicomponent approach include:

1) Avoidance of restraints/tethers, including belts, soft restraints, oxygen, IV catheters, and urinary catheters when possible.

2) Avoidance of medications at risk of causing or worsening delirium, such as anticholinergic medications and sedative medications.

3) Proactive treatment of pain and constipation.

4) Comprehensive geriatrics consultation.

We recommend a multicomponent intervention for delirium prevention in medical and surgical inpatients at moderate to high risk.⊗⊖ These interventions are simple and can be carried out by volunteers, nurses, allied health-care professionals, physicians, and even family members. We encourage hospital leadership to adopt this approach for all units caring for moderate-risk and high-risk patients (receiving pharmacotherapy, with hip fractures, from nursing homes, and in the ICU). Systematic implementation with continuous quality improvement is key in delirium prevention.

Pharmacologic Prevention

Despite testing multiple interventions, there is no convincing evidence of the benefit of any pharmacologic interventions for delirium prevention.

1. Antipsychotics: There have been a number of clinical trials testing the effectiveness of antipsychotic medications for delirium prevention in postoperative and ICU patients. Although several trials show a decreased incidence of delirium, there are significant concerns regarding adverse effects of antipsychotic medications and conversion to hypoactive delirium. Furthermore, antipsychotics do not prevent long-term complications of delirium. Overall, we do not recommend antipsychotic medications for delirium prevention.⊗⊖

2. Cholinesterase inhibitors: We recommend not to use cholinesterase inhibitors (eg, donepezil, rivastigmine) for prevention of delirium because clinical trials have not shown a benefit.⊗⊖

3. Melatonin: There is inconsistent evidence that melatonin or melatonergic drugs (ramelteon) may decrease the incidence of delirium in postoperative or medical inpatients. However, the largest clinical trial to date did not demonstrate any benefits of melatonin.⊖ There is insufficient evidence at this time to make a recommendation for melatonin for delirium prevention.

4. Gabapentin: We recommend not to use gabapentin for prevention of postoperative delirium.⊗⊖ A single large randomized controlled trial showed no reduction in delirium incidence with postoperative gabapentin, but there was a signal toward increased harm in those undergoing hip surgery.

5. Peripheral nerve block: There is insufficient evidence to recommend peripheral nerve block for delirium prevention. A single randomized controlled trial specifically looking at delirium incidence in patients with hip fracture had significant methodologic limitations including an increased use of meperidine in the placebo group.⊗○

6. Dexmedetomidine: There is inconsistent evidence to suggest the use of dexmedetomidine, a highly selective α-2 agonist, for delirium prevention in the ICU.⊙○

7. Ketamine: We recommend against using ketamine for the prevention of postoperative delirium.⊗⊖ A single large randomized controlled trial showed no reduction in delirium incidence but hallucinations and nightmares were significantly increased in the ketamine group.

8. Alternative strategies: **Bispectral index–guided anesthesia:** There are 2 moderately sized clinical trials showing a reduction in postoperative delirium when depth of anesthesia was monitored intraoperatively. One study was industry funded and the other did not state the method of delirium detection. Long-term outcomes were not reported. Given these limitations, individual hospitals may consider this intervention if available.⊙○

→ PROGNOSIS

Delirium is a well-established predictor of poor prognosis. It is associated with increased length of hospital stay, risk of dementia, functional impairment, institutionalization, and death. There is evidence that a multicomponent nonpharmacologic intervention can improve short-term outcomes including length of stay and need for long-term care.⊖ However, no study has shown improvement in long-term outcomes, even when delirium incidence was reduced.

4. Dementia

→ DEFINITION, ETIOLOGY, PATHOGENESIS

Dementia is a common syndrome of acquired cognitive deficits which interfere with daily function and are not due to other conditions such as delirium or severe depression. Most commonly dementia is due to neurodegenerative conditions such as Alzheimer disease (AD) or less frequently due to cerebrovascular disease, trauma, infections, and numerous other causes. In order to destigmatize the label of dementia, the latest edition of the American Psychiatric Association's *Diagnostic and Statistical Manual of Mental Disorders* (*DSM-5*) uses the term **major neurocognitive disorder** to replace dementia; however, the definition is essentially the same.

The formal definition of **dementia** is cognitive or behavioral symptoms that represent a decline from previous levels of function; interfere with daily function; are not explained by delirium or psychiatric illness; could be detected by history and cognitive testing; and include ≥2 of amnesia, agnosia, aphasia, executive dysfunction, and behavior change (eg, apathy, disinhibition). The gradual onset, progressive changes, irreversibility, and memory loss as essential features are absent from the current definition, as these features, which are typical of AD, are not necessarily present in other types of dementia.

Pathologic subtypes: In Canada and most of developed countries, **AD** is the most prevalent pathologic process causing dementia. Nearly 50% of cases of dementia are attributable to AD, and a further one-third is due to multiple pathologies, most commonly AD with cerebrovascular disease. The other principal neurodegenerative diseases are **frontotemporal dementia (FTD)** and **dementia with Lewy bodies (DLB)**. Nowadays pure **vascular dementia** is considered to be relatively uncommon. FTD is distinct pathologically and usually also clinically from AD. Genetic influences account for ~50% of FTD cases. DLB is related to Parkinson disease (PD), and a family history of PD may be present. Primary PD is also associated with high risk of developing dementia.

Mild cognitive impairment (MCI) refers to the period of asymptomatic disease that precedes the onset of symptoms of dementia and is associated with preserved daily function. For example, in the case of AD the onset of dementia is usually preceded by a period of mild memory deficits, which do not compromise daily function. This is known as **amnestic MCI** and in the *DSM-5* definition termed **minor neurocognitive disorder**.

Risk factors: While many of risk factors parallel those for cardiovascular and cerebrovascular disease (eg, diabetes mellitus, hypertension, smoking, prior stroke, physical inactivity), risk factors unique to dementia include repeated or severe head trauma, exposure to pesticides, fewer years of education, and use of anticholinergic drugs. The greatest risk factor by far is age, and the increasing prevalence of dementia is largely attributable to increasing life expectancy.

Genetic factors: Genetic influences are important in **early-onset Alzheimer disease (EOAD)**, in which autosomal dominant transmission may occur. EOAD accounts for <2% of all cases of dementia. Single gene mutations in amyloid precursor protein (*APP*) and presenilin (*PS1*, *PS2*) genes confer 100% probability of developing EOAD, as does Down syndrome (trisomy 21). Spontaneous mutations may occur but many cases of EOAD do not have these gene abnormalities. In the far more common **late-onset Alzheimer disease (LOAD)** genetic factors play a less obvious role and no deterministic gene abnormalities have so far been identified. For example, in the *APO E* gene system on chromosome 19 there are three alleles: ε2, ε3, and ε4. While the presence of ε2 lowers the risk for AD and ε3 is neutral, possessing 1 or (worse) 2 copies of ε4 increases the risk of LOAD.

→ CLINICAL FEATURES AND NATURAL HISTORY

1. AD: AD is a neurodegenerative condition characterized by neuronal death and accumulation of the toxic protein aggregates β-amyloid and tau.

The most common first symptom is impairment in memory. At first this usually affects recent or episodic memory and may go unnoticed by the individual. The cognitive decline is usually noticed first by spouses, other family members, and coworkers. Family members will often complain of the patient repeating questions, repeating stories, losing objects, and not being able to remember discrete conversations or events. Because the onset is insidious and progression is gradual, the date of onset is typically difficult to ascertain. Over time, other cognitive functions are affected: often language (especially word retrieval), executive function (the ability to plan and sequence complex tasks), visuospatial function (the ability to orient oneself in one's environment), and praxis (the ability to perform learned motor skills). As these deficits increase, difficulty is experienced in performing familiar tasks (eg, the electrician can no longer change a light bulb, the gourmet cook can no longer prepare a meal). Not being able to find appropriate words, becoming lost in familiar environments, and not being able to use household objects (eg, remote control) are also common complaints. As the disease progresses further, behavior problems such as apathy, irritability, and aggression may supervene.

In the final stages of the disease motor function may be affected. Swallowing difficulty, rigidity, and contractures may announce end-stage AD. The average duration from first symptoms to death is generally within 7 to 10 years, but in the Canadian Study of Health and Aging the average life expectancy was only 3.4 years. However, in this longitudinal study the average age of onset was 81 years (~10 years later than the usual onset). At age 81, the usual life expectancy is ~5 years.

Notwithstanding the more typical amnestic presentation of AD, several different clinical phenotypes exist (→Table 4-1), including a primarily language variant (logopenic primary progressive aphasia), frontal or executive variant, or visuospatial variant (posterior cortical atrophy).

2. FTD: In contrast to AD, the prominent early symptoms do not involve memory, but feature behavioral and/or language changes. This group of diseases may be as common as AD between the ages of 45 and 64 years, with an annual incidence of 15/100,000 in some studies. There are 3 principal variants of FTD: behavioral variant FTD (bvFTD), semantic dementia (SD), and progressive nonfluent aphasia (PNFA). The latter two are language variants, presenting with progressive aphasia instead of behavioral changes. While initially one typically sees changes of behavior or language, as the disease progresses combinations of both types of symptoms develop, as originally described by Arnold Pick, whose name the condition previously bore (→Table 4-2).

bvFTD is characterized by early onset of behavioral disinhibition (socially inappropriate behavior, impulsive actions); apathy or inertia (lack of goal--directed behaviors); loss of sympathy or empathy; obsessive/perseverative behaviors; hyperorality (binge eating, oral exploration of inedible objects), and

---

Table 4-1. Diagnostic criteria for probable Alzheimer disease

1. Insidious onset
2. Clear-cut history of worsening
3. Initial and prominent cognitive deficits on history and examination with either amnestic or nonamnestic presentation

Variants
Language variant: Progressive nonfluent aphasia
Visuospatial variant: Posterior cortical atrophy
Frontal executive variant: Frontal atrophy

AD is considered improbable in case of:
- Substantial evidence of cerebrovascular disease
- Core features of dementia with Lewy body present (complex visual hallucinations, early parkinsonism, fluctuating cognition)
- Prominent features of behavioral variant frontotemporal dementia (disinhibition, apathy, loss of empathy, hyperorality, executive dysfunction, perseverative behavior)
- Prominent features of semantic dementia or primary progressive aphasia
- Other neurologic or nonneurologic illness or drugs

Table 4-2. Diagnostic criteria for frontotemporal dementia

Early and progressive change in:
- **Personality**: Difficulty modulating behavior, inappropriate responses and activity (eg, disinhibition, apathy, poor insight and judgment, self-neglect)
or
- **Language**: Expression, severe naming difficulty or meaning (progressive expressive aphasia) contraction of language

---

a neuropsychologic profile displaying impaired executive function with intact episodic memory. When apathy is the most prominent feature, it may be difficult to distinguish from depression. Patients stop engaging in daily activities and may sit idle for hours a day watching television but usually they do not endorse depression symptoms. If disinhibition is present (eg, insulting strangers, inappropriate sexual behavior, stealing), the disease usually reaches the medical or legal system earlier than in cases where apathy predominates. Often the most concerning to caregivers is the lack of empathy, interrelatedness, and personal warmth. Traumatic or tragic events in the caregiver's life may not register with the patient, making it extremely challenging for the caregiver to handle. Loss of insight is typical, which makes explaining and managing the disease particularly difficult.

In aphasic variants in FTD (SD and PNFA) language deficits are the most prominent and principal cause of impaired daily activities at disease onset. Patients with aphasic variants may evolve to resemble bvFTD in the course of their disease and occasionally develop movement disorders, including progressive supranuclear palsy and corticobasal syndrome. PNFA is characterized by effortful halting speech, with spared single-word comprehension and object knowledge. These patients may develop mutism over time. By contrast, SD has spared speech production (motor and grammar) but has difficulties with confrontational naming, single-word comprehension, and objective knowledge. Patients with SD may describe a zebra as an animal, then later as a thing. They may suffer from semantic paraphasias and call objects by their incorrect names. The meaning of words and symbols may be lost.

Table 4-3. Diagnostic criteria for dementia with Lewy bodies

Dementia plus:

1) **Core features**:
   - Fluctuating cognition
   - Well-formed visual hallucinations
   - Spontaneous parkinsonism

2) **Suggestive features**:
   - REM sleep disorder
   - Severe neuroleptic sensitivity

REM, rapid eye movement.

Table 4-4. Vascular cognitive impairment: probable vascular dementia

1. Dementia is present
2. Deficits in daily function are independent of the motor/sensory sequelae of the vascular event
3. Cognitive impairment and imaging evidence of cerebrovascular disease and:
   1) A clear temporal relationship between a vascular event (eg, clinical stroke) and onset of cognitive deficits; or
   2) A clear relationship in the severity and pattern of cognitive impairment and presence of diffuse subcortical cerebrovascular disease
4. No history of gradually progressive cognitive deficits before or after stroke that suggests the presence of a nonvascular neurodegenerative disorder

FTD shares the underlying pathology with movement disorders, and the evolution of a clinical phenotype means that a patient may start out with one disorder and progress to look like a different disorder over time. For example, a patient with behavioral disinhibition and apathy, resembling a case of bvFTD, may evolve over time to develop rigidity and tremor, apraxia, and dystonia, and be better classified as with frontal features. Similarly, a person with PNFA may present with language difficulties, and then develop traits consistent with progressive supranuclear palsy. There is considerable clinical and pathophysiologic overlap among bvFTD, SD, PNFA, corticobasal syndrome, and progressive supranuclear palsy.

3. DLB: Lewy bodies, the aggregations of α synuclein that characteristically occur within the basal ganglia of individuals with PD, may also deposit within the cerebral cortex and other parts of the brain. Individuals with DLB exhibit hallucinations or delusions, fluctuations in the severity of symptoms, and spontaneous or drug-induced parkinsonism. The presentation with hallucinations and fluctuating attention renders the distinction from delirium particularly important. In many individuals finally diagnosed with DLB, a history of repeated, extensive investigations for the causes of delirium has occurred. Cognitively, disturbances in visuospatial performance are prominent in DLB: difficulties with clock drawing or completing the interlocking pentagons on the Mini Mental State Examination (MMSE) are clues to this diagnosis. DLB may be preceded by many years with rapid-eye movement sleep disorder, that is, acting out dreams, sometimes violently. Adverse reactions to neuroleptic agents including rigidity, bradykinesia and other extrapyramidal adverse effects are further clues to this diagnosis (→Table 4-3).

4. Vascular dementia (vascular cognitive impairment [VCI]; →Table 4-4): The concept of a vascular dementia has evolved considerably since the original descriptions of "multi-infarct dementia." Observations from the Nun Study of Aging and Alzheimer's Disease altered our understanding in that most dementias previously considered to be of vascular origin are actually due to the presence of cerebral vascular disease superimposed upon neurodegenerative conditions, such as AD. Individuals even with prominent pathologic changes of AD (neurofibrillary tangles and amyloid plaques) may appear cognitively normal in life, but the presence of even a single white matter stroke greatly increases the risk of that individual having a dementia.

5. Rapidly progressive dementia (RPD): This unusual condition is defined by a dementia which develops within 1 year from the individual being cognitively normal. There are many causes, including tumors; paraneoplastic syndromes, infections (eg, HIV); and metabolic, autoimmune, psychiatric, toxic, and vascular events. A significant portion of RPD is caused by neurodegenerative disease, such as AD. While the cause is not infrequently discovered by the usual diagnostic process (→below), causes such as Creutzfeldt-Jakob disease and anti-NMDA (N-methyl-D-aspartate-type) receptor encephalitis may be revealed by more elaborate investigations.

→ DIAGNOSIS

The process of history examination and basic laboratory testing will usually allow the type of dementia to be identified. Insidious onset with progressive memory decline points towards AD. Onset of progressive aphasia usually indicates FTD or a language variant of AD. Prominent apathy may indicate FTD or frontal variant AD but mandates exclusion of depression as a potential diagnosis. Abrupt onset in the absence of a new medication or intercurrent infection points towards a vascular or mixed etiology. Simple neuroimaging studies may be added if indications are present.

1. History: By far the most important diagnostic tool is a careful history including collateral data from family and others. The timing and onset of symptoms, type of symptoms, any precipitating events, and risk factors are all important data elements. The prescription of a new medication, onset of systemic disease (eg, heart failure, pulmonary, renal or hepatic failure, hypothyroidism, infection), as well as psychiatric, family, educational, and occupational history are all important. It is usually necessary to consult other health-care professionals for background history. Findings such as "poor historian," missing appointments, or poor adherence to prescribed medications are clues that should not be ignored.

2. Objective cognitive testing: Once the suspicion of a cognitive disorder is raised, physical examination and neurologic examination to detect focal signs together with brief cognitive tests are the next step. There are many **brief cognitive tests** in common use.

1) **MMSE**: While this widely used tool was originally designed to distinguish dementia from depression, it has been used extensively in clinical practice, epidemiologic surveys, and pharmacologic studies. The domains covered in the MMSE include orientation, short-term recall, basic language, and visuospatial construction. A standardized version has improved reliability. The MMSE is insensitive to the identification of MCI but declines at a fairly predictable rate during the progression of typical AD.

2) **Montreal Cognitive Assessment (MoCA)** (available at www.mocatest.org): This tool was introduced to detect mild cognitive impairment but has gained wide acceptance in a broad range of cognitive disorders. Although initially introduced as royalty-free, the creators began restricting access to those who participated in paid training sessions in 2019. Each item in the MoCA is derived from more established neuropsychologic tests and it is available in several versions and multiple languages. In addition to testing delayed recall and orientation, the language section is more comprehensive than the MMSE (phonemic fluency, sentence repetition), and executive function is tested with clock drawing, a short version of trail making test part B (connecting a sequence of alternating numbers and letters), and a 3-dimensional diagram. Attention is measured by digit span forward and backward as well as a finger-tapping exercise. A simple version of the categories test explores abstract thinking.

As part of the clinical assessment of mental status, simple bedside cognitive tests allow for measurement of decline or response to treatment of dementia.

Table 4-5. Indications for neuroimaging

– Age <65 years	– Anticoagulants or bleeding diathesis
– Relatively short clinical history	– Malignancy that might metastasize to brain
– Focal neurologic symptoms	– Atypical features (not suggesting Alzheimer disease)
– Focal neurologic signs	– In cases where finding of cerebrovascular disease
– History of head trauma	would significantly influence management

Extensive neurocognitive testing is usually reserved for younger patients who may need to apply for disability pensions or to determine whether an occupation is still feasible. Testing may also be appropriate for older patients who are still working, especially in medical, academic, and legal occupations. Unusual presentations of dementia may also benefit from neurocognitive testing and can add to the above measures when it is essential to determine if an individual with MCI is most likely to progress to dementia.

3. Laboratory tests: In all suspected cases of dementia or MCI we recommend 6 basic laboratory tests to be performed if not done recently: complete blood count (CBC), blood glucose level or glycated hemoglobin (HbA_{1c}), serum calcium, serum thyroid-stimulating hormone, electrolytes and serum B_{12} levels.◐○

4. Neuroimaging: Neuroimaging is appropriate for most individuals presenting with dementia but the yield of significant abnormalities is higher if indications for neuroimaging are present (→Table 4-5). Specific findings on imaging may help refine diagnosis. Medial temporal and hippocampal atrophy are characteristic of AD, frontotemporal atrophy suggests FTD, and atrophy of occipital and posterior parietal lobes supports the visuospatial presentation of AD. When performing computed tomography (CT) or magnetic resonance imaging (MRI) for suspected dementia, make sure to specify complex or 3 views (axial, coronal, sagittal) to obtain maximum information. In some cases a radionuclide scan may be helpful in distinguishing FTD from AD, especially where language deficits or behavioral symptoms predominate. A positron emission tomography (PET) scan with fluorodeoxyglucose (FDG) is optimal but usually not available outside the research setting. A single-photon emission computed tomography (SPECT) scan is a reasonable alternative. PET amyloid scanning is emerging as an accurate method of diagnosing AD but is not yet widely available.

5. Cerebral spinal fluid (CSF) analysis: CSF analysis for early diagnosis of AD is becoming more available. The typical findings in AD, even before the onset of dementia, include an elevated level of tau and depressed level of β-amyloid.

6. Screening: Present evidence does not support screening for cognitive impairment or dementia in any age group.●○

→ MANAGEMENT

General Considerations

1. Education and support: Education and support for patient, caregivers, and family comprise the cornerstone of management.◐○ Establishing the degree of risk to the individual and others is an important first step. Several items mandate urgent attention (→Table 4-6). Some of these may be easily addressed, for example, by disabling the stove or removing guns from the house.

Support and advocacy organizations such as the Alzheimer's Society of Canada (ASC) are extremely helpful to patients, relatives, and caregivers. The ASC website (www.alzheimer.ca) is particularly helpful and many local chapters offer educational programs and support activities. Referral to a local chapter of the ASC is suggested for all newly diagnosed individuals.

2. Driving: The issue of driving safety is important and contentious. In most provinces physicians are required to report to the Provincial Ministry of

Table 4-6. Clinically alarming features (red flags) in patients with cognitive decline	
Red flags	**Examples/clues**
Fire	Smoking, kitchen safety
Wandering	Increased unexplained time away from home, leaving home at night
Inability to summon help	Using telephone, understanding emergency response system, eg, Lifeline
Risk of falls/injuries	Abnormal gait, history of falls, bruises/injuries
Risk to others	Potential violence to spouse, caregiver, others, guns in home
Motor vehicle driving	Damage to vehicle, impaired judgment when driving
Narrow therapeutic index medications	Where missed or duplicated doses may have serious consequences (eg, insulin, oral hypoglycemic agents, anticoagulants, anticonvulsants, lithium, digoxin)

Transport individuals who have conditions that may threaten their driving safety. It may be necessary to arrange road assessments when driving safety is hard to assess in the office. If the individual has a severe dementia, the course of action is unequivocal. In individuals with MCI or early dementia the risk to driving safety is usually small but the clinical assessment can be further refined by an on-road or computer-aided test (eg, for Ontario visit the website of the Ministry of Transportation). In those with mild to moderate dementia the decision to report is made on an individual basis.

3. Future planning: It is important to consider future planning, for example, assigning powers of attorney for property and personal care, planning advance directives, and making a will. There are many initiatives that help maintain quality of life in patients with dementia. These include therapeutic and social day programs, individually tailored recreational therapies, and activities based on former hobbies and pastimes.

4. Coexisting conditions: It is important to address coexisting conditions. For example, poorly controlled endocrine and metabolic disorders may aggravate the cognitive deficits at present in an individual with dementia. Heart failure is an important contributor to cognitive deficits and optimal management of heart failure can significantly improve these manifestations. Attention is also directed towards medications that may aggravate cognitive symptoms. These include most sedatives, hypnotics, anxiolytics, and numerous medications with anticholinergic adverse effects, such as tricyclic antidepressants, antispasmodics, older antihistamines, and medications used for overactive bladder. Most narcotics also affect cognition, and many medications for diverse purposes have anticholinergic adverse effects.

Pharmacologic Therapy

Medications play a relatively minor role in the spectrum of management for dementing conditions (→Table 4-7).

1. Cholinesterase inhibitor (ChEI) cognitive enhancers have modest efficacy at best but in some individuals they show useful improvement or stabilization of symptoms over a number of months, sometimes extending into years. For this reason, most individuals with AD, mixed dementia, DLB, or PD should be offered a trial of a ChEI for 3 to 6 months.⊙⊙ If decline continues during the trial, switching to an alternative agent is occasionally helpful. If there is no evidence of improvement or stabilization, the ChEI should be tapered before discontinuation. Balanced against the modest benefits in cognition, daily activities, and possibly behavior, these drugs are expensive and can have significant adverse effects. Gastrointestinal disturbance occurs in ~10%

Table 4-7. Medications for dementia (Alzheimer disease, mixed, dementia with Lewy bodies)

Starting and maximum doses	Dosage	Comments
Donepezil		
Start: 5 mg daily (2.5 mg for very frail persons) **Max**: 10 mg daily	Increase to 10 mg daily after 4 weeks (in the very frail 2.5 mg daily for 2 weeks then 5 mg daily for 4 weeks; 10 mg later if tolerated)	GI adverse effects in ~10% of patients, syncope, falls, worsening cardiac conduction (avoid with severe bradycardia, heart blocks) night cramps, can disturb sleep
Galantamine ER		
Start: 8 mg daily **Max**: 32 mg daily	Increase to 16 mg daily after 4 weeks, then 24 mg daily after another 4 weeks if tolerated	GI adverse effects in ~10%, syncope, falls, worsening cardiac conduction (avoid with severe bradycardia, heart blocks)
Rivastigmine		
Oral **Start**: 1.5 mg bid (1.5 mg daily for very frail persons) **Max**: 6 mg bid	Increase to 3 mg bid after 4 weeks, 4.5 mg bid after another 4 weeks, then 6 mg bid after another 4 weeks if tolerated (in the very frail, 1.5 mg daily for 2 weeks, then 1.5 mg bid for 4 weeks, then 3 mg bid for 4 weeks, and increments of 1.5 mg bid each 4 weeks)	GI adverse effects in ~10%, syncope, falls, worsening cardiac conduction (avoid with severe bradycardia, heart blocks)
Transdermal patch **Start**: Exelon patch 5 (4.6 mg every 24 hours) **Max**: Exelon patch 15 (13.3 mg every 24 hours)	Starting dose patch 5, increase to patch 10 after 4 weeks	Transcutaneous patch delivers rivastigmine with much lower incidence of GI adverse effects
Memantine		
Start: 5 mg daily **Max**: 10 mg bid	After 1 week increase to 5 mg bid; after 1 more week 10 mg every morning, 5 mg every afternoon; after 1 more week 10 mg bid	Occasional headache, dizziness
Donepezil, galantamine, rivastigmine are cholinesterase inhibitors. Memantine is an NMDA receptor agonist.		
bid, 2 times a day; ER, extended release; GI, gastrointestinal.		

of patients, including nausea, anorexia, abdominal cramps, and looser bowel movements, and occasionally vomiting or severe diarrhea. Bradycardia and heart blocks develop on occasion and may result in falls and syncope. Caution is required in patients who are receiving β-blockers or nondihydropyridine calcium channel blockers (eg, diltiazem, verapamil), as bradycardia may be precipitated. Bifascicular and trifascicular blocks are contraindications to ChEIs. Right bundle branch or left anterior fascicular blocks are not considered contraindications providing there is no atrioventricular delay. These drugs may also precipitate bronchospasm and should be used with caution in individuals with reversible airways disease. Prior to considering ChEIs, electrocardiography (ECG) is recommended, together with evaluation of history for previous peptic ulceration, gastroesophageal reflux disease, or asthma.

2. Memantine is an NMDA receptor partial agonist with modest efficacy in moderate to severe degrees of AD. It is usually prescribed together with a ChEI as their actions are possibly complementary. It is debatable whether this drug has any real benefit over donepezil alone.◉

Neuropsychiatric Symptoms

Neuropsychiatric symptoms in dementia are common and often progressive. Depression, apathy, anxiety, and agitation are the most prevalent features. Management should start with nonpharmacologic strategies to address the cause of the symptoms with appropriate modification of activities, communication, and environment.◉◉ Comorbid depression should be treated as it often compounds the severity of irritability and apathy.◉◉ Caregiver education and counseling are also crucial. A thorough review of the patient's clinical status may reveal infection, organ failure, dehydration, constipation, pain, inappropriate medications, or insomnia as reversible causes of agitation. If symptoms persist despite nonpharmacologic means, consider a trial of an antidepressant, such as citalopram.◉◉ Atypical antipsychotics should be considered only when serious psychotic symptoms are present, as they are associated with an increased risk of stroke and death.◉◉ Also →Chapter 12.4.1.

End-of-Life Care in Dementia

Almost all causes of dementia are relentlessly progressive, and as the condition worsens decisions must be made about treatment of coexisting or superimposed illnesses. Decisions to continue or stop medications (eg, statins), offer surgical versus palliative treatment (eg, for severe osteoarthritis, symptomatic coronary artery disease), or initiate invasive care for acute infections (eg, ventilation for respiratory failure) can be very challenging. Decisions must be individualized, based wherever possible on the individual's advance directives, and considering the prognosis in advanced dementia. For example, in nursing home residents with advanced dementia, pneumonia or a febrile episode are associated with nearly 50% mortality within 6 months, while eating problems in this population are associated with nearly 40% mortality in 6 months.◉ One approach to weighing up the risks and benefits of planned treatments in frail individuals has been well described in the process entitled Palliative and Therapeutic Harmonization (PATH), which sets out a framework to approach decision-making in this context.◉

Specialist Clinic Management

Referral to a specialist clinic is needed when the diagnosis is unclear or if help with management is needed. Specialist clinics adopt a multidisciplinary approach and usually provide management support. Future planning, home and driving safety, community outreach, and follow-up are all parts of dementia care, as are pharmacotherapy and ultimately end-of-life care. Counseling, education, and caregiver support have been shown to significantly delay nursing home placement and reduce caregiver burnout.◉◉ Specialist clinics may also provide access to research studies.

➡ PREVENTION

Reduction of vascular risk factors appears to be the most promising approach to preventing dementia. For example, if one can delay or prevent strokes, it may be possible to delay or prevent the onset of mixed or vascular dementias. The only trial which shows this conclusively is the SYST-EUR study, which demonstrated that treatment of moderately severe systolic hypertension reduced the risk of dementia of all types by 50% over 5 years.◉◉ Epidemiologic studies suggest that those who are more active physically and mentally are less likely to experience dementia, but strong evidence for such claims is lacking. Restriction of heavy (but not moderate) alcohol use and striving for more education are some of the measures that might be helpful. There are some encouraging signs that the prevalence of dementia is beginning to decline in North America and Europe, which is thought to be due to more aggressive management of vascular risk factors.

4.1. Neuropsychiatric Symptoms in Dementia

➤ DEFINITION

Dementia is a clinical syndrome characterized by progressive cognitive decline and impairment in one or more cognitive domains sufficient to cause decline in daily function. The term "dementia" is subsumed under the newly named entity referred to in the fifth edition of the American Psychiatric Association's *Diagnostic and Statistical Manual of Mental Disorders* (*DSM-5*) as major neurocognitive disorders, which encompasses a group of acquired disorders. Mild neurocognitive disorder is a *DSM-5*–recognized term for the less severe level of cognitive impairment (also referred to as mild cognitive impairment) (MCI), considered to be a potential prodrome of Alzheimer disease or other neurodegenerative forms of dementia.

Individuals with MCI or dementia can present with prominent and disabling behavioral disturbances, termed **neuropsychiatric symptoms** (NPSs), previously denominated as behavioral and psychological symptoms of dementia (BPSD). These include agitation, depression, apathy, delusions, hallucinations, and sleep impairment. In some cases, they present as clusters, constituting syndromes such as dementia-associated psychotic or mood disturbances. These symptoms have serious adverse consequences for patients and caregivers, such as greater impairment in activities of daily living, more rapid cognitive decline, worse quality of life, earlier institutionalization, and greater caregiver depression. Therefore, the NPSs of dementia are serious conditions that are increasingly becoming a focus of attention.

In this chapter, we review the assessment and management of NPSs. Assessment, differential diagnosis, and management of cognitive symptoms in dementia: →Chapter 12.4.

➤ EPIDEMIOLOGY

NPSs can occur in over 90% of patients with dementia, as an isolated symptom or in symptom clusters, and are often the presenting problems in seeking care. They are associated with more rapid disease progression, worse outcomes, and significant distress to the patient and caregivers.

The NPSs in patients with dementia may result from a number of precipitants or causal factors, including neurobiologically related disease factors; patient's unmet needs (eg, too hot, too cold, hunger, incontinence, need to go to the bathroom); caregiver factors; environmental triggers; and interactions of the patient, caregiver, and environmental factors. It is likely that these potential causal factors are all relevant to differing degrees in an individual patient.

The cause of NPSs, while multifactorial, is likely due to regional brain degeneration. In late stages, NPSs may be common to all dementias, irrespective of etiology. Changes in the brain structure impact on brain biology at multiple levels, including neural and neurotransmitter levels. Behaviors may result from these changes affecting the brain function or from the challenges with communication and environment. The traditional view of these behaviors as "challenging" to manage is gradually being replaced with the more person--centered terminology of these being **responsive behaviors**, in recognition that the behavior represents the brain's attempts to communicate distress or unmet needs and should cue caregivers to determine potential triggers.

➤ CLINICAL FEATURES

NPSs constitute a heterogeneous range of reactions, psychiatric symptoms, and behaviors that may impact the safety and care of patients with MCI or dementia. The most common NPSs in dementia (→Table 4-8) and some of their key symptom presentations are further described below.

Table 4-8. Common neuropsychiatric symptoms in dementia	
– Apathy	– Sundowning
– Depression	– Illusions and hallucinations
– Elevated mood	– Delusions
– Irritability	– Sleep disturbances
– Mood lability	– Wandering
– Anxiety	– Pacing
– Disruptive vocalization	– Hoarding
– Aggression	– Inappropriate sexualized behavior
– Agitation	

1. Agitation is one of the most pervasive symptoms and can occur as a primary symptom or as secondary to other NPSs, including anxiety, depression, or psychosis. It may be associated with verbal (eg, repetitive vocalizations, shouting) or motor (eg, pacing, physical aggression, resistance to care) manifestations and can lead to injury, with significant implications for the safety of the patient and others. Sundowning refers to a specific pattern of agitation, with worsening of agitation in the late afternoon or early evening. Onset of sundowning has been associated with decreased light exposure, timing of medications, and dysfunctional sleep-wake cycles.

2. Apathy may manifest as deficits in thinking, diminished ability to initiate action, and cognitive and emotional blunting. It tends to occur early and increase over the course of the illness. It is important to distinguish from depression, which, unlike apathy, causes great suffering and distress to the patient. Often more distressing to the caregiver than the patient, apathy can be associated with diminished self-care and lead to increased social isolation.

3. Psychotic symptoms in patients with dementia, such as hallucinations and delusions, also frequently occur in delirium, which must be excluded. Visual hallucinations are highly suggestive of delirium but do also occur in neurodegenerative causes of parkinsonism, such as Parkinson disease, dementia with Lewy bodies, progressive supranuclear palsy, multiple system atrophy, and corticobasal degeneration syndrome (types of dementia: →Chapter 12.4). Paranoid delusions are the commonest, with themes of theft, infidelity, and misidentification syndromes as the most prominent. Psychotic symptoms can vary in intensity and severity, and if present without causing harm or distress to the patient or others, they may not require active pharmacologic treatment.

4. Depression has a high prevalence rate (15%-18%) in patients with dementia. Patients with dementia who have a past personal or family history of depression appear to be at greater risk for a major depressive episode, as do those who have suffered a stroke. Irritability and mood lability become more prevalent with the progression of dementia. Particularly, the apolipoprotein E ε 4 carriers with Alzheimer disease may have an increased risk of developing NPSs of depression and anxiety. Also →Chapter 12.5.

5. Disinhibition occurs in approximately one-third of patients and is more common with frontal lobe involvement. Sexually disinhibited or inappropriate behavior is often a source of great distress to caregivers. These behaviors can be caused by neurologic disorders, be associated with medication adverse effects (eg, dopamine agonists for Parkinson disease, benzodiazepines), be part of an undiagnosed bipolar disorder with mania, or occur as a symptom of the dementia. Dementia-related disinhibited behaviors are important to distinguish from mania or hypomania, as this will have significant treatment implications. In individuals with a past personal or family history of bipolar or depressive disorder, a circumscribed trial of a mood stabilizer, if helpful, may provide diagnostic information, but this should not be done routinely and should prompt a referral to a geriatric psychiatrist for diagnostic clarification and management.

6. Sleep-wake cycle disturbances are common and often associated with greater caregiver burden. Sleep disturbance is a common NPS in patients with dementia, who experience more sleep-wake cycle arousals and awakenings, diminished rapid eye movement sleep, and take more daytime naps, exacerbating the problem.

→ DIAGNOSIS

The diagnosis of NPSs includes a thorough evaluation of the following items:

1. An accurate **history** from both the patient and caregiver is an essential component to determine the cause or precipitant of the NPSs. Skill, patience, and flexibility are required to obtain accurate data. The clinician should face the patient directly and pay particular attention to eye contact, use unambiguous language, and speak in a calm, nonthreatening tone. Ongoing assessment for frustration or agitation of the patient is critical, as is recognizing when to switch topics or allow a break. The most important differential diagnosis is to exclude delirium as a cause for the behavioral change. Important elements of the history include:

1) Chronology and onset of the emergence of NPSs.

2) Sudden decline from baseline in function of instrumental and basic activities of daily living, suggesting delirium or acute cerebrovascular event.

3) Presence of a comorbid illness, especially signs and symptoms of delirium, vascular disease (risk factor for depression and agitation), infection, pain, and constipation.

4) Presence of past psychiatric episodes (eg, mood, psychosis, anxiety), which may represent a recurrence or relapse of underlying psychiatric disorder.

5) Presence of comorbid substance use disorder or withdrawal.

6) Medication adherence, changes, and withdrawal.

2. Physical examination, including a neurologic examination, is necessary to exclude infection, pain, constipation, and cerebrovascular or cardiovascular disease as a precipitant for the NPSs. A neurologic examination is important to exclude focal neurologic signs suggestive of stroke or subdural hematoma.

3. In patients with NPSs, the regular **mental status examination** should include a cognitive assessment, with a particular focus on change from previous testing. The most important task is to distinguish NPSs from delirium as a cause for the symptoms, particularly in cases of an acute change in attention. The presence of sadness, weepiness, agitation, suspiciousness or paranoia, disinhibition, or apathy should be documented. It can be challenging to distinguish depression as an NPS from a primary depressive disorder or a depressive episode of bipolar disorder. In both instances, severity as well as degree of distress and impairment of function guide treatment. The **cognitive assessment** may include the use of the Mini Mental State Examination (MMSE), which detects largely cortical deficits; however, the copyright restrictions make it less user-friendly (→Chapter 12.4). This should be supplemented by tests such as the Clock Drawing Test and the Montreal Cognitive Assessment (MoCA), which evaluates frontal-subcortical executive function as well. The MoCA is available in multiple languages, without cost, at www.mocatest.org. In advanced stages of the illness, many patients are unable to complete formal cognitive tests. In such cases, it is important to rely on observations of behavior, speech, and response to stimuli to determine the level of cognitive impairment, noting that a change from baseline is more significant than the absolute test scores.

4. When NPSs occur in existing cognitive impairment but cannot be explained by the typical course of the underlying dementia, a formal **neuropsychological assessment** can be a useful tool for helping to quantify impairment and for monitoring for change over time; however, it is resource-intensive, expensive,

Table 4-9. Neuropsychiatric Inventory (NPI) questionnaire domains

- Delusions
- Hallucinations
- Agitation
- Dysphoria
- Anxiety
- Apathy

- Irritability
- Euphoria
- Disinhibition
- Aberrant motor behavior
- Night-time behavior disturbances
- Appetite and eating abnormalities

Table 4-10. Laboratory examinations in the diagnosis of dementia

Basic screening investigations	– Complete blood count, thyroid-stimulating hormone, serum electrolytes, eGFR, serum calcium, and serum glucose – Screening for depression (eg, Geriatric Depression Scale)
Specific examinations (if justified)	– Heavy metal screens – VDRL test – Routine genetic markers (eg, apolipoprotein E) are not recommended
ECG	– Screening for vascular risk factors
Lumbar puncture	– For specific concerns (eg, infection, demyelinating diseases, CSF 14-3-3 protein in Creutzfeldt-Jakob disease) – CSF biomarkers of Alzheimer disease pathology (CSF aβ1-42 and tau) have no clinical utility in Canada but are part of research protocols
EEG	– Creutzfeldt-Jakob disease or dementia with seizures can be identified
Structural brain imaging (CT or MRI)	– CCCDTD4 recommends that structural neuroimaging is indicated in most but not required in all patients with cognitive impairment. (Details about recommendations for neuroimaging and specific clinical features: →Chapter 12.4) – Although more costly and less available, MRI is preferable to CT – CT or MRI should be undertaken in the assessment of cognitive impairment if the presence of unsuspected cerebrovascular disease would change the clinical management
Functional brain imaging (FDG-PET, SPECT)	– Where available, FDG-PET or PET amyloid imaging can be used for clinical purposes in patients with atypical dementias – 18F-florbetaben FDG-PET can be recommended for differential diagnosis purposes if the underlying pathologic process remains unclear after a baseline evaluation, preventing adequate clinical management. If FDG-PET is unavailable, a SPECT study can be recommended – PET amyloid imaging is not currently approved for clinical use in Canada. When available in the future, it must be considered as an adjunct to a comprehensive evaluation for complex atypical presentations when a more accurate clinical diagnosis is needed

CCCDTD4, 4th Canadian Consensus Conference on the Diagnosis and Treatment of Dementia; CSF, cerebrospinal fluid; CT, computed tomography; ECG, electrocardiography; EEG, electroencephalography; eGFR, estimated glomerular filtration rate; FDG-PET, 18F-fluorodeoxyglucose positron emission tomography; MRI, magnetic resonance imaging; PET, positron emission tomography; SPECT, single-photon emission computed tomography; VDRL, venereal disease research laboratory.

and not recommended on a routine basis. The most commonly used scale for detection of NPSs of dementia is the Neuropsychiatric Inventory (NPI), which assesses symptoms in 12 domains (details: →Table 4-9). The NPI-Clinician (NPI-C) version scale measures 14 domains and includes aberrant vocalization.

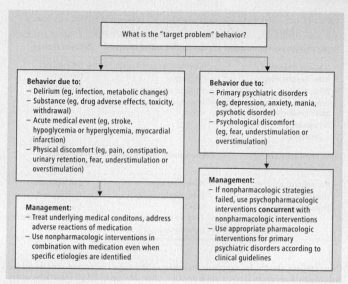

Figure 4-1. Identification of "target problem" behavior and its management.

Diagnostic Tests

In patients initially presenting with NPSs early in the course of dementia or where diagnostic clarification will impact on management, laboratory investigations are helpful to exclude other contributing or reversible factors. A summary of basic and more specific laboratory examinations performed to diagnose dementia: →Table 4-10; details: →Chapter 12.4.

Differential Diagnosis

The differential diagnoses to be considered in a patient with cognitive impairment exhibiting NPSs include delirium, neurologic diseases, infections, metabolic abnormalities, depression, psychotic disorders, and drug-related mood or psychotic syndromes.

→TREATMENT

The treatment of NPSs can have a significant impact on the quality of life of the patient, their families, and caregivers. Referral to a geriatric psychiatrist, where available, a psychiatrist, or a geriatrician should be considered in instances of refractory symptoms, which cause marked distress.

A useful approach to NPSs, which takes into account the likely precipitants or causal factors: →Figure 4-1.

1. Nonpharmacologic treatment: The first line of treatment should always be to identify and address the underlying cause or precipitant of the NPS whenever possible (eg, pain, infection, constipation). Symptomatic treatment consists of nonpharmacologic strategies (→Table 4-11) and should be the primary intervention for patients with dementia and NPSs, with clinicians and caregivers responding appropriately, knowledgeably, and promptly to address the patient's needs while searching for the most likely trigger. Since there are fewer risks associated with these treatments, it is recommended that they should always be considered first,🗹⊖ tailored to the individual patient, and

Table 4-11. Categories for specific nonpharmacologic interventions for neuropsychiatric symptoms

Sensory enhancement/relaxation	Social contact: real or simulated	Behavior therapy
– Massage and touch – Individualized music – White noise – Controlled multisensory stimulation (Snoezelen) – Art therapy – Aromatherapy	– Individualized social contact – Pet therapy – 1:1 social interaction – Simulated interactions/family videos	– Differential reinforcement – Stimulus control

Structured activities	Environmental modifications	Training and development
– Recreational activities – Outdoor walks – Physical activities	– Wandering areas – Natural/enhanced environments – Reduced stimulation – Light therapy	– Staff education – Staff support – Training programs for family caregivers

their impact should be carefully monitored through the use of standardized behavioral assessment tools such as the Cohen-Mansfield Agitation Inventory. Even when specific etiologies are identified, nonpharmacologic interventions should be utilized in combination with medication (→Figure 4-1). Family and caregivers are key collaborators and need to be involved in treatment planning.

2. Pharmacologic treatment: General prescribing principles: Prior to prescribing, in nonemergent situations it is imperative to inform patients or their substitute decision-makers of pertinent risks and warnings issued regarding medication (discussed below), to weigh the benefits versus the risks, and to document informed consent in the patient's chart. Age-related changes in pharmacodynamics and pharmacokinetics of psychotropic medications (eg, longer time to reach steady state, longer half-life, and longer elimination time) should be taken into consideration. Lower doses, cautious dose adjustments, and regular reassessment of the need for continuing the treatment in the geriatric patients should be considered. Geriatric patients with dementia are more vulnerable to adverse effects, including sedation, anticholinergic adverse effects, cognitive decline, extrapyramidal symptoms, and drug-drug interactions. Agitation, which is often the presenting symptom of an underlying mood, anxiety, or psychotic disorder, is the most common NPS requiring specific pharmacologic treatment after other treatments have failed. Below is a summary of the options that can be utilized for NPSs.

1) **Antidepressants**: The evidence for benefits of antidepressants in patients with dementia is modest; however, clinical guidelines suggest a trial of an antidepressant when there is a high index of suspicion for depression causing distress (despite not meeting criteria for major depressive disorder), while monitoring for adverse effects. Adverse events associated with antidepressants include hyponatremia, bleeds, falls, fragility, and osteoporotic fractures, and their rates are fairly low. It should be noted that at higher doses, selective serotonin reuptake inhibitors (SSRIs) can cause affective flattening and worsen apathy. In patients partially responsive to SSRIs or with prominent apathy, cautious use of low-dose psychostimulants (eg, methylphenidate, atomoxetine, modafinil) may be suggested, particularly in individuals who are both profoundly apathetic and medically ill.☺☺ Because psychostimulants can induce elevation of blood pressure and heart rate, irritability, agitation, and psychosis, a careful patient selection

is critical, especially in individuals with severe cardiovascular disease or other underlying cardiac conditions.

Antidepressants have limited evidence for efficacy,☺☺ especially beyond 12 weeks, in the treatment of NPSs of dementia of any type other than major depression, but there are clinical scenarios where a trial of an antidepressant may be appropriate. Patients with dementia may develop NPSs of apathy, social withdrawal, and sleep disturbance that may suggest the presence of depression but that are NPSs entirely due to dementia. Given the degree of suffering in untreated depression, a therapeutic trial with an antidepressant may be a reasonable diagnostic strategy in such cases. A low threshold for initiating antidepressant treatment should be considered in patients with preexisting history of depression or significant cerebrovascular disease. SSRIs are the preferred antidepressants in treating depression in patients with dementia and are generally well tolerated. Selection of an antidepressant is usually based upon the adverse-effect profile (particularly anticholinergic), drug-drug interactions, medical comorbidities, and cost.

SSRIs may also be useful in the management of agitation and psychosis in patients with Alzheimer disease, particularly if a poorly articulated depression is a likely precipitant of the NPS manifestation or cannot be excluded when no other cause is apparent.☺☺ Although having limited efficacy, the antidepressant citalopram has been shown to be as effective as risperidone, a second-generation antipsychotic (SGA), in the treatment of agitation due to dementia. Patients who are more likely to benefit from citalopram have moderate agitation and lower levels of cognitive impairment. Citalopram should be avoided in patients at increased risk for arrhythmias and discontinued in the case of a persistent QTc >500 ms. Because of the association of citalopram with cardiac QTc prolongation, use of this medication to treat agitation may be limited to a subgroup of patients with dementia. Health Canada and US Food and Drug Administration (FDA) recommend for citalopram a maximum daily dose of 20 mg for patients aged ≥60 years. The use of SSRIs for an indication of NPSs other than depression necessitates an ongoing assessment of benefits versus risks, and consideration for withdrawing the medications should be made periodically. Several other antidepressants were not found to be useful for agitation. However, sertraline at daily doses 25 to 100 mg can have a modest benefit on agitation.

Some evidence suggests that the NPSs in frontotemporal dementia may be caused by deficits in the serotoninergic system, in particular the repetitive behaviors. There is limited evidence of benefit for serotonergic antidepressant agents in these patients (→Table 4-12). Given the absence of evidence for using any other pharmacologic agents in this illness, a trial of an SSRI in these patients is warranted if the NPSs are causing distress.

2) **Cholinesterase inhibitors**: Cholinesterase inhibitors have only modest benefits overall for treatment of NPSs. In individuals with dementia due to Alzheimer disease or dementia with Lewy bodies, cholinesterase inhibitors may be used for treatment of apathy, anxiety, and depression, as well as disinhibition and aberrant motor symptoms. Cholinesterase inhibitors are not recommended as treatment for agitation in patients with dementia because they may worsen the agitation,⊗☺ particularly in patients with frontotemporal dementia.

3) **Anticonvulsant mood stabilizers**: Treatment with anticonvulsant mood stabilizers (eg, carbamazepine, valproic acid, gabapentin) in the patients with dementia and NPSs can be considered, but use of these agents should be limited. Carbamazepine can have significant adverse events (particularly in geriatric patients) such as sedation, hyponatremia, and cardiac toxicity, and is a strong enzymatic inducer, with a high likelihood of drug-drug interactions, making the risk-benefit ratio too high to be considered on a routine basis. Valproic acid is less recommended due to very limited efficacy on these symptoms. In general, anticonvulsants are not routinely used in the treatment of NPSs, unless the patient has a comorbid diagnosis of bipolar disorder.

Table 4-12. Pharmacologic agents used in the management of neuropsychiatric symptoms in dementia

Medication category	Daily dose	Adverse-effect monitoring	Comments
Second-generation antipsychotics (SGAs)			
Risperidone (LAI, ODT, liquid)	Initial: 0.25 mg once daily to bid Titration: 0.25-0.5 mg every 3-7 days Max: 2 mg	– Sedation – Postural hypotension – Falls – Anticholinergic adverse effects (dry mouth, constipation, confusion) – EPS, particularly par-kinsonian signs and symptoms (rigidity, bradykinesia, shuf-fling gait, masked facies, tremor) – Olanzapine and que-tiapine more sedating than risperidone or aripiprazole	– Best supported SGA for NPSs – Most likely SGA to cause EPS
Olanzapine (IM, ODT)	Initial: 2.5-5 mg at bedtime Titration: 2.5-5 mg every 3-7 days Max: 10 mg		– Most likely SGA to cause metabolic adverse effects – Availability in rapidly dis-solving preparation advan-tageous in noncompliance
Quetiapine	Initial: 12.5 mg bid Titration: 12.5-25 mg every 3-7 days Max: 150 mg		– Used for Parkinson disease dementia and dementia with Lewy bodies at lower doses due to high sensitivi-ty to EPS – In those with psychosis and Parkinson disease demen-tia, if possible, first reduce dopaminergic agents
Aripiprazole	Initial: 2-5 mg daily Titration: 2-5 mg every 3-7 days Max: 10 mg		– Most likely SGA to cause akathisia (restlessness)
First-generation antipsychotics (FGAs)			
Haloperidol (IM, IV, LAI, liquid)	Initial: 0.25 mg bid Titration: 0.5 mg bid every 3-7 days Max: 1.5 mg bid	– Haloperidol more likely to cause EPS than SGAs	– Gold standard for delirium – Can be given IM in ED when other formulations unavailable or IV in ICU; monitor ECG for QTc pro-longation, especially when dosage ≥3 mg/d
SSRI antidepressants			
Citalopram	Initial: 5-10 mg daily Titration: 10 mg every 7 days Max: 20 mg	– Headache – Nausea (give with food to ↓ GI upset) – Diarrhea – Sweating – Insomnia – Hyponatremia – Risk of GI bleed – QTc prolongation at higher doses of citalo-pram – Risk of falls, fractures, and osteoporosis	– Citalopram is the best supported SSRI for NPS; monitor ECG for QTc pro-longation, especially when dosage ≥20 mg/d – In FTD patients, SSRIs are first-line agents, particular-ly for repetitive behaviors
Escitalo-pram	Initial: 5 mg daily Titration: 5 mg every 7 days Max: 10 mg		
Sertraline	Initial: 25 mg daily Titration: 25 mg every 7 days Max: 100 mg		

Medication category	Daily dose	Adverse-effect monitoring	Comments
Anticonvulsants			
Carbamaze-pine	Initial: 50 mg daily Titration: 50 mg every 7-14 days, bid to tid Max: 500 mg	– Sedation – Ataxia/falls – Neutropenia – Hyponatremia – ↑ Liver function tests – Skin rash	– Risk of drug-drug interactions – Monitor drug level
Agents for sleep			
Lorazepam (IM, IV, liquid)	Initial: 0.25-0.5 mg at bedtime Titration: 0.25-0.5 mg every 3-7 days Max: 2 mg	BZPs: – Sedation – Confusion/cognitive impairment – Ataxia/falls – Disinhibition Trazodone: – Postural hypotension – Dry mouth – Constipation	– BZPs for short-term use only – BZPs carry risk of tolerance/dependence, falls, worsening cognition, and withdrawal upon discontinuation; their use should be limited to situations that may require rapid onset of action while under close observation – Trazodone can be used in FTD, in 25 mg bid to tid starting dose to 100-300 mg daily
Zopiclone	Initial: 3.75 mg at bedtime Titration: 3.75 mg every 3-7 days Max: 15 mg		
Trazodone	Initial: 25 mg at bedtime Titration: 25 mg every 3-7 days Max: 100 mg		
Cholinesterase inhibitors			
Donepezil	Initial: 2.5-5 mg daily Titration: 2.5-5 mg every 4-6 weeks Max: 10 mg (23 mg slow release)	– GI upset (nausea/vomiting/diarrhea) – Loss of appetite – ↓ GI adverse effects with patch – Insomnia, hypervivid dreams – Bradycardia – Urinary incontinence – Muscle cramps	– ChEIs are first-line agents for psychosis in Parkinson disease dementia and dementia with Lewy bodies – ChEIs can be beneficial in apathy – Take with food to minimize GI upset – Rotate patch site – In FTD, ChEIs are contraindicated
Rivastig-mine	Initial: 1.5 mg bid Titration: 1.5 mg every 4 weeks Max: 12 mg		
	Initial: 4.6 mg patch Titration: 9.5 mg every 4 weeks Max: 13.3 mg		
Galantam-ine	Initial: 8 mg daily Titration: 8 mg every 4 weeks Max: 24 mg		Extended-release formulation

bid, 2 times a day; BZP, benzodiazepine; ChEI, cholinesterase inhibitor; ECG, electrocardiogram; ED, emergency department; EPS, extrapyramidal symptoms; FGA, first-generation antipsychotic; FTD, frontotemporal dementia; GI, gastrointestinal; ICU, intensive care unit; IM, available as intramuscular formulation; IV, available as intravenous formulation; LAI, available as long-acting injectable formulation; NPS, neuropsychiatric symptom; ODT, available as orally dissolving/disintegrating tablet; SGA, second-generation antipsychotic; SSRI, selective serotonin reuptake inhibitor; tid, 3 times a day.

4) **Antipsychotics**: Psychosis and aggression in dementia requiring pharmacotherapy with antipsychotics may respond best to risperidone, olanzapine, and aripiprazole. The use of haloperidol should be limited to addressing agitation or psychosis in delirium only, using low doses for a brief period of time until symptoms clear. When the target problem behaviors are wandering, social withdrawal, vocalizing, pacing, touching, or incontinence, antipsychotics are not usually effective and are thus not recommended.

If the behavioral disturbances such as agitation or aggression are not part of a psychotic disorder or bipolar mania but rather nonspecific symptoms of dementia, antipsychotics have modest benefits at best. The serious adverse effects of these agents, such as increased risk of cerebrovascular events and mortality, necessitate the use of antipsychotic medications as a last resort to treat NPSs of dementia and **only** if nondrug therapies have failed to be effective **and** the patients' actions threaten themselves or others.◔◖ Notably, from 2005 onwards, regulatory agencies in North America, Europe, and Australia have issued black box warnings on the increased risk of cerebrovascular events and mortality in patients with dementia receiving either first-generation antipsychotics (FGAs) or SGAs. However, Health Canada indicates the use of an SGA, risperidone, for "the short-term symptomatic management of aggression or psychotic symptoms in patients with **severe** dementia of the Alzheimer type unresponsive to nonpharmacologic approaches and when there is a risk of harm to self or others." Common adverse events of antipsychotics include sedation; gait changes; increased risk of falls and fracture; extrapyramidal symptoms, including parkinsonism, dystonias, and akathisia (particularly with antipsychotics with high D_2 blockade, such as haloperidol, risperidone, and aripiprazole); and metabolic adverse effects of weight gain and dyslipidemia (higher risk in female patients, with olanzapine and quetiapine). Longer-term use of FGAs (and some SGAs) carries the risk of tardive dyskinesia, particularly in older female patients with dementia and comorbid depressive or bipolar disorders. Because there is no single most effective and safe treatment option, physicians prescribing antipsychotics to patients with dementia should trade off between the effectiveness and safety of these medications in the treatment of NPSs.◔◖

Most behavioral symptoms of dementia are intermittent and often do not persist for longer than 3 months. Therefore, when antipsychotic treatment is instituted, regular attempts to withdraw these medications are recommended.◔◖ Generally, stopping antipsychotics for patients with dementia does not cause problems, even in those with long-term use, and it is suggested that discontinuation programs should be incorporated into routine practice. Therefore, antipsychotics can be safely discontinued in specific cases without short-term worsening of behavioral symptoms. Predictors of successful discontinuation include lower daily doses of antipsychotics and lower baseline severity of behavioral symptoms. A small subgroup of patients with more severe NPSs at baseline may be unable to tolerate discontinuation of antipsychotics and will require long-term treatment. It remains uncertain whether discontinuation of antipsychotics leads to a decrease in mortality.

5) **Benzodiazepines**: Despite widespread use, there is a lack of evidence for prescribing benzodiazepines safely in older adults. The risks clearly outweigh the benefits, where large-scale studies consistently show that the risk of worsening cognition, falls, and hip fractures leading to hospitalization and death can more than double in older adults taking benzodiazepines. According to Choosing Wisely Canada, the use of benzodiazepines should be reserved for alcohol withdrawal symptoms in delirium tremens or severe generalized anxiety disorder unresponsive to other therapies; other acceptable indications would be neuroleptic malignant syndrome or catatonia. Outside of these specific indications, benzodiazepines should not be used as a first-line agent in treating agitation or other behavioral disturbances in patients with NPSs of dementia. Initiating (risk of dependence) or discontinuing (risk of

Table 4-13. Common neuropsychiatric symptom clusters in dementia and pharmacologic strategies

NPSs in dementia	Pharmacologic options	"Better-not-to-use" pharmacologic options
Agitation/ aggression	– Serotonergic antidepressants (eg, citalopram, sertraline, trazodone) – Shorter-acting BZPs (eg, lorazepam, oxazepam) – Anticonvulsants (eg, carbamazepine, valproic acid) if comorbid bipolar disorder – SGAs (eg, risperidone, olanzapine, quetiapine, aripiprazole) – FGAs (eg, haloperidol)	– Do not use SGAs/FGAs as first choice – Avoid highly anticholinergic FGAs/SGAs (eg, chlorpromazine, perphenazine, clozapine) – Avoid highly dopamine-blocking FGAs and SGAs in parkinsonism-related dementias (eg, haloperidol, risperidone) – Limit use of anticonvulsants (eg, carbamazepine, valproic acid) if no comorbid bipolar disorder – ChEIs may worsen agitation; do not use in FTD – Avoid BZDs/sedative-hypnotics as first choice
Apathy	– ChEIs (eg, donepezil, rivastigmine, galantamine) – Antidepressants – Psychostimulants (eg, methylphenidate, modafinil)	– FGAs/SGAs may worsen apathy – Antidepressants at high doses may worsen apathy
Psychosis	– ChEIs (eg, donepezil, rivastigmine, galantamine) – SGAs – FGAs	– Limit use of FGAs and most of SGAs (except quetiapine) in dementia with Lewy bodies and Parkinson disease dementia due to worsening of EPSs in dose-dependent fashion – Limit use of FGAs/SGAs in prolonged QTc syndrome (except aripiprazole)
Depression	– Antidepressants (eg, citalopram, escitalopram, sertraline, venlafaxine, bupropion, mirtazapine)	– Avoid highly anticholinergic antidepressants (eg, clomipramine, amitriptyline, doxepin)
Disinhibition	– Antidepressants (eg, citalopram, trazodone) – Antiandrogens (eg, medroxyprogesterone acetate) – GnRH analogues (eg, leuprolide) – SGAs/FGAs (eg, quetiapine, haloperidol)	– BZPs may worsen disinhibition – Dopamine agonists may worsen disinhibition
Sleep disturbances	– Antidepressants (eg, mirtazapine, trazodone) – Shorter-acting BZPs/sedative-hypnotics, if necessary, for a brief period of time (eg, lorazepam, oxazepam, temazepam, zopiclone)	– Avoid BZDs/sedative-hypnotics as first choice – Do not use long-acting BZPs (eg, diazepam, chlordiazepoxide, flurazepam) due to drug accumulation, active metabolites

BZP, benzodiazepine; ChEI, cholinesterase inhibitor; EPS, extrapyramidal symptom; FGA, first-generation antipsychotic; FTD, frontotemporal dementia; GnRH, gonadotropin-releasing hormone; NPS, neuropsychiatric symptom; SGA, second-generation antipsychotic.

withdrawal) sedative-hypnotics in hospital can have substantial impact on their long-term use. Short-term use, on demand use (as needed), or use as a chemical restraint of shorter-acting benzodiazepines, such as lorazepam (often in conjunction with haloperidol), can be considered to address severe agitation or aggression. In practice, many older adults present with NPSs who have been on benzodiazepines for decades and are likely to continue to need this class of drugs; however, the goal is to taper and use the lowest doses of short- or intermediate-acting agents (lorazepam, clonazepam) that are effective. Ultra-short-acting agents, such as alprazolam, are not recommended due to their amnestic and significant dependence effects.

A more comprehensive review of the common pharmacologic agents used in the management of NPSs in dementia: →Table 4-12.

Some common pharmacologic options to use versus "better-not-to-use" pharmacologic options for the main NPS clusters in dementia: →Table 4-13.

5. Depressive Disorders

→ DEFINITION, EPIDEMIOLOGY

The group of depressive disorders share a common set of symptoms including periods of either low mood or loss of pleasure (anhedonia) and are accompanied by sleep changes, feelings of guilt, low energy, poor concentration, appetite changes, psychomotor slowing or agitation, and suicidal ideation.

In the fifth edition of the American Psychiatric Association's *Diagnostic and Statistical Manual of Mental Disorders* (*DSM-5*), depressive disorders are classified into:

1) Major depressive disorder (MDD), single and recurrent episodes.
2) Persistent depressive disorder (previously "dysthymia").
3) Premenstrual dysphoric disorder.
4) Substance/medication-induced depressive disorder.
5) Depressive disorder due to another medical condition.
6) Other specified depressive disorder.
7) Unspecified depressive disorder.

MDD (or "depression," as it is commonly known) is a debilitating condition that affects many people worldwide. Average lifetime prevalence rates have been reported between 11.1% and 14.6%.

In terms of disability, unipolar depression (depression in the absence of hypomania or mania) was ranked as the first leading cause of years lost to disability (YLD) and the ninth highest leading cause of all disability-adjusted life years (DALYs) in the world in 2012 by the World Health Organization. Responsible for 2.8% of all DALYs, depression caused similar rates of disability when compared to road injury (2.9%) and HIV/AIDS (3.4%).

→ CLINICAL FEATURES AND DIAGNOSIS

Screening for Major Depressive Disorder

1. It is important to accurately recognize, diagnose, and treat depression.

2. Depressed patients do not always present with mood complaints. A substantial proportion of depressed patients present only with somatic complaints.◔

3. Goals of assessment include establishing rapport, evaluating for safety, assessing for comorbidities, and providing patient education.

Table 5-1. Screening for depression: 9-question Patient Health Questionnaire (PHQ-9)
Questions
Over the last 2 weeks, how often have you been bothered by any of the following problems?
1. Little interest or pleasure in doing things
2. Feeling down, depressed, or hopeless
3. Trouble falling or staying asleep, or sleeping too much
4. Feeling tired or having little energy
5. Poor appetite or overeating
6. Feeling bad about yourself or that you are a failure or have let yourself or your family down
7. Trouble concentrating on things, such as reading the newspaper or watching television
8. Moving or speaking so slowly that other people could have noticed. Or the opposite: being so fidgety or restless that you have been moving around a lot more than usual
9. Thoughts that you would be better off dead or of hurting yourself in some way
Each criterion is scored as "0" (not at all) to "3" (nearly every day). A total score ≥10 has a sensitivity of 88% and a specificity of 88% for major depression.

Table 5-2. Screening for depression: 2-stem questions instrument
During the past month, have you often been bothered by feeling down, depressed, or hopeless? During the past month, have you often been bothered by little interest or pleasure in doing things?
Answering "no" to both of these questions is effective in excluding depression.

4. Screening for depression can be done using several tools, which have been shown to be moderately but equally effective. They include:

1) Patient Health Questionnaire (PHQ-9): Examples of the PHQ-9 and 2-stem questionnaire: →Table 5-1, →Table 5-2. The 2-stem question instrument is a highly sensitive screen for depression (98% sensitivity, 86% specificity), however the 9-item questionnaire allows for assessing the response to treatment at follow-up visits by showing the change in the total score.

2) Quick Inventory of Depressive Symptomatology-Self Report (QIDS-SR).

3) Beck Depression Inventory first (BDI-I) or second (BDI-II) edition.

4) Zung Self-Rating Scale.

5) Center for Epidemiologic Studies-Depression (CES-D) scale.

5. For specific populations, other screening tools include the Geriatrics Depression Scale and the Edinburgh Postnatal Depression Scale.

Diagnosing Depression

According to the *DSM-5*, a diagnosis of MDD requires the presence of ≥5 symptoms, of which at least 1 must be either depressed mood or anhedonia. Additional symptoms may include sleep changes, feelings of worthlessness or guilt, low energy, poor concentration, appetite changes, psychomotor slowing or agitation, and suicidal ideation. These symptoms must continue for 2 weeks, cause significant distress or functional impairment, and not be better explained by other mental disorders, other medical disorders, or the effect of a substance. These criteria constitute a major depressive episode (MDE). One or more major depressive episodes make up MDD.

Differential diagnosis includes other psychiatric conditions, medical conditions, and substance use.

Mild depression is defined in the *DSM-5* as "few, if any, symptoms in excess of those required" for the diagnosis. The intensity of symptoms is "manageable" and there is "minor impairment" in functioning.

Moderate depression according to the *DSM-5* refers to situations where the intensity and impairment due to depressive symptoms fall between mild and severe.

Severe depression according to the *DSM-5* refers to situations where "the number of symptoms is substantially in excess of that required" for the diagnosis, the symptoms are "seriously distressing and unmanageable," and they "markedly interfere" with functioning.

Other Forms of Depression

Depressive symptoms occur in a number of mental disorders. In medical settings, adjustment disorder with depressed mood and MDD are the most commonly seen. Adjustment disorders occur in response to a stressor, with symptoms of marked distress or impaired functioning. Symptoms must develop within 3 months of the stressor occurring and should resolve within 6 months of the stressor ending.

Although MDD can also occur after a stressor, the key difference between MDD and adjustment disorder is whether the patient perceives their low mood would remit if the stressor were removed. In adjustment disorder the removal of the stressor would lead to remission of depressive symptoms. In MDD the removal of the stressor might improve symptoms marginally but not completely.

→ RISK FACTORS

Risk Factors in the Development of Depression

A number of risk factors have been identified in the development of depression. Risk factors include female sex, chronic medical conditions, sleep disorders, low socioeconomic status, recent bereavement, positive family history, childhood maltreatment history, and substance use. Further information about the strength of those associations: →Table 5-3.

In elderly patients, risk factors for depression include institutionalized living, dementia, female sex, chronic disease, and sensory impairment. It should be also noted that the elderly are at risk for suicide: in 2011, there were 517 deaths by suicide in Canada.

Depression due to a General Medical Condition

Some medical conditions cause symptoms that overlap with those of depression and can be said to mimic depression (eg, hypothyroidism), while others appear to increase the risk of developing depression or may have a joint factor that causes depression (eg, multiple sclerosis).

It is important to screen each patient for other simple causes of depressive symptoms that are plausible within each patient's own context and treat the underlying condition when possible. Treatment of depression should be considered when depressive symptoms appear to be interfering with functioning and persist despite treatment of the underlying medical condition.

Medical conditions that may be associated with depressive symptoms include anemia (particularly in the elderly), hypothyroidism, stroke, Parkinson disease, Huntington disease, Alzheimer disease, traumatic brain injury, multiple sclerosis, systemic lupus erythematosus, neoplasm, HIV, cytokine-induced sickness behavior, and delirium.

Medication-Induced Depression

In the literature, there are several reports of medications causing depression. However, most claims are not supported by high-quality evidence.

There is low-quality evidence suggesting that a variety of medications may cause or be associated with depressive symptoms, including barbiturates,

Table 5-3. Risk factors for development of depression

Individual	Psychologic
Chronic medical condition (9.3%-23.0% of patients with chronic physical disease have comorbid depression compared to 3.2% without chronic disease; $P<0.0001$) 　CHF (OR, 1.96; 95% CI, 1.23-3.11) 　HTN (OR, 2.00; 95% CI, 1.74-2.31) 　DM (OR, 1.96; 95% CI, 1.59-2.42) 　CAD (OR, 2.30; 95% CI, 1.94-2.68) 　CVA (OR, 3.15; 95% CI, 2.33-4.25) 　COPD (OR, 3.21; 95% CI, 2.72-3.79) 　ESRD (OR, 3.56; 95% CI, 2.61-4.87) 　Any chronic condition (OR, 2.61; 95% CI, 2.31-2.94) 　Migraine (RR, 1.53; 95% CI, 1.35-1.74) 　Headache (RR, 1.44; 95% CI, 1.32-1.56) 　Cancer (HR, 3.55; 95% CI, 2.79-4.52) 　Chronic lung disease (HR, 2.21; 95% CI, 1.64-2.79) 　Heart disease (HR, 1.45; 95% CI, 1.09-1.93) 　Arthritis (HR, 1.46; 95% CI, 1.11-1.92)	**Maltreatment in childhood** 　Emotional abuse (F/M: OR, 2.7/2.5; 95% CI, 2.3-3.2/1.9-3.2) 　Physical abuse (F/M: OR, 2.1/1.6; 95% CI, 1.8-2.4/1.4-1.9) 　Sexual abuse (F/M: OR, 1.8/1.6; 95% CI, 1.5-2.0/1.3-2.0) 　Witnessed interpersonal violence (F/M: OR, 2.1/1.5; 95% CI, 1.8-2.5/1.2-1.9)
Female sex (OR, 1.83; 95% CI, 1.43-2.35; $P<0.001$)	**Stressful life events**
Sleep disorder 　Insomnia (OR, 4.0; 95% CI, 2.2-7.0) 　Hypersomnia (OR, 2.9; 95% CI, 1.5-5.6)	Recent bereavement (10%-20% of bereaved population develop clinical depression)
Positive family history 　One parent affected (OR, 2.7; 95% CI, 2.1-3.5) 　Two parents affected (OR, 3.0; 95% CI, 2.2-4.1)	**Substance use and addictions** 　Ethanol (OR, 1.50; 95% CI, 1.17-1.92); $P<0.001$) 　Marijuana (OR, 1.41; 95% CI, 1.21-1.65; $P<0.001$) 　Other illicit drugs (OR, 1.65; 95% CI, 1.34-2.02, $P<0.001$)
Low socioeconomic status (low education/income/social status/combination) (OR, 1.81; 95% CI, 1.57-2.10, $P<0.001$)	

CAD, chronic artery disease; CHF, chronic heart failure; CI, confidence interval; COPD, chronic obstructive pulmonary disease; CVA, cerebrovascular accident; DM, diabetes mellitus; ESRD, end-stage renal disease; F, female; HR, hazard ratio; HTN, hypertension; M, male; OR, odds ratio; RR, relative risk.

vigabatrin, topiramate, flunarizine, glucocorticoids, mefloquine, efavirenz, and interferon α.

Because individual response to treatment varies between patients, if depressive symptoms are noted to occur temporally after initiation of a medication and remit when the medication is stopped, consider using another agent.

➡ TREATMENT

General Considerations

Please remember that **depression is not simply "the blues," and it is not a sign of a character flaw or weak will**. The compassionate clinician recognizes that patients with depression will not improve by being advised to "pull themselves together" or to "just get over it." **Depression is a serious illness with profound consequences that can—and should—be treated in this modern era.**

Be sure to listen attentively to your patient with compassion and sensitivity, and do not underestimate their complaints. Be advised that the safety of your patient is paramount, and thus, any declaration of suicidal ideation should be assessed carefully, and appropriate action taken when necessary.

It is important to note that there are multiple management options to treating depression, including psychotherapy, pharmacologic approaches, electroconvulsive therapy (ECT), or a combination of these modalities. The following is a more in-depth explanation of management approaches based on the severity of symptoms.

Appropriate management should be **individualized** to each patient according to:

1) The **nature** of the disorder (that is, confirm the diagnosis of depression, exclude other causes).

2) The **severity** of symptoms.

3) Any medical or psychiatric **comorbidities** (including the possibility of drug-drug interactions and pregnancy).

4) **Previous response** to treatment (in the patient or other family members).

5) The **existing support**, resources, preferences, and psychosocial environment of the patient.

The assessment of efficacy of pharmacologic treatment of depression is hampered by short duration of trials, large number of patients not completing studies, and confounding of treatment effect by spontaneous remissions. The treatment effect is also influenced by the various methods of measurement of depressive disorder and outcomes of interests adding to the limitations of the generalizability of trial findings. The overall body of evidence suggests shortening of depressive episodes and possibly prevention of recurrent episodes, especially among patients with previous recurrences. The suggestions include continuation of treatment for up to 12 months after remission and possibly longer or permanently after consecutive relapses. Such relapses are common, and after discontinuation of treatment about one-third of patients will experience relapse of symptoms within 1 year.

Management of Mild Depression

1. Self-care is recommended:

1) NEST-S: "**N**utrition, **e**xercise, **s**leep, **t**ime for self, and **s**ocial support" are effective in the management of mild depression.

2) Behavioral activation: Encourage physical activity.

2. Psychotherapy is effective and recommended in the management of mild depression:

1) **Cognitive behavioral therapy (CBT)**: CBT involves 12 to 16 sessions of psychotherapy treatment that identifies and treats maladaptive behaviors, cognitive distortions, negative schemas, and the cognitive triad of a negative view of self, the world, and the future in order to improve mood symptoms.◉◉

2) **Interpersonal therapy (IPT)**: Interpersonal therapy is a 12- to 16-session psychotherapy treatment that focuses on improving mood symptoms by identifying and working through distressing life events, which include complicated bereavement (grief), role disputes (interpersonal conflicts), and role transitions.◉◉

3) **Problem-solving therapy (PST)**: The theory behind problem-solving therapy is to improve mood by improving patients' problem-solving skills. The goal of this psychotherapy is to identify the patient's problems, consider various solutions, decide on the most appropriate solution, prepare a plan to carry out that solution, and assess whether the solution was effective.◉◯

4) **Self-management resources** such as workbooks and websites are suggested when low resources exist for traditional psychotherapy.

3. Free examples developed at Simon Fraser University (www.sfu.ca) include:

1) *Antidepressant Skills Workbook* (for adults).

2) *Antidepressant Skills at Work: Dealing with Mood Problems in the Workplace.*

3) *Positive Coping with Health Conditions.*

4) *Managing Depression: A Self-help Skills Resource for Women Living With Depression During Pregnancy, After Delivery, and Beyond.*

5) *Dealing with Depression* (for adolescents).

4. Free interactive websites include the MoodGYM training program.

5. Resources available at cost include:

1) Greenberger D, Padesky, C. *Mind Over Mood: Change How You Feel by Changing the Way You Think.* New York: Guilford Press; 1995.

2) Beating the Blues (website): www.beatingtheblues.co.uk.

Management of Moderate Depression

Combination therapy of **antidepressants and psychotherapy** is recommended to increase the probability of remission. First-line treatment may involve drugs from different classes: selective serotonin reuptake inhibitors (SSRIs), serotonin-norepinephrine reuptake inhibitors (SNRIs), noradrenergic and specific serotonergic antidepressants (NaSSAs), bupropion, and reversible inhibitors of monoamine oxidase A (RIMAs), with some suggestion that escitalopram and sertraline have the best balance between efficacy and acceptability.● Other useful modalities include different types of psychotherapy (CBT, IPT, PST), as outlined above.

Management of Severe Depression

1. Combination therapy of **antidepressants and psychotherapy** is recommended to increase the probability of remission.

2. **Major depressive episodes with psychotic features** can be treated with a combination of an antidepressant and an antipsychotic medication.

3. **ECT** should be considered for severe, treatment-resistant depression or depression with psychotic features.

Management of Depression in the Elderly

1. **Escitalopram and sertraline** are considered first-line antidepressant treatments for the elderly, especially for severe depression, because of efficacy and tolerance.

2. Moderate-intensity **exercise** (30-minute sessions 3 to 5 times a week for 3 to 4 months) is an effective adjunct for depression treatment in the elderly.

3. **Psychotherapy**: CBT, IPT, and PST have shown efficacy.

4. Be mindful of **adverse effects**, which may be exaggerated in the elderly (eg, polypharmacy interactions, any anticholinergic adverse effects). In general, elderly patients should be started on lower doses of psychotropic medications and dose escalation should occur slowly, with the goal of attaining a therapeutic dose.

Pharmacotherapy

1. **Choosing an antidepressant medication**: The choice of an antidepressant, when indicated, should be discussed with the patient. The selection should be based on the patient's preference, type of symptoms, adverse effect profile of the medication, comorbidities, and concomitant medication use. When selecting an antidepressant, most clinicians start with an SSRI, as this class is well tolerated and effective.

1) SSRIs, SNRIs, and newer antidepressants such as bupropion or mirtazapine are considered first-line medications for severe depression.

2) TCAs are considered second-line treatment and monoamine oxidase inhibitors (MAOIs) are considered third-line agents due to their adverse-effect profiles.

Table 5-4. Major adverse effects and interactions of different classes of antidepressant agents

Class	Examples	Major adverse effects
Selective serotonin reuptake inhibitors (SSRIs) (considered second generation)	Citalopram Escitalopram Fluoxetine Paroxetine Sertraline	Suicidal ideation, CNS, GI upset, weight gain, sexual dysfunction, hyponatremia, serotonin syndrome, bleeding risk (especially when combined with NSAIDs)
Fluvoxamine (considered second generation)	(belongs to SSRI class but is less commonly used for depression)	SSRI adverse effects ± palpitations, tachycardia, malaise, sedation
Serotonin-norepinephrine reuptake inhibitors (SNRIs) (considered second generation)	Desvenlafaxine Duloxetine Venlafaxine	GI, weight gain, CNS, sexual dysfunction, dermatologic
Noradrenergic and specific serotonergic antidepressants (NaSSAs) (considered second generation)	Mirtazapine	Increased appetite, weight gain, postural hypotension, drowsiness
Bupropion (considered second generation)		GI, CNS, dermatologic
Tricyclic antidepressants (TCAs) (considered first generation)	Amitriptyline Desipramine Imipramine Nortriptyline	Arrhythmias, CNS, sedation, anticholinergic, endocrine, hyponatremia, GI, weight gain; high lethality with overdose
Reversible inhibitors of monoamine oxidase A (RIMAs) (considered second generation)	Moclobemide	Sleep disturbances, CNS, GI, dermatologic
Monoamine oxidase inhibitor (MAOI) (considered first generation)	Phenelzine	Postural hypotension, sleep disturbances, CNS, GI, fetal malformations; can cause **hypertensive crisis** when combined with certain foods and medications, in particular other antidepressants (eg, during tapering course)

CNS, central nervous system; GI, gastrointestinal tract; NSAID, nonsteroidal anti-inflammatory drug.

A network meta-analysis comparing different antidepressants ranked the following antidepressants as the top 5 based on their efficacy and tolerability: mirtazapine, escitalopram, venlafaxine, sertraline, and citalopram.

Other treatment options exist, such as the addition of second-generation antipsychotics (eg, olanzapine, risperidone, aripiprazole) along with other classes of antidepressants. However, more complex treatment regimens should be used under the supervision of a psychiatrist.

2. Major adverse effects and interactions of antidepressant agents: →Table 5-4.

3. Suggestions for initiating antidepressant medications:

1) Before starting any antidepressant agent, consider completing **baseline liver function tests and a metabolic workup**, such as screening for diabetes mellitus, dyslipidemia, and thyroid disease.

Table 5-5. Dosing of common first-line medications shown to be effective in treating major depression (based on British National Formulary [BNF] 72)

Medication	Starting dose (mg/d)	Usual dose (mg/d)
Selective serotonin reuptake inhibitors		
Citalopram	20	20-40
Escitalopram	10	10-20
Fluoxetine	20	20-60
Paroxetine	20	20-50
Sertraline	50	50-200
Serotonin-norepinephrine reuptake inhibitors		
Venlafaxine, immediate release	75	75-375
Venlafaxine, extended release	75	75-375
Duloxetine	60	60-120
Norepinephrine-serotonin modulator		
Mirtazapine	15	15-45
Dopamine-norepinephrine reuptake inhibitor		
Bupropion, immediate release	150	300-450
Bupropion, sustained release	150	300-400
Bupropion, extended release	150	300-450

For some of these medications (such as tricyclic antidepressants), the upper dosing limit reflects **risk of toxicity** or need for plasma level assessment, whereas others (such as selective serotonin reuptake inhibitors) can be used safely at higher doses.

Elderly patients, patients with anxiety disorders, patients with liver disease or other major medical comorbidities should receive a **lower starting dose**.

Starting doses should be **increased gradually** until therapeutic dose is reached or the patient achieves remission.

2) Obtain an **electrocardiogram (ECG)** to determine any baseline arrhythmias as well as the QTc (which can be prolonged with psychotropic use) prior to initiation of a medication.

3) Consider **follow-up every 1 to 2 weeks** when titrating an antidepressant. The frequency can then be reduced to every 2 to 4 weeks when a therapeutic dose is reached, depending on the severity of depression and response to treatment.

4) In selecting the appropriate antidepressant agent, **patient comorbidities** should be taken into account along with any adverse effects of the medications. For example, mirtazapine is associated with increased appetite and weight gain, and therefore may be avoided in patients with obesity and diabetes mellitus.

4. Dosing of common first-line medications effective in treating major depression: →Table 5-5.

5. Assessing treatment response:

1) Initial treatment response: Most clinical trials define clinical response as a ≥50% reduction in the score on a depression rating scale, while clinical remission is defined as a score within the normal range of the scale. Improvement may begin **within 1 to 2 weeks of treatment**; however, it can take **>8 weeks** for response and/or remission.

2) Adjusting medication treatment:

   a) If there is **<20% improvement** on one of the depression scales **after 2 weeks**, consider increasing the dose of medication.

   b) If there is **≥20% improvement after 4 to 6 weeks** (but not remission), consider an additional 2 to 4 weeks of the same treatment.

   c) If there is **no further improvement**, consider other treatment strategies: nonpharmacologic interventions such as CBT and IPT; switching antidepressants; augmentation (combining an antidepressant with a second medication) under the supervision of a psychiatrist; ECT under the supervision of a psychiatrist.

6. Length of therapy: Pharmacotherapy should be **continued for at least 6 months** after remission. For those with recurrence of depression or risk factors for recurrence, treatment is recommended to be continued for **at least 2 years**. Depending on the number of recurrent episodes, longer treatment courses can be considered. Dosing should be continued at the **same effective dose**, not a reduced dose.

7. Switching antidepressant medications⟳: No difference exists between switching within the same class of medications versus switching to a different class of medications.

1) The technique for safe switching to a different class of antidepressant agents depends on **drug-drug interactions** and the pharmacologic properties of the medications. For example, when switching from SSRIs to MAOIs, withdraw SSRIs first and wait for 2 weeks (in the case of fluoxetine, wait for 5 to 6 weeks) before starting MAOIs.

2) If switching an SSRI to **venlafaxine**, cross-taper cautiously and start venlafaxine at a smaller dose of 37.5 mg.

3) If switching from **mirtazapine** to a **TCA**, withdraw mirtazapine first and then start the TCA.

4) When stopping antidepressants, consider reducing the dose gradually over 4 weeks.

8. Tapering medications: Abrupt discontinuation of antidepressant agents can lead to **withdrawal symptoms**. Common antidepressant withdrawal symptoms include nausea, headache, light-headedness, chills, body aches, insomnia, and neurologic symptoms such as paresthesias, and "electric shock--like" phenomena. When stopping antidepressants, consider reducing the dose gradually over 4 weeks if tolerated.

➔ PROGNOSIS

Remission is defined as a period of ≥2 months with no symptoms, or only 1 to 2 symptoms present to no more than a mild degree. It can be expected within 3 months for 60% of patients and within 1 year for 80% of patients, regardless of whether the depression is treated.

Decreased rates of remission are expected if the patient has a comorbid anxiety disorder, personality disorder, psychotic symptoms, or severe symptoms.

The **risk of recurrence is higher** in young patients, individuals with previous multiple episodes, and in patients whose previous episodes were considered severe.

6. Difficult Patient

→ DEFINITION

The term "difficult patient" does not denote a specific diagnostic entity and does not assign blame but rather reflects certain characteristics of the **interaction between the physician and the patient**.

A difficult patient is defined more by the physician's response than by specific criteria. The description "difficult patient encounter" is more accurate. Here we define "the difficult patient" as one towards whom the physician experiences strong negative emotions: anxiety, dread, fear, anger, frustration, irritation, despair, or hopelessness.

The concept of the difficult patient has emerged out of medical rather than psychiatric settings. We have chosen to present the discussion of the difficult patient within the psychiatry section of the *McMaster Textbook of Internal Medicine*, as key principles in psychiatric assessment and management are relevant to the care of these individuals.

Many medical and psychiatric conditions present intrinsic difficulties with diagnosis or treatment: cancer, diabetes, chronic obstructive pulmonary disease, schizophrenia. However, this is different from the concept of "difficult patient" or "difficult patient encounters" as used in the literature. Such patients cut across all diagnostic groups.

It is estimated that 15% to 20% of patient encounters in medical settings are perceived as "difficult."● Physicians may describe such patients as demanding with high expectations, emotionally draining and time-consuming, or requesting special treatment. The patients may appear angry, intimidating, or noncompliant.

Patient characteristics identified in studies included psychosomatic complaints, mild to moderate depression, and personality problems. Symptoms may be vague, and the patients may be perceived as overreacting to them. These patients had more physical symptoms, higher use of services, and worse functional status. They had frequently experienced recent stress and depressive or anxiety disorders.

Certain patient vulnerability factors may be predictive of difficult encounters, such as the presence of a comorbid psychiatric disorder, risky behaviors (eg, violence, substance abuse), high use of health-care services, and social determinants (isolation, lack of housing, finances, language barrier), in addition to illness complexity and chronicity.

In observational studies physicians involved in encounters perceived as difficult were less experienced, less disposed to dealing with the psychosocial aspects of medicine, and had a less open communicative style.

Difficult interactions may lead to physician and patient dissatisfaction, conflict, demoralization, patient complaints, higher liability claims, and poorer treatment outcomes.

→ ETIOLOGY AND PATHOGENESIS

Difficult encounters cut across all diagnoses and result from individual patient factors, physician factors, and organizational factors.

Patient Factors

All of us possess a unique range of personality traits and interpersonal patterns. These patterns develop as a result of inborn temperament combined with early attachment experiences and multiple social, genetic, and environmental factors. Some patterns are maladaptive. "**Personality disorder**" refers to problems in a person's way of viewing himself or herself and others, problems with emotional regulation, and in patterns of behavior. This in turn is associated with difficulties in relationships and social functioning.

In the present psychiatric diagnostic systems, the fifth edition of the American Psychiatric Association's *Diagnostic and Statistical Manual of Mental Disorders* (*DSM-5*) and the *International Classification of Diseases* (*ICD*), personalities are grouped into specific categories, although in actuality personality traits are dimensional and there is no absolute cutoff between "normal" and "abnormal."

Difficult patient encounters may reflect problems with the capacity to regulate emotions; feelings of shame, self-hatred, and mistrust of others; problems with empathy, that is, the ability to appreciate other people's experiences and motivations; inability to see things from the other person's point of view and not understanding the effects of one's own behavior on others; difficulty connecting with other people; problems with closeness to others; and insecure attachment behavior. Although we list them as patient factors, all of those traits may be present in clinicians as well (→Physician Factors, below).

The quality of childhood attachment with caregivers influences the development of neurocircuits involved in emotion regulation and is a major determinant of adult capacity for empathy and establishment of close relationships. Attachment status affects how patients interact with physicians and influences their responses to illness. Individuals with secure attachment tend to be trusting and positive in their approach to seeking help. They will more readily collaborate with the health-care team. Individuals with insecure attachment may be guarded and wary. They may not follow through with treatment and appointments.

Patients whose caregivers in childhood were distant or rejecting can develop "avoidant" attachment, which manifests as inability to establish a trusting relationship. Some may be fearful of dependency, intimacy, or rejection. This may present as active hostility and criticism of the health-care providers.

Certain personality types may have specific difficulties in medical settings. Physical illness may lead to an intensification of preexisting interpersonal difficulties as a result of fear and feelings of loss of control and helplessness. For example:

1) **Narcissistic patients** have problems with self-esteem and are hypersensitive to perceived rejection or mistreatment. They cannot see things from the other person's point of view because of impaired empathy. They may compensate for these deficits by an outward sense of superiority and feelings of entitlement. They may demand special treatment and complain forcefully if they perceive any shortcomings.

2) **Patients with antisocial or psychopathic personality traits** may be withholding or dishonest. They may have a hidden agenda. They may attempt to manipulate the physician by means of flattery or, failing that, threats. They may not conform to lawful and normative ethical behavior. They are orientated towards personal gratification. They lack concern for the feelings or suffering of others. They do not display feelings of empathy, guilt, or remorse. Their relationships with others are characterized by exploitation and may involve deceit, coercion, and intimidation to control others.

3) **Patients with borderline personality traits** are characterized by emotional dysregulation, with more intense mood reactivity and a slower return to baseline. This leads to impulsivity, frequent self-harm, and thoughts of suicide. Angry confrontations with clinical staff are common. Physicians may feel anxious because of the high levels of emotional arousal and the fear that the patient may become violent, elope, or attempt to self-harm.

Physician Factors

These factors may contribute as much or more to difficult encounters. Physician factors include personality traits, psychosocial orientation, and the impact of their own developmental experiences. Those include:

1) **Physician emotional factors**: Self-awareness is very important. Physicians need to become aware of the types of patients or situations that trigger their

discomfort, irritation, or anxiety. This is in part determined by patient factors but also by the physician's own past experiences. Physicians may respond to patients in a way that is not appropriate to the current context but reflects an emotional reaction based on the physician's early childhood. This is referred to as "countertransference." It is exactly the same phenomenon as the patient's transference but in the reverse direction. Transference and countertransference are the unconscious processes in which feelings, attitudes, and expectations from key childhood relationships are transferred or projected onto present relationships and encounters.

Difficult encounters may undermine the physician's own sense of competence and their own self-esteem. If the physician has narcissistic or perfectionistic traits, this can be more difficult and lead to an urge to avoid the patient. Overwork, burnout, and personal health problems may also be factors in the physician's response.

2) **Physician cognitive biases**: Cognitive biases are unconscious thinking modes that may lead to clinical error. Again, physician self-awareness is paramount, as cognitive biases may lead to an incorrect evaluation of the situation, misdiagnosis, and inappropriate management.

  a) Stereotyping is when the physician's thinking is preshaped by expectations that are triggered by other aspects of the patient's presentation.

  b) Anchoring is the tendency to fixate on specific features of the patient's presentation too early in the diagnostic process, leading to premature closure.

  c) Confirmation bias is the tendency to look for evidence that supports the physician's initial impressions while overlooking information that contradicts them. It is caused by an unconscious selective tendency to focus on certain data only. This can lead to erroneous conclusions about the patient's physical issues, behavior, or personality.

  d) Attribution error is the tendency to blame the patient when things go wrong. It may reflect the physician's difficulty in empathizing with the patient or fully appreciating the impact of their physical or psychiatric symptoms.

Patients may be experienced as "difficult" due to the direct effects of an underlying medical illness (eg, systemic lupus erythematosus, multiple sclerosis, hyperthyroidism), an adverse drug effect (eg, glucocorticoids, levodopa, antidepressants), an underlying psychiatric problem, or some combination. This needs to be carefully explored in a way that minimizes the cognitive biases that can result in serious medical errors.

Context

Organizational values and expectations impact on the physician-patient encounter. The prevailing organizational culture influences morale and team functioning.

Team members who become frustrated with particular patients may attempt to redefine the problem as "not my problem." Medical or psychiatry staff may try to label the patient problem as "supratentorial rather than organic," malingering, or a "low pain threshold." Staff may feel that the patient does not belong on a particular service and should be transferred.

These responses may be based on unconscious stigmatization of those with, for example, mental illness, addictions, and certain infections, or belonging to specific socioeconomic or cultural strata, and the false belief that patients are responsible for their symptoms. In the case of mental illness, but also particular medical conditions, some health professionals still cling to outdated ideas that certain illnesses (depression, alcoholism, obesity, carcinoma of the lung) are caused by weakness, personal inadequacy, or irresponsibility. This may result in clinical staff acting out in a punitive way towards the patient, leading to escalation of the problems.

→ TREATMENT AND INTERVENTIONS

Approaches to difficult patient encounters can be regarded as specific and generic. Specific treatment depends on a careful and thorough assessment of physical, psychiatric, psychosocial, and contextual aspects. The patient should be assessed for specific psychiatric disorders, with specific psychotropic medications targeting probable underlying psychiatric syndromes, such as anxiety or depression.

Psychiatric consultation is of value in assessing the contribution of psychiatric morbidity to the clinical presentation. To the extent that acute or chronic psychiatric illness is contributing to the problematic interactions, there may be appropriate evidence-based pharmacologic and psychotherapeutic interventions that are indicated.

Clinical Interview

Generic interventions cut across diagnoses and relate to the conduct of the clinical interview. The Calgary Cambridge guide to the medical interview provides a robust and evidence-based approach to communicating with patients. Below we have extracted some key points.

The following are some of the key areas adapted and emphasized for application to the difficult patient encounter:

1) Building the relationship: Greet the patient. Introduce yourself. Demonstrate respect and interest. Maintain appropriate eye contact, facial expression, posture, as well as pacing, volume, and tone of speech. Accept the legitimacy of patient's views and feelings; be nonjudgmental. Be empathic, communicate understanding and appreciation of the patient's feelings or predicament, express concern, understanding, and willingness to help.

2) Gathering information: Encourage the patient to tell the story of the problems. Use open and closed questioning technique, appropriately moving from open to closed. Listen attentively, allowing the patient to complete statements without interruption. Periodically summarize to verify understanding of what the patient has said. Explore:

   a) The patient's ideas and beliefs regarding the illness.

   b) The patient's concerns regarding each problem.

   c) The patient's expectations.

   Encourage the patient to express their feelings.

3) Explaining and planning: Achieve a shared understanding incorporating the patient's perspective. Provide opportunities and encourage the patient to ask questions, seek clarification, or express doubts. Elicit reactions and feelings regarding information given, acknowledge and address where necessary. Share your own thinking. Make suggestions rather than give directives. Encourage the patient to contribute their own suggestions and preferences. Negotiate a mutually acceptable plan.

4) Closing the encounter: Summarize the session briefly and clarify the plan of care. Check the patient's reactions and concerns about plans and treatments including acceptability.

We believe that adopting this approach will reduce physician uncertainty and avoidance, that empathy and engagement will reduce burnout and anxiety. In the inpatient setting, team support, debrief meetings, and consultation can also be used.

Psychopharmacology

In the context of difficult patient encounters it should be emphasized that drug treatment may not be appropriate. For use of medications for delirium, agitated patients, or depression, see appropriate chapters. In general, nonspecific agitation or anxiety can be treated in the short term with benzodiazepines. However, it should be noted that benzodiazepines can occasionally have a paradoxical effect with increased disinhibition and anger.

→ **PREVENTION OF DIFFICULT ENCOUNTERS**

1. It is of key importance to gain physician self-awareness of own feelings and biases.

2. Make adequate time for the encounter.

3. Use specific validated interview methods.

4. Develop an agreed treatment plan.

5. Treat underlying psychiatric and medical disorders.

7. Eating Disorders

→ **DEFINITIONS AND CLINICAL FEATURES**

Eating disorders are severe mental illnesses that include both psychiatric and physical symptoms. They can result in substantial morbidity and mortality. Early identification, treatment, and intervention are critically important.

The essential features of the 5 most common eating disorders are as follows:

1) **Anorexia nervosa (AN)**:
   a) Persistent restriction of caloric/food intake, often resulting in significantly low body weight.
   b) Intense fear of gaining weight or behaviors that interfere with weight gain.
   c) Disturbed body image.

2) **Bulimia nervosa (BN)**:
   a) Binge eating episodes.
   b) Inappropriate compensatory behaviors (eg, vomiting, fasting, excessive exercise).
   c) The binge eating and inappropriate compensatory behaviors both occur, on average, ≥ 1 a week for 3 months.

3) **Binge eating disorder (BED)**:
   a) Binge eating episodes in the absence of inappropriate compensatory behaviors.
   b) The binge eating occurs, on average, ≥ 1 a week for 3 months.

4) **Avoidant/restrictive food intake disorder (ARFID)**: The absence of body image disturbance and at least one of the following: failure to meet appropriate nutrition and/or energy needs resulting in significant weight loss (or failure to gain weight/grow as expected), significant nutritional deficiency, dependence on nutritional supplements or enteric feeding methods, marked interference with psychosocial functioning.

5) **Other specified feeding or eating disorders (OSFEDs)**: A mixture of any of the above symptoms but not meeting the full criteria for AN, BN, or BED.

→ **EPIDEMIOLOGY, PATHOGENESIS, NATURAL HISTORY**

The prevalence of AN is approximately 0.3% to 0.4% of the female population and is highest in 15-to-19-year-olds, accounting for 40% of all new cases. Less accurate data are available for males. Clinical samples in adult populations show a female to male patient ratio of 10:1, although the ratio in the general population is likely less extreme. BN is more common than AN, with a prevalence rate around 1%, again with a mainly female predominance. BN typically presents in late adolescence or early adulthood. BED is a new diagnosis in the fifth edition of the American Psychiatric Association's *Diagnostic and Statistical Manual of Mental Disorders (DSM-5)* and thus data are more limited, though the prevalence is estimated at about 1.6% in females and 0.8% in males. ARFID is a new diagnostic category. Recent literature from tertiary care pediatric eating disorder programs suggests that its prevalence is up to 14% of patients.

The pathogenesis of all the eating disorders is multifactorial, with developmental, biological, genetic, environmental, and psychosocial contributions. Genetic contributions appear particularly important for AN, with heritability estimates in the range of 50% to 85%. Many brain pathways are likely involved, including those that manage memory, reward, emotions, mood, fear, and attention. Malnutrition itself can alter or worsen cognition and may alter the brain's normal development when the onset of the eating disorder is in the prepubertal or adolescent years. The hypothalamic-pituitary axis is also affected by malnutrition and impacts various organs. Particularly important is the signaling system involved with hunger, energy intake, and satiety. Some early risk factors for an eating disorder include being anxious, sensitive, obsessive, perfectionistic, impulsive, or difficult to soothe.

AN has the highest mortality rate (10%-20%) of any psychiatric illness, with approximately half of deaths due to medical complications and the other half by suicide. The most common medical complications causing death include cardiac events and electrolyte disturbances. About 50% to 70% of patients with AN will recover, with the remainder experiencing a more chronic course. With BN and BED, a relapsing and remitting course of illness is common. For example, 10 years after initial presentation with BN ~10% of patients still have ongoing and chronic symptoms, 20% have subclinical levels of symptoms, and the remaining 70% have achieved recovery.

→ MEDICAL EVALUATION

The following recommendations apply to restrictive eating disorders and other eating disorders with significant purging behaviors.

History

History should include details of the present illness, with a focus on eating disorder symptoms as well as psychiatric and medical comorbidities:

1) Food/eating patterns, including restriction, fasting, acute refusal, food rituals, food allergies and subjective intolerances, 24-hour dietary recall.

2) Weight changes (amount and rate), highest and lowest weights (dates when these occurred), and thoughts and feelings about body shape, weight, and size.

3) Binging and purging (ask individually about each method of purging, eg, self-induced vomiting, use of ipecac, laxative misuse, diuretic misuse, complementary or alternative medicines, or purposeful omission or misuse of prescription medication for the purpose of weight loss).

4) Exercise, including quantity, quality, frequency, and type.

5) For females: Menstrual history, including menarche, usual pattern, any missed periods, last normal menstrual period, amenorrhea and duration of amenorrhea, menstrual threshold weight (weight at which the individual lost her menstrual period), and contraceptive use.

6) For males: Change in sexual function, including erectile dysfunction, loss of morning tumescence, or nocturnal emissions in teens.

7) Medication use/misuse.

8) Alcohol and substance use history.

9) Developmental and growth history.

10) Screen for psychiatric comorbidities, especially mood and anxiety disorders.

11) Suicide/self-harm and risk assessment.

Table 7-1. Symptoms, signs, and clinical findings in patients evaluated for eating disorders

General	Brain (neurologic/psychiatric)	Head and neck
– Weakness, fatigue, lethargy – Dizziness, syncope – Weight fluctuations: marked weight loss or gain – Arrested linear growth – Cold intolerance – Sweating/hot flashes	– Poor concentration and memory – Altered cognition – Insomnia – Features of depression, anxiety, obsessive-compulsive disorder – Social withdrawal – Irritability	– Dental enamel erosion and caries – Parotid enlargement (from self-induced vomiting) – Oral trauma and lacerations – Dry, cracked lips and tongue
Cardiac and pulmonary	**Gastrointestinal**	**Endocrine**
– Dysrhythmias – Palpitations – Chest pain – Shortness of breath – Edema – Dizziness – Orthostatic heart rate and blood pressure changes – Delayed capillary refill – Acrocyanosis	– Constipation or diarrhea – Gastroesophageal reflux – Abdominal discomfort/bloating – Delayed gastric emptying, early satiety – Hemorrhoids, prolapse – Hematemesis	– Amenorrhea or irregular menses – Delayed pubertal development – In diabetes, poor glucose control and possible diabetic ketoacidosis – Infertility
Renal/metabolic	**Dermatologic**	**Musculoskeletal**
– Renal calculi – Edema – Dehydration – Incontinence	– Dry skin – Carotenoderma – Hair loss or thinning – Brittle nails – Lanugo – Poor wound healing – Russell sign: calluses on the knuckles or dorsum of the hand due to self-induced vomiting	– Decreased bone mineral density/osteoporosis, risk of bone fractures – Fatigue – Muscle weakness – Cramps

12) Family history, including eating disorders, other mental illness, substance use, suicide, and medical conditions.

13) Review of systems (→Table 7-1).

Physical Examination

1. Vital signs, including oral temperature and orthostatic vital signs (heart rate and blood pressure).

2. Measurement of weight and height, determination of body mass index (BMI). In children and teens, a growth curve is needed to plot height, weight, and BMI, and to make comparisons with the previous growth pattern.

3. Mental status evaluation (→Chapter 12.11).

4. Focused physical examination (→Table 7-1).

5. Sexual maturity rating in adolescents (a scale of pubertal development based on secondary sexual characteristics, to be completed by a skilled pediatrician or other qualified clinician).

Table 7-2. Recommended blood testing in patients evaluated for eating disorders

CBC, differential count	Creatinine and urea	Pregnancy test (in women of childbearing age)
– Electrolytes: Sodium, potassium, chloride, bicarbonate – Extended electrolytes: Calcium, magnesium, phosphorous – Glucose	Liver function tests: AST, ALT, ALP, GGT, total protein, albumin, bilirubin	– TSH – LH, FSH, and estradiol in patients with amenorrhea
ESR and/or CRP	Amylase	Ferritin

ALP, alkaline phosphatase; ALT, alanine aminotransferase; AST, aspartate aminotransferase; CBC, complete blood count; CRP, C-reactive protein; ESR, erythrocyte sedimentation rate; FSH, follicle-stimulating hormone; GGT, γ-glutamyl transferase (transpeptidase); LH, luteinizing hormone; TSH, thyroid-stimulating hormone.

→ DIAGNOSIS

Diagnostic Tests

1. Blood tests (→Table 7-2).

2. Urinalysis.

3. Electrocardiography (ECG).

4. Consider dual-energy x-ray absorptiometry (DXA) to measure bone mineral density in females with long-standing amenorrhea (eg, >6 months).

Differential Diagnosis

Although most eating disorders are easily diagnosed, other medical and psychiatric conditions should be considered, particularly in patients with atypical presentations. Medical conditions that should be considered include:

1) Inflammatory bowel disease.

2) Irritable bowel syndrome.

3) Celiac disease.

4) Malabsorption.

5) Gastric dysmotility.

6) Gastroesophageal reflux.

7) Pregnancy.

8) Endocrine disorders:

    a) Diabetes mellitus.

    b) Addison disease.

    c) Hyperthyroidism.

9) Other:

    a) Central nervous system lesions (eg, vasculitis; hypothalamic/pituitary tumors).

    b) Chronic infection (eg, tuberculosis, HIV).

    c) Immunodeficiency.

    d) Collagen vascular disease.

    e) Malignancies.

Clinicians should also consider other psychiatric disorders, including:

1) Mood disorders.

2) Anxiety disorders.

3) Somatic symptom disorder (previously called somatization disorder).

4) Substance use disorders.

5) Psychotic disorders.

→ COMPLICATIONS

Acute Medical Complications

1. Metabolic complications, including hypokalemia as a result of vomiting or hyponatremia as a result of significant water loading, can be life-threatening. A common electrolyte disturbance seen with vomiting is hypochloremic metabolic alkalosis. Misuse of laxatives can also result in metabolic alkalosis, dehydration, and hypokalemia.

2. Dehydration is often secondary to restriction of fluids or vomiting.

3. Cardiovascular complications include ECG changes such as bradycardia, prolonged QTc, and other life-threatening dysrhythmias. Orthostatic heart rate and blood pressure changes are also common. Studies in patients with AN have shown loss of cardiac muscle, decrease in left ventricular wall thickness, and decreased cardiac output.

4. Peripheral edema can be a sign of metabolic abnormalities and refeeding syndrome including congestive heart failure.

5. Refeeding syndrome (→Tenets of Good Patient Care, below).

Chronic Medical Complications

1. Reduced bone mineral density can occur early in the course of the illness.

2. Brain imaging studies have shown grey and white matter reductions during the illness. In some of these studies, full recovery of these changes does not occur with weight restoration (the clinical significance of this finding is unknown).

3. In children and adolescents linear growth and pubertal development can be delayed, impaired, or both.

4. Exposure of the teeth and esophagus to gastric acid can result in dental enamel erosion and esophagitis and/or esophageal spasm, respectively.

5. Hematemesis in patients with BN may be indicative of Mallory-Weiss tears.

6. Binge eating has the potential to cause acute gastric dilatation and possible gastric rupture, although this is rare.

7. BED is associated with obesity, with the inherent increased morbidity and mortality.

→ TREATMENT AND MONITORING

Tenets of Good Patient Care

1. Interdisciplinary team: An interdisciplinary team is critical in the comprehensive treatment (medical complications, nutritional rehabilitation, psychiatric comorbidities) of individuals with eating disorders.

2. General approach to management: The initial goals in the management of an individual with a diagnosis of an eating disorder is nutritional rehabilitation including correction of acute medical complications, promotion of metabolic recovery, and restoration of a healthy body weight (if needed). Timely intervention may prevent long-term complications. The interdisciplinary team will need to decide on the treatment setting that is most appropriate for the individual patient. Various treatment settings for the management of an eating disorder include inpatient, day treatment, outpatient, or residential treatment.

3. General approach to inpatient management:

1) **Initial approach**:

    a) Medical stabilization and nutritional rehabilitation should occur first, on an internal medicine or a pediatric hospital ward, if necessary, with consultation from the psychiatric department, or on a specialized eating disorder unit.

b) If the patient has been admitted to a medical unit, transfer or referral to a specialized eating disorders program should be considered once the individual is medically stable.

c) Voluntary treatment is preferred. However, in some circumstances patients can be treated involuntarily if medical complications pose an immediate risk or if the patient lacks the capacity to consent to treatment due to their psychiatric illness. Consultation with the psychiatric department and adherence to local mental health legislation is necessary in these situations.

2) **Medical stabilization and medical monitoring**:

a) Monitor orthostatic heart rate and blood pressure daily and as indicated.

b) Continuous cardiac monitoring is preferred in patients who are medically unstable and performed as needed thereafter.

c) Ongoing blood testing including extended electrolytes should be performed daily during the first 4 to 5 days of refeeding. If blood test results are normal thereafter, it can be followed as indicated.

d) Fluid intake and output should be monitored and documented until the patient is medically stable.

e) Initially IV fluids should be used with caution and should not exceed doses of maintenance fluids. Aggressive resuscitation can result in congestive heart failure and edema.

f) New evidence suggests that inpatient nutritional rehabilitation in patients with AN can be more aggressive than previously recommended. Nutrition can be safely initiated at 1500 kcal/d in mildly and moderately malnourished patients and be increased by 250 calories per day to achieve a daily weight gain of ~0.2 to 0.4 kg/d.⊘⊖

3) **Refeeding syndrome**: Refeeding syndrome is a potentially life-threatening issue that can arise during refeeding of a severely malnourished individual. It involves a rapid shift in fluids and electrolytes for which the body cannot compensate. Clinically, refeeding syndrome consists of cardiovascular (congestive heart failure, peripheral and pulmonary edema; vital sign instability), neurologic (delirium), and metabolic complications associated with significant morbidity and mortality. Refeeding hypophosphatemia, the hallmark biochemical feature of refeeding syndrome, has been correlated with the degree of malnutrition on admission.

Close medical monitoring includes, but is not limited to, continuous cardiac monitoring, regular checking of electrolytes and extended electrolytes, and evaluation of mental status. The frequency of bloodwork can be adjusted up or down based on clinical judgement.

4) **Management of eating disorder behaviors**:

a) Close monitoring during meals is very important, resources permitting, to ensure the patient is completing their meals/snacks as prescribed.

b) Support patients by preventing behaviors driven by the eating disorder. For instance, mealtime support conducted by skilled staff or family members (who have been taught the methods of meal support) can be helpful to patients. An example of techniques used in meal support includes distracting the patient with conversation or listening to music, so they are less focused on the food itself. These techniques can be helpful in facilitating the patient to complete their entire meal.

c) Following meals, some patients may experience psychological and physical discomfort. They may be preoccupied with thoughts of purging and feelings of guilt. A period of support and distraction (for 30-60 minutes) following meals with restriction of the use of washrooms can help reduce these thoughts and urges and prevent these behaviors.

d) The activity level of individuals with an eating disorder on the inpatient unit should be kept to a minimum, in an effort to decrease energy expenditure. Initial clinical practice for patients who are medically unstable typically includes a short period of medical bed rest.

e) Physical restraint should be avoided.

f) Laxatives that were regularly used/misused by the patient should not be withdrawn abruptly, as this could cause severe constipation and obstruction.

4. General considerations for outpatient treatment: **Psychotherapy**:

1) Family-based therapy has the best evidence for adolescents with AN and is recommended as first-line treatment.⊘● Family-based treatment may also be helpful for adolescents with BN, although there is less evidence supporting this.

2) Other psychotherapies can be of benefit in BN and BED (eg, cognitive behavior therapy [CBT], interpersonal therapy).

3) Dialectical behavior therapy (DBT) is a specialized form of CBT that integrates mindfulness and acceptance strategies. It is primarily skills-based and can be helpful in those with extensive mood dysregulation, interpersonal difficulties, and impulsive behaviors (including self-harm, substance use, bingeing and purging).

5. Medications:

1) There is little clear evidence for the use of medications to treat the primary diagnosis of an eating disorder, especially for AN. Furthermore, there is even less clarity of evidence for use of medications with children and adolescents.

2) Fluoxetine has been suggested (especially at higher doses, ~60 mg/d) for individuals with BN to target the binge/purge behaviors once the decision to treat with pharmacotherapy has been reached.⊘● We recommend this treatment for at least an additional 6 to 12 months following the cessation of binge/purge symptoms and when there are no ongoing eating disorders/ body image cognitive distortions.

3) A low-dose atypical antipsychotic (such as olanzapine 2.5-5 mg or risperidone 0.5-1 mg) can be helpful in patients with severe distress. In our practice severe distress is more commonly seen in patients with AN compared with other eating disorders.

4) Benzodiazepines can also be used for agitation, but we suggest this should be at low doses and should be used minimally and with caution, as they have addiction potential; in younger patients, there is the possibility of a paradoxical reaction whereby the benzodiazepine worsens agitation.

8. Medical Care of the Seriously Mentally Ill

▷DEFINITIONS, ETIOLOGY, EPIDEMIOLOGY

Serious mental illness (SMI) is a term applied to those mental illnesses that either currently or in the previous year have been associated with serious functional impairment. SMI typically refers to cases of schizophrenia, bipolar disorder, and depression. The 12-month prevalence of SMI is estimated at 4% to 6% of the adult population.●

Compared with the general population, individuals with SMI have a 2-fold to 3-fold higher risk of death at a given age and their life expectancy is dramatically reduced. This difference is referred to as the "**mortality gap**," and it is estimated to be approximately 10 years for individuals with schizophrenia

Table 8-1. Minding the mortality gap in patients with serious mental illness

Patients with serious mental illness:
- Have elevated risk of dying from cardiovascular, respiratory, gastrointestinal, endocrine, infectious, genitourinary, neurologic, and neoplastic causes
- Have higher rates of suicide and accidental and violent deaths
- Have higher rates of obesity, hypertension, hyperlipidemia, hypercholesterolemia, diabetes, and metabolic syndrome
- Have higher rates of smoking
- Have more difficulty accessing services
- Have more difficulty adhering to medical treatments
- Are less likely to receive a comprehensive medical assessment
- Are less likely to receive screening tests
- Are less likely to receive specialty consultations and diagnostic tests

and is greater in men than in women.● The mortality gap has remained stable at these levels despite overall improvements in life expectancy for the general population. The purpose of this chapter is to heighten the awareness of physicians about this alarming situation so that the factors contributing to this problem can be appropriately addressed.

Individuals with SMI who present for medical care may receive poor or delayed treatment because physicians attribute their physical symptoms to their mental illness. This phenomenon is referred to as "**diagnostic overshadowing**," meaning that it may be difficult for physicians to recognize medical illness when they view the patient through the shadow cast by their mental illness.

SMIs are understood as being highly heritable disorders, with estimates of heritability ranging from over 80% for schizophrenia and bipolar disorder to 37% for major depression. For example, the risk of developing schizophrenia in people with a first-degree relative with schizophrenia is approximately 10-fold higher than in the general population.● Mental illnesses may be chronic and persisting or remitting and relapsing in their course. It is estimated that 75% of cases of mental illnesses in adults have their onset by the age of 24 years. The impact of SMI on physical health problems reflects the cumulative effects of a range of determinants of health over many decades. Addressing the mortality gap requires appreciation of a host of health determinants early in the course of SMI.

Our understanding of the outcome from mental illness has changed dramatically over the past 60 years since psychotropic medications were first introduced for the treatment of schizophrenia, bipolar disorder, and major depression. These illnesses are highly treatable with the expectation of high rates of remission. While relapses are common and often result in rehospitalization, their rates can be dramatically reduced by maintenance medications. Recent attention to illness self-management and relapse prevention has the potential to alter the course of these illnesses. Concurrent substance use disorders and developmental disorders compound problems with treatment adherence and together contribute to the challenge of managing medical comorbidity in this population.

→ CLINICAL CONSIDERATIONS

There are many factors that contribute to premature mortality (the mortality gap) observed in individuals with SMI (→Table 8-1):

1) **Causes of death**: Both men and women with schizophrenia are more likely to die as a result of a number of medical causes compared with the general population. When expressed as standardized mortality ratio (SMR), individuals with schizophrenia are twice as likely to die of natural causes, including cardiovascular diseases (SMR, 1.88), digestive diseases (SMR, 3.34),

endocrine diseases (SMR, 4.07), infectious diseases (SMR, 3.77), genito-urinary diseases (SMR, 2.90), respiratory diseases (SMR, 3.51), nervous diseases (SMR, 3.55), and neoplastic diseases (SMR, 1.33).

2) **Elevated risk factors for medical illness**: Individuals with schizophrenia are much more likely to smoke cigarettes relative to the general population (odds ratio, 5.3).● They are more likely to be heavy smokers with higher nicotine dependence scores and lower cessation rates. It has been estimated that persons with broadly defined mental illness consume over 40% of all cigarettes in the United States.◒

Individuals with schizophrenia have much higher rates of obesity, hypertension, hyperlipidemia and hypercholesterolemia, diabetes, and metabolic syndrome.● Increased rates of glucose intolerance and insulin resistance may be directly linked to schizophrenia. A combination of poor diet, sedentary behavior, obesity, and adverse effects of psychotropic medications over time compound this association. Most antipsychotics and mood stabilizers have the potential to cause weight gain, as do many antidepressant medications. Amongst antipsychotic agents, clozapine and olanzapine are considered to carry the greatest risk of weight gain.● Mean one-year weight gain from olanzapine in patients treated for their first episode of psychosis is estimated at 15.5 kg compared with 7.1 kg for those treated with haloperidol, a first-generation antipsychotic considered to have among the lowest risks of weight gain.◒ Antipsychotic medications may lead to abnormalities in glucose and lipid metabolism through molecular mechanisms that may be only partially accounted for by weight gain.

Current users of antipsychotic medications have been found to be at a significantly greater risk of sudden cardiac death, which has been found to be dose-related. The risk varies with first-generation antipsychotics (eg, haloperidol, perphenazine, chlorpromazine, thioridazine) from an incidence risk ratio of 1.31 with low doses to 2.42 with high doses; with second-generation antipsychotics (eg, risperidone, olanzapine, quetiapine, clozapine), the incidence risk ratio rises from 1.59 with low doses to 2.86 with high doses.◒ It is thought the increased risk of sudden cardiac death is likely due to ventricular arrhythmias such as torsades de pointes secondary to the blockade of potassium channels and prolonged cardiac repolarization. Antipsychotic medications vary substantially in the degree to which they cause QTc prolongation, as do antidepressants and mood stabilizing medications. Despite the cardiac risks associated with the use of antipsychotic medications in patients with schizophrenia, epidemiologic evidence suggests that long-term use may be associated with reduced mortality.○

Many antipsychotic medications have profound anticholinergic effects, which is also the case for antiparkinsonian medications and some antidepressant medications. These medications commonly lead to severe problems with constipation. Bowel obstruction and paralytic ileus are amongst the most common and severe complications of treatment for schizophrenia. In patients treated with clozapine, for example, severe constipation is associated with a very high mortality rate and is much more common than agranulocytosis or myocarditis—severe adverse events that receive more attention.

Poor Medical Care

Individuals with SMI are less likely to receive good medical care, and this is thought to contribute substantially to their reduced life expectancy. The phenomenon can be understood as involving factors attributable to the behavior of patients and of health providers.

Patients with SMI may be less inclined to seek care and may have lower adherence to medical treatments. Approaches that facilitate health care–seeking and support treatment adherence in individuals with cognitive and motivational deficits are essential. Patients may have reduced access to care as a result of poverty, differences in insurance coverage, as well as stigma and discrimination.

There are ways in which medical providers may contribute to the poor care received by some patients with SMI. It may be challenging to obtain a history from some patients with SMI if they are uncooperative or thought-disordered. Behavior that is bizarre or aggressive, poor hygiene, as well as active features of psychosis, mania, or depression may also interfere with a proper assessment. Assessment is also likely to be more difficult and time-consuming, which further limits the likelihood that physicians working with severe time constraints, such as in an emergency department, will carry out a comprehensive assessment.

Many physicians are uncomfortable working with patients who have SMI (→Chapter 12.6). This may be due to a perceived lack of knowledge about mental illness and its management, fear of violence, and the pervasive stigma associated with SMI. These factors likely contribute substantially to the lower intensity of care that patients with SMI often receive.◎ Patients with SMI are less likely to receive tests for diabetes monitoring, to have their blood pressure or cholesterol recorded during regular health visits, to have up-to-date cancer screening, and to receive chemotherapy, radiation, and surgery when diagnosed with cancer. Patients with schizophrenia who present with myocardial infarction have been found to be 50% less likely to see a cardiologist or to have a cardiac procedure and 56% more likely to die within 30 days of presentation. Similarly, patients with SMI who have been hospitalized for the treatment of infection have been reported to have a 30-day mortality rate that is approximately 50% higher than those without SMI.

When encountering patients with SMI, many physicians have difficulty separating physical illness from psychiatric illness and incorrectly assume that whatever physical complaints are being described can be explained by the person's psychiatric problems. This diagnostic overshadowing results in patients with SMI receiving care of lower intensity and quality. It is important to appreciate that patients with SMI not only have all of the same potential medical problems that are observed in those without mental illness, but they are expected to have many of these problems at a higher frequency and younger age.

Death from Unnatural Causes

Higher rates of suicide and accidental and violent deaths account for one-third of the excess mortality associated with schizophrenia; people with schizophrenia are 8 times as likely to die of unnatural causes and 16 times more likely to die by suicide in particular.◎

→ TREATMENT

Internists and family practitioners must be aware of the heightened risk of medical illness and the large reduction in life expectancy associated with having SMI. This awareness should lead to greater vigilance in ensuring that such patients receive a careful and comprehensive assessment notwithstanding the challenges they may present. Some experts recommend that individuals with SMI have a comprehensive physical assessment at least annually, including assessment of weight, waist circumference, pulse, blood pressure, and metabolic monitoring, as well as a review of bowel, cardiac, and respiratory functions. Electrocardiography (ECG) should be completed before administering an antipsychotic—or, if not feasible, early in the course of antipsychotic treatment—and then followed up when treatment has been stabilized. As it is very common for many individuals with SMI to be treated concurrently with multiple psychotropic medications, repeating ECG periodically should be considered, for example, when doses are increased or new medications are added. Communication with the patient's psychiatrist and mental health team about concurrent medical problems and their management is critically important.

Health promotion initiatives have been introduced to improve the health of individuals with SMI and may be available through local family health teams or mental health services. Initiatives to enhance physical activity together with dietary counseling may contribute to the management of obesity and associated metabolic problems. Smoking cessation programs have been of great benefit to many individuals with SMI. Treatment with varenicline, bupropion, and nicotine patches have been demonstrated to be of benefit in helping patients with SMI to discontinue smoking, and we recommend efforts to help patients with SMI to quit smoking⊘● (→Chapter 13.10). Lifestyle changes may be particularly challenging for patients with SMI who experience illness-related deficits in cognition, organization, and motivation. Early use of medications to address problems with hypertension, glucose intolerance, cholesterol and lipid abnormalities, as well as antipsychotic-induced weight gain (eg, metformin) should be given consideration.

→ SUMMARY

Individuals with SMI have dramatically lower life expectancies and a greatly increased risk of death due to a broad range of medical disorders. This can be understood as resulting from the confluence of a number of critical problems:

1) Lifestyle factors including poor diet, sedentary lifestyle, and high rates of obesity and smoking.

2) Adverse effects of antipsychotic and other psychotropic medications.

3) More limited access to health-care services, reduced health care–seeking behavior, and poor adherence to medical care.

4) Provision of lower-quality care.

The magnitude and complexity of this problem requires that internists and family practitioners be especially vigilant in assessing patients with SMI comprehensively, in guarding against the tendency to see physical symptoms as being due to mental illness, in ensuring that medical illness is identified early, and in confirming that the systems and supports are in place, so that patients with SMI are able to adhere to the recommended treatments.

9. Medical Practice and the Law

→ INTRODUCTION

The practice of medicine occurs in a complex matrix of ethical guidelines and legal structures that, although usually complementary, may sometimes come into conflict. The Canadian Medical Association's (CMA) *Code of Ethics* states: "Physicians should be aware of the legal and regulatory requirements that govern medical practice in their jurisdictions." This statement highlights the fact that many of the legal and regulatory requirements governing medical practice vary from province to province. Furthermore, the medical colleges of individual provinces and territories also provide standards and guidelines for their constituents (visit the website of the Royal College of Physicians and Surgeons of Canada).

Although a thorough treatment of the medical-legal issues that may affect medical practitioners in the course of their work is beyond the scope of this chapter, we have tried to highlight some key areas and to provide brief conceptual overviews as well as resources that can be accessed for more detailed, geographically relevant information. The specific issues we have elected to examine are ones that often present themselves in the practice of psychiatry but are also common in many other areas of medical practice. An excellent practical overview of this topic may be found in the *Medical-legal handbook for physicians in Canada*, a publication of the Canadian Medical Protective Association (CMPA).

→ INVOLUNTARY ADMISSION

Although more commonly encountered in the practice of psychiatry, the application of civil legislation for the purpose of involuntary hospitalization (often referred to as civil commitment) may occur in other areas, such as emergency departments or medical units. Although the specific criteria vary significantly throughout Canada, certain principles apply generally. Due to the serious nature of involuntary admission, every effort must be made to ensure that the appropriate legal criteria have been met, that the appropriate documentation has been completed, and that the patient is made aware of their legal rights in the situation. The process of involuntary admission can be extremely stressful and stigmatizing. Therefore, the application of any seclusion or restraint measures (physical or pharmacologic) is often experienced as very traumatic and should be done in the least restrictive or intrusive manner that permits the safe care of the individual.

Significant variation exists among provincial statutes in terms of the criteria that must be met to permit civil commitment. In addition to the presence of mental disorder, provinces vary with regard to requirements of the risk of harm to self and/or others, likelihood of mental or physical deterioration or impairment, and imminence or seriousness of these. For details regarding the requirements for involuntary hospitalization in specific locations, the reader is directed to review the relevant provincial or territorial statutes. These can be accessed through the Canadian Legal Information Institute.

→ CONSENT TO TREATMENT

The right of a capable person to accept or reject an offered treatment, being it for psychiatric or any other condition, is considered fundamental in the Canadian health-care system. Respect for this right is a responsibility as described in the CMA *Code of Ethics*. In addition to being an ethical requirement, consent is also mandated by legislation, although situations exist in which treatment may proceed based on a court order (eg, to restore fitness to stand trial) or an emergency basis (to prevent severe suffering or to manage imminent threat to life, limb, or health). In all other circumstances valid consent must be obtained from the patient or, in situations in which the patient has been determined to be incapable of providing consent for a particular treatment, from an appropriate substitute decision-maker (SDM). In order for the consent to be valid, it must meet certain criteria: the patient must be capable and the consent must be voluntary and properly informed. The Supreme Court of Canada in *Starson v Swayze* (2003 SCC 32) considered the issue of treatment capacity and in its decision indicated that 2 criteria are involved and both must be met in order for an individual to be considered capable:

1) The patient must be able to understand the information that is relevant to making a treatment decision.
2) The patient must be able to appreciate the reasonably foreseeable consequences of the decision or lack of one.

As in all cases, the physician is required to complete an appropriate assessment and document the results. Depending upon legislation in the place of practice, the appropriate forms must be completed and notifications, including rights of appeal, must take place. In addition to provincial legislation and college policies, the reader is directed to CMPA's *Consent: A guide for Canadian physicians*.

Consent is often implied either by the words or behavior of the patient or by the circumstances under which treatment is given. Physicians should be reasonably confident the actions of the patient imply permission for proposed examinations, investigations, and treatments. When there is doubt, it is preferable the consent be expressed, either orally or in writing. A patient may be incapable of consenting to a particular medical treatment but may be capable of consenting to other treatments for the same or another condition. The obligation to obtain consent must always rest with the physician who is to carry out the treatment or the investigative procedure. The patient must have been given an adequate explanation about the nature of the proposed treatment or investigation and its anticipated outcome as well as the significant risks involved and alternatives available. The ability to consent may fluctuate over time and thus must be monitored and reassessed as required. In circumstances where it has been determined that a patient is incapable to consenting to a particular treatment or investigation, an SDM may be appointed. SDMs must act in compliance with any prior capable wishes of the patient and, where these are not known, should be guided by the patient's best interests. The assignment of SDMs will take place according to appropriate legislative guidelines that exist in the physician's jurisdiction.

Psychiatric emergencies in medical settings often involve management of an agitated patient. In order to prevent harm to himself or herself or others, an agitated patient may be restrained using pharmacologic or physical means without obtaining consent. Once the patient is stabilized, capacity- and consent-related issues as well as involuntary hospitalization (civil commitment) should be considered as soon as possible.

CONFIDENTIALITY

Privacy is generally accepted as a fundamental human right. Confidentiality has been a cornerstone of ethical medical practice throughout history and is referred to in the Hippocratic oath. The confidentiality of health information, in addition to being an expectation within the CMA's *Code of Ethics* and the ethical guidelines of most provincial colleges, is also protected through privacy legislation. At the national level, the Personal Information Protection and Electronic Documents Act (PIPEDA) addresses the management of personal information by private sector organizations. The collection, storage, and use of personal health information is subject to provincial and territorial legislation with oversight by designated privacy commissioners.

Although a written consent to release personal health information should be obtained wherever possible, certain circumstances exist where this may not be required. In some statutes (eg, the Personal Health Information Protection Act in Ontario) physicians are entitled to assume that they have the patient's implied consent to share information within the patient's "circle of care" for the purpose of providing health care (visit the website of The College of Physicians and Surgeons of Ontario). Expressed consent is required in all other circumstances unless the release of information is mandated by statute. Such statutes also vary by province or territory but include such examples as the reporting of issues related to fitness to drive, reporting of certain communicable diseases, or reporting when a child is believed to be at risk of harm.

Provincial or territorial colleges publish lists of mandatory and permissive reportable circumstances, events, or clinical conditions.

The release of personal health information may also be permitted where it is necessary in order to protect the safety of members of the public. This issue is reviewed thoroughly in a position paper of the Canadian Psychiatric Association addressing the duty to protect. In the paper the authors make specific reference to the Supreme Court's position articulated in the decision in *Smith v Jones* ([1999] 1 SCR 455), which they recommend should be taken as a professional standard of practice. The Canadian Psychiatric Association takes the position "that its members have a legal duty to protect intended victims of their patients. This duty to protect may include informing intended victims or the police, or both, but may more easily be addressed in some circumstances by detaining and possibly treating the patient." The authors recommend that as part of the informed consent process patients should be warned of the limits of confidentiality. Furthermore, they specify that a duty to protect (warn or inform) exists (1) "in the event that risk to a clearly identifiable person or group of persons is determined"; (2) "when the risk of harm includes severe bodily injury, death, or serious psychological harm"; (3) "when there is an element of imminence, creating a sense of urgency."

→ MEDICAL MALPRACTICE

Malpractice is defined as an instance of negligence or incompetence on the part of a professional. Most civil actions against physicians are based in torts (civil wrongs), which are classified into intentional or unintentional. Intentional torts, such as assault or slander, are far less common than unintentional torts, such as negligence. These may be alleged actions or omissions on the part of the physician, which are claimed to have resulted in harm to the patient. In order for negligence to be proven, several elements must be established:

1) A duty of care to a patient: Accepting a patient establishes a duty of care. A physician is expected to exercise reasonable skill and judgment in coming to a diagnosis and recommending appropriate evaluation and treatment.

2) A breach of that duty of care: A physician is expected to perform to a standard that might reasonably be observed in a colleague under similar circumstances.

3) The patient must have suffered some harm or injury.

4) The harm has to be causally related, on the balance of probabilities, to the breach of duty of care.

→ MANAGING LEGAL ISSUES IN PRACTICE

The management of medical/legal issues in health-care settings is often challenging and complex. It is recommended that physicians involve professional colleges, administrators, or legal resources, such as hospital council and CMPA representatives, as required.

For a more comprehensive discussion of issues related to medical liability, the reader is referred to the CMPA.

10. Perinatal Depressive and Anxiety Disorders

→ INTRODUCTION

Pregnancy and the first year of the postpartum, commonly referred to as the perinatal period, are widely believed to be a time of bliss and joy. However, for many women the risk of depressive and/or anxiety disorders is elevated. These problems, if occur, are frequently not recognized or not managed appropriately. The lack of adequate treatment can increase the risk for obstetrical complications; negatively influence relationship with partners; impair maternal-infant attachment; result in poor breastfeeding outcomes; and result in behavioral, emotional, and cognitive problems in the offspring.

In this chapter we discuss the etiology of perinatal depressive and anxiety disorders as well as screening methods, outline recommended treatments, and discuss the consequences of untreated illness during this important period in life.

→ EPIDEMIOLOGY, ETIOLOGY, CLINICAL FEATURES

Epidemiology

The prevalence of major depressive episodes during pregnancy has been estimated to vary between 4% to 13% and 6.5% to 16% during the first 3 months of the postpartum period. ◔ Anxiety disorders are also very common during the perinatal period, with prevalence estimates ranging from 9% to 21% during pregnancy and 6% to 14% in the first 6 months postpartum. Of particular interest to women and clinicians is the fact that rates of generalized anxiety disorder and obsessive-compulsive disorder (OCD) are higher among pregnant and postpartum women relative to the general population.

Clinical Features and Screening

Identifying a major depressive episode (symptoms: →Chapter 12.5) throughout pregnancy and the postpartum is complicated by the fact that physiologic changes commonly occurring during the perinatal period can produce physical complaints resembling somatic symptoms of a major depressive episode (eg, affecting appetite, weight, sleep, and energy). As a result, it is important to complement the use of screening instruments with a clinical interview and careful judgement. Of these instruments, the Edinburgh Postnatal Depression Scale (EPDS), which focuses more on the neurocognitive symptoms of depression (eg, low mood, anhedonia), has the most evidence to support its ability to reliably and accurately identify probable cases of perinatal depression. In general, a score ≥12 during pregnancy is suggestive of depression. A score ≥10 in the postpartum period has also been suggested to be consistent with an elevated risk of a depressive episode.

Significantly less evidence exists to support the widespread use of any specific screening instrument for perinatal anxiety. Some research has suggested that a score ≥6 on the anxiety subscale of the EPDS is suggestive of an anxiety disorder. The Generalized Anxiety Disorder-7 (GAD-7) (available at mdcalc.com) has been recommended as well, with a score ≥13 suggesting the presence of generalized anxiety disorder among perinatal women. The Perinatal Obsessive-Compulsive Scale (POCS) is a useful screening tool for perinatal OCD as it contains items that are specific to addressing obsessions and compulsions relating to the fetus/newborn baby. This is important given that perinatal OCD often presents with a distinctive clinical picture and course where obsessions and compulsions are focused on the fetus and/or newborn baby.

The severity of depressive and anxiety disorders is defined according to the fifth edition of the American Psychiatric Association's *Diagnostic and Statistical Manual of Mental Disorders* (*DSM-5*).

Etiology and Risk Factors

A complex interactive etiologic pathway involving psychosocial, clinical, and biologic factors contributes to the development of perinatal depressive and anxiety disorders.

Psychosocial risk factors for perinatal depression and anxiety include a lack of partner or social support, history of abuse (especially a history of childhood sexual abuse), domestic violence, unplanned or unwanted pregnancy, and experiencing adverse life events and/or high levels of perceived stress during pregnancy. Potent clinical risk factors include a past history of mental illness (most notably a mood or anxiety disorder), prepregnancy obesity, previous or current pregnancy complications, history of miscarriage, having an emergency caesarean section, chronic medical conditions (eg, diabetes mellitus or hypertension/heart disease), adolescence, and sleep deprivation.

In terms of biologic risk factors, genetics appears to play a role in the etiology of postpartum depression (PPD). A family history of PPD is higher among women who develop perinatal depression and women with PPD also report to have more than expected first-degree relatives with a major depressive disorder (MDD).

Major changes occur in the hypothalamic gonadal, adrenal, and thyroid axes as well as in the systems regulating prolactin and oxytocin throughout the perinatal period. However, for most of these hormones, it is not their absolute levels that are related to the development of perinatal anxiety or depression but rather the abrupt change seen in the hormonal milieu. Levels of estrogen and progesterone increase gradually during pregnancy with a rapid and abrupt drop to prepregnancy levels immediately in the postpartum period. It has been suggested that this rapid drop in these reproductive hormones contributes to the development of PPD. This notion is supported by the known interplay between reproductive hormones and neurotransmitters involved in mental health disorders (eg, serotonin and dopamine). Recent studies have shown that estrogen modulates changes in neurotransmitter systems which in turn may influence maternal sensitivity, behavior, and attitude in the postpartum. One notable exception is hypothyroidism, which can directly contribute to the development and presentation of a depressive disorder perinatally. Hypothyroidism often occurs in the setting of postpartum thyroiditis, a common complication affecting close to 5% of all women in the postpartum period.

Sleep is frequently disrupted during pregnancy as well as in the postpartum. Women experience dramatic changes in sleep patterns and quality throughout the perinatal period. This includes frequent awakenings, fewer hours of total sleep, reduced sleep efficiency, shorter rapid eye movement sleep latency, and circadian phase shifts, all of which may lead to changes in mood.

→ MANAGEMENT

Treatment During Pregnancy

During pregnancy, women with depression and anxiety must make choices about treatment with psychotherapy and/or pharmacologic treatments in the absence of significant evidence and a complete lack of systematic studies comparing these interventions directly. Such decisions must take into account the risks associated with fetal exposure and those of untreated mental illness.

1. Mild to moderate MDD during pregnancy: Generally accepted first--line treatments for *DSM-5*–defined mild to moderate MDD during pregnancy include individual or group cognitive behavioral therapy (CBT) or interpersonal psychotherapy (IPT) (definitions of MDD severity: →Chapter 12.5). In acknowledgement of the importance of the need for rapid treatment effects and risks associated with depressive symptoms during pregnancy, previously effective antidepressants for individual women may also be considered very early in treatment decision-making (assuming that women understand the risks and benefits and prefer it upon balancing these against the risks of other treatments and untreated depression). Since selective serotonin-reuptake inhibitors (SSRIs) are effective across the range of severity of MDD, despite a relative absence of randomized clinical trials during pregnancy sertraline, citalopram, and escitalopram are the top choices, given their effectiveness and relative lack of known teratogenic effects. However, these antidepressants should be considered second-line treatments, behind CBT and IPT.◎◎ If patients are not able to tolerate antidepressant medications or are not willing to take them, referral to professionals able to deliver evidence-based psychotherapies is indicated. Before antidepressants are prescribed, bipolar disorder should be excluded by the clinician.

Based on the strength of evidence in the women's general population, combination treatment with sertraline, citalopram, and escitalopram plus CBT or IPT are accepted as second-line treatments. The remainder of the SSRIs (except paroxetine) and newer antidepressants are generally viewed as third-line therapies, given relatively less reproductive data and more limited use in perinatal clinical practice. Tricyclic antidepressants (with the exception of clomipramine) are also considered third line, along with mindfulness-based, psychodynamic, and supportive psychotherapies, bright light therapy, transcranial magnetic stimulation, and complementary/alternative treatments (including structured exercise such as walking and depression-specific acupuncture).

Despite increased risks of cardiovascular malformations (→below), paroxetine and clomipramine can be used in pregnancy but should be reserved for cases with very strong indications (eg, previous good response, ongoing stability on the medication, preference after consideration of risks and benefits). Monoamine oxidase inhibitors (MAOIs) are not recommended during pregnancy given their propensity to interact with certain analgesic and anesthetic agents. Early consultation with an anesthetist is recommended if MAOIs are used.

2. Severe MDD during pregnancy: For severe major depressive episodes, sertraline, citalopram, and escitalopram, alone or in combination with CBT or IPT, should be considered as first-line treatments given their efficacy in nonperinatal populations. The remaining SSRIs (except paroxetine), newer antidepressants, and tricyclic antidepressants are generally considered second line. Electroconvulsive therapy (ECT) is recommended as third-line treatment given its superior effectiveness and relative safety and tolerability in pregnancy. Combination pharmacotherapy can also be considered, but since its use in pregnancy is limited to sparse case reports, very little is known about its short-term and long-term risks to the fetus (which are likely to be in excess of monotherapy) and it should be used only if absolutely necessary.

3. Anxiety during pregnancy: Although there is far less evidence examining the effectiveness of treatment options for anxiety disorders during pregnancy, it is generally recommended that the first-line treatment for *DSM-5*–defined mild to moderate anxiety disorders is either individual or group CBT. Pregnant women with mild anxiety may also benefit from low-intensity psychological therapies such as facilitated self-help. In the case of pregnant women exhibiting severe anxiety disorders or among those who are not responding to psychological interventions and require rapid relief of symptoms, SSRIs may be considered: sertraline, citalopram, and escitalopram. In general, benzodiazepines are not a widely considered treatment option for women who have a mild to moderate anxiety disorder during pregnancy. Pregnant women with a severe anxiety disorder and are not responding to the recommended SSRIs mentioned above may benefit from a short-term use of benzodiazepines. Among these medications, only lorazepam has been recommended for use in perinatal women. If the patient has a past history or current substance abuse/dependence disorder, a short-term use of a neuroleptic (eg, quetiapine) could be considered instead. However, the prescription of any medication for women in the perinatal period must be accompanied by a discussion of the benefits and drawbacks of treatment as well as the risks of untreated mental illness to the mother, fetus/infant, partner, and other children in the household.

4. Augmenting agents for depressive and anxiety disorders during pregnancy: Although very little research has been conducted with pregnant or lactating women, certain antipsychotics have been considered as augmenting agents for those with treatment-resistant depressive or anxiety disorders. Based on randomized controlled trials consisting of general population samples, aripiprazole, quetiapine, olanzapine, and risperidone seem to be effective as augmenting agents for depression. Furthermore, adding quetiapine or risperidone may also augment the effect of antidepressants among those with OCD. However, it is important to be cautious with these second-generation antipsychotics, as they may cause weight gain and increase the risk for metabolic complications (eg, gestational diabetes and/or obesity) during pregnancy. In addition, the use of these second-generation antipsychotics may also cause sedation and extrapyramidal symptoms in women. In general, clozapine should not be used during pregnancy, given that it can cross the placenta and possibly cause agranulocytosis in the fetus/newborn. Furthermore, gestational use of clozapine has also been associated with floppy infant syndrome (ie, signs of hypotonia) and seizures in the infant.

Risks Associated With Treatment During Pregnancy

Research examining the risks associated with the use of psychotropic medications during pregnancy is limited by the fact that many variables that confound associations between medication exposure and offspring adverse effects (eg, maternal mental illness, substance misuse, poor prenatal care, maternal health problems) are not controlled for in observational studies of these links. As a result, in the absence of randomized controlled trials, the magnitude and nature of these risks are not completely understood.

1. Antidepressants during pregnancy: Among the evidence that does exist, there are suggestions that most antidepressant medications are not generally associated with an increased risk of major congenital malformations. A small increase in risk for cardiovascular malformations (odds ratio, ~1.5; not thought to be clinically relevant at the individual level) has been found with paroxetine.○ However, a number of these complications resolve spontaneously and do not pose significant functional impairment to the offspring. More recent work has linked fluoxetine to a small increase in cardiovascular malformations as well (relative risk, ~1.4). However, significant evidence has not accrued that supports increased risks with other SSRIs, bupropion, mirtazapine, serotonin-norepinephrine reuptake inhibitors (SNRIs), or tricyclic antidepressants except for clomipramine, which may be associated with an elevated risk of cardiovascular malformations. There may also be a modest link between gestational SSRI use and spontaneous abortion (odds ratio, ~1.5), but this may not be present for all agents.⊙○ Furthermore, SSRI use may also slightly increase the risk of preterm birth (odds ratio, ~1.2). However, it is important to note that neither these risks nor that of congenital malformations are in excess of the 2-fold increase in risk that is traditionally accepted as clinically significant. It is also important to point out that studies that have linked SSRIs to shortened gestational age and reduced birth weight show that the magnitude of these findings are 4 days and 74 grams, respectively, and may not be greater than the risks associated with untreated depression during this time.

After delivery infants exposed previously to SSRIs in the third trimester are at an increased risk for a syndrome of poor neonatal adaptation marked by jitteriness, irritability, tremor, respiratory distress, and excessive crying. Occurring in up to 10% to 30% of infants, these symptoms are time limited (typically resolving in 2-14 days) and not associated with an increased risk of mortality or long-term neurodevelopmental problems (and resolve with supportive care). This risk may be highest with paroxetine, venlafaxine, and fluoxetine. Limited data also suggest that SSRIs taken late (but not early) in pregnancy may also be associated with an increased risk for persistent pulmonary hypertension of the newborn (PPHN). The absolute risk is about 3/1000 infants (the risk in the general population is 2/1000) and 339 additional infants need to be exposed to an SSRI in the third trimester in order to produce one additional case of PPHN.○

The limited data that exist on the longer-term effects of fetal exposure to SSRIs report no lasting cognitive, emotional, or behavioral problems in the offspring. Finally, despite the fact that a small number of studies have suggested that fetal SSRI exposure may be associated with autism-spectrum disorder, these studies have significant methodological limitations (eg, lack of controlling for multiple confounds) and wide confidence intervals and require replication before they should be considered by patients and physicians.

2. Benzodiazepines during pregnancy: A past meta-analysis consisting of case-control studies has suggested that gestational use of benzodiazepines may increase the risk of the offspring in developing an oral cleft palate (odds ratio, ~1.8). In addition, the use of benzodiazepines during the third trimester and close to delivery may be associated with withdrawal symptoms (eg, irritability, restlessness, tremors) and signs of intoxication (eg, lethargy, respiratory distress, and hypothermia) in the neonate. Furthermore, gestational use of benzodiazepines has also been associated with floppy infant syndrome (ie, signs of hypotonia). Exposure to benzodiazepines during pregnancy may also be linked to other obstetrical complications including low birth weight, preterm birth, caesarean delivery, respiratory support for infants, and admission to neonatal intensive care units. Finally, there is a small number of studies suggesting that gestational exposure to benzodiazepines may be associated with delays in the infant during the postpartum period.

3. Antipsychotics during pregnancy: Two meta-analyses have suggested that antipsychotics may be associated with major congenital malformations including cardiovascular defects in the fetus/newborn. Exposure to antipsychotics during the third trimester may also increase the risk of extrapyramidal (eg, abnormal muscle movements) and withdrawal symptoms (eg, irritability, restlessness, and tremors) in the neonate. Additionally, gestational use of antipsychotics may also be associated with adverse obstetrical outcomes such as preterm birth, small for gestational age, and a decreased birth weight. Finally, a few prospective studies have suggested that there may also be a link between the use of antipsychotics during pregnancy and developmental delays in infants.

4. ECT during pregnancy: Like the studies examining the risks associated with psychotropic medications during gestation, those investigating adverse events from ECT use during pregnancy are small and methodologically limited. Indeed, most of these consist of case study designs with no control participants, small sample sizes, different ECT procedures, and varying periods of follow-up.

In addition to the general adverse effects that are commonly found in ECT treatment (eg, headaches, confusion, nausea), one systematic review of cases studies suggests that ECT use during the second or third trimester may lead to premature uterine contractions and preterm labor. Additionally, pregnant women undergoing ECT may frequently report vaginal bleeding as well as abdominal and pelvic pain. ECT use during pregnancy may also be linked with bradycardia and other cardiac arrhythmias in the fetus. Moreover, multiple reviews examining cases studies have noted that 3% to 8% of patients undergoing ECT during pregnancy report either abortions, stillbirths, or neonatal deaths.

Treatment During the Postpartum Period

1. Mild to moderate MDD in the postpartum period: This chapter outlines general treatment recommendations for women in the postpartum period who choose to breastfeed their infants. Those who do not should refer to general population guidelines for treating depressive disorders. For women with a *DSM--5*-defined mild to moderate major depressive episode who are breastfeeding, first-line treatments include CBT and IPT. As mentioned above, if these psychotherapies are not available in a given setting and women cannot or will not take an antidepressant, referral to other providers able to deliver CBT or IPT is warranted. Second-line agents include those for which data exist on the effectiveness during the postpartum period that minimize exposure during lactation and that poses the least known risk during the childbearing years (eg, sertraline, citalopram, and escitalopram).◔◔ Combination treatment with these agents plus CBT or IPT are also second line (owing mainly to the lack of studies examining their effectiveness). As in pregnancy, structured exercise (eg, walking) and depression-specific acupuncture are complementary and alternative therapies that have some evidence for efficacy and are accepted third-line treatments. Some evidence also supports the use of newer therapies like assisted internet behavioral activation and CBT as third-line options. While not extensively studied in the postpartum period, mindfulness-based, supportive, and psychodynamic psychotherapy have clinical support for their use.

Despite the presence of randomized controlled trial support for the efficacy in PPD, fluoxetine and paroxetine are third-line treatments. This is because fluoxetine has a long half-life and has been associated with higher rates of minor adverse reactions in breastfed infants, while paroxetine still poses a risk for cardiovascular malformations in potential subsequent pregnancies. The remainder of the new antidepressants are also third-line treatments for mild to moderate MDD because of the more limited clinical experience in lactating women. Tricyclic antidepressants, in particular nortriptyline, are also recommended at this level. Doxepin should be avoided if possible in the postpartum setting owing to reports of significant adverse reactions in breastfed infants. Finally, transcranial magnetic stimulation and bright light therapy may also be effective for the treatment of mild to moderate unipolar depressive episodes and are considered third line.

2. Severe MDD in the postpartum period: For severe PPD, sertraline, citalopram, and escitalopram are first-line choices, and third-line medications for mild to moderate depression (→above) are considered as second-line for women who are severely depressed. ECT is an extremely effective treatment that is listed as third line owing to its adverse-effect profile.

3. Postpartum anxiety: In terms of *DSM-5*–defined mild to moderate anxiety disorders in the postpartum period, first-line treatment is individual or group CBT. Facilitated self-help may also be useful in treating postpartum women with more mild anxiety. In postpartum women with severe anxiety or those who are not responding to psychological therapies, SSRIs may be considered as a treatment option: sertraline, citalopram, and escitalopram. As in during pregnancy, benzodiazepines should generally not be offered to lactating postpartum women with mild to moderate anxiety. A short-term use of lorazepam may be considered for those with severe levels of anxiety who are not responding to the SSRIs recommended above. If the patient has a history or current substance abuse/dependence disorder, a short-term use of a neuroleptic that has limited breastmilk passage like quetiapine might also be considered, although it is important to be aware that 2 breastfeeding patients using quetiapine reported mild delays in their infants.

4. Augmenting agents for postpartum depressive and anxiety disorders: Postnatal women with treatment-resistant depression may benefit from the following augmenting agents: aripiprazole, quetiapine, olanzapine, and risperidone. Quetiapine or risperidone may also enhance antidepressant therapy for postpartum OCD. In addition to being cognizant of the general adverse effects associated with antipsychotics (→above), clinicians should also monitor prolactin levels among women who choose to use antipsychotics as augmenting agents during the postpartum period. Clozapine should also not be used as an augmenting agent among lactating women because several adverse events have been reported among breastfed infants (more details on clozapine: →above).

Risks Associated With Treatments in the Postpartum Period

Breastfeeding is an individual decision made by women and should be supported by physicians as the use of most psychotropic medications while nursing is not an absolute contraindication to breastfeeding. However, monitoring by women and clinicians is required when breastfeeding is undertaken while taking psychotropic medications. Concerns about breastfeeding while taking medications often regard short-term adverse reactions and longer-term neurodevelopmental effects.

1. Antidepressant risks in breastfeeding: Exposure to antidepressants in breastfed infants is 5 to 10 times lower than exposure in utero. Serum levels in infants born preterm or those with liver and/or kidney impairment can be higher and consultation with a pediatrician can help guide decisions in these infants. It is generally believed that relative infant doses (RIDs) of medication <10% are generally safe (RID estimates infant drug exposure through breast milk using a known milk concentration and comparing it to a weight-adjusted therapeutic dose); all of the SSRIs and SNRIs tested to date appear to produce exposures below this threshold. Of the SSRIs, sertraline, fluvoxamine, and paroxetine have the lowest RID and milk-to-plasma (M/P) ratios. Just 1 to 2 minor infant reactions have been noted in case studies of >200 infants breastfed by mothers treated with sertraline and paroxetine. Citalopram and fluoxetine have had higher rates of infant reactions (4%-5%) but these are reversible and generally limited to short-lived increases in irritability, restlessness, somnolence, or insomnia. Given its relatively low RID, nortriptyline can be a useful choice if women prefer or require treatment with a tricyclic antidepressant.

Next to no data exists on the MAOIs during lactation. There is also a paucity of data on the long-term neurodevelopmental outcomes associated with breastfeeding on antidepressants. However, the limited existing evidence fails to support an increased risk of adverse long-term neurodevelopmental effects. This should be considered given the known risks associated with untreated depression in new mothers.

2. Benzodiazepine risks in breastfeeding: Low levels of benzodiazepines can be found in the breast milk of mothers who are taking these medications during the postpartum period. In one study <2% of exposed infants reported adverse events. The most common adverse events seen among exposed infants is sedation followed by lethargy, poor weight gain, apnea, and irritability.

3. Antipsychotics risks in breastfeeding: Data on most second-generation antipsychotics indicate a RID <10% and a M/P ratio <1, suggesting that they are generally safe for short-term use while breastfeeding infants. However, use of olanzapine postnatally has led to reports of adverse events in exposed infants. The most frequent adverse event seen is sedation/lethargy followed by irritability, tremors, insomnia, diarrhea, poor suckling, and possibly jaundice. Amisulpride should be avoided in general given its RID ~11% and M/P ratio ranges from 11 to 20, suggesting that it may not be safe to use during breastfeeding. Also, clozapine exhibits a high M/P ratio of 2.8 and there was 1 case reported of agranulocytosis in the exposed infant. Other women using clozapine as they breastfeed have also reported sedation and irregular vocal development in their exposed infants.

4. ECT risks in the postpartum: ECT in the postpartum poses some risks to the mother. Common adverse effects include transient memory loss, confusion, anterograde amnesia, and prolonged seizures. Among postpartum women with venous thromboembolism, it is recommended that ECT should be avoided in the first 6 weeks of the postnatal period, given that the procedure can displace thrombi. Although it is suggested that anesthetic drugs may pose minimal risks to breastfed infants, clinicians should consult with anesthetists in determining whether ECT is a viable option for breastfeeding mothers.

➔ CONSEQUENCES

Depression and anxiety disorders during pregnancy may not only cause impairment in functioning and affect interpersonal relationships but can increase the risk for adverse outcomes in the offspring. In its most severe form it can lead to suicide in mothers, one of the leading causes of maternal and neonatal mortality.

The mechanism for the association between mental distress during the perinatal period and adverse outcomes in the offspring is not fully understood. Dysregulation in the maternal-placental-fetal axis as well as irregular patterns of inflammation throughout pregnancy have been suggested to be common physiologic pathways. Environmental factors associated with depression and anxiety such as maternal smoking, drug or alcohol abuse, poor nutrition, and low socioeconomic status also play a role.

When untreated, MDD during pregnancy is associated with poorer nutrition and medical care as well as recreational substance misuse. In addition, it has been linked to an increased risk for poor obstetrical outcomes including preeclampsia, preterm delivery, low birth weight, poor head growth, low Apgar scores, smaller head circumference, and neonatal unit admission. Postnatally, depression during pregnancy is associated with increased rates of complications at delivery, decreased rates of breastfeeding, impaired mother-infant attachment, and cognitive, behavioral, and emotional problems in the offspring.

The deleterious effects of untreated PPD on women and their families are well known. PPD has been linked to impaired mother-infant attachment, negative parenting practices, poorer breastfeeding outcomes, relationship problems with their partner, paternal depression, as well as cognitive, emotional, and behavioral problems in the offspring. However, successful treatment of maternal depression during this period may reduce certain risks in the offspring.

As for untreated gestational anxiety, less is known, but it appears to be associated with several adverse obstetrical outcomes including preterm birth, low birth weight, small for gestational age, and a smaller head circumference for the neonate. Additionally, anxiety during pregnancy may increase the risk for a subsequent episode of PPD (odds ratio, ~2.5) and may also be associated with reduced rates of breastfeeding as well as behavioral, emotional, and cognitive problems in the offspring. In terms of postpartum anxiety, this may be linked with poorer breastfeeding outcomes as well as impaired bonding between the mother and the infant.

11. Psychiatric Examination

⇥ INTRODUCTION

The purpose of this chapter is to provide a framework for the nonpsychiatrist physician to collect a thoughtful and thorough psychiatric history and conduct a mental status examination. This should provide the physician with enough information to construct a differential diagnosis, institute initial management/treatment, and determine whether referral for psychiatric consultation is indicated.

Psychiatric assessment is based on detailed history and observation. Psychiatric history follows the basic format of a medical history, including identifying data and chief complaints. Once the chief complaint has been established, more targeted questions can be asked to determine if the described symptoms fit a cluster suggestive of a particular syndrome. All psychiatric histories should include an exploration of personal history and screening for harm to self and others. Suicide assessment is described in detail elsewhere (→Chapter 12.12). Observation (ie, mental status examination) is pivotal to adding information for diagnostic and management purposes.

The psychiatric interview touches upon very personal information; thus, privacy and confidentiality are of utmost importance. Given this, patients should be told a priori about the limits of confidentiality (eg, imminent risk to self or others, abuse of a child or elderly person, driving safety issues related to illness). In situations of mandatory reporting, the physician must take steps to ensure safety and meet reporting obligations (these can vary by jurisdiction; →Chapter 12.9).

Setting the stage is important for the psychiatric interview. The room should be quiet and afford privacy. Both interviewer and patient should feel safe. As the interviewer, try to sit at the same eye level as the patient. Even for a brief interview, give your patient your undivided attention. Given the potential for agitation with some psychiatric conditions, safety measures include consistently having an exit route from the interview room and ensuring that the patient is not seated between you and the exit. There are times when additional staff or security should be in the vicinity in case of increased risk of agitation or aggression.

The psychiatric interview is not substantively different from the typical medical interview, and the mental status examination mostly relies on careful observation. These skills can identify imminent risk issues and provide information to make appropriate psychiatric referrals with subsequent treatment of psychiatric illness in medical patients; this may lead to better outcomes with reduced morbidity, mortality, and readmission rates.

→ PSYCHIATRIC HISTORY

Introduce yourself to the patient! This is very important and sets the tone for the interview. It is also valuable to briefly explain the purpose of the interview. The introduction need not be lengthy and may entail something along the lines of: "Over the next X minutes I'll be asking you several questions. Some of these questions may be very private. I'm doing this to better understand you and how I may be able to help you."

Identifying Data

Ask the patient about the name, age, occupation, marital status, children, and place of residence. This is important to ask even if you know the information, particularly in hospitalized patients, as it is a preliminary screening test of cognition. If the patient cannot answer these questions, consider performing focused cognitive testing (→Chapter 12.4).

History of Presenting Illness

Ask an open-ended question to find out why the patient thinks they are seeing you and identify concerns from their perspective. This question also serves to evaluate insight. If you can resist interrupting for a few minutes, allow the patient to elaborate on their perception of symptoms or lack thereof. This uninterrupted listening is key to the mental status assessment, because it provides an opportunity to observe the organization of the patient's speech and the content of their thoughts. Once you have an idea of why they think you are seeing them, you can ask for elaboration, timelines, and details. There will be patients who talk at length because they are disorganized, manic, anxious, agitated, or intoxicated, for example. In these cases, you may need to interrupt and redirect the patient.

Asking about specific psychiatric symptoms is guided by both what the patient has already told you, your preexisting knowledge of the patient, and mental status examination observations you have already made. The questions discussed below capture most major symptoms of commonly encountered psychiatric syndromes.

Mood

When screening for depression, it is helpful to have the patients describe their mood using one word. The 2 best follow-up questions to screen for major depression are, "Have you felt down, hopeless, sad, or blue most days?" and "Have you realized you no longer find pleasure in things you once did?"

Key point: Some depressed patients will not identify their mood as sad or depressed. Elderly people in particular will often report somatic symptoms such as "tired" or "sore."

Patients in the midst of a classic manic episode are usually easy to diagnose, given their typical elated mood, pressured speech, grandiosity, and irritability. However, mania is more difficult to diagnose when patients are in the early stages of becoming manic or are partially treated. Screening for past episodes of mania can also be challenging. In fact, many patients who have had documented mania will not recall their symptoms. Helpful screening questions include, "Have you felt full of energy? Thinking of big plans? Have you ever had several days of not sleeping much but still felt full of energy?" and "Has your family ever noted you to be sped up, in thought and movement, with a notable change in mood?"

Key point: It is common for patients to have limited recollection of past manic and hypomanic events. If you are suspicious of bipolar illness, collateral history from the family, partners, or close friends is particularly useful.

Anxiety

Anxiety disorders, particularly panic and generalized anxiety disorders, are common and occur at higher rates in medically unwell patients, especially those with cardiac or respiratory illnesses. To screen for panic disorder, you can ask, "Do you ever feel suddenly panicked and have physical symptoms like a racing heart, sweating, or trouble catching your breath?" Note that in general a psychiatric diagnosis is a diagnosis of exclusion, and medical causes for symptoms need to first be ruled out. Generalized anxiety can be screened for by asking, "Do you worry about things all the time?" Everyone has worries, of course, but patients with generalized anxiety disorder are disabled by their anxiety and can usually identify this.

Psychosis

The key to conducting a reliable and valid psychosis assessment is to start with general, more open-ended questions and then becoming more targeted and specific. For example, when screening for paranoia it can be helpful to ask if the patient has had any concerns about people around them lately (eg, family, neighbors, copatients, staff), or if it has felt as if anyone has been more bothersome to them lately.

Hallucinations can be visual, auditory, olfactory, tactile/somatic, or gustatory. If you are aware of the possibility of psychosis, ask direct questions without judgment, such as, "Have you heard voices when there is no one around?" or "Have you ever seen things and thought maybe other people don't see them?" It is important to screen for command hallucinations, as the presence of such may increase the risk of harm to self and others. Visual hallucinations are more suggestive of an organic cause, particularly in the absence of auditory hallucinations or delusional thought content.

Similarly, when asking about delusions (fixed false beliefs), do so in an open and empathic way. For instance: "Have you felt that people are out to get you? Watching you? Or perhaps following you?" In hospitalized patients with psychotic symptoms be sure to ask about delusions involving staff, as this may interfere with care. Appropriate questions in this situation include, "Do you trust your nurses and doctors? Do you think they are looking out for your best interests?"

Cognition

Assessment of cognition relies on multiple sources of information such as collateral history and mental status examination. Often patients with neurocognitive disorders may not have full insight into their deficits. Cognitive changes may also occur with primary psychiatric illnesses. Nonetheless, in patients where you suspect a cognitive disorder it is important to screen for memory problems by asking, "Have you had problems with your memory or concentration?" Aphasia can be screened for by asking, "Do you have problems remembering words or using the wrong words?" Apraxia can be screened for by asking, "Do you find yourself having difficulties doing tasks you used to find easy, like turning on the television or brushing your teeth?"

Key point: If you suspect a cognitive disorder, you should screen for safety, such as leaving the stove on, driving, wandering, and forgetting to take medications or even taking double doses because the patients have forgotten they took their medication.

Review of Systems

It is also important to screen for symptoms common to a number of psychiatric disorders, such as disturbances to sleep, appetite, energy, and motivation. Specifically, one should ask about weight loss, quantify the amount lost, and establish if the loss was intentional (→Chapter 12.7). Sleep should be quantified as well. Depending on presentation, knowledge of the patient, and information already gathered, physical symptoms can be explored, such as pain, headache, seizures, and abnormal movements.

Past Psychiatric History

Past psychiatric history is a crucial part of psychiatric examination. It is important to document all past diagnoses, hospitalizations, courses of outpatient treatment, and medication trials, as well as suicide attempts and other dangerous behaviors. Assessing past suicide attempts: →Chapter 12.12.

Past Medical History

This part of examination is identical to the past medical history taken during a medical examination. Of particular note, infectious (eg, HIV), autoimmune (eg, lupus; medications such as prednisone), and neurologic illnesses (eg, seizures, migraine, movement disorders) should be explored, as these can often present with psychiatric symptoms. Ask about head injury and severity of any such injuries (eg, if the patient required neurosurgical intervention or hospitalization).

A full list of all medications, both prescription and over-the-counter, needs to obtained.

Substances

A screen of substance use and abuse may be the main clinical focus during the psychiatric history and deserves careful clinical attention. All substances of abuse should be documented including the amount used, route, period of time of use, last time used, adverse effects, withdrawal, and past substance abuse treatment. Smoking, including the amount and duration of use, should be assessed because of possible interactions with medications and increased risk of physical illness.

Family History

Family history of psychiatric illness should be explored. Specific diagnoses of family members, particularly first-degree relatives, are important. This information may guide diagnosis and treatment options for your patient. Family history of completed and attempted suicides should be explored, as suicide has significant heritability. Note that families often do not openly discuss psychiatric illnesses, and so general (rather than diagnosis-specific) questioning may be more helpful (eg, "Have you had any siblings, parents, cousins, aunts/uncles who may have had problems with their nerves/mood/functioning/behavior?").

Social History

Social history can be overwhelming, especially for nonpsychiatrists. It is impossible to gain more than a gist of someone's life story through 10 minutes of history taking. The interviewer should have an idea of the patient's work, love, and play. Important elements to understand are developments (eg, premorbid personality and any changes, how far along in school the patient got), trauma, and life events, such as marriage and losses. An exploration of recent stressors is often indicated.

→ MENTAL STATUS EXAMINATION

The second component of the psychiatric examination is the mental status examination. The mental status examination is the psychiatric equivalent of the physical examination. It provides information on areas such as emotions, speech, thoughts, perception, cognition, insight, and judgment **at the time of the assessment**. The mental status examination is performed mainly through observation of the patient while collecting the history in addition to specific questions. The core components of the mental status examination are listed below. Additionally, in all hospitalized patients presenting with psychiatric symptoms, a full physical examination, including a detailed neurologic assessment, is required.

1. General appearance, behavior and movements: Take note of dress, grooming, posture, and general health. Note if the patient can focus and shift attention appropriately. Are there any alterations in the level of consciousness? Also, be mindful of any abnormal movements such as tremor, chorea, dyskinesia, or parkinsonian slowing. It is important to test tone for rigidity and cogwheeling. Antipsychotic medications are a common cause of parkinsonism.

2. Speech: Take note of rate, rhythm, volume, tone, quality, and spontaneity. Depressed patients may have slow sparse speech, whereas hypomanic or manic patients typically have fast and pressured (difficult to interrupt) speech. Word-finding difficulties or substituting the wrong word is suggestive of a neurocognitive disorder.

3. Mood and affect: The assessment of mood and affect is helpful for psychiatric diagnosis. Mood is the subjective emotional state as described by the patient. Affect is the examiner's appreciation of the patient's emotional state in terms of quality (eg, anxious, sad, euthymic, euphoric), range (flat, blunted, restricted, or full), and stability (stable versus labile). Obviously, a patient who reports their mood as depressed needs a careful assessment of depression, while an anxious affect suggests an anxiety disorder. Furthermore, there may be discrepancies between the described mood and the affect. For instance, patients with apathy may have blunted affect and look depressed but describe their mood as normal.

4. Thought process: Take note of general coherence and stream. Abnormalities that should be noted include tangentiality (changing the topic), circumstantiality (inability to answer questions without giving excessive detail), thought-blocking (abrupt stop in a train of thought), flight of ideas (jumping from one idea to another), perseveration (repetition of words or ideas even when the interviewer tries to change the subject), and echolalia (repeating what the interviewer says).

5. Thought content: Take note of any delusional thoughts and their nature. There are many different types of delusions, including persecutory (paranoid, with the patient believing others are trying to harm or monitor him or her in some way), referential (believing radio, television, or printed media have messages directed to the patient), grandiose (believing there is something special about self), religious, and somatic, among others. Thought content can also include obsessional thoughts, ruminations (repetitive worries), and somatic preoccupations. Assessment of content also includes asking questions about the **current** risk (eg, thoughts of harm to self or others). Remember that patients sometimes endorse "paranoia" but are in fact describing situations of anxiety that make them more sensitive to their environment and others.

6. Perception: Describe the nature of any hallucinations. In the case of auditory hallucinations, describe any command hallucinations. Assessment of possible hallucinations includes actively asking the patient but also observing for objective signs (eg, if the patient appears to be responding to internal stimuli). Remember that a patient's endorsement of "voices" does not always mean they are having auditory hallucinations.

7. Cognition: If there are symptoms of a neurocognitive disorder elicited through the interview, performing the Montreal Cognitive Assessment (MoCA), available at www.mocatest.org, is a quick and sensitive tool for evaluating cognitive disorders. The MoCA can be used to evaluate for mild cognitive impairment, dementia, or delirium. At a more basic, bedside-screening level, you can ask for orientation, recall (say 3 words and have the patient repeat), memory (ask the patient to remember the 3 words and repeat them in 5 minutes), attention and concentration (spell "world" backwards), language (repeat a complex sentence), and specific tests for frontal lobe function such as similarities (how are an apple and orange alike?), abstraction (interpretation of proverbs), and verbal fluency (the FAS test, in which the patient names as many words that start with "f," "a," and "s" in one minute). When pressed for time, you can ask the patient to draw a clock face with hands at 10 past 11; a perfect clock makes a cognitive disorder unlikely.

Table 12-1. Risk factors for suicide

- Family history of suicide
- Family history of child maltreatment
- Previous suicide attempt
- History of mental disorders, particularly clinical depression
- History of alcohol and substance abuse
- Feelings of hopelessness
- Impulsive or aggressive tendencies
- Cultural and religious beliefs (eg, belief that suicide is noble resolution of a personal dilemma)
- Local epidemics of suicide
- Isolation, a feeling of being cut off from other people
- Barriers to accessing mental health treatment
- Loss (relational, social, work, or financial)
- Physical illness
- Easy access to lethal methods
- Unwillingness to seek help because of the stigma attached to mental health and substance abuse disorders or to suicidal thoughts

Source: Centers for Disease Control and Prevention. Risk Factors for Suicide. https://www.cdc.gov/violenceprevention/suicide/riskprotectivefactors.html. Accessed September 26, 2019.

12. Suicide Risk Assessment

→ DEFINITION, ETIOLOGY, PATHOGENESIS

Suicide is a deliberate action taken to intentionally end one's life. In 2009 there were 3890 completed suicides in Canada, a rate of 11.5 per 100,000 people. The suicide rate for males was 3 times higher than the rate for females (17.9 vs 5.3 per 100,000). Although suicide deaths affect almost all age groups, those aged 40 to 59 had the highest rates, with risk increased among individuals who are single, divorced, or widowed. Overall, suicide is the 9th leading cause of death, the 2nd leading cause in young adults aged 15 to 24 years.

Suicidal ideation is any thought about ending one's life, from vague and fleeting to intense and detailed. Passive suicidal ideation is the presence of thoughts about wanting or wishing to be dead, such as hoping to die from a terminal illness or to go to sleep and not wake up.

Serious thoughts of suicide, plans for suicide, and suicide attempts are surprisingly common in the general population. However, death by suicide is still a low-rate event and impossible to predict accurately. Although relatively uncommon, suicide has a lifelong and profound effect on the families, friends, and physicians of the person who dies by suicide.

Suicide risk factors (→Table 12-1) are associated with an overall increased risk of suicide but do not reflect the immediacy of this risk. Risk factors for patients in the emergency department or admitted to a psychiatric or nonpsychiatric (medical or surgical) unit include previous attempted suicide, especially if recent, treatment with antidepressants, presence of physical health problems (eg, chronic pain), poor health prognosis, social stressors, hopelessness, and substance abuse. Additional risk factors among inpatients include anxiety, agitation, delirium, and insomnia.

Warning signs are specific symptoms or behaviors that are acute or subacute in nature and which are associated with an elevated risk of suicide. Warning signs can be identified, explored further, and addressed with clinical and psychosocial interventions. Anxiety, psychomotor agitation, sleep problems, poor concentration, hopelessness, social isolation, and excessive or increasing use of alcohol or drugs are all worrisome factors that can be modified with prompt interventions. Difficulties with impulse control or anxiety in the context of depression can progress to suicidal behavior. On inpatient medical or surgical units the presence of warning signs should be a cue to exploring thoughts of suicide with the patient. Warning signs of particular concern in medical/surgical inpatients include both acute mental and motoric agitation.

Self-injurious behaviors (parasuicide) are deliberate, repetitive, impulsive actions to harm oneself without lethal intent. These behaviors are associated with difficulty expressing emotions and require psychiatric assessment and treatment. Self-injurious behaviors are a risk factor for suicide.

There are many theories proposed to understand suicidal ideation. It is associated with hopelessness, perception of having unsolvable problems, and wanting to escape one's problems. One theory proposes that suicide is the result of perceived burdensomeness, thwarted belongingness, and acquired capability (ie, the view that one's existence burdens family, friends, and/or society; belief that the need to belong is unmet; and circumstances).

→ CLINICAL FEATURES AND ASSESSMENT

Suicidal ideation is associated with depressive disorders, anxiety disorders, and other psychiatric illnesses. In a nonpsychiatric hospitalized setting, patients experiencing stresses, psychiatric illness, or physical distress may have thoughts of suicide. Patients identified as being at elevated risk or who have made a medically serious suicide attempt should have a full psychiatric evaluation.

It is essential that a suicide risk assessment be performed in a face-to-face interview. Patients are more likely to trust and share their thoughts of suicide with health-care providers showing empathy and listening nonjudgmentally.

All physicians should be able to screen for suicide. Include questions about depression and suicidal ideation during the review of systems if the topic has not yet been touched upon. Effective screening questions are, "Do you ever have thoughts that life is not worth living?" or "Do you ever wish you could go to sleep and not wake up?" A positive response to either of these nonjudgment questions leads naturally to questions exploring the nature of the patient's thoughts ("What sorts of thoughts have you had?"). The assessment needs to include questions about the frequency and intensity of thoughts of suicide, specific plans, protective factors, and any actions taken to prepare for death. It is important to explore any prior suicide attempt, especially if it has occurred within several weeks of the assessment. Clinicians should include assessment of agitation, anxiety, and hopelessness in their evaluation. It is important to understand that exploring the patient's thoughts of suicide will not increase the risk of an attempt while it may decrease the risk by giving the patient the possibility to share distressing thoughts. Seek collateral information from family members and health-care professionals involved in the patient's care.

A number of screening or clinical evaluation tools are available (eg, Suicide Risk Assessment Guide at the website of the Canadian Patient Safety Institute; Columbia-Suicide Severity Rating Scale; American Foundation for Suicide Prevention; SAFE-T at the website of SAMHSA-HRSA Center for Integrated Health Solutions). It is likely that none replaces careful clinical interview, thoughtful assessment, and reasonable level of clinician alertness, but they may be useful for ensuring all risk factors have been considered and for learning effective questions for risk assessment.

→ TREATMENT

1. General considerations: **Interventions depend on the evaluation of risk**. Patients who have made a medically severe suicide attempt or disclose active suicidal ideation and intent need prompt assessment by a mental health professional and a secure setting with no access to lethal means. Delirium and a history of impulsivity or addiction are factors that increase the risk of unpredictable behavior and risk of suicide for nonpsychiatric inpatients. These individuals also need a secure setting and close observation.

Factors to consider in determining intervention include the presence of suicidal ideation, changes in the level of ideation or intent, warning signs, risk factors, and collateral information. Interventions include pharmacotherapy, structured psychotherapy modalities, reducing access to lethal means, community-based crisis interventions, and hospitalization for higher-risk patients.

2. Hospitalization: A patient may be hospitalized for psychiatric reasons or for conditions requiring medical or surgical interventions. When elevated suicide risk is the determining factor, there is usually acute psychiatric illness requiring inpatient treatment and/or emotional dysregulation. Patients assessed as being at elevated risk of suicide may require involuntary commitment if they refuse to stay in hospital or require physical or chemical restraints to prevent harm to themselves or others. Nursing staff provide therapeutic care to suicidal patients. Engagement nursing (as opposed to simply observational nursing care) has been associated with increased patient and staff job satisfaction.

3. Pharmacotherapy: Treatment of suicidal ideation depends on the underlying stressors and psychiatric illness or illnesses. For patients at elevated risk of suicide, consider choosing a medication with low lethality in overdose and/or prescribing limited drug amounts (weekly dispensing).

For patients with bipolar disorder, there is evidence that lithium prophylaxis may be associated with reduced risk of suicide.⊘○ Clozapine, in comparison with olanzapine, is likely associated with a reduced risk of recurrent suicidal behavior in persons with schizophrenia considered to be at high risk for suicide.◐ Both should only be started after consultation with a psychiatrist, as each requires monitoring, has significant adverse effects, and is toxic in overdose.

4. Psychotherapy: Several talk therapies have been found effective in reducing the risk of suicide and/or suicidal ideation. Interventions found effective are generally structured manual-based therapies delivered in individual or group settings. Therapists are not available in all communities.

Dialectical behavior therapy (DBT) and the Collaborative Assessment and Management of Suicidality (CAMS) have been found effective for preventing suicide and are generally considered outpatient treatments. DBT is a year-long structured therapy that guides patients through the development of emotion regulation and distress tolerance skills as well as behavior skills to build a life worth living. Treatment includes individual and group sessions, phone coaching, and therapist consultation. Some inpatient settings offer DBT groups. CAMS is a briefer structured intervention that focuses on identifying factors leading to suicidal ideation and employs problem-solving strategies to address these. Patients must be carefully selected and be motivated to make changes in their lives to reduce their thoughts of suicide.

Skills for Safer Living is a 20-week outpatient psychotherapy group for people who have made 1 or more suicide attempts. Less well-known than DBT or CAMS, it uses peer leaders with lived experience.

5. Electroconvulsive therapy (ECT): While in specialized settings, patients at very high risk of suicide should be considered for ECT.

6. Secure hospital environment: Guidelines are available for providing secure inpatient settings that focus on minimizing environmental risks. Mental health units are now designed to reduce the risk of hanging from doors, windows, shower heads (ligature points) and to minimize access to lethal means (sharps and other medical equipment in locked areas only, elimination of plastic bags). Medical and surgical units are rarely designed to these standards. Additional staffing and vigilance may be required to minimize risk.

7. Access to means: Reducing access to lethal means is a harm-reduction strategy for suicide prevention. Patients expressing suicidal ideation should be asked about access to firearms, lethal medications, and other materials for suicide methods they are considering. It is impossible to make community settings safe but limited access to lethal means can reduce impulsive suicide attempts. Public health interventions focus on community-based approaches to reducing access to lethal means (eg, barriers at bridges and railway tracks). In the hospital, medical and surgical unit personnel may need to change practices to reduce access to lethal means to increase the safety of the hospital environment for a suicidal patient (eg, not storing sharps in the patient's room, removing cords).

8. Crisis support: A growing number of communities have access to crisis supports. This can include telephone crisis lines, drop-in centers for mental health support, and crisis outreach teams that assess people in their home or other community setting. Training for police results in fewer persons brought to emergency departments for assessment. Patients with suicidal thoughts managed in the community may benefit from a safety plan that describes actions, contacts, and strategies to cope should they develop active suicidal ideation.

→ PREVENTION

Suicide prevention is a public health issue with initiatives that can be targeted at individual, health-care system, community, or societal level. Population-based approaches include education initiatives, reduced access to lethal means, and stigma reduction. Primary interventions include training family doctors to better assess and treat depression and substance abuse treatment. Targeted interventions focus on groups at elevated risk of suicide such as lesbian, gay, bisexual, transgender, questioning/queer (LGBTQ) youth and aboriginal persons.

Many hospitals have implemented suicide prevention measures such as staff training, patient care protocols, and environmental reviews to minimize risks. Zero Suicide is a hospital-based quality improvement initiative to reduce suicide rates of registered inpatients. It includes a specific set of tools and strategies, many evidence-based, that a health-care organization can implement to reduce suicides in inpatient and outpatient populations (visit zerosuicide.sprc.org). The comprehensive approach to suicide prevention requires support from leadership, education of staff, assessment and treatment protocols, and measurement of indices associated with suicide prevention.

Suicide of a hospital inpatient on a psychiatric or nonpsychiatric unit is an uncommon but tragic event. Suicide of a hospital patient is a critical incident and should be explored in a death review that examines circumstances of the death and seeks to prevent similar deaths but does not find fault or assign blame. Physicians and other health-care providers who lose a patient to suicide should be offered support to cope with the loss in individual or group counseling.

1. Acute Bronchitis

→ **DEFINITION, ETIOLOGY, PATHOGENESIS**

Acute bronchitis is an acute respiratory infection characterized by a cough lasting <3 weeks. Diagnosis is established after excluding pneumonia.

Causes: Most frequently, respiratory viruses (influenza A and B viruses, parainfluenza viruses, respiratory syncytial virus, coronaviruses, adenoviruses, or rhinoviruses). Bacterial infections are found in <10% of patients and are most commonly caused by *Bordetella pertussis*, *Mycoplasma pneumoniae*, and *Chlamydophila pneumoniae*.

→ **CLINICAL FEATURES AND NATURAL HISTORY**

1. Symptoms: Fever, muscle pain, cough, production of mucous or purulent sputum. Wheezing may be observed in some patients.

2. Signs: Wheezes and rhonchi may be audible over the entire lungs. The disease usually resolves spontaneously.

→ **DIAGNOSIS**

Pneumonia must be excluded; features suggesting the absence of pneumonia include heart rates <100 beats/min, respiratory rates <24 breaths/min, body temperature (oral) <38°C, lack of signs indicative of infiltrates on physical examination.

In patients with suspected pneumonia, perform a chest radiograph. If symptoms persist >3 weeks and spirometry reveals features of obstruction, differential diagnosis should include asthma or chronic obstructive pulmonary disease. In equivocal cases, spirometry may be supplemented with a bronchial hyper-responsiveness test after the symptoms of infection have resolved.

→ **TREATMENT**

1. Symptomatic treatment: Antipyretics and cough suppressants may be used.⊙○

2. Do not use antibiotics unless pertussis is diagnosed.⊗●○

3. In patients with symptoms of acute bronchitis during an influenza epidemic, consider administration of antiviral agents active against influenza viruses within 48 hours of the onset of symptoms.⊙○

4. Inhaled β₂-agonists should likely be used only in patients with signs of bronchial obstruction (→Chapter 13.2).⊙○

2. Asthma

→ **DEFINITION, ETIOLOGY, PATHOGENESIS**

According to the 2019 Global Initiative for Asthma (GINA), asthma is "a heterogeneous disease, usually characterized by chronic airway inflammation. It is defined by the history of respiratory symptoms such as wheeze, shortness of breath, chest tightness, and cough that vary over time and in intensity, together with variable airflow limitation." Chronic inflammation is associated with airway hyperresponsiveness and recurrent symptoms that are often worse at night or early in the morning. Variable airflow limitation is caused by bronchial smooth muscle contraction, mucosal edema, and formation of "mucus plugs." In some patients irreversible airflow limitation may be caused by airway remodeling.

There are a number of different asthma phenotypes, the most common of which is **allergic asthma**. In such cases the binding of an allergen to which the patient is sensitized to specific IgE antibodies on the surface of mast cells leads to the release of mediators (including histamine, cysteinyl leukotrienes, and proteolytic enzymes), which cause airway obstruction. In some patients this early phase of allergic reaction is followed within 6 to 8 hours by a late-phase reaction in which mast cells, basophils, and other cells release cytokines and chemokines. This causes an increase in the influx of inflammatory cells, particularly eosinophils, to the airways. However, not all eosinophilic asthma can be shown to be associated with allergen sensitization. A preferred term for this phenotype is type 2 asthma, because the cytokines that cause the persistent airway inflammation originate from T-helper 2 (Th-2) cells or innate lymphoid cells type 2. The mechanisms of **non–type 2 asthma** are not as well understood, but the airway inflammatory cells are either neutrophils or are very scarce (paucigranulocytic). Repeated episodes of airway inflammation are believed to result in airway remodeling.

Factors triggering asthma symptoms and exacerbations or prolonging their course: Allergens, respiratory infections (predominantly of viral etiology), air pollutants (including tobacco smoke, household aerosols, paint fumes), exercise, stress, weather conditions, drugs (β-blockers, nonsteroidal anti-inflammatory drugs [NSAIDs]), food additives.

Factors increasing the risk of exacerbations: Uncontrolled asthma, excessive β_2-mimetic use (>1 canister of 200 doses per month), lack of inhaled corticosteroid (ICS) treatment, forced expiratory volume in 1 second (FEV_1) <60% of the predicted value, major psychological or socioeconomic problems, exposure to tobacco smoke, exposure to allergens (in allergic asthma), comorbidities, increased sputum or blood eosinophilia, pregnancy, intubation or treatment in the intensive care unit (ICU) due to asthma, ≥1 severe exacerbations in the previous 12 months.

Factors increasing the risk of fixed airflow limitation: Lack of ICS treatment, exposure to tobacco smoke or noxious inhaled agents, low FEV_1, chronic cough with sputum production.

→ CLINICAL FEATURES AND NATURAL HISTORY

1. Symptoms are variable in nature and consist of breathlessness, chest tightness, wheezing, and cough. They resolve spontaneously or after treatment. Cough can be the sole symptom. In some patients symptoms of other allergic diseases, most frequently allergic rhinitis, may coexist.

2. Signs: Wheezing and rhonchi (diffuse, bilateral, mainly expiratory) and a prolonged expiratory phase. These are sometimes observed only during forced expiration and may be absent in very severe exacerbations (silent chest).

3. Natural history: Asthma may occur at any age, but it most commonly develops in childhood; in such cases it is usually allergic. Asthma with onset in adulthood is more frequently nonallergic and often has a more severe course. Asthma exacerbations are severe, potentially life-threatening events, which usually develop over several days. Signs and symptoms of asthma may be absent in the periods between attacks or exacerbations.

→ DIAGNOSIS

Diagnostic Tests

1. Spirometry: Airflow obstruction measured by FEV_1 (however normal spirometry results do not exclude the diagnosis of asthma); positive reversibility test: improvement in FEV_1 >12% and >200 mL after an inhaled bronchodilator;

positive bronchial challenge (methacholine or histamine; sometimes indirect airway challenges such as exercise).

2. Peak expiratory flow (PEF): Mean diurnal PEF variability >10% (diurnal $PEF_{max} - PEF_{min}/PEF_{mean}$, averaged for 1 week) identifies asthma. Short-term PEF monitoring is used for assessing response to treatment, identifying factors triggering asthma attacks (eg, occupational factors), and establishing a baseline for action plans. Long-term monitoring is used in severe asthma or in patients with poor perception of symptoms.

3. Chest radiographs are usually normal. In patients with asthma exacerbation radiographs may reveal features of hyperinflation and certain complications of asthma exacerbations (eg, pneumothorax).

4. Pulse oximetry and (in acute severe exacerbations) **arterial blood gas measurements** may be performed to evaluate the severity of respiratory failure during exacerbations and to monitor their course. Notably, alveolar hyperventilation is usual in an acute severe exacerbation, so normal arterial partial pressure of carbon dioxide (arterial pCO_2) may be a sign of impending respiratory failure. Venous blood gases may also allow evaluation and follow-up of pH and pCO_2.

5. IgE-dependent allergic tests: Skin prick tests as well as total and specific serum IgE levels may identify allergens causing sensitization in patients with allergic asthma.

6. Measurement of exhaled nitric oxide (FeNO) levels is not recommended for the diagnosis of asthma but may prove helpful for disease monitoring in assessing adherence to ICSs.

7. Sputum examination: Sputum eosinophilia is a marker of eosinophil inflammation in the airways and can be useful in guiding management.

Diagnostic Criteria

None of asthma symptoms are specific. The diagnosis, based on medical history and symptoms, must include demonstration of expiratory airflow limitation and its excessive variability.

Domains contributing to diagnosis are:

1) Presence of variable respiratory symptoms (wheezes, dyspnea, chest tightness, cough, heavy breathing); often worse at night or on waking; worsening with viral infections; sometimes triggered by allergens, cold air, exercise, laughter.

2) Documented airflow limitation (at least once; a normal FEV_1/FVC ratio in adults >0.75-0.8) and its variability:

   a) >10% diurnal PEF variability (the greater the variability, the more likely the diagnosis of asthma).

   b) Documented bronchodilator reversibility testing: Minimum expected increase in FEV_1 after 200 to 400 µg of albuterol or equivalent >12% (or >200 mL) from baseline. The probability of asthma increases with further increase in bronchodilation.

   c) Improved airflow after 4 weeks of anti-inflammatory treatment (increase in FEV_1 by >12% and >200 mL or increase in PEF by 20%.

   d) Bronchoconstriction after exercise challenge testing (FEV_1 decrease by >10% and >200 mL from baseline); standard methacholine or histamine challenge test (FEV_1 decrease from baseline by ≥20%); or mannitol, hypertonic saline, or hyperventilation challenge test (FEV_1 decrease ≥15%).

   e) Excessive variations in FEV_1 between visits (>12% and >200 mL).

Classification of asthma: Currently, in daily practice asthma is classified according to the levels of asthma control (assessment covers the preceding 4 weeks):

1) **Well-controlled asthma:**

   a) Daytime symptoms ≤2 times a week.

   b) No nocturnal symptoms.

   c) Reliever medications needed ≤2 times a week.

   d) No activity limitation due to asthma.

2) **Partly controlled asthma**: 2 or 3 of the above criteria from point 1 fulfilled.

3) **Uncontrolled asthma**: 0 or 1 of the above criteria from point 1 fulfilled.

The future risk of exacerbations and fixed airflow limitation (→Definition, Etiology, Pathogenesis, above) as well as treatment issues (correct inhaler technique, adherence, adverse effects) should also be assessed. When the treatment level needed for asthma control is established (→Figure 2-1), it is used in the evaluation of the **severity of asthma**, which may be mild (controlled with treatment step 1 or 2), moderate (controlled with step 3 treatment), or severe (treatment step 4 or 5 necessary).

Differential Diagnosis

Differential diagnosis includes chronic obstructive pulmonary disease (COPD), vocal cord dysfunction, hyperventilation with panic attacks, heart failure, bronchiectasis, pulmonary embolism, and respiratory tract infections.

Less frequent conditions: Tumor of the respiratory tract, foreign body aspiration, tracheal stenosis after tracheostomy, bronchiolitis obliterans, acquired tracheobronchomalacia, hypereosinophilic syndromes. Also →Chapter 1.3; →Chapter 1.8.

Distinguishing between asthma and COPD may occasionally be difficult and even lead to a diagnosis of asthma-COPD overlap syndrome. Features favoring asthma include:

1) Younger age of onset.

2) Short-term variations in symptoms (over hours or days).

3) Symptoms worsening at night and early morning (as opposed to exertional).

4) Symptoms triggered in the short term by emotions, dust, allergens, or exercise (as opposed to chronic cough, sputum production, and dyspnea).

5) Variable versus persistent airflow limitation.

6) Lung function normal between symptoms (versus persistently abnormal).

7) General lack of progression of symptoms over time (seasonal variation likely) versus slow long-term progression.

8) Family history of asthma.

9) Lack of heavy exposure to COPD risk factors (mainly tobacco smoking).

10) Rapid response to bronchodilators and anti-inflammatory treatment (hours to days or short weeks) versus transient relief with short-acting bronchodilators.

11) Normal chest radiographs.

→ TREATMENT

Asthma cannot be cured, but with appropriate treatment it is usually possible to achieve and maintain good asthma control.

Education consists of informing the patient about the diagnosis and nature of the disease, available treatments, drug inhalation techniques, measures used to reduce exposure to the factors triggering asthma attacks and exacerbations, and monitoring of disease control. Patients should have a personal written asthma action plan covering controller treatment and measures to be taken in case of exacerbations.

Nonpharmacologic Interventions

1. Encourage the patient to engage in physical activity (inform about exercise-induced bronchoconstriction and methods of its prevention).

2. Actively help to cease tobacco smoking (counseling, pharmacotherapy; →Chapter 13.10).

3. Identify subjects with occupational exposures and provide counseling on the appropriate methods of prevention.

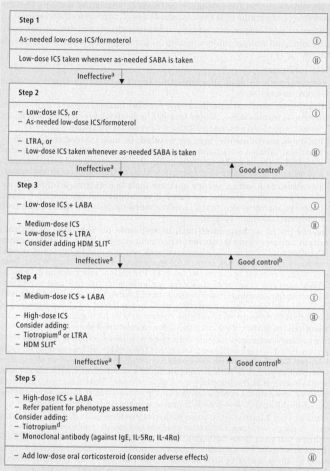

Step 1

| As-needed low-dose ICS/formoterol | ① |
| Low-dose ICS taken whenever as-needed SABA is taken | ② |

Ineffective[a] ↓

Step 2

| − Low-dose ICS, or
− As-needed low-dose ICS/formoterol | ① |
| − LTRA, or
− Low-dose ICS taken whenever as-needed SABA is taken | ② |

Ineffective[a] ↓   ↑ Good control[b]

Step 3

| − Low-dose ICS + LABA | ① |
| − Medium-dose ICS
− Low-dose ICS + LTRA
− Consider adding HDM SLIT[c] | ② |

Ineffective[a] ↓   ↑ Good control[b]

Step 4

| − Medium-dose ICS + LABA | ① |
| − High-dose ICS
Consider adding:
− Tiotropium[d] or LTRA
− HDM SLIT[c] | ② |

Ineffective[a] ↓   ↑ Good control[b]

Step 5

| − High-dose ICS + LABA
− Refer patient for phenotype assessment
Consider adding:
− Tiotropium[d]
− Monoclonal antibody (against IgE, IL-5Rα, IL-4Rα) | ① |
| − Add low-dose oral corticosteroid (consider adverse effects) | ② |

Notes: The preferred option for as-needed treatment for all patients is an inhaler containing low-dose ICS/formoterol. Another possibility is as-needed SABA.

[a] Uncontrolled symptoms, asthma exacerbations or risk factors for exacerbation, and/or risk factors for persistent airway obstruction. **Prior to increasing treatment intensity, make sure that the patient is compliant and uses a proper inhaler technique.**

[b] In patients with good asthma control for ≥3 months and low risk of exacerbations, indications for reducing treatment intensity should be evaluated (see text).

[c] In sensitized patients with allergic rhinitis and FEV_1 >70% predicted.

[d] In patients with a history of asthma exacerbations, use of tiotropium via soft-mist inhaler is recommended.

① First-line treatment. ② Second-line treatment.

HDM, house dust mite; ICS, inhaled corticosteroid; LABA, long acting β₂-agonist (inhaled); LTRA, leukotriene receptor antagonist; SABA, short acting β₂-agonist (inhaled); SLIT, sublingual immunotherapy.

Figure 2-1. Controller treatment of asthma in adults. *Based on the 2019 Global Initiative for Asthma (GINA) guidelines.*

4. Recommend allergen avoidance methods in sensitized patients (for the majority of indoor allergens these methods are of unproven effectiveness).

5. Schedule psychological counseling or mental health assessment when necessary.

6. Recommend annual flu vaccination in patients with moderate-to-severe asthma.

Pharmacotherapy

1. General principles of pharmacotherapy: The following classes of asthma medications are used:

1) **Controller medications**, used **on a regular basis** (long-term daily administration), include ICSs, inhaled long-acting β_2-agonists (LABAs), tiotropium, leukotriene modifiers, and sustained-release theophylline.

2) **Reliever medications**, used **as needed**, include inhaled rapid-onset β_2-agonists, inhaled anticholinergics, and rapid-onset $\beta2$-agonists together with ICS in the same device. This group also comprises oral corticosteroids and other drugs used for short periods of time to treat asthma exacerbations.

3) **Treatments used in severe asthma** include oral corticosteroids, monoclonal antibodies directed against IgE (omalizumab), interleukin 5 (IL-5) (mepolizumab or reslizumab), IL-5Rα (benralizumab), IL-4Rα (dupilumab), and bronchial thermoplasty.

The choice of asthma medications depends on the level of asthma control and previous treatment (treatment steps: →Figure 2-1). In patients with infrequent symptoms (≤2 times a month, without night symptoms), normal lung function, and no risk factors for exacerbations, only intermittent treatment with a reliever is suggested (step 1). Previously short-acting β_2-agonist (SABA) was the reliever of choice for patients with intermittent symptoms. More recently, a combination of a rapid-onset LABA (formoterol) together with ICS (budesonide) in the same device, used as a reliever, has been shown to be more effective at improving asthma control and reducing the risk of asthma exacerbations when compared to SABA as a reliever.◐●

In previously untreated patients with more frequent symptoms of asthma, it is recommended to start with step 2 treatment (preferably with a low-dose ICS).◐● However, as adherence with maintenance low-dose ICS is poor, an alternative treatment approach is with a combination of a rapid-onset LABA (formoterol) together with ICS (budesonide) used as a reliever. This treatment approach provides less asthma control but is equally effective at reducing exacerbation risk as maintenance low-dose ICS and at a lower daily ICS dose.◐●

Consider step 3 treatment in those with symptoms on most days or night symptoms ≥1 times per week. Controller medications result in clinical improvement within a few days from the beginning of treatment and their full therapeutic effects develop in 3 to 4 months. Frequent use of reliever medications (≥2 times/week) is an indicator of poor asthma control and need for intensification of controller treatment.

If ICS monotherapy is not providing good control, it is recommended that the preferred next treatment step consists in adding LABA to a low-dose ICS (step 3).◐● If asthma control is still not achieved, it is recommended to step up to a medium-dose or high-dose ICS/LABA (step 4).◐●

Patients who do not achieve asthma control with step 3 treatment need to be reevaluated for other conditions or factors responsible for severe asthma.

In patients maintaining adequate asthma control for ≥3 months, consider a step-down in treatment intensity, depending on treatment that achieved adequate asthma control:

1) ICS: Reduce the dose by 50% or (when a low dose was used) to once daily or to as-needed low-dose ICS/formoterol.

2) ICS + LABA: Reduce the ICS dose by 50% or to once daily (when a low dose was used) and continue LABA. LABA discontinuation is more likely to lead to deterioration.

3) ICS + formoterol (as maintenance and reliever treatment): Reduce the ICS dose (by 50% or to a low dose), continue maintenance and as-needed treatment.

4) ICS + second controller: Reduce the ICS dose by 50% and continue the second controller.

5) High-dose ICS + LABA + oral corticosteroid: Reduce the oral corticosteroid dose in a stepwise manner, then administer it every other day. A sputum-guided approach may be used in experienced centers.

In patients in whom adequate asthma control could not be achieved with step 3 treatment, reassess the patient for other diseases and causes of refractory asthma.

2. Controller medications (administered on a regular basis):

1) **ICS**: ICSs are the most effective and preferred asthma controller medications and should be the first choice for therapy.◕◕ Dosage: →Table 2-1. Local adverse effects include oral candidiasis, hoarseness, and cough due to throat irritation. Prevention of adverse effects: mouth rinsing after drug inhalation (use of spacers when administering drugs via a metered-dose inhaler [MDI]) or use of prodrugs (eg, ciclesonide). Long-term high-dose treatment may cause systemic adverse effects (→Chapter 5.1.2).

2) **LABA**: →Table 2-1. It is recommended that a regular LABA never be used without concomitant ICS therapy.◕◕ To prevent the use of LABA alone, the agents should be prescribed as a fixed combination inhaler containing LABA and ICS. The most frequent adverse effects of LABAs include tachycardia, muscle tremor, and hypokalemia.

3) **Leukotriene modifiers**: **Montelukast** 10 mg once daily, **zafirlukast** 20 mg bid. These are less effective than ICS monotherapy but have very infrequent adverse effects.

4) **Long-acting muscarinic antagonists**: **Tiotropium** via a soft-mist inhaler 5 µg once daily can be added in patients with a history of exacerbations despite a medium-dose or high-dose ICS + LABA treatment.

5) **Sustained-release theophylline** is less effective than inhaled drugs and more frequently causes significant adverse effects.

3. Reliever medications (administered as needed): **Rapid-onset short-acting inhaled β$_2$-agonists** (fenoterol, albuterol [INN salbutamol], terbutaline) (→Table 2-1) are used solely for asthma symptom relief or to prevent exercise-induced bronchoconstriction; they cause rapid symptomatic relief. The onset of action is after a few minutes, peak effect develops after ~15 minutes, and effect lasts for 4 to 6 hours. A fixed combination of the rapid-onset LABA formoterol with ICS in one inhaler may be used as a reliever medication in step 1 and 2 patients and both as a controller and a reliever medication for step 3 or higher patients.

4. Treatment used in severe asthma:

1) **Oral corticosteroids**: **Prednisone**, **prednisolone**, **methylprednisolone**. Used only for exacerbations and in patients with severe refractory asthma (step 5 treatment) because of serious adverse effects (→Chapter 5.1.2). For intensification of long-term controller treatment, usually 20 to 30 mg once daily in the morning is used; then taper off to the lowest dose providing good asthma control (this may be as low as 5 mg/d). Long-term treatment with oral corticosteroids warrants prevention of osteoporosis (→Chapter 14.13).

2) **Monoclonal antibodies** are used in patients with moderate or severe allergic or eosinophilic asthma that is not controlled with step 4 treatment (→Table 2-2). In appropriately selected patients these treatments have been shown to reduce severe exacerbation risk and may improve lung function. Evaluate the effectiveness of treatment after 4 to 6 months.

3) **Bronchial thermoplasty**: Consider this in selected patients with severe refractory asthma. Because long-term effects are unknown, the procedure should be used in clinical trials only.

Table 2-1. Inhaled asthma medications used in adults

Medication	Forms	Dosage
SABAs		
Fenoterol	MDI 100 μg	Reliever: 1-2 doses Maintenance: 1-2 doses qid
Albuterol (INN salbutamol)	MDI 100 μg DPI 100 and 200 μg Nebulizer solution 1, 2, and 5 mg/mL	Reliever: 1-2 doses Maintenance: 1-2 doses tid to qid 2.5-5 mg over 10 min (up to 40 mg/d in severe exacerbations)
Terbutaline	DPI 500 μg	Reliever: 1-2 doses
LABAs		
Formoterol	MDI 12 μg DPI 4.5, 9, and 12 μg	1-2 doses bid (maximum, 54 μg/d)
Salmeterol	MDI 25 μg DPI 50 μg	1-2 doses bid (maximum, 200 μg/d)
ICSs		
Beclomethasone	MDI 100 and 250 μg	50-100 μg bid (low dose) 100-200 μg bid (medium dose) >200 μg bid (high dose)
Budesonide	MDI 200 μg DPI 100, 200, and 400 μg Nebulizer solution 0.125, 0.25, and 0.5 mg/mL	100-200 μg bid (low dose) >200-400 μg bid (medium dose) >400 μg bid (high dose)
Ciclesonide	MDI 80 and 160 μg	80-160 μg once daily (low dose) >160-320 μg once daily (medium dose) >320 μg once daily (high dose)
Fluticasone (propionate)	MDI 50, 125, and 250 μg DPI 50, 100, 125, 250, and 500 μg Nebulizer solution 0.25 and 1 mg/mL	50-125 μg bid (low dose) >125-250 μg bid (medium dose) >250 μg bid (high dose)
Mometasone	MDI 400 μg	110-220 μg/d (low dose) >220-440 μg/d (medium dose) >440 μg/d (high dose)
Fixed combination of LABA + ICS in one inhaler		
Formoterol + budesonide	DPI 4.5 μg/80 μg, 4.5 μg/160 μg, 9 μg/320 μg	1-2 doses bid
Salmeterol + fluticasone propionate	MDI 25 μg/50, 125, or 250 μg DPI 50 μg/100, 250, or 500 μg	1-2 doses bid
Formoterol + beclomethasone	MDI 6 μg/100 μg	1-2 doses bid
Vilanterol + fluticasone furoate	DPI 25 μg/100 μg, 25 μg/200 μg	1 dose a day
Formoterol + mometasone	MDI 5 μg/50, 100, or 200 μg	1-2 doses bid

Medication	Forms	Dosage
Anticholinergics		
Ipratropium (short-acting)	MDI 20 µg Nebulizer solution (0.25 mg/mL)	In exacerbations (→Chapter 13.2)
Tiotropium (long--acting)	Soft mist inhaler 2.5 µg	1-2 doses daily

bid, 2 times a day; DPI, dry powder inhaler; ICS, inhaled corticosteroid; INN, international non-proprietary name; LABA, long-acting β_2-agonist; MDI, metered-dose inhaler; qid, 4 times a day; SABA, short-acting β_2-agonist; tid, 3 times a day.

Table 2-2. Currently available biologic agents used in asthma

Mechanism of action	Medication	Dosage
Anti-IgE monoclonal antibody	Omalizumab	75-600 mg SC (based on baseline serum IgE level), 1-4 injections every 2-4 weeks
Anti-IL-5 monoclonal antibodies	Mepolizumab	100 mg SC every 4 weeks
	Reslizumab	3 mg/kg IV every 4 weeks
Anti-IL-5 receptor monoclonal antibody	Benralizumab	30 mg SC every 4 weeks for 3 months, then every 8 weeks
Anti-IL-4 receptor monoclonal antibody	Dupilumab	200 or 300 mg SC every 2 weeks

IL, interleukin; IV, intravenous; SC, subcutaneous.

5. Allergen-specific immunotherapy is effective for the treatment of allergic rhinitis but is not generally recommended for the treatment of asthma. However, consider house dust mite sublingual immunotherapy (SLIT) for sensitized asthmatic patients with allergic rhinitis and an FEV_1 >70%.

Management of Exacerbations

1. Management depends on the severity of exacerbation. Assessment and treatment in primary care: →Figure 2-2.

2. Goals of treatment to be achieved as soon as possible:

1) **Relieve airway obstruction** using inhaled rapid-onset β_2-agonists.

2) **Relieve hypoxemia** using oxygen therapy.

3) **Reduce inflammation and prevent recurrent exacerbations** by early administration of systemic corticosteroids.

3. Treatment monitoring should be continuous or frequently repeated and include:

1) Evaluation of the severity of signs and symptoms and response to treatment.

2) Spirometry or PEF (if possible, measure the baseline value before initiation of treatment but only if this does not delay therapy; then repeat PEF until an evident response to treatment is achieved).

3) Respiratory rate.

4) Heart rate.

5) Measurement of hemoglobin oxygen saturation in arterial blood (pulse oximetry [SpO_2]); blood gases in patients with life-threatening asthma attacks or with SpO_2 <90%.

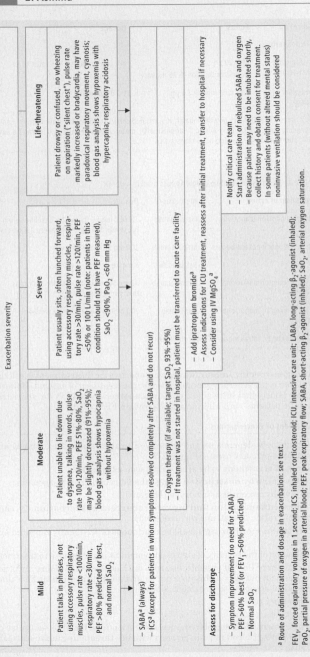

Exacerbation severity

Mild	Moderate	Severe	Life-threatening
Patient talks in phrases, not using accessory respiratory muscles, pulse rate <100/min, respiratory rate <30/min, PEF >80% predicted or best, and normal SaO$_2$	Patient unable to lie down due to dyspnea, talking in words, pulse rate 100-120/min, PEF 51%-80%, SaO$_2$ may be slightly decreased (91%-95%); blood gas analysis shows hypocapnia without hypoxemia	Patient usually sits, often hunched forward, using accessory respiratory muscles, respiratory rate >30/min, pulse rate >120/min, PEF <50% or 100 L/min (note: patients in this condition should not have PEF measured), SaO$_2$ <90%, PaO$_2$ <60 mm Hg	Patient drowsy or confused, no wheezing on expiration ("silent chest"), pulse rate markedly increased or bradycardia, may have paradoxical respiratory movement, cyanosis; blood gas analysis shows hypoxemia with hypercapnia; respiratory acidosis

– SABA[a] (always)
– ICS[a] (except for patients in whom symptoms resolved completely after SABA and do not recur)

– Oxygen therapy (if available; target SaO$_2$ 93%-95%)
– If treatment was not started in hospital, patient must be transferred to acute care facility

– Add ipratropium bromide[a]
– Assess indications for ICU treatment, reassess after initial treatment, transfer to hospital if necessary
– Consider using IV MgSO$_4$[a]

– Notify critical care team
– Start administration of nebulized SABA and oxygen
– Because patient may need to be intubated shortly, collect history and obtain consent for treatment. In some patients (without altered mental status) noninvasive ventilation should be considered

Assess for discharge

– Symptom improvement (no need for SABA)
– PEF >60% best (or FEV$_1$ >60% predicted)
– Normal SaO$_2$

[a] Route of administration and dosage in exacerbation: see text.

FEV$_1$, forced expiratory volume in 1 second; ICS, inhaled corticosteroid; ICU, intensive care unit; LABA, long-acting β$_2$-agonist (inhaled); PaO$_2$, partial pressure of oxygen in arterial blood; PEF, peak expiratory flow; SABA, short-acting β$_2$-agonist (inhaled); SaO$_2$, arterial oxygen saturation.

Figure 2-2. Management of asthma exacerbations depending on severity. *Based on the 2019 Global Initiative for Asthma (GINA) guidelines.*

Patients at high risk of fatal outcomes of asthma include those with a history of life-threatening asthma exacerbations requiring mechanical ventilation; patients who were hospitalized or needed urgent medical intervention due to asthma in the preceding year; patients who currently use or have recently discontinued oral corticosteroids; patients who do not currently take ICSs; patients who have required frequent as-needed inhalations of β_2-agonists; and patients with a psychiatric disorder or history of psychosocial problems.

Pharmacotherapy

1. Inhaled albuterol (→Table 2-1):

1) **Via an MDI** with a spacer: 4 to 10 doses of 100 µg every 20 minutes in mild and moderate exacerbations, up to 20 doses within 10 to 20 minutes in severe exacerbations. Later 2 to 6 doses every 3 or 4 hours in mild exacerbations, 6 to 10 doses every 1 to 2 hours in moderate exacerbations. In severe exacerbations more doses may be necessary.

2) **Via a nebulizer** (preferably oxygen-driven): This is usually not required except if the patient is not responding to commands. Doses of albuterol are 2.5 to 5 mg every 15 to 20 minutes, continuous nebulization 10 mg/h in severe exacerbations.

In very exceptional cases of patients in whom inhaled drug administration is impossible, use IV albuterol. Dosage: 4 µg/kg over 10 minutes, then a continuous infusion 0.1 to 0.2 µg/kg/min with continuous heart rate monitoring; alternatively administer 0.5 mg subcutaneously.

2. Oxygen should be administered as soon as possible in all patients with a severe asthma attack via nasal prongs or a mask to achieve SpO$_2$ 93% to 95% (partial pressure of oxygen in arterial blood [PaO$_2$] ≥60 mm Hg).

3. Systemic corticosteroids are used in all asthma exacerbations (except for the mildest cases), usually for 5 to 7 days. The first clinical effects are seen after 4 to 6 hours. Oral administration is as effective as the IV route if the patient is able to swallow the tablets and does not vomit (in such cases give an equivalent dose of IV corticosteroid). It is recommended to start a concomitant ICS as soon as the patient starts to improve. Dosage: oral **prednisone**, **prednisolone**, or **methylprednisolone** 1 mg/kg, up to 50 mg/d for 5 to 7 days, until satisfactory clinical improvement is achieved; IV **methylprednisolone**, dosage as above; IV **hydrocortisone** initial dose 100 to 200 mg, then 50 to 100 mg every 6 hours.

4. Other drugs:

1) **Ipratropium bromide** (→Table 2-1) should be added to albuterol in patients with moderate to severe exacerbations:

   a) Via an MDI: 4 to 8 doses of 20 µg repeated every 15 to 20 minutes; in severe exacerbation up to 20 doses within 10 to 20 minutes.

   b) Nebulized: 0.25 to 0.5 mg repeated every 15 to 20 minutes or continuous nebulization (combined with albuterol).

2) IV **magnesium sulfate** may be used in severe exacerbations if the patient is not responding to frequent administration of inhaled albuterol. Dosage: 1 to 2 g infused over 20 minutes.

3) IV **theophylline** should not be routinely used.

4) Antibiotics should only be used in case of bacterial respiratory tract infection.

Treatment of Respiratory Failure
→Chapter 13.16.1.

Follow-Up After Exacerbation
Before discharging the patient from the hospital, make sure they have learned the correct inhaler technique and arrange a follow-up visit (usually after 2-7 days). Educate the patient and modify the written asthma action plan when appropriate. Increase the dose of ICS for 2 to 4 weeks.

→ SPECIAL CONSIDERATIONS

Pregnancy

1. During pregnancy both deterioration and improvement of asthma control may occur. Poorly controlled asthma and fetal hypoxia are more dangerous than potential adverse drug reactions from asthma medications. Patient education is very important to ensure these medications are not stopped by the pregnant woman.

2. The principles of asthma controller treatment and management of exacerbations in pregnant patients are similar to those used for the general patient population. Preferred medications include ICSs (or oral corticosteroids if necessary, but efforts should be made to avoid these during the first trimester because of increased risk of cleft palate) and inhaled SABAs (data on the safety of LABAs is limited).

3. Women who were treated with prednisone in doses >7.5 mg/d for >2 weeks before delivery should receive IV hydrocortisone 50 to 100 mg every 6 to 8 hours during delivery. This is a pattern of practice based on a low quality of evidence.

4. Monitor blood glucose levels for 24 hours in the newborn if the mother received high doses of SABA during labor and delivery.

5. All asthma medications may be used in breastfeeding women.

Surgery

1. Prior to surgery asthma control and pulmonary function should be evaluated. Optimally the measurements should be performed early enough to allow for necessary intensification of treatment.

2. Patients undergoing surgical interventions associated with major perioperative stress (except for minor surgery and surgical procedures in local anesthesia) who were treated with systemic corticosteroids in doses ≥20 mg/d of prednisone or equivalent doses of other corticosteroids for ≥2 weeks in the preceding 6 months should receive IV hydrocortisone in the perioperative period (up to 24 hours after surgery) 50 to 100 mg every 8 hours with the first dose administered before surgery. This is a pattern of practice based on a low quality of evidence.

Special Forms of Asthma

1. Severe refractory asthma: In patients who require high-dose ICS + LABA (or systemic corticosteroids) to maintain control and in those who remain not fully controlled despite this therapy:

1) Confirm the diagnosis (→Differential Diagnosis, above).

2) Assess compliance.

3) Identify and treat comorbidities (rhinosinusitis, allergic bronchopulmonary aspergillosis, gastroesophageal reflux disease, obesity, obstructive sleep apnea syndrome, anxiety/depression).

4) Exclude exposure to tobacco smoke and other factors affecting asthma control and start available avoidance measures when appropriate.

Pharmacotherapy: Recommended high-dose ICS + LABA + additional controller (leukotriene modifier, theophylline, tiotropium) + systemic corticosteroids when necessary, in the lowest effective dose. Other treatment options in individuals with frequent exacerbations may include a trial of omalizumab in allergic patients or bronchial thermoplasty (while both are effective in some patients, high costs may limit their use). Bronchial thermoplasty is not recommended outside clinical trials.

2. Aspirin-induced asthma (AIA) or aspirin-exacerbated respiratory disease (AERD) is a specific type of asthma that occurs in ~10% of adult patients with asthma. AIA usually starts with persistent rhinitis, which leads to sinusitis and eventually to asthma. Nasal polyps and eosinophilia are frequent. Typical features of AIA are asthma attacks frequently associated with rhinorrhea, conjunctival irritation, and flushing of the head and neck developing within several minutes to hours following ingestion of aspirin (acetylsalicylic acid [ASA]) or other nonsteroidal anti-inflammatory drugs (NSAIDs). Analgesics safe for patients with AIA include acetaminophen (INN paracetamol) (single doses ≤1 g), salicylamide, and celecoxib. Despite avoidance of ASA and other NSAIDs, asthma persists and frequently has a severe course. The sole objective diagnostic method is aspirin challenge, which may only be performed in specialized centers that also provide desensitization.

3. Work-related asthma refers to occupational asthma (caused by conditions in the occupational environment) and work-exacerbated asthma (preexisting or concurrent asthma worsened by the occupational environment). Approximately 400 factors inducing occupational asthma or exacerbating asthma have been described. Two distinct types of occupational asthma have been identified:

1) **Immunologic**: Induced by allergens (IgE-dependent) or low-molecular--weight sensitizers (IgE-independent), most frequently develops insidiously, with variable latency periods. It is usually preceded by a complex of prodromal symptoms (eg, cough, rhinitis, or conjunctivitis).

2) **Nonimmunologic**: Called reactive airways dysfunction syndrome (RADS), induced by irritants, results from exposure to very high levels of chemical irritants and develops up to 24 hours after exposure without prodromal symptoms. It is characterized by severe long-standing nonspecific bronchial hyperresponsiveness.

Treatment is the same as in nonoccupational asthma. It is necessary to eliminate occupational exposure to the noxious factor. In some patients this leads to alleviation of symptoms and sometimes even to complete remission.

4. Exercise-induced bronchoconstriction: In patients with asthma bronchoconstriction can occur within 5 to 10 minutes after the end of exercise and resolves spontaneously in up to 30 to 45 minutes (it frequently develops in patients with poorly controlled asthma).

Diagnosis: An FEV_1 decrease ≥10% during exercise challenge or surrogate challenge (hyperventilation, inhalation of 4.5% sodium chloride or mannitol).

Management: SABA 15 minutes before exercise. In patients using SABAs daily, introduce regular controller treatment: ICS (with or without LABA), leukotriene modifier, or both. An appropriate warm-up before exercise may alleviate the symptoms. Patients exercising in cold weather may consider wearing a mask to warm the inhaled air.

5. Asthma-COPD overlap (ACO): ACO is diagnosed when features of asthma (variability in symptoms/lung function) and COPD (persistent airflow limitation) are present. Treatment: Smoking cessation, pulmonary rehabilitation, ICS + LABA.

3. Bronchiectasis

→ DEFINITION, ETIOLOGY, PATHOGENESIS

Bronchiectasis refers to a permanent abnormal dilation and destruction of bronchial walls, which involve both the major bronchi and bronchioles.

Classification:

1) **Congenital bronchiectasis** is associated with impaired mucociliary clearance (cystic fibrosis, Young syndrome [bronchiectases with normal ciliary structure, sinusitis, bronchitis, oligospermia, azoospermia], primary ciliary dyskinesia [50% of cases are due to Kartagener syndrome: bronchiectasis,

dextrocardia, sinusitis]), primary immunodeficiency, α_1-antitrypsin deficiency, other rare congenital diseases.

2) **Acquired bronchiectasis** develops in the course of severe infections (bacterial or measles), diseases causing pulmonary fibrosis (sarcoidosis, pneumoconioses, rheumatoid arthritis, idiopathic pulmonary fibrosis, ankylosing spondylitis, Sjögren syndrome, ulcerative colitis), inhalation of toxic gases, thermal injury, airway obstruction (irrespective of the cause, eg, neoplasm, foreign body), allergic bronchopulmonary aspergillosis, AIDS, postradiation lung injury, gastroesophageal reflux disease, and microaspiration of gastrointestinal contents.

→ CLINICAL FEATURES AND NATURAL HISTORY

1. Symptoms: Chronic cough with production of large amounts of sputum, usually purulent. In some cases, exertional dyspnea, wheezing, hemoptysis, recurrent lower respiratory tract infections, and low-grade fever may be present.

2. Signs: Fine and coarse rales, sometimes bronchial breath sounds, prolonged expiration, wheezes. Patients with advanced disease may develop cyanosis, clubbing of digits, and cachexia.

3. Natural history: The onset is insidious, with progressive development of productive cough followed by gradually developing respiratory failure.

→ DIAGNOSIS

Diagnostic Tests

1. Imaging studies: Chest radiographs may be normal in patients with early disease; in patients with advanced bronchiectasis, diffuse opacifications caused by atelectases, the finger-in-glove sign caused by dilated airways filled with mucous secretions, cystic air spaces (some with fluid levels), and pulmonary densities caused by fibrosis or inflammation may be observed. Bronchial wall thickening may produce a "tram tracks" pattern. **High-resolution computed tomography (HRCT)** is the gold standard test to confirm the diagnosis of bronchiectasis and is more sensitive and more specific than chest radiographs. Typical features include dilation of the airways and thickening of the bronchial walls, a lack of bronchial tapering, the presence of bronchial structures within <1 cm from the chest wall, and the "signet-ring sign."

2. Bronchoscopy is indicated in patients with unilateral bronchiectasis, a short history of symptoms, or hemoptysis.

3. Other studies to diagnose underlying conditions, including cystic fibrosis, immunodeficiency, abnormal mucociliary clearance, allergic bronchopulmonary aspergillosis.

4. Sputum microbiology is recommended for microscopy, culture, and sensitivity for bacteria, fungi, viruses, and mycobacteria. The most commonly encountered pathogens in bronchiectasis are *Haemophilus influenzae* and *Pseudomonas aeruginosa*, followed by *Streptococcus pneumoniae*, *Staphylococcus aureus*, nontuberculous mycobacteria, and enterococci.

5. Spirometry is recommended in all patients, at least yearly. Usually obstructive ventilation impairment is observed, the severity of which often correlates with the stage of the disease; in one-third to two-thirds of patients, bronchial hyperresponsiveness is observed.

6. Diagnostic workup of patients hospitalized for exacerbation: Sputum microbiology (optimally the sputum sample should be collected before the start of antimicrobial treatment), chest radiographs, pulse oximetry (or blood gases when indicated), blood cultures (in the case of fever), monitoring of the daily amounts of produced sputum.

Diagnostic Criteria

Diagnosis is confirmed by HRCT.

Differential Diagnosis

Other diseases associated with cough and sputum production (→Chapter 1.3).

→ TREATMENT

1. Chest physiotherapy and other approaches to facilitate the removal of bronchial secretions: postural drainage combined with vibration and chest percussion; nebulized hypertonic saline, oscillatory positive expiratory pressure devices, and controlled breathing exercises (such as pursed-lip breathing).

2. Antimicrobial treatment: In patients with acute infection, start from empiric therapy with antibiotics active against *H influenzae* and *S aureus*: amoxicillin/clavulanic acid. In patients with hypersensitivity to penicillins, administer macrolides (clarithromycin or azithromycin). In patients with severe bronchiectasis and chronic *H influenzae* colonization, use higher doses of antibiotics (eg, amoxicillin 1 g tid). In patients with *P aeruginosa* colonization, administer ciprofloxacin and, after the antimicrobial resistance pattern of the sputum cultures is obtained, start targeted antimicrobial treatment, typically for 2 to 3 weeks.

3. Other drugs are used to treat the underlying condition, if possible. Some patients may benefit from treatment with **mucolytics** or with **bronchodilators** (β_2-agonists, anticholinergics).

4. Surgical treatment is used in selected cases; typically partial lung resection (usually including a lobe or several segments) in patients with severe clinical course and bronchiectases located in a limited area, or in the case of a life--threatening hemorrhage. An alternative procedure in the case of hemorrhage is embolization of a bronchial artery.

4. Bronchiolitis Obliterans

→ DEFINITION, ETIOLOGY, CLINICAL FEATURES

Bronchiolitis obliterans refers to fibrosis of the bronchioles that leads to their narrowing and obliteration.

Causes: Connective tissue diseases (particularly rheumatoid arthritis [RA]); infections (viruses, mycoplasmas); inhalation of toxic substances (including nitrogen oxide, ammonia, welding fumes); drugs (gold salts, penicillamine); inflammatory bowel disease; complications of lung, heart, or bone marrow transplantation as a form of graft-versus-host disease (bronchiolitis obliterans syndrome [BOS]).

Symptoms: Exertional breathlessness and cough. Lung auscultation may demonstrate inspiratory crackles, wheeze, or occasional inspiratory squawk. The disease is often progressive and may lead to chronic respiratory failure.

→ DIAGNOSIS

The diagnostic gold standard traditionally has involved histopathologic evaluation of samples obtained from surgical lung biopsy. A working diagnosis is often established via a combination of clinical, physiologic, and radiographic features. The term BOS is generally reserved for patients after lung or hematopoietic stem cell transplantation who develop chronic lung allograft dysfunction characterized by spirometric evidence of airflow obstruction with no other identified causes. A diagnosis of BOS does not require surgical lung biopsy.

Diagnostic Tests

Spirometry reveals irreversible airway obstruction, but restriction or a mixed ventilatory defect can also be observed. Diffusing capacity of the lungs for carbon monoxide (DL_{CO}) is usually reduced. Chest radiographs are normal in one-third of patients; in some individuals signs of hyperinflation may be observed. Bronchiectases on radiographs are rare. High-resolution computed tomography (HRCT) may show mosaic perfusion, bronchiectases, and characteristic air trapping during expiration. Centrilobular nodules may also be observed. Bronchoscopy and bronchoalveolar lavage are nonspecific but may identify features of an alternative diagnosis, such as infection, malignancy, sarcoidosis, or hypersensitivity pneumonitis (the last two are usually associated with lymphocytic alveolitis).

→ TREATMENT

Treatment of bronchiolitis obliterans is often ineffective. Symptomatic treatment with an inhaled β-adrenergic agonist and systemic or inhaled glucocorticoid may be tried. In patients with BOS the intensity of immunosuppressive treatment may be increased (although the efficacy of this is questionable). Observational data suggest benefits of inhaled fluticasone, azithromycin, and montelukast (FAM) in slowing disease progression in hematopoietic stem cell transplant patients with early-onset BOS.⊘◯ In patients with RA, discontinue gold salts and penicillamine when used; a trial course of immunosuppression escalation, a high-dose oral glucocorticosteroid, or azithromycin may be attempted, although data to support such interventions are minimal.

5. Chronic Obstructive Pulmonary Disease (COPD)

→ DEFINITION, ETIOLOGY, PATHOGENESIS

According to the 2019 Global Initiative for Chronic Obstructive Lung Disease (GOLD) guideline, chronic obstructive pulmonary disease (COPD) is defined as "persistent airflow limitation that is usually progressive and associated with an enhanced chronic inflammatory response in the airways and the lung to noxious particles or gases" with the overall severity of disease increased by exacerbations and comorbidities. A rare (<1%) risk factor for COPD is hereditary α_1-antitrypsin deficiency. Exposure to noxious particles and gases in susceptible individuals triggers chronic airway inflammation (involving macrophages, neutrophils, and $CD8^+$ lymphocytes) and mucus hypersecretion. Inflammatory process, proteolysis (due to protease-antiprotease imbalance), and oxidative stress result in tissue damage, irreversible narrowing of the small bronchi, and destruction of the lung parenchyma. These changes in turn cause airflow limitation and lung hyperinflation, which when advanced may lead to gas exchange abnormalities, and in severe cases are followed by the development of pulmonary hypertension (due to hypoxic vasoconstriction, structural changes to the small pulmonary arteries, and loss of the pulmonary capillary bed) and cor pulmonale. Ventilation-perfusion mismatch caused by unequal ventilation and perfusion—with some alveoli being perfused but not ventilated, thus forming a nonanatomical venous shunt—leads to hypoxemia, while alveolar hypoventilation causes hypercapnia. Chronic inflammation, hypoxia, and physical inactivity cause **COPD systemic effects**, which include cachexia, skeletal muscle wasting, reduced bone density, anemia, and central nervous system abnormalities. **COPD comorbidities** (hypertension, ischemic heart disease, stroke, diabetes mellitus, anxiety, and depression) have adverse effects on the patient's health status and prognosis. COPD increases the risk of lung cancer.

The most frequent **causes of exacerbations of COPD** are respiratory tract infections (usually viral or bacterial), air pollution (eg, dusts, nitrogen dioxide, sulfur dioxide), or discontinuation of long-term treatment.

→ CLINICAL FEATURES AND NATURAL HISTORY

COPD is a progressive disease, particularly in the case of sustained exposure to noxious agents (mainly to cigarette smoke). It may have a variable course. The prevailing majority of patients have a multiple-year history of tobacco smoking.

1. Symptoms: Chronic cough that may be periodic or daily, frequently lasting the whole day, and in rare cases present exclusively at night; chronic sputum production, most profuse after awakening; dyspnea, which is exertional in the early stages of the disease and becomes more severe with time, leading to resting dyspnea in patients with severe disease. Unlike in asthma, the symptoms are usually characterized by low diurnal and day-to-day variation. Patients with severe COPD may complain of fatigue, anorexia, and weight loss, as well as depressed mood (or other symptoms of depression/anxiety).

2. Signs depend on the severity of the disease (in early COPD physical examination is normal, particularly when the patient is breathing quietly) as well as on the dominant role of the symptoms of bronchitis (wheezing, rhonchi) or of emphysema (patients with advanced emphysema may have an increased antero-posterior diameter of the chest [sometimes barrel chest], impaired diaphragmatic motion during respirations, hyperresonance on percussion, diminished breath sounds, prolonged expiratory phase [particularly at forced expiration]). In patients with severe COPD use of accessory muscles of ventilation, intercostal retractions during inspiration, "pursed-lip" breathing, and sometimes central cyanosis may be present; patients with decompensated cor pulmonale reveal signs and symptoms of chronic right ventricular failure (→Chapter 3.8.2); and patients with more advanced disease may develop cachexia, skeletal muscle wasting, and depression. Patients with a low respiratory drive ("blue bloaters") feel less shortness of breath and have good exercise tolerance despite hypoxemia. In patients with high respiratory drive ("pink puffers") blood gases are within normal limits due to hyperventilation at the cost of high respiratory effort, constant feeling of shortness of breath, and poor exercise tolerance.

3. Exacerbation: Acute worsening of the respiratory symptoms (dyspnea, sputum volume and/or purulence) that is beyond the usual day-to-day variations.

→ DIAGNOSIS

Diagnostic Tests

1. Lung function tests:

1) **Spirometry**: According to the 2019 GOLD guideline, a postbronchodilator (eg, albuterol 400 µg) ratio of forced expiratory volume in 1 second (FEV_1) to forced vital capacity (FVC) that is <0.7 confirms the presence of persistent airflow obstruction and, combined with appropriate clinical symptoms and risk factors, confirms the diagnosis of COPD. The severity of airway obstruction is classified on the basis of postbronchodilator FEV_1:

a) **Mild** (GOLD 1): ≥80% of the predicted value.

b) **Moderate** (GOLD 2): ≥50% to <80% of the predicted value.

c) **Severe** (GOLD 3): ≥30% to <50% of the predicted value.

d) **Very severe** (GOLD 4): <30% of the predicted value).

Do not perform routine spirometry in patients with exacerbations of COPD because the results are unreliable.

2) **Body plethysmography**, which may reveal increased residual volume (RV), functional reserve capacity (FRC), and total lung capacity (TLC), as well as an increased RV/TLC ratio in the case of hyperinflation and emphysema.

3) **Diffusing capacity of the lungs for carbon monoxide (DL_{CO})**, which is useful in patients with dyspnea disproportionate to the severity of airway obstruction. In patients with advanced emphysema DL_{CO} is reduced.

4) **Exercise tests** may reveal reduced exercise capacity in advanced COPD, which correlates with the general health status and prognosis:

a) Walking tests (6-minute walk test, shuttle walking test).

b) Cardiopulmonary exercise tests using a cycloergometer or treadmill.

c) Monitoring everyday activity with accelerometers or other devices.

2. Imaging studies: Chest radiographs reveal a flattened and depressed diaphragm, increased anteroposterior chest diameter and retrosternal space, and hyperlucency of the lungs. In patients with pulmonary hypertension reduced or absent vascular markings in the peripheral areas of the lungs and dilation of pulmonary arteries and the right ventricle are observed. **High-resolution computed tomography (HRCT)** is helpful in the case of diagnostic difficulties, as it allows for differentiation between various types of emphysema, assessment of its severity and location, and diagnosis of coexisting bronchiectasis.

3. Pulse oximetry and arterial blood gas measurements are performed to estimate the severity of COPD exacerbations, in chronic respiratory failure, and to monitor the safety of oxygen therapy (risk of increasing hypercapnia).

4. Sputum cultures (or tracheal aspirate cultures in intubated patients) are performed in patients with severe or prolonged exacerbations and an increased sputum volume or purulence.

5. Other tests:

1) **Complete blood count (CBC)**: Polycythemia (hematocrit often >55%) in patients with hypoxemia or normocytic normochromic anemia (anemia of chronic disease).

2) **Electrocardiography (ECG), echocardiography**: Features of cor pulmonale.

3) **Tests for α_1-antitrypsin deficiency** in patients <45 years of age, particularly nonsmokers or those with a family history significantly suggestive of the deficiency.

Diagnostic Criteria

COPD should be suspected in every patient who presents with (1) persistent dyspnea; (2) chronic cough; (3) chronic sputum production; and/or (4) exposure to risk factors for COPD.

According to the 2019 GOLD guideline, a postbronchodilator FEV_1/FVC ratio <0.7 in a proper clinical scenario confirms the diagnosis of COPD (→Diagnostic Tests, above).

Diagnostic Workup

It should be noted that there is only a weak correlation between FEV_1, symptoms, and impairment of the patient's health status. For this reason, formal assessment of symptoms is required, including asking about history of exacerbations and/or hospitalization within the last year. A comprehensive evaluation of patients with COPD that forms the basis for the choice of appropriate treatment includes:

1) Assessment of the current severity of symptoms using the COPD Assessment Test (CAT) (catestonline.org). This scale assesses 8 symptoms, each on

a 5-point scale (maximum, 40 points): frequency of cough, production of phlegm, chest tightness, dyspnea when walking on incline, limitation in household activities, confidence in leaving house, quality of sleep, and amount of energy. Scores ≥ 10 indicate severe symptoms, and scores >20 correspond to very severe symptoms. The clinical COPD questionnaire (CCQ) (available at ccq.nl) is another option. The modified Medical Research Council (mMRC) dyspnea scale (available at mdcalc.com) is also a possibility but limited to the assessment of dyspnea ($\rightarrow$Chapter 1.8).

2) Worsening of spirometric parameters of airflow limitation (based on FEV_1).

3) Risk of exacerbations estimated on the basis of:

a) The number and severity of exacerbations in the prior 12 months (<2 exacerbations, low risk; ≥ 2 exacerbations, high risk).

b) Hospitalization due to exacerbation in the last 12 months (hospitalization is associated with high risk).

c) Increased airflow obstruction (GOLD 1 and 2, lower risk; GOLD 3 and 4, higher risk).

In case of discrepancies in risk assessment using these methods, select the method that reveals a higher risk.

4) Comorbidities.

On the basis of symptoms, spirometric abnormalities, and the risk of exacerbations, **4 groups of patients with COPD** can be identified ($\rightarrow$Figure 5-1):

1) **Group A**: Mild symptoms, at most 1 exacerbation without hospital admission.

2) **Group B**: Increased symptoms, at most 1 exacerbation without hospital admission.

3) **Group C**: Mild symptoms but ≥ 2 exacerbations or ≥ 1 hospital admission.

4) **Group D**: Increased symptoms and ≥ 2 exacerbations or ≥ 1 hospital admission) can be identified.

Differential Diagnosis

Asthma, bronchiectasis, left ventricular failure, tuberculosis, lung cancer, and other causes of chronic cough; rarely obliterative bronchiolitis, airway tumor, foreign body in the airway, pulmonary hypertension, and tracheobronchomalacia.

Differential diagnosis of COPD exacerbations includes pulmonary embolism, pneumothorax, left ventricular failure, worsening of bronchiectasis or exacerbation of asthma, and lower respiratory tract infection.

Distinguishing between COPD and asthma may occasionally be difficult and even lead to a diagnosis of asthma-COPD overlap. Features favoring COPD include:

1) Older age of onset.

2) Lack of short-term variations in symptoms (over hours or days).

3) Persistence of symptoms (presence of bad days and good days is possible).

4) Chronic cough, sputum production, and dyspnea (rather than short-term triggers like emotions, dust, or allergens).

5) Persistent airflow limitation (rather than variable).

6) Persistent abnormal lung function.

7) Generally slow progression of symptoms over years.

8) No family history of asthma.

9) Heavy exposure to COPD risk factors (mainly tobacco smoking).

10) Transient relief with short-acting bronchodilators versus rapid response to bronchodilators and anti-inflammatory treatment (hours to days).

11) Persistent hyperinflation on chest radiographs (rather than normal between exacerbations).

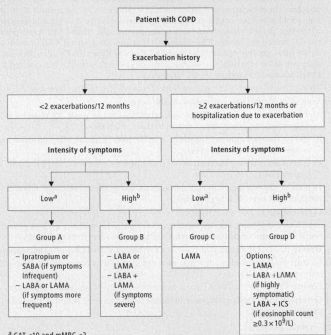

^a CAT <10 and mMRC <2.
^b CAT ≥10 and mMRC ≥2.

Note: Agents in each group are listed in alphabetical order, not in order of preference.

COPD, chronic obstructive pulmonary disease; ICS, inhaled corticosteroid; LABA, long-acting β₂-agonist (inhaled); LAMA, long-acting muscarinic agonist (inhaled); SABA, short-acting β₂-agonist (inhaled).

Figure 5-1. Classification of patients with chronic obstructive pulmonary disease and proposed initial pharmacologic treatment.

→ T R E A T M E N T

Management of Stable COPD

General Measures

1. Definitive smoking cessation as well as avoidance of passive smoking and exposure to outdoor and indoor air pollution. At each visit patients should be advised to quit smoking and offered assistance in obtaining counseling or starting pharmacotherapy (→Chapter 13.10).●●

2. Influenza vaccination (all patients) and **pneumococcal vaccination** (patients ≥65 years and younger patients with severe comorbidities, eg, heart disease).

3. Exercise is recommended in all grades of COPD.

4. Rehabilitation: In all patients with shortness of breath when walking at their own pace on the level.●● To be effective, rehabilitation should be continued for ≥4 weeks. Comprehensive rehabilitation programs include pulmonary rehabilitation, respiratory exercises, general exercise training, education of patients and their family/caregivers, smoking cessation programs, psychological support, psychosocial interventions, and nutrition counseling.

5. Treatment of patients with coexisting bronchiectasis is essentially similar but during exacerbations they may need a more aggressive and prolonged antibiotic therapy.

Pharmacotherapy

The choice of initial treatment depends on the severity of symptoms, spirometric category, and risk of exacerbation (→Figure 5-1). Management of patients with dyspnea despite current treatment: →Table 5-1. Management of patients with exacerbations despite current treatment: →Table 5-2. Patients with both dyspnea and exacerbations should be treated as those with exacerbations.

The patient's preferences should also be considered.

1. Bronchodilators are the mainstay of symptomatic treatment of COPD. They are administered either as needed or on a regular basis. The choice of individual agents depends, among others, on the individual response to treatment and comorbidities, particularly cardiovascular disease.

1) **Inhaled β_2-agonists**:

   a) Long-acting β_2-agonists (LABAs): **Formoterol** and **salmeterol** (duration of action, ~12 hours; agents and dosage: →Table 2-1), **indacaterol** (75, 150, or 300 μg once daily; duration of action, 24 hours); **vilanterol** (22 μg once daily; duration of action, ~24 hours; available only as a combination product with fluticasone furoate); **olodaterol** (2.5-5 μg once daily).

   b) Short-acting β_2-agonists (SABAs): **Fenoterol** and **albuterol** (INN salbutamol) (duration of action, 4-6 hours). Agents and dosage: →Table 2-1.

2) **Inhaled anticholinergics**:

   a) Long-acting muscarinic antagonists (LAMAs): **Tiotropium** (dry powder inhaler [DPI], 18 μg once daily); **glycopyrronium bromide** (44 μg once daily), **umeclidinium bromide** (55 μg once daily; duration of action, 24 hours); **aclidinium bromide** (322 μg bid; duration of action, ~12 hours). **LABA + LAMA combination products: Indacaterol + glycopyrronium bromide** (85 + 43 μg once daily), **vilanterol + umeclidinium bromide** (22 + 55 μg once daily). In comparison with LABAs, tiotropium results in similar or improved outcomes and may be the preferred agent for the initial monotherapy,⊘⊖ although a combination of ICS and LABA may provide a better quality of life improvement than the use of LAMA alone.⊖

   b) Short-acting muscarinic antagonists (SAMAs): **Ipratropium bromide** (duration of action, 6-8 hours; metered-dose inhaler [MDI] 20 μg/dose, 2-4 doses qid; solution for nebulization 0.25 mg/mL, 0.5-2 mL tid or qid). **SABA + SAMA combination products: Fenoterol + ipratropium** (MDI 50 + 20 μg/dose, 1-2 doses tid or qid; solution for nebulization 0.5 + 0.25 mg/mL, 1-2 mL tid or qid, as needed up to 4 mL), **albuterol + ipratropium** (solution for nebulization 2.5 + 0.5 mg/vial, 1 vial tid or qid).

3) **Extended-release theophylline**: Dosage: 150 to 375 mg bid. This is a second-line therapy due to its lower efficacy compared with that of inhaled agents as well as due to adverse effects (at daily doses ≥10 mg/kg) that include nausea and vomiting, tachycardia, arrhythmias, and seizures. Prevention of adverse effects involves monitoring of serum theophylline levels to maintain them in the range from 5 to 15 μg/mL. Metabolism of theophylline is induced—which means the dose should be increased—by fever, pregnancy, smoking, rifampin (INN rifampicin), and antiepileptic drugs, and it is inhibited—the dose should be decreased—by liver disease, heart failure, quinolones, macrolides, and cimetidine. Although the use of theophylline in resource-rich countries is limited, when added to bronchodilators

Table 5-1. Selected aspects of management of patients with COPD and persistent dyspnea despite treatment

Current treatment	Recommended follow-up
LABA or LAMA	LABA + LAMA
LABA + LAMA	– Consider changing inhaler type or drug – Look for alternative causes of dyspnea – Consider switching back to bronchodilator monotherapy – Consider LABA + LAMA + ICS
LABA + ICS	– LABA + LAMA + ICS or – LABA + LAMA[a]
LABA + LAMA + ICS	– Look for alternative causes of dyspnea – LABA + LAMA[a]

[a] Consider in case of recent pneumonia, lack of indications for ICS, or lack of response to ICS treatment

COPD, chronic obstructive pulmonary disease; ICS, inhaled corticosteroid; LABA, long-acting β_2-antagonist; LAMA, long-acting muscarinic agonist.

Table 5-2. Selected aspects of management of patients with COPD and exacerbations or hospitalization despite treatment

Current treatment	Suggested changes
LABA or LAMA	– LABA + LAMA or – LABA + ICS (consider in patients with eosinophil count $\geq 0.3 \times 10^9$/L or in those with eosinophil count $\geq 0.1 \times 10^9$/L and exacerbations [≥ 2/y or ≥ 1 hospitalization])
LABA + LAMA	– Eosinophil count $\geq 0.1 \times 10^9$/L: LABA + LAMA + ICS – Eosinophil count $< 0.1 \times 10^9$/L: Consider roflumilast[a] or azithromycin (in ex-smokers) or theophylline[b]
LABA + ICS	– LABA + LAMA + ICS or – LABA + LAMA (consider in case of recent pneumonia, lack of indications for ICS, or lack of response to ICS treatment)
LABA + LAMA + ICS	– Roflumilast[a] or azithromycin (in ex-smokers) or theophylline[b] or – LABA + LAMA (consider in case of recent pneumonia, lack of indications for ICS, or lack of response to ICS treatment)

[a] In patients with FEV$_1$ <50% and chronic cough with sputum production.
[b] Not used often in resource-rich countries.

COPD, chronic obstructive pulmonary disease; FEV$_1$, forced expiratory volume in 1 second; ICS, inhaled corticosteroid; LABA, long-acting β_2-antagonist; LAMA, long-acting muscarinic agonist.

(LAMA/LABA or ICS/LABA and LAMA) it may improve bronchodilation and reduce inflammation. It may be used in similar situations as roflumilast (→below), but these two agents should not be used together.

2. ICSs are used in COPD with decreasing frequency and not as monotherapy. When used (→Table 2-1), they are either combined with LABA or are part of the so-called triple therapy with LABA and LAMA. ICS may play a role in preventing exacerbations in high-risk patients (groups C and D). The GOLD guidelines suggest their use with LABA in patients having symptoms when treated with ≥1 long-acting bronchodilator and having elevated eosinophil counts $>0.3 \times 10^9$/L or $>0.1 \times 10^9$/L and hospitalization and/or >1 exacerbation per year. A once-daily triple therapy in a single inhaler combining fluticasone furoate 100 µg, umeclidinium 62.5 µg, and vilanterol 25 µg has recently become available for group D patients. There is concern about ICSs increasing the risk of pneumonia and reactivation of tuberculosis. ICSs should likely be withdrawn once the patient is stable.

3. Combination of inhalers from different classes: Numerous studies comparing effects of drugs from different classes are available and were recently summarized in a Cochrane network meta-analysis.◓ The relevant points are:

1) The LABA/LAMA combination is likely the most effective for reducing COPD exacerbations in populations at risk for exacerbation with the additive effect on bronchodilation and lung function. Several products contain LAMA and LABA in a single inhaler (aclidinium/formoterol, glycopyrronium/indacaterol, tiotropium/olodaterol, umeclidinium/vilanterol). The relative benefit of those drugs over 2-inhaler regimen and relative value against each other is not proven or not clear.

2) LAMA-containing inhalers may have an advantage over those without LAMA for preventing COPD exacerbations.

3) Combination therapies are likely more effective than monotherapies for improving symptom and quality-of-life scores.

4) ICS-containing inhalers are associated with an increased risk of pneumonia.

4. Roflumilast is a phosphodiesterase-4 (PDE-4) inhibitor; it may be considered as an add-on therapy (500 mg once daily) to 1 or 2 inhaled bronchodilators in group C or D patients with symptoms of chronic bronchitis. Do not use roflumilast in patients who are underweight or treated with theophylline.

5. Other agents:

1) In young patients with confirmed $α_1$-antitrypsin deficiency, consider $α_1$-antitrypsin augmentation therapy.

2) Morphine to control dyspnea in patients receiving palliative care (→Chapter 11.1).

3) Mucolytics: Avoid long-term use (except in selected patients with viscous bronchial secretions). In patients with moderate to severe COPD, ≥2 exacerbations in the last 2 years, and not treated with ICS, the use of carbocysteine or N-acetylcysteine may reduce the frequency of exacerbations. Antioxidants and respiratory stimulants are not recommended. Antitussives are contraindicated.

4) Vitamin D supplementation is used only in patients with documented deficiency (blood vitamin D concentration <50 nmol/L).

5) Azithromycin: To be considered in patients with moderate to severe COPD with ≥1 moderate or severe COPD exacerbations in the last year (this is used with the aim of reducing COPD exacerbations).

Long-Term Oxygen Therapy

This is usually necessary in patients with severe COPD and either of the following:

1) Partial pressure of oxygen in arterial blood (PaO_2) ≤55 mm Hg or hemoglobin oxygen saturation in arterial blood (SpO_2) ≤88%.

2) PaO_2 56 to 60 mm Hg or SpO_2 ~88% and symptoms of pulmonary hypertension, peripheral edema suggestive of congestive heart failure, or hematocrit >55%.

The target values are PaO_2 ≥60 mm Hg or SpO_2 ≥90%. The decision to use home oxygen therapy should be based on PaO_2 values confirmed 2 times over a 3-week period in a clinically stable awake patient.

Ventilatory Support

In patients with very severe COPD (group D), and particularly those with significant daytime hypercapnia despite optimal pharmacotherapy, consider noninvasive ventilation (NIV) combined with home oxygen therapy. NIV parameters should be adjusted to decrease partial pressure of carbon dioxide in arterial blood ($PaCO_2$) by ≥20%. In patients with coexisting obstructive sleep apnea, consider ventilatory support with continuous positive airway pressure (CPAP).

Surgical Treatment

1. Removal of large bullae (bullectomy): Consider this if the bulla extends over ≥50% of the lung volume and causes evident compression of the adjacent pulmonary parenchyma.

2. Lung volume reduction surgery (LVRS) may be considered in patients with FEV_1 >20% of the predicted value and emphysema that involves mainly upper lobes or in patients with low physical capacity after preoperative rehabilitation and homogenously distributed emphysema.

3. Lung transplantation: Criteria for referral for the lung transplantation waiting list according to GOLD guideline are a BODE (**b**ody-mass index, airflow **o**bstruction, **d**yspnea, and **e**xercise) index of 7 to 10 and ≥1 of the following:

1) History of exacerbation with acute hypercapnia ($PaCO_2$ >50 mm Hg).

2) Pulmonary hypertension and/or cor pulmonale despite oxygen therapy.

3) FEV_1 <20% of the predicted value and DL_{CO} <20% of the predicted value or homogeneous distribution of emphysema.

Palliative Care

Palliative care is aimed at improving the quality of life and daily functioning in terminally ill patients with severe COPD. It also includes spiritual support and end-of-life care decisions.

Management of Exacerbations

Medical history: Ask about duration of worsening or new symptoms, severity of airflow limitation (based on previous examinations), history of exacerbations (including hospitalizations and mechanical ventilation), comorbidities, as well as treatment used and any recent treatment modifications.

Treatment Setting

1. Indications for diagnostic or therapeutic hospital admission: Severe COPD or history of frequent exacerbations, significant worsening of symptoms (eg, rapid onset of resting dyspnea), alarming signs (eg, cyanosis, peripheral edema), no improvement with first-line treatment, severe comorbidities (eg, heart failure or onset of arrhythmia), uncertain diagnosis, advanced age, inadequate home care. Other patients can be treated at home.

2. Indications for admission to the intensive care unit (ICU) (the first 5 usually also include indication for endotracheal intubation and ventilatory support):

1) Respiratory arrest or irregular respirations.

2) Severe dyspnea (particularly when associated with evident involvement of accessory muscles of respiration and paradoxical motion of the abdominal wall or tachypnea >35 breaths/min) with poor response to initial acute treatment and NIV.

3) Altered mental status (confusion, somnolence, coma, agitation).

4) Persistent/worsening hypoxemia (PaO_2 <40 mm Hg), severe/worsening hypercapnia ($PaCO_2$ >60 mm Hg), or severe/worsening respiratory acidosis (pH <7.25) despite oxygen therapy and NIV.

5) Unavailability or intolerance of NIV.

6) Hemodynamic instability (need for vasoconstrictor use, bradycardia <50 beats/min with altered mental status).

7) Other severe complications (metabolic disturbances, sepsis, severe pneumonia, high-risk pulmonary embolism, barotrauma, pneumothorax, large pleural effusions, massive aspiration).

8) Inadequate supervision and expertise with the use of NIV in a non-ICU setting.

Assessment

In hospitalized patients: Arterial blood gases, CBC, electrolyte levels, renal and liver function tests, ECG, chest radiographs.

Microbiology of sputum (or tracheal aspirates in intubated patients) in case of (1) an infectious exacerbation not responding to initial antimicrobial therapy; (2) a severe exacerbation or risk factors for nonresponse to empirical antimicrobial therapy (prior treatment with antibiotics or oral corticosteroids, >4 exacerbations in the previous year, FEV_1 <30% of the predicted value, protracted exacerbation).

Do not perform spirometry in patients with a COPD exacerbation. In patients treated at home pulse oximetry is usually sufficient for SpO_2 measurements.

Pharmacotherapy

1. SABA (→Table 2-1): Up to 8 doses via an MDI with a spacer device every 1 to 2 hours or nebulized (eg, albuterol 2.5-5 mg every 4-6 hours). Drug doses and frequency of administration depend on response to treatment. In addition, you may use **ipratropium bromide** (2-8 doses via an MDI with a spacer device or 0.25-0.5 mg nebulized qid). β_2-Agonists and anticholinergics may be used in the form of a fixed combination (fenoterol + ipratropium) with administration of up to 8 doses via an MDI with a spacer device or 1 to 2.5 mL nebulized qid. IV theophylline is a second-line drug: administer 3 mg/kg in an injection followed by an infusion of 0.5 mg/kg/h (maximum total dose, 750 mg/d).

2. Corticosteroids⊘●: A reasonable regimen may consists of oral **prednisone** 40 mg/d (in patients unable to take oral medications, administer IV **hydrocortisone** 100 mg every 6-8 hours or **methylprednisolone** 40 mg/d) for 5 to 7 days rather than longer,⊘● even in patients with severe or very severe disease. Alternatively use nebulized budesonide 2 mg qid.

3. Antibiotics: Usually a 5-day to 10-day course is indicated in patients with suspected bacterial infection, that is, when sputum becomes more purulent, its production increases, and/or dyspnea increases as well, and in patients receiving ventilatory support (invasive or noninvasive). Measurements of procalcitonin levels may be helpful when considering the need for antimicrobial therapy; it is safe to use no antimicrobial therapy in patients with procalcitonin levels <0.25 µg/L, but in such cases the measurement may be repeated after 6 to 24 hours. The most frequent etiologic factors are *Haemophilus influenzae*, *Streptococcus pneumoniae*, and *Moraxella catarrhalis*.

1) In **patients at low risk of *Pseudomonas aeruginosa* infection**:

   a) And no risk factors for worsening of exacerbation (severe COPD, serious comorbidities, frequent exacerbations [>3 per year], prior antimicrobial therapy within 3 months), use **amoxicillin** (the first-choice antimicrobial agent).

   b) In other patients use **amoxicillin/clavulanic acid** (2 g/d).

   c) In patients with penicillin hypersensitivity use macrolides.

   d) Second-line antimicrobial agents: Fluoroquinolones with antistreptococcal activity (levofloxacin, moxifloxacin) or second-generation or third--generation cephalosporins.

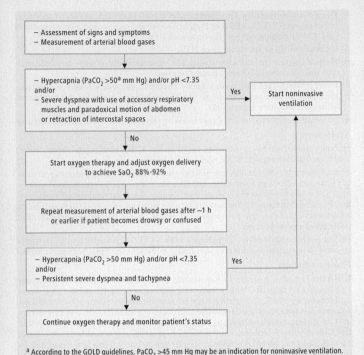

a According to the GOLD guidelines, $PaCO_2$ >45 mm Hg may be an indication for noninvasive ventilation.

COPD, chronic obstructive pulmonary disease; GOLD, Global Initiative for Chronic Obstructive Lung Disease; $PaCO_2$, partial pressure of carbon dioxide in arterial blood; SaO_2, arterial oxygen saturation.

Figure 5-2. Oxygen therapy in chronic obstructive pulmonary disease exacerbations.

2) In **patients at high risk of *P aeruginosa* infection** (recent hospitalization, frequent antimicrobial treatment [≥4 times a year], severe exacerbation, positive *P aeruginosa* cultures obtained during prior exacerbation or when clinically stable):

a) If oral treatment is possible use oral **ciprofloxacin**.

b) If parenteral treatment is necessary use parenteral **ciprofloxacin** or β-lactams active against *P aeruginosa* (eg, **ceftazidime**, **cefepime**).

Also →Chapter 13.14.

Oxygen Therapy and Supportive Treatment

1. Patients with respiratory failure should receive **oxygen therapy** (→Figure 5-2). In patients receiving optimal pharmacologic treatment and oxygen therapy who develop acidosis (pH ≤7.35) and/or increasing hypercapnia ($PaCO_2$ >45 mm Hg) or who have persistent dyspnea (particularly if severe, with involvement of accessory muscles of respiration and paradoxical motion of the abdominal wall or tachypnea >35 breaths/min), use ventilatory support, unless not indicated due to end-stage disease. Use NIV whenever possible; in other cases intubate the patient and continue ventilatory support.

2. Supportive treatment in hospitalized patients:

1) **Appropriate hydration** (with strict monitoring of fluid balance).

2) **Nutritional support**.

3) **Antithrombotic prophylaxis** (→Chapter 3.19.2).

4) **Procedures facilitating evacuation of airway secretions** (by cough stimulation and forced small-volume expirations). In patients who produce copious amounts of sputum or have lobar atelectasis, manual or mechanical chest percussion and postural drainage may be effective. In patients with atelectasis perform therapeutic bronchoscopy.

Conditions of Hospital Discharge

1. The patient (or caregiver) is able to appropriately administer prescribed medications.

2. The patient requires inhaled SABA administration not more frequently than every 4 hours.

3. The patient, who could walk before the admission, is currently able to walk around the room.

4. The patient can eat and sleep without frequently waking up due to dyspnea.

5. The patient's clinical condition (including blood gases) has been stable over the prior 12 to 24 hours.

6. Follow-up visits and home support (eg, nurse visits, oxygen delivery, meal preparation) have been arranged. The first follow-up visit is usually scheduled 4 to 6 weeks after discharge

Follow-Up Evaluation After Hospital Discharge

Follow-up evaluation:

1) Estimation of the severity of symptoms (the CAT or mMRC scale can be used).

2) Assessment of the patient's ability to manage in the community, exercise, and perform daily activities.

3) Spirometry.

4) Assessment of drug inhalation techniques.

5) Assessment of the patient's understanding of prescribed treatment.

6) Assessment of the need for long-term oxygen therapy or use of nebulized medications at home.

7) Assessment of comorbidities.

In patients who develop hypoxemia during exacerbations, arterial blood gases or pulse oximetry (or both) should be performed before and 3 months after hospital discharge.

→ COMPLICATIONS

Pulmonary hypertension and right ventricular failure, secondary polycythemia, anemia of chronic disease, cachexia, venous thromboembolism, depression, and anxiety. Also →Chapter 13.16.2.

→ SPECIAL CONSIDERATIONS

Asthma-COPD Overlap
→Chapter 13.2.

Surgery
COPD increases the risk of perioperative complications. It can be minimized by achieving optimal lung function before surgery, early mobilization after surgery, pulmonary physiotherapy, and effective treatment of pain. Lung function tests are required only before chest or cardiac surgery, but in patients with more severe COPD they are also indicated prior to other types of surgery.

Air Travel

Patients with FEV_1 <30% of the predicted value or requiring long-term oxygen therapy should consult a pulmonary medicine specialist before the flight. During air travel patients receiving long-term oxygen therapy should have oxygen administered via nasal prongs to maintain SpO_2 >85% (2-4 L/min). Most airlines provide oxygen on request, but this must be booked in advance.

→ **PROGNOSIS**

Prognosis can be improved mainly by smoking cessation. COPD exacerbations increase the risk of death. The main causes of death are cardiovascular disease, lung cancer, and respiratory failure.

→ **PREVENTION**

The most effective method of COPD prevention is nonsmoking. However, avoidance of exposure to air pollution and other risk factors is also important.

6. Cystic Fibrosis

→ **DEFINITION, ETIOLOGY, PATHOGENESIS**

Cystic fibrosis (CF) is a genetic disorder causing abnormal secretion of the exocrine glands, mainly affecting the respiratory and gastrointestinal (GI) systems. It is caused by mutations of the *CFTR* gene encoding CFTR (cystic fibrosis transmembrane conductance regulator; a cellular membrane protein that acts on chloride ion channels in epithelial cells). Synthesis of the defective protein affects the transmembrane transport of sodium and chloride, resulting in lumen dehydration and reduction in water content of exocrine secretions and mucus. High concentrations of sodium chloride inactivate the enzymes and proteins involved in local response to infection.

Abnormalities of the respiratory system include increased mucus secretion and retention with secondary chronic infections (DNA released from dead neutrophils increases the mucus viscosity) leading to mucus plugging, segmental atelectasis, bronchiectasis, and cysts (subpleural cysts frequently cause pneumothoraces).

Abnormalities of the GI system affect the pancreas and include retention of pancreatic secretions, activation of proteolytic enzymes, inflammation, and dilation of the pancreatic ducts with fibrosis (hence the name cystic fibrosis), resulting in pancreatic exocrine insufficiency and diabetes mellitus. Areas of steatosis and biliary cirrhosis are found in the liver. The presence of thick secretions in the intestines may cause any combination of abdominal pain, bowel obstruction, gastroenteritis, colitis, and distal intestinal obstruction syndrome (DIOS).

Effects on other organs include obliteration and hypoplasia of the vas deferens (resulting in male infertility). Impaired chloride reabsorption in the sweat glands leads to elevated sweat chloride levels and salty sweat. Chronic rhinosinusitis and nasal polyps are common.

→ **CLINICAL FEATURES AND NATURAL HISTORY**

1. Symptoms: Chronic cough is usually the presenting pulmonary symptom. It is associated with the production of thick purulent sputum (frequently upon awakening). Other symptoms include dyspnea, wheeze, chest congestion, nasal congestion with chronic purulent secretions, epistaxis, and hemoptysis.

The passage of bulky and foul-smelling stools (indicative of pancreatic insufficiency), flatulence, abdominal pain, bloating, and constipation with weight loss and failure to grow are common presenting features.

2. Physical findings: Rhonchi, rales, coarse breath sounds (upper lobe predominance), clubbing of digits, nasal polyps, and low body weight are common.

3. Natural history: The disease usually manifests in early childhood or infancy, uncommonly at a later age (in such cases it is associated with less severe and atypical symptoms). Typically the condition causes chronic destruction of the airways with subsequent involvement of the pulmonary parenchyma, ultimately leading to respiratory failure and death. Median age of survival (the age beyond which we expect 50% of babies with CF born today to live) in 2017 in Canada was 52.3 years.◓

4. Pulmonary exacerbations: Deterioration of performance status, worsening cough, increased production of purulent sputum, chest congestion, fever, and increased dyspnea are usually accompanied by varying progression of the auscultatory, spirometric, and radiographic abnormalities and new or increased pathogens appearing in the sputum.

→ DIAGNOSIS

Diagnosis is suggested by clinical symptoms or by the diagnosis of cystic fibrosis in siblings.

1. Diagnosis is confirmed by ≥1 of the following tests:

1) Sweat chloride [Cl] concentrations ≥60 mmol/L in 2 measurements carried out on different days.

2) Demonstration of a known mutation of both *CFTR* allele (this test is recommended in all patients and is crucial when [Cl]⁻ concentration measurements are not diagnostic).

3) Abnormal nasal transepithelial electrical potential difference or transepithelial potential difference in rectal mucosa biopsy.

2. Other diagnostic tests:

1) **Chest radiographs and high-resolution computed tomography (HRCT)** reveal pulmonary abnormalities (depending on the stage of the disease, the earliest and most severe lesions are usually observed in the upper lobes), including various combinations of airway thickening, dilation of the bronchi (bronchiectasis), subpleural cysts or bullae, peripheral circular or linear opacifications, recurrent consolidation or segmental atelectases with the "tree-in-bud" appearance, hilar lymphadenopathy, and pneumothorax.

2) **Lung function tests** can reveal obstructive respiratory flow pattern with significant hyperinflation (increased total lung capacity [TLC], functional residual capacity [FRC], residual volume [RV], and RV/TLC ratio). Repeat spirometry at every visit and full pulmonary function testing on a yearly basis is recommended.

3) **Sputum microbiology** (or less frequently bronchoalveolar lavage, throat swab): Bacterial infection is initially caused by *Staphylococcus aureus* or *Haemophilus influenzae* and later *Pseudomonas aeruginosa* (PsA). Less prevalent pathogens include *Achromobacter xylosoxidans*, *Stenotrophomonas maltophilia*, *Aspergillus species*, and *Burkholderia cepacia* complex. Sputum is usually sent every 3 to 6 months and with pulmonary exacerbations.

4) **Laboratory tests**:

   a) Reduced fecal levels of elastase 1, trypsin, and chymotrypsin with increased fecal excretion of fats (72-hour fecal fat collection).

   b) Increased serum liver enzyme levels (particularly alkaline phosphatase, γ-glutamyl transferase [transpeptidase]).

   c) Increased erythrocyte sedimentation rate, C-reactive protein, and white blood cell counts (especially during exacerbations).

d) Oral glucose tolerance test (repeat every year, as this allows for early diagnosis of CF-related diabetes mellitus).

e) Pulse oximetry, arterial blood gases (when hypoxemic), or both. Routine blood testing including fat-soluble vitamin levels (A, D, E, K) should be performed yearly.

5) **Ultrasonography** to assess the liver (suggested every 2 years).

6) **Bone densitometry** (suggested every 2 years).

7) **Incremental exercise testing** (cycle ergometry; 6-minute walk test) annually for patients who are dyspneic or have moderate to severe disease.

→ TREATMENT

Nonpharmacologic Management

1. Respiratory physiotherapy repeated systematically several times—usually twice—a day (postural drainage assisted by chest percussion or vibration, effective coughing techniques, and use of simple support devices [eg, Flutter, Acapella]) are recommended. Earlier physiotherapy studies compared to doing nothing demonstrated a variable improvement in pulmonary function, reduction of daily symptoms, increased sputum expectorated, and decreased future pulmonary exacerbations. The best evidence in current practice is usually seen with postural drainage with chest percussion and vibration or the use of Positive Expiratory Pressure (PEP) masks. During **exacerbations**, physiotherapy should be intensified (3-4 times a day), particularly in patients with atelectasis or mucus plugging. A regular exercise program is indicated in all patients, especially those who are dyspneic or have more severe disease.⊘○ Psychological assessment and counseling is important in that anxiety and/or depression is prevalent, especially in those with moderate to severe disease.

2. Nutritional management: Suggest a high-protein, high-fat (35%-40% of calories from fat), and high-calorie (130%-150% of normal daily requirement) diet, supplemented with enzyme preparations and vitamins (particularly fat-soluble vitamins A, D, E, and K) for patients with pancreatic insufficiency (85% of Canadian CF patients).

3. Immunoprophylaxis: All vaccines should be administered as in the general population, with particular emphasis on vaccination against pertussis and measles. Patients with liver disease should receive vaccination coverage against hepatitis A and B. All patients should be vaccinated against influenza every year.

4. Oxygen therapy: Recommended for patients who are hypoxemic (PaO_2 ≤55 mm Hg, SpO_2 <88%); it may also improve exercise performance in those who demonstrate hypoxemia with physical activities.

Pharmacotherapy

1. Mucolytics (individual or combined): Inhaled **dornase α** 2.5 mg once daily (especially in patients with moderate to severe disease); inhaled hypertonic (3-5 mL of 3%-7%) saline; inhaled dry powder mannitol 400 mg bid. An inhaled $β_2$-agonist must be administered before inhalation of mucolytics. Mannitol is currently approved in Australia and the UK.

2. Bronchodilators are commonly used before the administration of inhaled mucolytics, physiotherapy, inhaled saline solutions, or prior to exercising in patients who have shown postbronchodilator improvement of symptoms or spirometry results.

3. Inhaled glucocorticoids: Only in patients with coexistent asthma or allergic bronchopulmonary aspergillosis (ABPA).

4. Pancreatic enzymes (for pancreatic insufficient patients) should be administered with each meal at individually adjusted doses. In adults, the starting dose is 500 IU of lipase/kg per meal and 250 IU/kg with snacks. If necessary, increase the dose by 150 to 250 IU/kg per meal to a maximum of 2500 IU/kg per meal (do not exceed 7000-12,000 IU/kg/d).

5. Fat-soluble vitamins A, D, E, and K are recommended on a daily basis. Their doses should be adjusted on the basis of serum vitamin levels or evidence of end organ damage (CF-related liver or bone disease). The vitamins should be taken together with pancreatic enzymes.

6. Oral nonsteroidal anti-inflammatory drugs (NSAIDs): Azithromycin (a commonly used antibiotic, but in this instance used for its anti-inflammatory and purported immune-modulating properties) 250 or 500 mg (patients ≥36 kg body weight) 3 times/wk (particularly in patients with PsA infection).⊘◐ This may be beneficial long term in patients with more advanced lung disease and those who are prone to more frequent pulmonary exacerbations. Clinical effectiveness should be reevaluated every 6 to 12 months. Before the initiation of long-term treatment, sputum tests must be performed to exclude nontuberculous mycobacterial (NTB) infection. Repeat sputum testing for NTB should be performed every 6 months thereafter while receiving azithromycin. Ibuprofen given orally in high doses, maintaining a serum concentration of 50 to 100 µg/mL in patients with CF (6-18 years old), can slow the progression of lung disease. This is usually not recommended for the adult population.

7. Chronic antimicrobial treatment: Inhaled preservative-free tobramycin (300 mg nebulized bid for 1 month) is strongly recommended in patients aged ≥6 years for the eradication of PsA after the first documented culture of sputum or throat swab. For CF patients who are chronically infected with PsA, preservative-free tobramycin (300 mg nebulized bid) administered in 1-month cycles (on alternating months) has been shown to be effective in maintaining or improving lung function, reducing respiratory symptoms, and reducing the risk for future pulmonary exacerbations. Tobramycin via a dry powder inhaler (4 capsules or 112 mg bid) has shown similar results in comparison with tobramycin inhaled solution (TIS). Aztreonam lysine inhaled solution (75 mg nebulized tid) given in 1-month cycles (on alternating months) has shown similar results and is equally effective when compared with tobramycin. Colistin (polymyxin E), commercially manufactured as colistin sulfate or colistimethate sodium, has been used in an inhaled format for the chronic treatment of PsA infection in CF. When compared with placebo, it has demonstrated similar results to that of TIS. Older studies using inhaled colistimethate sodium (1 million IU bid) when compared with TIS appeared to be less effective; however, this may be due to a dose-dependent effect and/or type of colistin preparation used. More conventional dosing of colistimethate sodium would be 240 to 480 mg/d in divided dosing (bid). Colistimethate sodium via a dry powder inhaler (1,662,500 IU bid) has been shown to be comparable to TIS in this patient population. Liposomal amikacin (590 mg nebulized once daily) versus placebo has shown comparable results to TIS and has been shown to be noninferior in comparison to TIS. Levofloxacin inhaled solution (240 mg nebulized bid) has also been shown to be as effective as TIS short term. The new inhaled antibiotics (aztreonam lysine, liposomal amikacin, levofloxacin) are also delivered by a much more efficient nebulizer system, which reduces times of treatment and increases dosage/deposition into the airways. This is also true of the dry powder inhalers increasing ease of use and compliance long term. For patients with CF who have more frequent pulmonary exacerbations or more severe pulmonary impairment, the use of continuous inhaled and/or oral antipseudomonal antibiotics is often prescribed. Long-term administration of oral antibiotics for the treatment of chronic *Staphylococcus aureus* is not recommended.

8. CFTR modulators: CFTR modulators aim to improve CFTR function by targeting the underlying protein defect that causes CF. There are 2 classes of CFTR modulators: CFTR correctors and potentiators. Correctors are agents that increase the delivery and amount of functional CFTR protein to the cell surface, resulting in increased ion transport. Potentiators increase the ion channel activity of CFTR protein located at the cell surface, resulting in increased ion transport. Clinically significant improvements include an increase in lung function (forced expiratory volume in 1 second [FEV_1], by ~4%-7% in absolute terms), quality of life, and weight with a reduction in pulmonary exacerbations (by about 30%-40% in relative terms), respiratory symptoms, and sweat chloride concentration. The strength of any recommendations regarding their use reflects relative value placed on clinical benefits and on high cost of medication. Use is restricted to specific situations and prescribers (the cost may be as high as $250,000 per year).

1) **Ivacaftor** (trade name Kalydeco) is taken orally bid (150 mg for patients aged ≥6 years; 75 mg [weight >14 kg] or 50 mg [weight 7-14 kg] for those aged 12 months to 6 years). It is a CFTR potentiator that has been shown to be clinically effective in CF patients with at least one G55ID (class III) *CFTR* mutation.◕

2) **Lumacaftor/ivacaftor** (trade name Orkambi) is taken orally bid (patients aged 2-5 years: weight <14 kg, 1 package 100 mg/25 mg or weight >14 kg, 1 package 150 mg/188 mg; patients aged 6-11 years: 2 tablets 200 mg/250 mg bid; patients aged ≥12 years: 2 tablets 400 mg/250 mg). It is a combination CFTR corrector/potentiator that has been shown to be clinically effective in CF patients who are homozygous for F508del (50% CF patients; class II mutation).◕

3) **Tezacaftor/ivacaftor** (trade name Symdeko) taken orally (1 tablet [tezacaftor 100 mg/ivacaftor 150 mg] in the morning and 1 tablet [ivacaftor 150 mg] in the evening, 12 hours apart). It is a new combination CFTR corrector/potentiator that has been shown to be clinically effective in CF patients aged ≥12 years who are either homozygous or heterozygous for F508del mutation (50% CF patients are homozygous, 75% CF patients are heterozygous).◕

Additional combination CFTR correctors/potentiators are currently being studied in CF patients with similar or more encouraging results. Other therapeutic approaches under development and study focus on bypassing the defective CFTR protein to restore ion balance. This includes agents that may be used to block sodium hyperabsorption through the epithelial sodium channel.

Treatment of Pulmonary Exacerbations

1. Intensification of physiotherapy, particularly in patients with atelectasis. This should be performed in combination with the use of nebulized hypertonic saline tid to qid.

2. Pharmacotherapy:

1) Early treatment with an antibiotic (intravenous or oral, frequently plus inhaled, but not an inhaled antibiotic alone) for at least 10 days (on average 14-21 days). While waiting for sputum culture results, use combined empiric treatment to cover *H influenzae* and *S aureus* (semisynthetic penicillins or β-lactamase–resistant cephalosporins or clarithromycin) as well as PsA (oral ciprofloxacin and inhaled aminoglycoside or colistin). In patients with more severe exacerbations, administer intravenous β-lactams [eg, ceftazidime, piperacillin, ticarcillin] combined with an aminoglycoside. Alternatively, carbapenems (imipenem or meropenem) or aztreonam may be used. Clinical improvement is usually achieved no earlier than after 4 to 7 days of treatment.

2) Consider a short-term systemic glucocorticoid treatment (eg, prednisone 1 mg/kg/d or 40-50 mg/d for 7-10 days) in patients with severe exacerbations, and particularly with severe chronic obstructive pulmonary disease, allergic bronchopulmonary aspergillosis, or asthma.

3. Mechanical ventilation (usually noninvasive) is indicated in acute respiratory failure that is caused by a reversible cause or in patients with chronic respiratory failure awaiting lung transplantation.

4. Distal intestinal obstruction syndrome: Appropriate oral/intravenous hydration and laxatives (eg, polyethylene glycol), rectal suppositories, or contrast (eg, gastrografin) enema. In rare cases, colonoscopy or surgical intervention may be necessary.

Surgical Treatment

In patients with severe life-threatening hemoptysis, radiology-guided embolization and, if not effective or not available, lobectomy may be indicated. Refractory bronchopleural fistulas unresponsive to chest tube drainage may require surgical pleurodesis or bullectomy (or both). In chronic respiratory failure, early referral for lung transplantation should be considered. In patients with advanced liver disease, consider liver transplantation.

→ **FOLLOW-UP**

Every 3 months assess nutritional status, perform spirometry, SpO_2 measurement, and sputum microbiology. Ideally, all patients should be seen regularly at a CF center or, if unavailable, by a CF specialist at least twice a year. Follow-up chest radiographs should be repeated in cases of severe exacerbations, suspected complications, or rapid decline in pulmonary function. Annual blood testing should be performed with particular attention to assessing liver disease, CF-related diabetes mellitus, fat-soluble vitamins, and nutritional status. Annual full pulmonary function testing, incremental exercise testing, and bone densitometry should be considered in patients with moderate to severe lung disease.

→ **COMPLICATIONS**

Respiratory complications: Atelectasis, pneumothorax, hemoptysis, allergic bronchopulmonary aspergillosis, pulmonary hypertension.

Extrapulmonary complications: Cor pulmonale, diabetes mellitus, cholelithiasis or cholangitis, fatty liver disease, cirrhosis, acute pancreatitis, DIOS, gastroesophageal reflux disease, hypertrophic osteoarthropathy, osteopenia or osteoporosis, infertility.

7. Interstitial Lung Diseases

→ **INTRODUCTION**

Interstitial lung disease refers to a group of heterogeneous, noninfectious, and nonmalignant diseases that are characterized by diffuse inflammatory and/or fibrotic infiltration of the alveolar space or interstitial septum. Patients typically have a restrictive ventilatory defect, reduction in diffusion capacity of the lung for carbon monoxide (DL_{CO}), and variety of alveolar filling and interstitial changes on high-resolution computed tomography of the chest.

7.1. Diffuse Alveolar Hemorrhage

→ **DEFINITION, ETIOLOGY, PATHOGENESIS**

Diffuse alveolar hemorrhage (DAH) refers to the extravasation of blood from pulmonary capillaries with accumulation of erythrocytes in the alveolar spaces. There is no consensus classification for DAH. The underlying cause of DAH is generally reflected in the histopathologic pattern. One of 3 patterns may be observed:

1) **Pulmonary capillaritis**: Neutrophilic inflammation of the alveolar interstitium leads to vascular injury or necrosis and subsequent loss of the structural integrity of alveolar epithelial or capillary endothelial cells. Causes

of pulmonary capillaritis include systemic vasculitides (granulomatosis with polyangiitis and microscopic polyangiitis), anti-glomerular basement membrane [GBM] disease, rheumatic diseases (systemic lupus erythematosus [SLE], rheumatoid arthritis, mixed connective tissue disease, primary antiphospholipid syndrome), and drug reactions.

2) **Bland pulmonary hemorrhage:** This is characterized by hemorrhage into the alveolar space with no inflammation or destruction of the alveolar structures. Causes include anticoagulant therapy, thrombocytopenia, idiopathic pulmonary hemosiderosis, and mitral stenosis.

3) **Diffuse alveolar damage:** Edema of the alveolar walls with hyaline membranes. Causes include any infection causing acute respiratory distress syndrome, connective tissue diseases (polymyositis and SLE), drugs (amiodarone, amphetamine, nitrofurantoin, cocaine), acute interstitial pneumonia, radiation therapy, and pulmonary infarction.

→ **CLINICAL FEATURES AND NATURAL HISTORY**

Symptoms include dyspnea, cough, hemoptysis (an absent or late clinical finding in up to 33% of cases), or disease-specific complaints. DAH due to immunologic causes is usually preceded by a prodromal phase lasting >10 days, with symptoms including malaise, arthralgia, or manifestations of a preexisting immunologic disorder.

→ **DIAGNOSIS**

Diagnostic Tests

1. Chest radiography usually reveals patchy or disseminated opacities, which may follow a relapse-remitting or migratory pattern.

2. High-resolution computed tomography (HRCT) reveals ground-glass opacities or consolidations that reflect blood filling the alveoli. In patients with recurrent DAH, reticulation may appear, providing evidence of interstitial fibrosis.

3. Laboratory tests: Iron deficiency anemia is commonly encountered in chronic recurrent hemorrhage. Thrombocytopenia should be excluded. An underlying bleeding diathesis should be assessed with an evaluation of coagulation. Serum creatinine, urinalysis, and urine microscopy are of value, as the presence of renal dysfunction, hematuria, red blood cell (RBC) casts, or proteinuria is suggestive of a systemic vasculitis. A urine drug screen test may reveal evidence of culprit illicit drug use. Evaluation of specific autoantibodies, including antineutrophil cytoplasmic antibodies, anti-GBM antibodies, antinuclear antibodies, and extractable nuclear antigens may permit the diagnosis of an underlying systemic inflammatory process.

4. Pulmonary function tests: A transient increase in carbon dioxide diffusing capacity of the lungs (DL_{CO}) is a characteristic feature of DAH. Recurrent DAH is associated with a restrictive pattern and reduced DL_{CO}.

5. Bronchoscopy with bronchoalveolar lavage (BAL) is essential to the accurate identification of DAH. An increasing RBC presence on sequential samples is consistent with the diagnosis. Evidence of hemorrhage should ideally be confirmed in more than one bronchial segment. The presence of hemosiderin--laden macrophages provides evidence of chronic hemorrhage even when frank (clinically evident) bleeding is not apparent at the time of bronchoscopy. BAL also serves to exclude other causes of diffuse pulmonary infiltrates or hemoptysis.

→ **TREATMENT**

In severely ill patients with a suspected immunologic cause of DAH, promptly start high-dose IV glucocorticoid treatment (eg, methylprednisolone 500--1000 mg/d) for 3 days. Cytotoxic therapies including cyclophosphamide or rituximab should be considered in the setting of an underlying capillaritis (→Chapter 14.23). In the case of bleeding, coagulopathy, or thrombocytopenia, administer blood products and reversal agents as required. Attempt to achieve adequate oxygen saturation by administering oxygen or using assisted ventilation when necessary. Treat respiratory insufficiency (→Chapter 13.16.1) and pulmonary hemorrhage (rare; →Chapter 1.13).

7.2. Eosinophilic Lung Diseases

Eosinophilic lung diseases represent a heterogeneous group of conditions characterized by the accumulation of eosinophils in the alveoli and pulmonary parenchyma.

1. Eosinophilic pneumonia in the course of parasitic infections is likely the most common cause of eosinophilic pneumonia in the world and is mainly due to parasites that migrate through the lungs as they develop (*Ascaris lumbricoides*, *Strongyloides stercoralis*, and *Ancylostoma duodenale*).

Symptoms include cough, rhinitis, loss of appetite, night sweating, low-grade fever, or less frequently wheezing and dyspnea. Eosinophilia in the peripheral blood is common. Sputum should be examined for parasitic larvae. Identification of the worm or ova in stool is reliable only several weeks after infestation. Parasite-specific serologic assays may be of value. Eosinophilic pneumonia may also be caused by parasites present in the blood or tissues (*Toxocara canis*, *Trichinella spiralis*, and taeniasis).

2. Allergic bronchopulmonary aspergillosis (ABPA) is a distinct pulmonary syndrome due to the fungus *Aspergillus*. ABPA is characterized by asthma, eosinophilia, and bronchiectasis secondary to complex immune-mediated airway reactions to *Aspergillus* antigens. The disease commonly manifests in patients with established diagnoses of asthma and cystic fibrosis.

Symptoms of ABPA include symptoms of asthma, sometimes with fever and the expectoration of tenacious brown mucus plugs. Chest radiographs reveal damage to the large proximal airways with associated upper-lobe predominant bronchiectasis, mucus plugging, and consequent atelectasis. Acute flares of ABPA are characterized on imaging by fleeting pulmonary opacities due to eosinophilic pneumonia or mucus plugging with regional atelectasis.

Diagnostic criteria:

1) Atopic asthma or cystic fibrosis.
2) Positive skin prick test results with *Aspergillus fumigatus* antigens or elevated specific IgE against *A fumigatus*.
3) Serum IgE >1000 ng/mL.
4) Positive precipitation reaction with *A fumigatus* antigens.
5) Peripheral eosinophilia >0.5×10^9/L.
6) Pulmonary opacities consistent with ABPA.
7) Proximal bronchiectasis (not consistently seen in all patients).

Differential diagnosis includes other types of pulmonary eosinophilia, cryptogenic organizing pneumonia, eosinophilic vasculitis (particularly eosinophilic granulomatosis with polyangiitis [Churg-Strauss syndrome]), and poorly controlled asthma.

Treatment: Oral prednisone 0.5 mg/kg during exacerbations for 14 days followed by a weaning protocol for a total treatment course of 3 to 6 months. Long-term glucocorticoid maintenance therapy is reserved for patients with recurrent exacerbations or with progressive lung injury. Itraconazole can be used as a corticosteroid-sparing agent either as part of an up-front initial combination therapy or in patients demonstrating an inadequate response to corticosteroids alone.

3. Chronic eosinophilic pneumonia: An idiopathic process that most frequently affects middle-aged women. Approximately 50% and 60% of patients have a preceding history of asthma or atopy. The vast majority of patients are nonsmokers.

Symptoms include fever, night sweats, cough, and weight loss. The disease is characterized by a progressive onset of symptoms over weeks to months. Chest radiographs reveal upper-zone consolidations in the peripheral areas of the lungs (a "photographic negative of pulmonary edema"). Consolidations often do not correspond to anatomic pulmonary segments and are migratory in 25% of patients. Eosinophilia in the peripheral blood is frequent, and significant eosinophilia in the bronchoalveolar lavage (BAL) fluid is present.

Diagnosis is based on the clinical manifestations and presence of eosinophilia in serum and BAL; surgical lung biopsy is rarely necessary.

Treatment: Oral prednisone 0.5 mg/kg/d for 2 weeks followed by 0.25 mg/kg/d. Improvement is usually observed within 1 or 2 weeks of treatment initiation, with 80% of patients noting improvement by 48 hours. Continue treatment for ≥6 months while tapering the dose. Patients are at high risk of disease relapse with corticosteroid withdrawal.

4. Acute eosinophilic pneumonia: The etiology is unknown, although a strong association with the initiation of smoking or with numerous environmental exposures has been described.

Symptoms include acute-onset fever, dyspnea, cough, myalgias, and pleuritic pain, although it may also develop subacutely over a few weeks. Patients often develop respiratory failure and require ventilation. Chest radiographs initially reveal fine, disseminated parenchymal lesions that quickly (within hours to 2 days) progress to disseminated consolidations, which are commonly accompanied by pleural effusions. Eosinophilia is very high in BAL and pleural fluids, while eosinophil counts in the peripheral blood are usually normal.

Diagnosis is based on established criteria:

1) Acute onset of febrile respiratory manifestations (duration ≤1 month).
2) Bilateral diffuse opacities on chest radiography.
3) Hypoxemia with partial pressure of carbon dioxide in the arterial blood (PaO_2) on room air <60 mm Hg, and/or PaO_2/fraction of inspired oxygen (FiO_2) ≤300 mm Hg, and/or oxygen saturation on room air <90%.
4) Lung eosinophilia with >25% eosinophils in the BAL differential cell count.
5) Absence of infection or other known causes of eosinophilic lung disease (especially potential drug reactions).

Treatment: IV methylprednisolone 125 mg every 6 hours until the resolution of respiratory failure followed by prednisone 40 to 60 mg/d, which can be tapered over 2 to 4 weeks. Response is generally observed within 48 hours, allowing rapid weaning from mechanical ventilation if warranted.

5. Eosinophilic bronchitis is characterized by elevated sputum eosinophils and active airway inflammation in the absence of airway hyperresponsiveness. This disease is airway-centered and is a common mimicker of asthma.

Diagnosis is established in the presence of chronic cough, >3% eosinophils in induced sputum, and a negative methacholine challenge test.

Treatment: Inhaled corticosteroids.

6. Other: Chronic eosinophilic leukemia (→Chapter 7.8.9), eosinophilic granulomatosis with polyangiitis (Churg-Strauss syndrome).

7.3. Hypersensitivity Pneumonitis

→ DEFINITION, ETIOLOGY, PATHOGENESIS

Hypersensitivity pneumonitis (HP) is a complex syndrome resulting from repeated inhalational exposure to a wide variety of organic particles or chemical agents small enough to reach the alveoli (<5 μm). In susceptible individuals exposure to these antigens triggers an exaggerated immune response of the small airways and lung parenchyma (mediated by immune complexes, complement activation, and cellular immunity). More than 200 causative factors have been identified, including animal, insect, fungal, and bacterial proteins, and low-molecular-weight chemical compounds. The disease is typically characterized by a lymphocytic (CD8⁺-dominant) and granulomatous inflammation with a bronchiocentric distribution, although advanced fibrosis can be observed in chronic disease.

→ **CLINICAL FEATURES AND NATURAL HISTORY**

1. Acute/subacute HP is characterized by a flu-like syndrome and generally manifests a few hours after exposure. Symptoms include cough, dyspnea, fever, chills, arthralgia, and malaise. Signs include an accelerated respiratory rate, tachycardia, and bilateral crackles at the lung bases. Untreated disease resolves within a day to a few weeks. In the case of repeated exposure to the antigen (even at low levels), patients develop dyspnea on exertion, cough, and sometimes also a low-grade fever. In general, acute HP is nonprogressive and intermittent, with spontaneous improvement in the setting of antigen avoidance. Subacute HP may result from repeated low-level exposures and is characterized by slowly progressive dyspnea, fatigue, and cough that develops over weeks to months.

2. Chronic (irreversible) HP develops over months to years and can lead to pulmonary fibrosis. Many patients with chronic HP have no recognizable acute deterioration and present as slowly progressive pulmonary fibrosis. In the field of interstitial lung disease (ILD), this is one of the most difficult diagnoses to make. The classification of HP into distinct acute, subacute, and chronic forms can be misleading, as clinical manifestations frequently overlap. Nevertheless, symptoms of chronic HP typically include productive cough, weight loss, loss of appetite, and malaise, whereas signs include tachypnea, bilateral crackles at the lung bases, rarely clubbing, and signs of chronic respiratory insufficiency.

→ **DIAGNOSIS**

Obtaining a thorough medical history is the cornerstone of establishing a diagnosis of HP. History should include environmental exposures (occupational, pets/animals, birds, feather pillows/duvets, hobbies including woodworking and gardening, the use of humidifiers and saunas, basement flooding, and visible mold in the home), similar symptoms in household members/coworkers, and the course of the disease.

Diagnostic Tests

1. Laboratory tests: Patients with acute HP may have elevated white blood cell counts with neutrophilia, elevated serum C-reactive protein levels and erythrocyte sedimentation rate, and positive serum precipitating antibodies against the offending antigen. The finding of a specific IgG-precipitating antibody in the serum of a patient with suspected HP indicates exposure but does not indicate that the precipitating antibody is pathogenic. Hence, precipitating antibodies are neither sensitive nor specific. In patients with chronic HP precipitating antibodies are variably present, and mild elevations of immunoglobulin levels or acute phase markers may be apparent.

2. Imaging studies:

1) **Chest radiographs**: In patients with acute HP the findings may be normal. A fine micronodular pattern or diffuse ground-glass opacities can be observed. In chronic HP diffuse, irregular reticular patterns are typically observed in the middle and upper lung zones.

2) **High-resolution computed tomography (HRCT)**: In acute HP typical findings include diffuse, fine, poorly demarcated centrilobular nodules, focal air trapping, and a mosaic pattern caused by highly heterogeneous parenchymal density (a combination of ground-glass opacities and hypodense areas reflecting the air trapping). Distinctive HRCT findings in chronic HP include a combination of reticular, ground-glass, and centrilobular nodular opacities with associated signs of fibrosis, including traction bronchiectasis and occasionally honeycomb changes (→Chapter 13.7.4.1). It can often be difficult to differentiate chronic HP from idiopathic pulmonary fibrosis (IPF) on the basis of imaging studies alone, although the presence of air trapping and absence of a lower zone predominance are suggestive of chronic HP. Expiratory computed tomography (CT) images are very useful and should be part of the HRCT protocol.

3. Pulmonary function testing reveals a restrictive pattern (this may be minor in patients with early disease) with decreased carbon dioxide diffusing capacity of the lungs (DL_{CO}). The 6-minute walk test reveals a shortened walk distance and frequently resting or exertional hypoxemia (or both).

4. Bronchoscopy often reveals high cellularity of bronchoalveolar lavage (BAL) fluid and an increased proportion of lymphocytes with predominant $CD8^+$ cells. An elevated neutrophil count can also be observed in chronic fibrotic disease and is associated with poor prognosis.

5. Lung biopsy: Patients with acute HP do not require tissue confirmation, given the self-limited nature of their disease. Transbronchial biopsy can occasionally be diagnostic in the presence of bronchiocentric granulomatous inflammation. Surgical lung biopsy is indicated in patients who do not meet a sufficient number of clinical criteria for a definitive diagnosis and to exclude other disease entities that require different management, especially IPF.

Diagnostic Criteria

Three complementary findings support a diagnosis of HP:

1) Clinical and functional features of an underlying ILD.
2) Relevant history of exposure based on thorough clinical assessment, circulating specific antibodies, or both.
3) HRCT with typical findings suggestive of HP.

If the diagnosis is doubtful, perform BAL. The presence of BAL lymphocytosis and "typical" HRCT makes the diagnosis of HP confident even in the absence of a definitive antigen exposure. Lung biopsy is indicated in patients in whom a diagnosis has not been established and other diseases must be excluded; this decision is usually made in a specialized center.

→ **TREATMENT**

An accelerated decline in lung function has been demonstrated for most forms of HP with continued antigen exposure. Thus, early diagnosis and antigen avoidance are the mainstays of treatment. Pharmacologic therapy acts as an adjunct for patients with severe or progressive disease. It should be noted, however, that the use of glucocorticoids and other immunosuppressive agents in HP is primarily supported by anecdotal reports with little in the way of controlled trials.

1. Acute HP resolves without treatment in the majority of patients. In patients with severe symptoms use oral prednisone 0.5 mg/kg/d (40-60 mg/d) for 1 to 2 weeks, then taper the dose over 4 to 6 weeks. Treatment of respiratory insufficiency: →Chapter 13.16.1.

2. Chronic HP: In patients with severe subacute progressive or chronic disease, oral prednisone 0.5 mg/kg/d for 4 weeks followed by a taper to a maintenance dose over 2 months is suggested. After 6 months assess for clinical response and continue therapy only in patients with objective improvement (assessed by spirometry, DL_{CO}, plethysmography, and gas exchange at rest and during exercise). Cytotoxic agents such as azathioprine, mycophenolate mofetil, and cyclophosphamide have been used in patients with progressive refractory disease, but their efficacy is largely unproven and based on expert opinion. In patients with airflow obstruction or persistent cough, consider treatment with an inhaled corticosteroid or a β_2-agonist. Lung transplantation is reserved for patients with end-stage fibrosis.

7.4. Idiopathic Interstitial Pneumonias

7.4.1. Idiopathic Pulmonary Fibrosis

→ DEFINITION, ETIOLOGY, PATHOGENESIS

Idiopathic pulmonary fibrosis (IPF) is the most common form of chronic progressive fibrosing interstitial pneumonia of unknown cause, occurring primarily in older adults aged >60 years and limited to the lungs. Defined by a distinct radiographic and histologic pattern called usual interstitial pneumonia (UIP), IPF is characterized by a relentless progression of interstitial fibrosis and a progressive decline in gas exchange. The median survival from the time of diagnosis is approximately 3 to 5 years.

The incidence of disease increases with older age, with presentation typically occurring in the sixth and seventh decades of life. Cohort studies have shown that the majority of patients have a history of cigarette smoking and more men than women are affected.

A genetic predisposition is observed in 2% to 20% of patients. Hereditary disease is typically inherited as an autosomal dominant trait with incomplete penetrance. Mutations in the promoter region of *MUC5B* and genes associated with telomere maintenance and surfactant protein expression have been among the various genetic abnormalities reported. The precise genetic and host susceptibility factors that determine the phenotypic expression and clinical manifestations of sporadic IPF remain unknown.

→ CLINICAL FEATURES

IPF has an insidious onset and manifests as unexplained exertional dyspnea and dry cough, which progress over many months to years. Patients commonly have bibasilar crackles on chest auscultation, with nearly 25% of patients demonstrating evidence of clubbing. In later stages IPF patients can develop symptoms of cor pulmonale with progressive right ventricular dysfunction.

→ DIAGNOSIS

The radiographic and histologic UIP pattern can be observed in numerous fibrotic interstitial lung diseases (ILDs), including asbestosis, connective tissue disease–related interstitial lung disease (CTD-ILD), chronic hypersensitivity pneumonitis, and drug reactions. Hence, as proposed by the updated consensus statement on IPF, the establishment of a diagnosis of IPF requires:

1) Exclusion of other known causes of ILD (eg, chronic hypersensitivity pneumonitis, occupational environmental exposures, connective tissue diseases, and adverse drug reactions).
2) Confirmation of typical features of UIP on high-resolution computed tomography (HRCT) in patients not subjected to surgical lung biopsy.
3) Specific combinations of HRCT and histologic abnormalities suggestive of the UIP pattern in patients in whom surgical lung biopsy was performed.

Hence HRCT of the chest is an absolute necessity in the evaluation of ILD. The UIP pattern on HRCT includes basilar-predominant subpleural reticular changes, traction bronchiectasis, and honeycombing. Honeycombing is critical for making a diagnosis in the absence of a surgical lung biopsy. It is manifested on HRCT as clustered cystic airspaces, typically of comparable diameters on the order of 3 to 10 mm (→Figure 7-1).

In the absence of a diagnostic gold standard, accuracy is dependent on clinical, radiographic, and histopathologic correlation. This can be best accomplished with expert multidisciplinary discussion, particularly in instances of diagnostic uncertainty.

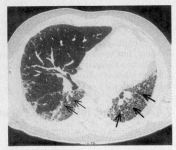

Figure 7-1. Idiopathic pulmonary fibrosis. A high-resolution computed tomography scan with reticular opacities, traction bronchiectasis (thin arrows), and honeycombing (thick arrows).

→ TREATMENT

In patients with mild to moderate disease, consider the use of oral pirfenidone 801 mg tid or nintedanib 150 mg bid.⊘⊖ Consider antacid therapy in all IPF patients.⊘⊖ Immunosuppressive therapy with prednisone and azathioprine should be avoided in the long-term management of IPF given an increased risk of hospitalization and death. Do not use anticoagulants in patients with IPF who have no other indications for antithrombotic prophylaxis. Use optimal symptomatic treatment (particularly oxygen therapy in patients with significant hypoxemia at rest) and consider pulmonary rehabilitation in the majority of patients. Consider enrolling patients in clinical studies that evaluate the use of novel therapeutic agents. Referral for lung transplantation should be considered in early stages of IPF. Listing for lung transplantation should be considered in the case of:

1) A decline in forced vital capacity (FVC) ≥10% during 6 months of follow-up.

2) A decline in diffusion capacity of the lung for carbon monoxide (DL_{CO}) ≥15% during 6 months of follow-up.

3) Desaturation to <88%, a distance <250 meters on the 6-minute walk test, or a decline >50 meters in the 6-minute walk distance over a 6-month period.

4) Pulmonary hypertension (on right heart catheterization or echocardiogram).

5) Hospitalization because of respiratory decline, pneumothorax, or acute exacerbation.

Acute Exacerbations

Acute exacerbations are serious events in IPF with an incidence of 5% to 15% per year and median survival <3 months. Clinical evaluation is required to exclude alternative causes of acute respiratory failure, including pneumonia, heart failure, pulmonary embolism, and other identifiable causes of acute lung injury. Even if there is a lack of evidence for infection, broad-spectrum antibiotic therapy is usually administered. Glucocorticoids are also often used, based on their potential to treat acute lung injury or organizing pneumonia, and are recommended for the treatment of acute exacerbations despite very limited evidence. Pulse doses of glucocorticoids (IV methylprednisolone 0.5-1 g daily for 3 days) are commonly used, while lower doses (prednisone 1 mg/kg) may be preferred in patients with a milder flare. Both strategies are typically followed by a rapid taper and cessation of prednisone within several weeks.

→ PROGNOSIS

The median survival from the time of diagnosis is 3 to 5 years. Significant heterogeneity, however, exists among individual patients, and the clinical course is variable and unpredictable. In some patients the disease is characterized by rapid progression and functional impairment, while others experience a protracted course punctuated by acute exacerbations. The risk of acute exacerbation increases with the severity of lung function impairment. Lung cancer develops in 10% to 15% of IPF patients.

7.4.2. Selected Other Types of Idiopathic Interstitial Pneumonia

1. Nonspecific interstitial pneumonia (NSIP): A common presentation includes dyspnea and cough of usually 6 to 7 months' duration in the sixth decade of life. In contrast to idiopathic pulmonary fibrosis (IPF), NSIP more commonly affects women and never-smokers. Diffuse crackles may be audible. Most patients have a restrictive ventilatory defect on pulmonary function tests. High-resolution computed tomography (HRCT) abnormalities include bilateral ground-glass opacities or irregular reticular opacities with traction bronchiectasis. NSIP can be idiopathic but is often associated with an underlying connective tissue disease, especially scleroderma. Connective tissue disease–related interstitial lung disease (CTD-ILD) is the leading cause of mortality in patients with scleroderma and is often characterized by a progressive decline in lung function.

Treatment: To date, no randomized clinical trial of treatment in idiopathic NSIP has been performed, but typical treatment includes glucocorticoids, with or without additional immunosuppressive agents. In patients with scleroderma-related interstitial lung disease (ILD), a randomized controlled trial demonstrated likely similar efficacy of both mycophenolate mofetil and cyclophosphamide.⊜ Furthermore, a recent randomized controlled trial has also demonstrated the clinical value of the tyrosine kinase inhibitor nintedanib in the management of scleroderma-related ILD.⊜

Prognosis: Prognosis is variable but it is generally better than in IPF.

2. Cryptogenic organizing pneumonia (COP; formerly termed bronchiolitis obliterans organizing pneumonia [BOOP]): This disorder can be idiopathic (referred to as COP) or secondary to drugs, connective tissue disease, or viral infections (then preferentially called "organizing pneumonia"). The onset of the disease can be similar to an acute viral flu-like infection, with cough, dyspnea, fever, malaise, loss of appetite, and weight loss. Symptoms are normally present for <2 months. Physical examination usually discloses focal sparse crackles but may be normal. Chest radiographs reveal unilateral or bilateral patchy consolidation. HRCT most often reveals patchy consolidations with subpleural or peribronchial localization and associated ground-glass opacities. Radiologic changes have a tendency to migrate, changing in size and location, even without treatment. Characteristic histologic features include intraluminal fibrotic buds seen in respiratory bronchioles, alveolar ducts, and alveoli.

Treatment: Glucocorticoid therapy (prednisone 0.75-1 mg/kg) results in a complete clinical, radiographic, and physiologic recovery in approximately two-thirds of patients. High-dose therapy has to be maintained for 4 to 8 weeks with a subsequent gradual taper over the following 9 to 12 months. In case of relapse prolong the treatment and consider addition of a second immunosuppressive agent.

3. Acute interstitial pneumonia (AIP): Classically described in previously healthy individuals, AIP is a rare fulminant lung injury that presents acutely (days to weeks). A prodromal flulike illness prior to disease onset is commonly encountered. Signs include fever, tachypnea, tachycardia, cyanosis, and diffuse crackles over the lungs. In the majority of patients respiratory failure develops rapidly and mechanical ventilation is required. Chest radiographs typically demonstrate diffuse bilateral air-space disease. HRCT features include bilateral multifocal or diffuse areas of consolidative changes and ground-glass opacities. A surgical lung biopsy may be required to confirm the diagnosis; however, the severity of illness often precludes this intervention. On histopathologic examination, AIP is characterized by a diffuse alveolar damage (DAD) pattern. AIP should be differentiated from severe infection or aspiration, acute respiratory distress syndrome, acute exacerbation of IPF, acute exacerbation of a connective tissue disease, or toxic drug reaction.

Treatment: Treatment is mainly symptomatic; mechanical ventilation may be required. Empiric antibiotic therapy is usually given due to the clinical/radiographic similarities of AIP with acute infection. Pulse-dose glucocorticoids are used in the early phase of the disease (eg, our practice is to use IV methylprednisolone 1 g once daily for 3 days followed by lower doses tapered according to the clinical response).

Prognosis: Mortality is estimated at 50%, with the majority of patients dying within 3 months of presentation. Survivors can experience disease relapse and a chronic progressive fibrotic ILD.

4. Respiratory bronchiolitis–associated interstitial lung disease (RB-ILD)/desquamative interstitial pneumonia (DIP): These diseases represent a distinct clinical entity, which is found almost exclusively in cigarette smokers between their third and sixth decades of life. The cardinal feature of RB-ILD is the accumulation of pigmented alveolar macrophages within the respiratory bronchioles with extension into alveolar ducts. DIP is characterized by the uniform filling of the alveolar spaces by cohesive clusters of pigmented alveolar macrophages and inflammatory cells. The presentation is insidious, with exertional dyspnea and persistent nonproductive cough. Coarse bibasilar crackles are frequently observed. Chest radiographs are often normal in RB-ILD, with only occasional bronchial wall thickening or reticular opacities. Key HRCT features of RB-ILD include patchy ground-glass opacities predominant in the upper lung zone and centrilobular nodularity. In DIP chest radiograph abnormalities are nonspecific and include middle- to lower-lung field air-space opacities. HRCT findings in DIP include basal ground-glass attenuation with tiny thin-walled cysts noted in the ground-glass areas in 60% of patients. RB-ILD and DIP are related conditions that may reflect different stages of the same process. As such, overlap between clinical, radiographic, and pathologic features is common.

Treatment: Smoking cessation is absolutely indicated and usually results in improvement of clinical symptoms, gas transfer, and radiographic abnormalities. Glucocorticoids can be considered for patients with recurrent or refractory disease despite ongoing smoking cessation.

7.5. Pneumoconiosis

Pneumoconioses represent a group of lung diseases caused by the inhalation of occupational inorganic dusts leading to progressive parenchymal lung disease.

1. Silicosis is a fibrotic lung disease attributable to the inhalation of crystalline silica, usually in the form of quartz. Silica dust penetrates to the pulmonary parenchyma, undergoes phagocytosis by macrophages, and causes lysis of the macrophages and the release of substances responsible for pulmonary fibrosis.

Three clinicopathologic types of silicosis have been described: chronic silicosis, accelerated silicosis, and silicoproteinosis. Chronic silicosis is the most common form, which usually follows decades of sustained exposure. Accelerated disease follows shorter, heavier exposures after 3 to 10 years. The pathogenic hallmarks are silicotic nodules, which can become confluent and lead to the development of progressive massive fibrosis. Silicoproteinosis follows intense exposure to fine dust of high silica content and shows pathologic features of alveolar proteinosis. Patients exposed to silica dust are also at increased risk of developing chronic obstructive pulmonary disease (COPD), lung cancer, mycobacterial infection, and immune-mediated diseases, such as scleroderma and rheumatoid arthritis. Occupations at risk of exposure include employment in tunnel and shaft construction, stone pits, metallurgical industry, pottery and porcelain manufacture, and production of heat-resistant and abrasive materials.

Chronic silicosis usually develops after >10 years of exposure and remains asymptomatic for a prolonged period. As fibrosis progresses, patients develop dyspnea and cough, sometimes accompanied by cor pulmonale and respiratory failure. It is important to note that the appearance of breathlessness or worsening bronchitic symptoms may be reflective of a separate disease associated with silica dust exposure, rather than silicosis itself, including COPD, tuberculosis, or lung cancer. The changes of chronic silicosis are irreversible and have a tendency to continued progression despite the discontinuation of the exposure. In acute silicosis, dyspnea may be disabling within months of exposure, followed by impaired gas exchange and respiratory failure.

Additional tests:

1) Chest radiography in chronic silicosis is characterized by fine, round nodular opacities that are usually dense and well demarcated, sometimes with calcifications. Lesions are usually bilateral with upper-lobe predominance. Enlargement of hilar lymph nodes with eggshell calcifications is strongly suggestive of the diagnosis.

2) High resolution computed tomography (HRCT) is useful in identifying early conglomeration or the infectious or malignant complications of silica dust exposure.

3) Pulmonary function tests have value in longitudinal assessment of disease progression. Patients with chronic silicosis often demonstrate a mixed ventilatory impairment with restriction and obstruction related to interstitial lung diseases (ILDs) and comorbid COPD, respectively. Functional impairment is often more closely associated with airflow obstruction than restriction.

Diagnosis is based on significant occupational exposure and radiologic changes.

Differential diagnosis:

1) Other diseases causing upper-lobe nodularity: Sarcoidosis, miliary tuberculosis, lymphangitic carcinomatosis, pulmonary Langerhans cell histiocytosis, respiratory bronchiolitis–associated ILD, or chronic hypersensitivity pneumonitis.

2) Lung tumors: Cancer, tuberculoma.

Treatment: Treatment is focused on stopping the exposure (personal protective equipment) and symptomatic management. Smoking cessation is critical. Lung transplantation should be considered in patients with accelerated and acute disease.

2. Coal workers' pneumoconiosis (CWP) involves focal fibrosis of the pulmonary parenchyma caused by inhalation of coal dust. Coal miners may also develop silicotic nodules when the coal is mined from hard rocks. Coal mining, even in the absence of CWP, is associated with chronic bronchitis and airflow obstruction. Progressive symptoms can develop with progressive fibrosis. Chest radiographs reveal nodules that are less sharply demarcated and less dense than those observed in silicosis; consolidations >3 mm and calcifications within the nodules occur less frequently. **Caplan syndrome** includes the rapid development of multiple pulmonary nodules 0.5 to 5 cm in diameter visible on chest radiographs accompanied by features of rheumatoid arthritis and positive rheumatoid factor in blood.

3. Asbestosis is a diffuse interstitial pulmonary fibrosis, frequently associated with pleural lesions, which is caused by the inhalation of asbestos fibers. Exposure is most often occupational and may occur in mining, milling, manufacturing, pipefitting, remote work with automobile brake pads, and applying or removing asbestos fiber products. Retention and clearance of fibers is inhomogeneous. Fibers <3 µm are cleared by alveolar macrophages, subsequently translocated to lymphatic channels, and eventually drained into the pleural space. Longer fibers are incompletely phagocytosed by macrophages and are retained in the lungs as asbestos bodies. The fibers induce inflammation that leads to fibrosis.

Clinical manifestations: Patients are normally asymptomatic for at least 20 to 30 years after the initial exposure. Determinants of disease include burden of exposure, duration of exposure, pattern of exposure, age of exposure (young age is associated with a longer fiber residence time), and type of fiber inhaled. Symptoms are similar to other types of interstitial fibrosis (dyspnea on exertion worsening with the progression of lesions; crackles at lung bases may be audible). Changes are irreversible and have a tendency to progress despite the discontinuation of exposure. Pleural changes related to exposure to asbestos may coexist with fibrosis or occur independently. They include nonmalignant lesions: limited pleural thickening (plaques that are usually located on the parietal pleura and have a tendency to develop calcifications) and diffuse pleural thickening (usually affecting the visceral pleura; depending on the extent, it may impair pulmonary function), as well as malignant lesions.

Additional tests:

1) Chest radiographs are crucial for diagnosis and reveal irregular basilar--predominant linear shadows. Subpleural parenchymal changes may be obscured by overlying asbestos-related pleural thickening or pleural calcification. Early fibrotic changes are better visualized by HRCT. Mediastinal lymphadenopathy and progressive massive fibrosis are not typically observed. In advanced disease the usual interstitial pneumonia (UIP) pattern (→Chapter 13.7.4.1) may be observed.

2) Pulmonary function tests reveal a restrictive pattern with decreased carbon dioxide diffusing capacity of the lungs (DL_{CO}) and static compliance.

3) Bronchoalveolar lavage using special staining may confirm the presence of asbestos bodies; however, this finding proves only the exposure to asbestos.

Diagnosis is based on radiologic features and the patient's history of occupational exposure. Differential diagnosis includes idiopathic pulmonary fibrosis, connective tissue disease–related ILD, hypersensitivity pneumonitis, or lymphangitic tumor spread.

Treatment is symptomatic only.

Complications: Asbestos exposure has been also linked to pleural plaques, pleural effusion, malignant mesothelioma, and lung cancer.

7.6. Rare Interstitial Lung Diseases

1. Pulmonary Langerhans cell histiocytosis (PLCH) is most commonly encountered in young adult smokers. Approximately 90% of PLCH patients smoke cigarettes or have a history of substantial second-hand smoke exposure. Langerhans cells are dendritic cells of the monocyte-macrophage lineage, which regulate mucosal airway immunity. The identification of mutations in the genes *BRAF* and *MAP2K1* in up to 50% of patients suggests that at least a proportion of PLCH cases represents a smoking-induced dendritic cell neoplasm with a prominent inflammatory component. The earliest lesion in PLCH is the peribronchial accumulation of Langerhans cells and other immune cells that lead to the typical radiographic and histologic patterns.

Symptoms: Cough and dyspnea on exertion, sometimes fever, weight loss, sweating, chest pain. Pneumothorax may be the first symptom. Pulmonary function tests usually reveal decreased carbon dioxide diffusing capacity of the lungs (DL_{CO}). Patients often have airflow obstruction (sometimes partially reversible) with hyperinflation, although a mixed pattern can be observed. Chest radiographs may initially be normal or show nodular opacities and/or a reticular pattern sparing supradiaphragmatic areas. High-resolution computed tomography (HRCT) reveals centrilobular nodules and multiform, irregular thin-walled cysts in the upper and middle lobes. A small proportion of patients may have symptoms due to a disease that is extrathoracic. Establishing a definite diagnosis requires the presence of clinical features and demonstration of Langerhans cells in tissue specimens (transbronchial or surgical lung biopsy). A probable diagnosis is based on clinical features and HRCT.

Differential diagnosis: Lymphangioleiomyomatosis (in young women), desquamative interstitial pneumonia, emphysema, lymphocytic interstitial pneumonia, Birt-Hogg-Dubé syndrome.

Treatment includes mandatory smoking cessation and follow-up with pulmonary function tests (repeated initially every 3-6 months, later every 6-12 months). Smoking cessation may promote disease stabilization/regression and sometimes complete resolution. Other patients experience a progressive decline despite smoking cessation. In patients with persistent symptoms or worsening pulmonary function test results despite successful smoking cessation, use oral prednisone (1 mg/kg/d for 1 month with the dose tapered over 5 months). If disease progression ensues consider the use of cladribine.☉◯ Diffuse lesions limited to the lungs and causing respiratory insufficiency may be an indication for lung transplantation.

2. Lymphangioleiomyomatosis (LAM): The disease can be sporadic or seen in the setting of tuberous sclerosis complex. Sporadic LAM is a rare disease that almost exclusively affects young women. Dysfunction of either the *TSC1* or *TSC2* gene leads to the proliferation of atypical smooth muscle cells around the bronchi, blood vessels, and lymphatic vessels, resulting in bronchial obstruction and the formation of parenchymal cysts.

Manifestations: Pneumothorax, chylothorax, progressive dyspnea on exertion, cough, sometimes hemoptysis, angiomyolipomas of the kidneys and other organs. Chest radiographs reveal lung hyperinflation and a reticular pattern (sometimes with nodular opacities and small cysts).

HRCT findings:

1) Characteristic features: Multiple (>10) bilateral thin-walled and well-defined cysts, normal or increased lung volume, absent signs of other interstitial diseases.

2) Features compatible with LAM: From 2 to 9 thin-walled and well-defined cysts <30 mm in diameter, other features as listed above.

Diagnostic criteria:

1) Definite LAM:
   a) Characteristic or compatible HRCT image + histologic features of LAM.
   b) Characteristic HRCT image + ≥1 of the following: Renal angiomyolipoma, thoracic or abdominal chylous effusion, lymphangioleiomyoma or a lymph node affected by LAM, definite or probable tuberous sclerosis complex.

2) Probable LAM:
   a) Characteristic HRCT image + typical clinical features.
   b) Compatible HRCT image + renal angiomyolipoma and thoracic or abdominal chylous effusion.

3) Possible LAM: Characteristic or compatible HRCT image.

Probable or possible LAM is confirmed by serum vascular endothelial growth factor (VEGF)-D levels >800 pg/mL.

Treatment: Bronchodilators are used for patients with reversible airflow obstruction. Pleurodesis can be performed following initial pneumothorax because of the high rate of ipsilateral recurrence. Estrogen-containing birth control pills and estrogen replacement therapy should be avoided. Counselling around pregnancy is required, given that pregnancy has been associated with an increased risk of spontaneous pneumothorax, chylothorax, and bleeding from renal angiomyolipomas. Counselling regarding air travel is also advised. The mammalian target of rapamycin (mTOR) inhibitor sirolimus 1 to 2 mg/d may be considered in patients with a forced expiratory volume in 1 second (FEV$_1$) <70%,⊘○ especially in the presence of rapid progression, renal angiomyolipoma >3 cm, large lymphangioleiomyoma, and thoracic or abdominal chylous effusion. Lung transplantation should be considered in patients with respiratory insufficiency (resting hypoxemia and VO$_{2max}$ <50% predicted).

3. Pulmonary alveolar proteinosis (PAP) is characterized by the progressive accumulation of an abnormal surfactant in the alveoli, which leads to impaired gas exchange and respiratory failure. Three forms are recognized: congenital, acquired, and secondary (associated with many secondary etiologies). Acquired disease is the most common and associated with a high prevalence of antibodies to granulocyte and macrophage colony-stimulating factor (GM-CSF) that are thought to be pathogenic.

Symptoms: Slowly progressive dyspnea and nonproductive cough; sometimes fatigue, weight loss, low-grade fever. Untreated patients are more susceptible to respiratory infections (nocardia, mycobacteria, and opportunistic fungi). The clinical course of acquired autoimmune disease follows 3 distinct patterns: progressive deterioration, stable disease, or spontaneous resolution. Chest radiographs reveal ground-glass opacities and consolidations with air bronchogram. HRCT shows areas of ground-glass opacities that are well demarcated from the normal lung parenchyma as well as thickening of the interlobular septa, which produces a "crazy paving" pattern. Positive serum and/or bronchoalveolar lavage (BAL) autoantibodies to GM-CSF (titers >1/400 or concentrations >5 µg/mL) are characteristic of acquired PAP.

Diagnosis is based on clinical features, radiologic features, and BAL fluid examination (a characteristic "milky" appearance; cytologic examination reveals a granular periodic acid Schiff [PAS] positive lipoproteinaceous material that is both extracellular and fills alveolar macrophages). Surgical lung biopsy is required for diagnosis in a minority of patients. Secondary causes of PAP need to be excluded.

Treatment: Whole-lung lavage under general anesthesia for patients with severe dyspnea and hypoxemia. Subcutaneous or inhaled administration of GM-CSF may be an option for adults who cannot undergo or who have not responded to whole-lung lavage. Rituximab can be considered in severe autoimmune cases not responsive to conventional therapy.

7.7. Sarcoidosis

→ **DEFINITION, ETIOLOGY, PATHOGENESIS**

Sarcoidosis is a multisystem inflammatory disorder of unknown etiology. Although the lung is the most commonly involved organ, with physiologic and/or radiographic abnormalities found in >90% of patients, granulomatous infiltration can occur in any organ system and result in chronic progressive dysfunction. Lymphocytes and macrophages accumulate in sites of the active inflammatory process, forming noncaseating granulomas. The presumable antigenic stimulus that initiates the disease process and promotes disease progression remains elusive.

→ **CLINICAL FEATURES AND NATURAL HISTORY**

Sarcoidosis is a worldwide disease, with the highest incidence noted in African Americans and Scandinavians. The disease can occur in both sexes, with a slight predominance in females. Seventy percent of patients are aged between 25 to 45 years.

1. Symptoms of organ involvement:

1) Dyspnea, cough, and chest pain (usually retrosternal, occasionally resembling angina).

2) Cutaneous changes: Erythema nodosum, lupus pernio (indurated, disfiguring infiltrations associated with discoloration of the skin of the nose, cheeks, lips, and ears), papular or maculopapular eruptions, subcutaneous nodules, fine ulcerations or areas of depigmentation or erythema, lesions similar to ichthyosis, alopecia.

3) Ocular involvement: Most frequently uveitis, conjunctivitis, and lacrimal gland involvement.

4) Enlarged, mobile, and painless peripheral lymph nodes (mostly cervical or supraclavicular).

5) Enlargement of the liver, less frequently of the spleen.

6) Arthralgia (hands and feet are classically most involved) and myalgia.

7) Central nervous involvement: Frequently cranial nerve involvement, in particular affecting the facial nerve, less frequently the optic or oculomotor nerves. It can also present with leptomeningitis, diabetes insipidus, hypopituitarism, spinal cord disease, polyneuropathy, and small fiber neuropathy.

8) Cardiac involvement: Symptoms of arrhythmias or conduction disturbances, symptoms of heart failure.

9) Features of pulmonary hypertension are present in 5% to 15% of all patients and in 70% of patients awaiting lung transplantation. Given its multifactorial nature, it is classified as group 5 pulmonary hypertension.

10) Head and neck disease: Nasal congestion, epistaxis, anosmia, hoarseness, stridor, and dysphagia.

11) Enlargement of one or both parotid glands, causing tenderness and edema (Heerfordt syndrome: parotid gland enlargement, fever, facial nerve palsy, and anterior uveitis).

12) Gastrointestinal involvement: Most often symptom-free but the esophagus, stomach, small intestine, and colon can be involved.

In many patients general symptoms are observed, including debilitating fatigue, weakness, loss of appetite, weight loss, and fever.

2. Natural history: In ~50% of patients spontaneous remission occurs within 2 years from the diagnosis and does so in many other cases within 5 years. After 5 years remission is much less likely, with many patients experiencing a chronic or progressive course. An acute onset with erythema nodosum, asymptomatic bilateral hilar lymph node enlargement, migratory polyarthralgia, and fever (Löfgren syndrome) is usually associated with a favorable prognosis. The course of the disease correlates with its onset: In >80% of patients with stage 1 radiographic changes (→Diagnostic Tests, below), the disease resolves without treatment. In stage 2 patients the lesions resolve in 40% of 70% of cases, and in stage 3 patients, in 10% to 20% of cases. Five-year mortality rates are reported to be between 1% and 7%. Most fatalities are related to advanced pulmonary fibrosis, central nervous system disease, or cardiac involvement. Pulmonary hypertension is the most robust predictor of mortality in patients who are candidates for lung transplantation.

→ DIAGNOSIS

Diagnostic Tests

1. Laboratory tests may reveal anemia (usually mild), leukopenia, hypercalcemia and hypercalciuria, increased serum angiotensin-converting enzyme levels, and hypergammaglobulinemia.

2. Electrocardiography (ECG): In patients with cardiac involvement ECG may reveal arrhythmia and conduction disturbances. However, normal ECG does not entirely exclude cardiac sarcoidosis.

3. Imaging studies: Chest radiographs most frequently reveal bilateral (hilar and paratracheal) lymph node enlargement; after several years lymph node calcifications may develop. Parenchymal lesions include nodular changes and reticular nodular changes, as well as upper-lobe volume loss and conglomerate mass formation in end-stage fibrosis. Disease staging on the basis of chest radiographs is as follows:

- Stage 0: Normal chest radiographs.
- Stage 1: Hilar and mediastinal lymph node enlargement.
- Stage 2: Hilar and mediastinal lymph node enlargement and parenchymal changes.
- Stage 3: Parenchymal changes, no lymph node enlargement.
- Stage 4: Pulmonary fibrosis.

The chest radiographic stages do not correspond to the chronologic progression of the disease but rather to the likelihood of future radiographic and symptomatic disease resolution.

High-resolution computed tomography (HRCT) of the chest reveals perilymphatic nodular lesions that are usually peribronchovascular, subpleural, and/or perifissural in distribution along with enlargement of hilar and mediastinal lymph nodes. Computed tomography (CT) is more sensitive and specific in evaluating parenchymal lung involvement than plain-film chest radiography.

4. Pulmonary function tests can identify different patterns of abnormalities, including a reduced carbon dioxide diffusing capacity of the lungs (DL_{CO}), restriction with reduced vital capacity, and commonly evidence of airflow obstruction related to small airway/endobronchial disease.

5. Bronchoscopy is done with the aim of performing lymph node biopsy (preferably using endobronchial ultrasonography), biopsy of bronchial mucosa, transbronchial lung biopsy, or bronchoalveolar lavage ($\geq 25\%$ of lymphocytes or a $CD4^+$:$CD8^+$ cell ratio >3.5).

6. Histologic examination reveals noncaseating granulomas in biopsy specimens of the bronchial mucosa, lung, or lymph nodes.

7. Other tests include contrast-enhanced magnetic resonance imaging (MRI) to assess for meningeal, brain, optic nerve, spinal cord, or cranial nerve involvement. Examination of cerebrospinal fluid (CSF) in patients with suspected central nervous system involvement identifies increased lymphocyte counts and protein levels in 80% of patients. Cardiac MRI and positron emission tomography (PET)/CT with ^{18}F-fluorodeoxyglucose (FDG) can be used to assess for evidence of active cardiac inflammation or cardiac fibrosis/scar indicative of chronic disease. PET/CT or whole-body gallium (^{67}Ga) scintigraphy can also be used to assess for systemic disease activity.

8. All patients should be referred for **ophthalmologic examination**.

Diagnostic Criteria

The diagnosis of sarcoidosis requires:

1) A compatible clinical and radiologic presentation.
2) Evidence of noncaseating granulomas.
3) Exclusion of other diseases capable of producing a similar clinical picture.

In the presence of a compatible clinical picture, the first step is to choose the site for a proper biopsy to confirm the presence of granulomatous inflammation. This confirmation is critical, taking into account the long-term nature and adverse-effect profile of potential treatments. Bronchoscopic lung biopsy, mediastinal lymph node biopsy, or both are recommended in most cases. A careful examination may disclose other extrapulmonary sites for biopsy, such as skin or superficial lymph nodes. Patients who present with a classic Löfgren syndrome do not require biopsy if resolution of the disease is rapid and spontaneous.

Differential Diagnosis

An essential component of the diagnosis of sarcoidosis is the exclusion of alternative possibilities, which can be difficult, given the heterogeneous presentation of individual patients:

1) Hilar and mediastinal lymph node enlargement: Lymphoid malignancies, metastatic neoplasm, and granulomatous inflammation as a result of inflammatory or infectious etiologies.

2) Disseminated lung changes: Berylliosis, silicosis, lymphangitic carcinomatosis, chronic hypersensitivity pneumonitis, and postprimary tuberculosis.

3) Diseases in which histologic examination may reveal granulomas: Tuberculosis, chronic beryllium disease, mycobacterial infections, fungal infections (including aspergillosis), hypersensitivity pneumonitis, granulomatosis with polyangiitis, lymphoma, a sarcoid-like reaction to adjacent malignancy, necrotizing sarcoid granulomatosis, lymphocytic interstitial pneumonia, and granulomatous-lymphocytic interstitial lung disease in patients with common variable immunodeficiency.

→ **TREATMENT**

1. Indications for treatment: The decision to treat either immediately or in follow-up is guided by the risk of severe dysfunction or irreversible damage to major organs, risk of death, or the presence of incapacitating symptoms. Most treatment protocols incorporate a period of observation without treatment whenever possible. The main indications for urgent treatment are cardiac involvement, eye disease that has not responded to topical therapy, symptomatic hypercalcemia, neurologic involvement, or severe disfiguring skin lesions. Parenchymal lung disease with severe functional impairment on presentation (vital capacity and/or DL_{CO} <50% predicted) and progressive pulmonary disease with functional deterioration in the last 6 to 12 months are considered by many experts to be treatment indications.

2. First-line treatment: Oral **corticosteroids**: Prednisone. Start with 0.5 mg/kg or 20 to 40 mg/d for 6 to 12 weeks with dose reduction thereafter to a maintenance dose of 5 to 10 mg/d over a period of 6 months. A minimum of 12 months of therapy is often advised to prevent relapse. Alternative immunosuppressive agents are considered in patients who fail to respond to corticosteroids or in whom a maintenance prednisone dose of >15 to 20 mg/d is required. Methotrexate is the first-choice add-on, with a target dose in the range of 15 to 20 mg/wk. Folic acid should be use in conjuncture with methotrexate to reduce the risk of toxicity and increase compliance. Agents such as azathioprine, mycophenolate mofetil, antimalarial drugs, and in severe refractory disease infliximab are considered if the initial second-line therapy fails. In patients with persistent cough, airflow obstruction, or both, consider inhaled corticosteroids.

3. Lung transplantation is reserved for patients with end-stage pulmonary fibrosis, especially in the presence of concomitant pulmonary hypertension.

→ **FOLLOW-UP**

For the first 2 years from diagnosis perform follow-up studies to assess organs previously involved using the least invasive methods. For pulmonary involvement perform chest radiography, spirometry, and DL_{CO} measurements every 3 to 6 months and then annually for ≥3 years from the discontinuation of treatment or induction of sustained remission. Monitor for new involvement of common target organs annually or sooner, depending on symptoms.

→ **COMPLICATIONS**

Complications depend on the organs involved and may include respiratory insufficiency, pulmonary hypertension, heart failure, sudden cardiac death, pulmonary aspergilloma, iris adhesions (leading to glaucoma, cataract, loss of vision), nephrocalcinosis, nephrolithiasis, renal failure, diabetes insipidus, hypothyroidism, and adrenal insufficiency. Close evaluation for adverse effects related to chronic corticosteroid and immunosuppressive therapy is also warranted (→Chapter 14.13).

8. Larynx Diseases

8.1. Laryngitis

→ **DEFINITION AND CLINICAL FEATURES**

Laryngitis refers to acute (lasting <3 weeks) or chronic (>3 weeks) inflammation of the vocal folds and surrounding tissues.

Causes:
1) **Acute laryngitis**: Infection (most frequently with respiratory viruses), vocal overuse, irritants (tobacco smoke).
2) **Chronic**: As a consequence of acute laryngitis, gastroesophageal reflux, fungal infection in patients treated with inhaled corticosteroids, benign lesions of laryngeal structures (nodules, papillomas, cysts, polyps, chondromas), and other rare causes (granulomatosis with polyangiitis, malignancy, tuberculosis, endemic mycoses).

Risk factors: Tobacco smoking, irritants, iatrogenic (eg, inhaled drugs or treatments causing dryness of the laryngeal mucosa, intubation), nasal congestion, alcohol use.

Signs and symptoms: Discomfort when speaking or swallowing, cough, hoarseness, sometimes stridor. The presence of concomitant fever is suggestive of intercurrent infection. In patients with fever, a toxic appearance, significant stridor, or dyspnea, always exclude bacterial tracheitis and epiglottitis.

→ **DIAGNOSIS**

The diagnosis of acute laryngitis is based on clinical features. Symptoms lasting >3 weeks are an indication for an ear, nose, and throat (ENT) consultation. In the diagnostic workup of chronic laryngitis laryngoscopy is necessary to exclude malignancy.

→ **TREATMENT**

Treatment is symptomatic and includes voice rest, air humidification, cessation of smoking, elimination of irritants, and oral nonsteroidal anti-inflammatory drugs. In the case of significant edema of vocal cords or urgent need for at least transient improvement of symptoms, you may consider a short course of oral glucocorticoids while seeking expert advice (in addition to adverse effects, glucocorticoids may mask the underlying process). Treatment of the underlying condition depends on etiology. Because the vast majority of acute laryngitis is caused by respiratory viruses, no specific treatment is indicated.

8.2. Voice Disorders: Functional and Organic Dysphonia

→ **DEFINITION, ETIOLOGY**

Dysphonia is the impaired ability to produce voice sounds. This is distinct from dysarthria, which is the impaired movement of muscles to produce speech, including the lips, tongue, vocal cords, and diaphragm. Dysphonia is subdivided into categories based on the presence or absence of an identifiable etiology, namely, organic versus functional dysphonia. Dysphonia can be assessed and described by the GRBAS system, which is a voice-rating scale. GRBAS is an auditory-perceptual evaluation of voice, which grades the degree of hoarseness based on roughness, breathiness, asthenia, and strain using a 0 to 3 scoring system, with 0 being normal and 3 being a high degree of dysfunction.

FUNCTIONAL DYSPHONIA

Functional dysphonia is diagnosed when no anatomical or organic cause can explain voice dysfunction. Functional dysphonia may be classified as one of the following:

1) **Psychogenic dysphonia**: Impaired voice due to a psychogenic rather than a physical origin. It is generally associated with anxiety. Psychogenic dysphonia may be a result of excessive laryngeal muscle tension to provide glottis closure.

2) **Vocal cord misuse**: This is caused by vocal overuse.

3) **Idiopathic vocal cord dysfunction**: A paradoxical adduction of the vocal folds during inspiration, causing dyspnea.

Treatment

Depending on etiology, treatment involves a combination of speech therapy, psychotherapy therapy, behavioral therapy, and hypnosis.

ORGANIC DYSPHONIA

Organic dysphonia includes several organic and anatomic pathologies. Given the vast differential diagnosis, organic dysphonia can be organized by system:

1) **Vascular**: Hemangiomas, arteriovenous malformation, lymphatic malformation.

2) **Infectious**: Laryngitis (viral, bacterial, and fungal).

3) **Trauma/toxin**: Arytenoid dislocation, neck trauma, caustic inhalation injury, laryngopharyngeal reflux.

4) **Autoimmune**: Connective tissue disorder (rheumatoid arthritis, systemic lupus erythematosus).

5) **Malignancy**: Laryngeal carcinoma (squamous cell carcinoma).

6) **Iatrogenic**: Postintubation neuropraxia; thyroid surgery; anterior cervical disc surgery; cardiothoracic, vascular, and neurologic procedures.

7) **Neoplasm**: Recurrent respiratory papillomatosis; benign laryngeal lesions (nodules, cysts, polyps); neoplasms of the skull base, mediastinum, esophagus, lung, and thyroid.

8) **Neurologic**: Stroke, myasthenia gravis, Parkinson disease.

9) **Endocrine**: Hypothyroidism (laryngeal myxedema).

10) **Congenital**: Congenital webs.

Diagnosis

Otolaryngology consultation is necessary. Diagnosis is based on nasolaryngoscopy for visualization or videostroboscopy for revealing mucosal wave abnormalities.

Ancillary Tests

Acoustic analysis, speech aerodynamic study, laryngeal electromyography, computed tomography (CT)/magnetic resonance imaging (MRI).

Treatment

Treat the underlying cause when discovered. Medical treatment rarely leads to resolution of symptoms; surgical treatment and voice therapy are generally

more appropriate. Guidelines from the American Academy of Otolaryngology-
-Head and Neck Surgery (AAO-HNS) suggest the following:

1) Recommend against prescribing antireflux medications without signs of acid reflux.

2) As an option, you may prescribe antireflux medications for hoarseness with signs of chronic laryngitis.

3) Recommend against prescribing routine oral glucocorticoids.

4) Recommend against prescribing routine antibiotics.

5) Perform laryngoscopy before suggesting voice therapy and speech language pathology.

6) Recommend surgery for laryngeal malignancy, benign lesions, or glottis insufficiency.

7) Educate patients on control and preventative measures.

9. Mediastinal Cysts and Tumors

→ **DEFINITION, ETIOLOGY, CLINICAL FEATURES**

Mediastinal cysts and tumors are usually detected incidentally on imaging or when investigating nonspecific complaints regarding a variety of structures in this area.

Classification based on localization:

1) **Anterior mediastinal mass**: Incidental anterior mediastinal lesions originate most frequently from the structures known as the 4 T's: thymus, thyroid, teratoma, and T-cell lymphoma. The most common thymic lesions are hyperplasia, cysts, and thymomas. Germ cell tumors include teratoma (most common), seminoma, nonseminomatous germ cell tumor, choriocarcinoma, and embryonal carcinoma. Other causes of anterior mediastinal mass include parathyroid adenoma, lymphoproliferative neoplasms, mesenchymal tumors, lipoma, liposarcoma, angiosarcoma, leiomyoma, and watery cysts (mediastinal lymphangioma).

2) **Middle mediastinal mass**: Lymphadenopathy: lymphoma, granulomatous disease (sarcoidosis, tuberculosis, silicosis, fungal infection); metastases of neoplasms of other organs; cysts: pericardial cysts, bronchial cysts; vascular lesions: aortic aneurysm, brachiocephalic trunk aneurysm, congenital vascular malformations; diaphragmatic hernia.

3) **Posterior mediastinal mass**: Neurogenic tumors; esophageal diseases: achalasia, cysts, cancer, diverticulum; lateral thoracic meningocele; thoracic duct cysts.

Symptoms: Most mediastinal tumors are asymptomatic. Symptoms are caused by mass effect and compression of other organs. They may include dyspnea, cough, stridor, continuous or periodic chest pain (referred to the chest wall), dysphagia, neuralgia, other neurologic symptoms (caused by compression of the spinal cord by a neurogenic tumor), and superior vena cava syndrome.

→ **DIAGNOSIS**

Chest radiography and computed tomography (CT), differentiation from metastases (of breast, lung, or gastric cancers), search for the primary lesion when necessary (in men examine the testes!), mediastinoscopy, and biopsy.

Imaging studies: Cystic lesions are commonly of thymic origin. Magnetic resonance imaging (MRI) is often useful for distinguishing between cysts and solid masses, particularly in posterior compartment masses, and for identifying necrosis and septations. Endoscopic ultrasonography is also helpful in differentiating cystic lesions from solid lesions and for collecting biopsy specimens. For noncystic lesions, if biopsy or surgery is not immediately decided upon, follow-up CT after 3 to 6 months is generally recommended to assess disease progression.

Tumor markers that should be considered:

1) Thymic masses: Acetylcholine receptor antibodies.

2) Suspected germ cell tumor: α-Fetoprotein (AFP) (ovarian and testicular germ cell tumor) and β human chorionic gonadotropin (β-hCG) (suspected choriocarcinoma).

3) Suspected germ cell tumor or lymphoma: Lactate dehydrogenase (LDH).

→ MANAGEMENT

Presence of an undiagnosed mediastinal mass usually requires consultation with a thoracic surgeon. For suspicious anterior mediastinal masses that are resectable, resection without biopsy is preferred to avoid tumor seeding. Core biopsy should be obtained whenever possible if it affects management (eg, if a lymphoma is suspected and the management is nonsurgical).

10. Nicotine Addiction

→ EPIDEMIOLOGY AND RISK FACTORS

According to the World Health Organization (WHO), tobacco use is the leading cause of preventable death and disease in the world, resulting in almost 6 million deaths each year. Despite recent decreases in the prevalence of smoking in high-income countries, the vast majority of smokers live in middle- or low-income countries, where 50% of men and 9% of women smoke daily, the numbers are increasing, and approximately half of smokers die from a smoking-related cause.

Health hazards of tobacco: Smoking reduces life expectancy by an average of 10 years.● It is a major cause of cancer (→Table 10-1) and respiratory disease, and a risk factor for osteoporosis and reproductive disorders. There is a clear dose-response relationship between smoking and risk of lung cancer.● Smoking also triples the odds of cardiovascular disease, and this risk increases linearly with the amount of cigarettes smoked.●

→ DIAGNOSIS

Nicotine is the main substance leading to physiologic dependence in smokers. Nicotine dependence has been classified by the WHO as a disorder caused by nicotine addiction (*International Classification of Diseases, Tenth Revision* [*ICD-10*] code F17). The fifth edition of *Diagnostic and Statistical Manual of Mental Disorders* (*DSM-5*) has changed the terminology for tobacco use disorder and defines it as the presence of 2 out of 11 criteria (→Figure 10-1) in the last year:

1) Tobacco often taken in larger amounts or over a longer period than was intended.

2) Persistent desire or unsuccessful efforts to cut down or control tobacco use.

3) A great deal of time spent in activities necessary to obtain or use tobacco.

4) Presence of craving, or a strong desire or urge to use tobacco.

5) Recurrent tobacco use resulting in failure to fulfill major obligations at work, school, or home.

6) Continued tobacco use despite persistent or recurrent social or interpersonal problems caused or exacerbated by the effects of tobacco.

7) Important social, occupational, or recreational activities given up or reduced because of tobacco use.

Table 10-1. Tobacco use and cancer risk

Cancer site	Average relative risk
Lung	15.0-30.0
Urinary tract	3.0
Upper aerodigestive tract (larynx,[a] oral cavity, oropharynx and hypopharynx,[a] esophagus)	2.0-10.0
Esophagus (adenocarcinoma)	1.5-2.5
Pancreas	2.0-4.0
Nasal cavity, paranasal sinuses	1.5-2.5
Stomach	1.5-2.0
Kidney	1.5-2.0
Uterine cervix	1.5-2.5
Myeloid leukemia	1.5-2.0

[a] Synergistic interaction with alcohol use.

Adapted from J Natl Cancer Inst. 2004;96(2):99-106.

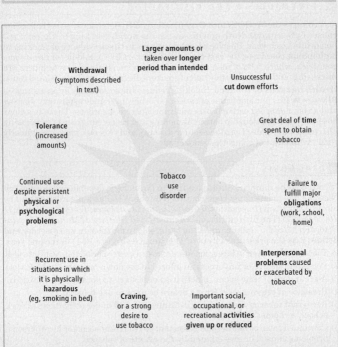

Figure 10-1. Criteria defining tobacco use disorder.

Table 10-2. Fagerström Test for Nicotine Dependence (FTND)		
Questions	**Answers**	**Score**
1. How soon after you wake up do you smoke your first cigarette?	Within 5 minutes	3
	6-30 minutes	2
	31-60 minutes	1
	After 60 minutes	0
2. Do you find it difficult to refrain from smoking in places where smoking is forbidden (eg, in church, at the library, in cinema)?	Yes	1
	No	0
3. Which cigarette would you hate most to give up?	The first one in the morning	1
	All others	0
4. How many cigarettes a day do you smoke?	≤10	0
	11-20	1
	21-30	2
	≥31	3
5. Do you smoke more frequently during the first hours after waking than during the rest of the day?	Yes	1
	No	0
6. Do you smoke if you are so ill that you are in bed most of the day?	Yes	1
	No	0
	Total	
Severity of nicotine dependence	**Score**	
	0-3, low dependence	
	4-6, moderate dependence	
	7-10, high dependence	

Source: Br J Addict. 1991;86(9):1119-27.

8) Recurrent tobacco use in situations in which it is physically hazardous (eg, smoking in bed).

9) Continued tobacco use despite persistent or recurrent physical or psychological problems that are caused or exacerbated by tobacco use.

10) Tolerance, defined by either a need for markedly increased amounts of tobacco to achieve desired effects or markedly diminished effects with continued use of the same amount of tobacco.

11) Withdrawal, manifested by the presence of the characteristic tobacco abstinence syndrome (eg, 4 of the following: irritability, anxiety, difficulty concentrating, increased appetite, restlessness, dysphoric mood, insomnia) or tobacco (or nicotine) taken to relieve or avoid tobacco withdrawal symptoms.

Signs and symptoms of nicotine withdrawal (selected, in isolation neither sensitive nor specific):

1) **Symptoms**: Craving for nicotine, obsessive thoughts about smoking, anxiety, tension, difficulty in relaxing, nervousness (irritability or aggression), discomfort, frustration, depression or depressed mood, impaired concentration, sleep disorders, and increased appetite.

2) **Signs**: Bradycardia, hypotension, decreased blood levels of cortisol and catecholamines, memory impairment, selective attention disturbances, weight gain.

Severity of dependence may be judged using a combination of several questions (→Table 10-2).

→ TREATMENT (SMOKING CESSATION)

Approach

Patients can stop smoking by themselves, but evidence supports psychosocial and pharmacologic interventions to assist cessation. Assessment of tobacco use is an iterative process and can be brief and pragmatic (→Figure 10-2).

General Measures

1. When talking with the patient, clearly emphasize the most important health consequences of smoking, highlight the benefits of smoking cessation that are relevant to the patient (→Table 10-3), and discuss potential difficulties in quitting and methods of coping with them (eg, discuss the symptoms and management of withdrawal).

2. Interventions should be positive and nonjudgmental.

3. Weight gain may be controlled by recommending adequate physical activity and a healthy diet. Exercise can also help to control cravings. Use of medication recommended for nicotine addiction in patients who have quit smoking delays but does not prevent weight gain.

4. Treatment modalities are selected on the basis of the patient's readiness to cease smoking, individual characteristics and preferences of the patient, amount of time dedicated to the patient, level of nicotine dependence, qualifications of the doctor or nurse, and the cost of the interventions.

5 A's Tobacco Cessation Strategy

1. Ask the patient about their smoking status (current, former, never) and record it in the medical chart.⊘⊖

2. Advise the patient to quit smoking. Strengthen their motivation by referring to personal health, the health of household members, being a role model for smoking family members or colleagues, the economic cost of smoking, esthetic concerns, and self-control.⊘⬤

3. Assess the patient's motivation to quit by noting on a scale from 1 to 10:

1) How important it is for him or her to quit at this time.

2) How confident they are that it would be possible to quit at this time.

3) How ready they are to quit.

Identifying the stage of change can help in adapting the interventions (→Table 10-4).

In the toolkit recommended by the WHO to deliver brief interventions in primary care, readiness to quit can be assessed using 2 questions:

1) Would you like to be a nontobacco user?

2) Do you think you have a chance of quitting successfully?

If responding with "no" to any of the questions or "unsure" to the first question, the patient is not ready to quit and needs additional interventions aimed at increasing their motivation to quit. In such patients, a brief motivational intervention called 5 R's can be used. The 5 elements addressed in this intervention are relevance (how quitting smoking is personally relevant), risks (what are the negative consequences of smoking relevant for the patient), rewards (what are the benefits of quitting smoking), roadblocks (what are the barriers to quitting and how they can be solved), and repetition (should be repeated at every visit of a patient not ready to quit).

4. Assist the patient in quitting:

1) Schedule multiple (4 or more) short (1-3 minutes) counselling sessions with occasional intensive interventions whenever possible. There is a dose--response effect for the number and length of counselling sessions.⬤

2) Use motivational interviewing (motivationalinterviewing.org).⊘⊖

3) Provide the patient with a combination of materials (self-help, web-based, individual, group, quitline).

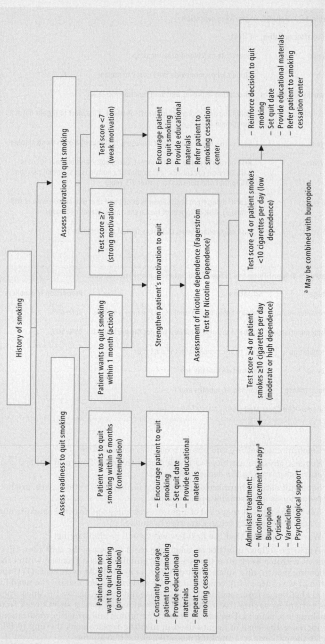

Figure 10-2. Smoking cessation algorithm.

Table 10-3. Benefits of smoking cessation

Time after quitting	Effect
20 min	Heart rate and blood pressure drop
12 h	Blood carbon monoxide level drops to normal
2 weeks to 3 months	Circulation improves and lung function increases
1-9 months	Coughing and shortness of breath decrease. Cilia start to regain normal function in the lungs
1 year	Excess risk of coronary heart disease is half that of a continuing smoker's
5 years	Risk of cancer of the mouth, throat, esophagus, and bladder is cut in half. Cervical cancer risk falls to that of a nonsmoker's. Stroke risk can fall to that of a nonsmoker's after 2-5 years
10 years	Risk of dying from lung cancer is about half that of a person who is still smoking. Risk of cancer of the larynx and pancreas decreases
15 years	Risk of coronary heart disease is that of a nonsmoker's

Table 10-4. Identifying the stage of the patient's motivation to quit

Stage	Situation	Proportion of smokers
Precontemplation	Not intending to quit smoking in the next 6 months	30%-45%
Contemplation	Maybe in the next 6 months but not the next month	35%-50%
Preparation	Tried to stop smoking in the past year	
Action	Stopped <6 months ago	
Maintenance	Stopped >6 months ago	

Based on Clin Chest Med. 1991;12(4):727-35.

4) Combine counselling and pharmacologic treatment.⊘●

5) Suggest physical activity⊘○ and a diet with ample fruit and fluids⊘○ to stay committed to the decision to quit.

6) Set a quit date if pharmacologic treatment is planned. In other cases, gradual reduction is a reasonable approach.⊘●

7) Advise the patient to get rid of cigarettes at home and to avoid smokers and situations that may trigger an urge to smoke.

8) Warn the patient that the first few weeks will be challenging.

5. Arrange follow-up visits or telephone calls to assess the quit plan (first contact within a week after the established quit date, second contact within the following month, and subsequent contacts as needed). At each visit: (1) if the attempt was successful, congratulate the patient and emphasize the need for total abstinence from smoking; (2) if the attempt was unsuccessful, encourage the patient by saying that relapses are common and even a short break from smoking is beneficial. Discuss the reasons for failure and prescribe medications or increase the dose of agents used in nicotine replacement therapy (NRT). Refer the patients to a smoking cessation clinic if available.

Table 10-5. Formulations, dosage, and principles for nicotine replacement therapy (NRT)

Formulation	Dosage	Comments
Short-acting Nicotine gum: 2 mg and 4 mg Nicotine lozenges: 1.5 mg, 2 mg, 4 mg Nicotine inhaler: 10 mg Nicotine spray: 1 mg/spray	The long-acting nicotine replacement should be adjusted to current nicotine intake and combined with short-acting replacement used as needed to reduce cravings	
Long-acting Nicotine 24-h transdermal system: 7 mg, 14 mg, 21 mg Nicotine 16-h transdermal system: 10 mg, 15 mg, 25 mg	**1 cigarette = 1-2 mg of nicotine** 21 mg for 6 weeks, 14 mg for 2 weeks, 7 mg for 2 weeks. Adjust for overdose symptoms or cravings	16-h patch can be used during daytime to minimize vivid dreams or insomnia

Table 10-6. Dosage of nonnicotine agents used in treatment of nicotine addiction

Agent	Dosage	
	Initial treatment	**Maintenance treatment**
Sustained-release bupropion tablets 150 mg	Treatment should be started 1-2 weeks before scheduled quit date. On days 1-3 use 1 tablet (150 mg) in the morning; from day 4 for 7-12 weeks from the date of smoking cessation use 150 mg bid	Treatment can be prolonged to 6 months according to patient preferences
Cytisine tablets 1.5 mg	Treatment should be started 1-5 days before the scheduled quit date Days 1-3: Use 1 tablet (1.5 mg) every 2 h (6×day) Days 4-12: 1 tablet every 2.5 h (5×day) Days 13-16: 1 tablet every 3 h (4×day) Days 17-20: 1 tablet every 5 h (3×day) Days 20-25: 1 to 2 tablets a day	–
Varenicline film-coated tablets 0.5 mg, 1 mg	Treatment should be started 1-2 weeks before scheduled quit date. On days 1-3 use 1 tablet (0.5 mg) once daily; days 4-7, 1 tablet (0.5 mg) bid; from day 8 for the next 11 weeks, 1 mg bid	In patients who quit smoking in the course of 12-week treatment you may consider using 1 mg bid for the next 12 weeks

bid, 2 times a day.

Pharmacotherapy

Formulations, dosage, and principles for NRT: →Table 10-5.

Dosage of nonnicotine agents used in treatment of nicotine addiction: →Table 10-6.

Smokers willing to quit should be offered pharmacologic therapy to reduce cravings and maximize their chances of prolonged abstinence. Pharmacotherapy interventions, including NRTs, bupropion (sustained release), varenicline, or cytisine—ideally in association with behavioral counselling—can increase the rate of tobacco abstinence in comparison to either used alone and are recommended.

1. NRTs are recommended for smoking cessation. Replacement therapies reduce cravings induced by abstinence or reduction and increase the rate of abstinence across different populations (patients with chronic obstructive lung disease, patients with psychiatric disorders, African Americans). Combined use of short-acting (gum, lozenges, inhalers) and long-acting (patches) NRT is more effective than monotherapy.◉ Contrary to the popular belief, smoking while on NRT does not appear to be harmful, and NRT can be used as part of the "reduce-to-quit" strategy. However, we suggest using NRT with caution in patients with unstable angina, recent myocardial infarction, or life-threatening arrhythmia. Replacement therapy should be matched to current nicotine consumption, considering that 1 cigarette equals 1-2 mg of nicotine. The dose can then be adjusted according to the frequency of cravings or adverse effects from nicotine overdose: hiccups, xerostomia, dyspepsia, nausea, heartburn, tachycardia, or sleep disorders. Temporomandibular articular pain from gum chewing can be relieved by intermittent chewing and parking the gum between the jaw and the cheek. Skin reaction from the patch is frequent and tends to attenuate after a few weeks of usage.

2. Sustained-release **bupropion** reduces nicotine reinforcement and cravings by blocking reuptake of dopamine and noradrenaline. We suggest it in smokers in the preparation phase with a set quit date.◉◉ It may be preferred in patients with depressive symptoms or patients worried about weight gain. The main contraindications to the use of bupropion are a past history of seizures of any etiology, head trauma, and eating disorders. The rate of de novo seizures is low (<0.5%) and generally associated with doses >450 mg. In the course of bupropion therapy, alcohol may be consumed in moderate amounts and not discontinued abruptly, as withdrawal-related seizure risk is increased. The other adverse reactions include insomnia, agitation, dry mouth, changes in behavior, hostility, agitation, depressed mood, suicidal ideations, and suicidal attempts.

3. Varenicline is a synthetic nicotinic receptor partial agonist that binds to receptors with a greater affinity than nicotine. Like bupropion, we suggest to use it for the first intention in motivated patients with a set quit date or in patients who have failed NRT alone.◉◉ Contraindications include pregnancy and end-stage renal failure. Although major studies have not demonstrated an increase in neuropsychiatric adverse events, mood disorders are more prevalent in smokers. Thus, we recommend to assess mood in all smokers with a simple questionnaire and use varenicline with caution in patients with psychiatric disorders. (For a sample questionnaire, you may consult the Suicide Risk Assessment Guide at the website of the Canadian Patient Safety Institute.) The most common adverse effects include moderate nausea that resolves in the course of treatment, abnormal dreams, insomnia, and headache.

4. Cytisine is a natural alkaloid and a nicotinic receptor partial agonist with a documented efficacy equivalent to NRT in healthy individuals. It is currently unavailable in North America, but it is available in some parts of Europe, and its low cost makes it an attractive choice when compared with other pharmacologic options.◉◉ Contraindications include hypersensitivity to cytisine, hypertension, pregnancy, and breastfeeding. Use cystine with caution in patients with advanced atherosclerosis or active peptic ulcer disease. Adverse effects include nausea, vomiting, pyrosis, xerostomia, pupil dilation, tachycardia, hypertension, fatigue, and malaise.

→ SPECIAL CONSIDERATIONS

Cardiovascular Diseases

Concerns have been raised regarding the safety of smoking cessation medications for patients with cardiovascular disease. Although caution is advised in patients with acute or severe coronary disease, the benefits of smoking cession generally outweigh the cardiac risks of bupropion or varenicline. NRT was associated with an increase in minor cardiovascular events such as tachycardia and arrhythmia but it does not increase the risk of major adverse cardiac events. Although the risks and benefits of these therapies should be adequately weighted in patients with acute or severe cardiac conditions, most patients risk more from continued tobacco use than from the medication.

Pregnancy

Cigarette smoking during pregnancy and early infancy is associated with multiple negative effects including low birth weight, increased preterm labor and pregnancy loss, sudden infant death syndrome, and childhood respiratory illnesses. Thus, all pregnant women should be advised to stop smoking and make their environment smoke-free.⊘○ Because of conflicting evidence of congenital defects associated with NRT, counselling should be considered the first line of therapy for smoking cessation in pregnant patients. NRT with gums or lozenges may be considered as a second line of therapy rather than continuous transcutaneous nicotine.

Electronic Cigarettes

In the last years, electronic nicotine delivery systems (ENDSs) have provided smokers with a new and attractive option to assist smoking cessation. ENDSs may be helpful in a harm-reduction strategy, but the evidence supporting their use is limited and their regulation needs to be strengthened to ensure public safety.⊘●

11. Obstructive Sleep Apnea

→ DEFINITION, ETIOLOGY, PATHOGENESIS

Obstructive sleep apnea (OSA) is a disease caused by recurrent episodes of upper airway collapse (causing apnea) or upper airway narrowing (causing hypopnea [a marked decrease in airflow]) at the level of the pharynx with normal function of the respiratory muscles. Apnea, hypopnea, or both cause episodes of nocturnal hypoxemia and arousals from sleep that lead to sleep fragmentation (patients are unaware of most of these episodes). This in turn causes daytime symptoms and in combination with repeated hypoxemia and an increase in sympathetic tone leads to an elevation in blood pressure and its complications.

Severe sleep apnea may occur in the absence of nighttime and daytime symptoms. Conversely, symptoms may occur with an apparently normal sleep study, particularly if nasal pressure monitoring is not done to detect flattening of the nasal pressure waveform, indicating increased upper airway resistance syndrome (UARS).

Apnea is a reduction of $\geq$90% in the amplitude of respirations lasting $\geq$10 seconds. **Hypopnea** is defined as a decrease of $\geq$30% in the pressure in the nasal cavity lasting $\geq$10 seconds and associated with a decrease of $\geq$3% in SpO_2 and/or associated with microarousal. The **apnea-hypopnea index (AHI)** is an index indicating the number of apneas and hypopneas per hour of sleep. **Respiratory event–related arousal (RERA)** is a disturbance of breathing lasting $\geq$10 seconds that does not meet the criteria for apnea or hypopnea and leads to arousal from sleep. The **respiratory disturbance index (RDI)** is the number of apneas, hypopneas, and RERAs per hour of sleep.

Factors contributing to pharyngeal obstruction during sleep include obesity (neck circumference >43 cm in men and >40 cm in women), long uvula, tonsillar and/or adenoidal hypertrophy, nasal septal deviation, turbinate enlargement, nasal polyps, alcohol consumption (particularly before bedtime), tobacco smoking, certain sedatives and hypnotics, hypothyroidism, and acromegaly.

→ **CLINICAL FEATURES AND NATURAL HISTORY**

1. Daytime symptoms: Sleepiness, morning headache, memory and concentration impairment, decreased libido, emotional disorders.

2. Nocturnal symptoms: Snoring (loud, irregular) and apneas, excessive sweating, arousal with a choking sensation, nocturia, palpitations, mouth dryness upon awakening.

3. Other symptoms: Overweight or obesity are observed in 70% of patients. Hypertension is observed in 50% of patients.

4. Sequelae: Untreated severe OSA increases the risk of cardiovascular diseases (hypertension, ischemic heart disease, arrhythmia, conduction disturbances, heart failure, stroke), increases perioperative risk, and likely increases the risk of death. Sleepiness and fatigue of drivers or operators from OSA of any severity increases accident risk.

→ **DIAGNOSIS**

A definitive diagnosis requires sleep study. Polysomnography (overnight monitoring of sleep [electroencephalography, electrooculogram, and electromyography]) together with the monitoring of airflow, respiratory effort (chest and abdomen respiratory movements), hemoglobin oxygen saturation in arterial blood (SpO_2), electrocardiography, body position, and limb movements is the gold standard. In patients without cardiorespiratory disease, potential respiratory muscle weakness (due to a neuromuscular condition), suspicion of sleep-related hypoventilation, chronic opioid medication use, or history of stroke or severe insomnia, the diagnosis can be made with home sleep apnea testing (involving at least recording of airflow, respiratory movement, and oximetry, or peripheral arterial tonometry with oximetry and actigraphy recording). However, when the home sleep apnea test is either negative or inconclusive and a clinical suspicion of significant OSA remains, polysomnography should be considered.

American Academy of Sleep Medicine diagnostic criteria:

1) At least 15 obstructed breathing events (apneas, hypopneas, RERAs) per hour of sleep (RDI ≥15; regardless of the presence or absence of symptoms).

2) RDI ≥5 in a patient with ≥1 of the following symptoms:

   a) Unintentional sleeping episodes, excessive daytime sleepiness, unrefreshing sleep, fatigue, or insomnia.

   b) Awaking with a feeling of apnea, dyspnea, or choking.

   c) The patient's partner reports habitual snoring or episodes of apnea during the patient's sleep.

During episodes of breathing disturbances it is necessary to confirm the presence of respiratory effort.

Classification of the severity of OSA based on the RDI:

1) RDI 5 to 15: Mild OSA.

2) RDI 15 to 30: Moderate OSA.

3) RDI >30: Severe OSA.

Daytime Sleepiness Assessment

The assessment of daytime sleepiness may be done using the Epworth Sleepiness Scale (www.epworthsleepinessscale.com). This scale asks the patient about the probability of falling asleep (or dozing) not related to tiredness in a number of normal daytime activities including:

1) Sitting or reading.

2) Watching TV.

3) Sitting inactive (eg, during meetings, in a theater).

4) Being a passenger in a car for over an hour.

5) Lying down in the afternoon.

6) Talking to somebody.

7) Sitting after eating lunch.

8) Being in a car while stopped for a few minutes.

The probability of falling asleep or dozing in each of those situations is scored from 0 (never), through slight (1), moderate (2), to high (3). Scores of ≤10 indicate normal daytime sleepiness, 11 to 12, mild sleepiness, 13 to 15, moderate sleepiness, and 16 to 24, severe excessive daytime sleepiness.

Screening for Severe OSA

Although the sleep study remains the gold standard in the diagnosis of OSA, an approach requiring such a test for screening for severe diseases has limitations due to major technology and resources requirements. Questionnaires, such as NoSAS score, STOP-Bang (www.stopbang.ca), or the Berlin questionnaire, are sometimes used to evaluate the need for sleep study; however, their sensitivity and specificity are limited. Some clinicians suggest that the STOP-Bang score may be used to identify patients at risk of severe OSA. Overnight oximetry screening with the following results may be used to identify those who are likely to have subsequent moderate or severe OSA on polysomnography and should undergo such a test:

1) An oxygen desaturation index >10 (ie, 10 per-hour episodes of a drop in SpO_2 by ≥4% for ≥10 seconds in comparison to preceding 120 seconds), or

2) More than 10% of total time with SpO_2 <90%, or

3) Lowest SpO_2 <85%.

This approach, although not fully tested, may limit the number of costly and time-consuming polysomnography studies, as a negative overnight oximetry study makes severe sleep apnea very unlikely. However, polysomnography or the home sleep study is mandatory to diagnose OSA and—in most if not all jurisdictions—to meet criteria for the continuous positive airway pressure (CPAP) funding as well as for screening patients in critical safety occupations.

Differential Diagnosis

Other causes of daytime sleepiness: central sleep apnea, obesity-hypoventilation syndrome, narcolepsy, periodic limb movement disorder, restless leg syndrome, and insomnia.

→ **TREATMENT**

1. Patient education: **Lifestyle changes**: Weight reduction in obese patients, sewing one or more golf balls into the back of the patient's pajamas (to prevent the patient from sleeping on the back; may not be effective), avoidance of alcohol consumption in the evening, avoidance of muscle relaxants, and cessation of tobacco smoking.

2. CPAP therapy (or its modifications: **auto-CPAP, bilevel positive airway pressure [BiPAP]**) is the method of choice for treating moderate or severe OSA, as well as mild OSA in patients with severe daytime symptoms. This treatment should be offered to reduce the severity of symptoms and prevent profound hypoxia in patients who experience it irrespective of symptoms. Although the effects of treatment on mortality and major cardiovascular morbidity were not clear in the SAVE trial, given the study population characteristics, low CPAP compliance, and improvement in quality of life, we recommend CPAP use for patients with severe OSA who can tolerate and comply with this treatment.●● CPAP provides upper airway patency by the use of a continuous positive pressure of 4 to 20 cm H_2O. In patients with daytime sleepiness persisting despite effective CPAP treatment, you may consider a trial of medication, including modafinil.●○

3. Oral devices: Most often these involve mandibular repositioning splints. These devices are suggested in patients with mild to moderate OSA in whom CPAP treatment is not feasible.●○

4. Surgical treatment may be considered as an adjunct to CPAP treatment (septoplasty, tonsillectomy, adenoidectomy, bariatric surgery) or in patients who do not tolerate CPAP (mandibular advancement, osteotomy of the hyoid bone). However, the effects of those treatments are not clear.○

5. Other methods: Implantation of a unilateral hypoglossal nerve stimulation device.

12. Pertussis

→ DEFINITION AND PATHOGENESIS

Pertussis (whooping cough) is an infectious disease of bacterial etiology, which classically manifests as prolonged bronchitis with episodes of a severe paroxysmal cough ("violent cough").

1. Etiologic agent: *Bordetella pertussis*, a gram-negative, aerobic bacillus that produces pertussis toxin (PT). The transmission route is via the upper respiratory tract droplets. PT induces necrosis of the respiratory epithelium (most prominent in the trachea), which results in abnormal secretion of respiratory mucus (making it very thick and viscous) and a powerful activation of the cough reflex.

2. Reservoir and transmission: Humans are the only host. The source of infection is sick individuals, including those previously vaccinated who eventually develop pertussis. The infection occurs mainly through inhalation of respiratory droplets expelled by a sick individual with cough.

3. Incubation and contagious period: The incubation period is 5 to 21 days (usually 7-14 days). Attack rates are high (up to 80%), particularly within the first 3 weeks of the disease (during the catarrhal and in the beginning of the paroxysmal phase).

→ CLINICAL FEATURES

Clinical manifestations resemble bronchitis with a chronic, paroxysmal cough. The clinical course and severity of signs and symptoms are variable (recurrent infections or infections in previously vaccinated individuals are milder and cause less typical clinical manifestations, with a dominant chronic atypical cough). Fever is most frequently mild or absent. Usually 3 phases may be distinguished:

1) **Catarrhal phase** (1-2 weeks): Flu-like symptoms, although fever is absent or low-grade. Cough appears at the end of this phase, initially at night, and later also during the day. It is dry at first and gradually becomes paroxysmal.

2) **Paroxysmal phase** (4-6 weeks): Attacks of a paroxysmal ("violent") cough within a single expiration, which terminate with a loud laryngeal stridor (a "whoop"; common in children, less frequent in adolescents and adults). The thick and viscous mucus is usually expectorated at the end of the episode (in children it may be swallowed and subsequently vomited). The episodes may be accompanied by edema and cyanosis of the face as well as facial and conjunctival petechiae. Newborns and young children may develop apnea and generalized seizures. Although the attacks of cough cause fatigue, between the episodes patients may appear quite well. Clinical manifestations in adults are usually dominated by a chronic atypical cough.

3) **Convalescent phase** (3-4 months): The cough gradually resolves, although periodic exacerbations may be observed, particularly after exercise or during subsequent infections.

Infants (particularly those <6 months of age) generally have an atypical presentation associated with a shorter catarrhal phase that ends with the onset of gagging and apneic episodes, which may be associated with bradycardia. These episodes can be prolonged and may be associated with cardiac arrest.

→ DIAGNOSIS

Pertussis may be suspected on the basis of clinical manifestations (particularly cough lasting >3 weeks); however, diagnosis must be based on results of serologic or microbiological testing. In most regions pertussis is considered a notifiable disease and must be reported to public health units. Laboratory tests are not necessary for the diagnosis in individuals who have typical clinical manifestations and had documented contact with a patient with laboratory--confirmed pertussis.

Diagnostic Tests

1. Serology (enzyme-linked immunosorbent assay [ELISA]): Positive serum antibodies against PT (validity of the test is limited due to difficulty in interpreting the results). Positive IgG titers in older children and adults reflect prior infection or vaccination. In patients who have not been vaccinated in the preceding 12 to 24 months, elevated levels of IgG against PT in ≥1 sample suggest a recent infection. Diagnosis is also likely based on an increase ≥100% or a decrease ≥50% in the antibody levels in the second serum sample collected 2 to 4 weeks after the first sample.

2. Microbiology:

1) The historic gold standard was *B pertussis* **culture** (eg, on Regan-Lowe or Bordet-Gengou medium) from secretions obtained by a nasopharyngeal aspirate or swab (use a Dacron or calcium alginate swab, not cotton swabs); however, it may yield up to 50% false-negative results (particularly in patients who have been vaccinated or treated with appropriate antibiotics).

2) **Molecular studies** (polymerase chain reaction [PCR]) that detect the genetic material of *B pertussis* in secretions have now become the most frequent means for the laboratory diagnosis of pertussis, given their rapid turnaround time and significantly improved sensitivity. Consult the local laboratory regarding accepted sample types for testing.

3. Complete blood count: White blood cell (WBC) counts between 20×10^9/L and 30×10^9/L with lymphocytes predominant in the differential blood count (although not pathognomonic, this feature is helpful in establishing diagnosis). WBC counts are often normal in adolescents and adults (particularly in the elderly). High WBC counts (ie, $>30 \times 10^9$/L) in infants have been associated with mortality.

Differential Diagnosis

Other causes of chronic cough, including *Bordetella parapertussis* and *Bordetella bronchiseptica* infections that can have a very similar presentation to *B pertussis*.

→ TREATMENT

Antimicrobial Treatment

In adolescents and adults start therapy within 3 weeks of the onset of cough. An early intervention at the onset of the catarrhal phase alleviates the course of pertussis. Therapy instituted in the paroxysmal phase shortens the contagious period but has no effect on the clinical manifestations of the disease. First-line agents are oral **macrolides**: azithromycin 500 mg on day 1 followed by 250 mg once daily on days 2 to 5; clarithromycin 500 mg bid for 7 days or erythromycin 500 mg qid for 14 days. In patients allergic to or intolerant of macrolides, use sulfamethoxazole 800 mg/trimethoprim 160 mg bid for 14 days.

Symptomatic Treatment and General Measures

Patients with chronic comorbidities and young infants will often require hospitalization (they may have a severe course of infection and are at high risk for complications). Oxygen therapy or ventilatory support may be necessary in severe cases.

→ COMPLICATIONS

Infants (particularly <6 months of age) and patients with chronic comorbidities (particularly neuromuscular) are at the highest risk for complications, which include:

1) **Pneumonia** (secondary, of bacterial etiology), atelectasis, pneumothorax.

2) **Neurologic complications** (predominantly in infants, rarely in adults): Apneic episodes, seizures, cerebral edema, intracranial hemorrhage, subdural hemorrhage, ischemic encephalopathy (severe cognitive impairment, focal neurologic symptoms, focal or generalized seizures lasting >24 hours). These complications may lead to irreversible sequelae (mental retardation, deafness, epilepsy).

3) **Other**: Hernia, rectal prolapse, urinary incontinence, rib fractures, damage of the lingual frenulum, subconjunctival hemorrhages.

→ PROGNOSIS

In neonates and infants, the course of pertussis is severe and associated with a high risk of death (~1% in patients <2 months, ~0.5% in patients 2-11 months of age) and complications. In older children and adults, the prognosis is good, but the disease is very exhausting and may lead to major impairment of general performance status. Neither vaccination nor exposure confer permanent immunity, but in such cases subsequent infections are usually milder.

→ PREVENTION

1. Vaccination is the key prevention method. Note that multiple studies have suggested that the duration of protection afforded by acellular pertussis vaccines appears to be shorter than that associated with the previous whole-cell pertussis vaccine, despite the more favorable adverse-effect profile of acellular vaccines.

2. Management of exposures: All close contacts who are unvaccinated or partially vaccinated should be offered age-appropriate vaccination schedules as soon as possible. Some authorities recommend **postexposure chemoprophylaxis** (following one of the regimens used for treatment) for all close contacts regardless of their vaccination status, although high-risk contacts (eg, infants) should always be provided with prophylaxis. The prophylactic regimen is the same as that recommended for a therapeutic course (→Antimicrobial Treatment, above).

3. Isolation: Patients receiving effective antimicrobial therapy should be isolated for 5 days after initiation of appropriate antibiotic therapy. Patients not receiving antimicrobial treatment should be isolated for 3 weeks from the onset of the paroxysmal cough.

13. Pleural Diseases

13.1. Pleural Effusion

→ DEFINITION AND CLINICAL FEATURES

Pleural effusion results from an imbalance between fluid formation and resorption within the pleural space. It may be transudative or exudative. Pleural effusion may be asymptomatic or manifest with dyspnea, trepopnea, orthopnea, cough, or chest pain, depending the on underlying conditions and degree of fluid accumulation. Signs of pleural effusion and differential diagnosis: →Chapter 1.22, Table 22-1. Diagnosis is based on results of imaging studies

Table 13-1. Light's criteria for distinguishing exudative from transudative pleural effusion		
Light's criteria	Sensitivity for exudate	Specificity for exudate
Exudative pleural effusion if meets ≥1 of:	98%	83%
Pleural fluid protein to serum protein ratio >0.5	86%	84%
Pleural fluid LDH to serum LDH ratio >0.6	90%	82%
Pleural fluid LDH >2/3 of ULN for serum LDH	82%	89%
Adapted from N Engl J Med. 2002;346(25):1971-7.		
LDH, lactate dehydrogenase; ULN, upper limit of normal.		

(chest radiographs, computed tomography [CT], ultrasonography) and analyses of pleural fluid. Also →Chapter 16.10.

→ DIAGNOSIS

If history and physical examination are suggestive of pleural effusion (decreased breath sound with dullness on percussion), further investigations are required to confirm the diagnosis. **Posteroanterior chest radiography** should be performed in the assessment of pleural effusion. Pleural effusions ≥200 mL normally exhibit an abnormal opacity with decreased lung volume on chest radiographs, but effusions of as little as 50 mL can cause blunting of the cost-ophrenic angle. To date, **ultrasonography** is the gold standard investigation to diagnose a pleural effusion. Ultrasonography detects fibrin and septations within the pleural space with greater sensitivity than CT. It also increases the success rate of thoracentesis while minimizing procedure-related complications. **Chest CT** with contrast is useful in the evaluation of exudative pleural effusions, providing critical findings that may be suggestive of a malignant effusion, me-sothelioma, complications of lung infection (parapneumonic effusion, empyema), and vascular or lymphatic obstruction.

Pleural fluid analysis is critical in characterizing the type of pleural effusion and guiding further investigations. Pleural effusion may appear serous, sero-sanguinous, bloody, purulent, or milky. Some presentations are associated with specific conditions, such as putrid purulent fluid in anaerobic empyema, milky fluid in chylothorax or pseudochylothorax, and bile-stained fluid in biliary-pleural fistula. Results of pleural fluid analysis are used to categorize pleural effusion as transudative and exudative using Light's criteria (→Table 13-1), which are highly sensitive for an exudative process (sensitivity, 98%; specificity, 83%). Pleural fluid differential cell counts are helpful in the differential diagnosis but not disease-specific (→Table 13-2). Neutrophil-predominant effusions are associated with acute processes, while effusion related to malignancy, tuberculosis, and cardiac failure are commonly lymphocytic. However, any long-standing pleural effusion over time tends to become populated by lymphocytes. Fluid cytology should be done in all patients with exudative effusions to evaluate for malignancy. Gram stain and culture should be considered for a newly diagnosed effusion.

13.1.1. Chylothorax

→ DEFINITION

Chylothorax is a pleural effusion caused by the leakage of lymphatic fluid into the pleural space from a ruptured thoracic duct or obstruction of the lymphatic vessels.

Table 13-2. Pleural fluid differential cell counts and possible associated diseases

Neutrophil predominance

- Parapneumonic effusion
- Pulmonary embolism
- Early tuberculous pleuritis
- Benign asbestos pleural effusion

Lymphocyte predominance

- Malignancy
- Tuberculous pleuritis
- Lymphoma
- Cardiac failure
- After coronary bypass graft
- Rheumatoid effusion
- Chylothorax
- Uremic pleuritis
- Sarcoidosis
- Yellow nail syndrome
- Pulmonary embolism

Eosinophilia (≥10% of nucleated cells)

- Parapneumonic effusion
- Drug-induced pleuritis
- Benign asbestos pleural effusion
- Eosinophilic granulomatosis with polyangiitis
- Lymphoma
- Pulmonary embolism
- Parasitic infestation
- Malignancy

Pleural eosinophilia is a relatively nonspecific finding.

Adapted from Thorax. 2010;65 Suppl 2:ii4-17.

Causes: Malignancy (most commonly lymphoma or metastases of other cancers); injury, including surgery (particularly of the esophagus), chest trauma, sometimes catheterization of the superior vena cava; lymphangioleiomyomatosis; obstruction of a vena cava; amyloidosis.

→ DIAGNOSIS

Diagnosis is made on the basis of pleural fluid analysis. The fluid is milky-white and odorless and contains chylomicrons. The level of triglycerides is usually >1.24 mmol/L (110 mg/dL), no cholesterol crystals are present, and the level of cholesterol is <2.59 mmol/L (100 mg/dL).

Chylothorax has to be differentiated from pseudochylothorax, which occurs very rarely and is a result of the accumulation of cholesterol in a chronic pleural effusion. Usually it develops in the course of a chronic pleural effusion, such as in tuberculosis or rheumatoid arthritis. The pleural fluid in pseudochylothorax has the same appearance as in chylothorax, but the level of cholesterol is >5.18 mmol/L (200 mg/dL), cholesterol crystals are present, and the level of triglycerides is usually <0.56 mmol/L (50 mg/dL).

→ T R E A T M E N T

Treatment includes pleural drainage and management of the underlying disturbances. Evaluation by a dietitian and instructions on a high-protein low-fat (<10 g/d) diet are recommended. Total parenteral nutrition to reduce lymph production and close the fistula between the lymph vessel and the pleural space can also be considered if oral therapy is insufficient. Somatostatin and octreotide can be used as adjunctive therapies. In two-thirds of patients chylothorax resolves after 12 to 14 days. A constant lymph outflow >500 mL/d is an indication for surgical treatment.

13.1.2. Exudative Pleural Effusion

→ E T I O L O G Y

Pleural exudate is caused by inflammation or malignancy, leading to high protein and lactate dehydrogenase (LDH) levels.

Causes: Pneumonia (most often bacterial, including tuberculosis; less commonly viral or parasitic pneumonia), malignancy (including ovarian fibroma or sex-cord stromal tumor [Meigs syndrome]), pulmonary embolism (usually serosanguineous fluid is present, almost always accompanied by pulmonary infarction), esophageal perforation, pancreatitis, injuries to lymphatic or vascular systems causing chylothorax or hemothorax, thoracic or abdominal surgery, autoimmune diseases (rheumatoid arthritis, systemic lupus erythematosus), drug-induced reactions (amiodarone, nitrofurantoin, phenytoin, methotrexate, carbamazepine, procainamide, propylthiouracil, penicillamine, cyclophosphamide, and bromocriptine), cardiac surgery, and thoracic irradiation.

13.1.2.1. Exudative Pleural Effusion Caused by Malignancy

→ E T I O L O G Y A N D P A T H O G E N E S I S

Malignant pleural exudate may be caused by primary neoplasms (mesothelioma) and metastatic cancers, most often related to lung cancer, breast cancer, colon cancer, or lymphoma, although metastatic gastric, pancreatic, renal, bladder, or ovarian effusions are also encountered.

In patients with suspected malignant etiology in whom analysis of pleural fluid did not establish the diagnosis, repeat pleural fluid analysis is recommended, followed by percutaneous pleural biopsy (preferably a core-needle biopsy guided by imaging studies) if the results of testing are nondiagnostic. If the diagnosis remains in doubt, consider thoracoscopy.

→ T R E A T M E N T

Treatment is most often palliative and directed towards symptom management.

1. Asymptomatic patients with small effusions should be monitored.

2. In **patients with progressive effusions**, perform therapeutic thoracentesis. In almost all patients the effusion recurs after ~1 week to 1 month. Repeated thoracentesis for palliative treatment of dyspnea should be considered only in patients with a very short life expectancy.

3. In **symptomatic patients with recurrent effusions**, either chemical pleurodesis (pleural drainage followed by intrapleural administration of a sclerosing agent) or an indwelling intrapleural catheter can be used as the first-line definitive intervention for relieving dyspnea.

4. In **symptomatic patients with unexpandable lung** (→Chapter 13.13.1.2.2), **failed pleurodesis**, or **loculated effusion**, an indwelling intrapleural catheter is recommended.

5. Less common treatment modalities include intrapleural administration of fibrinolytic agents to facilitate drainage in patients with multiloculated pleural effusions and pleuroperitoneal shunting (in patients with lung entrapment caused by malignant infiltration).

13.1.2.2. Exudative Pleural Effusion in the Course of Bacterial Pneumonia

→ DEFINITION, ETIOLOGY, PATHOGENESIS

Exudative pleural effusions are relatively common (up to 20%-40% of hospitalized patients may have parapneumonic effusion) but the development of empyema following a parapneumonic effusion is much less common with prompt antibiotic therapy and fluid drainage used as needed. Classification of pleural disease secondary to bacterial pneumonia:

1) **Uncomplicated parapneumonic effusion** is purely exudative and accompanies bacterial pneumonia, lung abscess, or infected bronchiectasis. In the course of a lung infection an increase in the pulmonary interstitial fluid volume is observed. This fluid moves across the adjacent visceral pleural to accumulate as an effusion. The effusion fluid is clear and has a pH >7.2, lactate dehydrogenase (LDH) levels <1000 U/L, and glucose levels >2.2 mmol/L. No bacteria are observed in cultures or Gram-stained specimens. Cell counts typically demonstrate an intense neutrophilic reaction, although a tuberculosis-related effusion can be associated with lymphocytosis.

2) **Complicated parapneumonic effusion** corresponds to bacterial invasion across the damaged pleural lining, which leads to an intense inflammatory response that results in fibrin deposition and the development of loculations in the pleural space. The pleural fluid, however, is not yet distinctly purulent. The effusion may be clear or cloudy, with a pH <7.2, LDH levels >1000 U/L, and glucose levels <2.2 mmol/L. Bacteria may be observed by direct smear or in cultures. Pleural drainage is usually necessary.

3) **Pleural empyema**: The effusion is purulent (cloudy and often foul-smelling). Biochemical analysis results are similar to those of complicated parapneumonic effusion (pH may be <7.0). Bacteria may be sometimes observed by direct smear or in cultures (these are predominantly aerobic gram-positive [streptococci and *Staphylococcus aureus*] or gram-negative bacteria [*Escherichia coli*, *Pseudomonas*, *Haemophilus*, and *Klebsiella*]; the prevalence of anaerobic infections has been increasing). **Causes** include complicated parapneumonic effusions and, less commonly, complications of thoracic surgery, chest trauma, esophageal perforation, thoracentesis, and subdiaphragmatic infection. Persistent purulent effusions lead to the formation of septa within the empyema and to fibrosis of the visceral pleura, which impairs lung expansion; they may also result in the formation of bronchopleural fistulas and lead to the development of sepsis, malnutrition, and cachexia.

→ TREATMENT

1. Antibiotic treatment: Empiric antibiotic therapy is indicated for most patients as soon as a diagnosis of parapneumonic effusion or empyema is suspected. Antibiotics should not be routinely delayed while awaiting thoracentesis. The exception to this rule includes only stable patients with chronic effusions, as the microbial nature of such infections often differs from those associated with an acute pneumonic process.

Initial antibiotic therapy should include an agent that targets anaerobic species, which are commonly the culprit. Therapy can be tailored on the basis of drug susceptibility results. Empiric therapy usually involves administration of antibiotics that are active against bacteria typically causing community-acquired infections and against anaerobes, for instance, ceftriaxone 1 g daily combined with metronidazole 500 mg tid. Alternative regimens include a combination of a β-lactam and β-lactamase inhibitor (piperacillin/tazobactam 4.5 g tid) or monotherapy with a carbapenem (meropenem 1 g tid). For patients with a penicillin allergy, ciprofloxacin 400 mg bid with metronidazole is also usually satisfactory. Aminoglycosides should be avoided due to their poor penetration into the pleural space. Antimicrobial treatment used alone is effective only in small uncomplicated parapneumonic effusions.

2. Pleural drainage: Indications include documented purulent or cloudy effusions; effusion with a pH <7.2; presence of microorganisms in a nonpurulent pleural fluid documented by a direct Gram-stained smear or culture; large effusions (>50% of hemithorax); loculated pleural effusion with thickened pleura; or sepsis from a pleural source.

3. Intrapleural administration of tissue plasminogen activator (tPA) 10 mg with deoxyribonuclease (DNase) 5 mg bid for 3 days is indicated for patients with complicated parapneumonic effusion or empyema if the antibiotic therapy and initial drainage have failed. It is important to administer both agents in combination rather than as monotherapy, as guided by randomized controlled trial data.🗹⊖

4. Surgical treatment (videothoracoscopic procedures, open pleural drainage, thoracotomy, decortication) should be considered in symptomatic patients with persistent pleural fluid collections who had no adequate response to attempts of drainage, antimicrobial therapy, and a treatment course of tPA/DNase. Video-assisted thoracoscopic surgery (VATS) is preferred to open thoracotomy given the associated reduction in hospital stay.

13.1.3. Hemothorax

→ DEFINITION

Hemothorax is the presence of blood in the pleural space due to injury (including thoracic surgery) when the hematocrit of the pleural fluid is ≥50% of the peripheral blood hematocrit. The hematocrit value is used to distinguish hemothorax from a bloody exudate, which is most frequently caused by malignancy or pulmonary infarction (these are associated with a low hematocrit).

Symptoms are the same as in the case of pleural effusion and sometimes may be accompanied by manifestations of blood loss (anemia, tachycardia, hypotension). Complications include bacterial infection, pleural empyema, and fibrothorax.

→ TREATMENT

Urgent pleural drainage. Indications for videothoracoscopy or thoracotomy include ineffective drainage, persistent bleeding (blood loss >400 mL/h for 2-3 hours or 200-300 mL/h for 6 hours), suspected cardiac tamponade, damage to major vessels, necrotic lesions in the pleura, chest wounds, and large air leak from chest tube drainage. The prompt removal of blood from the pleural space reduces the risk of fibrothorax.

13.1.4. Transudative Pleural Effusion

Definition and Etiology

Transudative pleural effusions accumulate in the pleural space as a result of increase in the hydrostatic pressure in the pleural capillaries (mainly in the parietal pleura), decrease in the osmotic or oncotic pressure, or less commonly as a result of fluid translocation from the peritoneal cavity.

A transudate is a clear pale-yellow fluid with low protein and lactate dehydrogenase (LDH) levels, pH usually >7.35, and low cell counts comprising mostly lymphocytes.

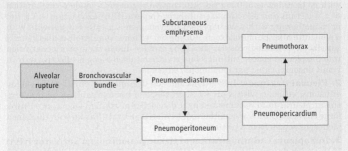

Figure 13-1. Pathophysiology of pneumomediastinum and associated complications.

Causes: Heart failure, cirrhosis, mitral stenosis, diseases of the pericardium, pulmonary embolism (rare), hypothyroidism, hypoalbuminemia, nephrotic syndrome, peritoneal dialysis, and urinothorax (presence of urine in the pleural cavity due to retroperitoneal leakage of urinoma).

→ TREATMENT

Treatment is limited to management of the underlying condition. In patients with cirrhosis and recurrent transudative pleural effusions, consider transjugular intrahepatic portosystemic shunt (TIPS).

13.2. Pneumomediastinum

→ DEFINITION, ETIOLOGY, CLINICAL FEATURES

Pneumomediastinum is the presence of air in the mediastinum. The most common cause by far is primary spontaneous pneumomediastinum, which results from alveolar rupture due to a sudden increase in alveolar pressure. Secondary pneumomediastinum may occur during mechanical ventilation, surgery, or diagnostic procedures, or it may be a result of chest trauma or severe asthma attack. Less commonly pneumomediastinum may be caused by tracheal, bronchial, or esophageal rupture.

Pathophysiology (→Figure 13-1, →Figure 13-2): After alveolar rupture, air penetrates through the peribronchovascular bundle to the mediastinum. Injury to the tracheo-bronchial wall or esophagus can cause air leak directly into the mediastinum. Continuous air leakage into the mediastinum may result in extension of air spreading into the neck and subcutaneous tissue (subcutaneous emphysema), pericardium

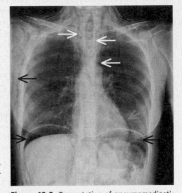

Figure 13-2. Presentation of pneumomediastinum and associated complications. A posteroanterior (PA) chest radiograph of a patient with extensive air leakage demonstrates pneumomediastinum (white arrows), subcutaneous emphysema (red arrows), pneumopericardium (blue arrow), and pneumoperitoneum (black arrows).

(pneumopericardium), pleural space (pneumothorax), or abdominal cavity (pneumoperitoneum). Of note, gas can also originate from gas-forming bacteria infecting the mediastinal soft tissues (mediastinitis).

Symptoms: Chest pain, which worsens with respiration and upon changes of body position; dyspnea; neck discomfort and crackles on compression of the neck and supraclavicular region (if air has entered tissues of the neck); or Hamman sign (audible precordial crunching or creaking sound synchronous with heartbeat, intensifying with inspiration and when lying on the left side).

→ **DIAGNOSIS**

Chest radiographs reveal linear radiolucent areas along the left margin of the cardiac silhouette and sometimes also the "continuous diaphragm" sign (a linear radiolucent area linking the hemidiaphragms under the cardiac silhouette; →Figure 13-3). Lateral chest radiographs reveal the presence of air behind the sternum and thin radiolucent areas highlighting the contour of the aorta, main pulmonary artery, and other mediastinal structures (→Figure 13-4). **Computed tomography (CT)** has greater sensitivity for identifying such abnormalities (→Figure 13-5). In primary spontaneous pneumomediastinum CT shows evidence of gas locules bilaterally, tracking upwards and downwards into the mediastinum. In secondary pneumomediastinum with tracheal or esophageal perforation, an air-fluid level and rim enhancement are also seen in the mediastinum, indicating infection. If tracheal, bronchial, or esophageal perforation is suspected based on history or imaging, **bronchoscopy** or **esophagoscopy** should be performed to evaluate the need for further surgical management (→Figure 13-6).

→ **MANAGEMENT**

In most patients medical treatment is sufficient, as air from the mediastinum is spontaneously evacuated into the subcutaneous tissue of the neck. In patients undergoing mechanical ventilation, chest tube drainage with suction is frequently required to manage pneumothorax. Lower tidal volumes and lower mean airway pressures should be implemented to prevent progression of pneumomediastinum from volutrauma and barotrauma.

13.3. Pneumothorax

→ **DEFINITION, ETIOLOGY, PATHOGENESIS**

Pneumothorax is the presence of air in the pleural space. The air enters the pleural space as a result of damage to the visceral pleura or parietal pleura, causing positive intrapleural pressure and compressing the lung. This in turn leads to impairment of gas exchange. **Classification**:

1) Based on the **cause**:

   a) **Spontaneous pneumothorax** is likely caused by rupture of an emphysematous bulla or subpleural alveoli. It may be **primary** (in previously healthy patients, ie, without any features of lung disease) or **secondary** (in the course of pulmonary diseases such as chronic obstructive pulmonary disease, cystic fibrosis, pulmonary Langerhans cell histiocytosis, or lymphangioleiomyomatosis).

   b) **Traumatic pneumothorax** is caused by chest trauma, both penetrating and nonpenetrating (stab wounds with a sharp object, fall from height, crush wounds, traffic accidents).

   c) **Iatrogenic pneumothorax** following thoracentesis, lung biopsy (percutaneous or transbronchial), catheterization of the large veins (a subclavian vein, less commonly an internal jugular vein), mechanical ventilation, or thoracic surgery.

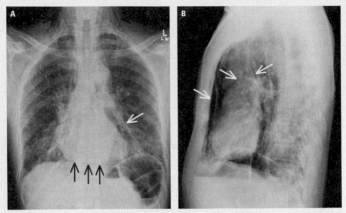

Figure 13-3. Posteroanterior (PA) chest radiography (**A**) and left lateral view (**B**) demonstrate pneumomediastinum (white arrows) and subcutaneous emphysema (red arrows). A linear radiolucent area (black arrows) linking the hemidiaphragms under the cardiac silhouette represents air in the mediastinal soft tissue (the "continuous diaphragm" sign).

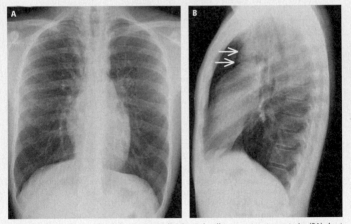

Figure 13-4. A patient with subtle pneumomediastinum, hardly seen on posteroanterior (PA) chest radiographs (**A**), that is identified on the basis of a thin radiolucent line highlighting the contour of the aorta (arrows) on the left lateral view (**B**). This finding represents air in the mediastinal soft tissue.

2) Based on the **mechanism**:
   a) **Closed pneumothorax**: A certain amount of air enters the pleural space and may be absorbed spontaneously after a few days (eg, as in the case of iatrogenic pneumothorax caused by thoracentesis).
   b) **Open pneumothorax**: Air passes into the pleural space through a hole in the chest and leaves it unrestricted. This may cause shifting of the mediastinum to the contralateral side, which in turn may lead to tension pneumothorax and cardiac arrest.

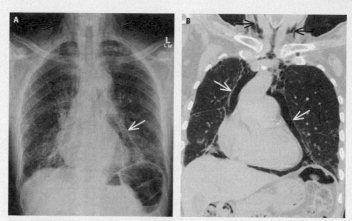

Figure 13-5. Posteroanterior (PA) chest radiograph (A) and computed tomography scan (B) demonstrate pneumomediastinum (white arrows) and subcutaneous emphysema (red arrows).

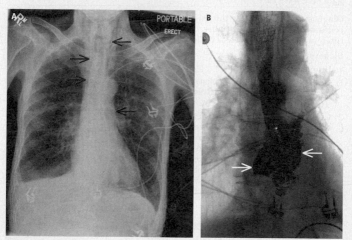

Figure 13-6. Chest radiography (A) shows pneumomediastinum (red arrows) along the paratracheal soft tissues and aorta. Contrast esophagography (B) reveals contrast leakage from the esophagus (white arrows), indicating pneumomediastinum secondary to esophageal rupture.

c) **Tension pneumothorax**: A one-way valve is formed in a hole through which air flows into the pleural space. During each inspiration air enters the pleural space but cannot leave it during expiration. As a consequence, the intrapleural pressure exceeds the atmospheric pressure and is constantly increasing, thereby causing not only ipsilateral compression of the lung but also contralateral displacement of the mediastinum, compression of the contralateral lung, compression of the large veins, decrease in the venous return, and reduction in cardiac output. These changes lead to sudden hypotension, hypoxemia, and potentially cardiac arrest. Tension pneumothorax is a life-threatening condition that requires immediate intervention.

3) Based on the **size** (pneumothorax diameter, ie, the distance between the chest wall and visceral pleura [lung margin] at the level of the pulmonary hilum on anteroposterior [AP] chest radiographs):

a) **Small pneumothorax** (<2 cm).

b) **Large pneumothorax** (≥2 cm).

→ CLINICAL FEATURES AND NATURAL HISTORY

The most common symptoms of pneumothorax are dyspnea, pleuritic chest pain, and cough, although some patients are asymptomatic. Signs (→Chapter 1.22) may be minor and include silent lung sounds, hypertympany on percussion on the side of the pneumothorax, or tracheal displacement to the contralateral side. Tension pneumothorax is usually accompanied by rapidly progressive dyspnea, hypotension, signs of hypoxemia (cyanosis, tachypnea, tachycardia), and in the event of further worsening of the pneumothorax also cardiac arrest. Pneumothorax may be accompanied by subcutaneous emphysema and pneumomediastinum.

→ DIAGNOSIS

Diagnosis is suggested by the patient's history and physical examination and confirmed with imaging studies. The size of a pneumothorax cannot be accurately estimated on the basis of signs and symptoms.

Diagnostic Tests

1. Imaging studies:

1) **Chest radiographs** demonstrate displacement of the lung edge away from the chest wall (→Figure 13-7).

2) **Computed tomography (CT) of the chest** is helpful in differentiating pneumothorax from an emphysematous bulla, especially in the setting of subcutaneous emphysema. Clinical data support the use of chest CT in the evaluation of incident pneumothorax to identify secondary causes (predisposing factors).○

3) **Ultrasonography** (using a 5-10 MHz probe placed in the midclavicular and anterior axillary lines): The findings of pleural sliding with respiration and the comet tail sign (a longitudinal artifact observed at the border of adherence of

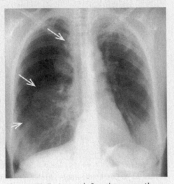

Figure 13-7. Large (≥2 cm) pneumothorax (arrows indicate the lung margin).

the layers of pleura in B-mode ultrasonography) exclude pneumothorax. In M-mode ultrasonography the normal lung shows a "seashore sign," which is a combination of a superficial layer of horizontal lines from the static chest wall and a deep layer of granular pattern caused by lung movement, while a pneumothorax shows a "barcode sign" or "stratosphere sign" (→Figure 13-8).

2. Pulse oximetry and arterial blood gas measurements may reveal decreased oxygen saturation (SpO_2) and hypoxemia (particularly in patients with a tension pneumothorax or large pneumothorax). In some cases hypercapnia and respiratory acidosis are seen (particularly in secondary pneumothorax).

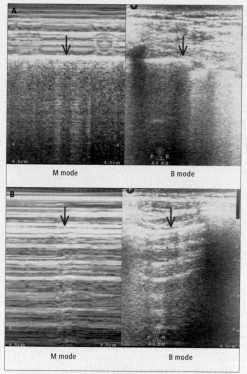

Figure 13-8. Pleural ultrasonography demonstrates the "seashore sign" in a healthy person (A) and the "barcode sign" in pneumothorax (B). Pleural lines are identified by arrows.

→ **TREATMENT**

Management of Life-Threatening Pneumothorax

Administer oxygen in all patients.

1. Tension pneumothorax: Immediately insert a catheter 4 to 5 cm long, 2 mm (14 gauge) or 1.7 mm (16 gauge) in diameter (as for a peripheral IV line) through the second intercostal space in the midclavicular line, along the upper edge of the third rib, into the pleural space. Leave it in place until a definitive drain is placed using traditional chest tube insertion or pig-tail catheterization.

2. Bilateral pneumothorax: Perform pleural drainage as required, starting from the larger pneumothorax. Usually this necessitates a higher level of care and observation than unilateral pneumothorax.

3. Pneumothorax with hemothorax requires urgent drainage or surgery.

Management of Non–Life-Threatening Pneumothorax

1. Primary spontaneous pneumothorax: Management algorithm: →Figure 13-9.

1) **Observation:** Observation is appropriate for patients with a small closed iatrogenic pneumothorax or primary spontaneous pneumothorax and with mild symptoms. You may consider outpatient treatment if a follow-up chest radiograph performed after 3 to 6 hours does not show an increase in the size

1321

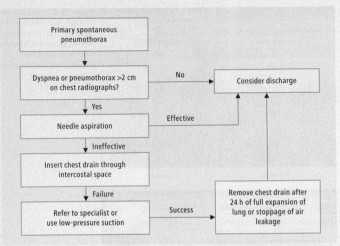

Figure 13-9. Treatment algorithm of primary spontaneous pneumothorax. *Adapted from Thorax.*
2010;65 Suppl 2:ii18-31.

of the pneumothorax; however, the patient should be asked to immediately
report to the hospital in case of worsening symptoms and should be informed
about the risk of recurrence. Other patients require hospitalization. If there
are no contraindications (eg, due to chronic hypercarbic respiratory failure),
administer oxygen at the rate of 10 L/min; this promotes reabsorption of air
from the pleural space. Perform follow-up chest radiographs and reassess
the need for hospitalization.

2) **Syringe aspiration through a catheter**: This may be used in primary
spontaneous and iatrogenic pneumothorax.☉☉ After thoracentesis (as in
pleural fluid collection) and inserting the catheter, remove up to 2.5 L of air
from the pleural space using a syringe connected to the catheter via a 3-way
stopcock. In case of ineffective aspiration (defined as removal of >2.5 L of
air, persistent breathlessness, or large pneumothorax on follow-up chest
radiographs), perform pleural drainage; aspiration may be repeated only in
patients in whom no technical difficulties were encountered during the procedure. In the case of secondary spontaneous pneumothorax, this technique
may be used only in patients with mild dyspnea and a small pneumothorax.
Aspiration through a catheter is not recommended in patients with recurrent
pneumothorax.

3) **Pleural drainage through the intercostal space**: Connect a drainage
tube inserted into the pleural space to a 3-chamber drainage set and leave
it until complete expansion of the lung or cessation of air leakage. If despite
the drainage the lung does not expand, a high-volume low-pressure suction
system may be applied to the drainage system.

4) **Surgical treatment**:

a) **Indications**: Second episode of spontaneous ipsilateral pneumothorax;
recurrence of pneumothorax on the contralateral side of the chest; bilateral spontaneous pneumothorax; persistent air leakage or incomplete
expansion of the lung after >5 days of pleural drainage; hemothorax;
occupations associated with an increased risk of pneumothorax (divers,
pilots, professional drivers, train engineers, sailors, deep sea fishermen,

glass factory workers, wind instrument players); cystic fibrosis (consider surgery after the first episode of pneumothorax).

b) **Types of procedures**: **Pleurodesis** (usually with the use of talc, which leads to obliteration of the pleural space), optimally in combination with videothoracoscopy; **pulmonary wedge resection and pleurectomy** (complete resection of the parietal pleura that leads to permanent obliteration of the pleural space and almost completely prevents recurrence of pneumothorax).

5) **Recommendations for patients with a history of pneumothorax**: Airlines recommend a 6-week interval between complete resolution of pneumothorax and air travel. A history of spontaneous pneumothorax is a permanent contraindication to diving (except for patients undergoing pleurectomy). Cessation of smoking reduces the risk of recurrent pneumothorax.

2. Management algorithm in secondary spontaneous pneumothorax:

1) **Hospitalization and supplemental oxygen**: All patients with secondary spontaneous pneumothorax should be considered for close observation with supplemental oxygen (→above). Asymptomatic patients with a pneumothorax <1 cm on AP chest radiographs may not require further active interventions.

2) **Drainage**: Needle aspiration may be tried in patients with mild symptoms and a small pneumothorax (<2 cm on AP chest radiographs) to avoid chest drain insertion. Otherwise, placement of a small-bore chest drain is recommended.

3) **Specialist consultation**: All patients with secondary spontaneous pneumothorax require early referral for evaluation and consideration of specialized definitive management. Patients with persistent air leak after 48 hours of chest drain insertion should be referred to a thoracic surgeon.

14. Pneumonia

14.1. Community-Acquired Pneumonia

→ DEFINITION, ETIOLOGY, PATHOGENESIS

Community-acquired pneumonia (CAP) is characterized by signs and symptoms of an acute lower respiratory tract infection and new-onset opacities observed on chest radiographs that cannot be explained otherwise (eg, by pulmonary edema or pulmonary infarct). For the purposes of this chapter, this definition does not apply to patients with cancer; immunocompromised individuals; persons hospitalized for pneumonia in oncology, hematology, palliative care, infectious diseases, or AIDS units; patients living in long-term care institutions; and patients hospitalized within the prior 14 days.

Etiologic agents: CAP can be caused by a large number of microbial species but most frequently by *Streptococcus pneumoniae*, *Haemophilus influenzae*, and *Mycoplasma pneumoniae*. In a large number of patients there may be dual infections, particularly where viruses (such as influenza) predispose to superinfection with bacteria such as *S pneumoniae* or *Staphylococcus aureus*. Pathogens may reach the lower respiratory tract as a result of microaspiration of upper respiratory tract secretions, aspiration of oral and upper respiratory tract secretions, inhalation of droplets produced by a coughing patient with viral infection, inhalation of a water aerosol containing *Legionella* organisms, or exposure to droplet nuclei, such as tuberculosis. Pneumonia may also be caused by fungi, viruses other than influenza or parainfluenza, or mycobacteria, which depend on epidemiologic exposure and host factors.

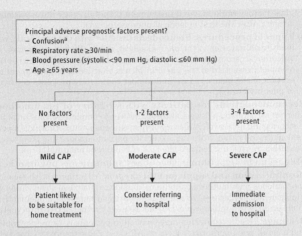

Principal adverse prognostic factors present?
– Confusion[a]
– Respiratory rate ≥30/min
– Blood pressure (systolic <90 mm Hg, diastolic ≤60 mm Hg)
– Age ≥65 years

No factors present	1-2 factors present	3-4 factors present
Mild CAP	**Moderate CAP**	**Severe CAP**
Patient likely to be suitable for home treatment	Consider referring to hospital	Immediate admission to hospital

[a] Defined as a score ≤8 on a 10-point scale (1 point awarded for each correct answer to questions about age, date of birth, current time, current year, name of the hospital, recognizing 2 persons [eg, doctor, nurse], address, year of the outbreak of World War II, name of a universally known individual [eg, president, prime minister], counting backwards from 20 to 1) or recent confusion with regard to people, place, or time.

CAP, community-acquired pneumonia.

Figure 14-1. Severity assessment of community-acquired pneumonia in the outpatient setting: **CRB-65 Score.** *Adapted from the 2009 British Thoracic Society guidelines.*

→ **CLINICAL FEATURES AND NATURAL HISTORY**

1. Symptoms typically have an acute onset and include fever, chills and sweating, pleuritic chest pain, cough with or without the production of purulent sputum, and dyspnea (in some patients). Elderly patients with CAP are more likely to have nonspecific symptoms, may not develop fever, and may develop confusion (→Figure 14-1).

2. Signs: Tachypnea, tachycardia, dull percussion over the area of inflammatory infiltrate, crackles, increased tactile fremitus, and sometimes bronchial breath sounds. In patients with pleural effusion, dull percussion, absence of tactile fremitus, and poorly audible breath sounds are observed.

→ **DIAGNOSIS**

Diagnostic Criteria

In patients treated on an outpatient basis or prior to hospitalization (in whom no laboratory test or radiologic results are available), the diagnosis of pneumonia is based on the following:

1) Signs and symptoms of acute lower respiratory tract infection: Cough and ≥1 additional manifestations of lower respiratory tract infection, such as dyspnea, pleuritic pain, or hemoptysis.

2) New local findings on examination of the chest.

3) One or more of the general signs and symptoms: Sweats, chills, myalgia, temperature ≥38°C.

4) No other explanations for the observed manifestations.

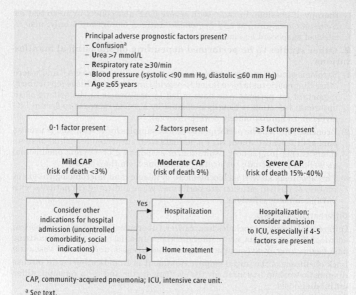

CAP, community-acquired pneumonia; ICU, intensive care unit.

[a] See text.

Figure 14-2. Severity assessment of community-acquired pneumonia in the inpatient setting: CURB-65 Score. *Adapted from the 2009 British Thoracic Society guidelines.*

Assessment of Disease Severity

To decide on an outpatient or inpatient treatment setting, use the **CRB-65 score** (→Figure 14-1) in outpatients and the **CURB-65 score** (→Figure 14-2) in hospitalized patients. Pulse oximetry can be considered in settings where emergency oxygen is used.

Diagnostic Tests

1. Studies to be performed in every patient on admission:

1) **Chest radiography**: Results reveal new infiltrates. There are no strong correlations between specific radiographic patterns and etiologic agents.

2) **Complete blood count (CBC) and differential blood count**: Leukocytosis with predominant neutrophils may be suggestive of a bacterial etiology.

3) **Serum levels of urea, electrolytes, bilirubin, aspartate aminotransferase, and alanine aminotransferase** may be used to help determine the severity of the systemic disease.

4) **Serum C-reactive protein (CRP) levels** (levels <20 mg/L suggest against the diagnosis of bacterial pneumonia; the increase is more pronounced in pneumococcal pneumonia with concomitant bacteremia than in pneumonia caused by viruses or *Mycoplasma* spp) or **procalcitonin levels** (also may be helpful in making the decision to discontinue antibiotic treatment).

5) **Measurement of blood oxygen levels**: Pulse oximetry (hypoxemia may be observed). In patients at risk of hypercapnia, patients with hemoglobin oxygen saturation in arterial blood (SpO_2) <92%, and patients with severe pneumonia, measure arterial blood gas levels.

6) **Microbiology**: Collect 2 sets of blood cultures and sputum specimens for culture in patients with moderate or severe CAP prior to starting antimicrobial

therapy, if possible. In those with severe CAP also collect urine to test for *S pneumoniae* antigen and *Legionella* antigen (serogroup 1 only; also in cases of suspected legionellosis).

2. Other studies to be performed depending on the clinical manifestations:

1) Serologic studies may be performed in patients with severe CAP and where other diagnostic tests have failed to provide an etiology. This is particularly important for patients who have failed to improve or in the setting of an outbreak. Infection is usually indicated by a 4-fold increase in serum IgG levels at an approximately 3-week interval.

2) Bronchoscopy may be performed to collect samples for testing and is used as part of differential diagnosis (in patients with suspected bronchial obstruction/stenosis, lung cancer, aspiration, or patients with recurrent pneumonia) as well as to evacuate respiratory secretions from the airway.

3) Thoracentesis as well as biochemical, cytologic, and microbiological examination of pleural effusion are performed when indicated (in patients with parapneumonic effusion).

Differential Diagnosis

Differential diagnosis includes lung cancer, tuberculosis, pulmonary embolism, eosinophilic pneumonia, acute interstitial pneumonia, cryptogenic organizing pneumonia, lung involvement in collagen tissue diseases, and systemic vasculitis.

Lack of efficacy of the initial empiric treatment is an indication for an intense diagnostic workup in search for the etiologic factor and for a repeated differential diagnosis.

→ TREATMENT

General Measures

1. Outpatient treatment: Smoking cessation, rest, drinking large quantities of fluids. Use acetaminophen (INN paracetamol) to control fever and pleuritic pain when present. Pulse oximetry may be useful for assessment of severity and oxygen requirement.

2. Hospital treatment:

1) Oxygen therapy with SpO_2 monitoring (in patients with chronic obstructive pulmonary disease [COPD], consider repeated arterial or venous blood gas measurements) with a target partial pressure of oxygen in arterial blood (PaO_2) ≥60 mm Hg and SpO_2 94% to 98% (88%-92% in patients with COPD and patients at risk of hypercapnia). If hypoxemia persists in spite of high-concentration oxygen therapy, consider high-flow oxygen therapy or mechanical ventilation.

2) Assess volume status and nutrition. Administer fluids and start nutrition therapy when indicated.

3) We suggest oral prednisone (50 mg once daily for 1 week), particularly in patients with CRP >150 mg/L, patients requiring mechanical ventilation, or patients with septic shock.⊘⊖

Antimicrobial Treatment

1. In patients who are referred to hospital with suspected CAP, consider starting antimicrobial treatment immediately in the case of severe illness or a risk of delay in reaching the hospital (>2 hours). In hospitalized patients, start antibiotic treatment as soon as possible after the diagnosis is established.

2. Choice of antimicrobial agent(s): Initial empiric treatment: →Figure 14-3; if the etiologic agent is known: →Table 14-1. In hospitalized patients, switch from IV to oral antibiotic when the patients are hemodynamically stable, improving clinically, and able to ingest medications. It should be noted that

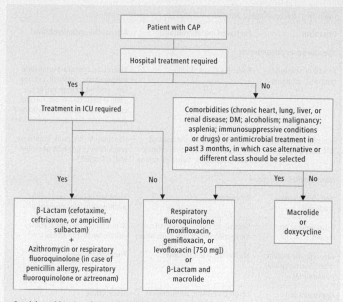

Special considerations for specific pathogens:

1. For patients without comorbidities in regions with a high rate (>25%) of infection with macrolide-resistant *Streptococcus pneumoniae* (MIC ≥16 µg/mL), use of an alternative agent is recommended, including respiratory fluoroquinolones.
2. Possible *Pseudomonas* infection: An antipneumococcal antipseudomonal β-lactam (piperacillin/tazobactam, cefepime, imipenem, or meropenem) plus (1) ciprofloxacin or levofloxacin (750 mg); (2) an aminoglycoside plus azithromycin; (3) or an aminoglycoside and an antipneumococcal fluoroquinolone (in case of penicillin allergy, substitute aztreonam for β-lactam).
3. Possible community-acquired methicillin-resistant *Staphylococcus aureus*: Add vancomycin or linezolid.

CAP, community-acquired pneumonia; DM, diabetes mellitus; ICU, intensive care unit; MIC, minimum inhibitory concentration.

Figure 14-3. Recommended empiric antibiotics in community-acquired pneumonia. *Adapted from Clin Infect Dis. 2007 Mar 1;44 Suppl 2:S27-72.*

European recommendations differ from current North American guidelines, as amoxicillin is the first-line therapy for mild CAP while ampicillin or penicillin IV and a macrolide is recommended for hospitalized cases, while amoxicillin and clavulanic acid and a macrolide are recommended for severe hospitalized cases.

3. Duration of treatment: In outpatients and the majority of hospitalized patients treatment is continued for a minimum of 5 days. The patient should be afebrile for 48 to 72 hours prior to discontinuing antibiotics. Key considerations are normalization of vital signs and oxygen saturation, return to normal mental status, and ability to maintain oral intake. Longer treatment should be considered if the expected improvement in symptoms does not occur during the first 3 days; in patients with severe CAP of undetermined etiology, it is continued for 10 days; and in patients with CAP caused by *Legionella pneumophila*, staphylococci, *Pseudomonas aeruginosa*, *Acinetobacter baumannii*, or gram-negative intestinal bacilli, for 14 to 21 days.

Table 14-1. Recommended antimicrobial therapy for specific pathogens

Organism	Preferred antimicrobial(s)	Alternative antimicrobial(s)
Streptococcus pneumoniae		
Penicillin nonresistant; MIC <2 µg/mL	Penicillin G, amoxicillin	Macrolide, cephalosporins (oral [cefpodoxime, cefprozil, cefuroxime, cefdinir, cefditoren] or parenteral [cefuroxime, ceftriaxone, cefotaxime]), clindamycin, doxycycline, respiratory fluoroquinolone[a]
Penicillin resistant; MIC ≥2 µg/mL	Agents chosen on the basis of susceptibility, including cefotaxime, ceftriaxone, fluoroquinolone	Vancomycin, linezolid, high-dose amoxicillin (3 g/d with penicillin MIC ≤4 µg/mL)
Haemophilus influenzae		
Non–β-lactamase producing	Amoxicillin	Fluoroquinolone, doxycycline, azithromycin, clarithromycin[b]
β-Lactamase producing	Second- or third-generation cephalosporin, amoxicillin-clavulanate	Fluoroquinolone, doxycycline, azithromycin, clarithromycin[b]
Mycoplasma pneumoniae/Chlamydophila pneumoniae	Macrolide, a tetracycline	Fluoroquinolone
Legionella spp	Fluoroquinolone, azithromycin	Doxycycline
Chlamydophila psittaci	A tetracycline	Macrolide
Coxiella burnetii	A tetracycline	Macrolide
Francisella tularensis	Doxycycline	Gentamicin, streptomycin
Yersinia pestis	Streptomycin, gentamicin	Doxycycline, fluoroquinolone
Bacillus anthracis (inhalation)	Ciprofloxacin, levofloxacin, doxycycline (usually with a second agent)	Other fluoroquinolones; β-lactam, if susceptible; rifampin; clindamycin; chloramphenicol
Enterobacteriaceae	Third-generation cephalosporin, carbapenem[c] (drug of choice if extended-spectrum β-lactamase producer)	β-Lactam/β-lactamase inhibitor,[d] fluoroquinolone
Pseudomonas aeruginosa	Antipseudomonal β-lactam[e] **plus** (ciprofloxacin or levofloxacin[f] or aminoglycoside)	Aminoglycoside **plus** (ciprofloxacin or levofloxacin[f])
Burkholderia pseudomallei	Carbapenem, ceftazidime	Fluoroquinolone, sulfamethoxazole/trimethoprim
Acinetobacter spp	Carbapenem	Cephalosporin-aminoglycoside, ampicillin/sulbactam, colistin
Staphylococcus aureus		
Methicillin susceptible	Antistaphylococcal penicillin[g]	Cefazolin, clindamycin
Methicillin resistant	Vancomycin or linezolid	Sulfamethoxazole/trimethoprim
Bordetella pertussis	Macrolide	Sulfamethoxazole/trimethoprim

Organism	Preferred antimicrobial(s)	Alternative antimicrobial(s)
Anaerobe (aspiration)	β-Lactam/β-lactamase inhibitor,[d] clindamycin	Carbapenem
Influenza virus	Oseltamivir or zanamivir	
Mycobacterium tuberculosis	Isoniazid plus rifampin plus ethambutol plus pyrazinamide	
Coccidioides spp	For uncomplicated infection in a normal host, no therapy generally recommended; for therapy, itraconazole, fluconazole	Amphotericin B
Histoplasmosis	Itraconazole	Amphotericin B
Blastomycosis	Itraconazole	Amphotericin B

Choices should be modified on the basis of susceptibility test results and advice from local specialists. Refer to local references for appropriate doses.

[a] Levofloxacin, moxifloxacin, gemifloxacin (not a first-line choice for penicillin susceptible strains); ciprofloxacin is appropriate for *Legionella* and most gram-negative bacilli (including *Haemophilus influenzae*).

[b] Azithromycin is more active in vitro than clarithromycin for *H influenzae*.

[c] Imipenem/cilastatin, meropenem, ertapenem.

[d] Piperacillin-tazobactam for gram-negative bacilli, ticarcillin/clavulanate, ampicillin/sulbactam or amoxicillin/clavulanate.

[e] Ticarcillin, piperacillin, ceftazidime, cefepime, aztreonam, imipenem, meropenem.

[f] 750 mg daily.

[g] Nafcillin, oxacillin flucloxacillin.

Source: Clin Infect Dis. 2007;44 Suppl 2:S27-72.

INN, international nonproprietary name; MIC, minimum inhibitory concentration.

→ FOLLOW-UP

1. Outpatients: Perform a follow-up examination after at most 48 hours. If no clinical improvement is observed, consider referring the patient for chest radiography and other diagnostic studies.

2. Hospitalized patients:

1) Monitor temperature, respiratory rate, pulse, blood pressure, mental status, and SaO_2. Initially perform these assessments at least twice a day, or more often in patients with severe pneumonia. In patients who receive an appropriate antibiotic, improvement should be observed within 24 to 48 hours.

2) In patients with clinical improvement, do not repeat chest radiographs prior to discharge. If the improvement has not been satisfactory, repeat chest radiographs.

3) If the initial empiric treatment has not been effective, make intensive efforts to identify the antibiotic-resistant pathogen(s) and repeat differential diagnosis.

4) Do not discharge patients who fulfill ≥2 of the following criteria during the prior 24 hours: temperature >37.5°C, respiratory rates ≥24/min, heart rates >100/min, systolic blood pressure ≤90 mm Hg, SpO_2 <90% (while on air), abnormal mental status, inability to eat without assistance. Consider a delayed discharge in those with a temperature >37.5°C.

5) In every patient schedule a follow-up visit within ~6 weeks. Chest radiographs should be repeated in all patients with persisting signs and symptoms and patients at a higher risk of developing cancer (particularly tobacco smokers and patients >50 years). Radiographic abnormalities, especially when extensive, resolve less rapidly than clinical features (typically within 4-8 weeks), particularly in elderly patients. If radiologic or clinical abnormalities persist after 6 weeks or recur in the same location, perform bronchoscopy.

→ COMPLICATIONS

1. Pleural effusion and empyema (→Chapter 13.13.1.2).

2. Lung abscess: A purulent collection located in the pulmonary parenchyma that most frequently develops as a consequence of pneumonia caused by staphylococci, anaerobic bacteria, *Klebsiella pneumoniae*, or *P aeruginosa*.

Signs and symptoms are the same as in pneumonia. Diagnosis is based on radiologic findings revealing an interstitial cavity with an air-fluid level.

Treatment: Antimicrobial agents and postural drainage. In rare cases not responding to treatment, surgical resection is used. As an initial empiric treatment, IV penicillin G (INN benzylpenicillin) 1.8 to 2.7 g (3-4.5 million IU) qid in combination with IV metronidazole 0.5 g qid can be used; IV clindamycin 600 mg qid; or IV amoxicillin/clavulanic acid 1.2 g tid to qid. If the etiologic agent and its resistance pattern are known, start targeted treatment. Treatment should be continued until the abscess cavity closes (usually within a few weeks).

→ SPECIAL CONSIDERATIONS

Pneumonia in Immunocompromised Patients

Diagnosis: This group of patients is particularly vulnerable to infections with mycobacteria, fungi (*Aspergillus fumigatus*, *Candida albicans*, *Pneumocystis jiroveci*), and viruses. The etiologic organism will differ depending on both host characteristics (specific immunologic defect) and epidemiologic exposures. Generally, diagnostic evaluations may include microscopic evaluation of sputum (this may help with the diagnosis of pneumocystosis and tuberculosis), sputum cultures, blood cultures, bronchoscopy and bronchoalveolar lavage, computed tomography (CT) scan imaging (eg, aspergillosis), or alternatively transbronchial lung biopsy specimens. Surgical lung biopsy may also be needed for some cases.

Treatment: Start treatment empirically, that is, prior to confirming microbiologic etiology, based on the nature of the immunocompromised state and knowledge of exposures. Prompt infectious diseases consultation is warranted.

14.2. Hospital-Acquired Pneumonia

→ DEFINITION, ETIOLOGY, PATHOGENESIS

Hospital-acquired pneumonia (HAP) is a pneumonia that develops after 48 hours of hospitalization in a patient who has not been intubated on admission. **Ventilator-associated pneumonia (VAP)** is a pneumonia that develops after >48 hours of starting mechanical ventilation. **Health care–associated pneumonia (HCAP)** is a pneumonia developing in patients who were hospitalized for ≥2 days within 90 days prior to the onset of the infection; residents of long-term care facilities; patients who received intravenous antibiotics, chemotherapy, or wound treatment within 30 days prior to the current infection; or patients who attended a hospital or hemodialysis clinic.

Etiologic agents:

1) **Within the first 4 days of admission** etiologic agents may be the same as in the case of community-acquired pneumonia (CAP) and may also include

gram-negative bacilli (*Escherichia coli*, *Klebsiella pneumoniae*, *Enterobacter* spp, *Proteus* spp, and *Serratia* spp).

2) **From day 5 onwards** etiologic agents are more likely to include multidrug--resistant strains, typically aerobic gram-negative bacilli: *Pseudomonas aeruginosa*, *E coli*, *K pneumoniae*, *Acinetobacter* spp, and more rarely *Legionella pneumophila*. The predominant gram-positive bacterium is *Staphylococcus aureus*, whose hospital strains may be methicillin-resistant.

The sources of pathogens are medical devices and the environment (air, water, equipment, clothing), but the pathogens can be also transmitted between the patient and the medical personnel or other patients.

→ CLINICAL FEATURES AND NATURAL HISTORY

Clinical features are the same as in CAP (→Chapter 13.14.1). Mortality rates in patients with HAP developing after surgery are ~20%. In patients treated in the intensive care unit, the mortality rates are 30% to 40%.

→ DIAGNOSIS

Diagnostic Tests

Diagnostic tests are the same as in CAP (→Chapter 13.14.1). Prior to any modification of antimicrobial treatment in patients with suspected HAP, collect samples from the lower respiratory tract material (obtained by endotracheal aspiration, bronchoalveolar lavage, or protected specimen brushing). Blood cultures should be performed in all patients with suspected VAP; a positive result may be indicative of pneumonia or an extrapulmonary infection.

Differential Diagnosis

Complications of an underlying condition, such as pulmonary embolism and pulmonary infarct (resulting from immobilization and deep vein thrombosis), sepsis (may be complicated by acute respiratory distress syndrome), or alveolar bleeding in the course of a systemic disease.

→ TREATMENT

Management of patients with HAP, VAP, and HCAP is similar.

General Measures

General measures are as in CAP (→Chapter 13.14.1).

Antimicrobial Treatment

Selection of antimicrobial agents: →Table 14-1. Management algorithm: →Figure 14-4.

1. Empiric treatment is modified on day 2 or 3 of therapy based on the clinical response and culture results. Start from intravenous antibiotics (in the case of fluoroquinolones and linezolid, you may switch to oral administration immediately after achieving clinical improvement):

1) **Patients hospitalized for <5 days without risk factors of drug resistance**: Treatment with one antibiotic: ceftriaxone, fluoroquinolone, ampicillin/sulbactam, or ertapenem.

2) **Patients hospitalized for ≥5 days at risk of drug resistance**: Combination treatment with a fluoroquinolone effective against *P aeruginosa* (ciprofloxacin) or an aminoglycoside and:

a) A cephalosporin effective against *P aeruginosa* (ceftazidime, cefepime); or

b) A carbapenem (imipenem, meropenem); or

c) A β-lactam with β-lactamase inhibitor (piperacillin + tazobactam, ticarcillin + clavulanic acid).

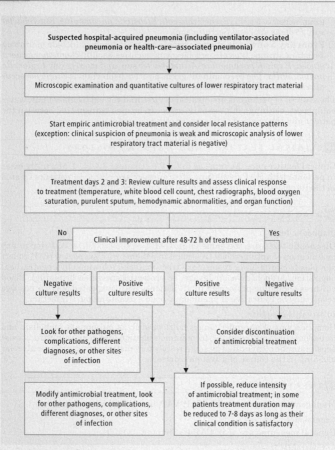

Figure 14-4. Management algorithm in patients with suspected hospital-acquired pneumonia.

3) In **patients with suspected *L pneumophila* infection**, administer a fluoroquinolone (eg, levofloxacin) or a macrolide instead of an aminoglycoside.

4) In **patients with methicillin-resistant *Staphylococcus aureus* (MRSA) risk factors**, add vancomycin or linezolid.

2. After identifying the etiologic agent, switch to targeted therapy when indicated. The duration of **combination treatment** should be as short as possible (up to 7 days, except for *P aeruginosa* infections). If the antimicrobial agents used in the empiric treatment were appropriate for the pathogens, attempt to shorten the total duration of treatment from 14 to 21 days down to as little as 7 days provided a good clinical response is achieved (this does not apply to HAP caused by *P aeruginosa*). In patients with pneumonia caused by *P aeruginosa*, combination treatment is used. In patients with *Acinetobacter* spp infection, use carbapenems, ampicillin + sulbactam, or colistin. In patients suspected to have infections caused by Enterobacteriaceae producing extended-spectrum β-lactamase (ESBL), carbapenems are recommended.

→ F O L L O W - U P

Assess the clinical response to antimicrobial treatment after 48 to 72 hours. Resolution of fever, a decrease in white blood cell counts, an increase in blood oxygen saturation, and an improved general condition confirm the effectiveness of treatment. If no improvement is observed, repeat microbiological tests and consider a different etiology (mycobacterial or fungal) or diagnoses other than pneumonia.

14.3. Pneumonia Caused by Specific Etiologic Agents

14.3.1. Influenza Pneumonia

→ D E F I N I T I O N   A N D   E T I O L O G Y

Influenza complicated by pneumonia rarely develops in otherwise healthy individuals. The risk is increased by chronic lung diseases (mainly chronic obstructive pulmonary disease), valvular heart disease, diabetes mellitus, nephrotic syndrome, immunosuppressive treatment, advanced age, and pregnancy. The same groups of patients are at high risk of infection with *Streptococcus pneumoniae*, which is a cause of pneumonia following initial infection with influenza.

→ D I A G N O S I S

Diagnosis is based on clinical features (manifestations of pneumonia with concomitant rhinitis and myalgia) and onset during an influenza season. Chest radiographs reveal bilateral, symmetric, diffuse opacities. The diagnosis may be confirmed by isolating the virus from sputum, bronchial secretions, or a pharyngeal swab, or by immunologic studies.

→ T R E A T M E N T

Symptomatic treatment and antiviral drugs (→Chapter 8.17.5).

14.3.2. Middle East Respiratory Syndrome

→ D E F I N I T I O N ,   E T I O L O G Y ,   P A T H O G E N E S I S

Middle East respiratory syndrome (MERS) is an infectious disease caused by a zoonotic coronavirus termed MERS-CoV that emerged in 2012 in Saudi Arabia. Cases of infection have been reported mainly in residents of and visitors to the Arabian Peninsula and Eastern Asia. **Transmission** is from animals (camels are the suspected source) to humans via unknown route; human-to-human transmission requires close person-to-person contact.

Clinical features range from asymptomatic infection to severe pneumonia with acute respiratory distress syndrome and sepsis. Initial symptoms include fever and cough, often with headache and muscle and joint pain; later patients develop dyspnea, sometimes nausea and vomiting, rarely abdominal pain and diarrhea.

→ D I A G N O S I S

Chest radiographs reveal unilateral or bilateral infiltrates, interstitial changes, and pleural fluid. Laboratory tests show leukopenia with lymphopenia, low platelet counts, and increased lactate dehydrogenase levels.

Diagnostic Tests

1. Polymerase chain reaction (bronchoalveolar lavage fluid, sputum, smear or aspirate from the nasal cavity or oropharynx).

2. Serology (serum sample collected in the first week of illness and 2-3 weeks later).

→ **TREATMENT**

No antiviral treatment is available. Administer oxygen or use mechanical ventilation when necessary. In the case of bacterial superinfection, administer antibiotics.

→ **PREVENTION**

While caring for the patient, wear a filtration mask (at least as effective as the N95 mask), gloves, gown, and protective goggles or face shield. The patient should be transferred to a hospital equipped with an isolation room complying with airborne infection isolation room (AIIR) standards.

14.3.3. Pneumonia Caused by *Aspergillus* spp (Invasive Aspergillosis)

→ **DEFINITION AND ETIOLOGY**

Invasive aspergillosis is most commonly caused by *Aspergillus fumigatus*, *Aspergillus flavus*, *Aspergillus niger*, or *Aspergillus terreus*. Risk factors include neutropenia, prior antibiotic treatment, and chronic pulmonary disease. **Clinical features** include fever, pleuritic pain, and hemoptysis. Chest radiographs may reveal peripheral solitary or multiple nodules, some of them with features of necrosis. CT scans reveal focal interstitial opacities surrounded by a cloud of a lower density image (halo sign).

→ **DIAGNOSIS**

The diagnosis of pneumonia is confirmed only if microscopic examination reveals the presence of fungi in lung biopsy specimens (in immunosuppressed patients also in bronchoalveolar lavage) and *Aspergillus* spp have been isolated in culture of the same specimen. An assay detecting *Aspergillus* spp antigen (galactomannan) in blood or bronchoalveolar lavage is useful in diagnostics. Using an optical density index (ODI) of 0.5 as a cutoff value, the sensitivity and specificity of the test to detect invasive aspergillosis is estimated to be ~80%. At a cutoff value of ODI 1.0, sensitivity is reduced to ~70% and specificity increased to ~90%. A positive sputum culture result is of low diagnostic value.

→ **TREATMENT**

Use IV **voriconazole** (6 mg/kg every 12 hours for 2 doses on day 1, followed by 4 mg/kg bid; after achieving clinical improvement, you may switch to oral administration [4 mg/kg bid] starting on day 7). Alternatively, you may use IV **amphotericin B** as a liposomal formulation 3 to 5 mg/kg/d, as a lipid complex 5 mg/kg/d, or as a colloidal dispersion 3 to 4 mg/kg/d; use of amphotericin deoxycholate 0.7 to 1 mg/kg/d (maximum, 1.5 mg/kg/d) is associated with a higher risk of nephrotoxicity and other adverse effects.

In patients with less severe disease and patients who have achieved clinical improvement, consider **itraconazole** (200 mg tid for 3 days followed by 200 mg bid for tablets; note that dose depends on the formulation and that absorption can be variable) or oral **voriconazole** 200 mg bid for 2 to 5 months. In patients with a single lesion (particularly those with hemoptysis) and patients with lesions adjacent to major blood vessels, the pericardium, penetrating into the pleural cavity, or infiltrating the ribs, surgical resection of the lesion may be indicated during antifungal treatment. In patients with resistance to or intolerance of amphotericin or azole antifungal agents, use **caspofungin** (70 mg/d IV; in patients with a body weight ≤80 kg administer 50 mg/d from day 2 of treatment), **micafungin** (100-150 mg/d IV), or **posaconazole** (start from 200 mg orally qid, after clinical stabilization of the patient change to 400 mg orally bid).

The antifungal therapy should be continued until all signs and symptoms of the infection have been resolved and will often be prolonged in patients with persistent immunologic impairment. Although the duration has not been well established, treatment is generally continued for a minimum of 6 to 12 weeks. Primary combination therapy is not routinely recommended based on the lack of clinical data but may be considered for individual patients.

14.3.4. Pneumonia Caused by Other Pathogens

→ TREATMENT

Treatment: →Table 14-1.

1. *Streptococcus pneumoniae*: The most common etiologic agent of community-acquired pneumonia (CAP). Sputum cultures are recommended in hospitalized patients, although they may be of limited use. Other methods of confirming the diagnosis include blood cultures (positive results in <25% of cases) and detection of the *Streptococcus pneumoniae* antigen in urine.

2. *Haemophilus influenza* and *Moraxella catarrhalis* may be a cause pneumonia, especially in patients with chronic lung disease.

3. *Staphylococcus aureus* causes <5% of CAP cases and ~30% of hospital--acquired pneumonia (HAP) cases; the disease usually has a severe course. The diagnosis is confirmed by microscopic examination of sputum samples, sputum cultures, and blood cultures. Patients with methicillin-resistant *Staphylococcus aureus* (MRSA) infection should be isolated. Infection with Panton-Valentine leukocidin-producing strain (PVL-SA) may lead to the formation of cavities in the lungs (necrotizing pneumonia) and multiple organ failure. Start targeted treatment as soon as results of microbiological studies are available.

4. *Klebsiella pneumoniae* and other gram-negative intestinal bacilli (*Escherichia coli*, *Proteus* spp): Radiologic features: →Chapter 13.14.1. The diagnosis is confirmed by blood or sputum cultures.

5. *Acinetobacter baumannii* usually causes HAP that is often severe and associated with leukopenia. Pleural effusions develop in 50% of patients.

6. Anaerobic bacteria are not a frequent cause of CAP and an uncommon cause of ventilator-associated pneumonia (VAP). They are of prime importance in patients with aspiration and may be associated with abscess formation. Detection can be difficult. Microscopic examination of sputum may be helpful.

7. Atypical pathogens:

1) *Mycoplasma pneumoniae*: The incubation period lasts 2 to 3 weeks. Patients rarely develop leukocytosis or lobar infiltrates. Occasionally hilar lymphadenopathy is observed. Features of hemolytic anemia may be present.

2) *Chlamydophila (Chlamydia) pneumoniae* typically causes pharyngitis that precedes CAP by ~2 weeks.

3) *Legionella pneumophila*: Air conditioning systems, air humidifiers, and tap water are potential sources of infection, which may cause headaches and disorientation. Diarrhea may also be observed. The infection may cause elevated serum levels of alanine aminotransferase, aspartate aminotransferase, creatine kinase; hyponatremia; albuminuria; and microscopic hematuria. The diagnosis is confirmed by detection of the *L pneumophila* antigen in urine.

14.3.5. Pneumonia Caused by *Pneumocystis jiroveci* (Pneumocystosis)

→ ETIOLOGY AND PATHOGENESIS

Pneumonia caused by *Pneumocystis jiroveci* (previously *Pneumocystis carinii*) (PCP) develops in patients with impaired cell-mediated immunity (most commonly in patients with AIDS). The incubation period lasts several weeks.

Clinical presentation: The most common manifestations include fever, dry cough, and dyspnea. In HIV-positive patients, the progression of symptoms may be very slow. White blood cell counts are normal, while lactate dehydrogenase levels are elevated. In patients with early disease, chest radiographs may frequently be normal; later they reveal bilateral, symmetric, ground-glass opacities. Carbon dioxide diffusing capacity of the lungs (DL_{CO}) is decreased.

DIAGNOSIS

Detection of trophozoites or cysts of *Pneumocystis jiroveci* in sputum (sensitivity, 60%), induced sputum, or bronchoalveolar lavage (sensitivity, 95%). In rare cases, lung biopsy (transbronchial or surgical) is necessary.

TREATMENT

Sulfamethoxazole/trimethoprim (trimethoprim 15-20 mg/kg/d) IV or orally in 3 or 4 divided doses for 3 weeks. In patients with a contraindication to sulfamethoxazole/trimethoprim with severe PCP, use intravenous pentamidine (4 mg/kg/d IV). For treatment of mild to moderate PCP in patients who are intolerant of sulfamethoxazole/trimethoprim, alternative regimens include clindamycin (600 mg/d orally in divided doses administered every 8 hours in combination with primaquine 30 mg/d orally), oral atovaquone 750 mg bid, trimethoprim (5 mg/kg orally tid) plus dapsone. In patients with partial pressure of oxygen in arterial blood (PaO_2) <70 mm Hg on room air, an alveolar-arterial (A-a) oxygen gradient ≥35 mm Hg, and/or evidence of hypoxemia (eg, room air oxygen saturation <92%), we suggest a glucocorticoid (oral prednisone 40 mg every 12 hours for 5 days followed by 40 mg/d for 6 days and 20 mg/d for the subsequent 10 days).◐◑

PREVENTION

In immunosuppressed patients and patients with HIV infection who have completed treatment, use sulfamethoxazole/trimethoprim (trimethoprim 80-160 mg orally daily or 160 mg orally 3 times/wk).

15. Pulmonary Hypertension

DEFINITION, ETIOLOGY, PATHOGENESIS

Pulmonary hypertension (PH) refers to an abnormal elevation in mean pulmonary artery pressure (mPAP) at the time of diagnostic right heart catheterization. A recent international task force has proposed a change in the definition from 25 mm Hg to 20 mm Hg with associated increased pulmonary vascular resistance (PVR). Increased mPAP may develop in the course of diseases of the heart, lungs, or pulmonary vessels.

Classification of PH based on pathology according to the European Society of Cardiology:

1) **Group 1: Pulmonary arterial hypertension (PAH)**:
   a) Idiopathic.
   b) Heritable.
   c) Drug-induced or toxin-induced.
   d) Associated with connective tissue disease, HIV infection, portal hypertension, congenital heart disease with left to right shunt, schistosomiasis.

e) PAH long-term responders to calcium channel blockers.

f) Pulmonary veno-occlusive disease (PVOD), pulmonary capillary hemangiomatosis, or both.

g) Persistent PH of the newborn.

2) **Group 2: PH due to left heart disease** (heart failure with preserved or reduced left ventricular ejection fraction; valvular disease; congenital/acquired cardiovascular condition leading to postcapillary PH).

3) **Group 3: PH due to lung diseases, hypoxia, or both** (chronic obstructive pulmonary disease [COPD], restrictive lung disease, other pulmonary diseases with mixed restrictive/obstructive pattern, hypoxia without lung disease [severe sleep-disordered breathing including obesity hypoventilation syndrome and exposure to high altitude], developmental lung disorders).

4) **Group 4: Chronic thromboembolic PH (CTEPH) and other pulmonary artery obstructions**.

5) **Group 5: PH with unclear or multifactorial etiology (or both)**:

a) Hematologic disorders (chronic hemolytic anemia, myeloproliferative neoplasms, splenectomy).

b) Systemic disorders (sarcoidosis, pulmonary Langerhans cell histiocytosis, lymphangioleiomyomatosis, neurofibromatosis).

c) Metabolic disorders (glycogen storage diseases, Gaucher disease, thyroid disorders).

d) Other: Pulmonary tumoral thrombotic microangiopathy, fibrosing mediastinitis, chronic renal failure treated with or without hemodialysis, segmental pulmonary hypertension.

→ CLINICAL FEATURES AND NATURAL HISTORY

1. Symptoms of isolated PH: Progressive limitation of exercise tolerance caused by dyspnea (the key symptom, regardless of etiology). Initial symptoms are mild and nonspecific. Resting dyspnea is often absent even in patients with advanced PH. Angina may be present, which is caused by right ventricular ischemia or by compression of the left main coronary artery by a significantly dilated pulmonary artery. Compression of the recurrent laryngeal nerve by dilated pulmonary arteries may cause hoarseness. Symptoms of the underlying condition are also seen (eg, heart failure or systemic disease, especially scleroderma). The World Health Organization (WHO) functional classification is determined on the basis of symptom severity (→Table 15-1).

2. Signs: Systolic parasternal heave, increased pulmonary component of the second heart sound, and murmur of tricuspid regurgitation. Features of right ventricular heart failure (→Chapter 3.8.2) and of the underlying condition.

3. Natural history: The disease is usually progressive, especially in patients with PAH (group 1).

→ DIAGNOSIS

Diagnosis includes confirmation of PH and determination of its cause.

Diagnostic Tests

1. Laboratory investigations: There are no laboratory features specific for isolated PH. The following tests may sometimes yield abnormal results, which are usually due to diseases associated with PH:

1) Arterial blood gas analysis may reveal moderate hypoxemia (this may be significant in patients with interstitial lung disease, congenital heart disease with shunt reversal, and in patients with a right-to-left shunt through a patent foramen ovale) or hypercapnia in patients with COPD or central abnormalities of respiratory function.

Table 15-1. The World Health Organization functional classification for treatment and monitoring of patients with pulmonary hypertension

Class	Description
I	Patients with pulmonary hypertension but without resulting limitation of physical activity. Ordinary physical activity does not cause undue dyspnea or fatigue, chest pain, or near syncope
II	Patients with pulmonary hypertension resulting in slight limitation of physical activity. They are comfortable at rest. Ordinary physical activity causes undue dyspnea or fatigue, chest pain, or near syncope
III	Patients with pulmonary hypertension resulting in marked limitation of physical activity. They are comfortable at rest. Less than ordinary activity causes undue dyspnea or fatigue, chest pain, or near syncope
IV	Patients with pulmonary hypertension with inability to carry out any physical activity without symptoms. These patients manifest signs of right-heart failure. Dyspnea, fatigue, or both may even be present at rest. Discomfort is increased by any physical activity

Source: Eur Heart J. 2016;37(1):67-119.

2) Antinuclear antibodies are found in approximately a third of patients with idiopathic PH. Anticentromere antibodies in the setting of scleroderma are particularly relevant.

3) HIV serology should be routinely measured.

4) Abnormal liver function tests are found in patients with PH associated with portal hypertension (portopulmonary hypertension).

2. Electrocardiography (ECG) is often normal in patients with early PH. In more advanced disease ECG reveals right axis deviation, P pulmonale, right bundle branch block, right ventricular hypertrophy, and right ventricular overload. Patients may also have arrhythmia (most frequently atrial tachycardia and atrial flutter).

3. Chest radiographs reveal dilation of the main pulmonary artery, lobar pulmonary arteries, right ventricle, and right atrium. Pulmonary congestion is seen in patients with PH due to left ventricular (LV) failure and in PVOD (without LV dysfunction documented on echocardiography). Features of interstitial lung disease or emphysema may also be seen.

4. Pulmonary function tests:

1) **Spirometry**: Results are often normal. Features of pulmonary restriction or obstruction are seen in patients with PH caused by interstitial lung disease or airway disease, respectively. Mild obstruction of the small airways may also be present.

2) **Plethysmography**: In the presence of restriction, interstitial lung disease should be considered and correlated with evidence of pulmonary fibrosis on high-resolution computed tomography (HRCT).

3) **Carbon dioxide diffusing capacity (DL_{CO})**: This may be decreased in patients with idiopathic PH and is particularly low in patients with concomitant parenchymal lung disease.

5. Echocardiography: The primary screening test used in the evaluation of PH. It has the advantage of identifying the etiology responsible for PH by evaluating for LV systolic and diastolic dysfunction, valvular heart disease, congenital heart disease, and other structural abnormalities. Features associated with PH include right ventricular dilation and right ventricular hypokinesis; in more advanced disease, right atrial enlargement, decreased dimensions and deformation of the LV and left atrium, and presence of pericardial effusion are also apparent. Doppler echocardiography, particularly when focused on the assessment of regurgitant jets through the right-heart valves, is used to estimate the pulmonary artery pressures.

6. Perfusion scintigraphy is critical in the evaluation of PH and should be considered in most patients. In the setting of CTEPH, ventilation-perfusion (V/Q) scans have exceptional sensitivity and a negative predictive value. As such, the use of V/Q imaging to exclude CTEPH is essential, given the dramatically different therapeutic approach and prognostic implications of CTEPH in comparison with other forms of PH. Identified perfusion defects should be correlated with computed tomography pulmonary angiogram (CTPA) to confirm the presence of intravascular filling defects.

7. Computed tomography (CT) of the chest demonstrating main pulmonary artery enlargement (≥29 mm), right ventricular dilation, right atrial dilation, or a main pulmonary artery to ascending aorta diameter ratio ≥1 is suggestive of PH. Unenhanced cuts can identify parenchymal lung disease and discriminate between group 3 and group 1 PH. Characteristic findings of PVOD can also be observed on CT. Contrast enhancement of the pulmonary vasculature is critical for the evaluation of CTEPH.

8. Catheterization of the right heart and main pulmonary artery is the gold standard in the hemodynamic assessment of pulmonary circulation and should be completed prior to the initiation of PAH-targeted therapies to provide critical diagnostic and prognostic information. In patients with idiopathic, heritable, or drug-induced PAH, perform acute vasoreactivity testing using a potent pulmonary artery vasodilator (nitric oxide, prostacyclin, or IV adenosine) to assess for vasodilator response, the presence of which has critical treatment and prognostic implications. Hemodynamic evaluation should be completed at dedicated centers of excellence with experience in managing patients with PAH.

9. Other studies depend on the suspected underlying condition.

Diagnostic Approach

The **probability of PH** is assessed using noninvasive techniques. Echocardiography is the primary screening test used in patients suspected to have PH. The probability of PH can be determined using the peak tricuspid regurgitation velocity to estimate right pulmonary artery systolic pressure and a formal evaluation of the size and function of the right-sided cardiac chambers as outlined below:

1) ≤2.8 m/s (tricuspid valve pressure gradient [TVPG] ≤31 mm Hg): Low probability.

2) 2.9 to 3.4 m/s (TVPG, 32-46 mm Hg): Intermediate probability.

3) >3.4 m/s: High probability.

The probability is increased (from low to intermediate and from intermediate to high) in the presence of other echocardiographic features of right ventricular or atrial overload (eg, a right ventricle to LV basal diameter ratio >1.0, flattening of the interventricular septum, pulmonary artery diameter >25 mm, inferior vena cava diameter indicating raised pressure). The echocardiographic probability of PH and clinical features are the basis for indications for cardiac catheterization, which is required to secure a formal diagnosis of PH.

In patients with no clear evidence suggesting a definite PH etiology that would qualify them to group 2, 3, or 5, the echocardiographic diagnosis should be confirmed by direct pressure and flow measurements during pulmonary artery catheterization (mean pressure at rest ≥20 mm Hg and PVR >3 Wood units). Cardiac catheterization is also useful in the differential diagnosis of PH. A pulmonary capillary wedge pressure >15 mm Hg is the key diagnostic criterion of PH caused by left-sided heart disease. Right atrial pressure, cardiac index, pulmonary vascular resistance, and mixed venous oxygen saturation are strong prognostic factors.

To establish prognosis and treatment, additionally assess the patient's WHO functional class (→Table 15-1), results of the 6-minute walk test, and serum B-type natriuretic peptide (BNP) levels.

→ TREATMENT

Treatment depends on the appropriate clinical classification of PH. Patients with both PAH and CTEPH are managed aggressively, as treatment has the potential to dramatically impact the clinical course and represents a cure for some patients. The treatment regimen for PAH has evolved dramatically over the last 25 years with the availability of targeted PAH therapies. Combination therapy, implemented in a goal-directed manner, has had a marked impact on disease course. **Given the potential benefits and toxicities of these therapies, their prescription and management should be orchestrated through an experienced PH center of excellence.**

1. PAH: Management should include acute vasoreactivity testing in patients with idiopathic, heritable, or drug-induced disease. In patients with vasoreactivity (~15% of patients with idiopathic PAH) start treatment with a calcium channel blocker. Other PAH patients are managed with PAH-specific therapies that typically should be used in combination to achieve optimal outcome. These agents primarily target endothelial cell dysfunction and include phosphodiesterase-5 (PDE-5) inhibitors, soluble guanylate cyclase stimulators, endothelin receptor antagonists, and/or agents targeting the prostacyclin pathways. Recent European guidelines suggest monotherapy in a minority of patients and only in specific situations.

2. PH due to left heart disease: Management involves treatment and optimization of the underlying cardiac condition. Randomized clinical trials have not shown a clear role for PAH-specific therapies in this patient population.

3. PH due to lung disease: Treatment of the underlying condition, oxygen therapy, consideration of lung transplantation.

4. CTEPH: Lifelong anticoagulation. In patients with WHO functional class II to IV, pulmonary endarterectomy is the gold-standard therapeutic intervention. Pulmonary endarterectomy is completed with curative intent with normalization of pulmonary hemodynamics in the majority of patients. In those who do not qualify for pulmonary endarterectomy because of distal surgically inaccessible disease or medical comorbidities, targeted medical therapy with the soluble guanylate cyclase stimulator riociguat with or without balloon pulmonary angioplasty (BPA) has therapeutic value.

General Measures

1. Patients with PH should be encouraged to be active within symptom limits. They should avoid excessive physical activity that leads to distressing symptoms, especially angina and syncope. Supervised exercise rehabilitation should be considered in deconditioned patients.

2. Dietary salt restriction, avoidance of excessive fluid intake.

3. Avoidance of pregnancy in women of child-bearing age.

4. Immunization against influenza and pneumococcal infection.

5. Psychosocial support though a multidisciplinary care team.

Pharmacologic Treatment

1. Anticoagulant treatment: Oral therapy may be considered in patients with idiopathic PAH, hereditary PAH, or PAH secondary to anorexigens, although the registry and randomized controlled trial data supporting this indication are weak and contradictory. Do not use anticoagulant treatment in patients with Eisenmenger syndrome or connective tissue disease because of the risk of bleeding. PH associated with LV dysfunction or lung disease is not an independent indication for anticoagulant treatment.

2. Oxygen therapy: Continuous supplemental oxygen therapy is recommended when partial pressure of oxygen in arterial blood (PaO_2) is ≤60 mm Hg.

3. Diuretics: These are used in case of right ventricular failure (→Chapter 3.8, Table 8-4).

4. Calcium channel blockers: Treatment exclusive to patients with documented hemodynamic evidence of pulmonary vasoreactivity (→Diagnostic Tests, above). Use **nifedipine** up to 240 mg/d, **diltiazem** up to 720 mg/d, or amlodipine up to 20 mg/d (agents: →Chapter 3.9, Table 9-4). Start from a standard dose and titrate upwards based on the patient's treatment tolerance.

5. "Targeted" treatment recommended in group 1 PAH: International guidelines recommend initiation of such therapies under the supervision of an expert treatment center. Agents are often used in combination in a goal-oriented fashion. Parenteral therapies are reserved for patients with the most advanced disease.

1) **PDE-5 inhibitors**: **Sildenafil** 20 mg tid, **tadalafil** 40 mg once daily (these are used in PAH). Common adverse effects include headache, flushing, dyspepsia, and visual disturbance. Concurrent use of organic nitrates in any form is contraindicated.

2) **Endothelin receptor antagonists**: **Bosentan** 62.5 to 125 mg bid, **ambrisentan** 5 to 10 mg once daily, **macitentan** 10 mg once daily. The most common adverse effect of endothelin receptor antagonists is increase in serum aminotransferase (monitor the levels during treatment); the increase is usually transient and asymptomatic, although it may warrant discontinuation of the drug. Ambrisentan and macitentan have lower hepatotoxicity.

3) **Prostanoids** are used in patients with severe disease as reflected by poor hemodynamic, functional, and clinical parameters. Without such intervention, the long-term prognosis in these patients is poor. **Epoprostenol** is administered by continuous IV infusion (using a central venous catheter and infusion pump). **Treprostinil**, a prostacyclin analogue, is administered by continuous subcutaneous infusion using a microinfusion pump and small abdominal subcutaneous catheter, IV, or orally. **Iloprost**, a prostacyclin analogue, is inhaled (6-9 times a day). **Selexipag** is a novel prostacyclin receptor agonist that can be administered orally.

4) **Riociguat** is a stimulator of soluble guanylyl cyclase approved by the US Food and Drug Administration for treatment of group 1 patients and the first-line agent in patients with CTEPH who do not qualify for pulmonary endarterectomy. Doses, ranging from 1 to 2.5 mg tid, are established individually. Do not use riociguat in combination with a PDE-5 inhibitor due to the high risk of hypotension and increased risk of death.

Invasive Treatment

1. Balloon atrial septostomy (BAS) is performed to create a septal defect to offload a failing right ventricle. This is a palliative procedure, sometimes also used as a bridging procedure before lung transplantation.

2. Bilateral lung transplantation or heart and lung transplantation is indicated in patients with unequivocal progression of PH despite using all available medical treatment measures.

3. CTEPH:

1) **Pulmonary endarterectomy** (treatment of choice in patients with symptomatic CTEPH) is the mechanical removal of thrombi attached to the endothelium of the proximal sections of pulmonary arteries.

2) **BPA** may be an alternative to surgical treatment mainly in patients who do not qualify for endarterectomy due to excessively distal location of lesions, very advanced age, or serious comorbidities.

→ **P R O G N O S I S**

Historically, the average survival time in patients with idiopathic PAH was 2 to 3 years and in those with functional class IV, <6 months. With the availability of targeted PAH therapies, the natural history of disease has been transformed, resulting in 5-year survival rates of 65%. Despite the availability of several effective therapeutic options, many patients are still at risk of substantial morbidity and premature mortality. In patients with evidence of vasoreactivity, the 5-year survival rate is 95%.

16. Respiratory Failure

→ **DEFINITION, ETIOLOGY, PATHOGENESIS**

Respiratory failure is a dysfunction of the respiratory system causing impaired pulmonary gas exchange and resulting in hypoxemia (a decrease in the partial pressure of arterial oxygen [PaO_2] <60 mm Hg [8 kPa] while breathing room air) or hypercapnia (an increase in the partial pressure of arterial carbon dioxide [$PaCO_2$] >45 mm Hg [6 kPa]). Respiratory failure is classified as hypoxemic respiratory failure or hypercapnic respiratory failure. It may be either acute or chronic.

Hypoxemia

1. Mechanisms of hypoxemia:

1) **Mismatch of alveolar ventilation and pulmonary perfusion**: Reduction of alveolar ventilation with an unchanged or slightly reduced pulmonary perfusion (eg, due to obstructive or interstitial lung disease, minor atelectases, or alveolar flooding) leads to lower partial pressure of oxygen in those areas of the lungs. Poorly oxygenated blood leaving the alveoli of those areas mixes in the pulmonary veins with oxygenated blood from well-ventilated areas of the lungs. This results in reduction in the oxygen content of the blood in the pulmonary veins, left atrium, left ventricle, and systemic arterial circulation.

2) **Shunting of poorly oxygenated blood**:

   a) **Intrapulmonary shunting of poorly oxygenated blood**: In the case of preserved perfusion of the nonventilated areas of the lung (eg, due to airway obstruction, major atelectases, or alveolar flooding), poorly oxygenated blood from these areas flows into the pulmonary veins and mixes with oxygenated blood flowing from the well-ventilated alveoli. Higher proportions of poorly oxygenated blood are associated with more severe hypoxemia.

   b) **Intracardiac shunting of poorly oxygenated blood** between the pulmonary and systemic circulations cause hypoxemia that responds poorly to oxygen therapy. It is the oxygen content (bound to hemoglobin plus dissolved oxygen) of deoxygenated blood that causes the hypoxemia. Since very little of the oxygen content of blood is affected by dissolved oxygen and hemoglobin cannot be saturated >100%, shunts are poorly responsive to oxygen therapy.

3) **Impaired alveolar-capillary diffusion**: This results from interstitial lung diseases, which cause thickening of the alveolar-capillary barrier that leads to impaired oxygen diffusion.

4) **Low inhaled partial pressure of oxygen**: This occurs at very high altitudes, where atmospheric pressure is relatively low.

2. Consequences of hypoxemia (acute and chronic):

1) Anaerobic metabolism is activated by tissue hypoxia, leading to lactic acidosis, cell death, multiorgan failure, and death (acute).

2) A compensatory physiologic response, including tachycardia, increased blood pressure, increased cardiac output, and hyperventilation. This can be transient, waning with persistent mild hypoxemia.

3) Pulmonary hypertension results from reflex vasoconstriction of the pulmonary arterioles and their increased resistance. It becomes persistent due to pulmonary vascular wall remodeling (acute and chronic).

4) Right ventricular failure caused by right ventricular overload and hypertrophy due to pulmonary hypertension secondary to hypoxemia in the course of diseases of the respiratory system (cor pulmonale; acute and chronic).

5) Cyanosis (acute and chronic).

6) Secondary polycythemia caused by chronic hypoxemia that stimulates the synthesis of erythropoietin in the kidney and thus increases erythropoiesis (chronic).

7) Clubbing of digits and hypertrophic osteoarthropathy (chronic).

Hypercapnia

1. Mechanism of hypercapnia: Alveolar hypoventilation: With inadequate ventilation, CO_2 accumulates in the lungs, reducing the pressure gradient across the alveolar-capillary membrane. This is the key factor in the development of hypercapnia, because CO_2 crosses the alveolar-capillary membrane approximately 20 times faster than O_2. Reduced permeability of this barrier and reduced lung perfusion both have much less effect on CO_2 removal than on oxygen uptake.

2. Causes of hypoventilation:

1) **Increased load on the respiratory system:**

   a) **Increased airway resistance:** Upper airway obstruction (foreign body, laryngeal edema or anaphylaxis, obstructive sleep apnea, loss of consciousness), lower airway obstruction (bronchial smooth muscle contraction and mucosal edema: chronic obstructive pulmonary disease [COPD], asthma, anaphylaxis; bronchial obstruction by secretions or tumor).

   b) **Reduced lung compliance:** Alveolar flooding (pulmonary edema, intra-alveolar bleeding), pneumonia, interstitial lung diseases, atelectasis, dynamic hyperinflation (most frequently in COPD); pleural effusion, pneumothorax.

   c) **Reduced chest wall compliance:** Severe obesity, elevation of the diaphragm (intestinal distention, ascites, paralysis of the diaphragm); chest wall deformity, circumferential burn eschar, or tumors.

   d) **Demand for increased minute ventilation (relative hypoventilation):** Shock, hypovolemia, sepsis, pulmonary embolism.

2) **Dysfunction of the nervous system or the respiratory muscles:**

   a) **Impaired activity of the central nervous system respiratory centers:** Drug overdose (opioids or sedatives), brainstem damage, central sleep apnea, myxedema coma.

   b) **Impaired nervous or neuromuscular conduction:** Cervical or thoracic spinal cord damage, phrenic nerve damage, Guillain-Barré syndrome, amyotrophic lateral sclerosis, muscle relaxants, myasthenic crisis, tetanus, botulism.

   c) **Impaired strength of respiratory muscles:** Respiratory muscle overload (increased work of breathing), electrolyte disturbances (low potassium, magnesium, or phosphate levels), acidosis, malnutrition, hypoxemia, shock, muscle diseases.

3) **Increased physiologic dead space ventilation:** Physiologic dead space (anatomic dead space and alveolar dead space) is the volume of inhaled gas that does not take part in gas exchange. It may increase as a consequence of:

   a) Increase in the volume of gas remaining in the conducting airways (anatomic dead space).

   b) Increased alveolar dead space, which occurs when alveolar pressure is greater than the perfusion pressure to alveolar units due to diminished perfusion to alveoli, overdistension (increased pressure) of compliant alveoli, or both.

4) **Increased production of carbon dioxide**: Any condition that increases metabolic demand will result in an increase in both oxygen consumption and carbon dioxide production. Unless there is an increase in minute ventilation, there will be a resultant hypercapnia.

3. Consequences of hypercapnia: Hypercapnia will stimulate ventilation via both central and peripheral chemoreceptors. However, in the absence of an appropriate increase in ventilation, hypercapnia will result in other significant effects:

1) **Respiratory acidosis**.

2) **Headache and altered mental status**: Confusion, pathologic somnolence, and hypercapnic coma, associated with cerebral vasodilation and increased intracranial pressure.

3) **Hypoxic respiratory drive**: Chronic respiratory failure with hypercapnia leads to a decreased sensitivity of the respiratory centers in the medulla and pons to increased $PaCO_2$. In such cases, the main impulses stimulating the respiratory centers originate from PaO_2 chemoreceptors located mainly in the carotid bodies and the aortic arch. In such patients, too aggressive oxygen therapy and too high PaO_2 inhibit the respiratory centers and cause hypoventilation, resulting in the worsening of hypercapnic respiratory failure, and thus leading to coma.

16.1. Acute Respiratory Failure

→ DEFINITION, ETIOLOGY, PATHOGENESIS

Acute respiratory failure develops suddenly (usually over hours or days to a few weeks) and is potentially reversible. This definition pertains to the timing of development rather than its cause, which may be due to any of the processes discussed in the chapter on respiratory failure.

Anatomical approach to acute hypoxemia:

1) **Diffuse lung parenchymal disease**:

   a) **Pulmonary edema** caused by increased hydrostatic pressure in the pulmonary vessels (left ventricular failure, fluid overload), increased permeability of the alveolar-capillary barrier (acute respiratory distress syndrome [ARDS]), drowning, lung reperfusion [after lung transplant or arterial embolectomy]); of unclear or complex mechanism (decompression [eg, pneumothorax], postobstructive [following the elimination of the cause of atelectasis], neurogenic, following stroke, after tocolytic therapy).

   b) **Alveolar bleeding**: Vasculitis and connective tissue diseases (including anti-glomerular basement membrane disease [formerly known as Goodpasture syndrome]), disorders of hemostasis (particularly disseminated intravascular coagulation).

2) **Focal lung parenchymal disease**: Severe pneumonia, atelectasis (resulting from airway obstruction by a foreign body, tumor, or exudate), pulmonary contusion.

3) **Pleural disease**: Pneumothorax (particularly tension or large pneumothorax), massive pleural effusions.

4) **Reduced pulmonary perfusion**: Pulmonary embolism, shock.

→ CLINICAL FEATURES AND NATURAL HISTORY

1. Symptoms: Dyspnea is a relatively uniform finding in acute respiratory failure. Depending on the cause, the following may also occur: cough, fever, chest pain, hemoptysis, and other symptoms.

2. Signs include signs of acute hypoxia (cyanosis, tachycardia, tachypnea) and acute hypercapnia (headache, altered mental status) as well as signs of the underlying condition. In more advanced states the use of accessory respiratory muscles and paradoxical movements of the chest wall and abdomen may be observed. Paradoxical abdominal indrawing on inspiration suggests that respiratory collapse is imminent. Untreated acute respiratory failure can be fatal.

→ **DIAGNOSIS**

1. Exclude other causes of dyspnea not related to respiratory failure (→Chapter 1.8).

2. Determine the cause of acute respiratory failure:

1) **Assess the respiratory system**: Inspect, palpate, and auscultate, looking for signs of upper airway obstruction, or parenchymal or pleural disease.

2) **Assess the cardiovascular system**: Assess for signs of cardiogenic pulmonary edema (→Chapter 3.8, Table 8-1), pulmonary embolism, or anaphylaxis.

3) **Exclude or confirm sepsis** (→Chapter 8.14), and if confirmed, determine its cause.

Diagnostic Tests

1. Pulse oximetry: Low SaO_2.

2. Blood tests:

1) **Arterial blood gas analysis**: Hypoxemia, hypercapnia (respiratory acidosis), and metabolic acidosis may be present in various combinations. Blood gas analysis provides measurement of blood pH, oxygen tension (PaO_2), carbon dioxide tension ($PaCO_2$), bicarbonate concentration, as well as the oxygen saturation of hemoglobin (SaO_2), allowing interpretation of oxygenation, ventilation, and acid-base balance. While an arterial blood gas (ABG) sample accurately reflects oxygenation and pulmonary gas exchange, central venous blood is more accurate at detecting the acid-base status and hypercapnia at the tissue level if severe hypoperfusion is present (ie, circulatory failure).◕ Peripheral venous blood gas (VBG) analysis is a simpler, less painful, and more convenient alternative to ABG. While it is likely sufficient to estimate arterial pH, VBG may not be sufficient to estimate arterial pCO_2, especially at highly abnormal values.◕ In the absence of circulatory failure or shock, venous pH, bicarbonate, and base excess have sufficient agreement with arterial values and, while the relationship between venous and arterial pCO_2 remains to a degree unpredictable, it may still be of value as a screening test for arterial hypercapnia or to monitor changes in respiratory function.◔◕

2) **Complete blood count (CBC) and biochemical tests**: Abnormalities may suggest specific etiologies (eg, leukocytosis, anemia, or eosinophilia; elevated serum brain natriuretic peptide or troponin, elevated D-dimers).

3. Microbiology: Because acute respiratory failure is frequently caused by infections, attempt to identify the etiologic agent (microbiological tests of respiratory secretions [eg, during flexible bronchoscopy], blood, or other clinically relevant material).

4. Imaging studies:

1) **Plain chest radiography**: Specific abnormalities may suggest the etiology (eg, various patterns of interstitial or air-space opacification in the lungs, volume loss, pneumothorax, pleural effusion).

2) **Chest ultrasonography or computed tomography (CT)** may further help in delineating the etiology of acute respiratory failure.

5. Electrocardiography (ECG) may reveal features of myocardial ischemia or pulmonary hypertension.

Diagnostic Criteria

Diagnostic criteria: →Chapter 13.16.1.1.

→ **TREATMENT**

1. Clearing the upper airway, as the situation requires: Noninstrumental (→Chapter 3.3); insertion of an oropharyngeal tube or other device; intubation; cricothyrotomy; tracheostomy (the procedure of choice in patients with massive laryngeal edema or prolonged mechanical ventilation).

2. Oxygen therapy with a high fraction of inspired oxygen (FiO_2 100%), as required. Consider the possibility of hypoxic respiratory drive.

3. High-flow nasal cannula compared with conventional oxygen therapy in the setting of acute hypoxemic respiratory failure decreases the need for noninvasive or invasive ventilation.⊘⊖ There is some evidence that it may be preferred to noninvasive ventilation maneuver in such situations.⊘⊖

4. Treatment of the underlying condition: Pharmacologic (eg, epinephrine for anaphylaxis, bronchodilators, antibiotics) or invasive (eg, decompression of pneumothorax, thoracentesis).

5. Mechanical ventilation:

1) Noninvasive positive pressure ventilation should be an early consideration for patients with an acute exacerbation of COPD⊘⬤ or cardiogenic pulmonary edema (in the absence of shock or an acute coronary syndrome).⊘⬤ It may also be considered in other situations of acute respiratory failure.

2) Invasive mechanical ventilation may be required.

6. Respiratory physiotherapy, including postural drainage.

7. Nutrition support to prevent malnutrition: →Chapter 13.16.2.

→ **COMPLICATIONS**

Consequences of hypoxemia and hypercapnia. More severe complications following intubation and mechanical ventilation: upper gastrointestinal tract bleeding due to stress ulcers or hemorrhagic gastritis (prevention: →Chapter 6.1.2.3.1), venous thromboembolism (prevention: →Chapter 3.19.2).

16.1.1. Acute Respiratory Distress Syndrome

→ **DEFINITION, ETIOLOGY, PATHOGENESIS**

1. According to the 2012 Berlin Definition, Acute respiratory distress syndrome (ARDS) is characterized by the following:

1) **Acuity of onset or new or worsening respiratory symptoms** within 1 week of a known clinical insult.

2) **Chest imaging abnormalities**: Bilateral opacities on plain radiographs or computed tomography (CT) scans not fully explained by effusions, lobar or lung collapse, or nodules.

3) **Origin of pulmonary edema**: Respiratory failure not fully explained by congestive heart failure or fluid overload. Patients with no risk factors for ARDS (→below) may require objective assessment (eg, echocardiography) to exclude hydrostatic edema.

4) **Hypoxemia**, as assessed in a ventilated patient by a ratio of PaO_2 to FiO_2 (in a healthy person breathing atmospheric air: PaO_2 = 97 mm Hg; FiO_2 = 0.21; PaO_2/FiO_2 = 470 mm Hg; at altitudes >1000 meters above the sea level use the formula: $PaO_2/FiO_2 \times$ atmospheric pressure in mm Hg/760). Based on this, ARDS is classified as one of the following:

   a) **Mild ARDS**: 200 mm Hg <PaO_2/FiO_2 ≤300 mm Hg with positive end--expiratory pressure (PEEP) or noninvasive continuous positive airway pressure (CPAP) ≥5 cm H_2O.

b) **Moderate ARDS**: 100 mm Hg <PaO_2/FiO_2 ≤200 mm Hg with PEEP ≥5 cm H_2O.

c) **Severe ARDS**: PaO_2/FiO_2 ≤100 mm Hg with PEEP ≥5 cm H_2O.

2. Causes (risk factors) of ARDS:

1) Direct lung injury: A direct insult to the lungs as a result of pneumonia, aspiration of gastric contents, pulmonary contusion, inhalation injury, near drowning.

2) Indirect lung injury: An indirect insult to the lungs as a result of sepsis, shock, acute pancreatitis, major burn injury, drug overdose, transfusion-related acute lung injury (TRALI), prolonged cardiopulmonary bypass. This list is incomplete and it is important to note that pneumonia, aspiration of gastric contents, and sepsis account for >85% of ARDS cases.

3. Pathogenesis of ARDS: An uncontrolled inflammatory process causing damage to the alveolar-capillary membrane with transfer of protein-rich fluid and cells from the vessels to the alveoli, destruction and impaired production of surfactant, collapse and edema of the alveoli (exudative phase); destruction of the alveolar septa by inflammatory cell infiltration, impaired gas exchange, reduced lung compliance, and eventually respiratory failure (with dominant hypoxemia) and (acute) pulmonary hypertension. Reparative processes begin within 2 to 3 weeks (proliferative phase) and regeneration of damaged cells or production of collagen by fibroblasts is possible at later stages (fibrotic phase).

→ DIAGNOSIS

→Chapter 13.16.1.

Diagnostic Criteria

→Definition, Etiology, Pathogenesis, above.

→ TREATMENT

→Chapter 13.16.1.

The initial treatment of patients with ARDS is the same as for other causes of acute respiratory failure. Two elements fundamental to the management of ARDS are treatment of the underlying disorder and supportive care, the mainstay of which is mechanical ventilation. Noninvasive ventilation may be considered in mild ARDS; with worsening severity, invasive ventilation is more appropriate.

Invasive Mechanical Ventilation in ARDS

Ventilatory management for ARDS focuses on preventing ventilator-induced lung injury with lung-protective ventilation and conservative fluid therapy to prevent excess lung water formation.

A lung-protective ventilation strategy that targets tidal volumes in the range of 4 to 8 mL/kg of predicted body weight is associated with higher survival rates than traditional tidal volumes in the range of 10 to 12 mL/kg.◐◖

Deceasing ventilator driving pressure may also prevent ventilator-induced lung injury. Driving pressure can be calculated as plateau pressure minus PEEP. Plateau pressure is measured as the pressure applied to small airways and alveoli during an inspiratory pause on the mechanical ventilator. During the inspiratory pause, gas flow (and therefore resistance) is zero; thus, the plateau pressure reflects respiratory system compliance for the tidal volume delivered. With progression of ARDS, maintaining stable (even low) tidal volume when confronted with decreasing compliance requires increases in driving pressure. Consequently, increased mechanical stress is applied to the still available functional lung. It is recommended that tidal volume be decreased in order to maintain a stable driving pressure. This single variable

Table 16-1. Strategies of PEEP/FiO$_2$ adjustment in patients with acute respiratory distress syndrome

Lower PEEP strategy

FiO$_2$	0.3-0.4	0.4-0.5	0.5-0.6	0.6-0.7
PEEP (cm H$_2$O)	5	5-8	8-10	8-10
FiO$_2$	0.7-0.8	0.8-0.9	0.9-1.0	1.0
PEEP (cm H$_2$O)	10-14	14	14-18	18-24

Higher PEEP strategy

FiO$_2$	0.3-0.4	0.4-0.5	0.5	0.5-0.8
PEEP (cm H$_2$O)	5-14	14-16	16-18	18-20
FiO$_2$	0.8-1.0	1.0		
PEEP (cm H$_2$O)	22	24		

Adapted from: ARDS Clinical Network. Mechanical ventilation protocol summary of low tidal volume used in the ALVEOLI study. http://www.ardsnet.org/files/ventilator_protocol_2008-07.pdf.

FiO$_2$, fraction of oxygen in the inspired air; PEEP, positive end-expiratory pressure.

is more strongly associated with survival than low tidal volume ventilation or higher PEEP.⊖

The relative benefit of a high PEEP versus a low PEEP strategy is not altogether clear; a higher PEEP strategy does not appear to be harmful and may improve survival in patients with moderate to severe ARDS⊘⊖ (→Table 16-1).

Esophageal pressure monitoring has long been considered for identifying an ideal PEEP strategy; however, titrating PEEP according to the esophageal pressure has yet to provide a clear benefit.⊗⊖ Prone ventilation improves ventilation-perfusion matching and keeps alveolar units open. It may reduce mortality in severe ARDS compared with conventional ventilation using relatively low PEEP.⊖ This strategy has not been tested against ventilation using higher PEEP strategies. Center-expertise in proning is another important consideration to avoid adverse complications, such as tube dislodgement or pressure ulceration. In our setting, in patients who will likely tolerate proning and in whom other treatments (PEEP, protected mode) have been optimized but the PaO$_2$/FiO$_2$ ratio remains <150 to 200 mm Hg, we use prone ventilation. The likelihood of benefit increases with the severity of hypoxia, relatively early application, and with duration of daily proning (likely >16 hours).⊘⊖

The use of extracorporeal membrane oxygenation (ECMO) requires consideration of not only overall incomplete evidence of its efficacy but also considerations of local expertise, resource use, and implication of transfer. In our setting, we consider the use of ECMO (and transfer) in patients with very severe refractory hypoxia, potentially reversible acute respiratory failure, and otherwise having a realistic chance for functional recovery.

Other Treatment Strategies

1. Volume status: Although it is important to distinguish ARDS from volume overload or heart failure, these entities may coexist in a significant number of patients. Consequently, a conservative fluid management strategy may improve lung function and shorten the duration of mechanical ventilation without compromising non-pulmonary organ function.⊘⊖ This may be best accomplished by avoiding fluid administration after reversal of shock.

2. Neuromuscular blockade: Although continuous neuromuscular blockade for severe ARDS has been common practice (the ACURASYS trial), early routine administration of such treatment in addition to a high PEEP strategy has not improved mortality in the most recent and largest trial and probably should be used more selectively.⊖

3. Glucocorticoids: Data on the use of glucocorticoids are imprecise and obtained in different populations; however, early (within 7 days) use of smaller doses of methylprednisolone (1 mg/kg) or higher doses (2 mg/kg) when started between 7 and 14 days is suggested.⊘⊖ Glucocorticoids should not be stopped abruptly but slowly tapered down over the course of 6 to 14 days.

Rescue Therapies in ARDS

In the most severe cases of ARDS with hypoxemia and/or hypercapnia refractory to mechanical ventilation, extracorporeal gas exchange techniques are sometimes used in experienced centers (best results are seen in influenza--associated severe ARDS in relatively young patients).

Other rescue therapies remain unproven. In particular, high-frequency oscillatory ventilation has been used as a rescue therapy; however, when used early, it is not superior to low-tidal volume ventilation and may cause harm.⊗⊖ The use of nitric oxide is also controversial, with most recent reviews and practice guidelines suggesting that it should not be used.⊗○

16.2. Chronic Respiratory Failure

→ DEFINITION, ETIOLOGY, PATHOGENESIS

Chronic respiratory failure develops progressively and is usually punctuated by acute exacerbations that may or may not be fully reversible.

Etiology:

1) Bronchial obstruction: Chronic obstructive pulmonary disease (COPD), bronchiectasis, cystic fibrosis, rarely asthma.

2) Chronic interstitial lung diseases, including idiopathic pulmonary fibrosis, sarcoidosis, pneumoconioses, postinfectious pulmonary fibrosis (eg, posttuberculosis or other pneumonias).

3) Primary and metastatic tumors of the respiratory system.

4) Chest deformities (eg, severe kyphoscoliosis).

5) Extreme obesity.

6) Neuromuscular diseases: Multiple sclerosis, Parkinson disease, chronic polyneuropathies, persistent posttraumatic damage of the phrenic nerves or the cervical or thoracic spinal cord, amyotrophic lateral sclerosis, chronic myopathies (muscular dystrophies).

7) Cardiovascular diseases: Chronic pulmonary embolism, cyanotic congenital heart disease, chronic congestive heart failure.

→ CLINICAL FEATURES

1. Symptoms:

1) Chronic progressive dyspnea on exertion or at rest with reduced exercise tolerance.

2) Somnolence and headache (in patients with hypercapnia).

3) Other symptoms of underlying conditions (eg, productive cough in COPD).

2. Signs:

1) Signs of hypoxemia (tachypnea, tachycardia, cyanosis, clubbing of digits, symptoms of right ventricular failure (→Chapter 3.8.2).

2) Signs of increased accessory respiratory muscle use—muscle hypertrophy, increased antero-posterior diameter of the chest and flattening of the diaphragms on chest radiograph (in COPD).

3) Vasodilatation due to hypercapnia—conjunctival injection and skin erythema.

4) Signs of the underlying condition.

▶ DIAGNOSIS

Diagnosis is based on the chronicity of signs, symptoms, and abnormalities on specific tests of pulmonary function (→Chapter 13.16). To determine the cause and severity, perform chest radiography, spirometry, arterial blood gas analysis, and other diagnostic tests as required, depending on the suspected underlying condition. To assess the consequences of chronic respiratory failure, measure complete blood count (look for polycythemia) and perform electrocardiography (ECG) and echocardiography (look for signs of pulmonary hypertension [→Chapter 13.15] and right ventricular failure [→Chapter 3.8.2]).

For those with chronic hypercapnic respiratory failure that is bordering on the need for chronic mechanical ventilation, a sleep study may be helpful. Hypoventilation worsens during sleep and nocturnal noninvasive ventilation may be indicated while avoiding complete ventilator dependency.

Differential Diagnosis

In differential diagnosis, consider other causes of chronic dyspnea (→Chapter 1.8).

▶ TREATMENT

1. Treatment of the underlying disease.

2. Oxygen therapy during acute exacerbations (in hospital) or long-term oxygen therapy (at home).

3. Rehabilitation: Respiratory physiotherapy (including postural drainage), general rehabilitation (eg, physical therapy, exercise), and education of the patient and family/caregivers are mainstays of treatment.

4. Nutrition support to prevent malnutrition is important. However, the role for a high fat/low carbohydrate diet in minimizing the production of CO_2 remains controversial.

5. Long-term mechanical ventilation in selected patients (mostly with neuromuscular diseases and COPD), at home (ideally with intermittent noninvasive ventilation) or in a clinical setting. Patients may initially require mechanical ventilation only while sleeping but over time progress to full-time chronic ventilation.

Note: It is often difficult to distinguish an acute exacerbation from a chronic progression to end-stage disease. In the latter situation, invasive treatments and mechanical ventilation have limited benefit and may cause unnecessary suffering. Ideally, a decision to undertake (or not) invasive support is discussed well in advance of end-stage disease, with both the patient and his or her caregivers, and a consultative body of physicians.

▶ COMPLICATIONS

1. Pulmonary hypertension. Treatment: Oxygen therapy.

2. Right ventricular heart failure (→Chapter 3.8.2). Treatment: Oxygen therapy, diuretic therapy (potassium and magnesium supplementation, as needed).

3. Secondary polycythemia and hyperviscosity: Treatment: Oxygen therapy.

4. Malnutrition and cachexia.

17. Subcutaneous Emphysema

Subcutaneous emphysema refers to the presence of air in the subcutaneous tissue. Most frequently it develops as a result of air leakage from a pneumothorax or pneumomediastinum into the subcutaneous tissue of the neck (less commonly the chest, head, or abdomen). On rare occasions it is caused by gastrointestinal (GI) perforation below the navel.

Signs and symptoms: Discomfort in the neck and chest, crackles on compression of the neck and supraclavicular region, features of pneumothorax or pneumomediastinum.

Chest radiographs reveal air in the subcutaneous tissue of the neck and chest (→Figure 17-1). This is accompanied by radiologic features of pneumothorax, pneumomediastinum, or perforation of the GI tract (air under a hemidiaphragm seen on plain abdominal radiographs). Differential diagnosis includes CO_2 insufflation for laparoscopic surgery.

In patients with subcutaneous emphysema associated with pneumomediastinum and not caused by esophageal, tracheal, or bronchial perforation, medical management (monitoring) is sufficient. Patients should be closely observed because the progression of subcutaneous emphysema towards the neck tissue can lead to upper airway obstruction. Subcutaneous emphysema coexisting with a pneumothorax

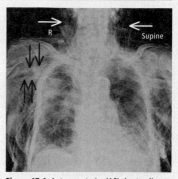

Figure 17-1. Anteroposterior (AP) chest radiography of a patient with a right-sided pneumothorax (with chest drain insertion) complicated by extensive subcutaneous emphysema. A large amount of air spreads into the subcutaneous tissue around the neck (white arrows) and pectoralis major muscles (black arrows).

requires the use of chest drainage to release the pneumothorax. Subcutaneous emphysema associated with the GI tract or airway perforation is an indication for urgent surgical intervention.

18. Tuberculosis and Other Mycobacterial Infections

This chapter is divided into subchapters to provide information on 3 related but discreet topics in tuberculosis (TB). A brief description of the topics is summarized below:

1) **Tuberculosis: Active Disease** refers to an active disease state that has resulted from infection with *Mycobacterium tuberculosis*. An individual

with active disease may present with systemic and/or respiratory symptoms. The disease can be pulmonary or extrapulmonary. If pulmonary disease is present, infection can be spread to others via airborne droplet nuclei. Since the disease is often present for several weeks or months before the onset of telltale signs or symptoms, transmission to susceptible individuals may occur before the illness is apparent. The gold standard for diagnosis of active TB disease is microbiological culture testing of sputum and other specimens yielded from affected sites. Treatment with combination drug therapy is usually highly successful in achieving cure.

2) **Tuberculosis: Latent Tuberculosis Infection** refers to a state of inactive infection due to *M tuberculosis* without the presence of the disease. An individual with latent TB infection is asymptomatic and cannot transmit infection to others. Individuals who become infected are at risk of progressing to active disease. About 5% of newly infected hosts (often those with immune dysfunction) are unable to contain the infection and therefore proceed to early disease progression within the first 18 to 24 months (**primary TB**). The rest of the infected hosts are classified as being in a state of latent TB infection. The majority of persons with latent TB infection will remain disease-free for life, but ~5% of all infected hosts will develop late disease progression with the development of active TB disease (**postprimary or reactivation TB**) sometime after 18 to 24 months of acquiring infection. Detection of latent TB infection occurs through targeted screening of high-risk groups using the TB skin test and/or the interferon γ release assay blood test. Treatment with preventative drug therapy is successful in reducing the risk of reactivation. The decision to treat latent TB infection is individualized and must balance the risk of reactivation with the risk of potential drug toxicities.

3) **Nontuberculous Mycobacteria (NTM) Diseases** refer to conditions related to mycobacterium other than the *M tuberculosis* complex, which are of unknown or lesser pathogenicity. NTM can exist as a contaminant or colonizer, or can cause disease. There are some shared features between the clinical presentation of active *M tuberculosis* disease and NTM disease. Unlike active TB, NTM organisms cannot be transmitted from human to human. The most common organ of involvement is the lung, although extrapulmonary sites can also be affected, especially in immune-deficient states. Detection is through microbiological culture, but clinical and radiographic assessments are necessary to differentiate between the states of colonization and disease. Combination drug therapy is used on selective individuals who manifest symptomatic disease of an advanced or progressive nature. The clinical response to therapy is often suboptimal.

18.1. Nontuberculous Mycobacterium Diseases

→ **DEFINITION, ETIOLOGY**

Mycobacterioses are caused by atypical mycobacteria: nontuberculous mycobacteria (NTM) and mycobacteria other than tuberculosis (MOTT). NTM species include *Mycobacterium avium* complex (MAC) (this comprises *Mycobacterium avium* and *Mycobacterium intracellulare*), *Mycobacterium fortuitum* complex, *Mycobacterium xenopi*, and *Mycobacterium kansasii*. Some species are associated with clinical disease, while others are rarely associated with disease. These strains are widely present in the environment, particularly in soil and water reservoirs. There is no evidence to suggest person-to-person transmission of NTM except for an isolated signal for a direct transmission of *Mycobacterium abscessus* between patients with cystic fibrosis in studies showing genetically distinct isolates in individuals attending shared clinics.○ Geologic factors account for regional variability in incidence and speciation. At-risk groups include HIV-positive individuals, patients treated with anti–tumor necrosis factor α agents, individuals with a history of tuberculosis (TB), and patients with pneumoconiosis, cystic fibrosis, bronchiectasis, chronic obstructive pulmonary disease, or alcohol dependence. Clinical syndromes can also occur in patients with no preexisting lung disease or apparent indicators of immune dysfunction. NTM infection is not transmitted between humans and therefore is not a disease that requires reporting to public health authorities. Although NTM disease is not caused by infection with *M tuberculosis* complex, it is often considered in conjunction with TB since both diseases (1) overlap with respect to several clinical presenting features and therapeutic agents; (2) have specimens processed at a common mycobacteriology laboratory with expertise in acid-fast bacillus (AFB) smear, culture, drug-sensitivity testing, and speciation; (3) are often treated in a TB clinic setting by a health-care team with expertise in mycobacteriosis.

→ CLINICAL FEATURES

The clinical features are similar to TB and typically include chronic, productive cough, sputum production (with or without hemoptysis), asthenia, and less frequently fever and sweating. The NTM diseases also yield specimens with similar laboratory characteristics to TB, including positive AFB stain and necrotizing granuloma formation. Nucleic acid amplification tests are a rapid method of differentiation between the two conditions; however, the gold standard for identification is culture.

The lesions are predominantly located in the lungs, although other sites include lymph nodes, skin, and bone/joint. In some cases, multiple organs are involved. In patients who are not significantly immunocompromised, pulmonary NTM may be associated with 2 patterns. One pattern is of multiple small nodules, bronchiectasis, and tree-in-bud densities (mainly in the right middle lobe or lingula) visible on high-resolution computed tomography (HRCT) of the chest, often found in middle-aged women without preexisting lung disease. The second pattern with cavitation in the upper lobes often occurs in the setting of preexisting lung disease such as chronic obstructive pulmonary disease, bronchiectasis, cystic fibrosis, and other abnormalities in pulmonary structure and mucus clearance. Patients with a single nodule or few nodules have no symptoms.

→ DIAGNOSIS

NTM organisms can be isolated from pulmonary specimens due to contamination, colonization, or disease. Clinical, radiographic, and microbiologic criteria are all equally important and all 3 must be met in order to make a diagnosis of NTM disease.

1. Clinical criteria:

1) Pulmonary symptoms (cough, sputum, hemoptysis, chest pain, dyspnea) and/or systemic symptoms (fever, weight loss, fatigue), **and**

2) Exclusion of other potential causes (such as *M tuberculosis* complex, other respiratory infections, sarcoidosis, malignancy).

3) Progressive symptoms, which increase the likelihood of an NTM disease.

2. Radiology:

1) Chest radiograph: Nodular or cavitary opacities, **or**

2) Computed tomography (CT) of the chest: Bronchiectasis with multiple small nodules or lung cavitation, **or** airspace disease (consolidation with ground--glass opacification).

3. Microbiological criteria:

1) Positive culture result from at least 2 sputum samples collected on separate occasions, **or**

2) Positive culture result from at least 1 bronchial wash or lavage, **or**

3) Transbronchial or other lung biopsy with mycobacterial histopathologic features (granulomatous inflammation or AFB) and positive culture of NTM,

or biopsy showing mycobacterial histopathologic features (granulomatous inflammation or AFB) and 1 or more sputum or bronchial washings that are culture-positive for NTM.

→ TREATMENT

Drug therapy for NTM lung diseases is not recommended for all patients. The decision to treat should be based on an individual assessment of the risks and benefits of therapy. Progression of clinical symptoms with compatible radiographic findings increases the likelihood of disease and may be an indication for a stronger recommendation for drug therapy. The long treatment period required to achieve a clinical effect is often poorly tolerated due to adverse effects and/or toxicities. Clinical outcomes for pulmonary NTM are suboptimal compared with treatment outcomes for *M tuberculosis* complex. Consultation with an expert in NTM disease is suggested, especially in complex cases where there is uncertainty about diagnosis of the disease, treatment indications, or management of drug therapy.

General principles of treatment:

1) **Asymptomatic patients** with a single or small number of randomly distributed incidental lung nodules due to NTM generally should not be treated unless there is significant radiographic progression with the development of symptoms.⊗○

2) **Combination therapy** with 3 or more drugs is recommended for the treatment of NTM disease. Macrolides are an important component included in drug regimens for many of the common NTM species. Patients with repeated isolation of NTM should not receive macrolide monotherapy for treatment of bacterial infections or for treatment of NTM, as this may foster resistance to this class of drugs, thereby limiting efficacy of future NTM treatment.⊗○

3) **Drug choices** are generally species-specific (→Table 18-1). Evidence to support the recommended treatment regimens to target the various NTM species is weak to moderate. Data to correlate results from drug-susceptibility testing with clinical response to treatment is lacking, except for identification of macrolide resistance in MAC and rifampin (INN rifampicin) resistance in *M kansasii*. For *M abscessus*, susceptibility testing against macrolides and a wider panel of antibiotics may be used as a guide for treatment.⊘○ Nebulized amikacin may be considered as an alternative to a parenteral aminoglycoside for longer-term therapy for *M avium*, *M xenopi*, and *M abscessus*.⊘○

4) The **duration of treatment** is ≥12 months from the first negative culture result; and when mycobacteriosis is diagnosed based on cultures of a material other than sputum, up to 18 months. Isolated pulmonary lesions and involved lymph nodes may be treated by surgical resection.

5) **Monitoring** while on drug therapy is important to assess clinical response, adverse effects, and drug toxicities. Medication schedules and regimens require frequent modifications if treatment is poorly tolerated or ineffective. Practices regarding regular monitoring for specific adverse reactions, such as liver toxicity (rifampin), optic neuritis (ethambutol), or nerve VIII and renal injury (aminoglycosides), are variable. Most clinicians recommend at least monthly monitoring of parameters appropriate to drug selection, which may include transaminases, visual assessment with an ophthalmologist or optometrist, audiograms, and/or creatinine levels.

18.2. Tuberculosis: Active Disease

→ DEFINITION, ETIOLOGY, PATHOGENESIS

Tuberculosis (TB) is an infectious disease caused by acid-fast bacilli belonging to the *Mycobacterium tuberculosis* complex, which includes *Mycobacterium tuberculosis*, *Mycobacterium bovis*, and *Mycobacterium africanum*. The pathogenesis of infection is as follows: mycobacteria are inhaled as droplet nuclei, which are phagocytized by macrophages, where intracellular multiplication of the bacilli occurs. Subsequently, destruction of the macrophages takes place and new cells become infected. Over the next 3 to 8 weeks the bacilli may migrate to both pulmonary and extrapulmonary sites via lymphatic and/or hematogenous channels. At the same time the patient develops a specific immune response mediated by CD4$^+$ Th1 cells, which activates further macrophages (mediated by interferon [IFN] γ and other mechanisms). This results in the formation of tuberculoid granulomas consisting of epithelioid and giant cells palisading around a central area of caseous necrosis at the sites of infection. Individuals are usually asymptomatic at this time but may demonstrate infection with a positive TB skin test (tuberculin skin test) (TST) and/or interferon γ release assay (IGRA) blood test. Lesions may heal spontaneously through fibrosis.

The majority of infected individuals will remain disease-free and in a state of latent tuberculosis infection (LTBI) for their lifetime. Approximately 5% of newly infected hosts (often those with immune dysfunction) are unable to contain the infection and therefore proceed to early disease progression within the first 18 to 24 months (**primary TB**, or **early disease progression**). Young children and individuals with impaired cell-mediated immunity are most at risk. Disseminated and central nervous system (CNS) TB can occur in infants as early as a few months after the onset of infection. Primary TB may present with complicated lymphadenopathy, pleural disease, or caseating pneumonia. Approximately 5% of individuals with LTBI will develop **postprimary or reactivation TB**, which occurs 18 to 24 months or more after having acquired the infection. The source for this **late disease progression** is the repository of infected macrophages, which are capable of harboring viable mycobacteria across a lifetime. Pulmonary upper lobe fibrocavitary disease is the most common presentation of reactivation TB, although atypical pulmonary findings or extrapulmonary disease are present in up to 30% of cases.

High-risk groups: The global burden of TB can be reduced by identifying high-risk groups to be targeted for screening, preventative therapy, and early disease detection/treatment. Reduction in immune function is the proposed mechanism for the following risk factors: HIV-positive, transplantation, end-stage renal disease, tumor necrosis factor α inhibitor therapy, diabetes mellitus, immunosuppressive drugs (≥15 mg prednisone/d), body mass index (≤20 kg/m^2), young age (<4 years). Other clinical risk factors include silicosis, malignancy (especially head and neck and hematologic), recent TB infection (≤2 years), fibronodular disease or granuloma (chest radiographs), heavy alcohol consumption (≥3 drinks/d), smoking (≥1 pack/d) (→Table 18-2). Exposure categories relevant for risk assessment include contact with an index case of active TB and origin from a country with a high disease incidence. Demographic and socioeconomic determinants have an influence on the impact of the above risk factors for any given population.

> **CLINICAL FEATURES AND NATURAL HISTORY**

Approximately 75% of active TB cases involve only the lungs. Extrapulmonary cases usually occur in a single remote site or may coexist with disease in the lungs. Multiple sites of involvement or dissemination often indicate a defect in host immunity. Clinical manifestations are highly varied. **General signs and symptoms** irrespective of the location of the lesions include fever, loss of appetite, weight loss, night sweats, and malaise. **Blood tests** are often normal but may reveal leukopenia or leukocytosis, anemia, elevated erythrocyte sedimentation rate, and very occasionally hyponatremia or hypercalcemia.

Pulmonary Tuberculosis

1. Symptoms: Chronic cough (initially nonproductive, subsequently associated with production of mucous or purulent sputum) and in some cases hemoptysis. Dyspnea develops in patients with advanced disease (such as caseating pneumonia or miliary TB), which may lead to respiratory insufficiency.

Table 18-1. Recommended treatment of nontuberculous mycobacterial disease[a]

Organism	Drugs	Duration
Mycobacterium avium complex lung disease (macrolide susceptible)	– Daily: clarithromycin 500 mg bid or azithromycin 250 mg; EMB 15 mg/kg (may use 25 mg/kg for initial 2 months); RMP (450-600 mg) or RBT (150-300 mg) ± aminoglycosides (SM or amikacin) intermittently (conditional recommendation, based on moderate evidence) – Thrice weekly[b] (may be considered for nonadvanced, nodular bronchiectatic pulmonary MAC): clarithromycin 500 mg bid or azithromycin 500 mg; EMB 25 mg/kg; RMP 600 mg (conditional recommendation, based on moderate evidence) – Clofazimine and FQNs may be useful (conditional recommendation, based on moderate evidence)	12 months after culture conversion to negative (conditional recommendation, based on moderate evidence)
MAC lymphadenitis (macrolide susceptible)	If antibacterial therapy is being considered: daily or thrice weekly clarithromycin or azithromycin plus EMB ± RMP (conditional recommendation, based on very weak evidence)	3-9 months (conditional recommendation, based on very weak evidence)
M xenopi lung disease	– Azithromycin or clarithromycin plus RMP plus EMB – Consider, in addition, moxifloxacin (or other FQNs), INH, SM, amikacin (conditional recommendation, based on very weak evidence)	12 months after culture-negative (conditional recommendation, based on very weak evidence)
M abscessus complex lung disease	Clarithromycin or azithromycin + amikacin, cefoxitin or imipenem (± tigecycline, linezolid, clofazimine) (conditional recommendation, based on moderate evidence)	2-6 months of combination IV and PO therapy (conditional recommendation, based on weak evidence)
M kansasii lung disease	– Daily RMP, EMB, INH – Consider clarithromycin or azithromycin, moxifloxacin, sulfamethoxazole, and aminoglycosides (strong recommendation, based on moderate evidence)	12 months after culture-negative (conditional recommendation, based on weak evidence)
M fortuitum lung disease	Based on in-vitro sensitivity testing: azithromycin or clarithromycin and RMP or EMB (± doxycycline, amikacin, imipenem, FQNs, sulfonamides, cefoxitin) (conditional recommendation, based on very weak evidence)	12 months after culture-negative for lung disease (conditional recommendation, based on very weak evidence)
M fortuitum skin/soft tissue	Based on in-vitro sensitivity testing: azithromycin or clarithromycin and RMP or EMB (± doxycycline, amikacin, imipenem, FQNs, sulfonamides, cefoxitin) (conditional recommendation, based on very weak evidence)	4 months for skin/soft tissue (6 months for severe disease) (conditional recommendation, based on weak evidence)

Organism	Drugs	Duration
M marinum skin/soft tissue	Clarithromycin, EMB ± RMP (conditional recommendation, based on weak evidence)	3-6 months (consider longer if deep structures involved) (conditional recommendation, based on weak evidence)
Disseminated MAC in HIV--infected patients Treatment	Clarithromycin 500 mg PO daily + EMB 15 mg/kg PO daily ± RBT 300 mg PO daily[c] (strong recommendation, based on very strong evidence)	Lifelong or until control of HIV viremia with rise of CD4 to $>100 \times 10^6$/L for at least 6 months and 12 months after culture-negative (strong recommendation, based on strong evidence)
Disseminated MAC in HIV--infected patients Prophylaxis Patients with CD4 $<50 \times 10^6$/L	Azithromycin 1200 mg weekly or RBT 300 mg a day or Clarithromycin 500 mg bid (strong recommendation, based on very strong evidence)	Lifelong or until control of HIV viremia with rise of CD4 to $>100 \times 10^6$/L for ≥6 months and 12 months after culture-negative (strong recommendation, based on strong evidence)

Suggested regimens for initial therapy of NTM disease should be modified, if needed, depending upon clinical circumstances such as drug intolerance, the presence of macrolide-resistant MAC, and lack of efficacy.

[a] More detailed recommendations and treatment guidance regarding other NTM species may be found elsewhere.

[b] Although directly observed therapy is recommended for intermittent therapy of TB, this is not so in NTM disease, because there is no public health consideration of contagion. Intermittent therapy for pulmonary NTM has been suggested to reduce toxic effects and sometimes costs of therapy and has been shown to be effective in many cases.

[c] Doses may need to be adjusted according to interactions with concurrent antiretroviral therapy.

Source: ©All Rights Reserved. Canadian Tuberculosis Standards, 7th Edition. The Public Health Agency of Canada, The Lung Association, and the Canadian Thoracic Society, 2014. Adapted and reproduced with permission from the Minister of Health, 2016.

EMB; ethambutol; FQNs, fluoroquinolones; HIV, human immunodeficiency virus; INH, isoniazid; IV, intravenous; MAC, *Mycobacterium avium* complex; NTM, nontuberculous mycobacterium; PO, oral; RBT, rifabutin; RMP, rifampin (INN rifampicin); SM, streptomycin.

2. Signs: The physical examination in pulmonary TB is usually normal except for patients with advanced disease. Examination should include looking for indicators of extrapulmonary involvement, such as lymphadenopathy, pleural effusion, or ascites.

3. Selected types of pulmonary TB:

1) **Miliary TB** is caused by hematogenous dissemination of mycobacteria. The disease has a severe clinical course with high-grade fever and dyspnea. Small nodules reminiscent of millet seeds are visible on chest radiographs (although radiographs may be normal in the initial 2-3 days of dissemination). Patients often develop hepatomegaly, splenomegaly, as well as various abnormalities in bone marrow, the ocular fundus, and CNS.

2) **Caseating pneumonia**: The dominant clinical features are those of toxemia with hectic high-grade fever, severe dyspnea, and frequent occurrence of hemoptysis. Sputum smears reveal very high mycobacteria counts if the contents of the cavities discharge into airways, which directly communicate with outside air during coughing.

Table 18-2. Risk factors for the development of active TB among people with a positive tuberculin skin test (presumed infected with *Mycobacterium tuberculosis*)

Risk factor	Estimated risk for TB relative to people with no known risk factors	Reference number
High risk		
AIDS	110-170	5
HIV infection	50-110	6, 7
Transplantation (related to immune-suppressant therapy)	20-74	8-12
Silicosis	30	13, 14
Chronic renal failure requiring hemodialysis	7-50	15-18, 46, 47
Carcinoma of head and neck	11.6	19
Recent TB infection (2 years)	15	20, 21
Abnormal chest radiographs: fibronodular disease	6-19	22-24
Moderate risk		
Tumor necrosis factor α inhibitors	1.5-5.8	25, 26, 43
Diabetes mellitus (all types)	2-3.6	27-29
Treatment with glucocorticoids (>15 mg/d prednisone)	4.9	30
Young age when infected (0-4 years)	2.2-5	31
Slightly increased risk		
Heavy alcohol consumption (>3 drinks/d)	3-4	32, 33
Underweight (<90% ideal body weight; for most people, this is a body mass index <20)	2-3	34
Cigarette smoker (1 pack/d)	1.8-3.5	35-38
Abnormal chest radiographs: granuloma	2	24, 39
Low risk		
Person with positive TST, no known risk factors, normal chest radiographs ("low-risk reactor")	1	40
Very low risk		
Person with positive 2-step TST (booster), no other known risk factors, and normal chest radiographs	0.5	Extrapolated from 40 and 1

Source: ©All Rights Reserved. Canadian Tuberculosis Standards, 7th Edition. The Public Health Agency of Canada, The Lung Association, and the Canadian Thoracic Society, 2014. Adapted and reproduced with permission from the Minister of Health, 2016.

AIDS, acquired immunodeficiency syndrome; HIV, human immunodeficiency virus; TB, tuberculosis; TST, tuberculin skin test.

Extrapulmonary Tuberculosis

1. Pleural TB typically presents with fever, nonproductive cough, dyspnea, and pleuritic pain. It is most commonly seen as a feature of primary TB but can also be a feature of TB reactivation, especially in the elderly. Pleural effusion is usually unilateral and is characterized by high cell counts (briefly showing neutrophilic predominance in the early stages but usually lymphocytic by the time fluid sampling takes place) as well as high protein and adenosine deaminase levels. Since the sensitivity of pleural fluid cultures is very low in primary TB and only ~30% in reactivation TB, open or closed pleural biopsy is often required for diagnosis.

2. Peripheral TB lymphadenitis affects predominantly children and young adults. Lymph nodes commonly involved include cervical (anterior and posterior) and supraclavicular lymph nodes, although disease in the axillary and inguinal sites may occur. Initially, the lymph nodes are enlarged, firm, and painless, with a normal appearance of the overlying skin. With time, gradual softening and formation of fistulas occurs. In ~50% of patients, TB lymphadenitis is accompanied by pulmonary lesions.

3. Genitourinary TB may present with sterile pyuria, gross hematuria, and mild symptoms of frequency, dysuria, and polyuria. Genitourinary TB in woman may manifest as pelvic pain and menstrual abnormalities and may lead to infertility. Men may develop prostatitis and epididymitis.

4. Bone and joint TB most frequently affects elderly patients. Tuberculous arthritis is usually a monoarthritis of the large joints presenting with arthralgia, edema, and limited mobility. Spinal or vertebral TB (Pott disease) presents with back pain and may lead to complications such as vertebral fractures and spinal cord compression.

5. CNS TB is a serious disease. Tuberculous meningitis most often occurs in children or in an immunocompromised host. The inflammatory process predominantly involves the base of the brain, damaging cranial nerves and leading to disturbances in cerebrospinal fluid circulation. Signs and symptoms include somnolence, headache, nausea, vomiting, and nuchal stiffness, often accompanied by paresis, pyramidal signs, and cerebellar signs. Altered mental status and seizures may also occur. Other types of CNS TB include tuberculoma, tuberculous abscess, cerebritis, and myelitis.

6. Abdominal TB can involve the intestines (often terminal ilium), peritoneum, and mesentery. Manifestations may include low-grade fever, weight loss, diarrhea, vomiting, abdominal pain, and ascites. Sometimes clinical features of appendicitis or intestinal obstruction are present.

7. Other types of extrapulmonary TB include ocular, pericardium, skin, breast, great vessels, and bone marrow TB. TB has the potential to cause disease in any organ.

→ DIAGNOSIS

Testing for active TB is indicated in anyone with clinical or radiographic indicators of TB. Every effort should be made to obtain a microbiological diagnosis. Acid-fast bacilli may be present on smear microscopy but could yield a false--positive result, especially in low-incidence regions with a high prevalence of nontuberculous mycobacterial infection/disease. Nucleic acid amplification test (NAAT) results are presumptive; thus, confirmation with culture is strongly recommended.◐ ● Sputum collection can be obtained by spontaneous expectoration or induction using a hypertonic NaCl solution. Bronchoscopy is used to obtain bronchial washings if the sputum sample cannot be collected, previous samples are smear-negative, or other diagnoses, such as lung cancer, are suspected. Gastric aspirate can be used for pediatric patients not capable of producing sputum. Consider microbiological (smear and culture) and histologic examination of biopsy specimens obtained from a suspicious lesion.

Criteria for TB diagnosis without a microbiological confirmation: Clinical judgment must be used when a suspect diagnosis of TB cannot be confirmed by a positive culture. The risks of treating TB on speculation include exposure to potential drug toxicities, conversion to drug-resistant TB without the benefit of drug-susceptibility test results, and neglect of an unrecognized disease that has masked as TB. If negative results for all microbiological tests are yielded despite a rigorous investigative process and there is no improvement after a trial of therapy with a broad-spectrum antibiotic, initiation of a trial for treatment for TB may be considered. This should be done with great caution after all feasible investigative options have been exhausted. The exception would be any patient for whom a delay in diagnosis could lead to a poor outcome, such as CNS or disseminated TB. Fluoroquinolones should be avoided during the investigative workup, as this class of drug is active against *M tuberculosis* and may result in a temporary clinical improvement and reduced sensitivity on smear and culture testing. Specimens from patients with extrapulmonary TB usually contain few mycobacteria, and the diagnosis is often based on histologic findings. A TB expert, if available, should be consulted if the diagnosis is uncertain.

HIV-positive patients: In HIV-infected individuals, the clinical presentation is often atypical, especially when the CD4 count is <250 μL. An increased incidence of extrapulmonary disease and a higher risk of dissemination are to be anticipated. In HIV-positive patients with early TB, the lesions are typical. However, in the advanced disease they may involve the lower and middle zones of the lungs. Cavities are rarely observed. Smear-negative disease is a common finding in HIV infection. The sensitivity of cultures increases with the number of evaluations performed, particularly if the examined material is induced sputum or lavage fluid obtained during bronchoscopy. In addition to sputum cultures, it may be necessary to perform blood cultures and biopsies of lymph nodes and bone marrow.

Diagnostic Tests

1. Chest radiography: In patients with primary TB, opacities are typically present in the middle and lower areas of the lungs and are accompanied by hilar and paratracheal lymphadenopathy. In patients with postprimary (reactivation) TB, opacities are found predominantly in the apical and posterior segments of the upper lobes and the upper segments of the lower lobes. In patients with advanced disease, cavities are often visible as radiolucent areas surrounded by an opaque rim. In some cases, infiltrates appear as solitary pulmonary nodules, which result from the encapsulation of caseous masses (tuberculomas). In immunocompromised patients, radiologic features may be atypical. Chest imaging is not specific for the diagnosis of TB and should not be used for this purpose alone ✖●; therefore, the diagnosis should be confirmed by microbiological testing.

2. Sputum smear microscopy: Tuberculous bacilli are identified with specific staining (Ziehl-Neelsen) using a bright light or florescence microscopy. Multiple samples are obtained to increase the diagnostic yield. Recent evidence supports that collection of 2 samples obtained on the same day has the same sensitivity (64%) and specificity (98%) compared with standard collection over multiple days. Collection of a total of 3 specimens (same day with 1 hour apart or multiple days) is recommended in Canada and other low-incidence settings where smear-negative TB is the most common presentation.◔● Specificity may be reduced in countries with a low incidence of TB and a high prevalence of nontuberculous mycobacterium.

3. Mycobacterial culture and phenotypic drug-sensitivity testing: Mycobacterial culture is the current gold-standard method for the detection of active TB disease with the highest sensitivity. Various solid or liquid culture medias exist and yield results in 2 to 8 weeks. The sensitivity of 3 sputum cultures is >90%. Drug-susceptibility test results are usually available within 1 week. They should be routinely performed in all first positive culture isolates obtained from each new case.

4. NAAT: Amplification of nucleic acids is a rapid method to assist with the diagnosis of TB and detection of drug resistance. Commercial government--approved assays, if available, are the most reliable. These tests are routinely used on smear-positive specimens and yield sensitivity and specificity >90%. Sensitivity in smear-negative specimens is only 50% to 70%, and thus NAAT testing is reserved for smear-negative cases that have a high pretest probability of active TB. In extrapulmonary specimens, sensitivity is lower. An automated, cartridge-based NAAT (Xpert MTB/RIF) can provide point-of-care testing to aid in the diagnosis of active TB and rifampin (INN rifampicin) resistance and has been shown to be a useful tool in developing countries with high TB prevalence. Data to support the accuracy for detection of TB disease and rifampin resistance in low-burden countries is lacking. It is therefore a conditional recommendation in Canada for all results generated by the Xpert MTB/RIF assay to be confirmed with government-approved commercial assays.◐◯

→ T R E A T M E N T

1. General principles of treatment:

1) **Early identification and treatment** of active TB is aimed at rapid killing of TB bacilli to effect rapid clinical improvement and to prevent transmission to others.

2) Treatment should be guided by the results of **drug-sensitivity testing** to effect cure and to prevent the emergence of drug resistance.

3) **Good adherence** to drug therapy and full completion of drug regimens are important for prevention of treatment failure and disease relapse.

4) A **treatment regimen** should always include at least 3 drugs during the first 2 months (initial intensive phase) and at least 2 drugs for another 4 to 7 months (continuation phase) that are effective against the mycobacteria isolated from the patient.

5) **Never add only one new drug** to an ineffective regimen.

6) Close supervision and monitoring is best accomplished with **directly observed therapy (DOT)**, which is recommended (if available) for individuals at risk of nonadherence or in those cases when treatment failure would have major implications for the individual or public health sector (drug resistance, disease relapse, pediatric disease, substance abuse, suspect nonadherence, mental health illness, homelessness).◐◯

7) Some patients may be considered for **intermittent, thrice-weekly therapy**, which is only recommended if administered by DOT and usually after having completed the first 2 months of daily therapy.◐◯ Intermittent therapy is not recommended for patients with multidrug-resistant TB (MDR-TB) or for persons with HIV infection.

8) **Reporting suspect or confirmed TB cases** to public health authorities is a requirement in many countries and is strongly recommended in others.

2. Anti-TB drugs: The drug regimens for TB therapy, as stated in this section, are consistent with Canadian and World Health Organization (WHO) guidelines. Flexibility in selection of drug choices and schedules is often required and related to drug intolerance or limited resources. All drug regimens must adhere to the general principles of treatment of active TB. If modifications in drug choices or schedules are required, referral to an expert in the management of TB is recommended.

1) **First-line (first-choice) agents** include isoniazid (INH), rifampin (RMP), pyrazinamide (PZA), and ethambutol (EMB). Drugs and dosage: →Table 18-3.

2) **Second-line (alternative) agents** include fluoroquinolones (FQNs), amikacin, streptomycin, ethionamide, capreomycin, cycloserine, para--aminosalicylic acid, kanamycin, and clarithromycin.

Table 18-3. Recommended drug doses for daily and intermittent therapy in adolescents and adults

	Daily		3 times a week	
	By weight	Maximum (mg)	By weight	Maximum (mg)
First-line drugs				
Isoniazid	5 mg/kg	300	10 mg/kg	600
Rifampin	10 mg/kg	600	10 mg/kg	600
Pyrazinamide	20-25 mg/kg	2000	30-40 mg/kg	4000
Ethambutol	15-20 mg/kg[a]	1600	25-40 mg/kg	2400
Second-line drugs				
Fluoroquinolones[b]: Moxi-floxacin		400		d
Fluoroquinolones[b]: Levo-floxacin		750-1000		d
Injectables: Amikacin[c]	15 mg/kg as a single dose[e]			d

[a] Optimal dosing is unclear. It is clear that eye toxicity is dose dependent, and its risk is higher at 25 mg/kg than at 15 mg/kg.

[b] Gatifloxacin is not recommended in Canada because of dysglycemia problems. This drug has been used in recent trials and is still used in some countries.

[c] Of the injectables, amikacin is preferred for use in Canada because of the ready availability of the drug, familiarity with its use by clinicians, nurses, and pharmacists, and the ability to measure serum drug concentration in many facilities. Streptomycin is not available in Canada but may be preferred in some low- and middle-income countries, as rates of toxicity are similar and costs may be lower.

[d] There are inadequate data from randomized trials on the use of fluoroquinolones or inject-ables as part of intermittent regimens. If these drugs are needed because of intolerance or resistance to first-line drugs, daily therapy is suggested.

[e] Initial dosage if renal function is normal. Dosing should be adjusted based on peak and trough serum levels in consultation with a pharmacist.

Source: ©All Rights Reserved. Canadian Tuberculosis Standards, 7th Edition. The Public Health Agency of Canada, The Lung Association, and the Canadian Thoracic Society, 2014. Adapted and reproduced with permission from the Minister of Health, 2016.

INN, international nonproprietary name.

3. Adjunctive use of glucocorticoids coupled with effective anti-TB thera-py is recommended for HIV noninfected patients with TB meningitis⊘● (IV dexamethasone 0.4 mg/kg daily for 2 weeks with the dose tapered over the next 8 weeks). Use of glucocorticoids for treatment of TB pericarditis may reduce death in HIV-negative patients but is of less certain efficacy in HIV-positive patients⊘○ (prednisone 1 mg/kg daily for 4 weeks with the dose tapered over the next 8 weeks). Replacement steroids may be used for TB-induced adrenal insufficiency, which can be associated with disseminated TB. Since evidence for use of steroids in other clinical scenarios is not robust, clinical judgment is reserved for the following: severe TB pleuritis and peritonitis with pleural effusion, life-threatening airway obstruction; lymph node TB with signs of compression of the adjacent organs; severe hypersensitivity reactions to anti-TB

Table 18-4. Adverse events of first-line and second-line drugs

	Common adverse events	Uncommon but important adverse events	Rank for probability of hepatitis[a]	Rank for probability of rash
First-line drugs				
Isoniazid	Rash, hepatitis, neuropathy	CNS toxicity, anemia	2	3
Rifampin	Drug interactions, rash	Hepatitis, influenza-like illness, neutropenia, thrombocytopenia	3	1
Pyrazinamide	Hepatitis, rash, arthralgia	Gout	1	2
Ethambutol	Eye toxicity	Rash	4	4
Second-line drugs				
Fluoroquinolones	Rash	Tendonitis, tendon rupture, QT interval prolongation		
Amikacin	Nephrotoxicity, ototoxicity			

[a] 1, most likely; 4, least likely.

Source: ©All Rights Reserved. Canadian Tuberculosis Standards, 7ᵗʰ Edition. The Public Health Agency of Canada, The Lung Association, and the Canadian Thoracic Society, 2014. Adapted and reproduced with permission from the Minister of Health, 2016.

CNS, central nervous system.

drugs that cannot be replaced with other agents; immune reconstitution inflammatory syndrome in patients with HIV infection.

4. Patients with new-onset TB:

1) Standard treatment for the **initial intensive phase** (first 2 months) for drug-sensitive (or expected drug-sensitive) TB includes combined use of INH, RMP, PZA, and EMB for 2 months. EMB can be discontinued as soon as drug-susceptibility tests indicate pansensitivity.

2) Standard treatment for the **continuation phase** (after the first 2 months and until treatment completion) for drug-sensitive TB includes combined use of INH and RMP for 4 more months for a total of 6 months of therapy. In patients with risk factors for relapse, the continuation phase should be prolonged to 7 months to provide a total of 9 months of therapy.◐● Risk factors for relapse include extensive disease and/or cavities on chest radiographs in the first 2 months of therapy, culture-positive after 2 months of therapy, or radiographic evidence for cavitation at treatment completion.

5. Monitoring adverse effects of anti-TB drugs: Monitoring for adverse effects of TB medications is important in order to detect adverse events, such as liver toxicity (INH, RMP, PZA), hypersensitivity reaction (RMP), optic neuritis (EMB), and neuropathy (INH) (→Table 18-4). Serious reactions should prompt stopping all potentially offending drugs with immediate initiation of 2 alternate TB medications. The evidence for standard baseline and follow-up monitoring schedules is weak. Most clinicians measure serum levels of liver enzymes, bilirubin, urea/blood urea nitrogen (BUN), creatinine, uric acid, and perform a complete blood count (CBC) when starting TB medications, and will schedule follow-up visits with liver enzyme measurements at least monthly thereafter. Hepatotoxic drugs must be discontinued in all patients with alanine aminotransferase (ALT) or aspartate aminotransferase (AST) levels ≥5 × upper limit of normal (ULN) and in patients with ALT and/or AST levels ≥3 × ULN who have gastrointestinal manifestations (jaundice, nausea, loss of appetite, abdominal distention, or abdominal pain). Advise patients to refrain from drinking alcohol while on INH, RMP, or PZA to reduce the risk of hepatic injury. When drug schedules must be altered due to adverse effects, consultation with a TB expert is advised to ensure that revised treatment schedules offer the best chance of treatment success with a minimal risk of further adverse reactions. If EMB is required beyond the first few weeks of drug therapy while awaiting drug susceptibility results, refer the patient for periodic ophthalmologic examinations.

6. Monitoring the clinical response to treatment: Methods to monitor response to therapy are based on expert opinion, and practices vary between institutions and countries. Microbiological testing of sputum is useful to assess the risk of transmitting infection to others and for early detection of treatment failure. Canadian experts suggest patients who are smear-positive at diagnosis should have sputum smears sent weekly until found to be negative. Thereafter, sputum cultures should be obtained at the end of the second month and near the end of drug therapy. If treatment failure is suspected, 2 sputum samples for smear and culture should be obtained and repeat drug-susceptibility testing should be requested on specimens that remain culture-positive. Clinical assessment should occur monthly with chest radiographs at 2 and 6 months.

7. Patients with a history of prior anti-TB treatment: Active TB in a patient who received prior therapy usually implies treatment failure, disease relapse, or in rare instances new reinfection (patients who are HIV-positive, immunocompromised). Consultation with a TB expert is advised. Drug-resistant TB should be suspected in patients who have previously been treated for active TB and therefore an expanded, empiric initial treatment regimen may be indicated (INH, RMP, PZA, EMB, and FQN). Rapid drug-susceptibility testing (subject to available resources) is recommended, so that drug resistance can either be excluded or promptly identified in order to provide appropriate and timely therapy. If drug resistance is ruled out, a standard 9-month course of drug therapy under DOT is recommended.

8. Treatment of drug-resistant TB: Drug-resistant mycobacterial strains may be resistant to only one drug or to multiple drugs. MDR-TB is resistance to at least INH and RMP. Pre-extensively drug-resistant TB (pre-XDR-TB) is resistance to INH and RMP plus either a FQN or one of the 3 injectable second-line drugs (amikacin, kanamycin, or capreomycin). Extensively drug-resistant TB (XDR-TB) is resistance to at least INH and RMP plus a FQN and one of the 3 injectable second-line drugs. There are recommended regimens for the management of drug-resistant TB; however, an individualized therapeutic approach based on drug-susceptibility test results, extent of disease, response to therapy, and drug tolerance is required. All treatment should be given by DOT. MDR-TB should be treated by a specialized health-care team with expertise in the management of drug-resistant tuberculosis.

1) **INH-resistant TB**: RMP + EMB + PZA daily for 6 to 9 months. A daily or thrice-weekly schedule after the first 2 months. In patients with extensive pulmonary lesions, add an FQN for the entire treatment and stop PZA after 2 months.

2) **RMP-resistant TB**: INH + EMB + a third-generation (levofloxacin) or fourth-generation (moxifloxacin) FQN daily for 12 to 18 months with PZA for the first 2 months. A daily or thrice-weekly schedule after the first 2 months. In patients with extensive pulmonary lesions, add a parenteral drug for the first 2 to 3 months.

3) **MDR-TB**: Assess drug sensitivity for all first-line and second-line drugs as a guide for individualized therapy. Use ≥4 anti-TB drugs of probable

effectiveness. Start selection using first-line drugs followed by second-line drugs with initial inclusion of PZA. In each case, use a third- or fourth--generation FQN plus a parenteral drug, with drug choices being made on the basis of sensitivity tests. In case of resistance to FQN, consider including linezolid and clofazimine. The new WHO guidelines recommend a standardized treatment regimen that is 9 to 12 months shorter as the first choice in patients with multidrug-resistant or rifampicin-resistant TB (MDR/RR-TB) strains not resistant to fluoroquinolones or second-line injectable agents.⊘ Although randomized trials to study the benefit of adjunctive therapy with vitamin D for the treatment of active TB have provided conflicting results, a recent meta-analysis indicated vitamin D accelerated the time to sputum conversion in a subgroup of patients with MDR pulmonary TB.⊘○

4) **XDR-TB**: The principles are similar to the treatment of MDR-TB. Consider the use of bedaquiline or high-dose INH. Another parenteral drug may be added (one with susceptibility to the TB strain, or one that has not been used before if the strain is resistant to all drugs from this group).

9. Treatment of TB in pregnant and breastfeeding women: INH, RMP, and EMB are considered safe in pregnancy. Therefore, use all 3 for initial treatments. Patients treated with INH should receive pyridoxine. PZA in pregnancy is recommended by the WHO, although there is some controversy regarding its safety. The use of PZA for pregnant women in Canada is restricted to those with extensive disease or intolerance to their first-line drugs. Breastfeeding is not contraindicated. Most second-line agents are not considered safe in pregnancy, which is related to toxic or teratogenic effects on the fetus, especially in the case of aminoglycosides (ototoxicity), FQN (bone growth), and ethionamide (teratogenic effects and increased risk of maternal nausea and vomiting). Sputum smear-positive mothers should be isolated from newborns until the smear results become negative. The infant must be urgently assessed to exclude active TB with a clinical examination, chest radiographs, cultures (which may include lumbar puncture), and abdominal ultrasound. A course of preventive treatment with INH is initiated for the infant if there is no evidence of active TB. Some countries recommend that the infant receive the BCG vaccine once the treatment has been completed.

10. Patients with renal failure: Use INH and RMP at standard doses (these are excreted predominantly with bile). Use EMB at a dose of 15 mg/kg and PZA at a dose of 25 mg/kg, both at a reduced frequency of 3 times a week (if undergoing hemodialysis, administer after dialysis).

11. Patients with liver failure: INH, RMP, and PZA may cause drug-induced hepatotoxicity.

1) **Acute liver failure**: Consider a brief delay in starting anti-TB treatment until liver function has been stabilized. If treatment is deemed necessary, use FQN + EMB + parenteral (amikacin) for 2 months and then FQN + EMB for a total of 18 months. If liver function has stabilized, RMP may be introduced with careful monitoring of liver parameters.

2) **Chronic liver failure:** Adjust treatment to the severity of liver failure and number of other coadministered hepatotoxic drugs.

12. Unconscious patients: In patients in whom enteral nutrition is administered via a gastrostomy or nasogastric tube, crushed oral anti-TB drugs can be given 2 to 3 hours before or after meals. Other options include intramuscular INH, intravenous RMP (when available), intravenous amikacin/intramuscular streptomycin, and intravenous FQN.

13. Patients after organ or bone marrow transplantation: Caution is necessary because of the possible interactions of rifamycins (RMP, rifabutin, rifapentine) with calcineurin inhibitors (cyclosporine [INN ciclosporin] and tacrolimus; doses of these agents should be increased 3- to 5-fold with concomitant monitoring of their blood levels) and with glucocorticoids (steroid dose may need to be increased by 50%).

14. HIV-positive patients: Treatment of TB in HIV-infected patients should be guided by a physician with expertise in the management of both diseases or in close collaboration with a physician expert in HIV care. A standard regime should be used, but with close attention of drug interactions between TB and antiretroviral treatment (ART). In the case of slow clinical or microbiological improvement, extend treatment to 9 months, or by at least an additional 4 months after obtaining sterile sputum culture results. In patients not receiving ART, the diagnosis of TB is an indication for starting such therapy. Initiate anti-TB treatment first and then add ART (efavirenz combined with 2 nucleoside reverse-transcriptase inhibitors after 2-8 weeks), depending on CD4 counts. Do not use RMP in patients treated with protease inhibitors, as it decreases blood levels of these drugs (substitute rifabutin to replace RMP after a 2-week washout period). Administration of ART in HIV-positive patients with TB may lead to immune reconstitution inflammatory syndrome, which may require treatment with glucocorticoids.

15. In patients treated with anti-TNF agents who develop TB in the course of therapy, anti-TNF treatment should be discontinued. It may be resumed no earlier than after one month of appropriate anti-TB treatment and confirmation of susceptibility of the mycobacteria to the drugs used.

→ **COMPLICATIONS**

Pneumothorax, bronchopleural fistula, pleural empyema, pleural fibrosis (fibrothorax), pulmonary hemorrhage, and amyloidosis.

→ **PREVENTION**

1. Rapid diagnosis and implementation of treatment for active TB.

2. Airborne precautions should be used for patients with suspect or confirmed respiratory TB who are admitted to hospital or assessed in ambulatory facilities.

3. Partnership with public health services who implement and set standards for TB surveillance, screening, isolation practices, and DOT.

4. Targeted screening and preventative therapy for LTBI: →Chapter 13.18.3.

5. Vaccination against TB (BCG): BCG is a live attenuated vaccine derived from *Mycobacterium bovis*. Policies and practices vary widely across the world. In the majority of countries, BCG vaccination is recommended either at birth or before 1 year of age. There is much debate about the efficacy of BCG in preventing development of TB infection, although most experts agree that the vaccine may prevent dissemination of the TB bacilli. In Canada, BCG is currently only recommended for infants in certain high-risk communities and also to be considered for travelling infants planning an extended stay in a country with a high incidence of TB.

18.3. Tuberculosis: Latent Tuberculosis Infection

→ **DEFINITION, ETIOLOGY, PATHOGENESIS**

Latent tuberculosis infection (LTBI) is an asymptomatic state where bacteria of the *Mycobacterium tuberculosis* complex may survive for years within small granulomas residing in the lung or in other sites after being seeded by lymphatic or hematologic spread. Even though tuberculosis (TB) bacteria thrive in an oxygen-rich environment, they are capable of surviving in a dormant, anaerobic state for extended periods.

Information on the pathogenesis of TB infection: →Chapter 13.18.2.

→ **DETECTION**

1. Screening: Targeted screening is used to detect individuals with LTBI who are at the highest risk of reactivation of TB and who would therefore benefit from preventative drug therapy. Screening of populations for LTBI is not justified in regions lacking the infrastructure to provide the monitoring and support required to ensure safe and complete administration of the medication. Tools used for screening include the tuberculin skin test (TST) and/or interferon γ release assay (IGRA). A positive result should be followed by a chest radiograph. The choice of which groups are to be selected for targeted screening is usually decided by public health authorities in conjunction with health-care professionals with expertise in the area of TB. The World Health Organization 2018 guidelines recommend systematic testing and treatment for LTBI in persons with HIV infection, child and adult contacts of patients with active pulmonary TB, or in patients with the following medical risk factors: anti–tumor necrosis factor α treatment, dialysis, preparing for organ or hematologic transplantation, silicosis. Systematic testing and treatment is to be considered for the following groups based on risks within the local and national context: prisoners, health-care workers, immigrants from high-burden countries, homeless persons, and illicit drug users.

Screening in HIV-positive individuals: Every patient with newly diagnosed HIV infection should be assessed with regard to TB exposure history and clinical features of TB. Testing for LTBI should be done in those with no prior history of TB infection or disease. Despite a lower threshold for diagnosis of LTBI (usually TST ≥5 mm), the results of TST are often negative, results of IGRA are often indeterminate, and positive results of a direct sputum examination are less frequent. A chest radiograph and sputum for smear and culture should be performed as part of the initial screen for HIV-infected patients with LTBI.

2. Diagnostic tests:

1) **TST** is a diagnostic aid used for identification of LTBI. It is an intradermal tuberculin (purified protein derivate) injection administered using the Mantoux technique. The reading, based on the diameter of skin induration, is measured 48 to 72 hours after administration. The interpretation of the reading depends on size of induration, positive predictive value, and risk of progressing to active disease, if the person is truly infected. Declaration of positivity is therefore dependent on several factors with a goal to identify individuals who would benefit from treatment for LTBI. The standard threshold in Canada for patients without mitigating features is ≥10 mm, but other countries may use a different value based on demographic and socioeconomic factors. The TST has no value for active TB detection. Induration at the test site can be observed in persons with *M tuberculosis* infection (test does not differentiate between LTBI and clinically overt active disease), individuals after BCG vaccination, and occasionally in persons with a history of exposure to nontuberculous mycobacteria. False-positive and false-negative reactions may occur. BCG vaccination can lower the specificity of the TST and may cause a false-positive reaction, especially if administered after 12 months of age.

2) **IGRAs based on interferon γ production by T cells**: The IGRA is an in-vitro blood test used for identification of latent LTBI. Like the TST, the IGRA should not be used for active TB disease detection in adults.◉◒ It may be reasonable to use the IGRA as a supplementary diagnostic aid for the investigation of children with suspected active TB under the age of 18 years. The assays have higher specificity than the TST, and the results are not influenced by BCG vaccination. Since comparison studies in similar populations do not provide strong evidence that the IGRA is preferred over the TST for prevention of active TB, either test may be used as a tool to detect LTBI.◉◒ IGRA assays are available in many countries, but access to IGRA testing in developing countries is inconsistent.

Table 18-5. Tuberculin skin test cut-off points for treatment of latent tuberculosis infection

TST result	Indication[a]
0-4 mm	– In general, this is considered negative and no treatment is indicated[b] – Close contacts in children <5 years of age should be treated pending results of repeat skin test 8 weeks after exposure[c]
≥5 mm	– HIV infection – Contact with infectious TB within the past 2 years – Fibronodular disease on chest radiographs (healed TB and not previously treated) – Organ transplantation (related to immune suppressant therapy)[d] – Tumor necrosis factor α inhibitors – Other immunosuppressive drugs, eg, glucocorticoids (equivalent of ≥15 mg/d of prednisone for 1 month or more; risk of TB disease increases with higher dose and longer duration) – End-stage renal disease
≥10 mm	All others, including the following specific situations: – TST conversion (within 2 years) – Diabetes, malnutrition (<90% ideal body weight), cigarette smoking, daily alcohol consumption (>3 drinks/d) – Silicosis – Hematologic malignancies (leukemia, lymphoma) and certain carcinomas (eg, head and neck)

[a] Age ≥35 years is not a contraindication to treatment of LTBI if the risk of progression to active TB disease is greater than the risk of serious adverse reactions to treatment.

[b] Treatment with isoniazid of people with HIV infection who were TST negative (0-4 mm) and/or anergic was of no benefit in several randomized trials. Other authorities suggest this treatment may be considered in the presence of HIV infection or other cause of severe immunosuppression and high risk of TB infection (contact with infectious TB, from high TB-incidence country or abnormal chest radiographs consistent with prior TB infection). Hence any decision to give treatment should be individualized in consultation with a TB expert.

[c] If first TST is negative, begin treatment immediately. Repeat TST 8 weeks after exposure to infectious TB case ended. Treatment can be stopped in a healthy child if repeat TST is negative (<5 mm induration). In children <6 months of age, the immune system may not be mature enough to produce a positive TST, even if the child is infected.

[d] LTBI therapy is often given to people in whom transplantation is planned but before the actual transplantation.

Source: ©All Rights Reserved. Canadian Tuberculosis Standards, 7th Edition. The Public Health Agency of Canada, The Lung Association, and the Canadian Thoracic Society, 2014. Adapted and reproduced with permission from the Minister of Health, 2016.

HIV, human immunodeficiency virus; LTBI, latent tuberculosis infection; TB, tuberculosis; TST, tuberculin skin test.

3) There are 2 **web-based tools** to assist with the interpretation TST and IGRA results:

a) An interactive algorithm, the Online TST/IGRA Interpreter, can provide a customized estimate of the positive predictive value of an individual's TST reading: www.tstin3d.com/en/calc.html.

b) The BCG World Atlas provides information on BCG vaccination policies in different countries: www.bcgatlas.org.

Table 18-6. Treatment regimens for LTBI recommended by the World Health Organization

Drug(s)	Duration	Schedule	Mode of administration	Level of evidence[a]
INH	6-9 months[b]	Daily	SAP	1
INH/RMP	3-4 months	Daily	SAP	1
INH/RPT[c]	3 months	Once weekly	DOP	1
RMP	3-4 months[d]	Daily	SAP	2

[a] Level 1, multiple randomized trials. Level 2, single randomized trial and/or multiple observational (cohort) studies.

[b] Canadian guidelines suggest 9 months as standard and 6 months as an acceptable alternative.

[c] Use this regimen with careful monitoring for hypersensitivity reactions, as these can be severe. RPT is only available in Canada through the Special Access Program.

[d] The Canadian standard is 4 months.

Based on: Latent tuberculosis infection: updated and consolidated guidelines for programmatic management. Geneva: World Health Organization; 2018 and Canadian Tuberculosis Standards, 7th Edition. The Public Health Agency of Canada, The Lung Association, and the Canadian Thoracic Society, 2014.

DOP, directly observed prophylaxis; INH, isoniazid; LTBI, latent tuberculosis infection; RMP, rifampin (international nonproprietary name: rifampicin); RPT, rifapentine; SAP, self-administered prophylaxis.

→ **TREATMENT**

1. General principles of treatment:

1) Always **exclude active TB** before starting drug treatment for LTBI. A history, physical examination, and chest radiograph are required to screen for active disease. If any features suspicious for active disease are detected, do further testing including sputum smear and culture. Other tests may be indicated.

2) The **decision to treat LTBI** should be individualized, with consideration of the risks of adverse events, such as hepatotoxicity, balanced against the risk of prior TB exposure and the risk of reactivation. Clinical factors, such as comorbid diseases (kidney/liver), immunosuppression, TB exposure status, fibronodular changes on chest imaging, or risk of drug-resistant LTBI, are to be strongly considered in the risk-benefit analysis. TST cut-points for treatment of LTBI in Canada: →Table 18-5.

2. Drug regimens for LTBI: The standard regimen of first choice is 9 months of daily self-administered isoniazid (INH) (5 mg/kg for adults, 10 mg/kg for children, with a maximum dose for all recipients of 300 mg/d). Pyridoxine 25 mg/d may be added to INH to offset the potential adverse effect of peripheral neuropathy for patients at risk of this complication. More recent studies have demonstrated noninferiority with 4 months of daily rifampin or 3 months of once-weekly rifapentine plus INH when compared with the standard 9-month INH regime. Other acceptable alternative daily self-administered regimen is 6 months INH. A summary of recommended regimens for LBTI treatment: →Table 18-6.

3. Monitoring during LTBI treatment: The goals of monitoring are to promote drug compliance and to detect and manage adverse effects. Since the evidence to guide follow-up schedules is weak, practice styles vary considerably. Many experts obtain baseline levels of transaminases and regular monthly testing in patients >35 years of age or those who have risk factors for liver disease. Patients on INH or rifampin are strongly advised against intake of alcohol, since this may increase the risk of hepatotoxicity.

1. Adult-Onset Still Disease

→ DEFINITION, ETIOLOGY, PATHOGENESIS

Adult-onset Still disease (AOSD) is a systemic form of juvenile idiopathic arthritis associated with fever, rash, lymphadenopathy, splenomegaly, serositis, and inflammation of multiple organs. The condition was first described in 1971 by Eric George Bywaters in a case series of adult patients with symptoms reminiscent of children with Still disease (now known as systemic juvenile idiopathic arthritis). It is classically characterized by spiking fevers, arthritis, and an evanescent salmon-colored rash. AOSD is a rare condition, with incidence rates ranging from 0.16 to 0.4/100,000 patient-years. The condition typically affects young adults, with a median age of onset of 36 years, and predominantly women. The exact etiology of AOSD is still unknown. It has been associated with a number of different human leukocyte antigens (HLAs), including HLA-Bw35, HLA-DR4, and HLA-DrW6; however, the strengths of these associations remain unclear. It is also proposed that a preceding infection may play a role in the etiology of AOSD, leading to an epigenetic effect.

→ CLINICAL FEATURES AND NATURAL HISTORY

AOSD develops after the age of 16. In adults the symptoms may be due to the first occurrence of the disease or a relapse. The course of AOSD may be self-limiting (lasting <1 year), relapsing (relapses may be very frequent), or chronic (symptoms are continuously present throughout the year). In some patients significant joint destruction occurs.

Symptoms (→Table 1-1):

1) Most frequent:
   a) **Fever** (>80% of cases; usually >39°C, most commonly in the evening or twice during a 24-hour period).

Table 1-1. Yamaguchi diagnostic criteria for adult-onset Still disease	
Major criteria	1) Fever ≥39°C persisting for ≥1 week
	2) Arthralgia persisting for ≥2 weeks
	3) Typical rash
	4) White blood cell count ≥10 × 10^9/L (>80% neutrophils)
Minor criteria	1) Sore throat
	2) Lymphadenopathy and/or splenomegaly
	3) Increased serum aminotransferase or lactate dehydrogenase levels (after other causes have been excluded)
	4) Negative IgM rheumatoid factor and antinuclear antibodies (immunofluorescence assay)
Exclusion criteria	1) Infections, in particular sepsis and infectious mononucleosis
	2) Malignancy, in particular lymphoma
	3) Other rheumatic diseases, in particular polyarteritis nodosa and vasculitis in the course of rheumatoid arthritis

For the diagnosis of adult-onset Still disease, ≥5 criteria must be met, including ≥2 major. In patients with any of the exclusion criteria, the diagnosis is excluded.
Sensitivity of the criteria is 80.6%, and specificity is 98.5%.

Source: J Rheumatol. 1992;19(3):424-30.

b) **Sore throat with features of inflammation** (>50%; frequently develops several days or weeks prior to other symptoms).

c) **Salmon-pink macular or maculopapular rash** (>80%; often transient, develops only during episodes of fever, rarely pruritic, most frequently located on the trunk and proximal limbs, less often on the face; it may be triggered by heat [eg, following a hot bath] or skin abrasion [eg, scratchy clothing]).

d) **Arthralgia** (>90%; worsens during febrile periods; occasionally arthritis, most commonly affecting the knees and wrists; approximately one-fourth of patients develop ankyloses of the involved joints).

e) **Myalgia** (>80%).

f) **Lymphadenopathy** (>50%; most frequently affecting the cervical lymph nodes; the lymph nodes may be tender; retroperitoneal lymphadenopathy may cause abdominal pain that is difficult to diagnose).

g) **Splenomegaly, hepatomegaly** (50%).

2) Less frequent: Symptoms of pleuritis or pericarditis, weight loss.

3) Rare: Pulmonary fibrosis, myocarditis or cardiac tamponade, hair loss, Sjögren syndrome, aseptic meningitis, peripheral neuropathy, amyloidosis, subacute glomerulonephritis and interstitial nephritis, hemolytic anemia, disseminated intravascular coagulation, macrophage activation syndrome, cataract, hearing impairment.

→ DIAGNOSIS

Diagnostic Tests

1. Laboratory tests: In periods of increased disease activity the following features are observed:

1) Elevated erythrocyte sedimentation rate (ESR) and plasma C-reactive protein (CRP) levels.

2) Leukocytosis (often >20 × 10^9/L) with >80% of neutrophils in the differential counts.

3) Thrombocytosis.

4) Anemia.

5) Hypoalbuminemia.

6) Very high serum ferritin levels (levels >3000 ng/mL are suggestive of AOSD [in adults, this is the second most frequent cause of ferritin levels >1000 ng/mL next to hemophagocytic syndrome: →Chapter 8.8.7; the increase correlates with the disease activity).

7) Elevated serum aminotransferase and lactate dehydrogenase (LDH) levels.

8) IgM rheumatoid factor (RF) and antinuclear antibodies (ANAs) (observed in <10% of patients; in diagnostic workup, negative RF and ANAs are suggestive of Still disease).

2. Synovial fluid: Synovial aspirate in AOSD is nonspecific, and features are consistent with inflammatory arthritis.

3. Imaging studies: Radiographs of the hands are usually nonspecific and not very helpful in establishing the diagnosis of AOSD. Radiographs of the involved joints may reveal periarticular osteopenia, narrowing of the joint space, erosions, as well as early development of ankylosis. In some patients, rapid destruction of 1 or both hip joints, less often of a knee joint, is observed. **Computed tomography (CT)** may demonstrate retroperitoneal lymphadenopathy.

Diagnostic Criteria

Most frequently diagnosis is based on the Yamaguchi diagnostic criteria (→Table 1-1).

Differential Diagnosis

The key categories of conditions in the differential diagnosis for AOSD are infections, malignancies, and autoimmune diseases. Potential infections to rule out include HIV, cytomegalovirus, Epstein-Barr virus, hepatitis B, hepatitis C, parvovirus B19, rubella, infective endocarditis, syphilis, and toxoplasmosis. Malignancies to exclude are primarily malignant lymphomas or any other metastatic disease. Potential autoimmune diseases, which may mimic AOSD, include systemic lupus erythematous, rheumatoid arthritis, systemic vasculitis, familial Mediterranean fever, hemophagocytic syndrome, and sarcoidosis.

→ TREATMENT

1. Nonsteroidal anti-inflammatory drugs (NSAIDs): Retrospective cohort studies have shown NSAIDs to be ineffective in controlling symptoms of AOSD, with >80% of patients failing to respond. In addition, up to 20% of patients experienced an adverse event. Therefore, NSAIDs are not an effective agent in controlling disease activity. They may be used as adjunctive therapy for arthritic symptoms, but high-quality evidence for their use in this role is lacking. NSAIDs could be tried alone in a mild form of the disease for a limited period of time.

2. Glucocorticoids: Retrospective cohort studies have shown that glucocorticoids at an oral dose of 0.5 to 1 mg/kg daily of prednisone (or an equivalent dose of methylprednisolone) may be used, as they were effective in controlling AOSD symptoms in up to 65% of patients.◯ Clinical improvement may be evident within hours of initiating therapy. Tapering usually begins within 4 to 6 weeks after initiating treatment. However, a large proportion of patients (40%-45%) become steroid-dependent and unable to completely taper off prednisone, which subjects them to many potential adverse effects, such as glucocorticoid-induced osteoporosis and avascular necrosis, among many others.

3. Disease modifying antirheumatic drugs (DMARDs): Adding a DMARD is critical, given the high percentage of patients who become steroid-dependent. Methotrexate is the drug suggested when selecting a steroid-sparing agent. Doses of oral methotrexate range from 7.5 mg/wk to 25 mg/wk. Although methotrexate is the most studied DMARD in the treatment of AOSD, the evidence for its use is still lacking, coming only from small retrospective cohorts. These small studies have shown that addition of methotrexate may achieve a partial or complete remission of AOSD and allows at least a majority of patients to either reduce their glucocorticoid dose, or to taper it off completely.◯ Methotrexate has been shown to have similar efficacy in patients with AOSD and primarily systemic or articular manifestations.

4. Interleukin-1 (IL-1) antagonists:

1) Anakinra is a recombinant IL-1 β-receptor antagonist given as a daily subcutaneous injection that might be considered in those resistant to the therapies described above. A number of case series have reported on the potential role that anakinra may play in patients with AOSD refractory to steroids, DMARDs, and in 1 case series, refractory to tumor necrosis factor (TNF)-α inhibitors. In addition, a small open randomized trial assessed the efficacy of anakinra as a steroid-sparing agent in patients with AOSD with active disease despite treatment with prednisolone ≥10 mg per day, with or without concomitant DMARD use.◯ Anakinra therapy typically has quick noticeable clinical improvements within days of initiating therapy. However, a number of cases of disease relapse have been reported several days after discontinuing anakinra.

2) Canakinumab is fully humanized monoclonal antibody against IL-1. Unlike anakinra, canakinumab has a much longer half-life (26 days vs 6 hours). The evidence for the drug is limited to a single case report of 2 patients successfully treated with canakinumab after failing to respond to glucocorticoids, methotrexate, and anakinra. Its cost for many is prohibitively high.

5. TNF-α inhibitors: Three available TNF-α inhibitors—infliximab, etanercept, and adalimumab—have been tried in patients with AOSD.

1) Infliximab is a chimeric monoclonal antibody against TNF-α. There are a number of small case series in which treatment with infliximab improved systemic and articular symptoms of AOSD, while also improving inflammatory markers (ESR, CRP) and ferritin levels. There are also case series suggesting infliximab may be used as a steroid-sparing agent in patients treated with prednisone and methotrexate. However, the evidence for infliximab in AOSD is limited to small retrospective case series and 1 prospective open-label trial consisting of only 4 patients.

2) Adalimumab is a fully human monoclonal antibody against TNF-α. Case reports and case series suggest that adalimumab may be effective in patients with AOSD and can be used as a steroid-sparing agent. The quality of evidence regarding the role of adalimumab role in the treatment of AOSD is limited to case reports and case series.

3) Etanercept is a recombinant molecule of fragments of soluble TNF-α receptor linked to the Fc portion of human IgG. A small prospective cohort study of 12 patients with AOSD with severe arthritic symptoms refractory to DMARDs who were treated with etanercept suggested a modest improvement in the arthritic symptoms, but most patients did not have a complete response. A number of other case reports and case series have reported that etanercept was able to achieve a partial response in patients with AOSD and primary chronic arthritic symptoms, but few were able to achieve disease remission. Like with the other TNF-α inhibitors, the quality of evidence for the role of etanercept role in the treatment of AOSD is poor, limited primarily to case reports, case series, and 1 small prospective open-label study. TNF-α inhibitors might be considered in those who do not respond to a more standard treatment with glucocorticoids and methotrexate.

6. Interleukin-6 (IL-6) antagonist: Tocilizumab is a fully humanized monoclonal antibody against IL-6 receptors, which was used in 1 prospective open-label trial of 14 patients with AOSD (who previously failed anakinra and at least 1 TNF-α inhibitor). After 6 months of therapy with tocilizumab, 57% of patients had remission of joint symptoms and 86% had resolution of the systemic symptoms. Another retrospective review consisted of 16 AOSD patients treated previously with at least 1 biologic before switching to tocilizumab.◯ All but one patient responded well after treatment with tocilizumab, and 2 patients were able to completely withdraw their glucocorticoid therapy. The effects were quite rapid, with a normalization of CRP levels by 7.1 weeks (mean), and ferritin levels by 5.8 weeks (mean). Overall, tocilizumab remains a promising option for patients with refractory AOSD with both systemic and articular manifestations. However, the quality of evidence is limited to case reports, case series, and 1 prospective open-label cohort study. As such, tocilizumab may be considered in patients failing therapy with glucocorticoids and methotrexate.

7. Intravenous immunoglobulins: Limited evidence from case reports and case series supports some benefit of IV immunoglobulins infusions in patients resistant to or unable to tolerate other forms of therapy.◯◯

→ **PROGNOSIS**

The natural history of AOSD can be quite variable. Some patients have a single systemic self-limited episode with symptoms improving within a few months and resolving by 1 year. Other patients have a polycyclic form of the disease, with multiple flares of the systemic and arthritic symptoms and clear periods of remission between the flares. Finally, the remaining patients have a form associated with chronic disease, where inflammatory arthritis is the predominant manifestation. These patients are prone to develop secondary osteoarthritis, with associated impact on health-related quality of life and disability.

Polyarthritis and arthritis affecting the large joints (shoulder, hip) at the onset of the disease are associated with an increased risk of developing chronic disease. AA amyloidosis is a rare complication of AOSD, which is attributed to chronic uncontrolled systemic inflammation. The incidence of AA amyloidosis is low, especially with appropriate therapies to decrease the level of inflammation. Death may occur due to infection, liver failure, amyloidosis (occurs in approximately a third of patients), respiratory failure, heart failure, or disseminated intravascular coagulation.

2. Algodystrophy (Complex Regional Pain Syndrome)

→ DEFINITION, ETIOLOGY, PATHOGENESIS

Complex regional pain syndrome (CRPS) type 1 is also termed algodystrophy, Sudeck atrophy, reflex sympathetic dystrophy, shoulder-hand syndrome, post-traumatic dystrophy, or posttraumatic osteoporosis.

CRPS is characterized by pain, perfusion abnormalities, atrophic changes, and functional impairment, which usually develop in response to a noxious stimulus. It mainly affects the limbs, involving areas that extend beyond those innervated by a single nerve.

The severity of symptoms is substantially higher than the strength of the stimulus would suggest. CRPS can manifest at any age (including childhood). CRPS tends to occur more frequently in women than in men.

Common **triggers** include:

1) Trauma (in up to 70% of patients; eg, in a third of patients following a Colles fracture).
2) Invasive procedures (eg, carpal tunnel release, arthroscopy, spine surgery).
3) Internal diseases (eg, myocardial infarction, pulmonary tuberculosis, cancer, pulmonary fibrosis).
4) Stroke or other brain injury with hemiplegia.

It may also be idiopathic (~20% of patients). The **pathogenesis** of CRPS remains unclear.

→ CLINICAL FEATURES AND NATURAL HISTORY

In most cases CRPS involves the wrists, while the knees, ankles, and feet are less common locations. An entire limb (shoulder-hand or hip-foot syndromes) or the face or trunk can sometimes be affected. The involvement is usually asymmetric; in patients with bilateral disease changes in the contralateral limb develop as the condition progresses.

Common **symptoms** include:

1) Severe, chronic, burning pain outside the area of trauma (not affecting muscles or joints).
2) Excessive sensitivity to mechanical, thermal, and painful stimuli.
3) Hyperesthesia (excessive physical sensory perception), allodynia (perception of pain with stimuli that do not normally cause pain) and hyperpathia (pain with mild stimuli, particularly repetitive ones).
4) Decreased sensitivity to stimuli with limb elevation, increased sensitivity with active and passive movement, changes in ambient temperature, and during emotional stress.

5) Locomotor symptoms including muscle weakness, impaired motion, tremor, muscle spasms, and contractures.

6) Atrophic dermatologic changes including skin atrophy, hyperkeratosis, changes in skin creases, fingertips, hair (thickening), and nails (thickening, whitening, browning, or furrowing).

7) Vascular and autonomic symptoms including pallor or erythema, warming or cooling of the affected extremity compared with the contralateral limb, edema (in >80% of patients; initially pitting, later indurated), and increased sweating.

Natural history: The Steinbrocker classification includes the following stages of CRPS (all of which may or may not manifest in a given patient):

1) **Stage 1** (acute) is usually 1 to 3 months in duration (but may last for up to 12 months) and includes pain, hyperesthesia, warming or cooling, and abnormal sweating. In most cases the disease resolves at this stage.

2) **Stage 2** (dystrophic) may last for 1 to 2 years and includes pain, atrophic changes of the skin, hair, and nails, as well as cooling of the skin.

3) **Stage 3** (atrophic or chronic) lasts for several years and includes skin atrophy, contractures, bone changes, and impaired limb function, which are usually irreversible.

→ D I A G N O S I S

Diagnostic Tests

1. Imaging studies: Radiographs of the affected limb typically demonstrate patchy osteoporosis that is most pronounced in periarticular areas and either forms a pattern of streaks or is irregular in appearance. Soft tissue edema is also visible. Bone marrow edema can be seen on magnetic resonance imaging (MRI) scanning.

2. Functional studies of the autonomic nervous system: Sympathetic blockade (eg, by administering IV phentolamine) is considered an accessory diagnostic test, with clinical improvement supporting the diagnosis of CRPS.

Diagnostic Criteria

To make the diagnosis of CRPS, all of the following criteria must be fulfilled:

1) Persistent pain without a clear cause or hyperesthesia extending beyond the area innervated by a single nerve and significantly more extensive than suggested by the triggering trauma.

2) Edema, vasomotor dysfunction, or sweating in the area of pain. These features do not need to occur at the time of establishing diagnosis (ie, a history of their occurrence is sufficient for diagnosis).

3) Exclusion of other known causes for the presenting symptoms.

Differential Diagnosis

Differential diagnosis should include:

1) CRPS type 2 (formerly termed causalgia, which includes symptoms [mainly pain] caused by nerve injury).

2) Inflammatory: Panniculitis, inflammatory arthritis.

3) Infectious: Cellulitis, osteomyelitis.

4) Vascular: Deep vein thrombosis.

5) Neoplastic.

6) Musculoskeletal: Fractures.

7) Neurogenic: Polyneuropathy.

In advanced CRPS it may be also important to exclude chronic vascular insufficiency and thoracic outlet syndrome.

➜ **TREATMENT**

No reliable data confirm the effectiveness of any treatment for CRPS type 1. Patient education is universally important. Psychotherapy has been shown to have some utility.

1. **Pharmacotherapy**:

1) **Anti-inflammatory treatment**: Oral or IV glucocorticoid regimens, dimethylsulfoxide cream, and IV free radical scavengers such as mannitol have been studied with small sample sizes, with most evidence not showing significant change in pain or composite CRPS scores.

2) **Bisphosphonate therapy**: Although the evidence is limited, benefits of bisphosphonates are best documented among all CRPS interventions.☺⊖ It is possible that these effects may be more likely in CRPS with accompanying bone mineral density loss (osteopenia or osteoporosis). Inhibition of bone resorption may lead to decrease in bone demineralization and associated benefits in pain and function.

3) **Calcitonin**: Effects are likely due to inhibition of bone resorption and possible β-endorphin–mediated analgesic action. Calcitonin has been shown to be potentially more effective than placebo and as effective as β-blockers, griseofulvin, oral acetaminophen (INN paracetamol), and IV bisphosphonates.

4) **N-methyl-D-aspartate (NMDA)-receptor antagonists**: Effects are possibly due to neuropathic pain modulatory action. Limited evidence suggests IV ketamine may provide short-term pain relief, although no sustained effect was found beyond 4 to 11 weeks after treatment.☺⊖

5) **Tadalafil**: Effects are possibly due to its vasodilatory action. Limited evidence suggests tadalafil may provide small but significant short-term CRPS-related pain relief, although with no significant change in function.☺⊖

6) **Systemic local anesthetic agents**: High-dose IV lidocaine may have a slightly larger analgesic effect compared with other agents such as diphenhydramine, at least in the short term.

2. **Epidural and IV regional blocks**: Epidural clonidine may provide immediate pain relief when CRPS-related pain is refractory to sympathetic blockade. IV regional blocks with atropine have generally not been found to be effective for sympathetically-maintained pain. IV regional blocks with bretylium or with lidocaine may provide longer duration of analgesia than lidocaine alone, and very limited evidence suggests ketanserin may be effective in reducing CRPS-related pain. IV regional blocks with droperidol and guanethidine have not been found to be effective, and the former has been associated with frequent adverse events.

3. **Botulinum toxin A sympathetic blockade**: This may effectively increase analgesic duration alongside local anesthesia compared with local anesthesia alone, although it is unclear what degree of pain relief can be attributed to this intervention.

4. **Neurostimulation**: No evidence is available supporting the effectiveness of repetitive transcranial magnetic stimulation. There is low-quality evidence supporting spinal cord stimulation in conjunction with physiotherapy for CRPS--related pain control and health-related quality of life but not for function.

5. **Physiotherapy**: Low-quality evidence suggests multimodal physiotherapy in conjunction with medical management may be more effective at reducing short-term (3 months) pain and long-term (12 months) impairment but not long-term pain, compared with social work plus medical management control arm.☺⊖ Physiotherapy may involve the use of heat or cold, depending on the phase of the disease and general condition of the patient. Limb elevation is used in patients with edema. Prevention of contractures is necessary.

6. **Other modalities** (for which evidence is very limited): Graded motor imagery and mirror therapy (physiotherapies), acupuncture (in conjunction

with rehabilitation therapy), gabapentin,⊗◯ sarpogrelate hydrochloride, local anesthetic sympathetic blockade, sympathectomy, pulsed electromagnetic field therapy, relaxation training, tactile discrimination training, stellate ganglion block under ultrasonography, manual lymphatic drainage with or without anti-inflammatory agents, physical therapy or exercise, and laser therapy.

→ PREVENTION

The following preventative strategies are generally recommended:
1) Avoidance of nerve damage during surgical procedures.
2) Early mobilization after surgery.
3) Physiotherapy.
4) Administration of vitamin C (500 mg/d for ~2 months) in patients after wrist fracture or before surgical treatment of foot fractures.

3. Amyloidosis

→ DEFINITION, ETIOLOGY, PATHOGENESIS

Amyloidosis is a group of diseases sharing the common feature of the extracellular accumulation of insoluble fibrous proteins called "amyloid" in tissues and organs. Etiology and pathogenesis are not fully understood.

Amyloidosis may be systemic (→below) or localized (eg, accumulation of amyloid β in Alzheimer disease and cerebral amyloid angiopathy). Types of amyloidosis differ with respect to the structure of proteins that form amyloid fibrils as well as clinical features and natural history of the disease.

1. AL amyloidosis (primary amyloidosis) occurs in patients with monoclonal gammopathies. Amyloid fibrils are formed by monoclonal immunoglobulin light chains.

2. AA amyloidosis (secondary, reactive amyloidosis) results from chronic inflammation (mainly rheumatoid arthritis, spondyloarthritis) or infection. The precursor of amyloid A is the acute-phase protein serum amyloid A (SAA).

3. Aβ_2-M amyloidosis is caused by long-term dialysis. The precursor of amyloid fibrils is β_2-microglobulin.

4. Familial amyloidosis is rare. The majority of different types of familial amyloidosis are autosomal dominant and caused by mutations in genes encoding various proteins. Most frequently this involves the transthyretin gene and leads to ATTR amyloidosis.

→ CLINICAL FEATURES AND NATURAL HISTORY

1. AL amyloidosis: Symptoms depend on the location and number of amyloid deposits.

2. AA amyloidosis: Features of the underlying condition and nephrotic syndrome causing progressive renal failure, diarrhea, malabsorption, and rarely features of cardiomyopathy.

3. Aβ_2-M amyloidosis: Carpal tunnel syndrome (usually the presenting symptom, often bilateral), joint pain and swelling (particularly affecting large joints), pathologic fractures.

4. ATTR amyloidosis: In all affected families the age of onset is similar. The presenting feature is peripheral sensory and motor neuropathy (starting in the lower extremities), cardiomyopathy (arrhythmia may be the only manifestation of cardiac involvement), or both; autonomic neuropathy usually presents with diarrhea and orthostatic hypotension.

→ DIAGNOSIS

Diagnostic Tests

1. Laboratory tests reveal proteinuria (the most frequent presenting feature; occurs in AA and AL amyloidosis as well as in some rare familial forms), elevated serum creatinine levels, elevated γ-glutamyl transferase (GGT) and alkaline phosphatase (ALP) liver isoenzyme levels (in AL amyloidosis), presence of a monoclonal protein and free light chains in serum or urine (in 90% of patients with AL amyloidosis).

2. Histologic examination: Usually biopsy specimens are collected from abdominal subcutaneous adipose tissue. Congo red staining and apple-green birefringence under polarized microscopy are part of the diagnostic algorithm.

3. Immunohistochemical studies are used to establish the type of amyloidosis.

Diagnostic Criteria

Diagnosis is based on clinical features, examination of biopsy specimens, and immunohistochemical studies. In patients with suspected amyloidosis and negative results of subcutaneous adipose tissue biopsy, perform biopsy of another organ, such as the kidney, liver, minor salivary glands in the lower lip, or gastrointestinal mucosa (eg, rectal or duodenal).

→ TREATMENT

1. Treatment of AL amyloidosis: Treatment of underlying monoclonal gammopathies.

2. Treatment of secondary amyloidosis (treatment in a specialized setting required):

1) Treatment of the underlying condition.

2) Specific treatment:

   a) Reducing the production of amyloid precursor proteins using anti-inflammatory and immunosuppressive drugs (the effectiveness of this approach has not been confirmed).

   b) Low-quality data suggest prevention of amyloid accumulation using oral colchicine 0.5 to 1 mg/d in monotherapy (in patients with a low erythrocyte sedimentation rate [ESR] and serum C-reactive protein [CRP] levels and no clinical features of amyloidosis) or in combination with cyclophosphamide (in patients with symptomatic amyloidosis).○

   c) Orthotopic liver transplantation in patients with familial ATTR amyloidosis was performed in selected cases to prevent organ damage, although progression of cardiac disease could still occur.○

3. Treatment of organ involvement depends on the location and symptoms.

4. Symptomatic treatment, as dictated by specific organ involvement.

→ PROGNOSIS

The estimated mean survival in patients with AA amyloidosis is ~10 years. Renal failure is the most common cause of death. Untreated patients with AL amyloidosis survive up to a year from the diagnosis. Cardiac involvement is a poor prognostic factor.

4. Antiphospholipid Syndrome

→ DEFINITION, ETIOLOGY, PATHOGENESIS

Antiphospholipid syndrome (APS) is a disease proposed to be caused by autoantibodies directed against protein-phospholipid complexes. It manifests as venous thrombosis, arterial thrombosis, and/or pregnancy morbidity. The etiology is unknown. Complications are attributed to procoagulant effects of antiphospholipid antibodies (APLAs): lupus anticoagulant (LA), anticardiolipin (aCL) antibodies, and anti–β_2-glycoprotein (GP) I antibodies. APS may be either **primary** (not related to any other disorder) or **secondary** (associated with another autoimmune disease, which in 30%-50% of cases is systemic lupus erythematosus [SLE]). Seronegative APS with clinical features of APS but no detectable serum antibodies has also been described.

→ CLINICAL FEATURES AND NATURAL HISTORY

Clinical manifestations depend on the vascular bed affected by thrombosis. Two-thirds of symptomatic patients have venous thrombosis.

1. Vascular thrombosis of the extremities is frequently bilateral, recurrent, and most commonly includes deep vein thrombosis (DVT). It can also involve vessels of the head and neck. Arterial thrombosis of the upper or lower extremities is rare; it causes symptoms of acute limb ischemia.

2. Vascular thrombosis of visceral organs may or may not be symptomatic and can affect any internal organ:

1) **Pulmonary involvement**: This manifests typically as pulmonary embolism, or rarely as pulmonary hypertension of thrombotic etiology or as diffuse alveolar hemorrhage secondary to small vessel capillaritis.

2) **Cardiac involvement**: The heart can be affected by thickening of the valve leaflets and impairment of the valvular function (mainly affecting the mitral valve, less commonly the aortic valve), small valvular vegetations (due to noninfective endocarditis, a risk factor for cerebrovascular accidents), or coronary artery thrombosis.

3) **Renal involvement**: >30% of patients develop renal thrombotic microangiopathy associated with hypertension, proteinuria of varying severity, microscopic hematuria, and mildly elevated serum creatinine levels. Symptomatic renal artery or vein thrombosis and renal infarcts are rare (<3% of patients).

4) **Involvement of other abdominal organs** is rare (<1% of patients) and may result in esophageal or intestinal ischemia or infarcts of the spleen, pancreas, or adrenal glands (causing Addison disease). Hepatic thrombosis may occur.

3. Vascular thrombosis of the central nervous system (~20% of patients) may cause ischemic stroke or transient ischemic attacks and is a leading cause of stroke in young patients. Recurrent strokes (including mild or asymptomatic microinfarcts manifesting as diffuse "white matter disease" on magnetic resonance imaging [MRI]) may lead to cognitive impairment or neuropsychiatric manifestations.

4. Thrombosis of the ocular vessels: Retinal artery or central retinal vein thrombosis can lead to transient loss of vision (amaurosis fugax) or optic neuritis.

5. Cutaneous manifestations: The most typical feature is livedo reticularis; less frequently observed manifestations are ischemic ulcers and cutaneous necrosis.

6. Musculoskeletal manifestations: About 40% of patients exhibit arthralgia; inflammatory arthritis is rare in the absence of SLE. Aseptic bone necrosis is rare.

7. Obstetric and fetal manifestations: Possible manifestations include fetal loss, premature birth, preeclampsia, placental insufficiency, and fetal growth retardation (→Table 4-1).

Table 4-1. Modified criteria for antiphospholipid antibody syndrome[a]

Clinical criteria

1. Vascular thrombosis: ≥1 episode of arterial, venous (excluding superficial veins), or small-vessel thrombosis affecting any tissue or organ confirmed by imaging studies, Doppler study, or histology; histologic features should reveal thrombosis without inflammation of the vessel wall

2. Pregnancy morbidity:
   1) ≥1 death of a morphologically normal fetus at ≥10 weeks' gestation (confirmed with ultrasonography or a direct examination)
   2) ≥1 preterm birth of a morphologically normal neonate before 34 weeks' gestation because of preeclampsia, eclampsia, or severe placental insufficiency
   3) ≥3 spontaneous miscarriages <10 weeks' gestation with no anatomic or chromosomal abnormalities

Laboratory criteria

1. Lupus anticoagulant detected in plasma on ≥2 occasions at a ≥12-week interval
2. IgG and/or IgM anticardiolipin antibodies present in the plasma or serum in a moderate or high titer (ie, >40 GPL or MPL units or >99th percentile) detected using a standardized ELISA method on ≥2 occasions at ≥12-week intervals
3. Anti–β_2-glycoprotein I antibodies in plasma or serum (in a titer >99th percentile) detected using a standardized ELISA method on ≥2 occasions at ≥12-week intervals

APS is diagnosed when ≥1 clinical and ≥1 laboratory criterion is fulfilled.
A **high-risk APLA profile** is defined as the presence of laboratory criterion 1; laboratory criteria 2 + 3; or persistently high APLA titers.

[a] The criteria must not be applied in patients with the onset of clinical manifestations of APS within <12 weeks or >5 years from the first detection of APLAs.

Adapted from J Thromb Haemost. 2006;4(2):295-306 and Ann Rheum Dis. 2019. doi: 10.1136/annrheumdis-2019-215213.

APS, antiphospholipid syndrome; APLA, antiphospholipid antibody; ELISA, enzyme-linked immunosorbent assay.

8. Catastrophic APS (CAPS): A subset of APS affecting <1% of individuals. CAPS is characterized by thrombosis in ≥3 organ systems occurring simultaneously or within a span of 1 week. The most common organ systems involved are kidneys, though involvement of virtually every organ system has been described. CAPS may be triggered by infections, surgical procedures, discontinuation of antithrombotic agents, subtherapeutic international normalized ratio (INR) levels on vitamin K antagonist (VKA) treatment, drugs, trauma, and stress. Symptoms depend on the site of thrombosis and include fever, dyspnea, abdominal pain, peripheral edema, cutaneous manifestations (purpura, livedo reticularis, necrosis), and altered mental status. Multisystem organ failure can ensue. Hematologic abnormalities can include thrombocytopenia, hemolytic anemia, and features of activation of the coagulation cascade. Mortality rates are as high as 50%.

→ DIAGNOSIS

Classification Criteria
Classification criteria: →Table 4-1.

Diagnostic Tests
1. Laboratory tests: APLAs are observed in >90% of patients (→Table 4-1). Lupus anticoagulant can cause prolongation of the activated partial

---

Table 4-2. Serologic features associated with a high risk for thrombosis in patients with positive antiphospholipid antibodies

- Lupus anticoagulant
- Lupus anticoagulant + aCL antibodies + anti-β_2-GPI antibodies
- Isolated positive aCL antibodies at medium-high titers (studied only in SLE)

A new definition of high-risk APLA profile: →Table 4-1

Adapted from Lupus. 2011;20(2):206-18.

aCL, anticardiolipin; anti-β_2-GPI, anti-β_2-glycoprotein I.

---

thromboplastin time (aPTT) in some assays; however, given the insensitivity, a prolonged aPTT is not diagnostic for the presence of lupus anticoagulant. Positive antinuclear antibodies are found in 45% of patients with primary APS. Mild thrombocytopenia (usually >50×10^9/L) is observed in ~30% of patients. Hemolytic anemia can occur.

2. Imaging studies: Results depend on the vascular bed affected by thrombosis.

Differential Diagnosis

1. Congenital and acquired thrombophilias (→Chapter 7.4.4).

2. Arterial thrombosis: Complications of atherosclerosis, vasculitis.

3. In case of prominent hematologic abnormalities: Thrombotic thrombocytopenic purpura (TTP), typical or atypical hemolytic-uremic syndrome (HUS), "HELLP syndrome" (Hemolysis, Elevated Liver enzymes, Low Platelet complicating pregnancy), sepsis, and disseminated intravascular coagulation (DIC).

→ TREATMENT

---

1. Acute thrombotic events: Treatment is the same as in patients without APS (CAPS: →below).

2. Primary prevention in patients with an APLA profile suggesting a high risk of thrombosis (→Table 4-2): Address cardiovascular risk factors; acetylsalicylic acid (ASA) may also be used, particularly in patients with SLE.⊘⊖ In patients with SLE and APLA, hydroxychloroquine is also recommended.⊘⊖ In patients with APLA and an increased risk of thrombosis (eg, surgery, immobility, puerperium), appropriate venous thromboembolism prophylaxis should be used.

3. Secondary prevention:

1) Patients with APLA (but without confirmed APS, for instance, low-titer positive aCL antibodies or lack of a second positive confirmatory antibody after 12 weeks) who present with a first episode of arterial or venous thrombosis should be treated as patients without APS.

2) Patients with a confirmed diagnosis of APS:

   a) Venous thrombosis: After initial treatment with heparin, start long-term (usually lifelong) treatment with a VKA. The target INR is 2.0 to 3.0.⊘⊖

   b) Isolated venous thromboembolism in the setting of a known transient precipitating risk factor and with a low-risk APLA profile (ie, negative lupus anticoagulant, low-titer aCL, or antibodies to β_2-GP I only): Start anticoagulation with VKA at a target INR of 2.0 to 3.0. A duration of treatment of 3 to 6 months only could be considered in this scenario.

   c) With a history of arterial thrombosis: Start long-term treatment. Depending on the individual risk of thrombosis, its complications (eg, APLA profile, additional cardiovascular risk factors, the first or subsequent thrombotic episode, risk of organ failure), and bleeding, you may consider: ASA + VKA (INR, 2.0-3.0) or a VKA with a target INR 2.0 to 3.0.

4. Treatment failure: First, verify that treatment failure occurred (therapeutic INR at the time of the event). If true failure has been confirmed, increase the intensity of the VKA therapy (target INR, 3.0-4.0) or switch to low-molecular-weight heparin (LMWH); in the case of arterial thrombosis, add ASA. The efficacy of direct oral anticoagulants (DOACs) in APS remains unclear but may be associated with increased harm compared with the use of warfarin.⊗◒

5. Thrombocytopenia: No treatment is indicated for mild thrombocytopenia without evidence of bleeding (platelet count >50 × 10^9/L). For symptomatic patients or patients with extreme thrombocytopenia (<20 × 10^9/L), consider treatment as in immune thrombocytopenia (→Chapter 7.4.3.1). For patients with an active systemic connective tissue disease, such as SLE, treat as SLE (→Chapter 14.21).

6. APS in pregnancy:

1) Patients with an uncomplicated pregnancy, no history of pregnancy morbidity, and an incidental finding of APLAs: No treatment or low-dose ASA.

2) Patients with a history of pregnancy morbidity and positive APLAs: Treatment depends on the type and level of the antibodies and may include ASA and LMWH. Referral to a specialist center is recommended.

7. CAPS: Treat the underlying cause if identified. Recommended first-line therapy is the combination of anticoagulation (typically with IV heparin), glucocorticoids, plasmapheresis, and/or intravenous immunoglobulin (IVIG).◒◯

8. Women with APS/APLAs should avoid the use of estrogens (in the form of oral contraceptive agents or hormone replacement therapy), as these may increase the risk of thrombosis⊗◯ (→Chapter 14.21).

→ PROGNOSIS

The prognosis depends on the location, severity, and frequency of thrombotic episodes and their complications. CAPS is a life-threatening condition. In secondary APS, the prognosis also depends on the underlying condition.

5. Calcium Pyrophosphate Dihydrate Deposition (CPPD) Disease

→ DEFINITION, ETIOLOGY, PATHOGENESIS

Calcium pyrophosphate dihydrate deposition (CPPD) disease, also known as **pseudogout** and **pyrophosphate arthropathy**, refers to a group of diseases caused by accumulation of calcium pyrophosphate dihydrate (CPP) crystals. CPPD disease most commonly occurs in articular fibrocartilage and hyaline cartilage. **Chondrocalcinosis** is caused by deposits of calcium salts (not only CPP) in joint cartilage; these are identified using imaging studies or during histologic examination.

The etiology of CPPD disease remains unknown. The disease may be familial with an autosomal dominant inheritance. **Secondary generalized (polyarticular) CPPD** may develop in patients with the following associated pathologies:

1) Endocrine disorders (thyrotoxicosis, hypothyroidism, hyperparathyroidism).

2) Hematologic disorders (hemochromatosis).

3) Electrolyte-related disorders (hypomagnesemia, hypophosphatemia).

4) Joint disorders (gout, previous joint injury).

5) Exogenous factors (persons receiving glucocorticoid therapy).

Localized CPPD may be associated with joint instability, prior resection of a joint meniscus, amyloid deposits, and biochemical abnormalities of cartilage matrix. This form of CPPD may be initiated by aging or injury and is mediated by factors such as transforming growth factor β.

CPP crystals formed in cartilage may move to synovium and synovial fluid and cause inflammation. The underlying mechanism is the same as in gout (→Chapter 14.8). Arthritis is often accompanied by degenerative lesions involving cartilage and bone.

→ CLINICAL FEATURES AND NATURAL HISTORY

CPPD disease rarely occurs before the age of 50 years. It is most frequently asymptomatic (isolated chondrocalcinosis or chondrocalcinosis coexisting with osteoarthritis) but may also cause symptoms of arthritis.

The following is a 6-phase classification for CPPD-related arthritis:

1) Acute CPP arthritis: Typically monoarticular, involving large joints (eg, knee).

2) Chronic CPP arthritis: Typically polyarticular, involving small and large joints.

3) Osteoarthritis with CPPD with an inflammatory component (chronic polyarticular arthritis with superimposed inflammatory acute arthritic episodes).

4) Osteoarthritis with CPPD without an inflammatory component (chronic polyarticular arthritis but without an inflammatory component).

5) Asymptomatic CPPD: Articular CPPD without signs or symptoms.

6) Pseudoneuropathic CPPD: Severe destructive arthropathy resembling neuropathic arthritis.

Episodes of acute CPPD arthritis are similar to those of gout, but symptoms develop less rapidly, over 6 to 24 hours, and pain is less severe. Joint pain lasts from 1 day to 4 weeks and most frequently affects the knees, with occasional involvement of shoulders, wrists, and the first metatarsophalangeal (MTP) joint of the foot.

Chronic CPPD arthritis may involve several joints concurrently and resemble rheumatoid arthritis. Episodes of acute arthritis may be superimposed on chronic arthritic disease.

CPPD-associated osteoarthritis most often affects the knee, although wrists, MTP joints, elbows, shoulders, hips, ankles, the tarsus, and the metatarsus may also be involved. Changes are typically symmetric. Unlike in osteoarthritis without CPPD, patients usually have narrowing of the lateral joint space of the knee and osteophytes and inflammation are more frequent. In addition to peripheral joints, CPPD may also involve the lumbar spine, causing symptoms similar to ankylosing spondylitis. Peripheral joint involvement may resemble joint changes caused by peripheral neuropathy (Charcot joints).

→ DIAGNOSIS

A complete history is of key importance and should include symptoms, chronicity and pattern of arthritis, associated conditions, and records of previous treatment. The accompanying physical examination should include a complete joint examination as well as close observation of the skin and examination for other extra-articular signs of inflammatory arthritis.

The diagnosis of CPPD disease requires the documented presence of CPP crystals in synovial fluid. CPPD can be diagnosed on the basis of joint lesions found on imaging studies and histologic examination; the absence of deposits on radiographs does not exclude the diagnosis.

Diagnostic Tests

1. Synovial fluid examination: Definitive diagnosis relies on the identification of CPP crystals based on synovial fluid examination. During an attack of acute arthritis, synovial fluid may be milky, slightly blood-stained, and inflammatory. CPP crystals are present in the sediment and are often visible in the cytoplasm of granulocytes, macrophages, or both. When carefully examined under polarized light microscopy, CPP crystals may reveal weakly positively birefringent rhomboid-shaped crystals (although the absence of birefringence does not exclude CPPD arthritis).

2. Radiography: CPP crystal deposits may be found in hyaline cartilage and fibrocartilage, tendons, ligaments, fascia, and joint capsules. Most often deposits present as punctate linear radiodense areas within the cartilage of the knee, hip, or elbow joints, and often also in the wrists. In the knee, triangular deposits are often seen within the menisci. In the spine, deposits may be found within the intervertebral cartilage. Radiographic examination of the knees, pelvis, and wrist should be conducted in all patients with suspected polyarticular CPPD. Plain radiographs are valuable to confirm a diagnosis of CPPD, but the absence of chondrocalcinosis should not be used to exclude the diagnosis.○

3. Ultrasonography and computed tomography (CT): Ultrasonography and other imaging modalities such as CT may detect small deposits that are sometimes missed by plain radiographs. Deposits may appear as hyperechoic streaks in hyaline cartilage and "shiny" punctate lesions in fibrocartilage. The diagnostic properties of the tests are, at best, moderate and their clinical utility is unclear.◑

4. Biochemistry: Blood tests may reveal elevated serum levels of calcium, parathyroid hormone, alkaline phosphatase, ferritin, iron, and total iron--binding capacity. Hypomagnesemia may be present. Serum erythrocyte sedimentation rate (ESR) and C-reactive protein (CRP) levels may be elevated, as with most inflammatory conditions, but they are of little diagnostic value, given their lack of specificity. Rheumatoid factor is positive in ~10% of CPPD patients.

Differential Diagnosis

The differential diagnosis of CPPD includes acute arthritis associated with gout (CPP may coexist with gout; 20% of patients with CPPD also have hyperuricemia), acute septic arthritis, osteoarthritis, rheumatoid arthritis (positive rheumatoid factor in ~10% of patients), Charcot joints, polymyalgia rheumatica, and Milwaukee shoulder syndrome (apatite-associated destructive arthritis).

→ TREATMENT

General Measures

As per the 2011 European League Against Rheumatism (EULAR) CPPD guidelines, optimal management requires both nonpharmacologic and pharmacologic treatments that are tailored to clinical features, general risk factors, and predisposing metabolic disorders.

No currently available treatment modifies CPP crystal formation or deposition.

In patients with secondary CPPD, treatment of the underlying condition is necessary. The goals of treatment include pain reduction and improved function of the affected joints.

Treatment of associated conditions (eg, hyperparathyroidism, hemochromatosis, hypomagnesemia) should be considered as part of the management plan for CPPD.

Treatment goals and strategies for CPPD with comorbid osteoarthritis are the same as without osteoarthritis.

Treatment of Acute Arthritis

1. Local therapy: Cold compresses (eg, ice packs, cool gel packs), temporary rest, synovial fluid aspiration, and intra-articular long-acting glucocorticoid injections may provide sufficient analgesia.

2. Initial systemic therapy: Systemic therapy with oral colchicine or non-steroidal anti-inflammatory drugs (NSAIDs) may provide rapid relief⊘○ but their use may be limited by toxicity and comorbidities in some patients.

3. Other systemic therapy: In patients not responding to intra-articular glucocorticoid injections, short-term oral or parenteral glucocorticoids in doses tapered over time are a reasonable alternative to colchicine and NSAIDs. Parenteral adrenocorticotropic hormone may also be considered in this setting.

Long-Term Treatment

1. Asymptomatic CPPD requires no treatment.

2. Frequent recurrences of acute arthritis: Low-dose colchicine in doses 0.5 to 1 mg/d or NSAIDs may be used to prevent relapses.

3. Chronic arthritis: Drugs that may be used are (in the order of choice): oral NSAIDs, low-dose colchicine (0.5-1 mg/d), or both; low-dose glucocorticoids; methotrexate; and hydroxychloroquine. Nevertheless, the efficacy of this approach is poorly documented.

4. Osteoarthritis associated with CPPD: Treatment is similar to that of osteoarthritis without CPPD. Note that intra-articular hyaluronic acid should not be used, as it may precipitate acute arthritis.

6. Erythema Nodosum

→ DEFINITION, ETIOLOGY, PATHOGENESIS

Erythema nodosum refers to inflammatory nodular lesions in the subcutaneous tissue characterized histologically by septal inflammation. Immune complexes are thought to play a role in the pathogenesis.

Causes of erythema nodosum:

1) **Infection**: Streptococci, *Mycobacterium tuberculosis*, *Mycobacterium leprae*, *Yersinia* spp, *Salmonella* spp, *Chlamydophila pneumoniae*, *Neisseria gonorrhoeae*, viruses (cytomegalovirus, hepatitis B virus, hepatitis C virus, Epstein-Barr virus, HIV), fungi.

2) **Drugs**: Antibiotics (particularly penicillin), sulfonamides, pyrazole derivatives.

3) **Diseases**: Sarcoidosis (one of the most frequent causes), inflammatory bowel disease, Sweet syndrome (acute febrile neutrophilic dermatosis), systemic connective tissue diseases (systemic lupus erythematosus, polymyositis/dermatomyositis, systemic sclerosis, systemic vasculitis syndromes).

4) **Pregnancy or oral contraceptives**.

→ CLINICAL FEATURES AND NATURAL HISTORY

Erythema nodosum occurs mainly in women (~90% of cases). The appearance of lesions is often accompanied by malaise, low-grade or high-grade fever, joint pain, arthritis, symptoms of upper respiratory tract infection, and gastrointestinal symptoms (abdominal pain, diarrhea). Nodules are most commonly located on the anterior lower leg (less frequently on the posterior lower leg), and less often on thighs, buttocks, shoulders, head, and trunk. The lesions are usually from 1 to 1.5 cm in diameter and may coalesce. Skin over the lesions is erythematous and warm but necrosis never occurs. The nodules are painful, persist for 2 to 9 weeks, and then resolve without scarring. Dark discoloration in the locations of the nodules usually persists for several weeks after they have resolved. Relapses occur in approximately half of the patients, most often in winter and spring.

→ DIAGNOSIS

Diagnostic Tests

1. Blood tests: With the appearance of the nodules, the tests reveal an elevated erythrocyte sedimentation rate (in 60%-85% of patients), leukocytosis with neutrophilia, and elevated serum immunoglobulin (a frequent feature) and aminotransferase levels.

2. Other studies are used depending on the cause. For instance, chest radiographs may reveal features typical for sarcoidosis.

Diagnostic Criteria

Diagnosis is based on clinical features. A skin biopsy is performed in exceptional cases, for instance, when the condition needs to be differentiated from idiopathic panniculitis (Weber-Christian disease).

Differential Diagnosis

Panniculitis, subcutaneous tissue changes directly caused by infection (most commonly staphylococcal), superficial vein thrombosis, cutaneous vasculitis (eg, urticarial vasculitis). Differential diagnosis also includes all the conditions that may cause erythema nodosum (→Definition, Etiology, Pathogenesis, above).

→ TREATMENT

1. Treatment of the underlying condition.

2. Symptomatic treatment: Nonsteroidal anti-inflammatory drugs (NSAIDs) may be used if local or systemic symptoms are judged to require treatment; if these are ineffective, short-term glucocorticoids may be used cautiously (note: they may be harmful, eg, in patients with tuberculosis).

7. Fibromyalgia

→ DEFINITION, ETIOLOGY, PATHOGENESIS

Fibromyalgia (FM) is a pain syndrome of unknown etiology manifesting as chronic widespread musculoskeletal pain that is frequently accompanied by fatigue and multiple somatic and psychosomatic complaints.

→ CLINICAL FEATURES AND NATURAL HISTORY

FM is 8 times more common in women than in men. It primarily affects white women between 35 and 55 years of age. Symptoms of FM include chronic widespread muscle and joint pain generalized to multiple body regions, chronic fatigue, cognitive symptoms, sleep disturbances, headaches, lower abdominal pain or cramping, and depression. Some rheumatologists question the concept of this disease.

FM is a common chronic condition and it is not typically degenerative or life-threatening. It is often associated with a high degree of disease burden,

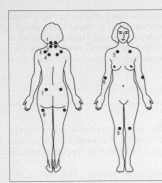

1 – Suboccipital muscle insertions
2 – Intertransverse spaces at C5–C7
3 – Midpoint of the upper border of the trapezius muscle
4 – Insertion of the supraspinatus muscle above the medial border of the scapular spine
5 – Second costochondral junctions
6 – 2 cm distal to the lateral epicondyle of the humerus
7 – Upper outer quadrants of buttocks
8 – Posterior to the trochanteric prominence
9 – Medial femoral condyle

Figure 7-1. Tender points in fibromyalgia (no longer part of the diagnostic criteria).

with few significant changes over time in the majority of patients. Complete remission, with full resolution of chronic pain, is rare.

DIAGNOSIS

Diagnostic Tests

No biochemical or radiographic investigations are diagnostic of FM. Diagnosis is made primarily on the basis of the clinical picture.

Diagnostic Criteria

To satisfy the modified 2016 FM criteria, the following 3 conditions must all be met:

1) Widespread pain index (WPI) ≥7 and symptom severity scale (SSS) score ≥5 **or** WPI 4 to 6 and SSS score ≥9.

2) Generalized pain (pain in ≥4 of 5 regions, including left and right upper and lower regions and the axial region) must be present. Jaw, chest, and abdominal pain are not included in the generalized pain definition.

3) Symptoms have been generally present for ≥3 months.

The new diagnostic criteria do not include a precise assessment of tender points (→Figure 7-1) and do not take into consideration secondary FM, which may occur in patients with other rheumatologic disorders. A diagnosis of FM may be valid irrespective of other diagnoses and it does not exclude the presence of other clinically important conditions. Unlike previous guidance regarding diagnosis, the new criteria have been standardized for both patients and health-care providers to encourage uniformity.

Differential Diagnosis

1. Rheumatologic diseases: Rheumatoid arthritis, systemic lupus erythematosus, polymyalgia rheumatica, myositis, myopathies, ankylosing spondylitis.

2. Neurologic disorders: Chronic neuropathic pain.

3. Endocrine disorders: Hypothyroidism.

TREATMENT

Treatment of FM is contentious. While practices vary significantly, the following treatment modalities are considered in recent practice guidelines:

1) The recommended nonpharmacologic therapies are **aerobic and strengthening exercises**. Other suggested treatments that may be tried include

cognitive behavioral therapy, acupuncture and hydrotherapy, meditative movement therapies (yoga, tai chi, qigong), and mindfulness therapy. Authors of the European League Against Rheumatism (EULAR) guidelines suggested against the use of biofeedback, hypnotherapy, and massage therapy.

2) Suggested pharmacologic treatments that could be tried for several weeks include low-dose amitriptyline (10-50 mg/d),⊘⊖ duloxetine or milnacipran (serotonin-norepinephrine reuptake inhibitors [SNRIs]), tramadol (although recent concerns have been raised about its overall safety),⊖ pregabalin (150-600 mg/d), and cyclobenzaprine (1-40 mg/d). The EULAR guidelines issued a strong recommendation against the use of growth hormone and sodium oxybate and suggestions against the use of capsaicin, monoamine oxidase inhibitors, nonsteroidal anti-inflammatory drugs, glucocorticoids, and selective serotonin reuptake inhibitors (SSRIs). No recommendations were issued regarding cannabinoids and antipsychotics.

8. Gout

→ DEFINITION, ETIOLOGY, PATHOGENESIS

Gout is a type of arthritis that is caused by the deposition of monosodium urate (MSU) crystals in synovial fluid. In addition, MSU can also be found in periarticular tissue, pinnae (as gouty tophi), kidneys (renal interstitium, tubes, and ureters), and at various other body sites.

Hyperuricemia is defined as serum uric acid levels >7 mg/dL (420 µmol/L). It may be either **primary** (due to an innate cause, such as a genetic abnormality of enzymes involved in purine metabolism) or **secondary** (due to an identifiable underlying pathology). Pathology involved in secondary hyperuricemia may be associated with:

1) **Increased production of urate**: Increased dietary purine intake (eg, meat, broth, some types of seafood) and tumor lysis syndrome (a common complication in solid organ transplant patients).

2) **Decreased excretion of urate**: Impaired renal excretion secondary to comorbid disorders (eg, patients with polycystic kidney disease, lead nephropathy), drugs (eg, diuretics, salicylates, pyrazinamide, ethambutol), and a ketogenic diet.

3) **Mixed etiology**: Alcohol use disorder (via accelerated adenosine triphosphate [ATP] degradation and increased lactic acid production), high dietary fructose intake (via accelerated ATP degradation and inhibition of uric acid secretion), and starvation (via increased purine conversion and impaired renal excretion).

Ultimately, however, it remains unclear what precise factors are directly responsible for the deposition of MSU crystals in synovial fluid and tissues in persons with hyperuricemia.

Crystal-induced arthritis may be acute or chronic. Recurrent acute episodes of arthritis (gouty attacks) and progression to chronic arthritis usually lead to progressive damage to articular cartilage and bone.

→ CLINICAL FEATURES AND NATURAL HISTORY

Gout is most prevalent in men >40 years of age and postmenopausal women. The natural history of gout can be divided into the following phases:

1) Asymptomatic hyperuricemia.

2) Episodes of acute gouty arthritis.

3) Periods of remission between attacks.

4) Chronic (tophaceous) gout.

Notably, the majority of patients with hyperuricemia never develop gout.

A different 4-phase classification proposal includes:

1) A high risk of gout (mostly hyperuricemia) without clinical features and without MSU crystal deposition in tissues detected by microscopy or imaging studies.

2) Asymptomatic hyperuricemia with MSU crystal deposition.

3) Acute flares of gout.

4) Tophaceous gout, chronic arthritis, and bone erosions detected by radiography.

Acute gouty arthritis manifests as sudden-onset very severe joint pain and swelling. The skin over the joint is erythematous, taut, and shiny. Epidermal desquamation develops early. Edema of subcutaneous tissue and effusions in large joints are seen. Symptoms most commonly affect the metatarsophalangeal (MTP) joint of the big toe (this is known as podagra; in ~95% of patients the joint is involved in the course of gout) and commonly occur in the early morning. Ankles, knees, and less frequently joints of the upper extremities may also be affected. Untreated acute gouty arthritis lasts from 10 days to 3 weeks and tends to resolve spontaneously. Factors triggering acute gouty arthritis include alcohol intake, fructose intake, consumption of large amounts of purine-rich foods (particularly meat), strenuous exercise, trauma, surgery, infection, low temperatures, and drugs (eg, thiazide or loop diuretics, cyclosporine [INN ciclosporin], low-dose acetylsalicylic acid [ASA]).

In patients with acute gouty arthritis recurrence may be expected after 6 months to 2 years, although the duration of remission varies. With time, gouty attacks may occur more frequently and patients gradually develop chronic polyarthritis (typically after 5-10 years). Urate deposits accumulate near the joints and in other tissues (gouty tophi) and may lead to renal failure. Approximately one--third of patients develop nephrolithiasis, which may manifest as renal colic, and 20% to 40% of patients have proteinuria. Hyperlipidemia, hyperglycemia, obesity, and hypertension often coexist with hyperuricemia, leading to an increased risk of cardiovascular diseases caused by atherosclerosis. Avascular necrosis of the femoral head is another potential complication of gout.

→ DIAGNOSIS

Diagnostic Criteria

The diagnosis of gout can be confirmed only on finding phagocytosed MSU crystals in synovial fluid obtained by joint aspiration or in gouty tophi. The clinical diagnosis of gout is suggested by symptoms of acute monoarthritis, most frequently affecting the first MTP joint, with periarticular erythema, which is most severe in the first 6 to 12 hours. Rapid improvement after the administration of colchicine supports the diagnosis of gout. In patients with chronic arthritis diagnosis is confirmed by joint changes found on radiographs.

Diagnostic Tests

Diagnostic tests include a combination of laboratory measures, synovial fluid analysis, imaging investigations and, at times, biopsies.

In patients with clinical presentations indicative of possible acute gout, synovial fluid analysis should be used as the diagnostic test of choice.

1. Laboratory tests: Elevated serum uric acid levels (although these may be normal during an acute gouty attack), often increased urinary urate excretion, hyperlipidemia, and elevated serum creatinine and glucose levels.

2. Synovial fluid: Inflammatory, containing MSU crystals. Cultures should always be ordered to exclude a coexisting bacterial infection. The American College of Physicians (ACP) recommends that clinicians use synovial fluid analysis when clinical judgment indicates that diagnostic testing is necessary in patients suspected of having acute gout.

3. Imaging studies: In patients with crystal deposits in cartilage and bone, **radiographs** may reveal narrowing of the joint space and well-defined bone erosions, sometimes with extensive osteolysis. When using **ultrasonography**, MSU crystals in synovial fluid may give a "snowstorm" appearance, while crystal deposits in articular cartilage may cause a "double outline." Crystals may also be seen in vessel walls. **Ultrasonography, computed tomography (CT), or magnetic resonance imaging (MRI)** may demonstrate MSU deposits in periarticular tissues (eg, tendons).

4. Biopsy: Histologic examination of periarticular tophi is performed to establish whether they are due to MSU deposition (MSU or uric acid crystal deposits may also be found in renal biopsy specimens). Biopsy material should be fixed in anhydrous ethanol, because all commonly used formaldehyde solutions may dissolve the crystals. Crystals may also be found in discharge from fistulae that can develop near gouty tophi.

Differential Diagnosis

1. Acute gouty arthritis: Acute arthritis caused by calcium pyrophosphate dihydrate (CPP) crystals (also termed pseudogout), arthritis associated with hyperlipidemia, infectious arthritis, reactive arthritis, trauma, hemarthrosis, serum sickness, early symptoms of other types of chronic arthritis and inflammatory osteoarthritis.

2. Chronic gouty arthritis: Rheumatoid arthritis, osteoarthritis.

→ TREATMENT

Treatment goals include rapid suppression of pain and inflammation in acute gout, preventing recurrence of gouty episodes, and inhibiting the evolution of chronic synovitis and associated connective tissue destruction.

General Measures

1. Provide patients with **information** about causes and consequences of gout and hyperuricemia, management of acute flares, lifestyle and dietary factors, activity, alcohol use, and urate-lowering therapies for prophylaxis. Before urate-lowering therapy is initiated, a discussion regarding benefits, harms, cost, values, and preferences should take place.

2. Weight reduction in overweight patients.

3. Low-purine diet: Avoidance of purine-rich products. Consumption of milk and low-fat dairy products is recommended.

4. Avoidance of alcohol (particularly beer), fructose, and tobacco.

5. Asymptomatic hyperuricemia is an indication for pharmacologic treatment in patients with serum uric acid levels >12 mg/dL (720 µmol/L), 24-hour urinary uric acid excretion >1100 mg, or as prevention of tumor lysis syndrome; in such instances, use allopurinol (→below).

6. An **individualized management strategy** with attention to concurrent comorbidities and medications.

7. Medication changes may be warranted in the presence of gout. For example, as per the 2016 European League Against Rheumatism (EULAR) guidelines, for patients on **loop or thiazide diuretics**, angiotensin receptor blockers (eg, losartan) or calcium channel blockers may be considered for hypertension, and statins or fibrates may be considered for hyperlipidemia.

Treatment of Acute Gouty Arthritis

1. Oral **colchicine**⊘☺: Moderate-quality evidence has shown that lower doses of colchicine (initially 1.2 mg followed by 0.6 mg after 1 hour) are as effective as higher doses for pain control and have fewer adverse effects. The recommended dose as per the 2016 EULAR guidelines is a loading dose of 1 mg followed 1 hour later by 0.5 mg on day 1.

Adverse effects of colchicine are primarily gastrointestinal (diarrhea, nausea, vomiting, abdominal cramping, and pain). Colchicine should be avoided in patients with severe renal impairment and in those receiving strong P-glycoprotein or CYP3A4 inhibitors (eg, cyclosporine, clarithromycin).

2. Oral **nonsteroidal anti-inflammatory drugs (NSAIDs)**⊘◌: Low-quality evidence has demonstrated a significant reduction in pain and subsequent gout flares with NSAIDs. NSAIDs at maximum doses have been recommended as the drugs of choice by the British Society for Rheumatology (BSR). Adverse effects are primarily gastrointestinal, ranging from minor (dyspepsia) to major (perforations, ulcers, and bleeding) complications. NSAIDs should be avoided in patients with severe renal impairment.

3. Glucocorticoids: Oral glucocorticoids have been also recommended by the ACP in patients without contraindications. They are a cost-effective alternative, with efficacy comparable with NSAIDs and fewer adverse effects. The recommended dose as per the 2016 EULAR guidelines is 30 to 35 mg daily of equivalent prednisolone dose for 3 to 5 days. Adverse effects include mood disorders, hyperglycemia, immunosuppression, and fluid retention.

Joint aspiration and injection of a glucocorticoid have also been recommended by the BSR as being highly effective in acute monoarticular gout and, potentially, as the treatment of choice for acute flares in patients with comorbidities.

4. Animal-derived **corticotropin**: Moderate-quality evidence shows pain reduction in patients with acute gout receiving parenteral corticotropin, with outcomes comparable to NSAIDs and glucocorticoids. Adverse effects are assumed to be similar to glucocorticoids.

5. In patients refractory to treatment, a combination of the above anti-inflammatory therapies (colchicine, NSAIDs, glucocorticoids) may be employed.

6. In some jurisdictions interleukin-1 (IL-1) inhibitors (canakinumab or anakinra) are approved for use in specialized settings in patients who are not controlled by usual treatments.

Long-Term Prophylaxis of Recurrent Gouty Attacks

1. Avoidance of triggering factors: As above.

2. Prophylactic colchicine: In patients with frequent attacks consider long-term treatment (ie, up to 6 months) with colchicine 0.5 to 1 mg/d (EULAR guidelines) or 0.6 to 1.2 mg/d (ACP guidelines).

3. Urate-lowering therapies: To reduce uric acid synthesis, the xanthine oxidase inhibitor allopurinol remains the first-line drug of choice, with febuxostat as an alternative. To increase urinary uric acid excretion, the uricosuric agents benzbromarone or probenecid as well as fenofibrate and losartan are indicated. Uric acid degradation (with pegloticase) is a further option.

As per the 2016 EULAR guidelines, urate-lowering therapy should be considered in all patients with a definite diagnosis of gout from their first presentation and is indicated in all patients with recurrent flares, tophi, urate arthropathy, or renal stones. The ACP recommends against initiating long-term urate-lowering therapy in most patients after a first gouty attack and in patients with infrequent attacks.

As per the 2016 EULAR guidelines, in gouty arthritis the target serum uric acid level is ≤6 mg/dL (360 µmol/L), and lower levels are recommended in tophaceous gout (≤5 mg/dL [300 µmol/L] but not ≤3 mg/dL [180 µmol/L]).

Because urate-lowering therapy may precipitate an acute gouty attack, start with low doses and for the first 6 to 12 months of treatment combine this with low-dose colchicine or an NSAID; if these are contraindicated or ineffective, glucocorticoids ≤10 mg/d can be used. The traditional advice was to wait 2 to 4 weeks until an acute gouty attack has resolved before starting uricosuric/

urate-lowering treatment; however, there is reasonable clinical suggestion that starting allopurinol immediately is unlikely harmful.◯ If an acute attack occurs during uricosuric/urate-lowering treatment, the drug should not be discontinued.

1) **Allopurinol**: There is moderate-quality evidence that allopurinol probably does not reduce the number of acute gouty attacks but does increase the proportion of individuals achieving target serum uric acid levels without serious adverse events.⊘◯ In patients with normal kidney function, the 2016 EULAR guidelines recommend starting allopurinol at 100 mg daily and increasing by 100 mg every 2 to 4 weeks as needed to reach the target serum uric acid level. In patients with renal impairment, the maximum dosage should be adjusted to creatinine clearance. Potential adverse effects include hypersensitivity reactions (fever, rash, hepatitis, eosinophilia, renal failure).

2) **Febuxostat**: A second-line drug used in patients not responding to allopurinol. Potential adverse effects include abdominal pain, diarrhea, and musculoskeletal pain. Febuxostat is contraindicated in patients with prior hypersensitivity reactions to allopurinol; the risk of adverse effects appears to be higher in patients with impaired kidney or liver function. Recent postmarketing trial evidence suggests that febuxostat may be associated with increased cardiovascular and all-cause mortality events compared with allopurinol. The US Food and Drug Administration suggests that it should be used only in patients in whom treatment with allopurinol has failed or is not tolerated and that clinicians should counsel patients about the drug's cardiovascular risk.◯

3) **Probenecid and benzbromarone**: Uricosurics, recommended in patients without an adequate response to allopurinol alone. Recommended dose ranges according to the 2016 EULAR guidelines are probenecid 1 to 2 g daily and benzbromarone 50 to 200 mg daily. Benzbromarone is more potent than probenecid. These agents are indicated in patients with hyperuricemia caused by impaired renal uric acid excretion (<700 mg/24 h). Contraindications include age >60 years, creatinine clearance <50 mL/min, and nephrolithiasis. Combination therapy with allopurinol and a uricosuric may be more effective than allopurinol alone.

4) **Pegloticase**: A recombinant uricase (an enzyme that degrades uric acid to easily excreted allantoin). The 2016 EULAR guidelines recommend pegloticase in patients with crystal-proven, severe, debilitating, chronic tophaceous gout and poor quality of life, where other drugs at maximal doses are unable to achieve the target serum uric acid level. Allergic reactions are a common adverse effect.

9. Infectious (Septic) Arthritis

→ **DEFINITION, ETIOLOGY, PATHOGENESIS**

Infectious arthritis is acute or chronic arthritis caused by microorganisms that have infected the synovium. The infection is most frequently blood-borne, direct (joint aspiration, arthroscopy, orthopedic surgery, trauma), or it spreads by continuity from adjacent tissues (infected skin ulcers, cellulitis, osteomyelitis).

Etiologic agents in adults are most commonly bacteria (*Staphylococcus aureus*, *Streptococcus pyogenes*, less frequently gram-negative pathogens, including *Neisseria gonorrhoeae*, *Neisseria meningitidis*) and less often viruses (rubella virus, hepatitis virus B and C, parvovirus B19, chikungunya virus, zika virus), fungi, and parasites.

Risk factors for bacterial arthritis include rheumatic diseases (rheumatoid arthritis [RA], systemic lupus erythematosus [SLE]), joint replacement surgery (particularly of the knee or hip), treatment with tumor necrosis factor (TNF)-α inhibitors, joint aspiration, advanced age, diabetes mellitus, immunosuppression (alcohol dependence, immunosuppressive treatment, HIV infection), IV drug use, renal or liver failure, and hemophilia.

→ CLINICAL FEATURES AND NATURAL HISTORY

Local manifestations: Pain, swelling, erythema, warming of the joint, and a decreased range of motion. Symptoms usually appear suddenly and progress rapidly. In some cases (tuberculosis, fungal infection, bacterial infection in individuals with RA or other connective tissue disorders, elderly patients, low virulence organisms) the course of infectious arthritis may be chronic and indolent. In 90% of patients bacterial arthritis affects only one joint, while in 10% of patients it affects multiple joints and is usually due to bacteremia. In prosthetic joint infections chronic joint loosening may develop.

General manifestations: Fever, rarely with chills or rigors; elderly patients are more frequently afebrile.

Features typical for specific etiologic factors:

1) **Nongonococcal bacterial arthritis**: Most frequently monoarthritis (usually of the knee). In ~20% of patients 2 to 3 joints are affected; septic polyarthritis is rare (it may develop, eg, in patients with RA or sepsis). In elderly patients symptoms may be minor. Joint aspirate cultures are positive in 70% of patients and blood cultures are positive in 24% to 76% of patients. In 30% to 50% of patients septic arthritis causes permanent joint damage.

2) **Gonococcal arthritis**: Migrating pain or polyarthritis (affecting knees, ankles, wrists), usually in young adults; rarely acute monoarthritis. Gonococcal arthritis frequently coexists with involvement of tendon sheaths and with cutaneous lesions (hemorrhagic bullae, papules, pustules). Joint aspirate cultures are positive in <25% of patients and blood cultures are rarely positive. The prognosis is good in >95% of patients.

3) **Viral arthritis**: Frequently polyarthritis (wrists and fingers), occasionally resembling RA (in parvovirus B19 infection). Patients may have coexisting cutaneous lesions (urticaria, erythema, petechiae) that resolve after 2 to 3 weeks. Viral arthritis mainly affects young women (it needs to be differentiated from SLE). Arthritis with associated fever is the main clinical sign of chikungunya infection and less commonly of zika infection, both of which should be considered in the differential diagnosis of patients who have traveled to tropical countries.

4) **Tuberculous arthritis**: Most commonly chronic arthritis affecting one large joint (the hip or knee). It is usually accompanied by osteomyelitis and myelitis. Joint aspirate cultures are positive in >80% of patients; synovial membrane biopsy is necessary for rapid diagnosis. This diagnosis is frequently delayed due to nonspecific symptoms and clinical course.

5) **Fungal arthritis**: Usually chronic monoarthritis, less commonly severe polyarthritis (sometimes accompanied by erythema nodosum).

→ DIAGNOSIS

Diagnostic Tests

1. Laboratory tests in most patients reveal significantly elevated erythrocyte sedimentation rate (ESR) and C-reactive protein (CRP) levels, leukocytosis (particularly in patients with bacterial arthritis), and hypochromic anemia (in patients with chronic arthritis, eg, tuberculous arthritis).

2. Synovial fluid examination: This should include macroscopic assessment (septic fluid is usually cloudy and yellow-grey or yellow-green) and cell counts (these are often $>25 \times 10^9$/L to 100×10^9/L, including >75% of neutrophils).

Gram-stained synovial fluid smears are used to guide empiric antimicrobial treatment (in patients with negative culture results this may be the only evidence of bacterial arthritis); cultures of synovial fluid should be performed (in patients with suspected gonococcal arthritis perform blood cultures and synovial fluid cultures as well as cultures/nucleic acid amplification test [NAAT] of swabs from the urethra, cervix, rectum, and throat). Synovial fluid must be examined for the presence of crystals.

3. Blood cultures or cultures of other specimens, depending on clinical features.

4. Molecular or serologic investigations depending on the suspected pathogen.

5. Imaging studies: In patients with early arthritis **radiographs** reveal soft tissue edema and features of effusion. After ~1 week they show periarticular osteoporosis and in severe cases also joint space narrowing (caused by destruction of articular cartilage). After ~2 weeks peripheral erosions are seen (due to destruction of subchondral bone by pannus). In patients with chronic arthritis, bony or fibrous adhesions may form. In prosthetic joint infections loosening of the prosthesis can be seen with chronic joint infection. **Ultrasonography** is used mainly to monitor the volume of effusions and to mark sites for aspiration. Occasionally **computed tomography (CT), magnetic resonance imaging (MRI), or scintigraphy** may be indicated.

Diagnostic Criteria

Diagnosis is based on clinical features, synovial fluid examination (macroscopic assessment, Gram staining, cultures), and blood cultures. In patients with gonococcal arthritis perform screening for other sexually transmitted diseases, including syphilis, *Chlamydia trachomatis*, and HIV infections.

Differential Diagnosis

Acute crystal-associated arthropathy (gout, pseudogout; differentiation from bacterial arthritis based solely on clinical examination is difficult, synovial fluid examination is conclusive; note that infectious arthritis may accompany gout), reactive arthritis (this may be acute monoarthritis, particularly following a genitourinary or respiratory tract infection), acute monoarthritis as part of noninfectious polyarthritis (RA [in RA exacerbations macroscopic features of synovial fluid may be similar to synovial fluid in infectious arthritis; perform cultures and withhold intra-articular administration of glucocorticoids], SLE, psoriatic arthritis), Lyme disease, hemarthrosis following joint trauma, rheumatic fever, subacute bacterial endocarditis, infections of periarticular tissues (eg, bursitis).

➡ TREATMENT

1. Bacterial arthritis: In patients with suspected bacterial arthritis start empiric antimicrobial therapy after obtaining appropriate specimens. Empiric coverage should include vancomycin and/or cefazolin, based on local antibiograms, for gram-positive cocci and ceftriaxone for gram-negative cocci.

1) **Nongonococcal bacterial arthritis**: If gram-positive organisms are found, use IV vancomycin 30 mg/kg/d (usually up to 2 g/d) in 2 to 3 divided doses if there is a high epidemiologic suspicion of methicillin-resistant *Staphylococcus aureus* (MRSA). In patients with low risk for MRSA, cefazolin 1 to 2 g every 8 hours could be used; if gram-negative organisms are found, use a third-generation IV cephalosporin (ceftazidime 1-2 g every 8 hours, ceftriaxone 2 g every 24 hours, or cefotaxime 2 g every 8 hours). In the case of gram-negative strains, use vancomycin in immunocompetent patients and add a third-generation cephalosporin in immunocompromised patients or patients with a history of joint trauma. Change antibiotics based on culture results. IV antimicrobial treatment is usually continued for 2 weeks and followed

by 2 weeks of oral treatment; exceptions to this regimen depend on clinical response, antibiotic bioavailability (eg, treatment with fluoroquinolones can be shorter and last 4-7 days), and culture results. Oral antimicrobial drugs with high bone penetration, such as quinolones or tetracyclines, started within 7 days of the beginning of therapy have been shown to be equivalent to longer parenteral therapy and likely either can be used.◐●

2) **Gonococcal arthritis**: Use ceftriaxone 1 g IM or IV or cefotaxime 1 g IV every 8 hours for 7 days; alternatively use ciprofloxacin 400 mg IV every 12 hours. Investigate and treat comorbid *Chlamydia trachomatis* infection as well as other sexually transmitted infections (eg, HIV, syphilis).

3) **Tuberculous arthritis**: The choice of drugs is as in pulmonary tuberculosis (→Chapter 13.18.2). Treatment should be continued for a minimum of 6 months but is often extended to 9 to 12 months.

4) **Infection following joint replacement surgery** usually warrants removal of the implant, either in 1-stage or 2-stage revision, and prolonged long-term antimicrobial therapy. In cases of a 1-stage revision with retained hardware, parenteral therapy combined with oral rifampin (INN rifampicin) 600 mg daily is added on for biofilm formation, followed by step-down to a highly bioavailable oral option, such as a quinolone, combined with rifampin for 3 to 6 months, based on clinical response. For patients with 2-stage revision, 6 weeks of therapy is recommended, followed by eventual long-term joint replacement.

2. Nonbacterial infection:

1) **Viral arthritis**: Nonsteroidal anti-inflammatory drugs (NSAIDs).

2) **Fungal arthritis**: In patients with candidiasis use fluconazole 400 mg/d (6 mg/kg/d) for ≥6 weeks or amphotericin B (lipid formulation) 3 to 5 mg/kg/d for ≥2 weeks, followed by fluconazole 400 mg/d for an additional 4 weeks. Alternative treatments include an IV echinocandin (caspofungin 50-70 mg/d, anidulafungin 100 mg/d, or micafungin 100 mg/d) or amphotericin B (deoxycholate) 0.5 to 1 mg/kg/d for ≥2 weeks, followed by fluconazole 400 mg/d for ≥6 weeks. Surgical debridement of the necrotic tissues is necessary; in case of osteomyelitis treatment should be extended to 6 to 12 months.

3. Source control: Open surgical debridement or repeated evacuation of joint effusion by joint aspiration using a large-bore needle and followed by lavage of the joint space may be required to obtain source control. Source control must be considered until negative culture results are obtained. Intra-articular administration of antimicrobial agents is not recommended. If joint aspirations are ineffective (ie, it is impossible to evacuate the entire volume of effusion), visually guided arthroscopic joint irrigation is recommended (particularly for knee or shoulder joint effusions) using high volumes of 0.9% saline. An alternative to arthroscopy is surgical arthrotomy with open drainage (this is the method of choice in patients with infectious arthritis of the hip).

4. For the first few days of treatment the joint should be immobilized in a splint (usually in extension). Beginning from day 3, passive mobilization should be started, followed by active mobilization after the resolution of pain; this promotes healing and regeneration of the cartilage and periarticular tissues as well as prevents contractures and adhesions within the joint.

5. Control pain using analgesics.

6. The risk of infectious arthritis and delayed wound healing after surgery (eg, joint replacement) is increased in patients treated with biologic agents (eg, anti-TNF agents, anti-interleukin (IL) 17 agents, anti-IL-6 agents, anti--CD20 antibodies) or Janus kinase (JAK) inhibitors (tofacitinib, baricitinib). According to the American College of Rheumatology (ACR), it is suggested to discontinue the drug and perform joint (hip, knee) replacement a week after the planned date for a consecutive dose and restart treatment after the wound has completely healed (2-4 weeks after surgery) when there are no signs of local or systemic infection.

10. Mixed Connective Tissue Disease (MCTD), Undifferentiated Connective Tissue Disease (UCTD), Overlap Syndromes

→ **ETIOLOGY, CLINICAL FEATURES**

Mixed connective tissue disease (MCTD) is a chronic systemic inflammatory condition with some features of systemic lupus erythematosus, systemic sclerosis, polymyositis/dermatomyositis, rheumatoid arthritis, and a high titer (>8 on the BioPlex assay) of antibodies against uridine-rich nuclear ribonucleoprotein (anti-U1 RNP).

→ **CLINICAL FEATURES**

MCTD often presents with nonspecific features, including malaise, Raynaud syndrome, and positive ANAs. Over the course of months to years patients may develop more specific features, such as hand swelling ("puffy hands") and organ involvement including arthralgia or arthritis, skin thickening, rashes, myalgia or myositis, as well as gastrointestinal, pulmonary, cardiac, and renal involvement.

Undifferentiated connective tissue disease (UCTD) refers to a group of symptoms and signs that suggest a connective tissue disease (CTD) but do not fulfil any specific CTD criteria. Often these patients will "evolve" over time to develop a diagnosable CTD.

→ **DIAGNOSIS**

Diagnostic Criteria

Diagnostic criteria for MCTD: →Table 10-1.

Overlap syndrome is diagnosed in patients fulfilling diagnostic criteria for ≥2 connective tissue diseases, such as systemic lupus erythematosus and myositis (→Table 10-2).

Diagnostic Tests

1. Antibodies to U1 RNP are found at high titers. Other antibodies are typically negative, including antibodies to Sm and to dsDNA. Complement levels are usually normal or rarely low (as found in active systemic lupus erythematosus). There may be an anemia, leukopenia, or thrombocytopenia. Inflammatory markers may be raised, and serum immunoglobulins can be very high.

2. Nail-fold capillaroscopy frequently shows dilated loops.

3. Other investigations are tailored to the internal organ involvement.

Differential Diagnosis

Differential diagnosis includes other systemic connective tissue diseases (→Table 10-3) and other conditions characterized by positive autoantibodies. Initially, early MCTD is most frequently diagnosed as rheumatoid arthritis, systemic lupus erythematosus, or UCTD (a combination of symptoms characteristic for systemic connective tissue diseases but not fulfilling the diagnostic criteria for any of them for ≥3 years; all patients are ANA-positive and typically also RNP-antibody positive).

→ **TREATMENT**

Treatment depends on the dominant symptoms and involves treating the internal organ manifestations of MCTD with immunosuppressive drugs and

Table 10-1. Diagnostic criteria for MCTD

Diagnostic criteria according to Alarcón-Segovia and Villareal

1. **Serologic criterion:** Positive antibodies to U1 RNP antibodies at a titer ≥1:1600
2. **Clinical criteria:** a) Edema of the hands; b) synovitis; c) myositis; c) Raynaud phenomenon; d) sclerodactyly

Diagnosis of MCTD: Fulfilled serologic criterion and ≥3 of the clinical criteria (coexisting edema of the hands, Raynaud phenomenon, and Sclerodactyly require an additional fulfillment of the criteria 2b or 2c).

Diagnostic criteria according to Kasukawa et al

1. **Common symptoms:** 1) Raynaud phenomenon; 2) swollen fingers or hands

2. **Positive antibodies to U1 RNP**

3. **Mixed findings:**
1) SLE-like findings: a) Polyarthritis; b) lymphadenopathy; c) facial erythema; d) pericarditis or pleuritis; e) leukopenia or thrombocytopenia
2) SSc-like symptoms: a) Sclerodactyly; b) pulmonary fibrosis, restrictive pattern on pulmonary function tests, or reduced DL_{CO}; c) hypomotility or esophageal dilation
3) Polymyositis-like symptoms: a) Muscle weakness; b) raised serum creatine kinase levels; c) myogenic pattern on electromyography

Diagnosis of MCTD: Presence of ≥1 common symptoms, serologic criterion, and ≥1 from each group of the mixed findings (1, 2, 3).

Adapted from: (1) Alarcón-Segovia D, Villarreal M. Classification and diagnostic criteria for mixed connective tissue disease. In: Kasukawa R, Sharp GC, eds. Mixed connective tissue disease and anti-nuclear antibodies. Amsterdam: Elsevier Science Publishers B.V. (Biomedical Division); 1987: 33-40; (2) Kasukawa R, Tojo T, Miyawaki S. Preliminary diagnostic criteria for classification of mixed connective tissue disease. In: Kasukawa R, Sharp GC, eds. Mixed connective tissue disease and anti--nuclear antibodies. Amsterdam: Elsevier Science Publishers B.V. (Biomedical Division); 1987: 41-7.

DL_{CO}, carbon dioxide diffusing capacity of the lungs; MCTD, mixed connective tissue disease; RNP, ribonucleoprotein; SLE, systemic lupus erythematosus; SSc, systemic sclerosis.

Table 10-2. Other connective tissue disease overlap syndromes

Syndrome	Features
SSc + PM (scleromyositis)	Serologic marker: Positive anti-PM/Scl antibodies in 24% of patients Clinical manifestations similar to antisynthetase syndrome; however, myositis and interstitial pneumonia are less frequent, the course is less severe, and the response to treatment is better
SLE + scleroderma	SLE with antibodies to histones and centromere: More frequent pulmonary, renal, and cardiac involvement SLE with anti-Scl-70 antibodies: Higher activity of the disease, more frequent pulmonary hypertension and renal involvement SLE with Raynaud phenomenon: More frequent anti-U1 RNP antibodies, dilated nail-fold capillaroscopy with "drop-outs" (typical for scleroderma)
SLE + RA (rhupus)	Destructive arthritis, rheumatoid nodules, positive RF and/or ACPAs; these most frequently precede features of SLE: leukopenia, thrombocytopenia, positive ANAs and anti-dsDNA, decreased levels of complement components

ACPA, anti-citrullinated protein antibody; dsDNA, double-stranded DNA; PM, polymyositis; RA, rheumatoid arthritis; RF, rheumatoid factor; RNP, ribonucleoprotein; SLE, systemic lupus erythematosus; SSc, systemic sclerosis.

Table 10-3. Features differentiating systemic connective tissue diseases					
Clinical symptom	SLE	RA	SSc	PM	MCTD
Pleuritis or pericarditis	++++	+	+	−	+++
Arthritis with joint destruction	±	++++	+	±	+
Raynaud phenomenon	++	−	++++	+	++++
Myositis	+	+	+	++++	+++
Sclerodactyly	±	−	++++	−	++
Skin thickening	−	−	+++	−	−
Interstitial lung disease	+	+	+++	++	+
Pulmonary hypertension	+	±	++	+	+++
Butterfly rash	++++				++
Oral ulcers	+++	−	−	−	++
Seizures or psychosis	+++	−	−	−	−
Nerve V neuropathy	+	−	++	−	+++
Peripheral polyneuropathy	++	++	±	−	++
Transverse myelitis	+++	+	−	−	++
Aseptic meningitis	+++	+	−	−	+++
Glomerulonephritis					
Proliferative	++++	−	−	−	+
Membranous	+++	−	−	−	++
Renovascular hypertension	+	−	++++	−	+++
Cutaneous (leukocytoclastic vasculitis on skin biopsy) or systemic vasculitis, including renal, neurologic, and pulmonary manifestations)	++	++	+	+	+
Noninflammatory vasculopathy	−	−	++++	−	+++
Impaired esophageal motility	±	±	++++	++	+++
Anti-RNP	++	−	+	+	++++
Anti-Sm	+++	−	−	−	−
Anti-dsDNA	++++	−	−	−	−
Anti-Scl-70, ACAs, anti-RNA polymerase III	−	−	+++	−	−
↓ levels of complement components	+++	−	−	−	+ or normal
Rheumatoid factor	++	+++	+	+	++
The number of pluses denotes the frequency.					

↓, decreased; ACA, anticentromere antibody; dsDNA, double-stranded DNA; MCTD, mixed connective tissue disease; PM, polymyositis; RA, rheumatoid arthritis; RNP, ribonucleoprotein; SLF, systemic lupus erythematosus; SSc, systemic sclerosis.

antifibrotics or with supportive therapies (depending on organ involvement), such as nonsteroidal anti-inflammatory drugs (NSAIDs), analgesics, or proton pump inhibitors (PPIs).

→ PROGNOSIS

The prognosis in patients with MCTD is more favorable than in those with systemic lupus erythematosus and systemic sclerosis. In some patients the clinical course is mild and remission occurs; some develop a distinct connective tissue disease; and in other cases signs and symptoms persist, warranting long-term immunosuppressive treatment. Nevertheless, MCTD sometimes leads to fatal complications, with the main causes of death in adult patients being pulmonary hypertension and heart failure.

11. Osteoarthritis

→ DEFINITION, ETIOLOGY, PATHOGENESIS

Osteoarthritis (OA) is caused by biological and mechanical factors that desta-bilize the complementary processes of degradation and formation of articular cartilage and the subchondral bony plate and eventually involves all tissues of the joint. OA is characterized by arthralgia, limited motion, crepitus, and secondary inflammatory changes of variable severity (eg, with joint effusion) not accompanied by systemic symptoms. OA may be classified as **primary OA** (more common; etiology is unknown) or **secondary OA** (caused by local damage and structural abnormalities of the joint or by systemic diseases). **Primary OA** typically affects weight-bearing joints (eg, facet joints of the spine, hips, knees) and hands (base of the thumbs, proximal interphalangeal [PIP] joints, distal interphalangeal [DIP] joints). **Secondary OA** should be suspected if atypical joints are affected (eg, shoulders, elbows, wrists, metacarpophalangeal [MCP] joints, and ankles).

Causes of secondary OA:

1) Acute or chronic joint trauma.
2) Congenital and developmental causes, such as avascular necrosis of the femoral head in children (Perthes disease), congenital hip dysplasia, slipped capital femoral epiphysis, differences in the length of lower extremities, var-us or valgus deformity of lower extremities, joint hypermobility syndrome, dysplasia of joints, dysplasia of bones.
3) Metabolic disorders: Alkaptonuria (ochronosis), hemochromatosis, Wilson disease, Gaucher disease.
4) Endocrine disorders: Acromegaly, thyrotoxicosis, diabetes mellitus, obesity, hypothyroidism.
5) Diseases caused by deposition of calcium salts: Chondrocalcinosis, hydroxy-apatite deposition disease.
6) Other bone and joint conditions: Fractures, avascular necrosis, infections, gout, rheumatoid arthritis and other inflammatory conditions, Paget disease, osteopetrosis, osteochondritis dissecans.
7) Neuropathic osteoarthropathy: Charcot joints.

Risk factors: Advanced age, female sex, overweight and obesity, genetic mutations (eg, affecting the type II collagen gene), mechanical factors (eg, oc-cupations requiring frequent knee-bending, professional sports, weakness of the adjacent muscles, prior trauma), proprioceptive dysfunction.

→ **CLINICAL FEATURES AND NATURAL HISTORY**

Clinical manifestations usually occur after the age of 45 years and are highly variable in severity. They do not always correlate with the degree of joint damage seen on imaging studies.

1. Joint pain is the dominant symptom. It is triggered by weight-bearing and/ or motion of the affected joint; in advanced OA, it may be severe and also occur at rest and at night. Pain can be worse during initial movements following a period of immobility and gradually improve with subsequent movements but then intensify with further use. Pain is usually relieved by rest. Associated periarticular soft-tissue involvement (eg, bursitis) can cause pain away from the joint line, whereas pain originating from the joint itself is usually maximal at the joint line.

2. Limited motion of the affected joints with secondary atrophy of local muscles.

3. Other features include transient stiffness lasting <30 minutes (early morning or after inactivity), absence of warmth, crepitus on movement, joint deformity, instability, and occasionally joint effusion.

OA progresses slowly, usually with periods of relapses and remissions. Joint damage is irreversible and the progression is independent of medical therapy. However, both pharmacologic and nonpharmacologic therapy can have beneficial effects on clinical manifestations. Disability depends on the location and severity of lesions.

1. OA of the hip: Pain is usually felt in the groin but may involve the anterior thigh and occasionally the lower back and buttocks. Pain can also radiate to the knee. Limited motion develops early in the course of the disease, usually with internal rotation being the first to be affected. Secondary inflammation of the insertions of the gluteal muscles in the greater trochanter and trochanteric bursitis may develop, causing pain in the lateral parts of the thigh, gluteal muscle atrophy, and relative limb shortening.

2. OA of the knee: Pain is located in the joint and the upper part of the lower leg and is usually worse with weight-bearing and ambulation. Flexion and extension of the joint may produce palpable crepitus. The axis of the limb is almost always abnormal, with varus deformity being more common than valgus deformity. Joint effusion and popliteal cyst (Baker cyst) are frequently seen. Joint outlines may be widened and deformed in advanced cases. Secondary changes include weakness and atrophy of the quadriceps muscles, enthesitis of the lateral collateral ligaments and knee flexors insertions, and pes anserine bursitis; these also cause pain. In patients with advanced OA of the knee, a flexion contracture of the knee can occur. OA can affect any or all compartments of the knee: medial (most common, may be accompanied by varus knee deformity), lateral (less common, may be accompanied by valgus knee deformity), and patellofemoral. Patients with patellofemoral OA may have more pain going downstairs than upstairs.

3. OA of the hands: Joint pain, brief morning stiffness (up to 30 minutes), and stiffness after periods of inactivity may occur, with limited correlation between symptom severity and imaging findings. Function can be affected, varying from mild to marked impairment. OA affects both hands, typically causing bony enlargement of the affected joints. The most frequently affected joints are DIP and PIP joints of the second to fifth digits as well as the base of the thumbs (the first carpometacarpal joint). Characteristic deformities are seen near to the DIP joints (Heberden nodes; →Chapter 1.11.2), PIP joints (Bouchard nodes; →Chapter 1.11.2), or both. Superimposed effusions as well as central joint erosions can occur; this is called erosive or inflammatory OA of the hands.

4. OA of the spine: Facet joint OA often coexists with degeneration of spinal ligaments and degenerative disc disease (loss of disc height, vertebral endplate changes, and osteophyte formation at the vertebral margins). A dominant

Table 11-1. Kellgren-Lawrence scale for radiographic classification of osteoarthritis

Grade	Description
0: Normal	
1: Questionable	Doubtful narrowing of joint space and possible osteophytic lipping
2: Mild	Definite osteophytes and possible narrowing of joint space
3: Moderate	Moderate multiple osteophytes, definite narrowing of joint space, some sclerosis, and possible deformity of bone ends
4: Severe	Large osteophytes, marked narrowing of joint space, severe sclerosis, and definite deformity of bone ends

Based on Ann Rheum Dis. 1957;16(4):494-502.

feature is paraspinal pain, which usually increases on movement. The type and location of lesions (intervertebral discs, facet joints, spinal ligaments) cannot be established on the basis of symptoms alone. Cervical facet OA can cause ipsilateral neck pain, which is aggravated by neck rotation or lateral flexion. Lumbar facet OA can produce localized lumbar pain, which may radiate unilaterally or bilaterally to the buttocks, groin, and thighs.

In patients with another noninflammatory disease, diffuse idiopathic skeletal hyperostosis (also known as Forestier disease), significant bony deposition occurs, with large osteophytes and calcification of spinal ligaments and entheses forming large bony bridges between vertebral bodies. Such soft-tissue calcification is not typical of OA. Pain is dull and of variable severity, and flexibility of the spine is significantly impaired.

5. OA may affect other joints, including the shoulder, acromioclavicular joints, ankle joints, sacroiliac joints, and temporomandibular joints. **OA of multiple joints** (so-called generalized OA) involves ≥3 of the joints listed above.

→ DIAGNOSIS

Diagnostic Tests

1. Joint radiographs reveal characteristic features: joint space narrowing caused by cartilage destruction, subchondral cysts (geodes) caused by bone destruction, sclerosis of the subchondral bony plate, and osteophytes at the joint margins. The severity of radiographic changes in patients with OA may be classified using the Kellgren-Lawrence scale (→Table 11-1).

2. Other imaging studies (computed tomography [CT], magnetic resonance imaging [MRI], ultrasonography, scintigraphy) may be useful in differentiating OA from other joint and bone disorders. MRI may reveal very early lesions, which precede clinical and radiographic manifestations.

Diagnostic Criteria

Diagnosis is based on symptoms accompanied by characteristic radiographic features. However, in the presence of typical signs and symptoms in the at-risk age group, OA can be diagnosed without radiography and/or laboratory investigations.

Differential Diagnosis

Clinical and radiographic features of OA are very characteristic and for that reason differentiating OA from other joint disorders is rarely necessary. However, conditions such as calcium pyrophosphate deposition disease, synovial osteochondromatosis, and avascular necrosis of the femoral head should be considered where appropriate. If secondary OA is suspected (causes: →Definition, Etiology, Pathogenesis, above), underlying etiologies should be evaluated. In patients with inflammatory OA of the hands, and particularly with erosions on radiographs, differential diagnosis should include rheumatoid arthritis, psoriatic arthritis, and gout.

→ **TREATMENT**

The **main goal of treatment** is pain relief and maintaining the best possible functional status.

Nonpharmacologic Management

1. Patient education.

2. Nutritional management to reduce body weight in overweight or obese patients.

3. Physiotherapy, mainly kinesiotherapy aimed at maintaining joint motion and muscle strength. This may also reduce pain severity.

4. Orthopedic aids, such as walking sticks, crutches, corrective shoe insoles, limb axis correction devices, knee joint stabilizers (including elastic bands), and external correction (medialization) of the patella.

5. Surgical treatment:

1) Arthroplasty is the key treatment modality in patients with severe pain or significant disability caused by OA of the hip or knee. It markedly improves the patient's quality of life.

2) Patellectomy, osteotomy to correct limb axis, and arthrodesis (joint fixation) are currently rarely performed.

Pharmacotherapy

1. Analgesics:

1) Start with oral **acetaminophen** (INN paracetamol) up to a maximum dose of 3 g/d (in long-term treatment use lower doses).🟢🔵

2) If acetaminophen is ineffective, administer a **nonsteroidal anti-inflammatory drug (NSAID)** at the lowest effective dose and for the shortest possible time (→Table 11-2; note the adverse effects and contraindications [eg, active peptic ulcer disease, severe renal or liver failure, drug hypersensitivity, bleeding]).🟢🔵 Suggested principles of choosing NSAIDs on the basis of the risk of gastrointestinal (GI) complications and cardiovascular risk are as follows:

   a) In patients with a low GI risk and low cardiovascular risk, you can use any NSAID.

   b) In patients with a low GI risk and high cardiovascular risk, use naproxen as the first-line agent. To achieve maximal gastric protection, you may add a proton pump inhibitor.

   c) In patients with a high GI risk and low cardiovascular risk, celecoxib is the agent of choice.

   d) In patients with a high GI risk and high cardiovascular risk, you can use nonpharmacologic management in combination with a medium-dose acetaminophen (up to 2 g/d).

   e) In patients receiving long-term acetylsalicylic acid treatment (eg, in prevention of myocardial infarction), avoid ibuprofen.

3) In patients in whom NSAIDs are contraindicated, not tolerated, or ineffective, one may try **opioids**, starting from weak opioids (→Chapter 1.20); note their adverse effects, such as somnolence and vertigo/dizziness, which may increase the risk of falls and fractures.🟢🔵

4) Topical agents, such as NSAIDs or capsaicin, can be used as alternatives or adjunctive therapy.

Table 11-2. Dosage of selected nonsteroidal anti-inflammatory drugs (alphabetical order; pattern of use differs among countries; maximum dose usually limited to a few days; please refer to local formularies)

Agent and formulation	Dosing	
	Usual	Maximum
Acemetacin		
Capsules	60 mg bid to tid	600 mg/d
Sustained-release capsules	90 mg once daily or bid	300 mg/d
Celecoxib[a]: capsules	200 mg once daily or 100 mg bid	200 mg bid
Dexibuprofen: coated tablets	200-400 mg tid	1.2 g/d
Dexketoprofen		
Coated tablets	25 mg tid	75 mg/d
PO granulate for suspension	25 mg tid	75 mg/d
Solution for IV/IM injections	50 mg every 8-12 hours	150 mg/d
Diclofenac[a]		
Tablets, capsules	50 mg every 8-12 hours	100 mg/d
Sustained-release tablets Modified-release tablets Sustained-release capsules Modified-release capsules	50-100 mg once daily or in 2 divided doses	100 mg/d
Suppositories, rectal capsules	50-100 mg/d in 2-3 divided doses	100 mg/d
Solution for IM injections	75 mg once daily	75 mg bid
Topical spray, gel, patch	Topically several times a day	
Etofenamate: topical gel, cream, spray	Topically several times a day	
Ibuprofen[a]		
Various PO formulations	Rheumatic diseases 400-800 mg tid to qid, analgesic treatment 200-400 mg 4-6 times/d	3.2 g/d
Cream, gel	Topically	
Indomethacin[a]		
Sustained-release tablets	75 mg once daily or bid	75 mg bid
Spray, ointment	Topically several times a day	
Ketoprofen[a,b]		
Tablets	100 mg once daily or bid	300 mg/d
Capsules	50 mg tid	300 mg/d
Modified-release tablets	150 mg once daily or in 2 divided doses	150 mg bid

Agent and formulation	Dosing	
	Usual	Maximum
Sustained-release tablets Sustained-release capsules	100-200 mg once daily	200 mg once daily
Suppositories	100 mg once daily or bid	300 mg/d
Gel	Topically bid	
Topical spray	3-4 doses once daily to tid	48 doses in 24 hours
Solution for IM injections	100 mg once daily to bid	200 mg/d
Mefenamic acid		
Tablets	250 mg qid	
Suppositories	500 mg once daily to tid	500 mg qid
Tiaprofenic acid: tablets	300 mg bid	
Tolfenamic acid: tablets	200 mg	400 mg
Meloxicam[a]		
Tablets	7.5-15 mg once daily	15 mg once daily
Suppositories	7.5-15 mg once daily	15 mg once daily
Solution for IM injections	15 mg once daily	15 mg once daily
Nabumetone: tablets	1-2 g once daily or 0.5-1 g bid	2 g/d
Naproxen[a]		
Tablets, PO suspension	250-500 mg bid	1.5 g/d
Suppositories	250-500 mg bid	1.5 g/d
Gel	Topically 2-6 times/d	
Nimesulide[c]: tablets, granulate for PO suspension	100 mg bid	
Piroxicam[d]: tablets, solution for IM injections	20 mg once daily or 10 mg bid	40 mg/d
Diethylamine salicylate: cream, gel	Topically tid or qid	

[a] Agents commonly used in Canada.

[b] One of the chapter's contributors preferred to specify ketoprofen should be used at the maximum dose only for up to several days.

[c] Not indicated in osteoarthritis; due to the risk of liver injury it should be used as a second-line agent at the lowest effective doses and for the shortest time possible (up to 15 days).

[d] One of the chapter's contributors preferred to remove piroxicam as an option due to its adverse effect profile.

bid, 2 times a day; IM, intramuscular; IV, intravenous; PO, oral; qid, 4 times a day; tid, 3 times a day.

2. Glucocorticoid injections: When analgesics are not sufficient, intra-articular glucocorticoid injections may be considered in patients with moderate-severe symptoms.⊘● Patients should be counselled about the potential risk of necrosis and infection (particular caution should be taken with hip injections). If repeat injections are required in the same joint, these should be done at least 3 to 4 months apart (maximum 3 times per year). No good quality data exist on a lifelong limit of injections and patterns of practice may vary.

3. Symptomatic slow-acting drugs in osteoarthritis (SYSADOA): Glucosamine and chondroitin are widely used but are of uncertain benefit; some trials suggest a small effect of pain improvement. In patients who wish to try these agents, we do not object, given their relative safety.⊘● If pain is not reduced and functional improvement is not achieved after 6 months, discontinuation of SYSADOA is justified.

4. Hyaluronic acid injections: A trial of intra-articular hyaluronate injections in patients who have had inadequate response to or intolerance of acetaminophen, NSAIDs, and intra-articular glucocorticoids may be considered.⊘● Note that in patients with OA, asymptomatic accumulation of calcium pyrophosphate crystals in joint cartilage may occur. In such cases, an injection of hyaluronic acid of high molecular weight may precipitate acute arthritis; therefore, medium-molecular-weight hyaluronic acid may be better tolerated. If effective, injections can be repeated every 6 months, although the efficacy of repeated courses and their frequency have not been adequately evaluated.

5. Serotonin and norepinephrine reuptake inhibitors (eg, duloxetine, milnacipran) also have analgesic effects via central pain modulation and may be tried in patients with chronic pain persisting despite the above-listed measures.

12. Osteonecrosis

→ DEFINITION, ETIOLOGY, PATHOGENESIS

Osteonecrosis (avascular necrosis of bone) is the end stage of various abnormalities of blood supply to the bone.

Causes:

1) **Trauma** (in ~50% of patients), particularly fractures of the proximal femur.

2) **Nontraumatic causes**: Glucocorticoid treatment (particularly involving oral and intra-articular administration; the risk depends on the daily dose and, to a lesser degree, on the duration of treatment and the cumulative dose), alcohol dependence (along with glucocorticoid treatment this accounts for the majority of cases of nontraumatic osteonecrosis), autoimmune diseases (particularly systemic lupus erythematosus, antiphospholipid syndrome, and rheumatoid arthritis), myeloproliferative neoplasms, irradiation, gout, sickle cell anemia, thrombophilia, decompression sickness, treatment with denosumab or IV bisphosphonates (osteonecrosis of the jaw, mostly due to long-term use in cancer patients with bony metastases; as an example, about 1 in 1000 multiple myeloma patients using bisphosphonates will be affected),◯ and other.

3) **Idiopathic osteonecrosis**: For instance, avascular necrosis of the femoral head in children (Legg-Calvé-Perthes disease).

Osteonecrosis most frequently affects the femoral head and less often involves the femoral condyles, the head of the humerus, or the proximal epiphysis of the tibia, talus, and carpal bones. Involvement may be bilateral, particularly in patients with osteonecrosis of the femoral head. Ischemia of the subchondral part of the trabecular bone leads to its necrosis, deformity of the articular surface, and secondary degenerative and proliferative changes of the joint.

→ CLINICAL FEATURES AND NATURAL HISTORY

Symptoms of osteonecrosis:

1) **Localized pain**: In patients with osteonecrosis of the femoral head pain is localized in the groin and buttock and referred to the inner thigh and knee. It is aggravated by weight-bearing upon walking but may also be present at rest and at night. Occasionally, the pain may precede radiologic features of necrosis by several weeks or even months. Chronic pain syndrome develops due to degenerative and proliferative changes.

2) **Short-lasting morning stiffness** (<60 minutes), which differentiates osteonecrosis from inflammatory conditions, such as rheumatoid arthritis (where the stiffness usually lasts >60 minutes). The range of motion is not limited until the joint space becomes narrowed and secondary degenerative and proliferative changes develop.

3) Patients with advanced avascular necrosis of the hip or knee have **limb shortening and gait abnormalities**.

→ DIAGNOSIS

The diagnosis of osteonecrosis is based on **imaging studies**. An accurate diagnosis is particularly important in the early stages of the disease, when medical treatment is possible in some patients.

In the early stages of osteonecrosis **radiography** reveals only minor osteopenia; in such cases magnetic resonance imaging (MRI) is the best diagnostic tool. In patients with more advanced disease radiography reveals changes in the trabecular bone, including osteolytic lesions (resorption of necrotic bone tissue), separated necrotic fragments of bone (sequestra), and osteosclerotic remodeling. With the progression of necrotic changes and collapse of the articular surface, patients develop joint space widening. Narrowing of the joint space and deformation of the articular surface appear in late stages of the disease (the "crescent sign" is pathognomonic for subchondral collapse), when secondary degenerative and proliferative changes develop.

Differential Diagnosis

Differential diagnosis mainly includes joint diseases (arthritis, degenerative and proliferative arthropathy), bone disorders (fractures, tumors, infections, metabolic bone diseases), entrapment syndromes (peripheral nerve entrapment), and, in patients with hip and thigh pain, atherosclerosis of the iliac arteries.

→ TREATMENT

1. Conservative management includes prevention of the collapse of articular surfaces and of the development of degenerative and proliferative changes (in the case of weight-bearing joints this is achieved by partial unweighting for 4-8 weeks with the use of crutches or a walking stick) as well as treatment of pain. Depending on the underlying cause, other therapies without clear evidence of efficacy are sometimes tried, including statins for glucocorticoid-induced disease and anticoagulants for thrombophilia-induced disease.

2. Surgical treatment: In patients with early osteonecrosis and preserved joint space, the aim of treatment is stopping the progression of changes. The best results are achieved by removal of necrotic bone fragments to reduce intraosseous pressure and simultaneous grafting of fragments of trabecular bone with blood vessels and sometimes with joint cartilage (such procedures are not always effective). In advanced disease, after joint space narrowing has developed, joint replacement is performed, especially in the case of involvement of hip or knee joints.

3. Bisphosphonate therapy: The benefit of this treatment is unproven and remains controversial.⊗◡

13. Osteoporosis

Osteoporosis is a systemic disease of the skeleton characterized by an elevated risk of bone fractures due to decreased bone strength. Bone strength depends on the mineral density and architecture of bones.

A **low-impact (fragility) fracture** is defined as a fracture caused by a force that normally does not cause fracture of a healthy bone (fall from a standing height or a spontaneous fracture). The cause of a low-impact fracture may be other than osteoporosis and involve, for instance, cancer.

Primary osteoporosis usually develops in postmenopausal women and less frequently in elderly men. **Secondary osteoporosis** results from various diseases or adverse effects of certain drugs, most frequently glucocorticoids.

Risk factors for osteoporosis:

1) **Genetic and demographic factors**: Family history (particularly hip fracture in a parent), advanced age, female sex, white or Asian populations, body mass index (BMI) <18 kg/m^2.

2) **Reproductive factors**: Deficiency of sex hormones (estrogen, testosterone) due to various etiologies, prolonged amenorrhea (late puberty, periods of estrogen deficiency), nulliparity, postmenopausal status (particularly premature, including patients after oophorectomy).

3) **Nutrition and lifestyle factors**: Low calcium intake (daily calcium requirements: children aged 1-10 years require ~800 mg elemental calcium; adolescents and adults, 1000-1200 mg; pregnant and breastfeeding women, postmenopausal women, and elderly persons, 1200-1300 mg), vitamin D deficiency (causes: →Chapter 4.2.1.2), low or excessive phosphate intake, protein deficiency or excessive protein intake, tobacco smoking, excessive alcohol or caffeine use, sedentary lifestyle.

4) **Coexisting conditions** (these may lead to secondary osteoporosis):

   a) Previous fractures, immobilization, sarcopenia (loss of mass, strength, and function of skeletal muscles related to age or comorbidities).

   b) Endocrinologic conditions: Hyperparathyroidism, Cushing syndrome (hyperadrenocorticism), thyrotoxicosis, acromegaly, diabetes mellitus, endometriosis, hyperprolactinemia, hypogonadism (primary or secondary), tumors secreting parathyroid hormone-related peptide (PTHrP), Addison disease.

   c) Gastrointestinal (GI) conditions: Malabsorption syndromes (most frequently celiac disease), patients after gastrectomy or small intestine resection, patients after bariatric surgery, inflammatory bowel disease (Crohn disease, ulcerative colitis), chronic liver disease with cholestasis (particularly primary biliary cholangitis in women) or without cholestasis, total parenteral nutrition.

   d) Renal conditions: Calcium-losing and phosphate-losing nephropathy, nephrotic syndrome, chronic kidney disease (CKD) (particularly in patients undergoing dialysis).

   e) Rheumatologic conditions: Rheumatoid arthritis (RA), ankylosing spondylitis (AS), psoriatic arthritis.

   f) Lung diseases: Chronic obstructive pulmonary disease, cystic fibrosis.

   g) Hematologic conditions: Multiple myeloma, myeloid leukemia, lymphoma, hemophilia, systemic mastocytosis, sickle cell anemia, thalassemia, amyloidosis.

   h) Other: Sarcoidosis, vitamin A toxicity.

5) **Drugs**: Glucocorticoids, high doses of thyroid hormones, antiepileptic drugs (phenobarbital, phenytoin, carbamazepine), heparin (in particular

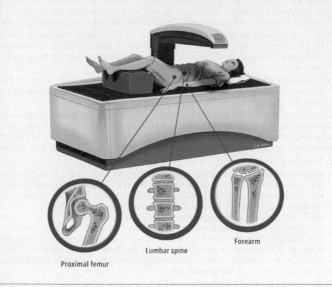

Figure 13-1. Dual-energy x-ray absorptiometry (DXA) showing the proximal femur, lumbar spine, and bones of the forearm. *Illustration courtesy of Dr Shannon Zhang.*

unfractionated heparin), vitamin K antagonists, cyclosporine (INN ciclosporin), high doses of immunosuppressive agents and other antimetabolites, bile acid sequestrants (eg, cholestyramine), gonadotropin-releasing hormone analogues, thiazolidinediones (pioglitazone), tamoxifen (in premenopausal women), aromatase inhibitors, androgen deprivation therapy, proton pump inhibitors (PPIs), selective serotonin reuptake inhibitors (SSRIs), serotonin-norepinephrine reuptake inhibitor (SNRIs), antiretroviral drugs.

→ DIAGNOSIS

Diagnostic Tests

1. Bone densitometry measures bone mineral density (BMD). It is particularly indicated in patients at increased risk of fractures but also used to monitor the disease and effectiveness of treatment. (The risk of fractures can be estimated using the fracture risk assessment tool FRAX BMI risk calculator adjusted for country or population; available online from the University of Sheffield.) The only recommended diagnostic method in osteoporosis is **dual-energy x-ray absorptiometry (DXA)** (→Figure 13-1), which is used to measure:

1) BMD of the proximal femur (femoral neck, shaft, Ward triangle, or greater trochanter; results are given separately for all the 3 sites or for the entire proximal femur [so-called total hip BMD]). Femoral neck and total hip BMDs are the recommended parameters for diagnosing osteoporosis, while fracture risk is determined by the femoral neck T score.

2) BMD of the lumbar spine (L1-L4; antero-posterior view). A falsely elevated spine T score may be caused by fracture of a vertebral body (detected by measurement of the lumbar spine); advanced degenerative changes of the spine (including vertebral bodies and facet joints), for instance, in Forestier disease

(diffuse idiopathic skeletal hyperostosis); significant atherosclerotic changes of the abdominal aorta; and calcification of spinal ligaments (eg, in AS). It is for this reason that femoral neck BMD is used for calculating fracture risk.

3) BMD of bones of the forearm. Densitometry of the bones of the forearm may be done if measurement of the proximal femur or of the spine is not possible, if the results are difficult to interpret, and in patients with hyperparathyroidism.

4) Total body BMD. This measurement may be performed in children and in adults but tends to be reserved for special circumstances, such as measuring body composition.

A typical printout of DXA results contains an image of the examined site and results of the following measurements: BMD in g/cm^2, T scores (standard deviation from values for healthy women aged 20-29 years), and Z scores (standard deviation from values for an age-matched and sex-matched reference population).

2. Imaging studies:

1) **Conventional plain radiography** has limited value in the assessment of osteoporosis, especially in the early stages of the disease. Plain radiographs will show decreased bone density if bone loss is >30% to 50%. Additional findings may include thinning of the cortex of long bones, loss of horizontal trabeculae, prominent supportive trabeculae, prominent laminae of vertebral bodies, and compression fractures. The technique used for detection and evaluation of fractures is radiographic morphometry. A compression fracture is defined as a decrease $\geq 20\%$ in the height of the vertebral body at any level as compared with the posterior vertebral height in the thoracic or lumbar region in the lateral view.

2) **Vertebral fracture assessment (VFA)** is a new technology using central DXA that permits imaging of the thoracic and lumbar spine to evaluate for the presence of vertebral fractures.

3) **Trabecular bone score (TBS)** is an indirect measure of bone structure derived from texture software developed for use with DXA. It is an independent predictor of fracture risk and has recently been incorporated into FRAX.

4) **Quantitative computed tomography (CT) and magnetic resonance imaging (MRI)** are useful in selected patients, particularly those with secondary osteoporosis. They provide information on the underlying bone quality and microarchitecture on top of volumetric BMD provided by DXA assessment.

3. Laboratory tests:

1) Increased levels of biochemical markers of bone turnover (these are not recommended for establishing the diagnosis but may be used for additional estimation of fracture risk and monitoring treatment effects).

2) Abnormalities associated with an underlying condition in patients with secondary osteoporosis: Perform appropriate tests to exclude secondary osteoporosis, including erythrocyte sedimentation rate (ESR); complete blood count (CBC); protein electrophoresis; serum levels of alkaline phosphatase (ALP), creatinine, parathyroid hormone (PTH), $25(OH)D_3$, calcium, and phosphate; as well as 24-hour urinary calcium excretion (assessment of calcium and phosphate metabolism: →Chapter 4.2.1, →Chapter 4.2.3).

Diagnostic Criteria

According to the World Health Organization (WHO) diagnostic criteria, osteoporosis is diagnosed on the basis of low BMD of the femoral neck (in clinical practice values for the proximal femur or lumbar spine are also used), with a T score ≤ -2.5 in postmenopausal women (T scores from -1.0 to > -2.5 are classified as osteopenia) and in men aged ≥ 50 years. In younger patients, additional risk factors are needed and usually secondary osteoporosis is diagnosed. In patients with continued skeletal growth, DXA must include Z scores instead of T scores.

While osteoporosis is defined by BMD measurement, the risk for fracture uses BMD and a number of risk factors, many defined in FRAX. BMD assessment alone is not sufficient to identify fracture risk, as certain patients will be undertreated or overtreated if decisions are based on BMD values alone. Therefore, it is necessary to calculate the absolute 10-year risk of fracture on the basis of risk factors present in the patient.

According to the WHO, the recommended tool for calculating individual risk in persons aged from 40 to 90 years is FRAX (available from the University of Sheffield). The calculator takes into consideration the following 12 parameters: age, sex, weight, height, prior fractures, prior hip fractures in a parent, current tobacco smoking, current treatment with glucocorticoids (for >3 months in a dose equivalent to ≥5 mg of prednisolone per day), RA, secondary osteoporosis, alcohol intake (≥3 units a day), and, if available, BMD of the femoral neck. Because the calculator does not take into account a number of other risk factors, the threshold for intervention should be lower in patients with multiple prior fractures, long-term high-dose glucocorticoid treatment, high levels of biochemical markers of bone turnover, as well as sarcopenia or a history of frequent falls. In younger individuals, including premenopausal women, and in patients receiving pharmacologic treatment for osteoporosis, FRAX is not useful.

Differential Diagnosis

1. Congenital bone fragility (eg, osteogenesis imperfecta).

2. Osteomalacia.

3. Secondary osteoporosis:

1) Drugs:

   a) Glucocorticoids.

   b) SSRIs, SNRIs.

   c) Aromatase inhibitors.

   d) PPIs.

   e) Androgen deprivation therapy.

2) Inflammatory disorders:

   a) RA.

   b) Inflammatory bowel disease.

   c) Chronic obstructive pulmonary disease.

4. Other metabolic bone disease:

1) Hyperparathyroidism.

2) Hyperthyroidism.

3) Cushing disease.

5. Malignancy:

1) Multiple myeloma.

2) Leukemia.

6. Chronic kidney and liver diseases.

→ TREATMENT

General Considerations

1. The **goal of treatment** is to prevent fractures. Therapeutic interventions should have proven efficacy in fracture prevention and not just in the prevention of further loss of BMD.

2. Indications for pharmacotherapy:

1) Postmenopausal women and men aged ≥50 years who are considered to be at high risk for fracture based on FRAX (including low-impact fracture at any age). Those at moderate risk for fracture may be considered for therapy

if additional fracture risk factors not used in FRAX are identified, such as falls or frailty.

2) In premenopausal women and men aged ≤50 years: A history of a low-impact fracture or a T score ≤−2.5.

3) Patients on glucocorticoids (>5 mg equivalent dose of prednisone) for >3 months.

3. Treatment:

1) Treatment or avoidance of modifiable risk factors for osteoporosis (→Definition, Etiology, Pathogenesis, above).

2) Ensuring optimal serum levels of $25(OH)D_3$ and adequate calcium intake through diet or calcium supplements.

3) Prevention of falls.

4) Drugs inhibiting bone resorption or stimulating bone formation.

5) Exercise, postfracture rehabilitation.

6) Treatment of pain, improvement of the quality of life.

Nonpharmacologic Management

1. Nutritional management: Optimal pharmacologic treatment requires adequate intake of calcium and vitamin D. Adequate sunlight exposure (~20 min/d) is also recommended.

The best dietary source of calcium (as well as phosphate) is milk and dairy products; low-fat dairy products contain the same amount of calcium as regular products. In persons with lactose intolerance, consumption of lactase-enriched milk or yoghurts should be recommended. About 1000 mg of elemental calcium is delivered with 3 or 4 glasses of milk, 700 mL of yoghurt, 100 to 120 g of hard cheese, or 1000 g of cottage cheese. Various products, such as cereals or fruit juices, are fortified with calcium. The absorption of calcium is inhibited by several foods, including spinach and other vegetables containing oxalate (eg, spinach, rhubarb), large amounts of cereals containing phytic acid (eg, wheat bran), and probably also tea (due to tannins and oxalates). If adequate dietary calcium intake cannot be provided, calcium supplements may be used.

An adequate intake of protein (~1.2 g/kg/d), potassium, and magnesium is necessary to maintain good functioning of the musculoskeletal system and to improve the healing of fractures.⊘●

2. Exercise:

1) Exercise involving resistance training appropriate for the individual's age and functional capacity as well as weight-bearing aerobic exercise are recommended for those with osteoporosis or at risk for osteoporosis.

2) Exercise to enhance core stability and thus to compensate for weakness or postural abnormalities is recommended for individuals who have had vertebral fractures.

3) Exercise that focuses on balance, such as tai chi, or on balance and gait training should be considered for those at risk of falls.

4) Use of hip protectors should be considered for older adults residing in long--term care facilities who are at high risk for fracture.

3. Prevention of falls: Elimination of all risk factors for falls, including correction of vision and improving physical mobility and muscle strength through adequate exercise.⊘● Recommend an appropriate, nonslippery footwear and avoidance of long-acting hypnotics. Gait aids, such as a walker or cane, may be useful in patients at high risk of falling.

Pharmacotherapy

1. Calcium supplements with calcium carbonate (these contain the highest proportion of elemental calcium [40%]) or other formulations such as calcium gluconate, calcium gluconolactobionate, and calcium lactogluconate. Calcium supplements should be taken orally with food at daily doses equivalent to 1 to

1.2 g of elemental calcium, depending on dietary calcium intake. It is debatable whether supplementation of calcium alone (particularly in high doses) or in combination with vitamin D_3 may increase the risk of cardiovascular events, although the weight of evidence does not support this concern. Obtaining calcium intake through diet is the preferable route.

2. Vitamin D (cholecalciferol): In adults without vitamin D deficiency, supplementation with cholecalciferol at 800 to 2000 IU/d should be used; in patients with vitamin D deficiency, the doses are much higher. In case of impaired hydroxylation of cholecalciferol, use oral **alfacalcidol** (in renal failure) or **calcitriol**, an active form of vitamin D (in severe renal and liver failure).

In obese patients with osteoporosis and inadequate exposure to sunlight or with a malabsorption syndrome, it may be necessary to increase the dose of cholecalciferol even to 4000 IU/d, and in case of severe vitamin D deficiency—$25(OH)D_3$ levels <10 ng/mL—a short course of cholecalciferol at a dose of 7000 to 10,000 IU/d may be required; in such patients serum levels of $25(OH)D_3$ should be monitored after ~3 months of treatment. Optimal levels are 30 to 50 ng/mL.

Contraindications include hypervitaminosis D, hypercalcemia, and severe liver failure.

Indications for and administration of calcium and vitamin D supplements in patients with CKD: →Chapter 9.2.

3. Bisphosphonates bind to hydroxyapatites in the bone, forming compounds resistant to enzymatic hydrolysis and causing the inhibition of osteoclastic bone resorption. Oral bisphosphonates are the drugs of choice in primary osteoporosis in postmenopausal women, in men, and in patients with glucocorticoid-induced osteoporosis. In patients with contraindications to oral bisphosphonates and in those who are noncompliant, consider IV bisphosphonates.

The optimal duration of bisphosphonate treatment has not been established. After 3 to 5 years, the effectiveness of treatment and adverse effects should be evaluated. Consider discontinuation of bisphosphonates after 3 to 5 years of treatment if the current risk of fractures is not high (ie, the patient has not had an osteoporotic fracture and the T score is >−2.5). However, high-risk patients should not be considered for a drug holiday, as the risk for fracturing outweighs the risk of potential adverse effects. After 2 or 3 years, reassess the risk on the basis of BMD and markers of bone turnover. If during this period the patient has had an osteoporotic fracture or their risk has increased, reintroduce bisphosphonate treatment; however, no data directly proving the benefits and safety of this management strategy are available.

The **key adverse effects** of oral bisphosphonates are related to the GI tract (eg, esophagitis or esophageal ulcers; adverse effects are less frequent in the case of weekly or monthly administration). In addition, absorption is poor if they are taken with anything but water. Therefore, the tablets should be taken on an empty stomach with plain water and the patient should remain upright for 30 minutes afterwards. Other adverse effects—associated particularly with IV administration—include bone, muscle, and joint pain; flu-like symptoms; rash; and decrease in serum calcium and phosphate levels.

Contraindications to oral bisphosphonates include hiatal hernia, gastroesophageal reflux disease, esophageal stenosis or dysmotility, active gastric or duodenal ulcer disease, inability to maintain an upright position for 30 to 60 minutes (relevant to oral preparations only), renal failure (creatinine clearance <35 mL/min), and hypocalcemia.

Agents:

1) Oral **alendronate** 10 mg once daily or 70 mg once weekly.

2) IV **zoledronic acid** 5 mg once a year.

3) Oral **ibandronate sodium** (INN ibandronic acid) 150 mg once a month or IV 3 mg every 3 months.

4) Oral **risedronate sodium** (INN risedronic acid) 5 mg once daily, 35 mg once a week, or 150 mg monthly.

4. Oral **strontium ranelate** (available in many countries; not approved for use in North America) in a dose 2 g/d (at bedtime, before sleep, ≥2 h after a meal) may be used in combination with calcium and vitamin D. Strontium ranelate inhibits bone resorption and probably also stimulates bone synthesis (this has not been proven to date). At the beginning of treatment, diarrhea may occur. Strontium ranelate is used in men and women with severe osteoporosis.

The agent is contraindicated in patients with ischemic heart disease, peripheral artery disease, cerebrovascular disease, uncontrolled hypertension, a history of venous thromboembolism, and in those who are immobilized. Strontium ranelate is not recommended in patients with creatinine clearance <30 mL/min.

5. Denosumab 60 mg subcutaneously every 6 months. This is a human monoclonal antibody against the receptor activator of nuclear factor κ-B ligand (RANKL), which prevents the activation of RANK on the cell surface of osteoclasts and their precursors. Denosumab inhibits the synthesis, function, and survival of osteoclasts, thus decreasing resorption of the compact and trabecular bone. It is recommended for osteoporosis in postmenopausal women and in men, and particularly in men with prostate cancer undergoing hormonal treatment who show loss of bone mass (thus being at increased fracture risk) and women with breast cancer where it may be beneficial in disease-free survival. Denosumab may be used in patients with renal failure as it is not excreted through the kidneys; however, these patients are at high risk for developing severe symptomatic hypocalcemia and should be monitored carefully. The effect on BMD may exceed the effect of bisphosphonates.○ After withdrawal of this drug, there may be a rapid loss of bone mass, so alternative treatment (eg, bisphosphonates) should be continued.

6. Teriparatide 20 µg subcutaneously once daily should be considered in those at high fracture risk. This is a recombinant 1-34 N-terminal fragment of the parathyroid hormone molecule. It is indicated in patients with severe osteoporosis and multiple fractures in whom bisphosphonates, strontium ranelate, and denosumab either cannot be used or are ineffective. It should not be used for >24 months (after this time use a bisphosphonate).

Contraindications include hypercalcemia, severe renal failure, other metabolic bone diseases, unexplained elevation in serum alkaline phosphatase levels, history of skeletal irradiation, malignant tumor of the musculoskeletal system, or bone metastases (an absolute contraindication).

7. Abaloparatide is a PTHrP that has recently been approved in the United States for the treatment of postmenopausal women with severe osteoporosis at high risk for fracture defined as a history of osteoporotic fractures, multiple risk factors for fracture, or those in whom other therapies are not tolerated or ineffective. The dose is 80 µg subcutaneously daily. Use for >2 years during a patient's lifetime is not recommended.

Warnings and precautions include orthostatic hypotension, hypercalcemia, kidney stones, and hypercalciuria. In addition there is a warning about a dose--dependent risk of osteosarcoma from rat studies (similar to teriparatide), and as a result abaloparatide should not be used in those at increased risk of osteosarcoma, including patients with Paget disease, unexplained elevations in alkaline phosphatase, prior radiation, or malignancy.

8. Romosozumab is a novel anabolic agent recently approved by the US Food and Drug Administration (FDA) for the treatment of osteoporosis. It is a monoclonal antibody that binds sclerostin. Sclerostin is produced by osteocytes and has a negative impact on osteoblastic activity and survival. Romosozumab decreases circulating sclerostin levels, and thus has an anabolic effect on bone formation. It has been shown to significantly reduce vertebral fractures at 12 months and 24 months of treatment (when crossed over to denosumab therapy at 12 months) compared with denosumab therapy; however, there has been no statistically significant reduction in nonvertebral fracture rates.

9. Other drugs reducing fracture risk:

1) Oral **raloxifene** 60 mg/d reduces the risk of vertebral fractures but at the same time increases the risk of deep vein thrombosis and incidence of hot flushes. It is a selective estrogen receptor modulator (SERM) and as such it also reduces the risk of breast cancer. It may be considered as treatment for osteoporosis in women with risk factors for breast cancer.

2) **Estrogen-progesterone (female sex hormones) replacement therapy** reduces the risk of vertebral and other fractures in postmenopausal women but at the same time increases the risk of breast cancer, uterine cancer, and deep vein thrombosis. It may be considered for the treatment or prevention of osteoporosis.

3) **Salmon calcitonin** is not recommended for the treatment of osteoporosis due to an increased risk of malignancy associated with its long-term use. The use of short-term regimens (maximum 2-4 weeks, 100 IU/d subcutaneously or IM) as analgesic therapy is acceptable in patients with fractures.

14. Paget Disease of Bone

→ **DEFINITION, ETIOLOGY, PATHOGENESIS**

Paget disease of bone (PDB) is a chronic metabolic bone disease of unknown etiology. Research suggests that mutations in sequestosome 1 increase the susceptibility to the development of PDB, and the potential role of paramyxovirus infection in causing the disease has been studied. PDB is characterized by a disruption in normal osteoclastic bone resorption and osteoblastic bone formation, which leads to disorganized bone remodeling, with vascularized foci of osteopenia interwoven with focal osteosclerosis and secondary myelofibrosis. Lesions with predominant osteolysis exhibit lower resistance to stress and deformities, whereas lesions with predominant bone formation show overgrowth and thickening of the bone, which result in increased susceptibility to fractures. Osteolytic and osteosclerotic lesions usually coexist.

→ **CLINICAL FEATURES AND NATURAL HISTORY**

Approximately 20% of patients have a solitary lesion. The lesions never involve an entire bone or the skeleton, but they may occur in any bone, most commonly in the pelvis, lumbar or thoracic spine (vertebral bodies), femur, skull, or tibia.

Signs and symptoms depend on the location and extent of the lesions and include pain, which may be caused by microfractures, secondary degeneration and expansion of bone, or mechanical stress of joints and the periarticular soft tissue (in 80% of symptomatic patients); warmth of the involved sites due to increased vascularity of the lesions; bone deformity (eg, the varus deformity or anterior bowing of the tibia, thickening of the bones of the skull); fractures of the long bones, usually of the femur, tibia, humerus, or forearm (these may be asymptomatic). There may be signs and symptoms related to compression of the cranial nerves or the medulla oblongata in patients with cranial involvement as well as the vascular steal syndrome (from the brain to a vascular lesion in the skull via the external carotid artery) compromising the cerebral perfusion and causing headaches, vision and hearing impairment, or ischemic stroke. One may encounter signs and symptoms of hyperkinetic circulation or even high-output heart failure, especially in patients with extensive (>35% of the skeleton) and highly vascular lesions.

→ DIAGNOSIS

Diagnostic Tests

1. Laboratory tests: Increased levels of serum alkaline phosphatase (ALP), a marker of bone formation, in 95% of patients (up to $7\times$ upper limit of normal [ULN]; levels correlate with the extent of lesions on scintigraphy). Other, more specific bone markers may be measured in those with underlying liver or hepatobiliary disease. Increased serum levels of N-terminal propeptide of type I collagen (PINP) and increased levels of markers of bone resorption (elevated levels of serum cross-linked C-terminal telopeptide of type I collagen [CTX] or cross-linked n-telopeptide of type I collagen [NTX]) correspond to the rate of bone turnover in PDB and may be used to determine the treatment response in those with the above-mentioned liver disorders. The use of these more specific markers should be weighed against their increased cost. Hypercalcemia and hypercalciuria (most commonly following a fracture and during periods of immobility) may be measured in those in whom abnormalities might be expected.

2. Imaging: **Radiography** reveals thickening and deformity of the outlines of long bones as well as coexisting osteolytic and osteosclerotic lesions. Radiologic changes evolve as osteolytic lesions progress with osteoblastic activity following, transforming the previously osteolytic bone into a mixed osteolytic-sclerotic bone, which finally is further transformed into a primarily sclerotic bone. In the spine the affected vertebral bodies manifest as a "picture frame" vertebra with an increased anteroposterior diameter and osteosclerotic vertebral body borders. An ivory vertebra is one that is predominantly sclerotic bone. Within the skull, thickening of the calvaria, loss of the periosteum, and thickening of the diploe and osteosclerotic lesions (the "cotton wool" appearance) are visible. Radiographs are recommended in suspected areas. **Bone scintigraphy** shows local uptake of radionuclide by the sites of intensive bone remodeling; compared with radiography, bone scintigraphy has higher sensitivity but lower specificity and will often identify asymptomatic lesions. Scintigraphy is recommended to determine the extent of the disease.

3. Bone biopsy and histology are indicated only in case of diagnostic uncertainty.

Diagnostic Criteria

Diagnosis is based on characteristic radiographic features and increased serum ALP levels; however, normal levels do not exclude PDB. In practice, PDB is suspected in patients with an increased serum ALP level or abnormal radiography results observed during a diagnostic workup performed for other reasons. Only 30% to 40% of patients have typical manifestations at diagnosis.

Differential Diagnosis

1. Focal lesions seen on radiography: Lymphoma, metastases (particularly prostate cancer), primary bone tumor (particularly osteolytic).

2. Focal uptake of radionuclide on scintigraphy: Osteomyelitis, arthritis, prior fracture, metastases, primary bone malignancy.

→ TREATMENT

Indications for Treatment

1. Treatment is indicated in **patients with active PDB** to prevent complications of the disease, which include hearing loss, osteoarthritis, paralysis, neoplasms, and congestive heart failure.

2. Hearing loss: Hearing loss was originally thought to be caused by the compression of nerve VIII. However, more recently it has been attributed to cochlear damage. There are no randomized controlled trials to demonstrate the benefits of anti-Paget therapy on hearing loss. In general, it is felt that treatment may prevent rapid hearing loss, but it does not reverse hearing loss.☺☹

3. Osteoarthritis: Treatment with analgesics such as nonsteroidal anti-inflammatory drugs (NSAIDs) is suggested in Paget disease and considered adjunctive treatment, as the agents do not deal with the underlying disease process. Treatment in those with joint pain, particularly of the hip and knee, and pagetic involvement of the adjacent bone often results in significant improvement in pain, and treatment prior to joint arthroplasty may be important in preventing bleeding at the site of surgery and for preventing loosening of the joint.

4. Paralysis: Paralysis may occur with vertebral body involvement. Treatment with an IV bisphosphonate or calcitonin is suggested to correct the vascular steal that may be occurring.

5. Neoplasm: The incidence of osteosarcomas complicating PDB is estimated at <1%. These cancers occur mostly in persons with long-standing polyostotic disease and affect patients in their seventh decade. Epidemiologic studies suggest that this late peak of osteosarcomas is absent in regions where PDB is infrequently reported. Whereas PDB has a predilection for the axial skeleton, skull, femurs, and tibias, pagetic osteosarcomas tend to spare the spine and are reported more commonly in the pelvis, femur, humerus, and skull.

Pharmacotherapy

1. Antiresorptive drugs relieve bone pain caused by the increased metabolic activity of the lesions and heal the lesions. Nevertheless, the long-term effect of the drugs on the disease progression is not known. Antiresorptive drugs have not been demonstrated to prevent complications of PDB.

1) **Aminobisphosphonates** are the drugs of choice. They are indicated mainly for bone pain due to the increased metabolic activity of the lesions, manifesting as elevated serum ALP levels. The first-line agent is zoledronic acid; it is recommended for symptomatic patients in a single IV dose of 5 mg. Second-line agents are alendronate sodium (INN alendronic acid) 40 mg/d for 6 months or risedronate sodium 30 mg/d for 2 months; they are recommended for patients intolerant of IV zoledronic acid or those who prefer an oral medication.☺☹ Caution with zoledronic acid should be given to those with renal insufficiency. Additionally, to prevent secondary hyperparathyroidism use calcium supplements 1000 mg/d and vitamin D_3 800 IU/d. In patients in whom serum ALP levels do not normalize despite good pain control, continue the antiresorptive therapy for several consecutive months (except for zoledronic acid, which may decrease the levels of bone markers for 5 years and may be administered again if there is an increase in ALP and worsening of symptoms during that period) and monitor the patient for complications. Although rare, in patients who relapse after initial zoledronic acid therapy, retreatment with another course may be able to reachieve a chemical and clinical response.☺☹

2) **Calcitonin** is used exclusively in patients in whom bisphosphonates are not tolerated, ineffective, or contraindicated, as the evidence for its use is derived only from observational studies.☺☹ The dose is 100 IU/d subcutaneously or IM; later it may be reduced to 50 to 100 IU every other day. Due to the increased risk of malignancy, treatment should be limited to 3 months (6 months in exceptional cases). After a careful analysis of risks and benefits, a repeated short-term treatment may be considered.

2. Analgesics: Opioids (dosage: →Chapter 1.20) and **NSAIDs** (dosage: →Chapter 14.11) relieve bone pain related to the increased metabolic activity but are used mainly in patients with pain related to complications, such as bone deformity and osteoarthritis, that cannot be controlled with antiresorptive therapy.

3. Surgery may be necessary for bone-related and joint-related complications.

→ **FOLLOW-UP**

Follow-up includes clinical assessment of pain and deformities and determination of ALP and one of PINP, CTX, or NTX levels for more specific measures when there is underlying hepatobiliary disease.⊘◉ Radiographic monitoring of the involved bones every 12 months may be used to evaluate treatment effectiveness or disease progression in patients not receiving treatment. Adequate pain control and normalization of ALP levels during treatment indicate remission, which may last for many years. After the administration of zoledronic acid, evaluate disease progression and treatment effects every 1 to 2 years after the normalization of bone markers, or every 6 to 12 months in the case of less potent bisphosphonates. An increase in the levels of markers of bone resorption by 20% to 30% above the ULN is an indication for retreatment.

15. Panniculitis

→ **DEFINITION, ETIOLOGY, PATHOGENESIS**

Panniculitis is an inflammatory reaction caused by necrosis of adipocytes. It mainly involves the subcutaneous tissue but may affect adipose tissue anywhere in the body and may also involve a number of systems and organs. Etiology is unknown. Triggering factors include trauma (including self-inflicted injury), external exposure to chemicals, biochemical disturbances (eg, increased activity of pancreatic enzymes), and infections. Panniculitis may be accompanied by other systemic connective tissue diseases (systemic lupus erythematosus), lymphoproliferative neoplasms, or histiocytosis.

→ **CLINICAL FEATURES AND NATURAL HISTORY**

The most common type of panniculitis is idiopathic neutrophilic lobular panniculitis (Weber-Christian disease). It usually occurs in white women. The key manifestations are very painful nodular lesions in the subcutaneous tissue, usually located on the limbs and less often on the trunk. An episode of the disease is commonly preceded by joint and muscle pain and low-grade fever. Subcutaneous lesions persist for several weeks and heal, leaving round, depressed scars. Less frequently, fistulae form with a sterile, oily discharge. Occasionally, arthritis, serositis, and nephritis occur, as well as liver and bone marrow injury. Subcutaneous lesions may coexist with pancreatic disorders (pancreatitis, pseudocyst, posttraumatic injury, ischemia). In some cases they are accompanied by arthritis, thus giving rise to a triad of symptoms: panniculitis, arthritis, pancreatitis.

→ **DIAGNOSIS**

Diagnostic Tests

1. Laboratory tests: In patients with an acute episode of panniculitis tests reveal a marked elevation in the erythrocyte sedimentation rate, leukocytosis with neutrophilia, anemia, occasionally proteinuria and increased red blood cell and white blood cell counts in urinary sediment, and elevated serum lipase levels (in patients with pancreatic involvement).

2. Histologic analysis of biopsy specimens collected from inflammatory lesions early in the course of the disease reveals necrosis of adipocytes, presence of macrophages containing phagocytosed lipids, thrombotic changes in vessels, and fibrosis at later stages.

3. Radiographs of the affected joints reveal joint space narrowing and osteolytic lesions.

Diagnostic Criteria

Diagnosis is based on typical histologic findings of lobular panniculitis. It is important to establish whether any other pathology apart from subcutaneous lesions is present that may be related to panniculitis (eg, panniculitis may be the presenting feature of pancreatic disease) and whether the disease is idiopathic or is part of another condition. Exclude intentional skin self-inflicted injury in patients with psychiatric disorders.

Differential Diagnosis

Erythema nodosum, subcutaneous tissue infection.

→ TREATMENT

Idiopathic panniculitis may be treated with nonsteroidal anti-inflammatory drugs. In severe episodes of the disease glucocorticoids or other immunosuppressive agents (cyclosporine [INN ciclosporin], cyclophosphamide) may be used.

16. Polymyalgia Rheumatica

→ DEFINITION, ETIOLOGY, PATHOGENESIS

Polymyalgia rheumatica (PMR) is an inflammatory disease of unknown etiology that affects individuals aged >50 years, women 4 times more frequently than men, with an incidence of 20 to 50 cases per 100,000 persons. It is characterized by pain and stiffness of the muscles of the neck, shoulder girdle, and/or pelvic girdle.

→ CLINICAL FEATURES AND NATURAL HISTORY

Pain in the muscles of the shoulder girdle, pelvic girdle, and neck, sometimes worsening at night, along with morning stiffness lasting ≥30 minutes are the classic symptoms of PMR. Initially the pain may be unilateral, but later it involves both sides symmetrically and can make it difficult or impossible for the patient to elevate the upper extremities. Arthritis is often present, most frequently involving the knees, sternoclavicular joints, and hips. Other symptoms may include pitting edema of the hands and feet as well as muscle weakness, which in more advanced disease may be followed by muscle atrophy and contractures. General symptoms may include low-grade fever, weight loss, and depression. In ~20% of patients PMR coexists with giant cell arteritis.

In the majority of cases symptoms resolve with treatment. Relapses are rare.

→ DIAGNOSIS

Diagnostic Tests

1. Blood tests: Elevated erythrocyte sedimentation rate (ESR) (usually >100 mm after 1 hour, very rarely normal or only slightly elevated), elevated acute-phase protein levels (C-reactive protein [CRP], fibrinogen), moderate normochromic or hypochromic anemia, thrombocytosis, eosinophilia, and/or mildly elevated serum liver enzyme levels (particularly alkaline phosphatase).

2. Imaging studies: Ultrasonography and **magnetic resonance imaging (MRI)** may reveal synovitis of the involved joints, bursitis, and inflammation of the tendon sheaths.

Diagnostic Criteria

Healey criteria for the diagnosis of PMR: All of the following are required for diagnosis:

1) Pain persisting for ≥1 month at ≥2 of the following sites: neck, shoulders, pelvic girdle.
2) Morning stiffness lasting >1 hour.
3) Prompt response to prednisone (20 mg/d).
4) Exclusion of other conditions that may account for symptoms (→Differential Diagnosis, below).
5) Age >50 years.
6) ESR >40 mm/h.

Differential Diagnosis

Differential diagnosis should include early stages of rheumatoid arthritis (especially in the elderly patients) and other types of arthritis, systemic connective tissue diseases (differentiated by multiorgan involvement, specific autoantibodies), polymyositis, and other myopathies (distinguished by muscle weakness and elevated muscle enzyme levels). Other considerations include fibromyalgia (ESR and CRP are not elevated), malignancy, osteoarthritis, neurologic disorders (eg, parkinsonism), bone diseases, infections, hypothyroidism, myalgia due to muscle overuse, and depression.

TREATMENT

1. Glucocorticoids: Oral prednisone 15 to 20 mg/d (or another glucocorticoid at an equivalent dose) should be administered, with clinical improvement expected within a few days (resolution of pain and stiffness, normalization of ESR and CRP levels).◐⊖ In exceptional cases, when no improvement has been observed after a week, the glucocorticoid may be continued for another week at a dose of 30 mg/d⊘○; however, if the patient still does not improve, the diagnosis should be reevaluated. Once symptoms begin to resolve, continue the treatment with prednisone, gradually tapering the dose down on an individual basis by monitoring clinical disease activity and decreasing ESR and CRP levels.◐○ For instance, after 2 to 3 weeks reduce the daily dose by 2.5 mg every 2 weeks down to 10 mg, and then to 7.5 mg, 5 mg, and 2.5 mg every 2 to 4 weeks to discontinuation. In patients with recurrent symptoms, return to the previous dose until remission is achieved, and subsequently taper the dose down less rapidly. Treatment may last ≥1 year and may commonly be extended to 2 years.⊘○ Note the importance of prophylaxis of osteoporosis in patients with PMR (→Chapter 14.13).◐⊖

2. In patients with contraindications to long-term glucocorticoid treatment and/or ≥2 relapses, some authors suggest the use of methotrexate 10 mg once weekly.⊘⊖

3. Nonsteroidal anti-inflammatory drugs (NSAIDs) may be useful and used in patients with persistent mild musculoskeletal symptoms in spite of a completed glucocorticoid treatment.⊘○

FOLLOW-UP

Monitor the patient for:

1) Efficacy of the glucocorticoid therapy and occurrence of adverse effects (monitor the blood pressure, blood glucose, and electrolyte levels).

2) Symptoms of giant cell arteritis (often temporal arteritis; →Chapter 14.23.6). The patient should be advised to immediately seek medical help upon observing any symptoms of visual disturbances, headache, scalp tenderness, or claudication of the jaw, as PMR coexists with giant cell arteritis in ~20% of patients.

17. Polymyositis and Dermatomyositis

→ DEFINITION, ETIOLOGY, PATHOGENESIS

Polymyositis (PM) is an acquired, idiopathic, inflammatory myopathy. Dermatomyositis (DM) is a type of myopathy associated with inflammatory cutaneous lesions. Both conditions may also cause inflammatory lesions of the heart, pulmonary interstitium, and in the case of DM, blood vessels.

The etiology of PM and DM is unknown; however, autoimmune processes are thought to play a major role in their pathogenesis, given the frequent presence of autoantibodies.

→ CLINICAL FEATURES AND NATURAL HISTORY

PM and DM are the most common idiopathic inflammatory myopathies in adults (although sporadic inclusion body myositis [sIBM] is more common in older men and women aged >50 years). sIBM will be only briefly considered in this chapter, as it is still unclear whether the associated T-cell–mediated inflammation is a primary factor or secondary phenomenon due to an underlying degenerative etiology. PM and DM affect women twice as frequently as men, with an incidence of between 1 to 8 cases per 1,000,000 per year (inclusion body myositis is ~3 times more common in men than women). PM and DM may occur at any age; however, the onset of DM is most often between the ages of 10 to 15 years for the juvenile form and 35 to 65 years for the later-onset form. PM is much more common in adulthood and is rarely diagnosed in those <20 years of age. PM can be idiopathic but is often associated with features of another connective tissue disease and is sometimes thus referred to as overlap myositis. The onset is usually acute (lasting a few days) to subacute (weeks) but can rarely have an indolent course over months to years.

1. General symptoms are fatigue, fever, and weight loss.

2. Symptoms of muscle involvement:

1) Usually symmetric weakness of muscles of the shoulder, hip, neck, and back, which leads to problems with such tasks as standing up from a sitting position, lifting heavy objects, brushing hair, lifting a head off a pillow or climbing stairs. The muscles may be tender and painful. Muscles may eventually undergo atrophy (especially myositis associated with antibodies against signal recognition particle [SRP]) and contribute to weight loss.

2) Respiratory muscle weakness, which may result in shortness of breath on exertion and occasionally respiratory failure.

3) Weakness of the muscles of the throat and upper esophagus are less common but can cause dysphagia and very rarely nasal dysarthria.

4) Involvement of extraocular muscles resulting in ophthalmoparesis and/or ptosis is so rare that its presence should warrant an investigation into alternate diagnoses.

3. Cutaneous manifestations occur in DM and PM. Their onset and severity may not be correlated with muscle involvement. Cutaneous manifestations may precede myositis or be the only sign of the disease in some cases of DM (clinically amyopathic dermatomyositis [CADM]; dermatomyositis *sine* myositis). CADM is often associated with antibodies against melanoma differentiation-associated gene 5 (MDA5/CADM-140). Erythematous lesions may be frequently accompanied by pruritus and/or skin photosensitivity.

1) DM: Periorbital violaceous erythema (heliotrope rash; →Figure 17-1) is a pathognomonic DM sign occurring in 30% to 60% of patients and is occasionally accompanied by lid edema (more common in juvenile DM). Erythematous rash on the upper chest (the V sign), on the neck and shoulders (the shawl sign; →Figure 17-2), or on the lateral thighs and hips (the holster sign) may also develop.

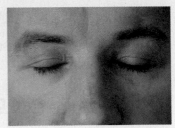

Figure 17-1. Polymyositis/dermatomyositis: Periorbital heliotrope rash.

2) DM: Gottron rash/sign is seen in ~70% of patients and is more commonly seen in DM (→Chapter 1.11, Figure 11-5). It consists of erythematous/violaceous eruptions on the extensor surfaces of finger joints (most frequently the proximal and distal interphalangeal and metacarpophalangeal joints with sparing between the joints but occasionally seen on wrists, elbows, knees, and ankles). Gottron papules are rarer and are a raised erythematous/violaceous coalescence of the Gottron rash.

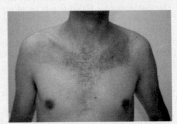

Figure 17-2. Polymyositis/dermatomyositis: Shawl sign and V-sign.

3) Other features seen in PM and DM: "Mechanic's hands" (→Figure 17-3), which is a thickening, desquamation, and cracking of the skin on the palmar surfaces of the fingers and the hand, more common in antisynthetase syndrome and in those with

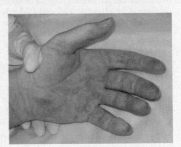

Figure 17-3. "Mechanic's hands."

interstitial lung disease (→below); erythema and periungual edema of the nail folds with petechiae and dilated capillary loops/telangiectasias; trophic ulcers due to coexisting cutaneous vasculitis; generalized erythroderma; inflammation of the subcutaneous tissue (panniculitis); livedo reticularis; and focal alopecia without scarring.

4. Cardiac manifestations are found with extensive testing in up to 70% of patients, usually in the form of tachycardia or bradycardia, but are rarely symptomatic. Signs and symptoms of heart failure are similarly rare.

5. Pulmonary manifestations: Symptoms of interstitial lung disease are seen in up to 30% of patients, predominantly in those with antisynthetase syndrome. Symptoms are mainly dry cough and worsening dyspnea progressing to chronic respiratory failure. In rare cases patients with dysphagia can develop aspiration pneumonia.

6. Gastrointestinal (GI) manifestations: Dysphagia is the most common feature, but patients may also have features of impaired esophageal, gastric, and intestinal motility, including gastroesophageal reflux. Dysphagia may persist after the proximal muscle weakness and CK elevation have resolved and may lead to the need for a feeding tube. In severe cases ulcerations and bleeding may occur. Consequently, proton pump inhibitors are often given simultaneously with glucocorticoids if the patient is symptomatic or has endoscopically determined esophagitis.

7. Joint manifestations: Symptoms of arthritis without erosions, or arthralgia, with a predilection for peripheral joints, mainly of the hands (in 20%-50% of patients). These features are more common in those with overlap myositis (ie, myositis associated with another connective tissue disorder, mixed connective tissue disease [MCTD], systemic lupus erythematosus [SLE], scleroderma).

8. Calcifications in the subcutaneous tissue, skeletal muscles, fasciae, and tendons are very rare with early treatment but may be of considerable size if treatment is delayed, especially in juvenile DM and some cases of PM with positive antibodies against SRP and antisynthetase antibody.

9. Raynaud phenomenon is seen in 10% to 15% of patients.

→ D I A G N O S I S

Diagnostic Tests

1. Laboratory tests:

1) **Blood tests**: Elevated plasma levels of muscle enzymes (creatine kinase [CK], aspartate aminotransferase [AST], alanine aminotransferase [ALT], lactate dehydrogenase [LDH], aldolase, myoglobin), hypergammaglobulinemia, increased erythrocyte sedimentation rate (ESR) and C-reactive protein (CRP) levels.

2) **Immunologic tests**: Autoantibodies are seen in 40% to 80% of patients and include antinuclear antibodies (ANAs); antibodies to double-stranded DNA (dsDNA), Ro, La, U1/U2 ribonucleoprotein (RNP), Ku, Sm; antibodies specifically associated with PM/DM (ie, antibodies to aminoacyl-tRNA synthetase [most commonly Jo-1]); and antibodies to SRP, transcription intermediary factor 1γ/α (TIF1γ/α, p155/140), MJ/nuclear matrix protein 2 (NXP-2), small ubiquitin-like modifier-1 (SUMO-1) activating enzyme (SAE), Mi-1, Mi-2, MDA5, PL7, PM/Scl75, PM/Scl100, Ku, Ej, and Oj. Other than the ANAs, most of the tests for the antibodies listed above are only available in specialty clinics but can be helpful from both a diagnostic and sometimes a prognostic perspective (→below).

2. Electromyography (EMG) usually shows spontaneous activity (fibrillations, positive sharp waves, pseudomyotonic discharges; more common in PM) with small, brief, early recruiting potentials in both PM and DM.

3. Histology:

1) **Muscle biopsy** typically shows a dense T-cell–mediated inflammatory reaction with inflammatory cells invading nonnecrotic fibers in PM. DM changes include perifascicular atrophy and B-cell infiltration often in the epimysium, perimysium, and/or blood vessels, with immunohistochemistry showing membrane attack complex (MAC) deposits around blood vessels. Electron microscopy frequently shows inflammatory cells in both DM and PM, but tubuloreticular inclusions in blood vessels are more commonly seen in DM and are thought to reflect a viral etiology and presence of interferon γ.

2) **Lung (surgical) biopsy** may reveal interstitial lung disease (various types have been observed), but this is rarely required, because typical features on chest radiography or high-resolution computed tomography (HRCT) and clinical symptoms are characteristic (the ground-glass appearance on chest radiographs and impaired carbon monoxide diffusion capacity [DL_{CO}]).

Table 17-1. Diagnostic criteria for polymyositis and dermatomyositis

1. Symmetric progressive muscle weakness affecting the muscles of the shoulder and hip
2. Histologic findings typical of myositis (see text)
3. Increased plasma creatine kinase levels
4. Electromyographic features of an irritative myopathy (active changes and myopathic potentials)
5. Typical cutaneous manifestations: Gottron sign, heliotrope rash, or rash on the anterior chest and shoulders

Diagnosis	Definite	Probable	Possible
	Number of symptoms		
PM	4	3	2
DM	3 or 4	2	1
	Plus typical cutaneous manifestations		

Adapted from N Engl J Med. 1975;292(7):344-7.

DM, dermatomyositis; PM, polymyositis.

---

4. Imaging studies: In the active phase, muscle **magnetic resonance imaging** (MRI) shows an increased signal intensity on fat-saturated, gadolinium--enhanced, T1-weighted, T2-weighted, or short tau inversion recovery (STIR) images; however, the findings are not pathognomonic for PM or DM. In the chronic phase, T1-weighted images may show atrophy of adipose tissue, muscle, or both. Imaging studies may facilitate the choice of an optimal site for muscle biopsy. **Chest radiographs** and **HRCT** may reveal interstitial lesions. **Radiographs of bones and joints** may reveal numerous calcifications, mainly within the subcutaneous tissue and muscles, as well as features of osteoporosis.

5. Electrocardiography (ECG) usually shows nonspecific ST-segment and T-wave abnormalities, sinus tachycardia, and less frequently first- or second--degree atrioventricular block.

Diagnostic Criteria

Diagnostic criteria: →Table 17-1.

Differential Diagnosis

Differential diagnosis should include:

1) **Idiopathic inflammatory myopathies other than PM/DM**: Myositis can be a presenting manifestation of several systemic connective tissue diseases, including SLE, rheumatoid arthritis, MCTD, Sjögren syndrome, and scleroderma (overlap myositis syndrome). The characteristic autoantibodies are important adjuncts to the history and physical examination in the diagnosis of these entities.

2) **Necrotizing autoimmune myopathies** often clinically resemble PM and are most commonly seen in association with statin use, with up to 50% showing T-cell infiltrates in addition to necrosis at some point in the disease course. These myopathies show canonical features of PM (usually there is no rash, as seen in DM) with high CK levels, classical EMG findings of PM, proximal weakness, and inflammation on biopsy. Many of the patients who develop necrotic autoimmune myopathy will show elevated titers for anti–HMG-CoA-reductase (HMGCR) antibodies.◉ Most (>90%) patients have a good clinical response to discontinuing the offending drug; however, if the CK elevation and weakness persist, then the addition of prednisone and, if needed, a disease-modifying agent to allow for glucocorticoid sparing (methotrexate being the most common) should be considered. Necrotizing

myopathies can also be associated with systemic connective tissue diseases, viral infections (eg, HIV), or malignancy. History, examination, and specific blood tests usually differentiate these entities from idiopathic PM.

3) **sIBM** is often mistaken for PM, and *vice versa*, in that sIBM shows hyperCKemia, T-cell infiltrates on biopsy, and EMG findings overlapping with PM. The differentiating features for sIBM are specific weakness of deep finger flexors as well as disproportionate weakness/atrophy of the quadriceps muscles and dysphagia in ~70% of cases, and often a very slow onset of symptoms that upon retrospect started many years earlier. Furthermore, the muscle biopsy in sIBM often shows the presence of inclusion bodies and/or mitochondrial alterations by modified Gomori trichrome staining or electron microscopy. The inclusion bodies can be seen in hereditary forms of inclusion body myositis (hIBM) but the clinical features are distinct (eg, the most common hIBM is due to mutations in the *GNE* gene and has an insidious onset of distal lower extremity weakness, with quadriceps sparing often starting in teenage years). Although CK levels in inclusion body myositis are often lower than those seen in PM or DM, a modest CK elevation (<1000 IU) cannot be used to exclude PM or DM. In contrast to PM/DM, there is a 3:1 male to female ratio in sIBM, and the disease is more common in those aged >50 years, with no juvenile cases. Unlike in PM and DM, there is no clinically meaningful response to immune suppression (IgG, prednisone).

4) **Other myopathies**: →Table 17-2.

Search for malignancy: →Follow-Up, below.

→ TREATMENT

Pharmacotherapy

1. Glucocorticoids: Oral prednisone 1 mg/kg/d (maximum, 60 mg). In patients with an acute onset or a severe course of the disease, IV methylprednisolone 0.5 to 1 g may be used as the initial treatment for 3 days in severe cases and in proportionately lower doses in less severe cases. After observing an improvement in the patient's condition (ie, increase in muscle strength and a substantial reduction in muscle enzymes; CK is all that is needed to follow the muscle damage; this is usually seen within 6 weeks), taper the dose, for instance, by ~10 mg a month down to 10 mg/d, and then taper more slowly (2.5 mg per month) until 5 mg/d, at which point tapering can continue at 1 mg/mo. If the CK level shows a consistent pattern of rising at a given dose and the patient starts to experience the return of symptoms, the dose should be increased by ≥50% and disease-modifying therapy should be introduced. If the prednisone dose is ≤5 mg/d, monotherapy can be considered due to the low risk of long-term adverse effects.

2. In case of either no satisfactory improvement within 6 weeks of starting treatment, a return of symptoms, or an increasing CK level (as described above), one should add a disease-modifying agent:

1) **Methotrexate**: Administer 10 to 25 mg/wk orally or parenterally (IM or subcutaneously) once a week, with folate 10 mg/wk or folinic acid (the same dose) the day after, for GI protection. Therapeutic effects may be observed up to 3 months after starting treatment. Start with a dose adjusted to the severity of the disease, for instance, 10 to 15 mg once weekly, and if the symptoms do not resolve, titrate the dose up by 5 mg every month. Monitor the complete blood count (CBC), γ-glutamyl transferase (GGT), bilirubin, and ALT monthly for 6 months and every 2 months thereafter. After a cumulative dose of 5 g, a referral to a gastroenterologist for consideration of transient elastography (FibroScan) or liver biopsy may be made.

2) **Azathioprine**: Therapeutic effects may be observed up to 4 months after starting treatment, and an increase in the mean corpuscular volume (MCV) >100 fL is often reflective of the optimal dose (1.5-2.5 mg/kg/d). Monitor the

Table 17-2. Myopathies and other disorders that can mimic polymyositis or dermatomyositis

Endocrine disorders	Hypothyroidism, hypercortisolemia, thyrotoxicosis, hypoparathyroidism, hyperparathyroidism Testing: Endocrine blood testing
Metabolic disorders	GSDs (primarily McArdle disease [type V] but also III, VII, and XV), lysosomal storage disease (Pompe, previously known as GSD II), mitochondrial myopathy (TK2, MELAS, and other mtDNA mutations), primary systemic carnitine deficiency Testing: Specific genetic testing (including mtDNA sequencing or nuclear--encoded gene testing, dry blood spot for Pompe disease, muscle histology and enzymatic testing (ie, PFK [GSD VII] and phosphorylase [GSD V])
Muscular dystrophy	Most common dystrophies to be mistaken for PM are Miyoshi myopathy due to dysferlin (*DYSF*) or *ANO5* mutations, dystrophinopathy (mainly Becker), other limb girdle MDs (eg, sarcoglycanopathy, caveolin-3). Because nearly every one of >70 types of MD will meet probable criteria for PM (proximal weakness, high CK, myopathic EMG), careful history and examination are essential (medial calf atrophy is characteristic of Miyoshi myopathy and not PM/DM), muscle biopsy (inflammation is common as a secondary finding in MD but invasion is of necrotic fibers unlike in PM where they are nonnecrotic; immunohistochemistry can be classic: patchy or absent dystrophin staining in Becker) Testing: Immunohistochemistry on muscle biopsy samples and specific genetic testing
Nerve disorders	Spinal muscular atrophy type III (EMG is usually characteristic, CK is not to minimally elevated), amyotrophic lateral sclerosis (weakness is usually asymmetric but CK can be elevated [usually <1000 IU], EMG shows active changes but recruitment is different than in PM [reduced and large, long vs small duration, brief and early recruiting in PM/DM]) Testing: Genetic testing for SMA; history, examination, and EMG for ALS (El-Escorial criteria)
Neuromuscular junction	LEMS can present with proximal weakness but EMG is not characteristic of PM/DM and CK is usually not elevated. Diagnosis is established with incremental CMAP response post contraction and presence of antibodies to P/Q-type voltage-gated calcium channels. MG usually presents with ocular and bulbar symptoms and only rarely proximal weakness; CK is not usually elevated and EMG is normal. Diagnosis is established by single-fiber EMG, decremental response of CMAP to repetitive stimulation, and presence of specific antibodies (antiacetylcholine receptor, anti-MuSK) Testing: EMG is suggestive but presence of antibodies is very specific
Infections	Viral, bacterial, parasitic (toxoplasmosis, trichinosis) Testing: Virology, bacterial culture, and PCR-based testing
Electrolyte disturbances	Decreased or increased plasma levels of sodium, potassium, calcium, magnesium, or phosphate Testing: Electrolyte analysis in blood
Granulomatous diseases	Sarcoidosis Testing: Noncaseating granulomas in muscle biopsy, low ACE levels in blood
Drugs	Lipid-lowering agents (statins, rarely fibrates), antimalarial agents (chloroquine and hydroxychloroquine), amiodarone, quinidine, cimetidine, cyclosporine (INN ciclosporin), danazol, D-penicillamine, interferon α, interleukin 2, colchicine, ε-aminocaproic acid, phenylbutazone, phenytoin, glucocorticoids (common: type 2 muscle fiber atrophy, especially with doses >10 mg), hydralazine, levodopa, penicillin, procainamide, rifampicin, sulfonamides, L-tryptophan, valproic acid, vincristine, some anti-HIV drugs (zidovudine, ddI, ddC)

Toxic substances	Acute exposure to carbon monoxide, alcohol, heroin, cocaine; history and specific testing will easily differentiate these from PM/DM

ACE, angiotensin-converting enzyme; ALS, amyotrophic lateral sclerosis; CK, creatine kinase; CMAP, compound muscle action potential; DM, dermatomyositis; EMG, electromyography; GSD, glycogen storage disease; INN, international nonproprietary name; LEMS, Lambert-Eaton myasthenic syndrome; MD, muscular dystrophy; MELAS, mitochondrial encephalomyopathy with lactic acidosis and stroke-like episodes; MG, myasthenia gravis; mtDNA, mitochondrial DNA; MuSK, muscle-specific kinase; PCR, polymerase chain reaction; PFK, phosphofructokinase; PM, polymyositis; SMA, spinal muscular atrophy; TK2, thymidine kinase 2.

CBC, GGT, bilirubin, and ALT monthly for 6 months and every 2 months thereafter. About 7% of patients will develop a flu-like illness within days of starting the agent (avoid the use of azathioprine with allopurinol or other xanthine oxidase inhibitors).

3) **Intravenous immunoglobulin (IVIG)**: This is often effective in combination with methylprednisolone (250-1000 mg/d) in severe disease and has been shown to be effective in lowering the steroid dose in both DM and PM.☕ Use a dose of 1 g/kg/d twice in 2 to 4 days or 0.4 g/kg/d for 5 consecutive days and then once a month for 3 to 7 months.

4) **Cyclosporine** (INN ciclosporin) in doses 2.5 to 5 mg/kg/d with prednisone was shown to be superior to prednisone alone. Cyclosporine is associated with a greater number of infections compared to prednisone alone. Renal function and blood pressure must be carefully monitored with cyclosporine use.

5) **Cyclophosphamide** 1 g IV once a month or 1 to 3 mg/kg orally once daily. This agent is generally only used in patients with severe interstitial pulmonary lesions not responding to standard therapy or in those with severe vasculitis.

6) **Mycophenolate mofetil** 2 to 3 g/d in case methotrexate, azathioprine, and cyclosporine are poorly tolerated or ineffective.

7) **Hydroxychloroquine** 200 mg bid or **chloroquine** 250 mg bid are indicated in patients with refractory cutaneous lesions.

8) **Biologic agents**: A variety of biologics have been tried primarily in juvenile DM, but their long-term safety and efficacy has not been determined. In the authors' experience, these agents are very rarely indicated (rituximab, abatacept, anti–tumor necrosis factor α drugs, and tocilizumab).

9) **Combination therapy**: Most patients are treated with a combination of a glucocorticosteroid and IVIG or another disease-modifying agent. In severe treatment-resistant cases one may consider the combination of methotrexate and azathioprine or one of available combinations with mycophenolate.

Rehabilitation

Exercise and physiotherapy are important measures to prevent issues and to restore physical function. In patients with acute disease mainly passive movements and stretching are recommended to prevent contractures. When subjective strength is improving and the CK level is closer to normal, the patient can start endurance and resistance exercises, initially at a low level and gradually increasing the intensity and duration as tolerated. In general, the suggested aerobic intensity is ≤65% of the maximal aerobic power; for resistance exercise, the number of suggested repetitions is >12; and the suggested intensity is ≤65% of the one-repetition maximum.

➔ FOLLOW-UP

Follow-up should involve periodic evaluation of muscle strength and plasma CK levels; for patients receiving disease-modifying agents, the CBC, liver function/damage tests (bilirubin, GGT, ALT; note that ALT will follow CK levels and is only relevant if disproportionate to CK); and in patients with interstitial lung disease, HRCT, pulmonary function tests, and the 6-minute walk test.

Assessment and monitoring for malignancy is important but need not be exhaustive (chest radiographs in smokers or those with respiratory symptoms, occult blood/colonoscopy [especially in those aged >50 years], mammography/breast examination, Papanicolaou test in women not immunized against human papillomavirus, abdominal and pelvic ultrasound in those with abdominal symptoms and women with altered periods, prostate examination [clinical and with prostate-specific antigen test] in men aged >50 years). The risk of cancer is highest within the first 3 years of the diagnosis of PM/DM but continues to be high even after 5 years. Other factors associated with an increased risk of malignancy include age >50 years, DM, severe skin involvement, and the presence of anti-155/140 kD (TIF1γ) antibodies.

➔ PROGNOSIS

The 5-year mortality rate for treated patients is between 20% and 35%, but for cancer-associated myositis the overall mortality rate (related to primary disease, drugs, or myositis complications) can be as high as 75%. A less favorable prognosis is also associated with advanced age and involvement of internal organs, particularly lungs, and the presence of antibodies to SRP. A more favorable prognosis is seen in PM cases associated with the Mi-2 antibody. The risk of malignancy is 4-fold to 6-fold greater than for aged-matched controls in adult patients with DM and 1.5-fold to 2-fold greater in patients with PM (including the increased risk of ovarian, breast, lung, intestinal, nose and throat, pancreatic, and bladder cancers as well as non-Hodgkin lymphomas).

18. Rheumatoid Arthritis

➔ DEFINITION, ETIOLOGY, PATHOGENESIS

Rheumatoid arthritis (RA) is a chronic systemic autoimmune connective tissue disease of unknown etiology characterized by symmetric polyarthritis and associated extra-articular and systemic manifestations. RA leads to impairment, disability, and premature death if treated inadequately. The onset and progression of the disease is considered to be related to the response of CD45RO+ T cells (memory cells) to an unknown antigen or antigens, exogenous or endogenous, in a genetically predisposed individual. Based on the presence or absence of autoantibodies (IgM rheumatoid factor [RF] and/or anti-citrullinated protein antibodies [ACPAs; also termed antibodies to cyclic citrullinated peptides]), the disease can be divided into seropositive RA and seronegative RA, respectively.

➔ CLINICAL FEATURES AND NATURAL HISTORY

RA affects women 3 times as often as men, with the peak age of onset occurring between 30 and 50 years. In ~70% of patients with RA, relapses and partial remissions are observed, leading to progressive joint destruction. In ~15% of patients the course of RA is mild, with moderate disease activity, involvement of a few joints, and slowly progressive joint destruction. In ~10% of patients remissions are prolonged, lasting up to several years. Very rarely, the course of the disease is episodic (so-called palindromic rheumatism) or self-limiting. Up to 25% of these seropositive patients will go on to develop RA in subsequent years. Usually the disease onset is insidious, over a few weeks to months;

however, in 10% to 15% of patients signs and symptoms develop rapidly over a few days (in these cases joint involvement may be asymmetric). In 75% of pregnant patients, symptoms improve in the first trimester and worsen after delivery. RA itself does not increase the risk of maternal or fetal complications.

1. Typical signs and symptoms: Symmetric pain and swelling of the joints of hands and feet, less frequently also of larger joints (eg, knee or shoulder). Morning joint stiffness of variable duration, usually lasting >1 hour.

2. Systemic manifestations: Low-grade fever, myalgia, fatigue, anorexia, and weight loss can occur. These usually precede the diagnosis.

3. Musculoskeletal manifestations: Early RA usually presents with a symmetric polyarthritis particularly affecting wrists, hands (metacarpophalangeal [MCP] and proximal interphalangeal [PIP] joints), and feet (metatarsophalangeal [MTP] joints), although the disease can present with large joint polyarthritis. The lumbar spine, distal interphalangeal (DIP) joints, and hip joints are unlikely to be involved in the inflammatory arthritis process. Joints of the upper extremities (particularly wrist joints) are affected more frequently than those of the lower extremities, although MTP joint involvement may be the first sign of RA. The onset of RA may be atypical, manifesting as monoarthritis or as palindromic rheumatism (pain and/or swelling in various joints lasting from a few hours to a few days and remitting spontaneously). Features occurring in the early stages of RA include heat (without erythema of the overlying skin), tenderness and swelling of joints and tendons, and joint effusions.

1) **Joints of the hand** (→Chapter 1.11.2): In patients with early RA, fusiform swelling of PIP and MCP joints and palmar erythema located on the thenar and hypothenar eminences may be observed. Deformities develop in patients with more advanced RA. Atrophy of the interosseous and lumbrical muscles may occur due to disuse or neuropathy. Ulnar deviation of digits is the most frequent deformity. In later stages patients may develop volar subluxation of the phalanges at the level of the MCP joints, hyperextension of the PIP joint with flexion of the DIP joint ("swan-neck deformity"), or flexion of the PIP joint with hyperextension of the DIP joint ("boutonnière deformity," caused by involvement of ligaments and tendons and muscle contractures), which lead to a significant impairment of finger movement. Wrist involvement includes dorsal or palmar swelling at the radiocarpal and carpal joints, swelling around the extensor carpi ulnaris tendon, and erosion of the ulnar styloid with interruption of the supporting ligaments, resulting in the "piano key" sign. The expanding synovium may compress the median nerve under the flexor retinaculum at the wrist, leading to carpal tunnel syndrome.

2) **Elbow**: Pain, swelling, and limited extension. Some patients may develop permanent flexion contractures.

3) **Shoulder**: Synovitis of the glenohumeral joint, subacromial-subdeltoid bursitis, rotator cuff tendonitis (causing subluxation), and atrophy of adjacent muscles. The acromioclavicular joint is rarely involved in RA (usually due to degenerative arthritis).

4) **MTP joints** are very frequently involved from the onset of the disease, causing toe deformities similar to those of the fingers.

5) **Ankle and midfoot joints** may be involved in progressive RA, often resulting in instability.

6) **Hip involvement** is uncommon in RA and is more commonly found in osteoarthritis. Hip synovitis presents with pain in the groin and progressive difficulty in walking.

7) **Knees** are frequently involved in patients with RA. Suprapatellar joint effusion results in a positive patellar tap test or swelling of the medial and/or lateral aspects of the joint, which increases upon compression of the suprapatellar region. A Baker cyst may develop (causing a palpable popliteal protrusion); increasing pressure of the accumulating effusion may lead to

a rupture of the Baker cyst, leakage of the synovial fluid into tissues of the lower leg, significant lower leg edema, and worsening of knee pain with concomitant contracture of the knee (this needs to be differentiated from deep vein thrombosis of the lower leg). When this is accompanied by blood tracking down to the ankle, a crescent sign may be seen (discoloration around the lateral malleolus).

8) **Spine**: The cervical spine can be affected, leading to subluxation, destruction of the cartilage of the intervertebral disc, and disc prolapse. Atlantoaxial subluxation is potentially dangerous and presents with pain referred to the occipital area, paresthesias within the shoulder girdle and the upper extremity, and spastic paraplegia in the case of spinal cord compression.

9) **Other joints**: Involvement of the temporomandibular joint (pain in the temporomandibular area, difficulty opening the mouth and eating), crico-arytenoid joint (hoarseness), and less commonly the sternoclavicular joint.

4. Extra-articular manifestations occur particularly in patients with severe, long-standing seropositive RA and include:

1) Painless **subcutaneous nodules** on extensor surfaces, in particular of the forearm but also in pressure areas (eg, buttocks), within tendons, and over the joints. Nodules may also develop within internal organs.

2) **Cardiovascular manifestations**: Atherosclerosis and thromboembolic events (cardiovascular events are a common cause of death in patients with RA), pericarditis (in advanced RA), pericardial effusion that can be clinically asymptomatic, myocardial and valvular lesions (nodules, cardiomyopathy), pulmonary hypertension.

3) **Pulmonary manifestations**: Pleuritis (effusion is often clinically asymptomatic), nodules in the lungs (which may undergo fibrosis, calcification, or infection, and may be mistaken for neoplastic lesions), obliterative bronchiolitis, pulmonary fibrosis.

4) **Ocular manifestations**: Dry conjunctiva in the course of secondary Sjögren syndrome, episcleritis, and rarely scleritis ("corneal melt").

5) **Renal manifestations** (mainly due to adverse effects of drugs used in RA treatment): Interstitial nephritis, pyelonephritis, secondary amyloidosis (complication of chronic active inflammation).

6) **Other**: Small- and medium-vessel vasculitis (this may lead to necrosis of distal digits, skin, and internal organs); involvement of the nervous system: carpal tunnel syndrome, polyneuropathy (particularly in the course of vasculitis), mononeuritis multiplex related to vasculitis, spinal nerve root compression due to destruction of cervical spine joints; submaxillary, cervical, axillary, and cubital lymphadenopathy; splenomegaly (with leukopenia [neutropenia] as part of Felty syndrome).

→ DIAGNOSIS

Diagnostic Tests

1. Laboratory tests: Elevated erythrocyte sedimentation rate (ESR) (>30 mm/h) and/or elevated C-reactive protein (CRP) levels, anemia (may be normocytic normochromic in anemia of chronic disease, microcytic hypochromic in iron deficiency anemia secondary to gastrointestinal blood loss, or macrocytic related to folate deficiency [methotrexate—MTX—use] or B_{12} deficiency [pernicious anemia can be associated with RA]), minor elevations in the white blood cell count with a normal differential count or leukopenia associated with disease-modifying antirheumatic drug (DMARD) use, thrombocytosis (in patients with highly active disease) or thrombocytopenia (adverse effect of drugs), elevated plasma α_1-globulin and α_2-globulin levels, positive serum IgM RF in ~75% of patients (high titers correlate with rapid joint destruction and presence of extra-articular features), ACPAs (sensitivity >50% and specificity

>98% in patients with RA; ~40% of patients with negative IgM RF have positive ACPAs, which are an adverse prognostic factor [similar to RF] and predict rapid joint destruction). A new test, 14-3-3η, is used in conjunction with the other autoantibodies and confers greater specificity and sensitivity. A triple antibody test is available commercially as "JOINTstat" (RF, ACPA, 14-3-3η).

2. Synovial fluid analysis: Features of inflammation. Other than when excluding infection, synovial fluid is not routinely examined in RA. If done, some clinicians consider testing for RF, which may be detected earlier than plasma RF. In some patients ragocytes may be observed (neutrophils, macrophages, monocytes, or synoviocytes with cytoplasmic inclusions of phagocytosed immune complexes).

3. Imaging studies: Radiographs of the affected joints reveal lesions that correlate with stage of the disease and may show 4 typical features: soft tissue swelling, joint space narrowing, periarticular osteopenia, and/or marginal erosions. **Ultrasonography** reveals synovial thickening, increased synovial vascularity, and effusions and erosions in small and large joints; joint erosions may be detected earlier by ultrasonography than by radiography. **Magnetic resonance imaging (MRI)** allows for early detection of synovitis, joint erosions, and bone marrow edema, which may precede synovitis. **Computed tomography (CT)** detects joint destruction earlier than radiographs and is the best method for visualizing bone cysts in patients with preserved or only slightly altered continuity of the bone cortex (in such cases the MRI signal of the cysts is normal and they may not be visualized); it is particularly useful in evaluating lesions in the cervical spine.

Diagnostic Workup

Basic laboratory investigations that should be undertaken include the ESR, CRP, IgM RF, ACPAs, complete blood count with a differential count, serum alanine aminotransferase (ALT), serum aspartate aminotransferase (AST), uric acid (if gout is suspected in the differential diagnosis), creatinine and electrolyte levels, urinalysis, synovial fluid analysis (to exclude other joint pathologies in patients with joint effusion [specifically infections or crystal arthropathies]), and radiographs of the hands, feet, or other affected joints. In patients with normal radiographs, ultrasonography with power Doppler and/or MRI could be performed to assess for early disease activity. Antinuclear antibody (ANA) levels are not useful in the clinical setting of probable RA but could be considered if a connective tissue disease such as lupus is in the differential diagnosis.

The diagnosis should also take into account disease activity (→Table 18-1) and functional capacity (assessed, eg, with the Health Assessment Questionnaire score or EuroQol tools).

Diagnostic Criteria

The American College of Rheumatology (ACR)/European League Against Rheumatism (EULAR) classification criteria are used: →Table 18-2.

Differential Diagnosis

The most likely alternative diagnosis is crystalline arthritis with "pseudo-RA." Other conditions that can mimic the joint pain of RA include spondyloarthritides encompassing psoriatic arthritis, and infective arthritis. Less commonly any of connective tissue diseases can present with arthritis; patients with connective tissue diseases develop arthralgia (pain but no inflammation in the joints) more frequently.

⇥ TREATMENT

Treat-to-Target Approach

The treatment target is clinical remission according to one of several criteria. The ACR/EULAR criteria (→Table 18-2) are frequently used. The target should be attained within 6 months; however, treatment should be modified

Table 18-1. Rheumatoid arthritis disease activity measures

Disease activity measure	Components	Interpretation of results
DAS[a]	In clinical practice DAS28 (including 28 joints: wrists, metacarpophalangeal joints, proximal interphalangeal joints, elbows, shoulders, knees) is used most commonly. Score is evaluated using a calculator that takes into account: 1) Number of swollen joints 2) Number of tender joints (including 28 joints: wrists, metacarpophalangeal joints, proximal interphalangeal joints, elbows, shoulders, knees) 3) ESR or CRP 4) Patient's global assessment of disease activity using VAS (0-100)	Score range: 0-9.4 **Interpretation:** <2.6: Remission ≤3.2: Low activity >3.2 and ≤5.1: Moderate activity >5.1: High activity **Evaluation of treatment response:** – Good: Change in activity ≥1.2 and low disease activity – Moderate: Change >0.6 and <1.2 and low or moderate disease activity, or change ≥1.2 and high or moderate disease activity – No response: Change <0.6 or <1.2 and high activity
SDAI	Takes into account same joints as DAS28 but does not require a calculator SDAI score = Number of tender joints + Number of swollen joints + Patient's global assessment of disease activity using VAS (0-10 cm) + Physician's global assessment of disease activity using VAS (0-10 cm) + Plasma CRP levels (0.1-10 mg/dL)	Score range: 0.1-86 **Interpretation:** Score ≤3.3: Remission ≤11: Low activity >11 and ≤26: Moderate activity >26: High activity **Evaluation of treatment response:** – Significant improvement: Change >21 – Moderate improvement: Change 10-21 – No improvement: Change ≤9
CDAI	Identical to SDAI but does not take CRP into account	Score range: 0.1-76 **Interpretation:** Score ≤2.8: Remission ≤10: Low activity >10 and ≤22: Moderate activity >22: High activity
ACR/ EULAR remission criteria	All must be fulfilled: – Tender joint count ≤1 – Swollen joint count ≤1 – Plasma CRP (mg/dL) ≤1 – Patient's global assessment of disease activity using VAS (0-10) ≤1 or SDAI ≤3.3	Criteria recommended by EULAR for assessment of effectiveness of treatment in clinical practice

In clinical practice, the CDAI is the most commonly performed measure of disease activity. Other measures are used mainly in research settings.

[a] www.das-score.nl/das28/en/

ACR, American College of Rheumatology; CDAI, Clinical Disease Activity Index; CRP, C-reactive protein; DAS, Disease Activity Score; ESR, erythrocyte sedimentation rate; EULAR, European League Against Rheumatism; SDAI, Simplified Disease Activity Index; VAS, visual analogue scale.

Table 18-2. The 2010 American College of Rheumatology/European League Against Rheumatism rheumatoid arthritis classification criteria

Target population (who should be tested)

Patients with:

1) ≥1 joint with definite clinical synovitis (swelling)

2) Synovitis not better explained by another disease[a]

The criteria are aimed at classification of newly presenting patients. In addition, patients with erosive disease typical of RA[b] or with long-standing disease, including those whose disease is inactive (with or without treatment), who based on retrospectively available data had previously fulfilled the 2010 criteria, should be classified as having RA.

Classification criteria for RA (score-based algorithm: add score of categories A-D; a score ≥6/10 is needed to classify a patient as having RA)[c].

A. Joint involvement[d]	Score
1 large joint[e]	0
2-10 large joints	1
1-3 small joints[f] (with or without involvement of large joints)	2
4-10 small joints (with or without involvement of large joints)	3
>10 joints[g] (including ≥1 small joint)	5

B. Serology (≥1 test result is needed for classification)[h]	Score
Negative RF and negative ACPAs	0
Low-positive RF or low-positive ACPAs	2
High-positive RF or high-positive ACPAs	3

C. Acute-phase reactants (≥1 test result is needed for classification)	Score
Normal CRP and normal ESR	0
Abnormal CRP or abnormal ESR	1

D. Duration of symptoms[i]	Score
<6 weeks	0
≥6 weeks	1

[a] Differential diagnosis may include conditions such as SLE, psoriatic arthritis, and gout. [b] Erosions (defined as disruptions of the bone cortex) revealed on radiographs of hands and feet in ≥3 individual joints among proximal interphalangeal joints, metacarpophalangeal joints, wrist joints (counted as 1 joint), and metatarsophalangeal joints. [c] Patients with a score <6/10 are not classifiable as having RA, however their status can be reassessed and the criteria may be fulfilled cumulatively over time. [d] Joint involvement refers to any swollen or tender joint on examination, which may be confirmed by imaging evidence of synovitis. Distal interphalangeal joints, first carpometacarpal joints, and first metatarsophalangeal joints are excluded from assessment (these are typically involved in osteoarthritis). [e] Large joints: Shoulders, elbows, hips, knees, and ankles. [f] Small joints: Metacarpophalangeal joints, proximal interphalangeal joints, second through fifth metatarsophalangeal joints, thumb interphalangeal joints, and wrists. [g] In this category ≥1 of the involved joints must be a small joint. Other joints can include any combination of large and additional small joints as well as other joints not specifically listed elsewhere (eg, temporomandibular, acromioclavicular, sternoclavicular). [h] Negative results refer to international unit values that are less than or equal to the ULN for the laboratory and assay. Low-positive results refer to international unit values that are higher than the ULN but 3 times the ULN for the laboratory and assay. High-positive results refer to international unit values that are 3 times the ULN for the laboratory and assay. [i] Duration of symptoms refers to the patient's self-report of the duration of signs or symptoms of synovitis (eg, pain, swelling, tenderness) of joints that are clinically involved at the time of assessment, regardless of treatment status.

Source: Ann Rheum Dis. 2010;69(9):1580-8.

ACPA, anti-citrullinated peptide antibody; CRP, C-reactive protein; ESR, erythrocyte sedimentation rate; RA, rheumatoid arthritis; RF, rheumatoid factor; SLE, systemic lupus erythematosus; ULN, upper limit of normal.

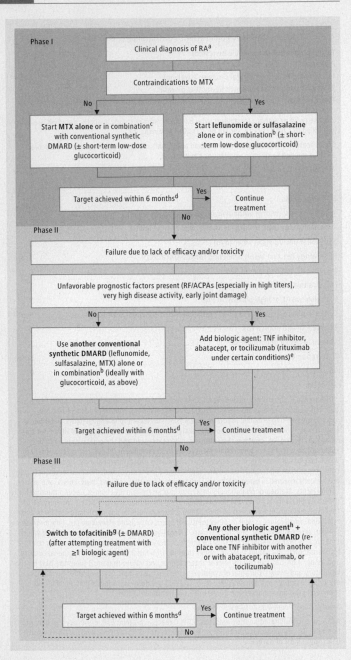

a 2010 ACR/EULAR classification criteria can be useful for early diagnosis.

b Combinations of leflunomide or sulfasalazine without MTX have not been well studied. They may include both these drugs with or without an antimalarial.

c The most common combination includes MTX, sulfasalazine, and hydroxychloroquine.

d The target is clinical remission according to the ACR/EULAR or, if remission is unlikely, at least low disease activity. The target should be reached within 6 months, but therapy should be adapted or changed if there is no improvement after 3 months.

e Mainly in patients with recent lymphoma, demyelinating disease, latent TB, contraindications to preventive pharmacotherapy, or living in areas where TB is endemic.

f Adalimumab, certolizumab, etanercept, golimumab, infliximab, or respective well-studied EMA/FDA-approved biosimilars.

g Where licensed.

h Efficacy and safety of treatment with biologic agents after failure of tofacitinib have not been studied to date.

Solid line (⟶), recommended.
Dotted line (·····▶), recommended after failure of a biologic agent (ideally 2 agents).
Dashed line (- - ▶), recommended after failure of 2 biologic agents, but efficacy and safety after failure of abatacept, rituximab, and tocilizumab have not been sufficiently studied

ACPA, anti-citrullinated peptide antibody; ACR, American College of Rheumatology; DMARD, disease-modifying antirheumatic drug; EMA, European Medicines Agency; EULAR, European League Against Rheumatism; FDA, Food and Drug Administration; MTX, methotrexate; RA, rheumatoid arthritis; RF, rheumatoid factor; TB, tuberculosis; TNF, tumor necrosis factor.

Figure 18-1. Management algorithm for rheumatoid arthritis. *Based on Ann Rheum Dis. 2017;76(6):960-977.*

if no improvement is observed after 3 months. The 2016 EULAR treatment algorithm: →Figure 18-1.

Pharmacotherapy

1. DMARDs are the mainstay of therapy in RA, as they prevent or delay joint damage. They should be introduced promptly after the diagnosis of RA is established.◉● DMARDs are classified as follows:

1) **Synthetic DMARDs:**

   a) **Conventional DMARDs**: MTX, leflunomide, sulfasalazine, gold salts, hydroxychloroquine.

   b) **Targeted DMARDs**: Tofacitinib (Janus kinase [JAK] 3 and 1 inhibitor), baricitinib (JAK 1 and 2 inhibitor).

2) **Biologic agents (biologics; biologic DMARDs):**

   a) **Innovator biologics**, including anticytokine agents targeting tumor necrosis factor (TNF)-α (etanercept, adalimumab, infliximab, certolizumab, golimumab), interleukin 6 (IL-6) (tocilizumab), interleukin 1 (IL-1) (anakinra), and other biologic drugs targeting noncytokine pathways (abatacept, rituximab).

   b) **Biosimilar agents**: For instance, biosimilar infliximab.

The choice of individual agents depends on disease activity and duration, prior treatment, prognostic factors (adverse prognostic factors include positive autoantibodies [RF and/or ACPAs, particularly in high titers], very high disease activity, early development of erosions), and comorbidities, as well as adverse effects and availability of the drugs (agents, dosage, contraindications, and treatment monitoring: →Table 18-3).

In patients with active RA, start with MTX 15 mg once weekly, titrate up to the optimal dose (usually 20-25 mg/wk, with 25 mg/wk being the maximum; →Table 18-3) over 2 to 6 weeks (target dose might be a little lower in patients with adverse effects of MTX), and continue for ≥8 weeks in combination with folic acid 5 mg 24 hours after MTX. Folic acid counteracts some of the adverse

Table 18-3. Disease-modifying antirheumatic drugs used in the treatment of rheumatoid arthritis

Drug	Dosage	Contraindications	Adverse reactions	Monitoring
Conventional (nonbiologic) DMARDs				
Hydroxychloroquine	200 mg PO once daily or bid	Retinal diseases; visual impairment; renal failure; porphyria; psoriasis; G6PD deficiency; untreated chronic hepatitis B or C with Child-Pugh class C	Retinal (macular) damage reversible after drug discontinuation; rash; abdominal pain, diarrhea, appetite loss, nausea; other (very rare): myopathy, blurred vision, visual impairment, abnormal cutaneous/mucosal pigmentation, peripheral neuropathy	Ophthalmic exam (fundoscopy and visual fields): before starting treatment, follow-up every 12 months. There is a maximum lifetime dose of 1000 g, which is reached after 7 years on 400 mg/d
Leflunomide	10-20 mg PO once daily	Infection[a]; leukopenia <3 ×10⁹/L; thrombocytopenia <50 ×10⁹/L; myelodysplasia; lymphoproliferative disorder treated in last ≤5 years; liver disease[b,c,d]; pregnancy and breastfeeding; severe or moderate renal impairment	Diarrhea, abdominal pain, nausea; rash; alopecia; liver damage; kidney damage; hypertension; teratogenicity (effective contraception necessary). In case of complications, drug has to be discontinued; elimination may be accelerated using cholestyramine (8 g tid for 11 days) or activated charcoal (50 g qid for 11 days). In women planning pregnancy and men planning to become fathers, levels of metabolite of leflunomide should be measured several times following accelerated elimination	CBC: before starting treatment, then every 2 weeks in initial 3 months of treatment, then every 2-3 months; after 6 months of treatment repeat every 3 months or less frequently. Serum creatinine: every 2 weeks until target drug dose is established, then every month. Serum ALT and AST: as above; in case of sustained increase in AST/ALT >3 × ULN, drug should be discontinued and liver biopsy considered to assess liver damage
Methotrexate	15-25 mg PO, IM, or SC once weekly; titrate dose to a max 25 mg; folic acid (5 mg/wk) or leucovorin (INN folinic acid) to be used concomitantly to prevent adverse effects (cytopenia, mouth ulceration, nausea)	As above + interstitial pneumonitis/pulmonary fibrosis; CrCl <30 mL/min	Elevated serum liver enzyme levels, liver fibrosis and cirrhosis (very rare); risk factors: alcohol consumption, obesity, diabetes, hepatitis B and C; pancytopenia due to bone marrow suppression and complications (dose-dependent); oral ulcers (in 30% of patients); nausea within 24-48 h of drug administration; interstitial lung disease (2%-6% of drug administration); teratogenicity (effective contraception necessary): methotrexate should be discontinued (in both women and men) 3 months before planned conception; milder adverse effects (due to folic acid deficiency): mucositis, alopecia, GI disturbances	As above + chest x-ray before starting treatment (results of studies performed in the previous year are acceptable) and in course of treatment if cough or dyspnea develop

	Dose	Contraindications	Adverse effects	Monitoring
Sulfasalazine	1.5 g PO bid (dose should be titrated up)	Hypersensitivity to sulfonamides and salicylate; after ileostomy; liver disease[b,c,e], renal failure; porphyria; G6PD deficiency; breastfeeding; considered safe in pregnancy	Majority of adverse effects occur within first few months of treatment and can be avoided by starting with low dose and titrating up gradually: loss of appetite, dyspepsia, nausea, vomiting, abdominal pain (30%); headache, vertigo/dizziness; fever; allergic skin (urticaria, photosensitivity) and joint reactions; hemolytic anemia (in patients with G6PD deficiency), very rarely aplastic anemia; granulocytopenia (1%-3%) may occur at any time of treatment (most commonly in first 3 months); elevated serum ALT/AST; interstitial lung disease (rare)	CBC, serum ALT, AST, and creatinine: as above
Biologic DMARDS: TNF inhibitors				
Adalimumab	20-40 mg SC every 1-2 weeks	Infection[a]; viral hepatitis[c,e]; pregnancy, breastfeeding; heart failure (NYHA class III/IV and EF ≤50%); multiple sclerosis or other demyelinating disease; lymphoproliferative disease treated in last ≤5 years[f]	Severe infections (including opportunistic infections); positive autoantibodies including ANAs, anti-dsDNA, anticardiolipin, and antichimeric; rarely drug-induced lupus (in which case treatment should be discontinued); cytopenias (mainly leukopenia); demyelination syndromes; optic neuritis (very rare) with symptoms resolving after drug discontinuation; reactivation of HBV infection; elevated serum ALT/AST	Before starting: chest x-ray and tuberculin skin test/IGRA test, CBC, serum ALT/AST and creatinine; tests for viral hepatitis; pneumococcal (periodic), influenza (annual), and hepatitis B (in patients at risk of infection) vaccinations recommended; live vaccines contraindicated but could be administered prior to starting DMARD or biologic treatment; in course of treatment patients should be monitored for symptoms of infection; in women mammography is recommended before starting treatment
Etanercept	25 mg SC twice a week or 50 mg/wk	As above	As above	
Infliximab	3-10 mg/kg IV, repeated after 2 and 6 weeks, then every 8 weeks, or 3-5 mg/kg every 4 weeks	As above	As above	

Drug	Dosage	Contraindications	Adverse reactions	Monitoring
Certolizumab	200 mg SC bid, repeated after 2 and 4 weeks, followed by maintenance dose 200 mg every 2 weeks	As above	As above	As above
Golimumab	50 mg SC once a month	As above	As above	As above
Other biologic DMARDs				
Abatacept	IV infusion over 30 min; body weight <60 kg: 500 mg, 60-100 kg: 750 mg, >100 kg: 1 g; subsequent doses to be administered 2 and 4 weeks after first infusion, then every 4 weeks	Infection[a]; viral hepatitis[c,e]; pregnancy and breastfeeding	Severe infections; probably causes progressive multifocal leukoencephalopathy (very rare)	Before starting: chest x-ray and tuberculin skin test/IGRA test, CBC, serum ALT/AST and creatinine, tests for viral hepatitis; pneumococcal (periodic), influenza (annual), and hepatitis B (in patients at risk of infection) vaccinations recommended; live vaccines contraindicated; in course of treatment patients should be monitored for symptoms of infection; in women mammography is recommended before starting treatment
Rituximab	1 g IV, 2 doses at 14-day interval; can be repeated every 6 months	Infection[a]; viral hepatitis[c,e]; pregnancy and breastfeeding	Allergic reactions, infections, probably causes progressive multifocal leukoencephalopathy (very rare), reactivation of HBV infection	As above + plasma immunoglobulin levels
Tocilizumab	8 mg/kg IV every 4 weeks or 162 mg SC weekly	Infection[a]; ALT/AST >5× ULN; viral hepatitis[c,g]; neutropenia <0.5×10⁹/L and thrombocytopenia <50×10⁹/L; pregnancy and breastfeeding	Infections, neutropenia, and thrombocytopenia, elevated ALT/AST (in particular during concomitant use of potentially hepatotoxic drugs, eg, DMARDs), dyslipidemia, intestinal perforation in patients with diverticulitis (infrequent)	As above (drug may suppress acute-phase reaction so patients should be very carefully monitored for features of infection) + ALT/AST every 4-8 weeks for first 6 months of treatment, then every 3 months; CBC after 4-8 weeks of treatment, then repeat when necessary

Targeted DMARDs

Tofacitinib	5 mg PO bid	Malignancy, current infection, pregnancy and breastfeeding	Headache, diarrhea, bacterial infections, herpes zoster infection	TB skin prick test and chest x-ray; CBC, ALT, AST, creatinine, and lipids; monitor for infection and malignancy
Baricitinib	2 mg PO daily	As tofacitinib	As tofacitinib	As tofacitinib

a Active bacterial infection, TB (active or latent in patients not receiving anti-TB prophylaxis), active infection with varicella zoster or herpes simplex virus, active severe fungal infection (in the case of biologic agents probably also febrile viral upper respiratory tract infection and poorly healing infected skin ulcers).

b ALT and/or AST levels >2×ULN.

c Acute hepatitis B or C.

d Chronic hepatitis B or C (regardless of treatment status and severity of liver disease).

e Chronic hepatitis B (unless treated and with Child-Pugh class A; sulfasalazine can be used in both class A and B) or chronic hepatitis C associated with Child-Pugh class B or C (etanercept is recommended as potentially safe in patients with chronic hepatitis C).

f Rituximab is recommended in patients with RA qualifying for a biologic agent and a history of treated lymphoproliferative malignancy or skin melanoma (anytime), as well as treated within the last 5 years nonmelanoma skin cancers or solid malignancies.

g Evidence is scarce regarding safety of tocilizumab in chronic viral hepatitis.

h Loading dose may be used to speed up the onset of effect; however, it is common practice to avoid it because of the risk of diarrhea and compliance issues. It is not recommended when leflunomide is used in combination therapy.

ANA, antinuclear antibody; ALT, alanine aminotransferase; AST, aspartate aminotransferase; bid, 2 times a day; CBC, complete blood count; CrCl, creatinine clearance; DMARD, disease-modifying antirheumatic drug; EF, ejection fraction; G6PD, glucose-6-phosphate dehydrogenase; GI, gastrointestinal; IM, intramuscular; IV, intravenous; HBV, hepatitis B virus; IGRA, interferon γ release assay; INN, international nonproprietary name; NYHA, New York Heart Association; PO, oral; qid, 4 times a day; RA, rheumatoid arthritis; SC, subcutaneous; TB, tuberculosis; tid, 3 times a day; TNF, tumor necrosis factor; ULN, upper limit of normal.

effects (such as aphthous ulceration, nausea, hair loss) of the antimetabolite, MTX. MTX may be used alone or in combination with other DMARDs as first--line management. In the case of contraindications to or intolerance of MTX, use oral leflunomide (10-20 mg daily) or oral sulfasalazine (up to 1.5 g bid), alone or in combination. In the initial treatment strategy, consider adding low-dose glucocorticoids (prednisone ≤7.5 mg/d or equivalent doses of methylprednisolone or prednisolone); these should be continued for the shortest period possible (<6 months); ensure prevention/treatment of osteoporosis (→Chapter 14.13). Often dual or triple therapy is initiated following diagnosis, with evidence supporting optimization of these therapies.

In the event that the goals of treatment are not achieved within 6 months despite the use of optimal doses of conventional synthetic DMARDs, no improvement is observed within 3 months, or drug adverse effects develop (in the case of MTX intolerance start by changing the route of administration from oral to IM or subcutaneous), consider the following:

1) Switch to or add another conventional DMARD, optimally in combination with short-term low-dose glucocorticoids.◐●

2) Add a biologic DMARD or targeted therapy (TNF inhibitor, rituximab, abatacept, tocilizumab, or JAK inhibitor◐●; →Figure 18-1).

Use all biologic DMARDs in combination with MTX (≥10 mg/wk) or other conventional DMARDs. If the treatment target of low disease activity or remission has not been achieved within 3 to 6 months, consider switching to another biologic DMARD combined with a conventional DMARD.

Once long-term remission has been achieved, you could discuss a careful reduction of the doses of conventional DMARDs with the patient. However, discontinuation of conventional DMARDs in patients in remission may result in a flare or exacerbation of RA and achieving a second remission is much more difficult. In selected cases (severe treatment-resistant RA or contraindications to conventional and/or biologic DMARDs) you may consider using azathioprine or cyclosporine (INN ciclosporin) (or, exceptionally, cyclophosphamide).

2. Oral **nonsteroidal anti-inflammatory drugs (NSAIDs)** should be used for acute control of signs and symptoms of inflammation. In patients with contraindications to or intolerance of NSAIDs, use acetaminophen (INN paracetamol) and/or weak opioids (eg, tramadol).

3. Intra-articular **glucocorticoids** may be considered when the disease (or its exacerbation) involves only one or a few joints (injections to a single joint can be repeated not more often than every 3 months). Before injection exclude any other reasons for the exacerbation of joint manifestations, such as infection or crystal-associated arthropathy. Doses depend on the size of the joint: methylprednisolone, 40 to 80 mg; betamethasone, 0.8 to 4 mg; dexamethasone, 0.2 to 6 mg.

Rehabilitation

Rehabilitation should be part of treatment in every phase of the disease:

1) **Physiotherapy** increases muscle strength, improves physical functioning, prevents contractures and deformities, and prevents disability. There is no clear evidence for beneficial effects of other therapies, including electrotherapy, laser therapy, thermotherapy, cryotherapy, massage, and balneotherapy.

2) **Psychological counseling**.

Surgical Treatment

Consider surgical treatment in the case of:

1) Severe pain and inflammation despite maximal intensity of medical treatment.

2) Joint destruction that limits the range of movement to an extent that causes significant disability.

Types of surgical interventions: synovectomy, reconstructive and corrective procedures, arthrodesis, and arthroplasty.

Synthetic DMARDs need not be stopped in the perioperative period; targeted DMARD tofacitinib should be stopped 7 days before surgery◉ It is recommended that biologic DMARDs are stopped within 2 half-lives prior to surgery and restarted after the surgical wound has healed with exact timing depending on the severity of underlying rheumatologic condition and probability of its deterioration.◯

Biologics should be stopped if the patient has an intercurrent infection.

19. Sjögren Syndrome

→ DEFINITION, ETIOLOGY, PATHOGENESIS

Sjögren syndrome is a chronic autoimmune condition of unknown etiology characterized by lymphocytic infiltrates in the exocrine glands, which result in their impaired secretion, and by inflammation of multiple organs and systems. Sjögren syndrome may be either **primary** (40% of cases) or **secondary** (in the course of other conditions, most frequently rheumatoid arthritis [RA]). This is the second most common connective tissue disease after RA, with a prevalence of 0.5% to 5%.

→ CLINICAL FEATURES

Over 90% of the patients are female. The peak age of onset is ~50 years.

1. Signs and symptoms of involvement of the exocrine glands (the sicca syndrome):

1) **Lacrimal glands**: Corneal and conjunctival dryness (keratoconjunctivitis sicca) perceived as a sandy or gritty feeling under the eyelids, burning, and itching; sensitivity to light, wind, cigarette smoke; conjunctival injection.

2) **Salivary glands**: Dry mouth (xerostomia), difficulty in chewing and swallowing, speech problems, loss of taste (dysgeusia), rapidly progressive caries, difficulty using dentures; enlargement of the parotid and/or submandibular salivary glands, stomatitis.

2. Extraglandular manifestations: General systemic symptoms such as fatigue, low-grade fever, myalgia, arthralgia, occasionally arthritis; symptoms of mild myopathy that may resemble RA (these may precede the onset of the sicca syndrome); Raynaud phenomenon (in ~40% of patients); lymphadenopathy (in 20% of patients); pulmonary manifestations (up to 20% of patients, usually causing minor symptoms or asymptomatic; rarely lymphocytic pneumonitis, nodular changes, or lymphoma); renal manifestations (up to 15% of patients; mainly interstitial nephritis, rarely renal tubular acidosis, occasionally nephrolithiasis and chronic kidney disease); pancreatitis, hepatomegaly; primary biliary cholangitis; vasculitis affecting small vessels of the skin and manifesting as purpura, urticaria, ulcerations; peripheral neuropathies; dry skin with pruritus (up to 55% of patients), autoimmune thyroiditis (frequent but usually asymptomatic).

→ DIAGNOSIS

Diagnostic Tests

1. Blood tests: Hypergammaglobulinemia (in 80% of patients), cryoglobulins (30%), antinuclear antibodies (ANAs) at a titer >1:80 (90%), anti-Ro/SSA (55%)

and anti-La/SSB (40%) antibodies, rheumatoid factor at a titer >1:40 (60%); anemia (25%), leukopenia (10%).

2. Imaging studies: Sialography reveals irregular dilations and strictures of the glandular ducts (a "cherry blossom" appearance). **Salivary scintigraphy** reveals a delayed uptake, decreased accumulation, and delayed excretion of the radiolabeled marker following stimulation. **Ultrasonography** (the most useful test) is used to assess the size and structure of the parotid and submandibular salivary glands, as well as to detect cysts or local lymphadenopathy.

3. Ophthalmologic examination: The Schirmer test is helpful in estimating tear production: a strip of filter paper 5×30 mm with a rounded edge at one end is placed under the lower eyelid in such a way that it does not touch the cornea. After 5 minutes, more than 5 mm of the filter paper should be moistened by tears. The rose Bengal stain (or a test using another dye) is used to assess the corneal surface.

4. Assessment of saliva production (without stimulation) using the Saxon test: The patient chews a piece of a sterile gauze (5×5 cm) for 2 minutes; the weight of the gauze should increase by ≥2.75 g.

5. Histologic examination of salivary gland biopsy specimens: Assessment of the number of lymphocytic infiltrates.

Diagnostic Criteria

Classification criteria: →Table 19-1.

Differential Diagnosis

Exclusion criteria: →Table 19-1.

Differential diagnosis should also include viral infections (eg, chronic parotitis, Epstein-Barr virus infection), amyloidosis, fibromyalgia, hyperlipoproteinemia (types IIa, IV, and V), age-related changes, and IgG4-related systemic disease (differentiated by increased levels of IgG4, absence of anti-Ro and anti-La antibodies). Symptoms of dry eye may be caused by blepharitis or conjunctivitis, infrequent blinking in neurologic or endocrine conditions, or lacrimal gland dysfunction. Xerostomia may occur in diabetes mellitus, hypercalcemia, or due to psychogenic factors. Perhaps the most common cause is the use of anticholinergic medications. Arthritis associated with primary Sjögren syndrome is typically nonerosive and should be differentiated from RA, and a combination of organ involvement with the presence of antibodies should be differentiated from systemic lupus erythematosus.

→ TREATMENT

1. Eye protection using **preservative-free ophthalmic preparations to replace deficient tears** (tear substitutes, artificial tears) in a form of solution or gel and soft contact lenses are helpful in mild disease. The addition of ocular 0.05% cyclosporine (INN ciclosporin) in patients with severe refractory disease may be tried. The symptoms of xerostomia are treated using artificial saliva preparations and sugar-free chewing gum; in patients with preserved residual function of the salivary glands, drugs stimulating production of saliva should be considered (eg, pilocarpine 5 mg every 6 hours⊘○; alternatively acetylcysteine in the case of contraindications to or intolerance of pilocarpine). Sips of water may be helpful, however if too frequent, they may increase the symptoms due to a loss of the mucus film and may also lead to nocturia, which increases fatigue due to sleep disruption. The patient should be advised to avoid alcohol and tobacco and instructed about the importance of good oral hygiene.

2. Among the **agents modifying the inflammatory process** the most frequently used are hydroxychloroquine 200 mg/d and chloroquine 250 mg/d. These have been used empirically, but their effectiveness has been questioned in a recent randomized controlled trial. As a result, we suggest that they not be used routinely.⊗○ Treatment of extraglandular manifestations is based

Table 19-1. Classification criteria for primary Sjögren syndrome according to ACR/EULAR guidelines

Clinical inclusion criteria (ocular and oral symptoms; ≥1 positive response to the following questions):

1) Have you had daily, persistent, troublesome dry eyes for >3 months?
2) Do you have a recurrent sensation of sand or gravel in your eyes?
3) Do you use tear substitutes >3 times a day?
4) Have you had a daily feeling of dry mouth for >3 months?
5) Do you frequently drink liquids to aid in swallowing dry food?
Or suspicion of Sjögren syndrome based on ESSDAI[a]

Clinical exclusion criteria: History of head and neck radiation therapy, active HCV infection (confirmed by PCR), AIDS, sarcoidosis, amyloidosis, graft-versus-host disease, IgG4-related disease

Classification criteria (histopathology, autoantibodies, ocular signs)	Points
Diagnosis of focal lymphocytic sialadenitis in a labial salivary gland[b] with a focus score count >1 foci/4 mm^2	3
Anti-Ro/SSA antibody positive	3
Ocular staining score[c] ≥5 or van Bijsterveld score[d] ≥4 in ≥1 eye	1
Schirmer test ≤5 mm/5 minutes in ≥1 eye[e]	1
Unstimulated whole saliva flow rate ≤0.1 mL/min[f]	1

Interpretation:
Patients with a total score ≥4 points meet the criteria for primary Sjögren syndrome (sensitivity, 96%; specificity, 95%)

[a] RMD Open. 2015;1(1):e000022.
[b] Arthritis Rheum. 2011 Jul;63(7):2021-30.
[c] Am J Ophthalmol. 2010 Mar;149(3):405-15.
[d] Arch Ophthalmol. 1969 Jul;82(1):10-4.
[e] Patients treated with anticholinergic drugs should be evaluated after a sufficient interval during which the drugs are withheld.
[f] J Am Dent Assoc. 2008 May;139 Suppl:35S-40S.

Adapted from Arthritis Rheumatol. 2017 Jan;69(1):35-45.

ACR, American College of Rheumatology; AIDS, acquired immunodeficiency syndrome; ESSDAI, EULAR Sjögren syndrome disease activity index; EULAR, European League Against Rheumatism; HCV, hepatitis C virus; PCR, polymerase chain reaction.

on **glucocorticoids** and other **immunosuppressants**, although anti-tumor necrosis factor treatments have not been shown to be clinically efficacious. In particularly resistant cases, rituximab is used; however, a recent study was not able to show alleviation of symptoms or disease activity over 24 weeks of follow-up. In secondary Sjögren syndrome, treat the underlying condition.

→ FOLLOW-UP

There is an increased risk of developing non-Hodgkin lymphoma compared to the general population, with an incidence of ~5%. Regular follow-up should be considered in individuals at high risk for the development of lymphoma. Predictors of lymphoma include purpura (cutaneous vasculitis), persisting or recurrent salivary gland enlargement and lymphadenopathy, monoclonal cryoglobulinemia, decreased serum levels of the C3 and/or C4 complement components, reduced levels of CD4+ cells, and a reduced ratio of CD4+/CD4- cells in the peripheral blood. The presence of structures resembling germinal centers within the lymphocytic infiltrates revealed by a minor salivary gland biopsy may be another predictor for lymphoma development.

20. Spondyloarthritides

The spondyloarthritides (SpAs) (also termed spondyloarthropathies) are a group of disorders with a predilection for inflammatory arthritis of the axial skeleton (sacroiliac joints and spine) and peripheral joints. SpAs include ankylosing spondylitis, psoriatic arthritis, reactive arthritis, juvenile-onset spondyloarthritis, arthritis associated with inflammatory bowel disease (enteropathic arthritis), arthritis associated with anterior uveitis, and undifferentiated spondyloarthritides. SpAs are characterized by inflammation of bones (osteitis), joints (arthritis), and peri-articular tissues, particularly entheses (enthesitis: inflammation of the sites where tendons or ligaments attach to the bone), as well as a number of extra-articular manifestations (such as psoriasis, anterior uveitis, and inflammatory bowel disease).

Spondyloarthritides can be broadly classified into:

1) **Axial SpAs**, which primarily affect the axial skeleton, typically the sacroiliac (SI) joints but often involving the spine itself.

2) **Peripheral SpAs**, which primarily manifest as peripheral arthritis (large and small joints), enthesitis, and dactylitis.

Of note, there is no single diagnostic feature for the SpA group as a whole or for any of the disease subsets. Diagnosis is therefore dependent on the assessment of symptoms and signs, laboratory investigations, and imaging studies, such as radiographs and magnetic resonance imaging (MRI). In patients with SpA serum IgM rheumatoid factor is negative, leading to the term "seronegative spondyloarthropathies," and HLA-B27 is frequently positive.

The term "nonradiographic axial spondyloarthritis" (nrAxSpA) refers to patients with clinical features of axial SpA but without adequate evidence of sacroiliitis on radiographs. Such patients would usually have positive findings on MRI.

Recent developments in the understanding of these diseases and introduction of new advanced therapies (biologic agents, Janus kinase inhibitors) underscore the need for specialist expertise in the diagnosis and management of SpAs.

20.1. Ankylosing Spondylitis

→ **DEFINITION, ETIOLOGY, PATHOGENESIS**

Ankylosing spondylitis (AS) is chronic and usually progressive arthritis that mainly affects the sacroiliac joints, intervertebral and costovertebral joints, entheses, annulus fibrosus, and ligaments of the spine and gradually leads to spinal fusion (ankylosis). Etiology is not completely understood but involves genetic and environmental factors. HLA-B27 is strongly associated with AS (75%-95% of patients) but is not necessary for diagnosis. Tumor necrosis factor (TNF) and interleukin 17 (IL-17) are major cytokines and targets of therapy.

→ **CLINICAL FEATURES AND NATURAL HISTORY**

The onset of AS is usually in late adolescence or young adulthood and very rarely after the age of 40 years. Traditionally men were thought to be more frequently affected. However, more recent studies have shown a 1:1 ratio of

Table 20-1. Assessment of SpondyloArthritis International Society (ASAS) criteria for inflammatory back pain

- Age at onset < 40 years
- Insidious onset
- Improvement with exercise
- No improvement with rest
- Pain at night (with improvement upon getting up)

Inflammatory back pain present if ≥4 criteria are present. Sensitivity, 79.6%; specificity 72.4%.

Adapted from Ann Rheum Dis. 2009;68(6):784-8.

males to females, especially in early disease and nonradiographic axial spondyloarthritis (nrAxSpA). The disease may follow a pattern of relapses and remissions but is generally chronic and progressive.

General symptoms: Low-grade fever, weight loss, fatigue.

Musculoskeletal manifestations: Inflammatory lower back pain is the most common initial presentation (→Table 20-1). Pain is worst at night and early in the morning, improves with activity, does not improve with rest, and is associated with significant morning stiffness. Pain can be constant with worsening at night/morning or intermittent and occurring in flares that last days, weeks, or months. Pain is usually dull, difficult to locate (but sometimes localized to the sacroiliac joints), and unilateral or bilateral. Pain and limitation of motion progressively worsen as the inflammatory process involves other areas of the spine. Involvement of the lumbar spine can eventually lead to loss of physiologic lordosis (flattening). Inflammation of the thoracic spine can cause upper back and chest pain that increases on inspiration and is referred to the front of the thorax along the ribs (this feature differentiates it from pleuritic pain). Eventually patients can develop increased kyphosis, decreased chest expansion, and paraspinal muscle atrophy. Inflammation of the cervical spine causes limitation and subsequent loss of motion and can lead to loss of lordosis. All of these eventually result in the classic stooped posture where the spine becomes rigid and kyphotic.

Many patients can develop peripheral arthritis, which potentially may affect any joint but most commonly involves the larger joints (hips, knees, shoulders). Other features include peri-articular inflammation, such as Achilles tendonitis, plantar fasciitis, and dactylitis.

Due to spinal rigidity and frequent comorbid osteoporosis, trauma can easily lead to spinal fracture, including fractures of the cervical spine.

Anterior uveitis affects up to 25% of patients with AS. It presents with pain, redness, visual impairment, and photophobia. It usually responds to topical glucocorticoids with resolution in 4 to 6 weeks. Recurrent, chronic, or inappropriately treated anterior uveitis can lead to synechiae, cataract formation, and glaucoma.

Cardiovascular manifestations are uncommon, occurring in <10% of patients, and can include aortic regurgitation, aortitis of the ascending aorta, conduction disturbances, and pericarditis.

Gastrointestinal manifestations are common. Up to 10% of patients develop overt inflammatory bowel disease. Up to 50% of patients can have subclinical inflammation affecting the distal small intestine and colon. Gastric or duodenal ulcers can occur; the use of nonsteroidal anti-inflammatory drug (NSAIDs) in the treatment of AS is a factor contributing to their development.

Other potential manifestations:

1) Fibrosis of the upper pulmonary lobes (apical fibrosis).
2) Proteinuria due to renal amyloid deposition or IgA nephropathy.

3) Neurologic symptoms in patients with atlantoaxial subluxation, atlantooccipital subluxation, or cervical vertebral fracture.

4) Depression is a consequence of pain, morning stiffness, and persisting fatigue, which interfere with daily activities.

Disease progression and risk of disability is variable. Poor prognostic factors include root joint involvement (hips, shoulders), positive HLA-B27, high C-reactive protein (CRP) level, and presence of syndesmophytes at baseline.

→ DIAGNOSIS

Diagnostic Tests

1. Laboratory tests: Elevated erythrocyte sedimentation rate (ESR) and CRP levels during active disease (~40% of patients with spinal involvement and ~60% of patients with peripheral arthritis), leukocytosis, mild normochromic anemia (in <15% of patients), hypergammaglobulinemia (frequently IgA); negative rheumatoid factor (RF), positive HLA-B27 (in 75%-95% of white patients versus 8% of the general population).

2. Imaging studies: Standard anteroposterior (AP) pelvis radiographs are adequate for radiographic assessment of sacroiliitis without the need for dedicated oblique sacroiliac (SI) joint views. Radiographs can be normal in early disease. Changes are graded as follows:

– Grade 0: Normal.

– Grade 1: Suspicious changes.

– Grade 2: Minimal abnormality (small localized areas with erosion or sclerosis without alteration in the joint width).

– Grade 3: Unequivocal abnormality (moderate or advanced sacroiliitis with ≥1 of erosions, evidence of sclerosis, widening, narrowing, or partial ankylosis).

– Grade 4: Total ankylosis of sacroiliac joints.

Conventional radiography of the sacroiliac joints is the first-choice imaging modality for the assessment of sacroiliitis as part of axial SpA. Imaging of the spine may reveal squaring of the vertebral bodies, syndesmophytes (bony bridging across vertebrae through calcification of annulus fibrosus), and complete fusion of the spine (bamboo spine). Ossification of ligament attachments (enthesophytes) may also be seen. Patients with long-standing disease may develop osteoporosis. In the peripheral joints narrowing of articular spaces with subsequent fusion of the joints may be found.

In patients with suspected axial spondyloarthritis (SpA) but normal radiographs **magnetic resonance imaging (MRI)** of the SI joints with or without the spine should be considered. MRI may reveal active inflammatory lesions (osteitis/bone marrow edema, enthesitis, capsulitis, synovitis) and structural lesions (bone erosion, new bone formation, sclerosis and fat infiltration). Active inflammatory lesions may predict response to biologic therapy but are not required for initiating such treatment.

Computed tomography (CT), ultrasonography, and scintigraphy are not recommended for diagnosing axial SpA. In patients with suspected peripheral SpA ultrasonography and MRI may be used to detect enthesitis, peripheral arthritis, tenosynovitis, and bursitis.

3. Synovial fluid analysis in patients with peripheral arthritis reveals features of inflammation.

4. Other studies, depending on indications (eg, high-resolution computed tomography [HRCT] of the chest in patients with pulmonary involvement).

Diagnostic Criteria

There are no diagnostic criteria. However, classification criteria are often adapted in clinical practice to establish diagnosis. According to the modified New York criteria (→Table 20-2), radiologic features are crucial for diagnosis.

Table 20-2. Modified New York diagnostic criteria for ankylosing spondylitis

Clinical criteria
1) Low back pain persisting for ≥3 months, reduced by exercise and not relieved by rest
2) Limited motion in the lumbar spine in coronal and sagittal planes
3) Limited chest expansion compared with normal values for age and sex

Radiologic criterion
Grade 3-4 unilateral or grade 2-4 bilateral sacroiliitis

Definite ankylosing spondylitis: The radiologic criterion and ≥1 of clinical criteria are fulfilled.
Probable ankylosing spondylitis: Three clinical criteria are fulfilled or the radiologic criterion alone is fulfilled.

Adapted from Arthritis Rheum. 1984;27(4):361-8.

The new Assessment of SpondyloArthritis International Society (ASAS) criteria (→Table 20-3) facilitate earlier diagnosis of SpA through the inclusion of MRI before development of structural damage on radiographs. These criteria also include a "clinical arm" that does not require any imaging modality but has lower specificity.

Differential Diagnosis

Scheuermann disease (juvenile kyphosis), other SpAs (→Table 20-4), rheumatoid arthritis, degenerative disc disease, malignancy, infections (eg, tuberculosis, brucellosis), metabolic bone diseases, diffuse idiopathic skeletal hyperostosis (DISH).

→ TREATMENT

Nonpharmacologic Management

1. Patient education: Advise the patient about the nature of the disease and importance of their active role in disease management and prevention of disability. Proper posture, deep breathing exercises, spinal extension and range-of-movement exercises, and maintenance of spinal alignment during sleep are all important. Avoidance of smoking is also significant, as smoking is associated with greater disease progression.

2. Physiotherapy is helpful for core strengthening, maintenance of spine and joint range of movement, and pain management.

Pharmacotherapy

1. NSAIDs are the first-line agents in patients with spinal pain and stiffness.◑● Agents and dosage: →Table 11-2.

2. Analgesics: Acetaminophen (INN paracetamol) and weak opioids (eg, tramadol) are used when NSAIDs are contraindicated, ineffective, or not tolerated.◑○

3. Glucocorticoids: Intra-articular injections are helpful for short-term management of active peripheral arthritis. SI joint injections (under imaging guidance) can be considered for sacroiliitis, especially when biologic therapy is contraindicated. Injections around the Achilles tendon should be avoided due to the risk of tendon rupture.

4. Disease-modifying antirheumatic drugs (DMARDs):
1) Conventional synthetic DMARDs (sulfasalazine, methotrexate, leflunomide) are not effective for the treatment of axial SpA.◑● However, they may be effective in peripheral arthritis, either as monotherapy or combination therapy, and can be tried for 3 to 6 months.
2) Biologic DMARDs are indicated in patients with active axial SpA with inadequate response to NSAIDs (or where NSAIDs are contraindicated).

Table 20-3. 2010 Assessment of SpondyloArthritis International Society (ASAS) criteria for classification of spondyloarthritis

Axial SpA (to be applied in patients with back pain present for ≥3 months and age of onset <45 years)

Sacroiliitis on imaging (MRI or radiography) and ≥1 other feature of SpA
or
Presence of HLA-B27 antigen and ≥2 other features of SpA

Features of SpA:
- Inflammatory back pain[a]
- Peripheral arthritis
- Enthesitis (heel)
- Uveitis
- Dactylitis
- Psoriasis
- Crohn disease or ulcerative colitis
- Good response to NSAIDs (resolution or significant improvement of back pain within 24-48 h of administration of a full dose)
- Family history of SpA
- HLA-B27
- Elevated serum CRP level (when other causes have been excluded)

Peripheral SpA

Arthritis, enthesitis, or dactylitis
and
≥1 of the following features of SpA:
- Anterior uveitis
- Psoriasis
- Crohn disease or ulcerative colitis
- Prior infection
- HLA-B27
- Sacroiliitis on imaging
or
≥2 of the following features of SpA:
- Arthritis
- Enthesitis
- Dactylitis
- Inflammatory back pain[a] (at any time in history)
- Family history of SpA

[a] Characterized by ≥4 of the following: (1) age of onset <40 years; (2) insidious onset; (3) reduced by exercise; (4) not relieved by rest; (5) present at night (decreases after getting up).

CRP, C-reactive protein; MRI, magnetic resonance imaging; NSAID, nonsteroidal anti--inflammatory drug; SpA, spondyloarthritis.

Tumor necrosis factor (TNF) inhibitors (etanercept, infliximab, adalimumab, golimumab, certolizumab) were the first class of biologics approved in SpA.⊘● IL-17 inhibitors (secukinumab, ixekizumab) were approved subsequently.⊘● Treatment with synthetic DMARDs is not required before or during biologic therapy for axial SpA.

In peripheral SpA biologic DMARDs are indicated in patients with inadequate response to synthetic DMARDs. Biologics are effective for peripheral arthritis, enthesitis, dactylitis, and psoriatic skin and nail disease.

Table 20-4. Differential diagnosis of arthritis

Features	Disease			
	PsA	RA	OA	AS
Sex	M:F 1:1	M:F 1:3	OA of hands and feet more common in women	M:F 3:1 (but 1:1 in nrAx-SpA)
Peripheral arthritis	Asymmetric	Symmetric	Varied	–
Involvement of distal interphalangeal joints	+	–	Heberden nodes	–
Sacroiliitis	Asymmetric	–	–	Symmetric
Stiffness	Morning stiffness of peripheral joints, cervical and lumbar spine	Morning stiffness	Stiffness associated with prolonged physical inactivity	Severe spinal stiffness
Enthesitis	+	–	–	+
Rheumatoid factor	–	+	–	–
HLA	B27, DR4	DR4	–	B27
Radiographic features	Erosions without osteopenia, "pencil--in-cup" deformity, juxta-articular new bone formation, large asymmetric syndesmophytes	Erosions, periarticular osteopenia	Osteophytes	Thin and symmetric syndesmophytes, vertebral osteopenia

AS, ankylosing spondylitis; F, female; M, male; nrAxSpA, nonradiographic axial spondyloarthritis; OA, osteoarthritis; PsA, psoriatic arthritis; RA, rheumatoid arthritis.

The choice of biologic agents is affected by concurrent extra-articular manifestations. All anti-TNF and anti-IL-17 agents are effective for psoriasis. With the exception of etanercept, anti-TNF agents are effective for inflammatory bowel disease and uveitis. Anti-IL-17 agents are not effective for the treatment of inflammatory bowel disease

Dosage, contraindications, and adverse effects of DMARDs: →Table 18-3.

Surgical Treatment

Consider hip arthroplasty in patients with severe pain or disability and radiographic features of joint destruction, regardless of the patient's age.⊘◯
Surgical correction of kyphosis (kyphoplasty) is rarely performed but can be considered in patients with severe kyphosis.⊘◯

→ FOLLOW-UP

Follow-up assessment of disease activity includes history, physical examination, CRP levels, and clinical tools such as the Bath Ankylosing Spondylitis Disease Activity Index (BASDAI) (available at qxmd.com). Repeat radiographs of the SI joints and/or spine may be considered for long-term monitoring of structural damage but often do not impact clinical decision-making. If uncertainty about disease activity exists (eg, other conditions confounding back pain or response to therapy), MRI of the sacroiliac joints and/or spine can be performed. MRI short tau inversion recovery (STIR) sequences are sufficient; contrast enhancement is not necessary. In peripheral SpA power Doppler ultrasonography or MRI can be considered if uncertainty exists after clinical assessment.

20.2. Enteropathic Arthritis

➜ DEFINITION, ETIOLOGY, PATHOGENESIS

Enteropathic arthritis is associated with inflammatory bowel disease (IBD): ulcerative colitis (UC) (→Chapter 6.1.3.7.2) and Crohn disease (CD) (→Chapter 6.1.3.7.1). Etiology is unknown.

➜ CLINICAL FEATURES AND NATURAL HISTORY

Peripheral arthritis is acute, migratory, asymmetric and most frequently involves the knees and ankles. It is generally nonerosive.

Types of peripheral joint involvement:

1) **Type 1**: Acute oligoarthritis (involvement of ≤5 joints) that may precede gastrointestinal manifestations or occur early in the disease course and is often associated with IBD flares, self-limiting (2-6 months), and frequently accompanied by extraintestinal features (eg, erythema nodosum). It affects 5% to 10% of patients with IBD.

2) **Type 2**: Polyarthritis (>5 joints) is usually independent of IBD activity, has a chronic course (months or years), and is associated with no extraintestinal features except for uveitis. It affects 3% to 4% of patients with IBD.

Spondyloarthritis with axial involvement: Inflammatory back pain (→Table 20-1) is the typical presentation of axial disease, occurring with or without peripheral arthritis. It is usually unrelated to bowel disease activity. From 10% to 20% of patients can develop clinical and radiographic features similar to ankylosing spondylitis (AS). Imaging studies can be negative in early spondyloarthritis. It is important to consider that arthralgia (in the absence of inflammatory arthritis) is very common in IBD, affecting about 10% of patients (as many as 50% in some studies).

Involvement of other organs in the course of IBD: →Chapter 6.1.3.7.2; →Chapter 6.1.3.7.1.

Natural history: Type 1 peripheral arthritis typically occurs early and is self-limiting (<6 months). Patients with type 2 peripheral arthritis may continue to have recurrent flares for many years. Axial enteropathic arthritis can cause disability and significantly impact quality of life. Peripheral enteropathic arthritis usually causes no permanent joint lesions or deformity.

➜ DIAGNOSIS

Diagnostic Tests

1. Laboratory tests: Markers of inflammation (elevated erythrocyte sedimentation rate [ESR] / C-reactive protein [CRP], thrombocytosis, anemia) can be confounded by bowel disease. Rheumatoid factor (RF) is usually negative. HLA-B27 is positive in 50% to 75% of patients with IBD-associated axial arthritis.

2. Synovial fluid examination: Findings are nonspecific and characteristic of inflammatory arthritis.

3. Imaging studies:

1) **Radiography**: Peripheral enteropathic arthritis is usually nonerosive, with <10% of patients having erosions of the affected joints. Radiographs may

show soft-tissue swelling, periarticular osteopenia, and mild periostitis. Radiographic features in axial involvement are similar to AS. Asymptomatic sacroiliitis can occur in up to 20% of patients.

2) **Magnetic resonance imaging (MRI)**: Similarly to AS, MRI can be used to assess for axial disease where radiographs are normal or to exclude inflammatory disease in mechanical back pain (when indicated).

Diagnostic Criteria

1. Diagnosis of UC or CD.

2. Features of peripheral arthritis or axial spondyloarthritis (diagnosis of axial spondyloarthritis often requires confirmation by imaging studies).

Differential Diagnosis

1. Peripheral enteropathic arthritis: Atypical rheumatoid arthritis, infectious arthritis, reactive arthritis, psoriatic arthritis.

2. Spondyloarthritis: Other spondyloarthritides.

→ **TREATMENT**

Treatment of the Underlying Condition

Many drugs used for IBD itself can benefit the articular manifestations. In addition, type 1 peripheral arthritis usually mirrors IBD disease activity and improves with improvement of the underlying IBD.

Treatment of Joint Involvement

1. Physiotherapy is helpful for the maintenance of functional capacity, particularly in patients with axial enteropathic arthritis.

2. Pharmacotherapy:

1) Use **acetaminophen (INN paracetamol)-based products** for pain control. Nonsteroidal anti-inflammatory drugs (NSAIDs) are generally avoided because of the potential risk of worsening IBD; however, NSAIDs (cyclooxygenase 1 [COX-1] and 2 [COX-2] inhibitors) can be used for arthritis if IBD is quiescent and in consultation with a gastroenterologist.

2) **Sulfasalazine** is the first-line disease-modifying antirheumatic drug (DMARD) in patients with peripheral enteropathic arthritis.◐◯ If it is ineffective or not tolerated, consider methotrexate or azathioprine. DMARDs are ineffective in patients with axial spondyloarthritis. Agents, dosage, contraindications, and adverse effects of DMARDs: →Table 18-3.

3) Intra-articular **glucocorticoids** can provide effective short-term relief in monoarthritis or oligoarthritis. Short-term systemic glucocorticoids may provide rapid short-term relief in patients with peripheral enteropathic arthritis.

4) **Anti–tumor necrosis factor (TNF) agents** (infliximab, adalimumab, golimumab, certolizumab) have beneficial effects on both intestinal manifestations and arthritis (axial and peripheral). Etanercept is ineffective for the treatment of IBD itself.

20.3. Psoriatic Arthritis

→ **DEFINITION, ETIOLOGY, PATHOGENESIS**

Psoriatic arthritis (PsA) is chronic inflammatory arthritis of unknown mechanism. It affects 10% to 40% of patients with psoriasis. It appears that genetic, immunologic, and environmental factors all contribute to the development of the disease. Compared with individuals with uncomplicated psoriasis, patients with PsA have an increased frequency of HLA-B7 and HLA-B27 and lower frequency of HLA-DR7 and HLA-Cw7. However, the frequency of HLA-B27 in PsA is not as high as it is in ankylosing spondylitis or reactive arthritis and many patients are HLA-B27–negative. While skin and joint diseases appear to have similar pathogenesis, these manifestations do not highly correlate in individual patients.

→ CLINICAL FEATURES AND NATURAL HISTORY

The onset of PsA is usually between the ages of 20 and 50 years but a juvenile form also occurs (usually between 9-12 years). Skin involvement generally precedes arthritis but arthritis can be the initial manifestation in ~10% of patients. There is no relationship between the severity of skin disease and degree of joint involvement. Skin involvement can be limited to minute plaques in or around the navel, intergluteal cleft, axillae, submammary folds, external genitalia, and scalp. The clinical course of PsA is highly variable, with periods of relapses and remissions. With time, the disease can lead to significant disability.

Periarticular involvement is common. This includes nail disease that is frequently associated with distal interphalangeal joint (DIP) involvement. Enthesitis (inflammation of the sites where tendons or ligaments attach to the bone) can occur with pain and swelling at the site. Achilles enthesitis is a common location. Dactylitis (inflammation of the joints, tendon sheaths, and other soft tissues of the toes or fingers) is usually episodic. It is commonly referred to as "sausage digits" due to the clinical appearance.

Extra-articular involvement can include psoriasis, anterior uveitis (iritis), and inflammatory bowel disease (IBD). Fatigue and depression are not uncommon.

Psoriatic arthritis can affect any joint in any pattern. Common symptoms include joint pain, swelling, warmth, and significant morning stiffness. Several common clinical patterns are recognized (the Moll and Wright classification):

1) **DIP-predominant arthritis**: The DIPs are primarily affected with pain, swelling, tenderness, and increasing deformity. Nails are frequently involved as the nail bed anchors in close proximity to the DIP. Other joints can be involved as well.

2) **Symmetric polyarthritis**: This affects large and small joints with a fairly symmetric pattern. It resembles rheumatoid arthritis, but DIP joints can be involved in psoriatic arthritis. Deformities similar to those in rheumatoid arthritis (RA) can occur, including boutonnière and swan-neck deformities (→Chapter 1.11.2).

3) **Asymmetric oligoarticular arthritis**: Asymmetric arthritis usually affecting <5 joints. Large joints (eg, knees) are commonly involved, but small joints can also be affected.

4) **Axial PsA**: This is similar to ankylosing spondylitis (but less symmetric on imaging) with inflammation of the joints of the spine and sacroiliac joints. It usually presents with inflammatory back pain (→Table 20-1). With time, limited range of motion of the cervical, thoracic, and lumbar spine can develop.

5) **Arthritis mutilans**: A very destructive form of psoriatic arthritis with significant osteolysis leading to bone resorption and joint destruction. Osteolysis of the phalanges leads to the formation of telescopic fingers (→Chapter 1.11.2).

The **course of PsA** is highly variable. In patients with severe PsA, particularly those with coexisting axial and peripheral joint involvement, deformities and disability can develop within a few years. Adverse prognostic factors include multiple joint involvement, elevated erythrocyte sedimentation rate (ESR)/C-reactive protein (CRP) levels, clinical or radiologic features of joint damage, and treatment failure. In patients with milder PsA periods of relapses and partial remissions are observed with gradually worsening limitation of joint motion. Quality of life is frequently severely impaired and may be worse than in RA because of coexisting skin/nail disease and other extra-articular manifestations (iritis, IBD).

Table 20-5. CASPAR criteria for classification of psoriatic arthritis

To meet the CASPAR criteria, the patient must have inflammatory articular disease (joint, spine, or enthesitis) plus ≥3 points from any of the following 5 categories:

1. Evidence of psoriasis:
   1) Evidence of current psoriasis (psoriatic lesions diagnosed by a rheumatologist or dermatologist): 2 points
   2) Personal history of psoriasis or family history of psoriasis (in a first-degree or second--degree relative): 1 point
2. Typical psoriatic nail dystrophy (onycholysis, pitting, and hyperkeratosis) observed on current physical examination: 1 point
3. Negative test result for rheumatoid factor (any assay except for the latex test), preferably using ELISA or nephelometry: 1 point
4. Current dactylitis (defined as swelling of an entire digit [so-called sausage digit]) or history of dactylitis recorded by a rheumatologist: 1 point
5. Radiographic evidence of juxta-articular new bone formation seen as ill-defined ossification near joint margins (excluding osteophyte formation) in the hand or foot: 1 point

Adapted from Arthritis Rheum. 2006;54(8):2665-73.

CASPAR, ClASsification criteria for Psoriatic ARthritis; ELISA, enzyme-linked immunosorbent assay.

➡ DIAGNOSIS

Diagnostic Tests

1. Laboratory tests: Elevated ESR/CRP can help in the assessment of clinical disease activity but these are not surrogate markers. Positive HLA-B27 is found in 60% to 70% of patients and therefore cannot be used to exclude the diagnosis of PsA.

2. Imaging studies:

1) **Radiographs** of peripheral joints reveal asymmetric involvement of the interphalangeal joints of the hands and feet and of large joints, erosions, new bone formation (at joint margins or along the periosteum). Osteolysis of the phalanges result in the classic "pencil-in-cup" deformity. Ankylosis of the joints of the hands and feet can be seen.

   Radiographs of the spine can reveal changes similar to ankylosing spondylitis, but changes can be asymmetric. Sacroiliitis (unilateral or bilateral) can be evidenced by joint space loss, sclerosis, erosions, and ankylosis. Syndesmophytes tend to be larger and more asymmetric than in ankylosing spondylitis (termed "chunky syndesmophytes").

2) **Power Doppler ultrasonography** is useful in detecting peripheral arthritis (synovitis) and enthesitis.

3) **Magnetic resonance imaging (MRI)** of the spine is useful for early sacroiliitis and spondylitis, showing bone marrow edema, erosions, and enthesitis.

3. Synovial fluid examination can be performed if there is diagnostic uncertainty. It typically reveals features of inflammation.

Diagnostic Criteria

There are no diagnostic criteria. However, the Classification of Psoriatic Arthritis (CASPAR) criteria are often adapted in clinical practice: →Table 20-5.

Differential Diagnosis

Differential diagnosis mainly includes RA, osteoarthritis, and other spondyloarthritides (→Table 20-4).

→ TREATMENT

The main goals of treatment are to prevent disease progression, achieve remission, and optimize long-term health-related quality of life. Assessment of disease activity must consider the many domains of psoriatic arthritis: peripheral arthritis, axial disease, enthesitis, dactylitis, and skin and nail disease. The level of disease activity is also crucial for determining therapy.

Treatment may involve the following:

1) Education of the patient and family or caregivers.

2) Rehabilitation, including physiotherapy and kinesiotherapy.

3) Pharmacologic treatment.

4) Orthopedic treatment (when indicated because of disability).

Pharmacotherapy

Pharmacologic therapy of PsA is based on the main domains involved and the level of disease activity.

1. Nonsteroidal anti-inflammatory drug (NSAIDs) are used as first-line drugs in mild peripheral arthritis, axial disease, enthesitis, and dactylitis. Agents and dosage: →Table 11-2.

2. Local **glucocorticosteroid** injections can be used for symptomatic treatment of peripheral arthritis, sacroiliitis, enthesitis, and dactylitis. Their role in sacroiliitis is mainly if there are contraindications to biologic therapy. Intra-articular injections are generally limited to 3 per joint per year. In patients with dactylitis injections can be delivered to tendon sheaths. Enthesitis can be treated with injections around the entheses. In general, injections around the Achilles tendon are avoided because of the risk of tendon rupture. In very symptomatic peripheral arthritis, systemic glucocorticoids (oral or IM) can be considered. There is a small risk of worsening skin disease on withdrawal, particularly in those who are not receiving concomitant disease-modifying antirheumatic drug (DMARD) therapy or in whom the dose of glucocorticoids is reduced too rapidly.

3. Oral small molecules (OSMs) include conventional synthetic DMARDs (methotrexate, sulfasalazine, leflunomide) and apremilast (a phosphodiesterase-4 [PDE-4] inhibitor). These agents are used in peripheral arthritis of varying severity (including patients with mild disease when NSAIDs or glucocorticoid injections are inadequate, not tolerated or contraindicated). They can also be helpful for skin and nail disease but have limited efficacy.

OSMs can be used as monotherapy or combination therapy in peripheral PsA. Methotrexate is the most frequent first-line agent.⊘○ Sulfasalazine or leflunomide can be used in combination with methotrexate in case of inadequate response or instead of methotrexate if it is contraindicated or not tolerated. In patients with inadequate response or intolerance of or contraindications to methotrexate, use sulfasalazine and/or leflunomide. Due to the cost, apremilast is often used as a second-line agent but can also be used as a first-line option.⊘● Dosage, contraindications, and adverse effects of DMARDs: →Table 18-3.

OSMs have no role in the treatment of axial PsA. Treatment is similar to AS (→Chapter 14.20.1).

4. Janus kinase (JAK) inhibitors (tofacitinib, baricitinib) are effective for the treatment of peripheral PsA and can be used as first-line or second-line agents.⊘●

5. Biologic agents are used in both peripheral arthritis and axial PsA. They can also be used for refractory enthesitis and dactylitis.

For peripheral PsA, biologics are initiated in patients with persistent moderate to high peripheral disease activity despite treatment with ≥1 OSMs administered at an optimal dose for 3 to 6 months. Tumor necrosis factor (TNF) inhibitors (adalimumab, etanercept, infliximab, golimumab, certolizumab) were the first class of biologics in PsA.🟢🟢 Ustekinumab (anti-interleukin 12/23 [anti-IL-12/23]) is also highly effective. Anti-IL-17 (secukinumab, ixekizumab) agents have also been approved.🟢🟢 In patients with very high disease activity, treatment with a JAK inhibitor or biologic agent may be considered as first-line treatment, without a prior trial of an OSM. In case of primary failure, it is best to switch classes (mechanisms) of biologics. In case of secondary failure after an initial response, one can switch within the same class or out of class.

For axial PsA, treatment is similar to AS (→Chapter 14.20.1), with biologics initiated if NSAIDs are contraindicated or after ≥1 NSAIDs in case of inefficacy or intolerance.

→ FOLLOW-UP

Assess the effects of treatment using a clinical evaluation tool, such as the swollen joint count, tender joint count, enthesitis scores, or number of dactylitic digits. Skin involvement is measured through body surface area (BSA) and Psoriasis Area Severity Index (PASI) (available at pasi.corti.li). The Bath Ankylosing Spondylitis Disease Activity Index (BASDAI) (available at qxmd.com) is a patient-reported questionnaire for gauging spine involvement. The Health Assessment Questionnaire (HAQ) provides a measure of overall function.

20.4. Reactive Arthritis

→ DEFINITION, ETIOLOGY, PATHOGENESIS

Reactive arthritis (ReA) is asymmetric arthritis, usually oligoarticular or polyarticular, that mostly affects the lower extremities. While the arthritis itself is sterile, ReA typically follows a preceding infection at a distant site, usually of the gastrointestinal or genitourinary tract (sexually acquired reactive arthritis [SARA]). The **most frequent organisms** include enteric gram-negative rods of Enterobacteriaceae family (*Salmonella* spp, *Yersinia* spp, *Campylobacter* spp, *Shigella* spp) and *Chlamydia* spp (*Chlamydia trachomatis, Chlamydia pneumoniae*). Less frequent organisms include *Clostridium difficile, Vibrio parahaemolyticus*, BCG vaccine strains of *Mycobacterium bovis* (following intravesical administration in treatment of bladder cancer), and *Mycoplasma* spp (eg, *Ureaplasma urealyticum*). The immune response to bacterial antigens plays a key role in the pathogenesis of ReA.

→ CLINICAL FEATURES AND NATURAL HISTORY

The preceding infection can occur up to 6 weeks prior to the onset of arthritis. The patient may not be able to recall it if the infectious symptoms were very mild.

1. General symptoms: Malaise, weakness, fever.

2. Musculoskeletal manifestations:

1) Acute-onset asymmetric oligoarthritis, often affecting the lower extremities (knees, ankles, feet). About 50% of patients can have upper limb involvement. Some develop polyarthritis of the small joints. A small proportion of patients can have arthritis lasting >6 months (termed chronic reactive arthritis).

2) Enthesitis can occur in 20% to 90% of patients. Common sites include the Achilles insertion and plantar fascia insertion on the calcaneus. Heel pain and difficulty walking are symptoms of Achilles tendonitis/enthesitis and plantar fasciitis.

3) Dactylitis frequency is variable but can affect up to 40% of patients.

4) Lower back pain (sacroiliac region and buttocks) and spinal pain/stiffness are symptoms of sacroiliitis and spondylitis. This can occur in up to 50% of patients.

3. Genitourinary manifestations:

1) Vesicles, erosions, or macules, mainly in the external urethral orifice, on the glans penis (termed circinate balanitis), and on the penile shaft. These lesions are more frequent in patients with SARA (up to 70%). They are painless (unless infected) and do not cause scarring.

2) Urethral discharge and dysuria (in men these may be accompanied by prostatitis, orchitis, epididymitis, and cystitis). Symptoms of urethritis or cystitis are present in ~80% of patients with SARA (especially in the case of *Chlamydia trachomatis* infection), while 10% to 30% of patients with enteric infection develop reactive urethritis.

3) Cervicitis or vaginitis in women with SARA is often asymptomatic.

4. Cutaneous and mucosal manifestations:

1) Vesicular lesions with scaling and hyperkeratosis of the soles, papular inflammatory lesions on palms and soles (keratoderma blennorrhagicum). This occurs in 10% to 30% of patients with SARA or less commonly in intestinal infections.

2) Yellowish or grey discolorations, thickening, furrows, and heaped-up hyperkeratosis (mainly in patients with chronic ReA).

3) Erythema nodosum, mainly in patients with *Yersinia* spp infection.

4) Painless shiny aphthous ulcers on the palate, tongue, and mucosa of the cheeks and lips.

5. Ocular manifestations:

1) Conjunctivitis, usually mild (erythema, lacrimation, rarely lid edema), is often an early manifestation of ReA. It usually resolves after a week but may persist for several months.

2) Acute anterior uveitis (in 10%-20% of patients with positive HLA-B27) causes unilateral eye pain with erythema, lacrimation, photophobia, and blurred vision. It usually resolves quickly with appropriate therapy.

6. Other signs and symptoms: Cardiac involvement (in <10% of patients, mainly those with chronic ReA) causing conduction disturbances and nonspecific ST and T changes found on electrocardiography (ECG); additional cardiac manifestations may include aortic regurgitation, pericarditis, myocarditis, and aortitis involving the ascending aorta. Other features may involve serositis, microscopic colitis, and meningitis (very rare).

The **natural history** of ReA is highly variable and probably depends on the infectious organism and the patient's genetic predisposition. Disease duration is typically 3 to 5 months, with most patients having either complete resolution or minimal disease activity within 6 to 12 months of presentation. However, 5% to 20% of patients may have more chronic persistent arthritis. Some patients with chronic ReA may develop features of another spondyloarthropathy, for instance, psoriatic arthritis, ankylosing spondylitis, or enteropathic arthritis. HLA-B27 has been associated with worse prognosis in some studies. Patients with the triad of postinfectious arthritis, urethritis, and conjunctivitis may also have a poorer prognosis.

→ DIAGNOSIS

Diagnostic Tests

1. Laboratory tests: Elevated erythrocyte sedimentation rate (ESR) and C-reactive protein (CRP) levels (common but not in all patients), mild leukocytosis, thrombocythemia, anemia, sterile pyuria (rare), positive HLA-B27 (varies widely; 30%-90% of patients).

2. Microbiological studies:

1) Gastrointestinal specimens: Stool cultures during acute diarrheal illness to test for *Salmonella*, *Shigella*, *Campylobacter*, and *Yersinia*. Cultures

are usually of little value as the diarrhea has usually resolved by the time arthritis develops.

2) Genitourinary specimens: First-catch urine and genital swab (cervical, urethral) testing can detect *C trachomatis* using nucleic acid amplification techniques.

3) Serologic testing is primarily used in epidemiologic studies and is less useful in clinical practice. In patients with *Yersinia* and *Salmonella* infections, serologic studies reveal a ≥4-fold increase in the specific IgG levels within a few weeks of infection.

3. Synovial fluid examination is performed mainly to exclude other causes of arthritis. Findings are nonspecific and characteristic of inflammatory arthritis. Synovial fluid culture is negative as ReA is not septic arthritis.

4. Imaging studies: In acute ReA findings on **radiographs** are usually limited to joint swelling. In patients with chronic ReA changes similar to other seronegative spondyloarthropathies (erosions, joint space loss, new bone formation) may be seen. In patients with axial disease radiographic sacroiliitis can be seen in some patients. **Magnetic resonance imaging (MRI)** of the spine (if clinically indicated) may reveal early changes (synovitis, enthesitis, osteitis).

Diagnostic Criteria

The diagnosis of ReA is based on establishing a relationship between the clinical features and a prior infection of the intestinal or genitourinary tract with organisms causing ReA. In patients with SARA a complete workup for sexually transmitted diseases (including gonorrhea) and investigation of the patient's sexual partners is indicated.

Differential Diagnosis

Other spondyloarthritides, septic arthritis, postinfectious arthritis (Lyme disease, postviral and poststreptococcal arthritis), crystal arthropathy, Behçet disease, sarcoidosis, trauma.

→ TREATMENT

Treatment of Arthritis and Enthesitis

1. Limitation of physical activity, particularly of walking in patients with arthritis of the lower extremities.

2. Physiotherapy aimed at reducing symptom severity, maintaining joint motion, and preventing muscle atrophy.

3. Pharmacologic treatment:

1) **Nonsteroidal anti-inflammatory drug (NSAIDs)** are the mainstay of treatment in early ReA (agents and dosage: →Table 11-2).

2) **Glucocorticoids** administered intra-articularly (after septic arthritis has been excluded) or systemically via oral or IM route (as in treatment of RA; →Chapter 14.18) can provide rapid relief.

3) **Disease-modifying antirheumatic drugs (DMARDs)** (agents, dosage, contraindications, adverse effects: →Table 18-3) are used if NSAIDs and glucocorticoids are ineffective in early disease or if arthritis becomes chronic.

   a) Conventional synthetic DMARDs: **Sulfasalazine** (moderate efficacy in patients with peripheral arthritis, ineffective in patients with axial arthritis or enthesitis).☺☹ When ineffective, use **methotrexate**.

   b) Biologic DMARDs: Infliximab, etanercept, adalimumab have been used with success in patients with severe ReA.

Treatment of Cutaneous and Mucosal Manifestations

1. Cutaneous lesions: Mild lesions require no treatment. In patients with moderate lesions use **keratolytic agents** (eg, topical salicylates), topical

glucocorticoids, or **calcipotriene** (INN calcipotriol) cream or ointment. In patients with severe lesions use **methotrexate** or **retinoids**.

2. Circinate balanitis: Use weak topical **glucocorticoids** (eg, hydrocortisone cream).

Treatment of Anterior Uveitis

Glucocorticoids in the form of eye drops (or oral in patients not responding to topical treatment) and mydriatics.

Treatment of Infection

1. Antimicrobial treatment is indicated only in patients with a documented active infection and is mainly used for *Chlamydia* spp infection. Antimicrobial treatment does not prevent the development of ReA.

2. *C trachomatis* **infection**: Early antimicrobial treatment in patients with *C trachomatis* urethritis (→Chapter 8.16.9) reduces the risk of recurrence and development of chronic ReA.

3. *C pneumoniae* **infection**: →Chapter 13.14.1.

4. *C difficile* **infection**: →Chapter 6.1.3.5.5.

21. Systemic Lupus Erythematosus (SLE)

→ DEFINITION, ETIOLOGY, PATHOGENESIS

Systemic lupus erythematosus (SLE) is a complex autoimmune disease leading to chronic inflammation of various organs and tissues. The etiology is unknown.

→ CLINICAL FEATURES AND NATURAL HISTORY

Women are affected 6 to 10 times more frequently than men. In almost two-thirds of patients disease onset is between the ages of 16 and 55 years, although it can also present initially in children or the elderly. The presenting symptoms may be nonspecific, such as fever, malaise, or weight loss. SLE usually presents as a multisystem disease, though disease manifestations can sometimes be limited to a single organ, such as the skin or kidneys. The course is typically relapsing-remitting in nature; however, a complete resolution of clinical and laboratory manifestations can occur.

1. Systemic manifestations: Fatigue, low-grade or high-grade fever, weight loss.

2. Cutaneous manifestations:

1) **Acute cutaneous lupus erythematosus (ACLE)** develops in 60% to 80% of patients with SLE; it may be limited to the face, involving the cheeks and nose ("butterfly rash": →Figure 21-1), or the lesions may be located on the forehead, around the eyes, or on the neck or chest. The lesions are frequently triggered by ultraviolet light, and the

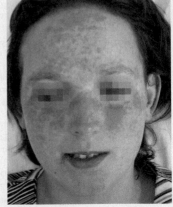

Figure 21-1. Systemic lupus erythematosus. Typical "butterfly" rash.

photosensitivity usually manifests within 24 hours of sun exposure. Rashes can persist from days to weeks. Acute cutaneous lupus can take several forms, including generalized erythroderma (→Figure 21-2), papular or vesicular lesions, or it may be severe and bullous in nature, resembling toxic epidermal necrolysis. In patients with active disease, ulcerations of the nasal and oral mucosa are frequently found. These ulcerations can be painful or painless.

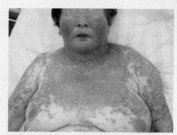

Figure 21-2. Systemic lupus erythematosus. Severe cutaneous manifestations following sunlight exposure.

2) **Subacute cutaneous lupus erythematosus (SCLE)** affects ~20% of patients with SLE and is a particular form of nonscarring photosensitive rash typically associated with anti-Sjögren syndrome A (anti-SSA) antibodies (also called anti-Ro antibodies). The lesions usually appear in one of 2 forms: circular, often raised, with a clear central area (→Figure 21-3); or scaly, psoriatic-like patches. As the lesions are typically associated with sun exposure, they are usually located on the neck, arms, and chest. While they do not cause scarring, they may be responsible for abnormal pigmentation or telangiectasia.

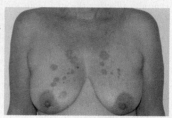

Figure 21-3. Subacute cutaneous lupus erythematosus. Circular lesions with erythema and swelling.

3) **Chronic cutaneous lupus erythematosus (CCLE)** is a noteworthy subgroup of cutaneous lupus, as it is often present in isolation, without any other systemic symptoms of lupus. Such patients are described as having isolated CCLE without having SLE. The most common variant of CCLE is discoid lupus erythematosus (DLE), which is characterized by erythematous or violaceous scaly plaques typically occurring on the head and neck, leading to follicular plugging, scarring, and localized alopecia

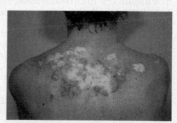

Figure 21-4. Discoid lupus erythematosus. Well--demarcated lesions with erythema, swelling, scarring, and central atrophy.

(→Figure 21-4). Early epidemiologic studies indicated that only 5% to 10% of patients with DLE would progress to fulfill the criteria for SLE, however, a more recent study has quoted a figure of >15%; incidence rates of SLE vary, depending on definition. Other CCLE rashes are hypertrophic (verrucous) lupus, lupus panniculitis (also called lupus profundus), chilblains lupus, and lupus erythematosus tumidus.

4) **Other, nonspecific cutaneous manifestations** include alopecia, lichen myxedematosus, atrophia maculosa cutis, and neutrophilic dermatoses.

5) **Vascular cutaneous manifestations** can be subdivided into those caused by true vasculitis (pathologic findings consistent with leukocytoclastic

vasculitis or panarteritis) and those classified as a nonspecific vasculopathy. Cutaneous leukocytoclastic vasculitis can present clinically as palpable purpura with or without ulcerative lesions or as urticarial vasculitis. Panarteritis can present similarly or with subcutaneous nodules resembling polyarteritis nodosa. Vasculopathy-type manifestations include Raynaud phenomenon (in 15%-40% of patients), livedo reticularis, cutaneous ulceration/necrosis, palmar erythema (particularly of the thenar and hypothenar eminences), fingertip erythema, nail-fold telangiectasias, erythromelalgia, splinter hemorrhages, Osler nodes, and Janeway lesions. The presence of cutaneous vascular lesions has been associated with a higher overall SLE disease activity. Skin ulcers, livedo reticularis, splinter hemorrhages, and fingertip erythema have been found to be associated with antiphospholipid antibodies.

3. Musculoskeletal manifestations: More than 80% of patients complain of arthralgia and/or myalgia, which are often migratory and of variable severity. A smaller number of patients develops a true inflammatory arthritis, typically affecting the small joints of the hands and/or feet; when the hands are affected, it usually involves the metacarpophalangeal (MCP), proximal interphalangeal (PIP), and wrist joints, and can be deforming. Although in these characteristics it can be indistinguishable from rheumatoid arthritis (RA), unlike RA it is nonerosive; this deforming, nonerosive arthritis is termed Jaccoud arthropathy. Tendonitis and tendon rupture as well as joint laxity are reported more frequently in patients with SLE than in the general population.

Patients with SLE can also develop generalized myositis, with elevated creatine kinase (CK) levels and inflammatory or necrotic changes on muscle biopsy, often similar to the changes found in dermatomyositis or polymyositis. Myositis is important to differentiate from myalgia, as only proven myositis warrants the introduction or augmentation of high-dose glucocorticoid and/or immunomodulatory therapy.

4. Renal manifestations (lupus nephritis): →Chapter 9.3.4.3.

5. Pulmonary manifestations: There are several different lung manifestations of SLE. Pleuritis with or without pleural effusion is a common manifestation occurring in up to 50% of patients. Pulmonary fibrosis of the nonspecific interstitial fibrosis pattern is a well-recognized SLE complication. Pulmonary hypertension can either occur in isolation or be associated with another pulmonary manifestation, such as venous thromboembolic disease. Diffuse alveolar hemorrhage can result secondary to interstitial lung disease with diffuse alveolar damage or autoimmune capillaritis. Shrinking lung syndrome, characterized by dyspnea, elevated hemidiaphragm(s), and restrictive findings on pulmonary function testing in the absence of parenchymal disease, is a rare but well-recognized complication. Pulmonary embolism occurs, particularly in patients with antiphospholipid antibodies. Acute interstitial pneumonitis can occur rarely (though mortality is high), and chronic fibrotic lung disease can result. Pulmonary complications of dysregulated immunity and immunomodulatory therapy should be considered in the differential diagnosis of patients presenting with respiratory symptoms and signs, including respiratory infections, as well as adverse effects of therapy, such as pneumonitis or interstitial lung disease secondary to methotrexate use.

6. Cardiovascular manifestations include pericarditis with pericardial effusion, myocarditis (rare, usually asymptomatic, found on echocardiography as global contractility impairment in patients with unexplained tachycardia or nonspecific ST-segment and T-wave abnormalities; it may cause conduction disturbances), valvular lesions possibly leading to valve dysfunction (often associated with antiphospholipid antibodies), noninfective (Libman-Sacks) endocarditis, hypertension (due to renal involvement or as a complication of glucocorticoid treatment), and increased risk of early development of coronary artery disease.

7. Nervous system manifestations (neuropsychiatric systemic lupus erythematosus [NPSLE]) are reported in 6% to 60% of patients, depending on the cohort and the NPSLE definition used. The American College of Rheumatology has described 19 neuropsychiatric syndromes, subdivided into central and peripheral nervous system disorders as follows:

1) **Central nervous system**:

    a) Aseptic meningitis.

    b) Cerebrovascular disease (ischemic stroke, transient ischemic attack).

    c) Demyelinating syndrome.

    e) Headache.

    f) Movement disorder (eg, chorea).

    g) Myelopathy.

    h) Seizure disorder.

    i) Acute confusional state.

    j) Anxiety disorder.

    k) Cognitive dysfunction.

    l) Mood disorder.

    m) Psychosis.

2) **Peripheral nervous system**:

    a) Acute inflammatory demyelinating polyneuropathy (Guillain-Barré syndrome).

    b) Autonomic disorder.

    c) Mononeuropathy (simplex or multiplex).

    d) Myasthenia gravis.

    e) Neuropathy, cranial.

    f) Plexopathy.

    g) Polyneuropathy.

To date, no laboratory or imaging findings specific to NPSLE have been described, and attribution of neurologic or psychiatric symptoms to SLE can be difficult. The most common abnormality on magnetic resonance imaging (MRI) in patients who present with NPSLE is nonspecific high T2-signal intensity lesions in white matter that can be focal or diffuse. These lesions have been found to be associated with antiphospholipid antibodies. Cerebrospinal fluid can show elevated protein levels with elevated IgG index. When patients present with neurologic, psychiatric, or neuropsychological findings, physicians have to consider and exclude alternative causes, such as infections, metabolic disturbances, and adverse effects of therapy.

8. Hematologic manifestations: Common hematologic abnormalities include leukopenia, lymphopenia, anemia, and thrombocytopenia (→Diagnostic Tests, below). Clinically, lymphadenopathy is common; lymph nodes are usually soft, painless, and not fixed to the surrounding tissues. Splenomegaly can be found. Secondary thrombotic thrombocytopenic purpura can rarely occur.

9. Gastrointestinal manifestations are relatively uncommon in SLE and can include dysphagia, hepatomegaly, or aseptic peritonitis. Mesenteric or other intra-abdominal thromboses can occur in association with antiphospholipid antibodies.

→ DIAGNOSIS

Diagnostic Criteria

Diagnosis is based on the typical clinical features and results of diagnostic tests. Negative antinuclear antibody (ANA) tests by immunofluorescence make the diagnosis of SLE much less likely (they are positive in >95% of patients), while

Table 21-1. 2019 EULAR/ACR classification criteria for systemic lupus erythematosus

Only one criterion, with the highest score, should count per each domain. It is sufficient to meet each criterion once and not necessarily simultaneously. Do not count a given criterion if it is likely explained by other conditions. Classification as SLE requires ≥10 points and ≥1 clinical criterion present.

Entry criterion: ANA titer ≥1/80[a]

Clinical domain	Criteria	Points	Comments
Fever	Fever >38.3°C	2	
Mucous membrane and skin	Acute cutaneous lupus	6	Observed by a clinician (direct examination or review of photographs)
	Subacute cutaneous or discoid lupus	4	
	Oral ulcers	2	
	Nonscarring alopecia	2	
Musculoskeletal	Joint involvement	6	≥2 joints involved with synovitis (swelling/effusion) **or** Tenderness and ≥30 min of morning stiffness
Serous membranes	Acute pericarditis	6	
	Pleural or pericardial effusion	5	On any of ultrasonography, radiography, CT, or MRI
Renal involvement	Renal biopsy class III or IV	10	
	Renal biopsy class II or V	8	
	Proteinuria >0.5 g/24 h	4	
Neurologic and psychiatric	Seizures	5	Generalized or partial/focal
	Psychosis	3	Delusions or hallucinations without insight and with absence of delirium
	Delirium	2	
Hematologic	Autoimmune hemolysis	4	Positive Coombs (direct antiglobulin) test **and** Low haptoglobin, elevated indirect bilirubin, elevated LDH
	Thrombocytopenia <100 × 10^9/L	4	
	Leukopenia <4 × 10^9/L	3	
SLE-specific antibodies	Anti-dsDNA or anti-Sm	6	
Antiphospholipid antibodies	Anti-cardiolipin, anti-β$_2$GPI, lupus anticoagulant	2	

| Complement protein | Low C3 and low C4 | 4 |
| | Low C3 or low C4 | 3 |

^a Testing using HEp-2 cells or equivalent.

Based on Arthritis Rheumatol. 2019;71(9):1400-1412.

ACR, American College of Rheumatology; ANA, antinuclear antibody; CT, computed tomography; dsDNA, double-stranded DNA; EULAR, European League Against Rheumatism; GPI, glycoprotein I; LDH, lactate dehydrogenase; MRI, magnetic resonance imaging; SLE, systemic lupus erythematosus.

positive anti–double-stranded DNA (dsDNA) or anti-Sm antibodies usually confirm the diagnosis. In 2019, new SLE classification criteria were published by the European League Against Rheumatism (EULAR) and American College of Rheumatology (ACR) (→Table 21-1). Please note that classification criteria are designed mostly to classify patients for research purposes and may clinically misclassify some patients diagnosed in routine clinical practice.

Diagnostic Tests

1. Laboratory tests:

1) **Serum biochemistry**:

   a) **Inflammatory markers**: Neither the erythrocyte sedimentation rate (ESR) nor C-reactive protein (CRP) is a reliable indicator of disease activity in SLE. In patients with polyclonal gammopathy, the ESR can be chronically elevated even in the absence of disease activity.

   b) **Hemoglobin**: An inflammatory anemia (anemia of chronic disease) is commonly found in patients with SLE, characterized by elevated ferritin levels with low serum iron, iron saturation, and total iron-binding capacity. Hemolytic anemia with a positive Coombs test result is characteristic of SLE and is an indication for systemic glucocorticoid and/or immunomodulatory therapy.

   c) **White blood cells**: Leukopenia (15%-20% of patients) and lymphopenia $<1.5 \times 10^9$/L are common in SLE and usually do not require specific therapy. Severe neutropenia may require therapy.

   d) **Platelets**: Thrombocytopenia is common and can be caused either by immunologic disturbances associated with SLE or by secondary antiphospholipid syndrome.

   e) **Creatinine**: Creatinine levels can be elevated in class III, IV, or V lupus nephritis.

   f) **Hypergammaglobulinemia**: Hypergammaglobulinemia is generally polyclonal. It may or may not be associated with active disease.

2) **Urinalysis**: Proteinuria is generally present in class III, IV, and V lupus nephritis; hematuria or pyuria can also be present, particularly in class III and IV nephritis. Urine sediment examination in class III and IV lupus nephritis can reveal dysmorphic erythrocyte, leukocyte, and erythrocyte casts.

3) **Immunology**: More than 95% of patients with SLE have ANAs, including extractable nuclear antigens (ENAs) by immunofluorescence or newer immunoassays (BioPlex). ANAs/ENAs represent a group of autoreactive antibodies directed against the nucleus. ENAs constitute antibodies to specific nuclear components, and these reactivities may predict clinical subtypes/phenotypes of lupus. The anti-dsDNA and anti-Sm antibodies are highly specific (95%-97%) for SLE diagnosis. Drug-induced SLE is associated with antihistone antibodies in >95% of people. Some autoantibodies are more specific to the involvement of certain organs, for instance: anti-dsDNA, lupus nephritis;

Table 21-2. Conditions associated with antinuclear antibodies

Conditions	Examples
Systemic connective tissue disorders	Systemic lupus erythematosus, scleroderma, Sjögren syndrome, polymyositis/dermatomyositis, mixed connective tissue disease, antiphospholipid syndrome, rheumatoid arthritis
Adverse drug reactions (including drug--induced lupus)	Chlorpromazine, methyldopa, hydralazine, propylthiouracil, procainamide, isoniazid, minocycline, D-penicillamine, quinidine, sulfonamides, nitrofurantoin, acebutolol
Chronic liver diseases	Autoimmune hepatitis, primary biliary cholangitis, primary sclerosing cholangitis, alcoholic liver disease
Chronic pulmonary diseases	Idiopathic pulmonary fibrosis, asbestosis, primary pulmonary hypertension
Infections	Tuberculosis, syphilis, chronic HCV/HBV infection, parasitic infestations
Malignancy	Lymphoma, leukemia, melanoma, ovarian cancer, breast cancer, lung cancer, colorectal cancer, prostatic cancer
Hematologic disorders	Immune thrombocytopenic purpura, autoimmune hemolytic anemia
Healthy individuals	More common in female patients, in pregnancy, and in advanced age
Other	Diabetes, Graves disease, Hashimoto thyroiditis, multiple sclerosis, subacute endocarditis, following organ transplantation

HBV, hepatitis B virus; HCV, hepatitis C virus.

anti-RNP, myositis; anti-SSA/anti-Ro, lymphopenia, lymphadenopathy, SCLE, sicca complex. Higher disease activity can correlate with low levels of C3 or C4 complement components and elevated levels of anti-dsDNA; in particular, all these can accompany activity of lupus nephritis. Antiphospholipid antibodies (anticardiolipin, anti–β_2-glycoprotein I, nonspecific inhibitor) are found in ~30% of patients with SLE.

2. **Biopsies**:
1) **Skin**: Skin biopsy samples taken from the areas with evident erythematous lesions or even from apparently healthy skin can reveal immunoglobulin and complement deposits along the border of the epidermis and dermis, although these may also occur in other skin conditions as well as in 20% of healthy individuals.
2) **Renal**: Kidney biopsy is indicated in the majority of patients with features of lupus nephritis. Biopsy results identify the type of glomerular lesions as well as the activity and chronic character of renal involvement, which has implications for both management and prognosis (→Chapter 9.3.4.3).

Differential Diagnosis

Other connective tissue diseases that can coexist or may be confused with SLE include Sjögren syndrome, systemic sclerosis, dermatomyositis/polymyositis, drug-induced SLE, mixed connective tissue disease (MCTD), and undifferentiated connective tissue disease (UCTD). However, depending on the specific clinical manifestations under consideration, differential diagnosis may be very broad and can include a variety of different conditions. For example, hematological abnormalities may be due to drug-induced lupus (causes: →Table 21-2), myeloproliferative disorders (particularly lymphomas), idiopathic thrombocytopenic purpura, microangiopathic hemolytic anemia, antiphospholipid syndrome, or infections. Facial rash may need to be differentiated from rosacea, seborrheic dermatitis, photodermatoses, and dermatomyositis. Conditions that may be associated with positive autoantibodies: →Table 21-2.

→ **TREATMENT**

General Considerations

The therapy of SLE varies based on specific clinical manifestations. While treatments of some specific manifestations of SLE (eg, lupus nephritis) have been reasonably well studied, management of many manifestations of SLE is hindered by a lack of high-quality comparative evidence. Thus, medication use in SLE is guided in many cases by uncontrolled studies, case series, and expert opinion. Guidance from a specialist physician with expertise in SLE management may be necessary.

1. Nonpharmacologic treatment: It is important for patients with SLE to avoid exposure to ultraviolet radiation by avoiding sunlight as well as tanning beds. Ultraviolet light is associated with both cutaneous SLE activity and increased overall SLE disease activity.

2. Pharmacologic treatment: Glucocorticoids are very effective for acute management of active SLE and are indicated in all patients with moderate or severe disease manifestations. However, given the potential adverse effects of glucocorticoids, concomitant use of other immunomodulatory agents is indicated in virtually all patients with SLE. The choice of medications and their dosage depends on predominant clinical features and disease activity.

1) **Antimalarials**: Hydroxychloroquine 6.5 mg/kg (usual maximum dose, 400 mg daily) or, if hydroxychloroquine is not tolerated, chloroquine 250 to 500 mg daily is indicated in all patients with SLE.◐◐ All patients taking antimalarial agents require screening for the rare risk of associated antimalarial-induced retinopathy. The timing of screening is variable, based on risk of retinopathy, and ranges from every 6 months to annually. Low-risk patients can generally be effectively screened by an optometrist. However, higher-risk patients and patients in whom a concern regarding hydroxychloroquine-induced retinopathy has been raised should be evaluated by an ophthalmologist.

2) **Methotrexate**: Methotrexate is often used to achieve disease control in patients in whom glucocorticoids cannot be tapered off, or for whom disease activity is incompletely controlled with glucocorticoids and hydroxychloroquine. Typical manifestations thought to be controlled by methotrexate include arthritis, cutaneous manifestations, and serositis. Typical doses range from 15 to 25 mg weekly administered orally or subcutaneously. Patients need to be monitored for liver enzyme elevation and cytopenias on a monthly basis or more frequently in higher-risk situations. Other adverse effects include potential development of interstitial lung disease or the risk of acute hypersensitivity pneumonitis. Methotrexate is teratogenic and should not be used in pregnant patients.

3) **Azathioprine**: Azathioprine is often used to achieve disease control in patients who are unable to taper off glucocorticoids or in whom disease activity is incompletely controlled with glucocorticoids and hydroxychloroquine. Typical manifestations thought to be controlled by azathioprine include cutaneous manifestations, serositis, and hematological abnormalities. It is also used as maintenance therapy for renal disease. Typical doses range from 1 to 3 mg/kg/d. Patients need to be monitored for cytopenias and liver enzyme elevation, initially every 2 weeks for 2 months, and monthly thereafter if no adverse events have been identified. Cytopenias can pose a particular risk in patients who have low or deficient thiopurine methyltransferase (TPMT) activity, and TMPT genotyping can be considered prior to the initiation of therapy with azathioprine.

4) **Mycophenolate mofetil (MMF)/mycophenolic acid**: MMF is the ester prodrug of mycophenolic acid. These agents are used to control disease in SLE, particularly in patients with active class III, IV, or severe class V lupus nephritis (→Chapter 9.3.4.3). It may have some benefit in the management of cutaneous manifestations and hematologic abnormalities in SLE, though there have been few studies addressing these particular manifestations. Doses differ depending on the agent used. When used for induction therapy for lupus nephritis, MMF is typically administered at 2 to 3 g/d in divided doses. Patients should be monitored for cytopenias on a monthly basis, or more frequently in higher-risk situations. Other adverse effects include elevation in cholesterol levels and gastrointestinal intolerance. The teratogenic potential of MMF is unknown, and at this time it is not recommended for use in pregnancy.

5) **Cyclophosphamide**: Cyclophosphamide was first introduced in the treatment of class III or IV lupus nephritis (→Chapter 9.3.4.3) in combination with glucocorticoids, either in pulse or daily dose regimens. Because of its potentially irreversible adverse effects on fertility, currently its use in SLE as a potent immunosuppressive agent is typically reserved for rapidly progressive nephritis unresponsive to MMF and for other severe, potentially life-threatening manifestations of SLE, including severe cutaneous vasculitis, diffuse alveolar hemorrhage, interstitial pneumonitis, NPSLE, or hematological manifestations, such as refractory autoimmune hemolytic anemia. Cyclophosphamide has a risk of causing cytopenias, particularly leukopenia. If it is being administered intravenously, a complete blood count should be performed at the time of white blood cell nadir at 7 to 10 days after administration and every 2 weeks thereafter. A repeat administration should not be given until the white blood cell count has recovered. For oral cyclophosphamide, the complete blood count should be monitored at least every 2 weeks or more frequently.

6) **Rituximab**: There has been controversy regarding the role of rituximab in SLE. At this time, use of rituximab is generally limited to special circumstances only.

7) **Belimumab**: Belimumab is a monoclonal antibody against anti–B lymphocyte-stimulating factor administered as an IV infusion. It has recently received an approval for use as an addition to the standard therapy for active nonrenal, nonneuropsychiatric SLE manifestations. Belimumab is used particularly to attempt to spare glucocorticoids in patients who have been unable to taper off glucocorticoids to an acceptable level.

Treatment of Specific Organ Manifestations

1. Cutaneous manifestations:

1) Avoidance of sunlight exposure: Protective clothing, sunscreens with a sun protection factor ≥15.

2) Topical treatment: Glucocorticoid ointments and creams (fluorinated glucocorticoids cause skin atrophy and should be used for short periods) or calcineurin inhibitors (eg, 0.1% tacrolimus).

3) Systemic treatment: Antimalarial agents, methotrexate, retinoids (eg, isotretinoin), other agents (eg, thalidomide, dapsone, mycophenolate mofetil, azathioprine), intravenous immunoglobulin (IVIG), and biological agents (eg, rituximab) may also be used.

2. Hematologic manifestations:

1) Autoimmune hemolytic anemia and autoimmune thrombocytopenia usually respond well to glucocorticoids. Other agents that may be effective include azathioprine, MMF, cyclosporine (INN ciclosporin), cyclophosphamide, IVIG, and rituximab. In treatment-resistant patients, splenectomy may be considered.

2) Leukopenia usually does not require treatment. In the case of granulocyte counts $<0.5 \times 10^9$/L, consider granulocyte colony-stimulating factor (G-CSF).

3) Thrombotic thrombocytopenic purpura: →Chapter 7.4.3.3.

4) Macrophage activation syndrome: →Special Considerations, below.

3. Arthralgia, myalgia, and arthritis: For arthralgia, myalgia, and arthritis, nonsteroidal anti-inflammatory drugs (NSAIDs) and antimalarial agents are the mainstays of therapy. For severe inflammatory arthritis in the acute phase, glucocorticoids are typically effective, and patients generally respond to doses of <15 mg of prednisone or equivalent daily. Methotrexate is often effective in patients with arthritis with incomplete response to antimalarial agents or dependence on prednisone.

4. Serositis: In patients with acute manifestations NSAIDs can be used for mild serositis, while glucocorticoids at a low to moderate dose (up to 40 mg/d, then the dose is tapered off) may be necessary for refractory symptoms or large associated effusions. Antimalarial agents, methotrexate, and azathioprine are also effective.

5. Renal manifestations: →Chapter 9.3.4.3.

6. NPSLE:

1) Neurologic symptoms in a patient with SLE should prompt a search for other underlying causes other than SLE itself; it is important to consider and exclude infection, drug reaction, and metabolic disturbances prior to instituting or amplifying immunosuppressive therapy.

2) The mainstay of therapy for active severe NPSLE symptoms, such as acute psychosis, seizures, myelopathy, peripheral neuropathy, or acute inflammatory demyelinating polyneuropathy, are high-dose glucocorticoids (a pulse of 500-1000 mg IV methylprednisolone once daily for 3 consecutive days, then 1 mg/kg to a maximum of 60 mg/d and subsequently tapered off) in combination with cyclophosphamide.

3) If the neurologic symptoms are thrombotic in origin, such as thrombotic stroke, and if they are associated with antiphospholipid antibodies (APLAs), antiplatelet and/or anticoagulant drugs may be the most appropriate management (→Chapter 14.4).

4) Adjunctive treatment can be used as appropriate to treat the individual NPSLE manifestations. For example, antiepileptic drugs are indicated in the management of seizures, and antipsychotic medications may be indicated in acute psychosis.

Treatment of Drug-Induced Lupus

1. Discontinue the drug that has caused the symptoms; in most cases, this will lead to the resolution of symptoms within a few days. The exception to this is hydralazine, in which case a more prolonged course of symptoms can occur.

2. In rare cases, depending on the severity of clinical manifestations, the use of NSAIDs and/or glucocorticoids and/or antimalarial agents for a limited time may be necessary.

3. Additional interventions:

1) Osteoporosis prophylaxis in patients treated with glucocorticoids.

2) Addressing cardiovascular risk factors, given the associated risk of early cardiovascular disease.

3) Vaccinations, particularly influenza and pneumococcal vaccines. Other vaccinations may be considered on the basis of an individual risk. Live vaccines are often contraindicated in patients with SLE due to the use of immunomodulatory agents.

4) Women of reproductive age require counseling about contraception and family planning. The following tenets should be considered:

   a) Estrogen-containing oral contraceptives do not increase disease activity in SLE in patients with well-controlled disease.●

   b) Estrogen-containing contraceptives should be avoided in patients with APLA due to the increased thrombosis risk.❸○

c) Many immunomodulatory agents used in SLE are teratogenic and must be stopped for an appropriate interval prior to any attempt at conception (depending on the medication, this interval can be <6 months).

Attempt at conception should ideally be made only after there has been clinical and serological quiescence of SLE activity for >6 months.◐○

5) In patients with persistently high titers of APLA, consider antiplatelet agents and/or hydroxychloroquine (→Chapter 14.4).

→ **FOLLOW-UP**

1. In patients with complete remission and no evidence of target organ damage or comorbidities, follow-up visits every 6 to 12 months are recommended. The remaining patients should be followed up more frequently.

2. Estimate the activity of SLE and diagnose recurrences on the basis of clinical symptoms, laboratory parameters (complete blood count, creatinine and albumin levels, proteinuria, urine sediment, C3 and C4 complement levels, and anti-dsDNA titers), and general SLE activity indices (eg, systemic lupus erythematosus disease activity index [SLEDAI]). These should be followed up every 3 to 12 months, depending on the clinical situation.

3. APLA levels should be measured before an intended pregnancy, surgery, or estrogen therapy.

4. Patients should undergo a diagnostic workup of hepatitis B virus, hepatitis C virus, cytomegalovirus, and tuberculosis infections based on the individual risk, particularly before starting an intensive immunosuppressive treatment.

→ **SPECIAL CONSIDERATIONS**

Macrophage Activation Syndrome

Macrophage activation syndrome (MAS) is one of the acquired forms of hemophagocytic lymphohistiocytosis (HLH) that occurs in patients with rheumatic disorders, most commonly with systemic idiopathic juvenile arthritis and in adults with SLE. It manifests with increased and prolonged activity of macrophages and T cells (particularly CD8+), leading to an uncontrolled inflammatory response. The manifestations include fever, hepatomegaly, splenomegaly, lymphadenopathy, cytopenias, elevated liver enzymes, disseminated intravascular coagulation, hypofibrinogenemia, hyperferritinemia, and hypertriglyceridemia.

Diagnosis is based on the general HLH criteria; however, these criteria have not been validated in patients with SLE. MAS requires differentiation from sepsis, malignancy, and exacerbations of SLE.

Treatment is controversial, and there is little evidence to guide therapy in this condition. Management typically consists of initially high-dose glucocorticoids, along with varying combinations of IVIG, cyclosporine, cyclophosphamide, tacrolimus, or etoposide. Poor prognostic factors include infection and CRP levels >50 mg/L.

Pregnancy

SLE does not affect fertility but it is associated with risks related to pregnancy and the health of both the mother and the child. It is recommended that female patients do not become pregnant until remission has been achieved. Flares occur in ~30% of pregnant patients with SLE; they are more likely to occur and can be more severe in patients in whom good control of disease activity was not achieved prior to conception. Antimalarial agents, glucocorticoids, and azathioprine are generally considered safe in pregnancy and are typically continued. NSAIDs have been associated with an increased risk of spontaneous abortion in the first trimester as well as with premature closure of the ductus arteriosus in the third trimester; however, they are generally considered safe in the second trimester. Obstetric complications and preeclampsia are mainly associated with APLA and lupus nephritis. The presence of anti-Ro and anti-La antibodies in the mother may cause neonatal lupus (in 3% of affected pregnancies) and is associated with cardiac conduction defects and congenital heart block. Patients with anti-Ro and/or anti-La antibodies should be followed by a high-risk obstetrical team and the fetus should be screened with fetal echocardiogram at intervals during pregnancy. Breastfeeding is possible, though care must be taken to use only medications compatible with breastfeeding.

Surgery

Before surgery disease activity should be assessed, as surgery may worsen the course of SLE. It is recommended to achieve remission before surgery, unless it cannot be postponed. The most rapid improvement can be achieved with perioperative administration of glucocorticoids.

→ PROGNOSIS

The most common causes of death in patients with early SLE include infections and severe target organ involvement (central nervous system, cardiovascular system, acute lupus pneumonitis, severe nephropathy); in patients with long--standing disease, these include complications of treatment (infections) and the effects of accelerated atherosclerosis as well as thromboembolism. With appropriate diagnosis and treatment, the 10-year overall survival rate is 80% to 98% depending on age at diagnosis, specific cohort studied, and country of origin, and the 20-year survival rate is ~65%. More than 40% to 50% of patients develop some degree of permanent target organ damage after 5 years of follow-up. In lupus nephritis, 10% to 30% of patients develop end-stage renal failure over 15 years despite treatment. Recurrence of SLE in transplanted kidneys is very rare (2%).

22. Systemic Sclerosis

→ DEFINITION, ETIOLOGY, PATHOGENESIS

Systemic sclerosis (SSc) is a connective tissue disease characterized by progressive fibrosis of skin and internal organs (leading to their failure), impairment of the structure and function of blood vessels, and abnormalities of the immune system. The etiology is unknown.

→ CLINICAL FEATURES AND NATURAL HISTORY

Women are affected 3 to 4 times more frequently than men. The incidence peaks between the ages of 30 and 50 years.

Clinical Forms

1. Limited cutaneous SSc (lcSSc) (formerly termed CREST [calcinosis, Raynaud phenomenon, esophageal dysmotility, sclerodactyly, telangiectasia] syndrome): The disease usually has a chronic course and often remains undiagnosed for several months to years after the onset of initial symptoms. Cutaneous involvement includes the face and **distal** parts of the upper and lower extremities. Thickening of the skin (scleroderma) has a tendency to remain at a constant, usually moderate level for many years; no correlation is observed between the severity of skin thickening and the extent of internal organ involvement. The gastrointestinal (GI) tract (particularly the esophagus) is most commonly affected, followed by interstitial lung disease and relatively rare cardiac involvement. Pulmonary hypertension may occur in lcSSc and should be assessed annually by echocardiography, even in asymptomatic patients. Primary biliary cholangitis is also associated with lcSSc. Patients with long-standing lcSSc may develop progressive dyspnea. This may indicate the development of pulmonary hypertension or pulmonary fibrosis and is associated with an adverse prognosis.

2. Diffuse cutaneous SSc (dcSSc): The course of the skin involvement is much more severe and acute than that in lcSSc; it is symmetric, diffuse, and includes the face, proximal parts of the extremities, and the trunk (occasionally sparing the fingers). Skin thickening usually progresses rapidly and peaks within 3 to 6 years. Organ involvement occurs almost simultaneously with skin thickening, with the lungs being affected most frequently, followed by the GI tract, heart, and kidneys. The rate and extent of internal organ involvement correlates with the severity and extent of skin thickening. Organ lesions developing in early dcSSc (conventionally defined as the first 3 years from the onset) are predictive of the subsequent course of the disease.

3. Systemic sclerosis without skin involvement (SSc sine scleroderma) is manifested by typical systemic features, such as pulmonary fibrosis, pulmonary hypertension, esophageal and other GI involvement, and renal involvement, along with serologic abnormalities, but without skin involvement.

4. Overlap syndromes with clinical features of SSc and other systemic connective tissue diseases, most commonly rheumatoid arthritis, dermatomyositis, systemic lupus erythematosus, or mixed connective tissue disease.

5. Early SSc: Raynaud phenomenon, puffy hands, capillaroscopy findings suggestive of SSc, and positive SSc-specific antinuclear antibodies (ANAs) (anticentromere [ACA], anti–Scl-70 [also known as antitopoisomerase I], antipolymerase III, anti-Th/To) with no or minimal skin thickening or internal organ involvement. This is now recognized as early disease using the new 2013 American College of Rheumatology (ACR)/European League Against Rheumatism (EULAR) criteria.

Organ Involvement

1. Raynaud phenomenon is observed in almost 100% of patients with lcSSc and in >90% of patients with dcSSc. It may precede the development of SSc by many years.

2. Cutaneous manifestations following 3 phases of development: edema, sclerosis, and atrophy; initially swollen digits (limited flexion), followed by flexion contractures; in lcSSc, pain related to damage-prone skin and poorly healing ulcers most commonly affecting fingertips; atrophy of the fingertips and nails, shortening of distal phalanges; a face with taut skin; a pinched, beak-like nose; thin lips surrounded by wrinkles (radial furrowing); reduced oral aperture, making it difficult to protrude the tongue; skin hyperpigmentation or hypopigmentation; telangiectasias, particularly on the face (and sometimes the mucosal surfaces); calcifications (most commonly of the skin of the fingers and extensor surfaces of the elbows and knees); pruritus; digital ulcers or digital pits.

3. Musculoskeletal involvement: Arthralgia or arthritis, usually symmetric, often severe; morning stiffness, usually affecting the fingers, wrists, elbows, and knees; transient episodes of joint swelling; limited joint movement caused by skin thickening; tendon rubs on movement caused by tendon involvement (tenosynovitis, particularly in dcSSc); muscle pain, muscle weakness (especially if there is associated myositis).

4. GI involvement: Sicca symptoms, gingivitis (causing tooth loss); gastroesophageal reflux disease (GERD) (due to impaired peristalsis and reduced function of the lower esophageal sphincter, which leads to gastroesophageal reflux), dysphagia (due to impaired esophageal motility and strictures). Bleeding from upper GI vascular lesions (gastric antral vascular ectasia [GAVE]) is the main cause of anemia in patients with SSc. Bloating and abdominal pain with alternating diarrhea and constipation are often associated with malabsorption (frequently due to bacterial overgrowth syndrome); symptoms of primary biliary cirrhosis may also occur (in <10%). Other GI features commonly found are severe constipation due to colonic hypomotility and fecal incontinence due to involvement of the anal sphincter.

5. Pulmonary involvement: Features of interstitial lung disease: dyspnea (initially on exertion, in advanced disease also at rest), chronic dry cough (patients frequently remain asymptomatic despite severe pulmonary involvement), basal crackles, occasionally pleural pain and pleural rub, tachypnea. Dry cough can be related to severe untreated GERD.

6. Cardiac involvement: Pulmonary arterial hypertension (progressive impairment of exercise tolerance, presyncope or syncope on exertion indicating advanced pulmonary hypertension and right ventricular failure) is the most common cardiac manifestation of SSc. Other features include angina (right ventricular ischemia caused by overload), symptoms of right ventricular failure and pulmonary hypertension (in advanced SSc), symptoms of left ventricular dysfunction (usually systolic), tachyarrhythmias, rarely bradyarrhythmias (palpitations, syncope), ischemic heart disease (most frequently caused by microcirculatory abnormalities), pericardial involvement (acute pericarditis, pericardial effusion, cardiac tamponade, constrictive pericarditis), acute myocarditis (rare).

7. Renal involvement: Symptoms are often mild and nonspecific even in patients with advanced lesions. **Scleroderma renal crisis** develops in 5% to 10% of patients with dcSSc (in 80% of cases, it occurs within the first 4 years of the disease) and is much less frequent (<2%) in patients with lcSSc. Positive anti-RNA polymerase III antibodies are a risk factor. Renal crisis manifests as rapidly increasing hypertension (this may be accompanied severe headache, visual disturbances, seizures, acute left ventricular failure) and features of renal failure; microangiopathic hemolytic anemia may occur (anemia, schistocytes, increased haptoglobin, reticulocytes, increased unconjugated bilirubin). In ~10% of cases, hypertension is absent; these are usually patients already receiving angiotensin-converting enzyme inhibitors (ACEIs) or calcium channel blockers, patients with previous low or low-normal blood pressure, or patients with heart disease. Risk factors for scleroderma renal crisis include dcSSc, male patients, glucocorticoids >15 mg;◔ the use of calcium channel blockers may be protective.◔

→ DIAGNOSIS

Diagnostic Tests

1. Laboratory tests:

1) **Blood tests**: A normal or mildly elevated erythrocyte sedimentation rate (ESR) (a significantly elevated ESR is usually associated with organ involvement or concomitant infection), anemia (usually mild, worsens in patients with malabsorption and progressive renal involvement), hypergammaglobulinemia (increased IgG and IgM levels), positive serum rheumatoid factor (in 20%-30% of patients), elevated serum B-type natriuretic peptide (BNP) or N-terminal pro—B-type natriuretic peptide (NT-proBNP) levels if heart failure and/or advanced pulmonary hypertension are suspected.

2) **Immunologic studies**: Positive ANAs (in 90% of patients), antitopoisomerase--I antibodies (Scl-70, typically in dcSSc [in 30% of patients]), ACAs typically in lcSSc (in 70%-80% of patients), antinucleolar antibodies (nucleolar immunofluorescence), for instance, to RNA polymerase I, RNA polymerase III, Th/To, fibrillarin.

2. Radiologic studies: Hand radiographs may reveal osteolysis of the distal phalanges (or total resorption of the distal phalanx in more advanced disease) and calcifications; less frequently, similar lesions are observed on feet radiographs. **Contrast-enhanced radiography of the GI tract** reveals impaired esophageal motility (in advanced SSc, dilation and pipe-like appearance of the entire esophagus), impaired motor function of the small intestine (alternating segments of strictures and dilations, hypersegmentation) and large intestine (diverticulosis, occasionally significant colonic distention). **Chest radiographs and high-resolution computed tomography (HRCT)** reveal features of interstitial lung disease, that is, ground-glass linear and reticular opacifications, mainly in the basal peripheral and subpleural areas of the lung, traction bronchiectases, and bronchial (honeycomb) cysts. **Magnetic resonance imaging (MRI) and single-photon emission computed tomography (SPECT)-CT** may be useful in the diagnosis of cardiac involvement.

3. Doppler echocardiography reveals features of pulmonary hypertension (increased right ventricular systolic pressure >35 mm Hg) (→Chapter 13.15), pericardial effusion, as well as systolic and diastolic dysfunction. Even in asymptomatic patients, echocardiography should be performed annually to facilitate early diagnosis and treatment of pulmonary hypertension.

4. Upper GI endoscopy: In the esophagus there are features of gastroesophageal reflux and telangiectasias; in the stomach, diffuse vascular lesions, particularly in the cardia, are observed (solitary or multiple telangiectasias described as a "watermelon stomach" or GAVE).

5. Pulmonary function tests may reveal a low carbon dioxide diffusing capacity of the lungs (DL_{CO}). If there is an isolated reduced DL_{CO}, or if there is a mismatch of DL_{CO} and forced vital capacity (FVC) (FVC%/DL_{CO}% >1.6), consider pulmonary hypertension as the cause and investigate with echocardiography. Even in asymptomatic patients, pulmonary function tests and echocardiography should be performed annually to facilitate early diagnosis and management of pulmonary fibrosis or pulmonary hypertension.

6. Nail-fold capillaroscopy reveals typical (though not pathognomonic) features of so-called megacapillaries or giant loops (more common in lcSSc) and avascular areas, known as "drop-outs" (predominantly in dcSSc).

7. Other studies:

1) **Stress tests** (6-minute walk test, cardio-respiratory exercise test; these may be used for monitoring the performance status of the patient and progression of SSc).

2) **Electrocardiography (ECG)** (arrhythmias and conduction disturbances).

3) **Cardiac catheterization** should be considered in patients with high right ventricular systolic pressure on echocardiography, those with symptoms or signs of right heart failure, and in those with isolated declining DL_{CO} on pulmonary function tests (diagnosis of pulmonary hypertension).

8. Skin biopsy is of limited use in patients with early SSc due to the high rate of false-negative results. In patients with typical clinical manifestations, the diagnosis is straightforward, which makes the skin biopsy unnecessary. Nevertheless, it is indicated in patients suspected of having other diseases characterized by skin thickening, such as eosinophilic fasciitis or scleredema or scleromyxedema.

Diagnostic Criteria

The 2013 ACR/EULAR classification criteria (→Table 22-1) are useful in both advanced and early SSc.

Differential Diagnosis

1. Early SSc: Raynaud phenomenon of a different etiology; other systemic connective tissue diseases, mainly undifferentiated connective tissue disease, mixed connective tissue disease, other overlap syndromes, dermatomyositis, rheumatoid arthritis.

2. Cutaneous manifestations: Skin thickening in the course of diffuse eosinophilic fasciitis (this is characterized by wood-like skin induration, peripheral blood eosinophilia, hypergammaglobulinemia, and elevated ESR; the etiology

Table 22-1. 2013 ACR/EULAR criteria for the classification of systemic sclerosis		
Criteria	**Score**	**Comments**
Skin thickening of the fingers of both hands extending proximal to the metacarpophalangeal joints	9	Sufficient criterion
Skin thickening of the fingers		
Puffy fingers[a]	2	If both are present, only the higher score counts
Sclerodactyly of the fingers[b]	4	
Fingertip lesions[c]		
Digital tip ulcers	2	If both are present, only the higher score counts
Fingertip pitting scars	3	
Telangiectasia[d]	2	
Abnormal nail-fold capillaries[e]	2	
Pulmonary arterial hypertension[f] and/or interstitial lung disease[g]	2	
Raynaud phenomenon[h]	3	
SSc-related autoantibodies:		
– Anticentromere	3	Maximum score: 3
– Antitopoisomerase I (anti-Scl 70)		
– Anti-RNA polymerase III		
Interpretation: The diagnosis of SSc can be made in patients with a total score ≥9.		

[a] A diffuse, usually nonpitting increase in soft tissue mass of the digits extending beyond the normal confines of the joint capsule, which affects the physiological contour of the fingers (normal digits are tapered distally with the tissues following the contours of the digital bone and joint structures).

[b] Skin hardening distal to the metacarpophalangeal joints but proximal to the proximal interphalangeal joints.

[c] Ulcers or scars distal to or at the proximal interphalangeal joint not thought to be due to trauma. Digital pitting scars are depressed areas at digital tips as a result of ischemia, rather than trauma or exogenous causes.

[d] Telangiectasia are visible, macular, dilated superficial blood vessels, which collapse upon pressure and fill slowly when pressure is released. Telangiectasias in a scleroderma-like pattern are round, well-demarcated, and found on hands, lips, inside of the mouth, and/or are large mat-like telangiectasias. Telangiectasias should be distinguished from rapidly filling spider angiomas with a central arteriole and from dilated superficial vessels.

[e] Abnormal nail-fold capillary patterns consistent with systemic sclerosis are enlarged capillaries and/or capillary loss with or without pericapillary hemorrhages at the nail fold. They may also be seen on the cuticle.

[f] Pulmonary arterial hypertension diagnosed by right-sided heart catheterization according to standard definitions.

[g] Interstitial lung disease: Pulmonary fibrosis seen on high-resolution CT or chest radiography, most pronounced in the basilar portions of the lungs, or occurrence of Velcro crackles on auscultation not due to another cause such as congestive heart failure.

[h] Raynaud phenomenon: Self-reported or reported by a physician, with at least a 2-phase color change in finger(s) and often toe(s) consisting of pallor, cyanosis, and/or reactive hyperemia in response to cold exposure or emotion; usually one phase is pallor.

The criteria are not applicable to patients with skin thickening sparing the fingers or to patients who have a scleroderma-like disorder that better explains their manifestations (eg, nephrogenic sclerosing fibrosis, generalized morphea, eosinophilic fasciitis, scleredema diabeticorum, scleromyxedema, erythromelalgia, porphyria, lichen sclerosis, graft-versus-host disease, diabetic cheiroarthropathy).

Adapted from Ann Rheum Dis. 2013;72(11):1747-55.

ACR, American College of Rheumatology; CT, computed tomography; EULAR, European League Against Rheumatism.

is unknown), localized scleroderma (discrete lesions with no symmetric skin changes on the extremities, no internal organ involvement or immunologic abnormalities), Buschke scleredema, scleromyxedema, lichen sclerosus et atrophicus, adipose tissue atrophy, skin thickening caused by other internal diseases (eg, chronic autoimmune hepatitis) or by chemical substances (including drugs that may cause scleroderma-like skin lesions, eg, bleomycin and contrast used in radiology), porphyria cutanea tarda, chronic graft-versus-host disease.

→ TREATMENT

General Considerations

1. No treatment can cure, effectively stop, or definitively delay the progression of SSc in the majority of patients; **organ-specific therapies** (→below) are used to improve the survival of patients with SSc. In highly selected patients with dcSSc and severe, rapidly progressive organ involvement but without significant cardiovascular involvement, autologous hematopoietic stem cell transplantation (HSCT) can be considered by specialized scleroderma teams.⊘⊖

2. Physiotherapy, kinesiotherapy (exercise, commonly preceded by paraffin therapy), **and occupational therapy** are used to improve or maintain the patient's physical capacity.

3. Because of the risk of scleroderma renal crisis, **do not use glucocorticoids** at a dose >15 mg/d (prednisone or prednisolone),⊗⊖ unless the use of glucocorticoids is indispensable because of life-threatening organ involvement. In such situations, a prophylactic calcium channel blocker may be considered along with close monitoring of plasma creatinine levels and blood pressure. Patients with dcSSc are particularly at risk within the first 5 years of disease. Do not use cyclosporine (INN ciclosporin), nonsteroidal anti-inflammatory drugs (NSAIDs), or drugs that may affect vascular tone, such as ephedrine, ergot derivatives, and β-blockers.

Treatment of Early dSSc

Make attempts to diagnose and treat organ involvement as early as possible. The extent of skin thickening (which may be measured in several areas, including the face, back, chest, arm, forearm, hand, fingers, abdomen, leg, foot) is called the **modified Rodnan skin score (mRss)**. This score correlates with internal organ involvement and may be useful in estimating the severity and dynamics of the disease. In patients with rapidly progressive skin lesions (particularly with mRss >15-20), consider **methotrexate** at a dose of up to 20 mg/wk, **mycophenolate mofetil**, or **cyclophosphamide** (dosage as in interstitial lung disease). In patients with severe rapidly progressive skin involvement, autologous HSCT could be considered by scleroderma specialist teams.⊘⊖ Calcium channel blockers may protect against digital ulcers and scleroderma renal crisis.⊘⊖

Treatment of Raynaud Phenomenon, Finger Ulcers, and Necrosis

Treatment consists mainly of extended-release formulations of **dihydropyridine calcium channel blockers**, such as nifedipine; other drugs: →Chapter 3.18.4.3. In patients with severe treatment-resistant SSc, and particularly in patients with poorly healing ulcers, intravenous **prostacyclins** (iloprost, alprostadil) are commonly used. The endothelin-1 receptor antagonist bosentan can prevent the development of new ulcers and could be considered.

Treatment of Interstitial Lung Disease

Also →Chapter 13.7.4.2.

Treatment of interstitial lung disease in the setting of scleroderma is best conducted by clinicians or teams experienced in both connective tissue and lung diseases. Below are some principles of treatment:

1) Either oral or IV **cyclophosphamide** can be used for 1 year, or oral **mycophenolate** for 2 years, with equivalent improvements in lung function.

Mycophenolate is often preferred due to fewer adverse reactions and is used also as maintenance therapy after cyclophosphamide.⊘● The cumulative dose of cyclophosphamide is lower if given by monthly IV infusion compared with daily oral dosing.

2) Cautious concomitant use of **glucocorticoids** may be considered (do not exceed doses equivalent to 15 mg/d of prednisone, if possible). Treatment with **azathioprine** or **rituximab** may also be considered.

3) Recently **nintedanib**, a tyrosine kinase inhibitor with antifibrotic effects, has been shown to limit the decline in pulmonary function in patients with systemic sclerosis and pulmonary fibrosis.⊘●

Treatment of Pulmonary Hypertension

→Chapter 13.15.

Treatment of Musculoskeletal Involvement

1. Arthralgia: Acetaminophen (INN paracetamol), **tramadol**.

2. Progressive polyarthritis or myositis: Methotrexate (doses as in rheumatoid arthritis), initial **glucocorticoid** treatment (<15 mg/d of prednisone) may be also considered. **Biologics** could be considered, in particular tumor necrosis factor (TNF) inhibitors, such as etanercept or adalimumab, or interleukin-6 (IL-6) receptor blockers, such as tocilizumab.

3. Myositis:

1) Mild or moderate: **Azathioprine** 2.5 mg/kg/d (maximum dose, 200 mg/d) orally or methotrexate (as above). Consider adding **glucocorticoids** at a dose equivalent to <15 mg/d of prednisone.

2) Severe: **Methylprednisolone** 3 to 4 pulses of 500 to 1000 mg IV (every day or every other day) followed by prednisone (a dose of 1 mg/kg/d may be required; patients should be counselled regarding the possibility of this inducing scleroderma renal crisis) and **azathioprine** or **methotrexate**.

Treatment of Gastrointestinal Involvement

Symptomatic treatment, that is, conservative measures, such as raising the head of the bed by 10 to 15 cm, and proton pump inhibitors (PPIs) (high doses are often required) in patients with GERD, prokinetic agents including domperidone 10 mg tid or prucalopride 2 mg once daily in patients with impaired motility, intermittent courses of antibiotics in patients with malabsorption due to bacterial overgrowth syndrome (empiric quinolones, amoxicillin/clavulanic acid, rifaximin).⊘○

Treatment of Cardiac Involvement

1. Pulmonary hypertension.

2. Arrhythmias, conduction abnormalities, heart failure: Symptomatic treatment.

3. Active myocarditis: Glucocorticoids (doses as in systemic lupus erythematosus); if ineffective, **cyclophosphamide** (doses as in interstitial lung disease).

Treatment of Scleroderma Renal Crisis

1. Elevated blood pressure >140/90 mm Hg, rise in blood pressure >20 mm Hg (either systolic or diastolic) higher than the patients' normal blood pressure, ≥2-fold increase in serum creatinine level, or proteinuria: Immediately start an ACEI (hospitalize if blood pressure >160/100 mm Hg). The dose of the ACEI should be titrated up to achieve a decrease in systolic blood pressure of 10 to 20 mm Hg over 24 hours, even if renal function is declining. If normalization of arterial pressure is not being achieved, add another antihypertensive agent, eg, an angiotensin receptor blocker, a calcium channel blocker, or a nitrate (particularly in patients with pulmonary edema).

2. Progressive renal failure: Renal replacement therapy (RRT). In half of the patients requiring RRT, renal function improves over 6 to 24 months to a degree that allows discontinuation of RRT.⊖ If kidney transplantation is being considered, it should be postponed for at least 2 years after the episode of scleroderma renal crisis.

3. The use of **calcium channel blockers** seems to be protective of scleroderma renal crisis and could be considered.⊘⊖

FOLLOW-UP

Suggested follow-up:

1) It is recommended that the patient is advised to **measure blood pressure** 3 times a week at home, particularly in the first 5 years of disease. At later stages of the disease, monthly blood pressure monitoring is probably sufficient (or more frequently if blood pressure is rising).

2) **Plasma creatinine levels, estimated glomerular filtration rate (eGFR), and urine dipstick test for proteinuria**: In early dcSSc these should be measured every 4 to 6 weeks; at later stages of the disease, every 3 to 6 months.

3) **ECG and Doppler echocardiography**: In early dSSc these should be performed every 6 to 12 months, and at later stages or in limited SSc every 12 to 24 months (depending on risk factors).

4) **Pulmonary function tests** (spirometry, DL_{CO}, postexertional pulse oximetry): In early dcSSc these tests should be performed every 6 to 12 months, and at later stages or in limited SSc every 12 months.

5) Other studies depend on symptoms and results of the above investigations and may include, for instance, the 6-minute walk test to monitor performance status. In early dcSSc monitor ESR, complete blood count, and serum creatine kinase, aspartate aminotransferase, and alanine aminotransferase levels every 12 months. Chest HRCT, contrast-enhanced radiographs of the GI, and endoscopy of the upper GI tract could be considered if clinically indicated. If disease progression is observed, the frequency of the follow-up studies could be increased.

PROGNOSIS

Prognosis depends on the presence and extent of internal organ involvement. More than half of all deaths in patients with SSc are related to pulmonary fibrosis, pulmonary hypertension, and renal involvement. Other causes of death are mainly infections, malignancy, and cardiovascular complications not directly related to SSc. In patients with cardiac involvement the average survival from the time of diagnosis is 9 years. Ten-year survival in patients with pulmonary involvement but without cardiac or renal involvement is 60%, and ~75% in patients without involvement of any of these organs. In patients with appropriately treated pulmonary hypertension 3-year survival rates are ~65%.

23. Vasculitis Syndromes

DEFINITION, ETIOLOGY, PATHOGENESIS

Vasculitides are a heterogeneous group of diseases in which blood vessel walls are damaged due to inflammation. This may result in bleeding and impaired blood flow, eventually leading to ischemia and necrosis of the associated tissues.

Table 23-1. Nomenclature of vasculitides adopted by the 2012 International Chapel Hill Consensus Conference	
Large-vessel vasculitis	Takayasu arteritis Giant cell arteritis
Medium-vessel vasculitis	Polyarteritis nodosa Kawasaki disease

Small-vessel vasculitis	ANCA-associated vasculitis:
	  – Microscopic polyangiitis
	  – Granulomatosis with polyangiitis (Wegener granulomatosis)
	  – Eosinophilic granulomatosis with polyangiitis (Churg-Strauss syndrome)
	Immune-complex small-vessel vasculitis:
	  – Anti–glomerular basement membrane (anti-GBM) disease
	  – Cryoglobulinemic vasculitis
	  – IgA vasculitis (Henoch-Schönlein purpura)
	  – Hypocomplementemic urticarial vasculitis (anti-C1q vasculitis)

Variable-vessel vasculitis	Behçet disease Cogan syndrome
Single-organ vasculitis	Cutaneous leukocytoclastic angiitis Cutaneous arteritis Primary central nervous system vasculitis Isolated aortitis Other
Vasculitis associated with systemic disease	Lupus vasculitis Rheumatoid vasculitis Sarcoid vasculitis Other
Vasculitis associated with probable etiology	Hepatitis C virus–associated cryoglobulinemic vasculitis Hepatitis B virus–associated vasculitis Syphilis-associated aortitis Drug-associated immune-complex vasculitis Drug-associated ANCA-associated vasculitis Cancer-associated vasculitis Other
Source: Arthritis Rheum. 2013;65(1):1-11.	
ANCA, antineutrophil cytoplasmic antibody.	

Vasculitis syndromes can be divided into **infectious vasculitis** (caused by direct invasion and proliferation of a pathogen in a vessel wall) and **noninfectious vasculitis**. According to the current nomenclature (2012), noninfectious vasculitides (→Table 23-1) can be categorized based on type/size of involved vessels, location of organ involvement, and underlying etiology:

1) **Type/size of involved vessels**: Large-vessel vasculitis, medium-vessel vasculitis, small-vessel vasculitis, and variable-vessel vasculitis.
2) **Location of organ involvement**: Single-organ vasculitides can be classified based on type of involved organ (eg, isolated aortitis, cutaneous arteritis).
3) **Underlying etiology**: Some vasculitides are associated with systemic disease (rheumatoid arthritis, sarcoidosis, systemic lupus erythematous) or

with another probable etiology. Probable etiologies include malignancy, viral infection (hepatitis B virus, hepatitis C virus, parvovirus B19, HIV), post--bacterial infection (syphilis), or drugs (eg, β-lactams, macrolides, selective serotonin reuptake inhibitors, anticonvulsants).

The most common type of vasculitis is small-vessel vasculitis, which is usually associated with immune complexes. Medium- and large-vessel vasculitides are less common, although giant cell arteritis is common in the elderly (12--25/100,000). Note that it is always necessary to establish whether vasculitis is primary or secondary (caused by underlying etiology).

Large-vessel vasculitis: Takayasu arteritis and giant cell arteritis. Large vessel vasculitides predominantly involve large arteries, such as the aorta, carotids, temporal artery, and subclavian arteries.

Medium-vessel vasculitis: Polyarteritis nodosa and Kawasaki disease. Medium-vessel vasculitides involve predominantly medium-sized arteries (in particular the main visceral arteries and their branches) but may affect arteries of any size.

Small-vessel vasculitis (→Table 23-1): These vasculitides mainly involve small parenchymal arteries, arterioles, capillaries, and venules. Small-vessel vasculitis can be further divided into antineutrophil cytoplasmic antibody (ANCA)-associated vasculitis and immune-complex vasculitis.

1) **ANCA-associated vasculitis** (eg, granulomatosis with polyangiitis [GPA], eosinophilic GPA [EGPA] [Churg-Strauss syndrome], microscopic polyangiitis [MPA]): These vasculitides contain few or absent immunoglobulin deposits in vessel walls. They are also often characterized by the presence of antibodies to myeloperoxidase (MPO ANCA, type of perinuclear ANCA [p-ANCA]) or to proteinase 3 (PR3 ANCA, type of cytoplasmic ANCA [c-ANCA]), although ANCA-negative patients are also observed. Both PR3 ANCA and MPO ANCA are detected using the enzyme-linked immunosorbent assay.

2) **Immune-complex vasculitis** (including anti-glomerular basement membrane disease): Moderate to severe immunoglobulin and/or complement deposition in vessel walls (often coexisting with glomerulonephritis).

23.1. Anti–Glomerular Basement Membrane Disease (Formerly Goodpasture Syndrome)

→ DEFINITION, ETIOLOGY

Anti–glomerular basement membrane (anti-GBM) disease is a vasculitis affecting glomerular capillaries and/or pulmonary capillaries, uniquely associated with the deposition antibodies to the GBM in the membrane. Pulmonary involvement leads to pulmonary hemorrhage, whereas renal involvement results in glomerulonephritis with necrosis and crescents. Historically, the eponym "Goodpasture syndrome" has referred to the combined pulmonary and renal manifestations of anti-GBM disease.

→ CLINICAL FEATURES AND NATURAL HISTORY

Clinical features:
1) **General symptoms**: Malaise, fever, arthralgia.
2) **Symptoms of pulmonary hemorrhage** (→Chapter 13.7.1) can include dyspnea, cough, hemoptysis, fever, respiratory failure, and shock.
3) **Symptoms of rapidly progressive glomerulonephritis**: Peripheral edema, hypertension. In 30% of patients the time between the onset of renal and pulmonary symptoms is from one week to one year.
4) **Other symptoms**: Nausea, vomiting, diarrhea.

The disease is usually rapidly progressive and leads to acute respiratory and renal failure. The main causes of death are pulmonary hemorrhage and respiratory failure. Long-term complications include chronic kidney disease, pulmonary fibrosis, and chronic respiratory failure.

➔ DIAGNOSIS

Diagnosis is based on the clinical features, positive circulating antibodies to the GBM, and characteristic histologic features of renal biopsy specimens.

Laboratory findings reveal elevations in the erythrocyte sedimentation rate and C-reactive protein levels, normocytic or microcytic hypochromic anemia, leukocytosis (often with eosinophilia), and signs of renal involvement (creatinine, active sediment [cellular casts], proteinuria <3 g/d in urinalysis), antibodies to the GBM (in 80%-90% of patients), myeloperoxidase (MPO) antineutrophil cytoplasmic antibody (ANCA) (in 10%-40%). Chest radiographs, high-resolution computed tomography, and bronchoalveolar lavage reveal abnormalities typical for pulmonary hemorrhage.

Differential Diagnosis

1. Other causes of pulmonary-renal syndrome (→Chapter 14.23.7).

2. Causes of diffuse alveolar hemorrhage other than vasculitis.

3. Other types of acute glomerulonephritis (→Chapter 9.3).

4. Renal vein thrombosis with pulmonary embolism.

5. Heart failure with renal failure.

➔ TREATMENT

Plasmapheresis (use repeatedly until complete removal of antibodies to the GBM) with cyclophosphamide and prednisone is the standard treatment for anti-GBM disease, particularly for improving renal outcomes.◉◉ In treatment of refractory disease, rituximab may be used.◉◉ In acute disease, assisted ventilation and renal replacement therapy are often necessary. From 60% to 90% of patients receiving appropriate treatment survive the acute phase of the disease. Treatment is less effective in patients presenting with renal failure. Up to 50% of patients eventually require renal replacement therapy.

23.2. Behçet Disease

➔ DEFINITION

Behçet disease is an immune-mediated small-vessel vasculitis that usually affects patients aged 20 to 40 years, more frequently men than women. The course of the disease is variable, with periods of relapses and remissions.

➔ CLINICAL FEATURES AND DIAGNOSIS

Clinical manifestations: Recurrent oral and/or genital aphthous ulcers with concomitant cutaneous, ophthalmic, joint, gastrointestinal (GI), and/or central nervous system (CNS) inflammatory lesions. Patients may have small-vessel vasculitis, arteritis, arterial aneurysms, and venous and arterial thromboangiitis and thrombosis.

Key clinical diagnostic criteria:

1) Painful oral aphthous ulcers, recurring ≥3 times over a 12-month period and healing spontaneously within 1 to 3 weeks; these are often the presenting symptom of the disease.

2) Presence of ≥2 of the following signs and symptoms: Recurrent genital ulcers; anterior and posterior uveitis or retinal vasculitis (in >80% of patients);

cutaneous lesions: erythema nodosum, acneiform eruptions, or vesicles; path-ergy, that is, hyperreactive skin leading to inflammatory lesions triggered by a minor trauma (eg, a needle prick causes the appearance of a pustule within 24-48 hours).

Other symptoms: Arthritis without erosions (in 50% of patients); CNS involve-ment (headache, features of brainstem and corticospinal tract damage, aseptic meningitis, mood disturbances, confusion); GI symptoms (abdominal pain, diarrhea); migrating superficial phlebitis; deep vein thrombosis.

→ TREATMENT

Behçet disease, like most other instances of vasculitis, is usually treated by rheumatologists. Treatment is based on severity of the disease and the specific organs involved.

1. Cutaneous lesions: First-line treatment for isolated lesions is with topi-cal glucocorticoids.◐◑ Other treatment options may include tacrolimus and antibiotics as well as colchicine (especially if there is erythema nodosum) and dapsone. In patients with severe lesions or in treatment-resistant patients, interferon α, methotrexate, azathioprine, and thalidomide may be used.◐◑ The general concern, as with all immunosuppressive drugs, is with the potential teratogenic effect.

2. Ocular involvement: According to the European League Against Rheumatism, in inflammatory eye disease affecting the posterior segment, treatment should include azathioprine and systemic glucocorticoids.◐◑ If there is severe eye disease, cyclosporine (INN ciclosporin) A or infliximab may be added to the treatment regimen, or treatment with interferon α may be considered (with or without glucocorticoids).◐◑

3. Treatment of internal organ involvement: There is no well-controlled evidence to guide treatment of major vessel, GI, or CNS involvement. Treatment might include oral glucocorticoids, interferon α, azathioprine, cyclosporine, and cyclophosphamide.◐◑ Cyclosporine A should probably be avoided in cases of CNS involvement (unless necessary due to severe ocular involvement) because of potential neurotoxicity.◐◑ Infliximab has been successfully used in treatment-resistant patients.

23.3. Cryoglobulinemic Vasculitis

→ DEFINITION, ETIOLOGY

Cryoglobulinemic vasculitis (CV) is characterized by cryoglobulin deposits that affect small vessels (mainly capillaries, venules, or arterioles) and circulate in the blood. Cryoglobulin deposits are monoclonal and polyclonal anti-IgG immunoglobulins of IgM class. They precipitate at low temperatures, can block blood vessels, and may eventually lead to gangrenous extremities. CV may be classified as idiopathic if the etiology is unknown or as secondary to other conditions. Most commonly CV is associated with hepatitis C virus (HCV) in-fection (~80% of patients) but can also be associated with lymphoproliferative or autoimmune diseases.

→ CLINICAL FEATURES AND NATURAL HISTORY

Clinical manifestations:

1) **General symptoms** include fatigue and low-grade fever.
2) **Cutaneous manifestations**: Palpable purpura in 90% of patients, usually on the lower extremities (cold triggers the appearance of new lesions), Raynaud phenomenon.

3) **Renal manifestations associated with glomerulonephritis**: Mainly peripheral edema and hypertension.

4) **Nervous system manifestations**: Peripheral polyneuropathy, cranial nerve involvement, central nervous system vasculitis.

5) **Other manifestations**: Arthralgia, myalgia. Less frequently, lymphadenopathy, hepatosplenomegaly, gastrointestinal symptoms.

In secondary CV **features of the underlying condition** may be observed. CV is frequently associated with exacerbations lasting 1 to 2 weeks followed by remissions lasting several days to months. With time, renal failure develops; renal involvement is associated with a less favorable prognosis. The most frequent cause of death is infection.

DIAGNOSIS

Diagnosis is based on the clinical manifestations and presence of cryoglobulins in the blood. Frequently, levels of complement component C4 (in 90% of patients) and total hemolytic activity of the complement complex (CH50) are markedly decreased. Rheumatoid factor is present in >70% of patients. The erythrocyte sedimentation rate may also be elevated. Histology results of skin biopsy specimens reveal features of leukocytoclastic angiitis, whereas renal biopsy shows proliferative membranous glomerulonephritis.

TREATMENT

In HCV-associated cryoglobulinemic vasculitis treatment with antiviral therapy is recommended.⊙● Traditionally, this is done with interferon α, although combination therapy with ribavirin may be superior and new interferon-free treatments for hepatitis C are also promising (such as sofosbuvir with or without ledipasvir; →Chapter 6.2.2.10.7).⊙○ Rituximab may also be of benefit in viral and nonviral cryoglobulinemic vasculitis.⊙● In patients with idiopathic CV treatment as in other small-vessel vasculitides is recommended⊙○ (→Chapter 14.23.7).

PROGNOSIS

Five-year survival rates in HCV-related and noninfectious vasculitis are similar (≥75%); in the former group, end-stage liver disease and infections are the most frequent causes of death, while in the latter, it is primarily infections. The main prognostic factors are severe liver fibrosis in HCV-related vasculitis, age >65 years, male sex, gastrointestinal and pulmonary involvement, and renal impairment in noninfectious vasculitis.

23.4. Cutaneous Leukocytoclastic Angiitis

DEFINITION

Cutaneous leukocytoclastic angiitis is an isolated cutaneous vasculitis with no internal organ involvement (also known as cutaneous small-vessel vasculitis; formerly hypersensitivity vasculitis). Secondary cutaneous leukocytoclastic vasculitis may be, among other causes, due to medications, infections, and malignancies.

CLINICAL FEATURES

Typically the disease manifests as fever, arthralgia, myalgia, and malaise. Cutaneous lesions usually cause no complaints but pruritus and burning sensation may occur. The lesions mainly involve the lower extremities, buttocks, and sites of prior trauma, as well as areas subject to pressure from tight clothing; they have a form of maculopapular rash, palpable purpura, urticaria, or ulcerating papules.

→ DIAGNOSIS

Diagnosis is based on results of histologic examination of skin biopsy specimens and exclusion of internal organ involvement.

Differential Diagnosis

Differential diagnosis includes thromboembolic events (eg, in the course of sepsis or disseminated intravascular coagulation), thrombotic thrombocytopenic purpura, other small-vessel vasculitides, and primary or secondary rash unrelated to vasculitis.

→ TREATMENT

1. Primary leukocytoclastic angiitis:

1) **General measures** (these are frequently sufficient): Keeping the involved area warm, avoiding exposure to cold and sunlight, limited physical activity.

2) **Antihistamines and nonsteroidal anti-inflammatory drugs** in the case of symptomatic cutaneous lesions or arthralgia may be helpful.

3) **Colchicine** 0.5 mg bid and/or **dapsone** 50 to 300 mg daily in patients with chronic, extensive, or painful skin lesions or persistent arthralgia may be effective.⊙○ The effects of treatment are observed within 2 weeks.

4) **Oral glucocorticoids** in patients with severe cutaneous lesions may be helpful.

5) **Azathioprine** 2 mg/kg/d in case the above-mentioned agents are ineffective (eg, when lesions recur after tapering down the dose of glucocorticoids).

2. Secondary leukocytoclastic angiitis: Treatment of the underlying condition or discontinuation of the offending drug. In the case of life-threatening symptoms, treatment is the same as in primary disease.

The primary disease usually resolves spontaneously within several weeks or months. In ~10% of patients the disease relapses after several months or years. The course of secondary disease depends on the underlying condition and usually resolves once the causative factor has been successfully treated.

23.5. Eosinophilic Granulomatosis with Polyangiitis (Churg-Strauss Syndrome)

→ DEFINITION, ETIOLOGY, PATHOGENESIS

Eosinophilic granulomatosis with polyangiitis (Churg-Strauss syndrome) (EGPA) is a necrotizing granulomatous inflammation with eosinophilic infiltration of various tissues and organs. In the respiratory tract, necrotizing inflammation affects predominantly small-sized and medium-sized vessels and is associated with concomitant asthma and eosinophilia. Nasal polyps as well as granulomatous and nongranulomatous extravascular inflammation (eg, nongranulomatous eosinophil-rich infiltrates of the lungs, myocardium, and gastrointestinal [GI] tract) are often observed.

→ CLINICAL FEATURES AND NATURAL HISTORY

1. Signs and symptoms:

1) **General symptoms**: Fever, weakness, anorexia, weight loss.

2) **Respiratory manifestations**: Asthma (in >95% of patients; usually severe), allergic rhinitis, often nasal polyps, acute or chronic sinusitis, pleural effusion, rarely hemoptysis due to alveolar bleeding.

3) **Nervous system manifestations**: Mononeuritis multiplex (in ~70% of patients), symmetric polyneuropathy (~60%), central nervous system symptoms (rare).

4) **Renal manifestations**: Glomerulonephritis (85%).

5) **Cardiovascular manifestations**: Eosinophilic endocarditis and/or myocarditis, vasculitis affecting coronary arteries (may lead to myocardial infarction), and pericarditis. Symptoms of heart failure and of secondary hypertension due to renal involvement.

6) **Cutaneous manifestations** (40%-70%): Palpable purpura. Less frequently subcutaneous nodules, urticaria, livedo reticularis, ulcerating papules.

7) **GI manifestations**: Eosinophilic gastroenteritis, intestinal ischemia, necrosis, and perforation due to vasculitis, manifesting as recurrent, often severe abdominal pain, diarrhea, and GI bleeding.

8) **Other manifestations** (rare): Obstructive uropathy (due to urethral narrowing or prostatic granulomas), myalgia, muscle weakness, arthralgia (usually without effusion), choroiditis.

2. Natural history:

1) **Prodromal phase**: In patients aged 20 to 40 years, allergic rhinitis is usually observed, sometimes with polyps and asthma (usually in patients >30 years).

2) **Eosinophilia phase**: Symptoms of eosinophilic infiltration of tissues, for instance, in the lungs and the GI tract.

3) **Vasculitis phase**: Usually within 3 years from the onset of symptoms (occasionally as late as after 30 years).

Vasculitis may resolve with time, while allergic symptoms may recur. The disease may also manifest with minor or atypical symptoms. The most frequent causes of death are cardiac complications (heart failure, myocardial infarction, cardiac arrest); less commonly, hemorrhage, renal failure, GI complications (perforation or hemorrhage), and respiratory failure.

→ DIAGNOSIS

Diagnostic Tests

1. Laboratory tests: Eosinophilia in peripheral blood (often >1.5×10^9/L), elevation in the erythrocyte sedimentation rate and C-reactive protein levels, normocytic anemia, features of renal involvement (microscopic hematuria, proteinuria), a positive myeloperoxidase (MPO) antineutrophil cytoplasmic antibody (ANCA) test result (in ~60% of patients).

2. Imaging studies: Radiographs and **computed tomography (CT)** reveal signs of chronic sinusitis and alveolar hemorrhage.

3. Pulmonary function tests: Features characteristic of asthma.

4. Histologic examination of samples of the involved organs (usually of the respiratory tract, skin, or kidneys): Patchy necrotizing vasculitis affecting small and medium vessels, necrotizing granulomatous inflammation with extensive eosinophilic infiltrates (nongranulomatous inflammation with eosinophilic infiltrates may also be present).

Diagnostic Criteria

Diagnostic criteria are based on the typical clinical features and histologic examination of the samples of the involved organs (if biopsy results are available). The Lanham classification criteria consist of asthma, peripheral blood eosinophilia (>1500 µL), and features of vasculitis involving ≥2 extrapulmonary organs.

Differential Diagnosis

Differential diagnosis should include other systemic vasculitides (will not present with peripheral blood eosinophilia), chronic severe asthma, pulmonary eosinophilias, and other causes of peripheral blood eosinophilia (→Chapter 7.8.9; in particular idiopathic eosinophilia, which is not associated with vasculitis).

→TREATMENT

In mild cases with no renal involvement, patients may be treated with **glucocorticoid monotherapy.**◐◐ In more severe cases, glucocorticoid therapy can be used in combination with cyclophosphamide according to the treatment regimen used in granulomatosis with polyangiitis.◐◐ Five-year survival rates are ~80%. In patients with refractory or relapsing disease, the addition of mepolizumab was associated with some benefit.◐

23.6. Giant Cell Arteritis

→DEFINITION, ETIOLOGY, PATHOGENESIS

Giant cell arteritis (GCA) is an inflammation of predominantly large- and medium-sized arteries that is frequently granulomatous and develops almost exclusively after the age of 50 years. It is characterized by involvement of the arteries branching from the aortic arch. Most often branches of the external carotid artery are involved, but any of the following arteries may be affected (in order of frequency): temporal arteries, vertebral arteries, posterior ciliary arteries, ophthalmic artery, internal carotid artery, external carotid artery, and central retinal artery. The name "temporal arteritis" is misleading, as temporal arteries are not always affected in patients with GCA and may be involved in patients with other vasculitides.

In general terms, large-vessel vasculitis (LVV) occurring in patients aged >50 years is usually diagnosed as or has a clinical form of GCA or more specifically, if temporal arteries are involved, of temporal arteritis. In younger people (<50 years and more so <40 years) the clinical presentation and diagnosis is usually that of Takayasu arteritis.

→CLINICAL FEATURES

The majority of patients have general symptoms, like low-grade or high-grade fever, fatigue, anorexia, and weight loss. Two-thirds of patients have severe headache, usually bilateral temporal or generalized, that is continuous, prevents them from sleeping, and does not resolve completely after the use of analgesics. Painful swelling of the temporal artery may also occur, which is clearly visible under the skin and often erythematous. In 30% of patients ocular symptoms develop, including diplopia and transient loss of vision (amaurosis fugax) progressing to a partial or total loss of vision due to the involvement of mainly ciliary arteries or the central retinal artery. Patients with the involvement of the visceral branches of the external carotid artery may have claudication and occasionally painful ulcerations of the tongue as well as claudication of the masseter muscles due to ischemia (jaw claudication). Neurologic manifestations such as transient ischemic attack or stroke, polyneuropathy, or mononeuropathy may be present. Arteritis may lead to the formation of an aneurysm and its rupture; one of the complications may be aortic dissection. Approximately 50% of patients have coexisting polymyalgia rheumatica.

Considering the risk of loss of vision, new-onset GCA should be regarded as an ophthalmologic emergency. Features indicating an increased risk of permanent loss of vision include amaurosis fugax (precedes permanent loss of vision in almost half of patients), jaw claudication, and abnormalities of a temporal artery found on physical examination.

→DIAGNOSIS

Diagnostic algorithm: →Figure 23-1.

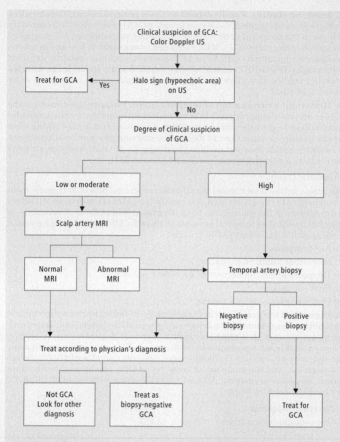

Probabilities listed below reflect clinical experience while following this algorithm:
1) US: About 2/10 patients will have a positive test result and no need for biopsy.
2) MRI: About 8/10 patients will have a negative test result and no need for biopsy.
3) No US, no MRI: Only patients with very low pretest probability should not be biopsied and by default do not have GCA. All other patients (with low, moderate, or high pretest probability) should be biopsied, because the end diagnosis of biopsy-negative GCA (based on clinical grounds and response to prednisone) carries a better prognosis.

GCA, giant cell arteritis; MRI, magnetic resonance imaging; US, ultrasonography.

Figure 23-1. Diagnostic algorithm for suspected giant cell arteritis involving temporal arteries.

Diagnostic Tests

1. Blood tests: Increased erythrocyte sedimentation rate (ESR) (usually >100 mm after 1 hour, but ESR within the reference range does not exclude the diagnosis of GCA, as <5% of patients have a normal ESR); elevated serum levels of acute phase proteins (C-reactive protein [CRP], fibrinogen); anemia of chronic disease; reactive thrombocytosis; a minor increase in liver function tests, particularly alkaline phosphatase (in ~30% of patients).

2. Imaging studies: Results depend on the location of lesions. Doppler ultrasonography and magnetic resonance imaging (MRI) may reveal inflammatory lesions in the temporal artery. Ultrasonography, conventional arteriography, computed tomography (CT), MRI, computed tomography (CTA) and magnetic resonance angiography (MRA), and ^{18}F-fluorodeoxyglucose positron emission tomography (FDG-PET) scanning may reveal lesions in the large arteries. Imaging studies also allow for detection of complications: aneurysms or arterial dissection.

3. Histologic examination of temporal artery biopsy specimens is the diagnostic gold standard, which in symptomatic patients may remain positive for months despite glucocorticoid treatment.⬤ It is usually performed within a few weeks (ideally no later than 14 days) after starting glucocorticoid treatment. A negative result does not exclude the diagnosis of GCA; however, patients rarely have a negative biopsy result and normal ESR.

Diagnostic Criteria

Diagnosis is based on clinical manifestations and results of diagnostic tests. Establishing the diagnosis of GCA is easy in typical cases with temporal artery involvement. If the patient has been diagnosed with a form of vasculitis, it may be classified as temporal arteritis in those fulfilling ≥3 of 5 the American College of Rheumatology (ACR) criteria:

1) Age ≥50 years.
2) New-onset localized headache.
3) Temporal artery tenderness or decreased pulsation.
4) ESR ≥50 mm/h.
5) Positive arterial biopsy results.

A diagnosis of temporal arteritis can be made in the setting of a high pretest probability supplemented by ultrasonography or MRI of a temporal artery and/or biopsy along with a rapid therapeutic response to prednisone. A positive biopsy result is not a prerequisite for diagnosis. This approach does not apply to and does not exclude the large-vessel presentation of aortitis/subclavian involvement, and the diagnosis of large-vessel GCA can be made with appropriate large-vessel imaging (CTA/MRA/PET) along with elevated ESR/CRP without the need for biopsy.

Differential Diagnosis

Other systemic vasculitides (→Chapter 14.23).

→ **T R E A T M E N T**

1. Glucocorticoids: Consensus-based guidelines suggest that treatment should be oral **prednisone** 1 mg/kg/d (maximum, 60 mg/d) or an equivalent dose of another glucocorticoid continued until the resolution of symptoms and normalization of ESR (usually within 2-4 weeks; assess ESR after 1 week of treatment).⊘⚪ In patients with ophthalmic symptoms IV **methylprednisolone** 500 to 1000 mg for 3 consecutive days may be used⊘⚪ (superiority of IV over oral administration of glucocorticoids has not been documented). Tapering is based on individual response to treatment. One possible method is to taper the dose of prednisone every 1 to 2 weeks by a maximum of 10% of the daily dose (usually up to 5-10 mg/d) and continue treatment for 1 to 2 years.⊘⚪ However, in many patients tapering of prednisone down to discontinuation is difficult. In case of recurring symptoms, use the last effective dose. Start osteoporosis prophylaxis (→Chapter 14.13).

2. In patients at high risk for complications of glucocorticoid treatment (eg, with diabetes mellitus or severe hypertension), consider adding oral **methotrexate** 7.5 to 15 mg/wk to reduce the glucocorticoid dose.⊘⚪

3. Tocilizumab has been recently shown to be more effective in comparison with prednisone.⊖ Another agent, **abatacept**, showed promising results.○

4. Long-term treatment with low-dose **acetylsalicylic acid** may be considered if the patient is deemed at risk for cardiovascular disease.

23.7. Granulomatosis with Polyangiitis

> DEFINITION, ETIOLOGY, PATHOGENESIS

Granulomatosis with polyangiitis (GPA), previously referred to as Wegener granulomatosis, is a granulomatous vasculitis that usually involves the upper and lower respiratory tracts, with associated necrotizing vasculitis affecting mainly small-sized and medium-sized vessels (ie, capillaries, venules, arterioles, arteries, and veins). GPA frequently leads to necrotizing glomerulonephritis, ocular vasculitis, pulmonary capillaritis with hemorrhage, and granulomatous and nongranulomatous extravascular inflammation.

GPA may also be limited to the upper or lower respiratory tract or to the eye. In these cases, features of systemic vasculitis may not be identified; however, in patients with clinical and histologic abnormalities identical to those seen in GPA, and particularly with a positive antineutrophil cytoplasmic antibody (ANCA) test result, the diagnosis of GPA should be made.

> CLINICAL FEATURES AND NATURAL HISTORY

Signs and symptoms:

1) **Upper respiratory tract manifestations**: Nasal congestion, mucosal ulcerations (may be painless), purulent and/or bloody nasal discharge or epistaxis, perforation of the nasal septum and destruction of the nasal cartilage resulting in a saddle nose deformity, symptoms of chronic sinusitis, hoarseness, features of upper airway obstruction caused by a developing subglottic stricture.

2) **Otitis media**, sometimes leading to hearing loss.

3) **Pulmonary manifestations** (present in ~90% of patients but asymptomatic in one-third): Cough and hemoptysis (may be severe in patients with diffuse alveolar hemorrhage), dyspnea, pleural pain.

4) **Renal manifestations**: Glomerulonephritis (in >70% of patients, frequently asymptomatic [abnormalities are observed mainly in the urinary sediment]; sometimes disease is limited to the kidneys). Concomitant involvement of the lungs and kidneys is known as **pulmonary-renal syndrome**.

5) **Ocular manifestations**: Episcleritis, scleritis, conjunctivitis, uveitis, dacryocystitis, rarely orbital pseudotumor with exophthalmos and diplopia, optic neuritis, ocular vasculitis (this may lead to irreversible loss of vision).

6) **Skin manifestations** (in 40%-60% of patients): Most frequently palpable purpura, less often ulcerating papules (particularly on the limbs) and subcutaneous nodules. Rarely necrosis.

7) **Musculoskeletal manifestations**: Myalgia and arthralgia. Less frequently other features of arthritis (occasionally symmetric but with no erosions or deformities).

8) **Nervous system manifestations** (in advanced disease): Most frequently mononeuritis multiplex, less often symmetric peripheral neuropathy. Rarely central nervous system involvement.

9) **Gastrointestinal manifestations**: Abdominal pain, diarrhea, bleeding from ulcerations.

10) **Genitourinary tract manifestations**: Bleeding from ulcerations.

11) **Cardiac manifestations**: Most frequently pericarditis with pericardial effusion. Rarely angina, endocarditis, or myocarditis.

GPA often starts with general symptoms (fever of unknown origin in ~50% of patients) and symptoms from the upper respiratory tract (70%), lungs (45%), and kidneys (<20%). The course is variable, ranging from indolent and mild (often without renal involvement) to rapidly progressive, life-threatening, and involving multiple organs.

→ DIAGNOSIS

Diagnostic Tests

1. Laboratory tests: Positive serum proteinase 3 (PR3) ANCA (in 80%-90% of patients; specificity, 98%). Additionally, there are often elevations in the erythrocyte sedimentation rate and C-protein levels, normocytic anemia, leukocytosis (in some cases $>20 \times 10^9$/L), thrombocytosis, and features of glomerulonephritis.

2. Imaging studies: **Radiographs** and **computed tomography (CT)** reveal features of chronic sinusitis, frequently accompanied by bone destruction. In the lungs, disseminated infiltrates (these may resolve or change their locations), necrotic nodules, and interstitial lesions (presenting as linear opacifications) are usually observed.

3. Histologic examination: Granulomatous inflammation, necrosis, and inflammatory lesions in vessel walls. Biopsy specimens are taken from an involved organ, ideally the upper respiratory tract or kidney. Usually it is difficult to establish the diagnosis of GPA solely on the basis of histology.

Diagnostic Criteria

Diagnostic criteria are based on the characteristic histologic features in a patient with typical pulmonary lesions and/or urinalysis findings and a positive ANCA test result (PR3 ANCA/cytoplasmic ANCA [c-ANCA]). In rare cases of patients with a limited form of the disease, ANCAs may be negative.

Differential Diagnosis

Differential diagnosis should include:

1) **Other causes of pulmonary-renal syndrome**: Microscopic polyangiitis (most frequently), eosinophilic granulomatosis with polyangiitis (Churg-Strauss syndrome), cryoglobulinemic vasculitis, IgA vasculitis (Henoch-Schönlein purpura; rare), other small-vessel vasculitides (eg, serum sickness), systemic lupus erythematosus, vasculitis associated with anti-glomerular basement membrane antibodies.
2) **Causes of alveolar hemorrhage other than vasculitis** (→Chapter 13.7.1).
3) Polyarteritis nodosa.
4) Glomerulonephritis with crescents and no immune deposits.

→ TREATMENT

General Considerations

1. Remission induction is started in the acute phase of the disease. After achieving remission, maintenance treatment is initiated.

2. Treatment depends on the category of vasculitis (according to the European Vasculitis Study categorization of ANCA-associated vasculitides), which may be:

1) **Localized**: Limited to the upper or lower respiratory tract with no systemic symptoms or other organ involvement.
2) **Early systemic**: Any other manifestations but with no organ or life-threatening features.
3) **Generalized**: Renal or other organ-threatening disease (creatinine level <500 µmol/L [5.6 mg/dL]).
4) **Severe**: Renal or other vital organ failure (creatinine level >500 µmol/L).

5) **Refractory disease**: Progression despite treatment with glucocorticoids and cyclophosphamide.

Treatment of Acute GPA (Remission Induction)

1. Generalized disease (including severe disease): In severe, newly--diagnosed disease (GPA as well as microscopic polyangiitis or eosinophilic granulomatosis with polyangiitis [Churg-Strauss syndrome]), remission induction therapy with a combination of cyclophosphamide and high-dose glucocorticoids is recommended.

1) **Cyclophosphamide** in IV pulses 15 mg/kg (maximum, 1200 mg/d). It is recommended that the first 3 pulses should be administered every 2 weeks and the subsequent 3 to 6 pulses every 3 weeks (for a total of 3-6 months). As an alternative, oral treatment at a dose of 2 mg/kg/d (maximum, 200 mg/d) may be used, but the IV route is preferred due to the lower toxicity and cumulative dose (the lifetime cumulative dose of cyclophosphamide should not be >25 g). In the case of renal failure and in elderly patients reduce the dose by 25% to 50%. In all patients we suggest prophylaxis of *Pneumocystis jirovecii* infection (sulfamethoxazole/trimethoprim 800/160 mg 1 tablet 3 times a week or 800/40 mg daily) to be continued until at least 3 months after cessation of cyclophosphamide.⊘○

2) **Glucocorticoids**: Prednisone 1 mg/kg/d orally or IV usually for 1 month is recommended, then the dose is tapered down. According to the British Society for Rheumatology, the maximum dose is 60 mg; another glucocorticoid at an equivalent dose may be used. In severe cases IV pulses of methylprednisolone 500 to 1000 mg/d may be used for the first 2 to 3 days in cases of life-threatening disease or major organ involvement.⊘○

3) As stated in the chapter on microscopic polyangiitis, **rituximab** (with high-dose glucocorticoids) is preferred over cyclophosphamide in patients at increased risk of infection or in younger patients who are planning a pregnancy, with the efficacy equal to that of cyclophosphamide.⊘● Administer 375 mg/m^2 once weekly for 4 weeks or 2 doses of 1 g in a 2-week interval.

4) **Plasmapheresis** is not recommended as a first-line therapy. Preliminary data from a large clinical trial of plasmapheresis in GPA did not show benefit but the full results of this are not expected until late 2019.○ In these cases, we suggest 7 plasma exchanges (60 mL/kg or 1 plasma volume exchange) within 14 days with albumin as the replacement fluid except in patients who are bleeding or are at high risk of bleeding.

2. Localized and early systemic disease (ie, without organ- or life--threatening features): Cyclophosphamide, which we prefer for its efficacy, may be replaced with oral methotrexate.⊘● Start from 15 mg/wk and administer it in combination with a glucocorticoid (dosage as above, or lower); the dose should be titrated up to 20 to 25 mg/wk over 1 to 2 months. Mycophenolate mofetil may also be used as an alternative to cyclophosphamide if methotrexate is not tolerated or contraindicated.⊘○

3. Refractory disease (remission cannot be achieved with conventional treatments or disease recurs): If cyclophosphamide is ineffective, rituximab may be used in combination with glucocorticoids for remission induction.⊘○ Other possible treatments include intravenous immunoglobulin, leflunomide, antithymocyte immunoglobulin, and anti-CD52 therapy.

4. End-stage renal disease: Renal replacement therapy (dialysis or transplantation).

Maintenance Treatment

Maintenance treatment is continued for ≥18 months (usually up to 5 years) after clinical remission has been achieved, particularly in patients with persistent PR3 ANCA positivity. In patients without persistent PR3 ANCA positivity, including patients with microscopic polyangiitis, maintenance treatment is usually shorter but should last ≥18 months.

1) **Azathioprine** 2 mg/kg/d or **methotrexate** 20 to 25 mg/wk. **Leflunomide** 20 mg/d or **mycophenolate mofetil** 2 to 3 g/d may also be used if the two former medications are not tolerated or contraindicated.◐◐ These treatments should probably be continued for a minimum of 18 months after achieving successful remission.◐○

2) **Rituximab** 500 mg every 4 to 6 months, assuming the cost is acceptable, is a preferred alternative to above treatment, particularly in patients with PR3 ANCA-positive GPA.◐◐

3) **Glucocorticoids**: The dose may be tapered (down to ≥15 mg/d over the first 2-3 months, then to ≤10 mg/d at around 3-6 months, and then down to discontinuation) in patients who continue to be in remission. In case of recurrence the dose can be increased again.

4) **Sulfamethoxazole/trimethoprim** 800/160 mg bid may be used as an adjunct to azathioprine and leflunomide or after stopping the maintenance immunosuppressive treatment.◐◐

Persistently elevated or increasing levels of ANCA are a risk factor for relapse.

→ PROGNOSIS

Treatment with cyclophosphamide achieves remission in >90% of patients and 8-year survival rates are >80%. Relapse usually occurs within a year from discontinuation of immunosuppressive treatment; in >50% of patients it occurs within 5 years. The most common causes of death are complications of the disease (renal or respiratory failure) or adverse effects of treatment (severe infection).

23.8. IgA Vasculitis (Henoch-Schönlein Purpura)

→ DEFINITION, ETIOLOGY

IgA vasculitis (IgAV) (formerly Henoch-Schönlein purpura) is a small-vessel vasculitis characterized by the presence of immune deposits (mainly IgA1), which involves small vessels (predominantly capillaries, venules, or arterioles). It primarily affects children (~75% cases in children aged 2-11 years), although it can also present in adults, where the prognosis is generally worse.

→ CLINICAL FEATURES AND NATURAL HISTORY

The onset of IgAV is acute. In most cases it develops within 1 to 2 weeks of a viral upper respiratory tract infection but sometimes follows a gastrointestinal (GI) infection. IgAV may also be associated with other diseases, for instance, liver disease, inflammatory bowel disease, or ankylosing spondylitis. IgAV characteristically involves a triad of palpable purpura, abdominal pain, and arthritis.

Signs and symptoms:

1) **Cutaneous manifestations** (in ~90% of patients): Macular rash or urticaria evolving into palpable purpura, usually located on the lower extremities and buttocks. Lesions develop in a single episode or are recurrent and accompany other symptoms.

2) **Joint manifestations**: Arthralgia involving mainly joints of the lower limbs (knees and ankles), occasionally with other symptoms of arthritis.

3) **GI manifestations**: Abdominal pain, usually diffuse, worsening after meals, and associated with intestinal vasculitis (most frequently affecting the small intestine). Occasionally bloody diarrhea.

4) **Renal manifestations**: Most frequently microscopic hematuria.

5) **Other manifestations**: Rarely, pulmonary (hemoptysis) and nervous system involvement (headache, seizures).

In children the disease tends to have a mild course, with a complete recovery observed within a few weeks or months. Cutaneous lesions resolve within 2 weeks. In adolescents and adults the course is more severe due to more frequent renal involvement; in ~30% of patients the disease progresses to renal failure.

→ **DIAGNOSIS**

Diagnosis is based on clinical symptoms and histologic examination of skin biopsy specimens (perivascular and vascular IgA deposits in small vessels). The disease may be limited to skin or kidneys (in the latter case IgA nephropathy is diagnosed). Kidney biopsy should only be considered in patients with severe proteinuria, hematuria, active sediment, or with renal failure.

→ **TREATMENT**

As most cases of IgAV are self-resolving, supportive therapy is the mainstay of treatment.⊘⊖ Symptomatic treatment is sufficient in patients without features of GI or renal involvement.

Early use of oral glucocorticoids (1-2 mg/kg prednisone per day for 2 weeks) may be used to improve joint and abdominal pain symptoms. Oral glucocorticoids do not prevent renal disease but can improve renal outcomes.⊖ Avoid nonsteroidal anti-inflammatory drugs (NSAIDs) in patients with renal involvement. In the case of cutaneous manifestations dapsone 100 mg/d may be administered. Also →Chapter 9.3.4.2.

In more severe cases particularly in rapidly progressive glomerulonephritis, glucocorticoids and immunosuppressive agents (azathioprine, cyclophosphamide, mycophenolate mofetil, or other), plasmapheresis, or IV immunoglobulin may be used.

→ **PROGNOSIS**

Prognosis is generally favorable, as most patients recover spontaneously. The primary cause of morbidity and mortality is due to renal consequences (~15% may develop long-term renal insufficiency).

23.9. Microscopic Polyangiitis

→ **DEFINITION, ETIOLOGY**

Microscopic polyangiitis (MPA) is a necrotizing vasculitis with few or no immunologic deposits, which usually affects small vessels (arterioles, capillaries, venules) and may involve small- and middle-sized arteries. It very frequently coexists with necrotizing glomerulonephritis and with pulmonary capillaritis. There is no inflammation extending beyond the blood vessels or granulomatous inflammation, distinguishing it from granulomatosis with polyangiitis.

→ **CLINICAL FEATURES AND NATURAL HISTORY**

The course of MPA may be indolent, with recurring general symptoms of fever, weight loss, myalgia, and arthralgia persisting for many months or years prior to the onset of organ-specific symptoms. Organ specific manifestations include:

1) **Cutaneous manifestations**: Palpable purpura (observed at presentation in ~50% of patients). These tend to favor the feet, lower legs, and buttocks.

2) **Renal manifestations**: There can be mild renal involvement or rapidly progressive glomerulonephritis.

3) **Nervous system manifestations**: Mononeuritis multiplex (~60%).
4) **Respiratory manifestations**: Lung involvement can present as diffuse alveolar hemorrhage.

→ **DIAGNOSIS**

Diagnosis is based on clinical manifestations and histologic examination of the skin, kidneys, or lung biopsies. A positive myeloperoxidase (MPO) antineutrophil cytoplasmic antibody (ANCA) (type of perinuclear ANCA [p-ANCA], present in ~70% of patients) or proteinase 3 (PR3) ANCA (type of cytoplasmic ANCA [c-ANCA], present in 45%) test result also suggests the diagnosis of microscopic polyangiitis.

Diagnostic Tests

Laboratory test results may reveal elevations in the erythrocyte sedimentation rate and C-reactive protein levels and features of glomerulonephritis. Chest radiographs, high-resolution computed tomography, and bronchoalveolar lavage reveal typical features of alveolar hemorrhage.

Differential Diagnosis

Polyarteritis nodosa (differences: only extraglomerular vessels of the kidneys are involved [no features of glomerulonephritis], pulmonary involvement usually does not occur, ANCA-negative); other causes of pulmonary-renal syndrome (→Chapter 14.23.7), cutaneous leukocytoclastic angiitis.

→ **TREATMENT**

Initial remission induction is recommended with cyclophosphamide and glucocorticoids.◐● Assuming the cost is acceptable, **rituximab** (with high-dose glucocorticoids) is preferred over cyclophosphamide in patients at increased risk of infection or in younger patients who are planning a pregnancy, with the efficacy equal to that of cyclophosphamide.◐● The dosage and long-term maintenance is the same as in granulomatosis with polyangiitis (→Chapter 14.23.7). Some patients may require long-term renal replacement therapy including dialysis or renal transplantation.

23.10. Polyarteritis Nodosa

→ **DEFINITION, ETIOLOGY**

Polyarteritis nodosa (PAN) is a necrotizing antineutrophil cytoplasmic antibody (ANCA)-negative vasculitis involving medium and small arteries. It can be distinguished from other vasculitides (mainly from microscopic polyangiitis) by the absence of pulmonary involvement, features of glomerulonephritis, or involvement of arterioles, capillaries, or venules. PAN is strongly associated with hepatitis B virus (HBV) infection (10%-80% of patients, according to various sources). A cutaneous form of PAN may also be associated with hepatitis C virus (HCV) infection. PAN usually affects patients aged 40 to 60 years and is more frequent in men than in women.

→ **CLINICAL FEATURES AND NATURAL HISTORY**

The onset of PAN is usually associated with **general symptoms** (fatigue, myalgia, arthralgia, weight loss, fever), which may persist for several months. Later signs and symptoms include:

1) **Cutaneous manifestations**: Palpable purpura (most frequent), livedo reticularis, ulcerations (on fingers, ankles, the anterior aspect of lower legs), subcutaneous nodules <2 cm in diameter (usually on the anterior aspect of lower extremities and dorsal aspect of feet).

2) **Nervous system manifestations**: Most frequently mononeuritis multiplex (usually fibular nerve palsy [foot drop]), less often symmetric peripheral neuropathy.

3) **Renal manifestations**: Hypertension related to extraglomerular vessel inflammation, features of renal failure. Rarely, it can lead to renal infarction (acute severe lumbar pain).

4) **Gastrointestinal manifestations**: Abdominal pain, most frequently due to intestinal ischemia from visceral vessel involvement (intestinal necrosis and perforation is rare).

Untreated disease has a fatal course and leads to death within 1 to 2 years. The cutaneous form (without internal organ involvement) has a mild course and may resolve spontaneously but frequently recurs.

→ DIAGNOSIS

Diagnosis is based on clinical manifestations and histologic findings from biopsies of the involved organs.

Diagnostic Tests

Laboratory test results often reveal elevations in the erythrocyte sedimentation rate and C-reactive protein levels as well as anemia (usually normocytic). In patients with renal involvement there can be elevated serum creatinine levels and rarely moderate proteinuria and microscopic hematuria. Angiography of the visceral arteries reveals dilations (microaneurysms) of medium arteries, for instance, kidney, liver, or intestinal arteries.

Differential Diagnosis

Other vasculitides, in particular granulomatosis with polyangiitis, microscopic polyangiitis, eosinophilic granulomatosis with polyangiitis (Churg-Strauss syndrome). ANCA testing is useful to help in the differentiation, as ANCA is negative in PAN.

→ TREATMENT

Remission induction is recommended with a combination of cyclophosphamide (intravenous or oral) and glucocorticoids.◐● Dosing is the same as in granulomatosis with polyangiitis (→Chapter 14.23.7).

In PAN associated with HBV infection, initial high-dose glucocorticoids (without cyclophosphamide) may be effective with tapering of the dose over 2 weeks. At the same time, the use of plasmapheresis followed by antiviral treatment may be of benefit.◐○ In the cutaneous form of PAN oral glucocorticoids alone may be of benefit. Hypertension requires aggressive antihypertensive treatment. As patients may have impaired renal arterial perfusion, angiotensin-converting enzyme inhibitors should be used with caution.

→ PROGNOSIS

In treated patients 5-year survival rates are ≤80%. In the cutaneous form of PAN the prognosis is good with only rare progression to systemic disease.

23.11. Takayasu Arteritis

→ DEFINITION, ETIOLOGY, PATHOGENESIS

Takayasu arteritis (TA) is a granulomatous vasculitis of large and medium vessels of unknown etiology that affects mostly the aorta and its branches. Less frequently, it may involve other arteries, such as the pulmonary arteries.

Typically, TA causes numerous segmental stenoses of the aortic branches. Thrombi may form in the stenotic segments and sometimes cause peripheral thromboembolism. Aneurysms usually occur distally to the stenosis. TA rarely leads to aortic dissection or rupture.

In general terms, large-vessel vasculitis occurring in patients aged >50 years is usually diagnosed as or has a clinical form of giant cell arteritis/temporal arteritis. In younger people (<50 years and more so <40 years) the clinical presentation and diagnosis is usually that of Takayasu arteritis.

→ CLINICAL FEATURES

Eighty to 90% of patients with TA are women. The age of onset is typically 10 to 40 years of age. The prevalence is highest in people of Asian descent.

1. Systemic manifestations: Early manifestations usually include influenza--like or rheumatic-like symptoms, such as low-grade fever, fatigue, myalgia, and arthralgia. Acute symptoms usually resolve spontaneously but may occur throughout the disease course.

2. Vascular manifestations: Patients with chronic disease develop symptoms of stenosis and arterial occlusion. Typical findings include weak or asymmetric pulses in the upper extremities ("pulseless disease") and bruits in the aorta and its main branches. With inflammation of the vasculature, pain and tenderness over the affected vessels may occur.

1) Aortic disease: The presenting manifestation may be an incidentally detected large thoracic aortic aneurysm. Patients may have audible bruits over stenoses within the aorta and a diastolic murmur of aortic regurgitation (an adverse prognostic factor). Heart failure from aortic insufficiency may occur.

2) Subclavian arteries: Stenosis or occlusion of a subclavian artery may lead to subclavian artery bruits, upper extremity claudication, and subclavian steal syndrome (reversal of ipsilateral vertebral artery flow leading to symptoms of vertebrobasilar ischemia). In patients with stenotic or occluded subclavian arteries, traditional blood pressure measurements are unreliable. A systolic blood pressure differential between the arms >10 mm Hg is abnormal. Systolic blood pressure should be measured on lower extremities with a Doppler device used for ankle-brachial index measurements.

3) Carotid and vertebral arteries: Manifestations depend on the location of stenosis and include dizziness, syncope, headache, visual disturbances, transient ischemic attacks, stroke, seizures, and claudication of the jaw.

4) Renal arteries: Patients commonly develop renal artery stenosis and resultant hypertension.

5) Gastrointestinal arteries: Abdominal pain, diarrhea, and gastrointestinal bleeding can occur from celiac and mesenteric artery involvement.

6) Pulmonary arteries: Dyspnea, hemoptysis, and chest pain can be evidence of pulmonary artery involvement.

7) Coronary arteries: Manifestations of myocardial ischemia may occur from coronary artery involvement or ostial narrowing.

→ DIAGNOSIS

Diagnostic Tests

1. Blood tests: Laboratory findings in patients with TA are not specific and reflect the underlying inflammation. A normochromic, normocytic anemia is common. Erythrocyte sedimentation rate and C-reactive protein can reflect disease activity, but values within reference ranges alone are not sensitive enough to exclude active disease. Other laboratory abnormalities may include an elevated fibrinogen concentration, hypoalbuminemia, polyclonal hypergammaglobulinemia, and an elevated interleukin-6 (IL-6) concentration (a newly proposed laboratory test that is not currently widely available).○

2. Imaging studies: Magnetic resonance angiography (MRA), computed tomography angiography (CTA), and angiography of the affected vessels demonstrate smooth luminal narrowing and possibly occlusion. CTA and MRA also have the added benefit of demonstrating wall thickening of the affected vessels. Positron emission tomography is being investigated as an imaging technique to monitor disease activity. Transthoracic echocardiogram is useful to assess for proximal aortic abnormalities and concomitant aortic insufficiency. Ultrasound of other affected vessels can also be useful if available.

Diagnostic Criteria

The American College of Rheumatology classification criteria for TA were designed to differentiate TA from other forms of vasculitis but are useful to help guide diagnosis. The classification requires that at least 3 of the following 6 criteria are met:

1) Disease onset at an age ≤40 years (note that many experts now use an age <50 years).

2) Claudication of any extremity (abnormal fatigue or discomfort with use, especially in the case of the upper extremities).

3) Weak or absent pulse in a brachial artery.

4) A systolic blood pressure differential between the arms ≥10 mm Hg.

5) Bruit over the subclavian artery or abdominal aorta.

6) Angiographic abnormalities not attributable to other causes, including stenosis or occlusion of the aorta, its branches, or proximal segments of the limb arteries.

Differential Diagnosis

Giant cell arteritis, aortic arch atherosclerosis, upper thoracic outlet syndrome, fibromuscular dysplasia of arteries, Behçet disease, Ehlers-Danlos syndrome, and ergotism.

⇒ TREATMENT

Pharmacotherapy

1. Glucocorticoids: Initial treatment for active disease with high-dose glucocorticoids (oral prednisone 1 mg/kg daily) for 3 months is suggested.⊘○ If inflammatory markers normalize, constitutional symptoms improve, and clinical findings do not progress, the dose can be tapered down at a maximum rate of 10% of the dose per week. Most patients will remain on low-dose glucocorticoids to prevent relapse.

2. Glucocorticoid-sparing agents: In the case of glucocorticoid failure or an inability to taper down the dose, the use of methotrexate, mycophenolate mofetil, azathioprine leflunomide, or cyclophosphamide is suggested.⊘○

3. Biologic agents: In patients with disease refractory to glucocorticoid-sparing agents or in those who relapse with attempts to discontinue glucocorticoids, the use of the anti–tumor necrosis factor α agent infliximab is suggested. In patients with disease refractory to infliximab, a trial of tocilizumab, an interleukin-6 receptor antibody, can be considered.⊘○

Surgical Treatment

Invasive treatment (surgical or endovascular) depends on the clinical features of organ ischemia. Restenosis following vascular interventions is common and can occur in as many as 50% of patients after 2 years.○ Surgery may be required in patients with aortic regurgitation.

1. Acetaminophen (Paracetamol)

➔ PATHOPHYSIOLOGY

Acetaminophen (INN paracetamol) poisoning is usually a result of an intentional (suicidal) overdose of oral formulations but may be also accidental from high doses taken for analgesia or due to accumulation of the drug in patients with severe liver disease. Ten-fold errors in the administration of parenteral acetaminophen have also resulted in toxicity.

In acute acetaminophen poisoning the liver is the critical organ with hepatocyte injury and necrosis. Acute kidney injury due to proximal renal tubule damage is less frequent, affecting 25% of patients with severe liver damage and 50% of patients with liver failure caused by acetaminophen poisoning.

Peak serum acetaminophen levels after oral ingestion of tablets or capsules occur after 2 to 4 hours. Hepatotoxicity can occur in adults who take a single dose of 6 to 7 g and toxicity may occur with ingestion of 150 mg/kg/d for ≥2 days.

➔ CLINICAL FEATURES AND DIAGNOSIS

Phase 1 (up to 24 hours from ingestion) is asymptomatic in most patients. Some individuals may have nausea and vomiting or, less frequently, abdominal pain, excessive sweating, pallor, and weakness. In very rare cases severe manifestations (coma, severe lactate acidosis) develop as early as on the first day from ingestion; this is characteristic for severe overdoses (75-100 g).

Phase 2 (24-72 hours): Pain or tenderness in the right upper abdominal quadrant, jaundice. Symptoms are accompanied by an increase in serum aminotransferase (alanine aminotransferase [ALT], aspartate aminotransferase [AST]) and bilirubin levels, international normalized ratio (INR), as well as hypoglycemia and metabolic acidosis.

Phase 3 (72-96 hours): Fulminant liver failure with encephalopathy and less frequently bleeding. An increase in serum creatinine levels is usually observed on days 2 to 5 from ingestion.

Phase 4 (death or organ regeneration): Death due to fulminant liver failure usually occurs on days 3 to 5 from ingestion. In surviving patients normalization of laboratory parameters and organ regeneration occur in 7 to 14 days from ingestion. Generally recovery of hepatic function is quite remarkable in survivors that do not need transplantation.

Diagnostic Studies

Serum acetaminophen levels should be measured not earlier than 4 hours from ingestion. If the level is drawn within 4 hours, it should be repeated at the 4-hour mark, unless it was nondetectable. If the level at 4 hours is borderline or there is suspected delayed absorption, measurement should be repeated at 8 hours. It is crucial to measure acetaminophen levels at 4 to 8 hours from ingestion and administer the antidote (N-acetylcysteine [NAC]), as its efficacy is highest in this period.

High anion gap metabolic acidosis can sometimes be associated with chronic acetaminophen toxicity, independent of hepatic damage, due to 5-oxoproline (pyroglutamic acid) accumulation. This is different from the lactic acidosis that may develop as a result of hepatic injury in acute overdose. Risk factors include chronic acetaminophen use (usually patients have serum values of acetaminophen well below the toxic range), female sex, malnutrition, chronic kidney disease, and pregnancy.

Other studies: Serum aminotransferase, urea/blood urea nitrogen (BUN), creatinine, bilirubin, lactate, and phosphate levels; INR; arterial blood gas analysis.

The Ontario Poison Center has recently changed its recommended management and testing protocol for acetaminophen poisoning. The current recommendations are as follows:

1) **On initial presentation of all patients with suspected acetaminophen overdose**:
   a) Acetaminophen level (≥4 hours after the end of ingestion).
   b) Acetylsalicylic acid (ASA) level.
   c) Venous or arterial blood gases, electrolytes (Na, K, Cl, HCO_3), glucose, BUN, creatinine, osmolality.
   d) AST, ALT, INR.
   e) Ethanol level, depending on clinical scenario.

2) **Sustained-release preparations or when opioid or anticholinergic drugs were ingested concurrently**: Repeat the acetaminophen level every 4 hours until it peaks, then repeat measurements every 12 hours until the level is undetectable (<66 µmol/L [10 µg/dL]).

3) **Patients receiving NAC**:
   a) Repeat venous gases, electrolytes, glucose, BUN, creatinine, AST, ALT, and INR every 12 hours.
   b) Repeat the acetaminophen level every 12 hours until it is undetectable.

4) **Patients determined to be at severe risk**:
   a) Lactate and lipase levels.
   b) Phosphate (PO_4) levels if liver enzymes are elevated.
   c) Repeat acetaminophen level, venous gases, electrolytes, glucose, BUN, creatinine, AST, ALT, and INR every 4 hours until the acetaminophen level peaks and then every 12 hours until it is undetectable.

→ **TREATMENT**

1. Decontamination: Administration of activated charcoal (1 g/kg in adults) within 1 to 2 hours. Activated charcoal can be administered after 2 hours if extended-release formulations of acetaminophen were ingested and repeat doses can be considered for massive ingestions. Gastric lavage may be used for massive ingestions in patients presenting within an hour of ingestion.

2. Antidote: NAC. IV administration is preferred because the duration of treatment is shorter compared with oral administration. Administration of NAC is associated with risk of a nonallergic anaphylactoid response (urticaria, angioedema, bronchospasm, or hypotension that typically resolve with stopping or slowing the infusion and providing supportive care). However, in patients with absolute indications for the treatment NAC is administered despite the adverse effects. The decision on the administration of NAC within 24 hours of poisoning is made based on a nomogram of acetaminophen blood levels (→Figure 1-1). The administration of NAC should be started when the measured drug level falls on or is above the curve. In patients admitted >24 hours from poisoning or in whom the time of poisoning cannot be established, start NAC administration immediately.

Based on recent literature suggesting safer administration and easier dosing strategies, the Ontario and Manitoba Poison Control Centre has changed its suggested dosing for NAC. The solution concentration has been standardized to minimize preparation errors and the loading dose is the same for both high--risk and low-risk (typical) patients.

A standard NAC solution of 30 mg/mL is prepared for all patients. At our site, this is prepared by adding 15,000 mg of NAC to achieve a total volume of 500 mL in a bag of 5% glucose (dextrose). The **loading dose** is 60 mg/kg/h for 4 hours (a maximum dose based on 100 kg). Maintenance dosing is continued for ≥12 hours or until the criteria for stopping are met.

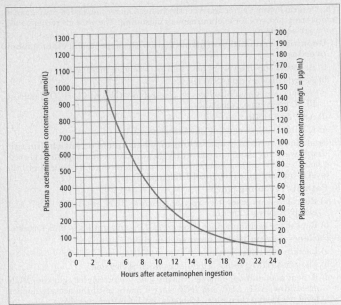

Figure 1-1. A decision-making nomogram for the use of antidotes in the treatment of acetaminophen overdose based on serum acetaminophen levels and time from ingestion. *Adapted from protocols by the Ontario Poison Centre.*

In a **typical scenario** after the loading dose infusion is continued at a rate of 6 mg/kg/h. In a **high-risk scenario** (patients with massive ingestion, evidence of liver dysfunction at presentation, or those needing hemodialysis) after the loading dose infusion is continued at 12 mg/kg/h.

Stopping criteria:

1) Acetaminophen level is nondetectable (<66 µmol/L [10 µg/dL]); and
2) AST/ALT levels are <100 IU/L (or decreasing and <50% of peak levels); and
3) INR is <2.0; and
4) The patient is well; and
5) A minimum of 12 hours (including the loading dose) of NAC has been given.

3. Methods of enhanced elimination: Hemodialysis. In patients with severe acetaminophen overdose (serum drug levels >5300 µmol/L [5.3 mmol/L]) associated with coma and metabolic acidosis, consider urgent hemodialysis; use a higher rate of NAC infusion (→above) for patients requiring dialysis. There are no established criteria for starting hemodialysis in patients with acetaminophen toxicity and it is not routinely used. Therefore, the decision to proceed with this intervention should be closely discussed with toxicology nephrology services.

4. Liver transplantation: Patients are qualified for transplantation using the King's College criteria (→Chapter 6.2.2.1).

2. Alcohols

Formulas and conversion tables used in the chapters discussing alcohols.

→ FORMULAS

Anion gap = Serum sodium (mEq/L) – [serum chloride (mEq/L) + serum bicarbonate (mEq/L)]
Note: mEq/L = mmol/L; an anion gap ≥12 is considered high (note normal values in your laboratory).

Osmolar gap = Measured osmolality (mOsm/L) – calculated osmolarity
Note: An osmolar gap >10 mOsm/L is considered high.

Calculated osmolarity (mOsm/L) = 2 × [sodium (mmol/L)] + [glucose (mmol/L)] + [urea (mmol/L)] + 1.25 × [ethanol (mmol/L)]

2.1. Ethyl Alcohol (Ethanol)

The contents of ethanol in alcoholic beverages are as follows: beer 4% to 9% by volume (ie, 4-9 mL of pure ethanol in a 100 mL beer), wine ≤16%, liqueurs and infusions 20% to 40%, and liquor (eg, vodka, gin, whiskey) ~40%. Ethanol is also used as an antiseptic (70%), in cosmetic products (eau de toilette, cologne; 70%), food flavorings (eg, vanilla, lemon extracts), mouthwash, pharmaceuticals (ie, elixirs), and as a household or industrial solvent. It is rapidly absorbed via the gastrointestinal (GI) tract, skin, and airways. Maximum blood levels are observed at 0.5 to 3 hours from ingestion, and ethanol is distributed in body water (volume of distribution, 0.5-0.7 L/kg). It is metabolized in the liver to acetaldehyde by alcohol dehydrogenase and is also cleared by microsomal ethanol-oxidizing systems. The average adult metabolizes 7 to 10 g of alcohol per hour. It is partially eliminated in unchanged form via the kidneys (2%-10%) and in exhaled air (>10%). It crosses the placenta and is excreted in breast milk.

Mechanism of toxicity: Ethanol is a central nervous system depressant. It has additive sedating effects when mixed with barbiturates, benzodiazepines, antidepressants, antipsychotics, or opioids. By inhibiting gluconeogenesis in the liver, it may cause hypoglycemia, especially in children or malnourished patients.

Toxic dose: Approximately 0.8 g/kg (1 mL/kg) of pure ethanol (roughly 3-4 drinks) will produce a blood ethanol concentration of 0.1 g/dL (equal to 100 mg/dL = 1 g/L = 0.1% = 21.7 mmol/L). In adults severe symptoms of ethanol intoxication may develop after ingestion of 1 to 1.5 mL/kg (50-100 mL) of pure alcohol. Death is usually associated with levels >80 to 90 mmol/L, but the lethal level may be much higher for chronic ethanol users.

→ CLINICAL FEATURES

1. Acute ethanol intoxication:
1) **Mild to moderate intoxication** leads to impaired judgment, disinhibition, agitation, and sometimes aggression. Patients may present with nausea, vomiting, abdominal pain, headache and vertigo, nystagmus, ataxia, diplopia, logorrhea (incoherent talkativeness), impaired concentration and posture, confusion, and slurred speech.
2) **Severe intoxication** may present with somnolence, coma, seizures, respiratory compromise, hypotension, bradycardia, hypothermia, and hypoglycemia. The pupils may be constricted, and patients are at risk of rhabdomyolysis from immobility.
3) **In patients treated with disulfiram**, the metabolism of ethanol is inhibited at the acetaldehyde stage and the accumulation of acetaldehyde results

in signs and symptoms of toxicity including nausea, vomiting, restlessness, anxiety, skin erythema, tremor, tachycardia, hypertension, and in severe cases hypotension and arrhythmias.

2. Chronic ethanol abuse may present with any number of complications including hepatic toxicity and cirrhosis, gastrointestinal bleeding, cardiomyopathy, alcoholic ketoacidosis, cerebral atrophy, cerebellar degeneration, peripheral neuropathy, and Wernicke encephalopathy or Korsakoff psychosis.

3. Coingestions of methanol, ethylene glycol, and isopropyl alcohol may occur with ethanol either accidentally or intentionally. It is also important to consider that alcohol may have been taken with other medications.

4. Alcohol withdrawal syndrome.

→ DIAGNOSIS

The clinical diagnosis of ethanol intoxication is often based on history, smell of alcohol or acetaldehyde, and presence of ataxia, nystagmus, and altered mental status. Alcohol increases the risk of falls and head trauma, hypothermia, and coingestion of other drugs or toxins.

Diagnostic Tests

1. Specific testing of blood ethanol levels can be measured directly in serum or plasma. There is only a rough correlation between blood ethanol levels and clinical presentation:

1) Up to 4 mmol/L (~20 mg/dL): Asymptomatic.
2) 4-10 mmol/L (~20-50 mg/dL): Behavioral and cognitive changes.
3) Above 10 mmol/L (>50 mg/dL): Toxic levels; alcohol intoxication (in some countries the toxic level is assumed at 21.7 mmol/L [100 mg/dL]).
4) Equal to or above 65 mmol/L (≥300 mg/dL): Usually profound coma.

Coma with an ethanol level <65 mmol/L (300 mg/dL) should prompt investigation of other causes.

2. Other suggested investigations in patients with severe ethanol intoxication include levels of electrolytes, glucose (due to the risk of hypoglycemia), urea/blood urea nitrogen, creatinine, aminotransferase, as well as prothrombin time/international normalized ratio, arterial blood gas analysis, or pulse oximetry and chest radiographs to exclude aspiration pneumonitis or pneumonia if aspiration is a possibility. Twelve-lead electrocardiography (ECG) or cardiac monitoring may reveal arrhythmia ("holiday heart"). Exclude other ingestions in comatose or delirious patients with a toxicology screen and measurement of acetaminophen (INN paracetamol) level. We suggest measuring toxic alcohol and salicylate levels if an anion gap is present. If biochemistry testing does not reveal a cause of altered mental status and ethanol level is not remarkable (<65 mmol/L or ~300 mg/dL in a comatose patient), we suggest a computed tomography (CT) scan of the head to exclude other pathology. Serum osmolarity and calculation of the osmolar gap may help identify other toxins (formulas: →Chapter 15.2) The contribution of ethanol to the osmolar gap is calculated as the level (in mmol/L) multiplied by 1.25. If a gap persists after calculating the ethanol level, and especially in the presence of an anion gap metabolic acidosis, diagnosis may include coingestion with toxic alcohols.

→ TREATMENT

1. Decontamination: There are no known methods of decontamination. Activated charcoal does not adsorb ethanol but may be of use if coingestion of other drugs or toxins is suspected.

2. Antidotes and specific therapies: There is no commercially available antidote to ethanol. Rehydration, glucose, and thiamine are used both for acute intoxication and treatment of alcoholic ketoacidosis. Thiamine is also used for the prevention and treatment of Wernicke-Korsakoff syndrome. We suggest **thiamine** replacement (100-300 mg daily IV or orally for 3-5 days) in patients with presumed chronic ethanol ingestion or malnutrition. The utility of thiamine in acute intoxication is less clear but there is little harm to administering it. There is unclear benefit of **multivitamin replacement** for acute ethanol ingestion but there would be little harm associated with its use. We suggest using multivitamins for patients with chronic alcoholism and risk factors for malnutrition.

3. Accelerated elimination: Hemodialysis is effective at removing ethanol but is rarely needed because most patients recover within a few hours with supportive care only.

4. Supportive care:

1) Protect the intoxicated person from aspiration of vomitus by placing them in the safe position (→Chapter 3.3, Figure 3-4) or intubating and assisting ventilation if needed.
2) Support basic vital functions and correct metabolic disturbances.
3) Watch for and correct hypothermia with gradual rewarming.

5. Management of alcohol withdrawal syndrome.

2.2. Ethylene Glycol

Ethylene glycol is a sweet-tasting, clear liquid with ethanol-like smell, used mainly as an automobile antifreeze, heat transfer liquid, and solvent, usually in the form of 95% solutions. It may be ingested as an ethanol substitute. Ethylene glycol is rapidly absorbed, not protein-bound, distributed in total body water, and metabolized in the liver by alcohol dehydrogenase. Approximately 22% of ethylene glycol is eliminated in an unchanged form in urine. The half-life is 3 hours. When coingested with ethanol, the elimination is purely renal and the half-life increases to 17 to 20 hours.

Mechanism of toxicity: Alcohol dehydrogenase converts ethylene glycol to glycolaldehyde, which leads to the formation of glycolic, glyoxylic, and oxalic acids. These metabolites may cause fatal toxicity by inducing a severe anion gap metabolic acidosis and renal injury (direct cytotoxic effect, formation of calcium oxalate crystals in renal tubules; usually resolves with no permanent sequelae). The organic acids and oxalate crystals are also damaging to other tissues. Lactic acidosis further worsens the metabolic acidosis.

Toxic dose: The minimum ethylene glycol serum concentration that causes serious toxicity is unknown, although serum levels >8 mmol/L (~50 mg/dL) are usually associated with symptoms of intoxication. If left untreated, the estimated lethal dose of 95% ethylene glycol (eg, antifreeze) is 1 to 1.5 mL/kg (~100 mL). Prompt recognition and early treatment can lead to survival in patients with much larger ingestions.

→ CLINICAL FEATURES

1. Symptoms of early poisoning are the same as in ethanol poisoning and may raise no suspicion of poisoning, particularly in persons with prior alcohol abuse.

2. Symptoms of late poisoning occur after a delay of 4 to 12 hours, when toxic metabolites appear, and include anion gap metabolic acidosis, Kussmaul breathing, nausea, vomiting, agitation, confusion, altered mental status that may progress to profound coma, seizures, anisocoria, hypotension, cardiac conduction problems or arrhythmias, oliguria progressing to anuria and acute kidney injury (reversible), and hypocalcemia (sometimes with tetany). Cerebral and pulmonary edema may also occur.

→ DIAGNOSIS

Clinical diagnosis is often based on symptoms, history of antifreeze ingestion, and a combined anion gap metabolic acidosis and osmolar gap (formulas: →Chapter 15.2). Examination of urine may reveal oxalate or hippurate crystals. Urine may fluoresce under a Wood lamp, as many antifreeze manufacturers add fluorescein to their products.

Diagnostic Tests

1. Specific testing of serum ethylene glycol levels >8 mmol/L (about 50 mg/dL) is usually associated with significant toxicity. However, lower levels do not exclude intoxication, as ethylene glycol may have already been metabolized. **Glycolic acid levels** may be a better measure of toxicity but are not readily available. Glycolic acid levels <10 mmol/L would suggest an alternative etiology in symptomatic patients. In the absence of laboratory testing for either ethylene glycol or glycolic acid, significant intoxication with ethylene glycol is unlikely in asymptomatic patients with a normal anion gap and osmolar gap.

2. Other suggested investigations include serum K, Na, Ca, glucose, urea/blood urea nitrogen, and osmolality (to calculate anion and osmolar gaps), creatinine, and aminotransferase levels; urinalysis with microscopy (oxalate crystals) and Wood lamp examination for the presence of fluorescein added to antifreeze; arterial blood gas analysis (in the setting of acidosis, blood ethylene glycol levels may be low, as the substance has already been metabolized; severity of the poisoning is estimated on the basis of the severity of acidosis and the anion gap), pulse oximetry, and electrocardiography (ECG) monitoring. High β-hydroxybutyrate levels may suggest alcoholic ketoacidosis as the cause or contributor to the anion gap.

→ TREATMENT

1. Decontamination: Gastric aspiration may only be useful within 30 minutes of ingestion of large volumes of polyethylene glycol. Activated charcoal would not adsorb ethylene glycol but may be useful for coingested toxins.

2. Antidotes and specific therapies:

1) **Ethanol and fomepizole** (dosage and administration: →Chapter 15.2.4) block ethylene glycol from being metabolized into toxic organic acids. We recommend their use if the ethylene glycol level is >3.2 mmol/L (20 mg/dL), or if the patient has an osmolar gap >10 mOsm/L and serum bicarbonate <20 mEq/L, pH <7.3, or oxalate crystals in urine.

2) **Vitamins**: Despite the lack of clinical evidence for benefit, there is little risk to administering either of these vitamin cofactors in ethylene glycol metabolism. We recommend continuing these agents until serum ethylene glycol is undetectable:

   a) **Pyridoxine (vitamin B$_6$)** may theoretically enhance the conversion of toxic glyoxylic acid to nontoxic glycine. It may be given in a dose of 50 mg IV or IM every 6 hours until ethylene glycol toxicity is resolved.

   b) **Thiamine (vitamin B$_1$)** 100 mg IV may be given every 12 hours (until serum toxic alcohol is undetectable) to theoretically minimize glyoxylic acid exposure.

3) **If toxic alcohol levels are unavailable** and the contents of the product ingested are unknown, we recommend treating for methanol toxicity as well (→Chapter 15.2.4).

3. Accelerated elimination: Hemodialysis can remove ethylene glycol and its toxic metabolites as well as correct electrolytes and acidosis and replace renal function in cases of ethylene glycol/oxalate-induced acute kidney injury. Indications for dialysis include:

1) Persistent acidosis (pH ≤7.3) and/or an osmolar gap >10.

2) Ethylene glycol ingestion accompanied by acute kidney injury or chronic kidney disease.

3) Ethylene glycol concentration >8 mmol/L (50 mg/dL).

4) Clinical worsening despite ethanol or fomepizole.

4. Treatment targets: Ethanol, fomepizole, or hemodialysis should be continued until the anion gap and osmolar gap are normalized and/or (if available) serum glycolic acid or ethylene glycol is cleared.

5. Supportive care is aimed at maintaining vital parameters and correcting any disturbances.

1) Ensure airway patency. Intubate and assist ventilation if necessary.

2) Observe for the development of coma, arrhythmia, kidney injury, and hypotension.

3) IV **calcium gluconate or calcium chloride** can be used to treat symptomatic hypocalcemia. Theoretically the administration of calcium may hasten calcium oxalate crystal formation, and this risk must be balanced against that of untreated hypocalcemia in asymptomatic patients.

4) **Sodium bicarbonate** infusion may be used to correct metabolic acidosis when pH is <7.3. It also has the advantage of increasing the renal elimination of glycolate and inhibiting precipitation of calcium oxalate crystals.

2.3. Isopropyl Alcohol

Isopropyl alcohol (isopropanol) is a solvent, antiseptic, and disinfectant often found in the home as a 70% solution (rubbing alcohol). It is sometimes used by alcohol abusers as a cheap substitute for ethanol. Unlike methanol and propylene glycol, isopropyl alcohol is not metabolized to toxic organic acids. It is well absorbed within 90 to 120 minutes and quickly distributes into body water. It is metabolized by alcohol dehydrogenase to acetone. Although rare and usually reported in children, toxicity may result from skin and inhalational exposure.

Mechanism of toxicity: Isopropyl alcohol is 2 to 3 times more potent a central nervous system (CNS) depressant than ethanol. Its metabolism to acetone (another CNS depressant) can prolong sedation or coma. Large ingestions may lead to respiratory arrest, hypotension due to vasodilation, and myocardial suppression. It is very irritating to the gastrointestinal mucosa and gastritis is common.

Toxic dose: Toxic ingestions have occurred at oral doses of 0.5 to 1 mL/kg of 70% isopropyl alcohol solution. Fatal ingestions have been reported with volumes of 200 to 250 mL, but this depends on individual tolerance and coingestions.

→ CLINICAL FEATURES

1. Isopropyl alcohol intoxication begins similar to ethanol intoxication with confusion, slurred speech, and postural instability, but with greater exposure (serum levels >25 mmol/L [150 mg/dL]) it can ultimately lead to coma, respiratory arrest, and hemodynamic instability. Acetone can contribute to CNS depression.

2. Gastric symptoms including pain and vomiting are more prevalent than with other alcohols, and severe gastritis may present with hematemesis.

→ DIAGNOSIS

The clinical diagnosis of isopropyl alcohol toxicity should be suspected with a history of ingestion, elevated osmolar gap, absence of a significant anion gap, and typical smell of isopropanol or acetone.

Diagnostic Tests

1. Specific testing for the isopropyl alcohol serum level is available from most toxicology laboratories. Acetone can be detected in blood within

1 hour and in urine within 3 hours of ingestion of isopropyl alcohol. When not available, the serum level may be estimated from the osmolar gap (formulas: →Chapter 15.2).

2. Other suggested investigations include electrolyte levels, blood glucose levels, blood urea nitrogen, osmolality (to calculate anion and osmolar gaps), as well as arterial blood gases. Ketones may be detected in blood and urine within 3 hours from ingestion. Oximetry and chest radiographs may be helpful for patients with a decreased level of consciousness or suspected aspiration.

→ **TREATMENT**

1. Decontamination: Since isopropyl alcohol is rapidly absorbed, gastric emptying procedures (like aspiration of stomach contents) are unlikely to offer benefit unless patients with large ingestions present within 20 to 30 minutes of ingestion.

2. Antidotes and specific therapies: There is no antidote. Ethanol and fomepizole are not necessary, as there are no toxic organic acids formed from isopropyl alcohol metabolism.

3. Accelerated elimination: Hemodialysis can remove isopropyl alcohol and acetone but most patients are successfully treated with supportive care alone. Dialysis is rarely necessary and reserved for massive ingestions (isopropyl levels >80 mmol/L [500 mg/dL]), in the presence of acute kidney injury, and if hypotension does not respond to fluid resuscitation and vasoactive medication.

4. Supportive care:

1) Ensure airway patency and intubate and assist ventilation if necessary.
2) Watch for and treat coma and hypotension.

2.4. Methyl Alcohol (Methanol)

Methanol (wood alcohol, wood spirits) is used in industry, in window cleaning products (particularly as a windshield-washing fluid), as fuel, and in paint thinners. It cannot be discerned by taste and smell from ethanol, which results in poisonings of persons consuming counterfeit alcohol products (containing methanol instead of ethanol). Methanol is rapidly absorbed from the gastrointestinal tract, distributed to the body water, and is not protein bound. Maximum blood levels are observed within 30 to 60 minutes from ingestion. Toxic methanol levels have also been reported after significant dermal exposure and concentrated inhalation. Methanol is metabolized by alcohol dehydrogenase about 10 times slower than ethanol. About 2% to 5% is excreted unchanged by the kidneys and 10% to 15% through breath.

Mechanism of toxicity: Methanol is a central nervous system (CNS) depressant that produces an inebriation similar to that of ethanol. Methanol is metabolized by alcohol dehydrogenase to formaldehyde, which is then converted to formic acid by aldehyde dehydrogenase. In methanol poisoning severe metabolic acidosis develops secondary to formic acid accumulation as well as lactate production due to inhibition of mitochondrial cytochrome c oxidase by formic acid. Formic acid accumulates in the optic nerve and can cause irreversible blindness from damage to the retina and optic nerve.

Toxic dose: The toxic dose depends on whether methanol was ingested alone or together with ethanol; in the former case, its toxicity is reduced. The consumption of as little as 10 mL of pure methanol may result in permanent loss of vision and as little as 30 mL may be lethal. Typically the lethal oral dose of pure methanol is in the range of 30 to 240 mL (20-150 g), with the median lethal dose being 100 mL (about 1-2 mL/kg). At the bedside, a toxic volume of methanol can be calculated (in mL) as 15×the patient's weight in kg divided by the% of methanol in the ingested fluid. For example, a toxic amount for a 100 kg patient who ingested a 50% methanol solution would be $(15 \times 100)/50 = 30$ mL.

→ CLINICAL FEATURES

1. Symptoms of early poisoning: Initially, before methanol is metabolized, it causes CNS depression and intoxication symptoms similar to those of ethanol. It may also cause gastritis.

2. Symptoms of late poisoning: After a latent period of 18 to 24 hours the metabolites of methanol accumulate and cause an anion gap metabolic acidosis. Visual disturbances, blindness, coma, and acute kidney injury with myoglobinuria may result. Patients describe visual disturbances as blurred vision, haze, or a "snowfield." Fundoscopic examination of these patients may reveal hyperemia of the optic disc or retinal edema. An afferent pupillary defect is a bad sign. Patients may have tachycardia, tachypnea, and altered mental status from advanced acidosis. With massive methanol overdoses, pulmonary edema and cardiovascular collapse may occur. Acute hemorrhagic pancreatitis is not uncommon in patients with methanol overdose. Some long-term survivors of methanol poisoning report parkinsonism-like extrapyramidal symptoms.

→ DIAGNOSIS

The clinical diagnosis of methanol intoxication is suggested by the history, symptoms (particularly visual changes), ocular physical examination, and an anion gap metabolic acidosis in the presence of an osmolar gap.

Diagnostic Tests

1. Specific testing for serum methanol, although not widely available, is helpful as methanol levels >6.25 mmol/L (about 20 mg/dL) are considered toxic; levels >12.5 mmol/L (40 mg/dL) are very serious. Optic nerve damage correlates with levels >20 mmol/L and usually occurs at levels >30 mmol/L (100 mg/dL). Levels >150 mg/dL are potentially lethal. If available, serum formate concentrations better reflect the degree of toxicity, since a low or normal methanol level may reflect nearly complete conversion to formic acid.

2. Other suggested investigations include measurement of levels of electrolytes (with anion gap calculation), blood glucose, blood urea nitrogen, creatinine, serum osmolarity (and osmolar gap calculation [formulas: →Chapter 15.2]), arterial blood gas, lactate level, ethanol level, and lipase (if pancreatitis is suspected). A large anion gap not accounted for by lactate may be a clue to a potential toxic alcohol ingestion. High β-hydroxybutyrate levels may suggest alcoholic ketoacidosis as the cause or contributor to the anion gap.

→ TREATMENT

1. Decontamination: There are no known methods of decontamination. Activated charcoal does not adsorb methanol but may be worthwhile if coingestion of other drugs or toxins is suspected. If ingestion of a large volume occurred within 20 to 30 minutes of presentation, aspiration of gastric contents may be performed.

2. Antidotes and specific therapies: By competitively inhibiting alcohol dehydrogenase and methanol metabolism, the amount of formaldehyde and formic acid produced can be limited. Therapy is indicated for patients with a methanol blood concentration >20 mg/dL (~6 mmol/L), and, when methanol levels are unavailable or delayed, should be used in patients with an anion gap metabolic acidosis and osmolar gap not accounted for by ethanol or a history of methanol ingestion with an osmolar gap >10 mOsm/L.

Note that both ethanol and fomepizole are reasonable first-line agents for toxic alcohol poisoning. Despite the higher direct cost of fomepizole, we suggest its use due to ease of administration and likely less need for monitoring.⊘○

1) **Ethanol**: Administer as early as possible, orally in a conscious patient or IV in an unconscious patient, to a target blood ethanol level of ≥20 mmol/L (>100 mg/dL, ie, 1%) but <40 mmol/L (~200 mg/dL). When given orally, start with a loading dose of 1 mL of 95% ethanol/kg followed by a maintenance dose of 0.1 to 0.2 mL of 95% ethanol/kg/h. If pharmaceutical-grade ethanol is unavailable, commercial alcohol (typically 40% alcohol, 80 proof) can be given as a loading dose of 2 mL/kg and a maintenance dose of 0.2 to 0.4 mL/kg/h. The loading dose will need to be adjusted if the patient has coingested ethanol and the maintenance dose doubled during dialysis. Parenterally ethanol is typically given as either a 5% or 10% solution of ethanol in 5% glucose (dextrose). The less concentrated solution is administered in a bolus at 15 mL/kg over 30 minutes followed by a maintenance dose of 2 to 4 mL/kg/h, and the higher concentration is given at half the bolus amount and half the maintenance rates. The maintenance rates will need to be doubled if the patient is on dialysis. Sometimes ethanol is added to the dialysate.

2) **Fomepizole (4-methylpyrazole, 4-MP)** is a competitive inhibitor of alcohol dehydrogenase and an easier-to-use antidote than ethanol, associated with greater convenience but also a higher cost. It is loaded at a dose of 15 mg/kg (up to 1.5 g for patients >100 kg) diluted in at least 100 mL of normal saline or 5% glucose and administered IV over 30 minutes. This is followed by 10 mg/kg every 12 hours for 4 doses and then increased to 15 mg/kg every 12 hours until methanol levels are <6 mmol/L (20 mg/dL). Since fomepizole is dialyzed, the dosing frequency is increased to every 4 hours during dialysis.

3) **Folic or folinic acid** (the latter preferred, especially in liver disease) can hasten the conversion of formate into carbon dioxide and water. A commonly suggested dose for either is 1 mg/kg (up to 50 mg) given IV every 4 hours.

4) **If toxic alcohol levels are unavailable** and the contents of the product ingested are unknown, we recommend treating for ethylene glycol toxicity as well (→Chapter 15.2.2).

3. Accelerated elimination: Hemodialysis is very efficient at removing methanol and formate. Indications for dialysis include:

1) A methanol level >15 mmol/L (50 mg/dL) and/or an osmolar gap >10.

2) Visual symptoms, coma, or seizures.

3) Acute kidney injury or concomitant renal failure.

4) Suspected methanol ingestion with metabolic acidosis (pH ≤7.15) or an anion gap >24 mmol/L.

5) Ongoing metabolic acidosis not responding to bicarbonate therapy.

Typical dialysis endpoints are a methanol level <6 mmol/L (20 mg/dL) and normalization of anion and osmolar gaps.

4. Supportive care aims to maintain vital parameters and correct any disturbances.

1) Ensure airway patency. Intubate and assist ventilation if necessary.

2) Treat coma (glucose, thiamine) and seizures (benzodiazepines) if they occur.

3) In the presence of acidosis, toxic organic acids are protonated into uncharged molecules, making them easier to penetrate tissues (like the retina) and less likely to be excreted in urine. Formate can be converted to formic acid (thus reducing retinal exposure) by treating metabolic acidosis (pH <7.3) with IV sodium bicarbonate dosed depending on results from ongoing blood gas measurement.

3. Anticholinergic Syndrome (Anticholinergic Toxicity)

→ DEFINITION AND ETIOLOGY

Acute anticholinergic syndrome refers to signs and symptoms caused by the inhibition of the effect of acetylcholine on muscarinic receptors.

Causes:

1) Belladonna alkaloids (atropine, scopolamine, hyoscine, hyoscyamine); jimson weed (*Datura stramonium*), nightshade plant (*Atropa belladonna*), henbane (*Hyoscyamus niger*).

2) Antihistamines and antihistamine sleep aids (diphenhydramine, dimenhydrinate, doxylamine).

3) Cholinolytic drugs used in the treatment of Parkinson disease (biperiden, benztropine [INN benzatropine]).

4) Tricyclic antidepressants (TCAs) (eg, amitriptyline, imipramine, clomipramine).

5) Antipsychotics (eg, olanzapine, clozapine).

6) Phenothiazines (eg, chlorpromazine, prochlorperazine, promethazine, thioridazine).

7) Eye drops (eg, cyclopentolate).

8) Illicit drugs (eg, heroin, which is often mixed with scopolamine).

→ CLINICAL FEATURES AND DIAGNOSIS

Diagnosis is based on signs and symptoms:

1) Central nervous system manifestations:

   a) Hallucinations; "Alice in Wonderland" hallucinations where people or objects appear larger or smaller.

   b) Confusion, delirium.

   c) Psychosis with paranoid delusions.

   d) Psychomotor agitation with jerky myoclonic or choreoathetotic movements (this can lead to rhabdomyolysis).

   e) Coma.

   f) Seizures (pure antimuscarinic agents do not cause seizures but other properties of drugs such as TCAs or antihistamines can have this effect).

2) Peripheral manifestations:

   a) Mydriasis leading to blurry vision.

   b) Vasodilation, diffuse erythema.

   c) Warm dry skin and dry mucosae.

   d) Hyperthermia.

   e) Tachycardia.

   f) Adynamic ileus.

   g) Urinary retention.

Diagnostic Tests

For some anticholinergic medications (particularly TCAs) blood level measurements are possible. While the presence of many nonprescription anticholinergic agents can be confirmed with comprehensive toxicology panels, routine hospital urine toxicology assays will not be useful.

Other diagnostic workup can include electrolytes, creatinine, blood glucose, blood gas analysis, creatine kinase, oximetry, and electrocardiography (ECG) or cardiac monitoring.

Diagnosis may be confirmed by resolution or improvement of symptoms during a slow (over 2-5 minutes) IV injection of 0.5 to 1 mg of **physostigmine salicylate**, a carbamate that reversibly inhibits acetylcholinesterase.

Differential Diagnosis

Psychiatric disorders, poisoning with sympathomimetics (presence of sweating and mydriasis with reaction to light is unlikely with anticholinergics) or hallucinogenic substances, alcohol withdrawal syndrome (including delirium tremens).

→**TREATMENT**

1. Decontamination can be attempted with oral **activated charcoal (AC)**. Because anticholinergic drugs impair gastric emptying and gut motility, AC may still be useful in delayed (>1 hour from ingestion) presentations. There is no role for hemodialysis or hemoperfusion.

2. Protect the agitated patient and other persons from injury. Sometimes physical or pharmacologic (high-dose sedatives) restraints are necessary. In exceptional cases patients may need endotracheal intubation and mechanical ventilation. Also →Chapter 12.1.

3. In severe poisoning monitor **cardiac function, blood pressure, and urine output** (to monitor for urinary retention). Watch for hyperthermia, coma, and rhabdomyolysis.

4. Antidote: In patients with agitated delirium use IV **physostigmine salicylate** 0.5 to 1 mg over 2 to 5 minutes; the dose may be repeated every 10 to 15 minutes up to a total dose of 2 mg. For patients requiring additional doses, discussion with a medical toxicologist is recommended. The drug is rarely used due to adverse effects (bradycardia and heart block) and is contraindicated in patients with seizure disorders, serious TCA overdose, or any patient with anticholinergic toxicity and a prolonged QRS complex on ECG. Caution should be used when considering physostigmine for patients with atrioventricular (AV) conduction disorders, parkinsonian syndrome, recent succinylcholine use, bronchospastic disease, and severe peripheral vascular disease. Patients must be in a setting with cardiac and respiratory monitoring and tools for resuscitation available. Atropine may be given to reverse any excessive muscarinic stimulation from physostigmine.

5. IV **diazepam** 10 mg in repeated doses every 3 to 5 minutes can be used for agitation if physostigmine cannot be used or is ineffective. Do not use phenothiazines or butyrophenones.

6. In the case of TCA-induced anticholinergic syndrome (caused by the TCA effect on muscarinic receptors), the effect of the drug through other mechanisms may cause widening of the QRS complex. In such patients a sodium bicarbonate injection followed by a continuous infusion should be administered. Our pattern is to give sodium bicarbonate until the QRS is normalized, pH is 7.5, or serum sodium levels are >150 mmol/L. The usual dose starts with 50 to 150 mmol (1-3 ampoules) and then is followed by 150 mmol of sodium bicarbonate in 1000 mL of 5% glucose (dextrose) at a rate of ~200 mL/h.

4. Benzodiazepines

→**PATHOPHYSIOLOGY**

Benzodiazepines are central nervous system (CNS) depressants. They are rapidly absorbed from the gastrointestinal tract, metabolized in the liver, and undergo minimal renal elimination in an unchanged form. The half-life of diazepam is between 40 and 70 hours. The therapeutic index of benzodiazepines is high. Moderate poisoning occurs after the administration of >10 times the therapeutic dose. Short-acting benzodiazepines (eg, midazolam, alprazolam) have a high potential for dependency. One of the undesirable effects of benzodiazepines—amnesia—is used for criminal purposes (mainly flunitrazepam; the so-called date rape drugs). Zaleplon (not currently sold in Canada), zopiclone, and zolpidem are the most commonly prescribed hypnotic drugs. Their mechanism of action and adverse effects are similar to those of benzodiazepines and overdose treatment is the same.

→ CLINICAL FEATURES AND DIAGNOSIS

1. Signs and symptoms of poisoning: Psychomotor retardation, slurred speech, unsteady gait, dizziness, ataxia, dyskinesia, diplopia, somnolence, coma, hyporeflexia, pinpoint pupils, hypotension, hypothermia.

2. Diagnostic tests: Urine qualitative tests for benzodiazepines, serum electrolyte levels, and arterial blood gas analysis. In patients with profound coma, check for other toxic substances in blood and urine (benzodiazepine poisoning may often be combined with ingestion of other substances, particularly alcohol). Computed tomography (CT) of the brain and blood glucose may be helpful, as the differential diagnosis of benzodiazepine overdose includes intracranial disorders and hypoglycemia.

→ TREATMENT

1. Decontamination: If <1 hour has elapsed from the ingestion of a very high dose of benzodiazepines, gastric lavage or activated charcoal (25-100 g) may be considered, but they carry the risk of aspiration in patients with decreased level of consciousness and the benefits are unclear, if any.⊗○

2. Antidote: IV flumazenil 0.5 to 2 mg. In unconscious patients with benzodiazepine poisoning administration of flumazenil usually results in full recovery of consciousness for a relatively short period of time (measured in minutes). Do not use flumazenil in patients treated with benzodiazepines for life-threatening indications (eg, epilepsy), patients receiving long-term benzodiazepine treatment (risk of withdrawal seizures), or in patients with suspected mixed poisoning with benzodiazepines and tricyclic or tetracyclic antidepressants. Flumazenil can precipitate arrhythmia and seizures and should not be used routinely.⊗○

3. Methods of enhanced elimination: None available.

4. Symptomatic treatment: Maintain vital functions and correct abnormalities. Invasive ventilation may be required. Manage hypothermia.

5. Cholinergic Syndrome (Cholinergic Toxicity)

→ DEFINITION AND ETIOLOGY

Acute cholinergic syndrome includes signs and symptoms caused by the stimulation of muscarinic and nicotinic receptors. This may be due to excess acetylcholine caused by the inhibition of enzymes like acetylcholinesterase (AChE), which degrades acetylcholine, or due to exogenous parasympathetic stimulants.

Causes:

1) Organophosphorus compounds (OPCs), like the pesticides malathion and parathion, inhibit red blood cell acetylcholinesterase and synaptic junctions as well as plasma cholinesterase (pseudocholinesterase).

2) Chemical warfare agents (tabun, sarin, soman, VX) also cause AChE inhibition.

3) Carbamates (eg, pyridostigmine) transiently inhibit AChE and lead to acetylcholine accumulation.

4) Cholinergic agents (eg, pilocarpine) or muscarine-containing mushrooms (like *Amanita muscaria* or *Clitocybe dealbata* [ivory funnel]) directly activate muscarinic acetylcholine receptors.

→ CLINICAL FEATURES AND DIAGNOSIS

Clinical features:

1) Stimulation of muscarinic receptors: Hypotension, skin erythema, miosis, visual disturbances, hypersalivation and lacrimation, severe bronchial hypersecretion (this may be confused with pulmonary edema), bronchoconstriction causing cough or dyspnea, excessive sweating, intestinal colic, vomiting, diarrhea, loss of bladder and bowel control, bradycardia, heart block, prolonged QTc.

2) Stimulation of nicotinic receptors (usually caused by carbachol, methacholine, or similar substances): Tremor, fasciculations, and muscle weakness up to paralysis (including the diaphragm), decreased tendon reflexes, tachycardia, hypertension.

Central nervous system (CNS) effects are more typical of OPCs and direct cholinergic agents, mostly because carbamates are less likely to cross the blood-brain barrier. CNS effects include restlessness, agitation, seizures, and coma leading to respiratory center depression.

Determination of red blood cell AChE activity or serum AChE or pseudocholinesterase activity is unreliable for the diagnosis of poisoning with pesticides, OPC-based chemical weapons, or carbamates. The degree of reduction of AChE activity is not directly proportional to poisoning severity; the activity may remain low for many weeks despite the resolution of poisoning symptoms and there is a large degree of variability in normal enzyme function between individuals. In the case of carbamates, the enzyme inhibition is reversible, making testing even less useful. Therefore, **diagnosis is typically based on history of exposure and characteristic findings** of nicotinic and muscarinic stimulation described above. The DUMBBELSS mnemonic is useful, standing for **d**iarrhea, **u**rinary incontinence, **m**iosis, **b**ronchospasm, **b**ronchorrhea, **e**mesis, **l**acrimation, **s**alivation, and **s**weating.

Initial workup should include blood gas analysis, electrolytes, creatinine, glucose, lactic acid, creatine kinase (CK), liver function tests, chest radiographs, and electrocardiography (ECG). The severity of respiratory muscle involvement can be assessed by spirometry and negative inspiratory assessment.

Differential Diagnosis

1. Excessive vagal stimulation (symptoms are short-lasting and weak).

2. Dyspnea associated with bronchorrhea and bronchoconstriction (pulmonary edema, asthma, toxic airway and lung injury by irritant gases).

3. Muscle weakness (myasthenia or pseudomyasthenic crisis).

4. Colic and diarrhea (acute gastrointestinal diseases).

→ TREATMENT

Health-care workers must take measures to protect themselves and other patients from cholinergic agents. Thus, **protective equipment, decontamination, and isolation** are a priority, often leading to patients being decontaminated outside of the hospital. However, airway protection and atropine administration should occur concurrently.

Decontamination is very important in cholinergic toxidromes. All contaminated clothing should be removed and the patient should be washed thoroughly with soap and water, including the hair and under the nails.

Patients should be treated in an intensive care unit (ICU) with airway maintenance and ventilation as needed.

1. Monitor cardiac and respiratory function.

2. Administer oxygen to improve tissue oxygenation before administering atropine. If intubation is required, avoid succinylcholine, as its effects will be prolonged.

3. Provide **antidotes**:

1) **Atropine** (muscarinic receptors antagonist): Administer 2 to 5 mg IV and repeat the dose every few minutes until reduction in bronchial hypersecretion and improvement of wheeze are achieved. Once bronchorrhea has resolved, atropine infusion may be helpful if frequent bolus doses are necessary. The dosing of atropine is aimed at stopping airway secretions but avoiding excessive atropine use, or "overatropinization" (tachycardia, urinary retention, excessively dry mouth). Delirium commonly develops as a result of the typical dosing required to reverse cholinergic toxicity. Atropine reverses only the muscarinic (and not nicotinic) effects. Glycopyrrolate can reverse peripheral muscarinic effects but does not help with CNS effects.

2) **Oximes**, like pralidoxime, that reactivate cholinesterase enzymes may have a role in OPC poisoning but not in carbamate poisoning (because their effects are short lived). If the nature of ingestion is unknown, oximes can be given empirically. **Pralidoxime** is initiated as a bolus dose of 30 to 50 mg/kg (1-2 g) and infused over 30 minutes. It can be repeated in 1 hour if fasciculations or weakness have not resolved. Given the short half-life of pralidoxime, an infusion of 8 to 20 mg/kg/h can be started after the initial bolus. Oximes should be administered in combination with atropine after response to atropine has been established.

4. In patients with severe agitation or seizures, administer IV **diazepam** 5 to 10 mg and repeat if necessary. In the ICU setting sedative infusions can be used for agitation or seizures.

5. Anticipate problems with bradycardia, hypotension, seizures, and altered level of consciousness.

6. Asymptomatic patients may have a delayed presentation and should be observed for 12 hours.

7. Patients who survive their initial presentation and treatment may develop proximal motor weakness with neck flexion and bulbar features 2 to 4 days after exposure. This "intermediate syndrome" can persist for 1 to 3 weeks. There are no specific therapies available apart from supportive care. Electromyography/nerve conduction studies may help to delineate this condition and follow its clinical progress.

8. Consultation with a poison center is important as cholinergic poisoning is rare in Canada and a variety of other treatments (magnesium, clonidine, fresh frozen plasma, exogenous hydrolases, and hemoperfusion) are currently being investigated.

6. Digoxin and Other Cardiac Glycosides

→ **PATHOPHYSIOLOGY**

Cardiac glycosides are a class of drugs that result in increased inotropy. Digoxin and digitoxin are the 2 commercially available cardiac glycosides. For the purposes of this chapter, we will focus on digoxin and its toxicity and management. Plant sources of cardiac glycosides include foxglove, oleander, lily of the valley, dogbane, yew needles, and milkweed.

The opening of the fast sodium channels in the myocytes is the first step in normal depolarization. This subsequently allows for a change in the resting membrane potential, leading to opening of the voltage-gated calcium channels. As calcium accumulates in the cell, further calcium is released from the sarcoplasmic reticulum, allowing for muscle contraction. The accumulated sodium and calcium are then released from the cell via the sodium potassium ATPase (Na-K-ATPase) and sodium-calcium antiporter (among other pathways).

The main **mechanism of action** of cardiac glycosides is a reversible inhibition of the Na-K-ATPase pump. This leads to sodium and subsequently calcium accumulation in the myocytes, causing augmentation of inotropy. Additionally, cardiac glycosides increase the vagal tone, resulting in reduced conduction through the sinoatrial (SA) and atrioventricular (AV) nodes.

Digoxin has a large volume of distribution and takes 6 hours to reach therapeutic levels when given orally. The biologic half-life is ~50 hours. The drug is predominantly excreted via the kidneys; the half-life in patients with anuria may be as long as 100 hours. This elimination is performed in part by the p-glycoproteins, which are inhibited by many other drugs, including other antiarrhythmic drugs (amiodarone, verapamil), antibiotics (macrolides), and antifungal agents.

Toxicity

Several factors predispose to digoxin toxicity, including concomitant use of drugs that inhibit the p-glycoprotein, hypokalemia (which increases the risks of arrhythmias in chronic dosing, as hypokalemia further interferes with the function of the Na-K-ATPase pump), hypercalcemia (further accumulation in the myocytes predisposing to arrhythmias), reduced renal function (related to decreased clearance and drug accumulation in blood). Acute-on-chronic overdoses (acute poisoning in patients receiving regular digoxin therapy) are usually more toxic than in drug-naive patients dose-for-dose.

The therapeutic range of digoxin is considered to be 0.8 to 2.0 ng/mL (1.0-2.6 nmol/L). Serum digoxin levels do not correlate well with systemic toxicity: Asymptomatic patients can have "toxic" levels, whereas other patients can have toxic manifestations with a normal serum digoxin level. However, concentrations >4 ng/mL (>5.1 nmol/L) correlate with severe toxic effects, both in acute and chronic poisonings. Therefore, clinical judgment is of critical importance when evaluating patients with symptoms and electrocardiographic (ECG) changes suggestive of digoxin toxicity, and there are absolute levels of digoxin that warrant therapy regardless of symptoms. A toxic effect may be caused by a single dose of 2 mg, serious effects may develop with 5 mg, and death may occur with 10 mg (all amounts are approximate and depend on clinical circumstances). Ingestion of just a few leaves of foxglove or oleander can lead to clinical toxicity.

Poor prognostic factors include age >55 years, male sex, underlying heart disease, high-degree AV block, hyperkalemia, and preexisting acute or chronic renal failure.

➔ CLINICAL FEATURES AND DIAGNOSIS

1. Signs and symptoms of poisoning:

1) Cardiac: Palpitations, dyspnea, syncope. Bradyarrhythmias include sinus bradycardia and second-degree or complete heart block. Tachyarrhythmias such as paroxysmal atrial tachycardia, accelerated junctional rhythm, and ventricular tachycardia (VT) and fibrillation may also occur.

2) Gastrointestinal: Nausea, abdominal pain, vomiting, and diarrhea. Mesenteric ischemia can occur with rapid IV infusions.

3) Other symptoms: Fatigue, hallucinations, dizziness, headaches, lethargy, abnormal vision, and a yellow or green rim perceived around sources of light (very rare).

2. Diagnostic and laboratory tests: Digoxin toxicity is a clinical diagnosis based on serum levels, exposure history, and clinical features along with ECG findings. The following laboratory and other investigations aid diagnosis:

1) **Serum digoxin concentration**: In patients with acute poisoning measured at admission and 6 hours after oral intake or 4 hours after IV intake. Serum concentration of glycosides may not correlate with the severity of poisoning, but a concentration >2 ng/mL (2.6 nmol/L) is considered toxic. Levels are not reliable, as they will be falsely elevated after administration of digitalis-
-specific antibodies.

2) **ECG and rhythm monitoring**: Several ECG changes are associated with digoxin effects or toxicity. These include scooping (bowl-shaped) and down-sloping of ST segments; flattened, biphasic, or inverted T waves; and PQ prolongation and QT shortening. Rhythm may show sinus bradycardia (in patients with atrial flutter or fibrillation ventricular rates may be very slow), first-degree AV block, ventricular premature beats (often in the form of bigeminy or trigeminy), and less commonly second-degree SA block and Mobitz type I (Wenckebach) second-degree AV block. Patients with more severe overdose may develop worsening of premature beats (clustered and multiform premature beats), worsening of sinus bradycardia, and in some cases AV junctional escape rhythm or characteristic types of arrhythmia: nonparoxysmal AV junctional tachycardia (with ventricular rates 60-130 beats/min that may easily be overlooked) and atrial tachycardia with AV block of various degrees. Patients with extremely high overdose may have third-degree AV block, third-degree SA block, VT (sometimes bidirectional, ie, with features of right bundle branch block and alternating left and right axis deviation), and ventricular fibrillation (VF).

3) **Electrolytes**: Due to the ability of digoxin to inhibit Na-K-ATPase in the skeletal muscle and myocardium, an increase in extracellular potassium occurs. Acute digoxin toxicity is often associated with hyperkalemia and the degree correlates with mortality. However, hypokalemia is of greater concern in chronic toxicity. Measuring levels of serum electrolytes (potassium, sodium, chloride) and extended electrolytes (magnesium, calcium, phosphate) along with blood gases (metabolic acidosis may be present), serum creatinine, and urea is important.

→ **T R E A T M E N T**

1. Discontinue the drug.

2. Decontamination: If ingestion of a toxic dose of digoxin (or oleander leaves, yew needles, or any amount of their infusion) occurred within 1 hour (according to some up 6-8 hours), consider gastric lavage with a suspension of activated charcoal.

3. Antidote: Fab fragments of digoxin-binding antibodies. Indicated in life-
-threatening arrhythmias (VT, VF, asystole, Mobitz type II or complete heart block, symptomatic bradycardia), hyperkalemia (serum potassium >5.5 mmol/L), evidence of end-organ dysfunction (otherwise unexplained reduced renal function or altered level of consciousness). Fab use is also recommended for absolute digoxin levels: >5.1 nmol/L in chronic toxicity and >10 nmol/L in acute ingestion/toxicity. When administering the antidote, closely monitor serum potassium levels, as there is a risk of serum potassium decreasing within 4 hours of administration. Patients with cardiac pacemakers may not have the findings mentioned above and in such cases serum potassium levels and end-organ damage may be the only criteria on the basis of which decision regarding Fab administration should be made.

Patients with renal failure need prolonged monitoring due to delayed/poor excretion of digoxin and antidote. Recurrent toxicity has rarely been described.

4. Methods of enhanced elimination: Dialysis and hemoperfusion are ineffective due to the large size and volume of distribution of digoxin. Repeat-dose activated charcoal or cholestyramine can be considered in cases of digitoxin toxicity (extensive enterohepatic recirculation) or in patients with impaired renal function and digoxin toxicity.

Symptomatic Treatment

1. Hypokalemia and hypomagnesemia: In patients with ventricular or supraventricular tachyarrhythmia without AV block, administer IV potassium to maintain potassium levels at the upper limits of normal (up to 0.5 mmol/min).

2. Treat **hyperkalemia** (>5.5 mmol/L).

3. In patients with **predominant bradyarrhythmia and conduction abnormalities**, consider atropine (0.5-2 mg IV). A temporary pacemaker may be required but should only be considered after failure of digoxin-specific antibodies, as pacing in the context of cardiac glycoside toxicity carries a high risk of triggering life-threatening arrhythmias.

4. Supraventricular tachycardia: Phenytoin. Cardioversion should be attempted only as a last resort and with low voltage (risk of treatment-resistant VT).

5. Ventricular tachyarrhythmia typically improves with administration of digoxin-specific antibodies but its resolution may be hastened by normalizing potassium and magnesium levels. If this does not lead to improvement, lidocaine, β-blockers, and further magnesium sulfate can be administered.

7. Lithium Toxicity

→ PATHOPHYSIOLOGY

Lithium is a univalent ion that has long been used in the treatment of psychiatric conditions, particularly bipolar disorder. The mechanism of action of lithium largely remains unknown but it is thought to be related to reduction in intracellular levels of inositol monophosphate and glycogen synthase kinase-3, which are signaling proteins involved in mood stabilization, neuroplasticity, and energy metabolism.

When given in a tablet form, the drug is highly absorbed through the gut and reaches peak levels within 1 to 2 hours or 4 to 6 hours following ingestion of immediate-release or sustained-release products, respectively. Plasma drug is highly non–protein-bound and has a small volume of distribution. The drug in its soluble form is univalent and handled entirely by the kidneys (very similar to sodium handling). The half-life is ~24 hours with a range typically between 14 and 30 hours. Glycogen synthase kinase-3 is also present in the principal cells of the nephrons, predominantly responsible for the action of arginine vasopressin (AVP). The epithelial sodium channel in the principal cells allows for the drug uptake into the cells, where it exerts its renal effects. In the presence of lithium in the principal cells, the cells are less receptive to the effects of AVP (the main mechanism of AVP is resorption of free water from that segment of the nephron), leading to volume loss.

Toxicity

Lithium tends to concentrate in the brain as well as kidneys, making these organs largely prone to acute and chronic toxicity. Volume depletion, chronic lithium use, advanced age, reduced glomerular filtration rate (GFR), and concomitant use of other nephrotoxic agents (nonsteroidal anti-inflammatory drugs [NSAIDs], angiotensin-converting enzyme inhibitor [ACEIs], thiazides) are among the major risk factors for toxicity. Acute toxicity typically occurs with doses >40 mg/kg (1 mEq/kg). In patients receiving long-term lithium therapy much lower doses can lead to clinically important toxicity, since tissues are already saturated with lithium. In patients with renal impairment even standard therapeutic doses can lead to lithium intoxication.

→ CLINICAL FEATURES

Lithium toxicity can be acute, acute-on-chronic, or chronic. **Acute and acute--on-chronic toxicity** present similarly and include gastrointestinal and neurologic dysfunction, rarely with cardiac dysfunction. Gastrointestinal manifestations include nausea, vomiting, and diarrhea. Neurologic manifestations are similar those present in chronic toxicity (→below). Prolongation of QT interval occurs rarely and may lead to arrhythmias.

Chronic toxicity usually presents with renal manifestations and/or neurologic dysfunction. Aside from its effects on the principal cells, lithium is thought to cause significant interstitial fibrosis, and this combination is likely a reason for the development of nephrogenic diabetes insipidus (NDI). Due to NDI, many patients have polyuria and, if compensated for, polydipsia. If other neurologic manifestations develop or the patient has restricted access to free water, severe hypernatremia due to significant reduction in total body free water content can occur.

Neurologic toxicity manifestations are broad and nonspecific. Presentation can vary and may include headaches, tremors, lethargy, ataxia, confusion, or agitation; and in extreme situations, seizures, rigidity, hyperpyrexia, status epilepticus, and death. A syndrome of irreversible lithium toxicity can develop, which may fail to improve despite drug cessation; this is called the SILENT syndrome (syndrome of irreversible lithium-effectuated neurotoxicity). It occurs due to demyelination at various levels of the central nervous system. The manifestations of SILENT syndrome include cerebellar and brainstem dysfunction, myopathy, nystagmus, blindness, extrapyramidal symptoms, and dementia. Lithium can precipitate or aggravate serotonin syndrome in the presence of other serotonergic drugs.

Some other rare manifestations may include both hypothyroidism and hyperthyroidism along with parathyroid cell hyperplasia causing hyperparathyroidism and hypercalcemia.

→ DIAGNOSIS

The diagnosis of acute or acute-on-chronic toxicity can be made based on history and physical examination in patients suspected to have lithium toxicity, which can be confirmed with measurements of lithium levels (if available). The diagnosis of chronic toxicity is predominantly made on the basis of clinical presentation but in most patients the severity of toxicity corresponds to serum drug levels.

If available, other toxicity screening including other drug levels and serum glucose should be obtained in addition to renal function, electrolyte levels, and electrocardiography (ECG). ECG abnormalities may include T-wave flattening or inversion, depression of ST segments, bradycardia, or heart block. Consider measuring levels of thyroid-stimulating hormone (TSH), calcium, and serum parathyroid hormone (PTH).

→ TREATMENT

General treatment of any toxicity includes management and stabilization of the airway, breathing, and circulation (ABC). Specific therapy involves reducing uptake from the gut, rapid removal via IV hydration, and/or hemodialysis. Discussion or consultation with a toxicology expert should be considered.

1. Gastrointestinal decontamination: Activated charcoal has no role in lithium toxicity as lithium particles cannot be removed/bound from the gut. For large ingestions of sustained-release products, whole bowel irrigation with 2 L/h of a bowel preparation agent may be administered until the rectal effluent is clear or ≥10 L is administered. Sodium polystyrene sulfonate may reduce the half-life of lithium but can induce hypokalemia; potassium levels should be closely monitored if this agent is used.

2. Hydration: The hallmark of lithium toxicity management is IV hydration to enhance lithium excretion through the kidneys. Target IV infusion rates can be approximately 2×the maintenance doses (eg, in a 75-kg patient use 200-250 mL/h of isotonic IV fluids). Caution should be taken in patients at high risk for volume overload (eg, with advanced chronic kidney disease or congestive heart failure). Serum sodium, lithium, and creatinine levels can be monitored serially to ensure normalization (if possible). In patients thought to be intravascularly depleted, crystalloid repletion with 1 to 2 L can be provided up front. Because of the risk of lithium-induced NDI, serum sodium levels should be followed and maintenance fluids may need to be switched to hypotonic fluids, such as half-normal (0.45%) saline. The goal of hydration is to enhance lithium elimination by establishing normal urine output. The use of diuretics is not recommended as only marginal gains in lithium excretion are obtained and many patients with lithium toxicity are dehydrated.

3. Renal replacement therapy: Hemodialysis is highly effective thanks to lithium being a small particle, not being protein-bound, and having a relatively small volume of distribution. Nephrology consultation should be obtained, where available, for assistance with decision-making and delivery of hemodialysis. Hemodialysis should be performed (if available) in patients with serum lithium levels >5.0 mmol/L; with serum levels of >4.0 mmol/L and renal impairment (creatinine >2 mg/dL [175 μmol/L]); or with serum levels >2.5 mmol/L and neurologic manifestations of seizures, coma, or conditions that prevent aggressive volume resuscitation (severe decompensated heart failure or advanced renal disease). Hemodialysis can also be considered (if available) in severe life-threatening situations (depressed level of consciousness, seizures, coma) regardless of the serum lithium level. Some patients do not meet any specific criteria, and in such situations toxicology and nephrology consultations are recommended. Because of equilibration of extracellular and intracellular lithium, a rebound in serum lithium levels can occur after cessation of a short session of hemodialysis. This may necessitate a longer session (6-8 h, depending on ingested quantity and initial serum levels) or another session. Lithium levels can be measured 2 to 4 hours after cessation of dialysis to assess for a rebound rise in serum levels. Continuous venovenous hemodiafiltration (CVVHDF) may be used, as it has the advantage of reducing the risk of rebound toxicity. However, CVVHDF provides limited lithium clearance and is not as efficient as hemodialysis in the case of massive ingestions.

4. Psychiatric consultation should be considered for further management of mood disorders, alternative mood stabilizing therapies, and/or suicidal attempts in patients with large ingestions.

5. NDI: Thiazides, amiloride, and indomethacin have been used for the treatment of nephrogenic diabetes insipidus. While these drugs may be used in the chronic management of lithium nephrotoxicity, they should not be used in patients with acute kidney injury or suspected intravascular volume depletion or dehydration. Also →Chapter 9.8.6.

8. Poisoned Patient: General Approach

→**INITIAL APPROACH**

First contact: As in all acutely ill patients, in individuals with poisoning the maintenance of airway, breathing, and circulation (ABC) is the priority. Decontamination, if applicable, is the next step that may even precede treatment (to avoid continuous patient's exposure and to avoid contaminating the hospital staff or the entire facility [eg, in the case of organophosphate overdose]). A detailed history and physical examination are frequently required to identify the offending agents. Some signs and symptoms of toxicity as well as syndromes or odors are specific for certain agents and aid in narrowing down differential diagnosis. Cardiac function should be monitored in all patients.

→DIAGNOSIS AND MANAGEMENT

1. Initial diagnostic workup:

1) Blood glucose levels.
2) Complete blood count (CBC), electrolyte levels, serum osmolality and creatinine.
3) Blood gas analysis (arterial or venous).
4) Electrocardiography (ECG).
5) Serum acetaminophen (INN paracetamol) and salicylate levels.
6) Urine drug screen (for certain toxins, if the history is suggestive).
7) Serum levels of alcohol and/or suspected drugs (if applicable).
8) Pregnancy testing if the history of pregnancy is unclear.

2. Decontamination methods:

1) **Ipecac:** Ipecac is no longer recommended by the European and North American toxicology associations (no evidence of efficacy).
2) **Activated charcoal (AC):** Current guidelines do not recommend routine AC administration. The potential benefit of this drug decreases rapidly if administered >60 minutes after ingestion of a toxin or poison. It may be of benefit if the poisoning involves drugs with delayed gastric emptying (eg, opioids, sustained-release drugs, or drug "packers" and "stuffers" [smuggling drugs in body cavities]). In the case of certain drugs patients may benefit from early and multiple doses of AC (eg, carbamazepine, acetylsalicylic acid [ASA], phenobarbital, theophylline). However, certain toxins are not affected by AC (acids, alkalis, metals, alcohol, hydrocarbons).

   The use of AC is not without risks, which include pulmonary aspiration in obtunded patients with oral or nasogastric tube administration.

   There is no supporting evidence for the use of cathartic drugs, such as sorbitol, with AC and they should be avoided.
3) **Whole-bowel irrigation (WBI):** WBI consists of rapid administration of polyethylene glycol electrolyte solution to produce liquid stools, allowing for elimination of tablets or drug packets from the gastrointestinal tract. It is not recommended routinely but may be helpful in situations involving sustained-release preparations or insertion of packs of drugs into body cavities. While WBI may be useful in clearing medication bezoars, it is contraindicated in patients with intestinal obstruction or bowel perforation.
4) **Gastric lavage (GL):** GL is a procedure where a large-bore orogastric tube is inserted with intent to aspirate tablets or fragments of pills from the stomach following an acute ingestion. This procedure requires airway protection and carries a risk of major complications including aspiration or esophageal rupture. It can be used in rare situations when experienced personnel are available and ingestion is potentially lethal.

→POISON CENTERS

Contact details of Canadian poison control centers: safemedicationuse.ca/tools_resources/poison_centres.html.

1. Abdominal Paracentesis

→ INDICATIONS

1. Diagnostic: A new diagnosis of ascites (either in an outpatient or inpatient setting), suspected spontaneous bacterial peritonitis, usually each hospitalization of a patient with cirrhosis and ascites (as this is frequently associated with spontaneous bacterial peritonitis that is asymptomatic or causes only minor symptoms).
2. Therapeutic: Initial treatment of large ascites (one-time fluid evacuation), ascites refractory to diuretics (repeated paracentesis is necessary).

→ CONTRAINDICATIONS

Disseminated intravascular coagulation or severe (symptomatic) bleeding disorder not responding to vitamin K and fresh-frozen plasma (FFP), acute abdominal conditions requiring urgent surgery. High international normalized ratio (INR) or low platelet counts associated with liver cirrhosis are not an absolute contraindication to paracentesis, but the threshold where correction may be required is not known. Infection overlying the paracentesis site (eg, cellulitis). Lack of patient cooperation or consent.

→ POTENTIAL COMPLICATIONS

Hematoma of the abdominal wall (1%), infection of the ascitic fluid, perforation of the bowel or urinary bladder, and hemoperitoneum (<1/1000 patients). In the case of therapeutic paracentesis, hypotension (caused by a blood volume shift to the decompressed visceral circulation), renal impairment, and electrolyte disturbances. Persistent leakage of ascitic fluid.

→ PATIENT PREPARATION

Obtain informed consent, documented as required in your institution. The patient should void prior to the procedure if a urinary catheter is not in place. It is mandatory to maintain good intravascular volume using infusion of a crystalloid or colloid (albumin). In most patients with asymptomatic coagulopathy, the administration of FFP or platelet concentrate is not necessary. Place the patient in a semirecumbent position (with the trunk elevated).

→ EQUIPMENT

Note: If available, a standard dedicated paracentesis kit may be preferred in most situations, especially with large-volume paracentesis. If not available, the following equipment can be used:
1) Equipment for surgical field preparation and infiltration anesthesia.
2) Catheter with a needle as for peripheral vein catheterization, bore 1.2 to 1.7 mm (18-16 gauge, 45 mm in length, allowing for fluid aspiration). A longer needle is necessary in patients with a thick abdominal wall (obesity or significant abdominal wall edema).
3) Three-way stopcock, drain tubing as for drip infusion, bottle for fluid collection (if not using a dedicated paracentesis kit).
4) Scalpel for skin incision if using a large-bore catheter.

→ SITE OF PARACENTESIS

Ultrasound guidance, when available, is preferred. A low-frequency abdominal probe or cardiac probe can be used to scan the abdomen to look for drainable fluid collections. Simple transudative ascites (high serum-ascites albumin gradient) is anechoic and can be contrasted with the hyperechoic bowel lying below; complex ascites can have a more complex echogenic appearance. Care should be taken to avoid a distended urinary bladder, which could be mistaken for ascites (as noted above, the patient should void if the bladder is not already decompressed with a Foley catheter). A drainable ascites pocket should have no overlying structures and be ≥3 cm deep. The site can be marked prior to skin preparation and draping.

If ultrasonography is not available, percuss the abdominal wall to verify the fluid level. The optimal paracentesis site usually lies 2 to 3 cm below the umbilicus or at a third of the length of the lower line connecting the anterior superior iliac spine with the umbilicus on the left side, less frequently on the right side.

→ PROCEDURE

1. Prepare the surgical field. Infiltrate the skin, subcutaneous tissue, and muscles down to the peritoneum using 1% or 2% lidocaine.

2. Pull the skin taut down and insert a syringe with a needle while aspirating continuously until the peritoneum is penetrated and fluid outflow is confirmed. Advance the catheter over the needle (or alternatively introduce the catheter over a guidewire as in pericardiocentesis). A 3-way stopcock can be used to control the drainage of fluid while collection setup is connected.

3. After diagnostic collection of 50 to 100 mL of fluid, or completion of therapeutic decompression using vacuum collection bottles, protect the puncture site with a sterile dressing.

→ AFTER THE PROCEDURE

Removal of larger amount of ascites may trigger a potentially harmful hemodynamic reaction (postparacentesis circulatory dysfunction), which is why volume replacement in such situations is considered standard practice. Our practice is to administer 6 to 8 g IV albumin in the form of a 20% to 25% solution for every liter of removed fluid over 4 to 5 L rather than using other volume expanders.◕

2. Arthrocentesis: Knee, Wrist, Ankle

Arthrocentesis refers to the aspiration of fluid from a joint cavity.

→ INDICATIONS

1. Diagnostic: Arthrocentesis is a useful tool in diagnosing causes of joint effusion and can therefore guide therapy. Potential etiologies include septic arthritis, hemarthrosis, crystal arthropathies, inflammatory arthropathies, and noninflammatory arthropathies.

2. Therapeutic: Decompression of joint effusion for pain relief, reducing septic burden in septic arthritis, and aspiration followed by intra-articular glucocorticoid administration for osteoarthritis and inflammatory arthritides.

→ CONTRAINDICATIONS

1. Absolute: Uncontrolled coagulopathy, superimposing skin or soft-tissue infection at the planned injection site.

2. Relative: Anticoagulation (especially with international normalized ratio [INR] >3.0, activated partial thromboplastin time [aPTT] > 2 × upper limit of normal), thrombocytopenia (platelet count <50 × 10^9/L), and infection in adjacent tissues.

→ POTENTIAL COMPLICATIONS

Septic arthritis, hemarthrosis, hematoma, joint cartilage injury, pain at the puncture site, adverse effects of local anesthetics or drugs administered intra--articularly (eg, glucocorticoids).

→ EQUIPMENT

1. Sterilizing solution.

2. Needles (we suggest 22-gauge 1 1/2-inch needles for most large joints and 25-gauge 5/8-inch needles for small joints [metacarpophalangeal, proximal interphalangeal, distal interphalangeal]).

3. Local anesthetic (skilled clinicians may skip this).

4. Sterile syringes for aspirate collection.

5. Dressing supplies.

→ PATIENT PREPARATION

Obtain informed consent. Explain the risks and benefits of arthrocentesis.

→ PROCEDURE

1. Knee: Medial approach (→Figure 2-1):

1) The patient is lying supine with the knee extended.

2) Palpate the medial parapatellar fossa, halfway between the superior and inferior poles of the patella. Place a mark in the soft spot, anticipating that the tip of the needle will be under the patella when it is advanced (a retracted pen is useful for impressing a mark).

3) Apply sterilizing solution in a circular fashion, starting at the injection site and moving outwards. Do not bring the swab back to the middle. Repeat 2 to 3 times (or more if needed).

4) Local anesthetic may be infiltrated using a small-bore needle (eg, 25 gauge), especially if a difficult or long procedure (large volume effusion) is anticipated. Skilled clinicians may skip this, as the discomfort of the actual procedure may be less than or equal to the pain of local anesthetic infiltration.

5) With the syringe/needle (eg, 22 gauge) held fairly horizontally, advance the needle aiming laterally. Once the needle is within subcutaneous tissue, withdraw the plunger a little to create negative syringe pressure as the needle is advanced. A "give" may be felt as the needle tip breaches the joint capsule or fluid may start flowing (if this does not happen, one should estimate the depth for the needle tip to be under the body of the patella). Aspirate as much fluid as possible, switching syringes as needed while keeping the needle in place. Medication can be administered through the same needle if needed.

2. Knee: Lateral approach (→Figure 2-1):

1) The patient is supine with the knee extended.

2) Palpate the lateral parapatellar groove under the superior 1/3 of the patella. Make an impression in the soft spot to mark the entry point.

3) Cleaning and local anesthetic use are as in the medial approach (→above).

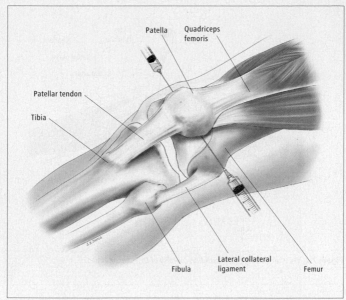

Figure 2-1. Knee arthrocentesis. Needle entry: medial approach underneath the mid point of the patella; lateral approach underneath the upper 1/3 of the patella. *Illustration courtesy of Dr Shannon Zhang.*

4) Follow other instructions as in the medial approach, advancing the syringe/needle (eg, 22 gauge) horizontally and aiming inferomedially (targeting the underside of the middle 1/3 of the patella).

3. Wrist (→Figure 2-2):

1) The patient is sitting or lying, with the forearm/hand prone and wrist slightly flexed (this can be achieved with a small rolled towel placed under the wrist).

2) Palpate distally along the middle of the wrist, just past Lister tubercle, and a soft spot in the radiocarpal joint space should be felt. Make an impression with a retracted pen.

3) Cleaning and local anesthetic use: →above.

4) With the syringe/needle (5/8-inch or 1-inch needle is usually sufficient) held fairly vertically, advance the needle downwards into the joint space. Once the capsule is breached, fluid may be aspirated. Intra-articular medications can be then administered if needed.

4. Ankle (→Figure 2-3):

1) The patient is lying supine with the knee extended and the ankle in a neutral position.

2) Palpate distally along the anteromedial aspect of the tibia until the soft spot between the tibia and the talus is found. This should be medial to the tibialis anterior tendon. Make an impression to mark the site of injection.

3) Cleaning and local anesthetic use: →above.

4) With the syringe/needle (1-inch or 1 1/2-inch) held almost parallel to the sole of the foot, advance the needle aiming posteriorly and slightly laterally (imagine the middle of the joint) until the capsule is breached or the needle

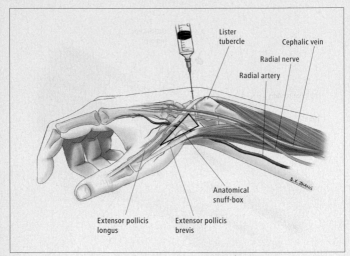

Figure 2-2. Wrist arthrocentesis. *Illustration courtesy of Dr Shannon Zhang.*

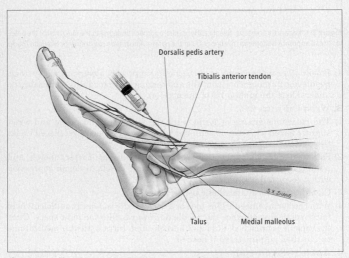

Figure 2-3. Ankle arthrocentesis. *Illustration courtesy of Dr Shannon Zhang.*

encounters the articular surface (in which case you should withdraw slightly). Apply negative pressure. Once the joint capsule is breached, fluid can be aspirated. Intra-articular medications can be administered through the same needle as needed.

3. Gastric Lavage

Gastric lavage should not be considered one of the routine decontamination methods in toxicology due to various potential complications, scarce evidence, and uncertain clinical effects. While studies in healthy volunteers and animals show decreased absorption of toxins and certain markers, high-quality clinical studies are lacking.

→ INDICATIONS

Gastric lavage may be considered within 1 hour of oral intake of a significant amount of a life-threatening toxic substance. It should be restricted to life--threatening exposure in either fully awake and cooperative patients or patients with a protected airway. Examples include recent ingestion of significant amounts of tricyclic antidepressants, labetalol, organophosphates, or toxic alcohols. If available, a local poison control center can provide guidance as to the appropriateness of gastric lavage with or without activated charcoal.

→ COMPLICATIONS

Aspiration, perforation of the gastrointestinal tract, rhythm disturbances.

→ CONTRAINDICATIONS

Poisoning with corrosives (risk of gastrointestinal perforation); poisoning with volatile substances, hydrocarbons, or detergents (high risk of aspiration); significant risk of gastrointestinal bleeding; unconscious patients (unless intubated); significant psychomotor agitation, patient refusal, lack of cooperation, or resistance.

→ PATIENT PREPARATION

The patient should be fully awake and cooperative to perform this procedure; otherwise, the patient's airway must be secured with endotracheal intubation. Ideally, proactive endotracheal intubation should be done because of the high risk of aspiration and respiratory compromise, either from the procedure or toxic ingestion.

→ EQUIPMENT

Large-bore nasogastric/orogastric tube coated with a lubricant gel (eg, lidocaine gel), funnel, bucket, 50 mL syringe.

→ PROCEDURE

1. Insert the nasogastric/orogastric tube into the stomach, then confirm placement (→Chapter 16.6). A fully awake patient should be placed in the left lateral decubitus position. An intubated patient may lie supine.

2. Introduce 200 to 300 mL of water at body temperature into the tube and then lower the tube into the bucket below the level of the stomach before water disappears from the funnel. This will cause the water to return (siphon phenomenon). Repeat until clear (watery) outflow is seen.

3. A single dose of activated charcoal (1 g/kg) can be administered into the stomach after completing gastric lavage as indicated. Exceptions include substances that are not adsorbed by activated charcoal (alcohols, mercury, lead, iron, caustics, and hydrocarbons.

Consider administration of repeated doses of activated charcoal (starting from 1 g/kg and followed by 0.5-1 g/kg every 2-4 hours) in patients who ingested life-threatening doses of quinine, dapsone, phenobarbital, carbamazepine, or theophylline.

4. Injections of Drugs and Other Substances

Before attempting any procedures described in these chapters, wash and disinfect your hands and wear disposable gloves.

4.1. Intramuscular Injections

→ CONTRAINDICATIONS

1. Absolute: Edema or inflammatory changes at the planned injection site, shock and peripheral hypoperfusion (except for the administration of epinephrine in patients with anaphylactic shock [→Chapter 2.2]), patients refusing consent to the procedure.

2. Relative: Muscle atrophy (this can impair absorption). Coagulopathy, thrombocytopenia, use of anticoagulants (risk of hematoma). Avoid IM injections in patients receiving long-term renal replacement therapy.

→ POTENTIAL COMPLICATIONS

Abscess and other infectious complications; irreversible nerve injury (most frequently of the sciatic nerve); reversible sensory abnormalities (in the area innervated by the sciatic nerve); aseptic muscle necrosis (most frequently seen after glucocorticoid injections); specific adverse effects of administered agents (eg, allergic reactions).

→ EQUIPMENT

Nonsterile disposable gloves; skin disinfectant (single-use alcohol swabs or single-use cotton swab with disinfectant solution); syringe; needle bore 0.8 to 0.9 mm (21 to 20 gauge); needle for drawing drug from ampoule (or a syringe prefilled with the drug, with or without a needle); sterile gauze and bandage; sharps container for disposal.

→ INJECTION SITE

1. Buttock: Place the patient on one side or supine with knees slightly flexed. Determine the injection site (defining gluteal quadrants is no longer recommended): Place the tip of the index finger on the anterior superior iliac spine and spread your fingers, moving the middle finger as far posteriorly as possible without displacing the index finger. While holding the index finger firmly in place, turn the hand so that your thenar rests on the greater trochanter of the patient's femur. The injection site should be within the lower third of the triangle formed by the index finger and the middle finger.

2. Arm: Injections into the lateral surface of the deltoid muscle are associated with a significant risk of nerve and vascular injury. If this site is chosen, have the patient relax their arm. By palpation, locate the acromion process. The injection site is 3 fingerbreadths below the acromion process, in the middle of the deltoid muscle.

3. Thigh: Place the patient supine. Place one hand on the greater trochanter and the other on the patient's knee on the lateral surface of the thigh, thumbs pointing towards each other. The injection site should be in the middle of the imaginary line connecting the thumbs.

→ PROCEDURE

1. Close the curtains to ensure privacy for the patient. Explain the planned procedure to the patient and confirm consent.

2. Prepare the medication, if necessary, by drawing the medication from the ampule or vial into the syringe using a sterile needle. It is unnecessary to clean the top of a sealed vial. Remove the needle used to draw up the drug from the syringe and replace with a sterile 20-gauge or 21-gauge needle.

3. Perform hand hygiene and don nonsterile disposable gloves.

4. Disinfect the planned injection site using a single-use alcohol swab or single--use cotton swab with disinfectant solution. Start over the planned injection site and work outwards. Allow the disinfectant to dry completely.

5. Using the nondominant hand to hold the skin around the injection site, insert the needle with a syringe attached into the skin at a 90° angle and deep enough to make the needle tip stay within the muscle. If the needle touches the bone, withdraw the needle ~1 cm.

6. Before injecting the drug, aspirate with the plunger to avoid intravascular administration. If blood is aspirated, withdraw the needle and prepare another drug dose using a new needle and syringe.

7. Immobilize the needle by holding the needle hub with one hand and slowly inject the drug, then withdraw the needle at a 90° angle to the skin.

8. Immediately cover the site with a clean dry cotton gauze and apply pressure. If bleeding occurs, protect the injection site with dressing.

9. Dispose of all sharps securely in a sharps container. Do not recap needles to avoid needle-stick injuries. Remove gloves and perform hand hygiene.

4.2. Intravenous Injections

Repeated IV drug injections are performed similarly to IV drug infusions via a peripheral IV catheter and, when necessary, via a central venous catheter. The procedure described below is a peripheral IV injection using an injection needle; this is most frequently performed when only one injection is planned or if an IV catheter is not available.

→ CONTRAINDICATIONS

Absolute: Patients refusing to consent for the procedure.

Relative: Avoid peripheral vein catheterization at sites of local infection, burns, in the veins of the upper limb with an arteriovenous fistula used for hemodialysis, or in the veins of a limb postmastectomy with lymph node dissection or lymphedema.

→ POTENTIAL COMPLICATIONS

Phlebitis, hematoma, infection, drug extravasation.

→ EQUIPMENT

Nonsterile disposable gloves; skin disinfectant (single-use alcohol swabs or single-use cotton swab with disinfectant solution); tourniquet; needle (usually bore 0.9 mm [20 gauge]); syringe; needle for drawing drug from ampoule; sterile gauze and bandage; sharps container for disposal.

→ INJECTION SITE

In adults the sites of IV injections are usually the forearm and outer surface of the hand or less commonly the outer surface of the foot. In urgent situations other sites can be used: veins of the cubital fossa and external jugular veins.

→ PROCEDURE

1. Close the curtains to ensure privacy for the patient. Explain the planned procedure to the patient and confirm consent.

2. Prepare the medication, if necessary, by drawing the medication from the ampoule or vial into the syringe using a sterile needle. It is unnecessary to clean the top of a sealed vial. Remove the needle used to draw up the drug from the syringe and replace with a sterile 20-gauge or 21-gauge needle.

3. Select a suitable superficial vein. This can also be done using ultrasonography, as when obtaining intravenous access.

4. Wrap a tourniquet (usually on the upper arm) to fill the peripheral veins. Visualizing and puncturing a vein can be facilitated by warming the limb and massaging (tapping) the planned injection site. Spread the skin taut below the planned injection site using a thumb or fingers of one hand. Alternatively ask the patient to open and close their fist several times.

5. Perform hand hygiene, and don nonsterile disposable gloves.

6. Clean and disinfect the planned injection site using a single-use alcohol swab or single-use cotton swab with disinfectant solution. Start over the planned injection site and work outwards. Allow the disinfectant to dry completely.

7. Spread the skin taut below the planned injection site using a thumb or fingers of one hand. Insert the needle with a syringe attached into the skin at a ~30° angle, simultaneously aspirating the syringe plunger.

8. When blood is seen in the syringe, release the tourniquet and inject the drug (this is usually done slowly), then withdraw the needle.

9. Compress the injection site with a sterile gauze immediately after the needle is removed to stop bleeding, then protect it with a small adhesive dressing.

10. Dispose of all sharps securely in a sharps container. Do not recap needles to avoid needle-stick injuries. Remove gloves and perform hand hygiene.

4.3. Subcutaneous Injections

→ CONTRAINDICATIONS

Absolute: Edema or inflammation at the planned injection site, shock and peripheral hypoperfusion (this can impair absorption), patients refusing consent to the procedure.

Relative: Coagulopathy, thrombocytopenia, use of anticoagulants (risk of hematoma).

→ POTENTIAL COMPLICATIONS

Phlebitis, hematoma, infection, drug extravasation.

→ EQUIPMENT

Nonsterile disposable gloves; skin disinfectant (single-use alcohol swabs or single-use cotton swab with disinfectant solution); syringe; short needle (bore up to 0.7 mm [22 gauge]); needle for drawing drug from ampoule (or a syringe prefilled with the drug, with or without a needle); sterile gauze and bandage; sharps container.

The abdomen or lateral thigh, alternatively the lateral arm.

1. Close the curtains to ensure privacy for the patient. Explain the planned procedure to the patient and confirm consent.

2. Prepare the medication, if necessary, by drawing the medication from the ampule or vial into the syringe using a sterile needle. It is unnecessary to clean the top of a sealed vial. Remove the needle used to draw up the drug from the syringe and replace with a sterile 20-gauge or 21-gauge needle.

3. Perform hand hygiene and don nonsterile disposable gloves.

4. Disinfect the planned injection site using the single-use alcohol swab or single-use cotton swab with disinfectant solution. Start over the planned injection site and work outwards. Allow the disinfectant to dry completely.

5. Grab and lift the skin using 2 or 3 fingers, elevating a skin fold that is ~2 cm thick.

6. Insert the needle at a 90° angle to the skin fold and aspirate by pulling the syringe plunger to avoid intravascular administration. If blood is aspirated, withdraw the needle and prepare another drug dose using a new needle and syringe.

7. Immobilize the needle by holding the needle hub with one hand and slowly inject the drug, then withdraw the needle at a 90° angle to the skin.

8. Immediately cover the site with clean dry cotton gauze and apply pressure. If bleeding occurs, protect the injection site with a dressing.

9. Dispose of all sharps securely in a sharps container. Do not recap needles to avoid needle-stick injuries. Remove gloves and perform hand hygiene.

Alternative technique: After inserting the needle, release the skin fold, hold the syringe with both hands, aspirate to confirm the needle tip is not in a vessel, and inject as per steps 7 to 9.

5. Lumbar Puncture

1. Diagnostic:
1) Suspected central nervous system (CNS) infection, particularly meningitis (the key indication for lumbar puncture).
2) Autoimmune CNS diseases.
3) Metabolic CNS diseases.
4) Certain types of neuropathy.
5) Suspected subarachnoid hemorrhage in a patient with negative computed tomography (CT) results.
6) Other CNS diseases where cerebrospinal fluid (CSF) examination can be useful for establishing the diagnosis (eg, neoplastic meningitis).
7) Intrathecal administration of a contrast agent.

2. Therapeutic:
1) Intrathecal administration of drugs when indicated: Antibiotics for CNS infection, cytotoxic drugs for CNS malignancy, anesthetics.

2) Emergency CSF evacuation in patients with elevated intracranial pressure (ICP) (eg, in communicating hydrocephalus; neurosurgical input is suggested prior to therapeutic drainage).

3) Relief of elevated intracranial pressure in certain diseases (eg, benign intracranial hypertension, cryptococcal meningitis).

→ CONTRAINDICATIONS

1. Absolute: Cerebral edema or tumor (a tumor not located in the posterior cranial fossa and not causing displacement of planes might be considered a relative contraindication).

2. Relative: Infection of the skin and subcutaneous tissue at the planned puncture site, developmental abnormalities of the spine and spinal cord (eg, dysraphia), coagulation abnormalities (international normalized ratio [INR] >1.5, activated partial thromboplastin time [aPTT] >2×upper limit of normal, or platelet count <50×10^9/L); suspected subarachnoid hemorrhage (in such cases perform CT of the head before lumbar puncture).

→ COMPLICATIONS

1. Post–lumbar puncture syndrome:

1) Postural headache that develops 24 to 48 hours following lumbar puncture, most frequently in the frontal or occipital area. It can be accompanied by nausea, vomiting, dizziness, tinnitus, visual disturbances, and signs suggestive of meningitis. The headache improves spontaneously within 1 to 2 days (occasionally it may take several weeks to resolve).

   Prevention: Use a smaller-bore needle (eg, 22-gauge instead of 18-gauge), direct the tip of the needle with its bevel towards the lateral portion of the spine (to make the needle separate the fibers of the dura mater instead of cutting through them), or use a needle that has a blunted, noncutting tip, termed "atraumatic needle." Bedrest after lumbar puncture or administration of intravenous fluids does not prevent the postpuncture headache.⊗⊖

   Treatment: Bed rest, oral analgesics (acetaminophen [INN paracetamol] with or without caffeine, opioids; do not use nonsteroidal anti-inflammatory drugs or other agents that impair platelet function). In patients that do not improve with drug treatment, epidural blood patching—involving injecting the patient's venous blood at the puncture site—has been shown to alleviate headache by sealing the dural tear.⊘⊖

2) Back pain at the lumbar puncture site.

3) Radicular pain that is most frequently referred to the lower extremities. The onset of the pain at the time of needle insertion is a sign of nerve root irritation. In such cases, withdraw the needle and change the direction of needle insertion.

2. Other (rare): Paraplegia caused by epidural hematoma (usually seen in patients who have received anticoagulants shortly before or after lumbar puncture); brain herniation into the foramen magnum (in patients with cerebral edema, tumor causing increased ICP, or large subarachnoid hemorrhage; this complication is frequently fatal); subarachnoid and/or subdural hemorrhage; injury to spinal ligaments or the vertebral periosteum; acute bacterial vertebral osteomyelitis; abscess; epidermoid cyst; sixth nerve palsy from a sudden decrease in ICP, which may result in traction of the sixth nerve.

→ PATIENT PREPARATION

1. Obtain informed consent from the conscious patient or substitute decision-maker, documented as per your institutional policy.

2. Assess the platelet count, INR, aPTT, and correct if abnormal. If the patient is treated with anticoagulants, discontinue them (→Chapter 3.1, Table 1-6).

3. Exclude elevated ICP (cerebral edema or tumor) on the basis of fundoscopy (look for papilledema) or CT of the head. CT should be performed in all patients with a history of immunodeficiency, previous CNS disease, or recent seizure (epilepsy), age >60 years, as well as patients with papilledema, altered mental status, or focal neurologic signs.⊘○

4. Place the patient in the lateral decubitus position, close to the edge of the examination table, with the patient's back facing you. Lower limbs should be flexed at knees and hips, knees pulled against the abdomen, head at maximum flexion towards the knees (→Figure 5-1). Avoid excessive flexion of the spine; it should form a single line in one plane. The back and shoulders should be aligned in a plane perpendicular to the table. The procedure can also be done in a cooperative patient in a sitting position and under fluoroscopic guidance in a prone position.

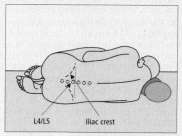

Figure 5-1. Appropriate patient positioning for lumbar puncture and location of the L4/L5 intercostal space.

→ EQUIPMENT

1. Equipment for surgical field preparation and optionally for infiltration anesthesia.

2. Sterile single-use lumbar puncture needle with a stylet, 22 gauge or 20 gauge, 8.75 cm in length (if only available, we recommend a newer pencil-point atraumatic needle in place of the traditional cutting-type needle).⊘● Optionally, you may use a smaller-bore needle inserted through a shorter larger-bore needle (an introducer needle); such a needle may be required for using an atraumatic needle if skin puncture is difficult.

3. Manometer for CSF pressure measurement.

4. Sterile test tubes labeled 1 to 4.

→ PUNCTURE SITE

The interspinous space, optimally the L4 and L5 or L3 and L4 but not above the L2 and L3 space to avoid the end of the spinal cord, in the midline passing in-between the spinous processes, slightly laterally to it. The line connecting the most proximal points of the iliac crests should cross the lumbar spine at the level of the L4 spinal process (→Figure 5-1).

→ PROCEDURE

1. Prepare the surgical field. If necessary, anesthetize the skin and subcutaneous tissue using a local anesthetic, for instance, EMLA cream or infiltration anesthesia using a 1% lidocaine solution (not necessary in an unconscious patient).

2. Slowly insert the needle with a stylet, directing it obliquely in the cranial direction and towards the umbilicus. Direct the bevel of the needle upwards, with a trajectory at the midsagittal plane. The puncture of the ligamentum flavum and the dura mater is perceived as loss of resistance accompanied by a "pop" (in adults the subdural space is located at a depth of 4-7 cm). After overcoming the resistance of the dura mater, remove the stylet. The needle is supposed to displace the nerve roots but may rarely irritate one of them. Drops of CSF should appear at the needle hub. If the patient is conscious, ask him or her to relax the lower limbs (reduce hip flexion). If CSF outflow is not seen, replace the stylet and gently advance the needle or turn it by 90°, then remove the stylet again. Do not apply intense pressure to overcome resistance to the needle. The absence of CSF may be caused by passing the needle beyond the subarachnoid space. Blood-staining of the fluid can result from injury to a spinal canal vein during the procedure; in such cases, CSF often becomes clear after a while. If this is not seen, repeat the lumbar puncture one intervertebral space above or below.

3. For accurate CSF pressure measurement (not always necessary), hold the needle in one hand and connect the CSF pressure-measurement device using the other hand (a normal pressure range is 7-15 [<20] cm H_2O, which usually corresponds to a CSF outflow rate of 20-60 drops per minute; the measurement result is reliable if the patient remains still and relaxed).

4. After measuring CSF pressure, collect the CSF to several sterile tubes for testing (usually 3-5 mL; after excluding cerebral edema, a maximum volume of 40 mL may be collected). Ideally the tubes should be collected sequentially. If blood in the CSF is due to a traumatic tap from the procedure, the amount of blood will decrease in the order the blood is collected (eg, most blood in the first tube, decreasing blood through the fourth tube).

5. Once the CSF is collected, reintroduce the stylet into the needle, withdraw the needle, and protect the skin with a sterile dressing. Complications such as nerve root herniation and post–dural puncture headache may occur with failure to reintroduce the stylet into the needle.

→ AFTER THE PROCEDURE

Patients are encouraged to ambulate after the procedure when possible.

6. Nasogastric or Orogastric Tube Insertion

→ INDICATIONS

Gastric content retention, intestinal obstruction, suspected upper gastrointestinal bleeding, enteral feeding, medication administration, or gastric dilation (eg, following ventilation with a self-inflating bag and face mask).

→ CONTRAINDICATIONS

Esophageal stricture, rupture, or recent esophageal variceal banding. Take special care or seek surgical consultation in patients with a recent gastric or esophageal surgery or procedure. Do not introduce a nasogastric tube in patients with limited nostril patency (most frequently due to septal deviation). In patients with severe facial trauma or basal skull fracture the decision to place the tube has to be made by appropriate surgical service.

→ POTENTIAL COMPLICATIONS

Insertion of the nasogastric or orogastric tube into the trachea, pharyngeal irritation, gastritis.

Additional complications of nasogastric tube insertion: Nasal mucosa injury, epistaxis, sinusitis.

→ **PATIENT PREPARATION**

Obtain informed consent. Place the patient in a supine or sitting position. Topical lidocaine spray or gel can be administered prior to procedure if available.

→ **EQUIPMENT**

Nasogastric/orogastric tube (thin tubes are used for feeding only; thick tubes are used for gastric decompression, especially in patients with gastrointestinal bleeding or bowel obstruction or ileus but can also be used for administering drugs or enteral feeds) Longer small-bowel feeding tubes can be used for postpyloric feeding, which may reduce the risk of pneumonia in critically ill patients without impact upon other outcomes.⊘⊖ Lubricant lidocaine gel; 60 mL slip-tip syringe; stethoscope; adhesive tape; nonsterile gloves.

→ **PROCEDURE**

Use topical anesthesia (lidocaine spray or jelly) if available to ensure maximal patient comfort during nasogastric tube insertion. Mark the distance from the tip of the nose (nasogastric tube) or from the mouth (orogastric tube) to the earlobe and distance from the ear to the stomach on the tube, so that the uppermost aspirating port is located at the level of the xiphoid process (in adults the cardia is usually located ~40 cm from the teeth). Coat the tip of the tube with lidocaine lubricant gel. For nasogastric tubes, gently insert the tube into the lowermost portion of the nostril perpendicular to the coronal plane. If this is unsuccessful, try to introduce the tube through the other nostril. For orogastric tubes, insert the tube backwards and downwards through the mouth and oropharynx. In conscious and cooperative patients ask them to flex the neck and swallow the tube. Insert the tube to the predetermined depth.

To assess placement, inject ~10 to 30 mL of air using a syringe and simultaneously auscultate the epigastrium. Gurgling sounds suggest correct tube positioning. Coughing, respiratory distress, hypoventilation, voice changes, or air outflow through the tube can all be signs of introducing the tube past the vocal cords. Secure the tube to the nose (nasogastric tube) or to the angle of the mouth (orogastric tube) using adhesive tape. If the tube is being used for feeding, confirm placement using radiography prior to administration of feeds or medications.

→ **AFTER THE PROCEDURE**

If the tube is used for feeding (enteral nutrition [EN]), we suggest to not monitor routinely for gastric residual volume (GRV) in patients with an endotracheal tube, as GRV measurements may lead to unnecessary withholding of EN due to perceived feeding intolerance.⊗⊖ In patients at high risk of vomiting and aspiration, measurements of GRV could be considered especially at EN initiation and progression; EN should be delayed if GRV is >500 mL/6 h. Patients should be upright (head of the bed at ≥30°) while nutrition is being administered. Flush and fill the tube regularly with clear water when not in use.

7. Pericardiocentesis

→ **PREFERRED METHOD**

Pericardiocentesis is most commonly performed percutaneously by needle drainage of pericardial fluid and insertion of a pericardial drain with or without echocardiographic guidance. Echocardiographic guidance is associated with relatively low complication and recurrence rates and a high success rate.● Surgical drainage may be preferable in certain situations, such as hemopericardium with clotted blood, concomitant surgical issues (eg, type A aortic dissection), or other conditions making needle drainage difficult or high risk (eg, posterior pericardial fluid collection, purulent effusion).

→ INDICATIONS

1. Therapeutic: Cardiac tamponade (a life-saving procedure).

2. Diagnostic: Pericardial effusion of unclear etiology if the fluid thickness on echocardiography (in diastole) is >20 mm.

→ CONTRAINDICATIONS

Cardiac tamponade with aortic dissection (emergency cardiac surgery is necessary). In the case of diagnostic pericardiocentesis, relative contraindications include uncompensated coagulopathy (international normalized ratio [INR] ≥1.5, activated partial thromboplastin time [aPTT] >1.5×upper limit of normal), anticoagulant treatment, platelet count <50×10^9/L, and predominantly posterior pericardial effusion.

→ POTENTIAL COMPLICATIONS

Perforation of the myocardium or coronary vessels, air embolism, pneumothorax, arrhythmia (usually bradycardia resulting from a vasovagal response), inadvertent puncture of the peritoneum or abdominal organs.

→ PATIENT PREPARATION

Obtain informed consent. Place the patient in a supine position. Studies include echocardiography and coagulation tests.

→ EQUIPMENT

1. Equipment for surgical field preparation and infiltration anesthesia.

2. Echocardiography or fluoroscopy equipment (if neither is available, transfer of the patient should be considered, if feasible).

3. Long needle with metal stylet (a Tuohy needle, thin-walled 18-gauge needle), central vein catheterization kit (a needle with a guidewire and a single-lumen catheter) or long sheathed angiocatheter and 3-way stopcock.

→ SITE OF PERICARDIOCENTESIS

Most frequently the apical or subcostal (subxiphoid) approach is used. The ideal entry site is the area with the largest fluid pocket on echocardiography that is closest to the skin.

→ PROCEDURE

1. Prepare the surgical field and use infiltration anesthesia of the skin.

2. Under sterile technique and guidance of echocardiography (bedside) or fluoroscopy (in the cardiac catheterization laboratory) insert the needle (a large-bore angiocatheter or needle used for central venous catheterization) connected to a syringe while aspirating continuously. The needle should be directed towards the largest pocket of pericardial fluid with the needle trajectory based on echocardiographic or fluoroscopic assessment. Needle placement in pericardial space can be confirmed by instillation of agitated saline and visualizing bubbles in pericardial space using echocardiography. Once the position is confirmed, fluid can be removed. If ongoing drainage is planned, insert a guidewire through the needle, withdraw the needle, insert a catheter over the guidewire, and remove the guidewire. Extended catheter drainage is associated with reduced rates of recurrence. Secure the catheter with a suture.

3. Drain the fluid in portions <1 L to help avoid acute right ventricular dilation or dysfunction. Maintain the drainage (catheter) until the aspirated fluid volume is <25 to 50 mL over 24 hours.

4. Collect samples for tests as in the case of pleural effusion (eg, cell count, gram stain, culture, acid-fast bacilli stain, lactate dehydrogenase, protein, cytology).

8. Pleural Drainage

Pleural drainage is performed to remove air, blood, or fluid from the pleural cavity, to achieve lung expansion, and to correct mediastinal shift that may cause hemodynamic abnormalities. The procedure described below uses a chest drain. Emergency decompression of tension pneumothorax: →Chapter 13.13.3. Decompression of pneumothorax using a syringe and catheter: →Chapter 13.13.3. Thoracentesis: →Chapter 16.10.

→ **INDICATIONS**

1. Pneumothorax:

1) Primary spontaneous pneumothorax persisting (>2 cm on chest radiography) after aspiration using a catheter and syringe. Note that a larger amount of aspirated air (>2.5 L) may indicate ongoing air leakage.

2) Secondary or iatrogenic spontaneous pneumothorax, excluding asymptomatic patients with a small (<2 cm) pneumothorax.

3) Tension pneumothorax.

4) Bilateral pneumothorax.

5) Hemorrhagic pneumothorax (hemopneumothorax).

6) Mechanical ventilation–induced pneumothorax.

7) Posttraumatic pneumothorax in patients with penetrating chest injuries.

2. Pleural effusion:

1) Malignant (drainage combined with pleurodesis: →Chapter 13.13.1.2.1).

2) Complicated parapneumonic effusion or empyema.

3) Hemothorax.

4) Pleural effusion following surgery, including thoracotomy, esophageal resection, or cardiac surgery.

→ **POTENTIAL COMPLICATIONS**

Subcutaneous emphysema; infection of the pleural cavity, skin, or intercostal tissues; incorrect tube positioning; lung injury; visceral injury; hemothorax; lung edema following expansion (re-expansion pulmonary edema); intercostal nerve injury; Horner syndrome (very rare).

→ **PATIENT PREPARATION**

1. Confirm the diagnosis of pneumothorax or pleural effusion using appropriate imaging. Studies include chest radiography (if pneumothorax or anatomy is

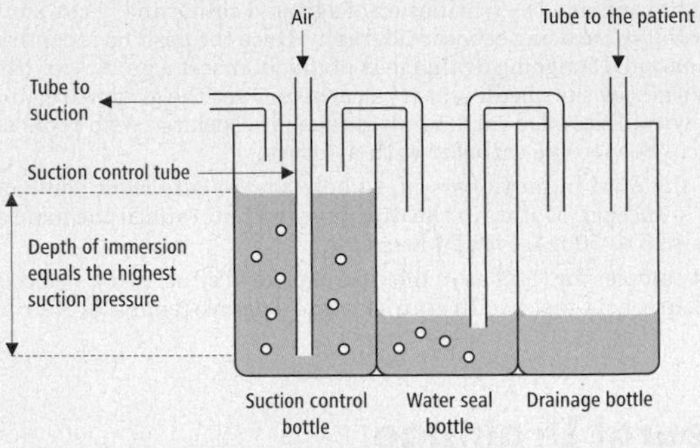

Figure 8-1. A 3-bottle chest drainage system.

doubtful, perform computed tomography [CT] of the chest) and ultrasonography of the pleural cavity. If time permits, prior to procedure obtain complete blood count (CBC) (including platelet count), international normalized ratio (INR), activated partial thromboplastin time (aPTT), and blood group and screen.

2. Obtain informed consent.

3. If the procedure is elective (which is rarely the case) and the patient is receiving anticoagulant treatment, discontinue vitamin K antagonists and wait for the INR to decrease to <1.5; discontinue direct oral anticoagulants (DOACs) as before surgery with a high risk of bleeding (→Chapter 3.1.3). The last prophylactic dose of low-molecular-weight heparin (LMWH) should be administered ≥12 hours before the procedure and the last therapeutic dose of LMWH should be administered ≥24 hours before the procedure.

4. Insert a peripheral venous catheter.

5. Place the patient lying on the side opposite the planned procedure with an upper limb elevated on the side of the procedure. In the event that an apical pneumothorax requires drainage, positioning the patient in the supine position with the head-of-bed elevated to 45° is appropriate.

→ EQUIPMENT

1. Equipment for surgical field preparation, infiltration anesthesia, and short general anesthesia if necessary.

2. Chest drain and needle (bore 0.7-0.9 mm [22-20 gauge]) with syringe (10 or 20 mL). Small-bore chest drains are sometimes packaged in kits containing a needle and guidewire (as for central vein catheterization). Pigtail catheters are preferred to large-bore chest tubes⊘⊖ as they are associated with significantly lower risk of complications during insertion and shorter duration of drainage and hospital stay than large-bore chest tubes. In most nontraumatic pneumothoraces we prefer small-bore tubes (<14 F) if a chest tube is used.

3. If the chest drain is to be inserted using surgical technique, equipment for skin incision and dissection of the intercostal space is necessary. This includes scalpel, surgical and anatomical forceps, and blunt curved hemostat.

4. Suturing equipment: Needle holder, 1.0 needle with thread.

5. Three-chamber chest suction unit (fill the suction pressure-regulating chamber [typically to a level of 10-20 cm] and the underwater valve chamber [to the mark] with a sterile fluid: →Figure 8-1), connecting tubing, and low-pressure suction unit if required (a central [wall or bedside panel vacuum port] or electric suction device).

→ SITE OF CHEST DRAIN INSERTION

Always insert the chest drain at the superior margin of the rib.

1. Pneumothorax: The fifth to eighth intercostal spaces in the mid-axillary line or the second intercostal space in the mid-clavicular line.

2. Nonencapsulated pleural effusion: The fifth to eighth intercostal spaces in the mid-axillary line.

3. Limited air or fluid collection: Depending on location determined using imaging studies and ultrasound guidance.

→ PROCEDURE

1. Use ultrasonography, if available, to guide chest tube insertion.

2. Prepare the surgical field and perform local anesthesia. IV conscious sedation is useful (→Chapter 16.9).

3. Puncture the pleural cavity using a syringe and needle (→Chapter 16.10) to confirm the presence of air or fluid.

4. To insert a small-bore chest drain, use the Seldinger technique (pass a guide-wire through the needle into the pleural cavity, withdraw the needle, dilate skin and intercostal soft tissue by a dilator, then remove the dilator, insert a chest drain over the guidewire, and finally remove the guidewire). When using larger-bore tubes, make a ~1.5 to 2 cm skin incision at the level of the upper edge of the rib and dissect the intercostal tissue. Once the pleural cavity is entered (ie, the parietal pleura is penetrated), place a mattress stay suture. In patients with pneumothorax advance the chest drain towards the apex of the lung; in patients with pleural effusion advance the chest drain towards the base of the lung. If the chest drain is fitted with a trocar, withdraw the trocar ~1 cm within the tube before attempting chest drain insertion. Chest drains used for pleural effusion should optimally be inserted under imaging guidance. After insertion do not evacuate >1.5 L of fluid per hour.

5. Connect the tube to the one-way valve suction unit (→Figure 8-1). If active suction devices are used, the negative pressure should be from −10 to −20 cm H_2O.

6. Secure the chest drain to the chest wall with suturing.

→ AFTER THE PROCEDURE

1. Check the position of the chest drain on chest radiography.

2. Monitor evacuated fluid volumes. Check for evacuation of air from the pleural cavity (this is evidenced by air bubbles in the suction unit chamber [usually the middle chamber] fitted with an underwater seal valve). Make sure the suction system is airtight. Do not clamp the chest drain when air bubbles are seen inside or a drain is inserted for the treatment of pneumothorax.

3. Tube removal:

1) **Indications**: No airflow in the chest drain, complete lung expansion confirmed by chest radiographs (also after conversion from active to passive suction [eg, disconnection of the 3-chamber collection from suction]) for a period of several hours. The volume of fluid drained from the pleural cavity should be <200 mL/24 h.

2) **Technique**: Cut the securing suture. Instruct the patient to perform the Valsalva maneuver (ie, forced expiration with closed airway). Withdraw the chest drain at the time of the maneuver using a quick motion and immediately tie the stay suture to seal the tube track.

9. Procedural Sedation and Analgesia

→ D E F I N I T I O N

Procedural sedation and analgesia is provided for the purpose of preventing or relieving discomfort, pain, and anxiety for patients who are undergoing short procedures associated with discomfort. Sedation is a drug-induced state of depressed consciousness, for most procedures (eg, endoscopies) preferably to a level at which the patient is still capable of a purposeful response to verbal or light tactile stimulation. For some procedures (elective intubation, cardioversion) short-term general anesthesia, making the patient unresponsive to pain stimulation, is usually required. The purpose of this chapter is to provide information relevant to the nonanesthesiologist who, for variety of reasons, may provide short-term procedural sedation.

Of note, "procedural sedation and analgesia" was previously referred to as "conscious sedation" (and still may continue to be called this way). The association of these two terms may be contradictory, as the effective sedation reduces consciousness.

→ M O N I T O R I N G

All sedative-hypnotic agents, alone or in combination, are capable of rendering the patient apneic and hypotensive. Therefore, patients who are receiving sedative agents must be appropriately monitored, a minimum requirement being pulse oximetry and blood pressure, preferably with an automatic blood pressure cuff. In general, the person responsible for monitoring and sedation should be different from the person performing the procedure.

Continuous capnography is mandated by the American Society of Anesthesia for all patients who receive procedural sedation and by the Canadian Anesthesiologists' Society for sedation to a Ramsay sedation score ≥4 (a score of 4 means the patient is asleep but responds purposefully to a loud verbal or light tactile stimulus). Capnography identifies apnea more rapidly than pulse oximetry, thereby allowing intervention to occur before the onset of hypoxia or severe hypercarbia. Supplemental oxygen should be delivered by a face mask or nasal prongs.

If flumazenil or naloxone is administered (→below), ≥2 hours of monitoring after the last dose of the reversal agent must be provided, due to the short half-life of the reversal agents compared with opioids and benzodiazepines.

→ P E R S O N N E L

In general, only an appropriately trained person should administer procedural sedation and analgesia, and training in airway management is an absolute requirement. The precise regulation differs in specific jurisdictions. An individual skilled in airway management (bag-valve-mask ventilation, endotracheal intubation) must be in attendance, along with appropriate airway management equipment and a source of oxygen and suction. The ability to manage hypotension with fluids and vasopressor medications and a "crash cart" containing advanced cardiac life support (ACLS) drugs, as well as naloxone and flumazenil, should be immediately available.

→ D R U G S

General Issues

Drug requirements vary widely between patients, making it difficult to define safe dosage for any one individual. Advancing age, body habitus, critical illness, dehydration, hemodynamic instability, and level of consciousness before the procedure are some of the factors that may contribute to cardiorespiratory instability with the administration of even small doses of sedatives and opioids. Titration to effect is therefore a key principle in the safe provision of conscious sedation.

Goals for sedative and analgesic management should be established and drugs appropriate to the achievement of these goals should be administered. For example, opioid agents are excellent analgesics but have little amnestic or anxiolytic effects in small doses. Commonly used sedative agents such as the benzodiazepines and propofol are excellent anxiolytics and hypnotics but provide no analgesia. It is therefore common practice to use a combination of medications to achieve the desired effect of anxiolysis and analgesia. For example, the benzodiazepine midazolam and the opioid fentanyl are commonly used in combination for procedural sedation. **It is imperative that it be understood that combining sedative agents with opioids will have at least an additive effect on level of consciousness, respiratory drive, and cardiovascular stability.**

Two other agents, of a different class than the opioids and benzodiazepines are dexmedetomidine, an α_2 agonist, and ketamine. The discussion of these agents is beyond the scope of this chapter.

Adverse effects other than the cardiorespiratory depression are characteristic of all sedative and opioid agents and are not discussed here. For example, a knowledge of the propofol infusion syndrome, a potentially fatal complication of long-term high-dose propofol infusion, must be appreciated by those who prescribe this drug in such a way.

Specific Drugs and Dosages

The following dosages are guidelines only.

1. Sedatives:

1) Benzodiazepines:

   a) Midazolam: 0.5 to 1 mg, repeated as necessary. Peak effect in 2 to 3 minutes.

   b) Lorazepam: 0.25 to 1 mg, repeated as necessary. Peak effect in 5 to 20 minutes.

   c) Diazepam: 2 mg, repeated as necessary. Peak effect in 2 to 5 minutes.

2) Propofol: 10 to 20 mg, repeated as necessary. Peak effect is rapid, in 90 to 100 seconds, or longer in older patients.

2. Opioids:

1) Fentanyl: 25 to 50 µg, repeated as necessary. Rapid onset. Half-life of 1.5 to 6 hours.

2) Morphine: 2 to 5 mg, repeated as necessary. Slower onset and longer half-life than fentanyl (3-7 hours).

3) Hydromorphone: 0.25 to 0.5 mg, repeated as necessary. Half-life of 1.5 to 3.5 hours.

3. Reversal agents:

1) Flumazenil may be used when reversal of sedating action of benzodiazepines is desired immediately. The starting dose is 0.2 mg IV over 15 seconds, which may be followed by a dose of 0.1 mg after 1 minute, repeated every minute up to a total dose of 1 mg (usually 0.3-0.6 mg is sufficient).

2) Naloxone may be used when reversal of sedating action of opioids (eg, fentanyl, morphine) is desired. The starting dose is 0.1 mg, 0.2 mg, 0.4 mg IV up to a cumulative dose of ~1 mg.

→ PATIENT PREPARATION

Obtain informed consent for the procedure. Maintain the patient in a fasting state (nothing by mouth for solids and fatty liquids for 6 hours and clear fluids for 2 hours). Insert a relatively large-bore (bore ≥1.2 mm [18 gauge]) peripheral IV catheter.

→ **EQUIPMENT**

1. Equipment for insertion of a peripheral venous catheter and drug administration, equipment for airway management, equipment for mechanical ventilation and oxygen therapy.

2. Cardiac monitor, pulse oximeter, automated blood pressure monitor, defibrillator.

3. Drugs for the management of hypotension (IV fluids, catecholamines; →Chapter 3.16), anaphylaxis (→Chapter 2.2), and for cardiopulmonary resuscitation (→Chapter 3.3).

→ **PROCEDURE**

1. Start monitoring blood pressure, heart rate, and hemoglobin oxygen saturation (SpO_2) before administering any drugs and continue until complete reversal of sedation. Measure blood pressure frequently and regularly (usually every 1-5 minutes). Administer oxygen as needed.

2. Titrate small incremental doses of sedative and/or opioid medications, continuously monitoring level of consciousness.

3. Maintain the airway (head tilt and chin lift; use an oropharyngeal airway if necessary), continue oxygen therapy, and ventilate with a self-inflating bag as required.

4. In case of achieving sedation beyond the targeted point (ie, deeper than planned), interrupt drug delivery, maintain the airway, and use reversal drugs as needed.

10. Thoracentesis

→ **GENERAL INDICATIONS**

1. Diagnostic analysis of pleural effusion:
1) Any new pleural effusion, except in the case of clinically suspected transudate due to heart failure, hypoalbuminemia, cirrhosis, end-stage renal failure, or in patients with small effusions; in such circumstances treat the underlying cause, reassess, and consider thoracentesis if effusion does not resolve with treatment.
2) Persistent effusion despite an adequate trial of therapy of the underlying disease, large unilateral effusions (particularly left-sided), symptoms of pleurisy, dyspnea or fever, or effusion of unknown etiology.

2. Treatment of pleural effusion: Symptomatic lung compression by a pleural effusion. Usually the volumes drained during one procedure should not exceed 1500 mL due to risk of reexpansion pulmonary edema (RPE). Although rare (<1%) and not clearly associated with the volume of fluid removed, the mortality rate of RPE is as high as 20%, which explains the conservative suggestion of drainage of ≤1500 mL at a time.⊘○ Repeat therapeutic thoracentesis may be done several hours later if there is no evidence of RPE and the patient remains symptomatic.

→ **CONTRAINDICATIONS**

1. Absolute: None.
2. Relative: International normalized ratio (INR) >1.5 and activated partial thromboplastin time (aPTT) >2×upper limit of normal, platelet counts

$<50 \times 10^9/\text{L}$, lack of operator experience, small effusions (increased risk of pneumothorax), or dermatitis/cellulitis at the planned thoracentesis site.

→ COMPLICATIONS

1. Early: Pain at the site of thoracentesis, pneumothorax, hemothorax, visceral injury, vasovagal reflex, procedure failure, adverse effects of local anesthetics and disinfectants.

2. Late: Skin infection at the site of thoracentesis, empyema and dissemination of cancer cells along the needle track (particularly in mesothelioma).

→ PATIENT PREPARATION

1. Obtain informed consent. The optimal patient position is sitting with arms supported (→Figure 10-1).

2. Tests: Review a recent chest radiograph; if available, use pleural ultrasonography immediately before or during thoracentesis (this is associated with lower failure rates and lower complication rates).◐◔

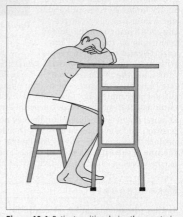

Figure 10-1. Patient position during thoracentesis.

→ EQUIPMENT

1. Surgical field preparation and local anesthesia.

2. Needle (bore 0.8 mm [21 gauge]) and a syringe (50-60 mL) in diagnostic thoracentesis. In the case of anticipated collection of higher fluid volumes, use a special thoracentesis kit including a syringe, large-bore thoracentesis catheter (bore 1.4-2 mm [14-18 gauge]) fitted with an aspiration needle, 3-way stopcock, pressure tubing, and bottle for collecting effusion fluid.

3. Syringes and tubes for fluid samples (as required depending on indications):

1) Chemistry (basic: protein, lactate dehydrogenase, pH, glucose, albumin [compared with serum values]; as needed: triglycerides, total cholesterol, amylase, adenosine deaminase): Dry tube, 2 to 5 mL of fluid.

2) Cell count and differential count: Dry ethylenediaminetetraacetic acid (EDTA) or heparinized tube, 2 to 3 mL of fluid. Hematocrit can be measured if a hemothorax is suspected (pleural fluid hematocrit >50% of the patient's peripheral blood hematocrit).

3) Cytology: Heparinized tube (1 mL), >30 to 50 mL of fluid. Fluid can be sent for flow cytometry if malignancy is suspected.

4) Microbiology: Sterile plastic container or transport culture medium. If infection is suspected, pleural fluid should additionally be sent in blood culture bottles (this increases diagnostic yield). If empyema is suspected a specific anaerobic culture medium should be prepared and pleural fluid should be immediately put into the medium (with tight seal) to minimize air exposure, which could result in lower yield of anaerobe growth. Acid-fast bacilli and tuberculosis culture should be performed when there is clinical suspicion of mycobacterial pleuritis.

→ SITE OF THORACENTESIS

Use bedside pleural ultrasonography for guidance, if available (→Figure 10-2). It is common practice to proceed with pleural fluid aspiration with the patient in the sitting position and the needle inserted posteriorly (→Figure 10-1). Palpate the intercostal space; with aseptic technique, perform thoracentesis at the ultrasonography--guided site at the superior margin of a rib to reduce the risk of injury to the neurovascular bundle. A lateral site is preferred using an ultrasonography-guided technique as the risk of intercostal vessel trauma increases

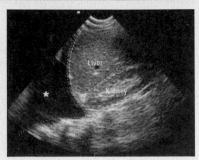

Figure 10-2. Ultrasonography of the right hypochondrium visualizing a pleural effusion (asterisk).

with more posterior or medial procedures. In the case of large free-flowing effusions, the percussion method can be used to identify the thoracentesis site (2 intercostal spaces below the upper limit of the dull percussion area) if ultrasonography is not available. Using this approach, the needle is inserted equidistant from the spinous process and the posterior axillary line.

Of note, the neurovascular bundle may not be entirely covered by the rib in this position and the triangle of safety (bordered anteriorly by the lateral edge of pectoralis major, laterally by the lateral edge of latissimus dorsi, inferiorly by the line of the fifth intercostal space, and superiorly by the base of the axilla) is considered a safer alternative by the British Thoracic Society.

→ PROCEDURE

1. Use ultrasonography, if available, to mark the thoracentesis site.

2. Prepare the surgical field; use sterile technique.

3. Perform infiltration anesthesia of the skin, subcutaneous tissues, and parietal pleura using 1% lidocaine without epinephrine (5-10 mL is usually sufficient).

4. Advance the thoracentesis needle, perpendicularly to the skin, with an overlying catheter. If one is available, towards the pleural effusion along the ultrasound--marked site (→Figure 10-3) while aspirating (constantly drawing back the syringe plunger).

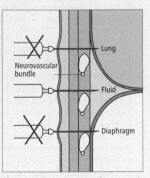

Figure 10-3. Appropriate thoracentesis approach.

5. After the fluid appears in the needle, advance the catheter further into the pleural cavity while withdrawing the needle during expiration (patient can be asked to hum during this process), then disconnect the syringe. Connect the catheter to a special kit or a 3-way stopcock draining into a bottle or a bag; if a needle without a catheter is used, connect it to a 50 or 60 mL syringe before performing thoracentesis.

6. Collect fluid samples in syringes and tubes.

Withdraw the needle or catheter (this is best done on expiration) and secure the site of thoracentesis using a small sterile dressing.

11. Vascular Access and Catheterization

11.1. Blood Sample Collection for Blood Gas Analysis

Blood gas analysis is testing the arterial or arterialized capillary blood (the latter is less reliable) or less frequently venous blood or blood obtained during cardiac catheterization to assess the acid-base balance and gas exchange.

➜ INDICATIONS

Diagnostics and monitoring of treatment in (1) respiratory failure; (2) acid--base disturbances.

11.1.1. Arterial Blood Gas Sampling

➜ CONTRAINDICATIONS

There are no absolute contraindications. Take special care in patients with significant coagulation abnormalities (eg, due to anticoagulant treatment), thrombocytopenia ($<30 \times 10^9$/L), or with a diastolic blood pressure >120 mm Hg.

➜ POTENTIAL COMPLICATIONS

Bleeding, bruising, arterial spasm and arterial wall dissection, thrombosis, arterial embolism.

➜ PATIENT PREPARATION

Obtain informed consent for the procedure. Place the patient in a supine position; a sitting position is optional in the case of upper extremity arterial blood sampling.

➜ PUNCTURE SITE

1. The **radial artery** in the palmar crease area, between the radial styloid process and the flexor carpi radialis tendon (the nondominant limb is preferred). It is recommended that the Allen test be performed before arterial puncture and particularly before arterial catheterization: Ask the patient to close their fist for 30 seconds, apply finger pressure to both forearm arteries (the ulnar artery and the radial artery; this is best done with the limb elevated), then release pressure on the ulnar artery. Repeat the test, this time releasing pressure on the radial artery. The capillary return time should be <5 seconds. The test is positive if the hand remains blanched after this time (this is a sign of impaired perfusion). Patients with positive results of the Allen test should not undergo arterial puncture on the affected limb. In emergencies it may not be possible to perform the Allen test; this should be documented in the medical chart.

2. The **femoral artery** distal to the inguinal ligament, most frequently in the inguinal crease (the artery is located lateral to the femoral vein and medial to the femoral nerve).

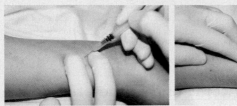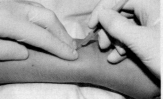

Figure 11-1. Techniques of radial artery puncture for arterial blood gas sampling.

3. The **brachial artery** in the elbow (this site is not recommended due to the risk of hematoma causing nerve compression; if used, the nondominant limb is preferred).

→ EQUIPMENT

1. Needle bore 0.5 to 0.6 mm (25-23 gauge) for radial artery puncture or 0.6 to 0.7 mm (23-22 gauge) for femoral or brachial artery puncture.

2. Heparinized syringe or insulin syringe flushed with heparin (optimally heparin should be drawn and then ejected via the needle that would subsequently be used for arterial puncture).

3. Stopper cap for sealing syringe (or needle) after sample collection.

4. Nonsterile disposable gloves; skin disinfectant (single-use alcohol swabs or single-use cotton swab with disinfectant solution); sharps disposal container; equipment for infiltration anesthesia if necessary.

→ PROCEDURE

1. Perform hand hygiene and wear disposable gloves. Clean and disinfect skin (as for peripheral venipuncture: →Chapter 16.4.2) and anesthetize with 1% lidocaine.

2. Hold the artery still between your fingertips and insert the needle at a 90° angle (a 45° angle is optional for the radial artery; →Figure 11-1).

3. After pulsatile blood outflow in the syringe is confirmed, draw ~1 mL of blood, gently pulling the syringe plunger. Take care not to aspirate air into the syringe. After sample collection, seal the syringe (or the needle) with a stopper cap and invert the syringe several times to mix the contents.

4. Apply compression to the artery until bleeding stops: for ≥5 minutes in the case of radial artery and for ≥10 to 15 minutes in the case of brachial or femoral arteries.

Blood gas analysis should be performed within 15 minutes. If this is not feasible, the blood sample can be stored in a refrigerator for ≤1 hour at ~4°C and transported to the laboratory on ice.

11.1.2. Arterialized Capillary Blood Sampling

→ PUNCTURE SITE

Fingertip or earlobe.

→ EQUIPMENT

Nonsterile disposable gloves; skin disinfectant (single-use alcohol swabs or single-use cotton swab with disinfectant solution); special blade or fine needle for puncturing skin; 2 special heparinized capillary tubes; 2 metal pins and

4 caps; magnet; sharps disposal container; equipment for infiltration anesthesia if necessary.

→ PROCEDURE

1. Warm (massage) the puncture site.

2. Puncture skin at a depth that ensures free outflow of a large drop of blood.

3. Fill the capillary tubes with blood; avoid introducing air bubbles inside.

4. Place the metal pins into the capillary tubes, close the tube ends tightly using plastic stopper caps, and mix the blood with the magnet.

Analysis should be performed immediately. If this is not feasible, the samples can be stored for ≤30 minutes on ice.

11.2. Peripheral Venous Blood Sampling

→ CONTRAINDICATIONS

As in IV injections (→Chapter 16.4.2).

→ POTENTIAL COMPLICATIONS

Phlebitis, hematoma, infection.

→ PATIENT PREPARATION AND VENIPUNCTURE SITE

As in IV injections.

→ EQUIPMENT

As in IV injections. However, special vacuum tubes or syringes with matching needles are most frequently used instead of standard needles and syringes. The contents of tubes or syringes used for blood sample collection as well as the label or cap color code vary depending on the planned tests; if unsure, check with the nursing staff or your laboratory to ensure you are using the correct tube types:

1) Empty tubes or tubes containing a coagulant (dry tube; "clot tube") are used for measurements of electrolytes, urea, creatinine, bilirubin, lipids, enzymes, and other serum proteins.

2) Tubes containing ethylenediaminetetraacetic acid (EDTA) or heparin are used for complete blood count (CBC).

3) Tubes containing sodium citrate are used for plasma coagulation tests, that, international normalized ratio (INR), activated partial thromboplastin time (aPTT), fibrinogen, and D-dimer levels. The usual citrate salt to blood sample volume ratio is 1:9.

4) Tubes containing sodium fluoride are used for plasma glucose.

5) Tubes containing lithium heparin are used for serum ammonia or whole blood electrolyte levels.

→ PROCEDURE

As in IV injections (→Chapter 16.4.2). In some blood collection systems a special needle is introduced into the vein and a vacuum tube or syringe is connected after blood appears in the needle hub. If many different tests are necessary, the needle is left in the vein while various tubes or syringes are being attached.

11.3. Peripheral Venous Catheter Placement

Peripheral venous catheter placement is the easiest method of obtaining vascular access for the administration of drugs or fluids. Drugs intended for IV administration should usually be appropriately diluted. Drugs can be administered IV as injections (bolus), intermittent infusions, or continuous IV infusions. Most parenteral nutrition formulas or other high-osmolarity substances (such as concentrated KCl solution) as well as drugs that may cause vein damage should not be administered via peripheral veins. Large-bore peripheral venous catheters allow for a more rapid administration of fluids and blood products compared with standard central venous catheters. Peripheral catheters are characterized by lower flow resistance, as they are shorter than central catheters and have an equal or larger bore.

⮕ POTENTIAL COMPLICATIONS

As in IV injections (→Chapter 16.4.2). Catheter-associated infections: →Chapter 8.8.

⮕ PATIENT PREPARATION AND PUNCTURE SITE

As in IV injections.

⮕ EQUIPMENT

As in IV injections, but a peripheral venous catheter is used instead of a needle. In adults the following catheter sizes are used: 22 gauge (blue, bore 0.8 mm), 20 gauge (pink, bore 1 mm), 18 gauge (green, bore 1.2 mm), 17 gauge (white, bore 1.4 mm), 16 gauge (grey, bore 1.7 mm), and 14 gauge (orange, bore 2 mm); 18-gauge and 20-gauge catheters are most frequently used. Larger catheters (14 or 16 gauge) allow for more rapid infusions. For intermittent infusions use an infusion kit containing infusion tubing fitted with a clamp and a sharp-tipped reservoir used to pierce the bottle/container with the infusion fluid or drug solution. Use a 3-way stopcock and drop counter when necessary. For continuous infusions use an infusion pump, infusion tubing, appropriate syringe (50, 20, or 10 mL; some infusion pumps accept only certain types of syringes), and 3-way stopcock.

⮕ PROCEDURE

1. Close the curtains to ensure privacy for the patient. Explain the planned procedure to the patient and confirm consent.

2. Select a suitable peripheral vein. The most commonly used veins are in the upper limbs: antecubital veins, forearm veins, and the dorsal venous network on the back of the hand. If locating a vein is difficult, ultrasonography can be used to identify a suitable peripheral vein. Using a linear probe on the shallowest depth setting, scan for small compressible vessels, ideally <1.5 cm from the skin surface. If the vein is not visible to the naked eye, you may need to cannulate the vein under direct guidance (step 6, below).

3. Wrap a tourniquet (usually on the upper arm) to fill the peripheral veins. Visualizing and puncturing a vein can be facilitated by warming the limb and massaging (tapping) the planned injection site. Alternatively ask the patient to open and close their fist several times.

4. Clean and disinfect your hands and wear disposable gloves.

5. Clean and disinfect the puncture site using a gauze swab soaked with a disinfectant solution or with prepackaged sterile swabs. Spray the skin

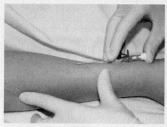
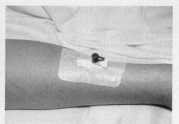

Figure 11-2. Peripheral venous catheterization.   **Figure 11-3.** Protecting the catheter with a dressing.

with a disinfectant solution from a distance of 20 to 30 cm and wait for ~1 to 1.5 minutes (unless the patient's condition requires immediate venous access).

6. Spread the skin taut below the planned injection site using a thumb or fingers of one hand. Insert the catheter with a needle into the skin at a ~30° angle (→Figure 11-2). If you are cannulating the vein under ultrasound guidance, cover the ultrasound machine with a clear waterproof dressing (eg, Tegaderm). Center the probe over the target vessel (check both long-axis and short-axis views to obtain a clear sense of the vessel location and course). Follow the needle tip until the catheter has entered the vessel.

7. When blood appears in the needle hub, hold the needle still with one hand and advance the catheter into the vessel with the other hand. Then withdraw the needle and release the tourniquet. If the needle has been introduced very slowly, blood may appear in the needle hub while the tip of the catheter (shorter than the needle) is still located outside the vessel. Advance the needle with the catheter by a further ~1 mm before immobilizing the needle and attempting to advance the catheter over the needle into the vessel lumen.

8. Confirm patency of the catheter by aspirating blood and injecting a small volume of 0.9% saline.

9. Attach the catheter to the skin using tape or a special dressing (→Figure 11-3).

10. Document date and time of catheter placement in appropriate medical records (or on the dressing).

11. Drug administration:

1) **Injection**: Maintaining sterile conditions, draw the drug into the syringe, dilute (if appropriate), and inject via the catheter (this is usually done slowly). Occasionally drugs can be injected using a plain injection needle (using the same technique as in blood sample collection with a plain needle and syringe; inject the drug after aspirating blood into the syringe). If only a portion of drug dose in the syringe has been administered and you presume that the remaining drug may need to be administered later, protect the syringe by placing a sterile needle covered with a needle cap and label the syringe (name of the drug, dose in mg/mL); check how long the diluted drug can be stored and in what storage conditions.

2) **Intermittent infusion**: Maintaining sterile conditions, dilute the drug in an infusion fluid (note the name and dose of the diluted drug on the container/bottle), prime the infusion set (infusion tubing with a reservoir) with the solution to expel any air, and fill the reservoir to half of its volume. Connect the tubing to the catheter (usually using a 3-way stopcock previously primed with an infusion fluid) and set the required infusion rate using the pump, valve, or drop counter.

3) **Continuous infusion**: Make sure that the syringe can be used with your infusion pump. Select an appropriate type of syringe from the menu (if applicable to pump model). Maintaining sterile conditions, prepare drug solution

in the syringe. Prime the infusion tubing using the prepared solution to expel any air, connect the tubing to the catheter (this is usually done with a 3-way stopcock), label the syringe, and carefully mount it in the infusion pump (drug name and total dose or strength in mg/mL must remain visible at all times). Then set the infusion rate and start the infusion (health-care institutions should provide tables for calculating desired doses of the most commonly used drugs for infusion rates in mL/h [or minutes]; alternatively you may program a modern infusion pump by inputting drug name, total dose, solution volume [or drug concentration], and the patient's body mass, and set the infusion rate expressed, eg, as µg/min/kg).

12. After every drug administration flush the catheter with 0.9% saline. Do not reuse Luer lock plugs. Replace the dressing if soaked. In patients with features of local inflammation, pain, or fever, remove the catheter immediately. Treatment of superficial thrombophlebitis: →Chapter 3.18.5.2.

13. After removing the catheter, disinfect the venipuncture site and apply compression. Cover the site with a small adhesive dressing to stop bleeding.

Management of Selected Emergencies